D0938785

Bailey & Scott's

# Diagnostic Microbiology

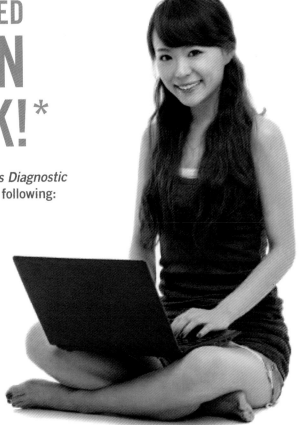

Bailey & Scott's

# Diagnostic Microbiology

## THIRTEENTH 13 EDITION

**Patricia M. Tille,** PhD, MLS(ASCP)

Program Director
Medical Laboratory Science
South Dakota State University
Brookings, South Dakota

3251 Riverport Lane
St. Louis, Missouri 63043

BAILEY & SCOTT'S DIAGNOSTIC MICROBIOLOGY                    ISBN: 978-0-323-08330-0
**Copyright © 2014 by Mosby, Inc., an affiliate of Elsevier Inc.**

---

**Notices**

Knowledge and best practice in this field are constantly changing. As new research and experience broaden our understanding, changes in research methods, professional practices, or medical treatment may become necessary.

Practitioners and researchers must always rely on their own experience and knowledge in evaluating and using any information, methods, compounds, or experiments described herein. In using such information or methods they should be mindful of their own safety and the safety of others, including parties for whom they have a professional responsibility.

With respect to any drug or pharmaceutical products identified, readers are advised to check the most current information provided (i) on procedures featured or (ii) by the manufacturer of each product to be administered, to verify the recommended dose or formula, the method and duration of administration, and contraindications. It is the responsibility of practitioners, relying on their own experience and knowledge of their patients, to make diagnoses, to determine dosages and the best treatment for each individual patient, and to take all appropriate safety precautions.

To the fullest extent of the law, neither the Publisher nor the authors, contributors, or editors, assume any liability for any injury and/or damage to persons or property as a matter of products liability, negligence or otherwise, or from any use or operation of any methods, products, instructions, or ideas contained in the material herein.

---

Previous editions copyrighted 2007, 2002, 1998, 1994, 1990, 1986, 1982, 1978, 1974, 1970, 1966, 1962
ISBN: 978-0-323-08330-0

*Publishing Director:* Andrew Allen
*Content Manager:* Ellen Wurm-Cutter
*Publishing Services Manager:* Julie Eddy
*Senior Project Manager:* Rich Barber
*Designer:* Teresa McBryan

Printed in China

Last digit is the print number:   9  8  7  6  5  4  3  2

*To my parents, whose memory continues to inspire me; to my husband David, whose love has helped me through all of life's ups and downs; to our four children and their significant others, Christina (Mike), Malissa, DJ (Alyssa), and Katie (Milan, Junior, and Julia), who are not only an inspiration and a joy, but continue to support me in my professional career and in my multiple roles as a mother, a mentor, and a friend. Not to forget my grandson, Aedan, who loved to sit on my lap and look at the pictures of my "bugs" every time I tried to work on this text. Lastly, the two new additions to the family: Jayce and Maja. To my mentors, who are too numerous to mention and have inspired me, challenged me, and continued to support me during my journey to continue to grow intellectually and professionally. Finally, to all my colleagues and friends who have provided materials, contributions, photos, and encouragement to complete this text. Without their assistance and influence, this new edition would have been an insurmountable undertaking.*

*In loving memory of: Richard "Dick" Duman 1945–2013*

# Reviewers

**Hassan A. Aziz, PhD, MLS(ASCP) CM**
Director and Associate Professor of Biomedical Science
Acting Coordinator of Graduate Program
College of Arts and Sciences
Qatar University
Doha, Qatar

**Asmita Bhakta, CLS, MT(ASCP)**
Instructor of Clinical Microbiology
Saddleback College
Mission Viejo, California

**Gloria Rudine Boyer, BS, MT(ASCP)**
Emory University Hospital
Atlanta, Georgia

**Lynda Britton, PhD, MLS(ASCP) CM**
Professor and Program Director
LSU Health Sciences Center
Shreveport, Louisiana

**Stacie A. Brown, PhD**
Texas State University
San Marcos, Texas

**Patricia Buchner, MS, CLS, ASCP**
Stanford Hospital and Clinics
Palo Alto, California
DeAnza College
Cupertino, California

**Louisiana A. Buckhanan BS, M(ASCP)**
Medical Technologist
Lakeland Healthcare
St. Joseph, Michigan

**Joyce A. Bulgrin, MSA, MT(ASCP)**
Senior Lecturer
School of Health Care Professions
University of Wisconsin—Stevens Point
Stevens Point, Wisconsin

**Delfina C. Dominguez, PhD, MLS(ASCP)**
Professor
The University of Texas at El Paso
El Paso, Texas

**Donna M. Duberg, MA, MS, MT(ASCP)SM**
Assistant Professor
Clinical Laboratory Science Department
Saint Louis University
St. Louis, Missouri

**Rosemary Duda, MLS(ASCP), MS, SM, I**
MLS Program Director
St. Margaret Hospital
Hammond, Indiana

**Maribeth L. Flaws, PhD, SM(ASCP)SI**
Associate Chairman and Associate Professor
Department of Medical Laboratory Science
Rush University Medical Center
Chicago, Illinois

**Linda J. Graeter, PhD, MLS(ASCP)**
Associate Professor
University of Cincinnati
Cincinnati, Ohio

**Theresa A. Greaves, MS, CLS, MT(ASCP)**
Professor
Ivy Tech Community College
South Bend, Indiana

**Michele G. Harms, MS, MLS(ASCP)**
Program Director
WCA Hospital School of Medical Technology
Jamestown, New York

**Rita M. Heuertz, PhD, MT(ASCP)**
Professor, Director of Departmental Research
Department of Clinical Laboratory Science
Doisy College of Health Sciences
Saint Louis University
St. Louis, Missouri

**Alissa Lehto-Hoffman, MT(ASCP)**
Education and Training Coordinator
Charge Technologist
South Bend Medical Foundation
Adjunct Professor
Ivy Tech Community College
South Bend, Indiana
Adjunct Professor
Andrews University
Berrien Springs, Michigan

**Jennifer A. Lichamer, MPH, CHES, IC, MT(ASCP)**
Instructor
Northern Illinois University
DeKalb, Illinois

**Patty Liddell, MS, MT(ASCP)SH**
Supervisor, Science Laboratories
Baptist College of Health Science
Memphis, Tennessee

**Kathleen Micklow, BSMT, M(ASCP), CIC**
Infection Preventionist
Einstein Healthcare Network
Philadelphia, Pennsylvania

**Paula C. Mister, MS, MT(ASCP), SM, ASCP CM**
Educational Coordinator, Clinical Microbiology
Johns Hopkins Hospital
Adjunct Faculty stevenson University
Community Colleges of Baltimore County
Baltimore, Maryland

**Michelle Moy, MAdEd, MT(ASCP)SC**
CLS Program Director
School of Continuing and Professional Studies
Institutes for Allied Health
Loyola University—Chicago
Chicago, Illinois

**Karen Peterson, MS, MT(ASCP)**
Education Coordinator
University of North Dakota
Grand Forks, North Dakota

**Lynn Poth, MS, MT(ASCP)**
Faculty
Saint Paul College
St. Paul, Minnesota

**Jody L. Provencher, MS, MT(ASCP)**
Medical Technologist
Albert Einstein Medical Center
Clinical Laboratory Instructor
Thomas Jefferson University
Philadelphia, Pennsylvania

**Jessica L. Reinhardt, MT, CLS (M, NCA)**
Microbiologist, Center for Aerobiological Sciences
U.S. Army Medical Research Institute of Infectious
   Diseases
Frederick, Maryland
Adjunct Instructor in Pathology
School of Medicine and Health Sciences
The George Washington University
Washington, D.C.

**Wanda C. Reygaert, PhD**
Associate Professor
Department of Biomedical Sciences
William Beaumont School of Medicine
Oakland University
Rochester, Michigan

**Lauren Roberts, MS, MT(ASCP)**
Microbiology Laboratory
St. Joseph's Hospital and Medical Center
Phoenix, Arizona

**John P Seabolt, EdD, MT(ASCP)SM**
Seaior Academic Coordinator
Biology Department
University of Kentucky
Lexington, Kentucky

**Cassandra Street, MT(ASCP), MMsc**
Emory University Hospital
Atlanta, Georgia

**Connie L. Wallace, BS, M(ASCP)**
Microbiologist
South Bend Medical Foundation
South Bend, Indiana

**James L. Vossler, MS, MLS(ASCP)SM CM**
Assistant Professor
SUNY Upstate Medical University
Syracuse, New York

# Contributors

**Hassan A. Aziz, PhD, MLS (ASCP) CM**
Director and Associate Professor of Biomedical Science
Acting Coordinator of Graduate Program
College of Arts and Sciences
Qatar University
Doha, Qatar

**Maribeth L. Flaws, PhD, SM (ASCP) SI**
Associate Chairman and Associate Professor
Department of Medical Laboratory Science
Rush University Medical Center
Chicago, Illinois

**Lynne S. Garcia, MS, CLS, FAAM**
Director, LSG & Associates
Santa Monica, California

**Laurie A. Gregg, MT (ASCP)**
Senior Microbiologist
Technical Supervisor Microbiology/Mycology/
    Parasitology
South Dakota Public Health Laboratory
Pierre, South Dakota

**April L. Harkins, PhD, MT (ASCP)**
Assistant Professor
Department of Clinical Laboratory Science
Marquette University
Milwaukee, Wisconsin

**Rita M. Heuertz, PhD, MT (ASCP)**
Professor, Director of Departmental Research
Department of Clinical Laboratory Science
Doisy College of Health Sciences
Saint Louis University
St. Louis, Missouri

**Danette M. Lipp Hoffman, BS, MT (ASCP)**
Sr. Microbiologist/Technical Supervisor, Virology
South Dakota Department of Health
South Dakota Public Health Laboratory
Pierre, South Dakota

**Denene Lofland, PhD, MT (ASCP)**
Assistant Professor
Medical Laboratory Science
Armstrong Atlantic State University
Savannah, Georgia

**Philip F. Meyer, DO**
Internal Medicine Physician
Avera Medical Group
Pierre, South Dakota

**Erik Munson, PhD, M (ASCP)**
Technical Director
Wheaton Franciscan Laboratory
Clinical Assistant Professor College of Health Sciences
University of Wisconsin—Milwaukee
Milwaukee, Wisconsin

**Wanda C. Reygaert, PhD**
Associate Professor
Department of Biomedical Sciences
William Beaumont School of Medicine
Oakland University
Rochester, Michigan

**Robyn Y. Shimizu, MT (ASCP)**
Department of Pathology and Laboratory Medicine
UCLA Health System
Los Angeles, California

**Patricia M. Tille, PhD, MLS (ASCP)**
Program Director
Medical Laboratory Science
South Dakota State University
Brookings, South Dakota

# Preface

This, the thirteenth edition of *Bailey and Scott's Diagnostic Microbiology*, is the first edition that I have had the great pleasure to edit and author with some amazing colleagues. Although as a clinical and research microbiologist, I have learned much during our preparation of this edition, the dynamics of infectious disease trends along with the technical developments available for diagnosing, treating, and controlling these diseases continues to present major challenges in the laboratory and medical care. In meeting these challenges, the primary goal for the thirteenth edition is to provide an updated and reliable reference text for practicing clinical microbiologists and technologists, while also presenting this information in a format that supports the educational efforts of all those responsible for preparing others for a career in diagnostic microbiology. Admittedly this is not an easy task. In the effort to achieve both purposes, we have had to make some difficult decisions, the results of which may from time to time dissatisfy either the practitioners or the educators. Nonetheless, by carefully reviewing the compliments and the criticisms of the twelfth edition readers and countless reviewers of the chapters for the new edition, I believe that the thirteenth edition provides a strong compromise for both a reference and a teaching text.

To align our goals with the reader's expectations and needs, we have kept the favorite features and made adjustments in response to important critical input from users of the text. Learning objectives, chapter review, the splitting of the large sections into manageable units in parasitology, mycology, and virology, and the addition of complex case studies constitute major changes to the text. The succinct presentation of each organism group's key laboratory, clinical, epidemiologic, and therapeutic features in tables and figures has been kept and updated, and new tables have been added. Regarding content, the major changes reflect the changes that the discipline of diagnostic microbiology continues to experience. The chapter that deals with molecular methods for identifying and characterizing microbial agents has been expanded and updated. Also, although the grouping of organisms into sections according to key features (e.g., Gram reaction, catalase or oxidase reaction, growth on MacConkey) has remained, changes regarding the genera and species discussed in these sections have been made. These changes, along with changes in organism nomenclature, were made to accurately reflect the changes that have occurred, and continue to occur, in bacterial taxonomy. Also, throughout the text, the content has been enhanced with new photographs and artistic drawings. Finally, although some classic methods for bacterial identification and characterization developed over the years (e.g., catalase, oxidase, Gram stain) still play a critical role in today's laboratory, others have given way to commercial identification systems. We realize that in a textbook such as this, a balance is needed for practicing and teaching diagnostic microbiology; our selection of identification methods that received the most detailed attention may not always meet the needs of both groups. However, we have tried to be consistent in selecting those methods that reflect the most current and common practices of today's clinical microbiology laboratories along with those that present historical information required within an educational program.

Finally, in terms of organization, the thirteenth edition is similar in many aspects to the twelfth edition, but some changes have been made. Various instructor ancillaries, specifically geared for the thirteenth edition, are available on the Evolve website, including a test bank, PowerPoints, and an electronic image collection. Student resources include a laboratory manual, review questions with answer key, and procedures.

We sincerely hope that clinical microbiology practitioners and educators find *Bailey & Scott's* thirteenth edition to be a worthy and useful tool to support their professional activities.

## ACKNOWLEDGMENTS

I would like to acknowledge the help of my colleagues at Elsevier who guided me through this project: Rich Barber, Senior Project Manager, and Ellen Wurm-Cutter, Content Manager.

Secondly, I would like to sincerely acknowledge and thank all the clinical microbiologists, scientists, clinicians, and educators who have over many years been my colleagues and who, through their contribution to the field and their communications and support, have made the writing of this edition possible.

Finally, but certainly not the least, my students—who keep me humble, laugh at my jokes, correct my spelling, and remind me that this work is transforming as they are the future of clinical diagnostics.

**Patricia M. Tille**

# Contents

# Microbial Taxonomy

## OBJECTIVES

1. Define classification, identification, species, genus, and binomial nomenclature.
2. Properly use binomial nomenclature in the identification of microorganisms, including syntax, capitalization, and punctuation.
3. Identify a microorganism's characteristics as either phenotypic or genotypic.
4. Describe how the classification, naming, and identification of organisms play a role in diagnostic microbiology in the clinical setting.

Taxonomy is the area of biologic science comprising three distinct but highly interrelated disciplines: classification, nomenclature (naming), and identification of organisms. Applied to all living entities, taxonomy provides a consistent means to classify, name, and identify organisms. This consistency allows biologists worldwide to use a common label for every organism studied within the multitude of biologic disciplines. The common language that taxonomy provides minimizes confusion about names, allowing more attention to be focused on other important scientific issues and phenomena. The importance of taxonomy is realized not only in phylogeny (the evolutionary history of organisms), but also in virtually every other biologic discipline, including microbiology.

In diagnostic microbiology, classification, nomenclature, and identification of microorganisms play a central role in providing accurate and timely diagnosis of infectious diseases. A brief, detailed discussion of the three major components of taxonomy is important for a thorough understanding of bacterial identification and application to diagnostic microbiology.

## CLASSIFICATION

Classification is a method for organizing microorganisms into groups or taxa based on similar morphologic, physiologic, and genetic traits. The hierarchical classification system consists of the following taxa designations:

- Species (specific epithet; lower case Latin adjective or noun)
- Genus (contains similar species)
- Family (contains similar genera)
- Order (contains similar families)
- Class (contains similar orders)
- Phylum (contains similar classes; equivalent to the Division taxa in botany)
- Kingdom (contains similar divisions or phyla)

## SPECIES

*Species* (abbreviated as sp., singular, or spp., plural) is the most basic of the taxonomic groups and can be defined as a collection of bacterial strains that share common physiologic and genetic features and differ notably from other microbial species. Occasionally, taxonomic subgroups within a species, called *subspecies*, are recognized. Furthermore, designations such as *biotype*, *serotype*, or *genotype* may be given to groups below the subspecies level that share specific but relatively minor characteristics. For example, *Klebsiella pneumoniae* and *Klebsiella oxytoca* are two distinct species within the genus *Klebsiella*. *Serratia odorifera* biotype 2 and *Treponema pallidum* subsp. *pallidum* are examples of a biotype and a subspecies designation. A biotype is considered the same species with the same characteristic genetic makeup that displays differential physiologic characteristics. Subspecies are typically environmentally isolated from the original species but do not display significant enough divergence to be classified as a biotype or a new species. Although these subgroups may have some taxonomic importance, their usefulness in diagnostic microbiology is limited.

## GENUS

*Genus* (plural, genera), the next taxon, contains different species that have several important features in common. Each species within a genus differs sufficiently to maintain its status as an individual species. Placement of a species within a particular genus is based on various genetic and phenotypic characteristics shared among the species. Microorganisms do not possess the multitude of physical features exhibited by higher organisms such as plants and animals. For instance, they rarely leave any fossil record, and they exhibit a tremendous capacity to intermix genetic material among supposedly unrelated species and genera. For these reasons, confidently establishing a microorganism's relatedness in higher taxa beyond the genus level is difficult. Although grouping similar genera into common families and similar families into common orders is used for classification of plants and animals, these higher taxa designations (i.e., division, class, order) are not useful for classifying bacteria.

## FAMILY

A *family* encompasses a group of organisms that may contain multiple genera and consists of organisms with a common attribute. The name of a family is formed by adding the suffix *-aceae* to the root name of the type genus; for example, the Streptococcaceae family type genus is *Streptococcus*. One exception to the rule in microbiology is the family Enterobacteriaceae; the type species is *Escherichia coli*. Bacterial (prokaryotic) type species or strains are determined according to guidelines published by the International Committee for the Systematics of Prokaryotes. Species definitions are distinguished using DNA profiling, including a nearly complete 16S rRNA sequence with less than 0-5% ambiguity in combination with phenotypic traits. Type species should also be described in detail using diagnostic and comparable methods that are reproducible.

## NOMENCLATURE

*Nomenclature* is the naming of microorganisms according to established rules and guidelines set forth in the International Code of Nomenclature of Bacteria (ICNB) or the Bacteriological Code (BC). It provides the accepted labels by which organisms are universally recognized. Because genus and species are the groups commonly used by microbiologists, the discussion of rules governing microbial nomenclature is limited to these two taxa. In this binomial (two name) system of nomenclature, every organism is assigned a genus and a species of Latin or Greek derivation. Each organism has a scientific "label" consisting of two parts: the genus designation, in which the first letter is always capitalized, and the species designation, in which the first letter is always lower case. The two components are used simultaneously and are printed in italics or underlined in script. For example, the streptococci include *Streptococcus pneumoniae, Streptococcus pyogenes, Streptococcus agalactiae,* and *Streptococcus bovis,* among others. Alternatively, the name may be abbreviated by using the upper case form of the first letter of the genus designation followed by a period (.) and the full species name, which is never abbreviated (e.g., *S. pneumoniae, S. pyogenes, S. agalactiae,* and *S. bovis*). Frequently an informal designation (e.g., staphylococci, streptococci, enterococci) may be used to label a particular group of organisms. These designations are not capitalized or italicized.

As more information is gained regarding organism classification and identification, a particular species may be moved to a different genus or assigned a new genus name. The rules and criteria for these changes are beyond the scope of this chapter, but such changes are documented in the *International Journal of Systemic and Evolutionary Microbiology*. In the diagnostic laboratory, changes in nomenclature are phased in gradually so that physicians and laboratorians have ample opportunity to recognize that a familiar pathogen has been given a new name. This is usually accomplished by using the new genus designation while continuing to provide the previous designation in parentheses; for example, *Stenotrophomonas (Xanthomonas) maltophilia* or *Burkholderia (Pseudomonas) cepacia.*

---

**BOX 1-1**   Role of Taxonomy in Diagnostic Microbiology

- Establishes and maintains records of key characteristics of clinically relevant microorganisms
- Facilitates communication among technologists, microbiologists, physicians, and scientists by assigning universal names to clinically relevant microorganisms. This is essential for:
  - Establishing an association of particular diseases or syndromes with specific microorganisms
  - Epidemiology and tracking outbreaks
  - Accumulating knowledge regarding the management and outcome of diseases associated with specific microorganisms
  - Establishing patterns of resistance to antimicrobial agents and recognition of changing microbial resistance patterns
  - Understanding the mechanisms of antimicrobial resistance and detecting new resistance mechanisms exhibited by microorganisms
  - Recognizing new and emerging pathogenic microorganisms
  - Recognizing changes in the types of infections or diseases caused by characteristic microorganisms
  - Revising and updating available technologies for the development of new methods to optimize the detection and identification of infectious agents and the detection of resistance to antiinfective agents (microbial, viral, fungal, and parasitic)
  - Developing new antiinfective therapies (microbial, viral, fungal, and parasitic)

---

## IDENTIFICATION

Microbial **identification** is the process by which a microorganism's key features are delineated. Once those features have been established, the profile is compared with those of other previously characterized microorganisms. The organism can then be assigned to the most appropriate taxa (classification) and can be given appropriate genus and species names (nomenclature); both are essential aspects of the role taxonomy plays in diagnostic microbiology and infectious diseases (Box 1-1).

### IDENTIFICATION METHODS

A wide variety of methods and criteria are used to establish a microorganism's identity. These methods usually can be separated into either of two general categories: genotypic characteristics and phenotypic characteristics. **Genotypic characteristics** relate to an organism's genetic makeup, including the nature of the organism's genes and constituent nucleic acids (see Chapter 2 for more information about microbial genetics). **Phenotypic characteristics** are based on features beyond the genetic level and include both readily observable characteristics and characteristics that may require extensive analytic procedures to be detected. Examples of characteristics used as criteria for bacterial identification and classification are provided in Table 1-1. Modern microbial taxonomy uses a combination of several methods to characterize

**TABLE 1-1** Identification Criteria and Characteristics for Microbial Classification

| Phenotypic Criteria Examples | Principles |
|---|---|
| Macroscopic morphology | Characteristics of microbial growth patterns on artificial media as observed when inspected with the unaided eye. Examples of such characteristics include the size, texture, and pigmentation of bacterial colonies. |
| Microscopic morphology | Size, shape, intracellular inclusions, cellular appendages, and arrangement of cells when observed with the aid of microscopic magnification. |
| Staining characteristics | Ability of an organism to reproducibly stain a particular color with the application of specific dyes and reagents. Staining is used in conjunction with microscopic morphology for bacterial identification. For example, the Gram stain for bacteria is a critical criterion for differential identification. |
| Environmental requirements | Ability of an organism to grow at various temperatures, in the presence of oxygen and other gases, at various pH levels, or in the presence of other ions and salts, such as NaCl. |
| Nutritional requirements | Ability of an organism to utilize various carbon and nitrogen sources as nutritional substrates when grown under specific environmental conditions. |
| Resistance profiles | Exhibition of a characteristic inherent resistance to specific antibiotics, heavy metals, or toxins by certain microorganisms. |
| Antigenic properties | Establishment of profiles of microorganisms by various serologic and immunologic methods for determining the relatedness among various microbial groups. |
| Subcellular properties | Establishment of the molecular constituents of the cell that are typical of a particular taxon, or organism group, by various analytic methods. Some examples include cell wall components, components of the cell membrane, and enzymatic content of the microbial cell. |
| Genotypic Criteria Examples | Principles |
| Deoxyribonucleic acid (DNA) base composition ratio | DNA comprises four bases (guanine, cytosine, adenine, and thymine). The extent to which the DNA from two organisms is made up of cytosine and guanine (i.e., G + C content) relative to their total base content can be used as an indicator of relatedness or lack thereof. For example, an organism with a G + C content of 50% is not closely related to an organism with a G + C content of 25%. |
| Nucleic acid (DNA and ribonucleic acid [RNA]) base sequence analysis, including hybridization assays. | The order of bases along a strand of DNA or RNA is known as the *base sequence*. The extent to which sequences are similar (homologous) between two microorganisms can be determined directly or indirectly by various molecular methods. The degree of similarity in the sequences may be a measure of the degree of organism relatedness, specifically, the ribosomal RNA (rRNA) sequences that remain stable in comparison to the genome as a whole. |

microorganisms thoroughly so as to classify and name each organism appropriately.

Although the criteria and examples in Table 1-1 are given in the context of microbial identification for classification purposes, the principles and practices of classification parallel the approaches used in diagnostic microbiology for the identification and characterization of microorganisms encountered in the clinical setting. Fortunately, because of the previous efforts and accomplishments of microbial taxonomists, microbiologists do not have to use several burdensome classification and identification schemes to identify infectious agents. Instead, microbiologists use key phenotypic and genotypic features on which to base their identification in order to provide clinically relevant information in a timely manner (see Chapter 13). This should not be taken to mean that the identification of all clinically relevant organisms is easy and straightforward. This is also not meant to imply that microbiologists can only identify or recognize organisms that have already been characterized and named by taxonomists. Indeed, the clinical microbiology laboratory is well recognized as the place where previously unknown or uncharacterized infectious agents are initially encountered, and as such it has an ever-increasing responsibility to be the sentinel for emerging etiologies of infectious diseases.

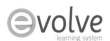 *Visit the Evolve site to complete the review questions.*

## BIBLIOGRAPHY

Brock TD, Madigan M, Martinko J, et al, editors: *Biology of microorganisms*, Englewood Cliffs, NJ, 2009, Prentice Hall.

Dworkin M, Falkow S, Rosenberg E, et al, editors: *The prokaryotes: a handbook on the biology of bacteria: ecophysiology, isolation, identification, applications*, vol 1-4, New York, 2006, Springer.

Garrity GM, editor: *Bergey's manual of systematic bacteriology*, ed 2, New York, 2001, Springer.

Stackebrandt E, Frederiksen W, Garrity GM, et al: Report on ad hoc committee for the re-evaluation of the species identification in bacteriology, *Int J Syst Evol Microbiol* 52:1043-1047, 2002.

# Bacterial Genetics, Metabolism, and Structure

## OBJECTIVES

1. Describe the basic structure and organization of prokaryotic (bacterial) chromosomes, including number, relative size, and cellular location.
2. Outline the basic processes and essential components required for genetic information transfer in replication, transcription, translation, and regulatory mechanisms.
3. Define mutation, recombination, transduction, transformation, and conjugation.
4. Describe how genetic alterations and diversity provide a mechanism for evolution and survival of microorganisms.
5. Differentiate environmental oxygenation and final electron acceptors (aerobes, facultative anaerobes, and strict anaerobes) in the formation of energy.
6. Compare and contrast the key structural elements, cellular organization, and types of organisms classified as prokaryotic and eukaryotic.
7. State the functions and biologic significance of the following cellular structures: the outer membrane, cell wall, periplasmic space, cytoplasmic membrane, capsule, fimbriae, pili, flagella, nucleoid, and cytoplasm.
8. Differentiate the organization and chemical composition of the cell envelope for a gram-positive and a gram-negative bacterium.

Microbial genetics, metabolism, and structure are the keys to microbial viability and survival. These processes involve numerous pathways that are widely varied, often complicated, and frequently interactive. Essentially, survival requires energy to fuel the synthesis of materials necessary to grow, propagate, and carry out all other metabolic processes (Figure 2-1). Although the goal of survival is the same for all organisms, the strategies microorganisms use to accomplish this vary substantially.

Knowledge regarding genetic, metabolic, and structural characteristics of microorganisms provides the basis for understanding almost every aspect of diagnostic microbiology, including:

- The mechanism or mechanisms by which microorganisms cause disease
- Developing and implementing optimum techniques for microbial detection, cultivation, identification, and characterization
- Understanding antimicrobial action and resistance
- Developing and implementing tests for the detection of antimicrobial resistance
- Designing strategies for disease therapy and control

Microorganisms vary significantly in many genetic and therefore physiologic aspects. A detailed consideration of these differences is beyond the scope of this textbook. Therefore, a generalized description of bacterial systems is used as a model to discuss microbial genetics, metabolism, and structure. Information regarding characteristics of fungi, parasites, and viruses can be found in subsequent chapters that discuss these specific taxonomic groups.

# BACTERIAL GENETICS

*Genetics*, the process of heredity and variation, is the starting point from which all other cellular pathways, functions, and structures originate. The ability of a microorganism to maintain viability, adapt, multiply, and cause disease is determined by the organism's genetic composition. The three major aspects of microbial genetics that require discussion include:

- The structure and organization of genetic material
- Replication and expression of genetic information
- The mechanisms by which genetic information is altered and exchanged among bacteria

## NUCLEIC ACID STRUCTURE AND ORGANIZATION

For all living entities, hereditary information resides or is encoded in nucleic acids. The two major classes of nucleic acids are deoxyribonucleic acid (DNA), which is the most common macromolecule that encodes genetic information, and ribonucleic acid (RNA). In some forms, RNA encodes genetic information for various viruses; in other forms, RNA plays an essential role in several of the genetic processes in prokaryotic and eukaryotic cells, including the regulation and transfer of information. Prokaryotic or "prenuclear" organisms do not have membrane bound organelles and the cells' genetic material is therefore not enclosed in a nucleus. Eukaryotic "true nucleus" are all of the organisms that have their genetic material enclosed in a nuclear envelope.

### Nucleotide Structure and Sequence

DNA consists of deoxyribose sugars connected by phosphodiester bonds (Figure 2-2, *A*). The bases that are covalently linked to each deoxyribose sugar are the key to the genetic code within the DNA molecule. The four bases include two purines, adenine (A) and guanine (G), and the two pyrimidines, cytosine (C) and thymine (T) (Figure 2-3). In RNA, uracil replaces thymine. The combined sugar, phosphate, and a base form a single unit referred to as a **nucleotide** (adenosine triphosphate [ATP], guanine triphosphate [GTP], cytosine triphosphate [CTP], and thymine triphosphate [TTP]). DNA and RNA are nucleotide polymers (i.e., chains or strands), and the order of bases along a DNA or RNA strand is known as the **base sequence.** This sequence provides the information that codes for the proteins that will be synthesized by microbial cells; that is, the sequence is the **genetic code**.

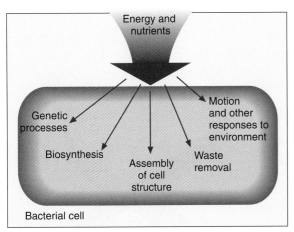

**Figure 2-1** General overview of bacterial cellular processes.

## DNA Molecular Structure

The intact DNA molecule is composed of two nucleotide polymers. Each strand has a 5' (prime) phosphate and a 3' (prime) hydroxyl terminus (see Figure 2-2, A). The two strands run antiparallel, with the 5' of one strand opposed to the 3' terminal of the other. The strands are also complementary, because the adenine base of one strand always binds to the thymine base of the other strand by means of two hydrogen bonds. Similarly, the guanine base of one strand always binds to the cytosine base of the other strand by means of three hydrogen bonds. As a result of the molecular restrictions of these base pairings, along with the conformation of the sugar-phosphate backbones oriented in antiparallel fashion, DNA has the unique structural conformation often referred to as a "twisted ladder" or double helix (see Figure 2-2, B). Additionally, the dedicated base pairs provide the format essential for consistent replication and expression of the genetic code. In contrast to DNA, which carries the genetic code, RNA rarely exists as a double-stranded molecule. The three major types of RNA (**messenger RNA [mRNA], transfer RNA [tRNA],** and **ribosomal RNA [rRNA]**) play key roles in gene expression.

## Genes and the Genetic Code

A DNA sequence that encodes for a specific product (RNA or protein) is defined as a **gene.** Thousands of genes in an organism encode messages or blueprints for the production of one or more proteins and RNA products that play essential metabolic roles in the cell. All the genes in an organism comprise the organism's *genome.* The size of a gene and an entire genome is usually expressed in the number of base pairs (bp) present (e.g., kilobases [$10^3$ bases], megabases [$10^6$ bases]).

Certain genes are widely distributed among various organisms while others are limited to particular species. Also, the base pair sequence for individual genes may be highly conserved (i.e., show limited sequence differences among different organisms) or be widely variable. As discussed in Chapter 8, these similarities and differences in gene content and sequences are the basis for the

development of molecular tests used to detect, identify, and characterize clinically relevant microorganisms.

## Chromosomes

The genome is organized into discrete elements known as **chromosomes.** The set of genes within a given chromosome is arranged in a linear fashion, but the number of genes per chromosome is variable. Similarly, although the number of chromosomes per cell is consistent for a given species, this number varies considerably among species. For example, human cells contain 23 pairs (i.e., diploid) of chromosomes whereas bacteria contain a single, unpaired (i.e., haploid) chromosome.

Bacteria are classified as prokaryotes; therefore, the chromosome is not located in a membrane-bound organelle (i.e., nucleus). The bacterial chromosome contains the genes essential for viability and exists as a double-stranded, closed, circular macromolecule. The molecule is extensively folded and twisted (i.e., supercoiled) in order to fit within the confined space of the bacterial cell. The linearized, unsupercoiled chromosome of the bacterium *Escherichia coli* is about 1300 μm long, but it fits within a cell $1 \times 3$ μm; this attests to the extreme compact structure of the supercoiled bacterial chromosome. For genes in the compacted chromosome to be expressed and replicated, unwinding or relaxation of the molecule is required.

In contrast to the bacterial chromosome, the chromosomes of parasites and fungi number more than one per cell, are linear, and are housed within a membrane-bound organelle (the nucleus) of the cell. This difference is a major criterion for classifying bacteria as *prokaryotic* organisms and fungi and parasites as *eukaryotes.* The genome topology of a virus may consist of DNA or RNA contained within a protein coat rather than a cell.

## Nonchromosomal Elements of the Genome

Although the bacterial chromosome represents the majority of the genome, not all genes in a given cell are confined to the chromosome. Many genes may also be located on plasmids and transposable elements. Both of these extrachromosomal elements are able to replicate and encode information for the production of various cellular products. Although considered part of the bacterial genome, they are not as stable as the chromosome and may be lost during cellular replication, often without any detrimental effects on the viability of the cell.

Plasmids exist as double-stranded, closed, circular, autonomously replicating extrachroosomal genetic elements ranging in size from 1 to 2 kilobases up to 1 megabase or more. The number of plasmids per bacterial cell varies extensively, and each plasmid is composed of several genes. Some genes encode products that mediate plasmid replication and transfer between bacterial cells, whereas others encode products that provide a specialized function, such as determinants of antimicrobial resistance or a unique metabolic process. Unlike most chromosomal genes, plasmid genes do not usually encode for products essential for viability. Plasmids, in whole or in part, may also become incorporated into the chromosome.

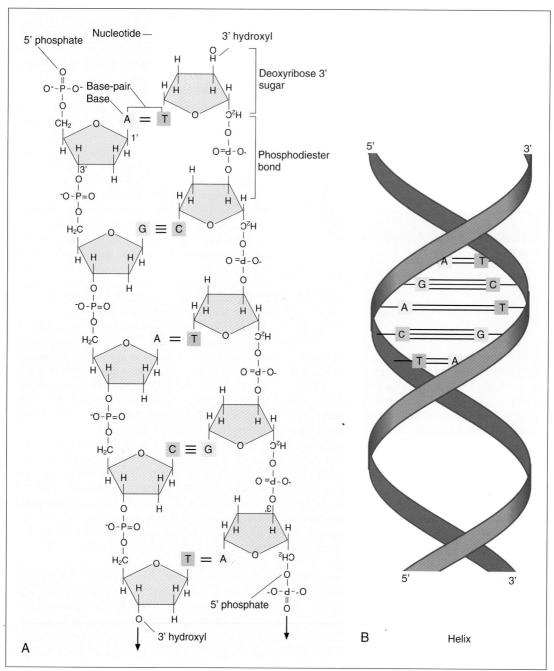

**Figure 2-2 A,** Molecular structure of DNA depicting nucleotide structure, phosphodiester bonds connecting nucleotides, and complementary base pairing (*A*, adenine; *T*, thymine; *G*, guanine; *C*, cytosine) between antiparallel nucleic acid strands. **B,** 5' and 3' antiparallel polarity and double helix configuration of DNA.

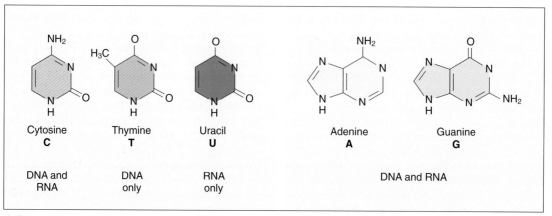

**Figure 2-3** Molecular structure of nucleic acid bases. Pyrimidines: cytosine, thymine, and uracil. Purines: adenine and guanine.

Transposable elements are pieces of DNA that move from one genetic element to another, from plasmid to chromosome or vice versa. Unlike plasmids, they are unable to replicate independently and do not exist as separate entities in the bacterial cell. The two types of transposable elements are **the simple transposon or insertion sequence (IS)** and the **composite** transposon. Insertion sequences are limited to containing the genes that encode information required for movement from one site in the genome to another. Composite transposons are a cassette (grouping of genes) flanked by insertion sequences. The internal gene imbedded in the insertion sequence encodes for an accessory function, such as antimicrobial resistance. Plasmids and transposable elements coexist with chromosomes in the cells of many bacterial species. These extrachromosomal elements play a key role in the exchange of genetic material throughout the bacterial microbiosphere, including genetic exchange among clinically relevant bacteria.

## REPLICATION AND EXPRESSION OF GENETIC INFORMATION

### Replication

Bacteria multiply by cell division, resulting in the production of two daughter cells from one parent cell. As part of this process, the genome must be replicated so that each daughter cell receives an identical copy of functional DNA. Replication is a complex process mediated by various enzymes, such as DNA polymerase and cofactors; replication must occur quickly and accurately. For descriptive purposes, replication may be considered in four stages (Figure 2-4):

1. Unwinding or relaxation of the chromosome's supercoiled DNA
2. Separation of the complementary strands of the parental DNA so that each may serve as a template (i.e., pattern) for synthesis of new DNA strands
3. Synthesis of the new (i.e., daughter) DNA strands
4. Termination of replication, releasing two identical chromosomes, one for each daughter cell

Relaxation of supercoiled chromosomal DNA is required so that enzymes and cofactors involved in replication can access the DNA molecule at the site where the replication process will originate (i.e., **origin of replication**). The origin of replication (a specific sequence of approximately 300 base pairs) is recognized by several initiation proteins, followed by the separation of the complementary strands of parental DNA. Each parental strand serves as a template for the synthesis of a new complementary daughter strand. The site of active replication is referred to as the **replication fork;** two bidirectional forks are involved in the replication process. Each replication fork moves through the parent DNA molecule in opposite directions so that replication is a bidirectional process. Activity at each replication fork involves

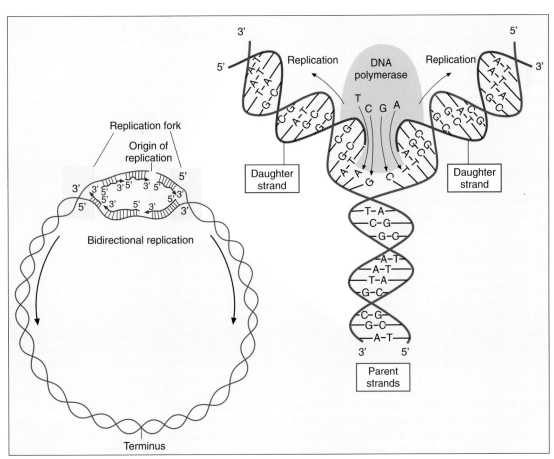

**Figure 2-4** Bacterial DNA replication depicting bidirectional movement of two replication forks from origin of replication. Each parent strand serves as a template for production of a complementary daughter strand and, eventually, two identical chromosomes.

different cofactors and enzymes, with **DNA polymerases** playing a central role. Using each parental strand as a template, DNA polymerases add nucleotide bases to each growing daughter strand in a sequence that is complementary to the base sequence of the template (parent) strand. The complementary bases of each strand are then held together by hydrogen bonding between nucleotides and the hydrophobic nature of the nitrogenous bases. The new nucleotides can be added only to the 3' hydroxyl end of the growing strand so that synthesis for each daughter strand occurs only in a 5' to 3' direction.

Termination of replication occurs when the replication forks meet. The result is two complete chromosomes, each containing two complementary strands, one of parental origin and one newly synthesized daughter strand. Although the time required for replication can vary among bacteria, the process generally takes approximately 20 to 40 minutes in rapidly growing bacteria such as *E. coli*. The replication time for a particular bacterial strain can vary depending on environmental conditions, such as the availability of nutrients or the presence of toxic substances (e.g., antimicrobial agents).

### Expression of Genetic Information

*Gene expression* is the processing of information encoded in genetic elements (i.e., chromosomes, plasmids, and transposons), which results in the production of biochemical molecules, including RNA molecules and proteins. The overall process of gene expression is composed of two complex steps, transcription and translation. Gene expression requires various components, including a DNA template representing a single gene or cluster of genes, various enzymes and cofactors, and RNA molecules of specific structure and function.

**Transcription.** Gene expression begins with transcription. During transcription the DNA base sequence of the gene (i.e., the genetic code) is converted into an mRNA molecule that is complementary to the gene's DNA sequence (Figure 2-5). Usually only one of the two DNA strands (the sense strand) encodes for a functional gene product. This same strand is the template for mRNA synthesis.

RNA polymerase is the enzyme central to the transcription process. The enzyme is composed of four protein subunits and a sigma factor. Sigma factors are required for the RNA polymerase to identify the appropriate site on the DNA template where transcription of mRNA is initiated. This initiation site is also known as the *promoter sequence*. The remainder of the enzyme functions to unwind the double-stranded DNA at the promoter sequence and use the DNA strand as a template to sequentially add ribonucleotides (ATP, GTP, uracil triphosphate [UTP], and CTP) to form the growing mRNA strand.

Transcription proceeds in a 5' to 3' direction. However, in mRNA, the TTP of DNA is replaced with UTP. TTP contains thymine, and UTP contains uracil. Both molecules contain a heterocyclic ring and are classified as pyrimidines. During synthesis and modification of these molecules, a portion of the molecules are dehydroxylated, forming a 2'-deoxy-nucleotide monophosphate. The dUMP (dehydroxylated uracil monophosphate) is then methylated, forming dTMP (dehydroxylated

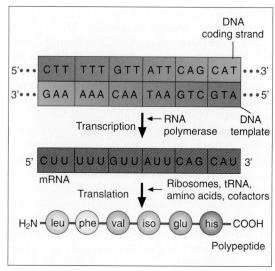

**Figure 2-5** Overview of gene expression components; transcription for production of mRNA and translation for production of polypeptide (protein).

thymine monophosphate). Following phosphorylation, thymine is only found in the final state as deoxythymidine and therefore cannot be incorporated into an RNA molecule. Synthesis of the single-stranded mRNA product ends when specific nucleotide base sequences on the DNA template are encountered. Termination of transcription may be facilitated by a rho (a prokaryotic protein) cofactor or an intrinsic termination sequence. Both of these mechanisms disrupt the mRNA-RNA polymerase template DNA complex.

In bacteria, the mRNA molecules that result from the transcription process are polycistronic, that is, they encode for several gene products. Frequently, polycistronic mRNA may encode several genes whose products (proteins) are involved in a single or closely related cellular function. When a cluster of genes is under the control of a single promoter sequence, the gene group is referred to as an *operon*.

The transcription process not only produces mRNA but also tRNA and rRNA. All three types of RNA have key roles in protein synthesis.

**Translation.** The next phase in gene expression, translation, involves protein synthesis. Through this process the genetic code in mRNA molecules is translated into specific amino acid sequences that are responsible for protein structure and function (see Figure 2-5).

Before addressing the process of translation, a discussion of the genetic code that is originally transcribed from DNA to mRNA and then translated from mRNA to protein is warranted. The code consists of triplets of nucleotide bases, referred to as *codons;* each codon encodes for a specific amino acid. Because there are 64 different codons for 20 amino acids, an amino acid can be encoded by more than one codon (Table 2-1). Each codon is specific for a single amino acid. Therefore, through translation, the codon sequences in mRNA direct which amino acids are added and in what order. Translation ensures that proteins with proper structure and function are

**TABLE 2-1** The Genetic Code as Expressed by Triplet-Base Sequences of mRNA*

| Codon | Amino Acid | Codon | Amino Acid | Codon | Amino Acid | Codon | Amino Acid |
|-------|------------|-------|------------|-------|------------|-------|------------|
| UUU | Phenylalanine | CUU | Leucine | GUU | Valine | AUU | Isoleucine |
| UUC | Phenylalanine | CUC | Leucine | GUC | Valine | AUC | Isoleucine |
| UUG | Leucine | CUG | Leucine | GUG | Valine | AUG (start)† | Methionine |
| UUA | Leucine | CUA | Leucine | GUA | Valine | AUA | Isoleucine |
| UCU | Serine | CCU | Proline | GCU | Alanine | ACU | Threonine |
| UCC | Serine | CCC | Proline | GCC | Alanine | ACC | Threonine |
| UCG | Serine | CCG | Proline | GCG | Alanine | ACG | Threonine |
| UCA | Serine | CCA | Proline | GCA | Alanine | ACA | Threonine |
| UGU | Cysteine | CGU | Arginine | GGU | Glycine | AGU | Serine |
| UGC | Cysteine | CGC | Arginine | GGC | Glycine | AGC | Serine |
| UGG | Tryptophan | CGG | Arginine | GGG | Glycine | AGG | Arginine |
| UGA | None (stop signal) | CGA | Arginine | GGA | Glycine | AGA | Arginine |
| UAU | Tyrosine | CAU | Histidine | GAU | Aspartic | AAU | Asparagine |
| UAC | Tyrosine | CAC | Histidine | GAC | Aspartic | AAC | Asparagine |
| UAG | None (stop signal) | CAG | Glutamine | GAG | Glutamic | AAG | Lysine |
| UAA | None (stop signal) | CAA | Glutamine | GAA | Glutamic | AAA | Lysine |

Modified from Brock TD et al, editors: *Biology of microorganisms,* Upper Saddle River, NJ, 2009, Prentice Hall.
*The codons in DNA are complementary to those given here. Thus, U is complementary to the A in DNA, C is complementary to G, G to C, and A to T. The nucleotide on the left is at the 5'-end of the triplet.
†AUG codes for N-formylmethionine at the beginning of messenger ribonucleic acid (mRNA) in bacteria.

produced. Errors in the process can result in aberrant proteins that are nonfunctional, underscoring the need for translation to be well controlled and accurate.

To accomplish the task of translation, intricate interactions between mRNA, tRNA, and rRNA are required. Sixty different types of tRNA molecules are responsible for transferring different amino acids from intracellular reservoirs to the site of protein synthesis. These molecules, which have a structure that resembles an inverted t, contain one sequence recognition site (anticodon) for binding to specific 3-base sequences (codons) on the mRNA molecule (Figure 2-6). A second site binds specific amino acids, the building blocks of proteins. Each amino acid is joined to a specific tRNA molecule through the enzymatic activity of aminoacyl-tRNA synthetases. Therefore, tRNA molecules have the primary function of using the codons of the mRNA molecule as the template for precisely delivering a specific amino acid for polymerization. **Ribosomes,** which are compact nucleoproteins, are composed of rRNA and proteins. They are central to translation, assisting with coupling of all required components and controlling the translational process.

Translation, diagrammatically shown in Figure 2-6, involves three steps: initiation, elongation, and termination. Following termination, bacterial proteins often undergo posttranslational modifications as a final step in protein synthesis.

Initiation begins with the association of ribosomal subunits, mRNA, formylmethionine tRNA ([f-met] carrying the initial amino acid of the protein to be synthesized), and various initiation factors (see Figure 2-6, *A*). Assembly of the complex begins at a specific 3- to 9-base (Shine-Dalgarno sequence) on the mRNA about 10 bp upstream of the AUG start codon. After the initial complex has been formed, addition of individual amino acids begins.

Elongation involves tRNAs mediating the sequential addition of amino acids in a specific sequence that is dictated by the codon sequence of the mRNA molecule (see Figure 2-6, *B* and *C,* and Table 2-1). As the mRNA molecule threads through the ribosome in a 5' to 3' direction, peptide bonds are formed between adjacent amino acids, still bound by their respective tRNA molecules in the P (peptide) and A (acceptor) sites of the ribosome. During the process, the forming peptide is moved to the P site, and the most 5' tRNA is released from the E (exit) site. This movement vacates the A site, which contains the codon specific for the next amino acid, so that the incoming tRNA–amino acid can join the complex (see Figure 2-6, *C*).

Because multiple proteins encoded on an mRNA strand can be translated at the same time, multiple ribosomes may be simultaneously associated with one mRNA molecule. Such an arrangement is referred to as a *polysome;* its appearance resembles a string of pearls.

Termination, the final step in translation, occurs when the ribosomal A site encounters a stop or nonsense codon that does not specify an amino acid (i.e., a "stop signal"; see Table 2-1). At this point, the protein synthesis complex disassociates and the ribosomes are available for another round of translation. After termination, most proteins must undergo modification, such as folding or enzymatic trimming, so that protein function,

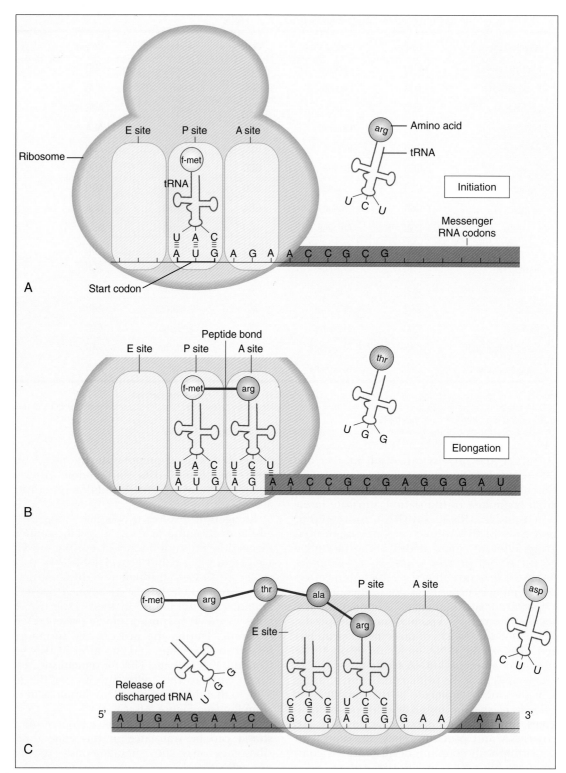

**Figure 2-6** Overview of translation in which mRNA serves as the template for the assembly of amino acids into polypeptides. The three steps include initiation **(A),** elongation (**B** and **C**), and termination (not shown).

transportation, or incorporation into various cellular structures can be accomplished. This process is referred to as *posttranslational modification.*

### Regulation and Control of Gene Expression

The vital role that gene expression and protein synthesis play in the survival of cells dictates that bacteria judiciously control these processes. The cell must regulate gene expression and control the activities of gene products so that a physiologic balance is maintained. Regulation and control are also key factors. These are highly complex mechanisms by which single-cell organisms are able to respond and adapt to environmental challenges, regardless of whether the challenges occur naturally or result from medical intervention (e.g., antibiotics).

Regulation occurs at one of three levels of information transfer from the gene expression and protein synthesis pathway: transcriptional, translational, or posttranslational. The most common is transcriptional regulation. Because direct interactions with genes and their ability to be transcribed to mRNA are involved, transcriptional regulation is also referred to as *genetic control*. Genes that encode enzymes involved in biosynthesis (anabolic enzymes) and genes that encode enzymes for biodegradation (catabolic enzymes) are used as examples of genetic control.

In general, genes that encode anabolic enzymes for the synthesis of particular products are repressed (i.e., are not transcribed and therefore are not expressed) in the presence of the gene end product. This strategy prevents waste and overproduction of products that are already present in sufficient supply. In this system, the product acts as a co-repressor that forms a complex with a repressor molecule. In the absence of co-repressor product (i.e., gene product), transcription occurs (Figure 2-7, *A*). When present in sufficient quantity, the product forms a complex with the repressor. The complex then binds to a specific base region of the gene sequence known as the *operator region* (Figure 2-7, *B*). This binding blocks RNA polymerase progression from the promoter sequence and inhibits transcription. As the supply of product (co-repressor) dwindles, an insufficient amount remains to form a complex with the repressor. The operator region is no longer bound to the repressor molecule. Transcription of the genes for the anabolic enzymes commences and continues until a sufficient supply of end product is again available.

In contrast to repression, genes that encode catabolic enzymes are usually induced; that is, transcription occurs only when the substrate to be degraded by enzymatic action is present. Production of degradative enzymes in the absence of substrates would be a waste of cellular energy and resources. When the substrate is absent in an inducible system, a repressor binds to the operator sequence of the DNA and blocks transcription of the genes for the degradative enzymes (Figure 2-7, *C*). In the presence of an inducer, which often is the target substrate for degradation, a complex is formed between inducer and repressor and results in the release of the repressor from the operator site, allowing transcription of the genes encoding the specific catabolic enzymes (Figure 2-7, *D*).

Certain genes are not regulated; that is, they are not under the control of inducers or repressors. These genes are referred to as *constitutive*. Because they usually encode for products that are essential for viability under almost all growth and environmental conditions, these genes are continuously expressed. Also, not all regulation occurs at the genetic level (i.e., transcriptional regulation). For example, the production of some enzymes may be controlled at the protein synthesis (i.e., translational) level. The activities of other enzymes that have already been synthesized may be regulated at a posttranslational level; that is, certain catabolic or anabolic metabolites may directly interact with enzymes either to increase or to decrease their enzymatic activity.

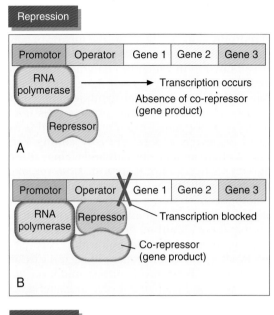

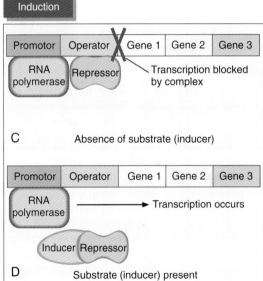

**Figure 2-7** Transcriptional control of gene expression. **A** and **B**, Gene repression. **C** and **D**, Induction.

Among different bacteria and even among different genes in the same bacterium, the mechanisms by which inducers and co-repressors are involved in gene regulation vary widely. Furthermore, bacterial cells have mechanisms to detect environmental changes. These changes can generate signals that interact with the gene expression mechanism, ensuring that appropriate products are made in response to the environmental change. In addition, several complex interactions between different regulatory systems are found within a single cell. Such diversity and interdependence are necessary components of metabolism that allow an organism to respond to environmental changes in a rapid, well-coordinated, and appropriate way.

## GENETIC EXCHANGE AND DIVERSITY

In eukaryotic organisms, genetic diversity is achieved by sexual reproduction, which allows the mixing of genomes through genetic exchange. Bacteria multiply by simple binary cell division in which two daughter cells result by division of one parent cell. Each daughter cell receives the full and identical genetic complement contained in the original parent cell. This process does not allow for the mixing of genes from other cells and leaves no means of achieving genetic diversity among bacterial progeny. Without genetic diversity and change, the essential ingredients for evolution are lost. However, microorganisms have been on earth for billions of years, and microbiologists have witnessed their ability to change as a result of exposure to chemicals (i.e., antibiotics). It is evident that these organisms are fully capable of evolving and altering their genetic composition.

Genetic alterations and diversity in bacteria are accomplished by three basic mechanisms: mutation, genetic recombination, and exchange between bacteria, with or without recombination. Throughout diagnostic microbiology and infectious diseases, there are numerous examples of the impact these genetic alteration and exchange mechanisms have on clinically relevant bacteria and the management of the infections they cause.

### Mutation

*Mutation* is defined as an alteration in the original nucleotide sequence of a gene or genes within an organism's genome; that is, a change in the organism's genotype. This alteration may involve a single DNA base in a gene, an entire gene, or several genes. Mutational changes in the sequence may arise spontaneously, perhaps by an error made during DNA replication. Alternatively, mutations may be induced by chemical or physical factors (i.e., mutagens) in the environment or by biologic factors, such as the introduction of foreign DNA into the cell. Alterations in the DNA base sequence can result in changes in the base sequence of mRNA during transcription. This, in turn, can affect the types and sequences of amino acids that will be incorporated into the protein during translation.

Depending on the site and extent of the mutation, various outcomes may affect the physiologic functions of the organism. For example, a mutation may be so devastating that it is lethal to the organism; the mutation, therefore, "dies" along with the organism. In other instances the mutation may be silent so that no changes are detected in the organism's observable properties (i.e., the organism's phenotype). Alternatively, the mutation may result in a noticeable alteration in the organism's phenotype, and the change may provide the organism with a survival advantage. This outcome, in Darwinian terms, is the basis for prolonged survival and evolution. Nonlethal mutations are considered stable if they are passed on from one generation to another as an integral part of the cell's genotype (i.e., genetic composition). Additionally, genes that have undergone stable mutations may also be transferred to other bacteria by one of the mechanisms of genetic exchange. In other instances, the mutation may be lost as a result of cellular repair mechanisms capable of restoring the original genotype and phenotype, or it may be lost spontaneously during subsequent cycles of DNA replication.

### Genetic Recombination

Besides mutations, bacterial genotypes can be altered through recombination. In this process, some segment of DNA originating from one bacterial cell (i.e., donor) enters a second bacterial cell (i.e., recipient) and is exchanged with a DNA segment of the recipient's genome. This is also referred to as *homologous recombination*, because the pieces of DNA that are exchanged usually have extensive homology or similarities in their nucleotide sequences. Recombination involves a number of binding proteins, with the RecA protein playing a central role (Figure 2-8, *A*). After recombination, the recipient DNA consists of one original, unchanged strand and a second strand from the donor DNA fragment that has been recombined.

Recombination is a molecular event that occurs frequently in many varieties of bacteria, including most of the clinically relevant species, and it may involve any portion of the organism's genome. However, the recombination event may go unnoticed unless the exchange of DNA results in a distinct alteration in the phenotype. Nonetheless, recombination is a major means by which bacteria may achieve genetic diversity and continue to evolve.

### Genetic Exchange

An organism's ability to undergo recombination depends on the acquisition of "foreign" DNA from a donor cell. The three mechanisms by which bacteria physically exchange DNA are transformation, transduction, and conjugation.

**Transformation.** Transformation involves recipient cell uptake of naked (free) DNA released into the environment when another bacterial cell (i.e., donor) dies and undergoes lysis (see Figure 2-8, *B*). This genomic DNA exists as fragments in the environment. Certain bacteria are able to take up naked DNA from their surroundings; that is, they are able to undergo transformation. Such bacteria are said to be *competent.* Among the bacteria that cause human infections, competence is a characteristic commonly associated with members of the genera *Haemophilus, Streptococcus,* and *Neisseria.*

Once the donor DNA, usually as a singular strand, gains access to the interior of the recipient cell, recombination with the recipient's homologous DNA can occur. The mixing of DNA between bacteria via transformation and recombination plays a major role in the development of antibiotic resistance and in the dissemination of genes that encode factors essential to an organism's ability to cause disease. Additionally, gene exchange by transformation is not limited to organisms of the same species, thus allowing important characteristics to be disseminated to a greater variety of medically important bacteria.

**Transduction.** Transduction is a second mechanism by which DNA from two bacteria may come together in one cell, thus allowing for recombination (see Figure 2-8, *C*). This process is mediated through viruses capable of infecting bacteria (i.e., bacteriophages). In their "life

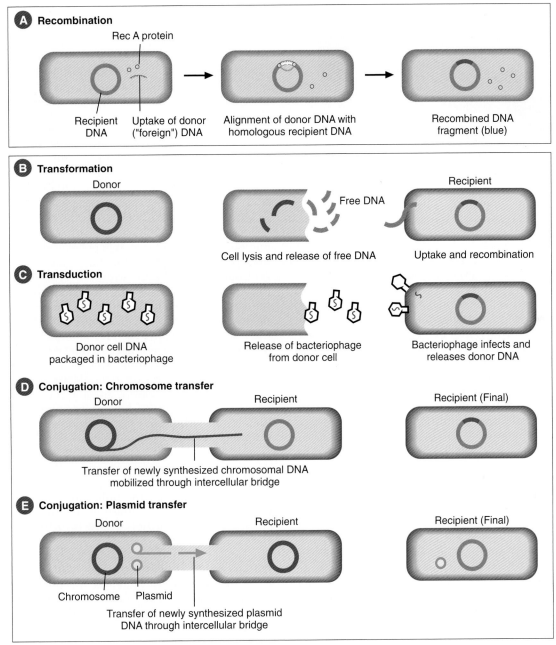

**A,** Genetic recombination. The mechanisms of genetic exchange between bacteria: transformation **(B),** transduction **(C),** and conjugational transfer of chromosomal **(D)** and plasmid **(E)** DNA.

cycle," these viruses integrate their DNA into the bacterial cell's chromosome, where viral DNA replication and expression occur. When the production of viral products is complete, viral DNA is excised (cut) from the bacterial chromosome and packaged within a protein coat. This virion contains bacterial and viral DNA. The newly formed recombinant virion, along with the additional multiple virions (virus particles), is released when the infected bacterial cell lyses. In transduction, the recombinant virion incorporates its own DNA but may also pick up a portion of the donor bacterium's DNA.

The bacterial DNA may be randomly incorporated with viral DNA (generalized transduction), or it may be incorporated along with adjacent viral DNA (specialized transduction). In either case, when the viruses infect another bacterial cell, they release their DNA contents, which includes the previously incorporated bacterial donor DNA. Therefore, the newly infected cell is the recipient of donor DNA introduced by the bacteriophage, and recombination between DNA from two different cells occurs.

**Conjugation.** The third mechanism of DNA exchange between bacteria is **conjugation.** This process occurs between two living cells, involves cell-to-cell contact, and requires mobilization of the donor bacterium's chromosome. The nature of intercellular contact is not well

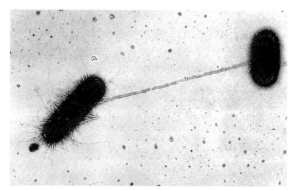

**Figure 2-9** Photomicrograph of *Escherichia coli* sex pilus between donor and recipient cell. (From Brock TD et al, editors: *Biology of microorganisms,* Upper Saddle River, NJ, 2009, Prentice Hall.)

characterized in all bacterial species capable of conjugation. However, in *E. coli*, contact is mediated by a sex pilus (Figure 2-9). The sex pilus originates from the donor and establishes a conjugative bridge that serves as the conduit for DNA transfer from donor to recipient cell. With intercellular contact established, chromosomal mobilization is undertaken and involves DNA synthesis. One new DNA strand is produced by the donor and is passed to the recipient (see Figure 2-8, *D*). The amount of DNA transferred depends on how long the cells are able to maintain contact, but usually only portions of the donor molecule are transferred. In any case, the newly introduced DNA is then available to recombine with the recipient's genome.

In addition to chromosomal DNA, genes encoded in extrachromosomal genetic elements, such as plasmids and transposons, may be transferred by conjugation (see Figure 2-8, *E*). Not all plasmids are capable of conjugative transfer, but for those that are, the donor plasmid usually is replicated so that the donor retains a copy of the plasmid transferred to the recipient. (See the discussion of the F plasmid in the section Cellular Appendages, later in the chapter.) Plasmid DNA may also become incorporated into the host cell's chromosome.

In contrast to plasmids, transposons do not exist independently in the cell. Except when they are moving from one location to another, transposons must be incorporated into the chromosome or plasmids or both. These elements are often referred to as "jumping genes" because of their ability to change location within and even between the genomes of bacterial cells. Transposition is the process by which these genetic elements excise from one genomic location and insert into another. Transposons carry genes that have products that help mediate the transposition process, in addition to genes that encode for other accessory characteristics, such as antimicrobial resistance. Homologous recombination between the genes of plasmids or transposons and the host bacterium's chromosomal DNA may occur.

Plasmids and transposons play a key role in genetic diversity and dissemination of genetic information among bacteria. Many characteristics that significantly alter the activities of clinically relevant bacteria are encoded and disseminated on these elements. Furthermore, as shown in Figure 2-10, the variety of strategies that bacteria can use to mix and match genetic elements provides them with a tremendous capacity to genetically adapt to environmental changes, including those imposed by human medical practices. A good example of this is the emergence and widespread dissemination of resistance to antimicrobial agents among clinically important bacteria. Bacteria have used their capacity for disseminating genetic information to establish resistance to many of the commonly prescribed antibiotics. (See Chapter 11 for more information about antimicrobial resistance mechanisms.)

# BACTERIAL METABOLISM

Fundamentally, bacterial metabolism involves all the cellular processes required for the organism's survival and replication. Familiarity with bacterial metabolism is essential for understanding bacterial interactions with human host cells, the mechanisms bacteria use to cause disease, and the basis of diagnostic microbiology; that is, the tests and strategies used for laboratory identification of infectious etiologies. Because metabolism is an extensive and complicated topic, this section focuses on processes typical of medically relevant bacteria.

For the sake of clarity, metabolism is discussed in terms of four primary, but interdependent, processes: fueling, biosynthesis, polymerization, and assembly (Figure 2-11).

## FUELING

Fueling is considered the utilization of metabolic pathways involved in the acquisition of nutrients from the environment, production of precursor metabolites, and energy production.

### Acquisition of Nutrients

Bacteria use various strategies for obtaining essential nutrients from the external environment and transporting these substances into the cell's interior. For nutrients to be internalized, they must cross the bacterial cell wall and membrane. These complex structures help protect the cell from environmental insults, maintain intracellular equilibrium, and transport substances into and out of the cell. Although some key nutrients (e.g., water, oxygen, and carbon dioxide) enter the cell by simple diffusion across the cell membrane, the uptake of other substances is controlled by membrane-selective permeability; still other substances use specific transport mechanisms.

Active transport is among the most common methods used for the uptake of nutrients such as certain sugars, most amino acids, organic acids, and many inorganic ions. The mechanism, driven by an energy-dependent pump, involves carrier molecules embedded in the membrane portion of the cell structure. These carriers combine with the nutrients, transport them across the membrane, and release them inside the cell. Group translocation is another transport mechanism that requires energy but differs from active transport in that

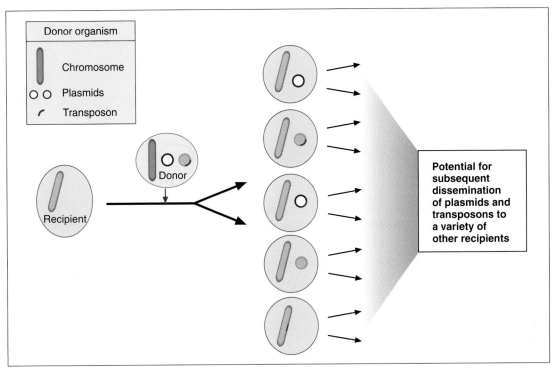

**Figure 2-10** Pathways for bacterial dissemination of plasmids and transposons, together and independently.

## Production of Precursor Metabolites

Once inside the cell, many nutrients serve as the raw materials from which precursor metabolites for subsequent biosynthetic processes are produced. These metabolites, listed in Figure 2-11, are produced through three central pathways; the Embden-Meyerhof-Parnas (EMP) pathway, the tricarboxylic acid (TCA) cycle, and the pentose phosphate shunt. These pathways and their relationship to one another are shown in Figure 2-12; not shown are the several alternative pathways (e.g., the Entner-Douder off pathway) that play key roles in redirecting and replenishing the precursors as they are used in subsequent processes.

The production efficiency of a bacterial cell resulting from these precursor-producing pathways can vary substantially, depending on the growth conditions and availability of nutrients. This is an important consideration because the accurate identification of medically important bacteria often depends heavily on methods that measure the presence of products and byproducts of these metabolic pathways.

## Energy Production

The third type of fueling pathway is one that produces energy required for nearly all cellular processes, including nutrient uptake and precursor production. Energy production is accomplished by the breakdown of chemical substrates (i.e., chemical energy) through the degradative process of catabolism coupled with oxidation-reduction reactions. In this process, the energy source molecule (i.e., substrate) is oxidized as it donates electrons to an electron-acceptor molecule, which is then reduced. The transfer of electrons is mediated through carrier molecules, such as nicotinamide-adenine-dinucleotide (NAD+) and nicotinamide-adenine-dinucleotide-phosphate (NADP+). The energy released by the oxidation-reduction reaction is transferred to phosphate-containing compounds, where high-energy phosphate bonds are formed. ATP is the most common of such molecules. The energy contained in this compound is eventually released by the hydrolysis of ATP under controlled conditions. The release of this chemical energy, coupled with enzymatic activities, specifically catalyzes each biochemical reaction in the cell and drives nearly all cellular reactions.

The two general mechanisms for ATP production in bacterial cells are substrate-level phosphorylation and electron transport, also referred to as *oxidative phosphorylation*. In substrate-level phosphorylation, high-energy phosphate bonds produced by the central pathways are donated to adenosine diphosphate (ADP) to form ATP (see Figure 2-12). Additionally, pyruvate, a primary intermediate in the central pathways, serves as the initial substrate for several other pathways to generate ATP by substrate level phosphorylation. These other pathways constitute fermentative metabolism, which does not require oxygen and produces various end products, including alcohols, acids, carbon dioxide, and hydrogen. The specific fermentative pathways and the end products produced vary with different bacterial species. Detection of these products is an important basis for laboratory identification of bacteria. (See Chapter 7 for more information on the biochemical basis for bacterial identification.)

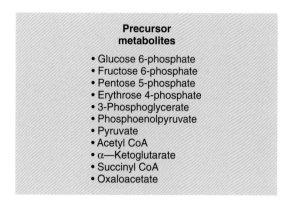

**Precursor metabolites**

- Glucose 6-phosphate
- Fructose 6-phosphate
- Pentose 5-phosphate
- Erythrose 4-phosphate
- 3-Phosphoglycerate
- Phosphoenolpyruvate
- Pyruvate
- Acetyl CoA
- α—Ketoglutarate
- Succinyl CoA
- Oxaloacetate

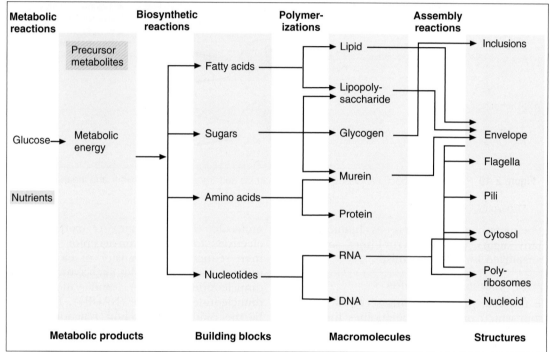

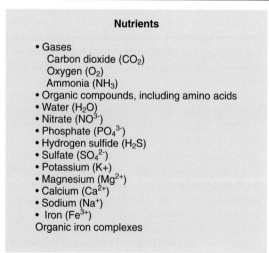

**Nutrients**

- Gases
  Carbon dioxide ($CO_2$)
  Oxygen ($O_2$)
  Ammonia ($NH_3$)
- Organic compounds, including amino acids
- Water ($H_2O$)
- Nitrate ($NO_3^-$)
- Phosphate ($PO_4^{3-}$)
- Hydrogen sulfide ($H_2S$)
- Sulfate ($SO_4^{2-}$)
- Potassium ($K+$)
- Magnesium ($Mg^{2+}$)
- Calcium ($Ca^{2+}$)
- Sodium ($Na^+$)
- Iron ($Fe^{3+}$)
Organic iron complexes

**Figure 2-11** Overview of bacterial metabolism, which includes the processes of fueling, biosynthesis, polymerization, and assembly. (Modified from Niedhardt FC, Ingraham JL, Schaechter M, editors: *Physiology of the bacterial cell: a molecular approach*, Sunderland, Mass, 1990, Sinauer Associates.)

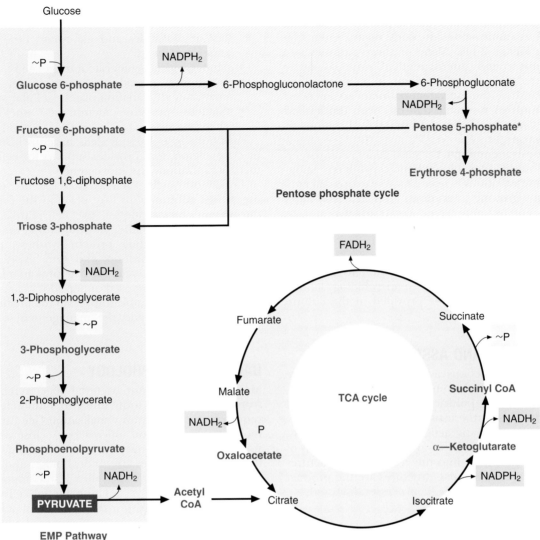

**Figure 2-12** Overview diagram of the central metabolic pathways (Embden-Meyerhof-Parnas [EMP], the tricarboxylic acid [TCA] cycle, and the pentose phosphate shunt). Precursor metabolites (see also Figure 2-11) that are produced are highlighted in red; production of energy in the form of ATP (~P) by substrate-level phosphorylation is highlighted in yellow; and reduced carrier molecules for transport of electrons used in oxidative phosphorylation are highlighted in green. (Modified from Niedhardt FC, Ingraham JL, Schaechter M, editors: *Physiology of the bacterial cell: a molecular approach,* Sunderland, Mass, 1990, Sinauer Associates.)

**Oxidative Phosphorylation.** Oxidative phosphorylation involves an electron transport system that conducts a series of electron transfers from reduced carrier molecules such as NADH2 and NADPH2, produced in the central pathways (see Figure 2-12), to a terminal electron acceptor. The energy produced by the series of oxidation-reduction reactions is used to generate ATP from ADP. When oxidative phosphorylation uses oxygen as the terminal electron acceptor, the process is known as *aerobic respiration. Anaerobic respiration* refers to processes that use final electron acceptors other than oxygen.

A knowledge of which mechanisms bacteria use to generate ATP is important for designing laboratory protocols for cultivating and identifying these organisms. For example, some bacteria depend solely on aerobic respiration and are unable to grow in the absence of oxygen (strictly aerobic bacteria). Others can use either aerobic respiration or fermentation, depending on the availability of oxygen (facultative anaerobic bacteria). For still others, oxygen is absolutely toxic (strictly anaerobic bacteria).

## BIOSYNTHESIS

The fueling reactions essentially bring together all the raw materials needed to initiate and maintain all other cellular processes. The production of precursors and energy is accomplished through catabolic processes and the degradation of substrate molecules. The three remaining pathways for biosynthesis, polymerization, and assembly depend on anabolic metabolism. In anabolic metabolism, precursor compounds are joined for the creation of larger molecules (polymers) required for assembly of cellular structures (see Figure 2-11).

Biosynthetic processes use the precursor products in dozens of pathways to produce a variety of building blocks, such as amino acids, fatty acids, sugars, and nucleotides (see Figure 2-11). Many of these pathways are highly complex and interdependent, whereas other pathway are completely independent. In many cases, the enzymes that drive the individual pathways are encoded on a single mRNA molecule that has been transcribed from contiguous genes in the bacterial chromosome (i.e., an operon).

As previously mentioned, bacterial genera and species vary extensively in their biosynthetic capabilities. Knowledge of these variations is necessary to use optimal conditions for growing organisms under laboratory conditions. For example, some organisms may not be capable of synthesizing an essential amino acid necessary as a building block for proteins. Without the ability to synthesize the amino acid, the bacterium must obtain the building block from the environment. Similarly, if the organism is cultivated in the microbiology laboratory, the amino acid must be provided in the culture medium.

## POLYMERIZATION AND ASSEMBLY

Various anabolic reactions assemble (polymerize) the building blocks into macromolecules, including lipids, lipopolysaccharides, polysaccharides, proteins, and nucleic acids. This synthesis of macromolecules is driven by energy and enzymatic activity in the cell. Similarly, energy and enzymatic activities also drive the assembly of various macromolecules into the component structures of the bacterial cell. Cellular structures are the product of all the genetic and metabolic processes discussed.

# STRUCTURE AND FUNCTION OF THE BACTERIAL CELL

Based on key characteristics, all cells are classified into two basic types: prokaryotic and eukaryotic. Although these two cell types share many common features, they have many important differences in terms of structure, metabolism, and genetics.

## EUKARYOTIC AND PROKARYOTIC CELLS

Among clinically relevant organisms, bacteria are single-cell prokaryotic microorganisms. Fungi and parasites are single-cell or multicellular eukaryotic organisms, as are plants and all higher animals. Viruses are dependent on host cells for survival and therefore are not considered cellular organisms but rather infectious agents.

A notable characteristic of eukaryotic cells, such as those of parasites and fungi, is the presence of membrane-enclosed organelles that have specific cellular functions. Examples of these organelles and their respective functions include:

- Endoplasmic reticulum—process and transport proteins

- Golgi body—modification of substances and transport throughout the cell, including internal delivery of molecules and exocytosis or secretion of other molecules
- Mitochondria—generate energy (ATP)
- Lysosomes—provide environment for controlled enzymatic degradation of intracellular substances
- Nucleus—provide membrane enclosure for chromosomes

Additionally, eukaryotic cells have an infrastructure, or cytoskeleton, that provides support for cellular structure, organization, and movement.

Prokaryotic cells, such as bacteria, do not contain organelles. All functions take place in the cytoplasm or cytoplasmic membrane of the cell. Prokaryotic and eukaryotic cell types differ considerably at the macromolecular level, including protein synthesis machinery, chromosomal organization, and gene expression. One notable structure present only in prokaryotic bacterial cells is a cell wall composed of peptidoglycan. This structure has an immeasurable impact on the practice of diagnostic bacteriology and the management of bacterial diseases.

## BACTERIAL MORPHOLOGY

Most clinically relevant bacterial species range in size from 0.25 to 1 µm in width and 1 to 3 µm in length, thus requiring microscopy for visualization (see Chapter 6 for more information on microscopy). Just as bacterial species and genera vary in their metabolic processes, their cells also vary in size, morphology, and cell-to-cell arrangements and in the chemical composition and structure of the cell wall. The bacterial cell wall differences provide the basis for the Gram stain, a fundamental staining technique used in bacterial identification schemes. This staining procedure separates almost all medically relevant bacteria into two general types: gram-positive bacteria, which stain a deep blue or purple, and gram-negative bacteria, which stain a pink to red (see Figure 6-3). This simple but important color distinction is due to differences in the constituents of bacterial cell walls that influence the cell's ability to retain differential dyes following treatment with a decolorizing agent.

Common bacterial cellular morphologies include cocci (circular), coccobacilli (ovoid), and bacillus (rod shaped), as well as fusiform (pointed end), curved, or spiral shapes. Cellular arrangements are also noteworthy. Cells may characteristically occur singly, in pairs, or grouped as tetrads, clusters, or in chains (see Figure 6-4 for examples of bacterial staining and morphologies). The determination of the Gram stain reaction and the cell size, morphology, and arrangement are essential aspects of bacterial identification.

## BACTERIAL CELL COMPONENTS

Bacterial cell components can be divided into those that make up the outer cell structure and its appendages (cell envelope) and those associated with the cell's interior. It is important to note that the cellular structures work together to function as a complex and integrated unit.

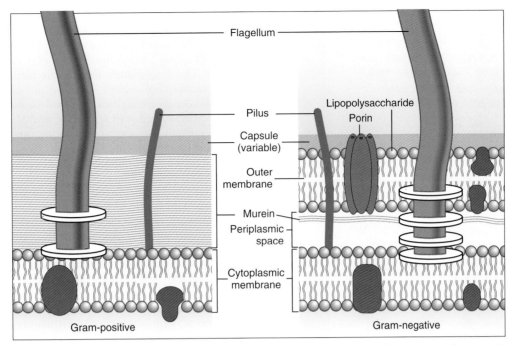

**Figure 2-13** General structures of the gram-positive and gram-negative bacterial cell envelopes. The outer membrane and periplasmic space are present only in the gram-negative envelope. The murein layer is substantially more prominent in gram-positive envelopes. (Modified from Niedhardt FC, Ingraham JL, Schaechter M, editors: *Physiology of the bacterial cell: a molecular approach,* Sunderland, Mass, 1990, Sinauer Associates.)

## Cell Envelope

As shown in Figure 2-13, the outermost structure, the cell envelope, comprises:

- An outer membrane (in gram-negative bacteria only)
- A cell wall composed of the peptidoglycan macromolecule (also known as the *murein layer*)
- Periplasm (in gram-negative bacteria only)
- The cytoplasmic or cell membrane, which encloses the cytoplasm

**Outer Membrane.** Outer membranes, which are found only in gram-negative bacteria, function as the cell's initial barrier to the environment. These membranes serve as primary permeability barriers to hydrophilic and hydrophobic compounds and contain essential enzymes and other proteins located in the periplasmic space. The membrane is a bilayered structure composed of lipopolysaccharide, which gives the surface of gram-negative bacteria a net negative charge. The outer membrane also plays a significant role in the ability of certain bacteria to cause disease.

Scattered throughout the lipopolysaccharide macromolecules are protein structures called *porins*. These water-filled structures control the passage of nutrients and other solutes, including antibiotics, through the outer membrane. The number and types of porins vary with bacterial species. These differences can substantially influence the extent to which various substances pass through the outer membranes of different bacteria. In addition to porins, other proteins (murein lipoproteins) facilitate the attachment of the outer membrane to the next internal layer in the cell envelope, the cell wall.

**Cell Wall (Murein Layer).** The cell wall, also referred to as the *peptidoglycan,* or *murein layer,* is an essential structure found in nearly all clinically relevant bacteria. This structure gives the bacterial cell shape and strength to withstand changes in environmental osmotic pressures that would otherwise result in cell lysis. The murein layer protects against mechanical disruption of the cell and offers some barrier to the passage of larger substances. Because this structure is essential for the survival of bacteria, its synthesis and structure are often the primary targets for the development and design of several antimicrobial agents.

The structure of the cell wall is unique and is composed of disaccharide-pentapeptide subunits. The disaccharides N-acetylglucosamine and N-acetylmuramic acid are the alternating sugar components (moieties), with the amino acid chain linked to N-acetylmuramic acid molecules (Figure 2-14). Polymers of these subunits cross-link to one another by means of peptide bridges to form peptidoglycan sheets. In turn, layers of these sheets are cross-linked with one another, forming a multilayered, cross-linked structure of considerable strength. Referred to as the *murein sacculus,* or sack, this peptidoglycan structure surrounds the entire cell.

A notable difference between the cell walls of gram-positive and gram-negative bacteria is the substantially thicker peptidoglycan layer in gram-positive bacteria (see Figure 2-13). Additionally, the cell wall of gram-positive bacteria contains teichoic acids (i.e., glycerol or ribitol phosphate polymers combined with various sugars, amino acids, and amino sugars). Some teichoic acids are linked to N-acetylmuramic acid, and others (e.g.,

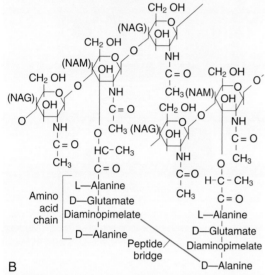

**Figure 2-14** Peptidoglycan sheet **(A)** and subunit **(B)** structure. Multiple peptidoglycan layers compose the murein structure, and different layers are extensively cross-linked by peptide bridges. Note that amino acid chains are only derived from NAM. *NAG,* N-acetylglucosamine; *NAM,* N-acetylmuramic acid. (Modified from Saylers AA, Whitt DD: *Bacterial pathogenesis: a molecular approach,* Washington, DC, 2010, American Society for Microbiology Press.)

lipoteichoic acids) are linked to the next underlying layer, the cellular membrane. Other gram-positive bacteria (e.g., mycobacteria) have waxy substances within the murein layer, such as mycolic acids. Mycolic acids make the cells more refractory to toxic substances, including acids. Bacteria with mycolic acid in the cell walls require unique staining procedures and growth media in the diagnostic laboratory.

**Periplasmic Space.** The periplasmic space typically is found only in gram-negative bacteria (whether it is present in gram-positive organisms is the subject of debate). The periplasmic space is bounded by the internal surface of the outer membrane and the external surface of the cellular membrane. This area, which contains the murein layer, consists of gellike substances that assist in the capture of nutrients from the environment. This space also contains several enzymes involved in the degradation of macromolecules and detoxification of environmental solutes, including antibiotics that enter through the outer membrane.

**Cytoplasmic (Inner) Membrane.** The cytoplasmic (inner) membrane is present in both gram-positive and gram-negative bacteria and is the deepest layer of the cell envelope. The cytoplasmic membrane is heavily laced with various proteins, including a number of enzymes

vital to cellular metabolism. The cell membrane serves as an additional osmotic barrier and is functionally similar to the membranes of several of eukaryotic cellular organelles (e.g., mitochondria, Golgi complexes, lysosomes). The cytoplasmic membrane functions include:

- Transport of solutes into and out of the cell
- Housing of enzymes involved in outer membrane synthesis, cell wall synthesis, and the assembly and secretion of extracytoplasmic and extracellular substances
- Generation of chemical energy (i.e., ATP)
- Cell motility
- Mediation of chromosomal segregation during replication
- Housing of molecular sensors that monitor chemical and physical changes in the environment

**Cellular Appendages.** In addition to the components of the cell envelope proper, cellular appendages (i.e., capsules, fimbriae, and flagella) are associated with or proximal to this portion of the cell. The presence of these appendages, which can play a role in the mediation of infection and in laboratory identification, varies among bacterial species and even among strains within the same species.

The capsule is immediately exterior to the murein layer of gram-positive bacteria and the outer membrane of gram-negative bacteria. Often referred to as the "slime layer," the capsule is composed of high-molecular-weight polysaccharides, the production of which may depend on the environment and growth conditions surrounding the bacterial cell. The capsule does not function as an effective permeability barrier or add strength to the cell envelope, but it does protect bacteria from attack by components of the human immune system. The capsule also facilitates and maintains bacterial colonization of biologic (e.g., teeth) and inanimate (e.g., prosthetic heart valves) surfaces through the formation of biofilms. A biofilm consists of a monomicrobic or polymicrobic group of bacteria housed in a complex polysaccharide matrix. (See Chapter 3 for further discussion of microbial biofilms.)

Fimbriae, or pili, are hairlike, proteinaceous structures that extend from the cell membrane into the external environment; some may be up to 2 μm long. Fimbriae may serve as adhesins that help bacteria attach to animal host cell surfaces, often as the first step in establishing infection. In addition, a pilus may be referred to as a *sex pilus;* this structure, which is well characterized in the gram-negative bacillus *E. coli,* serves as the conduit for the passage of DNA from donor to recipient during conjugation. The sex pilus is present only in cells that produce a protein referred to as the F factor. F-positive cells initiate mating or conjugation only with F-negative cells, thereby limiting the conjugative process to cells capable of transporting genetic material through the hollow sex pilus.

Flagella are complex structures, mostly composed of the protein flagellin, intricately embedded in the cell envelope. These structures are responsible for bacterial motility. Although not all bacteria are motile, motility plays an important role in survival and the ability of certain bacteria to cause disease. Depending on the bacterial species, flagella may be located at one end of the cell (monotrichous flagella) or at both ends of the cell (lophotrichous flagella), or the entire cell surface may be covered with flagella (peritrichous flagella).

## Cell Interior

Those structures and substances that are bounded internally by the cytoplasmic membrane compose the cell interior and include the cytosol, polysomes, inclusions, the nucleoid, plasmids, and endospores.

The cytosol, where nearly all other functions not conducted by the cell membrane occur, contains thousands of enzymes and is the site of protein synthesis. The cytosol has a granular appearance caused by the presence of many polysomes (mRNA complexed with several ribosomes during translation and protein synthesis) and inclusions (i.e., storage reserve granules). The number and nature of the inclusions vary depending on the bacterial species and the nutritional state of the organism's environment. Two common types of granules include glycogen, a storage form of glucose, and polyphosphate granules, a storage form for inorganic phosphates that are microscopically visible in certain bacteria stained with specific dyes.

Unlike eukaryotic chromosomes, the bacterial chromosome is not enclosed within a membrane-bound nucleus. Instead the bacterial chromosome exists as a nucleoid in which the highly coiled DNA is intermixed with RNA, polyamines, and various proteins that lend structural support. At times, depending on the stage of cell division, more than one chromosome may be present per bacterial cell. Plasmids are the other genetic elements that exist independently in the cytosol, and their numbers may vary from none to several hundred per bacterial cell.

The final bacterial structure to be considered is the endospore. Under adverse physical and chemical conditions or when nutrients are scarce, some bacterial genera are able to form spores (i.e., sporulate). Sporulation involves substantial metabolic and structural changes in the bacterial cell. Essentially, the cell transforms from an actively metabolic and growing state to a dormant state, with a decrease in cytosol and a concomitant increase in the thickness and strength of the cell envelope. The spore remains in a dormant state until favorable conditions for growth are again encountered. This survival tactic is demonstrated by a number of clinically relevant bacteria and frequently challenges our ability to thoroughly sterilize materials and food for human use.

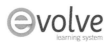

*Visit the Evolve site to complete the review questions.*

## BIBLIOGRAPHY

Brock TD, Madigan M, Martinko J, et al, editors: *Biology of microorganisms*, Upper Saddle River, NJ, 2009, Prentice Hall.

Joklik WK, Willett H, Amos B, et al, editors: *Zinsser microbiology*, Norwalk, Conn, 1992, Appleton & Lange.

Krebs JE, Goldstein ES, Kilpatrick ST: *Lewin's genes X*, Sandbury, Mass, 2011.

Moat AG, Foster JW: *Microbial physiology*, New York, 2002, Wiley-Liss.

Neidhardt FC, Ingraham JL, Schaecter M, editors: *Physiology of the bacterial cell: a molecular approach*, Sunderland, Mass, 1990, Sinauer Associates.

Ryan KJ, editor: *Sherris medical microbiology: an introduction to infectious diseases*, Norwalk, Conn, 2003, McGraw-Hill Medical.

Saylers AA, Wilson BA, Whitt DD, Winkler ME: *Bacterial pathogenesis: a molecular approach*, Washington, DC, 2010, American Society for Microbiology Press.

# Host-Microorganism Interactions

## OBJECTIVES

1. List the various reservoirs (environments) that facilitate host-microorganism interactions.
2. Define direct versus indirect transmission and provide examples of each.
3. Define and differentiate the interactions between the host and microorganism, including colonization, infection, normal (resident) flora, pathogens, opportunistic pathogens, and nosocomial infection.
4. List and describe the components involved in specific versus nonspecific immune defenses, including inflammation, phagocytosis, antibody production, and cellular responses.
5. Identify elements involved in the two arms of the immune system: humoral and cell-mediated immunity.
6. Provide specific examples of disease prevention strategies, including preventing transmission, controlling reservoirs and minimizing risk of exposure.
7. Differentiate between bacterial endotoxins and exotoxins and provide examples of each.
8. Given a patient history of an infectious process, identify and differentiate a sign versus a symptom.
9. Define and differentiate between an acute infectious process and one that is chronic and/or latent.

Interactions between humans and microorganisms are exceedingly complex and far from being completely understood. What is known about the interactions between these two living entities plays an important role in the practice of diagnostic microbiology and in the management of infectious disease. Understanding these interactions is necessary for establishing methods to reliably isolate specific microorganisms from patient specimens and for developing effective treatment strategies. This chapter provides the framework for understanding the various aspects of host-microorganism interactions. Box 3-1 lists a variety of terms and definitions associated with host-microorganism interactions.

Host-microorganism interactions should be viewed as bidirectional in nature. Humans use the abilities and natural products of microorganisms in various settings, including the food and fermentation industry, as biologic insecticides for agriculture; to genetically engineer a multitude of products; and even for biodegrading industrial waste. However, microbial populations share the common goal of survival with humans, using their relationship with humans for food, shelter, and dissemination, and they have been successful at achieving those goals. Which participant in the relationship is the user and which is the used becomes a fine and intricate balance of nature. This is especially true when considering the microorganisms most closely associated with humans and human disease.

The complex relationships between human hosts and medically relevant microorganisms are best understood by considering the sequential steps in the development of microbial-host associations and the subsequent development of infection and disease. The stages of interaction (Figure 3-1) include (1) the physical encounter between host and microorganism; (2) colonization or survival of the microorganism on an internal (gastrointestinal, respiratory, or genitourinary tract) or external (skin) surface of the host; (3) microbial entry, invasion, and dissemination to deeper tissues and organs of the human body; and (4) resolution or outcome.

## THE ENCOUNTER BETWEEN HOST AND MICROORGANISM

### THE HUMAN HOST'S PERSPECTIVE

Because microorganisms are found everywhere, human encounters are inevitable, but the means of encounter vary widely. Which microbial population a human is exposed to and the mechanism of exposure are often direct consequences of a person's activity or behaviors. Certain activities carry different risks for an encounter, and there is a wide spectrum of activities or situations over which a person may or may not have absolute control. For example, acquiring salmonellosis because one fails to cook the holiday turkey thoroughly is avoidable, whereas contracting tuberculosis as a consequence of living in conditions of extreme poverty and overcrowding may be unavoidable. The role that human activities play in the encounter between humans and microorganisms cannot be overstated, because most of the crises associated with infectious disease could be avoided or greatly reduced if human behavior and living conditions could be altered.

#### Microbial Reservoirs and Transmission

Humans encounter microorganisms when they enter or are exposed to the same environment in which the microbial agents live or when the infectious agents are brought to the human host by indirect means. The environment, or place of origin, of the infecting agent is referred to as the reservoir. As shown in Figure 3-2, microbial reservoirs include humans, animals, water, food, air, and soil. The human host may acquire microbial agents by various means referred to as the modes of transmission. The mode of transmission is direct when the host directly contacts the microbial reservoir and is indirect when the host encounters the microorganism by an intervening agent of transmission.

The agents of transmission that bring the microorganism from the reservoir to the host may be a living entity, such as an insect, in which case they are called *vectors*, or

---

**BOX 3-1** Definitions of Selected Epidemiologic Terms

**Carrier:** A person who harbors the etiologic agent but shows no apparent signs or symptoms of infection or disease

**Common source:** The etiologic agent responsible for an epidemic or outbreak originates from a single source or reservoir

**Disease incidence:** The number of new diseases or infected persons in a population

**Disease prevalence:** The percentage of diseased persons in a given population at a particular time

**Endemic:** A disease constantly present at some rate of occurrence in a particular location

**Epidemic:** A larger than normal number of diseased or infected individuals in a particular location

**Etiologic agent:** A microorganism responsible for causing infection or infectious disease

**Mode of transmission:** The means by which etiologic agents are brought in contact with the human host (e.g., infected blood, contaminated water, insect bite)

**Morbidity:** The state of disease and its associated effects on the host

**Morbidity rate:** The incidence of a particular disease state

**Mortality:** Death resulting from disease

**Mortality rate:** The incidence in which a disease results in death

**Nosocomial infection:** Infection for which the etiologic agent was acquired in a hospital or long-term health care center or facility

**Outbreak:** A larger than normal number of diseased or infected individuals that occurs over a relatively short period

**Pandemic:** An epidemic that spans the world

**Reservoir:** The origin of the etiologic agent or location from which it disseminates (e.g., water, food, insects, animals, other humans)

**Strain typing:** Laboratory-based characterization of etiologic agents designed to establish their relatedness to one another during a particular outbreak or epidemic

**Surveillance:** Any type of epidemiologic investigation that involves data collection for characterizing circumstances surrounding the incidence or prevalence of a particular disease or infection

**Vector:** A living entity (animal, insect, or plant) that transmits the etiologic agent

**Vehicle:** A nonliving entity that is contaminated with the etiologic agent and as such is the mode of transmission for that agent

---

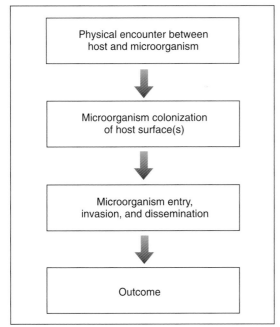

**Figure 3-1** General stages of microbial-host interaction.

they may be a nonliving entity, referred to as a *vehicle* or fomite. Additionally, some microorganisms may have a single mode of transmission, whereas others may spread by various methods. From a diagnostic microbiology perspective, knowledge about an infectious agent's mode of transmission is often important for determining optimum specimens for isolation of the organism and for implementing precautions that minimize the risk of laboratory-acquired infections (see Chapters 4 and 80 for more information regarding laboratory safety).

## Human and Microbe Interactions

Humans play a substantial role as microbial reservoirs. Indeed, the passage of a neonate from the sterile environment of the mother's womb through the birth canal, which is heavily colonized with various microbial agents, is a primary example of one human directly acquiring a microorganism from another human serving as the reservoir. This is the mechanism by which newborns first encounter microbial agents. Other examples in which humans serve as the microbial reservoir include acquisition of "strep" throat through touching; hepatitis through blood transfusions; gonorrhea, syphilis, and acquired immunodeficiency syndrome through sexual contact; tuberculosis through coughing; and the common cold through sneezing. Indirect transfer can occur when microorganisms from one individual contaminate a vehicle of transmission, such as water (e.g., cholera), that is then ingested by another person. In the medical setting, indirect transmission of microorganisms from one human host to another by means of contaminated medical devices helps disseminate infections in hospitals. Hospital-acquired, health care–, or long-term care–associated infections are referred to as *nosocomial infections.*

## Animals as Microbial Reservoirs

Infectious agents from animal reservoirs can be transmitted directly to humans through an animal bite (e.g., rabies) or indirectly through the bite of insect vectors that feed on both animals and humans (e.g., Lyme disease and Rocky Mountain spotted fever). Animals may

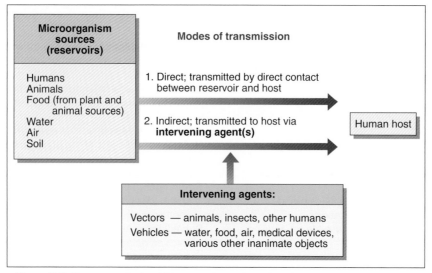

**Figure 3-2** Summary of microbial reservoirs and modes of transmission to humans.

also transmit infectious agents by acquiring or depositing them in water and food supplies. For example, beavers are often heavily colonized with parasites that cause infection of the human gastrointestinal tract. These parasites may be encountered and subsequently acquired when stream water becomes contaminated by the beaver and is used by the vacationing camper. Alternatively, animals used for human food carry numerous bacteria (e.g., *Salmonella* and *Campylobacter*) that, if not destroyed through appropriate cooking during preparation, can cause severe gastrointestinal illness.

Many other infectious diseases are encountered through direct or indirect animal contact, and information regarding a patient's exposure to animals is often a key component in the diagnosis of these infections. Some microorganisms primarily infect animal populations and on occasion accidentally encounter and infect humans. When a human infection results from such an encounter, it is referred to as *a zoonotic infection.*

### Insects as Vectors

The most common role of insects (arthropods) in the transmission of infectious disease is as vectors rather than as reservoirs. A wide variety of arthropods transmit viral, parasitic, and bacterial disease from animals to humans, whereas others transmit microorganisms between human hosts without an intermediate animal reservoir. Malaria, a deadly disease, is a prime example of an infectious disease maintained in the human population by the feeding and survival of an insect vector, the mosquito. Still other arthropods may themselves be agents of disease. These include organisms such as lice and scabies, which are spread directly between humans and cause skin irritations but do not penetrate the body. Because they are able to survive on the skin of the host without gaining access to internal tissues, they are referred to as *ectoparasites.* In addition, nonfungal infections (e.g., tetanus) may result when microbial agents in the environment, such as endospores, are mechanically introduced by the vector as a result of a bite, scratch, or other penetrating wound.

### The Environment as a Microbial Reservoir

The soil and natural environmental debris are reservoirs for countless types of microorganisms. Therefore, it is not surprising that these also serve as reservoirs for microorganisms that can cause infection in humans. Many of the fungal agents (see Part V: Mycology) are acquired by inhalation of soil and dust particles containing microorganisms (e.g., San Joaquin Valley fever). Other, nonfungal infections (e.g., tetanus endospores) may result when microbial agents in the environment are introduced into the human body as a result of a penetrating wound.

## THE MICROORGANISM'S PERSPECTIVE

Clearly, numerous activities can result in human encounters with many microorganisms. Because humans are engaged in all of life's complex activities, the tendency is to perceive the microorganism as having a passive role in the encounter process. However, this assumption is a gross oversimplification.

Microorganisms are also driven by survival, and the environment of the reservoirs they occupy must allow their metabolic and genetic needs to be fulfilled. Reservoirs maybe inhabited by hundreds or thousands of different species of microorganisms. Yet human encounters with the reservoirs, either directly or indirectly do not result in all species establishing an association with the human host. Although some species have evolved strategies that do not involve the human host to ensure survival, others have included humans to a lesser or greater extent as part of their survival tactics. Therefore, the latter type of organism often has mechanisms that enhance its chances for human encounter.

Depending on factors associated with both the human host and the microorganism involved, the encounter may have a beneficial, disastrous, or inconsequential impact on each of the participants.

# MICROORGANISM COLONIZATION OF HOST SURFACES

## THE HOST'S PERSPECTIVE

Once a microbe and the human host are brought into contact, the outcome of the encounter depends on what happens during each step of interaction (see Figure 3-1), beginning with colonization. The human host's role in microbial colonization, defined as the persistent survival of microorganisms on a surface of the human body, is dictated by the defenses that protect vital internal tissues and organs against microbial invasion. The first defenses are the external and internal body surfaces that are in direct contact with the external environment and are the anatomical regions where the microorganisms will initially come in contact with the human host. These surfaces include:

- Skin (including conjunctival epithelium covering the eye)
- Mucous membranes lining the mouth or oral cavity, the respiratory tract, the gastrointestinal tract, and the genitourinary tract

Because body surfaces are always present and provide protection against all microorganisms, skin and mucous membranes are considered constant and nonspecific protective mechanisms. As is discussed later in this text, other protective mechanisms are produced in response to the presence of microbial agents (inducible defenses), and some are directed specifically at particular microorganisms or (specific defense mechanisms).

### Skin and Skin Structures

Skin serves as a physical and chemical barrier to microorganisms; its protective characteristics are summarized in Table 3-1 and Figure 3-3. The acellular, outermost layer of the skin, along with the tightly packed cellular layers underneath, provide an impenetrable physical barrier to all microorganisms, unless damaged. Additionally, these layers continuously shed, thus dislodging bacteria that have attached to the outer layers. The skin is also a dry and cool environment; this is incompatible with the growth requirements of many microorganisms, which thrive in a warm, moist environment.

The follicles and glands of the skin produce various natural antibacterial substances, including sebum and sweat. However, many microorganisms can survive the conditions of the skin. These bacteria are known as *skin colonizers,* and they often produce substances that may be toxic and inhibit the growth of more harmful microbial agents. Beneath the outer layers of skin are various host cells that protect against organisms that breach the surface barriers. These cells, collectively known as *skin-associated lymphoid tissue,* mediate specific and nonspecific responses directed at controlling microbial invaders.

### Mucous Membranes

Because cells that line the respiratory tract, gastrointestinal tract, and genitourinary tract are involved in numerous functions besides protection, they are not covered with a hardened, acellular layer as is the skin surface.

**TABLE 3-1** Protective Characteristics of the Skin and Skin Structures

| Skin Structure | Protective Activity |
|---|---|
| Outer (dermal) layers | • Act as physical barrier to microbial penetration<br>• Sloughing of outer layers removes attached bacteria.<br>• Provide dry, acidic, and cool conditions that limit bacterial growth |
| Hair follicles, sweat glands, sebaceous glands | • Produce acids, alcohols, and toxic lipids that limit bacterial growth |
| Eyes/conjunctival epithelium | • Flushing action of tears removes microorganisms.<br>• Tears contain lysozyme that destroys bacterial cell wall.<br>• Mechanical blinking of the eyelid removes microorganisms. |
| Skin-associated lymphoid tissue | • Mediates specific and nonspecific protection mechanisms against microorganisms that penetrate outer tissue layers |

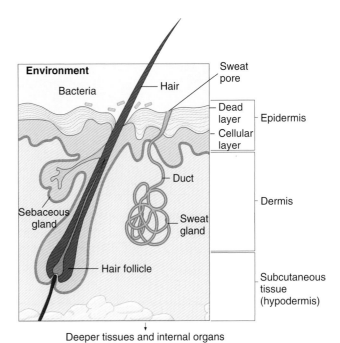

**Figure 3-3** Skin and skin structures.

However, the cells that compose these membranes still exhibit various protective characteristics (Table 3-2 and Figure 3-4).

**General Protective Characteristics.** Mucus is a major protective component of the membranes. This substance serves to trap bacteria before they can reach the outer surface of the cells, lubricates the cells to prevent damage that promotes microbial invasion, and contains specific chemical (i.e., antibodies) and nonspecific antibacterial substances. In addition to the chemical properties and

**TABLE 3-2** Protective Characteristics of Mucous Membranes

| Mucous Membrane | Protective Activity |
|---|---|
| Mucosal cells | • Rapid sloughing for bacterial removal<br>• Tight intercellular junctions prevent bacterial penetration. |
| Goblet cells | • Mucus production: Protective lubrication of cells; bacterial trapping; contains specific antibodies with specific activity against bacteria<br>• Provision of antibacterial substances to mucosal surface:<br>   ○ Lysozyme (degrades bacterial cell wall)<br>   ○ Lactoferrin (competes for bacterial iron supply)<br>   ○ Lactoperoxidase (production of substances toxic to bacteria) |
| Mucosa-associated lymphoid tissue | • Mediates specific responses against bacteria that penetrate outer layer |

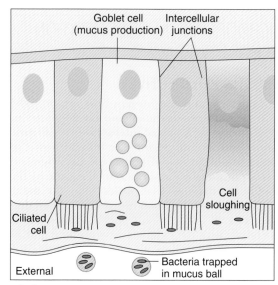

**Figure 3-4** General features of mucous membranes highlighting protective features such as ciliated cells, mucus production, tight intercellular junctions, and cell sloughing.

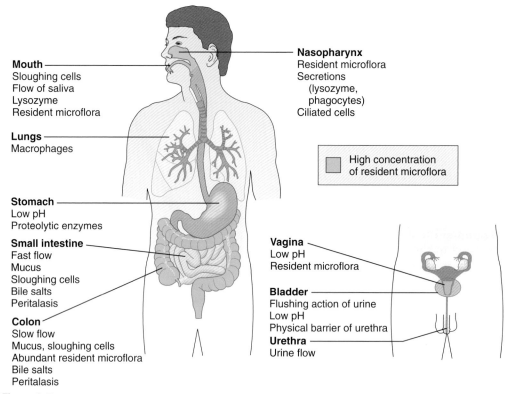

**Mouth**
Sloughing cells
Flow of saliva
Lysozyme
Resident microflora

**Lungs**
Macrophages

**Stomach**
Low pH
Proteolytic enzymes

**Small intestine**
Fast flow
Mucus
Sloughing cells
Bile salts
Peritalasis

**Colon**
Slow flow
Mucus, sloughing cells
Abundant resident microflora
Bile salts
Peritalasis

**Nasopharynx**
Resident microflora
Secretions
 (lysozyme,
 phagocytes)
Ciliated cells

High concentration of resident microflora

**Vagina**
Low pH
Resident microflora

**Bladder**
Flushing action of urine
Low pH
Physical barrier of urethra
**Urethra**
Urine flow

**Figure 3-5** Protective characteristics associated with the mucosal linings of different internal body surfaces.

physical movement of the mucus and trapped microorganisms mediated by ciliary action, rapid cellular shedding and tight intercellular connections provide effective barriers to infection. As is the case with the skin, specific cell clusters, known as *mucosa-associated lymphoid tissue,* exist below the outer cell layer and mediate specific protective mechanisms against microbial invasion.

**Specific Protective Characteristics.** Besides the general protective properties of mucosal cells, the mucosal linings throughout the body have characteristics specific to each anatomic site (Figure 3-5).

The mouth, or oral cavity, is protected by the flow of saliva that physically carries microorganisms away from cell surfaces and also contains antibacterial substances, such as antibodies (IgA) and lysozyme that participate in the destruction of bacterial cells. The mouth is also heavily colonized with protective microorganisms that produce substances that hinder successful invasion by harmful organisms.

In the gastrointestinal tract, the low pH and proteolytic (protein-digesting) enzymes of the stomach prevent the growth of many microorganisms. In the small intestine, protection is provided through the presence of bile salts, which disrupt bacterial membranes, and by peristaltic movement and the fast flow of intestinal contents, which hinder microbial attachment to mucosal cells. Although the large intestine also contains bile salts, the movement of bowel contents is slower, permitting a higher concentration of microbial agents the opportunity to attach to the mucosal cells and inhabit the gastrointestinal tract. As in the oral cavity, the high concentration of normal microbial inhabitants in the large bowel also contributes significantly to protection.

In the upper respiratory tract, nasal hairs keep out large airborne particles that may contain microorganisms. The cough-sneeze reflex significantly contributes to the removal of potentially infective agents. The cells lining the trachea contain cilia (hairlike cellular projections) that move microorganisms trapped in mucus upward and away from the delicate cells of the lungs (see Figure 3-4); this is referred to as the *mucociliary escalator*. These barriers are so effective that only inhalation of particles smaller than 2 to 3 μm have a chance of reaching the lungs.

In the female urogenital tract, the vaginal lining and the cervix are protected by heavy colonization with normal microbial inhabitants and a low pH. A thick mucus plug in the cervical opening is a substantial barrier that keeps microorganisms from ascending and invading the more delicate tissues of the uterus, fallopian tubes, and ovaries. The anterior urethra of males and females is naturally colonized with microorganisms, and a stricture at the urethral opening provides a physical barrier that, combined with a low urine pH and the flushing action of urination, protects against bacterial invasion of the bladder, ureters, and kidneys.

## THE MICROORGANISM'S PERSPECTIVE

As previously discussed, microorganisms that inhabit many surfaces of the human body (see Figure 3-5) are referred to as *colonizers*, or *normal flora* (also referred to as normal microbiota). Some are transient colonizers, because they are able to survive, but do not multiply, on the surface and are frequently shed with the host cells. Others, called *resident flora*, not only survive but also thrive and multiply; their presence is more persistent.

The body's normal flora varies considerably with anatomic location. For example, environmental conditions, such as temperature and oxygen availability, differ considerably between the nasal cavity and the small bowel. Only microorganisms with the metabolic capability to survive under the physiologic conditions of the anatomic location are inhabitants of those particular body surfaces.

Knowledge of the normal flora of the human body is extremely important in diagnostic microbiology,

especially for determining the clinical significance of microorganisms isolated from patient specimens. Organisms considered normal flora are frequently found in clinical specimens. This may be a result of contamination of normally sterile specimens during the collection process or because the colonizing organism is actually involved in the infection. Microorganisms considered as normal colonizers of the human body and the anatomic locations they colonize are addressed in Part VII.

### Microbial Colonization

Colonization may be the last step in the establishment of a long-lasting, mutually beneficial (i.e., commensal), or harmless, relationship between a colonizer and the human host. Alternatively, colonization may be the first step in the process for the development of infection and disease. Whether colonization results in a harmless or damaging infection depends on the characteristics of the host and the microorganism. In either case, successful initial colonization depends on the microorganism's ability to survive the conditions first encountered on the host surface (Box 3-2).

To avoid the dryness of the skin, organisms often seek moist areas of the body, including hair follicles, sebaceous (oil, referred to as *sebum*) and sweat glands, skin folds, underarms, the genitals or anus, the face, the scalp, and areas around the mouth. Microbial penetration of mucosal surfaces is mediated by the organism becoming embedded in food particles to survive oral and gastrointestinal conditions or contained within airborne particles to aid survival in the respiratory tract. Microorganisms also exhibit metabolic capabilities that assist in their survival. For example, the ability of staphylococci to thrive in relatively high salt concentrations enhances their survival in and among the sweat glands of the skin.

Besides surviving the host's physical and chemical conditions, colonization also requires that microorganisms attach and adhere to host surfaces (see Box 3-2). This can be particularly challenging in places such as the

---

**BOX 3-2** Microbial Factors Contributing to Colonization of Host Surfaces

**Survival Against Environmental Conditions**
- Localization in moist areas
- Protection in ingested or inhaled debris
- Expression of specific metabolic characteristics (e.g., salt tolerance)

**Achieving Attachment and Adherence to Host Cell Surfaces**
- Pili
- Adherence proteins
- Biofilms
- Various protein adhesins

**Other Factors**
- Motility
- Production of substances that compete with host for acquisition of essential nutrients (e.g., siderophores for capture of iron)
- Ability to coexist with other colonizing microorganisms

mouth and bowel, in which the surfaces are frequently washed with passing fluids. Pili, the rodlike projections of bacterial envelopes, various molecules (e.g., adherence proteins and adhesins), and biochemical complexes (e.g., biofilm) work together to enhance attachment of microorganisms to the host cell surface. Biofilm is discussed in more detail later in this chapter. (For more information concerning the structure and functions of pili, see Chapter 2.)

In addition, microbial motility with flagella allows organisms to move around and actively seek optimum conditions. Finally, because no single microbial species is a lone colonizer, successful colonization also requires that a microorganism be able to coexist with other microorganisms.

# MICROORGANISM ENTRY, INVASION, AND DISSEMINATION

## THE HOST'S PERSPECTIVE

In most instances, to establish infection, microorganisms must penetrate or circumvent the host's physical barriers (i.e., skin or mucosal surfaces); overcoming these defensive barriers depends on both host and microbial factors. When these barriers are broken, numerous other host defensive strategies are activated.

### Disruption of Surface Barriers

Any situation that disrupts the physical barrier of the skin and mucosa, alters the environmental conditions (e.g., loss of stomach acidity or dryness of skin), changes the functioning of surface cells, or alters the normal flora population can facilitate the penetration of microorganisms past the barriers and into deeper host tissues. Disruptive factors may vary from accidental or intentional (medical) trauma that results in surface destruction to the use of antibiotics that remove normal, protective, colonizing microorganisms (Box 3-3). It is important to note that a number of these factors are related to medical interventions and procedures.

### Responses to Microbial Invasion of Deeper Tissues

Once surface barriers have been bypassed, the host responds to microbial presence in the underlying tissue in various ways. Some of these responses are nonspecific, because they occur regardless of the type of invading organism; other responses are more specific and involve the host's immune system. Both nonspecific and specific host responses are critical if the host is to survive. Without them, microorganisms would multiply and invade vital tissues and organs, resulting in severe damage to the host.

**Nonspecific Responses.** Some nonspecific responses are biochemical; others are cellular. Biochemical factors remove essential nutrients, such as iron, from tissues so that it is unavailable for use by invading microorganisms. Cellular responses are central to tissue and organ defenses, and the cells involved are known as *phagocytes.*

***Phagocytes.*** Phagocytes are cells that ingest and destroy bacteria and other foreign particles. The two

---

**BOX 3-3** Factors Contributing to Disruption of the Skin and Mucosal Surface

**Trauma**
- Penetrating wounds
- Abrasions
- Burns (chemical and fire)
- Surgical wounds
- Needle sticks

**Inhalation**
- Noxious or toxic gases
- Particulate matter
- Smoking

**Implantation of Medical Devices**

**Other Diseases**
- Malignancies
- Diabetes
- Previous or simultaneous infections
- Alcoholism and other chemical dependencies

**Childbirth**

**Overuse of Antibiotics**

---

major types of phagocytes are polymorphonuclear leukocytes, also known as PMNs or neutrophils, and macrophages. Phagocytes ingest bacteria by a process known as *endocytosis* and engulf them in a membrane-lined structure called a *phagosome* (Figure 3-6). The phagosome is then fused with a second structure, the lysosome. When the lysosome, which contains toxic chemicals and destructive enzymes, combines with the phagosome, the bacteria trapped within the structure, referred to as a **phagolysosome,** are neutralized and destroyed. This destructive process must be carried out inside membrane-lined structures; otherwise the noxious substances contained within the phagolysosome would destroy the phagocyte itself. This is evident during the course of rampant infections when thousands of phagocytes exhibit "sloppy" ingestion of the microorganisms and toxic substances spill from the cells, damaging the surrounding host tissue. This process is referred to as phagocytosis.

Although both PMNs and macrophages are phagocytes, these cell types differ. PMNs develop in the bone marrow and spend their short lives (usually a day or less) circulating in blood and tissues. Widely dispersed in the body, PMNs usually are the first cells on the scene of bacterial invasion. Macrophages also develop in the bone marrow but first go through a cellular phase in which they are called *monocytes.* Macrophages circulating in the bloodstream are called *monocytes.* When deposited in tissue or at a site of infection, monocytes transform into mature macrophages. In the absence of infection, macrophages usually reside in specific organs, such as the spleen, lymph nodes, liver, or lungs, where they live for days to several weeks, awaiting encounters with invading bacteria. In addition to the ingestion and destruction of bacteria, macrophages play an important role in mediating immune system defenses (see Specific Responses—The Immune System later in this chapter).

In addition to the inhibition of microbial proliferation by phagocytes and by biochemical substances such as

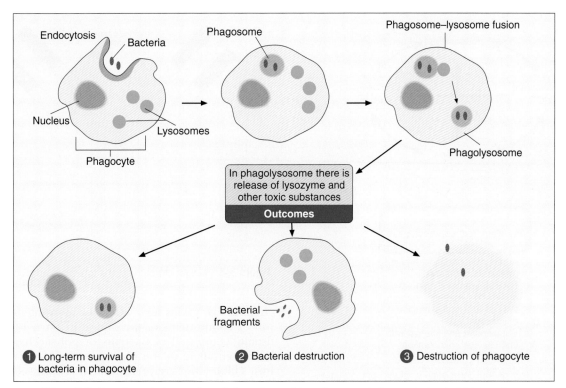

**Figure 3-6** Overview of phagocyte activity and possible outcomes of phagocyte-bacterial interactions.

lysozyme, microorganisms are "washed" from tissues during the flow of lymph fluid. The fluid carries infectious agents through the lymphatic system, where they are deposited in tissues and organs (e.g., lymph nodes and spleen) heavily populated with phagocytes. This process functions as an efficient filtration system.

**Inflammation.** Because microbes may survive initial encounters with phagocytes (see Figure 3-6), the inflammatory response plays an extremely important role as a primary mechanism against microbial survival and proliferation in tissues and organs. Inflammation has both cellular and biochemical components that interact in various complex ways (Table 3-3).

The complement system is composed of a coordinated group of proteins activated by the immune system or as a result of the presence of invading microorganisms. On activation of this system, a cascade of biochemical events occurs that attracts (chemotaxis) and enhances the activities of more phagocytes. Because PMNs and macrophages are widely dispersed throughout the body, signals are needed to attract and concentrate these cells at the point of invasion, and serum complement proteins provide many of these signals. Cytokines are chemical substances, or proteins secreted by a cell, that have effects on the activities of other cells. Cytokines draw more phagocytes toward the infection and activate the maturation of monocytes to macrophages.

Additional protective functions of the complement system are enhanced by the coagulation system, which works to increase blood flow to the area of infection and also can effectively wall off the infection through the production of blood clots and barriers composed of cellular debris.

**TABLE 3-3** Components of Inflammation

| Component | Functions |
|---|---|
| Phagocytes (polymorphonuclear neutrophils [PMNs], dendritic cells, and macrophages) | • Ingest and destroy microorganisms |
| Complement system (coordinated group of serum proteins) | • Attracts phagocytes to site of infection (chemotaxis)<br>• Helps phagocytes recognize and bind to bacteria (opsonization)<br>• Directly kills gram-negative bacteria (membrane attack complex) |
| Coagulation system (wide variety of proteins and other biologically active compounds) | • Attracts phagocytes to site of infection<br>• Increases blood and fluid flow to site of infection<br>• Walls off site of infection, physically inhibiting the spread of microorganisms |
| Cytokines (proteins secreted by macrophages and other cells) | • Multiple effects that enhance the activities of many different cells essential to nonspecific and specific defensive responses |

The manifestations of inflammation are evident and familiar to most of us and include the following:
• Swelling—caused by increased flow of fluid and cells to the affected body site

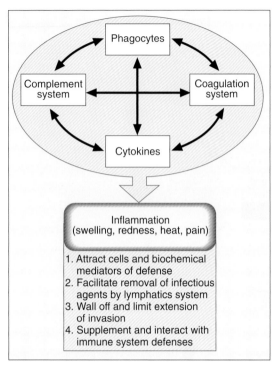

**Figure 3-7** Overview of the components, signs, and functions of inflammation.

- Redness—results from vasodilation of blood vessels and increased blood flow at the infection site
- Heat—results from increased cellular metabolism and energy production in the affected area
- Pain—due to tissue damage and pressure on nerve endings from increased flow of fluid and cells

On a microscopic level, the presence of phagocytes at the infection site is an important observation in diagnostic microbiology. Microorganisms associated with these host cells are frequently identified as the cause of a particular infection. An overview of inflammation is depicted in Figure 3-7.

## SPECIFIC RESPONSES—THE IMMUNE SYSTEM

The immune system provides the human host with the ability to mount a specific protective response to the presence of the invading microorganism. In addition to this specificity, the immune system has a "memory." When a microorganism is encountered a second or third time, an immune-mediated defensive response is immediately available. It is important to remember that nonspecific (i.e., phagocytes, inflammation) and specific (i.e., the immune system) host defensive systems are interdependent in their efforts to limit the spread of infection.

### Components of the Immune System

The central molecule of the immune response is the antibody. *Antibodies,* also referred to as *immunoglobulins,* are specific glycoproteins produced by plasma cells (activated B cells) in response to the presence of a molecule recognized as foreign to the host (referred to as an *antigen*). In the case of infectious diseases, antigens are

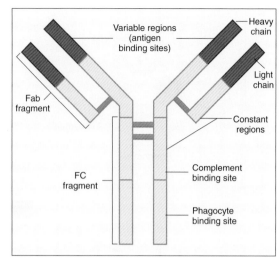

**Figure 3-8** General structure of the IgG class antibody molecule.

chemicals or toxins secreted by the invading microorganism or components of the organism's structure and are usually composed of proteins or polysaccharides. Antibodies circulate in the plasma or liquid portion of the host's blood and are present in secretions such as saliva. These molecules have two active areas: the antigen binding site (Fab region) and the phagocyte and complement binding sites (Fc region) (Figure 3-8).

Five major classes of antibody have been identified: IgG, IgA, IgM, IgD, and IgE. Each class has distinctive molecular configurations. IgM is the largest and first antibody produced when an invading microorganism is initially encountered; production of the most abundant antibody, IgG, follows. IgA is secreted in various body fluids (e.g., saliva and tears) and primarily protects body surfaces lined with mucous membranes. Increased IgE is associated with various parasitic infections and various allergies. IgD is attached to the surface of specific immune system cells and is involved in the regulation of antibody production. As is discussed in Chapter 10, our ability to measure specific antibody production is a valuable tool for the laboratory diagnosis of infectious diseases.

Regarding the cellular components of the immune response, there are three major types of cells: B lymphocytes, T lymphocytes, and natural killer cells (Box 3-4). B lymphocytes originate from stem cells and develop into B cells in the bone marrow before being widely distributed to lymphoid tissues throughout the body. These cells primarily function as antibody producers (plasma cells). T lymphocytes also originate from bone marrow stem cells, but they mature in the thymus and either directly destroy infected cells (cytotoxic T cells) or work with B cells (helper T cells) to regulate antibody production. Natural killer cells are a subset of T cells. There are different types of natural killer cells, with the most prevalent referred to as invariant natural killer T cells (NKT). NKT cells develop in the thymus from the same precursor cells as other T lymphocytes. Each of the three cell types is strategically located in lymphoid tissue throughout the body to maximize the chances of encountering invading microorganisms that the lymphatic system drains from the site of infection.

**B Lymphocytes (B Cells)**
**Location:** Lymphoid tissues (lymph nodes, spleen, gut-associated lymphoid tissue, tonsils)
**Function:** Antibody-producing cells
**Subtypes:**
  B lymphocytes: Cells waiting to be stimulated by an antigen
  Plasma cells: Activated B lymphocytes that secrete antibody in response to an antigen
  B-memory cells: Long-lived cells preprogrammed to antigen for subsequent exposure

**T Lymphocytes (T Cells)**
**Location:** Circulate and reside in lymphoid tissues (lymph nodes, spleen, gut-associated lymphoid tissue, tonsils)
**Functions:** Multiple (see different subtypes)
**Subtypes:**
  Helper T cells ($T_H$): Interact with B cells to facilitate antibody production
  Cytotoxic T cells ($T_C$): Recognize and destroy host cells that have been invaded by microorganisms
  Suppressor T cells ($T_S$): Mediate regulatory responses within the immune system

**Natural Killer Cells (NK Cells)**
**Function:** Similar to that of cytotoxic T cells; however, NK cells do not require the presence of an antigen to stimulate function

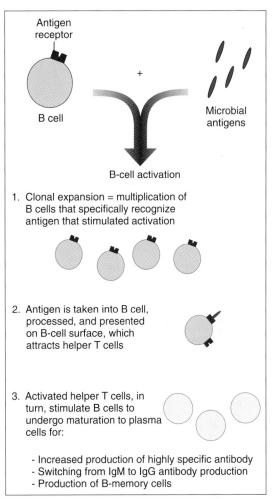

**Figure 3-9** Overview of B-cell activation that is central to antibody-mediated immunity.

**Two Branches of the Immune System.** The immune system provides immunity that generally can be divided into two branches:
- Antibody-mediated immunity, or humoral immunity
- Cell-mediated immunity, or cellular immunity

Antibody-mediated immunity is centered on the activities of B cells and the production of antibodies. When B cells encounter a microbial antigen, they become activated and a series of events is initiated. These events are mediated by the activities of helper T cells and the release of cytokines. Cytokines mediate clonal expansion, and the number of B cells capable of recognizing the antigen increases. Cytokines also activate the maturation of B cells into plasma cells that produce antibodies specific for the antigen. The process results in the production of B-memory cells (Figure 3-9). B-memory cells remain quiescent in the body until a second or subsequent exposure to the original antigen occurs. With secondary exposure, the B-memory cells are preprogrammed to produce specific antibodies immediately upon encountering the original antigen.

Antibodies protect the host in a number of ways:
- Helping phagocytes to ingest and kill microorganisms through a coating mechanism referred to as *opsonization*
- Neutralizing microbial toxins detrimental to host cells and tissues
- Promoting bacterial clumping (agglutination) that facilitates clearing from the infection site
- Inhibiting bacterial motility
- Viral neutralization; blocking the virus from entering the host cell
- Combining with microorganisms to activate the complement system and inflammatory response

Because a population of activated specific B cells is a developmental process as a result of the exposure to microbial antigens, antibody production is delayed when the host is first exposed to an infectious agent. This delay in the primary antibody response underscores the importance of nonspecific response defenses, such as inflammation, that work to hold the invading organisms in check while antibody production begins. This also emphasizes the importance of B-memory cell production. By virtue of this memory, any subsequent exposure or secondary *(anamnestic)* response to the same microorganism results in rapid production of protective antibodies so that the body is spared the delays characteristic of the primary exposure.

Some antigens, such as bacterial capsules and outer membranes, activate B cells to produce antibodies without the intervention of helper T cells. However, this activation does not result in the production of B-memory cells, and subsequent exposure to the same bacterial antigens does not result in a rapid host memory response.

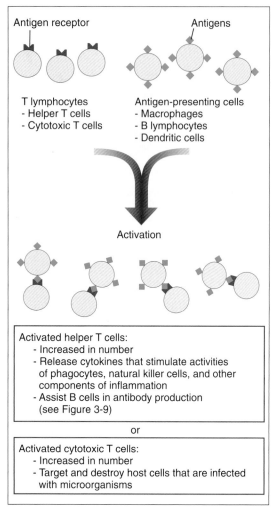

**Figure 3-10** Overview of T-cell activation that is central to cell-mediated immunity.

The primary cells involved in cell-mediated immunity are T lymphocytes (cytotoxic T cells) that recognize and destroy human host cells infected with microorganisms. This function is extremely important for the destruction and elimination of infecting microorganisms. Some pathogens (e.g., viruses, tuberculosis, some parasites, and fungi) are able to survive in host cells, protected from antibody interaction. Antibody-mediated immunity targets microorganisms outside human cells, whereas cell-mediated immunity targets microorganisms inside human cells. However, in many instances these two branches of the immune system overlap and work together.

Like B cells, T cells must be activated. Activation is accomplished by T-cell interactions with other cells that process microbial antigens and present them on their surface (e.g., macrophages, dendritic cells, and B cells). The responses of activated T cells are very different and depend on the subtype of T cell (Figure 3-10). Activated helper T cells work with B cells for antibody production (see Figure 3-9) and facilitate inflammation by releasing cytokines. Cytotoxic T cells directly interact with and destroy host cells containing microorganisms or other infectious agents, such as viruses. The activated T-cell subset, helper or cytotoxic cells, is controlled by an

extremely complex series of biochemical pathways and genetic diversity within the major histocompatibility complex (MHC). MHC molecules are present on cells and form a complex with the antigen to present them to the T cells. The two primary classes of major histocompatibility molecules are MHC I and MHC II. MHC I molecules are located on every nucleated cell in the body and are predominantly responsible for the recognition of endogenous proteins expressed from within the cell. MHC II molecules are located on specialized cell types, including macrophages, dendritic cells, and B cells, for the presentation of extracellular molecules or exogenous proteins.

In summary, the host presents a spectrum of challenges to invading microorganisms, from physical barriers, including the skin and mucous membranes, to the interactive cellular and biochemical components of inflammation and the immune system. All these systems work together to minimize microbial invasion and prevent damage to vital tissues and organs resulting from the presence of infectious agents.

## THE MICROORGANISM'S PERSPECTIVE

Given the complexities of the human host's defense systems, it is no wonder that microbial strategies designed to survive these systems are equally complex.

### Colonization and Infection

Many of our body surfaces are colonized with a wide variety of microorganisms without apparent detriment. In contrast, an infection involves the growth and multiplication of microorganisms that result in damage to the host. The extent and severity of the damage depend on many factors, including the microorganism's ability to cause disease, the site of the infection, and the general health of the individual infected. Disease results when the infection produces notable changes in human physiology associated with damage or loss of function to one or more of the body's organ systems.

### Pathogens and Virulence

Microorganisms that cause infections and/or disease are called *pathogens*, and the characteristics that enable them to cause disease are referred to as *virulence factors*. Most virulence factors protect the organism against host attack or mediate damaging effects on host cells. The terms *pathogenicity* and *virulence* reflect the degree to which a microorganism is capable of causing disease. Pathogenicity specifically refers to the organism's ability to cause disease, whereas virulence refers to the measure or degree of pathogenicity of an organism. An organism of high pathogenicity is very likely to cause disease, whereas an organism of low pathogenicity is much less likely to cause infection. When disease does occur, highly virulent organisms often severely damage the human host. The degree of severity decreases with diminishing virulence of the microorganism.

Because host factors play a role in the development of infectious diseases, the distinction between a pathogenic and nonpathogenic organism or colonizer is not always clear. For example, many organisms that colonize our skin usually do not cause disease (i.e., exhibit low pathogenicity) under normal circumstances. However, when damage to the skin occurs (see Box 3-3) or when the skin is disrupted in some other way, these organisms can gain access to deeper tissues and establish an infection.

Organisms that cause infection when one or more of the host's defense mechanisms are disrupted or malfunction are known as *opportunistic pathogens,* and the infections they cause are referred to as *opportunistic infections.* On the other hand, several pathogens known to cause serious infections can be part of a person's normal flora and never cause disease. However, the same organism can cause life-threatening infection when transmitted to other individuals. The reasons for these inconsistencies are not fully understood, but such widely different results undoubtedly involve complex interactions between microorganism and human. Recognizing and separating **pathogenic** from **nonpathogenic organisms** present one of the greatest challenges in interpreting diagnostic microbiology laboratory results.

## Microbial Virulence Factors

Virulence factors provide microorganisms with the capacity to avoid host defenses and damage host cells, tissues, and organs in a number of ways. Some virulence factors are specific for certain pathogenic genera or species, and substantial differences exist in the way bacteria, viruses, parasites, and fungi cause disease. Knowledge of a microorganism's capacity to cause specific types of infections plays a major role in the development of diagnostic microbiology procedures used for isolating and identifying microorganisms. (See Part VII for more information regarding diagnosis by organ system.)

**Attachment.** Whether humans encounter microorganisms in the air, through ingestion, or by direct contact, the first step of infection and disease development, a process referred to as *pathogenesis,* is microbial attachment to a surface (exceptions being instances in which the organisms are directly introduced by trauma or other means into deeper tissues).

Many of the microbial factors that facilitate attachment of pathogens are the same as those used by nonpathogenic colonizers (see Box 3-2). Most pathogenic organisms are not part of the normal microbial flora, and attachment to the host requires that they outcompete colonizers for a place on the body's surface. Medical interventions, such as the overuse of antimicrobial agents, result in the destruction of the normal flora, creating a competitive advantage for the invading pathogenic organism.

**Invasion.** Once surface attachment has been secured, microbial invasion into subsurface tissues and organs (i.e., infection) is accomplished by disruption of the skin and mucosal surfaces by several mechanisms (see Box 3-3) or by the direct action of an organism's virulence factors. Some microorganisms produce factors that force mucosal surface phagocytes (M cells) to ingest them and then release them unharmed into the tissue below the surface. Other organisms, such as staphylococci and streptococci, are not so subtle. These organisms produce an array of enzymes (e.g., hyaluronidases, nucleases, collagenases) that hydrolyze host proteins and nucleic acids,

---

> **BOX 3-5** Microbial Strategies for Surviving Inflammation
>
> **Avoid Killing by Phagocytes (Polymorphonuclear Leukocytes)**
> - Producing a capsule, thereby inhibiting phagocytes' ability to ingest them
>
> **Avoid Phagocyte-Mediated Killing**
> - Inhibiting phagosome-lysosome fusion
> - Being resistant to destructive agents (e.g., lysozyme) released by lysosomes
> - Actively and rapidly multiplying within a phagocyte
> - Releasing toxins and enzymes that damage or kill phagocytes
>
> **Avoid Effects of the Complement System**
> - Using a capsule to hide surface molecules that would otherwise activate the complement system, including the formation of a complex protein polysaccharide matrix referred to as a biofilm
> - Producing substances that inhibit the processes involved in complement activation
> - Producing substances that destroy specific complement proteins

destroying host cells and tissues. This destruction allows the pathogen to "burrow" through minor openings in the outer surface of the skin and into deeper tissues. Once a pathogen has penetrated the body, it uses a variety of strategies to survive attack by the host's inflammatory and immune responses. Alternatively, some pathogens cause disease at the site of attachment without further penetration. For example, in diseases such as diphtheria and whooping cough, the bacteria produce toxic substances that destroy surrounding tissues. The organisms generally do not penetrate the mucosal surface they inhabit.

**Survival Against Inflammation.** If a pathogen is to survive, the action of phagocytes and the complement components of inflammation must be avoided or controlled (Box 3-5). Some organisms, such as *Streptococcus pneumoniae,* a common cause of bacterial pneumonia and meningitis, avoid phagocytosis by producing a large capsule that inhibits the phagocytic process. Other pathogens may not be able to avoid phagocytosis but are not effectively destroyed once internalized and are able to survive within phagocytes. This is the case for *Mycobacterium tuberculosis,* the bacterium that causes tuberculosis. Still other pathogens use toxins and enzymes to attack and destroy phagocytes before the phagocytes attack and destroy them.

The defenses offered by the complement system depend on a series of biochemical reactions triggered by specific microorganism molecular structures. Therefore, microbial avoidance of complement activation requires that the infecting agent either mask its activating molecules (e.g., via production of a capsule that covers bacterial surface antigens) or produce substances (e.g., enzymes) that disrupt critical biochemical components of the complement pathway.

Any single microorganism may possess numerous virulence factors, and several may be expressed simultaneously. For example, while trying to avoid phagocytosis, an

- Pathogen multiplies and invades so quickly that damage to host is complete before immune response can be fully activated, or organism's virulence is so great that the immune response is insufficient.
- Pathogen invades and destroys cells involved in the immune response.
- Pathogen survives unrecognized in host cells and avoids detection by immune system.
- Pathogen covers its antigens with a capsule or biofilm so that an immune response is not activated.
- Pathogen changes antigens so that immune system is constantly fighting a primary encounter (i.e., the memory of the immune system is neutralized).
- Pathogen produces enzymes (proteases) that directly destroy or inactivate antibodies.

**BOX 3-7** Summary of Bacterial Toxins

**Endotoxins**
- General toxin common to almost all gram-negative bacteria
- Composed of lipopolysaccharide portion of cell envelope
- Released when gram-negative bacterial cell is destroyed
- Effects on host include:
  - Disruption of clotting, causing clots to form throughout the body (i.e., disseminated intravascular coagulation [DIC])
  - Fever
  - Activation of complement and immune systems
  - Circulatory changes that lead to hypotension, shock, and death

**Exotoxins**
- Most commonly associated with gram-positive bacteria
- Produced and released by living bacteria; do not require bacterial death for release
- Specific toxins target specific host cells; the type of toxin varies with the bacterial species.
- Some kill host cells and help spread bacteria in tissues (e.g., enzymes that destroy key biochemical tissue components or specifically destroy host cell membranes).
- Some destroy or interfere with specific intracellular activities (e.g., interruption of protein synthesis, interruption of internal cell signals, or interruption of neuromuscular system).

organism may also excrete other enzymes and toxins that destroy and penetrate tissue and produce other factors designed to interfere with the immune response. Microorganisms may also use host systems to their own advantage. For example, the lymphatic and circulatory systems used to carry monocytes and lymphocytes to the site of infection may also serve to disperse the organism throughout the body.

**Survival Against the Immune System.** Microbial strategies to avoid the defenses of the immune system are outlined in Box 3-6. Again, a pathogen can use more than one strategy to avoid immune-mediated defenses, and microbial survival does not necessarily require devastation of the immune system. The pathogen may merely need to "buy" time to reach a safe area in the body or to be transferred to the next susceptible host. Also, microorganisms can avoid much of the immune response if they do not penetrate the surface layers of the body. This strategy is the hallmark of diseases caused by microbial toxins.

**Microbial Toxins.** *Toxins* are biochemically active substances released by microorganisms that have a particular effect on host cells. Microorganisms use toxins to establish infections and multiply within the host. Alternatively, a pathogen may be restricted to a particular body site from which toxins are released to cause systemic damage throughout the body. Toxins also can cause human disease in the absence of the pathogens that produced them. This common mechanism of food poisoning involves ingestion of preformed bacterial toxins (present in the food at the time of ingestion) and is referred to as *intoxication*, a notable example of which is botulism.

*Endotoxin* and *exotoxin* are the two general types of bacterial toxins (Box 3-7). Endotoxin is a component of the cellular structure of gram-negative bacteria and can have devastating effects on the body's metabolism, the most serious being endotoxic shock, which often results in death. The effects of exotoxins produced by grampositive bacteria tend to be more limited and specific than the effects of gram-negative endotoxin. The activities of exotoxins range from enzymes produced by many staphylococci and streptococci that augment bacterial

invasion by damaging host tissues and cells to highly specific activities (e.g., diphtheria toxin inhibits protein synthesis, and cholera toxin interferes with host cell signals). Examples of other highly active and specific toxins are those that cause botulism and tetanus by interfering with neuromuscular functions.

## Genetics of Virulence: Pathogenicity Islands

Many virulence factors are encoded in genomic regions of pathogens known as pathogenicity *islands (PAIs)*. These are mobile genetic elements that contribute to the change and spread of virulence factors among bacterial populations of a variety of species. These genetic elements are thought to have evolved from lysogenic bacteriophages and plasmids and are spread by horizontal gene transfer (see Chapter 2 for information about bacterial genetics). PAIs are typically comprised of one or more virulence-associated genes and "mobility" genes (i.e., integrases and transposases) that mediate movement between various genetic elements (e.g., plasmids and chromosomes) and among different bacterial strains. In essence, PAIs facilitate the dissemination of virulence capabilities among bacteria in a manner similar to the mechanism diagrammed in Figure 2-10; this also facilitates dissemination of antimicrobial resistance genes (see Chapter 11). PAIs are widely disseminated among medically important bacteria. For example, PAIs have been identified as playing a role in virulence for each of the following organisms:

*Helicobacter pylori*
*Pseudomonas aeruginosa*
*Shigella* spp.

*Yersinia* spp.
*Vibrio cholerae*
*Salmonella* spp.
*Escherichia coli* (enteropathogenic, enterohemorrhagic or serotoxigenic, (verotoxigenic) uropathogenic, enterotoxigenic, enteroinvasive, enteroaggregative, meningitis-sepsis associated; see Chapter 20).
*Neisseria* spp.
*Bacteroides fragilis*
*Listeria monocytogenes*
*Staphylococcus aureus*
*Streptococcus* spp.
*Enterococcus faecalis*
*Clostridium difficile*

**Biofilm Formation.** Microorganisms typically exist as a group or community of organisms capable of adhering to each other or to other surfaces. A variety of bacterial pathogens, along with other microorganisms, are capable of forming biofilms, including *S. aureus, P. aeruginosa,* and *Candida albicans.* A **biofilm** is an accumulation of microorganisms embedded in a polysaccharide matrix. Pathogenic microorganisms use the formation of biofilm to adhere to implants and prosthetic devices. For example, nosocomial infections with *Staphylococci* spp. associated with implants have become more prevalent. Interestingly, biofilm-forming strains have a much more complex antibiotic resistance profile, indicating failure of the antibiotic to penetrate the polysaccharide layer. In addition, some of the cells in the sessile or stationary biofilm may experience nutrient deprivation and therefore exist in a slow-growing or starved state, displaying reduced susceptibility to antimicrobial agents. These organisms also have demonstrated a differential gene expression, compared to their planktonic or free-floating counter parts. The biofilm-forming communities are able to adapt and respond to changes in their environment, similar to a multicellular organism.

Biofilms may form from the accumulation of a single microorganism (monomicrobic aggregation) or from the accumulation of numerous species (polymicrobic aggregation). It is widely accepted that the cells in a biofilm are physiologically unique from the planktonic cells and are referred to as *persister cells.* During biofilm accumulation, the cells reach a critical mass that results in alteration in metabolism and gene expression. This is accomplished through a mechanism of signaling between cells or organisms through chemical signals or inducer molecules, such as acyl homoserine lactone (AHL) in gram-negative bacteria or oligopeptides in gram-positive bacteria. These signals are capable of interspecies and intraspecies communication.

Microbial biofilm formation is important to many disciplines, including environmental science, industry, and public health. Biofilm formation affects the efficient treatment of wastewater; it is essential for the effective production of beer, which requires aggregation of yeast cells; and it affects bioremediation for toxic substances such as oil. It has been reported that approximately 65% of hospital-acquired infections are associated with biofilm formation. Box 3-8 provides an overview of pathogenic organisms associated with biofilm formation in human infections.

---

**BOX 3-8** Biofilms and Human Infections

These pathogenic organisms have been associated with biofilm formation in human infections.

**Artificial Prosthetics and Indwelling Devices**
- *Candida albicans*
- Coagulase-negative staphylococci
- *Enterococci* spp.
- *Klebsiella pneumoniae*
- *Pseudomonas aeruginosa*
- *Staphylococcus aureus*
- *Streptococci* spp.

**Food-Borne Contamination**
- *Listeria monocytogenes*

---

# OUTCOME AND PREVENTION OF INFECTIOUS DISEASES

## OUTCOME OF INFECTIOUS DISEASES

Given the complexities of host defenses and microbial virulence, it is not surprising that the factors determining outcome between these two living entities are also complicated. Basically, outcome depends on the state of the host's health, the virulence of the pathogen, and whether the host can clear the pathogen before infection and disease cause irreparable harm or death (Figure 3-11).

The time from exposure to an infectious agent and the development of a disease or infection depends on host and microbial factors. Infectious processes that develop quickly are referred to as *acute infections,* and those that develop and progress slowly, sometimes over a period of years, are known as *chronic infections.* Some pathogens, particularly certain viruses, can be clinically silent inside the body without any noticeable effect on the host before suddenly causing a severe and acute infection. During the silent phase, the infection is said to be latent. Again, depending on host and microbial factors, acute, chronic, or latent infections can result in any of the outcomes detailed in Figure 3-11.

Medical intervention can help the host fight the infection but usually is not instituted until after the host is aware that an infectious process is underway. The clues that an infection is occurring are known as the *signs* and *symptoms* of disease and result from host responses (e.g., inflammatory and immune responses) to the action of microbial virulence factors (Box 3-9). **Signs** are measurable indications or physical observations, such as an increase in body temperature (fever) or the development of a rash or swelling. **Symptoms** are indictors as described by the patient, such as headache, aches, fatigue, and nausea. The signs and symptoms reflect the stages of infection. In turn, the stages of infection generally reflect the stages in host-microorganism interactions (Figure 3-12).

Whether medical procedures contribute to controlling or clearing an infection depends on key factors, including:

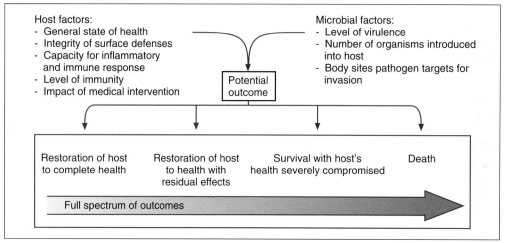

**Figure 3-11** Possible outcomes of infections and infectious diseases.

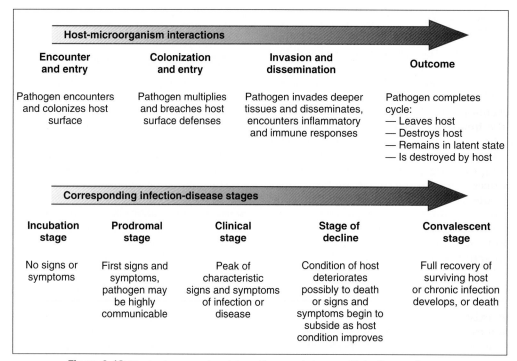

**Figure 3-12** Host-microorganism interactions and stages of infection or disease.

---

**BOX 3-9** Signs and Symptoms of Infection and Infectious Diseases

- General or localized aches and pains
- Headache
- Fever
- Fatigue
- Swollen lymph nodes
- Rashes
- Redness and swelling
- Cough and sneezes
- Congestion of nasal and sinus passages
- Sore throat
- Nausea and vomiting
- Diarrhea

---

- The severity of the infection, which is determined by host and microbial interactions already discussed
- Accuracy in diagnosing the pathogen or pathogens causing the infection
- Whether the patient receives appropriate treatment for the infection (which depends on accurate diagnosis)

## PREVENTION OF INFECTIOUS DISEASES

The treatment of an infection is often difficult and not always successful. Because much of the damage may already have been done before appropriate medical intervention is provided, the microorganisms gain too much of a "head start." Another strategy for combating

**Preventing Transmission**
- Avoid direct contact with infected persons or take protective measures when direct contact will occur (e.g., wear gloves, wear condoms).
- Block the spread of airborne microorganisms by wearing masks or isolating persons with infections transmitted by air.
- Use sterile medical techniques.

**Controlling Microbial Reservoirs**
- Sanitation and disinfection
- Sewage treatment
- Food preservation
- Water treatment
- Control of pests and insect vector populations

**Minimizing Risk Before or Shortly After Exposure**
- Immunization or vaccination
- Cleansing and use of antiseptics
- Prophylactic use of antimicrobial agents

infectious diseases is to stop infections before they start (i.e., disease prevention). As discussed at the beginning of this chapter, the first step in any host-microorganism relationship is the encounter and exposure to the infectious agent. Therefore, strategies to prevent disease involve interrupting or minimizing the risk of infection when exposures occur. As outlined in Box 3-10, interruption of encounters may be accomplished by preventing transmission of the infecting agents and by controlling or destroying reservoirs of human pathogens. Interestingly, most of these measures do not really involve medical practices but rather social practices and policies.

### Immunization

Medical strategies exist for minimizing the risk of disease development when exposure to infectious agents occurs. One of the most effective methods is **vaccination,** also referred to as *immunization.* This practice takes advantage of the specificity and memory of the immune system. The two basic approaches to immunization are active immunization and passive immunization. With active immunization, modified antigens from pathogenic microorganisms are introduced into the body and cause an immune response. If or when the host encounters the pathogen in nature, the memory of the immune system ensures minimal delay in the immune response, thus affording strong protection. With passive immunization, antibodies against a particular pathogen that have been produced in one host are transferred to a second host, where they provide temporary protection. The passage of maternal antibodies to the newborn is a key example of natural passive immunization. Active immunity is generally longer lasting, because the immunized host's own immune response has been activated. However, for complex reasons, naturally acquired active immunity has had limited success for relatively few infectious diseases, necessitating the development of vaccines. Successful immunization has proven effective against many infectious diseases, including diphtheria, whooping cough (pertussis), tetanus, influenza, polio, smallpox, measles, hepatitis, and certain *Streptococcus pneumoniae* and *Haemophilus influenzae* infections.

Prophylactic antimicrobial therapy, the administration of antibiotics when the risk of developing an infection is high, is another common medical intervention for preventing infection.

### Epidemiology

To prevent infectious diseases, information is required regarding the sources of pathogens, the mode of transmission to and among humans, human risk factors for encountering the pathogen and developing infection, and factors that contribute to good and bad outcomes resulting from the exposure. *Epidemiology* is the science that characterizes these aspects of infectious diseases and monitors the effect diseases have on public health. Fully characterizing the circumstances associated with the acquisition and dissemination of infectious diseases gives researchers a better chance of preventing and eliminating these diseases. Additionally, many epidemiologic strategies developed for use in public health systems also apply in long-term care facilities (i.e., nursing homes, hospitals, assisted living centers) for the control of infections acquired within the facility (i.e., nosocomial infections; for more information on infection control, see Chapter 80).

The field of epidemiology is broad and complex. Diagnostic microbiology laboratory personnel and epidemiologists often work closely to investigate problems. Therefore, familiarity with certain epidemiologic terms and concepts is important (see Box 3-1).

Because the central focus of epidemiology is on tracking and characterizing infections and infectious diseases, this field heavily depends on diagnostic microbiology. Epidemiologic investigations cannot proceed unless researchers first know the etiologic or causative agents. Therefore, the procedures and protocols used in diagnostic microbiology to detect, isolate, and characterize human pathogens are essential for patient care and also play a central role in epidemiologic studies focused on disease prevention and the general improvement of public health. In fact, microbiologists who work in clinical laboratories are often the first to recognize patterns that suggest potential outbreaks or epidemics.

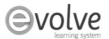 *Visit the Evolve site to complete the review questions.*

## CASE STUDY 3-1

An 8-year-old boy presents to the emergency department (ED) with right upper abdominal pain associated with vomiting, headache, and fever. The boy had been seen in the ED approximately 1.5 months previously for a sore throat, cough, and headache. After the first visit to the ED, the patient was treated with amoxicillin. The boy was born in northern Africa in a refugee camp. He and his family had emigrated from Africa approximately 8 months ago. Generally the boy appears to be in good health. His immunizations are current, and he has no allergies. He currently resides with his parents and three siblings, who all appear to be in good health. His mother speaks very little English.

The attending physician orders an abdominal computed tomography (CT) scan and identifies a mass in the left hepatic lobe. There appears to be no evidence of gastrointestinal bleeding. The attending physician orders a complete work-up on the patient, including a complete blood count, microbiology tests, chemistry, coagulation, and a hepatitis panel. The laboratory results indicate some type of infection and inflammatory condition. The patient has an elevated white blood cell (WBC) count that correlates with his erythrocyte sedimentation rate (ESR) and C-reactive protein (CRP) level. The ESR and the CRP level are clear indicators of an inflammatory process.

### QUESTIONS

1. Identify and differentiate the patient's signs and symptoms.
2. Explain whether this patient likely has an acute or a chronic infection.

## BIBLIOGRAPHY

Atlas RM: *Principles of microbiology,* St Louis, 2006, Mosby.

Brock TD, Madigan M, Martinko J, et al, editors: *Biology of microorganisms,* Upper Saddle River, NJ, 2009, Prentice Hall.

Dobrindt U: Genomic islands in pathogenic and environmental microorganisms, *Nat Rev Microbiol* 2:414, 2002.

Engleberg NC, DiRita V, Dermody TS: *Schaechter's mechanisms of microbial disease,* Baltimore, Md, 2007, Lippincott Williams & Wilkins.

Hu T, Gimferrer I, Alberola-Ila J: Control of early stages in invariant natural killer T-cell development, *Immunology* 134;1-7, 2011.

Karunakaran E, Mukherjee J, Ramalingam B, Biggs CA: Biofilmology: a multidisciplinary review of the study of microbial biofilms, *Appl Microbiol Biotechnol* 90:1869, 2011.

Simões LC, Lemos M, Pereira AM et al: Persister cells in a biofilm treated with a biocide, *Biofouling* 27:4, 403, 2011.

Murray PR, editor: *Medical microbiology,* ed 5, St Louis, 2008, Mosby.

Ryan KJ, editor: *Sherris medical microbiology: an introduction to infectious diseases,* Norwalk, Conn, 2003, McGraw-Hill Medical.

Schmidt H, Hensel M: Pathogenicity islands in bacterial pathogenesis, *Clin Microbiol Rev* 17:14, 2004.

CHAPTER

4

# Laboratory Safety

## OBJECTIVES

1. Define and differentiate sterilization, disinfection, and antiseptic.
2. List the factors that influence the effectiveness of disinfectants in the microbiology laboratory.
3. Describe the methods used for the disposal of hazardous waste, including physical and chemical methods, and the material and/or organisms effectively eliminated by each method.
4. Define a chemical hygiene plan and describe the purpose of the methods and items that are elements of the plan, including proper labeling of hazardous materials, training programs, and material safety data sheets.
5. Name the four types of fire extinguishers and the specific flammables that each is effective in controlling.
6. Describe the process of Universal or Standard Precautions in the microbiology laboratory, including handling of infectious materials, personal hygiene, use of personal protective equipment, handling of sharp objects, and hand-washing procedures.
7. Define Biosafety Levels 1 through 4, including the precautions required for each, and identify a representative organism for each.
8. Outline the basic guidelines for packing and shipping infectious substances.
9. Describe the management and response required during a biologic or chemical exposure incident in the laboratory.

Microbiology laboratory safety practices were first published in 1913 in a textbook by Eyre. They included admonitions such as the necessity to (1) wear gloves, (2) wash hands after working with infectious materials, (3) disinfect all instruments immediately after use, (4) use water to moisten specimen labels rather than the tongue, (5) disinfect all contaminated waste before discarding, and (6) report to appropriate personnel all accidents or exposures to infectious agents.

These guidelines are still incorporated into safety programs in the diagnostic microbiology laboratory. Safety programs also have been expanded to include not only the proper handling of biologic hazards encountered in processing patient specimens and handling infectious microorganisms, but also fire safety; electrical safety; the safe handling, storage, and disposal of chemicals and radioactive substances; and techniques for safely lifting or moving heavy objects. In areas of the country prone to natural disasters (e.g., earthquakes, hurricanes, snowstorms), safety programs include disaster preparedness plans that outline the steps to take in an emergency. Although all microbiologists are responsible for their own health and safety, the institution and supervising personnel are required to provide safety training to

familiarize microbiologists with known hazards in the workplace and to prevent exposure. Laboratory safety is considered an integral part of overall laboratory services, and federal law in the United States mandates pre-employment safety training, followed by quarterly safety in-services. Safety training regulations are enforced by the United States Department of Labor Occupational Safety and Health Administration (OSHA). Regulations and requirements may vary based on the type of laboratory and updated regulations. It is recommended that the laboratory review these requirements as provided by OSHA (www.osha.gov).

Microbiologists should be knowledgeable, properly trained, and equipped with the proper protective materials and working controls while performing duties in the laboratory if the safety regulations are internalized and followed without deviation. Investigation of the causes of accidents indicates that unnecessary exposures to infectious agents occur when individuals become sloppy in performing their duties or when they deviate from standardized safety precautions.

## STERILIZATION AND DISINFECTION

**Sterilization** is a process that kills all forms of microbial life, including bacterial spores. **Disinfection** is a process that destroys pathogenic organisms, but not necessarily all microorganisms or spores. Sterilization and disinfection may be accomplished by physical or chemical methods.

### METHODS OF STERILIZATION

The physical methods of sterilization include:
- Incineration
- Moist heat
- Dry heat
- Filtration
- Ionizing (gamma) radiation

**Incineration** is the most common method of treating infectious waste. Hazardous material is literally burned to ashes at temperatures of 870° to 980°C. Incineration is the safest method to ensure that no infective materials remain in samples or containers when disposed. Prions, infective proteins, are not eliminated using conventional methods. Therefore incineration is recommended. Toxic air emissions and the presence of heavy metals in ash have limited the use of incineration in most large U.S. cities.

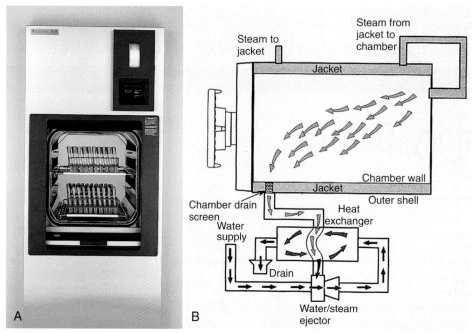

**Figure 4-1** Gravity displacement type of autoclave. **A,** Typical Eagle Century Series sterilizer for laboratory applications. **B,** Typical Eagle 3000 sterilizer piping diagram. The arrows show the entry of steam into the chamber and the displacement of air. (Courtesy AMSCO International, a subsidiary of STERIS Corp., Mentor, Ohio.)

**Moist heat** (steam under pressure) is used to sterilize biohazardous trash and heat-stable objects; an autoclave is used for this purpose. An autoclave is essentially a large pressure cooker. Moist heat in the form of saturated steam under 1 atmosphere (15 psi [pounds per square inch]) of pressure causes the irreversible denaturation of enzymes and structural proteins. The most commonly used steam sterilizer in the microbiology laboratory is the gravity displacement type (Figure 4-1). Steam enters at the top of the sterilizing chamber; because steam is lighter than air, it displaces the air in the chamber and forces it out the bottom through the drain vent. The two common sterilization temperatures are 121°C (250°F) and 132°C (270°F). Items such as media, liquids, and instruments are usually autoclaved for 15 minutes at 121°C. Infectious medical waste, on the other hand, is often sterilized at 132°C for 30 to 60 minutes to allow penetration of the steam throughout the waste and the displacement of air trapped inside the autoclave bag. Moist heat is the fastest and simplest physical method of sterilization.

**Dry heat** requires longer exposure times (1.5 to 3 hours) and higher temperatures than moist heat (160° to 180°C). Dry heat ovens are used to sterilize items such as glassware, oil, petrolatum, or powders. Filtration is the method of choice for antibiotic solutions, toxic chemicals, radioisotopes, vaccines, and carbohydrates, which are all heat sensitive. Filtration of liquids is accomplished by pulling the solution through a cellulose acetate or cellulose nitrate membrane with a vacuum. Filtration of air is accomplished using high-efficiency particulate air (HEPA) filters designed to remove organisms larger than 0.3 μm from isolation rooms, operating rooms, and biologic safety cabinets (BSCs). The ionizing radiation used in microwaves and radiograph machines is composed of short wavelength and high-energy gamma rays. Ionizing radiation is used for sterilizing disposables such as plastic syringes, catheters, or gloves before use. The most common chemical sterilant is ethylene oxide (EtO), which is used in gaseous form for sterilizing heat-sensitive objects. Formaldehyde vapor and vapor-phase hydrogen peroxide (an oxidizing agent) have been used to sterilize HEPA filters in BSCs. Glutaraldehyde, which is sporicidal (kills spores) in 3 to 10 hours, is used for medical equipment such as bronchoscopes, because it does not corrode lenses, metal, or rubber. Peracetic acid, effective in the presence of organic material, has also been used for the surface sterilization of surgical instruments. The use of glutaraldehyde or peracetic acid is called *cold sterilization.*

## METHODS OF DISINFECTION

### Physical Methods of Disinfection

The three physical methods of disinfection are:
- Boiling at 100°C for 15 minutes, which kills vegetative bacteria
- Pasteurizing at 63°C for 30 minutes or 72°C for 15 seconds, which kills food pathogens without damaging the nutritional value or flavor
- Using nonionizing radiation such as ultraviolet (UV) light

UV rays are long wavelength and low energy. They do not penetrate well, and organisms must have direct surface exposure, such as the working surface of a BSC, for this form of disinfection to work.

### Chemical Methods of Disinfection

**Chemical** disinfectants comprise many classes, including:
- Alcohols
- Aldehydes

- Halogens
- Heavy metals
- Quaternary ammonium compounds
- Phenolics

Chemicals used to destroy all life are called *chemical sterilants,* or *biocides;* however, these same chemicals, used for shorter periods, act as disinfectants. Disinfectants used on living tissue (skin) are called *antiseptics.*

A number of factors influence the activity of disinfectants, including:

- Types of organisms present
- Temperature and pH of process
- Number of organisms present (microbial load)
- Concentration of disinfectant
- Amount of organics present (blood, mucus, pus)
- Nature of surface to be disinfected (e.g., potential for corrosion; porous or nonporous surface)
- Length of contact time
- Type of water available (hard or soft)

Resistance to disinfectants varies with the type of microorganism. Bacterial spores, such as *Bacillus* spp., are the most resistant, followed by mycobacteria (acid-fast bacilli); nonenveloped viruses (e.g., poliovirus); fungi; vegetative (nonsporulating) bacteria (e.g., gram-negative rods); and enveloped viruses (e.g., herpes simplex virus), which are the most susceptible to the action of disinfectants. The Environmental Protection Agency (EPA) registers chemical disinfectants used in the United States and requires manufacturers to specify the activity level of each compound at the working dilution. Therefore, microbiologists who must recommend appropriate disinfectants should check the manufacturer's cut sheets (product information) for the classes of microorganisms that will be killed. Generally, the time necessary for killing microorganisms increases in direct proportion to the number of organisms (microbial load). This is particularly true of instruments contaminated with organic material such as blood, pus, or mucus. The organic material should be mechanically removed before chemical sterilization to decrease the microbial load. This is analogous to removing dried food from utensils before placing them in a dishwasher, and it is important for cold sterilization of instruments such as bronchoscopes.

The type of water and its concentration in a solution are also important. Hard water may reduce the rate of killing of microorganisms. In addition, 70% ethyl alcohol is more effective as a disinfectant than 95% ethyl alcohol because the increased water ($H_2O$) hydrolyzing bonds in protein molecules make the killing of microorganisms more effective.

Ethyl or isopropyl alcohol is nonsporicidal (does not kill spores) and evaporates quickly. Therefore, its use is limited to the skin as an antiseptic or on thermometers and injection vial rubber septa as a disinfectant.

Because of their irritating fumes, the aldehydes (formaldehyde and glutaraldehyde) are generally not used as surface disinfectants.

The halogens, especially chlorine and iodine, are frequently used as disinfectants. Chlorine is most often used in the form of sodium hypochlorite (NaOCl), the compound known as household bleach. The Centers for Disease Control and Prevention (CDC) recommends that tabletops be cleaned after blood spills with a 1 : 10 dilution of bleach.

Iodine is prepared either as a tincture with alcohol or as an iodophor coupled to a neutral polymer (e.g., povidone-iodine). Both iodine compounds are widely used antiseptics. In fact, 70% ethyl alcohol, followed by an iodophor, is the most common compound used for skin disinfection before drawing blood specimens for culture or surgery.

Because mercury is toxic to the environment, heavy metals containing mercury are no longer recommended, but an eye drop solution containing 1% silver nitrate is still placed in the eyes of newborns to prevent infections with *Neisseria gonorrhoeae.*

Quaternary ammonium compounds are used to disinfect bench tops or other surfaces in the laboratory. However, surfaces grossly contaminated with organic materials, such as blood, may inactivate heavy metals or quaternary ammonium compounds, thus limiting their utility.

Finally, phenolics, such as the common laboratory disinfectant Amphyl, are derivatives of carbolic acid (phenol). The addition of detergent results in a product that cleans and disinfects at the same time, and at concentrations of 2% to 5%, these products are widely used for cleaning bench tops.

The most important point to remember when working with biocides or disinfectants is to prepare a working solution of the compound exactly according to the manufacturer's package insert. Many think that if the manufacturer says to dilute 1 : 200, they will be getting a stronger product if they dilute it 1 : 10. However, the ratio of water to active ingredient may be critical, and if sufficient water is not added, the free chemical for surface disinfection may not be released.

## CHEMICAL SAFETY

In 1987, the U.S. Occupational Safety and Health Administration (OSHA) published the Hazard Communication Standard, which provides for certain institutional educational practices to ensure that all laboratory personnel have a thorough working knowledge of the hazards of the chemicals with which they work. This standard has also been called the "employee right to know." It mandates that all hazardous chemicals in the workplace be identified and clearly marked with a National Fire Protection Association (NFPA) label stating the health risks, such as carcinogen (cause of cancer), mutagen (cause of mutations in deoxyribonucleic acid [DNA] or ribonucleic acid [RNA]), or teratogen (cause of birth defects), and the hazard class, for example, corrosive (harmful to mucous membranes, skin, eyes, or tissues), poison, flammable, or oxidizing (Figure 4-2).

Each laboratory should have a chemical hygiene plan that includes guidelines on proper labeling of chemical containers, manufacturers' material safety data sheets (MSDSs), and the written chemical safety training and retraining programs. Hazardous chemicals must be inventoried annually. In addition, laboratories are required to maintain a file of every chemical they use and a corresponding MSDS. The manufacturer provides the MSDS for every hazardous chemical; some manufacturers also provide letters for nonhazardous chemicals, such as saline, so that these can be included with the other MSDSs. The MSDSs include information on the nature of the chemical, the precautions to take if the chemical is spilled, and disposal recommendations. The sections in the typical MSDS include:

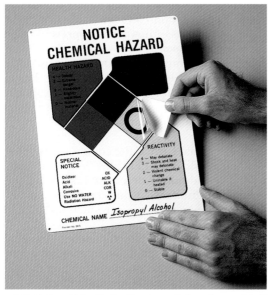

**Figure 4-2** National Fire Protection Association diamond indicating a chemical hazard. This information can be customized (as shown here for isopropyl alcohol) by applying the appropriate self-adhesive polyester numbers to the corresponding color-coded hazard area. (Courtesy Lab Safety Supply, Janesville, Wisconsin.)

- Substance name
- Name, address, and telephone number of manufacturer
- Hazardous ingredients
- Physical and chemical properties
- Fire and explosion data
- Toxicity
- Health effects and first aid
- Stability and reactivity
- Shipping data
- Spill, leak, and disposal procedures
- Personal protective equipment
- Handling and storage

Employees should become familiar with the location and organization of MSDS files in the laboratory so that they know where to look in the event of an emergency.

Fume hoods (Figure 4-3) are provided in the laboratory to prevent inhalation of toxic fumes. Fume hoods protect against chemical odor by exhausting air to the outside, but they are not HEPA-filtered to trap pathogenic microorganisms. It is important to remember that a BSC (discussed later in the chapter) is not a fume hood.

Work with toxic or noxious chemicals should always be done wearing nitrile gloves, in a fume hood, or when wearing a fume mask. Spills should be cleaned up using a fume mask, gloves, impervious (impenetrable to moisture) apron, and goggles. Acid and alkaline, flammable, and radioactive spill kits are available to assist in rendering any chemical spills harmless.

# FIRE SAFETY

Fire safety is an important component of the laboratory safety program. Each laboratory is required to post fire

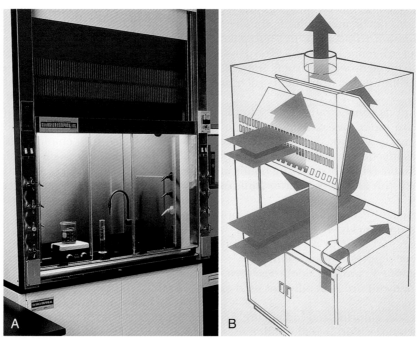

**Figure 4-3** Fume hood. **A,** Model ChemGARD. **B,** Schematics. Arrows indicate airflow through cabinet to outside vent. (Courtesy the Baker Co., Sanford, Maine.)

evacuation plans that are essentially blueprints for finding the nearest exit in case of fire. Fire drills conducted quarterly or annually, depending on local laws, ensure that all personnel know what to do in case of fire. Exit paths should always remain clear of obstructions, and employees should be trained to use fire extinguishers. The local fire department is often an excellent resource for training in the types and use of fire extinguishers.

Type A fire extinguishers are used for trash, wood, and paper; type B extinguishers are used for chemical fires; and type C extinguishers are used for electrical fires. Combination type ABC extinguishers are found in most laboratories so that personnel need not worry about which extinguisher to reach for in case of a fire. However, type C extinguishers, which contain carbon dioxide ($CO_2$) or another dry chemical to smother flames, are also used, because this type of extinguisher does not damage equipment.

The important actions in case of fire and the order in which to perform tasks can be remembered with the acronym RACE:

1. **R**escue any injured individuals.
2. **A**ctivate the fire alarm.
3. **C**ontain (smother) the fire, if feasible (close fire doors).
4. **E**xtinguish the fire, if possible.

## ELECTRICAL SAFETY

Electrical cords should be checked regularly for fraying and replaced when necessary. All plugs should be the three-prong, grounded type. All sockets should be checked for electrical grounding and leakage at least annually. No extension cords should be used in the laboratory.

## HANDLING OF COMPRESSED GASES

Compressed gas cylinders ($CO_2$, anaerobic gas mixture) contain pressurized gases and must be properly handled and secured. When leaking cylinders have fallen, tanks have become missiles, resulting in loss of life and destruction of property. Therefore, gas tanks should be properly chained (Figure 4-4, *A*) and stored in well-ventilated areas. The metal cap, which is removed when the regulator is installed, should always be in place when a gas cylinder is not in use. Cylinders should be transported chained to special dollies (Figure 4-4, *B*).

## BIOSAFETY

Individuals are exposed in various ways to laboratory-acquired infections in microbiology laboratories, such as:

- Rubbing the eyes or nose with contaminated hands
- Inhaling aerosols produced during centrifugation, mixing with a vortex or spills of liquid cultures
- Accidentally ingesting microorganisms by putting pens or fingers in the mouth
- Receiving percutaneous inoculation (i.e., through puncture from an accidental needle stick)
- Manipulating and/or opening bacterial cultures in liquid media or on plates, creating potentially hazardous aerosols outside of a biosafety hood

Risks from a microbiology laboratory may extend to adjacent laboratories and to the families of those

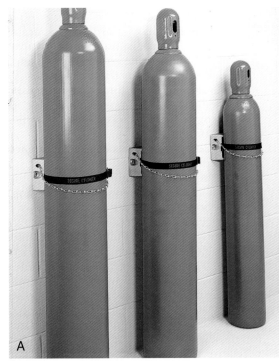 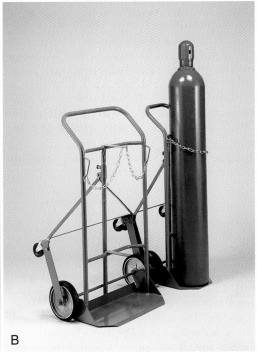

**Figure 4-4 A,** Gas cylinders chained to the wall. **B,** Gas cylinder chained to a dolly during transportation. (Courtesy Lab Safety Supply, Janesville, Wisconsin.)

who work in the microbiology laboratory. For example, Blaser and Feldman[1] noted that 5 of 31 individuals who contracted typhoid fever from proficiency testing specimens did not work in a microbiology laboratory. Two patients were family members of a microbiologist who had worked with *S. enterica* subsp. Typhi; two were students whose afternoon class was in the laboratory where the organism had been cultured that morning; and one worked in an adjacent chemistry laboratory.

In the clinical microbiology laboratory, shigellosis, salmonellosis, tuberculosis, brucellosis, and hepatitis are frequently acquired laboratory infections. Additional infections have been reported from agents such as *Coxiella burnetii, Francisella tularensis, Trichophyton mentagrophytes,* and *Coccidioides immitis.* Viral agents transmitted through blood and body fluids cause most of the infections in non–microbiology laboratory workers and in health care workers in general. These include hepatitis B virus (HBV), hepatitis C virus (HCV), hepatitis D virus (HDV), and human immunodeficiency virus (HIV). Interestingly, males and younger employees (17 to 24 years old) are involved in more laboratory-acquired infections than females and older employees (45 to 64 years old). It is important to note that laboratory-associated infections are not a new phenomena and are based primarily on voluntary reporting. Therefore, such incidents are widely underreported because of fears of repercussions associated with such events.

# EXPOSURE CONTROL PLAN

The laboratory director and supervisor is legally responsible for ensuring that an **Exposure Control Plan** has been implemented and that the mandated safety guidelines are followed. The plan identifies tasks that are hazardous to employees and promotes employee safety through use of the following:
- Employee education and orientation
- Appropriate disposal of hazardous waste
- Standard (formerly Universal) Precautions
- Engineering controls and safe work practices, as well as appropriate waste disposal and use of BSCs
- Personal protective equipment (PPE), such as laboratory coats, shoe covers, gowns, gloves, and eye protection (goggles, face shields)
- Postexposure plan for investigating all accidents and a plan to prevent recurrences

# EMPLOYEE EDUCATION AND ORIENTATION

Each institution should have a safety manual that is reviewed by all employees and a safety officer who is knowledgeable about the risks associated with laboratory-acquired infections. The safety officer should provide orientation for new employees and quarterly continuing education updates for all personnel. Initial training and all retraining should be documented in writing. Hand washing should be emphasized for all laboratory personnel. The mechanical action of rubbing the hands together and soaping under the fingernails is the most important part of the process. In the laboratory, unlike in hospital areas such as operating rooms, products containing antibacterial agents are not more effective than ordinary soap.

All employees should also be offered, at no charge, the HBV vaccine and annual skin tests for tuberculosis. For employees whose skin tests are already positive or who have previously been vaccinated with bacillus Calmette-Guérin (BCG), the employer should offer chest radiographs upon employment, although follow-up annual chest radiographs are no longer recommended by the CDC.

# DISPOSAL OF HAZARDOUS WASTE

All materials contaminated with potentially infectious agents must be decontaminated before disposal. These include unused portions of patient specimens, patient cultures, stock cultures of microorganisms, and disposable sharp instruments, such as scalpels and syringes with needles. It is recommended that syringes with needles not be accepted in the laboratory; staff members should be required to submit capped syringes to the laboratory. Infectious waste may be decontaminated by use of an autoclave, incinerator, or any one of several alternative waste-treatment methods. Some state or local municipalities permit blood, serum, urine, feces, and other body fluids to be carefully poured into a sanitary sewer. Infectious waste from microbiology laboratories is usually autoclaved on site or sent for incineration.

In 1986 the EPA published a guide to hazardous waste reduction to limit the amount of hazardous waste generated and released into the environment. These regulations call for the following:
- Substituting less hazardous chemicals when possible; for example, substituting ethyl acetate for ether in ova and parasite concentrations and Hemo-de in place of xylene for trichrome stains
- Developing procedures that use less of a hazardous chemical; for example, substituting infrared technology for radioisotopes in blood culture instruments
- Segregating infectious waste from uncontaminated (paper) trash
- Substituting miniaturized systems for identification and antimicrobial susceptibility testing of potential pathogens to reduce the volume of chemical reagents and infectious waste

Recently, several alternative waste-treatment machines were developed to reduce the amount of waste buried in landfills. These systems combine mechanical shredding or compacting of the waste with chemical (sodium hypochlorite, chlorine dioxide, peracetic acid), thermal (moist heat, dry heat), or ionizing radiation (microwaves, radio waves) decontamination. Most state regulations for these units require at least a sixfold reduction in vegetative bacteria, fungi, mycobacteria, and enveloped viruses and at least a fourfold reduction in bacterial spores.

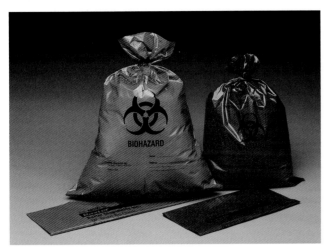

**Figure 4-5** Autoclave bags. (Courtesy Allegiance Healthcare, McGaw Park, Illinois.)

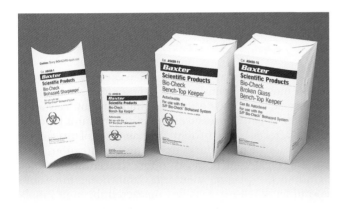

A

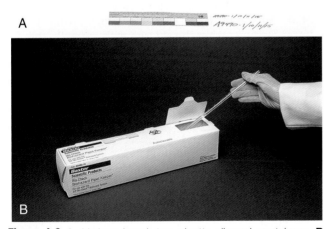

B

**Figure 4-6 A,** Various bench-top pipette discard containers. **B,** Bench-top serologic pipette discard container. (Courtesy Allegiance Healthcare, McGaw Park, Illinois.)

Infectious waste (agar plates, tubes, reagent bottles) should be placed into two leak-proof, plastic bags for sturdiness (Figure 4-5); this is known as **double bagging.** Pipettes, swabs, and other glass objects should be placed into rigid cardboard containers (Figure 4-6) before disposal. Broken glass is placed in thick boxes lined with plastic biohazard bags (Figure 4-7); when full, the box is incinerated or autoclaved. Sharp objects, including

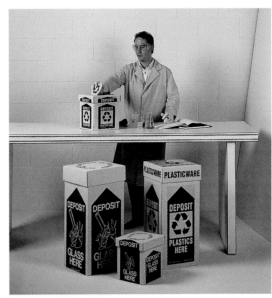

**Figure 4-7** Cartons for broken glass. (Courtesy Lab Safety Supply, Janesville, Wisconsin.)

scalpels and needles, are placed in sharps containers (Figure 4-8) and then autoclaved or incinerated.

# STANDARD PRECAUTIONS

In 1987 the CDC published guidelines known as Universal Precautions to reduce the risk of HBV transmission in clinical laboratories and blood banks. In 1996 these safety recommendations became known as **Standard Precautions.** These precautions require that blood and body fluids from every patient be treated as potentially infectious. The essentials of Standard Precautions and safe laboratory work practices are as follows:

- Do not eat, drink, smoke, or apply cosmetics (including lip balm).
- Do not insert or remove contact lenses.
- Do not bite nails or chew on pens.
- Do not mouth-pipette.
- Limit access to the laboratory to trained personnel only.
- Assume all patients are infectious for all blood-borne pathogens.
- Use appropriate barrier precautions to prevent skin and mucous membrane exposure, including wearing gloves at all times and masks, goggles, gowns, or aprons if splash or droplet formation is a risk.
- Thoroughly wash hands and other skin surfaces after removing gloves and immediately after any contamination.
- Take special care to prevent injuries with sharp objects, such as needles and scalpels.

Standard Precautions should be followed for handling blood and body fluids, including all secretions and excretions submitted to the microbiology laboratory (e.g., serum, semen, all sterile body fluids, saliva from dental procedures, and vaginal secretions). Standard

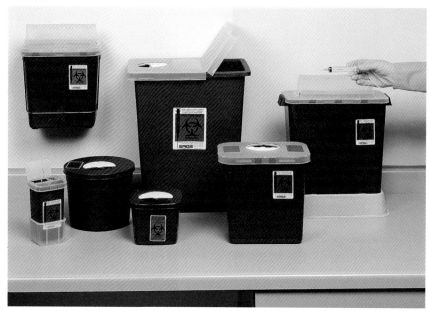

**Figure 4-8** Sharps containers. (Courtesy Lab Safety Supply, Janesville, Wisconsin.)

Precautions applies to blood and all body fluids, except sweat. Practice of Standard Precautions by health care workers handling all patient material lessens the risks associated with such specimens.

Mouth-pipetting is strictly prohibited. Mechanical devices must be used for drawing all liquids into pipettes. Eating, drinking, smoking, and applying cosmetics are strictly forbidden in work areas. Food and drink must be stored in refrigerators in areas separate from the work area. All personnel should wash their hands with soap and water after removing gloves, after handling infectious material, and before leaving the laboratory area. In addition, it is good practice to store sera collected periodically from all health care workers so that, in the event of an accident, a seroconversion (acquisition of antibodies to an infectious agent) can be documented (see Chapter 10).

All health care workers should follow Standard Precautions whether working inside or outside the laboratory. When collecting specimens outside the laboratory, individuals should follow these guidelines:

- Wear gloves and a laboratory coat.
- Deal carefully with needles and lancets.
- Discard sharps in an appropriate, puncture-resistant container.
- Never recap needles by hand; if necessary, special safety devices are available. (Manufacturers are now producing needles with built in safety devices to prevent accidental needle sticks).

# ENGINEERING CONTROLS

## LABORATORY ENVIRONMENT

The biohazard symbol should be prominently displayed on laboratory doors and any equipment (refrigerators, incubators, centrifuges) that contain infectious material.

The air-handling system of a microbiology laboratory should move air from lower to higher risk areas, never the reverse. Ideally, the microbiology laboratory should be under negative pressure, and air should not be recirculated after passing through microbiology. The selected use of BSCs for procedures that generate infectious aerosols is critical to laboratory safety. Infectious diseases, including the plague, tularemia, brucellosis, tuberculosis, and legionellosis, may be contracted through inhalation of infectious particles present in a droplet of liquid. Because blood is a primary specimen that may contain infectious virus particles, subculturing blood cultures by puncturing the septum with a needle should be performed behind a barrier to protect the worker from droplets. Several other common procedures used to process specimens for culture, notably mincing, grinding, vortexing, and preparing direct smears for microscopic examination, are known to produce aerosol droplets. These procedures must be performed in a BSC.

The microbiology laboratory poses many hazards to unsuspecting and untrained people; therefore, access should be limited to employees and other necessary personnel (biomedical engineers, housekeepers). Visitors, especially young children, should be discouraged. Certain areas of high risk, such as the mycobacteriology and virology laboratories, should be closed to visitors. Custodial personnel should be trained to discriminate among the waste containers, dealing only with those that contain noninfectious material. Care should be taken to prevent insects from infesting any laboratory area. Mites, for example, can crawl over the surface of media, carrying microorganisms from colonies on a plate to other areas. Houseplants can also serve as a source of insects and should be carefully observed for infestation, if they are not excluded altogether from the laboratory environment. A pest control program should be in place to control rodents and insects.

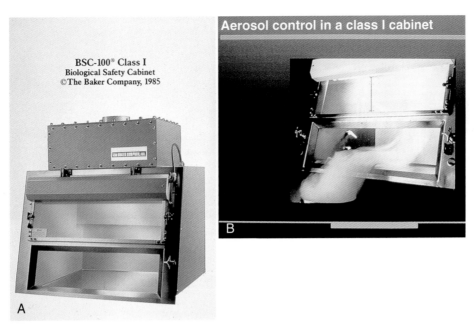

**Figure 4-9** Class I biologic safety cabinet. **A,** Model BSC-100. **B,** Schematics showing airflow. (Courtesy the Baker Co., Sanford, Maine.)

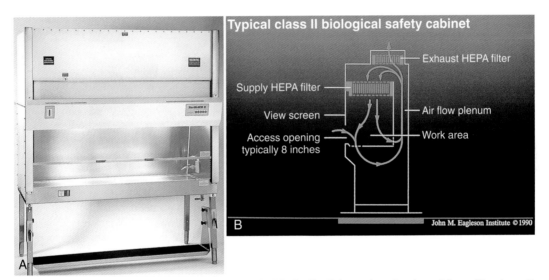

**Figure 4-10** Class II biologic safety cabinet. **A,** Model SterilGARD II. **B,** Schematics showing airflow. (Courtesy the Baker Co., Sanford, Maine.)

## BIOLOGIC SAFETY CABINET

A BSC is a device that encloses a workspace in such a way as to protect workers from aerosol exposure to infectious disease agents. Air that contains the infectious material is sterilized, either by heat, ultraviolet light or, most commonly, by passage through a HEPA filter that removes most particles larger than 0.3 μm in diameter. These cabinets are designated as class I through 3, according to the effective level of biologic containment. Class I cabinets allow room (unsterilized) air to pass into the cabinet and around the area and material within, sterilizing only the air to be exhausted (Figure 4-9). They have negative pressure, are ventilated to the outside, and are usually operated with an open front.

Class II cabinets sterilize air that flows over the infectious material, as well as air to be exhausted. The air flows in "sheets," which serve as barriers to particles from outside the cabinet and direct the flow of contaminated air into the filters (Figure 4-10). Such cabinets are called **vertical laminar flow BSCs.** Class II cabinets have a variable sash opening through which the operator gains access to the work surface. Depending on their inlet flow velocity and the percent of air that is HEPA filtered and recirculated, class II cabinets are further differentiated into type A or B. A class IIA cabinet is self-contained, and 70% of the air is recirculated. The exhaust air in class IIB cabinets is discharged outside the building. A class IIB cabinet is selected if radioisotopes, toxic chemicals, or carcinogens will be used.

Because they are completely enclosed and have negative pressure, class III cabinets afford the most protection to the worker. Air coming into and going out of the

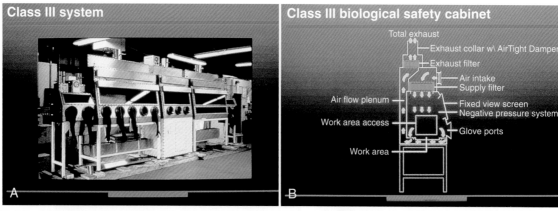

**Figure 4-11** Class III biologic safety cabinet. **A,** Custom-built class III system. **B,** Schematics with arrows showing airflow through cabinet. (Courtesy the Baker Co., Sanford, Maine.)

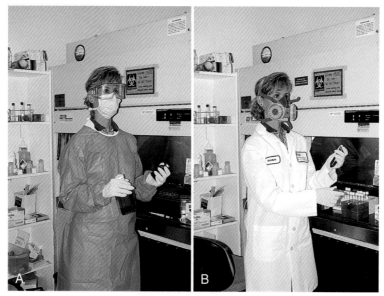

**Figure 4-12** Personal protective equipment. **A,** Microbiologist wearing a laboratory gown, gloves, goggles, and face mask. **B,** Microbiologist wearing a laboratory coat, gloves, and respirator with high-efficiency particulate air (HEPA) filters (pink cartridges) for cleaning up spills of *Mycobacterium tuberculosis*.

cabinet is filter sterilized, and the infectious material within is handled with rubber gloves that are attached and sealed to the cabinet (Figure 4-11).

Most hospital clinical microbiology laboratory scientists use class IIA cabinets. Routine inspection and documentation of adequate function of these cabinets are critical factors in an ongoing quality assurance program. It is important to the proper operation of laminar flow cabinets that an open area for 3 feet from the cabinet be maintained during operation of the air-circulating system; this ensures that infectious material is directed through the HEPA filter. BSCs must be certified initially, whenever moved more than 18 inches, and annually thereafter.

## PERSONAL PROTECTIVE EQUIPMENT

OSHA regulations require that health care facilities provide employees with all **personal protective equipment**

necessary to protect them from hazards encountered during the course of work (Figure 4-12). PPE usually includes plastic shields or goggles to protect workers from droplets, disposal containers for sharp objects, holders for glass bottles, trays in which to carry smaller hazardous items (e.g., blood culture bottles), handheld pipetting devices, impervious gowns, laboratory coats, disposable gloves, masks, safety carriers for centrifuges (especially those used in the Acid Fast Bacteriology (AFB) laboratory), and HEPA respirators.

HEPA respirators are required for all health care workers, including phlebotomists, who enter the rooms of patients with tuberculosis, as well as workers who clean up spills of pathogenic microorganisms (see Chapter 80). All respirators should be fit-tested for each individual so that each person is assured that his or hers is working properly. Males must shave their facial hair to achieve a tight fit. Respirators are evaluated according to guidelines of the National Institute for Occupational

Safety and Health (NIOSH), a branch of the CDC. N95 or P100 disposable masks (available from 3M, St. Paul, Minnesota) are commonly used in the clinical laboratory.

Microbiologists should wear laboratory coats over their street clothes, and these coats should be removed before leaving the laboratory. Most exposures to blood-containing fluids occur on the hands or forearms, so gowns with closed wrists or forearm covers and gloves that cover all potentially exposed skin on the arms are most beneficial. If the laboratory protective clothing becomes contaminated with body fluids or potential pathogens, it should be sterilized in an autoclave immediately and cleaned before reusing. The institution or a uniform agency should clean laboratory coats; it is no longer permissible for microbiologists to launder their own coats. Alternatively, disposable gowns may be used. Obviously, laboratory workers who plan to enter an area of the hospital where patients at special risk of acquiring infection are present (e.g., intensive care units, the nursery, operating rooms, or areas in which immunosuppressive therapy is being administered) should take every precaution to cover their street clothes with clean or sterile protective clothing appropriate to the area visited. Special impervious protective clothing is advisable for certain activities, such as working with radioactive substances or caustic chemicals. Solid-front gowns are indicated for those working with specimens being cultured for mycobacteria. Unless large-volume spills of potentially infectious material are anticipated, impervious laboratory gowns are not necessary in most microbiology laboratories.

## POSTEXPOSURE CONTROL

All laboratory accidents and potential exposures must be reported to the supervisor and safety officer, who will immediately arrange to send the individual to employee health or an outside occupational health physician. Immediate medical care is of foremost importance; investigation of the accident should take place only after the employee has received appropriate care. If the accident is a needle stick injury, for example, the patient should be identified and the risk of the laboratorian acquiring a blood-borne infection should be assessed. The investigation helps the physician determine the need for prophylaxis, such as hepatitis B virus immunoglobulin (HBIG) or an HBV booster immunization in the event of exposure to hepatitis B. The physician also is able to discuss the potential for disease transmission to family members, such as after exposure to a patient with *Neisseria meningitidis.* Follow-up treatment also should be assessed, such as the drawing of additional sera at intervals of 6 weeks, 3 months, and 6 months for HIV testing. Finally, the safety committee, or at least the laboratory director and safety officer, should review the events of the accident to determine whether it could have been avoided and to delineate measures to prevent future accidents. The investigation of the accident and corrective action should be documented in an incident report.

# CLASSIFICATION OF BIOLOGIC AGENTS BASED ON HAZARD

*Classification of Etiological Agents on the Basis of Hazard,* from the CDC, served as a reference for assessing the relative risks of working with various biologic agents until the CDC, together with the National Institutes of Health (NIH), produced the manual *Biosafety in Microbiological and Biomedical Laboratories.* The fifth edition of this manual is currently available on the CDC website (www.cdc.gov/biosafety/publications/bmbl5/BMBL.pdf). In general, patient specimens pose a greater risk to laboratory workers than do microorganisms in culture, because the nature of etiologic agents in patient specimens is initially unknown.

Biosafety Level (BSL-1) agents include those that have no known potential for infecting healthy people and are well defined and characterized. These agents are used in laboratory teaching exercises for undergraduate, secondary educational training and teaching laboratories for students in microbiology. BSL-1 agents include *Bacillus subtilis* and *Naegleria gruberi;* in addition, exempt organisms under the NIH guidelines are representative microorganisms in this category. Precautions for working with BSL-1 agents include standard good laboratory technique, as described previously.

BSL-2 agents are those most commonly being sought in clinical specimens and used in diagnostic, teaching, and other laboratories. They include all the common agents of infectious disease, as well as HIV, hepatitis B virus, *Salmonella* organisms, and several more unusual pathogens. For the handling of clinical specimens suspected of harboring any of these pathogens, BSL-2 precautions are sufficient. Specimens expected to contain prions (PrPSc), abnormal proteins associated with neurodegenerative diseases, including spongiform encephalitis, should be handled using BSL-2 procedures. This level of safety includes the principles outlined previously, provided the potential for splash or aerosol is low. If splash or aerosol is probable, the use of primary containment equipment is recommended, as are limiting access to the laboratory during working procedures, training laboratory personnel in handling pathogenic agents, direction by competent supervisors, and performing aerosol-generating procedures in a BSC. Employers must offer hepatitis B vaccine to all employees determined to be at risk of exposure.

BSL-3 procedures have been recommended for the handling of material suspected of harboring organisms unlikely to be encountered in a routine clinical laboratory and for such organisms as *Mycobacterium tuberculosis, Coxiella burnetii,* the mold stages of systemic fungi, and for some other organisms when grown in quantities greater than that found in patient specimens. These precautions, in addition to those undertaken for BSL-2 agents, consist of laboratory design and engineering controls that contain potentially dangerous material by careful control of air movement and the requirement that personnel wear protective clothing and gloves, for instance. Those working with BSL-3 agents should have

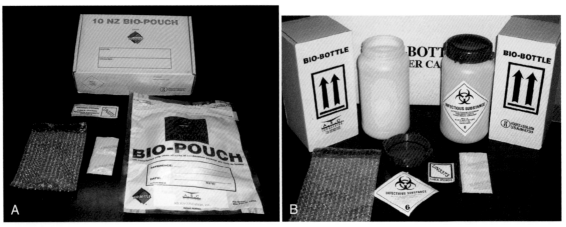

**Figure 4-13 A,** The Bio-Pouch (lower right) is made of laminated, low-density polyethylene, which is virtually unbreakable. The label for shipping a diagnostic specimen is shown (UN 3373). **B,** The Bio-Bottle is made of high-density polyethylene and is used as the secondary container. This packaging is used for both infectious substances (the class 6 label is shown) with the UN 3373 label. (Courtesy Air Sea Containers, Miami, Florida.)

baseline sera specimens stored for comparison with acute sera that can be drawn in the event of unexplained illness. BSL-3 organisms are primarily transmitted by infectious aerosol.

BSL-4 agents are exotic agents that are considered high risk and cause life-threatening disease. They include Marburg virus or Congo-Crimean hemorrhagic fever. Personnel and all materials must be decontaminated before leaving the facility, and all procedures are performed under maximum containment (special protective clothing, class III BSC). Most of the facilities that deal with BSL-4 agents are public health or research laboratories. As mentioned, BSL-4 agents pose life-threatening risks and are transmitted via aerosols; in addition, no vaccine or therapy is available for these organisms.

# MAILING BIOHAZARDOUS MATERIALS

In March 2005, the requirements for packaging and shipping of biologic material were significantly revised in response to an international desire to ensure reasonable yet safe and trouble-free shipment practices for infectious material. Before this date, clinical specimens submitted for infectious disease diagnosis, as well as isolates of any microorganism, were considered an "infectious substance" and packaged and labeled under UN 6.2 dangerous goods regulations. Infectious substances now are classified as category A, B, or C organisms. A category A specimen is an infectious substance capable of causing disease in healthy humans and animals; it is assigned to division UN 6.2, UN 2814, UN 2900, or UN 3373. Category B includes infectious substances that are not included in category A and are assigned to UN 3373. Only the category A organisms or specimens listed in Table 4-1 must be shipped as dangerous goods. The UN created the designation UN 3373 so that non–category A specimens or cultures can be packed and shipped as diagnostic or clinical specimens. The proper shipping name for a UN 3371 specimen is "biological substance, category B."

The use of the former shipping names for diagnostic or clinical specimens is no longer permitted. If the laboratory director is unsure whether a patient has symptoms of a category A agent, it is prudent to ship the specimen as an infectious substance rather than a biologic substance. Figure 4-13, *A*, shows triple packaging for both diagnostic, clinical or infectious substances in a pouch; Figure 14-13, *B*, shows triple packaging for diagnostic, clinical, or infectious substances in a rigid bottle.

Packaging must meet the requirements of the International Air Transport Association (IATA) and the International Civil Aviation Organization (IACO). Packaging instructions are available in the annual IATA regulations under 620 (dangerous goods). All air and ground shippers, such as the U.S. Postal Service (USPS), the U.S. Department of Transportation (DOT), and Federal Express (Fed Ex) have adopted IATA standards.

Training in the proper packing and shipping of infectious material is a key feature of the regulations. Every institution that ships infectious materials, whether a hospital or (physician office laboratory (POL), is required to have appropriately trained individuals; training may be obtained through carriers, package manufacturers, and special safety training organizations. The **shipper** is the individual (institution) ultimately responsible for safe and appropriate packaging. Any fines or penalties are the shipper's responsibility.

Infectious specimens or isolates should be wrapped with absorbent material and placed inside a plastic biohazard bag, called a *primary receptacle*. The primary receptacle is then inserted into a secondary container, most often a watertight, hard plastic mailer. The secondary container is capped and placed inside an outer, tertiary container that protects it from physical and water damage (see Figure 4-13, *B*). A UN class 6 label on the outer box confirms that the packaging meets all the required standards. The package must display the UN Packaging Specification Marking and must be labeled with a specific hazard label as an infectious substance. A packing list and a Shippers Declaration for Dangerous Goods Form must

**TABLE 4-1** Examples of Infectious Substances Included in Category A

| UN Number and Proper Shipping Name | Microorganisms |
|---|---|
| UN 2814—Infectious Substance Affecting Humans | *Bacillus anthracis* (cultures only)*<br>*Brucella abortus* (cultures only)*<br>*Brucella melitensis* (cultures only)*<br>*Brucella suis* (cultures only)*<br>*Burkholderia mallei—Pseudomonas mallei*-Glanders (cultures only)*<br>*Burkholderia pseudomallei—Pseudomonas pseudomallei* (cultures only)*<br>*Chlamydia psittaci*—avian strains (cultures only)<br>*Clostridium botulinum* (cultures only)<br>*Coccidioides immitis* (cultures only)<br>*Coxiella burnetii* (cultures only)<br>Crimean-Congo hemorrhagic fever virus*<br>Dengue virus (cultures only)<br>Eastern equine encephalitis virus (cultures only)*<br>*Escherichia coli,* verotoxigenic (cultures only)<br>Ebola virus*<br>Flexal virus<br>*Francisella tularensis* (cultures only)*<br>Guanarito virus<br>Hantaan virus<br>Hantaviruses causing hantavirus pulmonary syndrome<br>Hendra virus*<br>Hepatitis B virus (cultures only)<br>Herpes B virus (cultures only)<br>Human immunodeficiency virus (cultures only)<br>Highly pathogenic avian influenza virus (cultures only)<br>Japanese encephalitis virus (cultures only)<br>Junin virus<br>Kyasanur Forest disease virus<br>Lassa virus*<br>Machupo virus<br>Marburg virus*<br>Monkeypox virus*<br>*Mycobacterium tuberculosis* (cultures only)<br>Nipah virus*<br>Omsk hemorrhagic fever virus<br>Poliovirus (cultures only)<br>Rabies virus (cultures only)<br>*Rickettsia prowazekii* (cultures only)*<br>*Rickettsia rickettsii* (cultures only)*<br>Rift Valley fever virus*<br>Russian spring-summer encephalitis virus (cultures only)<br>Sabia virus<br>*Shigella dysenteriae* type 1 (cultures only)<br>Tick-borne encephalitis virus (cultures only)<br>Variola virus<br>Venezuelan equine encephalitis virus (cultures only)*<br>West Nile virus (cultures only<br>Yellow fever virus (cultures only)<br>*Yersinia pestis* (cultures only) |
| UN 2900—Infectious Substance Affecting Animals | African swine fever virus (cultures only)*<br>Avian paramyxovirus type 1—Velogenic Newcastle disease virus (cultures only)<br>Classical swine fever virus (cultures only)<br>Foot and mouth disease virus (cultures only)<br>Lumpy skin disease virus (cultures only)<br>*Mycoplasma mycoides*—Contagious bovine pleuropneumonia (cultures only)*<br>Peste des petits ruminants virus (cultures only)*<br>Rinderpest virus (cultures only)*<br>Sheep-pox virus (cultures only)*<br>Goatpox virus (cultures only)<br>Swine vesicular disease virus (cultures only)*<br>Vesicular stomatitis virus (cultures only)* |

This table is not exhaustive. Infectious substances, including new or emerging pathogens, that do not appear in the table but that meet the same criteria must be assigned to category A. In addition, if doubt exists as to whether a substance meets the criteria, it must be included in category A.
*An infectious agent also designated as a "select agent" that has the potential to pose a severe threat to public health and safety.

accompany the air bill or ground form. Diagnostic or clinical specimens are packaged similarly, but a UN specification marking is not required and it is not necessary to fill out a shippers declaration.

Shippers should note that some carriers have additional requirements for coolant materials, such as ice, dry ice, or liquid nitrogen. Because the shipper is liable for appropriate packaging, it is best to check with individual carriers in special circumstances and update the instructions yearly when the new IATA Dangerous Goods Regulations are published.

Shipping and packaging regulations from the Code of Federal Regulations can be found at the website www.gpoaccess.gov/cfr/. IATA regulations can be found at the website www.iata.org. International importation or exportation of biologic agents requires a permit from the CDC. Information on importing and exporting a variety of materials may be found at www.cdc.gov/ncidod/srp/specimens/shipping-packing.html.

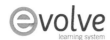 **Visit the Evolve site to complete the review questions.**

# BIBLIOGRAPHY

Blaser MJ, Feldman RA: Acquisition of typhoid fever from proficiency testing specimens, *N Engl J Med* 303:1481, 1980.

Centers for Disease Control: Update: Universal precautions for prevention of transmission of human immunodeficiency virus, hepatitis B virus, and other blood-borne pathogens in health care settings, *MMWR Morb Mortal Wkly Rep* 37:377, 1988.

Centers for Disease Control: Recommendations for prevention of HIV transmission in health-care settings, *MMWR Morb Mortal Wkly Rep* 36:3S, 1987.

Denys GA, Gary LD, Snyder JW (Sewell DL, coordinating editor): *Cumitech 40: packing and shipping of diagnostic specimens and infectious substances*, Washington, DC, 2003, ASM Press.

Eyre JWH: *Bacteriologic technique*, Philadelphia, 1913, WB Saunders.

Fleming DO, Hunt DL: *Biological safety: principles and practices*, ed 3, Washington, DC, 2000, ASM Press.

Hospital Infection Control Practices Advisory Committee: Guideline for isolation precautions in hospitals, *Infect Control Hosp Epidemiol* 17:53, 1996.

International Air Transport Association: *Dangerous goods regulations*, ed 46, Montreal, 2005, International Air Transport Association.

Jamison R, Noble MA, Proctor EM et al (Smith JA, coordinating editor): *Cumitech 29: laboratory safety in clinical microbiology*, Washington, DC, 1996, American Society for Microbiology.

Clinical and Laboratory Science Institute: *Clinical laboratory safety: approved guideline GP17-A2*, Wayne, Pa, 2004, National Committee for Clinical Laboratory Standards.

National Committee for Clinical Laboratory Standards: *Protection of laboratory workers from instrument biohazards and infectious disease transmitted by blood, body fluids and tissue: approved guideline M29-A*, Wayne, Pa, 1997, National Committee for Clinical Laboratory Standards.

National Committee for Clinical Laboratory Standards: *Protection of laboratory workers from occupationally acquired infections: approved standard, M29-A2*, Wayne, Pa, 2001, National Committee for Clinical Laboratory Standards.

Occupational Safety and Health Administration: Occupational exposure to blood-borne pathogens: final rule, *Fed Regist* 56:64175, 1991.

Occupational Safety and Health Administration: Occupational exposure to blood-borne pathogens: correction July 1, 1992, 29 CFR Part 1910, *Fed Regist* 57:127: 29206, 1991.

Occupational Safety and Health Administration: Draft guidelines for preventing the transmission of tuberculosis in health care facilities, *Fed Regist* 58:52810, 1993.

Sewell DL: Laboratory-associated infections and biosafety, *Clin Microbiol Rev* 8:389, 1995.

United States Department of Health and Human Services: *Biosafety in microbiological and biomedical laboratories*, ed 5, Washington, DC, 2009, US Government Printing Office.

United States Environmental Protection Agency: *EPA guide for infectious waste management*, Publication EPA/530-SW-86-014, Washington, DC, 1986, US Environmental Protection Agency.

# Specimen Management

## OBJECTIVES

1. State four critical parameters that should be monitored in the laboratory from specimen collection to set up and describe the effects each may have on the quality of the laboratory results (e.g., false negatives or positives, inadequate specimen type, incorrect sample).
2. Identify the proper or improper labeling of a specimen, and determine adequacy of a specimen given a patient scenario.
3. Define and differentiate backup broth, nutritive media, and differential and selective media.
4. Describe the oxygenation states (atmospheric conditions) associated with anaerobic, facultative anaerobic, capnophilic, aerobic, and microaerophilic organisms. Provide an example for each.

In the late 1800s, the first clinical microbiology laboratories were organized to diagnose infectious diseases such as tuberculosis, typhoid fever, malaria, intestinal parasites, syphilis, gonorrhea, and diphtheria. Between 1860 and 1900, microbiologists such as Pasteur, Koch, and Gram developed the techniques for staining and the use of solid media for isolation of microorganisms that are still used in clinical laboratories today. Microbiologists continue to look for the same organisms that these laboratorians did, as well as a whole range of others that have been discovered, for example, *Legionella*, viral infections, nontuberculosis acid-fast bacteria, and fungal infections. Microbiologists work in public health laboratories, hospital laboratories, reference or independent laboratories, and physician office laboratories (POLs). Depending on the level of service and type of testing of each facility, in general a microbiologist will perform one or more of the following functions:

- Cultivation (growth), identification, and antimicrobial susceptibility testing of microorganisms
- Direct detection of infecting organisms by microscopy
- Direct detection of specific products of infecting organisms using chemical, immunologic, or molecular techniques
- Detection of antibodies produced by the patient in response to an infecting organism (serology)

This chapter presents an overview of issues involved in infectious disease diagnostic testing. Many of these issues are covered in detail in separate chapters.

## GENERAL CONCEPTS FOR SPECIMEN COLLECTION AND HANDLING

Specimen collection and transportation are critical considerations, because results generated by the laboratory are limited by the quality and condition of the specimen upon arrival in the laboratory. Specimens should be obtained to preclude or minimize the possibility of introducing contaminating microorganisms that are not involved in the infectious process. This is a particular problem, for example, in specimens collected from mucous membranes that are already colonized with an individual's endogenous or "normal" flora; these organisms are usually contaminants but may also be opportunistic pathogens. For example, the throats of hospitalized patients on ventilators may frequently be colonized with *Klebsiella pneumoniae*; although *K. pneumoniae* is not usually involved in cases of community-acquired pneumonia, it can cause a hospital-acquired respiratory infection in this subset of patients. Use of special techniques that bypass areas containing normal flora when feasible (e.g., covered brush bronchoscopy in critically ill patients with pneumonia) prevents many problems associated with false-positive results. Likewise, careful skin preparation before procedures such as blood cultures and spinal taps decreases the chance that organisms normally present on the skin will contaminate the specimen.

## APPROPRIATE COLLECTION TECHNIQUES

Specimens should be collected during the acute (early) phase of an illness (or within 2 to 3 days for viral infections) and before antibiotics are administered, if possible. Swabs generally are poor specimens if tissue or needle aspirates can be obtained. It is the microbiologist's responsibility to provide clinicians with a collection manual or instruction cards listing optimal specimen collection techniques and transport information. Information for the nursing staff and clinicians should include the following:

- Safety considerations
- Selection of appropriate anatomic site and specimen
- Collection instructions including type of swab or transport medium
- Transportation instructions including time and temperature
- Labeling instructions including patient demographic information (minimum of two patient identifiers)
- Special instructions such as patient preparation
- Sterile versus nonsterile collection devices
- Minimal acceptable quality

Instructions should be written so that specimens collected by the patient (e.g., urine, sputum, or stool) are handled properly. Most urine or stool collection kits contain instructions in several languages, but nothing substitutes for a concise set of verbal instructions. Similarly, when distributing kits for sputum collection, the microbiologist should be able to explain to the patient the difference between spitting in a cup (saliva) and producing good lower respiratory secretions from a deep cough (sputum). General collection information is shown in Table 5-1. An in-depth discussion of each type of specimen is found in Part VII.

**TABLE 5-1** Collection, Transport, Storage, and Processing of Specimens Commonly Submitted to a Microbiology Laboratory*

| Specimen | Container | Patient Preparation | Special Instructions | Transportation to Laboratory | Storage before Processing | Primary Plating Media | Direct Examination | Comments |
|---|---|---|---|---|---|---|---|---|
| **Abscess (also Lesion, Wound, Pustule, Ulcer)** Superficial | Aerobic swab moistened with Stuart's or Amie's medium | Wipe area with sterile saline or 70% alcohol | Swab along leading edge of wound | < 2 hrs | 24 hrs/RT | BA, CA, Mac, CNA optional | Gram | Add CNA if smear suggests mixed gram-positive and gram-negative flora |
| Deep | Anaerobic transporter | Wipe area with sterile saline or 70% alcohol | Aspirate material from wall or excise tissue | < 2 hrs | 24 hrs/RT | BA, CA, Mac, CNA Anaerobic BBA, LKV, BBE | Gram | Wash any granules and "emulsify" in saline |
| **Blood or Bone Marrow Aspirate** | Blood culture media set (aerobic and anaerobic bottle) or Vacutainer tube with SPS | Disinfect venipuncture site with 70% alcohol and disinfectant such as Betadine | Draw blood at time of febrile episode; draw two sets from right and left arms; do not draw more than three sets in a 24-hr period; draw ≥20 ml/set (adults) or 1-20 ml/set (pediatric) depending on patient's weight | Within 2 hrs/RT | Must be incubated at 37°C on receipt in laboratory | Blood culture bottles may be used. BA, CA BBA-anaerobic | Direct gram Stain from positive blood culture bottles | Other considerations: brucellosis, tularemia, cell wall–deficient bacteria, leptospirosis, or AFB |
| **Body Fluids** Amniotic, abdominal, ascites (peritoneal), bile, joint (synovial), pericardial, pleural | Sterile, screw-cap tube or anaerobic transporter or direct inoculation into blood culture bottles | Disinfect skin before aspirating specimen | Needle aspiration | < 15 min | Plate as soon as received Blood culture bottles incubate at 37°C on receipt in laboratory | May use an aerobic and anaerobic blood culture bottle set for body fluids BA, CA, thio CNA, Mac (Peritoneal) BBA, BBE, LKV anaerobic | Gram (vaginal fluid is recommended) | May need to concentrate by centrifugation or filtration —stain and culture sediment |
| Bone | Sterile, screw-cap container | Disinfect skin before surgical procedure | Take sample from affected area for biopsy | Immediately/RT | Plate as soon as received | BA, CA, Mac, thio | Gram | May need to homogenize |

**TABLE 5-1** Collection, Transport, Storage, and Processing of Specimens Commonly Submitted to a Microbiology Laboratory—cont'd

| Specimen | Container | Patient Preparation | Special Instructions | Transportation to Laboratory | Storage before Processing | Primary Plating Media | Direct Examination | Comments |
|---|---|---|---|---|---|---|---|---|
| **Cerebrospinal Fluid** | Sterile, screw-cap tube | Disinfect skin before aspirating specimen | Consider rapid testing (e.g., Gram stain; cryptococcal antigen) | < 15 min | < 24 hrs Routine Incubate at 37°C except for viruses, which can be held at 4°C for up to 3 days | BA, CA (Routine) BA, CA, thio (shunt) | Gram—best sensitivity by cytocentrifugation (may also want to do AO if cytocentrifuge not available) | Add thio for CSF collected from shunt |
| **Ear** Inner | Sterile, screw-cap tube or anaerobic transporter | Clean ear canal with mild soap solution before myringotomy (puncture of the ear drum) | Aspirate material behind drum with syringe if ear drum intact; use swab to collect material from ruptured ear drum | < 2 hrs | 24 hrs/RT | BA, CA, Mac (add thio if prior antimicrobial therapy) BBA-(anaerobic) | Gram | Add anaerobic culture plates for tympanocentesis specimens |
| Outer | Aerobic swab moistened with Stuart's or Amie's medium | Wipe away crust with sterile saline | Firmly rotate swab in outer canal | < 2 hrs/RT | 24 hrs/RT | BA, CA, Mac | Gram | |
| **Eye** Conjunctiva | Aerobic swab moistened with Stuart's or Amie's medium | | Sample both eyes; use swab premoistened with sterile saline | < 2 hrs/RT | 24 hrs/RT | BA, CA, Mac | Gram, AO, histologic stains (e.g., Giemsa) | Other considerations: Chlamydia trachomatis, viruses, and fungi |
| Aqueous/ vitreous fluid | Sterile, screw cap tube | | | < 15 min/RT | Set up immediately on receipt | BA, Mac, 7H10, Ana | Gram/AO | |
| Corneal scrapings | Bedside inoculation of BA, CA, SDA, 7H10, thio | Clinician should instill local anesthetic before collection | | < 15 min/RT | Must be incubated at 28°C (SDA) or 37°C (everything else) on receipt in laboratory | BA, CA, SDA, 7H10, Ana, thio | Gram/AO The use of 10-mm frosted ring slides assists with location of specimen due to the size of the specimen | Other considerations: Acanthamoeba spp., herpes simplex virus and other viruses, Chlamydia trachomatis, and fungi |

Continued

**TABLE 5-1** Collection, Transport, Storage, and Processing of Specimens Commonly Submitted to a Microbiology Laboratory—cont'd

| Specimen | Container | Patient Preparation | Special Instructions | Transportation to Laboratory | Storage before Processing | Primary Plating Media | Direct Examination | Comments |
|---|---|---|---|---|---|---|---|---|
| **Foreign Bodies** | | | | | | | | |
| IUD | Sterile, screw-cap container | Disinfect skin before removal | | < 15 min/RT | Plate as soon as received | Thio | | |
| IV catheters, pins, | Sterile, screw-cap container | Disinfect skin before removal | Do not culture Foley catheters; IV catheters are cultured quantitatively by rolling the segment back and forth across agar with sterile forceps four times; ≥15 colonies are associated with clinical significance | < 15 min/RT | Plate as soon as received if possible store < 2 hrs 4° C | BA, Thio prosthetic valves | | |
| **GI Tract** | | | | | | | | |
| Gastric aspirate | Sterile, screw-cap tube | Collect in early AM before patient eats or gets out of bed | Most gastric aspirates are on infants or for AFB | < 15 min/RT | Must be neutralized with sodium bicarbonate within 1 hr of collection | BA, CA, Mac, HE, CNA, EB | Gram/AO | Other considerations: AFB |
| Gastric biopsy | Sterile, screw-cap tube (normal saline < 2 hrs transport medium recomended) | | Rapid urease test or culture for *Helicobacter pylori* | < 1 hr/RT | 24 hrs/4° C | Skirrow's, BA, BBA | H&E stain optional: Immunostaining | Other considerations: urea breath test Antigen test (*H. pylori*) |
| Rectal swab | Swab placed in enteric transport medium | | Insert swab ~ 2.5 cm past anal sphincter; feces should be visible on swab | Within 24 hrs/RT | < 48 hrs/RT or store 4° C | BA, Mac, XLD HE, Campy, EB | Methylene blue for fecal leukocytes | Other considerations: *Vibrio, Yersinia enterocolitica, Escherichia coli* 0157:H7 |

**TABLE 5-1** Collection, Transport, Storage, and Processing of Specimens Commonly Submitted to a Microbiology Laboratory—cont'd

| Specimen | Container | Patient Preparation | Special Instructions | Transportation to Laboratory | Storage before Processing | Primary Plating Media | Direct Examination | Comments |
|---|---|---|---|---|---|---|---|---|
| Stool culture | Clean, leak-proof container; transfer feces to enteric transport medium (Cary-Blair) if transport will exceed 1 hr | | Routine culture should include Salmonella, Shigella, and Campylobacter; specify Vibrio, Aeromonas, Plesiomonas, Yersinia, Escherichia coli O157:H7, if needed Follow-up may include Shiga toxin assay as recommended by CDC | Within 24 hrs/RT Unpreserved < 1 hr/RT | 72 hrs/4° C | BA, Mac, XLD, HE, Campy, EB, optional: Mac-S; Chromogenic agar | Methylene blue for fecal leukocytes Optional: Shiga toxin testing | See considerations in previous rectal swabs Do not perform routine stool cultures for patients whose length of stay in the hospital exceeds 3 days and whose admitting diagnosis was not diarrhea; these patients should be tested for Clostridium difficile |
| O&P | O&P transporters (e.g., 10% formalin and PVA) | Collect three specimens every other day at a minimum for outpatients; hospitalized patients (inpatients) should have a daily specimen collected for 3 days; specimens from inpatients hospitalized more than 3 days should be discouraged | Wait 7-10 days if patient has received antiparasitic compounds, barium, iron, Kaopectate, metronidazole, Milk of Magnesia, Pepto-Bismol, or tetracycline | Within 24 hrs/RT | Indefinitely/RT | | Liquid specimen should be examined for the presence of motile organisms | |
| **Genital Tract** FEMALE Bartholin cyst | Anaerobic transporter | Disinfect skin before collection | Aspirate fluid; consider chlamydia and GC culture | < 2 hrs | 24 hrs/RT | BA, CA, Mac, TM, Ana | Gram | |

*Continued*

**TABLE 5-1**   Collection, Transport, Storage, and Processing of Specimens Commonly Submitted to a Microbiology Laboratory—cont'd

| Specimen | Container | Patient Preparation | Special Instructions | Transportation to Laboratory | Storage before Processing | Primary Plating Media | Direct Examination | Comments |
|---|---|---|---|---|---|---|---|---|
| Cervix | Swab moistened with Stuart's or Amie's medium | Remove mucus before collection of specimen | Do not use lubricant on speculum; use viral/chlamydial transport medium, if necessary; swab deeply into endocervical canal | < 2 hrs/RT | 24 hrs/RT | BA, CA, Mac, TM | Gram | |
| Cul-de-sac | Anaerobic transporter | | Submit aspirate | < 2 hrs/RT | 24 hrs/RT | BA, CA, Mac, TM, Ana | Gram | |
| Endometrium | Anaerobic transporter | | Surgical biopsy or transcervical aspirate via sheathed catheter | < 2 hrs/RT | 24 hrs/RT | BA, CA, Mac, TM, Ana | Gram | |
| Urethra | Swab moistened with Stuart's or Amie's medium | Remove exudate from urethral opening | Collect discharge by massaging urethra against pubic symphysis or insert flexible swab 2-4 cm into urethra and rotate swab for 2 seconds; collect at least 1 hr after patient has urinated | < 2 hrs/RT | 24 hrs/RT | BA, CA, TM | Gram | Other considerations: Chlamydia, Mycoplasma |
| Vagina | Swab moistened with Stuart's or Amie's medium or JEMBEC transport system | Remove exudate | Swab secretions and mucous membrane of vagina | < 2 hrs/RT | 24 hrs/RT | BA, TM Culture is not recommended for the diagnosis of bacterial vaginosis; inoculate selective medium for group B Streptococcus (LIM broth) if indicated on pregnant women | Gram | Examine Gram stain for bacterial vaginosis, especially white blood cells, clue cells, gram-positive rods indicative of Lactobacillus, and curved, gram-negative rods indicative of Mobiluncus spp. |

**TABLE 5-1** Collection, Transport, Storage, and Processing of Specimens Commonly Submitted to a Microbiology Laboratory—cont'd

| Specimen | Container | Patient Preparation | Special Instructions | Transportation to Laboratory | Storage before Processing | Primary Plating Media | Direct Examination | Comments |
|---|---|---|---|---|---|---|---|---|
| MALE | | | | | | | | |
| Prostate | Swab moistened with Stuart's or Amie's medium or sterile, screw-cap tube | Clean glans with soap and water | Collect secretions on swab or in tube | < 2 hrs/RT for swab; immediately if in tube/RT | Swab: 24 hrs/RT; tube: plate secretions immediately | BA, CA, Mac, TM, CNA | Gram | |
| Urethra | Swab moistened with Stuart's or Amie's medium or JEMBEC transport system | | Insert flexible swab 2-4 cm into urethra and rotate for 2 seconds or collect discharge on JEMBEC transport system | < 2 hrs/RT for swab; within 2 hrs for JEMBEC system | 24 hrs/RT for swab; put JEMBEC at 37° C immediately on receipt in laboratory | BA, CA, TM | Gram | Other considerations: Chlamydia, Mycoplasma |
| **Hair, Nails, or Skin Scrapings (for fungal culture)** | Clean, screw-top tube | Nails or skin: wipe with 70% alcohol | Hair: collect hairs with intact shaft Nails: send clippings of affected area Skin: scrape skin at leading edge of lesion | Within 24 hrs/RT | Indefinitely/RT | SDA, IMAcg, SDAcg | CW | |
| **Respiratory Tract** LOWER BAL, BB, BW | Sterile, screw-top container | | Anaerobic culture appropriate only if sheathed (protected) catheter used | < 2 hrs/RT | 24 hrs/4° C | BA, CA, Mac, CNA | Gram and other special stains as requested (e.g., Legionella DFA, acid-fast stain) | Other considerations: quantitative culture for BAL, AFB, Legionella, Nocardia, Mycoplasma, Pneumocystis, cytomegalovirus |

*Continued*

**TABLE 5-1** Collection, Transport, Storage, and Processing of Specimens Commonly Submitted to a Microbiology Laboratory—cont'd

| Specimen | Container | Patient Preparation | Special Instructions | Transportation to Laboratory | Storage before Processing | Primary Plating Media | Direct Examination | Comments |
|---|---|---|---|---|---|---|---|---|
| Sputum, tracheal aspirate (suction) | Sterile, screw-top container | Sputum: have patient brush teeth and then rinse or gargle with water before collection | Sputum: have patient collect from deep cough; specimen should be examined for suitability for culture by Gram stain; induced sputa on pediatric or uncooperative patients may be watery because of saline nebulization | < 2 hrs/RT | 24 hrs/4° C | BA, CA, Mac PC OFPBL-cystic fibrosis | Gram and other special stains as requested (e.g., Legionella DFA, acid-fast stain) | Other considerations: AFB, *Nocardia* |
| UPPER Nasopharynx Nose | Swab moistened with Stuart's or Amie's medium | | Insert flexible swab through nose into posterior nasopharynx and rotate for 5 seconds; specimen of choice for *Bordetella pertussis* | < 2 hrs/RT | 24 hrs/RT | BA, CA BA, chromogenic agar | | Other considerations: add special media for *Corynebacterium diphtheriae*, pertussis, *Chlamydia*, and *Mycoplasma* |
| Pharynx (throat) | Swab moistened with Stuart's or Amie's medium | | Swab posterior pharynx and tonsils; routine culture for group A *Streptococcus (S. pyogenes)* only | < 2 hrs/RT | 24 hrs/RT | BA or SSA | | Other considerations: add special media for *C. diphtheriae*, *Neisseria gonorrhoeae*, and epiglottis (*Haemophilus influenzae*) |
| **Tissue** | Anaerobic transporter or sterile, screw-cap tube | Disinfect skin | Do not allow specimen to dry out; moisten with sterile, distilled water if not bloody | < 15 min/RT | 24 hrs/RT | BA, CA, Mac, CNA, Thio Anaerobic: BBA, LKV, BBE | Gram | May need to homogenize |

**TABLE 5-1** Collection, Transport, Storage, and Processing of Specimens Commonly Submitted to a Microbiology Laboratory—cont'd

| Specimen | Container | Patient Preparation | Special Instructions | Transportation to Laboratory | Storage before Processing | Primary Plating Media | Direct Examination | Comments |
|---|---|---|---|---|---|---|---|---|
| **Urine** | | | | | | | | |
| Clean-voided midstream (CVS) | Sterile, screw-cap container Containers that include a variety of chemical urinalysis preservatives may also be used | Females: clean area with soap and water, then rinse with water; hold labia apart and begin voiding in commode; after several mL have passed, collect midstream Males: clean glans with soap and water, then rinse with water; retract foreskin; after several mL have passed, collect midstream | | Preserved within 24 hrs/RT unpreserved < 2 hrs/RT | 24 hrs/4° C | BA, Mac Optional: Chromogenic agar | Check for pyuria, Gram stain not recommended | Plate quantitatively at 1:1000; consider plating quantitatively at 1:100 if patient is female of childbearing age with white blood cells and possible acute urethral syndrome |
| Straight catheter (in and out) | Sterile, screw-cap container | Clean urethral area (soap and water) and rinse (water) | Insert catheter into bladder; allow first 15 mL to pass; then collect remainder | < 2 hrs/RT preserved < 24 hrs/RT | 24 hrs/4° C | BA, Mac | Gram or check for pyuria | Plate quantitatively at 1:100 and 1:1000 |
| Indwelling catheter (Foley) | Sterile, screw-cap container | Disinfect catheter collection port | Aspirate 5-10 mL of urine with needle and syringe | < 2 hrs/4° C (preserved < 24 hrs/RT) | 24 hrs/4° C | BA, Mac | Gram or check for pyuria | Plate quantitatively at 1:1000 |
| Suprapubic aspirate | Sterile, screw-cap container or anaerobic transporter | Disinfect skin | Needle aspiration above the symphysis pubis through the abdominal wall into the full bladder | Immediately/RT | Plate as soon as received | BA, Mac, Ana, Thio | Gram or check for pyuria | Plate quantitatively at 1:100 and 1:1000 |

7H10, Middlebrook 7H10 agar; *AFB*, acid-fast bacilli; *AM*, morning; *Ana*, anaerobic agars as appropriate (see Chapter 41); *AO*, acridine orange stain; *BA*, blood agar; *BAL*, bronchial alveolar lavage; *BB*, bronchial brush; *BBA*, brucella blood agar; *BBE*, Bacteroides bile esculin agar; *BW*, bronchial wash; *CA*, chocolate agar; *Campy*, selective Campylobacter agar; *CNA*, Columbia agar with colistin and nalidixic acid; *CW*, calcofluor white stain; *DFA*, direct fluorescent antibody stain; *EB*, enrichment broth; *GC*, *Neisseria gonorrhoeae*; transport using JEMBEC system with modified Thayer-Martin; *GI*, gastrointestinal; *Gram*, Gram stain; *HBT*, human blood-bilayer Tween agar; *HE*, Hektoen enteric agar; *hrs*, hours; *IMAcg*, inhibitory mold agar with chloramphenicol and gentamicin; *IUD*, intrauterine device; *LKV*, laked blood agar with kanamycin and vancomycin; *Mac*, MacConkey agar; *Mac-S*, MacConkey-sorbitol; *mL*, milliliters; *OFPBL*, oxidative-fermentative polymixin B-bacitracin-lactose-agar; *O&P*, ova and parasite examination; *PC*, Pseudomonas cepacia agar; *PVA*, polyvinyl alcohol; *RT*, room temperature; *SDA*, Sabouraud dextrose agar; *SDAcg*, Sabouraud dextrose agar with cycloheximide and gentamicin; *SPS*, sodium polyanethol sulfonate; *SSA*, group A streptococcus selective agar; *thio*, thioglycollate broth; *TM*, Thayer-Martin agar; *XLD*, xylose lysine deoxycholate agar.
*Specimens for viruses, chlamydia, and mycoplasma are usually submitted in appropriate transport media at 4° C to stabilize respective microorganisms.

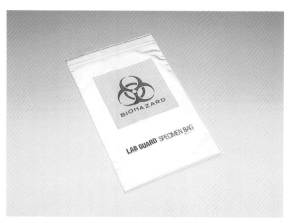

**Figure 5-1** Specimen bag with biohazard label, separate pouch for paperwork, and self-seal. (Courtesy Allegiance Healthcare Corp., McGaw Park, Ill.)

## SPECIMEN TRANSPORT

Ideally, specimens should be transported to the laboratory within 2 hours of collection. All specimen containers should be leak-proof, and the specimens should be transported within sealable, leak-proof, plastic bags with a separate section for paperwork; resealable bags or bags with a permanent seal are common for this purpose. Bags should be marked with a biohazard label (Figure 5-1). Many microorganisms are susceptible to environmental conditions such as the presence of oxygen (anaerobic bacteria), changes in temperature (*Neisseria meningitidis*), or changes in pH (*Shigella*). Thus, use of special preservatives or holding media for transportation of specimens delayed for more than 2 hours is important to ensure organism viability (survival).

## SPECIMEN PRESERVATION

Preservatives, such as boric acid for urine or polyvinyl alcohol (PVA) and buffered formalin for stool for ova and parasite (O&P) examination, are designed to maintain the appropriate colony counts (for urines) or the integrity of trophozoites and cysts (for O&Ps), respectively. Other transport, or holding, media maintain the viability of microorganisms present in a specimen without supporting the growth of the organisms. This maintains the organisms in a state of suspended animation so that no organism overgrows another or dies out. Stuart's medium and Amie's medium are two common holding media. Sometimes charcoal is added to these media to absorb fatty acids present in the specimen that could kill fastidious (fragile) organisms such as *Neisseria gonorrhoeae* or *Bordetella pertussis*.

Anticoagulants are used to prevent clotting of specimens such as blood, bone marrow, and synovial fluid, because microorganisms will otherwise be bound up in the clot. The type and concentration of anticoagulant is very important because many organisms are inhibited by some of these chemicals. Sodium polyanethol sulfonate (SPS) at a concentration of 0.025% (w/v) is usually used, because *Neisseria* spp. and some anaerobic bacteria are particularly sensitive to higher concentrations. Because

the ratio of specimen to SPS is so important, it is necessary to have both large (adult-size) and small (pediatric-size) tubes available, so organisms in small amounts of bone marrow or synovial fluid are not overwhelmed by the concentration of SPS. SPS is also included in blood culture collection systems. Heparin is also a commonly used anticoagulant, especially for viral cultures, although it may inhibit growth of gram-positive bacteria and yeast. Citrate, ethylenediaminetetraacetic acid (EDTA), or other anticoagulants should not be used for microbiology, because their efficacy has not been demonstrated for a majority of organisms. It is the microbiologist's job to make sure the appropriate anticoagulant is used for each procedure. The laboratory generally should not specify a color ("yellow-top") tube for collection without specifying the anticoagulant (SPS), because at least one popular brand of collection tube (Vacutainer, Becton, Dickinson and Company) has a yellow-top tube with either SPS or trisodium citrate/citric acid/dextrose (ACD); ACD is not appropriate for use in microbiology.

### Specimen Storage

If specimens cannot be processed as soon as they are received, they must be stored (see Table 5-1). Several storage methods are used (refrigerator temperature [4°C], ambient [room] temperature [22°C], body temperature [37°C], and freezer temperature [either –20° or –70°C]), depending on the type of transport media (if applicable) and the etiologic (infectious) agents suspected. Specimens should never be stored in the refrigerator and should remain at room temperature. Urine, stool, viral specimens, sputa, swabs, and foreign devices such as catheters should be stored at 4°C. Serum for serologic studies may be frozen for up to 1 week at –20°C, and tissues or specimens for long-term storage should be frozen at –70°C.

## SPECIMEN LABELING

Specimens should be labeled with the patient's name, identifying number (hospital number) or birth date, date and time of collection, and source. Enough information must be provided on the specimen label so that the specimen can be matched up with the requisition when it is received in the laboratory.

## SPECIMEN REQUISITION

The specimen (or test) requisition is an order form that is sent to the laboratory along with a specimen. Often the requisition is a hard (paper) copy of the physician's orders and the patient's demographic information (e.g., name and hospital number). Sometimes, however, if a hospital information system offers computerized order entry, the requisition is transported to the laboratory electronically. The requisition should contain as much information as possible regarding the patient history and diagnosis. This information helps the microbiologist to work up the specimen and determine which organisms are significant in the culture. A complete requisition should include the following:
- The patient's name
- Hospital number

- Age or date of birth
- Sex
- Collection date and time
- Ordering physician
- Exact nature and source of the specimen
- Diagnosis (may be ICD-9-CM code)
- Current antimicrobial therapy

## REJECTION OF UNACCEPTABLE SPECIMENS

Criteria for specimen rejection should be set up and distributed to all clinical practitioners. In general, specimens are unacceptable if any of the following conditions apply:

- The information on the label does not match the information on the requisition or the specimen is not labeled at all (patient's name or source of specimen is different).
- The specimen has been transported at the improper temperature.
- The specimen has not been transported in the proper medium (e.g., specimens for anaerobic bacteria submitted in aerobic transports).
- The quantity of specimen is insufficient for testing (the specimen is considered quantity not sufficient [QNS]).
- The specimen is leaking.
- The specimen transport time exceeds 2 hours postcollection or the specimen is not preserved.
- The specimen was received in a fixative (formalin), which, in essence, kills any microorganism present.
- The specimen has been received for anaerobic culture from a site known to have anaerobes as part of the normal flora (vagina, mouth).
- The specimen is dried.
- Processing the specimen would produce information of questionable medical value (e.g., Foley catheter tip).

It is an important rule to always talk to the requesting physician or another member of the health care team before discarding unacceptable specimens. In some cases, such as mislabeling of a specimen or requisition, the person who collected the specimen and filled out the paperwork can come to the laboratory and correct the problem; a mislabeled specimen or requisition should not be identified over the telephone. However, correction of mislabeled specimens must be completed at the discretion of the laboratories standard operating procedures. Frequently, it may be necessary to do the best possible job on a less than optimal specimen, if it would be impossible to collect the specimen again because the patient is taking antibiotics, the tissue was collected at surgery, or the patient would have to undergo a second invasive procedure (bone marrow or spinal tap). A notation regarding improper collection should be added to the final report in this instance, because only the primary caregiver is able to determine the validity of the results.

## SPECIMEN PROCESSING

Depending on the site of testing (hospital, independent lab, physician's office lab) and how the specimens are transported to the laboratory (in-house, courier, or driver), microbiology samples may arrive in the laboratory in large numbers or as single tests. Although batch processing may be possible in large independent laboratories, most often hospital testing is performed as specimens arrive. When multiple specimens arrive at the same time, priority should be given to those that are most critical, such as cerebrospinal fluid (CSF), tissue, blood, and sterile fluids. Urine, throat, sputa, stool, or wound drainage specimens can be saved for later. Acid-fast, viral, and fungal specimens are usually batched for processing at one time. When a specimen is received with multiple requests but the amount of specimen is insufficient to do all of them, the microbiologist should call the clinician to prioritize the testing. Anytime a laboratory staff member contacts the physician or nurse, the conversation and agreed-upon information should be documented to ensure proper follow-up. On arrival in the laboratory, the time and date received should be recorded.

## GROSS EXAMINATION OF SPECIMEN

All processing should begin with a gross examination of the specimen. Areas with blood or mucus should be located and sampled for culture and direct examination. Stool should be examined for evidence of barium (i.e., chalky white color), which would preclude O&P examination. Notations should be made on the handwritten or electronic work card regarding the status of the specimen (e.g., bloody, cloudy, clotted) so that if more than one person works on the sample, the results of the gross examination are available for consultation.

## DIRECT MICROSCOPIC EXAMINATION

All appropriate specimens should have a direct microscopic examination. The direct examination serves several purposes. First, the quality of the specimen can be assessed; for example, sputa can be rejected that represent saliva and not lower respiratory tract secretions by quantitation of white blood cells or squamous epithelial cells present in the specimen. Second, the microbiologist and clinician can be given an early indication of what may be wrong with the patient (e.g., 4+ gram-positive cocci in clusters in an exudate). Third, the workup of the specimen can be guided by comparing what grows in culture to what was seen on the original smear. A situation in which three different morphotypes (cellular types) are seen on direct Gram stain but only two grow out in culture, for example, alerts the microbiologist to the fact that the third organism may be an anaerobic bacterium. Or there are more than three organisms on the culture plate that were not visible on Gram stain, indicating possible contamination. Gram stains are also layered with cells and debris. Organisms that appear on the surface of white blood cells may actually be ingested organisms that are no longer viable or capable of growth. It is imperative that the Gram stain results and specimen culture correlate to the type of specimen to ensure accurate information is provided to the clinician.

Direct examinations are usually not performed on throat, nasopharyngeal, or stool specimens but are

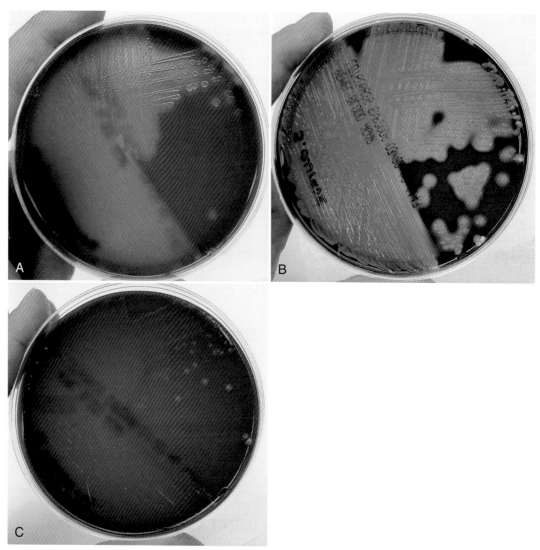

**Figure 5-2** Examples of various types of hemolysis on blood agar. **A,** *Streptococcus pneumoniae* showing alpha (α)-hemolysis (i.e., greening around colony). **B,** *Staphylococcus aureus* showing beta (β)-hemolysis (i.e., clearing around colony). **C,** *Enterococcus faecalis* showing gamma (γ)-hemolysis (i.e., no hemolysis around colony).

indicated from most other sources due to the presence of abundant normal microbiota.

The most common stain in bacteriology is the Gram stain, which helps the clinician to visualize rods, cocci, white blood cells, red blood cells, or squamous epithelial cells present in the sample. The most common direct fungal stains are KOH (potassium hydroxide), PAS (periodic-acid Schiff), GMS (Grocott's methenamine silver stain), and calcofluor white. The most common direct acid-fast stains are AR (auramine rhodamine), ZN (Ziehl-Neelsen), and Kinyoun. Chapter 6 describes the use of microscopy in clinical diagnosis in more detail.

## SELECTION OF CULTURE MEDIA

Primary culture media are divided into several categories. The first are nutritive media, such as blood or chocolate agars. Nutritive media support the growth of a wide range of microorganisms and are considered nonselective because, theoretically, the growth of most organisms

is supported. Nutritive media can also be differential, in that microorganisms can be distinguished on the basis of certain growth characteristics evident on the medium. Blood agar is considered both a nutritive and differential medium because it differentiates organisms based on whether they are alpha (α)-, beta (β)-, or gamma (γ)-hemolytic (Figure 5-2). Selective media support the growth of one group of organisms, but not another, by adding antimicrobials, dyes, or alcohol to a particular medium. MacConkey agar, for example, contains the dye crystal violet, which inhibits gram-positive organisms. Columbia agar with colistin and nalidixic acid (CNA) is a selective medium for gram-positive organisms because the antimicrobials colistin and nalidixic acid inhibit gram-negative organisms. Selective media can also be differential media if, in addition to their inhibitory activity, they differentiate between groups of organisms. MacConkey agar, for example, differentiates between lactose-fermenting and nonfermenting gram-negative rods by the color of the colonial growth (pink or clear,

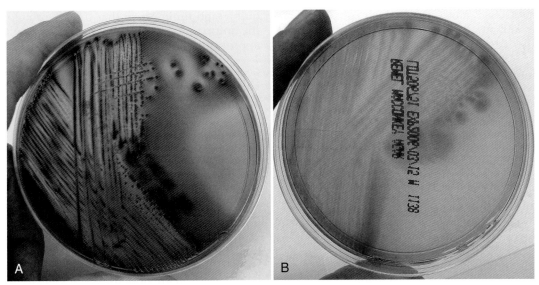

**Figure 5-3** MacConkey agar. **A,** *Escherichia coli,* a lactose fermenter. **B,** *Pseudomonas aeruginosa,* a nonlactose fermenter.

respectively); this is shown in Figure 5-3. In some cases (sterile body fluids, tissues, or deep abscesses in a patient on antimicrobial therapy), backup broth (also called supplemental or enrichment broth) medium is inoculated, along with primary solid (agar) media, so small numbers of organisms present may be detected; this allows detection of anaerobes in aerobic cultures and organisms that may be damaged by either previous or concurrent antimicrobial therapy. Thioglycollate (thio) broth, brain-heart infusion broth (BHIB), and tryptic soy broth (TSB) are common backup broths.

Selection of media to inoculate for any given specimen is usually based on the organisms most likely to be involved in the disease process. For example, in determining what to set up for a CSF specimen, one considers the most likely pathogens that cause meningitis (*Streptococcus pneumoniae, Haemophilus influenzae, Neisseria meningitidis, Escherichia coli,* group B *Streptococcus*) and selects media that will support the growth of these organisms (blood and chocolate agar at a minimum). Likewise, if a specimen is collected from a source likely to be contaminated with normal flora, for example, an anal fistula (an opening of the surface of the skin near the anus that may communicate with the rectum), one might want to add a selective medium, such as CNA, to suppress gram-negative bacteria and allow gram-positive bacteria and yeast to be recovered.

Routine primary plating media and direct examinations for specimens commonly submitted to the microbiology laboratory are shown in Table 5-1. Chapter 7 on bacterial cultivation reemphasizes the strategies described here for selection and use of bacterial media.

## SPECIMEN PREPARATION

Many specimens require some form of initial treatment before inoculation onto primary plating media. Such procedures include homogenization (grinding) of tissue; concentration by centrifugation or filtration of large volumes of sterile fluids, such as ascites (peritoneal) or pleural (lung) fluids; or decontamination of specimens, such as those for legionellae or mycobacteria. Swab specimens are often vortexed (mixed) in 0.5 to 1 mL of saline or broth for 10 to 20 seconds to dislodge material from the fibers.

## INOCULATION ON SOLID MEDIA

Specimens can be inoculated (plated) onto solid media either quantitatively by a dilution procedure or by means of a quantitative loop, or semiquantitatively using an ordinary inoculating loop. Urine cultures and tissues from burn victims are plated quantitatively; everything else is usually plated semiquantitatively. Plates inoculated for quantitation are usually streaked with a 1:100 or 1:1000 loop. Plates inoculated for semiquantitation are usually streaked out in four quadrants. Detailed methods for streaking solid media are provided in Chapter 7, Figure 7-9. Semiquantitation is referred to as streaking for isolation, because the microorganisms present in the specimen are successively diluted out as each quadrant is streaked until finally each morphotype is present as a single colony. Numbers of organisms present can subsequently be graded as 4+ (many, heavy growth) if growth is out to the fourth quadrant, 3+ (moderate growth) if growth is out to the third quadrant, 2+ (few or light growth) if growth is in the second quadrant, and 1+ (rare) if growth is in the first quadrant. This tells the clinician the relative numbers of different organisms present in the specimen; such semiquantitative information is usually sufficient for the physician to be able to treat the patient.

## INCUBATION CONDITIONS

Inoculated media are incubated under various temperatures and environmental conditions, depending on the organisms suspected, for example, 28° to 30°C for fungi and 35° to 37°C for most bacteria, viruses, and acid-fast bacillus. A number of different environmental conditions exist. Aerobes grow in ambient air, which contains 21% oxygen ($O_2$) and a small amount (0.03%) of carbon dioxide ($CO_2$). Anaerobes usually cannot grow in the presence of $O_2$, and the atmosphere in anaerobe jars, bags, or chambers is composed of 5% to 10% hydrogen ($H_2$), 5% to 10% $CO_2$, 80% to 90% nitrogen ($N_2$), and 0% $O_2$. Capnophiles, such as *Haemophilus influenzae* and *Neisseria gonorrhoeae*, require increased concentrations of $CO_2$ (5% to 10%) and approximately 15% $O_2$. This atmosphere can be achieved by a candle jar (3% $CO_2$) or a $CO_2$ incubator, jar, or bag. Microaerophiles (*Campylobacter jejuni, Helicobacter pylori*) grow under reduced $O_2$ (5% to 10%) and increased $CO_2$ (8% to 10%). This environment can also be obtained in specially designed jars or bags.

# SPECIMEN WORKUP

One of the most important functions that a microbiologist performs is to decide what is clinically relevant regarding specimen workup. Considerable judgment is required to decide what organisms to look for and report. It is essential to recognize what constitutes indigenous (normal) flora and what constitutes a potential pathogen. Indiscriminate identification, susceptibility testing, and reporting of normal flora can contribute to unnecessary use of antibiotics and potential emergence of resistant organisms. Because organisms that are clinically relevant to identify and report vary by source, the microbiologist should know which ones cause disease at various sites. Part VII contains a detailed discussion of these issues.

## EXTENT OF IDENTIFICATION REQUIRED

As health care continues to change, one of the most problematic issues for microbiologists is the extent of culture workup. Microbiologists still rely heavily on definitive identification, although shortcuts, including the use of limited identification procedures in some cases, are becoming commonplace in most clinical laboratories (see CLSI document M35-A2 for information on abbreviated identification of organisms). Careful application of knowledge of the significance of various organisms in specific situations and thoughtful use of limited approaches will keep microbiology testing cost effective and the laboratory's workload manageable, while providing for optimum patient care.

Complete identification of a blood culture isolate, such as *Clostridium septicum* as opposed to a genus identification of *Clostridium* spp., will alert the clinician to the possibility of malignancy or other disease of the colon. At the same time, a presumptive identification of *Escherichia coli* if a gram-negative, spot indole-positive rod is recovered with appropriate colony morphology on Mac-Conkey agar (flat, lactose-fermenting colony that is precipitating bile salts) is probably permissible from an uncomplicated urinary tract infection. In the final analysis, culture results should always be compared with the suspected diagnosis. The clinician should be encouraged to supply the microbiologist with all pertinent information (e.g., recent travel history, pet exposure, pertinent radiograph findings) so that the microbiologist can use the information to interpret culture results and plan appropriate strategies for workup.

## COMMUNICATION OF LABORATORY FINDINGS

To fulfill their professional obligation to the patient, microbiologists must communicate their findings to those health care professionals responsible for treating the patient. This task is not as easy as it may seem. This is nicely illustrated in a study in which a group of physicians was asked whether they would treat a patient with a sore throat given two separate laboratory reports—that is, one that stated, "many group A Streptococcus," and one that stated, "few group A Streptococcus." Although group A Streptococcus (*Streptococcus pyogenes*) is considered significant in any numbers in a symptomatic individual, the physicians said that they would treat the patient with many organisms but not the one with few organisms. Thus, although a pathogen (group A *Streptococcus*) was isolated in both cases, one word on the report (either *many* or *few*) made a difference in how the patient would be handled.

In communicating with the physician, the microbiologist can avoid confusion and misunderstanding by not using jargon or abbreviations and by providing reports with clear-cut conclusions. The microbiologist should not assume that the clinician is fully familiar with laboratory procedures or the latest microbial taxonomic schemes. Thus, when appropriate, interpretive statements should be included in the written report along with the specific results. One example would be the addition of a statement, such as "suggests contamination at collection," when more than three organisms are isolated from a clean-voided midstream urine specimen.

Laboratory newsletters should be used to provide physicians with material such as details of new procedures, nomenclature changes, and changes in usual antimicrobial susceptibility patterns of frequently isolated organisms. This last information, discussed in more detail in Chapter 12 is very useful to clinicians when selecting empiric therapy. Empiric therapy is based on the physician determining the most likely organism causing a patient's clinical symptoms and then selecting an antimicrobial that, in the past, has worked against that organism in a particular hospital or geographic area. Empiric therapy is used to start patients on treatment before the results of the patient's culture are known and may be critical to the patient's well-being in cases of life-threatening illnesses.

Positive findings should be communicated to the clinician in a timely manner, and all verbal reports should be followed by written confirmation of results. Results should be legibly handwritten or generated electronically in the laboratory information system (LIS).

## CRITICAL (PANIC) VALUES

Certain critical results must be communicated to the clinician immediately. Each clinical microbiology laboratory, in consultation with its medical staff, should prepare a list of these so-called panic values. Common panic values include the following:

- Positive blood cultures
- Positive spinal fluid Gram stain or culture
- *Streptococcus pyogenes* (group A *Streptococcus*) in a surgical wound
- Gram stain suggestive of gas gangrene (large boxcar-shaped gram-positive rods)
- Blood smear positive for malaria
- Positive cryptococcal antigen test
- Positive acid-fast stain
- Detection of a select agent (e.g., Brucella) or other significant pathogen (e.g., Legionella, vancomycin-resistant *S. aureus,* or other antibiotic-resistant organisms as outlined by the facility and infection control policies).

## EXPEDITING RESULTS REPORTING: COMPUTERIZATION

Before widespread computerization of clinical microbiology laboratories, results were communicated via handwritten reports and couriers delivered hard copies that were pasted into the patient's chart. Today, microbiology computer software is available that simplifies and speeds up this task.

Central processing units (CPUs), disks, tape drives, controllers, printers, video terminals, communication ports, modems, and other types of hardware support running the software. The hardware and software together make up the complete LIS. Many LIS systems are, in turn, interfaced with a hospital information system (HIS). Between the HIS and LIS, most functions involved in ordering and reporting laboratory tests can be handled electronically. Order entry, patient identification, and specimen identification can be handled using the same type of bar coding that is commonly used in supermarkets. The LIS also takes care of results reporting and supervisory verification of results, stores quality control data, allows easy test inquiries, and assists in test management reporting by storing, for example, the number of positive, negative, and unsatisfactory specimens. Most large systems also are capable of interfacing (communicating) with microbiology instruments to automatically download (transfer) and store data regarding positive cultures or antimicrobial susceptibility results. Results of individual organism antibiograms (patterns) can then be retrieved monthly so hospital-wide susceptibility patterns can be studied for the emergence of resistant organisms or other epidemiologic information. Many vendors of laboratory information systems are now writing software for microbiology to adapt to personal computers (PCs) so that large CPUs may no longer be needed. This brings down the cost of microbiology systems so that even smaller laboratories are able to afford them. Today, small systems can be interfaced with printers or electronic facsimile machines (faxes) as well as access through smart phones or tablets for quick and easy reporting and information retrieval, further improving the quality of patient care.

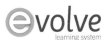 *Visit the Evolve site to complete the review questions.*

## BIBLIOGRAPHY

Lee A and McLean S: The laboratory report: a problem in communication between clinician and microbiologist? *Med J Aust* 2:858, 1977.
Versalovic J: Manual of clinical microbiology, ed 10, Washington, D.C., 2011, ASM Press.

# Approaches to Diagnosis of Infectious Diseases

# Role of Microscopy

## OBJECTIVES

1. Explain the role of microscopy in the identification of etiologic agents including bacteria, fungi, viruses, and parasites.
2. List the four types of microscopy available for diagnostic evaluation, explain their basic principles, and list a clinical application for each.
3. Define the three main principles of light microscopy, magnification, resolution, and contrast.
4. List the staining techniques used to aid in the visualization of bacteria, explain the chemical principle and limitations for each, and provide an example of a clinical application for each stain.
5. Include the following stains: Gram stain, the Kinyoun stain, the Ziehl-Neelsen stain, the Calcofluor white stain, the Acridine orange stain, and the Auramine-Rhodamine stain.
6. Explain the chemical principle for fluorescent dyes in microscopy, and list two examples routinely used in the clinical laboratory.
7. Describe the purpose and method for Kohler illumination.

The basic flow of procedures involved in the laboratory diagnosis of infectious diseases is as follows:

1. Direct examination of patient specimens for the presence of etiologic agents
2. Growth and cultivation of the agents from these same specimens
3. Analysis of the cultivated organisms to establish their identification and other pertinent characteristics such as susceptibility to antimicrobial agents

For certain infectious diseases, this process may also include measuring the patient's immune response to the infectious agent.

Microscopy is the most common method used both for the detection of microorganisms directly in clinical specimens and for the characterization of organisms grown in culture (Box 6-1). Microscopy is defined as the use of a microscope to magnify (i.e., visually enlarge) objects too small to be visualized with the naked eye so that their characteristics are readily observable. Because most infectious agents cannot be detected with the unaided eye, microscopy plays a pivotal role in the laboratory. Microscopes and microscopic methods vary, but only those of primary use in diagnostic microbiology are discussed.

The method used to process patient specimens is dictated by the type and body source of specimen (see Part VII). Regardless of the method used, some portion of the specimen usually is reserved for microscopic examination. Specific stains or dyes applied to the specimens, combined with particular methods of microscopy, can detect etiologic agents in a rapid, relatively inexpensive, and productive way. Microscopy also plays a key role in the characterization of organisms that have been cultivated in the laboratory (for more information regarding cultivation of bacteria, see Chapter 7).

The types of microorganisms to be detected, identified, and characterized determine the most appropriate types of microscopy to use. Table 6-1 outlines the four types of microscopy used in diagnostic microbiology and their relative utility for each of the four major types of infectious agents. Bright-field microscopy (also known as light microscopy) and fluorescence microscopy have the widest use and application within the clinical microbiology laboratory. Dark field and electron microscopes are not typically found within a clinical laboratory and are predominantly used in reference or research settings. Which microorganisms can be detected or identified by each microscopic method also depends on the methods used to highlight the microorganisms and their key characteristics. This enhancement is usually achieved using various dyes or stains.

## BRIGHT-FIELD (LIGHT) MICROSCOPY

### PRINCIPLES OF LIGHT MICROSCOPY

For light microscopy, visible light is passed through the specimen and then through a series of lenses that bend the light in a manner that results in magnification of the organisms present in the specimen (Figure 6-1). The total magnification achieved is the product of the lenses used.

#### Magnification

In most light microscopes, the objective lens, which is closest to the specimen, magnifies objects 100× (times), and the ocular lens, which is nearest the eye, magnifies 10×. Using these two lenses in combination, organisms in the specimen are magnified 1000× their actual size when viewed through the ocular lens. Objective lenses of lower magnification are available so that those of 10×, 20×, and 40× magnification power can provide total magnifications of 100×, 200×, and 400×, respectively. Magnification of 1000× allows for the visualization of fungi, most parasites, and most bacteria, but it is not sufficient for observing viruses, which require magnification of 100,000× or more (see Electron Microscopy in this chapter).

## Resolution

To optimize visualization, other factors besides magnification must be considered. Resolution, defined as the extent to which detail in the magnified object is maintained, is also essential. Without it everything would be magnified as an indistinguishable blur. Therefore, resolving power, which is the closest distance between two objects that when magnified still allows the two objects to be distinguished from each other, is extremely important. The resolving power of most light microscopes allows bacterial cells to be distinguished from one another but usually does not allow bacterial structures, internal or external, to be detected.

To achieve the level of resolution desired with 1000× magnification, oil immersion must be used in conjunction with light microscopy. Immersion oil has specific optical and viscosity characteristics designed for use in microscopy. Immersion oil is used to fill the space between the objective lens and the glass slide onto which the specimen has been affixed. When light passes from a material of one refractive index to a material with a different refractive index, as from glass to air, the light bends. Light of different wavelengths bend at different angles creating a less distinct distorted image. Placing immersion oil with the same refractive index as glass between the objective lens and the coverslip or slide decreases the number of refractive surfaces the light must pass through during microscopy. The oil enhances resolution by preventing light rays from dispersing and changing wavelength after passing through the specimen. A specific objective

---

**BOX 6-1** Applications of Microscopy in Diagnostic Microbiology

- Rapid preliminary organism identification by direct visualization in patient specimens
- Rapid final identification of certain organisms by direct visualization in patient specimens
- Detection of different organisms present in the same specimen
- Detection of organisms not easily cultivated in the laboratory
- Evaluation of patient specimens for the presence of cells indicative of inflammation (i.e., phagocytes) or contamination (i.e., squamous epithelial cells)
- Determination of an organism's clinical significance; bacterial contaminants usually are not present in patient specimens at sufficiently high numbers ($\times 10^5$ cells/mL) to be seen by light microscopy
- Provide preculture information about which organisms might be expected to grow so that appropriate cultivation techniques are used
- Determine which tests and methods should be used for identification and characterization of cultivated organisms
- Provide a method for investigating unusual or unexpected laboratory test results

---

**TABLE 6-1** Microscopy for Diagnostic Microbiology

| Organism Group | Bright-Field Microscopy | Fluorescence Microscopy | Dark-Field Microscopy | Electron Microscopy |
|---|---|---|---|---|
| Bacteria | + | + | ± | − |
| Fungi | + | + | − | − |
| Parasites | + | + | − | ± |
| Viruses | − | + | − | ± |

+, Commonly used; ±, limited use; −, rarely used.

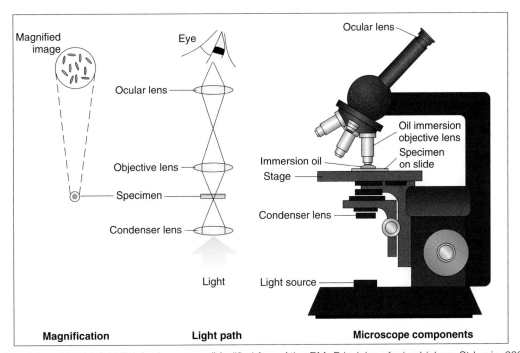

| Magnification | Light path | Microscope components |

**Figure 6-1** Principles of bright-field (light) microscopy. (Modified from Atlas RM: *Principles of microbiology,* St Louis, 2006, Mosby.)

lens, the oil immersion lens, is designed for use with oil; this lens provides 100× magnification on most light microscopes.

Lower magnifications (i.e., 100× or 400×) may be used to locate specimen samples in certain areas on a microscope slide or to observe microorganisms such as some fungi and parasites. The 1000× magnification provided by the combination of ocular and oil immersion lenses usually is required for optimal detection and characterization of bacteria.

### Contrast

The third key component to light microscopy is contrast, which is needed to make objects stand out from the background. Because microorganisms are essentially transparent, owing to their microscopic dimensions and high water content, they cannot be easily detected among the background materials and debris in patient specimens. Lack of contrast is also a problem for the microscopic examination of microorganisms grown in culture. Contrast is most commonly achieved by staining techniques that highlight organisms and allow them to be differentiated from one another and from background material and debris. In the absence of staining, the simplest way to improve contrast is to reduce the diameter of the microscope aperture diaphragm increasing contrast at the expense of the resolution. Setting the controls for bright field microscopy requires a procedure referred to as setting the Kohler illumination (see Procedure 6-1 on the Evolve site).

## STAINING TECHNIQUES FOR LIGHT MICROSCOPY

### Smear Preparation

Staining methods are either used directly with patient specimens or are applied to preparations made from microorganisms grown in culture. A direct smear is a preparation of the primary clinical sample received in the laboratory for processing. A direct smear provides a mechanism to identify the number and type of cells present in a specimen, including white blood cells, epithelial cells, and predominant organism type. Occasionally an organism may grow in culture that was not seen in the direct smear. There are a variety of potential reasons for this, including the possibility that a slow-growing organism was present, the patient was receiving antibiotic treatment to prevent growth of the organism, the specimen was not processed appropriately and the organisms are no longer viable, or the organism requires special media for growth. Preparation of an indirect smear indicates that the primary sample has been processed in culture and the smear contains organisms following purification or growth on artificial media. Indirect smears may include preparation from solid or semisolid media or broth. Care should be taken to ensure the smear is not too thick when preparing the slide from solid media. In addition, smear from a liquid broth should not be diluted. Liquid broth cultures result in smears that more clearly and accurately represent the native cellular morphology and arrangement in

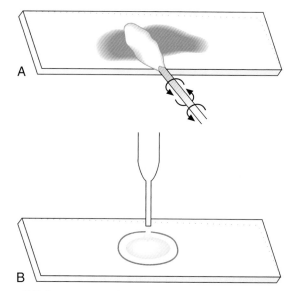

**Figure 6-2** Smear preparations by swab roll **(A)** and pipette deposition **(B)** of patient specimen on a glass slide.

comparison to smears from solid media. Details of specimen processing are presented throughout Part VII, and in most instances the preparation of every specimen includes the application of some portion of the specimen to a clean glass slide (i.e., "smear" preparation) for subsequent microscopic evaluation.

Generally, specimen samples are placed on the slide using a swab that contains patient material or by using a pipette into which liquid specimen has been aspirated (Figure 6-2). Material to be stained is dropped (if liquid) or rolled (if on a swab) onto the surface of a clean, dry, glass slide. To avoid contamination of culture media, once a swab has touched the surface of a nonsterile slide, it should not be used for subsequently inoculating media.

A slide may also be presterilized to avoid contaminating the swab when only a single specimen is received for processing of slides and cultures. Sterilization can be performed by thoroughly flaming the slide using a Bunsen burner and allowing it to cool before use. The slide may be alternately dipped in absolute ethanol and flamed, allowing the alcohol to burn off and thereby killing contaminating organisms. These techniques, although useful, may be limited by increasing safety regulations and the removal of open flame equipment such as Bunsen burners within the clinical laboratory.

For staining microorganisms grown in culture, a sterile loop or needle may be used to transfer a small amount of growth from a solid medium to the surface of the slide. This material is emulsified in a drop of sterile water or saline on the slide. For small amounts of growth that might become lost in even a drop of saline, a sterile wooden applicator stick can be used to touch the growth; this material is then rubbed directly onto the slide, where it can be easily seen. The material placed on the slide to be stained is allowed to air-dry and is affixed to the slide by placing it on a slide warmer (60° C) for at least 10 minutes or by flooding it with 95% methanol for 1 minute. Smears should be air-dried completely prior to heat fixing to prevent the distortion of cell shapes prior to staining. To examine organisms grown in liquid medium, an aspirated sample of the broth culture is applied to the slide, air-dried, and fixed before staining.

A squash or crush prep may be used for tissue, bone marrow aspirate, or other aspirated sample. The aspirate may be placed in the anticoagulant ethylenediaminetetraacetic acid (EDTA) tube and inverted several times to mix contents. This prevents clotting of the aspirated material. To prepare the slide, place a drop of the aspirate on a slide and then gently place a second slide on top, pressing the two slides together and crushing or squashing any particulate matter. Gently slide or pull the two slides apart using a horizontal motion. Air-dry the slides before staining.

Smear preparation varies depending on the type of specimen being processed (see the chapters in Part VII that discuss specific specimen types) and on the staining methods to be used. Nonetheless, the general rule for smear preparation is that sufficient material must be applied to the slide so that chances for detecting and distinguishing microorganisms are maximized. At the same time, the application of excessive material that could interfere with the passage of light through the specimen or that could distort the details of microorganisms must be avoided. Finally, the staining method to be used is dictated by which microorganisms are suspected in the specimen.

As listed in Table 6-1, light microscopy has applications for bacteria, fungi, and parasites. However, the stains used for these microbial groups differ extensively. Those primarily designed for examination of parasites and fungi by light microscopy are discussed in Chapters 47 and 60, respectively. The stains for microscopic examination of bacteria, the Gram stain and the acid-fast stains, are discussed in this chapter.

## Gram Stain

The Gram stain is the principal stain used for microscopic examination of bacteria and is one of the most important bacteriologic techniques within the microbiology laboratory. Gram staining provides a mechanism for the rapid presumptive identification of pathogens, and it gives important clues related to the quality of a specimen and whether bacterial pathogens from a specific body site are considered normal flora colonizing the site or the actual cause of infection. Nearly all clinically important bacteria can be detected using this method, the only exceptions being those organisms that exist almost exclusively within host cells (e.g., chlamydia), those that lack a cell wall (e.g., mycoplasma and ureaplasma), and those of insufficient dimension to be resolved by light microscopy (e.g., spirochetes). First devised by Hans Christian Gram during the late nineteenth century, the Gram stain can be used to divide most bacterial species into two large groups: those that take up the basic dye, crystal violet (i.e., gram-positive bacteria), and those that allow the crystal violet dye to wash out easily with the decolorizer alcohol or acetone (i.e., gram-negative bacteria).

**Procedure Overview.** Although modifications of the classic Gram stain that involve changes in reagents and timing exist, the principles and results are the same for all modifications. The classic Gram stain procedure entails fixing clinical material to the surface of the microscope slide, either by heating or by using methanol. Methanol fixation preserves the morphology of host cells, as well as bacteria, and is especially useful for examining bloody specimen material. Slides are overlaid with 95% methanol for 1 minute; the methanol is allowed to run off, and the slides are air-dried before staining. After fixation, the first step in the Gram stain is the application of the primary stain crystal violet. A mordant, Gram's iodine, is applied after the crystal violet to chemically bond the alkaline dye to the bacterial cell wall. The decolorization step distinguishes gram-positive from gram-negative cells. After decolorization, organisms that stain gram-positive retain the crystal violet and those that are gram-negative are cleared of crystal violet. Addition of the counterstain safranin will stain the clear gram-negative bacteria pink or red (Figure 6-3). See Procedure 6-2 on the Evolve site for detailed methodology, expected results, and limitations.

**Principle.** The difference in composition between gram-positive cell walls, which contain thick peptidoglycan with numerous teichoic acid cross-linkages, and gram-negative cell walls, which consist of a thinner layer of peptidoglycan, and the presence of an outer lipid bilayer that is dehydrated during decolorization, accounts for the Gram staining differences between these two major groups of bacteria. Presumably, the extensive teichoic acid cross-links contribute to the ability of gram-positive organisms to resist alcohol decolorization. Although the gram-positive organisms may take up the counterstain, their purple appearance will not be altered.

Gram-positive organisms that have lost cell wall integrity because of antibiotic treatment, dead or dying cells, or action of autolytic enzymes may allow the crystal violet to wash out with the decolorizing step and may appear gram-variable, with some cells staining pink and others staining purple. However, for identification purposes, these organisms are considered to be truly gram-positive. On the other hand, gram-negative bacteria rarely, if ever, retain crystal violet (e.g., appear purple) if the staining procedure has been properly performed. Host cells, such as red and white blood cells (phagocytes), allow the crystal violet stain to wash out with decolorization and should appear pink on smears that have been correctly prepared and stained.

**Gram Stain Examination.** Once stained, the smear is examined using the 10× objective (100× magnification). The microbiologist should scan the slide looking for white blood cells, epithelial cells, debris, and larger organisms such as fungi or parasites. Next the smear should be examined using the oil immersion (1000× magnification) lens. When clinical material is Gram stained (e.g., the direct smear), the slide is evaluated for the presence of bacterial cells as well as the Gram reactions, morphologies (e.g., cocci or bacilli), and arrangements (e.g., chains, pairs, clusters) of the cells seen (Figure 6-4). This information often provides a preliminary diagnosis regarding the infectious agents and frequently is used to direct initial therapies for the patient.

The direct smears should also be examined for the presence of inflammatory cells (e.g., phagocytes) that are

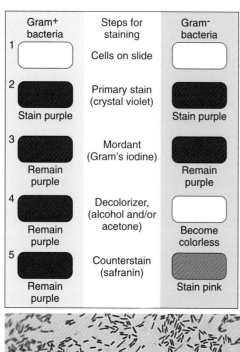

| Gram+ bacteria | Steps for staining | Gram- bacteria |
|---|---|---|
| 1 | Cells on slide | |
| 2 **Stain purple** | Primary stain (crystal violet) | **Stain purple** |
| 3 **Remain purple** | Mordant (Gram's iodine) | **Remain purple** |
| 4 **Remain purple** | Decolorizer, (alcohol and/or acetone) | **Become colorless** |
| 5 **Remain purple** | Counterstain (safranin) | **Stain pink** |

1 Fix material on slide with methanol or heat. If slide is heat fixed, allow it to cool to the touch before applying stain.
2 Flood slide with crystal violet (*purple*) and allow it to remain on the surface without drying for 10 to 30 seconds. Rinse the slide with tap water, shaking off all excess.
3 Flood the slide with iodine to increase affinity of crystal violet and allow it to remain on the surface without drying for twice as long as the crystal violet was in contact with the slide surface (20 seconds of iodine for 10 seconds of crystal violet, for example). Rinse with tap water, shaking off all excess.
4 Flood the slide with decolorizer for 10 seconds or less (optimal decolorization depends on chemical used) and rinse off immediately with tap water. Repeat this procedure until the blue dye no longer runs off the slide with the decolorizer. Thicker smears require more prolonged decolorizing. Rinse with tap water and shake off excess.
5 Flood the slide with counterstain and allow it to remain on the surface without drying for 30 seconds. Rinse with tap water and gently blot the slide dry with paper towels or bibulous paper or air dry. For delicate smears, such as certain body fluids, air drying is the best method.
6 Examine microscopically under an oil immersion lens at 1000x for phagocytes, bacteria, and another cellular material.

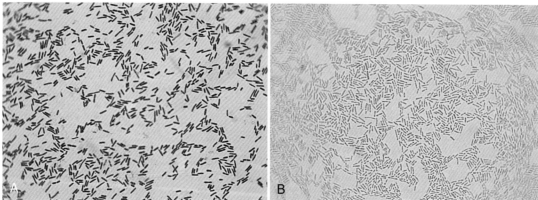

**Figure 6-3** Gram stain procedures and principles. **A,** Gram-positive bacteria observed under oil immersion appear purple. **B,** Gram-negative bacteria observed under oil immersion appear pink. (Modified from Atlas RM: *Principles of microbiology,* St Louis, 2006, Mosby.)

key indicators of an infectious process. Noting the presence of other host cells, such as squamous epithelial cells in respiratory specimens, is also helpful because the presence of these cells may indicate contamination with organisms and cells from the mouth (for more information regarding interpretation of respiratory smears, see Chapter 71). Observing background tissue debris and proteinaceous material, which generally stain gramnegative, also provides helpful information. For example, the presence of such material indicates that specimen material was adequately affixed to the slide. Therefore, the absence of bacteria or inflammatory cells on such a smear is a true negative and not likely the result of loss of specimen during staining (Figure 6-5). Other ways that Gram stain evaluations of how direct smears are used are discussed throughout the chapters of Part VII that deal with infections of specific body sites.

Several examples of Gram stains of direct smears are provided in Figure 6-6. Basically, whatever is observed is also recorded and is used to produce a laboratory report for the physician. The report typically includes the following (see Procedure 6-2):

- The presence of host cells and debris.
- The Gram reactions, morphologies (e.g., cocci, bacilli, coccobacilli), and arrangement of bacterial cells present. Note: Reporting the absence of bacteria and host cells can be equally as important.
- Optionally, the relative amounts of bacterial cells (e.g., rare, few, moderate, many) may be provided. However, it is important to remember that to visualize bacterial cells by light microscopy, a minimum concentration of $10^5$ cells per 1 mL of specimen is required. This is a large number of bacteria for any normally sterile body site and to describe the quantity as rare or few based on microscopic observation may be understating their significance in a clinical specimen. On the other hand, noting the relative amounts seen on direct smear may be useful laboratory information to correlate smear results with the amount of growth observed subsequently from cultures.

Although Gram stain evaluation of direct smears is routinely used as an aid in the diagnosis of bacterial infections, unexpected but significant findings of other infectious etiologies may be detected and cannot be

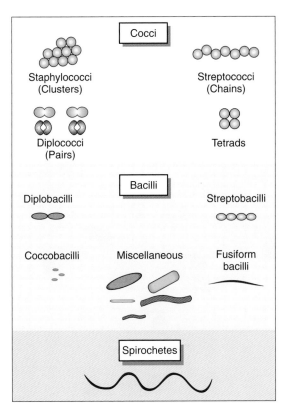

**Figure 6-4** Examples of common bacterial cellular morphologies, Gram staining reactions, and cellular arrangements.

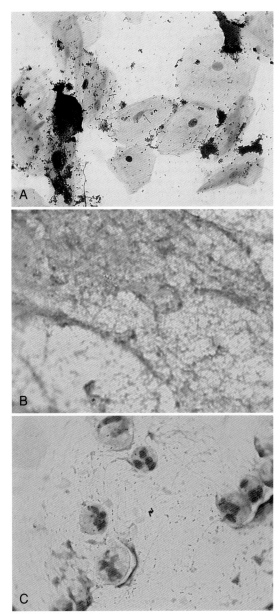

**Figure 6-5** Gram stains of direct smears showing squamous cells and bacteria **(A)**, proteinaceous debris **(B)**, and proteinaceous debris with polymorphonuclear leukocytes and bacteria **(C).**

ignored. For example, fungal cells and elements generally stain gram-positive, but they may take up the crystal violet poorly and appear gram-variable (e.g., both pink and purple) or gram-negative. Because infectious agents besides bacteria may be detected by Gram stain, any unusual cells or structures observed on the smear should be evaluated further before being dismissed as unimportant (Figure 6-7).

**Gram Stain of Bacteria Grown in Culture.** The Gram stain also plays a key role in the identification of bacteria grown in culture. Similar to direct smears, indirect smears prepared from bacterial growth are evaluated for the bacterial cells' Gram reactions, morphologies, and arrangements (see Figure 6-4). If growth from more than one specimen is to be stained on the same slide, a wax pencil may be used to create divisions. Drawing a "map" of such a slide allows different Gram stain results to be recorded in an organized fashion (Figure 6-8). The smear results will be used to determine subsequent testing for identifying and characterizing the organisms isolated from the patient specimen.

## Acid-Fast Stains

The acid-fast stain is the other commonly used stain for light-microscopic examination of bacteria.

**Principle.** The acid-fast stain is specifically designed for a subset of bacteria whose cell walls contain long-chain fatty (mycolic) acids. Mycolic acids render the cells resistant to decolorization, even with acid alcohol decolorizers. Thus, these bacteria are referred to as being acid-fast. Although these organisms may stain slightly

or poorly as gram-positive, the acid-fast stain takes full advantage of the waxy content of the cell walls to maximize detection. Mycobacteria are the most commonly encountered acid-fast bacteria, typified by *Mycobacterium tuberculosis*, the etiologic agent of tuberculosis. Bacteria lacking cell walls fortified with mycolic acids cannot resist decolorization with acid alcohol and are categorized as being non–acid-fast, a trait typical of most other clinically relevant bacteria. However, some degree of acid-fastness is a characteristic of a few nonmycobacterial bacteria, such as *Nocardia* spp., and coccidian parasites, such as *Cryptosporidium* spp.

**Procedure Overview.** The classic acid-fast staining method, Ziehl-Neelsen, is depicted in Figure 6-9 and outlined in Procedure 6-3 on the Evolve site. The procedure requires heat to allow the primary stain (carbolfuchsin)

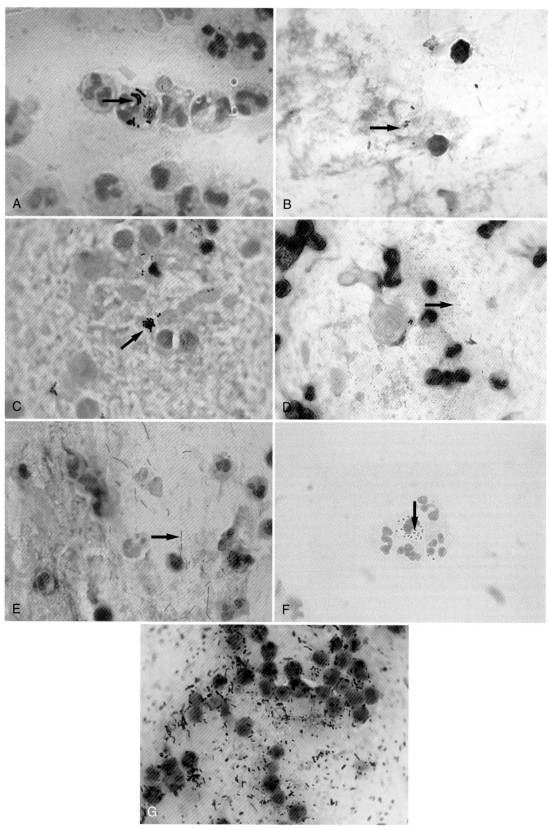

**Figure 6-6** Gram stain of direct smears showing polymorphonuclear leukocytes, proteinaceous debris, and bacterial morphologies (*arrows*), including gram-positive cocci in chains **(A)**, gram-positive cocci in pairs **(B)**, gram-positive cocci in clusters **(C)**, gram-negative coccobacilli **(D)**, gram-negative bacilli **(E)**, gram-negative diplococci **(F)**, and mixed gram-positive and gram-negative morphologies **(G)**.

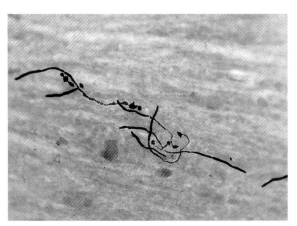

**Figure 6-7** Gram stains of direct smears can reveal infectious etiologies other than bacteria, such as the yeast *Candida tropicalis.*

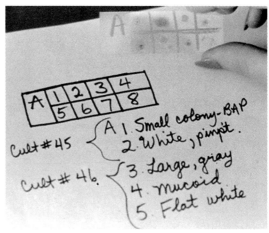

**Figure 6-8** Example of a slide map for staining several bacterial colony samples on a single slide.

| Acid-fast–positive bacilli | Steps for staining | Acid-fast–negative bacilli |
|---|---|---|
| 1 | Cells on slide | |
| 2 Stain red | Primary stain (carbolfuchsin red) | Stain red |
| 3 Remain red | Decolorizer (HCl, alcohol) | Become colorless |
| 4 Remain red | Counterstain (methylene blue) | Stain blue |

1 Fix smears on heated surface (60°C for at least 10 minutes).

2 Flood smears with carbolfuchsin (primary stain) and heat to almost boiling by performing the procedure on an electrically heated platform or by passing the flame of a Bunsen burner underneath the slides on a metal rack. The stain on the slides should steam. Allow slides to sit for 5 minutes after heating; do not allow them to dry out. Wash the slides in distilled water (note: tap water may contain acid-fast bacilli). Drain off excess liquid.

3 Flood slides with 3% HCl in 95% ethanol (decolorizer) for approximately 1 minute. Check to see that no more red color runs off the surface when the slide is tipped. Add a bit more decolorizer for very thick slides or those that continue to "bleed" red dye. Wash thoroughly with water and remove the excess.

4 Flood slides with methylene blue (counterstain) and allow to remain on surface of slides for 1 minute. Wash with distilled water and stand slides upright on paper towels to air dry. Do not blot dry.

5 Examine microscopically (see **A** and **B** below), screening at 400× magnification and confirm all suspicious (i.e., red) organisms at 1000× magnification using an oil-immersion lens.

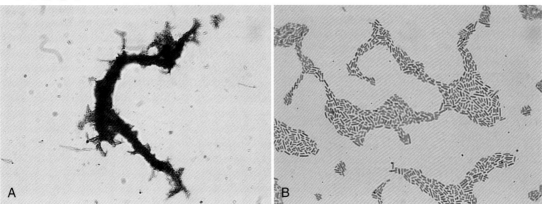

**Figure 6-9** The Ziehl-Neelsen acid-fast stain procedures and principles. **A,** Acid-fast positive bacilli. **B,** Acid-fast negative bacilli. (Modified from Atlas RM: *Principles of microbiology,* St Louis, 2006, Mosby.)

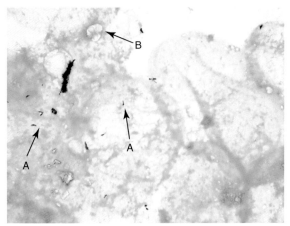

**Figure 6-10** Acid-fast stain of direct smear to show acid-fast bacilli staining deep red (*arrow A*) and non–acid-fast bacilli and host cells staining blue with the counterstain methylene blue (*arrow B*).

to enter the wax-containing cell wall. A modification of this procedure, the Kinyoun acid-fast method (see Procedure 6-4 on the Evolve site), does not require the use of heat or boiling water, minimizing safety concerns during the procedure. Because of a higher concentration of phenol in the primary stain solution, heat is not required for the intracellular penetration of carbolfuchsin. This modification is referred to as the "cold" method. Another modification of the acid-fast stain that is used for identifying certain nonmycobacterial species is described and discussed in Part III, Section 14. When the acid-fast–stained smear is read with 1000× magnification, acid-fast–positive organisms stain red. Depending on the type of counterstain used (e.g., methylene blue or malachite green), other microorganisms, host cells, and debris stain a blue to blue-green color (Figures 6-9 and 6-10).

As with the Gram stain, the acid-fast stain is used to detect acid-fast bacteria (e.g., mycobacteria) directly in clinical specimens and provide preliminary identification information for suspicious bacteria grown in culture. Because mycobacterial infections are much less common than infections caused by other non–acid-fast bacteria, the acid-fast stain is only performed on specimens from patients highly suspected of having a mycobacterial infection. That is, Gram staining is a routine part of most bacteriology procedures, whereas acid-fast staining is reserved for specific situations. Similarly, the acid-fast stain is applied to bacteria grown in culture when mycobacteria are suspected based on other growth characteristics (for more information regarding identification of mycobacteria, see Chapter 43).

## PHASE CONTRAST MICROSCOPY

Instead of using a stain to achieve the contrast necessary for observing microorganisms, altering microscopic techniques to enhance contrast offers another approach. Phase contrast microscopy utilizes beams of light passing through the specimen that are partially deflected by the different densities or thicknesses (i.e., refractive indices) of the microbial cells or cell structures in the specimen.

The greater the refractive index of an object, the more the beam of light is slowed, which results in decreased light intensity. These differences in light intensity translate into differences that provide contrast. Therefore, phase microscopy translates differences in phases within the specimen into differences in light intensities that result in contrast among objects within the specimen being observed.

Smear preparations and permanent staining is used to visualize cellular structures from nonliving or dead microorganisms. Because staining is not part of phase contrast microscopy, this method offers the advantage of allowing observation of viable microorganisms. The method is not commonly used in most aspects of diagnostic microbiology, but it is used to identify medically important fungi grown in culture (for more information regarding the use of phase contrast microscopy for fungal identification, see Chapter 60).

## FLUORESCENT MICROSCOPY

### PRINCIPLE OF FLUORESCENT MICROSCOPY

Certain dyes, called fluors or fluorochromes, can be raised to a higher energy level after absorbing ultraviolet (excitation) light. When the dye molecules return to their normal, lower energy state, they release excess energy in the form of visible (fluorescent) light. This process is called fluorescence, and microscopic methods have been developed to exploit the enhanced contrast and detection that this phenomenon provides.

Figure 6-11 depicts diagrammatically the principle of fluorescent microscopy in which the excitation light is emitted from above (epifluorescence). An excitation filter passes light of the desired wavelength to excite the fluorochrome that has been used to stain the specimen. A barrier filter in the objective lens prevents the excitation wavelengths from damaging the eyes of the observer. When observed through the ocular lens, fluorescing objects appear brightly lit against a dark background.

The color of the fluorescent light depends on the dye and light filters used. For example, use of the fluorescent dyes acridine orange, auramine, and fluorescein isothiocyanate (FITC) requires blue excitation light, exciter filters that select for light in the 450- to 490-λ wavelength range and a barrier filter for 515-λ. Calcofluor white, on the other hand, requires violet excitation light, an exciter filter that selects for light in the 355- to 425-λ wavelength range and a barrier filter for 460-λ. Which dye is used often depends on which organism suspected and the fluorescent method used. The intensity of the contrast obtained with fluorescent microscopy is an advantage it has over the use of chromogenic dyes (e.g., crystal violet and safranin of the Gram stain) and light microscopy.

### STAINING TECHNIQUES FOR FLUORESCENT MICROSCOPY

Based on the composition of the fluorescent stain reagents, fluorescent staining techniques may be divided into two general categories: fluorochroming, in which a

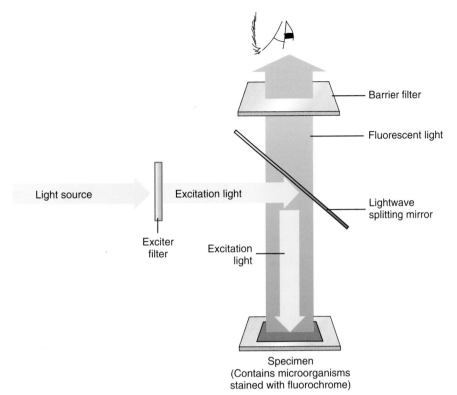

**Figure 6-11** Principle of fluorescent microscopy. Microorganisms in a specimen are stained with a fluorescent dye. On exposure to excitation light, organisms are visually detected by the emission of fluorescent light by the dye with which they have been stained (i.e., fluorochroming) or "tagged" (i.e., immunofluorescence).

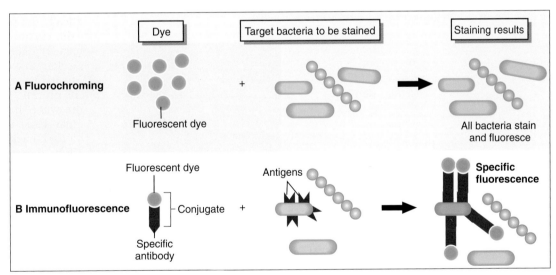

**Figure 6-12** Principles of fluorochroming and immunofluorescence. Fluorochroming **(A)** involves nonspecific staining of any bacterial cell with a fluorescent dye. Immunofluorescence **(B)** uses antibodies labeled with fluorescent dye (i.e., a conjugate) to specifically stain a particular bacterial species.

fluorescent dye is used alone, and immunofluorescence, in which fluorescent dyes have been linked (conjugated) to specific antibodies. The principal differences between these two methods are outlined in Figure 6-12.

## Fluorochroming

In fluorochroming a direct chemical interaction occurs between the fluorescent dye and a component of the bacterial cell; this interaction is the same as occurs with the stains used in light microscopy. The difference is that use of a fluorescent dye enhances contrast and amplifies the observer's ability to detect stained cells tenfold greater than would be observed by light microscopy. For example, a minimum concentration of at least $10^5$ organisms per milliliter of specimen is required for visualization by light microscopy, whereas by fluorescent microscopy that number decreases to $10^4$ per milliliter. The most common fluorochroming

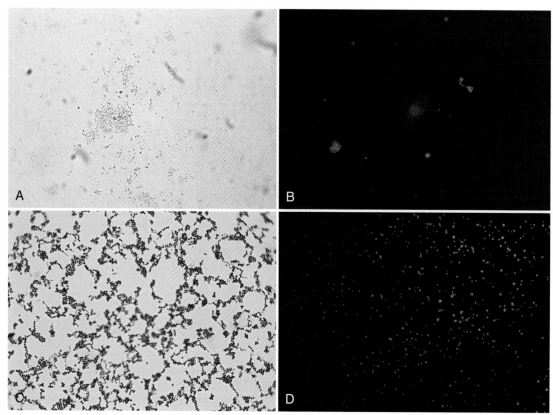

**Figure 6-13** Comparison of acridine orange fluorochroming and Gram stain. Gram stain of mycoplasma demonstrates the inability to distinguish cell wall-deficient organisms from amorphous gram-negative debris **(A)**. Staining the same specimen with acridine orange confirms the presence of nucleic acid–containing organisms **(B)**. Gram stain distinguishes between gram-positive and gram-negative bacteria **(C)**, but all bacteria stain the same with the nonspecific acridine orange dye **(D)**.

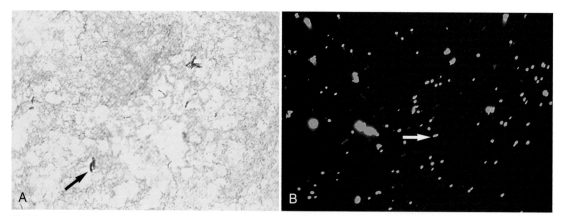

**Figure 6-14** Comparison of the Ziehl-Neelsen–stained **(A)** and auramine-rhodamine–stained **(B)** *Mycobacterium* spp. (*arrows*).

methods used in diagnostic microbiology include acridine orange stain, auramine-rhodamine stain, and calcofluor white stain.

**Acridine Orange.** The fluorochrome acridine orange binds to nucleic acid. This staining method (see Procedure 6-4) can be used to confirm the presence of bacteria in blood cultures when Gram stain results are difficult to interpret or when the presence of bacteria is highly suspected but none are detected using light microscopy. Because acridine orange stains all nucleic acids, it is nonspecific. Therefore, all microorganisms and host cells will stain and give a bright orange fluorescence. Although this stain can be used to enhance detection, it

does not discriminate between gram-negative and gram-positive bacteria. The stain is also used for detection of cell wall–deficient bacteria (e.g., mycoplasmas) grown in culture that are incapable of retaining the dyes used in the Gram stain (Figure 6-13) (see Procedure 6-5 on the Evolve site).

**Auramine-Rhodamine.** The waxy mycolic acids in the cell walls of mycobacteria have an affinity for the fluorochromes auramine and rhodamine. As shown in Figure 6-14, these dyes will nonspecifically bind to nearly all mycobacteria. The mycobacterial cells appear bright yellow or orange against a greenish background. This fluorochroming method can be used to enhance

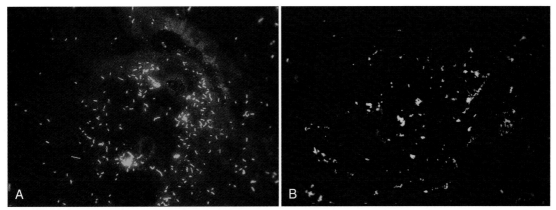

**Figure 6-15** Immunofluorescence stains of *Legionella* spp. **(A)** and *Bordetella pertussis* **(B)** used for identification.

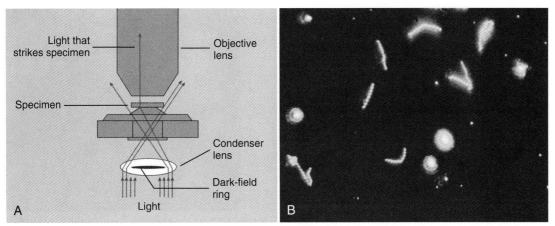

**Figure 6-16** Dark-field microscopy. Principal **(A)** and dark-field photomicrograph showing the tightly coiled characteristics of the spirochete *Treponema pallidum* **(B)**. (From Atlas RM: *Principles of microbiology,* St Louis, 2006, Mosby.)

detection of mycobacteria directly in patient specimens and for initial characterization of cells grown in culture.

**Calcofluor White.** The cell walls of fungi will bind the stain calcofluor white, which greatly enhances fungal visibility in tissue and other specimens. This fluorochrome is commonly used to directly detect fungi in clinical material and to observe subtle characteristics of fungi grown in culture (for more information regarding the use of calcofluor white for the laboratory diagnosis of fungal infections, see Chapter 60). Calcofluor white may also be used to visualize some parasites such as microsporidia.

## Immunofluorescence

As discussed in Chapter 3, antibodies are molecules that have high specificity for interacting with microbial antigens. That is, antibodies specific for an antigen characteristic of a particular microbial species will only combine with that antigen. Therefore, if antibodies are conjugated (chemically linked) to a fluorescent dye, the resulting dye-antibody conjugate can be used to detect, or "tag," specific microbial agents (see Figure 6-12). When "tagged," the microorganisms become readily detectable by fluorescent microscopy. Thus, immunofluorescence combines the amplified contrast provided by fluorescence with the specificity of antibody-antigen binding.

This method is used to directly examine patient specimens for bacteria that are difficult or slow to grow (e.g.,

*Legionella* spp., *Bordetella pertussis,* and *Chlamydia trachomatis*) or to identify organisms already grown in culture. FITC, which emits an intense, apple green fluorescence, is the fluorochrome most commonly used for conjugation to antibodies (Figure 6-15). Immunofluorescence is also used in virology (Chapter 66) and to some extent in parasitology (Chapter 47).

Fluorescent in situ hybridization using peptide nucleic acid probes is a powerful technique used in the clinical laboratory and is discussed in further detail in Chapter 8.

Two additional types of microscopy, dark-field microscopy and electron microscopy, are not commonly used to diagnose infectious diseases. However, because of their importance in the detection and characterization of certain microorganisms, they are discussed here.

## DARK-FIELD MICROSCOPY

Dark-field microscopy is similar to phase contrast microscopy in that it involves the alteration of microscopic technique rather than the use of dyes or stains to achieve contrast. By the dark-field method, the condenser does not allow light to pass directly through the specimen but directs the light to hit the specimen at an oblique angle (Figure 6-16, *A*). Only light that hits objects, such as microorganisms in the specimen, will be deflected upward into the objective lens for visualization. All other light that passes through the specimen will miss the objective, thus making the background a dark field.

This method has greatest utility for detecting certain bacteria directly in patient specimens that, because of their thin dimensions, cannot be seen by light microscopy and, because of their physiology, are difficult to grow in culture. Dark-field microscopy is used to detect spirochetes, the most notorious of which is the bacterium *Treponema pallidum*, the causative agent of syphilis (for more information regarding spirochetes, see Chapter 46). As shown in Figure 6-16, *B*, spirochetes viewed using dark-field microscopy will appear extremely bright against a black field. The use of dark-field microscopy in diagnostic microbiology has decreased with the advent of reliable serologic techniques for the diagnosis of syphilis.

# ELECTRON MICROSCOPY

The electron microscope uses electrons instead of light to visualize small objects and, instead of lenses, the electrons are focused by electromagnetic fields and form an image on a fluorescent screen, like a television screen. Because of the substantially increased resolution this technology allows, magnifications in excess of 100,000× compared with the 1000× magnification provided by light microscopy are achieved.

Electron microscopes are of two general types: the transmission electron microscope (TEM) and the scanning electron microscope (SEM). TEM passes the electron beam through objects and allows visualization of internal structures. SEM uses electron beams to scan the surface of objects and provides three-dimensional views of surface structures (Figure 6-17). These microscopes are powerful research tools, and many new morphologic features of bacteria, bacterial components, fungi, viruses, and parasites have been discovered using electron microscopy. However, because an electron microscope is a major capital investment and is not needed for the laboratory diagnosis of most infectious diseases (except for certain viruses and microsporidian parasites), few laboratories employ this method.

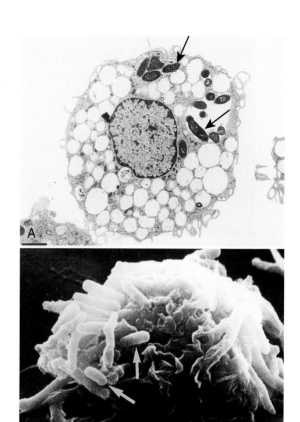

**Figure 6-17 A,** Transmission electron micrograph showing *Escherichia coli* cells internalized by a human mast cell (*arrows*). **B,** Scanning electron micrograph of *E. coli* interacting with the surface of human mast cell (*arrows*). (**A** and **B** Courtesy SN Abraham, Washington University School of Medicine, St Louis.)

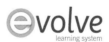 *Visit the Evolve site to complete the review questions.*

# BIBLIOGRAPHY

Atlas RM: *Principles of microbiology,* St Louis, 2006, Mosby.

# Traditional Cultivation and Identification

## OBJECTIVES

1. Define bacterial cultivation and list the three most important purposes for bacterial cultivation.
2. Define bacterial media; list the four general types of media and explain the general biochemical principle for each type.
3. List the environmental conditions that are crucial in supporting bacterial in vitro growth and explain how each factor is controlled and monitored.
4. Explain the most common bacterial streaking technique, the principle associated with the technique, and how colonies are enumerated using this technique.
5. Identify the key criteria used in characterizing and reporting bacterial culture growth pertaining to the phenotypic results; differentiate genotypic and phenotypic characteristics.
6. Explain the use and chemical principle of the following enzymatic tests used in preliminary bacterial identification: catalase test, oxidase test, urease test, indole test, PYR test, and hippurate hydrolysis.
7. Define and differentiate bacterial susceptibility and resistance; give an example in how these are used to assist in the identification bacteria.
8. List the three assays used to measure metabolic pathways and provide an example of each.
9. Describe the steps required to develop "rapid" identification schemes and explain how these differ from conventional schemes.
10. List the four basic identification components common to all commercially available multitest systems.

D irect laboratory methods such as microscopy provide preliminary information about the bacteria involved in an infection, but bacterial growth is usually required for definitive identification and characterization. This chapter presents the various principles and methods required for bacterial cultivation and identification.

## PRINCIPLES OF BACTERIAL CULTIVATION

This section focuses on the principles and practices of bacterial cultivation, which has three main purposes:
- To grow and isolate all bacteria present in a clinical specimen
- To determine which of the bacteria that grow are most likely causing infection and which are likely contaminants or colonizers
- To obtain sufficient growth of clinically relevant bacteria to allow identification, characterization, and susceptibility testing

Cultivation is the process of growing microorganisms in culture by taking bacteria from the infection site (i.e., the in vivo environment) by some means of specimen collection and growing them in the artificial environment of the laboratory (i.e., the in vitro environment). Once grown in culture, most bacterial populations are easily observed without microscopy and are present in sufficient quantities to allow laboratory identification procedures to be performed.

The successful transition from the in vivo to the in vitro environment requires that the nutritional and environmental growth requirements of bacterial pathogens be met. The environmental transition is not necessarily easy for bacteria. In vivo they are utilizing various complex metabolic and physiologic pathways developed for survival on or within the human host. Then, relatively suddenly, they are exposed to the artificial in vitro environment of the laboratory. The bacteria must adjust to survive and multiply. Of importance, their survival depends on the availability of essential nutrients and appropriate environmental conditions.

Although growth conditions can be met for most known bacterial pathogens, the needs of certain clinically relevant bacteria are not sufficiently understood to allow for development of in vitro laboratory growth conditions. Examples include *Treponema pallidum* (the causative agent of syphilis) and *Mycobacterium leprae* (the causative agent of leprosy).

## NUTRITIONAL REQUIREMENTS

As discussed in Chapter 2, bacteria have numerous nutritional needs that include different gases, water, various ions, nitrogen, sources for carbon, and energy. The source for carbon and energy is commonly supplied in carbohydrates (e.g., sugars and their derivatives) and proteins.

### General Concepts of Culture Media

In the laboratory, nutrients are incorporated into culture media on or in which bacteria are grown. If a culture medium meets a bacterial cell's growth requirements, then that cell will multiply to sufficient numbers to allow visualization by the unaided eye. Of course, bacterial growth after inoculation also requires that the medium be placed in optimal environmental conditions.

Because different pathogenic bacteria have different nutritional needs, various types of culture media have been developed for use in diagnostic microbiology. For certain bacteria, the needs are relatively complex, and exceptional media components must be used for growth. Bacteria with such requirements are said to be fastidious. Alternatively, the nutritional needs of most clinically important bacteria are relatively basic and straightforward. These bacteria are considered nonfastidious.

### Phases of Growth Media

Growth media are used in either of two phases: liquid (broth) or solid (agar). In some instances (e.g., certain

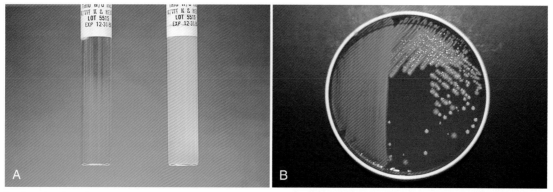

**Figure 7-1 A,** Clear broth indicating no bacterial growth (*left*) and turbid broth indicating bacterial growth (*right*). **B,** Individual bacterial colonies growing on the agar surface following incubation.

blood culture methods), a biphasic medium that contains both a liquid and a solid phase may be used.

In broth media, nutrients are dissolved in water, and bacterial growth is indicated by a change in the broth's appearance from clear to turbid (i.e., cloudy). The turbidity, or cloudiness, of the broth is due to light deflected by bacteria present in the culture (Figure 7-1). More growth indicates a higher cell density and greater turbidity. At least $10^6$ bacteria per milliliter of broth are needed for turbidity to be detected with the unaided eye.

In addition to amount of growth present, the location of growth within thioglycollate broth indicates the type of organism present based on oxygen requirements. Strict anaerobes will grow at the bottom of the broth tube, whereas aerobes will grow near the surface. Microaerophilic organisms will glow slightly below the surface where oxygen concentrations are lower than atmospheric concentrations. In addition, facultative anaerobes and aerotolerant organisms will grow throughout the medium, as they are unaffected by the variation in oxygen content.

A solid medium is a combination of a solidifying agent added to the nutrients and water. Agarose, the most common solidifying agent, has the unique property of melting at high temperatures ($\geq95^\circ$ C) but re-solidifying only after its temperature falls below $50^\circ$ C. The addition of agar allows a solid medium to be prepared by heating to an extremely high temperature, which is required for sterilization and cooling to $55^\circ$ C to $60^\circ$ C for distribution into petri dishes. On further cooling, the agarose-containing medium forms a stable solid gel referred to as agar. The petri dish containing the agar is referred to as the agar plate. Different agar media usually are identified according to the major nutritive components of the medium (e.g., sheep blood agar, bile esculin agar, xylose-lysine-desoxycholate agar).

With appropriate incubation conditions, each bacterial cell inoculated onto the agar medium surface will proliferate to sufficiently large numbers to be observable with the unaided eye (see Figure 7-1). The resulting bacterial population is considered to be derived from a single bacterial cell and is known as a *pure* colony. In other words, all bacterial cells within a single colony are the same genus and species, having identical genetic and phenotypic characteristics (i.e., are derived from a single

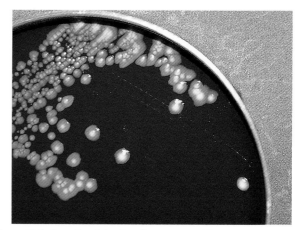

**Figure 7-2** Growth of *Legionella pneumophila* on the enrichment medium buffered charcoal-yeast extract (BCYE) agar, used specifically to grow this bacterial genus.

clone). Pure cultures are required for subsequent procedures used to identify and characterize bacteria. The ability to select pure (individual) colonies is one of the first and most important steps required for bacterial identification and characterization.

### Media Classifications and Functions

Media are categorized according to their function and use. In diagnostic bacteriology there are four general categories of media: enrichment, nutritive, selective, and differential.

Enrichment media contain specific nutrients required for the growth of particular bacterial pathogens that may be present alone or with other bacterial species in a patient specimen. This media type is used to enhance the growth of a particular bacterial pathogen from a mixture of organisms by providing specific nutrients for the organism's growth. One example of such a medium is buffered charcoal-yeast extract agar, which provides L-cysteine and other nutrients required for the growth of *Legionella pneumophila*, the causative agent of legionnaires' disease (Figure 7-2).

Enrichment media may also contain specialized enrichment broths used to enhance the growth of

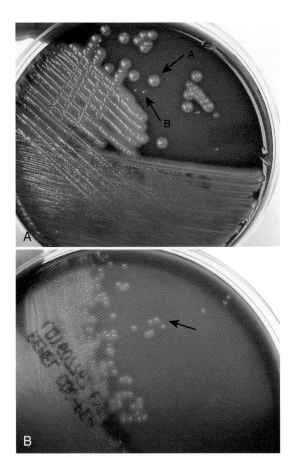

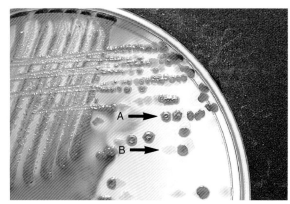

**Figure 7-4** Differential capabilities of MacConkey agar as gram-negative bacilli capable of fermenting lactose appear deep purple (*arrow A*), whereas those not able to ferment lactose appear light pink or relatively colorless (*arrow B*).

**Figure 7-3** **A,** Heavy mixed growth of the gram-negative bacillus *Escherichia coli* (*arrow A*) and the gram-positive coccus Enterococcus spp. (*arrow B*) on the nonselective medium sheep blood agar (SBA). **B,** The selective medium phenylethyl-alcohol agar (PEA) only allows the enterococci to grow (*arrow*).

organisms present in low numbers. Broths may be used to ensure growth of an organism when no organisms grow on solid media following initial specimen inoculation. Enrichment broths used in the clinical laboratory often include thioglycollate for the isolation of anaerobes, LIM broth for selective enrichment of group B streptococci, and gram-negative (GN) broth for the selective enrichment of enteric gram-negative organisms.

Nutritive media or supportive media contain nutrients that support growth of most nonfastidious organisms without giving any particular organism a growth advantage. Nutrient media include tryptic soy agar, or nutrient agar plates for bacteria or Sabouraud's dextrose agar for fungi. Selective media contain one or more agents that are inhibitory to all organisms except those "selected" by the specific growth condition or chemical. In other words, these media select for the growth of certain bacteria to the disadvantage of others. Inhibitory agents used for this purpose include dyes, bile salts, alcohols, acids, and antibiotics. An example of a selective medium is phenylethyl alcohol (PEA) agar, which inhibits the growth of aerobic and facultatively anaerobic gram-negative rods and allows gram-positive cocci to grow (Figure 7-3). Selective and inhibitory chemicals included

within nutritive media prevent the overgrowth of normal flora or contaminating organisms that would prevent the identification of pathogenic organisms. However, it is important to note that the use of selective media does not ensure that the inhibited organisms are not present in small quantity and may simply be too small to see.

Differential media employ some factor (or factors) that allows colonies of one bacterial species or type to exhibit certain metabolic or culture characteristics that can be used to distinguish it from other bacteria growing on the same agar plate. One commonly used differential medium is MacConkey agar, which differentiates between gram-negative bacteria that can and cannot ferment the sugar lactose (Figure 7-4).

Of importance, many media used in diagnostic bacteriology provide more than one function. For example, MacConkey agar is both differential and selective or *combination media* because it will not allow most gram-positive bacteria to grow. Another example is sheep blood agar. This is the most commonly used nutritive medium for diagnostic bacteriology because it allows many organisms to grow. However, in many ways this agar is also differential because the appearance of colonies produced by certain bacterial species is readily distinguishable, as indicated in Figure 5-2. Figure 7-5 shows differential hemolytic patterns by various organisms.

### Summary of Artificial Media for Routine Bacteriology

Various broth and agar media that have enrichment, selective, or differential capabilities and are used frequently for routine bacteriology are listed alphabetically in Table 7-1. Anaerobic bacteriology (Section 13), mycobacteriology (Section 14), and mycology (Chapter 60) use similar media strategies; details regarding these media are provided in the appropriate chapters.

Of the dozens of available media, only those most commonly used for routine diagnostic bacteriology are summarized in this discussion. Part VII discusses which media should be used to culture bacteria from various clinical specimens. Similarly, other chapters throughout Part III discuss media used to identify and characterize specific organisms.

**TABLE 7-1** Plating Media for Routine Bacteriology

| Medium | Components/Comments | Primary Purpose |
|---|---|---|
| Bile esculin agar (BEA) | Nutrient agar base with ferric citrate. Hydrolysis of esculin by group D streptococci imparts a brown color to medium; sodium desoxycholate inhibits many bacteria | Differential isolation and presumptive identification of group D streptococci and enterococci |
| Bile esculin azide agar with vancomycin | Contains azide to inhibit gram-negative bacteria, vancomycin to select for resistant gram-positive bacteria, and bile esculin to differentiate enterococci from other vancomycin-resistant bacteria that may grow | Selective and differential for cultivation of vancomycin-resistant enterococci from clinical and surveillance specimens |
| Blood agar | Trypticase soy agar, Brucella agar, or beef heart infusion with 5% sheep blood | Cultivation of nonfastidious microorganisms, determination of hemolytic reactions |
| Bordet-Gengou agar | Potato-glycerol–based medium enriched with 15%-20% defibrinated blood; contaminants inhibited by methicillin (final concentration of 2.5 μm/mL) | Isolation of *Bordetella pertussis* and *Bordetella parapertussis* |
| Brain heart infusion agar or broth | Dextrose, pork brain and heart dehydrated infusions. | Cultivation of fastidious organisms. |
| Buffered charcoal-yeast extract agar (BCYE) | Yeast extract, agar, charcoal, and salts supplemented with L-cysteine HCl, ferric pyrophosphate, ACES buffer, and α-ketoglutarate | Enrichment for *Legionella* spp. Supports the growth of *Francisella* and *Nocardia* spp. |
| Buffered charcoal-yeast extract (BCYE) agar with antibiotics | BCYE supplemented with polymyxin B, vancomycin, and ansamycin, to inhibit gram-negative bacteria, gram-positive bacteria, and yeast, respectively | Enrichment and selection for *Legionella* spp. |
| *Burkholderia cepacia* selective agar | Bile salts, gentamycin, ticarcillin, polymixin B, Peptone, yeast extract | For recovery of *B. Cepacia* from cystic fibrosis patients |
| Campy-blood agar | Contains vancomycin (10 mg/L), trimethoprim (5 mg/L), polymyxin B (2500 U/L), amphotericin B (2 mg/L), and cephalothin (15 mg/L) in a Brucella agar base with sheep blood | Selective for *Campylobacter* spp. |
| Campylobacter thioglycollate broth | Thioglycollate broth supplemented with increased agar concentration and antibiotics | Selective holding medium for recovery of *Campylobacter* spp. Incubated at 4° C for cold-enrichment. |
| CDC anaerobe 5% sheep blood agar | Tryptic soy broth, 5% sheep blood and added nutrients | Improved growth of obligate, slow-growing anaerobes |
| Cefoperazone, vancomycin, amphotericin (CVA) medium | Blood-supplemented enrichment medium containing cefoperazone, vancomycin, and amphotericin to inhibit growth of most gram-negative bacteria, gram-positive bacteria, and yeast, respectively | Selective medium for isolation of *Campylobacter* spp. |
| Cefsulodin-irgasan-novobiocin (CIN) agar | Peptone base with yeast extract, mannitol, and bile salts; supplemented with cefsulodin, irgasan, and novobiocin; neutral red and crystal violet indicators | Selective for *Yersinia* spp.; may be useful for isolation of *Aeromonas* spp. |
| Chocolate agar | Peptone base, enriched with solution of 2% hemoglobin or IsoVitaleX (BBL) | Cultivation of fastidious microorganisms such as *Haemophilus* spp., *Brucella* spp. and pathogenic *Neisseria* spp. |
| Chromogenic media | Organism-specific nutrient base, selective supplements and chromogenic substrate | Chromogenic media are designed to optimize growth and differentiate a specific type of organism. Chromagars are routinely used in the identification of yeasts, methicillin-resistant *Stapylococcus aureus* (MRSA), and a variety of other organisms. |
| Columbia colistin-nalidixic acid (CNA) agar | Columbia agar base with 10 mg colistin per liter, 15 mg nalidixic acid per liter, and 5% sheep blood | Selective isolation of gram-positive cocci |
| Cystine-tellurite blood agar | Infusion agar base with 5% sheep blood; reduction of potassium tellurite by *Corynebacterium diphtheriae* produces black colonies | Isolation of *C. diphtheriae* |
| Eosin methylene blue (EMB) agar (Levine) | Peptone base containing lactose; eosin Y and methylene blue as indicators | Isolation and differentiation of lactose-fermenting and non–lactose-fermenting enteric bacilli |

**TABLE 7-1** Plating Media for Routine Bacteriology—cont'd

| Medium | Components/Comments | Primary Purpose |
|---|---|---|
| Gram-negative broth (GN) | Peptone base broth with glucose and mannitol; sodium citrate and sodium desoxycholate act as inhibitory agents | Selective (enrichment) liquid medium for enteric pathogens |
| Hektoen enteric (HE) agar | Peptone base agar with bile salts, lactose, sucrose, salicin, and ferric ammonium citrate; indicators include bromthymol blue and acid fuchsin | Differential, selective medium for the isolation and differentiation of *Salmonella* and *Shigella* spp. from other gram-negative enteric bacilli |
| Loeffler's medium | Animal tissue (heart muscle), dextrose, eggs and beef serum, and sodium chloride | Isolation and growth of *Corynebacterium* |
| MacConkey agar | Peptone base with lactose; gram-positive organisms inhibited by crystal violet and bile salts; neutral red as indicator | Isolation and differentiation of lactose fermenting and non–lactose-fermenting enteric bacilli |
| MacConkey sorbitol agar | A modification of MacConkey agar in which lactose has been replaced with D-sorbitol as the primary carbohydrate | For the selection and differentiation of *E. coli* 0157:H7 in stool specimens |
| Mannitol salt agar | Peptone base, mannitol, and phenol red indicator; salt concentration of 7.5% inhibits most bacteria | Selective differentiation of staphylococci |
| New York City (NYC) agar | Peptone agar base with cornstarch, supplemented with yeast dialysate, 3% hemoglobin, and horse plasma; antibiotic supplement includes vancomycin (2 µg/mL), colistin (5.5 µg/mL), amphotericin B (1.2 µg/mL), and trimethoprim (3 µg/mL) | Selective for *Neisseria gonorrhoeae*; also supports the growth of *Ureaplasma urealyticum* and some *Mycoplasma* spp. |
| Phenylethyl alcohol (PEA) agar | Nutrient agar base. Phenylmethanol inhibits growth of gram-negative organisms | Selective isolation of aerobic gram-positive cocci and bacilli and anaerobic gram-positive cocci and negative bacilli |
| Regan Lowe | Charcoal agar supplemented with horse blood, cephalexin, and amphotericin B | Enrichment and selective medium for isolation of *Bordetella pertussis* |
| Salmonella-Shigella (SS) agar | Peptone base with lactose, ferric citrate, and sodium citrate; neutral red as indicator; inhibition of coliforms by brilliant green and bile salts | Selective for *Salmonella* and some *Shigella* spp. |
| Schaedler agar | Peptone and soy protein base agar with yeast extract, dextrose, and buffers; addition of hemin, L-cystine, and 5% blood enriches for anaerobes | Nonselective medium for the recovery of anaerobes and aerobes. Selective for Campylobacter and Helicobacter spp. |
| Selenite broth | Peptone base broth; sodium selenite toxic for most Enterobacteriaceae | Enrichment of isolation of *Salmonella* spp. |
| Skirrow agar | Peptone and soy protein base agar with lysed horse blood; vancomycin inhibits gram-positive organisms; polymyxin B and trimethoprim inhibit most gram-negative organisms | Selective for *Campylobacter* spp. |
| Streptococcal selective agar (SSA) | Contains crystal violet, colistin, and trimethoprim-sulfamethoxazole in 5% sheep blood agar base | Selective for *Streptococcus pyogenes* and *Streptococcus agalactiae* |
| Tetrathionate broth | Peptone base broth; iodine and potassium iodide, bile salts, and sodium thiosulfate inhibit gram-positive organisms and Enterobacteriaceae | Selective for *Salmonella* and *Shigella* spp. except *S. typhi*. |
| Thayer-Martin agar (modified Thayer Martin) | Blood agar base enriched with hemoglobin and supplement B; contaminating organisms inhibited by colistin, nystatin, vancomycin, and trimethoprim | Selective for *N. gonorrhoeae* and *N. meningitidis*. Supports the growth of *Francisella* and *Brucella* spp. |
| Thioglycollate broth | Pancreatic digest of casein, soy broth, and glucose enrich growth of most microorganisms; includes reducing agents thioglycolate, cystine, and sodium sulfite; semisolid medium with a low concentration of agar reducing oxygen diffusion in the medium | Supports growth of anaerobes, aerobes, microaerophilic, and fastidious microorganisms |
| Thiosulfate citrate-bile salts (TCBS) agar | Peptone base agar with yeast extract, bile salts, citrate, sucrose, ferric citrate, and sodium thiosulfate; bromthymol blue acts as indicator | Selective and differential for *Vibrio* spp. |
| Todd-Hewitt broth supplemented with antibiotics (LIM) | Todd-Hewitt, an enrichment broth for streptococci, is supplemented with nalidixic acid and gentamicin or colistin for greater selectivity; thioglycollate and agar reduce redox potential | Selection and enrichment for *Streptococcus agalactiae* in female genital specimens |

*Continued*

**TABLE 7-1** Plating Media for Routine Bacteriology—cont'd

| Medium | Components/Comments | Primary Purpose |
|---|---|---|
| Trypticase soy broth (TSB) | All-purpose enrichment broth that can support the growth of many fastidious and nonfastidious bacteria | Enrichment broth used for subculturing various bacteria from primary agar plates |
| Xylose lysine desoxycholate (XLD) agar | Yeast extract agar with lysine, xylose, lactose, sucrose, and ferric ammonium citrate; sodium desoxycholate inhibits gram-positive organisms; phenol red as indicator | Isolation and differentiation of *Salmonella* and *Shigella* spp. from other gram-negative enteric bacilli |

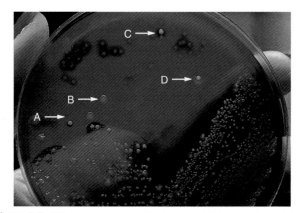

**Figure 7-5** Different colony morphologies exhibited on sheep blood agar by various bacteria, including alpha-hemolytic streptococci (*arrow A*), gram-negative bacilli (*arrow B*), beta-hemolytic streptococci (*arrow C*), and *Staphylococcus aureus* (*arrow D*).

**Brain-Heart Infusion.** Brain-heart infusion (BHI) is a nutritionally rich medium used to grow various microorganisms, either as a broth or as an agar, with or without added blood. Key ingredients include infusion from several animal tissue sources, added peptone (protein), phosphate buffer, and a small concentration of dextrose. The carbohydrate provides a readily accessible source of energy for many bacteria. BHI broth is often used as a major component of the media developed for culturing a patient's blood for bacteria (see Chapter 69), for establishing bacterial identification, and for certain tests to determine bacterial susceptibility to antimicrobial agents (see Chapter 12).

**Chocolate Agar.** Chocolate agar is essentially the same as blood agar except that during preparation the red blood cells are lysed when added to molten agar base. The cell lysis provides for the release of intracellular nutrients such as hemoglobin, hemin ("X" factor), and the coenzyme nicotinamide adenine dinucleotide (NAD or "V" factor) into the agar for utilization by fastidious bacteria. Red blood cell lysis gives the medium a chocolate-brown color from which the agar gets its name. The most common bacterial pathogens that require this enriched medium for growth include *Neisseria gonorrhoeae*, the causative agent of gonorrhea, and *Haemophilus* spp., which cause infections usually involving the respiratory tract and middle ear. Neither of these species is able to grow on sheep blood agar.

**Columbia CNA with Blood.** Columbia agar base is a nutritionally rich formula containing three peptone sources

and 5% defibrinated (whole blood with fibrin removed to prevent clotting) sheep blood. This supportive medium can also be used to help differentiate bacterial colonies based on the hemolytic reactions they produce. CNA refers to the antibiotics colistin (C) and nalidixic acid (NA) that are added to the medium to suppress the growth of most gram-negative organisms while allowing gram-positive bacteria to grow, thus conferring a selective property to this medium. Colistin disrupts the cell membranes of gram-negative organisms and nalidixic aid blocks DNA replication in susceptible organisms.

**Gram-Negative (GN) Broth.** A selective broth, gram-negative (GN) broth is used for the cultivation of gastrointestinal pathogens (i.e., *Salmonella* spp. and *Shigella* spp.) from stool specimens and rectal swabs. The broth contains several active ingredients, including sodium citrate and sodium desoxycholate (a bile salt), that inhibit gram-positive organisms and the early multiplication of gram-negative, nonenteric pathogens. The broth also contains mannitol as the primary carbon source. Mannitol is the favored energy source for many enteric pathogens, but it is not utilized by many other nonpathogenic enteric organisms. To optimize its selective nature, GN broth should be subcultured 6 to 8 hours after initial inoculation and incubation. After this time, the nonenteric pathogens begin to overgrow the pathogens that may be present in very low numbers.

**Hektoen Enteric (HE) Agar.** Hektoen enteric (HE) agar contains bile salts and dyes (bromthymol blue and acid fuchsin) to selectively slow the growth of most nonpathogenic gram-negative bacilli found in the gastrointestinal tract and allow *Salmonella* spp. and *Shigella* spp. to grow. The medium is also differential because many nonenteric pathogens that do grow will appear as orange to salmon-colored colonies. This colony appearance results from the organism's ability to ferment the lactose in the medium, resulting in the production of acid, which lowers the medium's pH and causes a change in the pH indicator bromthymol blue. *Salmonella* spp. and *Shigella* spp. do not ferment lactose, so no color change occurs and their colonies maintain the original blue-green color of the medium. As an additional differential characteristic, the medium contains ferric ammonium citrate, an indicator for the detection of $H_2S$, so that $H_2S$-producing organisms, such as *Salmonella* spp., can be visualized as colonies exhibiting a black precipitate (Figure 7-6).

**MacConkey Agar.** MacConkey agar is the most frequently used primary selective and differential agar. This medium contains crystal violet dye to inhibit the growth of gram-positive bacteria and fungi, and it allows many

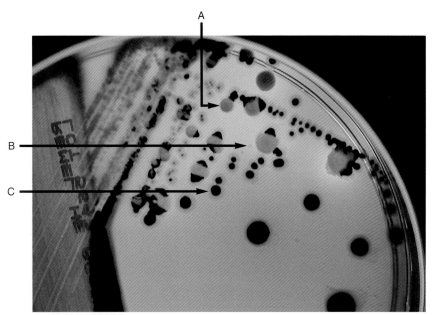

**Figure 7-6** Differential capabilities of HE agar for lactose-fermenting, gram-negative bacilli (e.g., *Escherichia coli, arrow A*), non–lactose-fermenters (e.g., *Shigella* spp., *arrow B*), and H₂S producers (e.g., *Salmonella* spp., *arrow C*).

types of gram-negative bacilli to grow. The pH indicator, neutral red, provides this medium with a differential capacity. Bacterial fermentation of lactose results in acid production, which decreases medium pH and causes the neutral red indicator to give bacterial colonies a pink to red color. Non–lactose-fermenters, such as *Shigella* spp., remain colorless and translucent (see Figure 7-4).

**Phenylethyl Alcohol (PEA) Agar.** Phenylethyl alcohol (PEA) agar is essentially sheep blood agar that is supplemented with phenylethyl alcohol to inhibit the growth of gram-negative bacteria. Five percent sheep blood in PEA provides nutrients for common gram-positive cocci such as enterococci, streptococci, and staphylococci (see Figure 7-3). PEA agar, although it contains sheep blood, should not be used in the interpretation of hemolytic reactions.

**Sheep Blood Agar.** Most bacteriology specimens are inoculated to sheep blood agar plates because this medium supports growth for all but the most fastidious clinically significant bacteria. Additionally, the colony morphologies that commonly encountered bacteria exhibit on this medium are familiar to most clinical microbiologists. The medium consists of a base containing a protein source (e.g., tryptones), soybean protein digest (containing a slight amount of natural carbohydrate), sodium chloride, agar, and 5% sheep blood.

Certain bacteria produce extracellular enzymes that lyse red blood cells in the agar (hemolysis). This activity can result in complete clearing of the red blood cells around the bacterial colony (beta hemolysis) or in only partial lysis of the cells to produce a greenish discoloration around the colony (alpha hemolysis). Other bacteria have no effect on the red blood cells, and no halo is produced around the colony (gamma or nonhemolytic). Microbiologists often use colony morphology and the degree or absence of hemolysis as criteria for determining

what additional steps will be necessary for identification of a bacterial isolate. To read the hemolytic reaction on a blood agar plate accurately, the technologist must hold the plate up to the light and observe the plate with the light coming from behind (i.e., transmitted light).

**Modified Thayer-Martin Agar.** Modified Thayer-Martin (MTM) agar is an enrichment and selective medium for the isolation of *Neisseria gonorrhoeae*, the causative agent of gonorrhea, and *Neisseria meningitidis*, a life-threatening cause of meningitis from specimens containing mixed flora. The enrichment portion of the medium is the basal components and the chocolatized blood, while the addition of antibiotics provides a selective capacity. The antibiotics include colistin to inhibit other gram-negative bacteria, vancomycin to inhibit gram-positive bacteria, and nystatin to inhibit yeast. The antimicrobial trimethoprim is also added to inhibit *Proteus* spp., which tend to swarm over the agar surface and mask the detection of individual colonies of the two pathogenic *Neisseria* spp. A further modification, Martin-Lewis agar, substitutes ansamycin for nystatin and has a higher concentration of vancomycin.

**Thioglycollate Broth.** Thioglycollate broth is the enrichment broth most frequently used in diagnostic bacteriology. The broth contains many nutrient factors, including casein, yeast and beef extracts, and vitamins, to enhance the growth of most medically important bacteria. Other nutrient supplements, an oxidation-reduction indicator (resazurin), dextrose, vitamin K1, and hemin have been used to modify the basic thioglycollate formula. In addition, this medium contains 0.075% agar to prevent convection currents from carrying atmospheric oxygen throughout the broth. This agar supplement and the presence of thioglycolic acid, which acts as a reducing agent to create an anaerobic environment deeper in the tube, allow anaerobic bacteria to grow.

Gram-negative, facultatively anaerobic bacilli (i.e., those that can grow in the presence or absence of oxygen) generally produce diffuse, even growth throughout the broth, whereas gram-positive cocci demonstrate flocculation or clumps. Strict aerobic bacteria (i.e., require oxygen for growth), such as *Pseudomonas* spp., tend to grow toward the surface of the broth, whereas strict anaerobic bacteria (i.e., those that cannot grow in the presence of oxygen) grow at the bottom of the broth (Figure 7-7).

**Xylose-Lysine-Desoxycholate (XLD) Agar.** As with HE agar, xylose-lysine-desoxycholate (XLD) agar is selective and differential for *Shigella* spp. and *Salmonella* spp. The salt, sodium desoxycholate, inhibits many gram-negative bacilli that are not enteric pathogens and inhibits gram-positive organisms. A phenol red indicator in the medium detects increased acidity from carbohydrate (i.e., lactose, xylose, and sucrose) fermentation. Enteric pathogens, such as *Shigella* spp., do not ferment these carbohydrates, so their colonies remain colorless (i.e., the same approximate pink to red color of the un-inoculated medium). Even though they often ferment xylose, colonies of Salmonella spp. are also colorless on XLD, because of the decarboxylation of lysine, which results in a pH increase that causes the pH indicator to turn red. These colonies often exhibit a black center that results from *Salmonella* spp. producing H$_2$S. Several of the nonpathogenic organisms ferment one or more of the sugars and produce yellow colonies (Figure 7-8).

### Preparation of Artificial Media

Nearly all media are commercially available as ready-to-use agar plates or tubes of broth. If media are not purchased, laboratory personnel can prepare agars and broths using dehydrated powders that are reconstituted in water (distilled or deionized) according to manufacturer's recommendations. Generally, media are reconstituted by dissolving a specified amount of media powder, which usually contains all necessary components, in water. Boiling is often required to dissolve the powder, but specific manufacturer's instructions printed in media package inserts should be followed exactly. Most media require sterilization so that only bacteria from patient specimens will grow and not contaminants from water or the powdered media. Broth media are

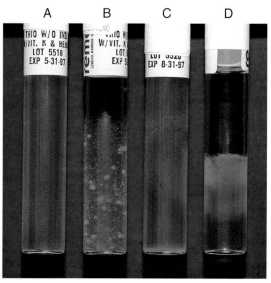

**Figure 7-7** Growth characteristics of various bacteria in thioglycollate broth. **A,** Facultatively anaerobic gram-negative bacilli (i.e., those that grow in the presence or absence of oxygen) grow throughout broth. **B,** Gram-positive cocci demonstrating flocculation. **C,** Strictly aerobic organisms (i.e., those that require oxygen for growth), such as *Pseudomonas aeruginosa*, grow toward the top of the broth. **D,** Strictly anaerobic organisms (i.e., those that do not grow in the presence of oxygen) grow in the bottom of the broth.

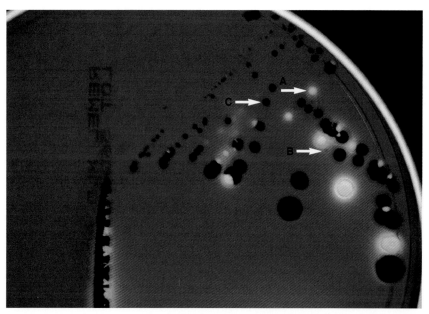

**Figure 7-8** Differential capabilities of xylose-lysine-desoxycholate (XLD) agar for lactose-fermenting, gram-negative bacilli (e.g., *Escherichia coli*, *arrow A*), non–lactose-fermenters (e.g., *Shigella* spp., *arrow B*), and H$_2$S producers (e.g., *Salmonella* spp., *arrow C*).

distributed to individual tubes before sterilization. Agar media are usually sterilized in large flasks or bottles capped with either plastic screw caps or plugs before being placed in an autoclave.

**Media Sterilization.** The timing of autoclave sterilization should start from the moment the temperature reaches 121°C and usually requires a minimum of 15 minutes. Once the sterilization cycle is completed, molten agar is allowed to cool to approximately 50°C before being distributed to individual petri plates (approximately 20 to 25 mL of molten agar per plate). If other ingredients are to be added (e.g., supplements such as sheep blood or specific vitamins, nutrients, or antibiotics), they should be incorporated when the molten agar has cooled, just before distribution to plates.

Delicate media components that cannot withstand steam sterilization by autoclaving (e.g., serum, certain carbohydrate solutions, certain antibiotics, and other heat-labile substances) can be sterilized by membrane filtration. Passage of solutions through membrane filters with pores ranging in size from 0.2 to 0.45 µm in diameter will not remove viruses but does effectively remove most bacterial and fungal contaminants. Finally, all media, whether purchased or prepared, must be subjected to stringent quality control before being used in the diagnostic setting (for more information regarding quality control see Chapter 79).

**Cell Cultures.** Although most bacteria grow readily on artificial media, certain pathogens require factors provided by living cells. These bacteria are obligate intracellular parasites that require viable host cells for propagation. Although all viruses are obligate intracellular parasites, chlamydiae, rickettsiae, and rickettsiae-like organisms are bacterial pathogens that require living cells for cultivation.

The cultures for growth of these bacteria comprise layers of living cells growing on the surface of a solid matrix such as the inside of a glass tube or the bottom of a plastic flask. The presence of bacterial pathogens within the cultured cells is detected by specific changes in the cells' morphology. Alternatively, specific stains, composed of antibody conjugates, may be used to detect bacterial antigens within the cells. Cell cultures may also detect certain bacterial toxins (e.g., *Clostridium difficile* cytotoxin). Cell cultures are most commonly used in diagnostic virology. Cell culture maintenance and inoculation is addressed in Chapter 66.

## ENVIRONMENTAL REQUIREMENTS

Optimizing the environmental conditions to support the most robust growth of clinically relevant bacteria is as important as meeting the organism's nutritional needs for in vitro cultivation. The four most critical environmental factors to consider include oxygen and carbon dioxide ($CO_2$) availability, temperature, pH, and moisture content of medium and atmosphere.

### Oxygen and Carbon Dioxide Availability

Most clinically relevant bacteria are aerobic, facultatively anaerobic, or strictly anaerobic. Aerobic bacteria use oxygen as a terminal electron acceptor and grow well in room air. Most clinically significant aerobic organisms are actually facultatively anaerobic, being able to grow in the presence (i.e., aerobically) or absence (i.e., anaerobically) of oxygen. However, some bacteria, such as *Pseudomonas* spp., members of the *Neisseriaceae* family, *Brucella* spp., *Bordetella* spp., and *Francisella* spp., are strictly aerobic and cannot grow in the absence of oxygen. Other aerobic bacteria require only low levels of oxygen (approximately 20%) and are referred to as being microaerophilic, or microaerobic. Anaerobic bacteria are unable to use oxygen as an electron acceptor, but some aerotolerant strains will still grow slowly and poorly in the presence of oxygen. Oxygen is inhibitory or lethal for strictly anaerobic bacteria.

In addition to oxygen, the availability of $CO_2$ is important for growth of certain bacteria. Organisms that grow best with higher $CO_2$ concentrations (i.e., 5% to 10% $CO_2$) than is provided in room air are referred to as being capnophilic. For some bacteria, a 5% to 10% $CO_2$ concentration is essential for successful cultivation from patient specimens.

### Temperature

Bacterial pathogens generally multiply best at temperatures similar to those of internal human host tissues and organs (i.e., 37°C). Therefore, cultivation of most medically relevant bacteria is done using incubators with temperatures maintained in the 35°C to 37°C range. For others, an incubation temperature of 30°C (i.e., the approximate temperature of the body's surface) may be preferable, but such bacteria are encountered relatively infrequently so that use of this incubation temperature occurs only when dictated by special circumstances.

Recovery of certain organisms can be enhanced by incubation at other temperatures. For example, the gastrointestinal pathogen *Campylobacter jejuni* is able to grow at 42°C. Therefore, incubation at this temperature can be used as an enrichment procedure. Other bacteria, such as *Listeria monocytogenes* and *Yersinia enterocolitica*, can grow at 4°C to 43°C but grow best at temperatures between 20° and 40°C. Cold enrichment has been used to enhance the recovery of these organisms in the laboratory.

### pH

The pH scale is a measure of the hydrogen ion concentration in the environment, with a pH value of 7 being neutral. Values less than 7 indicate the environment is acidic; values greater than 7 indicate alkaline conditions. Most clinically relevant bacteria prefer a near neutral pH range, from 6.5 to 7.5. Commercially prepared media are buffered in this range so that checking their pH is rarely necessary.

### Moisture

Water is provided as a major constituent of both agar and broth media. However, when media are incubated at the temperatures used for bacterial cultivation, a large portion of water content can be lost by evaporation. Loss of water from media can be deleterious to bacterial growth in two ways: (1) less water is available for essential bacterial metabolic pathways and (2) with a loss of water, there is a relative increase in the solute concentration of the media. An increased solute concentration can osmotically shock the bacterial cell and cause lysis. In addition, increased atmospheric humidity enhances the growth of certain bacterial species. For these reasons, measures such as sealing agar plates to trap moisture or using humidified incubators are utilized to ensure appropriate moisture levels are maintained throughout the incubation period.

### Methods for Providing Optimum Incubation Conditions

Although heating blocks and temperature-controlled water baths may be used occasionally, incubators are the primary laboratory devices used to provide the environmental conditions required for cultivating microorganisms. The conditions of incubators can be altered to accommodate the type of organisms to be grown. This section focuses on the incubation of routine bacteriology cultures. Conditions for growing anaerobic bacteria (Section 13), mycobacteria (Section 14), fungi (Chapter 59), and viruses (Chapter 65) are covered in other areas of the text.

Once inoculated with patient specimens, most media are placed in incubators with temperatures maintained between 35° and 37° C and humidified atmospheres that contain 3% to 5% $CO_2$. It is important to note that some media that contain pH indicators may not be placed in $CO_2$ incubators. The presence of $CO_2$ will acidify the media, causing the pH indicator to change color and thereby disrupt the differential properties of the media (e.g., Hektoen-Enteric agar and MacConkey agar). Incubators containing room air may be used for some media, but the lack of increased $CO_2$ may hinder the growth of certain bacteria.

Various atmosphere-generating systems are commercially available and are used instead of $CO_2$-generating incubators. For example, a self-contained culture medium and a compact $CO_2$-generating system can be used for culturing fastidious organisms such as *Neisseria gonorrhoeae*. A tablet of sodium bicarbonate is dissolved by the moisture created within an airtight plastic bag and releases sufficient $CO_2$ to support growth of the pathogen. As an alternative to commercial systems, a candle jar can also generate a $CO_2$ concentration of approximately 3% and has historically been used as a common method for cultivating certain fastidious bacteria. The burning candle, which is placed in a container of inoculated agar plates that is subsequently sealed, uses just enough oxygen before it goes out (from lack of oxygen) to lower the oxygen tension and produce $CO_2$ and water by combustion. Other atmosphere-generating systems are available to create conditions optimal for cultivating specific bacterial pathogens (e.g., *Campylobacter* spp. and anaerobic bacteria).

Finally, the duration of incubation required for obtaining good bacterial growth depends on the organisms being cultured. Most bacteria encountered in routine bacteriology will grow within 24 to 48 hours. Certain anaerobic bacteria may require longer incubation, and mycobacteria frequently take weeks before detectable growth occurs.

# BACTERIAL CULTIVATION

The process of bacterial cultivation involves the use of optimal artificial media and incubation conditions to isolate and identify the bacterial etiologies of an infection as rapidly and as accurately as possible.

## ISOLATION OF BACTERIA FROM SPECIMENS

The cultivation of bacteria from infections at various body sites is accomplished by inoculating processed specimens directly onto artificial media. The media are summarized in Table 7-1 and incubation conditions are selected for their ability to support the growth of the bacteria most likely to be involved in the infectious process.

To enhance the growth, isolation, and selection of etiologic agents, specimen inocula are usually spread over the surface of plates in a standard pattern so that individual bacterial colonies are obtained and semiquantitative analysis can be performed. A commonly used streaking technique is illustrated in Figure 7-9. Using this method, the relative numbers of organisms in the original specimen can be estimated based on the growth of colonies past the original area of inoculation. To enhance isolation of bacterial colonies, the loop should be flamed for sterilization between the streaking of each subsequent quadrant.

Streaking plates inoculated with a measured amount of specimen, such as when a calibrated loop is used to quantify colony-forming units (CFUs) in urine cultures, is accomplished by spreading the inoculum down the center of the plate. Without flaming the loop, the plate is then streaked side to side across the initial inoculum to evenly distribute the growth on the plate (Figure 7-10). This facilitates counting colonies by ensuring that individual bacterial cells will be well dispersed over the agar surface. Typically a calibrated loop of 1 µL is used for urine cultures. However, in situations where a lower count of bacteria may be present such as a suprapubic aspiration, a 10 µL loop may be needed to identify the lower count of organisms. The number of colonies identified on the plate is multiplied by the dilution factor in order to determine the number of colony-forming units per millimeter in the original specimen ($10^3$ for a 1 µL loop and $10^2$ for a 10 µL loop). In addition, to standardize the interpretation of colony count, a laboratory should have guidelines for the reporting of organisms based on the number and types of organisms present. A sample standardized method is outlined in Procedure 73-1.

### Evaluation of Colony Morphologies

The initial evaluation of colony morphologies on the primary plating media is extremely important. Laboratorians can provide physicians with early preliminary information regarding the patient's culture results. This information is also important for deciding how to proceed for definitive organism identification and characterization.

**Type of Media Supporting Bacterial Growth.** As previously discussed, different media are used to recover particular

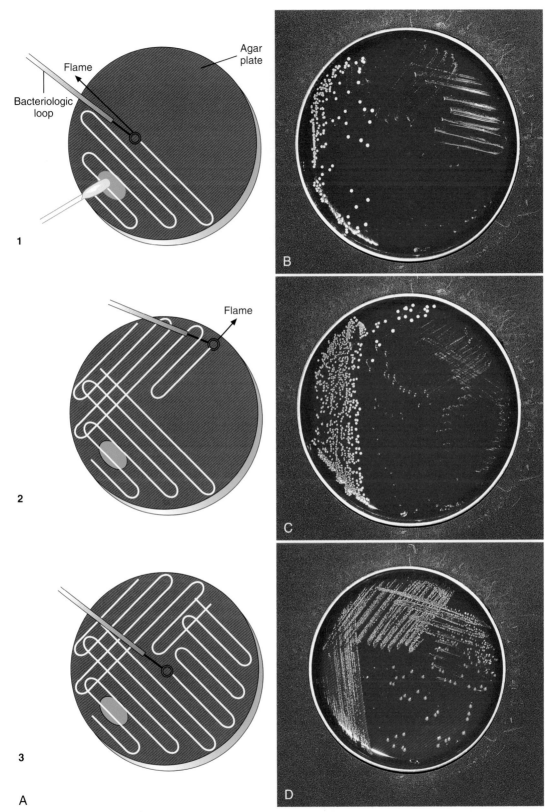

**Figure 7-9  A,** Dilution streak technique for isolation and semiquantitation of bacterial colonies. **B,** Actual plates show sparse, or 1+ bacterial growth that is limited to the first quadrant. **C,** Moderate, or 2+ bacterial growth that extends to the second quadrant. **D,** Heavy, or 3+ to 4+ bacterial growth that extends to the fourth quadrant.

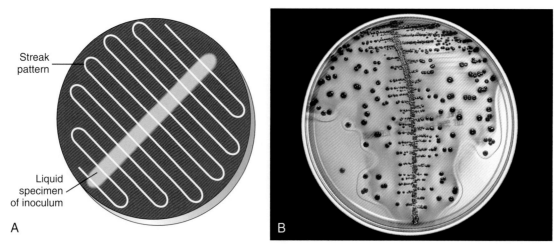

**Figure 7-10 A,** Streaking pattern using a calibrated loop for enumeration of bacterial colonies grown from a liquid specimen such as urine. **B,** Actual plate shows well-isolated and dispersed bacterial colonies for enumeration obtained with the calibrated loop streaking technique.

**TABLE 7-2** Semi-Quantitation Grading Procedure for Bacterial Isolates on Growth Media

| | NUMBER OF COLONIES VISIBLE IN EACH QUADRANT | | | |
|---|---|---|---|---|
| Score | #1 (Initial Quadrant) | #2 | #3 | #4 |
| 1+ | Less than 10 | | | |
| 2+ | Less than 10 | Less than 10 | | |
| 3+ | Greater than 10 | Greater than 10 | Less than 10 | |
| 4+ | Greater than 10 | Greater than 10 | Greater than 10 | Greater than 5 |

Note: This is a general guideline. Individual laboratories may vary in the methods used for quantitation.

bacterial pathogens. In other words, the media selected for growth is a clue to the type of organism isolated (e.g., growth on MacConkey agar indicates the organism is most likely a gram-negative bacillus). Yeast and some gram-positive cocci are capable of limited growth on MacConkey agar. The incubation conditions that support growth may also be a preliminary indicator of which bacteria have been isolated (e.g., aerobic versus anaerobic bacteria).

**Relative Quantities of Each Colony Type.** The predominance of a bacterial isolate is often used as one of the criteria, along with direct smear results, organism virulence, and the body site from which the culture was obtained, for establishing the organism's clinical significance. Several methods are used for semiquantitation of bacterial quantities including many, moderate, few or a numerical designation (4+, 3+, 2+) based on the number of colonies identified in each streak area (Table 7-2).

**Colony Characteristics.** Noting key features of a bacterial colony is important for any bacterial identification;

success or failure of subsequent identification procedures often depends on the accuracy of these observations. Criteria frequently used to characterize bacterial growth include the following:
- Colony size (usually measured in millimeters or described in relative terms such as pinpoint, small, medium, large)
- Colony pigmentation
- Colony shape (includes form, elevation, and margin of the colony [Figure 7-11])
- Colony surface appearance (e.g., glistening, opaque, dull, dry, transparent)
- Changes in agar media resulting from bacterial growth (e.g., hemolytic pattern on blood agar, changes in color of pH indicators, pitting of the agar surface; for examples, see Figures 7-3 through 7-8)
- Odor (certain bacteria produce distinct odors that can be helpful in preliminary identification)

Many of these criteria are somewhat subjective, and the adjectives and descriptive terms used may vary among different laboratories. Regardless of the terminology used, nearly every laboratory's protocol for bacterial identification begins with some agreed-upon colony description of the commonly encountered pathogens.

Although careful determination of colony appearance is important, it is unwise to place total confidence on colony morphology for preliminary identification. Bacteria of one species often exhibit colony characteristics that are nearly indistinguishable from those of many other species. Additionally, bacteria of the same species exhibit morphologic diversity. For example, certain colony characteristics may be typical of a given species, but different strains of that species may have different morphologies.

**Gram Stain and Subcultures.** Isolation of individual colonies during cultivation not only is important for examining morphologies and characteristics but also is necessary for timely performance of Gram stains and subcultures.

The Gram stain and microscopic evaluation of cultured bacteria are used with colony morphology to decide which identification steps are needed. To avoid

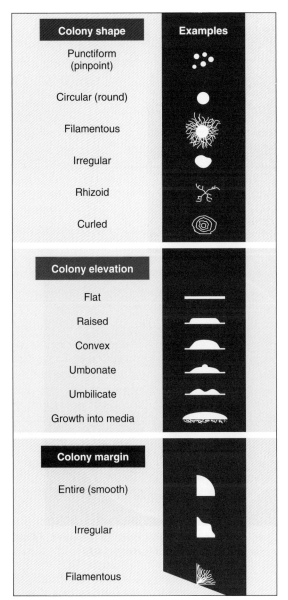

| Colony shape | Examples |
|---|---|
| Punctiform (pinpoint) | |
| Circular (round) | |
| Filamentous | |
| Irregular | |
| Rhizoid | |
| Curled | |

| Colony elevation | |
|---|---|
| Flat | |
| Raised | |
| Convex | |
| Umbonate | |
| Umbilicate | |
| Growth into media | |

| Colony margin | |
|---|---|
| Entire (smooth) | |
| Irregular | |
| Filamentous | |

**Figure 7-11** Colony morphologic features and descriptive terms for commonly encountered bacterial colonies.

confusion, organisms from a single colony are stained. In many instances, staining must be performed on all different colony morphologies observed on the primary plate. In other cases, staining may not be necessary because growth on a particular selective agar provides dependable evidence of the organism's Gram stain morphology (e.g., gram-negative bacilli essentially are the only clinically relevant bacteria that grow well on Mac-Conkey agar).

Following characterization of growth on primary plating media, all subsequent procedures for definitive identification require the use of pure cultures (i.e., cultures containing one strain of a single species). If sufficient inocula for testing can be obtained from the primary media, then a subculture is not necessary, except as a precaution to obtain more of the etiologic agent if needed and to ensure that a pure inoculum has been

used for subsequent tests (i.e., a "purity" check). However, frequently the primary media do not yield sufficient amounts of bacteria in pure culture and a subculture step is required (Figure 7-12).

Using a sterile loop, a portion of an isolated colony is taken and transferred to the surface of a suitable enrichment medium that is then incubated under conditions optimal for the organism. When making transfers for subculture, it is beneficial to flame the inoculating loop between streaks to each area on the agar surface. This avoids over inoculation of the subculture media and ensures individual colonies will be obtained. Once a pure culture is available in a sufficient amount, an inoculum for subsequent identification procedures can be prepared.

## PRINCIPLES OF IDENTIFICATION

Microbiologists use various methods to identify organisms cultivated from patient specimens. Although many of the principles and issues associated with bacterial identification discussed in this chapter are generally applicable to most clinically relevant bacteria, specific information regarding particular organism groups is covered in the appropriate chapters in Part III.

The importance of accurate bacterial identification cannot be overstated because identity is central to diagnostic bacteriology issues, including the following:

- Determining the clinical significance of a particular pathogen (e.g., is the isolate a pathogen or a contaminant?)
- Guiding physician care of the patient
- Determining whether laboratory testing for detection of antimicrobial resistance is warranted
- Determining the type of antimicrobial therapy that is appropriate
- Determining whether the antimicrobial susceptibility profiles are unusual or aberrant for a particular bacterial species
- Determining whether the infecting organism is a risk for other patients in the hospital, the public, or laboratory workers (i.e., is the organism one that may pose problems for infection control, public health, or laboratory safety?)
- Collecting epidemiologic data to monitor the control and transmission of organisms

The identification of a bacterial isolate requires analysis of information gathered from laboratory tests that provide characteristic profiles of bacteria. The tests and the order in which they are used for organism identification are often referred to as an identification scheme. Identification schemes can be classified into one of two categories: (1) those based on genotypic characteristics of bacteria and (2) those based on phenotypic characteristics. Certain schemes rely on both genotypic and phenotypic characteristics. Additionally, some tests, such as the Gram stain, are an integral part of many schemes used for identifying a wide variety of bacteria, whereas other tests may only be used in the identification scheme for a single species such as the fluorescent antibody test for identification of *Legionella pneumophila*.

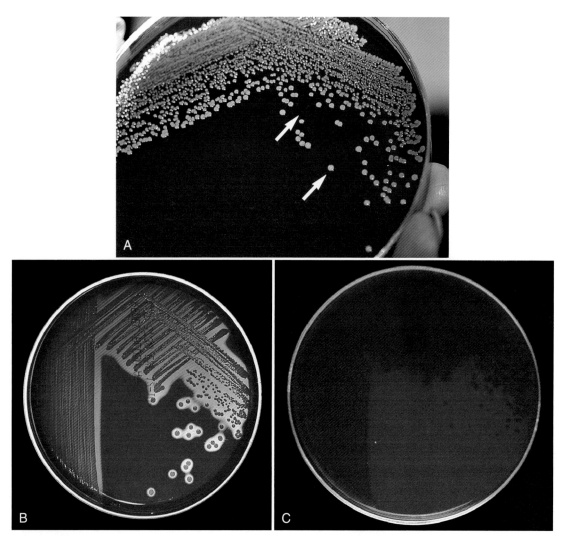

**Figure 7-12** Mixed bacterial culture on sheep blood agar **(A)** requires subculture of individually distinct colonies (*arrows*) to obtain pure cultures of *Staphylococcus aureus* (beta hemolysis evident) **(B)** and *Streptococcus pneumoniae* (alpha hemolytic) **(C)**.

## ORGANISM IDENTIFICATION USING GENOTYPIC CRITERIA

Genotypic identification methods involve characterization of some portion of a bacterium's genome using molecular techniques for DNA or RNA analysis. This usually involves detecting the presence of a gene, or a part thereof, or an RNA product that is specific for a particular organism. In principle, the presence of a specific gene or a particular nucleic acid sequence unique to the organism is interpreted as a definitive identification of the organism. The genotypic approach is highly specific and often very sensitive. Specificity refers to the percentage of patients without disease that will test negative for the presence of the organism. Sensitivity indicates the percentage of patients in whom the organism is present who actually test positive. With the ever-expanding list of molecular techniques being developed, the genetic approach to organism identification will continue to grow and become more integrated into diagnostic microbiology laboratory protocols (for more information regarding molecular methods, see Chapter 8).

## ORGANISM IDENTIFICATION USING PHENOTYPIC CRITERIA

Phenotypic criteria are based on observable physical or metabolic characteristics of bacteria—that is, identification is through analysis of gene products rather than through the genes themselves. The phenotypic approach is the classic approach to bacterial identification, and most identification strategies are still based on bacterial phenotype. Other characterizations are based on the antigenic makeup of the organisms and involve techniques based on antigen-antibody interactions (for more information regarding immunologic diagnosis of infectious diseases, see Chapter 10). However, most of the phenotypic characterizations used in diagnostic bacteriology are based on tests that establish a bacterial isolate's morphology and metabolic capabilities. The most commonly used phenotypic criteria include the following:
- Microscopic morphology and staining characteristics
- Macroscopic (colony) morphology, including odor and pigmentation
- Environmental requirements for growth

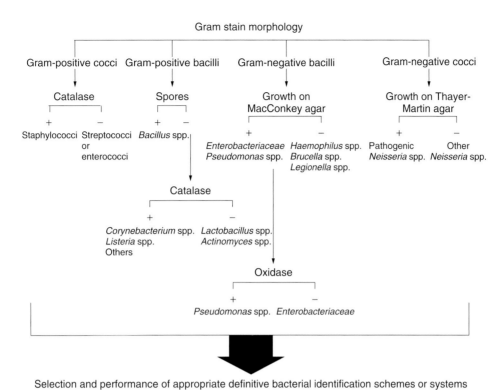

**Figure 7-13** Flowchart example of a bacterial identification scheme (not applicable to anaerobic organisms).

- Resistance or susceptibility to antimicrobial agents
- Nutritional requirements and metabolic capabilities

## Microscopic Morphology and Staining Characteristics

Microscopic evaluation of bacterial cellular morphology, as facilitated by the Gram stain or other enhancing methods discussed in Chapter 6, provides the most basic and important information on which final identification strategies are based. Based on these findings, most clinically relevant bacteria can be divided into four distinct groups: gram-positive cocci, gram-negative cocci, gram-positive bacilli, and gram-negative bacilli (Figure 7-13). Some bacterial species are morphologically indistinct and are described as "gram-negative coccobacilli," "gram-variable bacilli," or pleomorphic (i.e., exhibiting various shapes). Still other morphologies include curved or rods and spirals.

Even without staining, examination of a wet preparation of bacterial colonies under oil immersion (1000× magnification) can provide clues as to possible identity. For example, a wet preparation prepared from a translucent, alpha-hemolytic colony on blood agar may reveal cocci in chains, a strong indication that the bacteria are probably streptococci. Also, the presence of yeast, whose colonies can closely mimic bacterial colonies but whose cells are generally much larger, can be determined (Figure 7-14).

In most instances, schemes for final identification are based on the cellular morphologies and staining characteristics of bacteria. To illustrate, an abbreviated identification flowchart for commonly encountered bacteria is

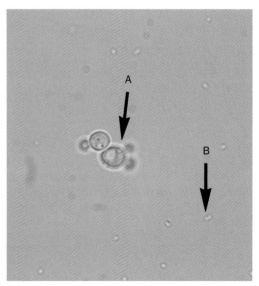

**Figure 7-14** Microscopic examination of a wet preparation demonstrates the size difference between most yeast cells, such as those of *Candida albicans* (*arrow A*), and bacteria, such as *Staphylococcus aureus* (*arrow B*).

shown in Figure 7-13 (more detailed identification schemes are presented throughout Part III); this flowchart simply illustrates how information about microorganisms is integrated into subsequent identification schemes that are based on the organism's nutritional requirements and metabolic capabilities. In certain cases, staining characteristics alone are used to definitively identify a bacterial species. Examples are mostly restricted to the use of fluorescent-labeled specific antibodies and fluorescent microscopy to identify organisms such as *Legionella pneumophila* and *Bordetella pertussis*.

## Macroscopic (Colony) Morphology

Evaluation of colony morphology includes considering colony size, shape, odor, color (pigment), surface appearance, and any changes that colony growth produces in the surrounding agar medium (e.g., hemolysis of blood in blood agar plates). A characteristic odor can be utilized in supporting an identification of an organism such as *Pseudomonas aeruginosa* described as having a fruity or grapelike smell. (Note: Smelling plates in a clinical setting can be dangerous and is strongly discouraged.)

Although these characteristics usually are not sufficient for establishing a final or definitive identification, the information gained provides preliminary information necessary for determining what identification procedures should follow. However, it is unwise to place too much confidence on colony morphology alone for preliminary identification of isolates. Microorganisms often grow as colonies whose appearance is not that different from many other species, especially if the colonies are relatively young (i.e., less than 14 hours old). Therefore, unless colony morphology is distinctive or unless growth occurs on a particular selective medium, other characteristics must be included in the identification scheme.

## Environmental Requirements for Growth

Environmental conditions required for growth can be used to supplement other identification criteria. However, as with colony morphologies, this information alone is not sufficient for establishing a final identification. The ability to grow in particular incubation atmospheres most frequently provides insight about the organism's potential identity. For example, organisms growing only in the bottom of a tube containing thioglycollate broth are not likely to be strictly aerobic bacteria, thus eliminating these types of bacteria from the list of identification possibilities. Similarly, anaerobic bacteria can be discounted in the identification schemes for organisms that grow on blood agar plates incubated in an ambient (room) atmosphere. An organism's requirement, or preference, for increased carbon dioxide concentrations can provide hints for the identification of other bacteria such as *Streptococcus pneumoniae*, *Haemophilus influenzae*, and *Neisseria gonorrhoeae*.

In addition to atmosphere, the ability to survive or even thrive in temperatures that exceed or are well below the normal body temperature of 37° C may be helpful for organism identification. The growth of *Campylobacter jejuni* at 42° C and the ability of *Yersinia enterocolitica* to survive at 0° C are two examples.

## Resistance or Susceptibility to Antimicrobial Agents

The ability of an organism to grow in the presence of certain antimicrobial agents or specific toxic substances is widely used to establish preliminary identification information. This is accomplished by using agar media supplemented with inhibitory substances or antibiotics (for examples, see Table 7-1) or by directly measuring an organism's resistance to antimicrobial agents that may be used to treat infections (for more information regarding antimicrobial susceptibility testing, see Chapter 12).

As discussed earlier in this chapter, most clinical specimens are inoculated to several media, including some selective or differential agars. Therefore, the first clue to identification of an isolated colony is the nature of the media on which the organism is growing. For example, with rare exceptions, only gram-negative bacteria grow well on MacConkey agar. Alternatively, other agar plates, such as Columbia agar with CNA, support the growth of gram-positive organisms to the exclusion of most gram-negative bacilli. Certain agar media can be used to differentiate even more precisely than simply separating gram-negative and gram-positive bacteria. Whereas chocolate agar will support the growth of all aerobic microorganisms including *Neisseria* spp., the antibiotic-supplemented Thayer-Martin formulation will almost exclusively support the growth of the pathogenic species *N. meningitidis* and *N. gonorrhoeae*.

Directly testing a bacterial isolate's susceptibility to a particular antimicrobial agent may be a very useful part of an identification scheme. Many gram-positive bacteria (with a few exceptions, such as certain Enterococci, *Lactobacillus*, *Leuconostoc*, and *Pediococcus* spp.) are susceptible to vancomycin, an antimicrobial agent that acts on the bacterial cell wall. In contrast, most clinically important gram-negative bacteria are resistant to vancomycin. Therefore, when organisms with uncertain Gram stain results are encountered, susceptibility to vancomycin can be used to help establish the organism's Gram "status." Any zone of inhibition around a vancomycin-impregnated disk after overnight incubation is usually indicative of a gram-positive bacterium (Figure 7-15). With few exceptions (e.g., certain *Chryseobacterium*, *Moraxella*, or *Acinetobacter* spp. isolates may be vancomycin susceptible), truly gram-negative bacteria are resistant to vancomycin. Conversely, most gram-negative bacteria are susceptible to the antibiotics colistin or polymyxin, whereas gram-positive bacteria are frequently resistant to these agents.

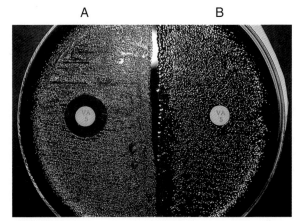

**Figure 7-15 A,** Zone of growth inhibition around the 5-μg vancomycin disk is indicative of a gram-positive bacterium. **B,** The gram-negative organism is not inhibited by this antibiotic, and growth extends to the edge of the disk.

## Nutritional Requirements and Metabolic Capabilities

Determining the nutritional and metabolic capabilities of a bacterial isolate is the most common approach used for determining the genus and species of an organism. The methods available for making these determinations share many commonalties but also have some important differences. In general, all methods use a combination of tests to establish the enzymatic capabilities of a given bacterial isolate as well as the isolate's ability to grow or survive the presence of certain inhibitors (e.g., salts, surfactants, toxins, and antibiotics).

**Establishing Enzymatic Capabilities.** As discussed in Chapter 2, enzymes are the driving force in bacterial metabolism. Because enzymes are genetically encoded, the enzymatic content of an organism is a direct reflection of the organism's genetic makeup, which, in turn, is specific for individual bacterial species.

**Types of Enzyme-Based Tests.** In diagnostic bacteriology, enzyme-based tests are designed to measure the presence of one specific enzyme or a complete metabolic pathway that may contain several different enzymes. Although the specific tests most useful for the identification of particular bacteria are discussed in Part III, some examples of tests commonly used to characterize a wide spectrum of bacteria are reviewed here.

**Single Enzyme Tests.** Several tests are commonly used to determine the presence of a single enzyme. These tests usually provide rapid results because they can be performed on organisms already grown in culture. Of importance, these tests are easy to perform and interpret and often play a key role in the identification scheme. Although most single enzyme tests do not yield sufficient information to provide species identification, they are used extensively to determine which subsequent identification steps should be followed. For example, the catalase test can provide pivotal information and is commonly used in schemes for gram-positive identifications. The oxidase test is of comparable importance in identification schemes for gram-negative bacteria (see Figure 7-13).

**Catalase Test.** The enzyme catalase catalyzes the release of water and oxygen from hydrogen peroxide ($H_2O_2$ + catalase => $H_2O$ + $O_2$); its presence is determined by direct analysis of a bacterial culture (see Procedure 13-8). The rapid production of bubbles (effervescence) when bacterial growth is mixed with a hydrogen peroxide solution is interpreted as a positive test (i.e., the presence of catalase). Failure to produce effervescence or weak effervescence is interpreted as negative. If the bacterial inoculum is inadvertently contaminated with red blood cells when the test inoculum is collected from a sheep blood agar plate, weak production of bubbles may occur, but this should not be interpreted as a positive test.

Because the catalase test is key to the identification scheme of many gram-positive organisms, interpretation must be done carefully. For example, staphylococci are catalase-positive, whereas streptococci and enterococci are negative; similarly, the catalase reaction differentiates *Listeria monocytogenes* and corynebacteria (catalase-positive) from other gram-positive, non–spore-forming bacilli (see Figure 7-13).

**Oxidase Test.** Cytochrome oxidase participates in electron transport and in the nitrate metabolic pathways of certain bacteria. Testing for the presence of oxidase can be performed by flooding bacterial colonies on the agar surface with 1% tetramethyl-p-phenylenediamine dihydrochloride. Alternatively, a sample of the bacterial colony can be rubbed onto filter paper impregnated with the reagent (see Procedure 13-33). A positive reaction is indicated by the development of a purple color. If an iron-containing wire is used to transfer growth, a false-positive reaction may result; therefore, platinum wire or wooden sticks are recommended. Certain organisms may show slight positive reactions after the initial 10 seconds have passed; such results are not considered definitive.

The test is initially used for differentiating between groups of gram-negative bacteria. Among the commonly encountered gram-negative bacilli, *Enterobacteriaceae*, *Stenotrophomonas maltophilia*, and *Acinetobacter* spp. are oxidase-negative, whereas many other bacilli, such as *Pseudomonas* spp. and *Aeromonas* spp., are positive (see Figure 7-13). The oxidase test is also a key reaction for the identification of *Neisseria* spp. (oxidase-positive).

**Indole Test.** Bacteria that produce the enzyme tryptophanase are able to degrade the amino acid tryptophan into pyruvic acid, ammonia, and indole. Indole is detected by combining with an indicator, aldehyde ([4-dimethylamino] benzaldehyde, hydrochloric acid, and penta-1-01, also referred to as Kovac's), which results in a blue color formation (see Procedure 13-20). This test is used in numerous identification schemes, especially to presumptively identify *Escherichia coli*, the gram-negative bacillus most commonly encountered in diagnostic bacteriology.

**Urease Test.** Urease hydrolyzes the substrate urea into ammonia, water, and carbon dioxide. The presence of the enzyme is determined by inoculating an organism to broth or agar containing urea as the primary carbon source followed by detecting the production of ammonia (see Procedure 13-41). Ammonia increases the pH of the medium so its presence is readily detected using a pH indicator. Change in medium pH is a common indicator of metabolic process and, because pH indicators change color with increases (alkalinity) or decreases (acidity) in the medium's pH, they are commonly used in many identification test schemes. The urease test helps identify certain species of *Enterobacteriaceae*, such as *Proteus* spp., and other important bacteria such as *Corynebacterium urealyticum* and *Helicobacter pylori*.

**PYR Test.** The enzyme L-pyrroglutamyl-aminopeptidase hydrolyzes the substrate L-pyrrolidonyl-β-naphthylamide (PYR) to produce a β-naphthylamine. When the β-naphthylamine combines with a cinnamaldehyde reagent, a bright red color is produced (see Procedure 13-36). The PYR test is particularly helpful in identifying gram-positive cocci such as *Streptococcus pyogenes* and *Enterococcus* spp., which are positive, whereas other streptococci are negative.

**Hippurate Hydrolysis.** Hippuricase is a constitutive enzyme that hydrolyzes the substrate hippurate to produce the amino acid glycine. Glycine is detected by oxidation with Ninhydrin reagent, which results in the production of a deep purple color (see Procedure 13-19). The hippurate test is most frequently used in the

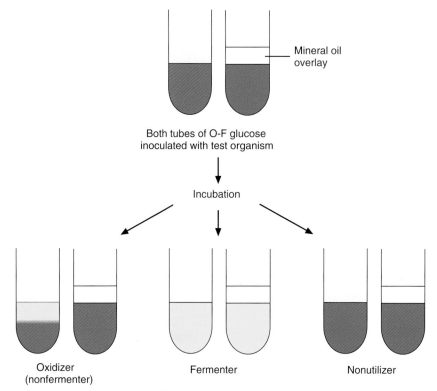

Both tubes of O-F glucose
inoculated with test organism

Incubation

Oxidizer
(nonfermenter)    Fermenter    Nonutilizer

**Figure 7-16** Principle of glucose oxidative-fermentation (O-F) test. Fermentation patterns shown in O-F tubes including examples of oxidative, fermentative, and nonutilizing bacteria.

identification of *Gardnerella vaginalis, Streptococcus agalactiae, Campylobacter jejuni,* and *Listeria monocytogenes.*

**Tests for Presence of Metabolic Pathways.** Several identification schemes are based on determining what metabolic pathways an organism uses and the substrates processed by these pathways. In contrast to single enzyme tests, these pathways may involve several interactive enzymes. The presence of an end product resulting from these interactions is measured in the testing system. Assays for metabolic pathways can be classified into three general categories: carbohydrate oxidation and fermentation, amino acid degradation, and single substrate utilizations.

**Oxidation and Fermentation Tests.** As discussed in Chapter 2, bacteria use various metabolic pathways to produce biochemical building blocks and energy. For most clinically relevant bacteria, this involves utilization of carbohydrates (e.g., sugar or sugar derivatives) and protein substrates. Determining whether substrate utilization is an oxidative or fermentative process is important for the identification of several different bacteria.

Oxidative processes require oxygen; fermentative ones do not. The clinical laboratory determines how an organism utilizes a substrate by observing whether acid byproducts are produced in the presence or absence of oxygen. In most instances, the presence of acid byproducts is detected by a change in the pH indicator incorporated into the medium. The color changes that occur in the presence of acid depend on the type of pH indicator used.

Oxidation-fermentation determinations are usually accomplished using a special semi-solid medium

(oxidative-fermentative [O-F] medium) that contains low concentrations of peptone and a single carbohydrate substrate such as glucose. The organism to be identified is inoculated into two glucose O-F tubes, one of which is then overlaid with mineral oil as a barrier to oxygen. Common pH indicators used for O-F tests, and the color changes they undergo with acidic conditions, include bromcresol purple, which changes from purple to yellow; Andrade's acid fuchsin indicator, which changes from pale yellow to pink; phenol red, which changes from red to yellow; and bromthymol blue, which changes from green to yellow.

As shown in Figure 7-16, when acid production is detected in both tubes, the organism is identified as a glucose fermenter because fermentation can occur with or without oxygen. If acid is only detected in the open, aerobic tube, the organism is characterized as a glucose-oxidizer. As a third possibility, some bacteria do not use glucose as a substrate and no acid is detected in either tube (a nonutilizer). The glucose fermentative or oxidative capacity is generally used to separate organisms into major groups (e.g., *Enterobacteriaceae* are fermentative; *Pseudomonas* spp. are oxidative). However, the utilization pattern for several other carbohydrates (e.g., lactose, sucrose, xylose, maltose) is often needed to help identify an organism's genus and species.

**Amino Acid Degradation.** Determining the ability of bacteria to produce enzymes that either deaminate, dihydrolyze, or decarboxylate certain amino acids is often used in identification schemes. The amino acid substrates most often tested include lysine, tyrosine, ornithine, arginine, and phenylalanine. (The indole test for tryptophan cleavage is presented earlier in this chapter.)

Decarboxylases cleave the carboxyl group from amino acids so that amino acids are converted into amines; lysine is converted to cadaverine, and ornithine is converted to putrescine. Because amines increase medium pH, they are readily detected by color changes in a pH indictor indicative of alkalinity. Decarboxylation is an anaerobic process that requires an acid environment for activation. The most common medium used for this test is Moeller decarboxylase base, whose components include glucose, the amino acid substrate of interest (i.e., lysine, ornithine, or arginine), and a pH indicator.

Organisms are inoculated into the tube medium that is then overlaid with mineral oil to ensure anaerobic conditions (see Chapter 13). Early during incubation, bacteria utilize the glucose and produce acid, resulting in a yellow coloration of the pH indicator. Organisms that can decarboxylate the amino acid then begin to attack the substrate and produce the amine product, which increases the pH and changes the indicator back from yellow to purple (if bromcresol purple is the pH indicator used; red if phenol red is the indicator). Therefore, after overnight incubation, a positive test is indicated by a purple color and a negative test (i.e., lack of decarboxylase activity) is indicated by a yellow color. With each amino acid tested, a control tube of the glucose-containing broth base without amino acid is inoculated. The standard's (control) color is compared with that of the tube containing the amino acid following incubation.

Because it is a two-step process, the breakdown of arginine is more complicated than lysine or ornithine. Arginine is first dehydrolyzed to citrulline, which is subsequently converted to ornithine. Ornithine is then decarboxylated to putrescine, which results in the same pH indicator changes as just outlined for the other amino acids.

Unlike decarboxylation, deamination of the amino acid phenylalanine occurs in air. The presence of the end product (phenylpyruvic acid) is detected by the addition of 10% ferric chloride, which results in the development of a green color. Agar slant medium is commercially available for this test.

Lysine iron agar media is a combination media utilized for the identification of decarboxylation and deamination in a single tube. Dextrose is incorporated in the media in a limited concentration of 0.1%. The organism is then stabbed into the media approximately within 3 mm above the bottom of the tube. When removing the inoculating needle from the stab, the slant of the medium is streaked. Organisms capable of dextrose fermentation will produce acid resulting in a yellow butt. Organisms that decarboxylate lysine will produce alkaline products that will return the yellow color to the original purple color of the media. Hydrogen sulfide–positive organisms produce gas that reacts with iron salts, ferrous sulfate, and ferric ammonium citrate in the media, producing a black precipitate. It is important to note that *Proteus* spp. are capable of deaminating lysine in the presence of oxygen, resulting in a red color change on the slant of the medium.

**Single Substrate Utilization.** Whether an organism can grow in the presence of a single nutrient or carbon source provides useful identification information. Such tests entail inoculating organisms to a medium that contains a single source of nutrition (e.g., citrate, malonate, or acetate) and, after incubation, observing the medium for growth. Growth is determined by observing the presence of bacterial colonies or by using a pH indicator to detect end products of metabolic activity.

**Establishing Inhibitor Profiles.** The ability of a bacterial isolate to grow in the presence of one or more inhibitory substances can provide valuable identification information. Examples regarding the use of inhibitory substances are presented earlier in this chapter.

In addition to the information gained from using inhibitory media or antimicrobial susceptibility testing, other more specific tests may be incorporated into bacterial identification schemes. Because most of these tests are used to identify a particular group of bacteria, their protocols and principles are discussed in the appropriate chapters in Part III. A few examples of such tests include the following:
- Growth in the presence of various NaCl concentrations (identification of *Enterococci* and *Vibrio* spp.)
- Susceptibility to Optochin and solubility in bile (identification of *Streptococcus pneumoniae*)
- Ability to hydrolyze esculin in the presence of bile (identification of *Enterococci* spp. in combination with NaCl)
- Ethanol survival (identification of Bacillus spp.)

# PRINCIPLES OF PHENOTYPE-BASED IDENTIFICATION SCHEMES

As shown in Figure 7-13, growth characteristics, microscopic morphologies, and single test results are used to categorize most bacterial isolates into general groups. However, the definitive identification to species requires use of schemes designed to produce metabolic profiles of the organisms. Identification systems usually consist of four major components (Figure 7-17):
- Selection and inoculation of a set (i.e., battery) of specific metabolic substrates and growth inhibitors
- Incubation to allow substrate utilization to occur or to allow growth inhibitors to act
- Determination of metabolic activity that occurred during incubation
- Analysis of metabolic profiles and comparison with established profile databases for known bacterial species to establish definitive identification

## SELECTION AND INOCULATION OF IDENTIFICATION TEST BATTERY

The number and types of tests that are selected for inclusion in a battery depends on various factors, including the type of bacteria to be identified, the clinical significance of the bacterial isolate, and the availability of reliable testing methods.

1. Selection and inoculation of tests

- Number and type of tests selected depend on type of organism to be identified, clinical significance of isolates, and availability of reliable methods
- Identification systems must be inoculated with pure cultures

2. Incubation for substrate utilization

- Duration depends on whether bacterial multiplication is or is not required for substrate utilization (i.e., growth-based test vs. a non–growth-based test)

3. Detection of metabolic activity (substrate utilization)

- Colorimetry, fluorescence, or turbidity are used to detect products of substrate utilization
- Detection is done visually or with the aid of various photometers

4. Analysis of metabolic profiles

- Involves conversion of substrate utilization profile to a numeric code (see Figure 7-18)
- Computer-assisted comparison of numeric code with extensive taxonomic data base provides most likely identification of the bacterial isolate
- For certain organisms for which identification is based on a few tests, extensive testing and analysis are not routinely needed

**Figure 7-17** Four basic components of bacterial identification schemes and systems.

### Type of Bacteria to Be Identified

Certain organisms have such unique features that relatively few tests are required to establish identity. For example, *Staphylococcus aureus* is essentially the only gram-positive coccus that appears microscopically in clusters, is catalase-positive, and produces coagulase. Therefore, identification of this common pathogen usually requires the use of only two tests coupled with colony and microscopic morphology. In contrast, identification of most clinically relevant gram-negative bacilli, such as those of the Enterobacteriaceae family, requires establishing metabolic profiles often involving 20 or more tests.

### Clinical Significance of the Bacterial Isolate

Although a relatively large number of tests may be required to identify a particular bacterial species, the number of tests actually inoculated may depend on the clinical significance of an isolate. For instance, if a gram-negative bacillus is mixed with five other bacterial species in a urine culture, it is likely to be a contaminant. In this setting, multiple tests to establish species identity are not

warranted and should not routinely be performed. However, if this same organism is isolated in pure culture from cerebrospinal fluid, the full battery of tests required for definitive identification should be performed.

### Availability of Reliable Testing Methods

Because of an increasing population of immunocompromised patients and the increasing multitude of complicated medical procedures, isolation of uncommon or unusual bacteria is occurring more frequently. Because of the unusual nature exhibited by some of these bacteria, reliable testing methods and identification criteria may not be established in most clinical laboratories. In these instances, only the genus of the organism may be identified (e.g., *Bacillus* spp.), or identification may not go beyond a description of the organism's microscopic morphology (e.g., gram-positive, pleomorphic bacilli, or gram-variable, branching organism). When such bacteria are encountered and are thought to be clinically significant, they should be sent to a reference laboratory whose personnel are experienced in identifying unusual organisms.

Although the number of tests included in an identification battery may vary and different identification systems may require various inoculation techniques, the one common feature of all systems is the requirement for inoculation with a pure culture. Inoculation with a mixture of bacteria produces mixed and often uninterpretable results. To expedite identification, cultivation strategies (described earlier in this chapter) should focus on obtaining pure cultures as soon as possible. Furthermore, positive and negative controls should be ran in parallel with most identification systems as a check for purity of the culture used to inoculate the system.

## INCUBATION FOR SUBSTRATE UTILIZATION

The time required to obtain bacterial identification depends heavily on the length of incubation needed before the test result is available. In turn, the duration of incubation depends on whether the test is measuring metabolic activity that requires bacterial growth or whether the assay is measuring the presence of a particular enzyme or cellular product that can be detected without the need for bacterial growth.

### Conventional Identification

Because the generation time (i.e., the time required for a bacterial population to double) for most clinically relevant bacteria is 20 to 30 minutes, growth-based tests usually require hours of incubation before the presence of an end product can be measured. Many conventional identification schemes require 18 to 24 hours of incubation, or longer, before the tests can be accurately interpreted. Although the conventional approach has been the standard for most bacterial identification schemes, the desire to produce results and identifications in a more timely fashion has resulted in the development of rapid identification strategies.

### Rapid Identification

In the context of diagnostic bacteriology, the term *rapid* is relative. In some instances a rapid method is one that provides a result the same day that the test was inoculated. Alternatively, the definition may be more precise, whereby *rapid* is only used to describe tests that provide results within 4 hours of inoculation. It is important to note that rapid identification still requires overnight incubation of culture media from the primary specimen. Pure culture isolates grown on culture media are required for use in rapid identification systems.

Two general approaches have been developed to obtain more rapid identification results. One has been to vary the conventional testing approach by decreasing the test substrate medium volume and increasing the concentration of bacteria in the inoculum. Several conventional methods, such as carbohydrate fermentation profiles, use this strategy for more rapid results.

The second approach uses unique or unconventional substrates. Particular substrates are chosen, based on their ability to detect enzymatic activity at all times. That is, detection of the enzyme does not depend on multiplication of the organism (i.e., not a growth-based test) so that delays caused by depending on bacterial growth

are minimized. The catalase, oxidase, and PYR tests discussed previously are examples of such tests, but many others are available as part of commercial testing batteries.

Still other rapid identification schemes are based on antigen-antibody reactions, such as latex agglutination tests, that are commonly used to quickly and easily identify certain beta-hemolytic streptococci and S. *aureus* (for more information regarding these test formats, see Chapter 10).

### Matrix-Assisted Laser Desorption Ionization Time of Flight Mass Spectrometry (MALDI-TOF)

MALDI-TOF is an advanced chemical technique that uses laser excitation to ionize chemical functional groups that are included in the proteins of an organism. MALDI-TOF has the potential to significantly reduce turnaround time and identification rates, while at the same time reducing the cost of consumables in the microbiology laboratory. The organism is either applied directly onto a plate from a pure culture or prepared as a protein extract prior to application. The sample is then mixed with a chemical matrix. The laser is applied to the sample and the matrix absorbs the energy transferring heat to the sample proteins and creating ions, this is essentially the desorption and ionization process. These ions are then separated in a tube referred to as a flight tube. The lighter the ions, the faster they will travel in the tube. The ions are then measured using a detector, and a protein spectrum for the specific organism is then created as a mass spectrum using a mass-to-charge ratio and signal intensity. Typically the proteins that are detected efficiently would include small relatively abundant proteins such as ribosomal proteins. This new organism protein profile can then be compared to other organisms included in a computerized database. As of this writing, there are a few commercially available MALDI-TOF systems including MALDI Biotyper (Bruker Daltonics Inc, Fremont, CA) and Vitek MS (BioMerieux, Etoile France). However, clinical identification of microorganisms including bacteria, fungi, and viruses is limited to the size of the current data base. The technique is also limited to the identification of organisms following pure colony isolation and is not useful on specimens containing contaminating microbiota or multiple species. More clinical data are needed before this technique becomes widely accepted within the microbiology laboratory.

## DETECTION OF METABOLIC ACTIVITY

The accuracy of an identification scheme heavily depends on the ability to reliably detect whether a bacterial isolate has utilized the substrates composing the identification battery. The sensitivity and strength of the detection signal can also contribute to how rapidly results are available. No matter how quickly an organism may metabolize a particular substrate, if the end products are slowly or weakly detected, the ultimate production of results will still be "slow."

Detection strategies for determining the end products of different metabolic pathways use one of the following: colorimetry, fluorescence, or turbidity.

## Colorimetry

Several identification systems measure color change to detect the presence of metabolic end products. Most frequently the color change is produced using pH indicators included in the media. Depending on the byproducts to be measured and the testing method, additional reagents may need to be added to the reaction before the results are interpreted. An alternative to the use of pH indicators is the oxidation-reduction potential indicator tetrazolium violet. Organisms are inoculated into wells that contain a single, utilizable carbon source. Metabolism of that substrate generates electrons that reduce the tetrazolium violet, producing a purple color (positive reaction) that can be spectrophotometrically detected. In a third approach, the substrates themselves may be chromogenic so that when they are "broken down" by the organism, the altered substrate produces a color.

Some commercial systems use a miniaturized modification of conventional biochemical batteries, with the color change being detectable with the unaided eye. Alternatively, in certain automated systems, a photoelectric cell measures the change in the wavelength of light transmitted through miniaturized growth cuvettes or wells, thus eliminating the need for direct visual interpretation by laboratory personnel. Additionally, a complex combination of dyes and filters may be used to enhance and broaden the scope of substrates and color changes that can be used in such systems. These combinations hasten identification and increase the variety of organisms that can be reliably identified.

## Fluorescence

There are two basic strategies for using fluorescence to measure metabolic activity. In one approach, substrate-fluorophore complexes are used. If a bacterial isolate processes the substrate, the fluorophore is released and assumes a fluorescent configuration. Alternatively, pH changes resulting from metabolic activity can be measured by changes in fluorescence of certain fluorophore markers. In these pH-driven, fluorometric reactions, pH changes result in either the fluorophore becoming fluorescent or, in other instances, fluorescence being quenched or lost. To detect fluorescence, ultraviolet light of appropriate wavelength is focused on the reaction mixture and a special kind of photometer, a fluorometer, measures fluorescence.

## Turbidity

Turbidity measurements are not commonly used for bacterial identifications but do have widespread application for determining growth in the presence of specific growth inhibitors, including antimicrobial agents, and for detecting bacteria present in certain clinical specimens.

Turbidity is the ability of particles in suspension to refract and deflect light rays passing through the suspension such that the light is reflected back into the eyes of the observer. The optical density (OD), a measurement of turbidity, is determined in a spectrophotometer. This instrument compares the amount of light that passes through the suspension (the percent transmittance) with the amount of light that passes through a control suspension without particles. A photoelectric sensor, or photometer, converts the light that impinges on its surface to an electrical impulse, which can be quantified. A second type of turbidity measurement is obtained by nephelometry or light scatter. In this case, the photometers are placed at angles to the suspension, and the scattered light, generated by a laser or incandescent bulb, is measured. The amount of light scattered depends on the number and size of the particles in suspension.

## ANALYSIS OF METABOLIC PROFILES

The metabolic profile obtained with a particular bacterial isolate is essentially the phenotypic fingerprint, or signature, of that organism. Typically, the profile is recorded as a series of pluses (+) for positive reactions and minuses (−) for negative or nonreactions (Figure 7-18). Although this profile by itself provides little information, microbiologists can compare the profile with an extensive identification database to establish the identity of that specific isolate.

## Identification Databases

Reference databases are available for clinical use. These databases are maintained by manufacturers of identification systems and are based on the continuously updated taxonomic status of clinically relevant bacteria. Although microbiologists typically do not establish and maintain their own databases, an overview of the general approach provides background information.

The first step in developing a database is to accumulate many bacterial strains of the same species. Each strain is inoculated to an identical battery of metabolic tests to generate a positive-negative test profile. The cumulative results of each test are expressed as a percentage of each genus or species that possesses that characteristic. For example, suppose that 100 different known *E. coli* strains and 100 known *Shigella* spp. strains are tested in four biochemicals, yielding the results illustrated in Table 7-3. In reality, many more strains and tests would be performed. However, the principle—to generate a database for each species that contains the percentage probability for a positive result with each test in the battery—is the same.

Manufacturers develop databases for each of the identification systems they produce for diagnostic use (e.g., *Enterobacteriaceae*, gram-positive cocci, nonfermentative gram-negative bacilli). Because the data are based on organism "behavior" in a particular commercial system, the databases cannot and should not be applied to interpret profiles obtained by other testing methods.

**TABLE 7-3** Generation and Use of Genus-Identification Database Probability: Percentage of Positive Reactions for 100 Known Strains

| Organism | BIOCHEMICAL PARAMETER | | | |
| | Lactose | Sucrose | Indole | Ornithine |
|---|---|---|---|---|
| *Escherichia* | 91 | 49 | 99 | 63 |
| *Shigella* | 1 | 1 | 38 | 20 |

| Test/ substrate | Test results (− or +) | Binary code conversion (0 or 1) | Octal code conversion* ||||
|---|---|---|---|---|---|---|
|  |  |  | Octal value | Octal score | Octal triplet total | Octal profile |
| 1 ONPG | + | 1 | × 1 | 1 |  |  |
| 2 Arginine dihydrolase | − | 0 | × 2 | 0 | 5 |  |
| 3 Lysine decarboxylase | + | 1 | × 4 | 4 |  |  |
| 4 Ornithine decarboxylase | + | 1 | × 1 | 1 |  |  |
| 5 Citrate utilization | − | 0 | × 2 | 0 | 1 |  |
| 6 H$_2$S production | − | 0 | × 4 | 0 |  |  |
| 7 Urea hydrolysis | − | 0 | × 1 | 0 |  |  |
| 8 Tryptophane deaminase | − | 0 | × 2 | 0 | 4 |  |
| 9 Indole production | + | 1 | × 4 | 4 |  |  |
| 10 VP test | − | 0 | × 1 | 0 |  |  |
| 11 Gelatin hydrolysis | − | 0 | × 2 | 0 | 4 | 5144572 (*E. coli*) |
| 12 Glucose fermentation | + | 1 | × 4 | 4 |  |  |
| 13 Mannitol fermentation | + | 1 | × 1 | 1 |  |  |
| 14 Inositol fermentation | − | 0 | × 2 | 0 | 5 |  |
| 15 Sorbitol fermentation | + | 1 | × 4 | 4 |  |  |
| 16 Rhamnose fermentation | + | 1 | × 1 | 1 |  |  |
| 17 Sucrose fermentation | + | 1 | × 2 | 2 | 7 |  |
| 18 Melibiose fermentation | + | 1 | × 4 | 4 |  |  |
| 19 Amygdalin fermentation | − | 0 | × 1 | 0 |  |  |
| 20 Arabinose fermentation | + | 1 | × 2 | 2 | 2 |  |
| 21 Oxidase production | − | 0 | × 4 | 0 |  |  |

*As derived from API 20E (bioMérieux, Inc.) for identification of *Enterobacteriaceae*.

**Figure 7-18** Example of converting a metabolic profile to an octal profile for bacterial identification.

Furthermore, most databases are established with the assumption that the isolate to be identified has been appropriately characterized using adjunctive tests. For example, if a *S. aureus* isolate is mistakenly tested using a system for identification of *Enterobacteriaceae*, the database will not identify the gram-positive cocci because the results obtained will only be compared with data available for enteric bacilli. This underscores the importance of accurately performing preliminary tests and observations, such as colony and Gram stain morphologies, before selecting a particular identification battery.

### Use of the Database to Identify Unknown Isolates

Once a metabolic profile has been obtained with a bacterial isolate of unknown identity, the profile must be converted to a numeric code that will facilitate comparison of the unknown's phenotypic fingerprint with the appropriate database.

To exemplify this step in the identification process, a binary code conversion system that uses the numerals 0 and 1 to represent negative and positive metabolic reactions, respectively, is used as an example (although other strategies are now used). As shown in Figure 7-18, using binary code conversion, a 21-digit binomial number (e.g., 101100001001101111010, as read from top to bottom in the figure) is produced from the test result. This number is then used in an octal code conversion scheme to produce a mathematic number (octal profile [see Figure 7-18]). The octal profile number is used to generate a numerical profile distinctly related to a specific bacterial species. As shown in Figure 7-18, the octal profile for the unknown organism is 5144572. This

profile would then be compared with database profiles to determine the most likely identity of the organism. In this example, the octal profile indicates the unknown organism is *E. coli*.

**Confidence in Identification.** Once metabolic profiles have been translated into numeric scores, the probability that a correct correlation with the database has been made must be established—that is, how confident can the laboratorian be that the identification is correct. This is accomplished by establishing the percentage probability, which is usually provided as part of most commercially available identification database schemes.

For example, unknown organism X is tested against the four biochemicals listed in Table 7-3 and yields results as follows: lactose (+), sucrose (+), indole (−), and ornithine (+). Based on the results of each test, the percentage of known strains in the database that produced positive results are used to calculate the percentage probability that strain X is a member of one of the two genera (*Escherichia* or *Shigella*) given in the example (Table 7-4). Therefore, if 91% of *Escherichia* spp. are lactose-positive (see Table 7-3), the probability that X is a species of *Escherichia* based on lactose alone is 0.91. If 38% of *Shigella* spp. are indole positive (see Table 7-3), then the probability that X is a species of *Shigella* based on indole alone is 0.62 (1.00 [all *Shigella*] − 0.38 [percent positive *Shigella*] = 0.62 [percent of all *Shigella* that are indole negative]). The probabilities of the individual tests are then multiplied to achieve a calculated likelihood that X is one of these two genera. In this example, X is more likely to be a species of *Escherichia*, with a probability of 357:1 (1 divided by 0.0028; see Table 7-4). This is still a

**TABLE 7-4** Generation and Use of Genus-Identification Database Probability: Probability That Unknown Strain X Is a Member of a Known Genus Based on Results of Each Individual Parameter Tested

| Organism | BIOCHEMICAL PARAMETER | | | |
|---|---|---|---|---|
| | Lactose | Sucrose | Indole | Ornithine |
| X | + | + | − | + |
| *Escherichia* | 0.91 | 0.49 | 0.01 | 0.63 |
| *Shigella* | 0.01 | 0.01 | 0.62 | 0.20 |

Probability that X is *Escherichia* = 0.91 × 0.49 × 0.01 × 0.63 = 0.002809.
Probability that X is *Shigella* = 0.01 × 0.01 × 0.62 × 0.20 = 0.000012.

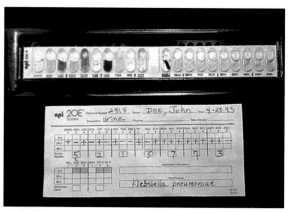

**Figure 7-19** Biochemical test panel (API; bioMérieux, Inc., Hazelwood, MO). The test results obtained with the substrates in each cupule are recorded, and an organism identification code is calculated by octal code conversion on the form provided. The octal profile obtained then is matched with an extensive database to establish organism identification.

very unlikely probability for correct identification, but only four parameters were tested, and the indole result was atypical. As more parameters are added to the formula, the importance of just one test decreases and the overall pattern prevails.

With many organisms being tested for 20 or more reactions, computer-generated databases provide the probabilities. As more organisms are included in the database, the genus and species designations and probabilities become more precise. Also, with more profiles in a data base, the unusual patterns can be more readily recognized and, in some cases, new or unusual species may be discovered.

The most common commercial suppliers of multicomponent identification systems are driven by patent information technology and data management systems that automatically provide analysis and outcome of the metabolic process and identification.

# COMMERCIAL IDENTIFICATION SYSTEMS

## ADVANTAGES AND EXAMPLES OF COMMERCIAL SYSTEM DESIGNS

Commercially available identification systems have largely replaced compilations of conventional test media and substrates prepared in-house for bacterial identification. This replacement has mostly come about because the design of commercial systems has continuously evolved to maximize the speed and optimize the convenience with which all four identification components shown in Figure 7-17 can be achieved. Because laboratory workload has increased, conventional methodologies have had difficulty competing with the advantages of convenience and updated databases offered by commercial systems. Table 13-1 lists and describes the most common manual and automated bacterial identification systems available.

Some of the simplest multi-test commercial systems consist of a conventional format that can be inoculated once to yield more than one result. By combining reactants, for example, one substrate can be used to determine indole and nitrate results; indole and motility results; motility, indole, and ornithine decarboxylase; or

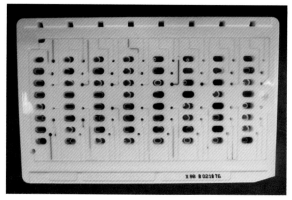

**Figure 7-20** Vitek cards composed of multiple wells containing dried substrates that are reconstituted by inoculation with a bacterial suspension (bioMérieux, Inc., Hazelwood, MO). Test results in the card wells are automatically read by the manufacturer's reading device.

other combinations. Alternatively, conventional tests have been assembled in smaller volumes and packaged so that they can be inoculated easily with one manipulation instead of several. When used in conjunction with a computer-generated database, species identifications are made relatively easily.

Another approach is to have substrates dried in plastic cupules that are arranged in series on strips into which a suspension of the test organism is placed (Figure 7-19). For some of these systems, use of a heavy inoculum or use of substrates whose utilization is not dependent on extended bacterial multiplication allows results to be available after 4 to 6 hours of incubation.

Still other identification battery formats have been designed to more fully automate several aspects of the identification process. One example is the use of "cards" that are substantially smaller than most microtiter trays or cupule strips (Figure 7-20). Analogous to the microtiter tray format, these cards contain dried substrates in tiny wells that are resuspended upon inoculation.

Commercial systems are often categorized as either automated or manual. As shown in Table 13-1, various aspects of an identification system can be automated, and these usually include, in whole or in part, the inoculation steps, the incubation and reading of tests, and the analysis of results. However, no strict criteria exist that state how many aspects must be automated for a whole system to be classified as automated. Therefore, whether a system is considered automated can be controversial. Furthermore, regardless of the lack or level of automation, the selection of an identification system ultimately depends on system accuracy and reliability, whether the system meets the needs of the laboratory, and limitations imposed by laboratory financial resources.

### Overview of Commercial Systems

Various multitest bacterial identification systems (as listed in Table 13-1) are commercially available for use in diagnostic microbiology laboratories, and the four basic identification components outlined in Figure 7-17 are common to them all. However, different systems vary in their approach to each component. The most common variations involve the following:

- Types and formats of tests included in the test battery
- Method of inoculation (manual or automated)
- Required length of incubation for substrate utilization; this usually depends on whether utilization requires bacterial growth
- Method for detecting substrate utilization and whether detection is manual or automated

- Method of interpreting and analyzing results (manual or computer assisted), and if computer assisted, the extent to which assistance is automated

The general features of some commercial identification systems are summarized in Table 13-1. More specific information is available from the manufacturers.

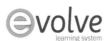 *Visit the Evolve site to complete the review questions.*

## BIBLIOGRAPHY

Alatoom AA, Cunningham SA, Ihde SM, et al: Comparison of direct colony method versus extraction method for identification of gram-positive cocci by use of Bruker Biotype matrix-assisted laser desorption ionization-time of flight mass spectrometry, *J Clin Microbiol* 49:2868, 2011.

Atlas RM, Parks LC, editors: *Handbook of microbiological media*, Boca Raton, FL, 1993, CRC Press.

Clinical Laboratory Standards and Institute (National Committee for Clinical Laboratory Standards): *Abbreviated identification of bacteria and yeast;* Approved Guidelines M35-A2, Wayne, PA, 2008, NCCLS.

Saffert RT, Cunnigham SA, Ihde SM, et al: Comparison of Bruker Biotyper Matrix-Assisted Laser Desorption Ionization-Time of Flight Mass Spectrometer to BD Phoenix Automated Microbiology System for Identification of Gram-Negative Bacilli, *J Clin Microbiol* 49:887, 2011.

Versalovic J. *Manual of clinical microbiology*, 10th ed., Washington D.C., 2011, ASM Press.

# Nucleic Acid–Based Analytic Methods for Microbial Identification and Characterization

## OBJECTIVES

1. Explain the importance of molecular testing in the microbiology laboratory. Also, list the three categories of molecular testing and provide a brief explanation of the methodology for each type.
2. Outline the four-step process in nucleic acid hybridization.
3. Explain the methodology for peptide nucleic acid fluorescent in situ hybridization (PNA FISH) and provide an example of a clinical application.
4. List the three types of nucleic acid extraction; also, compare and contrast the advantages, disadvantages, and outcomes for each.
5. Compare direct molecular hybridization detection with amplified direct detection.
6. Outline the three major steps in polymerase chain reaction (PCR) and describe the critical parameters of each step, including reagents, temperature, time, and interfering substances.
7. Define reverse transcription polymerase chain reaction (RT-PCR); also, explain how and why it is used and the methodology that differentiates it from a traditional PCR test.
8. Explain real-time PCR and list the four potential advantages this procedure has over conventional PCR.
9. Define palindrome, blunt and staggered cuts, and restriction endonuclease.
10. Describe how restriction endonucleases are used in epidemiologic applications and strain typing in molecular diagnostics.
11. Define pulsed-field gel electrophoresis (PFGE) and restriction fragment length polymorphism (RFLP) and state an application for each.

The principles of bacterial cultivation and identification discussed in Chapter 7 focus on phenotypic methods. These methods analyze readily observable bacterial traits and "behavior." Although these strategies are the mainstay of diagnostic bacteriology, notable limitations are associated with the use of phenotypic methods. These limitations are as follows:

- Inability to grow certain fastidious pathogens
- Inability to maintain viability of certain pathogens in specimens during transport to laboratory
- Extensive delay in cultivation and identification of slowly growing pathogens
- Lack of reliable methods to identify certain organisms grown in vitro
- Use of considerable time and resources in establishing the presence and identity of pathogens in specimens

The explosion in molecular biology over the past 20 years has provided alternatives to phenotypic strategies used to identify organisms in the diagnostic microbiology laboratory. These alternatives have the potential to avert some of the aforementioned limitations. Applications of molecular diagnostics in microbiology provide for the qualitative and quantitative detection of organisms, microbial identity testing, and genotyping for drug

resistance. The detection and manipulation of nucleic acids (deoxyribonucleic acid [DNA] and ribonucleic acid [RNA]) allows microbial genes to be examined directly (i.e., **genotypic methods**) rather than by analysis of their products, such as enzymes (i.e., **phenotypic methods**). Additionally, non–nucleic acid–based analytic methods that detect phenotypic traits undetectable by conventional strategies (e.g., cell wall components) have been developed to enhance bacterial detection, identification, and characterization. For laboratory diagnosis of infectious diseases to remain timely and effective, strategies that integrate conventional, nucleic acid–based, and analytic techniques must continue to evolve.

Several analytical methods using microbial DNA or RNA can detect, identify, and characterize infectious etiologies. Although technical aspects may differ, all molecular procedures involve the direct manipulation and analysis of nucleic acid sequences rather than the analysis of gene products. Furthermore, because nucleic acids are common to all living entities, most methods are adaptable for the diagnosis of viral, fungal, parasitic, or bacterial infections. This chapter discusses the general principles and applications of molecular diagnostics. It is intended to be an overview, and additional methods are included in upcoming chapters.

## OVERVIEW OF MOLECULAR METHODS

Because molecular diagnostic tests are based on the consistent and somewhat predictable nature of DNA and RNA, understanding these methods requires a basic understanding of nucleic acid composition and structure. Therefore, a review of the section Nucleic Acid Structure and Organization, in Chapter 2, is recommended.

The molecular methods included in this chapter are classified into one of three categories: (1) hybridization, (2) amplification, or (3) sequencing and enzymatic digestion of nucleic acids.

### SPECIMEN COLLECTION AND TRANSPORT

Proper specimen collection, transport, and processing are essential in all areas of the diagnostic laboratory to ensure accurate results. Nucleic acids are isolated from human, bacterial, viral, and fungal sources in the diagnostic laboratory. The quality and quantity of specimen, as well as maintaining the integrity of the nucleic acid, is essential to obtaining an accurate result in molecular diagnostics.

Depending on the type of specimen, separation and storage may affect the integrity of the sample. Unlike traditional culture, molecular diagnostics does not always require the detection of viable organisms. The timing and collection devices used for molecular testing remain critical to the successful detection of nucleic acids. For example, plastic swabs are recommended for collection of bacteria, viruses, and mycoplasmas from mucosal membranes. The organisms are more easily removed from the plastic shafts than from other materials such as wooden shafts or wire. This provides an increase in yield from the swab. In addition, calcium alginate swabs with aluminum shafts have been reported to interfere with amplification of nucleic acids. In addition, some molecular test kits include transport devices that contain lysing agents to improve isolation from samples that contain cellular debris as well as buffers or transport media that will maintain the integrity of the nucleic acids. In molecular diagnostics, it is essential that the specimen be collected and placed in the proper container or media recommended by the manufacturer of the assay.

## NUCLEIC ACID HYBRIDIZATION METHODS

Hybridization methods are based on the ability of two nucleic acid strands with complementary base sequences (i.e., they are **homologous**) to bond specifically with each other and form a double-stranded molecule, also called a **duplex** or **hybrid.** This duplex formation is driven by the hydrophobic structure and hydrogen bonding

pattern of the nucleotides, which ensure that the base adenine always bonds to thymine (two hydrogen bonds), whereas the bases guanine and cytosine (three hydrogen bonds) always form a bonding pair (see Figure 2-2). Because hybridization requires nucleic acid sequence homology, a positive hybridization reaction between two nucleic acid strands, each from a different source (i.e., intermolecular), indicates genetic relatedness between the two organisms that donated each of the nucleic acid strands for the hybridization reaction. Hybridization reactions may also occur within the same molecule (intramolecular hybridization). Intramolecular hybridization is used to differentiate sequences with electrophoretic separation.

Hybridization assays require detection or identification of two nucleic acid strands; one strand (the **probe**) originates from an organism or nucleic acid sequence of known identity, and the other strand (the **target**) originates from an unknown organism (Figure 8-1). Positive hybridization identifies the unknown organism as being the same as the probe-source organism or sequence. With a negative hybridization test result, the organism remains undetected or unidentified. The single-stranded nucleic acid components used in hybridization may be either

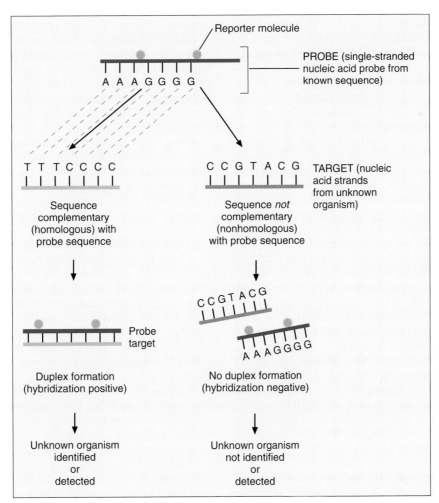

**Figure 8-1** Principles of nucleic acid hybridization. Identification of an unknown organism is established by positive hybridization (i.e., duplex formation) between a nucleic acid strand from the known sequence (i.e., the probe) and a target nucleic acid strand from the organism to be identified. Failure to hybridize indicates lack of homology between the probe and the target nucleic acid.

RNA or DNA; therefore, DNA-DNA, DNA-RNA, and even RNA-RNA duplexes may form, depending on the specific design of the hybridization assay. Hybridization assays may be classified as either nonamplified or amplified. A nonamplified assay requires three steps: preparation of the test sample (nucleic acid), hybridization, and signal detection. Amplified assays include an additional step; initial hybridization is followed by a target amplification and then by signal detection. Amplified assays allow detection of as little as a single organism or nucleic acid sequence in the sample material.

### Hybridization Steps and Components

The basic steps in a hybridization assay include:

1. Production and labeling of single-strand nucleic acid probe
2. Preparation of single-strand target nucleic acid
3. Mixture and hybridization of target and probe nucleic acid
4. Detection of hybridization

**Production and Labeling of Probe Nucleic Acid.** In keeping with the requirement of complementation for hybridization, the probe design (i.e., probe length and the sequence of nucleic acid bases) depends on the sequence of the intended target nucleic acid. Therefore, the selection and design of a probe depends on the intended use. For example, if a probe is to be used to recognize only gram-positive bacteria, its nucleic acid sequence must be specifically complementary to a nucleic acid sequence common only to gram-positive bacteria and not to gram-negative bacteria. Even more specific probes can be designed to identify a particular bacterial genus or species, virulence, or an antibiotic-resistance gene present in certain strains in a given species.

In the past, probes were produced through a labor-intensive process involving recombinant DNA and cloning techniques with the nucleic acid sequence of interest. More recently, probes have been chemically synthesized using instrumentation, a service that is commercially available. The base sequence of potential target genes, sequence patterns, or gene fragments for probe design is easily accessed using computer on-line services for nucleic acid sequence information (e.g., GENBANK, National Center for Biological Information). In short, the design and production of nucleic acid probes is now relatively easy. Although probes may be hundreds to thousands of bases long, oligonucleotide probes (i.e., those 20 to 50 bases long) usually are sufficient for detection of most clinically relevant targets.

All hybridization tests must have a means to detect or measure the hybridization reaction. This is accomplished with the use of a **"reporter"** molecule attached to the single-stranded nucleic acid probe. Probes may be labeled with a variety of molecules, but most commonly, radioactive (e.g., 32P, 3H, 125I, or 35S), biotin-avidin, digoxigenin, fluorescent, or chemiluminescent labels are used (Figure 8-2).

Radioactive labels are directly incorporated through chemical modification into the probe molecule. With the use of radioactively labeled probes, hybridization is detected by the emission of radioactivity from the probe-target complex (see Figure 8-2, *A*). Quantification of the complexes may be achieved through scintillation counting or densitometry. Although this is a highly sensitive method for detecting hybridization, the requirements for radioactive training, monitoring, licensing, and disposal of radioactive waste have limited the use of radioactive labeling in the diagnostic setting.

Biotinylation is a nonradioactive alternative for labeling nucleic acid probes that involves the chemical incorporation of biotin. Biotin labels are classified as indirect, based on the need for a secondary complex formation. Biotin-labeled probe-target nucleic acid duplexes are detected using avidin, a biotin-binding protein conjugated with an enzyme, such as horseradish peroxidase. When a chromogenic substrate is added, the peroxidase produces a colored product that can be detected visually or spectrophotometrically (see Figure 8-2, *B*).

Other nonradioactive labels are based on principles similar to those of biotinylation. For example, with digoxigenin-labeled probes, hybridization is detected using antidigoxigenin antibodies conjugated with an enzyme. Successful duplex formation means the enzyme is present; therefore, with the addition of a chromogenic substrate, color production, resulting in color formation, is interpreted as positive hybridization. Alternatively, the antibody may be conjugated with fluorescent dyes that can be directly detected without a secondary enzymatic reaction to produce a colored or fluorescent end product.

Chemiluminescent reporter molecules can be chemically linked directly to the nucleic acid probe without using a conjugated antibody. These molecules (e.g., acridinium or isoluminol) emit light during hybridization between the chemiluminescent-labeled probe and target nucleic acid. The light is detected using a luminometer (see Figure 8-2, *C*).

Fluorescent labels and fluorimetric reporter groups (e.g., fluorescein and rhodamine) are also considered direct nucleic acid probes. In addition to direct detection probes, fluorimetric reporter groups may be complexed with avidin, digoxigenin, or secondary antibodies, creating a secondary labeling process with additional fluorophores.

**Preparation of Target Nucleic Acid.** Because hybridization is driven by complementary binding of a homologous nucleic acid sequence between probe and target, the target nucleic acid must have a single strand and the base sequence integrity must be maintained. Failure to meet these requirements results in negative hybridization reactions as a result of factors such as target degradation, insufficient target yield, and the presence of interfering substances such as organic chemicals (i.e., false-negative results).

Because the relatively rigorous procedures for releasing nucleic acid from the target microorganism can be deleterious to the molecule's structure, obtaining target nucleic acid and maintaining its appropriate conformation and sequence can be difficult. The steps in target preparation vary, depending on the organism source of the nucleic acid and the nature of the environment from which the target organism is being prepared (i.e., laboratory culture media; fresh clinical material, such as fluid, tissue, or stool; and fixed or preserved clinical material). Generally, target preparation steps involve enzymatic

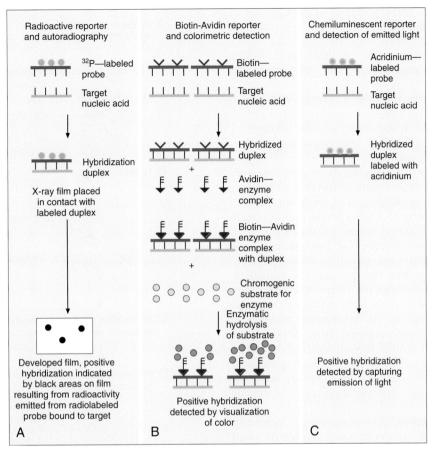

**Figure 8-2** Reporter molecule labeling of nucleic acid probes and principles of hybridization detection. Use of probes labeled with a radioactive reporter, with hybridization detected by autoradiography **(A)**; probes labeled with biotin-avidin reporter, with hybridization detected by a colorimetric assay **(B)**; probes labeled with chemiluminescent reporter (i.e., acridinium), with hybridization detected by a luminometer to detect emitted light **(C)**.

and/or chemical destruction of the microbial envelope to release target nucleic acid, the removal of contaminating molecules such as cellular components (protein), stabilization of target nucleic acid to preserve structural integrity and, if the target is DNA, denaturation to a single strand, which is necessary for binding to complementary probe nucleic acid. Nucleic acid extraction procedures are optimized to ensure a high degree of purity, integrity, and yield of the desired nucleic acid.

Nucleic acid extractions may be classified as organic or nonorganic extractions. Organic extractions use phenol, chloroform, or isoamyl alcohol to disrupt the cellular membranes and denature and remove proteins. After chemical treatment with the organic solution, the mixture is centrifuged, which results in the separation or phasing of the cellular material layered over the top of the organic molecules and waste along the bottom of the tube. The aqueous phase, containing the desired nucleic acid, is then extracted from the organic phase, and the resulting nucleic acid is precipitated using a buffered solution. Nonorganic extractions rely on protein precipitations and nucleic acid precipitations without the use of organic chemicals. Cell membranes and proteins are denatured with a detergent, and the proteins are precipitated with a salt solution. Nonorganic extractions are fast, easy, and do not require the disposal of hazardous organic materials.

DNA isolation is not as technically demanding as RNA extraction methods. RNA may be degraded rapidly by RNAse enzymes. RNAse enzymes are very stable, ubiquitous in the environment, and elevated in certain tissues, such as the placenta, liver, and some tumors. Guanidinium isothiocyanate may be used to denature and inactivate RNAse to preserve the nucleic acid sample before analysis.

Two primary physical methods are available for nucleic acid extraction: liquid-phase extraction, which requires a large sample volume, and solid-phase extraction, which requires a smaller sample volume. Solid-phase extractions are typically simpler than liquid-phase extractions, providing for ease of operation, processing of large batches, high reproducibility, and adaptability to automation. Solid-phase extractions use solid support columns constructed of fibrous or silica matrices, magnetic beads, or chelating agents to bind the nucleic acids.

**Mixture and Hybridization of Target and Probe.** Designs for mixing target and probe nucleic acids are discussed later, but some general concepts regarding the hybridization reaction require consideration.

The ability of the probe to bind the correct target depends on the extent of base sequence homology between the two nucleic acid strands and the environment in which probe and target are brought together. Environmental conditions set the **stringency** for a hybridization reaction, and the degree of stringency can determine the outcome of the reaction. Hybridization stringency is most affected by:

- Salt concentration in the hybridization buffer (stringency increases as salt concentration decreases)
- Temperature (stringency increases as temperature increases)
- Concentration of destabilizing agents (stringency increases with increasing concentrations of formamide or urea)

With greater stringency, a higher degree of base-pair complementarity is required between probe and target to obtain successful hybridization (i.e., less tolerance for deviations in base sequence). Under less stringent conditions, strands with less base-pair complementarity (i.e., strands having a higher number of mismatched base pairs within the sequence) may still hybridize. Therefore, as stringency increases, the specificity of hybridization increases and as stringency decreases, specificity decreases. For example, under high stringency a probe specific for a target sequence in *Streptococcus pneumoniae* may only bind to target prepared from this species (high specificity), but under low stringency the same probe may bind to targets from various streptococcal species (lower specificity). Therefore, to ensure accuracy in hybridization, reaction conditions must be carefully controlled.

**Detection of Hybridization.** The method of detecting hybridization depends on the reporter molecule used for labeling the probe nucleic acid and on the hybridization format (see Figure 8-2). Hybridization using radioactively labeled probes is visualized after the reaction mixture is exposed to radiographic film (i.e., **autoradiography**). Hybridization with nonradioactively labeled probes is detected using colorimetry, fluorescence, or chemiluminescence, and detection can be somewhat automated using spectrophotometers, fluorometers, or luminometers, respectively. The more commonly used nonradioactive detection systems (e.g., digoxigenin, chemiluminescence, fluorescence) are able to detect approximately $10^4$ target nucleic acid sequences per hybridization reaction.

## Hybridization Formats

Hybridization reactions can be done using either a solution format or solid support format.

**Solution Format.** In the solution format, probe and target nucleotide strands are placed in a liquid reaction mixture that facilitates duplex formation; hybridization occurs substantially faster than with a solid support format. However, before duplex formation can be detected, the hybridized, labeled probes must be separated from the nonhybridized, labeled probes (i.e., "background noise"). Separation methods include enzymatic digestion (e.g., S1 nuclease) of single-stranded probes and precipitation of hybridized duplexes, use of hydroxyapatite or charged magnetic microparticles that preferentially bind duplexes, or chemical destruction of the reporter molecule (e.g., acridinium dye) attached to unhybridized probe nucleic acid. After the duplexes have been "purified" from the reaction mixture and the

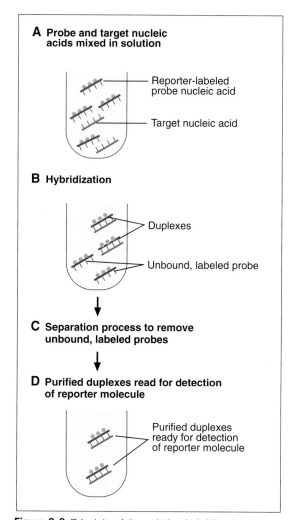

**Figure 8-3** Principle of the solution hybridization format.

background noise minimized, hybridization detection can proceed by the method appropriate for the type of reporter molecule used to label the probe (Figure 8-3).

**Solid Support Format.** Either probe or target nucleic acids may be attached to a solid support matrix and still be capable of forming duplexes with complementary strands. Various solid support materials and common solid formats exist, including filter hybridizations, southern or northern hybridizations, sandwich hybridizations, and in situ hybridizations.

**Filter (membrane) hybridization** has several variations. Filter hybridizations are often referred to as "dot blots." The target sample, which can be previously purified DNA, the microorganism containing the target DNA, or the clinical specimen containing the microorganism of interest, is affixed to a membrane (e.g., nitrocellulose or nylon fiber filters). To identify specimens, samples are usually oriented on the membrane using a template or grid. The membrane is chemically treated, causing release of the target DNA from the microorganism and denaturing the nucleic acid to single strands. The membrane is then submerged in a solution containing labeled nucleic acid probe and incubated, allowing hybridization to occur. After a series of incubations and washings to remove unbound probe, the membrane

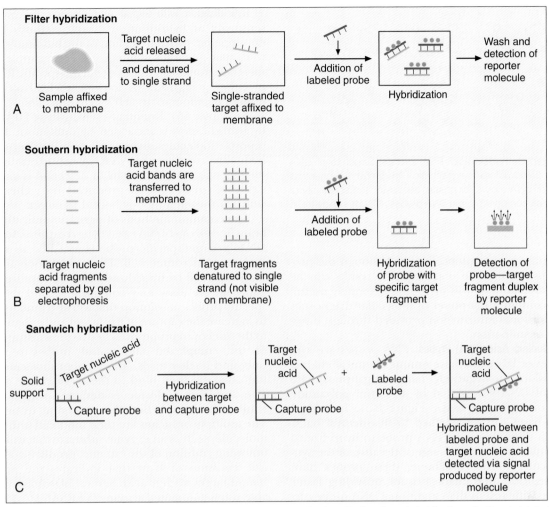

**Figure 8-4** Principle of solid support hybridization formats. **A,** Filter hybridization. **B,** Southern hybridization. **C,** Sandwich hybridization.

is processed for detection of duplexes (Figure 8-4, *A*). An advantage of this method is that a single membrane can hold several samples for exposure to the same probe.

**Southern hybridization** is another method that uses membranes as the solid support. In this instance, the nucleic acid target is purified from the organisms and digested with specific enzymes to produce several fragments of various sizes (Figure 8-4, *B*) (also see Enzymatic Digestion and Electrophoresis of Nucleic Acids later in this chapter). The nucleic acid fragments, which carry a net negative charge, are subjected to an electrical field, forcing them to migrate through an agarose gel matrix (i.e., **gel electrophoresis**). Because fragments of different sizes migrate through the porous agarose at different rates, they can be separated by molecular size. When electrophoresis is complete, the nucleic acid fragments are stained with the fluorescent dye **ethidium bromide** so that fragment "banding patterns" can be visualized on exposure of the gel to ultraviolet (UV) light. For southern hybridization, the target nucleic acid bands are transferred to a membrane that is submerged in solution, allowing for hybridization of the nucleic acid probe. After hybridization, the southern hybridization membrane is used to detect the specific target nucleic acid fragment carrying the base sequence by using

radiolabeled, fluorescent, or substrate-labeled detection. The complexity, time, and labor intensity of the procedure precludes its common use in most diagnostic settings.

With **sandwich hybridizations** two probes are used. One probe is attached to the solid support, is not labeled, and via hybridization "captures" the target nucleic acid from the sample to be tested. The presence of this duplex is then detected using a labeled second probe that is specific for another portion of the target sequence (Figure 8-4, *C*). Sandwiching the target between two probes decreases nonspecific reactions but requires a greater number of processing and washing steps. For such formats, plastic microtiter wells coated with probes have replaced filters as the solid support material, thereby facilitating the use of these multiple-step procedures for testing a relatively large number of specimens.

**In Situ Hybridization.** **In situ hybridization** allows a pathogen to be identified in the context of the pathologic lesion being produced. This method uses patient cells or tissues as the solid support phase. Tissue specimens thought to be infected with a particular pathogen are processed in a manner that maintains the structural integrity of the tissue and cells, yet allows the nucleic acid of the pathogen to be released and denatured to a single

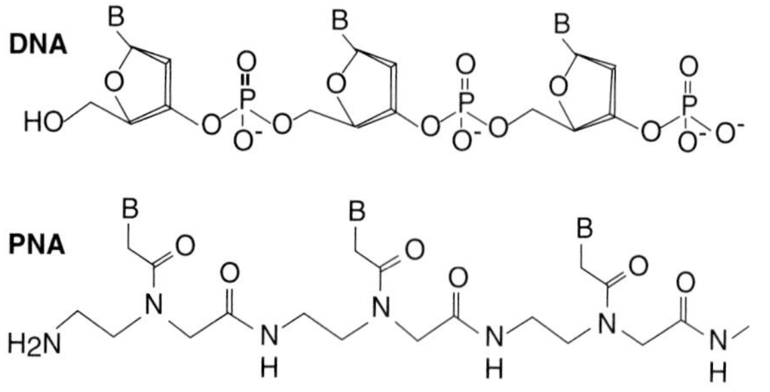

**Figure 8-5** Peptide nucleic acid (PNA) probes. Structure of DNA compared to the structure of a synthetic PNA probe; the chemical modification of DNA allows for greater sensitivity and specificity of the PNA probes compared to the DNA probes. (Courtesy AdvanDx, Woburn, Mass.)

strand with the base sequence intact. Although the processing steps required to obtain quality results can be technically demanding, this method is extremely useful, because it combines the power of molecular diagnostics with the additional information provided through histopathologic examination.

**Peptide Nucleic Acid (PNA) Probes.** PNA probes are synthetic pieces of DNA that have unique chemical characteristics in which the negatively charged sugar-phosphate backbone of DNA is replaced by a neutral polyamide backbone of repetitive units (Figure 8-5). Individual nucleotide bases can be attached to this neutral backbone, which then allows the PNA probe to hybridize to complementary nucleic acid targets. Because of the synthetic structure of the backbone, these probes have improved hybridization characteristics, providing faster and more specific results than traditional DNA probes. In addition, because these probes are not degraded by ubiquitous enzymes, such as nucleases and proteases, they provide a longer shelf-life in diagnostic applications. PNA FISH is a novel fluorescent in situ hybridization (FISH) technique that uses PNA probes to target species-specific ribosomal RNA (rRNA) sequences. Upon penetration of the microbial cell wall, the fluorescent-labeled PNA probes hybridize to multicopy rRNA sequences within the microorganisms, resulting in fluorescent cells. Recently, AdvanDx (Woburn, Massachusetts) introduced in vitro diagnostic kits (using PNA FISH), which have been approved by the U.S. Food and Drug Administration (FDA). These kits can be used to directly identify *S. aureus* and *C. albicans* and to differentiate *Enterococcus faecalis* from other enterococci in blood cultures. In brief, a drop from a positive blood culture bottle is added to a slide containing a drop of fixative solution. After fixation, the fluorescent-labeled PNA probe is added and allowed to hybridize; slides are washed and air dried. After the addition of a mounting medium and a coverslip, the slides are examined under a fluorescent microscope using a special filter set. Identification is based on the presence of bright green, fluorescent-staining organisms (Figure 8-6, *A* and *B*). For negative results, only slightly red-stained background material is observed (Figure 8-6, *C* and *D*). Multiple studies have been done to evaluate the efficacy of the PNA FISH kits for identifying *S. aureus* and *C. albicans* in positive blood cultures. The kits have demonstrated high sensitivity and specificity.

**Hybridization with Signal Amplification.** To increase the sensitivity of hybridization assays, methods have been developed in which detection of the binding of the probe to its specific target is enhanced. For example, one commercially available kit uses genotype-specific RNA probes in either a high-risk or low-risk cocktail to detect the human papillomavirus (HPV) DNA in clinical specimens (see Chapter 66). Essentially, sensitivity of HPV detection by hybridization is increased by multimeric layering of reporter molecules, increasing their number on an antibody directed toward DNA-RNA hybrids using chemiluminescence; thus, sensitivity of detection is enhanced by virtue of greater signal produced (i.e., chemiluminescence) for each antibody bound to target.

Two common methods of signal amplification include branched DNA (bDNA) and hybrid capture. In branched DNA, a target-specific probe is attached to a substrate such as a microtiter well. The complementary target is then captured by hybridization to the capture probe. In addition, the assay may contain a second set of target-specific probes in solution that will also bind to the target to increase the capture of the target and enhance binding to the anchored probes attached to the substrate. Washing of the complexed target and probes removes any unbound nucleic acids. An amplifier molecule added to the assay will then bind to the target-probe complexes. The amplifier molecule is designed similar to a tree trunk, with multiple branches extending from the trunk. The multiple branches are then modified with a reporter molecule, such as an enzyme substrate that will emit light following addition of the enzyme, producing a characteristic emission of light that indicates the presence of bound target nucleic acid. Several bDNA assays are available using automated systems (VERSANT™ 440 Molecular System, Siemens Healthcare Diagnostics, Deerfield, IL) for the detection of viral nucleic acid such as hepatitis B (HBV) DNA, hepatitis C (HCV), RNA, and HIV-1 RNA.

Hybrid capture differs from bDNA assays in that the hybridization occurs in solution using nucleic acid-specific probes followed by a bound universal capture antibody. The target nucleic acid is denatured, separating double-stranded DNA molecules. The denatured nucleic acids are then hybridized with a target-specific RNA probe. The DNA-RNA hybrids are then captured with an antihybrid antibody that contains a chemiluminescent reporter molecule (i.e., alkaline phosphatase). The light emitted is then measured using a luminometer. A variety of hybrid capture assays are FDA-approved for the detection of *Chlamydia trachomatis*, *Neisseria gonnorrhoeae*, cytomegalovirus, and human papillomavirus (Qiagen, Germantown, MD).

## AMPLIFICATION METHODS—PCR BASED

Although hybridization methods are highly specific for organism detection and identification, they are limited by their sensitivity; that is, without sufficient target nucleic acid in the reaction, false-negative results occur. Therefore, many hybridization methods require "amplifying" of target nucleic acid by growing target organisms to greater numbers in culture. The requirement for cultivation detracts from the potential for faster detection and identification of the organism using molecular methods.

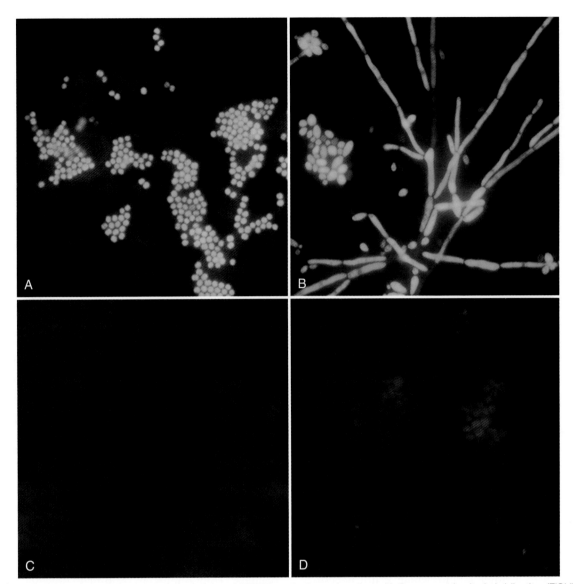

**Figure 8-6** Using a fluorescent-tagged peptide nucleic acid (PNA) probe in conjunction with fluorescent in situ hybridization (FISH), *Staphylococcus aureus* **(A)** or *Candida albicans* **(B)** was directly identified in blood cultures. A drop from the positive blood culture bottle is added to a slide containing a drop of fixative solution, which keeps the cells intact. After fixation, the appropriate fluorescent-labeled PNA probe is added. The PNA probe penetrates the microbial cell wall and hybridizes to the ribosomal RNA (rRNA). Slides are examined under a fluorescent microscope. If the specific target is present, bright green, fluorescent-staining organisms are present. Blood cultures negative for either *S. aureus* **(C)** or *C. albicans* **(D)** by PNA FISH technology are shown. (Courtesy AdvanDx, Woburn, Mass.)

Therefore, the development of molecular amplification techniques that do not rely on organism multiplication has contributed greatly to faster diagnosis and identification while enhancing sensitivity and maintaining specificity. For purposes of discussion, amplification methods are divided into two major categories: methods that use polymerase chain reaction (PCR) technology and assays that are not PCR based.

## Overview of PCR and Derivations

The most widely used target nucleic acid amplification method is the **polymerase chain reaction (PCR).** This method combines the principles of complementary nucleic acid hybridization with those of nucleic acid replication applied repeatedly through numerous cycles. This method is able to amplify a single copy of a nucleic acid target, often undetectable by standard hybridization

methods, and multiply to $10^7$ or more copies in a relatively short period. This provides ample target that can be readily detected by numerous methods.

Conventional PCR involves 25 to 50 repetitive cycles, with each cycle comprising three sequential reactions: denaturation of target nucleic acid, primer annealing to single-strand target nucleic acid, and extension of primer-target duplex.

**Extraction and Denaturation of Target Nucleic Acid.** For PCR, nucleic acid is first **extracted** (released) from the organism or a clinical sample potentially containing the target organism by heat, chemical, or enzymatic methods. Numerous manual methods are available to accomplish this task, including a variety of commercially available kits that extract either RNA or DNA, depending on the specific target of interest. Other commercially available kits are designed to extract nucleic acids from specific

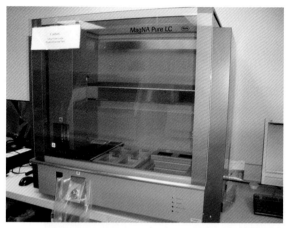

**Figure 8-7** The MagNaPure LC System from Roche Applied Science has been on the market since 1999. It is a fully automated nucleic acid extractor, capable of isolating DNA, RNA and viral nucleic acid from a variety of samples: blood, cells, plasma/serum, or tissue. Based on a magnetic bead technology, it is designed to automate nucleic acid purification and PCR set up. The new Mag-NaPure LC 2.0 is equipped with an integrated computer, LCD monitor with touch screen, and Laboratory Information Management System (LIMS) network compatibility.

types of clinical specimens, such as blood or tissues. Most recently, automated instruments (e.g., the Roche Mag-NaPure) have been introduced to extract nucleic acid from various sources, such as bacteria, viruses, tissue, and blood (Figure 8-7).

Once extracted, target nucleic acid is added to the reaction mix containing all the necessary components for PCR (primers, nucleotides, covalent ions, buffer, and enzyme) and placed into a thermal cycler to undergo amplification (Figure 8-8). For PCR to begin, target nucleic acid must be in the single-stranded conformation for the second reaction, primer annealing, to occur. Denaturation to a single strand, which is not necessary for RNA targets, is accomplished by heating to 94°C (Figure 8-9). Of note, for many PCR procedures, especially those involving commonly encountered bacterial pathogens, disruption of the organism to release DNA is done in one step by heating the sample to 94°C.

**Primer Annealing.** Primers are short, single-stranded sequences of nucleic acid (i.e., oligonucleotides usually 20 to 30 nucleotides long) selected to specifically hybridize (**anneal**) to a particular nucleic acid target, essentially functioning like probes. As noted for hybridization tests, the abundance of available gene sequence data allows for the design of primers specific for a number of microbial pathogens and their virulence or antibiotic resistance genes. Thus, primer nucleotide sequence design depends on the intended target, such as unique nucleotide sequences, genus-specific genes, species-specific genes, virulence genes, or antibiotic-resistance genes.

Primers are designed in pairs that flank the target sequence of interest (see Figure 8-9). When the primer pair is mixed with the denatured target DNA, one primer anneals to a specific site at one end of the target sequence of one target strand, and the other primer anneals to a specific site at the opposite end of the other,

complementary target strand. Usually primers are designed to amplify an internal target nucleic acid sequence of 50 to 1000 base pairs. The annealing process is conducted at 50° to 58°C or higher. Annealing or hybridization of primers is optimized according to the nucleic acid sequence. The nucleic acid sequence of the primer determines the optimal annealing melting temperature (Tm) for the primers. The melting temperature is defined as the temperature at which 50% of the primers are hybridized to the appropriate complementary sequence. Because of the complementary binding of nucleotides, the melting temperature may be determined for a known nucleotide sequence. The melting temperature is calculated according to a simple formula:

$$2 \times (A+T) + 4 \times (G+C)$$

Primer pairs should be optimally designed to anneal within 1 to 2 degrees of each other to maintain the specificity of the amplification reaction. Once the duplexes have been formed, the last step in the cycle (amplification), which mimics the DNA replication process, begins.

**Extension of Primer-Target Duplex.** Annealing of primers to target sequences provides the necessary template format that allows the DNA polymerase to add nucleotides to the 3' **terminus** (end) of each primer and extend sequence complementary to the target template (see Figure 8-9). Taq polymerase is the enzyme commonly used for primer extension, which occurs at 72°C. This enzyme is used because of its ability to function efficiently at elevated temperatures and to withstand the denaturing temperature of 94°C through several cycles. The ability to allow primer annealing and extension to occur at elevated temperatures without detriment to the polymerase increases the stringency of the reaction, thus decreasing the chance for amplification of nontarget nucleic acid (i.e., nonspecific amplification).

The three reaction steps in PCR occur in the same tube containing the mixture of target nucleic acid, primers, components to optimize polymerase activity (i.e., buffer, cation [MgCl2], salt), and deoxynucleotides. To minimize the time lag required to alter the reaction temperature between denaturation, annealing, and extension over several cycles, automated programmable **thermal cyclers** are used. These cyclers hold the reaction vessel and carry the PCR mixture through each reaction step at the precise temperature and for the optimal duration.

As shown in Figure 8-9, for each target sequence originally present in the PCR mixture, two double-stranded fragments containing the target sequence are produced after one cycle. At the beginning of the second cycle of PCR, denaturation produces four templates to which the primers will anneal. After extension at the end of the second cycle, there will be four double-stranded fragments containing target nucleic acid. Therefore, with completion of each cycle, there is a doubling or logarithmic increase of target nucleic acid, and after the completion of 30 to 40 cycles, $10^7$ to $10^8$ target copies will be present in the reaction mixture.

Although it is possible to detect one copy of a pathogen's gene in a sample or patient specimen by PCR technology, detection is dependent on the ability of the

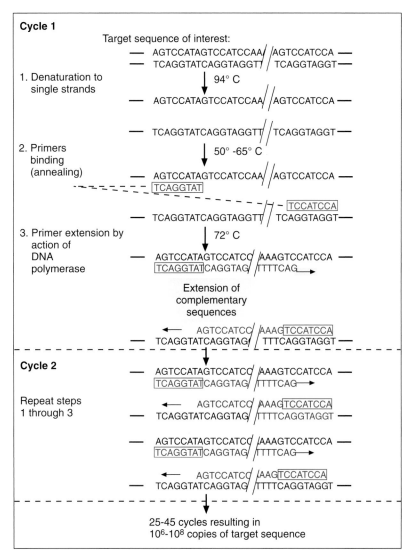

**Figure 8-8** Overview of polymerase chain reaction. The target sequence is denatured to single strands, primers specific for each target strand sequence are added, and DNA polymerase catalyzes the addition of deoxynucleotides to extend and produce new strands complementary to each of the target sequence strands (cycle 1). In cycle 2, both double-stranded products of cycle 1 are denatured and subsequently serve as targets for more primer annealing and extension by DNA polymerase. After 25 to 30 cycles, at least $10^7$ copies of target DNA may be produced. (Modified from Ryan KJ, Champoux JJ, Drew WL et al: *Sherris medical microbiology: an introduction to infectious diseases,* Norwalk, Conn, 1994, The McGraw-Hill Companies, Inc.)

primers to locate and anneal to the single target copy and on optimum PCR conditions. Nonetheless, PCR has proved to be a powerful amplification tool to enhance the sensitivity of molecular diagnostic techniques.

**Detection of PCR Products.** The specific PCR amplification product containing the target nucleic acid of interest is referred to as the **amplicon.** Because PCR produces an amplicon in substantial quantities, any of the basic methods previously described for detecting hybridization can be adopted for detecting specific amplicons. Detection involves using a labeled probe specific for the target sequence in the amplicon. Therefore, solution or solid-phase formats may be used with reporter molecules that generate radioactive, colorimetric, fluorometric, or chemiluminescent signals. Probe-based detection of amplicons serves two purposes: it allows visualization of the PCR product, and it provides specificity by ensuring that

the amplicon is the target sequence of interest and not the result of nonspecific amplification.

When the reliability of PCR for a particular amplicon has been well established, hybridization-based detection may not be necessary; confirming the presence of the correct-size amplicon may be sufficient. This is commonly accomplished by subjecting a portion of the PCR mixture, after amplification, to gel electrophoresis. After electrophoresis, the gel is stained with ethidium bromide to visualize the amplicon and, using molecular weight–size markers, the presence of amplicons of appropriate size (the size of the target sequence amplified depends on the primers selected for PCR) is confirmed (Figure 8-10).

**Derivations of the PCR Method.** The powerful amplification capacity of PCR has prompted the development of several modifications that enhance the utility of this methodology, particularly in the diagnostic setting. Specific examples include multiplex PCR, nested PCR, quantitative PCR, RT-PCR, arbitrary primed PCR, and PCR for nucleotide sequencing.

**Multiplex PCR** is a method by which more than one primer pair is included in the PCR mixture. This approach offers a couple of notable advantages. First, strategies including internal controls for PCR have been developed. For example, one primer pair can be directed at sequences present in all clinically relevant bacteria (i.e., the control or universal primers), and the second primer pair can be directed at a sequence specific for the particular gene of interest (i.e., the test primers). The control amplicon should always be detectable after PCR; absence of the internal control indicates that PCR

conditions were not met, and the test must be repeated. When the control amplicon is detected, absence of the test amplicon can be more confidently interpreted to indicate the absence of target nucleic acid in the specimen rather than a failure of the PCR assay (Figure 8-11).

Another advantage of multiplex PCR is the ability to search for different targets using one reaction. Primer pairs directed at sequences specific for different organisms or genes can be put together, avoiding the use of multiple reaction vessels and minimizing the volume of specimen required. For example, multiplexed PCR assays containing primers to detect viral agents that cause meningitis or encephalitis (e.g., herpes simplex virus, enterovirus, West Nile virus) have been used in a single reaction tube. A limitation of multiplex PCR is that mixing different primers can cause some interference in the amplification process. Optimizing multiplex PCR conditions can be difficult, especially as the number of different primer pairs included in the assay increases.

**Nested PCR** involves the sequential use of two primer sets. The first set is used to amplify a target sequence. The amplicon obtained is then used as the target sequence for a second amplification using primers internal to those of the first amplicon. The advantage of this approach is extreme sensitivity and confirmed specificity without the need for using probes. Because production of the second amplicon requires the presence of the first amplicon, production of the second amplicon automatically verifies the accuracy of the first amplicon. The problem encountered with nested PCR is that the procedure requires open manipulations of amplified DNA that is readily, albeit inadvertently, aerosolized and capable of contaminating other reaction vials.

**Arbitrary primed PCR** uses short (random) primers not specifically complementary to a particular sequence of a target DNA. Although these primers are not specifically directed, their short sequence (approximately 10 nucleotides) ensures that they randomly anneal to multiple sites in a chromosomal sequence. On cycling, the

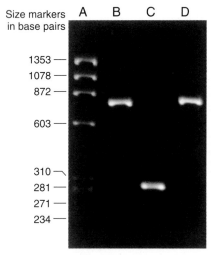

**Figure 8-9** Use of ethidium bromide–stained agarose gels to determine the size of PCR amplicons for identification. Lane A shows molecular-size markers, with the marker sizes indicated in base pairs. Lanes B, C, and D contain PCR amplicons typical of the enterococcal vancomycin-resistance genes vanA (783 kb), vanB (297 kb), and vanC1 (822 kb), respectively.

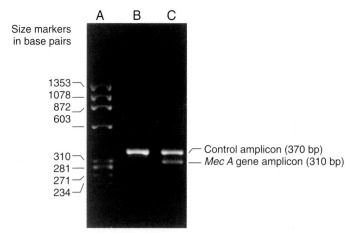

**Figure 8-10** Ethidium bromide–stained gels containing amplicons produced by multiplex PCR. Lane A shows molecular-size markers, with the marker sizes indicated in base pairs. Lanes B and C show amplicons obtained with multiplex PCR consisting of control primers and primers specific for the staphylococcal methicillin-resistance gene mecA. The presence of only the control amplicon (370 bp) in Lane B indicates that PCR was successful, but the strain on which the reaction was performed did not contain mecA. Lane C shows both the control and the mecA (310 bp) amplicons, indicating that the reaction was successful and that the strain tested carries the mecA resistance gene.

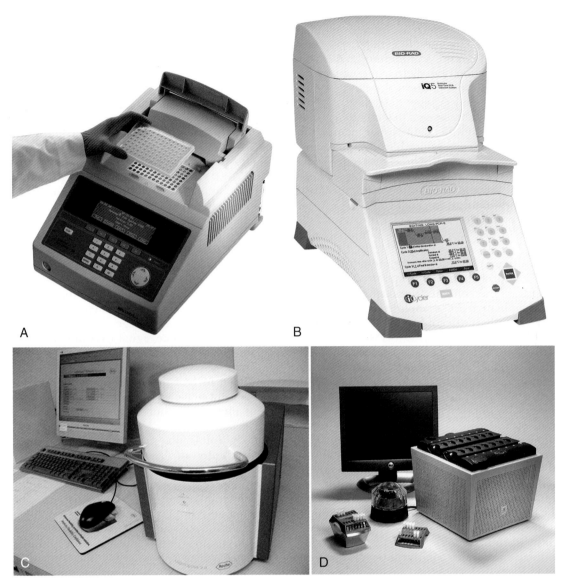

**Figure 8-11** Examples of real-time PCR instruments. **A,** Applied Biosystems. **B,** iCycler. **C,** Light Cycler. **D,** SmartCycler. (**A** copyright © 2012 Life Technologies Corporation. Used under permission. www.lifetechnologies.com; **B** courtesy Bio-Rad Laboratories, Hercules, Calif; **D** courtesy Cepheid, Sunnyvale, Calif.)

multiple annealing sites result in the amplification of multiple fragments of different sizes. Theoretically, strains with similar nucleotide sequences have similar annealing sites and thus produce amplified fragments (i.e., amplicons) of similar sizes. Therefore, by comparing fragment migration patterns after agarose gel electrophoresis, the examiner can judge strains or isolates to be the same, similar, or unrelated.

**Quantitative PCR** is an approach that combines the power of PCR for the detection and identification of infectious agents with the ability to quantitate the actual number of targets originally in the clinical specimen. The ability to quantitate "infectious burden" has tremendous implications for studying and understanding the disease state (e.g., acquired immunodeficiency syndrome [AIDS]), the prognosis of certain infections, and the effectiveness of antimicrobial therapy.

The PCR methods discussed thus far have focused on amplification of a DNA target. **Reverse transcription**

**PCR (RT-PCR)** amplifies an RNA target. Because many clinically important viruses have genomes composed of RNA rather than DNA (e.g., the human immunodeficiency virus [HIV], hepatitis B virus), the ability to amplify RNA greatly facilitates laboratory-based diagnostic testing for these infectious agents. Reverse transcription includes a unique initial step that requires the use of the enzyme **reverse transcriptase** to direct the synthesis of DNA from the viral RNA template, usually within 30 minutes. Once the DNA has been produced, relatively routine PCR technology is applied to obtain amplification.

### Real-Time PCR

Most conventional PCR-based tests used in clinical laboratories were developed in-house and required dedicated laboratory space to control or reduce cross-contamination that produced false-positive results. Conventional PCR assays also require multiple manipulations, including initial amplification of target nucleic acid, detection of amplified product by gel electrophoresis, and confirmation by an alternative method, such as Southern blotting or chemiluminescence techniques. In general, a conventional PCR assay would require a minimum of at least 4 to 6 hours from completion of nucleic acid extraction to placement of the sample into a thermal cycler to begin amplification to subsequent product detection.

Real-time automated instruments that combine target nucleic acid amplification with qualitative or quantitative measurement of amplified product have become commercially available (Table 8-1). These instruments are noteworthy for four reasons:

1. The instruments combine thermocycling or target DNA amplification with the ability to detect amplified target by fluorescently labeled probes as the hybrids are formed (i.e., detection of amplicon in real time).
2. Because both amplification and product detection can be accomplished in one reaction vessel without ever exposing the contents, the major concern of cross-contamination of samples with amplified product associated with conventional PCR assays is reduced.
3. The instruments are not only able to measure amplified product (amplicon) as it is made, but also, because of this capability, they are able to quantitate the amount of product and thereby determine the number of copies of target in the original specimen.
4. The time required to complete a real-time PCR assay is significantly reduced compared to conventional PCR-based assays, because the time required for amplification is reduced by heat and air exchange instead of a conventional heat block, and post-PCR detection of amplified product is eliminated by the use of fluorescent probes.

Several instruments (also referred to as *platforms*) are available for amplification in conjunction with real-time detection of PCR-amplified products (Figure 8-11). Each instrument has unique features that permit some flexibility, such that a clinical laboratory can fulfill its specific needs in terms of specimen capacity, number of targets simultaneously detected, detection format, and time for analysis. Nevertheless, all instruments have amplification (i.e., thermal cycling) capability, as well as an excitation or light source, an emission detection source, and a computer interface to selectively monitor the formation of amplified product.

As with conventional PCR, nucleic acid must first be extracted from the clinical specimen before real-time amplification. In principle, real-time amplification is accomplished in the same manner as previously described for conventional PCR-based assays in which denaturation of double-strand nucleic acid followed by primer annealing and extension (elongation) are performed in one cycle. However, it is the detection process that discriminates real-time PCR from conventional PCR assays. In real-time PCR assays, accumulation of amplicon is monitored as it is generated. Monitoring of amplified target is made possible by the labeling of primers, oligonucleotide probes (oligoprobes) or amplicons with molecules capable of fluorescing. These labels produce a change in

fluorescent signal that is measured by the instrument following their direct interaction with or hybridization to the amplicon. This signal is related to the amount of amplified product present during each cycle and increases as the amount of specific amplicon increases.

Currently, a range of fluorescent chemistries is used for amplicon detection; the more commonly used chemistries can be divided into two categories: (1) those that involve the nonspecific binding of a fluorescent dye (e.g., SYBER Green I) to double-stranded DNA and (2) fluorescent probes that bind specifically to the target of interest. SYBER Green I chemistry is based on the binding of SYBER Green I to a site referred to as the **DNA minor groove** (where the strand backbones of DNA are closer together on one side of the helix than on the other), which is present in all double-stranded DNA molecules. Once bound, fluorescence of this dye increases more than 100-fold. Therefore, as the amount of double-stranded amplicon increases, the fluorescent signal or output increases proportionally and can be measured by the instrument during the elongation stage of amplification. A major disadvantage of this particular means of detection is that the signal cannot discriminate specific versus nonspecific amplified products.

Three different chemistries commonly used to detect amplicon in real time (Figure 8-12) involve additional fluorescence-labeled oligonucleotides or probes. Sufficient amounts of fluorescence are released after cleavage of the probe (hydrolysis probes) or during hybridization of one (molecular beacon) or two oligonucleotides (hybridization probes) to the amplicon.

Introduction of these additional probes increases the specificity of the PCR product. Also, some real-time PCR instruments (e.g., Light Cycler; Roche Applied Science, Indianapolis, Indiana) can detect multiple targets (multiplex PCR) by using different probes labeled with specific fluorescent dyes, each with a unique emission spectra.

Some real-time PCR instruments also have the ability to perform melting curve analysis. This type of analysis of amplified products confirms the identification (i.e., specificity) of the amplified products and/or identifies nonspecific products. Melting curve analysis can be performed with assays using hybridization probes and molecular beacons but not hydrolysis probes, because hydrolysis probes are destroyed during the amplification process. The underlying basis of melting curve analysis is the ability of the double-stranded DNA to become single strand upon heating (referred to as *melting* or *denaturation*). The **melting temperature, or Tm,** as previously described, is the temperature at which the DNA becomes single strand ("melts") and is dependent on its base sequence (stretches of double-stranded DNA with more cytosines and guanines require more heat [energy] to break the three hydrogen bonds between these two bases, in contrast to adenine and thymidine base pairing, which has only two hydrogen bonds). Because the Tm of the probe is specific, being primarily based on probe-target base composition, amplification products can be confirmed as correct by its melting characteristics or Tm. Of significance, the Tm can also be used to distinguish base pair differences (e.g., genotypes, mutations, or

**TABLE 8-1**   Examples of Automation and Instrumentation Available for the Molecular Microbiology Research and Clinical Laboratory

|  | Instrument | Manufacturer | Comments |
|---|---|---|---|
| **Traditional Thermal Cyclers** | Veriti Thermal Cycler | Applied Biosystems; Life Technologies, Carlsbad, CA | End-point thermal cycler; FDA-approved for IVD use |
|  | GeneAmp 9700 PCR system | Applied Biosystems; Life Technologies, Carlsbad, CA | Interchangeable sample block modules for flexibility |
| **Real-Time Instruments** | 7500 System Fast | Applied Biosystems; Life Technologies, Carlsbad, CA | IVD applications available in certain countries |
|  | Quant Studio 12K Flex System | Applied Biosystems: Life Technologies, Carlsbad, CA | Taqman array and Open array; no IVD currently available |
|  | CFX Systems | Bio-Rad, Hercules, CA | Various well formats for flexibility |
|  | LightCycler 2.0 | Roche Diagnostics, Indianapolis, IN | Real-time PCR platform; infectious disease testing available |
|  | SmartCycler System | Cepheid, Sunnyvale, CA | Real-time platform; expandable up to 96 independent tests |
| **Isothermal Instrument** | Illumipro-10 | Meridian Bioscience, Inc. | Automated isothermal amplification and detection. Reduced hands-on time; approximately 2 minutes. FDA approved. |
| **Sequencing** | 3500 Series Genetic Analyzers | Applied Biosystems; Life Technologies, Carlsbad, CA | CE-IVD labeled |
|  | 5500W Series Genetic Analysis Systems | Applied Biosystems; Life Technologies, Carlsbad, CA | Research use only; flow chip design |
| **Semi-Automated** | COBAS Amplicor | Roche Diagnostics; Indianapolis, IN | Real-time PCR platform; FDA approved infectious disease testing available. |
|  | INFINITI Plus Analyzer | Autogenomics, Vista, CA | Post-amplification, microarray closed analytical system |
|  | Filmarray | Biofire Diagnostics Inc., Salt Lake City, UT | Respiratory panel for 20 different infectious agents, FDA-approved. Approximately 2 minutes hands-on time. Uses multiplex nested PCR, coupled with film-array detection. |
| **Fully Automated** | Cobas Ampliprep | Roche Diagnostics; Indianapolis, IN | Automated extraction, isolation, and real-time PCR platform |
|  | Panther System | Gen-Probe/Hologic, San Diego, CA | Fully automated platform with primary tube sampling to detection. Endpoint and real-time transcription-mediated amplification. FDA-approved testing available. |
|  | Verigene | Nanosphere, Northbrook, IL | Automated extraction, isolation, and detection. Some FDA cleared microbiology assays available. |
|  | GeneXpert and GeneXpert Infinity | Cepheid, Sunnyvale, CA | Fully automated, extraction, real-time detection in closed system. Fully automated expanded walkaway infinity system. |
| **Amplification and Mass Spectrometry** | Abbott PLEX-ID System | Ibis Biosciences | Stand-alone or integrated system that includes extraction and processing. Uses PCR platform and high-resolution mass spectrometry. |

**Note:** This table is intended to provide an overview of the various types of instruments available for molecular microbiology testing and is not intended to be all inclusive. Molecular diagnostic instrumentation, technology, and testing platforms are rapidly evolving.

polymorphisms) in target DNA, thus forming the basis for many genetic testing assays, because base pair mismatches resulting from mutations alter the Tm.

With respect to real-time PCR assays, because fluorescence of single-labeled probes is reversible by breaking the hydrogen bonds between the probe and target (i.e., denaturation), the Tm can be determined by measuring fluorescence. In real-time PCR thermal cyclers, melting curve analysis is performed once amplification is finished. The temperature of the reaction vessel is lowered below

the established annealing temperature of the hybridization probe or molecular beacon; this step allows the probe or beacon to anneal to its target and to other similar DNA sequences in the reaction. As the temperature is slowly raised, the hybridization probes or molecular beacon that were hybridized to the target separate (melt), and the fluorescent signal decreases (Figure 8-13).

Finally, as with conventional PCR, real-time PCR assays also have the ability to quantitate the amount of target in a clinical sample. For quantitative analysis, amplification

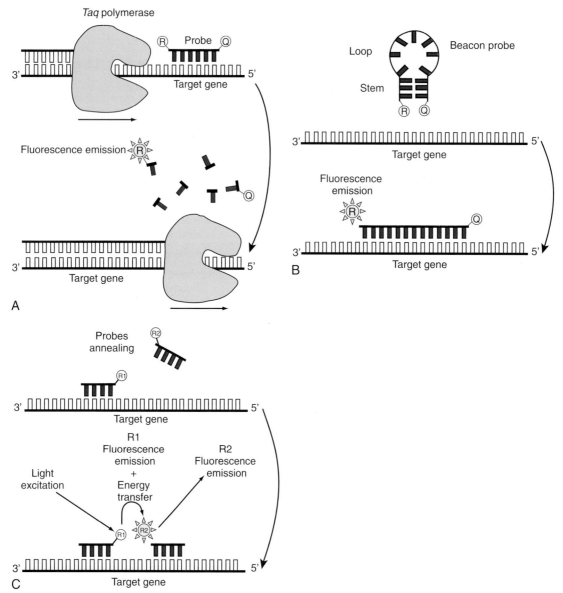

**Figure 8-12** Fluorogenic probes (probes with an attached fluorophore, a fluorescent molecule that can absorb light energy and then be elevated to an excited state and released as fluorescence in the absence of a quencher) commonly used for detection of amplified product in real-time PCR assays. **A,** Hydrolysis probe. In addition to the specific primers for amplification, an oligonucleotide probe with a reporter fluorescent dye (R) and a quencher dye (Q) at its 5' and 3' ends, respectively, is added to the reaction mix. During the extension phase, the quencher (the molecule that can accept energy from a fluorophore and then dissipate the energy, resulting in no fluorescence) can quench the reporter fluorescence when the two dyes are close to each other *(a).* Once amplification occurs and the fluorogenic probe binds to amplified product, the bound probe is degraded by the 5'-3' exonuclease activity of Taq polymerase; therefore, quenching is no longer possible, and fluorescence is emitted and then measured *(b).* **B,** Molecular beacon. Molecular beacons are hairpin-shaped molecules with an internally quenched fluorophore that fluoresces once the beacon probe binds to the amplified target and the quencher is no longer in proximity to the fluorophore. These probes are designed such that the loop portion of the molecule is a sequence complementary to the target of interest *(a).* The "stem" portion of the beacon probe is formed by the annealing of complementary arm sequences on the respective ends of the probe sequence. In addition, a fluorescent moiety (R) and a quencher moiety (Q) at opposing ends of the probe are attached *(a).* The stem portion of the probe keeps the fluorescent and quencher moieties in proximity to one another, quenching the fluorescence of the fluorophore. When it encounters a target molecule with a complementary sequence, the molecular beacon undergoes a spontaneous conformational change that forces the stem apart, thereby causing the fluorophore and quencher to move away from each other and leading to restoration of fluorescence *(b).* **C,** Fluorescent resonant energy transfer (FRET) or hybridization probes. Two different hybridization probes are used, one carrying a fluorescent reporter moiety at its 3' end (designated R1) and the other carrying a fluorescent dye at its 5' end (designated R2) *(a).* These two oligonucleotide probes are designed to hybridize to amplified DNA target in a head-to-tail arrangement in very close proximity to one another. The first dye (R1) is excited by a filtered light source and emits a fluorescent light at a slightly longer wavelength. Because the two dyes are so close to each other, the energy emitted from R1 excites R2 attached to the second hybridization probe, which emits fluorescent light at an even longer wavelength *(b).* This energy transfer is referred to as FRET. Selection of an appropriate detection channel on the instrument allows the intensity of light emitted from R2 to be filtered and measured. (Modified from Mocellin S, Rossi CR, Pilati P et al: Quantitative real-time PCR: a powerful ally in cancer research, *Trends Mol Med* 9:189, 2003.)

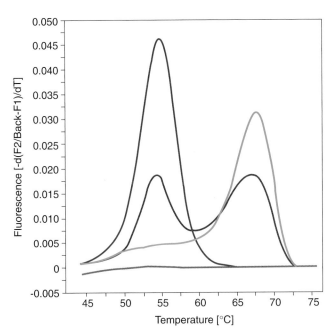

**Figure 8-13** Melting curve analyses performed using the LightCycler HSV1/2 Detection Kit. DNA was extracted and subjected to real-time PCR using the LightCycler to detect the presence of herpes simplex virus (HSV) DNA. After amplification, melting curve analysis was performed in which amplified product was cooled to below 55°C and the temperature then was raised slowly. The Tm is the temperature at which half of the DNA is single strand and is specific for the sequence of the particular DNA product. The specific melting temperature is determined at 640 nm (channel F2 on the cycler) for the clinical samples and the positive and negative controls. For illustration purposes, melting curve analyses are "overlaid" relative to one another in this figure for three clinical samples and the HSV-1 and HSV-2 positive or "template" control. The clinical specimens containing HSV-1 DNA *(red line)* or HSV-2 *(green line)* result in a melting peak at 54°C (the Tm) or 67°C (the Tm), respectively. The LightCycler positive or template control containing HSV-1 and HSV-2 DNA, displayed as a purple line, shows two peaks at 54°C and 67°C, respectively. The clinical sample that is negative *(brown line)* for both HSV-1 and HSV-2 shows no peaks.

curves are evaluated. As previously discussed, amplification is monitored either through the fluorescence of double-stranded DNA–specific dyes (e.g., SYBER Green 1) or by sequence-specific probes; thus during amplification, a curve is generated. During real-time PCR, there are at least three distinct phases for these curves: (1) an initial lag phase in which no product is detected, (2) an exponential phase of amplified product detected, and a (3) plateau phase. The number of targets in the original specimen can be determined with precision when the number of cycles needed for the signal to achieve an arbitrary threshold (the portion of the curve where the signal begins to increase exponentially or logarithmically) is determined. This segment of the real-time PCR cycle is within the linear amplification portion of the reaction where conditions are optimal and fluorescence accumulates in proportion to the amplicon.

With most instrument analyses, the value used for quantitative measurement is the PCR cycle number in which the fluorescence reaches a threshold value of 10 times the standard deviation of baseline fluorescence emission; this cycle number is referred to as the **threshold cycle (CT)** or **crossing point** and is inversely proportional to the starting amount of target present in the clinical sample (see Mackay in the Bibliography). In other words, the CT is the cycle number in which the fluorescent signal rises above background (the threshold value previously defined) and is dependent on the amount of target at the beginning of the reaction. Thus, to quantitate the target in a clinical specimen, a standard curve is generated in which known amounts of target are prepared and then subjected to real-time PCR, along with the clinical sample containing an unknown amount of target. A standard curve is generated using the CT values for each of the known amounts of target amplified. By taking the CT value of the clinical specimen and using the standard curve, the amount of target in the original sample can be determined (Figure 8-14). Quantitative nucleic acid methods are used to monitor response to therapy, detect the development of drug resistance, and predict disease progression.

The introduction of commercially available analyte-specific reagents (ASRs) followed soon after the introduction of real-time PCR. ASRs represent a new regulatory approach by the FDA in which reagents in this broad category (e.g., antibodies; specific receptor proteins; ligands; oligonucleotides, such as DNA or RNA probes or primers; and many reagents used in in-house PCR assays) can be used in multiple diagnostic applications. ASR-labeled reagents carry the "For Research Use Only" label, and the manufacturer is prohibited from promoting any applications for these reagents or providing recipes for using the reagents. On a cautionary note, because they have not been cleared by the FDA, ASR assays cannot be reimbursed by Medicare carriers. Because rulings vary on a state-by-state basis, laboratory supervisors should check into Medicare reimbursement before developing and introducing an ASR assay. A laboratory designated as high complexity according to the Clinical Laboratory Improvement Amendment (CLIA) must take full responsibility for developing, validating, and offering the diagnostic assay using these reagents. This new regulation essentially allows for new diagnostic methods to become available more quickly, particularly methods targeted toward smaller patient populations. It is important to note that because good manufacturing practices are mandated, ASRs provide more standardized products for the performance of amplification assays. ASRs are available for a number of organisms, such as beta-hemolytic group A and B streptococci, methicillin-resistant *S. aureus* (MRSA), *Bordetella pertussis,* vancomycin-resistant enterococci, hepatitis A virus, and Epstein-Barr virus. Molecular kits such as the IDI-MRSA and IDI-StrepB (Benton Dickinson Diagnostics, Franklin Lakes, N.J.) for direct detection in clinical specimens of MRSA and beta-hemolytic group B streptococci, respectively, have received FDA clearance.

## DIGITAL PCR

Digital PCR (dPCR) is an emerging real-time method that is a modification of the traditional polymerase chain

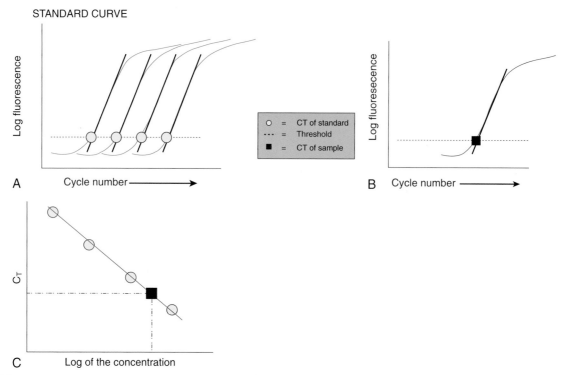

**Figure 8-14** Quantitation using real-time PCR. **A,** In the example, four samples containing known amounts of target are amplified by real-time PCR. The inverse log of their fluorescence is plotted against the cycle number and their respective $C_T$ is determined; the fewer the number of targets, the greater the $C_T$ value. **B,** Similarly, the clinical specimen is also amplified by real-time PCR, and its $C_T$ value is determined. **C,** The log of the nucleic acid concentration and the respective $C_T$ value for each specimen containing a known amount of target or nucleic acid are plotted to generate a standard curve. Knowing the $C_T$ value of the clinical specimen allows the concentration of target in the original sample to be determined.

reaction. In traditional PCR, multiple target sequences are amplified in a single-reaction cuvette or well. Digital PCR separates individual nucleic acid samples within a single specimen into separate regions or droplets. Each region or droplet within the sample will either contain no molecule, a single molecule, or a negative or positive reaction. Therefore, the quantitation of the amplification is based on counting the regions that contain a positive amplified product. The quantitation is not based on exponential amplification in comparison to the starting quantity of the target and therefore eliminates errors associated with rate of amplification changes that are affected by interfering substances and the use of a standard curve. Digital PCR provides a possible resolution for the detection of infectious agents or pathogens that are present in very low numbers in biological samples.

## AMPLIFICATION METHODS: NON–PCR-BASED

Although PCR was developed first and numerous PCR-based assays are available, rapid, sensitive, and specific detection of infectious agents by nucleic acid amplification can be achieved by a number of methods other than PCR. These amplification formats can be divided into two broad categories: those that amplify the signal used to detect the target nucleic acid and those that directly amplify the target nucleic acid but are not PCR based. Examples of signal amplification methods used in infectious disease diagnostics are listed in Table 8-2.

**TABLE 8-2** Examples of Commercially Available Signal Amplification Methods

| Method | Manufacturer |
|---|---|
| Branched DNA (bDNA) | Siemens Healthcare Diagnostics, Deerfield, IL |
| Invader assays | Hologic, Marlborough, MA |
| Signal-mediated amplification of RNA (SMART) | Cytocell Technologies, Ltd, Cambridge, U.K. |
| Hybrid capture | Qiagen, Germantown, MD |

### Isothermal Amplification

Loop-mediated isothermal amplification (LAMP) uses four primers and proceeds using a constant temperature coupled to a strand displacement reaction. This technology was developed by the Eiken Chemical Company, Japan. In addition to LAMP, there are other isothermal methods that have been developed that also use strand displacement for amplification. Strand displacement requires four primers, two for each strand of the parent double helix. One primer binds downstream of the other. The downstream primer contains a restriction endonuclease site on the 5' tail. DNA polymerase I (exonuclease deficient), extends from both primers and incorporates a modified nucleotide (2'-deoxyadenosine 5'-O-(1-thiotriphosphate). During the extension, the newly synthesized strand that is extended from the downstream primer is displaced by the new molecule that is being synthesized by the second primer that is upstream or outside of the first primer. A subsequent set of primers is then capable of binding to the new strand, producing additional amplification product. This amplification product is then used in the second stage of the amplification. In the second step of the reaction, the restriction endonuclease nicks 5′ end of the original downstream primer that is incorporated into the displaced strand. The complementary strand cannot be nicked, because the modified nucleotide that has been incorporated into the strand blocks restriction digestion, and the restriction site therefore is inactive. Once the restriction site has been cleaved, a new double strand region that contains the primer/probe provides for a new cycle of amplification.

Additional isothermal amplifications include nucleic-acid based sequencing (NABS) and transcription-mediated amplification. Both methods are used for the isothermal amplification of RNA. These methods are used for the amplification of viral RNA, *Mycobacterium* spp. antibiotic resistance determinants, and detection of bacteria. The assays use a reverse transcriptase (RT) to copy the target RNA into a complementary DNA molecule (cDNA). An enzyme, either RNase H or a RT molecule with RNase activity, degrades the RNA molecule in the RNA-DNA hybrid. The remaining cDNA molecule is replicated into double-stranded DNA molecules by the DNA polymerase activity of the polyermase (i.e., T7 bacteriophage RNA polymerase). The RT uses a promoter that was incorporated into the cDNA engineered into the primer for the first amplification of the cDNA. The RT then transcribes anti-sense RNA molecules from the cDNA molecules. The resulting anti-sense RNA amplicons then continue the cycle for increased amplification of the target sequence.

A relatively new helicase-dependent method uses DNA helicase to separate DNA double-stranded molecules to generate single-stranded templates for amplification. Helicase-dependent amplification is also an isothermal method.

### Probe Amplification

In a probe amplification assay, the amplified product no longer contains the target nucleic acid sequence. The amplification product is engineered to contain a sequence for detection that was present in the initial primer/probe used for the amplification reaction. The invader assays (Hologic-GenProbe, Madison, WI), is an isothermal system that can be used to amplify DNA or RNA. The reaction requires two synthetic oligonucleotides, the probe, and what is referred to as the invader oligo. The invader oligo binds to the target, with the primary probe binding to the target, creating a one-base pair overlap between the invader and the probe. The cleavase enzyme then cleaves the primary probe, releasing it along with one nucleotide. This released structure is referred to as a flap. The number of flaps released corresponds to the amount of target nucleic acid present in the sample. During the primary reaction, a secondary reaction occurs. The flaps combine with a fluorescent resonance energy transfer (FRET) probe and generates

a single that can be measured in real-time. Invader chemistry has also been incorporated into a new InvaderPLUS system that incorporates a PCR reaction, followed by an invader reaction, resulting in a combination target amplification followed by a signal amplification to improve the detection of nucleic acid present in low numbers in the initial specimen.

A number of other non-PCR-based technologies have been successfully used to detect a variety of infectious agents (Table 8-3). As with PCR, these applications are able to amplify DNA, RNA, mRNA, and rRNA targets; to have multiplex capabilities; and to be qualitative or quantitative. To learn more about these alternative target amplification methods, refer to additional reading and articles authored by Ginocchio.

## SEQUENCING AND ENZYMATIC DIGESTION OF NUCLEIC ACIDS

The nucleotide sequence of a microorganism's genome is the blueprint for the organism. Therefore, molecular methods that elucidate some part of a pathogen's genomic sequence provide a powerful tool for diagnostic microbiology. Other methods, either used independently or in conjunction with hybridization or amplification procedures, can provide nucleotide sequence information to detect, identify, and characterize clinically relevant microorganisms. These methods include nucleic acid sequencing and enzymatic digestion and electrophoresis of nucleic acids.

### Nucleic Acid Sequencing

Nucleic acid sequencing involves methods that determine the exact nucleotide sequence of a gene or gene fragment obtained from an organism. Although explaining the technology involved is beyond the scope of this text, nucleic acid sequencing will powerfully affect clinical microbiology for some time to come. To illustrate, nucleotide sequences obtained from a microorganism can be compared with an ever-growing gene sequence database for:

- Detecting and classifying previously unknown human pathogens
- Identifying various known microbial pathogens and their subtypes
- Determining which specific nucleotide changes resulting from mutations are responsible for antibiotic resistance
- Identifying sequences or cassettes of genes that have moved from one organism to another
- Establishing the relatedness between isolates of the same species

Before the development of rapid and automated methods, DNA sequencing was a laborious task only undertaken in the research setting. However, determining the sequence of nucleotides in a segment of nucleic acid from an infectious agent can be done rapidly using amplified target from the organism and an automated DNA sequencer. Because sequence information can now be rapidly produced, DNA sequencing has entered the arena of diagnostic microbiology. Identification of

**TABLE 8-3** Examples of Non-Polymerase Chain Reaction–Based Nucleic Amplification Tests

| Amplification Method | Manufacturer/Name | Method Overview | Examples Of Commercially Available Assays | Additional Comments |
|---|---|---|---|---|
| Nucleic acid sequence-based amplification (NASBA) | bioMérieux Inc. NucliSens technology: nucleic acid release, extraction, NASBA amplification, product detection. | 1. Isothermal amplification achieved through coordination of three enzymes (avian mycloblastosis, RNAseH, T7 RNA polymerase) in conjunction with two oligonucleotide primers specific for the target sequence.<br>2. Amplification based on primer extension and ribonucleic acid (RNA) transcription. | NucliSens HIV-1 QT NucliSens CMV pp67 NucliSens EasyQ HIV-1 NucliSens EasyQ enterovirus | 1. Can be adapted to real-time format using molecular beacons<br>2. Can develop in-house assays<br>3. Automated extraction available (NucliSens extractor)<br>4. EasyQ System comprises an incubator, analyzer, and a computer. |
| Transcription-mediated amplification (TMA) | Gen-Probe Hologic/Gen-Probe: Sample processing, amplification, target detection by hybridization protection or dual kinetic assays for *Chlamydia trachomatis* and *Neisseria gonorrhoeae*. Also, ASRs for hepatitis C virus (HCV), Bayer Inc., Tarrytown, NY; Gen-Probe/Chiron Corp.: TMA for screening donated blood products for human immunodeficiency virus type 1 ( HIV-1) and HCV. | 1. Autocatalytic, isothermal amplification using reverse transcriptase and T7 RNA polymerase and 2 primers complementary to the target.<br>2. Exponential extension of RNA (up to 10 billion amplicons within 10 minutes). | Gen-Probe: *Mycobacterium tuberculosis* Direct Test; APTIMA Combo 2 for dual detection of *C. trachomatis* and *N. gonorrhoeae*; Bayer ASR reagents for HCV; Gen-Probe/Chiron: Procleix HIV-1/HCV | 1. Second-generation TMA assays of Gen-Probe better at removing interfering substances<br>• Less labor intensive<br>• Uses target capture after sample lysis using an intermediate capture oligomer<br>• TMA performed directly on captured target<br>2. Fully Automated Systems PANTHER eliminates batch testing<br>• TGRIS DTS system, 1000 samples in 13.5 hours<br>• Instruments handle specimen processing through amplification and detection. |
| Strand displacement amplification (SDA) | BD ProbeTec ET System: SDA coupled with homogeneous real-time detection. | 1. Isothermal process in which a single-stranded target is first generated.<br>2. Exponential amplification of target. | BDProbe Tec ET System for *C. trachomatis* and *N. gonorrhoeae*; panel assays for *Mycoplasma pneumoniae*, *Chlamydophila pneumoniae*, and *Legionella pneumoniae*; Chlamydiaceae: assay that detects *C. trachomatis*, *C. pneumophila*, and *C. psittaci*; D ProbeTec *M. tuberculosis* Direct | 1. Reagents dried in separate disposable microwell strips<br>2. All assays have internal control to monitor for inhibition<br>3. Automated system for sample processing: BD Viper Sample Processor |

microorganisms using PCR in conjunction with automated sequencing is slowly making its way into clinical microbiology laboratories; presently, such molecular analyses are limited for the most part to research-oriented laboratories. It is becoming quite clear that combinations of phenotypic and genotypic characterization are most successful in identifying a variety of microorganisms for which identification is difficult such as the speciation of Nocardia, mycobacteria, and organisms that commercial automated instruments fail to identify or correctly

identify. Recently, Perkin Elmer Applied Biosystems Division (now Applera, Foster City, California) has introduced MicroSeq kit-based reagents in conjunction with automated sequencing that allows analysis of a sequence of either the bacterial 16S rRNA gene or the D2 expansion segment region of the nuclear large-subunit rRNA gene of fungi. Of significance, the MicroSeq sequence libraries contain accurate and rigorously verified sequence data; an important component for successful sequencing in the identification of organisms is an accurate and complete sequence database. In addition, the ability to create customized libraries for specific sequences of interest is possible by the availability of flexible software.

# POST-AMPLIFICATION AND TRADITIONAL ANALYSIS

## NUCLEIC ACID ELECTROPHORESIS

Traditional gel electrophoresis utilizes an electric current, a buffer, and a porous matrice of agarose or polyacrylamide for the separation of nucleic acid molecules according to size. As the electrical current is applied to the system, the negatively charged nucleic acids will migrate toward the positive pole or anode. Electrophoresis may utilize a horizontal or vertical gel apparatus or a small tube or capillary system. Capillary electrophoresis utilizes a thin glass silica capillary tube for faster separation and detection using fluorescent detection. Agarose is a polysaccharide polymer that is extracted from seaweed. It is relatively inexpensive and easy to use. Polyacrylamide is typically a mixture of acrylamide and a cross-linking methylene bisacrylamide. Polyacrylamide is a more porous or highly cross-linked gel that provides for a higher resolution of smaller fragments and single-stranded molecules. Despite the higher resolving power of acrylamide gels, it is important to note that in the powder form and unpolymerized form, acrylamide is neurotoxic, and proper safety precautions should be used during handling.

In addition to varying systems and matrices, different buffers may be used for the separation of nucleic acids. The two most common buffering systems include Trias acetate or Tris borate buffers. Tris borate EDTA (TBE, 0.089 M Tris-base, 0.089 boric acid, 0.0020 M EDTA) has a greater buffering capacity. However, TBE has a tendency to precipitate during storage and generates heat during electrophoresis. Excessive heating during electrophoresis can result in distorted patterns and make detection or interpretation of migration patterns difficult. Tris acetate EDTA (TAE, 0.04 M Tris-base, 0.005 M sodium acetate, 0.002 M EDTA) provides for faster migration or separation during electrophoresis. Denaturing agents such as detergents, formamide, or urea may be added to the buffers that break the hydrogen bonds between complementary sequences on DNA or RNA molecules that may alter migration patterns.

### Pyrosequencing

Traditional nucleic acid sequencing is based on chain-termination and the addition of a labeled nucleotide (TTP, GTP, ATP, CTP, or UTP) that is then detected using a radiolabeled or fluorescent tag. Pyrosequencing is a newer method that incorporates a luminescent signal (generation of a pyrophosphate) when nucleotides are added to the growing nucleic acid strand. The reaction incorporates a sequencing primer that hybridizes to the single-stranded target. The hybrids are incubated with DNA polymerase, ATP sulfurylase, luciferase, and apyrase along with the substrates adenosine-5′-phosphosulfate and luciferin. A single dNTP (deoxynucleotide triphospate) is added to the reaction. As the polymerase extends the target from the primer, the dNTP is incorporated, releasing a pyrophosphate (PPi). The ATP sulfurylase then converts the PPi to ATP, which drives the conversion of luciferin to oxyluciferin, generating light. The amount of light generated is proportional to the amount of the specific nucleotide incorporated, generating a report or pyrogram. The Apyrase degrades the ATP and unincorporated dNTPs, turning off the light and regenerating the reaction mixture. The next dNTP is added, repeating the process for each subsequent nucleotide. Pyrosequencing is useful for identifying drug-resistant mutations and identification of viral, bacterial, or fungal nucleic acids.

### High-Density DNA Probes

An alternative to gel-based sequencing has been the introduction of the high-density oligonucleotide probe array. This technology was developed recently by Affymetrix (Santa Clara, California). The method relies on the hybridization of a fluorescent-labeled nucleic acid target to large sets of oligonucleotides synthesized at precise locations on a miniaturized glass substrate that may include glass or "chip" or siliconized wafer. The hybridization pattern of the probe to the various oligonucleotides is then used to gain primary structure information about the target (Figure 8-15). Hybridization high-density microarrays in combination with sequence-independent amplification (PCR) have also been used to identify pathogens. This technology has been applied to a broad range of nucleic acid sequence analysis problems, including pathogen identification and classification, polymorphism detection, and drug-resistant mutations for viruses (e.g., HIV) and bacteria.

### Low- to Moderate-Density Arrays

Improved technology in molecular diagnostics has resulted in the development of low- to moderate-density microarray platforms that are less expensive than high-density arrays. This has allowed many laboratories to incorporate this new and powerful technology into the daily operations of the diagnostic microbiology laboratory. These microarrays utilize layered film, gold-plated electrodes, and electrochemical detection or gold-nanoparticles for the detection of target sequences. There are currently three FDA-approved platforms available in the United States: the INFINITI analyzer (Autogenomics, Vista, CA), the eSensor XT-8 system, (GenMark Diagnostics, Carlsbad, CA), and the Verigene system (Nanosphere Inc., Northbrook, IL). These instruments are closed-system, random access, completely automated systems, making the detection of nucleic acids relatively simple and free from the hazards of contamination by other circulating nucleic acids or amplification products.

### Enzymatic Digestion and Electrophoresis of Nucleic Acids

Enzymatic digestion and electrophoresis of DNA fragments are not as specific as sequencing or specific amplification assays in identifying and

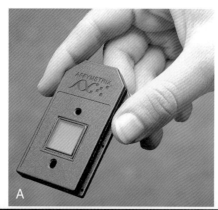

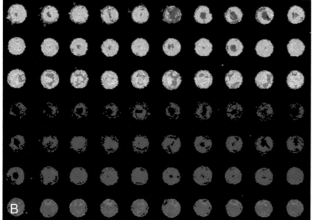

**Figure 8-15** Overview of high-density DNA probes. High-density oligonucleotide arrays are created using light-directed chemical synthesis that combines photolithography and solid-phase chemical synthesis. Because of this sophisticated process, more than 500 to as many as 1 million different oligonucleotide probes may be formed on a chip; an array is shown in **A.** Nucleic acid is extracted from a sample and then hybridized within seconds to the probe array in a GeneChip Fluidics Station. The hybridized array **(B)** is scanned using a laser confocal fluorescent microscope that looks at each site (i.e., probe) on the chip, and the intensity of hybridization is analyzed using imaging processing software.

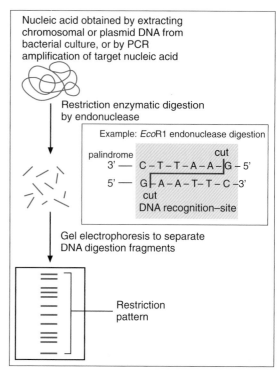

**Figure 8-16** DNA enzymatic digestion and gel electrophoresis to separate DNA fragments resulting from the digestion. An example of a nucleic acid recognition site and enzymatic cut produced by EcoR1, a commonly used endonuclease, is shown in the inset.

characterizing microorganisms. However, enzyme digestion-electrophoresis procedures still provide valuable information for the diagnosis and control of infectious diseases.

Enzymatic digestion of DNA is accomplished using any of a number of enzymes known as **restriction endonucleases.** Each specific endonuclease recognizes a specific nucleotide sequence (usually 4 to 8 nucleotides in length), known as the enzyme's **recognition,** or **restriction, site.** Restriction sites are often palindromic sequences; in other words, the two strands have the same sequence, which run antiparallel to one another. Once the recognition site has been located, the enzyme catalyzes the digestion of the nucleic acid strand at that site, causing a break, or **cut,** in the nucleic acid strand (Figure 8-16).

The number and size of fragments produced by enzymatic digestion depend on the length of nucleic acid being digested (the longer the strand, the greater the likelihood of more recognition sites and thus more fragments), the nucleotide sequence of the strand being digested, and the particular enzyme used for digestion. For example, enzymatic digestion of a bacterial plasmid whose nucleotide sequence provides several recognition sites for endonuclease A, but only rare sites for endonuclease B, will produce more fragments with endonuclease A. Additionally, the size of the fragments produced will depend on the number of nucleotides between each of endonuclease A's recognition sites present on the nucleic acid being digested.

The DNA used for digestion is obtained by various methods. A target sequence may be obtained by amplification via PCR, in which case the length of the DNA to be digested is relatively short (e.g., 50 to 1000 bases). Alternatively, specific procedures may be used to cultivate the organism of interest to large numbers (e.g., $10^{10}$ bacterial cells) from which plasmid DNA, chromosomal DNA, or total cellular DNA may be isolated and purified for endonuclease digestion.

After digestion, fragments are subjected to agarose gel electrophoresis, which allows them to be separated according to their size differences as previously described for Southern hybridization (see Figure 8-4, *B*). During electrophoresis all nucleic acid fragments of the same size comigrate as a single band. For many digestions, electrophoresis results in the separation of several different fragment sizes (Figure 8-17). The nucleic acid bands in the agarose gel are stained with the fluorescent dye ethidium bromide, which allows them to be visualized on exposure to UV light. Stained gels are photographed for a permanent record (see Figure 8-17; also Figures 8-18 and 8-19).

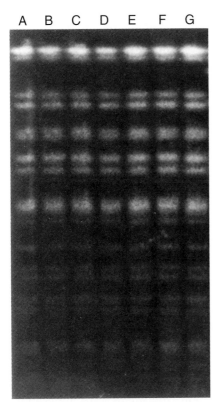

**Figure 8-17** Restriction fragment length polymorphisms of vancomycin-resistant *Enterococcus faecalis* isolates in Lanes A through G as determined by pulsed-field gel electrophoresis. All isolates appear to be the same strain.

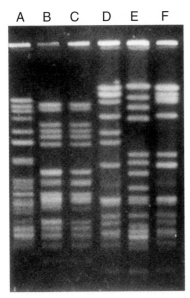

**Figure 8-18** Although antimicrobial susceptibility profiles indicated that several methicillin-resistant *S. aureus* isolates were the same strain, restriction fragment length polymorphism analysis using pulsed-field gel electrophoresis (Lanes A through F) demonstrates that only isolates B and C were the same.

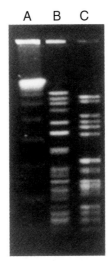

**Figure 8-19** Restriction patterns generated by pulsed-field gel electrophoresis for two *Streptococcus pneumoniae* isolates, one that was susceptible to penicillin (Lane B) and one that was resistant (Lane C), from the same patient. Restriction fragment length polymorphism analysis indicates that the patient was infected with different strains. Molecular-size markers are shown in Lane A.

One variation of this method, known as **ribotyping,** involves enzymatic digestion of chromosomal DNA followed by Southern hybridization using probes for genes that encode ribosomal RNA. Because all bacteria contain ribosomal genes, a hybridization pattern will be obtained with almost any isolate, but the pattern will vary depending on the arrangement of genes in a particular strain's genome.

Regardless of the method, the process by which enzyme digestion patterns are analyzed is referred to as **restriction enzyme analysis (REA).** The patterns obtained after gel electrophoresis are referred to as **restriction patterns,** and differences between microorganism restriction patterns are known as **restriction fragment length polymorphisms (RFLPs).** Because RFLPs reflect differences or similarities in nucleotide sequences, REA methods can be used for organism identification and for establishing strain relatedness within the same species (see Figures 8-17 to 8-19).

## APPLICATIONS OF NUCLEIC ACID–BASED METHODS

Categories for the application of molecular diagnostic microbiology methods are the same as those for conventional, phenotype-based methods:
- Direct detection of microorganisms in patient specimens
- Identification of microorganisms grown in culture
- Characterization of microorganisms beyond identification

## DIRECT DETECTION OF MICROORGANISMS

Nucleic acid hybridization and target or probe amplification methods are the molecular techniques most commonly used for direct organism detection in clinical specimens.

## Advantages and Disadvantages

When considering the advantages and disadvantages of molecular approaches to direct organism detection, comparison with the most commonly used conventional method (i.e., direct smears, culture, and microscopy) is helpful.

**Specificity.** Both hybridization and amplification methods are driven by the specificity of a nucleotide sequence for a particular organism. Therefore, a positive assay indicates the presence of an organism but also provides the organism's identity, potentially precluding the need for follow-up culture. Although molecular methods may not be faster than microscopic smear examinations, the opportunity to avoid delays associated with culture can be a substantial advantage.

However, for many infectious agents, detection and identification are only part of the diagnostic requirement. Determination of certain characteristics, such as strain relatedness or resistance to antimicrobial agents, is often an important diagnostic or epidemiologic component that is not possible without the availability of culture. For this reason, most molecular direct detection methods target organisms for which antimicrobial susceptibility testing is not routinely needed (e.g., *Chlamydia* sp.) or for which reliable cultivation methods are not widely available (e.g., *Ehrlichia* sp.).

The high specificity of molecular techniques also presents a limitation in what can be detected with any one assay; that is, most molecular assays focus on detecting the presence of only one or two potential pathogens. Even if tests for those organisms are positive, the possibility of a mixed infection involving other organisms has not been ruled out. If the tests are negative, other procedures may be needed to determine whether additional pathogens are present. In contrast, smear examination and cultivation procedures can detect and identify a broader selection of possible infectious etiologies. Of importance, Gram-stained smear results are often needed to determine the clinical relevance of finding a particular organism upon culture or detection using molecular assays. However, given the rapid development of molecular technology, protocols that widen the spectrum of detectable organisms in any particular specimen are becoming available. ASRs for real-time PCR that can detect as many as six to seven organisms are commercially available. Finally, a concern always associated with any amplification-based assay is the possibility for cross contamination between samples and/or by amplified byproduct. Thus, it is of utmost importance for any laboratory performing these assays to employ measures to prevent false-positive results.

**Sensitivity.** Hybridization-based methods are not completely reliable in directly detecting organisms. The quantity of target nucleic acid may be insufficient, or the patient specimen may contain substances that interfere with or cross-react in the hybridization and signal-generating reactions. One approach developed by Gen-Probe (San Diego, California) to enhance sensitivity has been to use DNA probes targeted for bacterial ribosomal RNA, of which there are up to 10,000 copies per cell. Essentially, amplification is accomplished by the choice of a target that exists within the cell as multiple copies rather than as a single copy.

**Amplification Techniques Enhance Sensitivity.** As was discussed with direct hybridization methods, patient specimens may contain substances that interfere with or inhibit amplification reactions such as PCR. Nonetheless, the ability to amplify target or probe nucleic acid to readily detectable levels has provided an invaluable means of overcoming the lack of sensitivity characteristic of most direct hybridization methods.

Besides the potential for providing more reliable test results than direct hybridization (i.e., fewer false-negative results), amplification methods have other advantages that include:

- Ability to detect nonviable organisms that are not retrievable by cultivation-based methods
- Ability to detect and identify organisms that cannot be grown in culture or are extremely difficult to grow (e.g., hepatitis B virus and the agent of Whipple's disease)
- More rapid detection and identification of slow-growing organisms (e.g., mycobacteria, certain fungi)
- Ability to detect previously unknown agents directly in clinical specimens by using broad-range primers (e.g., use of primers that anneal to a region of target DNA conserved among all bacteria)
- Ability to quantitate infectious agent burden in patient specimens, an application that has particular importance for managing HIV, cytomegalovirus (CMV), and hepatitis B and hepatitis C infections.

Despite these significant advantages, limitations still exist, notably the ability to find only the organisms toward which the primers have been targeted. Additionally, no cultured organism is available if subsequent characterization beyond identification is necessary. As with hybridization, the first limitation may eventually be addressed using broad-range amplification methods to screen specimens for the presence of any organism (e.g., bacteria, fungi, parasite). Specimens positive by this test would then be processed further for a more specific diagnosis. The second limitation is more difficult to overcome and is one reason culture methods will remain a major part of diagnostic microbiology for some time to come.

An interesting consequence of using highly sensitive amplification methods is the effect on clinical interpretation of results. For example, if a microbiologist detects organisms that are no longer viable, can he or she assume the organisms are or were involved in the infectious process being diagnosed? Also, amplification may detect microorganisms present in insignificant quantities as part of the patient's normal or transient flora, or as an established latent infection, that have nothing to do with the current disease state of the patient.

Finally, as previously mentioned, an underlying complication in the development and application of any direct detection method is that various substances in patient specimens can interfere with the reagents and conditions required for optimum hybridization or amplification. Specimen interference is one of the major issues that must be addressed in the design of any useful direct method for molecular diagnosis of infectious diseases.

## Applications for Direct Molecular Detection of Microorganisms

Given their inherent advantages and disadvantages, molecular direct detection methods are most useful when:

- One or two pathogens cause the majority of infections (e.g., *Chlamydia trachomatis* and *Neisseria gonorrhoeae* as common agents of genitourinary tract infections)
- Further organism characterization, such as antimicrobial susceptibility testing, is not required for management of the infection (e.g., various viral agents)
- Either no reliable diagnostic methods exist or they are notably suboptimal (e.g., various bacterial, parasitic, viral, and fungal agents)
- Reliable diagnostic methods exist but are slow (e.g., *Mycobacterium tuberculosis*)
- Quantitation of infectious agent burden that influences patient management (e.g., AIDS) is desired

A large number and variety of commercially available molecular systems and products for the detection and identification of infectious organisms are now available. These include automated or semiautomated systems. Many of these systems and products are mentioned throughout this textbook. Additionally, many direct detection assays have been developed by diagnostic manufacturers and research laboratories associated with academic medical centers. Therefore, direct molecular diagnostic methods based on amplification will continue to expand and enhance our understanding and diagnosis of infectious diseases. However, as with any laboratory method, their ultimate utility and application will depend on their accuracy, potential impact on patient care, advantages over currently available methods, and resources required to establish and maintain their use in the diagnostic setting.

## IDENTIFICATION OF MICROORGANISMS GROWN IN CULTURE

Once organisms are grown in culture, hybridization, amplification, or RFLP analysis may be used to establish identity. Because the target nucleic acid is already amplified via microbial cultivation, sensitivity is not usually a problem for molecular identification methods. Additionally, extensive nucleotide sequence data are available for most clinically relevant organisms, providing the required information to produce highly specific probes and primers. With neither specificity nor sensitivity as problems in this setting, other criteria regarding the application of molecular identification methods must be considered.

The criteria often considered in comparing molecular and conventional methods for microbial identification include speed, accuracy, and cost. For slow-growing organisms, such as mycobacteria and fungi, growth-based identification schemes can take weeks to months to produce a result. Molecular-based methods can identify these microorganisms almost immediately after sufficient

inoculum is available, clearly demonstrating a speed advantage over conventional methods. *Mycobacteria* spp. may take up to several months to correctly identify. A molecular test is available that amplifies the DNA coding sequence for the 16s subunit of the rRNA, which is a genetic characteristic common to all species of mycobacteria. This provides a screening method indicating the presence of a *Mycobacterium* species. This procedure may then be followed by amplification of a insertion sequence (S6110) that is unique and specific for *M. tuberculosis*. Additional species may be identified using the differential restriction digestion patterns for the hsp65 gene present in all mycobacteria. On the other hand, phenotypic-based methods used to identify frequently encountered bacteria, such as *S. aureus* and beta-hemolytic streptococci, can usually provide highly accurate results within minutes and are less costly and time-consuming than any currently available molecular method. However, this is rapidly changing. Real-time PCR–based methods are commercially available for screening of MRSA upon admission to a long-term care or hospital facility. This identification provides for immediate isolation of carriers, preventing the spread of nosocomial infections throughout the facility.

Although many of the phenotype-based identification schemes are highly accurate and reliable, in some situations phenotypic profiles may yield uncertain identifications and molecular methods are providing an alternative for establishing a definitive identification. This is especially the case when a common pathogen exhibits unusual phenotypic traits (e.g., optochin-resistant *Streptococcus pneumoniae*).

## CHARACTERIZATION OF MICROORGANISMS BEYOND IDENTIFICATION

Situations exist in which characterizing a microbial pathogen beyond identification provides important information for patient management and public health. In such situations, knowledge regarding an organism's virulence, resistance to antimicrobial agents, or relatedness to other strains of the same species can be extremely important. Although various phenotypic methods have been able to provide some of this information, the development of molecular technologies has greatly expanded our ability to generate this information in the diagnostic setting. This is especially true with regard to antimicrobial resistance and strain relatedness.

### Detection of Antimicrobial Resistance

As are all phenotypic traits, those that render microorganisms resistant to antimicrobial agents are encoded on specific genes (for more information regarding antimicrobial resistance mechanisms, see Chapter 11). Therefore, molecular methods for gene amplification or hybridization can be used to detect antimicrobial resistance. In many ways, phenotypic methods for resistance detection are reliable and are the primary methods for antimicrobial susceptibility testing (see Chapter 12). However, the complexity of emerging resistance mechanisms often challenges the ability of commonly used susceptibility testing methods to detect clinically important resistance to antimicrobial agents. As with molecular identification previously described, *Mycobacterium* sp. resistant to rifampin and isoniazid may be identified by the presence of the rpoB and katG genes.

Methods such as PCR play a role in the detection of certain resistance profiles that may not always readily be detected by phenotypic methods. Two such examples include detection of the van genes, which mediate vancomycin resistance among enterococci (see Figure 8-17), and the mec gene, which encodes resistance among staphylococci to all currently available drugs of the beta-lactam class (see Figure 8-18). Undoubtedly, conventional and molecular methods will both continue to play key roles in the characterization of microbial resistance to antimicrobial agents.

## Investigation of Strain Relatedness/Pulsed-Field Gel Electrophoresis

An important component of recognizing and controlling disease outbreaks inside or outside of a hospital is identification of the reservoir and mode of transmission of the infectious agents involved. Strain typing provides a mechanism for monitoring the spread of drug-resistant pathogens, the evaluation of multiple isolates from a single patient, differentiation of relapse from a new infection, and applications in epidemiology and infection control. Infection control measures often require establishing relatedness among the pathogens isolated during the outbreak. For example, if all the microbial isolates thought to be associated with a nosocomial infection outbreak are shown to be identical or at least very closely related, then a common source or reservoir for those isolates must be identified. If the etiologic agents are not the same, other explanations for the outbreak must be investigated (see Chapter 80). Because each species of a microorganism comprises an almost limitless number of strains, identification of an organism to the species level is not sufficient for establishing relatedness. **Strain typing,** the process used to establish the relatedness among organisms belonging to the same species, is required.

Although phenotypic characteristics (e.g., biotyping, serotyping, antimicrobial susceptibility profiles) historically have been used to type strains, these methods often are limited by their inability to consistently discriminate between different strains, their labor intensity, or their lack of reproducibility. In contrast, certain molecular methods do not have these limitations and have enhanced strain-typing capabilities. The molecular typing methods either directly compare nucleotide sequences between strains or produce results that indirectly reflect similarities in nucleotide sequences among "outbreak" organisms. Indirect methods usually involve enzymatic digestion and electrophoresis of microbial DNA to produce RFLPs for comparison and analysis.

Several molecular methods have been investigated for establishing strain relatedness (Table 8-4). The method chosen primarily depends on the extent to which the following four criteria proposed by Maslow and colleagues are met:

- **Typeability:** The method's capacity to produce clearly interpretable results with most strains of the bacterial species to be tested

**TABLE 8-4** Examples of Methods to Determine Strain Relatedness

| Method | Advantages/Limitations |
|---|---|
| Plasmid analysis | Simple to implement but cannot often discriminate because many bacterial species have few or no plasmids |
| Multilocus enzyme electrophoresis | Provides only an estimate of overall genetic relatedness and diversity (protein-based) |
| Multilocus sequence typing | Data are electronically portable and used as non–culture-based typing method; labor intensive and expensive |
| Pulsed-field gel electrophoresis | Highly discriminatory but it is difficult to resolve bands of similar size and interlaboratory reproducibility is limited |
| Randomly amplified polymorphic DNA | High discriminatory power but poor laboratory interlaboratory and intralaboratory reproducibility due to short random primer sequences and low PCR annealing temperatures |
| Repetitive sequence–based PCR | *Manual system:* Useful for strain typing, but low rates of interlaboratory reproducibility; suboptimal turnaround times (TATs) for both manual and automated systems. *Automated system:* Increased reproducibility and decreased TATs. |
| Ribotyping and PCR ribotyping | Difficult to distinguish among different subtypes |

- **Reproducibility:** The method's capacity to repeatedly obtain the same typing profile result with the same bacterial strain
- **Discriminatory power:** The method's ability to produce results that clearly allow differentiation between unrelated strains of the same bacterial species
- **Practicality:** The method should be versatile, relatively rapid, inexpensive, technically simple, and provide readily interpretable results

The last criterion, practicality, is especially important for busy clinical microbiology laboratories that provide support for infection control and hospital epidemiology.

Among the molecular methods used for strain typing, pulsed-field gel electrophoresis (PFGE) meets most of Maslow's criteria for a good typing system and is frequently referred to as the microbial typing "gold standard." This method is applicable to most of the commonly encountered bacterial pathogens, particularly those frequently associated with nosocomial infections and outbreaks such as staphylococci (MRSA), enterococci (vancomycin-resistant enterococci), and gram-negative pathogens, including *Escherichia coli*, and *Klebsiella, Enterobacter,* and *Acinetobacter* spp. For these reasons, PFGE has been widely accepted among microbiologists, infection control personnel, and infectious disease specialists as a primary laboratory tool for epidemiology.

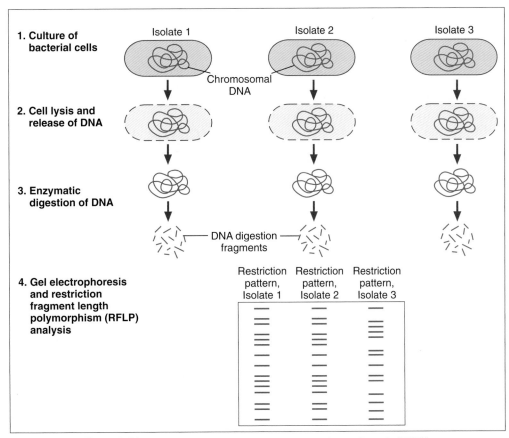

**Figure 8-20** Procedural steps for pulsed-field gel electrophoresis (PFGE).

PFGE uses a specialized electrophoresis device to separate chromosomal fragments produced by enzymatic digestion of intact bacterial chromosomal DNA. Bacterial suspensions are first embedded in agarose plugs, where they are carefully lysed (lysozyme) to release intact chromosomal DNA; the interfering contaminating proteins are then removed by treating the sample with Proteinase K; the DNA is then digested using restriction endonuclease enzymes. Enzymes that have relatively few restriction sites on the genomic DNA are selected so that 10 to 20 DNA fragments ranging in size from 10 to 1000 kb are produced (Figure 8-20). Because of the large DNA fragment sizes produced, resolution of the banding patterns requires the use of a **pulsed electrical field** across the agarose gel that subjects the DNA fragments to different voltages from varying angles at different time intervals.

Although comparison and interpretation of RFLP profiles produced by PFGE can be complex, the basic premise is that strains with the same or highly similar digestion profiles share substantial similarities in their nucleotide sequences and therefore are likely to be most closely related. For example, in Figure 8-19, isolates 1 and 2 have identical RFLP patterns, whereas isolate 3 has only 7 of its 15 bands in common with either isolates 1 or 2. Therefore, isolates 1 and 2 would be considered closely related, if not identical, whereas isolate 3 would not be considered related to the other two isolates.

One example of PFGE application for the investigation of an outbreak is shown in Figure 8-17. After SmaI endonuclease enzymatic digestion of DNA from seven vancomycin-resistant *E. faecalis* isolates, RFLP profiles show that the resistant isolates are probably the same strain. Such a finding strongly supports the probability of clonal dissemination of the same vancomycin-resistant strain among the patients from which the organisms were isolated.

The discriminatory advantage that PFGE profiles have over phenotype-based typing methods is demonstrated in Figure 8-18. Because all six methicillin-resistant *S. aureus* isolates exhibited identical antimicrobial susceptibility profiles, they were initially thought to be the same strain. However, PFGE profiling established that only isolates B and C were the same.

PFGE can also be used to determine whether a recurring infection in the same patient is due to insufficient original therapy, possibly as a result of developing antimicrobial resistance during therapy, or to acquisition of a second, more resistant, strain of the same species. Figure 8-19 shows restriction patterns obtained by PFGE with *S. pneumoniae* isolated from a patient with an unresolved middle ear infection. The PFGE profile of isolate B, which was fully susceptible to penicillin, differs substantially from the profile of isolate C, which was resistant to penicillin. The clear difference in PFGE profiles between the two strains indicates that the patient was most likely reinfected with a second, more resistant, strain. Alternatively, the patient's original infection may have been a mixture of both strains, with the more resistant one being lost during the original culture workup. In any case, this application of PFGE demonstrates that the method not only is useful for investigating outbreaks or strain dissemination involving several patients, it also gives us the ability to investigate questions regarding reinfections, treatment failures, and mixed infections involving more than one strain of the same species.

## Automation and Instrumentation

Molecular diagnostics has traditionally required extensive hands-on technical expertise to process specimens, extract the nucleic acids, amplify, and detect the target sequence. Technological advances in instrumentation and detection has rapidly changed the diagnostic microbiology laboratory. Traditional amplification instruments are still available; however, real-time amplification and detection as well as fully automated closed systems are rapidly replacing these instruments. See Table 8-1 for an overview and sample of instrumentation available for use in the molecular microbiology laboratory.

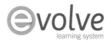 *Visit the Evolve site to complete the review questions.*

# BIBLIOGRAPHY

Buckingham L: *Molecular diagnostics, fundamentals, methods, and clinical applications*, ed 2, Philadelphia, 2012, FA Davis.

Chapin K, Musgnug M: Evaluation of three rapid methods for the direct detection of *Staphylococcus aureus* from positive blood cultures, *J Clin Microbiol* 41:4324, 2003.

Cockerill FR: Application of rapid-cycle real-time polymerase chain reaction for diagnostic testing in the clinical microbiology laboratory, *Arch Pathol Med* 127:1112, 2003.

Fontana C, Favaro M, Pelliccioni M et al: Use of the MicroSeq 5000 16S rRNA gene-based sequencing for identification of bacterial isolates that commercial automated systems failed to identify correctly, *J Clin Microbiol* 43:615, 2005.

Forbes BA: Introducing a molecular test into the clinical microbiology laboratory, *Arch Pathol Med* 127:1106, 2003.

Ginocchio CC: Life beyond PCR: alternative target amplification technologies for the diagnosis of infectious diseases. Part I, *Clin Microbiol Newls* 26:121, 2004.

Ginocchio CC: Life beyond PCR: alternative target amplification technologies for the diagnosis of infectious diseases. Part II, *Clin Microbiol Newls* 26:129, 2004.

Goering RV: Molecular strain typing for the clinical laboratory: current application and future direction, *Clin Microbiol Newsl* 22:169, 2000.

Haanpera M, Huovinen P, Jalava J: Detection and quantification of macrolide resistance mutations at positions 2058 and 2059 of the 23s rRNA gene by pyro-sequencing, *Antimicrob Agent Chemother* 49:457-460, 2005.

Hall L, Wohlfiel S, Roberts GD: Experience with the MicroSeq D2 large-subunit ribosomal DNA sequencing kit for identification of commonly encountered clinically important yeast species, *J Clin Microbiol* 41:5009, 2003.

Healy M, Huong J, Bittner T et al: Microbial DNA typing by automated repetitive-sequenced-based PCR, *J Clin Microbiol* 43:199, 2005.

Hindson BJ, Ness KD, Masquelier DA, et al: High-throughput droplet digital PCR system for absolute quantitation of DNA copy number, *Anal Chem* 83(22):8604-8610, 2011.

Kirchgesser M, vonFelten C, Kalin C et al: The new MagNa Pure LC 2.0 system: new design and improved performance combined with a proven nucleic acid isolation technique, Roche Applied Science, *Biochemica* 3:20, 2008.

Mackay IM: Real-time PCR in the microbiology laboratory, *Clin Microbiol Infect* 10:190, 2004.

Maslow JN, Mulligan ME, Arbeit RD: Molecular epidemiology: application of contemporary techniques to the typing of microorganisms, *Clin Infect Dis* 17:153, 1993.

Nolte FR, Caliendo AM: Molecular detection and identification of microorganisms. In Murray PR, Baron EJ, Pfaller MA et al, editors: *Manual of clinical microbiology*, ed 9, Washington, DC, 2007, American Society for Microbiology.

Oliviera K, Brecher SM, Durbin A et al: Direct identification *of Staphylococcus aureus* from positive blood culture bottles, *J Clin Microbiol* 41:889, 2003.

Persing DH, editor: *PCR protocols for emerging infectious diseases*, Washington, DC, 1996, American Society for Microbiology.

Persing DH et al, editors: *Diagnostic molecular microbiology: principles and applications*, Washington, DC, 1993, American Society for Microbiology.

Tenover FC, Arbeit RD, Goering RV et al: Interpreting chromosomal DNA restriction patterns produced by pulsed-field gel electrophoresis: criteria for bacterial strain typing, *J Clin Microbiol* 33:2233, 1995.

Versalovic J: *Manual of clinical microbiology*, ed 10, Washington, D.C., 2011, ASM Press.

Vincent M, Xy Y, Kong H: Helicase-dependent isothermal amplification, *Embo Rep* 5:795-800, 2004.

Wang D, Urisman A, Liu YT, et al: Viral discovery and sequence recovery using DNA microarrays, *PLOS Biol* 1:2, 2003.

Wetmur, JG: DNA probes: applications of the principles of nucleic acid hybridization, *Crit Rev Biochem Mol Biol* 26:227, 1991.

# Immunochemical Methods Used for Organism Detection

## OBJECTIVES

1. List the reasons a laboratory or clinician would use immunochemical tests to diagnose disease.
2. Define a polyclonal antibody and a monoclonal antibody and explain the difference between the two.
3. Explain how monoclonal antibodies are produced. How has their development affected immunochemical testing?
4. Define the four types of immunochemical testing—precipitation, particle agglutination, immunofluorescent assays, and enzyme immunoassays—and provide a clinical application for each.
5. Explain the difference between a direct fluorescent antibody (DFA) test and an indirect fluorescent antibody (IFA) test and explain how each is used in the clinical laboratory.
6. Explain the function of the hypoxanthine, aminopterin, and thymidine (HAT) medium in hybridoma production.

The diagnosis of an infectious disease by culture and biochemical techniques can be hindered by several factors. These factors include the inability to cultivate an organism on artificial media, such as *Treponema pallidum,* the agent that causes syphilis, or the fragility of an organism and its subsequent failure to survive transport to the laboratory, such as with respiratory syncytial virus and varicella-zoster virus. Another factor, the fastidious nature of some organisms (e.g., *Leptospira* or *Bartonella* spp.) can result in long incubation periods before growth is evident. In addition, administration of antimicrobial therapy before specimen collection, such as with a patient who has received partial treatment, can impede diagnosis. In these cases, detecting a specific product of the infectious agent in clinical specimens is very important, because this product would not be present in the specimen in the absence of the agent. This chapter discusses the direct detection of microorganisms in patient specimens using immunochemical methods and the identification of microorganisms by these methods once they have been isolated on laboratory media. Chapter 10 discusses the diagnosis of infectious diseases using serological methods.

## PRODUCTION OF ANTIBODIES FOR USE IN LABORATORY TESTING

Immunochemical methods use antigens and antibodies as tools to detect microorganisms. **Antigens** are substances recognized as "foreign" in the human body. Antigens are usually high-molecular-weight proteins or carbohydrates that elicit the production of other proteins, called **antibodies,** in a human or animal host (see Chapter 3). Antibodies attach to the antigens and aid the host in removing the infectious agent (see Chapters 3

and 10). Antigens may be part of the physical structure of the pathogen, such as the bacterial cell wall, or they may be a chemical produced and released by the pathogen, such as an enzyme or a toxin. Each antigen contains a region that is recognized by the immune system. These regions are referred to as **antigenic determinants** or **epitopes.** Figure 9-1 shows the multiple molecules within group A *Streptococcus (Streptococcus pyogenes)* that are recognized by the immune system as antigenic.

## POLYCLONAL ANTIBODIES

Because an organism contains many different antigens, the host response produces many different antibodies to these antigens; these antibodies are heterogenous and are called **polyclonal antibodies.** Polyclonal antibodies used in immunodiagnosis are prepared by immunizing animals (usually rabbits, sheep, or goats) with an infectious agent and then isolating and purifying the resulting antibodies from the animal's serum. Antibody idiotype variation is due to alterations in the nucleotide sequence during antibody production. Individual animals are able to produce different antibodies with different **idiotypes** (antigen binding sites). This variation in antigen binding sites creates a lack of uniformity in polyclonal antibody reagents and requires continual monitoring and comparisons of different antibody reagent lots for specificity and avidity (strength of binding) in any given immunochemical test system.

## MONOCLONAL ANTIBODIES

**Monoclonal antibodies** are antibodies that are completely characterized and highly specific. The ability to create an immortal cell line that produces large quantities of a monoclonal antibody has revolutionized immunologic testing. Monoclonal antibodies are produced by the fusion of a malignant single antibody-producing myeloma cell with an antibody-producing plasma B cell, forming a **hybridoma cell.** Clones of the hybridoma cells continuously produce specific monoclonal antibodies. One technique for the production of a clone of cells is illustrated in Figure 9-2.

The process starts with immunization of a mouse with the antigen for which an antibody is to be produced. The animal responds by producing many antibodies to the epitope (antigenic determinant) injected. The mouse's spleen, which contains antibody-producing plasma cells, is removed and emulsified to separate antibody-producing cells. The cells are then placed into individual wells of a microdilution tray. Viability of cells is maintained by fusing them with cells capable of continuously propagating, or immortal cells of the multiple myeloma. A multiple myeloma is a disease that produces a malignant tumor containing antibody-producing plasma cells.

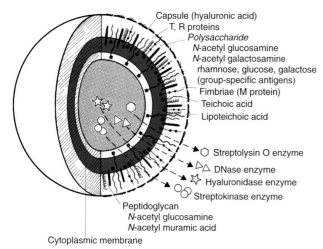

**Figure 9-1** Group A *Streptococcus (Streptococcus pyogenes)* contains many antigenic structural components and produces various antigenic enzymes, each of which may elicit a specific antibody response from the infected host.

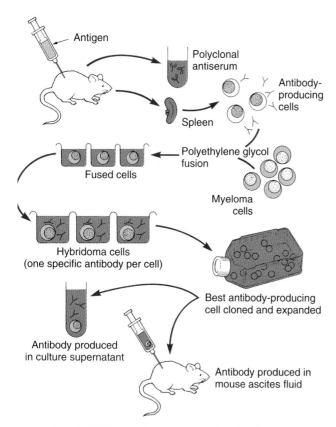

**Figure 9-2** Production of a monoclonal antibody.

Myeloma tumor cells used for hybridoma production are deficient in the enzyme hypoxanthine phosphoribosyl transferase. This defect leads to their inability to survive in a medium containing hypoxanthine, aminopterin, and thymidine (HAT medium). Antibody-producing spleen cells, however, contain the enzyme. Thus, fused hybridoma cells survive in the selective medium and can be recognized by their ability to grow indefinitely in the

medium. Unfused antibody-producing lymphoid cells die after several multiplications in vitro because they are not immortal, and unfused myeloma cells die in the presence of the toxic enzyme substrates. The only surviving cells are true hybrids.

The growth medium supernatant from the microdilution tray wells in which the hybridoma cells are growing is then tested for the presence of the desired antibody. Many such cell lines are usually examined before a suitable antibody is identified. The antibody must be specific enough to bind the individual antigenic determinant to which the animal was exposed, but not so specific that it binds only the antigen from the particular strain of organism with which the mouse was first immunized. When a good candidate antibody-producing cell is found, the hybridoma cells are either grown in cell culture in vitro or are reinjected into the peritoneal cavities of many mice, where the cells multiply and produce large quantities of antibody in the ascitic (peritoneal) fluid. Ascitic fluid can be removed from mice many times during the animals' lifetime, providing a continual supply of antibody formed to the originally injected antigen. Polyclonal and monoclonal antibodies are both used in commercial systems to detect infectious agents.

# PRINCIPLES OF IMMUNOCHEMICAL METHODS USED FOR ORGANISM DETECTION

Numerous immunologic methods are used for the rapid detection of bacteria, fungi, parasites, and viruses in patient specimens, and many of the same reagents often can be used to identify these organisms grown in culture. The techniques fall into four categories: precipitation tests, particle agglutination tests, immunofluorescence assays, and enzyme immunoassays.

## PRECIPITATION TESTS

The classic method of detecting soluble antigen (i.e., antigen in solution) is the Ouchterlony method, a **double immunodiffusion** precipitation method.

### Double Immunodiffusion

In the double immunodiffusion method, small circular wells are cut in an agarose gel, a gelatin-like matrix derived from agar, which is a chemical purified from the cell walls of brown algae. The agarose forms a porous material through which molecules can readily diffuse. The patient specimen containing antigen is placed in a well, and antibody directed against the antigen is placed in the adjacent well. Over 18 to 24 hours, the antigen and antibody diffuse toward each other, producing a visible precipitin band (a lattice structure or visible band) at the point in the gel where the antigen and antibody are in equal proportion (**zone of equivalence**). If the concentration of antibody is significantly higher than that of the antigen, no lattice forms and no precipitation reaction occurs; this is known as **prozone effect.** Conversely, if excess antigen prevents lattice formation,

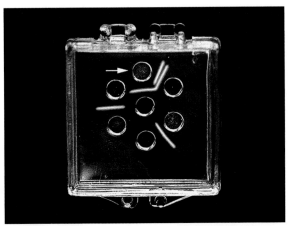

**Figure 9-3** Exo-Antigen Identification System (Immuno-Mycologics, Inc., Norman, Okla.) The center well is filled with a 50× concentrate of an unknown mold. The arrow identifies well 1; wells 2 to 6 are shown clockwise. Wells 1, 3, and 5 are filled with anti-*Histoplasma.* anti-*Blastomyces,* and anti-*Coccidioides* reference antisera, respectively. Wells 2, 4, and 6 are filled with *Histoplasma* antigen, *Blastomyces* antigen, and *Coccidioides* antigen, respectively. The unknown organism can be identified as *Histoplasma capsulatum* based on the formation of line(s) of identity (arc) linking the control band(s) with one or more bands formed between the unknown extract (center well) and the reference antiserum well (well 1).

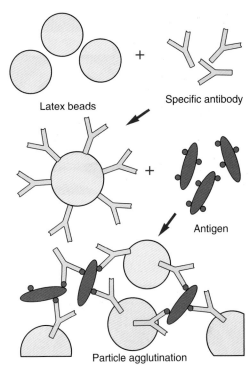

**Figure 9-4** Alignment of antibody molecules bound to the surface of a latex particle and latex agglutination reaction.

resulting in no band formation, the effect is termed **post-zone.** Immunodiffusion is currently used to detect exo-antigens produced by the systemic fungi to confirm their presence in culture (Figure 9-3). However, the technique is extremely time-consuming and is no longer used regularly in the clinical laboratory for antigen detection in patient specimens.

## PARTICLE AGGLUTINATION

Numerous procedures have been developed to detect antigen by means of the agglutination (clumping) of an artificial carrier particle, such as a latex bead, with antibody bound to the surface.

### Latex Agglutination

Antibody molecules can be bound in random alignment to the surface of latex (polystyrene) beads (Figure 9-4). The number of antibody molecules bound to each latex particle is large, resulting in a high number of exposed potential antigen binding sites. Antigen present in a specimen binds to the combining sites of the antibody exposed on the surfaces of the latex beads, forming cross-linked aggregates of latex beads and antigen. The size of the latex bead (0.8 μm or larger) enhances the ease with which the agglutination reaction is visualized. Levels of bacterial polysaccharides detected by latex agglutination have been shown to be as low as 0.1 ng/mL.

Because the pH, osmolarity, and ionic concentration of the solution influence the amount of binding that occurs, conditions under which latex agglutination

procedures are carried out must be carefully standardized. Additionally, some constituents of body fluids, such as rheumatoid factor, have been found to cause false-positive reactions in the latex agglutination systems available. To counteract this problem, some agglutination methods require specimens to be pretreated by heating at 56°C or with ethylenediaminetetraacetic acid (EDTA) before testing. Commercial test systems are usually performed on cardboard cards or glass slides; manufacturer's recommendations should be followed precisely to ensure accurate results.

Depending on the procedure, some reactions are reported as positive or negative and other reactions are graded on a 1+ to 4+ scale, with 2+ usually the minimum amount of agglutination visible in a positive sample without the aid of a microscope. Control latex (coated with antibody from the same animal species from which the specific antibody was made) is tested alongside the test latex. If the patient specimen or the culture isolate reacts with both the test and control latex, the test is considered nonspecific and the results therefore are invalid.

Latex tests are very popular in clinical laboratories for detecting antigen to *Cryptococcus neoformans* in cerebrospinal fluid or serum (Figure 9-5) and to confirm the presence of beta-hemolytic *Streptococcus* from culture plates (Figure 9-6). Latex tests are continually being developed for a variety of organisms. Some examples of additional latex tests are available for the detection of *Clostridium difficile* toxins A and B, rotavirus, and *Escherichia coli* 0157:H7 from suspect colonies of *E coli.*

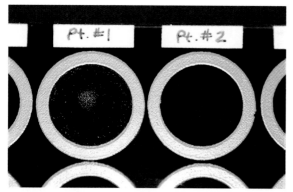

**Figure 9-5** Cryptococcal Antigen Latex Agglutination System (CALAS) (Meridian Diagnostics, Inc., Cincinnati, Ohio.) Patient 1 shows positive agglutination; patient 2 is negative.

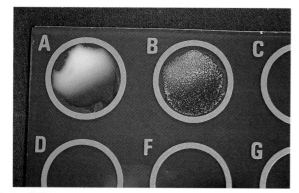

**Figure 9-6** Streptex (Remel, Inc., Lenexa, Kan.) Colony of beta-hemolytic *Streptococcus* agglutinates with group B *Streptococcus* (*Streptococcus agalactiae*) latex suspension.

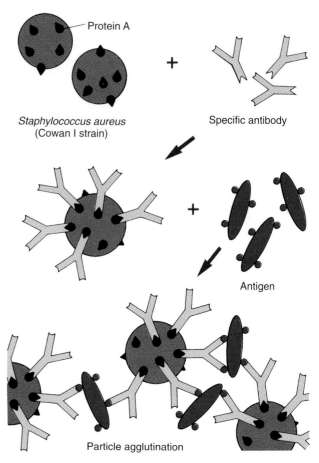

**Figure 9-7** Coagglutination.

## Coagglutination

Similar to latex agglutination, coagglutination uses antibody bound to a particle to enhance the visibility of the agglutination reaction between antigen and antibody. In this case the particles are killed and treated *S. aureus* organisms (Cowan I strain), which contain a large amount of an antibody-binding protein, protein A, in their cell walls. In contrast to latex particles, these staphylococci bind only the base of the heavy chain portion of the antibody, leaving both antigen-binding ends free to form complexes with specific antigen (Figure 9-7). Several commercial suppliers have prepared coagglutination reagents for identification of streptococci, including Lancefield groups A, B, C, D, F, G, and N; *Streptococcus pneumoniae; Neisseria meningitidis;* and *Haemophilus influenzae* types A to F grown in culture. The coagglutination reaction is highly specific and demonstrates reduced sensitivity in comparison to commercially prepared latex agglutination systems. Therefore, coagglutination is not usually used for direct antigen detection.

## IMMUNOFLUORESCENT ASSAYS

Immunofluorescent assays are frequently used for detecting bacterial and viral antigens in clinical laboratories. In these tests, antigens in the patient specimens are immobilized and fixed onto glass slides with formalin, methanol, ethanol, or acetone. Monoclonal or polyclonal antibodies conjugated (attached) to fluorescent dyes are applied to the specimen. After appropriate incubation, washing, and counterstaining (staining of the background with a nonspecific fluorescent stain such as rhodamine or Evan's blue), the slide is viewed using a microscope equipped with a high-intensity light source (usually halogen) and filters to excite the fluorescent tag. Most kits used in clinical microbiology laboratories use fluorescein isothiocyanate (FITC) as the fluorescent dye. FITC fluoresces a bright apple-green (Figure 9-8).

Fluorescent antibody tests are performed using either a direct fluorescent antibody (DFA) or and indirect fluorescent antibody (IFA) technique (Figure 9-9). In the DFA technique, FITC is conjugated directly to the specific antibody. In the IFA technique, the antigen-specific antibody is unlabeled, and a second antibody (usually raised against the animal species from which the antigen-specific antibody was harvested) is conjugated to the FITC. The IFA is a two-step, or sandwich, technique. The IFA technique is more sensitive than the DFA method, although the DFA method is faster because it involves a single incubation.

The major advantage of immunofluorescent microscopy assays is the ability to visually assess the adequacy of

**Figure 9-8** Legionella (Direct) Fluorescent Test System (Scimedx Corp., Denville, N.J.). *Legionella pneumophila* serogroup 1 in sputum.

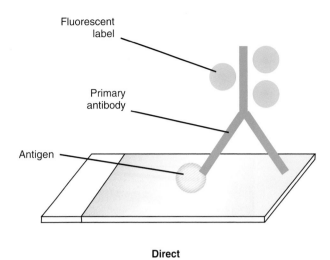

**Direct**

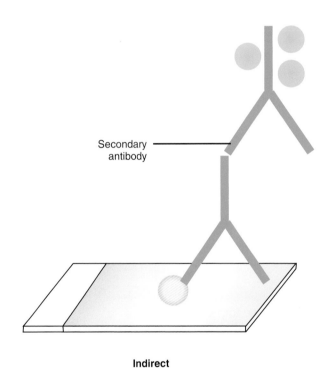

**Indirect**

**Figure 9-9** Direct and indirect fluorescent antibody tests for antigen detection.

a specimen. This is a major factor in tests for the identification of chlamydial elementary bodies or respiratory syncytial virus (RSV) antigens. Microbiologists can discern whether the specimen was collected from the columnar epithelial cells at the opening of the cervix in the case of the *Chlamydia* DFA test or from the basal cells of the nasal epithelium in the case of RSV. Reading immunofluorescent assays requires extensive training and practice for laboratory personnel to become proficient. Finally, fluorescence dyes fade rapidly over time, requiring digital imaging to maintain archives of the results. For this reason, some antibodies have been conjugated to other markers instead of fluorescent dyes. These colorimetric labels use enzymes, such as horseradish peroxidase, alkaline phosphatase, and avidin-biotin, to detect the presence of antigen by converting a colorless substrate to a colored end product. The advantage of these tags is that they allow the preparation of permanent mounts, because the reactions do not fade with storage and visualization does not require a fluorescent microscope.

In clinical specimens, fluorescent antibody tests are commonly used to detect infected cells that harbor *Bordetella pertussis; T. pallidum; L. pneumophila; Giardia, Cryptosporidium, Pneumocystis,* and *Trichomonas* spp.; herpes simplex virus (HSV), cytomegalovirus, varicella-zoster virus, RSV, adenovirus, influenza virus, and parainfluenza virus.

## ENZYME IMMUNOASSAYS

Enzyme immunoassay (EIA), or enzyme-linked immunosorbent assay (ELISA), was developed during the 1960s. The basic method consists of antibodies bonded to enzymes; the enzymes remain able to catalyze a reaction, yielding a visually discernible end product while attached to the antibodies. Furthermore, the antibody binding sites remain free to react with their specific antigen. The use of enzymes as labels has several advantages. First, the enzyme itself is not changed during activity; it can catalyze the reaction of many substrate molecules, greatly amplifying the reaction and enhancing detection. Second, enzyme-conjugated antibodies are stable and can be stored for a relatively long time. Third, the formation of a colored end product allows direct observation of the reaction or automated spectrophotometric reading.

The use of monoclonal antibodies has helped increase the specificity of currently available ELISA systems. New ELISA systems are continually being developed for detection of etiologic agents or their products. In some instances, such as detection of RSV, human immunodeficiency virus (HIV), and certain adenoviruses, ELISA systems may even be more sensitive than culture methods.

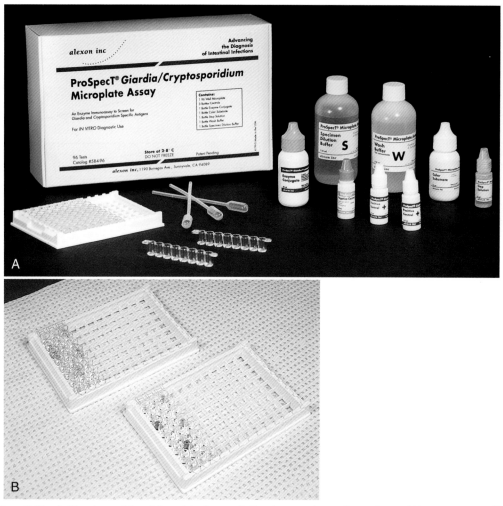

**Figure 9-10** ProSpecT Giardia/Cryptosporidium Microplate Assay. **A,** Breakaway microwell cupules and kit components. **B,** Positive (yellow) changing to blue following the addition of the stop reagent. The negative reactions remain clear. (Courtesy Remel, Inc., Lenexa, Kan.)

### Solid-Phase Immunoassay

Most ELISA systems developed to detect infectious agents consist of antibody firmly fixed to a solid matrix, either the inside of the wells of a microdilution tray or the outside of a spherical plastic or metal bead or some other solid matrix (Figure 9-10). Such systems are called *solid-phase immunosorbent assays (SPIA)*. If antigen is present in the specimen, stable antigen-antibody complexes form when the sample is added to the matrix. Unbound antigen is thoroughly removed by washing, and a second antibody against the antigen is then added to the system. This antibody has been complexed to an enzyme such as alkaline phosphatase or horseradish peroxidase. If the antigen is present on the solid matrix, it binds the second antibody, forming a sandwich with antigen in the middle. After washing has removed unbound, labeled antibody, the addition and hydrolysis of the enzyme substrate causes the color change and completes the reaction. The visually detectable end point appears wherever the enzyme is present (Figure 9-11). Because of the expanding nature of the reaction, even minute amounts of antigen (greater than 1 ng/mL) can be detected. These systems require a specific enzyme-labeled antibody for each antigen tested. However, it is simpler to use an indirect assay in which a second, unlabeled antibody is used to bind to the antigen-antibody complex on the matrix. A third antibody, labeled with enzyme and directed against the nonvariable Fc portion of the unlabeled second antibody, can then be used as the detection marker for many different antigen-antibody complexes (Figure 9-12). ELISA systems are important diagnostic tools for hepatitis Bs (surface) and hepatitis Be (early) antigens and HIV p24 protein, all indicators of early, active, acute infection.

### Membrane-Bound SPIA

The flow-through and large surface area characteristics of nitrocellulose, nylon, and other membranes have been exploited to enhance the speed and sensitivity of ELISA reactions. An absorbent material below the membrane pulls the liquid reactants through the membrane and helps to separate nonreacted components from the antigen-antibody complexes bound to the membrane; washing steps are also simplified. Membrane-bound SPIA systems are available for several viruses (Figure 9-13), group A beta-hemolytic streptococci

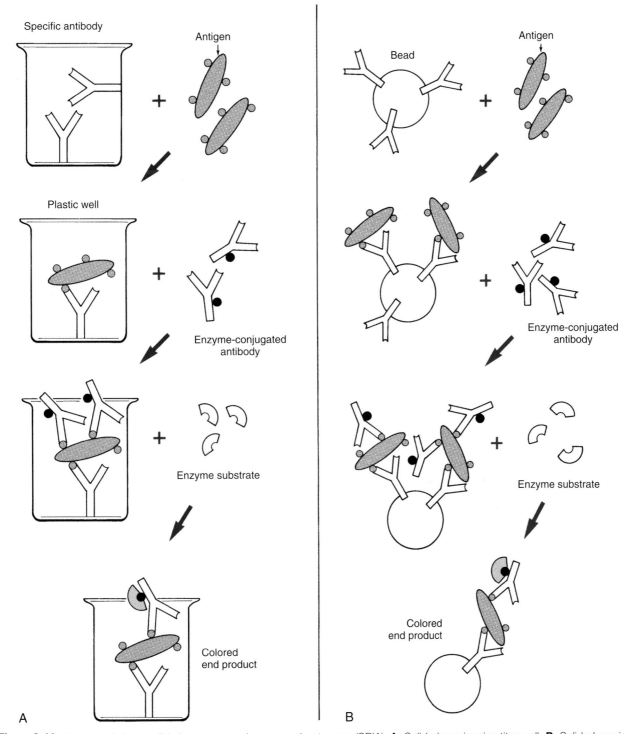

**Figure 9-11** Principle of direct solid-phase enzyme immunosorbent assay (SPIA). **A,** Solid phase is microtiter well. **B,** Solid phase is bead.

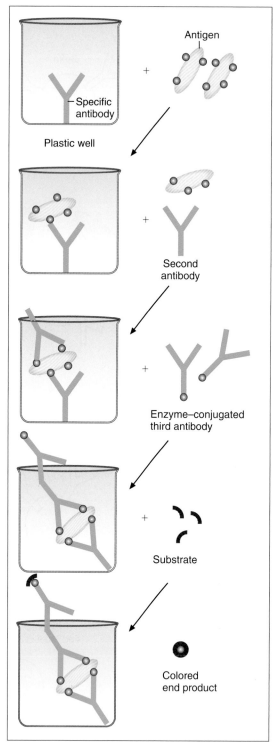

**Figure 9-12** Principle of indirect solid-phase enzyme immunosorbent assay (SPIA).

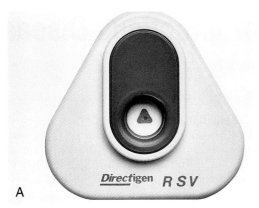
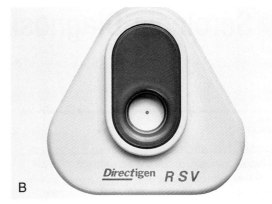

**Figure 9-13** Directigen respiratory syncytial virus (RSV) membrane-bound cassette. **A,** Positive reaction. **B,** Negative reaction. (Courtesy Becton Dickinson Diagnostic Systems, Sparks, Md.)

antigen directly from throat swabs, and group B streptococcal antigen in vaginal secretions. In addition to their use in clinical laboratories, these assays are expected to become more prevalent for home testing systems.

## OTHER IMMUNOASSAYS

Several other methods, including radioimmunoassay (RIA) and fluorescent immunoassay (FIA), are similar to ELISA except that radionucleotides (usually 125I or 14C) are substituted for enzymes in RIA and fluorochromes are substituted for enzymes in FIA. Although RIA was formerly the key method for antigen detection for numerous infectious agents, including hepatitis B virus, it has been largely replaced by ELISA

testing, which does not require use of radioactive substances.

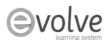 *Visit the Evolve site to complete the review questions.*

## BIBLIOGRAPHY

Benjamini E, Sunshine G, Leskowitz S: *Immunology: a short course,* ed 6, New York, 1999, Wiley-Liss.

Gaur S, Kesarwala H, Gavai M et al: Clinical immunology and infectious diseases, *Pediatr Clin North Am* 41:745, 1994.

James K: Immunoserology of infectious diseases, *Clin Microbiol Rev* 3:132, 1990.

# Serologic Diagnosis of Infectious Diseases

## OBJECTIVES

1. Define the two categories of human specific immune response, cell mediated and antibody mediated, including the definition of T cells and B cells and their role in the responses.
2. List the five classes of antibodies, define their roles in infectious disease, and explain the three antibody functions.
3. Explain the following serologic tests, giving consideration to their clinical applications: bacterial agglutination, particle agglutination, and flocculation tests.
4. Describe a cross reaction and explain why it occurs and how it may affect antibody testing.
5. In defining hemagglutination and neutralization assays, explain their similarity in testing, along with their disparities.
6. Explain how the difference in the size and structure of the IgM antibody is important to its activity and function.
7. Explain what the complement fixation test is and describe the two-step reaction.
8. Explain the principle of the Western blot assay and why it is used as a confirmatory test for many assays.

Immunochemical methods are used as diagnostic tools for serodiagnosis of infectious disease. An understanding of how these methods have been adapted for this purpose requires a basic working knowledge of the components and functions of the immune system. **Immunology** is the study of the components and functions of the immune system. The immune system is the body's defense mechanism against invading "foreign" antigens. One of the functions of the immune system is distinguishing "self" from "nonself" (i.e., the proteins or antigens from foreign substances). (Chapter 3 presents a more in-depth discussion of the host's response to foreign substances.) This chapter is intended to provide a brief overview and review of immunology. The complexity and detail required to fully understand immunology and serology are beyond the scope of this text.

## FEATURES OF THE IMMUNE RESPONSE

The host, or patient, has physical barriers, such as intact skin and ciliated epithelial cells, and chemical barriers, such as oils produced by the sebaceous glands and lysozyme found in tears and saliva, to prevent infections by foreign organisms. In addition, **natural (innate) immunity,** which is not specific, activates **chemotaxis,** the process by which phagocytes are recruited to a site of invasion and engulf organisms entering the host. **Acquired active immunity** is the specific response of the host to an infecting organism.

The human specific immune responses are simplistically divided into the following two categories: cell-mediated and antibody-mediated.

**Cell-mediated** immune responses are carried out by special lymphocytes of the T-cell (thymus derived) class. T cells proliferate and differentiate into various effector T cells, including cytotoxic and helper cells. **Cytotoxic T lymphocytes** specifically attack and kill microorganisms or host cells damaged or infected by pathogens. Helper cells promote the maturation of B cells by producing activator cytokines that induce the B cells to produce antibodies and attach to and kill invading organisms. Although diagnosis of certain diseases may be aided by measuring the cell-mediated immune response to the pathogen, such tests entail skin tests performed by physicians or in vitro cell function assays performed by specially trained immunologists. These tests are usually not within the repertoire of clinical microbiology laboratories.

**Antibody-mediated** immune responses are produced by specific proteins generated by lymphocytes of the B-cell (bone marrow derived) class. Because these proteins exhibit immunologic function and fold into a globular structure in the active state, they are also referred to as **immunoglobulins.** Antibodies are either secreted into the blood or lymphatic fluid (and sometimes other body fluids) by activated B lymphocytes (plasma cells), or they remain attached to the surface of the lymphocyte or other cells. Because the cells involved in this category of immune response primarily circulate in the blood, this type of immunity is also called **humoral immunity.** For purposes of determining whether a patient's body has produced an antibody against a particular infectious agent, the serum (or occasionally the plasma) is examined for the presence of the antibody. The study of the diagnosis of disease by measuring antibody levels in serum is referred to as **serology.**

## CHARACTERISTICS OF ANTIBODIES

Immunocompetent humans are able to produce antibodies specifically directed against almost all the antigens with which they may come into contact throughout their lifetimes and that the body recognizes as "foreign." Antigens may be part of the physical structure of a pathogen or a chemical produced and released by the pathogen, such as an exotoxin. One pathogen may contain or produce many different antigens that the host recognizes as foreign. Infection with one agent may cause the production of a number of different antibodies. In addition, some antigenic determinants on a pathogen may not be available for recognition by the host until the pathogen has undergone a physical change. For example, until a pathogenic bacterium has been digested by a human polymorphonuclear (PMN) leukocyte, certain antigens deep in the cell wall are not detected by the host immune system. Once the bacterium has been broken down, these new antigens are released and the specific

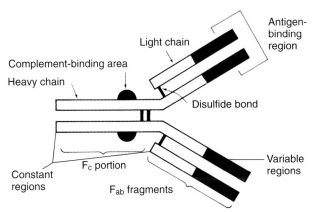

**Figure 10-1** Structure of immunoglobulin G. The heavy chains determine the antibody class (IgG, IgA, IgD, IgE, or IgM). The Fab fragment containing the variable regions determines the antibody binding specificity. The Fc portion (or function cells) binds to various immune cells to activate specific functions in the immune system.

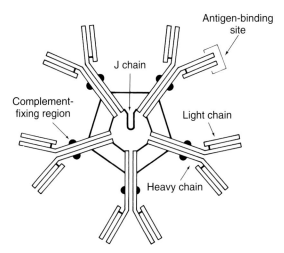

**Figure 10-2** Structure of immunoglobulin M.

antibodies can be produced. For this reason, a patient may produce different antibodies at different times during the course of a single disease. The immune response to an antigen also matures with continued exposure, and the antibodies produced become more specific and more **avid** (able to bind more tightly).

Antibodies function by (1) attaching to the surface of pathogens and making the pathogens more amenable to ingestion by phagocytic cells (**opsonizing antibodies**); (2) binding to and blocking surface receptors for host cells (**neutralizing antibodies**); or (3) attaching to the surface of pathogens and contributing to their destruction by the lytic action of complement (**complement-fixing antibodies**). Routine diagnostic serologic methods are used to measure primarily two antibody classes, IgM and IgG; however, antibodies are categorized into five classes: immunoglobulin G (IgG), immunoglobulin M (IgM), immunoglobulin A (IgA), immunoglobulin D (IgD), and immunoglobulin E (IgE). IgA, also referred to as *secretory antibody,* is the predominant class of antibody in saliva, tears, and intestinal secretions. IgD is attached to the surface of B cells and is involved in immune regulations. IgE levels increase as a result of infections caused by several parasites or in response to allergic reactions.

The basic structure of an antibody molecule comprises two mirror images, each composed of two identical protein chains (Figure 10-1). At the terminal ends are the antigen binding sites, or variable regions, which specifically attach to the antigen against which the antibody was produced. Depending on the specificity of the antibody, antigens of some similarity, but not total identity, to the inducing antigen may also be bound; this is called a **cross reaction.** The complement binding site is found in the center of the molecule in a structure similar for all antibodies of the same class and is referred to as the **constant region.** IgM is produced as a first response to many antigens, although the levels remain high transiently. Thus, the presence of IgM usually indicates recent or active exposure to an antigen or infection. IgG, on the other hand, may persist long after an infection has run its course.

The IgM antibody type (Figure 10-2) consists of five identical proteins (pentamer), with the basic antibody structures linked at the bases with 10 antigen binding sites on the molecule. IgG consists of one basic antibody molecule (monomer) that has two binding sites (see Figure 10-1). The differences in the size and conformation between these two classes of immunoglobulins result in differences in activities and functions.

### Features of the Humoral Immune Response Useful in Diagnostic Testing

Immunocompetent individuals produce both IgM and IgG antibodies in response to most pathogens. In most cases, IgM is produced by a patient after the first exposure to a pathogen and is no longer detectable within a relatively short period. For serologic diagnostic purposes, it is important to note that IgM is unable to cross the placenta. Therefore, any IgM detected in the serum of a newborn must have been produced by the infant and indicates an infection in utero. The larger number of binding sites on IgM molecules provides for more rapid clearance of the offending pathogen, even though each individual antigen binding site may not be the most efficient for binding to the antigen. Over time, the cells producing IgM switch to production of IgG. IgG is the highest circulating antibody in the human body.

IgG is often more specific for the antigen (i.e., it has higher avidity). IgG has two antigen binding sites, but it can also bind complement. Complement is a complex series of serum proteins that is involved in modulating several functions of the immune system, including cytotoxic cell death, chemotaxis, and opsonization. When IgG is bound to an antigen, the base of the molecule (Fc portion) is exposed in the environment. Structures on this Fc portion attract and bind the cell membranes of phagocytes, increasing the chances of engulfment and destruction of the pathogen by the host cells. A second exposure to the same pathogen induces a faster and greater IgG response and a much lesser IgM response. Several B lymphocytes retain memory of the pathogen, allowing a more rapid response and a higher level of

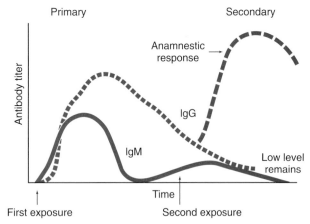

**Figure 10-3** Relative humoral response to antigen stimulation over time.

antibody production than the primary exposure or response. This enhanced response is called the **anamnestic response.** B-cell memory is not perfect. Occasional clones of memory cells can be stimulated through interaction with an antigen that is similar but not identical to the original antigen. Therefore, the anamnestic response may be polyclonal and nonspecific. For example, reinfection with cytomegalovirus may stimulate memory B cells to produce antibody against Epstein-Barr virus (another herpes family virus), which the host encountered previously, in addition to antibody against cytomegalovirus. The relative humoral responses are diagrammatically represented in Figure 10-3.

### Interpretation of Serologic Tests

In serology, a change in antibody titer is a central concept for the diagnosis and monitoring of disease progression. The titer of antibody is the reciprocal of the highest dilution of the patient's serum in which the antibody is still detectable. Patients with large amounts of antibody have high titers, because antibody is still detectable at very high dilutions of serum. Serum for antibody levels should be drawn during the acute phase of the disease (when it is first discovered or suspected) and again during convalescence (usually at least 2 weeks later). These specimens are called **acute** and **convalescent sera.** For some infections, such as legionnaires' disease and hepatitis, titers may not rise until months after the acute infection, or they may never rise. Therefore, changes in titer must be carefully correlated with the patient's signs and symptoms of the specific disease or suspected infectious agent.

Patients with intact humoral immunity develop increasing amounts of antibody to a pathogen over several weeks. If it is the patient's first exposure to the pathogenic organism and the specimen has been obtained early enough, no or very low titers of antibody are detected at the onset of disease. In the case of a second exposure, the patient's serum usually contains measurable antibody during the initial phase of the disease, and the antibody level quickly increases as a result of the anamnestic response. For most pathogens, an increase in the patient's titer of two doubling dilutions

(e.g., from a positive result of 1:8 to a positive result of 1:32) is considered to be diagnostic of current infection. This is defined as a **fourfold rise in titer.**

For many infections, accurate results used for diagnosis are achieved when acute and convalescent sera are tested concurrently in the same test system. Variables inherent in the procedures and laboratory error can cause a difference of one doubling (or twofold) dilution in the results obtained from a same sample tested concurrently in different laboratories. Unfortunately, a certain proportion of infected patients never demonstrate a rise in titer, necessitating the use of other diagnostic tests. Because the delay inherent in testing paired acute and convalescent sera results in diagnostic information arriving too late to affect the initial therapy, increasing numbers of early (IgM) serologic testing assays are being commercially evaluated. Moreover, it is sometimes more realistic to see a fourfold fall in titer between acute and convalescent sera when samples are tested concurrently in the same system. This is a result of the sera being collected late in the course of an infection, when antibodies have already begun to decrease.

## SERODIAGNOSIS OF INFECTIOUS DISEASES

With most diseases, a spectrum of responses may be seen in infected humans, such that a person may develop antibody from a subclinical infection or after colonization by an agent without actually having symptoms of the disease. In these cases, the presence of antibody in a single serum specimen or a similar titer of antibody in paired sera may merely indicate past contact with the agent and cannot be used to accurately diagnose recent disease. Therefore, in the vast majority of serologic procedures for diagnosis of recent infection, testing of both acute and convalescent sera is the method of choice. Except for detecting the presence of IgM, testing of a single serum may be recommended in certain cases. *Mycoplasma pneumoniae* and viral influenza B infections are examples in which high titers may indicate recent infection. IgM levels may be diagnostic if the infecting or disease-causing agent is extremely rare, such as rabies or exposure to botulism toxin, and people without disease or prior immunization would have no chance of developing an immune response.

The prevalence of antibody to an etiologic agent of disease in the population correlates with the number of people who have come into contact with the agent, not the number who actually develop disease. For most diseases, only a small proportion of infected individuals actually develop symptoms; others develop protective antibodies without experiencing signs and symptoms of the disease. In a number of circumstances, serum is tested to determine whether a patient is immune; that is, whether the patient has antibody to a particular agent either in response to a past infection or to immunization. These tests can be performed with a single serum sample. The results of the tests must be correlated with the actual immune status of individual patients to determine the

**TABLE 10-1** Noninclusive Overview of Tests Available for Serodiagnosis of Infectious Diseases

| Test | Sera Needed | Interpretation | Application |
|---|---|---|---|
| IgM | Single, acute (collected at onset of illness) | Newborn, positive: in utero (congenital) infection<br>Adult, positive: primary or current infection<br>Adult, negative: no infection or past infection | Newborn: STORCH* agents; other organisms<br>Adults: any infectious agent |
| IgG | Acute and convalescent (collected 2-6 weeks after onset) | Positive: fourfold rise or fall in titer between acute and convalescent sera tested at the same time in the same test system<br>Negative: no current infection or past infection, or patient is immunocompromised and cannot mount a humoral antibody response, or convalescent specimen collected before increase in IgG (Lyme disease, *Legionella* sp.) | Any infectious agent |
| IgG | Single specimen collected between onset and convalescence | Adult, positive: adult evidence of infection at some unknown time except in certain cases in which a single high titer is diagnostic (rabies, *Legionella*, *Ehrlichia* spp.).<br>Newborn, positive: maternal antibodies that crossed the placenta<br>Newborn, negative: patient has not been exposed to microorganism or patient has a congenital or acquired immune deficiency or specimen collected before increase in IgG (Lyme disease or *Legionella* sp.) | Any infectious agent |
| Immune status evaluation | Single specimen collected at any time | Positive: previous exposure<br>Negative: no exposure | Rubella testing for women of childbearing age, syphilis testing may be required in some states to obtain a marriage license, cytomegalovirus testing for transplant donor and recipient |

*STORCH, Syphilis, *Toxoplasma,* rubella virus, cytomegalovirus, herpes simplex virus.

level of detectable antibody present, in order to determine whether the individual has developed a true immunity to infection or a secondary reinfection. For example, sensitive tests can detect the presence of very tiny amounts of antibody to the rubella virus. Certain people, however, may still be susceptible to infection with the rubella virus with such small amounts of circulating antibody, and a higher level of antibody may be required to ensure protection from disease.

Alternatively, depending on the etiologic agent, even low levels of antibody may protect a patient from pathologic effects of disease and not prevent a second reinfection. For example, a person previously immunized with killed poliovirus vaccine who becomes infected with pathogenic poliovirus experiences multiplication of the virus in the gut and virus entry into the circulation. Damage to the central nervous system is blocked by humoral antibody in the circulation. As more sensitive testing methods are developed and these types of problems become more common, microbiologists must work closely with clinicians to develop guidelines for interpreting serologic test results in relation to the immune status of individual patients. Moreover, patients may respond to an antigenic stimulus by producing cross-reacting antibodies. These antibodies are nonspecific and may cause misinterpretation of serologic tests.

Table 10-1 provides a brief list of representative serologic tests available for immunodiagnosis of infectious diseases, the specimen required, interpretation of positive and negative test results, and examples of applications of each technique. Because serologic assays are rapidly evolving, this table is not intended to be all-inclusive.

# PRINCIPLES OF SEROLOGIC TEST METHODS

Antibodies can be detected in many ways. In some cases, antibodies to an agent may be detected in more than one way, but the different antibody detection tests may not be measuring the same antibody. For this reason, the presence of antibodies to a particular pathogen, as detected by one method, may not correlate with the presence of antibodies to the same agent as detected by another test method. Moreover, different test methodologies have varying degrees of sensitivity in detecting antibodies. However, because IgM is produced at an initial higher level during a patient's first exposure to an infectious agent, the detection of specific IgM can help the clinician a great deal in establishing a diagnosis. Most of the serologic test methods can be adapted for analysis of IgM.

## SEPARATING IGM FROM IGG FOR SEROLOGIC TESTING

IgM testing is especially helpful for diseases that have nonspecific clinical presentations, such as toxoplasmosis, and for conditions that require rapid therapeutic decisions. For example, rubella infection in pregnant women can lead to congenital defects in the unborn fetus, such as cataracts, glaucoma, mental retardation, and deafness. Therefore, pregnant women who are exposed to rubella virus and develop a mild febrile illness can be tested for the presence of anti-rubella IgM. In addition, identification of IgM within the amniotic fluid of a pregnant mother is diagnostic of neonatal infection. Because IgG can readily cross the placenta, newborns carry titers of IgG passed from the mother to the fetus during the first 2 to 3 months of life until the infant produces his or her own antibodies. This is the only form of natural passive immunity. Accurate serologic diagnosis of infection in neonates requires either demonstration of a rise in titer (which takes time to occur) or the detection of specific IgM directed against the putative agent. Because the IgM molecule does not cross the placental barrier, any IgM would have to be of fetal origin and diagnostic of neonatal infection. Agents difficult to culture or those that adult females would be expected to have encountered during their lifetimes, such as *Treponema pallidum,* cytomegalovirus, herpes virus, *Toxoplasma* sp., or rubella virus, are organisms that may cause an infection and elevation of fetal IgM. The names of some of these agents have been grouped together with the acronym **STORCH** (syphilis, *Toxoplasma* sp., rubella, cytomegalovirus, and herpes). These tests should be ordered separately, depending on the clinical illness of a newborn suspected of having one of these diseases. In many instances, however, infected babies display no clinical signs or symptoms of infection. Furthermore, in many cases serologic tests yield false-positive or false-negative results. Therefore, multiple considerations, including the patient history and the clinical signs and symptoms, must be included in the serodiagnosis of neonatal infection, and in many cases culture is still the most reliable diagnostic method.

Several methods have been developed to measure specific IgM in sera that may also contain IgG. In addition to using a labeled antibody specific for IgM as the marker or the IgM capture sandwich assays, the immunoglobulins can be separated from each other by physical means. Centrifugation through a sucrose gradient, performed at very high speeds, has been used in the past to separate IgM, which has a greater molecular weight than IgG.

Other available IgM separation systems use the presence of certain proteins on the surface of staphylococci (protein A) and streptococci (protein G expressed by group C and G streptococci) that bind the Fc portion of IgG. A simple centrifugation step separates the particles and their bound immunoglobulins from the remaining mixture, which contains the bulk of the IgM. Other methods use antibodies to remove IgM from sera containing both IgG and IgM. An added bonus of IgM separation systems is that **rheumatoid factor,** IgM antibodies produced by some patients against their own IgG, often binds to the IgG molecules being removed from the serum. Consequently, these IgM antibodies are removed along with the IgG. Rheumatoid factor can cause nonspecific reactions and interfere with the results in a variety of serologic tests.

## METHODS OF ANTIBODY DETECTION

### Direct Whole Pathogen Agglutination Assays

Basic tests for antibody detection measure the antibody produced by a host to determinants on the surface of a bacterial agent in response to infection. Specific antibodies bind to surface antigens of the bacteria in a thick suspension and cause the bacteria to clump in visible aggregates. Such antibodies are called **agglutinins,** and the test is referred to as **bacterial agglutination.** Electrostatic and additional chemical interactions influence the formation of aggregates in solutions. Because most bacterial surfaces have a negative charge, they tend to repel each other. Performance of agglutination tests in sterile physiologic saline (0.9% sodium chloride in distilled water), which contains free positive ions, enhances the ability of antibody to cause aggregation of bacteria. Although bacterial agglutination tests can be performed on the surface of both glass slides and in test tubes, tube agglutination tests are often more sensitive, because a longer incubation period can be used, allowing more antigen and antibody to interact. The small volume of liquid used for slide tests requires a rather rapid reading of the result, before the liquid evaporates, causing erroneous results.

Examples of bacterial agglutination tests include assays for antibodies to *Francisella tularensis* and *Brucella* spp., which are part of a panel referred to as **febrile agglutinin tests.** Bacterial agglutination tests are often used to diagnose diseases in which the bacterial agent is difficult to cultivate in vitro. Diseases diagnosed by this technique include tetanus, yersiniosis, leptospirosis, brucellosis, and tularemia. The reagents necessary to perform many of these tests are commercially available, singly or as complete systems. Because most laboratories are able to culture and identify the causative agent, agglutination tests for certain diseases, such as typhoid fever, are seldom used today. Furthermore, the typhoid febrile agglutinin test (called the **Widal test**) is often positive in patients with infections caused by other bacteria because of cross-reacting antibodies or a previous immunization against typhoid. Appropriate specimens from patients suspected of having typhoid fever should be cultured for the presence of salmonellae.

Whole cells of parasites, including *Plasmodium* and *Leishmania* spp., or *Toxoplasma gondii,* have also been used for direct detection of antibody by agglutination. In addition to using the actual infecting bacteria or parasites as the agglutinating particles, certain bacteria may be agglutinated by antibodies produced against another infectious agent. Many patients infected with one of the rickettsiae produce antibodies capable of nonspecifically agglutinating bacteria of the genus *Proteus,* specifically *Proteus vulgaris.* The **Weil-Felix test** detects these cross-reacting antibodies. Because newer, more specific serologic methods of diagnosing rickettsial disease have become more widely available, the use of the *Proteus* agglutinating test is no longer offered in many laboratories.

## Particle Agglutination Tests

Numerous serologic procedures have been developed to detect antibody via the agglutination of an artificial carrier particle with antigen bound to its surface. As noted in Chapter 9, similar systems using artificial carriers coated with antibodies are commonly used for detection of microbial antigens. Either artificial carriers (e.g., latex particles or treated red blood cells) or biologic carriers (e.g., whole bacterial cells) can carry an antigen on their surface capable of binding with antibody. The size of the carrier enhances the visibility of the agglutination reaction, and the artificial nature of the system allows the antigen bound to the surface to be extremely specific.

The results of particle agglutination tests depend on several factors, including the amount and avidity of antigen conjugated to the carrier, the time of incubation with the patient's serum (or other source of antibody), and the microenvironment of the interaction (including pH and protein concentration). Commercial tests have been developed as systems, complete with their own diluents, controls, and containers. For accurate results, a serologic test kit should be used as a unit, without modification or mixing from another kit. In addition, tests developed for use with cerebrospinal fluid, for example, should not be used with serum unless the package insert or the technical representative has certified such use.

Treated animal red blood cells have also been used as carriers of antigen for agglutination tests; these tests are called **indirect hemagglutination,** or **passive hemagglutination** tests, because it is not the original red blood cell antigens, but rather the passively attached antigens, that are bound by antibody. The most widely used indirect assays include the microhemagglutination test for antibody to *T. pallidum* (*MHA-TP,* so called because it is performed in a microtiter plate), the hemagglutination treponemal test for syphilis (HATTS), the passive hemagglutination tests for antibody to extracellular antigens of streptococci, and the rubella indirect hemagglutination tests, all of which are available commercially. Certain reference laboratories, such as the Centers for Disease Control and Prevention (CDC), also perform indirect hemagglutination tests for antibodies to some clostridia, *Burkholderia pseudomallei, Bacillus anthracis, Corynebacterium diphtheriae, Leptospira* sp., and the agents of several viral and parasitic diseases.

Complete systems for the use of latex or other particle agglutination tests are available commercially for accurate and sensitive detection of antibody to cytomegalovirus, rubella virus, varicella-zoster virus, the heterophile antibody of infectious mononucleosis, teichoic acid antibodies of staphylococci, antistreptococcal antibodies, mycoplasma antibodies, and others. Latex tests for antibodies to *Coccidioides, Sporothrix, Echinococcus,* and *Trichinella* spp. are available, although they are not widely used because of the uncommon occurrence of the corresponding infection or its limited geographic distribution. Use of tests for *Candida* antibodies has not yet shown results reliable enough for accurate diagnosis of disease.

## Flocculation Tests

In contrast to the aggregates formed when particulate antigens bind to specific antibody, the interaction of soluble antigen with antibody may result in the formation of a precipitate, a concentration of fine particles, usually visible only because the precipitated product is forced to remain in a defined space within a matrix. Variations of precipitation and flocculation are widely used for serologic studies.

In **flocculation tests** the precipitin end product forms macroscopically or microscopically visible clumps. The Venereal Disease Research Laboratory test, known as the **VDRL,** is the most widely used flocculation test. Patients infected with pathogenic treponemes, most commonly *T. pallidum,* the agent of syphilis, form an antibody-like protein called **reagin** that binds to the test antigen, cardiolipin-lecithin–coated cholesterol particles, causing the particles to flocculate. Reagin is not a specific antibody directed against *T. pallidum* antigens, therefore the test is highly sensitive but not highly specific; however, it is a good screening test, detecting more than 99% of cases of secondary syphilis.

The VDRL is the single most useful test available for testing cerebrospinal fluid in cases of suspected neurosyphilis, although it may be falsely positive in the absence of disease. Performance of the VDRL test requires scrupulously clean glassware and attention to detail, including numerous daily quality control checks. In addition, the reagents must be prepared fresh immediately before the test is performed, and patients' sera must be inactivated (complement inactivation) by heating for 30 minutes at 56°C before testing. Because of this complexity, the VDRL has been replaced in many laboratories by a qualitatively comparable test, the **rapid plasma reagin (RPR) test.**

The RPR test is commercially available as a complete system containing positive and negative controls, the reaction card, and the prepared antigen suspension. The antigen, cardiolipin-lecithin–coated cholesterol with choline chloride, also contains charcoal particles to allow for macroscopically visible flocculation. Sera can be tested without heating, and the reaction takes place on the surface of a specially treated cardboard card, which is then discarded (Figure 10-4). The RPR test is

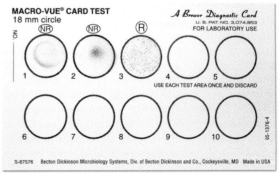

**Figure 10-4** MACRO-VUE RPR card test. *R,* Reactive (positive) test indicated by the diffuse degree of clumping. *NR,* non-reactive (negative test), indicated by a smooth suspension or non-diffuse slight roughness as demonstrated here as a peripheral roughness in well 1 or somewhat centric roughness in well 2. (Courtesy Becton Dickinson Diagnostic Systems, Sparks, Md.)

not recommended for testing of cerebrospinal fluid. All procedures are standardized and clearly described in product inserts, and these procedures should be strictly followed. Overall, the RPR appears to be a more specific screening test for syphilis than the VDRL, and it is not as technically complex. Several modifications have been made, such as the use of dyes to enhance visualization of results and the use of automated techniques.

Conditions and infections other than syphilis can cause a patient's serum to yield a positive result in the VDRL or RPR test; these are referred to as **biologic false-positive tests.** Autoimmune diseases, such as systemic lupus erythematosus and rheumatic fever, in addition to infectious mononucleosis, hepatitis, pregnancy, and old age have been known to cause false-positive reactions. The results of screening tests should always be considered presumptive until confirmed with a specific treponemal test.

### Immunodiffusion Assays

The Ouchterlony double immunodiffusion assay, which closely resembles the precipitation test, is used to detect antibodies directed against fungal cell components (see Chapter 9). Whole-cell extracts or other antigens of the suspected fungus are placed in wells in an agarose plate, and the patient's serum and a positive control serum are placed in adjoining wells. If the patient has produced specific antibody against the fungus, precipitin lines become visible in the agarose between the homologous (identical) antigen and antibody wells; the patient's sample identity, with similar lines from the control serum, helps confirm the results. The type and thickness of the precipitin bands may have both prognostic and diagnostic value. Antibodies against the pathogenic fungi *Histoplasma, Blastomyces, Coccidioides,* and *Paracoccidioides* spp., as well as some opportunistic fungi, are routinely detected by immunodiffusion. The test usually requires at least 48 hours, but additional time may be required for the bands to become visible.

### Hemagglutination Inhibition Assays

Many human viruses can bind to surface structures on red blood cells from different species. For example, rubella virus particles can bind to human type O, goose, or chicken erythrocytes and cause agglutination of the red blood cells. Influenza and parainfluenza viruses agglutinate guinea pig, chicken, or human O erythrocytes; many arboviruses agglutinate goose red blood cells; adenoviruses agglutinate rat or rhesus monkey cells; mumps virus binds red blood cells of monkeys; and herpes virus and cytomegalovirus agglutinate sheep red blood cells. Serologic tests for the presence of antibodies to these viruses exploit the agglutinating properties of the virus particles. Patients' sera that have been treated with kaolin or heparin-magnesium chloride (to remove nonspecific inhibitors of red cell agglutination and nonspecific agglutinins of the red cells) are added to a system containing the suspected virus. If antibodies to the virus are present, they form complexes and block the binding sites on the viral surfaces. When the proper red cells are added to the solution, all of the virus particles are bound by antibody, preventing the virus from agglutinating the red cells. Thus, the patient's serum is positive for hemagglutination-inhibiting antibodies. As for most serologic procedures, a fourfold increase in the titer is considered diagnostic. The hemagglutination inhibition tests for most agents are performed at reference laboratories. Rubella antibodies, however, are often detected with this method in routine diagnostic laboratories. Several commercial rubella hemagglutination inhibition test systems are available.

### Neutralization Assays

Antibody that inhibits the infectivity of a virus by blocking the host cell receptor site is called a **neutralizing antibody.** The test serum is mixed with a suspension of infectious viral particles of the same type as the virus suspected in a patient's infection. A control suspension of viruses is mixed with normal serum. The viral suspensions are then inoculated into a cell culture system that supports growth of the virus. The control cells display evidence of viral infection. If the patient's serum contains antibody to the virus, that antibody binds the viral particles and prevents them from invading the cells in culture; the antibody has neutralized the "infectivity" of the virus. These tests are technically demanding and time-consuming and are performed in reference laboratories.

Antibodies to bacterial toxins and other extracellular products that display measurable activities can be tested in a similar fashion. The ability of a patient's serum to neutralize the erythrocyte-lysing capability of streptolysin O, an extracellular enzyme produced by *Streptococcus pyogenes* during infection, has been used for many years as a test for identifying a previous streptococcal infection. After pharyngitis with streptolysin O–producing strains, most patients show a high titer of the antibody to streptolysin O (i.e., antistreptolysin O [ASO] antibody). Streptococci also produce the enzyme deoxyribonuclease B (DNase B) during infections of the throat, skin, or other tissue. A neutralization test that prevents activity of this enzyme, the anti–DNase B test, has also been used extensively as an indicator of recent or previous streptococcal disease. However, the use of particle agglutination tests (latex or indirect hemagglutination) for the presence of antibody to many of the streptococcal enzymes has replaced the use of these neutralization tests in many laboratories.

### Complement Fixation Assays

One of the classic methods of demonstrating the presence of antibody in a patient's serum is the complement fixation (CF) test. This test consists of two separate systems. The first (the test system) consists of the antigen suspected of causing the patient's disease and the patient's serum. The second (the indicator system) consists of a combination of sheep red blood cells, complement-fixing antibody (IgG) raised against the sheep red blood cells in another animal, and an exogenous source of complement (usually guinea pig serum). When these three components are mixed together in optimum concentrations, the anti-sheep erythrocyte antibody binds to the surface of the red blood cells, and the complement then binds to the antigen-antibody complex, ultimately causing lysis

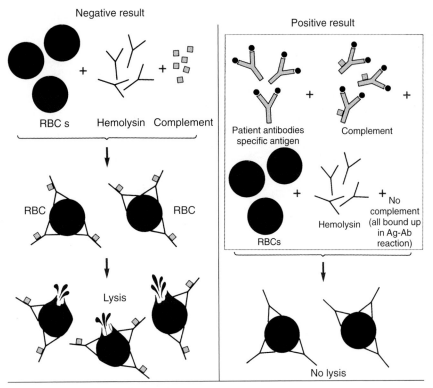

**Figure 10-5** Complement fixation test.

(bursting) of the red blood cells. For this reason the anti-sheep red blood cell antibody is also called **hemolysin.** For the CF test, these two systems are tested in sequence (Figure 10-5). The patient's serum is first added to the putative antigen; then the limiting amount of complement is added to the solution. If the patient's serum contains antibody to the antigen, the resulting antigen-antibody complexes bind all the complement added. In the next step, the sheep red blood cells and the hemolysin (indicator system) are added. The patient's complement is available to bind to the sheep cell–hemolysin complexes and cause lysis if the complement has not been bound by a complex formed with antibody from the patient's serum. A positive result, meaning the patient has complement-fixing antibodies, is revealed by failure of the red blood cells to lyse in the final test system. Lysis of the indicator cells indicates lack of antibody and a negative CF test result.

Although this test requires many manipulations, takes at least 48 hours to complete both stages, and often yields nonspecific results, it has been used for many years to detect many types of antibodies, particularly antiviral and antifungal antibodies. Many new systems have gradually been introduced to replace the CF test, because they demonstrate improved recovery of pathogens or their products and provide more sensitive and less demanding procedures for detecting antibodies, such as particle agglutination, indirect fluorescent antibody tests, and enzyme-linked immunosorbent assay (ELISA). CF tests are performed chiefly for diagnosis of unusual infections and are done primarily in laboratories.

## Enzyme-Linked Immunosorbent Assays

ELISA tests available for the detection of antibodies to infectious agents are sensitive and specific. As described in depth in Chapter 9, the presence of a specific antibody is detected by the ability of a second antibody, conjugated to a colored or fluorescent marker, to bind to the target antibody, which is bound to its homologous antigen. (Various enzyme-substrate systems, including the use of avidin-biotin to bind marker substances, are also discussed in Chapter 9.) The antigen to which the antibodies bind, if antibodies are present in the patient's sera, is either attached to the inside of the wells of a microtiter plate, adherent to a filter matrix, or bound to the surface of beads or plastic paddles. Advantages of ELISA tests include ease of performance on many serum samples at the same time and easy detection of the colored or fluorescent end products with appropriate instrumentation, removing the element of subjectivity inherent in so many serologic procedures. Disadvantages include the need for special equipment, the fairly long reaction times (often hours instead of minutes for particle agglutination tests), the relative end point of the test (which relies on measuring the amount of a visible end product that is not dependent on the original antigen-antibody reaction itself but on a second enzymatic reaction, compared to a directly quantitative result), and the requirement for batch processing to ensure cost effectiveness.

Commercial microdilution or solid-phase matrix systems are available to detect antibody specific for hepatitis virus antigens, herpes simplex viruses 1 and 2, respiratory syncytial virus (RSV), cytomegalovirus, human immunodeficiency virus (HIV), rubella virus (both IgG

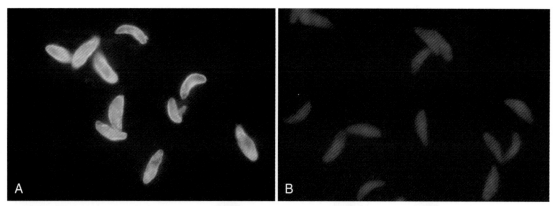

**Figure 10-6** Indirect fluorescent antibody tests for *Toxoplasma gondii,* IgG antibodies. **A,** Positive reaction. **B,** Negative reaction. (Courtesy Meridian, Cincinnati, Ohio.)

and IgM), mycoplasmas, chlamydiae, *Borrelia burgdorferi, Entamoeba histolytica,* and many other agents.

The introduction of membrane-bound ELISA components has improved sensitivity and ease of use dramatically. Slot-blot and dot-blot assays force the target antigen through a membrane filter, causing it to become affixed in the shape of the hole (a dot or a slot). Several antigens can be placed on one membrane. When test (patient) serum is layered onto the membrane, specific antibodies, if present, bind to the corresponding dot or slot of antigen. Addition of a labeled second antibody and subsequent development of the label allows visual detection of the presence of antibodies based on the pattern of antigen sites. Cassette-based membrane-bound ELISA assays, designed for testing a single serum, can be performed rapidly (often within 10 minutes). Commercial kits to detect antibodies to *Helicobacter pylori, Taxoplasma gondii,* and some other infectious agents are available.

Antibody capture ELISAs are particularly valuable for detecting IgM in the presence of IgG. Anti-IgM antibodies are fixed to the solid phase; therefore, only IgM antibodies, if present in the patient's serum, are bound. In a second step, specific antigen is added in a sandwich format and a second antigen-specific labeled antibody is added. Toxoplasmosis, rubella, and other infections are diagnosed using this technology, typically in research settings.

### Indirect Fluorescent Antibody Tests and Other Immunomicroscopic Methods

Indirect fluorescent antibody determination (IFA) is a widely applied method of detecting diverse antibodies (see Chapter 9). For these types of tests, the antigen against which the patient makes antibody (e.g., whole *Toxoplasma* organisms or virus-infected tissue culture cells) is affixed to the surface of a microscope slide. The patient's serum is diluted and placed on the slide, covering the area in which antigen was placed. If present in the serum, antibody binds to the specific antigen. Unbound antibody is then removed by washing the slide. In the second stage of the procedure, a conjugate of antihuman globulin directed specifically against IgG or IgM and a fluorescent dye (e.g., fluorescein) is placed on the slide. This labeled marker for human antibody binds

to the antibody already bound to the antigen on the slide and serves as a detector, indicating binding of the antibody to the antigen when viewed under a fluorescence microscope (Figure 10-6). Commercially available test kits include slides coated with the antigen, positive and negative control sera, diluent for the patients' sera, and the properly diluted conjugate. As with other commercial products, IFA systems should be used as units, without modification of the manufacturer's instructions. Commercially available IFA tests include those for antibodies to *Legionella* species, *B. burgdorferi, T. gondii,* varicella-zoster virus, cytomegalovirus, Epstein-Barr virus capsid antigen, early antigen and nuclear antigen, herpes simplex viruses types 1 and 2, rubella virus, *M. pneumoniae, T. pallidum* (the **fluorescent treponemal antibody absorption test [FTA-ABS]**), and several rickettsiae. Most of these tests, if performed properly, give extremely specific and sensitive results. Proper interpretation of IFA tests requires experienced and technically competent technologists. These tests can be performed rapidly and are cost effective.

### Radioimmunoassays

Radioimmunoassay (RIA) is an automated method of detecting antibodies that usually is performed in the chemistry section of the laboratory rather than in the serology section. RIA tests were originally used to detect antibody to hepatitis B viral antigens. Radioactively labeled antibody competes with the patient's unlabeled antibody for binding sites on a known amount of antigen. A reduction in radioactivity of the antigen–patient antibody complex, compared with the radioactive counts in a control test with no antibody, is used to quantitate the amount of patient antibody bound to the antigen. The development of new marker substances, such as ELISA systems, chemiluminescence, and fluorescence, resulted in the production of diagnostic tests as sensitive as RIA without the hazards associated with the use and disposal of radioactive reagents.

### Fluorescent Immunoassays

Fluorescent immunoassays (FIA) were developed in response to the inconveniences associated with RIA (i.e., radioactive substances and expensive scintillation

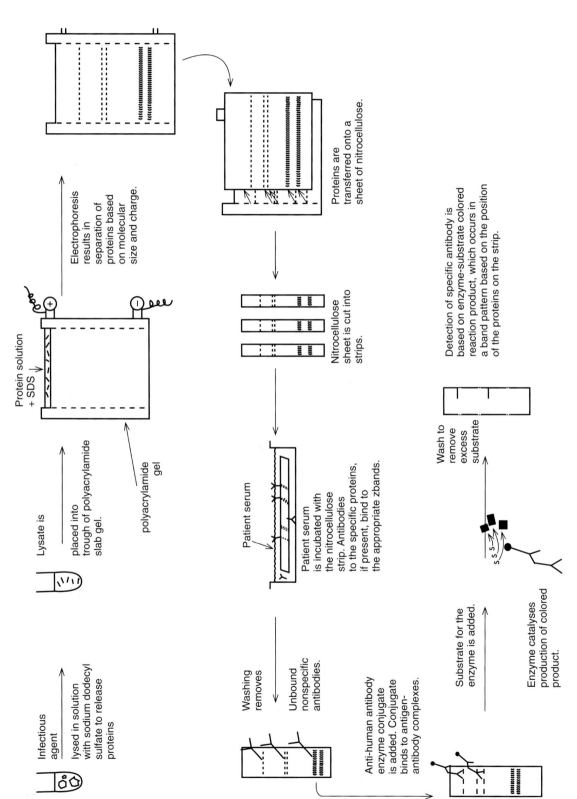

Infectious agent

lysed in solution with sodium dodecyl sulfate to release proteins

Lysate is placed into trough of polyacrylamide slab gel.

Protein solution + SDS

polyacrylamide gel

Electrophoresis results in separation of proteins based on molecular size and charge.

Proteins are transferred onto a sheet of nitrocellulose.

Nitrocellulose sheet is cut into strips.

Patient serum

Patient serum is incubated with the nitrocellulose strip. Antibodies to the specific proteins, if present, bind to the appropriate zbands.

Washing removes

Unbound nonspecific antibodies.

Anti-human antibody enzyme conjugate is added. Conjugate binds to antigen-antibody complexes.

Substrate for the enzyme is added.

Enzyme catalyses production of colored product.

Wash to remove excess substrate

Detection of specific antibody is based on enzyme-substrate colored reaction product, which occurs in a band pattern based on the position of the proteins on the strip.

**Figure 10-7** Diagram of Western blot immunoassay system.

counters). These tests, which use fluorescent dyes or molecules as markers instead of radioactive labels, are based on the same principle as RIA. The primary difference is that the competitive antibody in RIA systems is labeled with a radioisotope, and in FIA the antigen is labeled with a compound that fluoresces under the appropriate light emission source. Binding of patient antibody to a fluorescent-labeled antigen can reduce or quench the fluorescence, or binding can cause fluorescence by allowing conformational change in a fluorescent molecule. Measurement of fluorescence is a direct measurement of antigen-antibody binding and is not dependent on a second marker, as in ELISA tests. Systems are commercially available to measure antibody developed against numerous infectious agents, as well as against self-antigens (autoimmune antibodies).

### Western Blot Immunoassays

Requirements for the detection of very specific antibodies have driven the development of the Western blot immunoassay (Figure 10-7). The method is based on the electrophoretic separation of major proteins of an infectious agent in a two-dimensional agarose (first dimension) and acrylamide (second dimension) matrix. A suspension of the organism is mechanically or chemically disrupted, and the solubilized antigen suspension is placed at one end of a polyacrylamide (polymer) gel. Under the influence of an electrical current, the proteins migrate through the gel. Most bacteria or viruses contain several major proteins that can be recognized based on their position in the gel after electrophoresis. Smaller proteins travel faster and migrate farther in the lanes of the gel. The protein bands are transferred from the gel to a nitrocellulose or other type of thin membrane, and the membrane is treated to immobilize the proteins. The membrane is then cut into many thin strips, each carrying the pattern of protein bands. When patient serum is layered over the strip, antibodies bind to each of the protein components represented by a band on the strip. The pattern of antibodies present can be used to determine whether the patient has a current infection or is immune to the agent (Figure 10-8). Antibodies against microbes with numerous cross-reacting antibodies, such as *T. pallidum, B. burgdorferi*, herpes simplex virus types 1 and 2, and HIV, are identified more specifically using this technology than a single method that is used to identify a single antibody type. For example, the CDC defines an ELISA or immunofluorescence assay as a first-line test for Lyme disease antibody, but positive or equivocal results must be confirmed by a Western blot test.

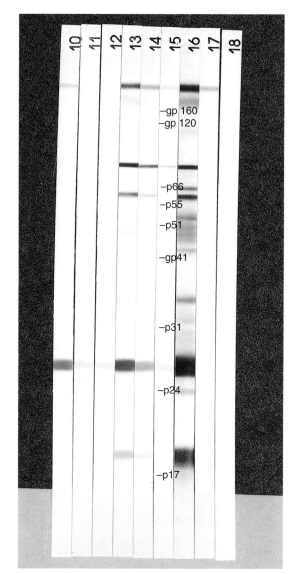

**Figure 10-8** Human immunodeficiency virus type 1 (HIV-1) Western blot immunoassay. Samples are characterized as positive, indeterminate, or negative based on the bands found to be present in significant intensity. A positive blot has any two or more of the following bands: p24, gp41, and/or gp120/160. An indeterminate blot contains some bands but not the definitive ones. A negative blot has no bands present. Lane 16 shows antibodies from a control serum binding to the virus-specific proteins (*p*) and glycoproteins (*gp*) transferred onto the nitrocellulose paper. (Courtesy Calypte Biomedical Corp., Pleasanton, Calif.)

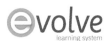 *Visit the Evolve site to complete the review questions.*

# Principles of Antimicrobial Action and Resistance

## OBJECTIVES

1. List the five general categories of antimicrobial actions.
2. Define antibiotic and antimicrobial.
3. Define and differentiate bactericidal and bacteriostatic agents.
4. Compare and contrast the following terms: biologic versus clinical resistance, environmentally mediated versus microorganism-mediated resistance and intrinsic versus acquired resistance.
5. Describe the basic structure and chemical principle for the mechanism of beta-lactam antimicrobials.
6. List common β-lactam antibiotics and provide an example of a common pathogen susceptible to these agents
7. Describe the chemical principle for the mechanism of resistance to β-lactam antibiotics.
8. Describe the chemical principle for the mechanisms of glycopeptide agents.
9. List common glycopeptides and provide an example of a common pathogen susceptible to these agents.
10. List examples of cell membrane inhibitors, inhibitors of protein synthesis, inhibitors of deoxyribonucleic acid (DNA) or ribonucleic acid (RNA) synthesis, and metabolic inhibitors. Provide an example of a common pathogen susceptible to each of the agents listed.
11. List five general mechanisms for antimicrobial resistance and provide an example for each.
12. Describe how the dissemination of antimicrobial resistance affects diagnostic microbiology, including effects on sensitivity testing, therapeutics, and organism identification.

Medical intervention in an infection primarily involves attempts to eradicate the infecting pathogen using substances that actively inhibit or kill the organism. Some of these substances are obtained and purified from other microbial organisms and are known as **antibiotics.** Others are chemically synthesized. Collectively, these natural and synthesized substances are referred to as **antimicrobial agents.** Depending on the type of organisms targeted, these substances are also known as *antibacterial, antifungal, antiparasitic,* or *antiviral agents.*

Because antimicrobial agents play a central role in the control and management of infectious diseases, understanding their mode of action and the mechanisms of microorganisms to circumvent antimicrobial activity is important, especially because diagnostic laboratories are expected to design and implement tests that measure a pathogen's response to antimicrobial activity (see Chapter 12). Much of what is discussed here regarding

antimicrobial action and resistance is based on antibacterial agents, but the principles generally apply to almost all antiinfective agents. More information about antiparasitic, antifungal, and antiviral agents can be found in Parts IV, V, and VI, respectively.

## ANTIMICROBIAL ACTION

### PRINCIPLES

Several key steps must be completed for an antimicrobial agent to successfully inhibit or kill an infecting microorganism (Figure 11-1). First, the agent must be in an active form. This is ensured through the pharmacodynamic design of the drug, which takes into account the route by which the patient receives the agent (e.g., orally, intramuscularly, intravenously). Second, the antibiotic must also be able to achieve sufficient levels or concentrations at the site of infection so that it has a chance to exert an antibacterial effect (i.e., it must be in anatomic approximation with the infecting bacteria). The ability to achieve adequate levels depends on the pharmacokinetic properties of the agent, such as rate of absorption, distribution, metabolism, and excretion of the agent's metabolites. Table 11-1 provides examples of various anatomic limitations characteristic of a few commonly used antibacterial agents. Some agents, such as ampicillin and ceftriaxone, achieve therapeutically effective levels in several body sites, whereas others, such as nitrofurantoin and norfloxacin, are limited to the urinary tract. Therefore, a knowledge of the site of infection can substantially affect the selection of the antimicrobial agent for therapeutic use.

The remaining steps in antimicrobial action relate to direct interactions between the antibacterial agent and the bacterial cell. The antibiotic is attracted to and maintains contact with the cell surface. Because most targets of antibacterial agents are intracellular, uptake of the antibiotic to some location inside the bacterial cell is required. Once the antibiotic has achieved sufficient intracellular concentration, binding to a specific target occurs. This binding involves molecular interactions between the antimicrobial agent and one or more biochemical components that play an important role in the microorganism's cellular metabolism. Adequate binding of the target results in disruption of cellular processes, leading to cessation of bacterial cell growth and,

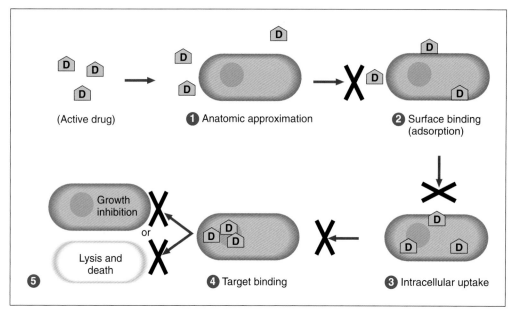

**Figure 11-1** The basic steps required for antimicrobial activity and strategic points for bacterial circumvention or interference (marked by X) of antimicrobial action, leading to resistance.

**TABLE 11-1** Anatomic Distribution of Some Common Antibacterial Agents

|  | Serum-Blood* | Cerebrospinal Fluid | Urine |
|---|---|---|---|
| Ampicillin | + | + | + |
| Ceftriaxone | + | + | + |
| Vancomycin | + | ± | + |
| Ciprofloxacin | + | ± | + |
| Gentamicin | + | − | + |
| Clindamycin | + | − | − |
| Norfloxacin | − | − | + |
| Nitrofurantoin | − | − | + |

+, Therapeutic levels generally achievable at that site; ±, therapeutic achievable levels moderate to poor; −, therapeutic levels generally not achievable at that site.
*Serum-blood represents a general anatomic distribution.

**BOX 11-1** Bacteriostatic and Bactericidal Antibacterial Agents*

**Generally Bacteriostatic**
Chloramphenicol
   Erythromycin and other macrolides
   Clindamycin
   Sulfonamides
   Trimethoprim
   Tetracyclines
   Tigecycline
   Linezolid
   Quinupristin/dalfopristin

**Generally Bactericidal**
Aminoglycosides
   β-lactams
   Vancomycin
   Daptomycin
   Teicoplanin
   Telavancin
   Quinolones (e.g., ciprofloxacin, levofloxacin)
   Rifampin
   Metronidazole

*The bactericidal and bacteriostatic nature of an antimicrobial may vary depending on the concentration of the agent used and the bacterial species targeted.

depending on the antimicrobial agent's mode of action, cell death. Antimicrobial agents that inhibit bacterial growth but generally do not kill the organism are known as **bacteriostatic agents.** Effectively reducing the growth rate of an organism provides adequate protection in individuals whose immune system is capable of removing the agent of infection. Agents that usually kill target organisms are said to be **bactericidal** (Box 11-1). Bacteriocidal agents are more effective against organisms that are more difficult to control in combination with the host's immune system.

The primary goal in the development and design of antimicrobial agents is to optimize a drug's ability to efficiently achieve all steps outlined in Figure 11-1 while minimizing toxic effects on human cells and physiology. Different antibacterial agents exhibit substantial specificity in terms of their bacterial cell targets, that is, their mode of action. For this reason, antimicrobial agents are frequently categorized according to their mode of action.

**TABLE 11-2** Summary of Mechanisms of Action for Commonly Used Antibacterial Agents

| Antimicrobial Class | Mechanism of Action | Spectrum of Activity |
|---|---|---|
| Aminoglycosides (e.g., gentamicin, tobramycin, amikacin, streptomycin, kanamycin) | Inhibit protein synthesis by binding to 30S ribosomal subunit | Gram-positive and gram-negative bacteria; not anaerobic bacteria |
| β-lactams (e.g., penicillin, ampicillin, mezlocillin, piperacillin, cefazolin, cefotetan, ceftriaxone, cefotaxime, ceftazidime, aztreonam, imipenem) | Inhibit cell wall synthesis by binding enzymes involved in peptidoglycan production (i.e., penicillin-binding proteins [PBPs]) | Both gram-positive and gram-negative bacteria, but spectrum may vary with the individual antibiotic. |
| Chloramphenicol | Inhibits protein synthesis by binding 50S ribosomal subunit | Gram-positive and gram-negative bacteria |
| Fluoroquinolones (e.g., ciprofloxacin, ofloxacin, norfloxacin) | Inhibit DNA synthesis by binding DNA gyrase and topoisomerase IV | Gram-positive and gram-negative bacteria, but spectrum may vary with individual antibiotic |
| Glycylglycines (e.g., tigecycline) | Inhibition of protein synthesis by binding to 30S ribosomal subunit | Wide spectrum of gram-positive and gram-negative species including those resistant to tetracycline |
| Ketolides (e.g., telithromycin) | Inhibition of protein synthesis by binding to 50S ribosomal subunit | Gram-positive cocci including certain macrolide-resistant strains and some fastidious gram-negatives (e.g., *H. influenzae* and *M. catarrhalis*) |
| Lipopeptides (e.g., daptomycin) | Binding and disruption of cell membrane | Gram-positive bacteria including those resistant to beta-lactams and glycopeptides |
| Nitrofurantoin | Exact mechanism uncertain; may have several bacterial enzyme targets and directly damage DNA | Gram-positive and gram-negative bacteria |
| Oxazolidinones (e.g., linezolid) | Bind to 50S ribosomal subunit to interfere with initiation of protein synthesis | Wide variety of gram-positive bacteria, including those resistant to other antimicrobial classes |
| Polymyxins (e.g., polymyxin B and colistin) | Disruption of cell membrane | Gram-negative bacteria, poor activity against most gram-positive bacteria |
| Rifampin | Inhibits RNA synthesis by binding DNA-dependent, RNA polymerase | Gram-positive and certain gram-negative (e.g., *N. meningitidis*) bacteria |
| Streptogramins (e.g., quinupristin/dalfopristin) | Inhibit protein synthesis by binding to two separate sites on the 50S ribosomal subunit | Primarily gram-positive bacteria |
| Sulfonamides | Interfere with folic acid pathway by binding the enzyme dihydropteroate synthase | Gram-positive and many gram-negative bacteria |
| Tetracycline | Inhibits protein synthesis by binding 30S ribosomal subunit | Gram-positive and gram-negative bacteria, and several intracellular bacterial pathogens (e.g., chlamydia) |
| Trimethoprim | Interferes with folic acid pathway by binding the enzyme dihydrofolate reductase | Gram-positive and many gram-negative bacteria |

## MODE OF ACTION OF ANTIBACTERIAL AGENTS

The interior of the bacterial cell has several potential antimicrobial targets. However, the processes or structures most frequently targeted are cell wall (peptidoglycan) synthesis, the cell membrane, protein synthesis, metabolic pathways, and DNA and RNA synthesis (Table 11-2).

### Inhibitors of Cell Wall Synthesis

The bacterial cell wall, also known as the *peptidoglycan,* or *murein,* layer, plays an essential role in the life of the bacterial cell. This fact, combined with the lack of a similar structure in human cells, has made the cell wall the focus of attention for the development of bactericidal agents that are relatively nontoxic for humans.

**β-Lactam (Beta-Lactam) Antimicrobial Agents.** β-lactam antibiotics have a four-member, nitrogen-containing, β-lactam ring at the core of their structure (Figure 11-2). The antibiotics differ in ring structure and attached chemical groups. This drug class comprises the largest group of antibacterial agents, and dozens of derivatives are available for clinical use. Types of β-lactam agents include penicillins, cephalosporins, carbapenems, and monobactams. The popularity of these agents results from their bactericidal action and lack of toxicity to humans; also, their molecular structures can be manipulated

| Beta-lactam class | Examples | Base molecular structure |
|---|---|---|
| Penicillins | Penicillin<br>Ampicillin<br>Piperacillin<br>Mezlocillin | 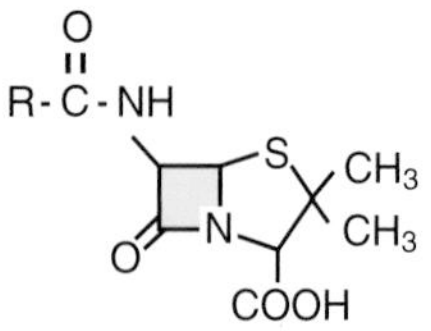 |
| Cephalosporins | Cefazolin<br>Cefuroxime<br>Cefotetan<br>Cefotaxime<br>Ceftriaxone<br>Ceftazidime<br>Cefepime | 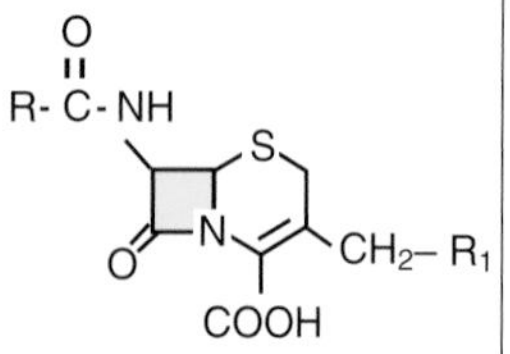 |
| Monobactams | Aztreonam | 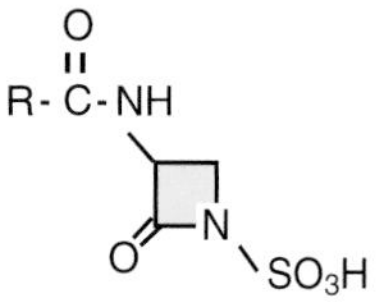 |
| Carbapenems | Imipenem<br>Meropenem<br>Doripenem | 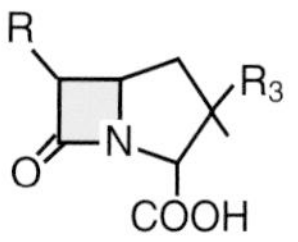 |

**Figure 11-2** Basic structures and examples of commonly used β-lactam antibiotics. The core β-lactam ring is highlighted in yellow in each structure. (Modified from Salyers AA, Whitt DD, editors: *Bacterial pathogenesis: a molecular approach,* Washington, DC, 1994, ASM Press.)

to achieve greater activity for wider therapeutic applications.

The β-lactam ring is the key to the mode of action of these drugs. It is structurally similar to acyl-D-alanyl-D-alanine, the normal substrate required for synthesis of the linear glycopeptide in the bacterial cell wall. The β-lactam binds the enzyme, inhibiting transpeptidation and cell wall synthesis. Most bacterial cells cannot survive once they have lost the capacity to produce and maintain their peptidoglycan layer. The enzymes essential for this function are anchored in the cell membrane and are referred to as **penicillin-binding proteins (PBPs).** Bacterial species may have four to six different types of PBPs. The PBPs involved in cell wall cross-linking (i.e., transpeptidases) are often the most critical for survival. When β-lactams bind to these PBPs, cell wall synthesis is essentially halted. Death results from osmotic instability caused by faulty cell wall synthesis, or binding of the β-lactam to PBP may trigger a series of events that leads to autolysis and death of the cell.

Because nearly all clinically relevant bacteria have cell walls, β-lactam agents act against a broad spectrum of gram-positive and gram-negative bacteria. However, because of differences among bacteria in their PBP content, natural structural characteristics (e.g., the outer membrane present in gram-negative but not gram-positive bacteria), and their common antimicrobial resistance mechanisms, the effectiveness of β-lactams against different types of bacteria can vary widely. Gram-positive bacteria secrete β-lactamase into the environment, whereas beta-lactamases produced by gram-negative bacteria remain in the periplasmic space, providing increased protection from the antimicrobial. In addition, any given β-lactam drug has a specific group or type of bacteria against which it is considered to have the greatest activity. The type of bacteria against which a particular antimicrobial agent does and does not have activity is referred to as that drug's **spectrum of activity.** Many factors contribute to an antibiotic's spectrum of activity, and knowledge of this spectrum is the key to many aspects of antimicrobial use and laboratory testing.

A common mechanism of bacterial resistance to β-lactams is the production of enzymes (i.e., β-lactamases) that bind and hydrolyze these drugs. Just as there is a variety of β-lactam antibiotics, there is a variety of β-lactamases. The β-lactamases are grouped into four major categories; classes A, B, C, and D. Classes A and D are considered serine peptidases; class C comprises cephalosporinases; and class B, which requires zinc, is called a *metallo-β-lactamase.* β-lactamase genes should be located on plasmids or transposons, within an integron, or within the chromosome of the organism. An integron is a large cassette region that contains antibiotic resistance genes and the enzyme integrase, which is required for movement of the cassette from one genetic element to another. In addition, the antimicrobial may be constitutively produced, continuously produced, or it may be induced by the presence of a β-lactam.

Bacteria normally susceptible to β-lactams have developed several resistance mechanisms against the antimicrobials. These include genetic mutations in the PBP coding sequence, altering the structure and reducing the binding affinity to the drug; genetic recombination, resulting in a PBP structure resistant to binding of the drug; overproduction of normal PBP, resulting in overload of the drug; and acquiring a new genetic coding sequence for PBP from another organism with a lower affinity to the drug. These acquired types of β-lactam resistance are more commonly found in gram-positive bacteria.

To circumvent the development of antimicrobial resistance, β-lactam combinations comprised of a β-lactam with antimicrobial activity (e.g., ampicillin, amoxicillin, piperacillin) and a beta-lactam without activity capable of binding and inhibiting β-lactamases (e.g., sulbactam, clavulanate, tazobactam) have been developed. The binding β-lactam "ties up" the β-lactamases produced by the bacteria and allows the other β-lactam in the combination to exert its antimicrobial effect. Examples of these β-lactam/β-lactamase inhibitor combinations include ampicillin/sulbactam, amoxicillin/clavulanate, and piperacillin/tazobactam. Such combinations are effective only against organisms that produce β-lactamases that are bound by the inhibitor; they have little effect on resistance that is mediated by altered PBPs (see Mechanisms of Antibiotic Resistance later in this chapter).

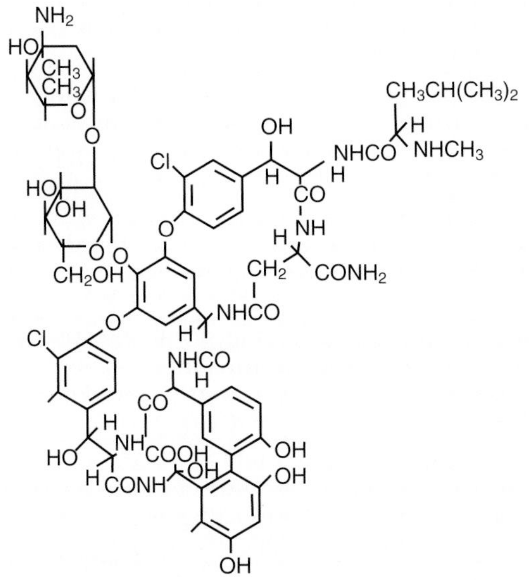

**Figure 11-3** Structure of vancomycin, a non–β-lactam antibiotic that inhibits cell wall synthesis. (Modified from Salyers AA, Whitt DD, editors: *Bacterial pathogenesis: a molecular approach,* Washington, DC, 1994, ASM Press.)

**Glycopeptides and Lipopeptides.** Glycopeptides are the other major class of antibiotics that inhibit bacterial cell wall synthesis by binding to the end of the peptidoglycan, interfering with transpeptidation. This is a different mechanism from that of the β-lactams, which bind directly to the enzyme. Two such antibiotics, vancomycin and teicoplanin, are large molecules and function differently from β-lactam antibiotics (Figure 11-3). With glycopeptides, the binding interferes with the ability of the PBP enzymes, such as transpeptidases and transglycosylases, to incorporate the precursors into the growing cell wall. With the cessation of cell wall synthesis, cell growth stops and death often follows. Because glycopeptides have a different mode of action, the resistance to β-lactam agents by gram-positive bacteria does not generally hinder their activity. However, because of their relatively large size, they cannot penetrate the outer membrane of most gram-negative bacteria to reach their cell wall precursor targets. Therefore, this agent is usually ineffective against gram-negative bacteria. Teicoplanin is approved for use throughout the world but is not currently available in the United States. When vancomycin is used, its levels should be monitored because the potential for toxicity.

Oritavancin and telavancin, which are lipoglycopeptides, are structurally similar to vancomycin. They are semisynthetic molecules that are glycopeptides that contain hydrophobic chemical groups. However, change in the molecular structure of the lipoglycopeptides provides a mechanism by which they can bind to the bacterial cell membrane, increasing the inhibition of cell wall synthesis. In addition, the lipoglycopeptides increase cell permeability and cause depolarization of the cell membrane potential. These agents also inhibit the transglycosylation process necessary for cell wall synthesis by complexing with the D-alanyl-D-alanine residues. The lipoglycopeptides' spectrum of activity is comparable to that of vancomycin but also includes vancomycin-intermediate *Staphylococcus aureus* (VISA).

The lipopeptide daptomycin is the most recently developed antimicrobial capable of exerting its antimicrobial effect by binding and disrupting the cell membrane of gram-positive bacteria. The drug binds to the cytoplasmic membrane and inserts its hydrophobic tail into the membrane, disrupting the permeability and resulting in cell death. Daptomycin has potent activity against gram-positive cocci, including those resistant to other agents such as beta-lactams and glycopeptides (e.g., methicillin-resistant *S. aureus* [MRSA], vancomycin-resistant enterococci [VRE], and vancomycin-resistant *S. aureus* [VRSA]). Because of the molecule's size, daptomycin is unable to penetrate the outer membrane of gram-negative bacilli and thus is ineffective against these organisms.

Several other cell wall–active antibiotics have been discovered and developed over the years, but toxicity to the human host has prevented their widespread clinical use. One example is bacitracin, which inhibits the recycling of certain metabolites required for maintaining peptidoglycan synthesis. Because of potential toxicity, bacitracin is usually only used as a topical antibacterial agent and internal consumption is generally avoided.

### Inhibitors of Cell Membrane Function
Polymyxins (polymyxin B and colistin) are cyclic polypeptide agents that disrupt bacterial cell membranes. The polymyxins act as detergents, interacting with the phospholipids in the cell membranes and increasing permeability. This disruption results in leakage of macromolecules and ions essential for cell survival. Because their effectiveness varies with the molecular makeup of the bacterial cell membrane, polymyxins are not equally effective against all bacteria. Most notably, they are more effective against gram-negative bacteria, whereas activity against gram-positive bacteria tends to be poor. Furthermore, human host cells also have membranes, therefore polymyxins pose a risk of toxicity. The major side effects are neurotoxicity and nephrotoxicity. Although toxic, the polymyxins are often the antimicrobial agents of last resort when gram-negative bacilli (e.g., *Pseudomonas aeruginosa, Acinetobacter* spp.) that are resistant to all other available agents are encountered.

### Inhibitors of Protein Synthesis
Several classes of antibiotics target bacterial protein synthesis and severely disrupt cellular metabolism. Antibiotic classes that act by inhibiting protein synthesis include aminoglycosides, macrolide-lincosamide-streptogramins (MLS group), ketolides (e.g., telithromycin) chloramphenicol, tetracyclines, glycylglycines (e.g., tigecycline), and oxazolidinones (e.g., linezolid). Although these antibiotics are generally categorized as protein synthesis inhibitors, the specific mechanisms by which they inhibit protein synthesis differ significantly.

**Aminoglycosides and Aminocyclitols.** Aminoglycosides (aminoglycosidic aminocyclitol) inhibit bacterial protein

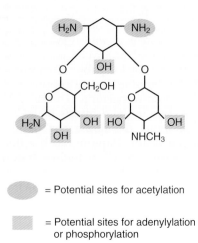

**Figure 11-4** Structure of the commonly used aminoglycoside gentamicin. Potential sites of modification by adenylating, phosphorylating, and acetylating enzymes produced by bacteria are highlighted. (Modified from Salyers AA, Whitt DD, editors: *Bacterial pathogenesis: a molecular approach,* Washington, DC, 1994, ASM Press.)

synthesis by irreversibly binding to protein receptors on the organism's 30S ribosomal subunit. This process interrupts several steps, including initial formation of the protein synthesis complex, accurate reading of the messenger RNA (mRNA) code, and formation of the ribosomal-mRNA complex. The structure of a commonly used aminoglycoside, gentamicin, is shown in Figure 11-4. Other aminoglycosides include tobramycin, amikacin, streptomycin, and kanamycin. The spectrum of activity of aminoglycosides includes a wide variety of aerobic gram-negative and certain gram-positive bacteria, such as *S. aureus.* Bacterial uptake of the aminoglycosides is accomplished by using them in combination with cell wall–active antibiotics, such as β-lactams or vancomycin. Anaerobic bacteria are unable to uptake these agents intracellularly and therefore are typically not inhibited by aminoglycosides. Aminoglycosides are associated with toxicity, and blood levels should be monitored during therapy. The major toxicities are nephrotoxicity and auditory or vestibular toxicity.

**Macrolide-Lincosamide-Streptogramin (MLS) Group.** The most commonly used antibiotics in the MLS group are the macrolides (e.g., erythromycin, azithromycin, clarithromycin, and clindamycin, which is a lincosamide). Protein synthesis is inhibited by drug binding to the 23sRNA on the bacterial 50S ribosomal subunit and subsequent disruption of the growing peptide chain by blocking of the translocation reaction. Macrolides are generally bacteriostatic, but they may be bactericidal if the infective dose of the organism is low and the drug is used in high concentrations. Primarily because of uptake difficulties associated with the outer membranes of gram-negative bacteria, the macrolides and clindamycin generally are not effective against most genera of gram-negative organisms. However, they are effective against gram-positive bacteria, mycoplasmas, treponemes, and rickettsiae. Quinupristin-dalfopristin is a dual streptogramin that

targets two sites on the 50S ribosomal subunit. Toxicity is generally low with macrolides, although hearing loss and reactions with other medications may occur.

The lincosamides, clindamycin and lincomycin, bind to the 50s ribosomal subunit and prevent elongation by interfering with the peptidyl transfer during protein synthesis. They may exhibit bacteriocidal or bacteriostatic activity. The spectrum of activity depends on the bacterial species, the size of the inoculum, and the drug concentration. Lincosamides are effective against gram-positive cocci.

Streptogramins are naturally occurring cyclic peptides including quinupristin-dalfopristin. The streptogramins enter the bacterial cells through passive diffusion and bind irreversibly to the 50s subunit of the bacterial ribosome inducing a conformational change in the ribosome structure. Alteration of the ribosome structure interferes with peptide bond formation during protein synthesis, disrupting elongation of the growing peptide. The streptogramins are able to enter most tissues and are effective against gram-positive and some gram-negative organisms. The drugs have low toxicity; localized phlebitis is the major complication of intravenous infusion.

**Ketolides.** This group of compounds consists of chemical derivatives of erythromycin A and other macrolides. As such, they act by binding to the 23s rRNA of the 50S ribosomal subunit, inhibiting protein synthesis. The key difference between the only currently available ketolide, telithromycin, and the macrolides is that telithromycin maintains activity against most macrolide-resistant gram-positive organisms and does not induce a common macrolide resistance mechanism (i.e., macrolide-lincosamide-streptogramin-B [MLSB] methylase), the alteration of the ribosomal target. Ketolides are effective against respiratory pathogens and intracellular bacteria. The agents are particularly effective against gram-positive and some gram-negative bacteria, as well as *Mycoplasma, Mycobacteria, Chlamydia,* and *Rickettsia* spp. and *Francisella tularensis.* Ketolides have low toxicity, and the major side effect are gastrointestinal symptoms, including diarrhea, nausea, and vomiting.

**Oxazolidinones.** Oxazolidinones, currently represented by linezolid, are a relatively new class of synthetic antibacterial agents available for clinical use. Linezolid is a synthetic agent that inhibits protein synthesis by specifically interacting with the 23S rRNA in the 50S ribosomal subunit, interfering with the binding of the transfer RNA (tRNA) for formylated-methionine. This action inhibits initiation of translation of any mRNA, thereby preventing protein synthesis. Therefore, linezolid is not expected to be affected by resistance mechanisms that affect other drug classes. Linezolid is effective against most gram-positive bacteria and mycobacteria. Toxicity is generally low, resulting in gastrointestinal symptoms, including diarrhea and nausea.

**Chloramphenicol.** Chloramphenicol inhibits the addition of amino acids to the growing peptide chain by reversibly binding to the 50S ribosomal subunit, inhibiting transpeptidation. This antibiotic is highly active against a wide variety of gram-negative and gram-positive bacteria; however, its use has dwindled because of drug toxicity and the development of new effective and safer agents, mostly of the beta-lactam class. Bone marrow toxicity is the major side effect associated with chloramphenicol treatment.

**Tetracyclines.** The tetracyclines are considered broad-spectrum bacteriostatic antibiotics. They inhibit protein synthesis by binding reversibly to the 30S ribosomal subunit, interfering with the binding of the tRNA–amino acid complexes to the ribosome, preventing peptide chain elongation. Tetracyclines have a broad spectrum of activity that includes gram-negative bacteria, gram-positive bacteria, several intracellular bacterial pathogens (e.g., *Chlamydia* and *Rickettsia* spp.), and some protozoa. Infections caused by *Neisseria gonorrhoeae*, mycoplasma, and spirochetes may be successfully treated with these drugs. Toxicity includes upper gastrointestinal effects, such as esophageal ulcerations, nausea, vomiting, and epigastric distress. In addition, cutaneous phototoxicity may also develop, resulting in disease, including photoallergic immune reactions.

**Glycylglycines.** These agents are semi-synthetic tetracycline derivatives. Tigecycline is the first agent of this class approved for clinical use. Similar to the tetracyclines, tigecycline inhibits protein synthesis by reversibly binding to the 30S ribosomal subunit. However, tigecycline has the advantage of being refractory to the most common tetracycline resistance mechanisms expressed by gram-negative and gram-positive bacteria. The most common side effects are nausea, vomiting, and diarrhea.

## Inhibitors of DNA and RNA Synthesis

The primary antimicrobial agents that target DNA metabolism are the fluoroquinolones and metronidazole.

**Fluoroquinolones.** Fluoroquinolones, also often simply referred to as quinolones, are derivatives of nalidixic acid, an older antibacterial agent. The structures of two quinolones, ciprofloxacin and ofloxacin, are shown in Figure 11-5. These agents bind to and interfere with DNA gyrase enzymes involved in the regulation of bacterial DNA supercoiling, a process essential for DNA replication, recombination, and repair. The newer fluoroquinolones also inhibit topoisomerase IV. Topoisomerase IV functions very similarly to DNA gyrase, unlinking DNA

after replication. The fluoroquinolones are potent bactericidal agents and have a broad spectrum of activity that includes gram-negative and gram-positive organisms. The fluoroquinolones target the DNA gyrase in gram-negative organisms and topoisomerase IV in gram-positive organisms. Because these agents interfere with DNA replication and therefore cell division, the drugs are bacteriocidal. However, the spectrum of activity varies with the individual quinolone agent. Toxicity varies with a variety of factors. Tendinitis and rupture of the Achilles tendon have been associated with fluoroquinolone treatment in the general population, and the risk is greater in older patients.

**Metronidazole.** The exact mechanism of metronidazole's antibacterial activity is related to the presence of a nitro group in the chemical structure. The nitro group is reduced by a nitroreductase in the bacterial cytoplasm, generating cytotoxic compounds and free radicals that disrupt the host DNA. Activation of metronidazole requires reduction under conditions of low redox potential, such as are found in anaerobic environments. Therefore, this agent is most potent against anaerobic and microaerophilic organisms, notably those that are gram negative. The drug is also effective in the treatment of protozoans, including *Trichomonas* and *Giardia* spp. and *Entamoeba histolytica*. Because susceptibility testing is not routinely performed on anaerobes, resistance is underreported. An emerging resistance to metronidazole is creating difficulties associated with bacterial diagnostics and treatments. Toxicity is low. Adverse side effects generally include mild gastrointestinal symptoms.

**Rifamycin.** Rifamycins, which include the drug rifampin (also known as *rifampicin*), are semisynthetic antibiotics that bind to the enzyme DNA-dependent RNA polymerase and inhibit synthesis of RNA. Because rifampin does not effectively penetrate the outer membrane of all gram-negative bacteria, activity against these organisms is decreased compared to the drug's activity in gram-positive bacteria. In addition, spontaneous mutation, resulting in the production of rifampin-insensitive RNA polymerases, occurs at a relatively high frequency of mutation. Therefore, rifampin is typically used in

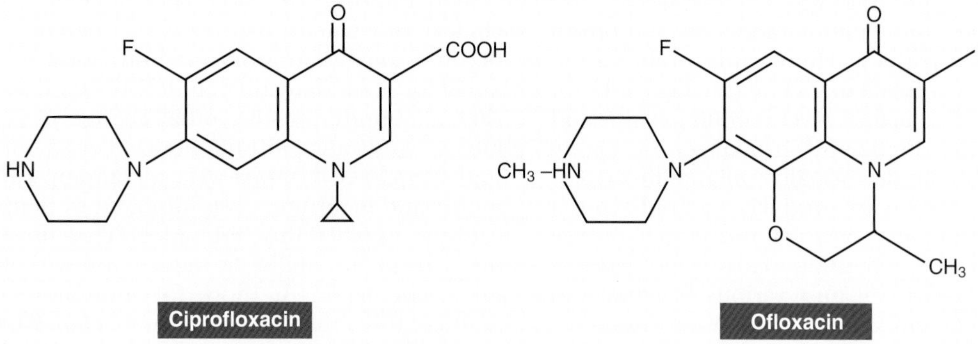

**Figure 11-5** Structures of the fluoroquinolones ciprofloxacin and ofloxacin. (Modified from Katzung BG: *Basic and clinical pharmacology,* Norwalk, Conn, 1995, Appleton & Lange.)

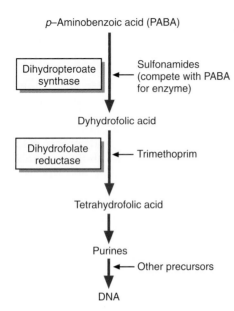

p–Aminobenzoic acid (PABA)

Dihydropteroate synthase ← Sulfonamides (compete with PABA for enzyme)

Dyhydrofolic acid

Dihydrofolate reductase ← Trimethoprim

Tetrahydrofolic acid

Purines

← Other precursors

DNA

**Figure 11-6** Bacterial folic acid pathway indicating the target enzymes for sulfonamide and trimethoprim activity. (Modified from Katzung BG: *Basic and clinical pharmacology,* Norwalk, Conn, 1995, The McGraw-Hill Companies, Inc.)

combination with other antimicrobial agents. Rifampin's side effects include gastrointestinal symptoms and hypersensitivity reactions.

### Inhibitors of Other Metabolic Processes

Antimicrobial agents that target bacterial processes other than those already discussed include sulfonamides, trimethoprim, and nitrofurantoin.

**Sulfonamides.** The bacterial folic acid pathway produces precursors required for DNA synthesis (Figure 11-6). Sulfonamides target and bind to one of the enzymes, dihydropteroate synthase, and disrupt the folic acid pathway. Several different sulfonamide derivatives are available for clinical use. These agents are active against a wide variety of bacteria, including the gram-positive and gram-negative (except *P. aeruginosa*) species. Sulfonamides are moderately toxic, causing vomiting, nausea, and hypersensitivity reactions. Sulfonamides are also antagonistic for several other medications, including warfarin, phenytoin, and oral hypoglycemic agents.

**Trimethoprim.** Like the sulfonamides, trimethoprim targets the folic acid pathway. However, it inhibits a different enzyme, dihydrofolate reductase (see Figure 11-6). Trimethoprim is active against several gram-positive and gram-negative species. Frequently, trimethoprim is combined with a sulfonamide (usually sulfamethoxazole) into a single formulation to produce an antibacterial agent that can simultaneously attack two targets on the same folic acid metabolic pathway. This drug combination can enhance activity against various bacteria and may help prevent the emergence of bacterial resistance to a single agent. Toxicity is typically mild. Adverse side effects include gastrointestinal symptoms and allergic skin rashes. Patients with acquired immunodeficiency

syndrome (AIDS) develop side effects more often than healthy individuals.

**Nitrofurantoin.** Nitrofurantoin consists of a nitro group on a heterocyclic ring. The mechanism of action of nitrofurantoin is diverse and multifaceted. This agent may have several targets involved in bacterial protein and enzyme synthesis. Nitrofurantoin is converted by bacterial nitroreductases to reactive intermediates that bind bacterial ribosomal proteins and rRNA, disrupting synthesis of RNA, DNA, and proteins. Nitrofurantoin is used to treat uncomplicated urinary tract infections and has good activity against most of the gram-positive and gram-negative bacteria that cause infections at that site. Toxicity primarily consists of gastrointestinal symptoms, including diarrhea, nausea, and vomiting. Chronic pulmonary conditions may develop, including irreversible pulmonary fibrosis.

# MECHANISMS OF ANTIBIOTIC RESISTANCE

## PRINCIPLES

Successful bacterial resistance to antimicrobial action requires interruption or disturbance of one or more steps essential for effective antimicrobial action (see Figure 11-1). These disturbances or resistance mechanisms can occur as a result of various processes, but the end result is partial or complete loss of antibiotic effectiveness. Different aspects of antimicrobial resistance mechanisms discussed include biologic versus clinical antimicrobial resistance, environmentally mediated antimicrobial resistance, and microorganism-mediated antimicrobial resistance.

## BIOLOGIC VERSUS CLINICAL RESISTANCE

The development of bacterial resistance to antimicrobial agents to which they were originally susceptible requires alterations in the cell's physiology or structure. **Biologic resistance** refers to changes that result in observably reduced susceptibility of an organism to a particular antimicrobial agent. When antimicrobial susceptibility has been lost to such an extent that the drug is no longer effective for clinical use, the organism has achieved clinical resistance.

It is important to note that biologic resistance and **clinical resistance** do not necessarily coincide. In fact, because most laboratory methods used to detect resistance focus on detecting clinical resistance, microorganisms may undergo substantial change in their levels of biologic resistance without notice. For example, for some time *Streptococcus pneumoniae*, a common cause of pneumonia and meningitis, was inhibited by penicillin at concentrations of 0.03 μg/mL or less. The clinical laboratory focused on the ability to detect strains requiring 2 μg/mL of penicillin or more for inhibition; this was the defined threshold for resistance required for interference with effective treatment using penicillin. However, although no isolates were being detected that required more than 2 μg/mL of penicillin for inhibition, strains were developing biologic resistance that required penicillin concentrations 10 to 50 times higher than 0.03 μg/mL for inhibition.

From a clinical laboratory and public health perspective, it is important to realize that biologic development of antimicrobial resistance is an ongoing process. Our inability to reliably detect all these processes with current laboratory procedures and criteria should not be misinterpreted as evidence that no changes in biologic resistance are occurring.

## ENVIRONMENTALLY MEDIATED ANTIMICROBIAL RESISTANCE

Antimicrobial resistance is the result of nearly inseparable interactions involving the drug, the microorganism, and the environment in which they coexist. Characteristics of the antimicrobial agents, other than the mode and spectrum of activity, include important aspects of each drug's pharmacologic attributes. However these factors are beyond the scope of this text. Microorganism characteristics are discussed in subsequent sections of this chapter (see Microorganism-Mediated Antimicrobial Resistance). The environmental impact on antimicrobial activity is considered here, and its importance cannot be overstated.

**Environmentally mediated resistance** is defined as resistance directly resulting from physical or chemical characteristics of the environment that either directly alter the antimicrobial agent or alter the microorganism's normal physiologic response to the drug. Examples of environmental factors that mediate resistance include pH, anaerobic atmosphere, cation concentrations, and thymidine content.

Several antibiotics are affected by the pH of the environment. For instance, the antibacterial activities of erythromycin and aminoglycosides diminish with decreasing pH, whereas the activity of tetracycline decreases with increasing pH.

Aminoglycoside-mediated shutdown of bacterial protein synthesis requires intracellular uptake across the cell membrane. Most of the aminoglycoside uptake is driven through oxidative processes in the cell. In the absence of oxygen, uptake (and hence the activity of the aminoglycoside) is substantially diminished.

Aminoglycoside activity is also affected by the concentration of cations in the environment, such as calcium and magnesium (Ca++ and Mg++). This effect is most notable with *P. aeruginosa*. As shown in Figure 11-1, an important step in antimicrobial activity is the adsorption of the antibiotic to the bacterial cell surface. Aminoglycoside molecules have a net positive charge, and as is true for most gram-negative bacteria, the outer membrane of *P. aeruginosa* has a net negative charge. This electrostatic attraction facilitates attachment of the drug to the surface before internalization and subsequent inhibition of protein synthesis (Figure 11-7). However, calcium and magnesium cations compete with the aminoglycosides for negatively charged binding sites on the cell surface. If the positively charged calcium and magnesium ions outcompete aminoglycoside molecules for these sites,

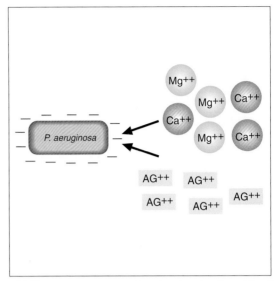

**Figure 11-7** Cations (Mg++ and Ca++) and aminoglycosides (AG++) compete for the negatively charged binding sites on the outer membrane surface of *Pseudomonas aeruginosa*. Such competition is an example of the impact that environmental factors (e.g., cation concentrations) can have on the antibacterial activity of aminoglycosides.

the amount of the drug taken up is decreased and antimicrobial activity is diminished. For this reason, aminoglycoside activity against *P. aeruginosa* tends to decrease as environmental cation concentrations increase.

The presence of certain metabolites or nutrients in the environment may also affect antimicrobial activity. For example, enterococci are able to use thymine and other exogenous folic acid metabolites to circumvent the activities of the sulfonamides and trimethoprim, which are folic acid pathway inhibitors (see Figure 11-6). In essence, if the environment supplies other metabolites for the microorganism, the activities of antibiotics that target pathways for producing those metabolites are greatly diminished, if not entirely lost. In the absence of the metabolites, full susceptibility to the antibiotics may be restored.

Information about environmentally mediated resistance is used to establish standardized testing methods that minimize the impact of environmental factors, allowing more accurate determination of microorganism-mediated resistance mechanisms (see the following discussion). It is important to note that in vitro, testing conditions are not established to recreate the in vivo physiology of infection, but rather are set to optimize detection of resistance expressed by microorganisms.

## MICROORGANISM-MEDIATED ANTIMICROBIAL RESISTANCE

**Microorganism-mediated resistance** refers to antimicrobial resistance that results from genetically encoded traits of the microorganism. Organism-based resistance can be divided into two subcategories, intrinsic or inherent resistance and acquired resistance.

**TABLE 11-3** Examples of Intrinsic Resistance to Antibacterial Agents

| Natural Resistance | Mechanism |
| --- | --- |
| Anaerobic bacteria versus aminoglycosides | Lack of oxidative metabolism to drive uptake of aminoglycosides |
| Gram-positive bacteria versus aztreonam (β-lactam) | Lack of penicillin-binding proteins (PBPs) that bind and are inhibited by this β-lactam antibiotic |
| Gram-negative bacteria versus vancomycin | Lack of uptake resulting from inability of vancomycin to penetrate outer membrane |
| *Pseudomonas aeruginosa* versus sulfonamides, trimethoprim, tetracycline, or chloramphenicol | Lack of uptake resulting from inability of antibiotics to achieve effective intracellular concentrations |
| *Klebsiella* spp. versus ampicillin (a β-lactam) targets | Production of enzymes (β-lactamases) that destroy ampicillin before the drug can reach the PBP |
| Aerobic bacteria versus metronidazole | Inability to anaerobically reduce drug to its active form |
| Enterococci versus aminoglycosides | Lack of sufficient oxidative metabolism to drive uptake of aminoglycosides |
| Enterococci versus all cephalosporin antibiotics | Lack of PBPs that effectively bind and are inhibited by these lactams |
| Lactobacilli and *Leuconostoc* sp. versus vancomycin | Lack of appropriate cell wall precursor target to allow vancomycin to bind and inhibit cell wall synthesis |
| *Stenotrophomonas maltophilia* versus imipenem (a beta-lactam) | Production of enzymes (β-lactamases) that destroy imipenem before the drug can reach the PBP targets |

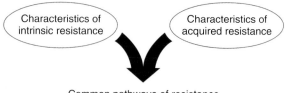

Common pathways of resistance

1. Enzymatic degradation or modification of the antimicrobial agent
2. Decreased uptake or accumulation of the antimicrobial agent
3. Altered antimicrobial target
4. Circumvention of the consequences of antimicrobial action
5. Uncoupling of antimicrobial agent-target interactions and subsequent effects on bacterial metabolism
6. Any combination of mechanisms 1 through 5

**Figure 11-8** Overview of common pathways bacteria use to effect antimicrobial resistance.

### Intrinsic Resistance

Antimicrobial resistance resulting from the normal genetic, structural, or physiologic state of a microorganism is referred to as **intrinsic resistance** (Table 11-3). Such resistance is considered a natural and consistently inherited characteristic associated with the vast majority of strains in a particular bacterial group, genus, or species. Therefore, this resistance pattern may be predictable, leading to identification of the organism. Intrinsic resistance profiles are useful for determining which antimicrobial agents should be included in the battery of drugs tested against specific types of organisms. For example, referring to the information given in Table 11-3, aztreonam would not be included in antibiotic batteries tested against gram-positive cocci. Similarly, vancomycin would not be routinely tested against gram-negative bacilli. As is discussed in Chapter 7, intrinsic resistance profiles are also useful markers to aid the identification of certain bacteria or bacterial groups.

### Acquired Resistance

Antibiotic resistance resulting from altered cellular physiology and structure caused by changes in a microorganism's genetic makeup is known as **acquired resistance.** Unlike intrinsic resistance, acquired resistance may be a trait associated with specific strains of a particular organism group or species. Therefore, the presence of this type of resistance in any clinical isolate is unpredictable. This unpredictability is the primary reason laboratory methods are necessary to detect resistance patterns in clinical isolates.

Because acquired resistance mechanisms are all genetically encoded, the methods for acquisition involve genetic change or exchange. Therefore, resistance may be acquired by:

- Successful genetic mutation
- Acquisition of genes from other organisms via gene transfer mechanisms
- A combination of mutational and gene transfer events

### COMMON PATHWAYS FOR ANTIMICROBIAL RESISTANCE

Whether resistance is intrinsic or acquired, bacteria share similar pathways or strategies to effect resistance to antimicrobial agents. Of the pathways listed in Figure 11-8, those that involve enzymatic destruction or alteration of the antibiotic, decreased intracellular uptake or accumulation of drug, and altered antibiotic target are the most common. One or more of these pathways may be expressed by a single cell successfully avoiding and protecting itself from the action of one or more antibiotics.

## Resistance to Beta-Lactam Antibiotics

As discussed earlier, bacterial resistance to beta-lactams may be mediated by enzymatic destruction of the antibiotics (β-lactamase); altered antibiotic targets, resulting in low affinity or decreased binding of antibiotic to the target PBPs; or decreased intracellular uptake or increased cellular efflux of the drug (Table 11-4). All three pathways play an important role in clinically relevant antibacterial resistance, but bacterial destruction of β-lactams through the production of β-lactamases is by far the most common method of resistance. Extended spectrum β-lactamases are derived from β-lactamases and confer resistance to both penicillins and cephalosporins; carbapenemases are active against carbapenem drugs, such as imipenem. β-lactamases open the drug's β-lactam ring, and the altered structure prevents subsequent effective binding to PBPs; consequently, cell wall synthesis is able to continue (Figure 11-9).

Staphylococci are the gram-positive bacteria that most commonly produce beta-lactamase; approximately 90% or more of clinical isolates are resistant to penicillin as a result of enzyme production. Rare isolates of enterococci also produce β-lactamase. Gram-negative bacteria, including Enterobacteriaceae, *P. aeruginosa*, and *Acinetobacter* spp., produce dozens of different β-lactamase types that mediate resistance to one or more of the β-lactam antibiotics.

Although the basic mechanism for β-lactamase activity shown in Figure 11-9 is the same for all types of these enzymes, there are distinct differences. For example, β-lactamases produced by gram-positive bacteria, such as staphylococci, are excreted into the surrounding environment, where the hydrolysis of β-lactams takes place before the drug can bind to PBPs in the cell membrane (Figure 11-10). In contrast, β-lactamases produced by gram-negative bacteria remain intracellular, in the periplasmic space, where they are strategically positioned to hydrolyze beta-lactams as they traverse the outer membrane through water-filled, protein-lined porin channels (see Figure 11-10). β-lactamases also vary in their spectrum of substrates; that is, not all β-lactams are susceptible to hydrolysis by every β-lactamase. For example, staphylococcal β-lactamase can readily hydrolyze penicillin and penicillin derivatives (e.g., ampicillin, mezlocillin, and piperacillin); however, it cannot effectively hydrolyze many cephalosporins or imipenem.

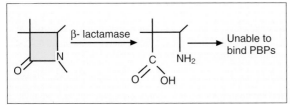

**Figure 11-9** Mode of β-lactamase enzyme activity. The enzyme cleaves the β-lactam ring, and the molecule can no longer bind to penicillin-binding proteins (PBPs) and is no longer able to inhibit cell wall synthesis. (Modified from Salyers AA, Whitt DD, editors: *Bacterial pathogenesis: a molecular approach,* Washington, DC, 1994, ASM Press.)

Various molecular alterations in the β-lactam structure have been developed to protect the β-lactam ring against enzymatic hydrolysis. This development has resulted in the production of more effective antibiotics in this class. For example, methicillin and the closely related agents oxacillin and nafcillin are molecular derivatives of penicillin that by the nature of their structure are not susceptible to staphylococcal β-lactamases. These agents are the mainstay of antistaphylococcal therapy. Similar strategies have been applied to develop penicillins and cephalosporins that are more resistant to the variety of β-lactamases produced by gram-negative bacilli. Even with this strategy, it is important to note that among common gram-negative bacilli (e.g., Enterobacteriaceae, *P. aeruginosa*, and *Acinetobacter* spp.), the list of molecular types and numbers of β-lactamases continues to emerge and diverge, thus challenging the effectiveness of currently available β-lactam agents.

Another therapeutic strategy has been to combine two different β-lactam moieties. One of the β-lactams (the β-lactamase inhibitor) has little or no antibacterial activity but avidly and irreversibly binds to the β-lactamase, rendering the enzyme incapable of hydrolysis; the second β-lactam, which is susceptible to β-lactamase activity, exerts its antibacterial activity. Examples of β-lactam/β-lactamase inhibitor combinations include ampicillin/sulbactam, amoxicillin/clavulanic acid, and piperacillin/tazobactam.

Altered targets also play a key role in clinically relevant β-lactam resistance (see Table 11-4). Through this pathway the organism changes, or acquires from another organism, genes that encode altered cell wall–synthesizing enzymes (i.e., PBPs). These "new" PBPs continue their function even in the presence of a β-lactam antibiotic, usually because the beta-lactam lacks sufficient affinity for the altered PBP. This is the mechanism by which staphylococci are resistant to methicillin and all other β-lactams (e.g., cephalosporins and imipenem). Methicillin-resistant *S. aureus* produces an altered PBP called *PBP2a*. PBP2a is encoded by the gene *mecA*. Because of the decreased binding between β-lactam agents and PBP2a, cell wall synthesis proceeds. Therefore, strains exhibiting this mechanism of resistance must be challenged with a non–β-lactam agent, such as vancomycin, another cell wall–active agent. Changes in PBPs are also responsible for ampicillin resistance in *Enterococcus faecium* and in the widespread β-lactam resistance observed in *S. pneumoniae* and viridans streptococci.

Because gram-positive bacteria do not have outer membranes through which β-lactams must pass before reaching their PBP targets, decreased uptake is not a pathway for β-lactam resistance among these bacteria. However, diminished uptake can contribute significantly to β-lactam resistance seen in gram-negative bacteria (see Figure 11-10). Changes in the number or characteristics of the outer membrane porins through which β-lactams pass contribute to absolute resistance (e.g., *P. aeruginosa* resistance to imipenem). Additionally, porin changes combined with the presence of certain β-lactamases in the periplasmic space may result in clinically relevant levels of resistance.

**TABLE 11-4** Summary of Resistance Mechanisms for Beta-Lactams, Vancomycin, Aminoglycosides, and Fluoroquinolones

| Antimicrobial Class | Resistance Pathway | Specific Mechanism | Examples |
|---|---|---|---|
| β-lactams (e.g., penicillin, ampicillin, mezlocillin, piperacillin, cefazolin, cefotetan, ceftriaxone, cefotaxime, ceftazidime, aztreonam, imipenem) | Enzymatic destruction | β-lactamase enzymes destroy β-lactam ring, thus antibiotic cannot bind to penicillin-binding protein (PBP) and interfere with cell wall synthesis (see Figure 11-9) | Staphylococcal resistance to penicillin; resistance of Enterobacteriaceae and *Pseudomonas aeruginosa* to several penicillins, cephalosporins, and aztreonam |
| | Altered target | Mutational changes in original PBPs or acquisition of different PBPs that do not bind β-lactams sufficiently to inhibit cell wall synthesis | Staphylococcal resistance to methicillin and other available β-lactams<br>Penicillin and cephalosporin resistance in *Streptococcus pneumoniae* and viridans streptococci |
| | Decreased uptake | Porin channels (through which β-lactams cross the outer membrane to reach PBPs of gram-negative bacteria) change in number or character so that β-lactam uptake is substantially diminished | *P. aeruginosa* resistance to imipenem |
| Glycopeptides (e.g., vancomycin) | Altered target | Alteration in the molecular structure of cell wall precursor components decreases binding of vancomycin so that cell wall synthesis is able to continue | Enterococcal and *Staphylococcus aureus* resistance to vancomycin |
| | Target overproduction | Excess peptidoglycan | Vancomycin-intermediate staphylococci |
| Aminoglycosides (e.g., gentamicin, tobramycin, amikacin, streptomycin, kanamycin) | Enzymatic modification | Modifying enzymes alter various sites on the aminoglycoside molecule so that the ability of drug to bind the ribosome and halt protein synthesis is greatly diminished or lost | Gram-positive and gram-negative resistance to aminoglycosides |
| | Decreased uptake | Porin channels (through which aminoglycosides cross the outer membrane to reach the ribosomes of gram-negative bacteria) change in number or character so that aminoglycoside uptake is substantially diminished | Aminoglycoside resistance in a variety of gram-negative bacteria |
| | Altered target | Mutational changes in ribosomal binding site diminish ability of aminoglycoside to bind sufficiently and halt protein synthesis | Enterococcal resistance to streptomycin (may also be mediated by enzymatic modifications) |
| Quinolones (e.g., ciprofloxacin, ofloxacin, levofloxacin, norfloxacin, lomefloxacin) | Decreased uptake | Alterations in the outer membrane diminish uptake of drug and/or activation of an "efflux" pump that removes quinolones before an intracellular concentration sufficient to inhibit DNA metabolism can be achieved | Gram-negative and staphylococcal (efflux mechanism only) resistance to various quinolones |
| | Altered target | Changes in the DNA gyrase subunits decrease ability of quinolones to bind this enzyme and interfere with DNA processes | Gram-negative and gram-positive resistance to various quinolones |
| Macrolides (e.g., erythromycin, azithromycin, clarithromycin) | Efflux | Pumps drug out of cell before target binding | Various streptococci and staphylococci |
| | Altered target | Enzymatic alteration of ribosomal target reduces drug binding | Various streptococci and staphylococci |

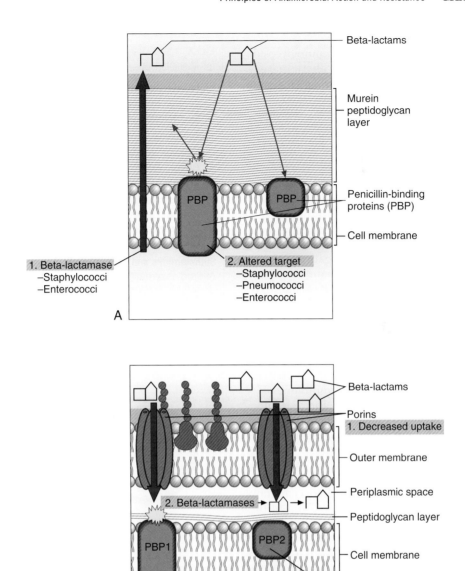

**Figure 11-10** Diagrammatic summary of β-lactam resistance mechanisms for gram-positive and gram-negative bacteria. **A,** Among gram-positive bacteria, resistance is mediated by β-lactamase production and altered PBP targets. **B,** In gram-negative bacteria, resistance can also be mediated by decreased uptake through the outer membrane porins.

## Resistance to Glycopeptides

To date, acquired, high-level resistance to vancomycin has been commonly encountered among enterococci, rarely among staphylococci, and not at all among streptococci. The mechanism involves the production of altered cell wall precursors unable to bind vancomycin with sufficient avidity to allow inhibition of peptidoglycan-synthesizing enzymes. The altered targets are readily incorporated into the cell wall, allowing synthesis to progress (see Table 11-4). A second mechanism of resistance to glycopeptides, described only among staphylococci to date, results in a lower level of resistance; this mechanism is thought to be mediated by overproduction of the peptidoglycan layer, resulting in excessive binding of the glycopeptide molecule and diminished ability of the drug to exert its antibacterial effect.

Because enterococci have high-level vancomycin resistance genes and also the ability to exchange genetic information, the potential for spread of vancomycin resistance to other gram-positive genera poses a serious threat to public health. In fact, the emergence of vancomycin-resistant *S. aureus* clinical isolates has been documented. In all instances the patients were previously infected or colonized with enterococci. Resistance to vancomycin by enzymatic modification or destruction has not been described.

## Resistance to Aminoglycosides

Analogous to beta-lactam resistance, aminoglycoside resistance is accomplished by enzymatic, altered target, or decreased uptake pathways (see Table 11-4). Gram-positive and gram-negative bacteria produce several different aminoglycoside-modifying enzymes. Three general types of enzymes catalyze one of the following modifications of an aminoglycoside molecule (see Figure 11-4):

- Phosphorylation of hydroxyl groups
- Adenylation of hydroxyl groups
- Acetylation of amine groups

Once an aminoglycoside has been modified, its affinity for binding to the 30S ribosomal subunit may be sufficiently diminished or totally lost, allowing protein synthesis to occur.

Aminoglycosides enter the gram-negative cell by passing through outer membrane porin channels. Therefore, porin alterations may also contribute to aminoglycoside resistance among these bacteria. Although some mutations that resulted in altered ribosomal targets have been described, this mechanism of resistance is rare in bacteria exposed to commonly used aminoglycosides.

## Resistance to Quinolones

Enzymatic degradation or alteration of quinolones has not been fully described as a key pathway for resistance. Resistance is most frequently mediated either by a decrease in uptake or in accumulation or by production of an altered target (see Table 11-4). Components of the gram-negative cellular envelope can limit quinolone access to the cell's interior location where DNA processing occurs. Other bacteria, notably staphylococci, exhibit a mechanism by which the drug is "pumped" out of the cell, thus keeping the intracellular quinolone concentration sufficiently low to allow DNA processing to continue relatively unaffected. This "efflux" process, therefore, is a pathway of diminished accumulation of drug rather than of diminished uptake.

The primary quinolone resistance pathway involves mutational changes in the targeted subunits of the DNA gyrase. With a sufficient number or substantial major changes in molecular structure, the gyrase no longer binds quinolones, so DNA processing is able to continue.

## Resistance to Other Antimicrobial Agents

Bacterial resistance mechanisms for other antimicrobial agents involve modifications or derivations of the recurring pathway strategies of enzymatic activity, altered target, or decreased uptake (Box 11-2).

# EMERGENCE AND DISSEMINATION OF ANTIMICROBIAL RESISTANCE

The resistance pathways that have been discussed are not necessarily new mechanisms that have recently evolved among bacteria. By definition, antibiotics originate from microorganisms. Therefore, antibiotic resistance mechanisms have always been part of the evolution of bacteria as a means of survival among antibiotic-producing competitors. However, with the introduction of antibiotics

---

**BOX 11-2** Bacterial Resistance Mechanisms for Miscellaneous Antimicrobial Agents

**Chloramphenicol**
Enzymatic modification (chloramphenicol acetyltransferase)
Decreased uptake

**Tetracyclines**
Diminished accumulation (efflux system)
Altered or protected ribosomal target
Enzymatic inactivation

**Macrolides (i.e., Erythromycin) and Clindamycin**
Altered ribosomal target
Diminished accumulation (efflux system)
Enzymatic modification

**Sulfonamides and Trimethoprim**
Altered enzymatic targets (dihydropteroate synthase and dihydrofolate reductase for sulfonamides and trimethoprim, respectively) that no longer bind the antibiotic

**Rifampin**
Altered enzyme (DNA-dependent RNA polymerase) target

---

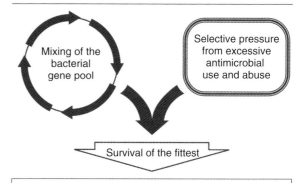

1. Emergence of "new" genes (e.g., methicillin-resistant staphylococci, vancomycin-resistant enterococci)

2. Spread of "old" genes to new hosts (e.g., penicillin-resistant *Neisseria gonorrhoeae*)

3. Mutations of "old" genes resulting in more potent resistance (e.g., beta-lactamase–mediated resistance to advanced cephalosporins in *Escherichia coli* and *Klebsiella* spp.)

4. Emergence of intrinsically resistant opportunistic bacteria (e.g., *Stenotrophomonas maltophilia*)

**Figure 11-11** Factors contributing to the emergence and dissemination of antimicrobial resistance among bacteria.

---

into medical practice, clinically relevant bacteria have adopted resistance mechanisms as part of their survival strategy. As a result of the increased use of antimicrobial agents, a survival of the fittest strategy has been documented as bacteria adapt to the pressures of antimicrobial attack (Figure 11-11).

All bacterial resistance strategies are encoded on one or more genes. These resistance genes are readily shared between strains of the same species, between species of different genera, and even between more distantly related bacteria. When a resistance mechanism arises, either by mutation or gene transfer, in a particular bacterial strain or species, it is possible for this mechanism to be passed on to other organisms using commonly described paths of genetic communication (see Figure 2-10). Therefore, resistance may spread to a wide variety of clinically relevant bacteria, and any single organism may acquire multiple genes and become resistant to the full spectrum of available antimicrobial agents. For example, strains of enterococci and *P. aeruginosa* already exist for which there are few effective therapeutic choices. Also, a gene encoding a single, very potent resistance mechanism may mediate multiple resistances. One such example is the *mecA* gene, which encodes staphylococcal resistance to methicillin and to all other beta-lactams currently available for use against these organisms; this leaves vancomycin as the only available and effective cell wall–inhibiting agent.

In summary, antibiotic use, coupled with the formidable repertoire bacteria have for thwarting antimicrobial activity and their ability to genetically share these strategies, drives the ongoing process of resistance emergence and dissemination (see Figure 11-11). This has been manifested by the emergence of new genes of unknown origin (e.g., methicillin-resistant staphylococci and vancomycin-resistant enterococci), the movement of old genes into new bacterial hosts (e.g., penicillin-resistant *N. gonorrhoeae* [PPNG]), mutations in familiar resistance genes that result in greater potency (e.g., beta-lactamase–mediated resistance to cephalosporins in *Escherichia coli*), and the emergence of new pathogens for which the most evident virulence factor is intrinsic or natural resistance to many of the antimicrobial agents used in the hospital setting (e.g., *Stenotrophomonas maltophilia*).

Because of the ongoing nature of the emergence and dissemination of resistance, reliable laboratory procedures to detect drug resistance serve as crucial aids to managing patients' infections and as a means of monitoring changing resistance trends among clinically relevant bacteria.

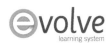

*Visit the Evolve site to complete the review questions.*

---

## CASE STUDY 11-1

A 40-year-old Michigan resident with diabetes, peripheral vascular disease, and chronic renal failure was receiving dialysis. The previous history was significant for multiple courses of antimicrobial therapy, including vancomycin, for the treatment of a chronic foot ulcer and methicillin-resistant *Staphylococcus aureus* (MRSA) bacteremia. In June 2002, a culture of the dialysis catheter site demonstrated growth of *S. aureus*. The isolate was resistant to oxacillin (minimum inhibitory concentration [MIC] greater than16 μg/mL) and vancomycin (MIC greater than 128 μg/mL). A subsequent culture from the chronic foot ulcer revealed vancomycin-resistant *S. aureus,* vancomycin-resistant *Enterococcus faecalis,* and *Klebsiella oxytoca.*

### QUESTIONS

1. Should the *S. aureus* isolate from the dialysis catheter site be reported as methicillin resistant?
2. What is the most likely mechanism by which the *S. aureus* isolate from the dialysis catheter site became resistant to vancomycin?

---

## BIBLIOGRAPHY

Higgins DL, Chang R, Debabov D et al: Telavancin: a multifunctional lipoglycopeptide, disrupts both cell wall synthesis and cell membrane integrity in methicillin-resistant staphylococcus aureus, *Antimicrob Agents Chemother* 49:1127, 2005.

Garau J: Other antimicrobials of interest in the era of extended-spectrum beta-lactamases: fosfomycin, nitrofurantoin and tigecycline, *Clin Microbiol Infect* 14:198, 2008.

Livermore DM: Linezolid in vitro: mechanism and antibacterial spectrum, *J Antimicrob Chemother* 51:ii9, 2003.

Mayers DL: *Antimicrobial drug resistance,* vol 1, New York NY, 2009, Springer.

Versalovic J: *Manual of clinical microbiology,* ed 10, Washington, DC, 2011, ASM Press.

Zhanel GG, Calic D, Schweizer F et al: New lipoglycopeptides: a comparative review of dalbavancin, oritavancin, and telavancin, *Drugs* 70:860, 2010.

## OBJECTIVES

1. List the relevant factors considered for control and standardization of antimicrobial susceptibility testing.
2. Describe testing conditions (medium, inoculum size, incubation conditions, incubation duration, controls, and purpose) for the broth dilution, agar dilution, and disk diffusion methods.
3. Define a McFarland standard and explain how it is used to standardize susceptibility testing.
4. Explain how end points are determined for the broth dilution, agar dilution, and disk diffusion methods.
5. Define the minimal inhibitory concentration (MIC) break point and identify the types of testing used to determine an MIC.
6. Define peak and trough levels and describe the clinical application for the data associated with each level.
7. Define the susceptible, intermediate, and resistant interpretive categories of antimicrobial susceptibility testing.
8. Outline the basic principles for agar screens, disk screens, and the "D" test for antimicrobial resistance detection, including method, application, and clinical utility.
9. Explain the principle and purpose of the chromogenic cephalosporinase test.
10. Compare and contrast molecular methods to detect resistance mechanisms versus traditional susceptibility testing, including clinical utility, effectiveness, and specificity.
11. Restate the principle of the minimal bactericidal concentration, time-kill assay, serum bactericidal test, and synergy test.
12. Define synergy and indifferent and antagonistic interactions in drug combinations.
13. Define and describe the purpose of drug susceptibility testing as it relates to the use of predictor drugs and organismal identification.
14. List the criteria for determining when to perform susceptibility testing.
15. Describe the purpose of reviewing susceptibility profiles and provide examples of profiles requiring further evaluation.

As discussed in Chapter 11, most clinically relevant bacteria are capable of acquiring and expressing resistance to antimicrobial agents commonly used to treat infections. Therefore, once an organism is isolated in the laboratory, characterization frequently includes tests to detect antimicrobial resistance. In addition to identifying the organism, the antimicrobial susceptibility profile often is a key component of the clinical laboratory report produced for the physician. The procedures used to produce antimicrobial susceptibility profiles and detect resistance to therapeutic agents are referred to as *antimicrobial susceptibility testing (AST) methods*. The methods applied for profiling aerobic and facultative anaerobic bacteria are the focus of this chapter; strategies for when and how these methods should be applied are also considered. Procedures for antimicrobial susceptibility testing of clinical isolates of

anaerobic bacteria and mycobacteria are discussed in Chapters 41 and 43, respectively.

## GOAL AND LIMITATIONS

The primary goal of antimicrobial susceptibility testing is to determine whether the bacterial isolate is capable of expressing resistance to the therapeutic antimicrobial agents selected for treatment. Because intrinsic resistance is usually known for most organisms, testing for instrinsic resistance usually is not necessary and organism identification is sufficient. In essence, antimicrobial susceptibility tests are assays designed to determine the extent of acquired resistance in any clinically important organism for which the antimicrobial susceptibility profile is unpredictable.

### STANDARDIZATION

For laboratory tests to accurately determine organism-based resistances, the potential influence of environmental factors on antibiotic activity should be minimized (see Chapter 11). This is not to suggest that environmental resistance does not play a clinically relevant role; however, the major focus of the in vitro tests is to measure an organism's expression of resistance. To control the impact of environmental factors, the conditions for susceptibility testing are extensively standardized. Standardization serves three important purposes:

- It optimizes bacterial growth conditions so that inhibition of growth can be attributed to the antimicrobial agent against which the organism is being tested and is not the result of limitations of nutrient, temperature, or other environmental conditions that may hinder the organism's growth.
- It optimizes conditions for maintaining antimicrobial integrity and activity; thus, failure to inhibit bacterial growth can be attributed to organism-associated resistance mechanisms rather than environmental drug inactivation.
- It maintains reproducibility and consistency in the resistance profile of an organism, regardless of the microbiology laboratory performing the test.

Standard conditions for antimicrobial susceptibility testing methods have been established based on numerous laboratory investigations. The procedures, guidelines, and recommendations are published in documents from the Subcommittee on Antimicrobial Susceptibility Testing of the Clinical and Laboratory Standards Institute (CLSI). The CLSI documents that describe various methods of antimicrobial susceptibility testing are continuously updated and may be obtained by contacting

CLSI, 940 W. Valley Road, Suite 1400, Wayne, Pennsylvania, 19087. **http://www.clsi.org**

The standardized components of antimicrobial susceptibility testing include:

- Bacterial inoculum size
- Growth medium (most frequently a Mueller-Hinton base)
  - pH
  - Cation concentration
  - Blood and serum supplements
  - Thymidine content
- Incubation atmosphere
- Incubation temperature
- Incubation duration
- Antimicrobial concentrations

## LIMITATIONS OF STANDARDIZATION

Although standardization of in vitro conditions is essential, the use of standard conditions imparts some limitations. Most notably, the laboratory test conditions cannot reproduce the in vivo environment at the infection site where the antimicrobial agent and bacteria will actually interact. Factors such as the bacterial inoculum size, pH, cation concentration, and oxygen tension can differ substantially, depending on the site of infection. Additionally, several other important factors play key roles in the patient outcome and are not taken into account by susceptibility testing. Some of these factors include:

- Antibiotic diffusion into tissues and host cells
- Serum protein binding of antimicrobial agents
- Drug interactions and interference
- Status of patient defense and immune systems
- Multiple simultaneous illnesses
- Virulence and pathogenicity of infecting bacterium
- Site and severity of infection

Despite these limitations, antimicrobial resistance can substantially alter the rates of morbidity and mortality in infected patients. Early and accurate recognition of resistant bacteria significantly aids the selection of antimicrobial therapy and optimal patient management. Thus, in vitro susceptibility testing provides valuable data that are used in conjunction with other diagnostic information to guide patient therapeutic options. Additionally, as discussed later in this chapter, in vitro susceptibility testing provides the data to track resistance trends among clinically relevant bacteria.

# TESTING METHODS

## PRINCIPLES

Three general methods are available to detect and evaluate antimicrobial susceptibility:

- Methods that directly measure the activity of one or more antimicrobial agents against a bacterial isolate
- Methods that directly detect the presence of a specific resistance mechanism in a bacterial isolate
- Special methods that measure complex antimicrobial-organism interactions

The method used depends on factors such as clinical need, accuracy, and convenience. Given the complexities of antimicrobial resistance patterns, a laboratory may commonly use methods from more than one category.

## METHODS THAT DIRECTLY MEASURE ANTIMICROBIAL ACTIVITY

Methods that directly measure antimicrobial activity involve bringing the antimicrobial agents of interest and the infecting bacterium together in the same in vitro environment to determine the impact of the drug's presence on bacterial growth or viability. The level of impact on bacterial growth is measured, and the organism's resistance or susceptibility to each agent is reported to the clinician. Direct measures of antimicrobial activity are accomplished using:

- Conventional susceptibility testing methods such as broth dilution, agar dilution, and disk diffusion
- Commercial susceptibility testing systems
- Special screens and indicator tests

### Conventional Testing Methods: General Considerations

Some general considerations apply to all three methods, including inoculum preparation and selection of antimicrobial agents.

**Inoculum Preparation.** Properly prepared inocula are the key to any antimicrobial susceptibility testing method. Inconsistencies in inoculum preparation may lead to inconsistencies and inaccuracies in susceptibility test results. The two important requirements for correct inoculum preparation are use of a pure culture and use of a standard-sized inoculum.

Interpretation of results obtained with a mixed culture is not reliable and can substantially delay reporting of results. Pure inocula are obtained by selecting four or five colonies of the same morphology, inoculating them into a broth medium, and allowing the culture to achieve active growth (i.e., midlogarithmic phase), as indicated by observable turbidity in the broth. For most organisms this requires 3 to 5 hours of incubation. Alternatively, four to five colonies 16 to 24 hours of age may be selected from an agar plate and suspended in broth or 0.9% saline solution to achieve a turbid suspension.

Use of a standard inoculum size is as important as culture purity and is accomplished by comparing the turbidity of the organism suspension with a turbidity standard. McFarland turbidity standards, prepared by mixing 1% sulfuric acid and 1.175% barium chloride to obtain a solution with a specific optical density, are commonly used. The 0.5 McFarland standard, which is commercially available, provides an optical density comparable to the density of a bacterial suspension of $1.5 \times 10^8$ colony forming units (CFU) per milliliter. Pure cultures are grown or are prepared directly from agar plates to match the turbidity of the 0.5 McFarland standard (Figure 12-1). The newly inoculated bacterial suspension and the McFarland standard are compared by examining turbidity against a dark background. Alternatively, any one of various commercially available instruments capable of measuring turbidity may be used to standardize the

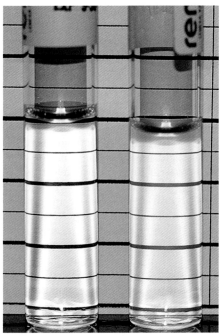

**Figure 12-1** Bacterial suspension prepared to match the turbidity of the 0.5 McFarland standard. Matching this turbidity provides a bacterial inoculum concentration of 1 to $2 \times 10^8$ CFU/mL. The McFarland standard on the right indicates the correct turbidity required for testing.

---

**BOX 12-1** Criteria for Antimicrobial Battery Content and Use

**Organism Identification or Group**
Antimicrobials to which the organism is intrinsically resistant are routinely excluded from the test battery (e.g., vancomycin versus gram-negative bacilli). Similarly, certain antimicrobials were developed specifically for use against particular organisms, but not against others (e.g., ceftazidime for use against *Pseudomonas aeruginosa* but not against *Staphylococcus aureus*); such agents should be included only in the appropriate battery.

**Acquired Resistance Patterns Common to Local Microbial Flora**
If resistance to a particular agent is common, the utility of the agent may be sufficiently limited and routine testing is not warranted. More potent antimicrobials are then included in the test battery. Conversely, more potent agents may not need to be in the test battery if susceptibility to less potent agents is highly prevalent.

**Antimicrobial Susceptibility Testing Method Used**
Depending on the testing method, some agents do not reliably detect resistance and should not be included in the battery.

**Site of Infection**
Some antimicrobial agents, such as nitrofurantoin, achieve effective levels only in the urinary tract and should not be included in batteries tested against bacterial isolates from other body sites (i.e., the agent must be able to achieve anatomic approximation; see Figure 11-1).

**Availability of Antimicrobial Agents in the Formulary**
Antimicrobial test batteries are selected for their ability to detect bacterial resistance to agents used by the medical staff and accessible in the pharmacy.

---

inoculum. If the bacterial suspension does not match the standard's turbidity, the suspension may be further diluted or supplemented with more organisms as needed.

**Selection of Antimicrobial Agents for Testing.** The antimicrobial agents chosen for testing against a particular bacterial isolate are referred to as the **antimicrobial battery** or **panel.** A laboratory may use different testing batteries, but the content and application of each battery are based on specific criteria. Although the criteria listed in Box 12-1 influence the selection of the panel's content, the final decision should not be made by the laboratory independently; input from the medical staff (particularly infectious diseases specialists) and the pharmacy is imperative.

CLSI publishes up-to-date tables listing potential antimicrobial agents recommended for inclusion in batteries for testing against specific organisms or organism groups. Two tables are of particular interest: Table 1, "Suggested Groupings of U.S. FDA–Approved Antimicrobial Agents That Should Be Considered for Routine Testing and Reporting on Nonfastidious Organisms by Clinical Microbiology Laboratories," and Table 1A, "Suggested Groupings of U.S. FDA–Approved Antimicrobial Agents That Should Be Considered for Routine Testing and Reporting on Fastidious Organisms by Clinical Microbiology Laboratories." Because revisions are made annually, laboratory protocols should be reviewed and modified accordingly (see the Bibliography). Further considerations about antibiotics that may be used for a specific organism or group are presented later in this chapter and in various chapters in Part III of this text.

Testing profiles are considered for each of the common organism groupings:
- Enterobacteriaceae
- *Pseudomonas aeruginosa* and *Acinetobacter* spp.
- *Staphylococcus* spp.
- *Enterococcus* spp.
- *Streptococcus* spp. (not including *S. pneumoniae*)
- *Streptococcus pneumoniae*
- *Haemophilus influenzae*
- *Neisseria gonorrhoeae*

## Conventional Testing Methods: Broth Dilution

Broth dilution testing involves challenging the organism of interest with antimicrobial agents in a liquid environment. Each antimicrobial agent is tested using a range of concentrations, commonly expressed as micrograms ($\mu$g) of active drug per milliliter (mL) of broth (i.e., $\mu$g/mL). The concentration range examined for a particular drug depends on specific criteria, including the safest therapeutic concentration possible in a patient's serum. Therefore, the concentration range examined often varies from one drug to the next, depending on the pharmacologic properties of the antimicrobial agent. Additionally, the concentration range may be based on the level of drug required to reliably detect a particular resistance mechanism. In this case, the test concentration for a drug may vary depending on the organism and its associated resistances. For example, to detect clinically

**TABLE 12-1** Summary of Broth Dilution Susceptibility Testing Conditions

| Organism Groups | Test Medium | Inoculum Size (CFU/mL) | Incubation Conditions | Incubation Duration |
|---|---|---|---|---|
| Enterobacteriaceae | Mueller-Hinton | $5 \times 10^5$ | 35°C; air | 16-20 hr |
| Staphylococci (to detect methicillin-resistant staphylococci) | Mueller-Hinton plus 2% NaCl | | 30°-35°C; air | 24 hr |
| *Streptococcus pneumoniae* and other streptococci | Mueller-Hinton plus 2%-5% lysed horse blood | $5 \times 10^5$ | 35°C; 5%-10% $CO_2$ | 20-24 hr |
| *Haemophilus influenzae* | *Haemophilus* test medium | $5 \times 10^5$ | 35°C; 5%-10% $CO_2$ | 20-24 hr |
| *Neisseria meningitidis* | Mueller-Hinton plus 2%-5% lysed horse blood | $5 \times 10^5$ | 35°C; 5%-7% carbon dioxide ($CO_2$) | 24 hr |

significant resistance to cefotaxime in *S. pneumoniae*, the dilution scheme uses a maximum concentration of 2 $\mu g$/mL; however, to detect cefotaxime resistance in *Escherichia coli*, the required maximum concentration is 16 $\mu g$/mL or higher.

Typically, the range of concentrations examined for each antibiotic is a series of doubling dilutions (e.g., 16, 8, 4, 2, 1, 0.5, 0.25 $\mu g$/mL); the lowest antimicrobial concentration that completely inhibits visible bacterial growth, as detected visually or with an automated or semiautomated method, is recorded as the **minimal inhibitory concentration (MIC)**.

**Procedures.** The key features of broth dilution testing procedures are shown in Table 12-1. Because changes are made in these procedural recommendations, the CLSI M07 series, "Methods for Dilution Antimicrobial Susceptibility Tests for Bacteria that Grow Aerobically," should be consulted annually.

***Medium and Antimicrobial Agents.*** With in vitro susceptibility testing methods, certain conditions must be altered when examining fastidious organisms to optimize growth and facilitate expression of bacterial resistance. For example, the Mueller-Hinton preparation is the standard medium used for most broth dilution testing, and conditions in the medium (e.g., pH, cation concentration, thymidine content) are well controlled by commercial manufacturers. However, media supplements or different media are required to obtain good growth and reliable susceptibility profiles for bacteria such as *S. pneumoniae* and *H. influenzae*. Although staphylococci are not considered fastidious organisms, media supplemented with sodium chloride (NaCl) enhance the expression and detection of methicillin-resistant isolates (see Table 12-1).

Broth dilution testing is divided into two general categories: microdilution and macrodilution. The principle of each test is the same; the only difference is the volume of broth in which the test is performed. For microdilution testing, the total broth volume is 0.05 to 0.1 mL; for macrodilution testing, the broth volumes are usually 1 mL or greater. Because most susceptibility test batteries require testing of several antibiotics at several different concentrations, the smaller volume used in microdilution allows this to be conveniently accomplished in a single microtiter tray (Figure 12-2).

The need for multiple large test tubes in the macrodilution method makes that technique substantially cumbersome and labor intensive when several bacterial isolates are tested simultaneously. For this reason, macrodilution is rarely used in most clinical laboratories, and subsequent comments about broth dilution focuses on the microdilution approach.

A key component of broth testing is proper preparation and dilution of the antimicrobial agents incorporated into the broth medium. Most laboratories that perform broth microdilution use commercially supplied microdilution panels in which the broth is already supplemented with appropriate antimicrobial concentrations. Therefore, antimicrobial preparation and dilution are not commonly carried out in most clinical laboratories (the details of this procedure are outlined in the CLSI M07-A6 document). In most instances, each antimicrobial agent is included in the microtiter trays as a series of doubling twofold dilutions. To ensure against loss of antibiotic potency, the antibiotic microdilution panels are stored at −20°C or lower, if possible, and are thawed immediately before use. Once thawed the panels should never be refrozen, which may result in substantial loss of antimicrobial action and potency. Alternatively, the antimicrobial agents may be lyophilized or freeze dried with the medium or drug in each well; upon inoculation with the bacterial suspension, the medium and drug are simultaneously reconstituted to the appropriate concentration.

***Inoculation and Incubation.*** Standardized bacterial suspensions that match the turbidity of the 0.5 McFarland standard (i.e., $1.5 \times 10^8$ CFU/mL) usually serve as the starting point for dilutions ultimately achieving the required final standard bacterial concentration of $5 \times 10^5$ CFU/mL in each microtiter well. It is essential to prepare the standard inoculum from a fresh, overnight, pure culture of the test organism. Inoculation of the microdilution panel is accomplished using manual or automated multiprong inoculators calibrated to deliver the precise volume of inoculum to each well in the panel simultaneously (see Figure 12-2).

Inoculated trays are incubated under optimal environmental conditions to optimize bacterial growth without interfering with the antimicrobial activity (i.e., avoiding environmentally mediated results). For the most

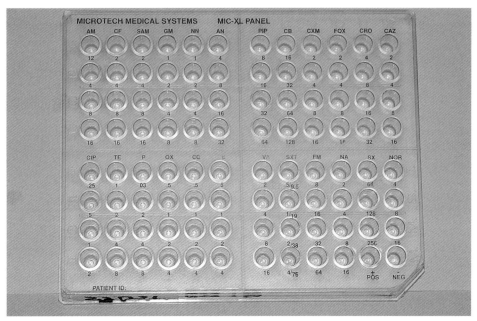

**Figure 12-2** Microtiter tray used for broth microdilution testing. Doubling dilutions of each antimicrobial agent in test broth occupies one vertical row of wells.

commonly tested bacteria (e.g., Enterobacteriaceae, *P. aeruginosa*, staphylococci, and enterococci), the environmental condition consists of room air at 35°C (see Table 12-1). Fastidious bacteria, such as *H. influenzae*, require incubation in 5% to 10% carbon dioxide ($CO_2$). Similarly, incubation durations for some organisms may need to be extended beyond the usual 16 to 20 hours (see Table 12-1). However, prolonged incubation times beyond recommended limits should be avoided, because antimicrobial deterioration may result in false or elevated resistance patterns. This is a primary factor that limits the ability to perform accurate testing with some slow-growing bacteria.

***Reading and Interpretation of Results.*** After incubation, the microdilution trays are examined for bacterial growth. Each tray should include a growth control that does not contain antimicrobial agent and a sterility control that was not inoculated. Once growth in the growth control and no growth in the sterility control wells have been confirmed, the growth profiles for each antimicrobial dilution can be established and the MIC determined. The detection of growth in microdilution wells is often augmented through the use of light boxes and reflecting mirrors. When a panel is placed in these devices, bacterial growth, manifested as light to heavy turbidity or a button of growth on the well bottom, is more reliably visualized (Figure 12-3).

When the dilution series for each antibiotic is inspected, the microdilution well containing the lowest drug concentration that completely inhibits visible bacterial growth is recorded as the MIC. Once the MICs for the antimicrobials in the test battery for an organism have been recorded, they are usually translated into one of the **interpretive categories,** specifically **susceptible, intermediate,** or **resistant** (Box 12-2). The interpretive criteria for these categories are based on extensive studies that correlate the MIC with serum-achievable levels for each antimicrobial agent, particular resistance mechanisms, and successful therapeutic outcomes. The interpretive criteria for an array of antimicrobial agents are published in the CLSI M07 series document, "Methods for Dilution Antimicrobial Susceptibility Tests for Bacteria that Grow Aerobically (M100 supplements)." For example, using these standards, an isolate of *P. aeruginosa* with an imipenem MIC of less than or equal to 4 $\mu$g/mL would be classified as susceptible; one with an MIC of 8 $\mu$g/mL would be classified as intermediate; and one with an MIC of 16 $\mu$g/mL or greater would be classified as resistant to imipenem.

After the MICs are determined and their respective and appropriate interpretive categories assigned, the laboratory may report the MIC, the category, or both. Because the MIC alone will not provide most physicians with a meaningful interpretation of data, either the category result with or without the MIC is usually reported.

In some settings, the full range of antimicrobial dilutions is not used; only the concentrations that separate the categories of susceptible, intermediate, and resistant are used. The specific concentrations that separate or define the different categories are known as **breakpoints,** and panels that only contain these antimicrobial concentrations are referred to as **breakpoint panels.** In this case, only category results are produced; precise MICs are not available, because the full range of dilutions is not tested.

***Advantages and Disadvantages.*** Broth dilution methods provide data for both quantitative results (i.e., MIC) and qualitative results (i.e., category interpretation). Whether this is an advantage is the subject of debate. On one hand, the MIC can be helpful in establishing the level of resistance of a particular bacterial strain and can substantially affect the decision to treat a

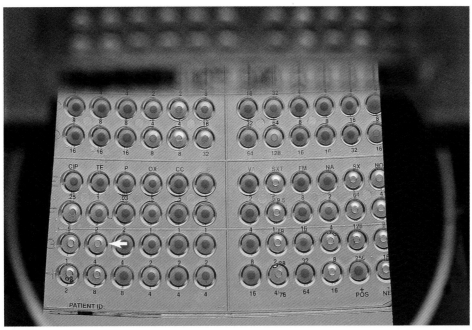

**Figure 12-3** Bacterial growth profiles in a broth microdilution tray. The wells containing the lowest concentration of an antibiotic that completely inhibits visible growth *(arrow)* are recorded in micrograms per milliliter (μg/mL) as the minimal inhibitory concentration (MIC).

**BOX 12-2** Definitions of Susceptibility Testing Interpretive Categories*

**Susceptible**
Indicates that the antimicrobial agent in question may be an appropriate choice for treating the infection caused by the organism. Bacterial resistance is absent or at a clinically insignificant level.

**Intermediate**
Indicates a number of possibilities, including:
- The potential utility of the antimicrobial agent in body sites where it may be concentrated (e.g., the urinary tract) or if high concentrations of the drug are used
- Possible effectiveness of the antimicrobial agent against the isolate, but possibly less so than against a susceptible isolate.
- Use as an interpretive safety margin to prevent relatively small changes in test results from leading to major swings in interpretive category (e.g., resistant to susceptible or vice versa)

**Resistant**
Indicates that the antimicrobial agent in question may not be an appropriate choice for treatment, either because the organism is not inhibited with serum-achievable levels of the drug or because the test result highly correlates with a resistance mechanism that indicates questionable successful treatment.

*Although these definitions are adapted from CLSI guideline M7-A3, Methods for Dilution Antimicrobial Susceptibility Tests for Bacteria that Grow Aerobically, they are commonly applied to results obtained by various susceptibility testing methods.

patient with a specific antimicrobial agent. For example, the penicillin MIC for *S. pneumoniae* may determine whether penicillin or alternative agents will be used to treat a patient with meningitis. On the other hand, for most antimicrobial susceptibility testing methods, a category report is sufficient and the actual MIC data are superfluous. This is one reason other methods (e.g., disk diffusion) that focus primarily on producing interpretive categories have been maintained among clinical microbiologists.

## Conventional Testing Methods: Agar Dilution

With agar dilution the antimicrobial concentrations and organisms to be tested are brought together on an agar-based medium rather than in liquid broth. Each doubling dilution of an antimicrobial agent is incorporated into a single agar plate; therefore, testing of a series of six dilutions of one drug requires the use of six plates, plus one positive growth control plate without antibiotic. The standard conditions and media for agar dilution testing are shown in Table 12-2. The surface of each plate is inoculated with $1 \times 10^4$ CFU (Figure 12-4). This method allows examination of one or more bacterial isolates per plate. After incubation the plates are examined for growth; the MIC is the lowest concentration of an antimicrobial agent in agar that completely inhibits visible growth. The same MIC breakpoints and interpretive categories used for broth dilution are applied for interpretation of agar dilution methods. Similarly, test results may be reported as the MICs only, the category only, or both.

The preparation of agar dilution plates (see CLSI M07-A6 series document, "Methods for Dilution Antimicrobial Susceptibility Tests for Bacteria That Grow

**TABLE 12-2** Summary of Agar Dilution Susceptibility Testing Conditions

| Organism Groups | Test Medium | Inoculum Size (CFU/spot) | Incubation Conditions | Incubation Duration |
|---|---|---|---|---|
| Enterobacteriaceae | Mueller-Hinton | $1 \times 10^4$ | 35°C; air | 16-20 hr |
| Enterococci | | | | |
| Staphylococci (to detect methicillin-resistant staphylococci) | Mueller-Hinton plus 2% NaCl | | 30°-35°C; air | 24 hr |
| *Neisseria meningitidis* | Mueller-Hinton plus 5% sheep blood | $1 \times 10^4$ | 35°C; 5%-7% carbon dioxide ($CO_2$) | 24 hr |
| *Streptococcus pneumoniae* | Agar dilution not recommended method for testing this organism | | | |
| Other streptococci | Mueller-Hinton plus 5% sheep blood | $1 \times 10^4$ | 35°C; air, $CO_2$ may be needed for some isolates | 20-24 hr |
| *Neisseria gonorrhoeae* | GC agar plus supplements | $1 \times 10^4$ | 35°C; 5%-X% $CO_2$ | 24 hr |

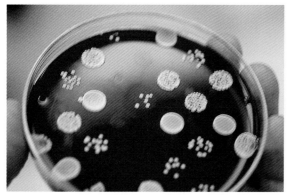

**Figure 12-4** Growth pattern on an agar dilution plate. Each plate contains a single concentration of antibiotic. Growth is indicated by a spot on the agar surface. No spot is seen for isolates inhibited by the concentration of antibiotic incorporated into the agar of that particular plate.

Aerobically") is sufficiently labor intensive to preclude the use of this method in most clinical laboratories in which multiple antimicrobial agents must be tested, even though several isolates may be tested per plate. As with broth dilution, the standard medium is the Mueller-Hinton preparation, but supplements and substitutions are made as needed to facilitate growth of more fastidious organisms. In fact, one advantage of this method is that it provides a means for determining MICs for *N. gonorrhoeae*, which does not grow sufficiently in broth to be tested by broth dilution methods.

## Conventional Testing Methods: Disk Diffusion

As more antimicrobial agents were created to treat bacterial infections, the limitations of the macrobroth dilution method became apparent. Before microdilution technology became widely available, it became clear that a more practical and convenient method of testing multiple

antimicrobial agents against bacterial strains was needed. Out of this need the disk diffusion test was developed, emerging from the landmark study by Bauer et al.[1] in 1966. These investigators standardized and correlated the use of antibiotic-impregnated filter paper disks (i.e., antibiotic disks) with MICs using many bacterial strains. With the disk diffusion susceptibility test, antimicrobial resistance is detected by challenging bacterial isolates with antibiotic disks placed on the surface of an agar plate that has been seeded with a lawn of bacteria (Figure 12-5).

When disks containing a known concentration of antimicrobial agent are placed on the surface of a freshly inoculated plate, the agent immediately begins to diffuse into the agar and establish a concentration gradient around the paper disk. The highest concentration is closest to the disk. Upon incubation, the bacteria grow on the surface of the plate except where the antibiotic concentration in the gradient around each disk is sufficiently high to inhibit growth. After incubation, the diameter of the zone of inhibition around each disk is measured in millimeters (see Figure 12-5).

To establish reference inhibitory zone–size breakpoints to define the susceptible, intermediate, and resistant categories for each antimicrobial agent/bacterial species combination, hundreds of strains are tested. The inhibition zone sizes obtained are then correlated with MICs obtained by broth or agar dilution, and a regression analysis is completed comparing the zone size in millimeters against the MIC (Figure 12-6). As the MICs of the bacterial strains tested increase (i.e., the more resistant bacterial strains), the corresponding inhibition zone sizes (i.e., diameters) decrease. Using Figure 12-6 to illustrate, horizontal lines are drawn from the MIC resistant breakpoint and the susceptible MIC breakpoint, 8 µg/mL and 2 µg/mL, respectively. Where the horizontal lines intersect the regression line, vertical lines are drawn to delineate the corresponding inhibitory zone size breakpoints (in millimeters). Using this approach,

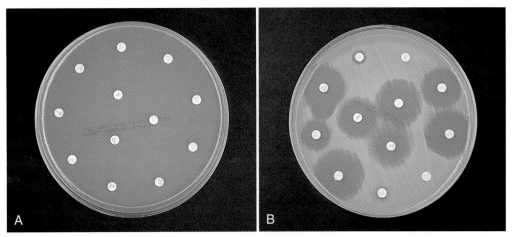

**Figure 12-5 A,** Disk diffusion method: antibiotic disks are placed on the agar surface just after inoculation of the surface with the test organism. **B,** Zones of growth inhibition around various disks are apparent after 16 to 18 hours of incubation.

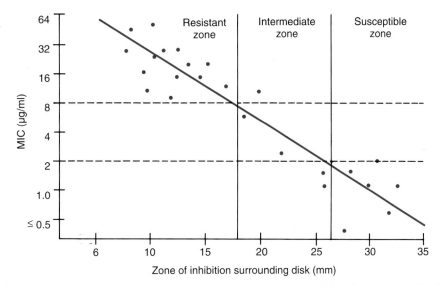

**Figure 12-6** Example of a regression analysis plot to establish zone-size breakpoints to define the categorical limits for susceptible, intermediate, and resistant for an antimicrobial agent. In this example, the maximum achievable serum concentration of the antibiotic is 8 $\mu$g/mL. Disk inhibition zones less than or equal to 18 mm in diameter indicate resistance; zones greater than or equal to 26 mm in diameter indicate susceptibility; the intermediate category is indicated by zones ranging from 19 to 25 mm in diameter.

zone size interpretive criteria have been established for most of the commonly tested antimicrobial agents and are published in the CLSI M02 series, "Performance Standards for Antimicrobial Disk Susceptibility Tests."

**Procedures.** The key features of disk diffusion testing procedures are summarized in Table 12-3, with more details and updates available through CLSI.

***Medium and Antimicrobial Agents.*** The Mueller-Hinton preparation is the standard agar-base medium used for testing of most bacterial organisms, although certain supplements and substitutions are required for testing of fastidious organisms. In addition to factors such as the pH and cation content, the depth of the agar medium can affect test accuracy and must be carefully controlled. Because antimicrobial agents diffuse in all

directions from the surface of the agar plate, the thickness of the agar affects the antimicrobial drug concentration gradient. If the agar is too thick, the antimicrobial agent diffuses down through the agar as well as outward, resulting in smaller zone sizes; if the agar is too thin, the inhibition zones are larger. For many laboratories that perform disk diffusion testing, commercial manufacturers are reliable sources for properly prepared and controlled Mueller-Hinton plates.

The appropriate concentration of drug for each disk is predetermined and set by the U.S. Food and Drug Administration (FDA). The disks are available from various commercial sources and should be stored at the recommended temperature in a desiccator until used. Inappropriate storage can lead to deterioration of the

**TABLE 12-3** Summary of Disk Diffusion Susceptibility Testing Conditions

| Organism Groups | Test Medium | Inoculum Size (CFU/mL) | Incubation Conditions | Incubation Duration |
|---|---|---|---|---|
| Enterobacteriaceae | Mueller-Hinton agar | Swab from $1.5 \times 10^8$ | 35°C; air | 16-18 hr |
| *Pseudomonas aeruginosa* | Mueller-Hinton agar | Swab from $1.5 \times 10^8$ suspension | 35°C; air | 16-18 hr |
| Enterococci | Mueller-Hinton agar | Swab from $1.5 \times 10^8$ suspension | 35°C; air | 16-18 hr (24 hr for vancomycin) |
| Staphylococci (to detect methicillin-resistant staphylococci) | Mueller-Hinton agar | Swab from $1.5 \times 10^8$ suspension | 30°-35°C; air | 24 hr |
| *Streptococcus pneumoniae* and other streptococci | Mueller-Hinton agar plus 5% sheep blood | Swab from $1.5 \times 10^8$ suspension | 35°C; 5%-7% carbon dioxide ($CO_2$) | 20-24 hr |
| *Haemophilus influenzae* | *Haemophilus* test medium | Swab from $1.5 \times 10^8$ suspension | 35°C; 5%-7% $CO_2$ | 16-18 hr |
| *Neisseria gonorrhoeae* | GC agar plus supplements | Swab from $1.5 \times 10^8$ suspension | 35°C; 5%-7% $CO_2$ | 20-24 hr |

antimicrobial agents and result in misleading zone size results.

To ensure equal diffusion of the drug into the agar, the disks must be placed flat on the surface and be firmly applied to ensure adhesion. This is most easily accomplished by using any one of several disk dispensers that are available through commercial disk manufacturers. With these dispensers, all disks in the test battery are simultaneously delivered to the inoculated agar surface and are adequately spaced to minimize the chances for inhibition zone overlap and significant interactions between antimicrobials. In most instances, a maximum of 12 antibiotic disks may be applied to the surface of a single 150-mm Mueller-Hinton agar plate (see Figure 12-5).

***Inoculation and Incubation.*** Before disk placement, the plate surface is inoculated using a swab that has been submerged in a bacterial suspension standardized to match the turbidity of the 0.5 McFarland turbidity standard, equivalent to $1.5 \times 10^8$ CFU/mL. The surface of the plate is swabbed in three directions to ensure even and complete distribution of the inoculum over the entire plate. Within 15 minutes of inoculation, the antimicrobial disks are applied and the plates are inverted for incubation to prevent the accumulation of moisture on the agar surface, which would interfere with the interpretation of test results.

Most organisms are incubated at 35°C in room air, but increased $CO_2$ is used for testing of specific fastidious bacteria (see Table 12-3). Similarly, the incubation time may be increased beyond 16 hours to enhance detection of certain resistance patterns (e.g., methicillin resistance in staphylococci and vancomycin resistance in enterococci) and to ensure accurate results in general for fastidious organisms such as *N. gonorrhoeae*.

The dynamics and timing of antimicrobial agent diffusion required for establishing a concentration gradient, in addition to growth of the organisms over 18 to 24 hours, are critical for reliable results. Therefore,

incubation of disk diffusion plates beyond the allotted time should be avoided, and disk diffusion generally is not an acceptable method for testing slow-growing organisms that require extended incubation such as mycobacteria and anaerobes.

***Reading and Interpretation of Results.*** Before results with individual antimicrobial agent disks are read, the plate is examined to confirm that a confluent lawn of growth has been obtained (see Figure 12-5). If growth between inhibitory zones around each disk is poor and nonconfluent, the test should not be interpreted and should be repeated. The lack of confluent growth may be due to insufficient inoculum. Alternatively, a particular isolate may have undergone mutation, and growth factors supplied by the standard medium are no longer sufficient to support robust growth. In the latter case, medium supplemented with blood and/or incubation in $CO_2$ may enhance growth. However, caution in interpreting results is required when extraordinary measures are used to obtain good growth and the standard medium recommended for testing a particular type of organism is not used. Plates should also be examined for purity. Mixed cultures are evident through the appearance of different colony morphologies scattered throughout the lawn of bacteria (Figure 12-7). Mixed cultures require purification and repeat testing.

A dark background and reflected light are used to examine a disk diffusion plate (Figure 12-8). The plate is situated so that a ruler or caliper can be used to measure the inhibition zone diameters for each antimicrobial agent. Certain motile organisms, such as *Proteus* spp., may swarm over the surface of the plate and complicate clear interpretation of the zone boundaries. In these cases, the swarming haze is ignored and zones are measured at the point where growth is obviously inhibited. Similarly, hazes of bacterial growth may be observed when testing sulfonamides and trimethoprim as a result of the organism population going through several doubling generations before inhibition; the resulting haze of

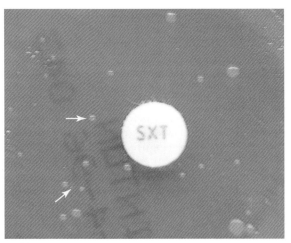

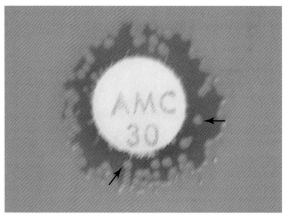

**Figure 12-7** Disk diffusion plate inoculated with a mixed culture, as evidenced by the various colonial morphologies *(arrows)* appearing throughout the lawn of growth.

**Figure 12-9** Bacterial growth is visible inside the zone of inhibition *(arrows)*. This may indicate inoculation with a mixed culture. However, emergence of resistant mutants of the test isolate is a more likely reason for this growth pattern.

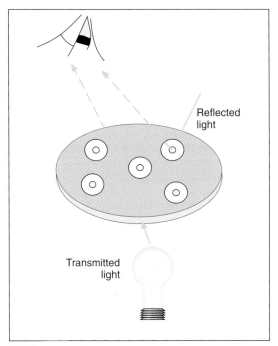

**Figure 12-8** Examination of a disk diffusion plate by transmitted and reflected light.

growth should be ignored for disk interpretation with these agents.

In instances not involving swarming organisms or the testing of sulfonamides and trimethoprim, hazes of growth that occur in more obvious inhibition zones should not be ignored. In many instances, this is the only way clinically relevant resistance patterns are manifested by certain bacterial isolates when tested using the disk diffusion method. Key examples in which this may occur include cephalosporin resistance among several species of Enterobacteriaceae, methicillin resistance in staphylococci, and vancomycin resistance in some enterococci. In fact, the haze produced by some staphylococci and

enterococci can best be detected using transmitted rather than reflected light. In these cases, the disk diffusion plates are held in front of the light source when methicillin and vancomycin inhibition zones are read (see Figure 12-8). Still other significant resistances may be subtly evident and appear as individual colonies in an obvious zone of inhibition (Figure 12-9). When such colonies are seen, purity of the test isolate must be confirmed. If purity is confirmed, the individual colonies are variants or resistant mutants of the same species, and the test isolate should be considered resistant.

Once zone sizes have been recorded, interpretive categories are assigned. Interpretive criteria for antimicrobial agent/organism combinations that may be tested by disk diffusion are provided in the CLSI-M2 series, "Performance Standards for Antimicrobial Disk Susceptibility Tests (M100 supplements)." The definitions of susceptible, intermediate, and resistant are the same as those used for dilution methods (see Box 12-2). For example, using the CLSI interpretive standards, an *E. coli* isolate that produces an ampicillin inhibition zone diameter of 13 mm or less is classified as resistant; if the zone is 14 to 16 mm, the isolate is considered intermediate to ampicillin; if the zone is 17 mm or greater, the organism is categorized as susceptible.

Unlike MICs, inhibition zone sizes are used to produce a category interpretation and have no clinical utility. Therefore, when testing is performed by disk diffusion, only the category interpretation of susceptible, intermediate, or resistant is reported.

***Advantages and Disadvantages.*** Two important advantages of the disk diffusion test are convenience and user friendliness. Up to 12 antimicrobial agents can be tested against one bacterial isolate with minimal use of extra materials and devices. Because the results are generally accurate and commonly encountered bacteria are reliably tested, the disk diffusion technique is still among the most frequently used methods for antimicrobial susceptibility testing. The major disadvantages of this method are the lack of interpretive criteria for organisms not included in Table 12-3 and the inability to provide more precise data about the level of an organism's resistance or susceptibility, as can be obtained using MIC methods.

## Commercial Susceptibility Testing Systems

The variety and widespread use of commercial susceptibility testing methods reflect the key role resistance detection plays in the responsibilities of clinical microbiology laboratories. In many instances, the commercial methods are variations of the conventional dilution or disk diffusion methods, and their accuracies have been evaluated by comparison of results with those obtained by conventional methods. Additionally, many of the media and environmental conditions standardized for conventional methods are maintained with the use of commercial systems. The goal of detecting resistance is the same for all commercial methods, but the principles and practices vary with respect to:

- Format in which bacteria and antimicrobial agents are brought together
- Extent of automation for inoculation, incubation, interpretation, and reporting
- Method used for detection of bacterial growth inhibition
- Speed with which results are produced
- Accuracy

Accuracy is an extremely important aspect of any susceptibility testing system and is addressed in more detail later in this chapter.

**Broth Microdilution Methods.** Several systems have been developed that provide microdilution panels already prepared and formatted according to the guidelines for conventional broth microdilution methods (e.g., BBL Sceptor, BD Microbiology Systems, Cockeysville, Maryland; Sensititre, Trek Diagnostics Systems, Inc., Westlake, Ohio; MicroScan touch SCAN-SR, Dade Behring, Inc., West Sacramento, California). These systems enable laboratories to perform broth microdilution without having to prepare their own panels.

The systems may differ to some extent regarding the volume in the test wells, how inocula are prepared and added, the availability of different supplements for the testing of fastidious bacteria, the types of antimicrobial agents and dilution schemes, and the format of medium and antimicrobial agents (e.g., dry-lyophilized or frozen). Furthermore, the degree of automation for inoculation of the panels and the devices available for reading results vary among the different products. In general, these commercial panels are designed to receive the standard inoculum and are incubated using conditions and durations recommended for conventional broth microdilution. They are growth-based systems that require overnight incubation, and CLSI interpretive criteria apply for interpretation of most results. Reading of these panels is frequently augmented by the availability of semiautomated reading devices.

**Agar Dilution Derivations.** One commercial system (Spiral Biotech Inc., Bethesda, Maryland) uses an instrument to apply antimicrobial agent to the surface of an already prepared agar plate in a concentric spiral fashion. Starting in the center of the plate, the instrument deposits the highest concentration of antibiotic and from that point drug application proceeds to the periphery of the plate. Diffusion of the drug in the agar establishes a concentration gradient from high (center of plate) to low (periphery of plate). Starting at the periphery of the plate, bacterial inocula are applied as a single streak perpendicular to the established gradient in a spoke-wheel fashion. After incubation, the distance is measured between the point where growth is noted at the edge of the plate to the point where growth is inhibited toward the center of the plate (Figure 12-10). This value is used to calculate the MIC for the antimicrobial agent against each of the bacterial isolates on the plate.

**Diffusion in Agar Derivations.** One test has been developed that combines the convenience of disk diffusion with the ability to generate MIC data. The Etest (bioMérieux, Durham, North Carolina) uses plastic strips; one side of the strip contains the antimicrobial agent concentration gradient, and the other contains a numeric scale that indicates the drug concentration (Figure 12-11). Mueller-Hinton plates are inoculated as for disk diffusion, and the strips are placed on the inoculum lawn. Several strips may be placed radially on the same plate so that multiple antimicrobials may be tested against a single isolate. After overnight incubation, the plate is examined and the number present at the point where the border of growth inhibition intersects the E-strip is taken as the MIC (Figure 12-11). The same MIC interpretive criteria used for dilution methods, as provided in CLSI guidelines, are used with the Etest value to assign an interpretive category of susceptible, intermediate, or resistant. This method provides a means of producing MIC data in situations in which the level of resistance can be clinically relevant (e.g., penicillin or cephalosporins against *S. pneumoniae*).

Another method (BIOMIC, Giles Scientific, Inc., New York, New York) combines the use of conventional disk diffusion methodology with video digital analysis to automate interpretation of inhibition zone sizes. Automated zone readings and interpretations are combined with computer software to produce MIC values and to allow for data manipulations and evaluations for detecting unusual resistance profiles and producing antibiogram reports.

**Automated Antimicrobial Susceptibility Test Systems.** The automated antimicrobial susceptibility test systems available for use in the United States include the Vitek Legacy and Vitek 2 systems (bioMérieux, Inc., Durham, North Carolina), the MicroScan WalkAway system (Dade International, Sacramento, California), and the Phoenix system (BD Microbiology Systems, Cockeysville, Maryland). These different systems vary with respect to the extent of automation of inoculum preparation and inoculation, the methods used to detect growth, and the algorithms used to interpret and assign MIC values and categorical findings (i.e., susceptible, intermediate, resistant).

For example, the Vitek 2 AST inoculum is automatically introduced by a filling tube into a miniaturized, plastic, 64-well, closed card containing specified concentrations of antibiotics (Figure 12-12). Cards are incubated in a temperature-controlled compartment. Optical readings are performed every 15 minutes to measure

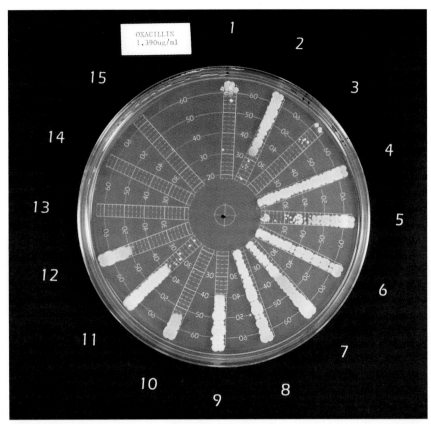

**Figure 12-10** Growth patterns on a plate containing an antibiotic gradient (the concentration decreases from the center of the plate to the periphery) applied by the Spiral Gradient instrument. The distance from the point where growth is noted at the edge of the plate to the point where growth is inhibited toward the center of the plate is measured. This value is used in a formula to calculate the MIC of the antimicrobial agent against each of the bacterial isolates streaked on the plate. (Courtesy Spiral Biotech, Inc., Bethesda, Md.)

the amount of light transmitted through each well, including a growth control well. Algorithmic analysis of the growth kinetics in each well is performed by the system's software to derive the MIC data. The MIC results are validated with the Advanced Expert System (AES) software, a category interpretation is assigned, and the organism's antimicrobial resistance patterns are reported. Resistance detection is enhanced with the sophisticated AES software, which can recognize and report resistance patterns using MICs. In summary, this system facilitates standardized susceptibility testing in a closed environment with validated results and recognition of an organism's antimicrobial resistance mechanism in 6 to 8 hours for most clinically relevant bacteria (Figure 12-13).

The MicroScan WalkAway system uses the broth microdilution panel format manually inoculated with a multiprong device. Inoculated panels are placed in an incubator-reader unit, where they are incubated for the required time and then the growth patterns are automatically read and interpreted. Depending on the microdilution tray used, bacterial growth may be detected using spectrophotometry or fluorometry (Figure 12-14).

Spectrophotometric analyzed panels require overnight incubation, and the growth patterns may be read manually as described for routine microdilution testing. Fluorometric analysis is based on the degradation of fluorogenic substrates by viable bacteria. The fluorogenic approach can provide susceptibility results in 3.5 to 5.5 hours. Either full dilution schemes or breakpoint panels are available. In addition to speed and facilitation of workflow, the automated systems provide increasingly powerful computer-based data management that can be used to evaluate the accuracy of results, manage larger databases, and interface with the pharmacy to improve and advance the utility of antimicrobial susceptibility testing data.

The Phoenix system provides a convenient, albeit manual, gravity-based inoculation process. Growth is monitored in an automated fashion based on a redox indicator system with results available in 8 to 12 hours. Supplemental testing (e.g., confirmatory extended spectrum beta-lactamase [ESBL] test for *E. coli*) is included in each panel, reducing the need for additional or repeat testing. Interpretation of results is augmented by a rules-based data management expert system.

## Alternative Approaches for Enhancing Resistance Detection

Although the various conventional and commercial antimicrobial susceptibility test methods provide accurate results in most cases, certain clinically relevant resistance mechanisms can be difficult to detect. In these instances supplemental tests and alternative approaches are

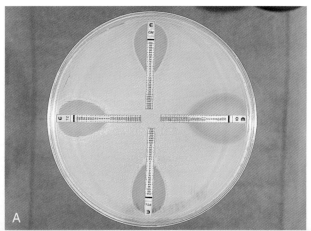

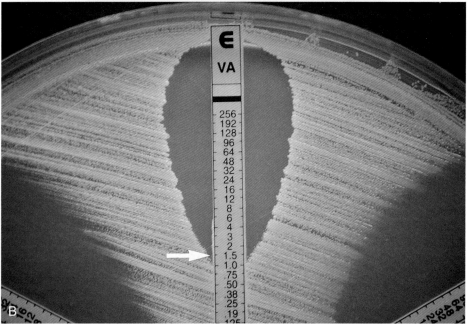

**Figure 12-11** The Etest® strip uses the principle of a predefined antibiotic gradient on a plastic strip to generate an MIC value. It is processed in the same way as the disk diffusion. **A,** Individual antibiotic strips are placed on an inoculated agar surface. **B,** After incubation, the MIC is read where the growth/inhibition edge intersects the strip graduated with an MIC scale across 15 dilutions (arrow). Several antibiotic strips can be tested on a plate. (Courtesy bioMérieux*, Marcy l'Etoile, France.)

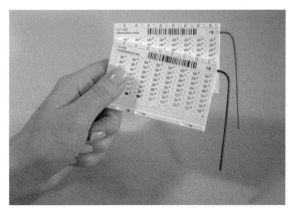

**Figure 12-12** The VITEK® 2 antimicrobial susceptibility test card contains 64 wells with multiple concentrations of up to 22 antibiotics. The antibiotic is rehydrated when the organism suspension is introduced into the card during the automated filling process. (Courtesy bioMérieux*, Marcy l'Etoile, France.)

needed to ensure reliable detection of resistance. Also, as new and clinically important resistance mechanisms emerge and are recognized, a "lag time" will occur, during which conventional and commercial methods are being developed to ensure accurate detection of new resistance patterns. During such lag periods, special tests may be used until more conventional or commercial methods become available. Key examples of such alternative approaches are discussed in this section.

**Supplemental Testing Methods.** Table 12-4 highlights some of the features of supplemental tests that may be used to enhance resistance detection. For certain strains of staphylococci, conventional and commercial systems may have difficulty detecting resistance to oxacillin and

---

*2013/Photos: bioMérieux/ BIOMERIEUX, the blue logo, Etest, Testremsa, VITEK are registered trademarks belonging to bioMérieux or one of its subsidiaries or one of its companies.

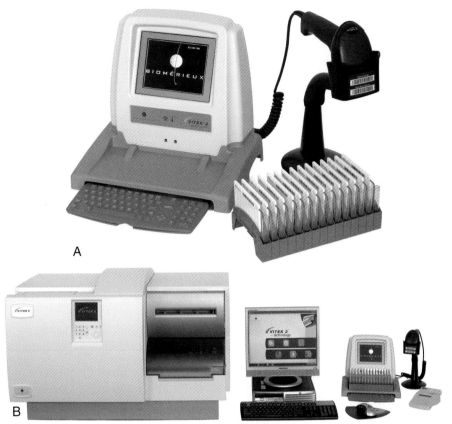

**Figure 12-13** The components of the VITEK® 2 system consist of the instrument housing; the sample processing and reader/incubator; the computer workstation, which provides data analysis, storage, and epidemiology reports; the Smart Carrier Station, which is the direct interface between the microbiologist on the bench and the instrument; and a bar code scanner to facilitate data entry. (Courtesy bioMérieux*, Marcy l'Etoile, France.)

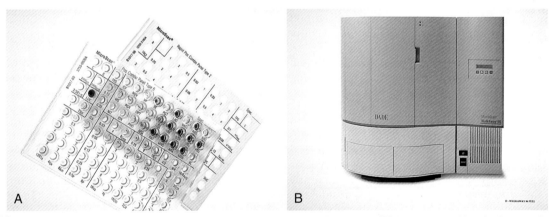

**Figure 12-14** Microdilution tray format **(A)** used with the MicroScan WalkAway instrument **(B)** for automated incubation, reading, and interpretation of antimicrobial susceptibility tests. (Courtesy Dade International, Sacramento, Calif.)

the related drugs methicillin and nafcillin. The oxacillin agar screen provides a backup test that may be used when other methods provide equivocal or uncertain profiles. Growth on the screen correlates highly with the presence of oxacillin (or methicillin) resistance, and no growth is strong evidence that an isolate is susceptible. This is an

*2013/Photos: bioMérieux/ BIOMERIEUX, the blue logo, Etest, Testremsa, VITEK are registered trademarks belonging to bioMérieux or one of its subsidiaries or one of its companies.

important determination; strains that are classified as resistant are considered resistant to all other currently available beta-lactam antibiotics, indicating the need for therapy to include the use of vancomycin. The agar screen plates can be made in-house, and are available commercially (e.g., Remel, Lenexa, Kansas; BBL, Cockeysville, Maryland). Additionally, other commercial tests designed to detect oxacillin resistance more rapidly (i.e., 4 hours) have been developed and may provide another approach to supplemental testing (e.g., Crystal MRSA ID System, BBL, Cockeysville, Maryland). In addition to the

**TABLE 12-4** Supplemental Methods for Detection of Antimicrobial Resistance

| Test | Purpose | Conditions | Interpretation |
|------|---------|-----------|----------------|
| Oxacillin agar screen | Detection of staphylococcal resistance to penicillinase-resistant penicillins (e.g., oxacillin, methicillin, or nafcillin) | Medium: Mueller-Hinton agar plus 6 $\mu$g oxacillin/mL plus 4% NaCl<br>Inoculum: Swab or spot from $1.5 \times 10^8$ standard suspension<br>Incubation: 30°-35°C 24 hr, up to 48 hr for non–*Staphylococcus aureus* | Growth = Resistance<br>No growth = Susceptible |
| Vancomycin agar screen | Detection of enterococcal resistance to vancomycin | Medium: Brain-heart infusion agar plus 6 $\mu$g vancomycin/mL Inoculum: Spot of $10^5$-$10^6$ CFU<br>Incubation: 35°C, 24 hr | Growth = Resistance<br>No growth = Susceptible |
| Aminoglycoside screens | Detection of acquired enterococcal high-level resistance to aminoglycosides that would compromise synergy with a cell wall–active agent (e.g., ampicillin or vancomycin) | Medium: Brain-heart infusion broth: 500 $\mu$g/mL gentamicin; 1000 $\mu$g/mL streptomycin Agar: 500 $\mu$g/mL gentamicin; 2000 $\mu$g/mL streptomycin<br>Inoculum: Broth; $5 \times 10^5$ CFU/mL agar; $10^6$ CFU/spot<br>Incubation: 35°C, 24 hr; 48 hr for streptomycin, only if no growth at 24 hr | Growth = Resistance<br>No growth = Susceptible |
| Oxacillin disk screen | Detection of *Streptococcus pneumoniae* resistance to penicillin | Medium: Mueller-Hinton agar plus 5% sheep blood plus 1 $\mu$g oxacillin disk<br>Inoculum: as for disk diffusion<br>Incubation: 5%-7% $CO_2$ 35° C; 20-24 hr | Inhibition zone $\leq$20 mm: penicillin susceptible Inhibition zone <20 mm: penicillin resistant, intermediate, or susceptible; further testing by MIC method is needed |
| D test | Differentiate clindamycin resistance among *S. aureus* resulting from efflux (*msrA* gene or MLSB resistance) | Approximation of clindamycin and erythromycin disk to look for blunting of clindamycin zone | Blunting of clindamycin zone to give "D" pattern, indicating inducible clindamycin resistance |

*CFU,* Colony forming units; *MIC,* minimum inhibitory concentration; *MLSB,* macrolide-lincosamide-streptogramin-B.

agar screen, 30-$\mu$g cefoxitin disks have been developed for disk diffusion to improve the detection of oxacillin-resistant staphylococci (CLSI M100-22). According to this method, cefoxitin inhibitory zones less than or equal to 24 mm indicate oxacillin resistance in staphylococci. The cefoxitin disk test is especially helpful in detecting oxacillin resistance in coagulase-negative staphylococci.

Similarly, reduced staphylococcal susceptibility to vancomycin (i.e., MICs from 4 to 16 $\mu$g/mL) can be difficult to detect by disk diffusion and some commercial methods. Although the therapeutic relevance of staphylococci with vancomycin MICs in this range is currently uncertain, the diminished susceptibility is outside the normal MIC range for susceptible strains; therefore, this phenotype needs to be detected. The agar screen used for this purpose is outlined in Table 12-4 and is essentially the same as that outlined for enterococci, also in Table 12-4. Strains that grow on the screen should be tested by broth microdilution to obtain a definitive MIC value.

Similarly, detection of enterococcal resistance to vancomycin can be difficult by some conventional and commercial methods, and the agar screen may be helpful in confirming the resistance pattern (see Table 12-4). However, as a screen, not all enterococcal isolates capable of growth are resistant to vancomycin at clinically relevant levels. Therefore, strains detected using this method should also be characterized using a broth microdilution method to determine the isolate's MIC.

Aminoglycosides also play a key role in therapy for serious enterococcal infections, and acquired high-level resistance, which essentially destroys the therapeutic value of these drugs for combination therapy with ampicillin or vancomycin, is not readily detected by conventional methods. Therefore, screens using high concentrations of aminoglycosides (see Table 12-4) have been developed and are available commercially (e.g., Remel, Lenexa, Kansas; or BBL, Cockeysville, Maryland).

With the emergence of penicillin resistance in *S. pneumoniae*, the penicillin disk diffusion test became insufficiently sensitive to detect subtle but significant changes in susceptibility to penicillin. To address this issue, the oxacillin disk screen described in Table 12-4 is useful but has a notable limitation. Although organisms identified with zones greater than or equal to 20 mm can be accurately characterized as penicillin susceptible, the penicillin susceptibility status of those with zones less than 20 mm remains uncertain, and an MIC value must be determined through an additional test.

With regard to macrolide (e.g., erythromycin, azithromycin, clarithromycin) and lincosamide (e.g., clindamycin) resistance among staphylococci, interpretation of in vitro results can also be complicated by the different underlying mechanisms of resistance that have very different therapeutic implications. Isolates that produce a profile of resistance to a macrolide (e.g., erythromycin) and susceptibility to clindamycin may do so as a result of two different resistance mechanisms. If this profile is the result of the efflux (*msrA* gene) mechanism, the isolate can be considered susceptible to clindamycin. However, if this profile resulted from the inducible macrolide-lincosamide-streptogramin-B (MLSB) mechanism, which results in an altered ribosomal target, clindamycin-resistant mutants may readily arise during therapy with this agent. Currently such strains should be reported as resistant to clindamycin. The D test that is used to distinguish between these two different resistance mechanisms is outlined in Table 12-4.

Undoubtedly, as complicated resistance mechanisms requiring laboratory detection continue to emerge, screening and supplemental testing methods will continue to be developed. Some of these will be maintained as the primary method for detecting a particular resistance mechanism, whereas others may tend to fade away as adjustments in conventional and commercial procedures enhance resistance detection and preclude the need for a supplemental test.

**Predictor Antimicrobial Agents.** Another approach that may be used to ensure accuracy in resistance detection is the use of "predictor" antimicrobial agents in the test batteries. The basic premise of this approach is to use antimicrobial agents (**predictor drugs**) that are the most sensitive indicators of certain resistance mechanisms. The profile obtained with such a battery is used to deduce the underlying resistance mechanism. A susceptibility report then is produced based on the likely effect the resistance mechanisms would have on the antimicrobials being considered for therapeutic use. The use of predictor drugs is not a new concept, and this approach has been taken in a number of cases, such as the following:

- Staphylococcal resistance to oxacillin is used to determine and report resistance to all currently available beta-lactams, including penicillins, cephalosporins, and carbapenems.
- Enterococcal high-level gentamicin resistance predicts resistance to nearly all other currently available aminoglycosides, including amikacin, tobramycin, netilmicin, and kanamycin.
- Enterococcal resistance to ampicillin predicts resistance to all penicillin derivatives.

## METHODS THAT DIRECTLY DETECT SPECIFIC RESISTANCE MECHANISMS

As an alternative to detecting resistance by measuring the effect of antimicrobial presence on bacterial growth, some strategies focus on assaying for the presence of a particular mechanism. When the presence or absence of the mechanism is established, the resistance profile of the organism can be generated without having to test several different antimicrobial agents. The utility of this approach, which can involve phenotypic and genotypic methods, depends on the presence of a particular resistance mechanism as being a sensitive and specific indicator of clinical resistance.

### Phenotypic Methods

The most common phenotypic-based assays test for the presence of β-lactamase enzymes in the clinical bacterial

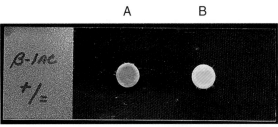

**Figure 12-15** The chromogenic cephalosporin test allows direct detection of β-lactamase production. When the β-lactam ring of the cephalosporin substrate in the disk is hydrolyzed by the bacterial inoculum, a deep pink color is produced **(A)**. Lack of color production indicates the absence of β-lactamase **(B)**.

isolate of interest. Less commonly used tests detect the chloramphenicol-modifying enzyme chloramphenicol acetyltransferase.

**β-Lactamase Detection.** β-lactamases play a key role in bacterial resistance to beta-lactam agents, and detection of their presence can provide useful information (see Chapter 11). Various assays are available to detect β-lactamases, but the most useful in clinical laboratories is the chromogenic cephalosporinase test. β-lactamases exert their effect by opening the β-lactam ring (see Figure 11-9). When a chromogenic cephalosporin is used as the substrate, this process results in a colored product. The Cefinase disk is an example of a commercially available chromogenic test (BD Microbiology Systems, Cockeysville, Maryland). The disk incorporates nitrocefin as the substrate (Figure 12-15).

Useful application of tests to directly detect β-lactamase production is limited to organisms producing enzymes whose spectrum of activity is known. This also must include the β-lactams commonly considered for therapeutic eradication of the organism. Examples of useful applications include detection of:

- *N. gonorrhoeae* resistance to penicillin
- *H. influenzae* resistance to ampicillin
- Staphylococcal resistance to penicillin

The actual utility of this approach, even for the organisms listed, is decreasing. As β-lactamase–mediated resistance has become widespread among *N. gonorrhoeae*, *H. influenzae*, and staphylococci, other agents not affected by the β-lactamases have become the therapeutic antimicrobials of choice. Therefore, the need to know the β-lactamase status of these bacterial species has become substantially less urgent. Whereas several Enterobacteriaceae and *P. aeruginosa* produce β-lactamases, the effect of these enzymes on the various β-lactams depends on which enzymes are produced. Therefore, even though such organisms would frequently produce a positive β-lactamase assay, very little, if any, information would be gained about which antimicrobial agents are affected. It is recommended that detection of β-lactam resistance among these organisms be accomplished using conventional and commercial systems that directly evaluate antimicrobial agent/organism interactions.

**Chloramphenicol Acetyltransferase Detection.** Chloramphenicol modification by chloramphenicol acetyltransferase (CAT) is one mechanism by which bacteria may express resistance to this agent. This, coupled with the substantially diminished use of chloramphenicol in today's clinical settings, significantly limits the utility of the CAT detection test. Commercial assays provide a convenient method for establishing the presence of this enzyme. If positive, chloramphenicol resistance can be reported, but a negative test result does not rule out resistance that may be mediated by other mechanisms, such as decreased uptake.

### Genotypic Methods

The genes that encode many of the clinically relevant acquired resistance mechanisms are known, as is all or part of their nucleotide sequences. This has allowed for the development of molecular methods involving nucleic acid hybridization and amplification for the study and detection of antimicrobial resistance (for more information on molecular methods for the characterization of bacteria, see Chapter 8). The ability to definitively determine the presence of a particular gene that encodes antimicrobial resistance has several advantages. However, as with any laboratory procedure, certain disadvantages and limitations also exist.

From a research and development perspective, molecular methods are extremely useful for more thoroughly characterizing the resistances of bacterial collections used to establish and evaluate conventional standards recommended by CLSI. Phenotype-based commercial susceptibility testing methods and systems, both automated and nonautomated, can also be evaluated.

Molecular methods also may be directly applied in the clinical setting as an important backup resource to investigate and arbitrate equivocal results obtained by phenotypic methods. For example, the clinical importance of accurately detecting methicillin resistance among staphylococci, coupled with the inconsistencies of phenotypic methods, is problematic. In doubtful situations, molecular detection of the *mec* gene encoding methicillin resistance can be applied to definitively establish an isolate's methicillin resistance. Similarly, doubt raised by equivocal phenotypic results obtained with potentially vancomycin-resistant enterococci can be definitively resolved by establishing the presence and classification of *van* genes that mediate this resistance.

Although molecular methods have been and will continue to be extremely important in antimicrobial resistance detection, numerous factors still complicate their use beyond supplementing phenotype-based susceptibility testing protocols. These factors include the following:

- Use of probes or oligonucleotides for specific resistance genes. Resistance mediated by divergent genes or totally different mechanisms could be missed (i.e., the absence of one gene may not guarantee antimicrobial susceptibility).
- Phenotypic resistance to a level that is clinically significant for any one antimicrobial agent may be due to a culmination of processes that involve enzymatic modification of the antimicrobial, decreased uptake, altered affinity of the drug's target, or some combination of these mechanisms (i.e., the presence of one gene does not guarantee resistance).

- The presence of a gene encoding resistance does not provide information about the status of the control genes necessary for expression of resistance; that is, although present, the genes may be silent or nonfunctional, and the organism may be incapable of expressing the resistance encoded by the gene.
- From a clinical laboratory perspective, it may be impractical to adopt molecular methods specific for only a few resistance mechanisms when the vast majority of the susceptibility testing still will be accomplished using phenotypic-based methods. Items to consider before adopting molecular tests may include (but are not limited to) clinical efficacy, space, personnel, and financial management.

Even though adoption of molecular methods for routine antimicrobial susceptibility testing poses challenges, these methods will continue to enhance the ability to detect antibiotic resistance.

## SPECIAL METHODS FOR COMPLEX ANTIMICROBIAL/ORGANISM INTERACTIONS

Certain in vitro tests have been developed to investigate aspects of antimicrobial activity not routinely addressed by commonly used susceptibility testing procedures. Specifically, these are tests designed to measure bactericidal activity (i.e., bacterial killing) or to measure the antibacterial effect of combination therapy with antimicrobial agents.

These tests are often labor intensive, fraught with the potential for technical problems, frequently difficult to interpret, and of uncertain clinical utility. For these reasons, their use should be substantially limited. Also, they should be done only if expert microbiology and infectious disease consultants are available.

### Bactericidal Tests

Bactericidal tests are designed to determine the ability of antimicrobial agents to kill bacteria. The killing ability of most drugs is already known, and they are commonly classified as bacteriostatic or bactericidal agents. However, many variables, including the concentration of antimicrobial agent and the species of targeted organism, can influence this classification. For example, beta-lactams, such as penicillin, typically are bactericidal against most gram-positive cocci but are usually only bacteriostatic against enterococci. If bactericidal tests are clinically appropriate, they should be applied only to evaluate antimicrobials typically considered to be bactericidal (e.g., beta-lactams and vancomycin) and not to agents known to be bacteriostatic (e.g., macrolides).

Key clinical situations in which achieving bactericidal activity is of greatest clinical importance include severe and life-threatening infections, infections in an immunocompromised patient, and infections in body sites where assistance from the patient's own defenses is minimal (e.g., endocarditis or osteomyelitis). Based on research trials in animal models and clinical trials in humans, the most effective therapy for these types of infections is often already known. However, occasionally the laboratory may be asked to substantiate that bactericidal activity is being achieved or is achievable. The methods available for this include minimal bactericidal concentration (MBC) testing, time-kill studies, and serum-cidal testing. Regardless of the method used, the need to interpret the results cautiously, with the understanding of uncertain clinical correlation and the potential for substantial technical artifacts, cannot be overemphasized.

**Minimal Bactericidal Concentration.** The MBC test involves continuation of the procedure for conventional broth dilution testing. After incubation and determination of the antimicrobial agent's MIC, an aliquot from each tube or well in the dilution series demonstrating inhibition of visible bacterial growth is subcultured to an enriched agar medium (usually sheep blood agar). After overnight incubation, the plates are examined and the CFUs determined. With the volume of the aliquot and the number of CFUs obtained, the number of viable cells per milliliter for each antimicrobial dilution can be calculated. This number is compared with the known CFU/mL in the original inoculum. The antimicrobial concentration resulting in a 99.9% reduction in CFU/mL compared with the organism concentration in the original inoculum is recorded as the MBC.

Although the clinical significance of MBC results is uncertain, applications of this information include considering whether treatment failure could be occurring as the result of an organism's MBC exceeding the serum-achievable level for the antimicrobial agent. Alternatively, if an antibiotic's MBC is greater than or equal to 32 times higher than the MIC, the organism may be tolerant to the drug. **Tolerance,** a phenomenon most commonly associated with bacterial resistance to beta-lactam antibiotics, reflects an organism's ability to be inhibited by an agent that is usually bactericidal. Although the physiologic basis of tolerance has been studied in several bacterial species, the actual clinical relevance of this phenomenon has not been well established.

**Time-Kill Studies.** Another approach to examining bactericidal activity involves exposing a bacterial isolate to a concentration of antibiotic in a broth medium and measuring the rate of killing over a specified period. By this time-kill analysis, samples are taken from the antibiotic-broth solution immediately after addition of the inoculum and at regular intervals afterward. Each time-sample is plated to agar plates; after incubation, CFU counts are performed as described for MBC testing. The number of viable bacteria from each sample is plotted over time to determine the rate of killing. Generally, a 1000-fold decrease in the number of viable bacteria in the antibiotic-containing broth after a 24-hour period, compared with the number of bacteria in the original inoculum, is interpreted as bactericidal activity. Although time-kill analysis is frequently used in the research environment to study the in vitro activity of antimicrobial agents, the labor intensity and technical specifications of the procedure preclude its use in most clinical microbiology laboratories to determine the proper treatment of a patient's infection.

**Serum Bactericidal (Schlichter Test).** The serum bactericidal test (SBT) is analogous to the MIC-MBC test except the medium used is the patient's serum containing the therapeutic antimicrobial agents the patient has been receiving. Using the patient's serum to detect bacteriostatic and bactericidal activity also allows observation of the antibacterial impact of factors other than the antibiotics (e.g., antibodies and complement).

Two serum samples are required for each test. One is collected just before the patient is to receive the next antimicrobial dose; this is the **trough specimen.** The other sample is collected when the serum antimicrobial concentration is highest; this is the **peak specimen.** The appropriate time to collect the peak specimen varies with the pharmacokinetic properties of the antimicrobial agents and the route by which they are being administered. Peak levels for intravenously, intramuscularly, and orally administered agents are generally obtained 30 to 60 minutes, 60 minutes, and 90 minutes after administration, respectively. The trough and peak levels should be collected for the same dose and tested simultaneously.

Serial twofold dilutions of each specimen are prepared and inoculated with the bacterial isolate from the patient (final inoculum of $5 \times 10^5$ CFU/mL). Dilutions are incubated overnight. The highest dilution that inhibits visibly detectable growth is the serum-static titer (e.g., 1:8, 1:16, 1:32). Aliquots of known size are then taken from each dilution at or below the serum-static titer (i.e., dilutions that inhibited bacterial growth) and are plated on sheep blood agar plates. After incubation, the CFUs per plate are counted, and the serum dilution resulting in a 99.9% reduction in the CFU/mL, compared with the original inoculum, is recorded as the serum-cidal titer. For example, if a bacterial isolate showed a serum-static titer of 1:32, the tubes containing dilutions of 1:2, 1:4, 1:8, 1:16, and 1:32 would be subcultured. If the 1:8 dilution was the highest dilution to yield a 99.9% decrease in CFUs, the serum-cidal titer would be recorded as 1:8.

The SBT was originally developed to assist in the prediction of the clinical efficacy of antimicrobial therapy for staphylococcal endocarditis. Peak serum-cidal titers of 1:32 to 1:64 or greater have been thought to correlate with a positive clinical outcome. However, even though the test is performed on the patient's serum, many differences go unaccounted for between the in vitro test environment and the in vivo site of infection. Therefore, although the test is used to evaluate whether effective bactericidal concentrations are being achieved, the predictive clinical value for staphylococcal endocarditis or any other infection caused by other bacteria is still uncertain.

Details regarding the performance of these bactericidal tests are provided in the CLSI document M26-A, "Methods for Determining Bactericidal Activity of Antimicrobial Agents."

## Tests for Activity of Antimicrobial Combinations

Therapeutic management of bacterial infections often requires simultaneous use of more than one antimicrobial agent. Some of the reasons for use of multiple therapies include:

- Treating polymicrobial infections caused by organisms with different antimicrobial resistance profiles
- Achieving more rapid bactericidal activity than may be achieved with any single agent

- Achieving bactericidal activity against bacteria for which no single agent is lethal
- Minimizing the emergence of resistant organisms during therapy

Testing the effectiveness of antimicrobial combinations against a single bacterial isolate is referred to as **synergy testing.** When combinations are tested, three outcome categories are possible:

- **Synergy:** the activity of the antimicrobial combination is substantially greater than the activity of the single most active drug alone
- **Indifference:** the activity of the combination is no better or worse than the single most active drug alone
- **Antagonism:** the activity of the combination is substantially less than the activity of the single most active drug alone (an interaction to be avoided)

The checkerboard assay and the time-kill assay are two basic methods of synergy testing. In the checkerboard method, MIC panels are set up containing two antimicrobial agents serially diluted independently and in combination. After inoculation and incubation, the MICs obtained with the individual agents and the various combinations are recorded. By calculating the MIC ratios obtained with individual and combined agents, the drug combination in question is classified as synergistic, indifferent, or antagonistic.

With the time-kill assay, the same procedure described for testing bactericidal activity is used, except that the killing curve obtained with a single agent is compared with the killing curve obtained with antimicrobial combinations. Synergy is indicated when the combination exhibits killing that is greater by 100-fold or more than the most active single agent tested alone after 24 hours of incubation. Killing rates between the most active agent and the combination that are similar are interpreted as indifference. Antagonism is evident when the combination appears less active than the most active single agent.

The decision to use more than one antimicrobial agent may be based on antimicrobial resistance profiles or identification of particular bacterial pathogens reported by the clinical microbiology laboratory. However, the decision regarding which antimicrobial agents to combine should not rely on the results of complex synergy tests performed in the clinical laboratory. Most clinically useful antimicrobial combinations have been investigated in a clinical research setting and are well described in the medical literature. These data should be used to guide the decision for combination therapy. The technical difficulties associated with performing and interpreting synergy tests, which at most would be performed only rarely in the clinical laboratory, precludes their utility in the diagnostic setting.

# LABORATORY STRATEGIES FOR ANTIMICROBIAL SUSCEPTIBILITY TESTING

The clinical microbiology laboratory is responsible for maximizing the positive impact that susceptibility testing information can have on the use of antimicrobial agents to treat infectious diseases. However, meeting this responsibility is difficult because of demands for more efficient use of laboratory resources, the increasing complexities of important bacterial resistance profiles, and the continued expectations for high-quality results. To ensure quality in the midst of dwindling resources and expanding antimicrobial resistance, strategies for antimicrobial susceptibility testing must be carefully developed. These strategies should target relevance, accuracy, and communication (Figure 12-16).

# RELEVANCE

Antimicrobial susceptibility testing should be performed only when sufficient potential exists for providing clinically useful and reliable information about antimicrobial agents appropriate for the bacterial isolate in question.

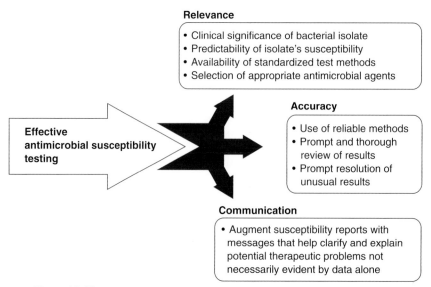

**Relevance**
- Clinical significance of bacterial isolate
- Predictability of isolate's susceptibility
- Availability of standardized test methods
- Selection of appropriate antimicrobial agents

**Effective antimicrobial susceptibility testing**

**Accuracy**
- Use of reliable methods
- Prompt and thorough review of results
- Prompt resolution of unusual results

**Communication**
- Augment susceptibility reports with messages that help clarify and explain potential therapeutic problems not necessarily evident by data alone

**Figure 12-16** Goals of effective antimicrobial susceptibility testing strategies.

Therefore, for the sake of relevance, two questions must be addressed:

- When should testing be performed?
- Which antimicrobial agents should be tested?

## WHEN TO PERFORM A SUSCEPTIBILITY TEST

The first issue that must be resolved is whether antimicrobial susceptibility testing is appropriate for a particular isolate. Although the answer may not always be clear, the issue must always be addressed. The decision to perform susceptibility testing depends on the following criteria:

- Clinical significance of a bacterial isolate
- Predictability of a bacterial isolate's susceptibility to the antimicrobial agents most commonly used against them, often referred to as the **drugs of choice**
- Availability of reliable standardized methods for testing the isolate

### Determining Clinical Significance

Performing tests and reporting antimicrobial susceptibility data on clinically insignificant bacterial isolates are a waste of resources and, more important, can mislead physicians, who depend on laboratory information to assist in establishing the clinical significance of a bacterial isolate. Useful criteria for establishing the clinical importance of a bacterial isolate include:

- Detection and/or the abundance of the organism on direct Gram stain of a patient's specimen, preferably in the presence of white blood cells, and growth of an organism with the same morphology in culture
- Known ability of the bacterial species isolated to cause infection at the body site from which the specimen was obtained (see Part VII)
- Whether the organism is generally considered either an epithelial or mucosal colonizer or is generally considered a pathogen
- Body site from which the organism was isolated (normally sterile or a typically colonized site)

Although these criteria are helpful and heavily depend on the capacity of the bacterial species isolated to cause disease, the final designation of clinical significance often still requires dialog between the laboratory and physician.

Reporting susceptibility results for organisms with questionable clinical importance may be incorrectly interpreted by the clinician as a indicator of clinical significance. Therefore, using criteria such as those listed should be included in the laboratory's antimicrobial susceptibility testing strategy.

### Predictability of Antimicrobial Susceptibility

If the organisms are clinically significant, what are the chances they could be resistant to the antimicrobial agents commonly used to eradicate them? Unfortunately, the increasing dissemination of resistance among clinically relevant bacteria has diminished the number of bacteria for which antimicrobial susceptibility can be confidently predicted based on identification without the need to perform testing. Table 12-5 categorizes many of

**TABLE 12-5** Categorization of Bacteria According to Need for Routine Performance of Antimicrobial Susceptibility Testing*

| Need for Testing | Bacteria |
|---|---|
| Testing commonly required | Staphylococci<br>*Streptococcus pneumoniae*<br>Viridans streptococci[†]<br>Enterococci<br>Enterobacteriaceae<br>*Pseudomonas aeruginosa*<br>*Acinetobacter* spp. |
| Testing occasionally required[‡] | *Haemophilus influenzae*<br>*Neisseria gonorrhoeae*<br>*Moraxella catarrhalis*<br>Anaerobic bacteria |
| Testing rarely required | Beta-hemolytic streptococci (groups A, B, C, F, and G)<br>*Neisseria meningitidis*<br>*Listeria monocytogenes* |

*Based on the assumption that the organism is clinically significant. Table includes bacteria for which standardized testing procedures are available, as outlined and recommended by the Clinical and Laboratory Standards Institute.
[†]Viridans streptococci require testing when implicated in endocarditis or isolated in pure culture from a normally sterile site with a strong suspicion of being clinically important.
[‡]Testing required if an antimicrobial to which the organisms are frequently resistant is still considered for use (e.g., penicillin for *Neisseria gonorrhoeae*).

the commonly encountered bacteria according to the need to perform testing to detect resistance.

Acquired resistance to various antimicrobial agents dictates that susceptibility testing be performed on all clinically relevant isolates of several bacterial groups, genera, and species. For other organisms, such as *H. influenzae* and *N. gonorrhoeae*, resistance to the original drugs of choice (ampicillin, penicillin, and recently ceftriaxone) has become widespread, and more potent antibiotics (e.g., ceftriaxone), for which no resistance has been described, have become the drugs of choice. Therefore, although testing used to be routinely indicated to detect ampicillin and penicillin resistance, testing for resistance to currently recommended antimicrobials for these organisms is not routinely necessary. The possible exception to this is the relatively recent emergence of fluoroquinolone resistance in *N. gonorrhoeae* that may warrant testing of clinical isolates.

One notable exception to the widespread emergence of resistance has been the absence of penicillin resistance among beta-hemolytic streptococci. Because susceptibility to penicillin is extremely predictable among these organisms, testing against penicillin provides little, if any, information that is not already provided by accurate organism identification. However, if the patient cannot tolerate penicillin, alternative agents, such as erythromycin, may be considered. Erythromycin resistance among beta-hemolytic streptococci has been well documented, and susceptibility testing in this instance would be indicated.

The recommendations outlined in Table 12-5 are guidelines. In any clinical setting, exceptions will arise that must be considered in consultation with the physician. Also, these guidelines are for providing data used for the management of a single patient's infection. When susceptibility testing is performed as a means of gathering surveillance data for the monitoring of emerging resistance (see Accuracy and Antimicrobial Resistance Surveillance later in this chapter), the guidelines may not necessarily apply.

### Availability of Reliable Susceptibility Testing Methods

If a reliable, standardized method for testing a particular bacterial genus or species does not exist, the ability to produce accurate and meaningful data is substantially compromised. Although standard methods exist for most of the commonly encountered bacteria (see Tables 12-1 to 12-3), clinically relevant isolates of bacterial species for which standard testing methods do not exist are encountered. In these instances, the dilemma stems from the conflict between the laboratory's urge to contribute in some way by providing data and the lack of confidence in producing interpretable and accurate information.

Many organisms not listed in Table 12-5 grow on the media and under the conditions recommended for testing commonly encountered bacteria. However, the ability to grow and the ability to detect important antimicrobial resistance patterns are not the same thing. For example, the gram-negative bacillus *Stenotrophomonas maltophilia* grows extremely well under most susceptibility testing conditions, but the results obtained with beta-lactam antibiotics can be widely variable and seriously misleading. This organism produces potent beta-lactamases that seriously compromise the effectiveness of most beta-lactams, yet certain isolates may appear susceptible by standard in vitro testing criteria. Therefore, even though testing may provide an potential answer, the answer may be incorrect.

Given the uncertainty surrounding the testing of bacteria for which standardized methods are lacking, two approaches may be used. One is to not perform testing, but rather to provide physicians with information based on clinical studies published in the medical literature about the antimicrobial agents generally accepted as the drugs of choice for the bacterial species in question. This approach is best handled when the laboratory medical director and infectious disease specialists are involved. The other option is to provide the literature information and perform the test to the best of the laboratory's ability. In this case, results must be accompanied by a message indicating that testing was performed by a nonstandardized method and results should be interpreted with caution. When such tests are undertaken, customized antimicrobial batteries, including the agents most commonly used to eradicate the bacterial species of interest, need to be assembled and used. Recently CLSI has published the document M45 to provide guidelines for the testing of certain less frequently encountered bacteria.

### SELECTION OF ANTIMICROBIAL AGENTS FOR TESTING

Selection of relevant antimicrobial agents is based on the criteria outlined in Box 12-1. These criteria should be

carefully considered when antimicrobial agents are selected to avoid cluttering reports with superfluous information, to minimize the risk of confusing physicians, and to substantially decrease the waste of time and resources in the clinical microbiology laboratory.

Antimicrobial agents that may be considered for inclusion in batteries to be tested against certain bacterial groups are provided in Table 12-6. The list is not exhaustive but is useful for illustrating some points about the development of relevant testing batteries. For example, with all the penicillins, cephalosporins, and other beta-lactam antibiotics available for testing, only penicillin and oxacillin need to be tested against staphylococci. The information acquired with these two agents reflects the general effectiveness of any other beta-lactam. In essence, these drugs are predictor agents, as discussed earlier in this chapter. Similarly, ampicillin can be used independently as an indicator of enterococcal susceptibility to various penicillins, and because of intrinsic resistance, cephalosporins should never be tested against these organisms.

In contrast to the relatively few agents that may be included in testing batteries for gram-positive cocci, several potential choices exist for use against gram-negative bacilli. This is mostly due to the commercial availability of several β-lactams with similar activities against Enterobacteriaceae and the general inability of one β-lactam to serve as a reliable predictor drug for other β-lactams. For example, an organism resistant to cefazolin may or may not be resistant to cefotetan, and an organism resistant to cefotetan may or may not be resistant to ceftazidime. With the lack of potential for selecting a predictor drug in these instances, more agents must be tested. However, in some instances overlap in activities does exist, so some duplication of effort can be avoided. For example, the spectra of activity of ceftriaxone and cefotaxime are sufficiently similar to allow the use of one in the testing battery.

Many scenarios exist in which the spectrum of activity and other criteria listed in Box 12-1 are considered for the sake of designing the most relevant and useful testing batteries. These criteria should be considered in consultation with patients' physicians and the pharmacy staff.

## ACCURACY

Susceptibility testing strategies focused on production of accurate results have two key components:
- Use of methods that produce accurate results
- The application of real-time review of results prior to reporting

### Use of Accurate Methodologies

Because of the complexities of the various resistance mechanisms, no one method, conventional, automated, or molecular, is sufficient for detection of all clinically relevant resistance patterns. Therefore, the selection of testing methods and careful consideration of how different methods are most effectively used together is necessary to ensure accurate and reliable detection of resistance.

**TABLE 12-6** Selection of Antimicrobial Agents for Testing Against Common Bacterial Groups*

| Antimicrobial Agents | Enterobacteriaceae | Pseudomonas aeruginosa | Staphylococci | Enterococci | Streptococcus pneumoniae | Viridans Streptococci |
|---|---|---|---|---|---|---|
| **Penicillins** | | | | | | |
| Penicillin | − | − | + | − | + | + |
| Oxacillin | − | − | + | − | − | − |
| Ampicillin | + | − | − | + | − | − |
| Piperacillin/ tazobactam | + | + | − | − | − | − |
| **Cephalosporins** | | | | | | |
| Cefazolin | + | − | − | − | − | − |
| Cefotetan | + | − | − | − | − | − |
| Ceftriaxone | + | − | − | − | + | + |
| Cefotaxime | + | − | − | − | + | + |
| Ceftazidime | + | + | − | − | − | − |
| **Other Beta-Lactams** | | | | | | |
| Aztreonam | + | + | − | − | − | − |
| Imipenem | + | + | − | − | ± | − |
| **Glycopeptides** | | | | | | |
| Vancomycin | − | − | + | + | + | + |
| **Aminoglycosides** | | | | | | |
| Gentamicin | + | + | ± | +[†] | − | − |
| Tobramycin | + | + | − | − | − | − |
| Amikacin | + | + | − | − | − | − |
| **Quinolones** | | | | | | |
| Ciprofloxacin | + | + | + | − | + | |
| Levofloxacin | + | + | + | − | + | + |
| **Other Agents** | | | | | | |
| Erythromycin | − | − | + | − | + | + |
| Clindamycin | − | − | + | − | + | + |
| Trimethoprim- sulfamethoxazole | + | − | + | − | + | −, ± |
| Tigecycline | + | − | + | + | ± | + |
| Daptomycin | − | − | + | + | ± | ± |
| Linezolid | − | − | + | + | ± | + |
| Telithromycin | − | − | + | − | + | |

+, May be selected for inclusion in testing batteries (not all agents with + need to be selected); ±, may be selected in certain situations; −, selection for testing is not necessary or not recommended.
*Not all available antimicrobial agents are included. Selection recommendation is based on non–urinary tract infections.
[†]Gentamicin testing against enterococci requires use of high-concentration disks or a special screen (see Table 12-4).

Microbiologists must be aware of the strengths and weaknesses of the primary susceptibility testing methods in the laboratory for detecting relevant resistance patterns and know when adjunct or supplemental testing is necessary. This awareness is accomplished by reviewing studies published in peer-reviewed journals focusing on the performance of antimicrobial testing systems and periodically challenging one's own system with organisms that have been thoroughly characterized with respect to their resistance profiles (e.g., proficiency testing programs). Furthermore, accurate and relevant testing not only means using various conventional methods or even using a mixture of automated, conventional, and screening methods, but also encompasses the potential application of molecular techniques and predictor drugs.

Testing of *S. pneumoniae* provides one example of the need to be aware of testing limitations and the importance of implementing supplemental tests. Not long ago, routine susceptibility testing of *S. pneumoniae* was considered unnecessary. However, with the emergence of beta-lactam resistance, testing has become imperative. As the need for testing emerged, the inability of conventional tests, such as penicillin disk diffusion, to detect resistance became apparent. Fortunately, a test that uses the penicillin derivative oxacillin was developed and widely used as a reliable screen for detecting resistance to penicillin. However, this test is only a screen because the level of penicillin intermediate resistance (i.e., the MIC) can vary greatly among nonsusceptible isolates, and some strains that appear resistant by the screen may actually be susceptible. Because the level of resistance can affect therapeutic decisions, another method that allows for MIC determinations should be used to test these organisms. Additionally, the emergence of cephalosporin (i.e., ceftriaxone or cefotaxime) resistance requires the use of tests for the detection of resistance to these agents.

Other important examples in which more than one method is required to obtain complete and accurate susceptibility testing data for certain organism groups or species include vancomycin-resistant enterococci, methicillin-resistant staphylococci, and extended spectrum, beta-lactamase–producing Enterobacteriaceae. In addition, molecular methods also may be used in the clinical setting as an important backup resource to investigate and arbitrate equivocal results obtained by phenotypic methods. However, multiple testing protocols are not routinely necessary for every organism encountered in the clinical laboratory. In most laboratories, one conventional or commercial method is likely to be the mainstay for testing, with additional testing available as a supplement when necessary.

## REVIEW OF RESULTS

In addition to selecting one or more methods to accurately detect resistance, the strengths and weaknesses of the testing systems must be continuously monitored. This is primarily accomplished by carefully reviewing the susceptibility data produced daily. In the past, establishing and maintaining aggressive and effective monitoring programs often have been prohibitively labor intensive. However, the speed and flexibility afforded by computerization of results review and reporting greatly facilitate the administration of such quality assurance programs, even in laboratories with modest resources. Effective computer programs may be a part of the general laboratory information system (or, in some cases, such programs are available through the commercial susceptibility testing system). Because automated expert data review greatly facilitates the review process and enhances data accuracy, this feature should be seriously considered when selecting an antimicrobial susceptibility testing system.

Susceptibility profiles must be scrutinized manually or with the aid of computers according to what profiles are likely, somewhat likely, somewhat unlikely, and nearly impossible. This awareness not only pertains to profiles exhibited by organisms in a particular institution, but also to those exhibited by clinically relevant bacteria in general. The unusual resistance profiles must be discovered and evaluated expeditiously to determine whether they are due to technical or clerical errors or are truly indicative of an emerging resistance problem. The urgency of making this determination is twofold. First, if the profile results from laboratory error, it must be corrected and the physician notified so the patient is not subjected to ineffective or inappropriate antimicrobial therapy. Second, if the profile is valid and presents a threat to the patient and to others (e.g., the emergence of vancomycin-resistant staphylococci), immediate notification of infection control and infectious disease personnel is warranted.

### Components of Results Review Strategies

Any laboratory strategy for monitoring the accuracy of results and the emergence of resistance must have two components:
- Data review—a mechanism for recognizing new or unusual susceptibility profiles
- Resolution—the application of protocols for determining whether an unusual profile is a result of an error (technical or clerical) or accurately reflects the emergence of a new resistance mechanism

Both components must be integrated into the review process to ensure efficient and timely use of resources.

**Data Review.** Recognition of unusual resistance profiles is primarily accomplished by carefully reviewing the daily laboratory susceptibility data. Examples of unusual susceptibility profiles for gram-positive and gram-negative bacteria are given in Table 12-7. The examples are a mixture of profiles that clearly demonstrate a likely error (i.e., clindamycin-resistant, erythromycin-susceptible staphylococci); profiles that have rarely been encountered but if observed require immediate attention (i.e., vancomycin resistance in staphylococci); and profiles that have been described but may not be common (i.e., imipenem resistance in Enterobacteriaceae).

The data review process for evaluation of profiles should not be the responsibility of a single person in the laboratory. Furthermore, the process requires checks and balances that do not impede the workflow or increase the time required to get the results to the physicians. The way this is established varies, depending on a particular laboratory's division of labor and workflow, but several key aspects must be considered:
- The identification of the organism must be known. To evaluate the accuracy of a susceptibility profile, identification and susceptibility data must be simultaneously analyzed in a timely fashion. Without knowing the organism's identification, it is frequently difficult to determine whether the susceptibility profile is unusual.
- Susceptibility results should be analyzed and reported as early in the day as possible. The workflow should allow time for corrective action for errors found during data review so that corrected, or substantiated, results can be provided to physicians as soon as possible.

**TABLE 12-7** Examples of Susceptibility Testing Profiles Requiring Further Evaluation

| Organism | Susceptibility Profile |
|---|---|
| Staphylococci | Vancomycin intermediate or resistant<br>Clindamycin resistant; erythromycin susceptible<br>Linezolid resistant<br>Daptomycin resistant |
| Viridans streptococci | Vancomycin intermediate or resistant |
| *Streptococcus pneumoniae* | Vancomycin intermediate or resistant |
| Beta-hemolytic streptococci | Penicillin intermediate or resistant |
| Enterobacteriaceae | Imipenem resistant |
| *Enterobacter/Citrobacter/ Serratia/Morganella/ Providencia/Klebsiella* | Susceptible to ampicillin or cefazolin |
| Enterococci | Vancomycin resistant, high level of aminoglycoside resistance by disk diffusion |
| *Pseudomonas aeruginosa* | Amikacin resistant; gentamicin or tobramycin susceptible |
| *Stenotrophomonas maltophilia* | Imipenem susceptible; trimethoprim/ sulfamethoxazole resistant |
| *Neisseria gonorrhoeae* | Ceftriaxone resistant |
| *Neisseria meningitidis* | Penicillin resistant |

Modified from Courvalin P: Interpretive reading of antimicrobial susceptibility tests, *Am Soc Microbiol News* 58:368, 1992.

- Two or more tiers of data review should be used. The first tier is at the bench level, where technologists are simultaneously reading the results and evaluating an organism's susceptibility profile for appropriateness. When unusual profiles are found, the technologist should be able to initiate troubleshooting protocols (see the next section). To prevent the release of erroneous and potentially dangerous information, results should not be reported at this point. Review at this level, which is greatly facilitated by automated expert review systems, maintains proficiency among technologists in relationship to the nuances of susceptibility profiles and important resistance patterns. The second tier is at the level of supervisory or laboratory director. The purpose of review at this level is to track and monitor the efficiency of the first tier, to take ultimate responsibility for the accuracy of results, to provide constructive and educational feedback to the technologists performing the first-line review, and to provide guidance for resolution of the unusual profiles. Again, a computer-based review process that searches all reports for predefined unusual profiles (similar to those outlined in Table 12-7) can greatly enhance the efficiency and accuracy of the second level of review.
- The review process must be flexible and updated. Because bacterial capabilities for antimicrobial resistance profiles change, laboratory resistance detection systems can become outdated. Therefore,

the list of unusual profiles requires periodic review and updating.

**Resolution.** The importance of having strategies for resolving unusual profiles cannot be overstated. However, developing detailed procedures for every contingency is not possible or practical. Most resolution strategies should focus on certain general approaches, with supervisory or laboratory director consultation always being among the options available to technologists. Although the steps taken to investigate and resolve an unusual profile often depend on the organism and antibiotics involved, most protocols for resolution should include one or more of the following approaches:

- Review data for possible clerical error.
- Determine whether susceptibility panel and identification system were inoculated with same isolate.
- Reexamine test panel or plate for reading error (e.g., misreading of actual zone of inhibition).
- Confirm purity of inoculum and proper inoculum preparation.
- For commercial systems, determine whether manufacturer's recommended procedures were followed.
- Confirm accuracy of organism identification.
- Confirm resistance by using a second method or screening test.

Often a quick review of the data recording and interpretation aspects, or purity of culture, will reveal the reason an unusual profile was obtained. Other times more extensive testing, perhaps by more than one method, may be needed to establish the validity of an unusual or unexpected resistance profile.

## ACCURACY AND ANTIMICROBIAL RESISTANCE SURVEILLANCE

Antimicrobial resistance surveillance involves tracking the susceptibility profiles produced by the bacteria encountered in a particular institution and in a specific geographic location (i.e., regionally, nationally, or internationally). For laboratories that serve a particular institution or group of institutions, periodic publication of an antibiogram report containing susceptibility data is the extent of the surveillance program. These reports, which may be further organized in various ways (e.g., according to hospital location, site of infection, outpatient or inpatient, duration of hospital stay), provide valuable information for monitoring emerging resistance trends among the local microbial flora. Such information is also helpful for establishing **empiric therapy** guidelines (i.e., therapy that is instituted before knowledge of the infecting organism's identification or its antimicrobial susceptibility profile), detecting areas of potential inappropriate or excessive antimicrobial use, and contributing data to larger, more extensive surveillance programs.

Data that have been validated through a results review and resolution program not only enhance the reliability of laboratory reports for patient management, but also strengthen the credibility of susceptibility data used for resistance surveillance and antibiogram profiling. Therefore, meeting the need for each institution to scrutinize susceptibility profiles daily can be accomplished by establishing a results review and resolution format that ensures the accuracy for patient management, detects emerging resistance patterns quickly, and maintains accuracy of the data included in the summary antibiogram reports.

# COMMUNICATION

Susceptibility testing profiles produced for each bacterial isolate are typically reported to the physician as a listing of the antimicrobial agents, with each agent accompanied by the category interpretation of susceptible, intermediate, or resistant. In most instances, this reporting approach is sufficient. However, as resistance profiles and their underlying mechanisms become more varied and complex, laboratory personnel must ensure that the significance of susceptibility data is clearly and accurately communicated to clinicians in a way that optimizes both patient care and antimicrobial use. In many situations, passively communicating the susceptibility data to the physician without adding comments or appropriately amending the reports is no longer sufficient.

For example, methicillin-resistant staphylococci are to be considered cross-resistant to all β-lactams, but in vitro results occasionally may indicate susceptibility to certain cephalosporins, β-lactam/β-lactamase inhibitor combinations, or imipenem. Simply reporting these findings without editing such profiles to reflect probable resistance to all beta-lactams would be seriously misleading. As another example, serious enterococcal infections often require combination therapy, including both a cell wall–active agent (ampicillin or vancomycin) and an aminoglycoside (i.e., gentamicin). This important information would not be conveyed in a report that simply lists the agents and their interpretive category results. Such an approach can leave the false impression that a "susceptible" result for any single agent indicates that one drug used alone provides appropriate therapy. Therefore, an explanatory note that clearly states the recommended use of combination therapy should accompany the enterococcal susceptibility report.

To prevent misinterpretations that may result by providing only antimicrobial susceptibility data, strategies must consider organism antimicrobial combinations that may require reporting of supplemental messages to the physician. Consultations with infectious disease specialists and other members of the medical staff are an important part of determining when such messages are needed and what the content should include. Finally, if a laboratory does not have the means to reliably relay these messages, either by computer or by paper, a policy of direct communication with the attending physician by telephone or in person should be established.

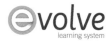 *Visit the Evolve site to complete the review questions.*

---

## CASE STUDY 12-1

A 28-year-old man presented to the emergency department (ED) complaining of painful urination and purulent urethral discharge. The patient was empirically treated with singles doses of ciprofloxacin and azithromycin before discharge. A subsequent nucleic acid amplification test showed a positive result for *Neisseria gonorrhoeae*. Two days later the patient returned to the ED because his symptoms had not resolved. A culture was collected and submitted to the microbiology laboratory. The etiologic agent was identified as *N. gonorrhoeae*. Antimicrobial susceptibility testing yielded the following results: ceftriaxone—susceptible; ciprofloxacin—resistant; tetracycline—susceptible.

**QUESTIONS**

1. Why don't clinical laboratories routinely perform antimicrobial susceptibility tests for *N. gonorrhoeae*?
2. Why would the physician be interested in culture and antimicrobial susceptibility test results on the patient's specimen?
3. If susceptibility testing is not routinely performed, how is resistance to fluoroquinolones and other antimicrobial agents monitored with *N. gonorrhoeae*?

---

# REFERENCE

1. Bauer AW, Kirby WM, Sherris JC et al: Antibiotic susceptibility testing by a single disc method, *Am J Clin Pathol* 45:49, 1966.

# BIBLIOGRAPHY

Clinical and Laboratory Standards Institute: *Methods for determining bactericidal activity of antimicrobial agents: tentative guideline M26-A*, Villanova, Pa, 1999, CLSI.

Clinical and Laboratory Standards Institute: *Methods for dilution antimicrobial susceptibility testing for bacteria that grow aerobically: M07-A8*, Wayne, Pa, 1999, CLSI.

Clinical and Laboratory Standards Institute: *Methods for antimicrobial dilution and disk susceptibility testing of infrequently isolated or fastidious bacteria: approved guideline—M45-A2*, Wayne, Pa, 1999, CLSI.

Clinical and Laboratory Standards Institute: *Analysis and presentation of cumulative antimicrobial susceptibility test data: approved guideline—M39-A3*, Wayne, Pa, 2013, CLSI.

Clinical and Laboratory Standards Institute: *Performance standards for antimicrobial disk susceptibility testing: M02-A10*, Wayne, Pa, 2013, CLSI.

Clinical and Laboratory Standards Institute: *Performance standards for antimicrobial susceptibility testing: M100-S21*, Wayne, Pa, 2013, CLSI.

Courvalin P: Interpretive reading of antimicrobial susceptibility tests, *Am Soc Microbiol News* 58:368, 1992.

Ohnishi M, Saika T, Hoshira S et al: Ceftraizone-resistant *Neisseria gonorrhoeal*, Japan, *Emerging Infectious Diseases* 17(1):148-9, 2011.

Stefaniuk E, Baraniak A, Gniadkowski M et al: Evaluation of the BD Phoenix Automated Identification and Susceptibility Testing System in clinical microbiology laboratory practice, *Eur J Clin Microbiol Infect Dis* 22:479, 2003.

Steward CD, Raney PM, Morrell AK et al: Testing for induction of clindamycin resistance in erythromycin-resistant isolates of *Staphylococcus aureus*, *J Clin Microbiol* 43:1716, 2005.

# Principles of Identification

# Overview of Bacterial Identification Methods and Strategies

## OBJECTIVES

*This chapter provides an overview of the traditional biochemical methods used to identify microorganisms. The student should study these detailed technical procedures in conjunction with specific chapters in this section to develop a clear understanding of the full process from specimen collection to identification. General objectives for the methods presented in this chapter include the following:*

1. State the specific diagnostic purpose for each test methodology.
2. Briefly describe the test principle associated with each test methodology.
3. Outline limitations and explain ways to trouble-shoot or report results in the event the test result indicates a false positive or false negative or is equivocal.
4. State the appropriate quality control organisms and results used with each testing procedure.

## ▤ RATIONALE FOR APPROACHING ORGANISM IDENTIFICATION

It is challenging to determine how most effectively to present and teach diagnostic microbiology in a way that is sufficiently comprehensive and yet not excessively cluttered with rare and seldom-needed facts about bacterial species uncommonly encountered. Approximately 530 different bacterial species or taxa are reported by clinical microbiology laboratories across the United States (Figure 13-1). Yet 95% of the bacterial identifications reported are distributed across only 27 of these taxa. This is an indication of how infrequently the other 500 or more taxa are identified and reported. Therefore, although the chapters in Part III, Bacteriology, are intended to be comprehensive in terms of the variety of bacterial species presented, it is helpful to keep in perspective which taxa are most likely to be encountered in the clinical environment. The relative frequencies with which the common bacterial species and organism groups are reported in clinical laboratories are presented in Figure 13-2.

Historically, most chapters in microbiology texts have been organized by genus name; however, they failed to provide information and processes needed to understand what is involved in analyzing information from the clinical specimen to the identification of the correct

genus. Many texts (including this one) provide flow charts containing algorithms or identification schemes for organism workup. Although these are helpful, one must be aware of the limitations of flow charts. In some cases they may be too general to be helpful; that is, they may lack sufficient detail to be useful for discriminating among key microbial groups and species. In other cases, they may be too esoteric to be of practical use in routine clinical practice (e.g., identification schemes based on cellular analysis of fatty acid analysis). In addition, many other criteria that must be incorporated into the identification process are too complex to be included in most flow charts. Thus, flow charts are only one of many tools used in the field of diagnostic microbiology.

Also, as discussed later in this chapter, organism taxonomy and profiles continuously change. Detailed flow charts are at risk of quickly becoming outdated. Furthermore, as is evident throughout the chapters in Part III, diagnostic microbiology is full of exceptions to rules, and flow charts are not constructed in a manner that readily captures many of the important exceptions.

To meet the challenges of bacterial identification processes beyond what can be portrayed in flow charts, the chapters in Part III have been arranged to guide the student through the entire workup of a microorganism, beginning with initial culture of the specimen. In most instances, the first information a microbiologist uses in the identification process is the macroscopic description of the colony, or **colony morphology.** This includes the type of hemolysis (if any), pigment (if present), size, texture (opaque, translucent, or transparent), adherence to agar, pitting of agar, and many other characteristics (see Chapter 7). After careful observation of the colony, the Gram stain is used to separate the organism into a variety of broad categories based on Gram stain reaction and the cellular morphology of gram-positive or gram-negative bacteria (e.g., gram-positive cocci, gram-negative rods; see Chapter 6). For gram-positive organisms, the catalase test should follow the Gram stain, and testing on gram-negative organisms should begin with the oxidase test. These simple tests, plus growth on Mac-Conkey agar, if the isolate is a gram-negative rod or coccobacillus, help the microbiologist assign the organism to one of the primary categories (organized here as subsections). Application of the various identification methods and systems outlined in this chapter generate

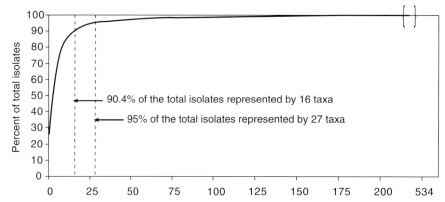

**Figure 13-1** Data demonstrating that more than 500 different bacterial species or taxa are reported from clinical laboratories across the United States. However, 95% of the isolates reported are distributed among only 27 different taxa, and more than 90% are represented by 16 different taxa. (Source: TSN Database—USA).

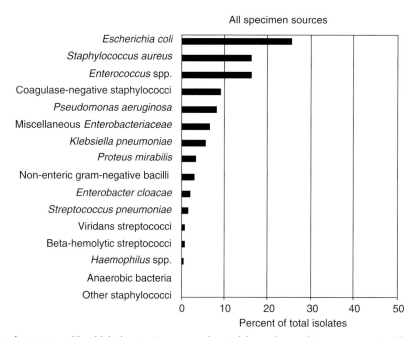

**Figure 13-2** Relative frequency with which the most common bacterial species and taxa are reported by clinical laboratories.

the data and criteria discussed in each chapter for the definitive identification of clinically relevant bacteria. Most of the procedures described in the following chapters can be found at the end of this chapter. In this chapter, each procedure includes a photograph of positive and negative reactions. Chapter 6 includes photographs of some commonly used bacteriologic stains. In addition, Table 13-1 lists several commonly used commercial identification systems for a variety of the microorganisms discussed in the following pages.

Because diagnostic microbiology is centered around the identification of organisms based on common phenotypic traits shared with known members of the same genus or family, microbiologists "play the odds" every day by finding the best biochemical "fit" and assigning the most

probable identification. For example, the gram-negative rod known as CDC group EF-4a may be considered with either MacConkey-positive or MacConkey-negative organisms, because it grows on MacConkey agar 50% of the time. Therefore, although CDC group EF-4a has been arbitrarily assigned to the section on oxidase-positive, MacConkey-positive, gram-negative bacilli and coccobacilli in this text, it is also included in the discussion of oxidase-positive, MacConkey-negative, gram-negative bacilli and coccobacilli. This example clearly demonstrates the limitations of solely depending on flow charts for the identification process.

The identification process often can be arduous and a drain on resources. Laboratorians must make every effort to identify only those organisms most likely to be

**TABLE 13-1** Examples of Commercial Identification Systems for Various Organisms

| Organism Group | System Type | Manufacturer | Incubation Time |
|---|---|---|---|
| Enterobacteriaceae | Manual: | | |
| | API 20E | bioMérieux* | 24-48 hr |
| | API Rapid 20E | bioMérieux | 4 hr |
| | Crystal Enteric/Nonfermenter | Becton Dickinson Diagnostic Systems† | 18 hr |
| | RapID ONE | Remel‡ | 4 hr |
| | Automated: | | |
| | GNI | bioMérieux | 4-13 hr |
| | GNI+ | bioMérieux | 2-12 hr |
| | NEG ID Type 2 | Dade MicroScan§ | 15-42 hr |
| | Rapid NEG ID Type 3 | Dade MicroScan | 2.5 hr |
| | Sensititre AP80 | Trek Diagnostic Systems¶ | 5-18 hr |
| *Enterococcus* spp. and *Streptococcus* spp. | Manual: | | |
| | API 20 Strep | bioMérieux | 4-24 hr |
| | RapID STR | Remel | 4 hr |
| | Crystal Gram-Positive ID | Becton Dickinson Diagnostic Systems | 18 hr |
| | Automated: | | |
| | GPI | bioMérieux | 2-15 hr |
| | Pos ID2 | Dade MicroScan | 18-48 hr |
| | Sensititre AP90 | Trek Diagnostic Systems | 24 hr |
| *Haemophilus* spp. | Manual: | | |
| | API NH | bioMérieux | 2 hr |
| | RapID NH | Remel | 4 hr |
| | NHI | bioMérieux | 4 hr |
| | Crystal *Neisseria/Haemophilus* | Becton Dickinson Diagnostic Systems | 4 hr |
| | Automated: | | |
| | HNID | Dade MicroScan | 4 hr |
| *Neisseria* spp. and *Moraxella catarrhalis* | Manual: | | |
| | API NH | bioMérieux | 2 hr |
| | RapID NH | Remel | 4 hr |
| | NHI | bioMérieux | 4 hr |
| | Crystal *Neisseria/Haemophilus* | Becton Dickinson Diagnostic Systems | 4 hr |
| | Automated: | | |
| | HNID | Dade MicroScan | 4 hr |
| Nonenteric gram-negative rods | Manual: | | |
| | API 20NE | bioMérieux | 24-48 hr |
| | Crystal Enteric/Nonfermenter | Becton Dickinson Diagnostic Systems | 18-20 hr |
| | RapID NF Plus | Remel | 4 hr |
| | Automated: | | |
| | GNI | bioMérieux | 2-18 hr |
| | NEG ID Type 2 | Dade MicroScan | 15-42 hr |
| | Sensititre AP80 | Trek Diagnostic Systems | 5-18 hr |

*Continued*

**TABLE 13-1** Examples of Commercial Identification Systems for Various Organisms—cont'd

| Organism Group | System Type | | Manufacturer | Incubation Time |
|---|---|---|---|---|
| *Staphylococcus* spp. | Manual: | | | |
| | | API STAPH | bioMérieux | 24 hr |
| | | Crystal Gram-Positive | Becton Dickinson Diagnostic Systems | 18-24 hr |
| | Automated: | | | |
| | | GPI | bioMérieux | 2-15 hr |
| | | Pos ID2 | Date MicroScan | 24-48 hr |
| Coryneform rods | Manual: | | | |
| | | API Coryne | bioMérieux | 24 hr |
| | | RapID CB Plus | Remel | 4 hr |
| | | Crystal Gram-Positive | Becton Dickinson Diagnostic Systems | 18-24 hr |
| | Automated: | | | |
| | | GPI | bioMérieux | 2-15 hr |

*Durham, N.C.: www.bioMerieux-Vitek.com
†Sparks, Md.: www.bectondickinson.com
‡Lenexa, Kan.: www.remelinc.com
§West Sacramento, Calif.: www.dadebehring.com
¶Westlake, Ohio: www.trekds.com

involved in the infection process. To that end, the chapters in Part III have also been designed to provide guidance for determining whether a clinical isolate is relevant and requires full identification. Furthermore, the clinical diagnosis and the source of the specimen can help determine which group of organisms to consider. For example, if a patient has endocarditis or the specimen source is blood and a small, gram-negative rod is observed on Gram stain, the microbiologist should consider a group of gram-negative bacilli known as the HACEK (Aggregatibacter [formerly the *aphrophilus* group of *Haemophilus* and *Actinobacillus*], *Cardiobacterium hominis*, *Eikenella corrodens*, and *Kingella* spp.), which are not commonly encountered in clinical specimens. Similarly, if a patient has suffered an animal bite, the microbiologist should think of *Pasteurella multocida* if the isolate is gram negative and *Staphylococcus hyicus* and *Staphylococcus intermedius* if the organism is gram positive. Finally, in consideration of an isolate's clinical relevance, each chapter also provides information on whether antimicrobial susceptibility testing is indicated and, if needed, the way it should be performed.

# FUTURE TRENDS OF ORGANISM IDENTIFICATION

Several dynamics are involved in clinical microbiology and infectious diseases that continue to challenge bacterial identification practices. For instance, new species associated with human infections will continue to be discovered, and well-known species may change their characteristics, affecting the criteria used to identify them. For these reasons, identification schemes and strategies for both conventional methods and commercial systems must be continually reviewed and updated. Also, although most identification schemes are based on the phenotypic characteristics of bacteria, the use of molecular and advanced chemical methods (e.g., matrix-assisted laser desorption/ionization time-of-flight mass spectrometry) to detect, identify, and characterize bacteria continues to expand and play a greater role in diagnostic microbiology. In addition, phenotypic, molecular, and advanced chemical methods increasingly will become incorporated into simpler automated systems.

## PROCEDURE 13-1

## Acetamide Utilization

### Purpose
Differentiate microorganisms based on the ability to use acetamide as the sole source of carbon.

### Principle
Bacteria capable of growth on this medium produce the enzyme acylamidase, which deaminates acetamide to release ammonia. The production of ammonia results in an alkaline pH, causing the medium to change color from green to royal blue.

Media: NaCl (5 g), NH4H2PO4 (1 g), K2HPO4 (1 g), agar (15 g), bromthymol blue indicator (0.8 g), per 1000 mL, acetamide (10 g), pH 6.8.

### Method
1. Inoculate acetamide slant with a needle using growth from an 18- to 24-hour culture. Do not inoculate from a broth culture, because the growth will be too heavy.

2. Incubate aerobically at 35°-37°C for up to 4 days. If equivocal, the slant may be reincubated for 2 additional days.

### Expected Results
Positive: Deamination of the acetamide, resulting in a blue color (Figure 13-3, A).
Negative: No color change (Figure 13-3, B).

### Limitations
Growth without a color change may indicate a positive test result. If further incubation results in no color change, repeat test with less inoculum.

### Quality Control
Positive: *Pseudomonas aeruginosa* (ATCC 27853)—growth; blue color
Negative: *Escherichia coli* (ATCC 25922)—no growth; green color

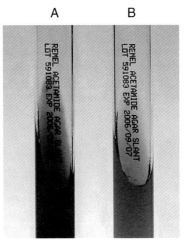

**Figure 13-3** Acetamide utilization. **A,** Positive. **B,** Negative.

## PROCEDURE 13-2

## Acetate Utilization

### Purpose
Differentiate organisms based on ability to use acetate as the sole source of carbon. Generally used to differentiate *Shigella* sp. from *Escherichia coli*.

### Principle
This test is used to differentiate an organism capable of using acetate as the sole source of carbon. Organisms capable of using sodium acetate grow on the medium, resulting in an alkaline pH, turning the indicator from green to blue.

Media: NaC2H3O2 (2 g); MgSO4 (0.1 g); NaCl (5 g); NH4H2PO4 (1 g); agar (20 g); bromthymol blue indicator (0.8 g), per 1000 mL, pH 6.7.

### Method
1. With a straight inoculating needle, inoculate acetate slant lightly from an 18- to 24-hour culture. Do not inoculate from a broth culture, because the growth will be too heavy.
2. Incubate at 35°-37°C for up to 7 days.

### Expected Results
Positive: Medium becomes alkalinized (blue) as a result of the growth and use of acetate (Figure 13-4, A).
Negative: No growth or growth with no indicator change to blue (Figure 13-4, B).

### Limitations
Some strains of *E. coli* may use acetate at a very slow rate or not at all, resulting in a false negative reaction in the identification process.

### Quality Control
Positive: *Escherichia coli* (ATCC 25922)—growth; blue
Negative: *Shigella sonnei* (ATCC 25931)—small amount of growth; green

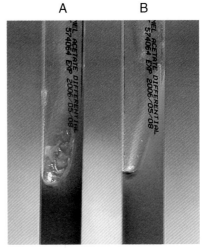

**Figure 13-4** Acetate utilization. **A,** Positive. **B,** Negative.

# Bacitracin Susceptibility

## Purpose

This test is used for presumptive identification and differentiation of beta-hemolytic group A streptococci (*Streptococcus pyogenes*–susceptible) from other beta-hemolytic streptococci. It is also used to distinguish staphylococci species (resistant) from micrococci (susceptible).

## Principle

The antibiotic bacitracin inhibits the synthesis of bacterial cell walls. A disk (TaxoA) impregnated with a small amount of bacitracin (0.04 units) is placed on an agar plate, allowing the antibiotic to diffuse into the medium and inhibit the growth of susceptible organisms. After incubation, the inoculated plates are examined for zones of inhibition surrounding the disks.

## Method

1. Using an inoculating loop, streak two or three suspect colonies of a pure culture onto a blood agar plate.
2. Using heated forceps, place a bacitracin disk in the first quadrant (area of heaviest growth). Gently tap the disk to ensure adequate contact with the agar surface.
3. Incubate the plate for 18 to 24 hours at 35°-37°C in ambient air for staphylococci and in 5% to 10% carbon dioxide ($CO_2$) for streptococci differentiation.
4. Look for a zone of inhibition around the disk.

## Expected Results

Positive: Any zone of inhibition greater than 10 mm; susceptible (Figure 13-5, *A*).
Negative: No zone of inhibition; resistant (Figure 13-5, *B*).

## Limitations

Performance depends on the integrity of the disk. Proper storage and expiration dates should be maintained.

## Quality Control

Positive: *Streptococcus pyogenes* (ATCC19615)—susceptible
*Micrococcus luteus* (ATCC10240)—susceptible
Negative: *Streptococcus agalactiae* (ATCC27956)—resistant
*Staphylococcus aureus* (ATCC25923)—resistant

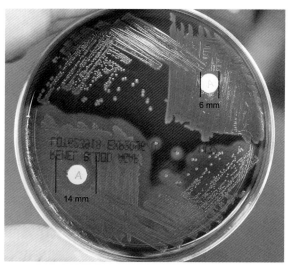

**Figure 13-5** Bacitracin (A disk) Susceptibility. Any zone of inhibition is positive *(Streptococcus pyogenes)*; growth up to the disk is negative *(Streptococcus agalactiae)*.

## Bile Esculin Test

### Purpose
This test is used for the presumptive identification of enterococci and organisms in the *Streptococcus bovis* group. The test differentiates enterococci and group D streptococci from non–group D viridans streptococci.

### Principle
Gram-positive bacteria other than some streptococci and enterococci are inhibited by the bile salts in this medium. Organisms capable of growth in the presence of 4% bile and able to hydrolyze esculin to esculetin. Esculetin reacts with Fe3+ and forms a dark brown to black precipitate.

Media: Beef extract (11 g), enzymatic digest of gelatin (34.5 g), esculin (1 g), ox bile (2 g), ferric ammonium citrate (0.5 g), agar (15 g), per 1000 mL, pH 6.6.

### Method
1. Inoculate one to two colonies from an 18- to 24-hour culture onto the surface of the slant.
2. Incubate at 35°-37°C in ambient air for 48 hours.

### Expected Results
Positive: Growth and blackening of the agar slant (Figure 13-6, *A*)
Negative: Growth and no blackening of medium (Figure 13-6, *B*)
No growth (not shown)

### Limitations
As a result of nutritional requirements, some organisms may grow poorly or not at all on this medium.

### Quality Control
Positive: *Enterococcus faecalis* (ATCC19433)—growth; black precipitate
Negative: *Escherichia coli* (ATCC25922)—growth; no color change
*Streptococcus pyogenes* (ATCC19615)—no growth; no color change

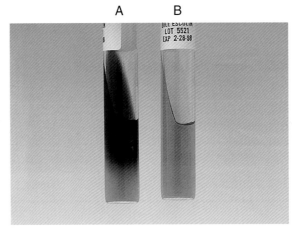

**Figure 13-6** Bile esculin agar. **A,** Positive. **B,** Negative.

## Bile Solubility Test

### Purpose
This test differentiates *Streptococcus pneumoniae* (positive–soluble) from alpha-hemolytic streptococci (negative–insoluble).

### Principle
Bile or a solution of a bile salt (e.g., sodium desoxycholate) rapidly lyses pneumococcal colonies. Lysis depends on the presence of an intracellular autolytic enzyme, amidase. Bile salts lower the surface tension between the bacterial cell membrane and the medium, thus accelerating the organism's natural autolytic process.

### Method
1. After 12 to 24 hours of incubation on 5% sheep blood agar, place 1 to 2 drops of 10% sodium desoxycholate on a well-isolated colony.
   *Note:* A tube test is performed with 2% sodium desoxycholate.
2. Gently wash liquid over the colony without dislodging the colony from the agar.
3. Incubate the plate at 35°-37°C in ambient air for 30 minutes.
4. Examine for lysis of colony.

### Expected Results
Positive: Colony disintegrates; an imprint of the lysed colony may remain in the zone (Figure 13-7, *A*).
Negative: Intact colonies (Figure 13-7, *B*).

### Limitations
Enzyme activity may be reduced in old cultures. Therefore, negative results with colonies resembling *S. pneumoniae* should be further tested for identification with alternate methods.

### Quality Control
Positive: *Streptococcus pneumoniae* (ATCC49619)—bile soluble
Negative: *Enterococcus faecalis* (ATCC29212)—bile insoluble

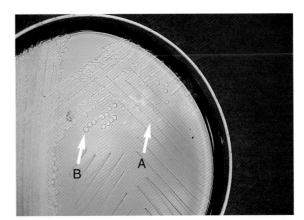

**Figure 13-7** Bile solubility (desoxycholate) test. **A,** Colony lysed. **B,** Intact colony.

## Butyrate Disk

### Purpose
This is a rapid test to detect the enzyme butyrate esterase, to aid identification of *Moraxella (Branhamella) catarrhalis.*

### Principle
Organisms capable of producing butyrate esterase hydrolyze bromochlorindolyl butyrate. Hydrolysis of the substrate in the presence of butyrate esterase releases indoxyl, which in the presence of oxygen spontaneously forms indigo, a blue to blue-violet color.

### Method
1. Remove a disk from the vial and place on a glass microscope slide.
2. Add 1 drop of reagent-grade water. This should leave a slight excess of water on the disk.
3. Using a wooden applicator stick, rub a small amount of several colonies from an 18- to 24-hour pure culture onto the disk.
4. Incubate at room temperature for up to 5 minutes.

### Expected Results
Positive: Development of a blue color during the 5-minute incubation period (Figure 13-8, *A*).
Negative: No color change (Figure 13-8, *B*).

### Limitations
Incubation longer than 5 minutes may result in a false-positive reaction.

False-negative reactions may occur if the inoculum is too small. If the organism is negative, repeat with a larger inoculum and follow-up with additional methods.

### Quality Control
Positive: *Moraxella catarrhalis* (ATCC25240)—formation of blue color
Negative: *Neisseria gonorrhoeae* (ATCC43069)—no color change

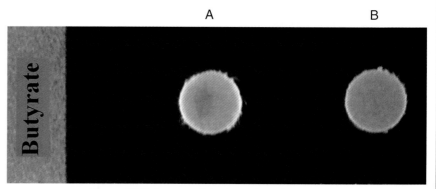

**Figure 13-8** Butyrate disk. **A,** Positive. **B,** Negative.

## CAMP Test

### Purpose
The Christie, Atkins, and Munch-Peterson (CAMP) test is used to differentiate group B streptococci (*Streptococcus agalactiae*–positive) from other streptococcal species. *Listeria monocytogenes* also produces a positive CAMP reaction.

### Principle
Certain organisms (including group B streptococci) produce a diffusible extracellular hemolytic protein (CAMP factor) that acts synergistically with the beta-lysin of *Staphylococcus aureus* to cause enhanced lysis of red blood cells. The group B streptococci are streaked perpendicular to a streak of *S. aureus* on sheep blood agar. A positive reaction appears as an arrowhead zone of hemolysis adjacent to the place where the two streak lines come into proximity.

### Method
1. Streak a beta-lysin–producing strain of *S. aureus* down the center of a sheep blood agar plate.
2. Streak test organisms across the plate perpendicular to the *S. aureus* streak within 2 mm. (Multiple organisms can be tested on a single plate).
3. Incubate overnight at 35°-37°C in ambient air.

### Expected Results
Positive: Enhanced hemolysis is indicated by an arrowhead-shaped zone of beta-hemolysis at the juncture of the two organisms (Figure 13-9, *A*).
Negative: No enhancement of hemolysis (Figure 13-9, *B*).

### Limitations
A small percentage of group A streptococci may have a positive CAMP reaction. The test should be limited to colonies with the characteristic group B streptococci morphology and narrow zone beta-hemolysis on sheep blood agar.

### Quality Control
Positive: *Streptococcus agalactiae* (ATCC13813)—enhanced arrowhead hemolysis
Negative: *Streptococcus pyogenes* (ATCC19615)—beta-hemolysis without enhanced arrowhead formation

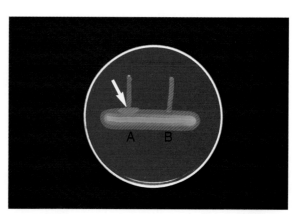

**Figure 13-9** CAMP test. **A,** Positive; arrowhead zone of beta-hemolysis *(at arrow)*, typical of group B streptococci. **B,** Negative; no enhancement of hemolysis.

## Catalase Test

### Purpose
This test differentiates catalase-positive micrococcal and staphylococcal species from catalase-negative streptococcal species.

### Principle
Aerobic and facultative anaerobic organisms produce two toxins during normal metabolism, hydrogen peroxide ($H_2O_2$) and superoxide radical ($O2-$). These bacteria have two enzymes that detoxify the products of normal metabolism. One of these enzymes, catalase, is capable of converting hydrogen peroxide to water and oxygen. The presence of the enzyme in a bacterial isolate is evidenced when a small inoculum introduced into hydrogen peroxide (30% for the slide test) causes rapid elaboration of oxygen bubbles. The lack of catalase is evident by a lack of or weak bubble production.

### Method
1. Use a loop or sterile wooden stick to transfer a small amount of colony growth to the surface of a clean, dry glass slide.
2. Place a drop of 30% hydrogen peroxide ($H_2O_2$) onto the medium.
3. Observe for the evolution of oxygen bubbles (Figure 13-10).

### Expected Results
Positive: Copious bubbles are produced (Figure 13-10, *A*).
Negative: No or few bubbles are produced (Figure 13-10, *B*).

### Limitations
Some organisms (enterococci) produce a peroxidase that slowly catalyzes the breakdown of $H_2O_2$, and the test may appear weakly positive. This reaction is not a truly positive test.

False positives may occur if the sample is contaminated with blood agar.

### Quality Control
Positive: *Staphylococcus aureus* (ATCC25923)
Negative: *Streptococcus pyogenes* (ATCC19615)

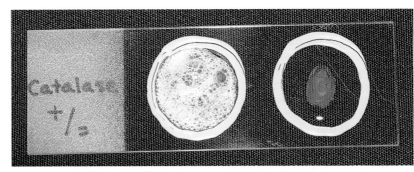

**Figure 13-10** Catalase test. **A,** Positive. **B,** Negative.

## Cetrimide Agar

### Purpose
This test is primarily used to isolate and purify *Pseudomonas aeruginosa* from contaminated specimens.

### Principle
The test is used to determine the ability of an organism to grow in the presence of cetrimide, a toxic substance that inhibits the growth of many bacteria by causing the release of nitrogen and phosphorous, which slows or kills the organism. *P. aeruginosa* is resistant to cetrimide.

Media: Enzymatic digest of gelatin (20 g), MgCl2 (1.4 g), K2SO4 (10 g), cetrimide (cetyltrimethylammonium bromide) (0.3 g), agar (13.6), pH 7.2.

### Method
1. Inoculate a cetrimide agar slant with 1 drop of an 18- to 24-hour brain-heart infusion broth culture.
2. Incubate at 35°-37°C for up to 7 days.
3. Examine the slant for bacterial growth.

### Expected Results
Positive: Growth, variation in color of colonies (Figure 13-11, *A*).
Negative: No growth (Figure 13-11, *B*).

### Limitations
Some enteric organisms will grow and exhibit a weak yellow color in the media. This color change is distinguishable from the production of fluorescein.

Additional testing is necessary to confirm a diagnosis of *P. aeruginosa*.

### Quality Control
Positive: *Pseudomonas aeruginosa* (ATCC27853)—growth and color change; yellow-green to blue-green colonies
Negative: *Escherichia coli* (ATCC25922)—no growth and no color change

A                                      B

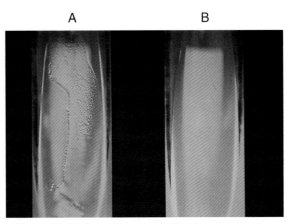

**Figure 13-11** Cetrimide agar. **A,** Positive. **B,** Negative.

# Citrate Utilization

### Purpose

The purpose of this test is to identify organisms capable of using sodium citrate as the sole carbon source and inorganic ammonium salts as the sole nitrogen source. The test is part of a series referred to as IMViC (indole, methyl red, Voges-Proskauer, and citrate), which is used to differentiate Enterobacteriaceae from other gram-negative rods.

### Principle

Bacteria that can grow on this medium produce an enzyme, citrate-permease, capable of converting citrate to pyruvate. Pyruvate can then enter the organism's metabolic cycle for the production of energy. Bacteria capable of growth in this medium use the citrate and convert ammonium phosphate to ammonia and ammonium hydroxide, creating an alkaline pH. The pH change turns the bromthymol blue indicator from green to blue.

Media: $NH_4H_2PO_4$ (1 g), $K_2HPO_4$ (1 g), NaCl (5 g), sodium citrate (2 g), $MgSO_4$ (0.2 g), agar (15 g), bromthymol blue (0.08 g), per 1000 mL, pH 6.9.

### Method

1. Inoculate Simmons citrate agar lightly on the slant by touching the tip of a needle to a colony that is 18 to 24 hours old. Do not inoculate from a broth culture, because the inoculum will be too heavy.
2. Incubate at 35°-37°C for up to 7 days.
3. Observe for growth and the development of blue color, denoting alkalinization.

### Expected Results

Positive: Growth on the medium, with or without a change in the color of the indicator. Growth typically results in the bromthymol blue indicator turning from green to blue (Figure 13-12, *A*).

Negative: Absence of growth (Figure 13-12, *B*).

### Limitations

Some organisms are capable of growth on citrate and do not produce a color change. Growth is considered a positive citrate utilization test, even in the absence of a color change.

### Quality Control

Positive: *Enterobacter aerogenes* (ATCC13048)—growth, blue color

Negative: *Escherichia coli* (ATCC25922)—little to no growth, no color change

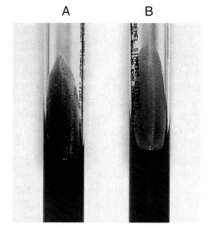

**Figure 13-12** Citrate utilization. **A,** Positive. **B,** Negative.

## Coagulase Test

### Purpose

The test is used to differentiate *Staphylococcus aureus* (positive) from coagulase-negative staphylococci (negative).

### Principle

*S. aureus* produces two forms of coagulase, bound and free. Bound coagulase, or "clumping factor," is bound to the bacterial cell wall and reacts directly with fibrinogen. This results in precipitation of fibrinogen on the staphylococcal cell, causing the cells to clump when a bacterial suspension is mixed with plasma. The presence of bound coagulase correlates with free coagulase, an extracellular protein enzyme that causes the formation of a clot when *S. aureus* colonies are incubated with plasma. The clotting mechanism involves activation of a plasma coagulase-reacting factor (CRF), which is a modified or derived thrombin molecule, to form a coagulase-CRF complex. This complex in turn reacts with fibrinogen to produce the fibrin clot.

### Method

#### A. Slide Test (Detection of ?)

1. Place a drop of coagulase plasma (preferably rabbit plasma with ethylenediaminetetraacetic acid [EDTA]) on a clean, dry, glass slide.
2. Place a drop of distilled water or saline next to the drop of plasma as a control.
3. With a loop, straight wire, or wooden stick, emulsify a portion of the isolated colony being tested in each drop, inoculating the water or saline first. Try to create a smooth suspension.
4. Mix well with a wooden applicator stick.
5. Rock the slide gently for 5 to 10 seconds.

### Expected Results

Positive: Macroscopic clumping in 10 seconds or less in coagulated plasma drop and no clumping in saline or water drop (Figure 13-13, *A*, left side).

Negative: No clumping in either drop.

*Note:* All negative slide tests must be confirmed using the tube test (Figure 13-13, *B*, right side).

#### B. Tube Test

1. Emulsify several colonies in 0.5 mL of rabbit plasma (with EDTA) to give a milky suspension.
2. Incubate tube at 35°-37°C in ambient air for 4 hours.
3. Check for clot formation.

### Expected Results

Positive: Clot of any size (Figure 13-13, *A*, left side).

Negative: No clot (Figure 13-13, *B*, right side).

### Limitations

#### Slide Test

Equivocal: Clumping in both drops indicates that the organism autoagglutinates and is unsuitable for the slide coagulase test.

#### Tube Test

1. Test results can be positive at 4 hours and then revert to negative after 24 hours.
2. If negative at 4 hours, incubate at room temperature overnight and check again for clot formation.

### Quality Control

Positive: *Staphylococcus aureus* (ATCC25923)
Negative: *Staphylococcus epidermidis* (ATC12228)

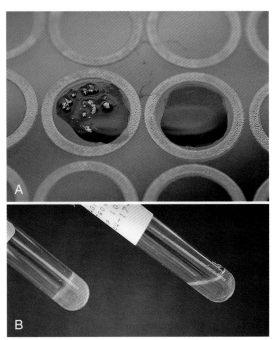

**Figure 13-13** Coagulase test. **A,** Slide coagulase test for clumping factor. Left side is positive; right side is negative. **B,** Tube coagulase test for free coagulase. Tube on the left is positive, exhibiting clot. Tube on the right is negative.

## Decarboxylase Tests (Moeller's Method)

### Purpose
This test is used to differentiate decarboxylase-producing Enterobacteriaceae from other gram-negative rods.

### Principle
This test measures the enzymatic ability (decarboxylase) of an organism to decarboxylate (or hydrolyze) an amino acid to form an amine. Decarboxylation, or hydrolysis, of the amino acid results in an alkaline pH and a color change from orange to purple.

Media: Peptic digest of animal tissue (5 g), beef extract (5 g), bromcresol purple (0.1 g), cresol red (0.005 g), dextrose (0.5 g), pyridoxal (0.005 g), amino acid (10 g), pH 6.0.

### Method
#### A. Glucose-Nonfermenting Organisms
1. Prepare a suspension (≥McFarland No. 5 turbidity standard) in brain-heart infusion broth from an overnight culture (18 to 24 hours old) growing on 5% sheep blood agar.
2. Inoculate each of the three decarboxylase broths (arginine, lysine, and ornithine) and the control broth (no amino acid) with 4 drops of broth.
3. Add a 4-mm layer of sterile mineral oil to each tube.
4. Incubate the cultures at 35°-37°C in ambient air. Examine the tubes at 24, 48, 72, and 96 hours.

#### B. Glucose-Fermenting Organisms
1. Inoculate tubes with 1 drop of an 18- to 24-hour brain-heart infusion broth culture.
2. Add a 4-mm layer of sterile mineral oil to each tube.

3. Incubate the cultures for 4 days at 35°-37°C in ambient air. Examine the tubes at 24, 48, 72, and 96 hours.

### Expected Results
Positive: Alkaline (purple) color change compared with the control tube (Figure 13-14, A).
Negative: No color change or acid (yellow) color in test and control tube. Growth in the control tube.

### Limitations
The fermentation of dextrose in the medium causes the acid color change. However, it would not mask the alkaline color change brought about by a positive decarboxylation reaction (Figure 13-14, B). An uninoculated tube is shown in Figure 13-14, C.

### Quality Control
Positive:
    Lysine—*Klebsiella pneumoniae* (ATCC33495)
    Ornithine—*Enterobacter aerogenes* (ATCC13048)
    Arginine—*Enterobacter cloacae* (ATCC13047)
Base—
Negative:
    Lysine—*Enterobacter cloacae* (ATCC13047)
    Ornithine—*Klebsiella pneumoniae* (ATCC13883)
    Arginine—*Klebsiella pneumoniae* (ATCC33495)
    Base—*Klebsiella pneumoniae* (ATC33495)

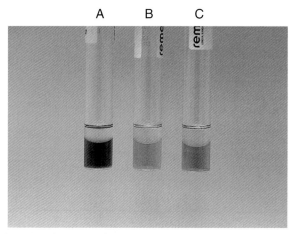

**Figure 13-14** Decarboxylase tests (Moeller's method). **A,** Positive. **B,** Negative. **C,** Uninoculated tube.

## DNA Hydrolysis (DNase Test Agar)

### Purpose
This test is used to differentiate organisms based on the production of deoxyribonuclease. It is used to distinguish *Serratia* sp. (positive) from *Enterobacter* sp., *Staphylococcus aureus* (positive) from other species, and *Moraxella catarrhalis* (positive) from *Neisseria* sp.

### Principle
The test is used to determine the ability of an organism to hydrolyze DNA. The medium is pale green because of the DNA–methyl green complex. If the organism growing on the medium hydrolyses DNA, the green color fades and the colony is surrounded by a colorless zone.

Media: Pancreatic digest of casein (10 g), yeast extract (10 g), deoxyribonucleic acid (2 g), NaCl (5 g), agar (15 g), methyl green (0.5 g), pH 7.5.

### Method
1. Inoculate the DNase agar with the organism to be tested and streak for isolation.
2. Incubate aerobically at 35°-37°C for 13 to 24 hours.

### Expected Results
Positive: When DNA is hydrolyzed, methyl green is released and combines with highly polymerized DNA at a pH of 7.5, turning the medium colorless around the test organism (Figure 13-15, *A* and *B*).

Negative: If no degradation of DNA occurs, the medium remains green (Figure 13-15, *C*).

### Limitations
Agar must be inoculated with a suspension of a young broth culture (4 hours old) or an 18- to 24-hour colony in 1-2 mL of saline.

### Quality Control
Positive: *Staphylococcus aureus* (ATCC25923)
Negative: *Escherichia coli* (ATCC25922)

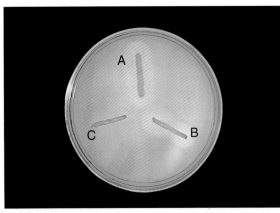

**Figure 13-15** DNA hydrolysis. **A,** Positive, *Staphylococcus aureus*. **B,** Positive, *Serratia marcescens*. **C,** Negative.

## Esculin Hydrolysis

### Purpose
This test is used for the presumptive identification and differentiation of Enterobacteriaceae.

### Principle
This test is used to determine whether an organism is able to hydrolyze the glycoside esculin. Esculin is hydrolyzed to esculetin, which reacts with Fe3+ and forms a dark brown to black precipitate.

Media: NaCl (8 g), $K_2HPO_4$ (0.4 g), $KH_2PO_4$ (0.1 g), esculin (5 g), ferric ammonium citrate (0.5 g), agar (15 g), per 1000 mL, pH 7.0.

### Method
1. Inoculate the medium with 1 drop of a 24-hour broth culture.
2. Incubate at 35°-37°C for up to 7 days.
3. Examine the slants for blackening and, under the ultraviolet rays of a Wood's lamp, for esculin hydrolysis.

### Expected Results
Positive: Blackened medium (Figure 13-16, *A*), which would also show a loss of fluorescence under the Wood's lamp.

Negative: No blackening and no loss of fluorescence under the Wood's lamp, or slight blackening with no loss of fluorescence under the Wood's lamp. An uninoculated tube is shown in Figure 13-16, *B*.

### Limitations
This medium is a nonselective agar. The bile esculin hydrolysis test presented in Procedure 13-4 is a selective differential method.

### Quality Control
Positive: *Enterococcus faecalis* (ATCC29212)
Negative: *Escherichia coli* (ATCC25922)

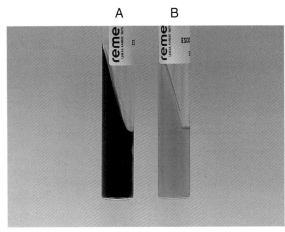

**Figure 13-16** Esculin hydrolysis. **A,** Positive, blackening of slant. **B,** Uninoculated tube.

**PROCEDURE 13-15**

## Fermentation Media

### Purpose

Fermentation media are used to differentiate organisms based on their ability to ferment carbohydrates incorporated into the basal medium. Andrade's formula is used to differentiate enteric bacteria from coryneforms, and bromocresol purple is used to distinguish enterococci from streptococci.

### Principle

Carbohydrate fermentation is the process microorganisms use to produce energy. Most microorganisms convert glucose to pyruvate during glycolysis; however, some organisms use alternate pathways. A fermentation medium consists of a basal medium containing a single carbohydrate (glucose, lactose, or sucrose) for fermentation. However, the medium may contain various color indicators, such as Andrade's indicator, bromocresol, or others. In addition to a color indicator to detect the production of acid from fermentation, a Durham tube is placed in each tube to capture gas produced by metabolism.

Basal media: Pancreatic digest of casein (10 g), beef extract (3 g), NaCl (5 g), carbohydrate (10 g), specific indicator (Andrade's indicator [10 mL, pH 7.4] or bromocresol purple [0.02 g, pH 6.8]).

### Method

*A. Peptone Medium with Andrade's Indicator (for Enterics and Coryneforms)*

1. Inoculate each tube with 1 drop of an 18- to 24-hour brain-heart infusion broth culture.
2. Incubate at 35°-37°C for up to 7 days in ambient air.
   *Note:* Tubes are held only 4 days for organisms belonging to the Enterobacteriaceae family.
3. Examine the tubes for acid (indicated by a pink color) and gas production.
4. Tubes must show growth for the test to be valid. If no growth in the fermentation tubes or control is seen after 24 hours of incubation, add 1 to 2 drops of sterile rabbit serum per 5 mL of fermentation broth to each tube.

### Expected Results

Positive: Indicator change to pink with or without gas formation in Durham tube (Figure 13-17, *A,* left and middle).

Negative: Growth, but no change in color. Medium remains clear to straw colored (Figure 13-17, *A,* right).

*B. Broth (Brain Heart Infusion Broth May Be Substituted) with Bromcresol Purple Indicator (for Streptococci and Enterococci)*

1. Inoculate each tube with 2 drops of an 18- to 24-hour brain-heart infusion broth culture.
2. Incubate 4 days at 35°-37°C in ambient air.
3. Observe daily for a change of the bromcresol purple indicator from purple to yellow (acid).

### Expected Results

Positive: Indicator change to yellow (Figure 13-17, *B,* left).

Negative: Growth, but no change in color. Medium remains purple (Figure 13-17, *B,* right).

### Limitations

Readings after 24 hours may not be reliable if no acid is produced. No color change or a result indicating alkalinity may occur if the organism deaminates the peptone, masking the evidence of carbohydrate fermentation.

### Quality Control

*Note:* Appropriate organisms depend on which carbohydrate has been added to the basal medium. An example is given for each type of medium.

*A. Peptone Medium with Andrade's Indicator*
Dextrose:
 Positive, with gas: *Escherichia coli* (ATCC25922)
 Positive, no gas: *Shigella flexneri* (ATCC12022)

*B. Brain-Heart Infusion Broth with Bromocresol Purple Indicator*
Dextrose:
 Positive, with gas: *Escherichia coli* (ATCC25922)
 Negative, no gas: *Moraxella osloensis* (ATCC10973)

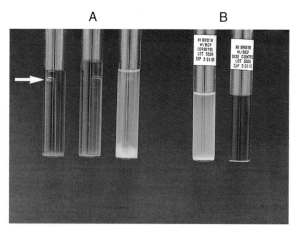

**Figure 13-17** Fermentation media. **A,** Peptone medium with Andrade's indicator. The tube on the left ferments glucose with the production of gas (visible as a bubble *[arrow]* in the inverted [Durham] tube); the tube in the middle ferments glucose with no gas production; and the tube on the right does not ferment glucose. **B,** Heart infusion broth with bromocresol purple indicator. The tube on the left is positive; the tube on the right is negative.

**PROCEDURE 13-16**

## Flagella Stain (Wet Mount Technique)

### Purpose
This technique is used to visualize the presence and arrangement of flagella for the presumptive identification of motile bacterial species.

### Principle
Flagella are too thin to be visualized using a bright field microscope with ordinary stains, such as the Gram stain, or a simple stain. A wet mount technique is used for staining bacterial flagella, and it is simple and useful when the number and arrangement of flagella are critical to the identification of species of motile bacteria. The staining procedures require the use of a mordant so that the stain adheres in layers to the flagella, allowing visualization.

### Method
1. Grow the organism to be stained at room temperature on blood agar for 16 to 24 hours.
2. Add a small drop of water to a microscope slide.
3. Dip a sterile inoculating loop into sterile water.
4. Touch the loopful of water to the colony margin briefly (this allows motile cells to swim into the droplet of water).
5. Touch the loopful of motile cells to the drop of water on the slide. *Note:* Agitating the loop in the droplet of water on the slide causes the flagella to shear off the cell.
6. Cover the faintly turbid drop of water on the slide with a cover slip. A proper wet mount has barely enough liquid to fill the space under a cover slip. Small air spaces around the edge are preferable.
7. Examine the slide immediately under 40× to 50× for motile cells. If motile cells are not seen, do not proceed with the stain.
8. If motile cells are seen, leave the slide at room temperature for 5 to 10 minutes. This allows the bacterial cells time to adhere either to the glass slide or to the cover slip.
9. Gently apply 2 drops of RYU flagella stain (Remel, Lenexa, Kansas) to the edge of the cover slip. The stain will flow by capillary action and mix with the cell suspension. Small air pockets around the

edge of the wet mount are useful in aiding the capillary action.
10. After 5 to 10 minutes at room temperature, examine the cells for flagella.
11. Cells with flagella may be observed at 100× (oil) in the zone of optimum stain concentration, about halfway from the edge of the cover slip to the center of the mount.
12. Focusing the microscope on the cells attached to the cover slip rather than on the cells attached to the slide facilitates visualization of the flagella. The precipitate from the stain is primarily on the slide rather than the cover slip.

### Expected Results
Observe the slide and note the following:
1. Presence or absence of flagella
2. Number of flagella per cell
3. Location of flagella per cell
   a. Peritrichous (Figure 13-18, *A*)
   b. Lophotrichous
   c. Polar (Figure 13-18, *B*)
4. Amplitude of wavelength
   a. Short
   b. Long
5. Whether or not "tufted"

### Limitations
Even with a specific stain, visualization of flagella requires an experienced laboratory scientist and is not considered an entry-level technique.

### Quality Control
Peritrichous: *Escherichia coli*
Polar: *Pseudomonas aeruginosa*
Negative: *Klebsiella pneumoniae*

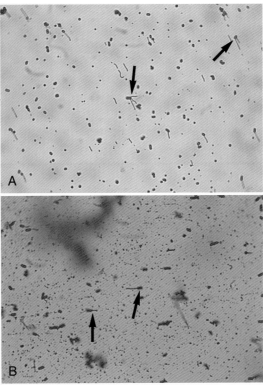

**Figure 13-18** **F**lagella stain (wet mount technique). **A,** *Alcaligenes* spp., peritrichous flagella *(arrows)*. **B,** *Pseudomonas aeruginosa,* polar flagella *(arrows)*.

## Gelatin Hydrolysis

### Purpose
The production of gelatinases capable of hydrolyzing gelatin is used as a presumptive test for the identification of various organisms, including *Staphylococcus* sp., Enterobacteriaceae, and some gram-positive bacilli.

### Principle
This test is used to determine the ability of an organism to produce extracellular proteolytic enzymes (gelatinases) that liquefy gelatin, a component of vertebrate connective tissue.

Nutrient gelatin medium differs from traditional microbiology media in that the solidifying agent (agar) is replaced with gelatin. When an organism produces gelatinase, the enzyme liquefies the growth medium.

Media: Enzymatic digest of gelatin (5 g), beef extract (3 g), gelatin (120 g), per 1000 mL, pH 6.8.

### Method
1. Inoculate the gelatin deep with 4 to 5 drops of a 24-hour broth culture.
2. Incubate at 35°-37°C in ambient air for up to 14 days. *Note:* Incubate the medium at 25°C if the organism grows better at 25°C than at 35°C.
3. Alternatively, inoculate the gelatin deep from a 24-hour-old colony by stabbing four or five times, 0.5 inch into the medium.
4. Remove the gelatin tube daily from the incubator and place at 4°C to check for liquefaction. Do not invert or tip the tube, because sometimes the only discernible liquefaction occurs at the top of the deep where inoculation occurred.
5. Refrigerate an uninoculated control along with the inoculated tube. Liquefaction is determined only after the control has hardened (gelled).

### Expected Results
Positive: Partial or total liquefaction of the inoculated tube (the control tube must be completely solidified) at 4°C within 14 days (Figure 13-19, *A*).
Negative: Complete solidification of the tube at 4°C (Figure 13-19, *B*).

### Limitations
Some organisms may grow poorly or not at all in this medium
Gelatin is liquid above 20°C; therefore determination of results must be completed following refrigeration.

### Quality Control
Positive: *Bacillus subtilis* (ATCC9372)
Negative: *Escherichia coli* (ATCC25922)
Uninoculated control tube: medium becomes solid after refrigeration.

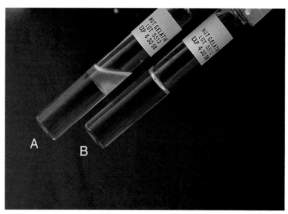

**Figure 13-19** Gelatin hydrolysis. **A,** Positive; note liquefaction at top of tube. **B,** Uninoculated tube.

## Growth at 42°C

### Purpose
This test is used to differentiate a pyocyanogenic pseudomonads from other *Pseudomonas* sp.

### Principle
The test is used to determine the ability of an organism to grow at 42°C. Several *Pseudomonas* species have been isolated in the clinical laboratory that are capable of growth at elevated temperatures.

### Method
1. Inoculate two tubes of trypticase soy agar (TSA) with a light inoculum by lightly touching a needle to the top of a single 13- to 24-hour-old colony and streaking the slant.
2. Immediately incubate one tube at 35°C and one at 42°C.
3. Record the presence of growth on each slant after 18 to 24 hours.

### Expected Results
Positive: Good growth at both 35°and 42°C (Figure 13-20, *A*).
Negative: No growth at 42°C (Figure 13-20, *B*), but good growth at 35°C.

### Quality Control
Positive: *Pseudomonas aeruginosa* (ATCC10145)
Negative: *Pseudomonas fluorescens* (ATCC13525)

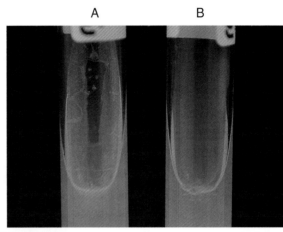

**Figure 13-20** Growth at 42°C. **A,** Positive; good growth. **B,** Negative; no growth.

## Hippurate Hydrolysis

### Purpose
Production of the enzyme hippuricase is used for the presumptive identification of a variety of microorganisms.

### Principle
The end products of hydrolysis of hippuric acid by hippuricase include glycine and benzoic acid. Glycine is deaminated by the oxidizing agent ninhydrin, which is reduced during the process. The end products of the ninhydrin oxidation react to form a purple-colored product. The test medium must contain only hippurate, because ninhydrin might react with any free amino acids present in growth media or other broths.

### Method
1. Add 0.1 mL of sterile water to a 12 ×75 mm plastic test tube.
2. Make a heavy suspension of the organism to be tested.
3. Using heated forceps, place a rapid hippurate disk in the mixture.
4. Cap and incubate the tube for 2 hours at 35°C; use of a water bath is preferred.

5. Add 0.2 mL ninhydrin reagent and reincubate for an additional 15 to 30 minutes. Observe the solution for the development of a deep purple color.

### Expected Results
Positive: Deep purple color (Figure 13-21, *A*).
Negative: Colorless or slightly yellow pink color (Figure 13-21, *B*).

### Limitations
A false-positive result may occur if incubation with ninhydrin exceeds 30 minutes.

### Quality Control
Positive: *Streptococcus agalactiae* (ATCC12386)
Negative: *Streptococcus pyogenes* (ATCC19615)

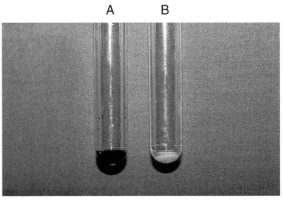

**Figure 13-21** Hippurate hydrolysis. **A,** Positive. **B,** Negative.

## Indole Production

### Purpose
This test is used to identify organisms that produce the enzyme tryptophanase.

### Principle
The test is used to determine an organism's ability to hydrolyze tryptophan to form the compound indole. Tryptophan is present in casein and animal protein. Bacteria with tryptophanase are capable of hydrolyzing tryptophan to pyruvate, ammonia, and indole. Kovac's reagent (dimethylamine-benzaldehyde and hydrochloride), when added to the broth culture, reacts with the indole, producing a red color. An alternative method uses Ehrlich's reagent. Ehrlich's reagent has the same chemicals as the Kovac preparation, but it also contains absolute ethyl alcohol, making it flammable. Ehrlich's reagent is more sensitive for detecting small amounts of indole. (The spot indole test is described in Procedure 13-39.)

Media: Casein peptone (10 g), NaCl (5 g), tryptophan (10 g), per 1000 mL.

### Method
#### A. Enterobacteriaceae
1. Inoculate tryptophane broth with 1 drop from a 24-hour brain-heart infusion broth culture.
2. Incubate at 35°-37°C in ambient air for 48 hours.
3. Add 0.5 mL of Kovac's reagent to the broth culture.

#### B. Other Gram-Negative Bacilli
1. Inoculate tryptophane broth with 1 drop of a 24-hour broth culture.

2. Incubate at 35°-37°C in ambient air for 48 hours.
3. Add 1 mL of xylene to the culture.
4. Shake the mixture vigorously to extract the indole and allow it to stand until the xylene forms a layer on top of the aqueous phase.
5. Add 0.5 mL of Ehrlich's reagent down the side of the tube.

### Expected Results
Positive: Pink- to wine-colored ring after addition of appropriate reagent (Figure 13-22, *A*).
Negative: No color change after addition of the appropriate reagent (Figure 13-22, *B*).

### Limitations
Ehrlich's method may also be used to differentiate organisms under anaerobic conditions.

### Quality Control
#### A. Kovac's Method
Positive: *Escherichia coli* (ATCC25922)
Negative: *Klebsiella pneumoniae* (ATCC13883)

#### B. Ehrlich's Method
Positive: *Haemophilus influenzae* (ATCC49766)
Negative: *Haemophilus parainfluenzae* (ATCC76901)

#### C. Ehrlich's Method (Anaerobic)
Positive: *Porphyromonas asaccharolytica* (ATCC25260)
Negative: *Bacteroides fragilis* (ATCC25285)

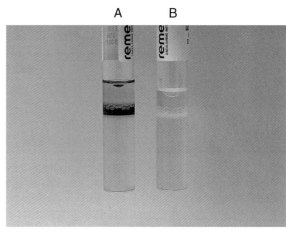

A      B

**Figure 13-22** Indole production. **A**, Positive. **B**, Negative.

## Leucine Aminopeptidase (LAP) Test

### Purpose
The LAP test is used for the presumptive identification of catalase-negative gram-positive cocci.

### Principle
The LAP disk is a rapid test for the detection of the enzyme leucine aminopeptidase. Leucine-beta-naphthylamide–impregnated disks serve as a substrate for the detection of leucine aminopeptidase. After hydrolysis of the substrate by the enzyme, the resulting beta-naphthylamine produces a red color upon addition of cinnamaldehyde reagent.

### Method
1. Before incubation, slightly dampen the LAP disk with reagent-grade water. Do not supersaturate the disk.
2. Using a wooden applicator stick, rub a small amount of several colonies of an 18- to 24-hour pure culture onto a small area of the LAP disk.
3. Incubate at room temperature for 5 minutes.
4. After this incubation period, add 1 drop of cinnamaldehyde reagent.

### Expected Results
Positive: Development of a red color within 1 minute after adding cinnamaldehyde reagent (Figure 13-23, *A*; swab test is depicted)
Negative: No color change or development of a slight yellow color (Figure 13-23, *B*).

### Limitations
The test result depends on the integrity of the substrate-impregnated disk.

### Quality Control
Positive: *Enterococcus faecalis* (ATCC29212)—red color
Negative: *Aerococcus viridans* (ATCC11563)—no color change

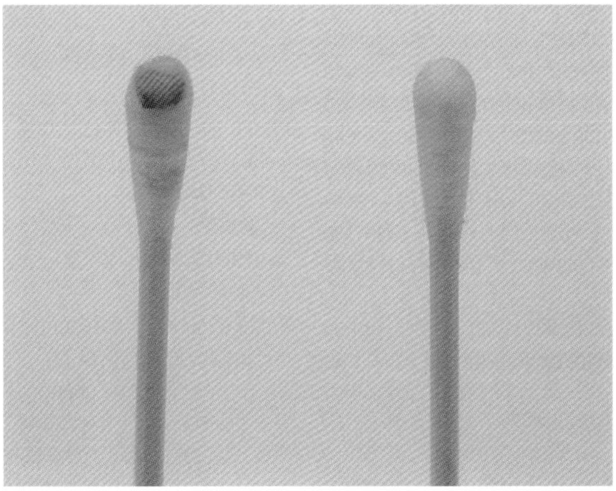

**Figure 13-23** LAP test. **A,** Positive. **B,** Negative.

## Litmus Milk Medium

### Purpose

This test differentiates microorganisms based on various metabolic reactions in litmus milk, including fermentation, reduction, clot formation, digestion, and the formation of gas. Litmus milk is also used to grow lactic acid bacteria.

### Principle

This test is used to determine an organism's ability to metabolize litmus milk. Fermentation of lactose is demonstrated when the litmus turns pink as a result of acid production. If sufficient acid is produced, casein in the milk is coagulated, solidifying the milk. With some organisms, the curd shrinks and whey is formed at the surface. Some bacteria hydrolyze casein, causing the milk to become straw colored and resemble turbid serum. Additionally, some organisms reduce litmus, in which case the medium becomes colorless in the bottom of the tube.

Media: Powdered skim milk (100 g), litmus (0.5 g), sodium sulphite (0.5 g), per 1000 mL, pH 6.8.

### Method

1. Inoculate with 4 drops of a 24-hour broth culture.
2. Incubate at 35°-37°C in ambient air.
3. Observe daily for 7 days for alkaline reaction (litmus turns blue), acid reaction (litmus turns pink), indicator reduction, acid clot, rennet clot, and peptonization. Multiple changes can occur over the observation period.
4. Record all changes.

### Quality Control

Fermentation: *Clostridium perfringens* (ATCC13124)—gas production
Acid: *Lactobacillus acidophilus* (ATCC11506)— clot formation
Peptonization: *Pseudomonas aeruginosa* (ATCC27853)—clearing
Appearance of Indicator (Litmus Dye)

### Limitations

Litmus media reactions are not specific and should be followed up with additional tests for definitive identification of microorganisms.

### Expected Results

Appearance of Indicator (Litmus Dye)

| Color | pH Change to ... | Record |
|---|---|---|
| Pink, mauve (Figure 13-24, *A*) | Acid | Acid (A) |
| Blue (Figure 13-24, *B*) | Alkaline | Alkaline (K) |
| Purple (identical to uninoculated control) (Figure 13-24, *C*) | No change | No change |
| White (Figure 13-24, *D*) | Independent of pH change; result of reduction of indicator | Decolorized |

### Appearance of Milk

| Consistency of Milk | Occurs When pH Is ... | Record |
|---|---|---|
| Coagulation or clot (Figure 13-24, *E*) | Acid or alkaline | Clot |
| Dissolution of clot with clear, grayish, watery fluid and a shrunken, insoluble pink clot (Figure 13-24, *F*) | Acid | Digestion |
| Dissolution of clot with grayish, watery fluid and a clear, shrunken, insoluble blue clot | Alkaline | Peptonization |

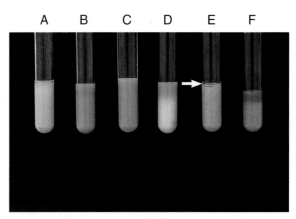

**Figure 13-24** Litmus milk. **A,** Acid reaction. **B,** Alkaline reaction. **C,** No change. **D,** Reduction of indicator. **E,** Clot. (Note separation of clear fluid from clot at *arrow*.) **F,** Peptonization.

## Lysine Iron Agar (LIA)

### Purpose

This test is used to differentiate gram-negative bacilli based on decarboxylation or deamination of lysine and the formation of hydrogen sulfide ($H_2S$).

### Principle

Lysine iron agar contains lysine, peptones, a small amount of glucose, ferric ammonium citrate, and sodium thiosulfate. The medium has an aerobic slant and an anaerobic butt. When glucose is fermented, the butt of the medium becomes acidic (yellow). If the organism produces lysine decarboxylase, cadaverine is formed. Cadaverine neutralizes the organic acids formed by glucose fermentation, and the butt of the medium reverts to the alkaline state (purple). If the decarboxylase is not produced, the butt remains acidic (yellow). If oxidative deamination of lysine occurs, a compound is formed that, in the presence of ferric ammonium citrate and a coenzyme, flavin mononucleotide, forms a burgundy color on the slant. If deamination does not occur, the LIA slant remains purple. Bromocresol purple, the pH indicator, is yellow at or below pH 5.2 and purple at or above pH 6.8.

Media: Enzymatic digest of gelatin (5 g), yeast extract (3 g), dextrose (1 g), L-lysine (10 g), ferric ammonium citrate (0.5 g), sodium thiosulfate (0.04 g), bromocresol purple (0.02 g), agar (13.5 g), per 1000 mL, pH 6.7.

### Method

1. With a straight inoculating needle, inoculate LIA (Figure 13-25, *E*) by twice stabbing through the center of the medium to the bottom of the tube and then streaking the slant.

2. Cap the tube tightly and incubate at 35°-37°C in ambient air for 18 to 24 hours.

### Expected Results

Alkaline slant/alkaline butt (K/K)—lysine decarboxylation and no fermentation of glucose (Figure 13-25, *A*)

Alkaline slant/acid butt (K/A)—glucose fermentation (Figure 13-25, *C*)

*Note:* Patterns shown in Figure 13-25, *A* and *C,* can be accompanied by a black precipitate of ferrous sulfide (FeS), which indicates production of $H_2S$ (Figure 13-25, *B*).

Red slant/acid butt (R/A)—lysine deamination and glucose fermentation (Figure 13-25, *D*)

### Limitations

*Proteus* sp. that produce hydrogen sulfide will not blacken the medium. Additional testing, such as triple sugar iron agar, should be used as a follow-up identification method.

### Quality Control

Alkaline slant and butt: $H_2S$ positive: *Citrobacter freundii* (ATCC8090)

Alkaline slant and butt: *Escherichia coli* (ATCC25922)

Alkaline slant and butt: $H_2S$ positive: *Salmonella typhimurium* (ATCC14028)

Red slant, acid butt: *Proteus mirabilis* (ATCC12453)

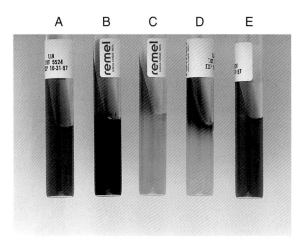

**Figure 13-25**  Lysine iron agar. **A,** Alkaline slant/alkaline butt (K/K). **B,** Alkaline slant/alkaline butt, $H_2S$ positive (K/K $H_2S$+). **C,** Alkaline slant/acid butt (K/A). **D,** Red slant/acid butt (R/A). **E,** Uninoculated tube.

# Methyl Red/Voges-Proskauer (Mrvp) Tests

## Purpose
The combination test methyl red (MR) and Voges-Proskauer (VP) differentiates members of the Enterobacteriaceae family.

## Principle
This test is used to determine the ability of an organism to produce and maintain stable acid end products from glucose fermentation, to overcome the buffering capacity of the system, and to determine the ability of some organisms to produce neutral end products (e.g., 2,3-butanediol or acetoin) from glucose fermentation. The methyl red detects mixed acid fermentation that lowers the pH of the broth. The MR indicator is added after incubation. Methyl red is red at pH 4.4 and yellow at pH 6.2. A clear red is a positive result; yellow is a negative result; and various shades of orange are negative or inconclusive. The VP detects the organism's ability to convert the acid products to acetoin and 2,3-butanediol. Organisms capable of using the VP pathway produce a smaller amount of acid during glucose fermentation and therefore do not produce a color change when the methyl red indicator is added. A secondary reagent is added, alpha-naphthol, followed by potassium hydroxide (KOH); a positive test result is indicated by a red color complex.

Media: Peptic digest of animal tissue (3.5 g), pancreatic digest of casein (3.5 g), dextrose (5 g), KPO$_4$ (5 g), per 1000 mL, pH 6.9.

## Method
1. Inoculate MRVP broth with 1 drop from a 24-hour brain-heart infusion broth culture.
2. Incubate at 35°-37°C for a minimum of 48 hours in ambient air. Tests should not be made with cultures incubated less than 48 hours, because the end products build up to detectable levels over time. If results are equivocal at 48 hours, repeat the tests with cultures incubated at 35°-37°C for 4 to 5 days in ambient air; in such instances, duplicate tests should be incubated at 25°C.
3. Split broth into aliquots for MR test and VP test.

### A. MR (Methyl Red) Test
1. Add 5 or 6 drops of methyl red reagent per 5 mL of broth.
2. Read reaction immediately.

## Expected Results
Positive: Bright red color, indicative of mixed acid fermentation (Figure 13-26, *A*).
Weakly positive: Red-orange color.
Negative: Yellow color (Figure 13-26, *B*).

### B. VP (Voges-Proskauer) Test (Barritt's Method) for Gram-Negative Rods
1. Add 0.6 mL (6 drops) of solution A (alpha-naphthol) and 0.2 mL (2 drops) of solution B (KOH) to 1 mL of MRVP broth.
2. Shake well after addition of each reagent.
3. Observe for 5 minutes.

## Expected Results
Positive: Red color, indicative of acetoin production (Figure 13-26, *C*).
Negative: Yellow color (Figure 13-26, *D*).

### C. VP (Voges-Proskauer) Test (Coblentz Method) for Streptococci
1. Use 24-hour growth from blood agar plate to heavily inoculate 2 mL of MRVP broth.

2. After 6 hours of incubation at 35°C in ambient air, add 1.2 mL (12 drops) of solution A (alpha-naphthol) and 0.4 mL (4 drops) solution B (40% KOH with creatine).
3. Shake the tube and incubate at room temperature for 30 minutes.

## Limitations
The MR test should not be read before 48 hours, because some organisms will not have produced enough products from the fermentation of glucose.
MR-negative organisms may also not have had sufficient time to convert those products and will appear MR positive.
MR-VP testing should be used in conjunction with other confirmatory tests to differentiate organisms among the Enterobacteriaceae.

## Quality Control
Methyl red—Voges-Proskauer
MR positive/VP negative: *Escherichia coli* (ATCC25922)
MR negative:/VP positive: *Enterobacter aerogenes* (ATCC13048)

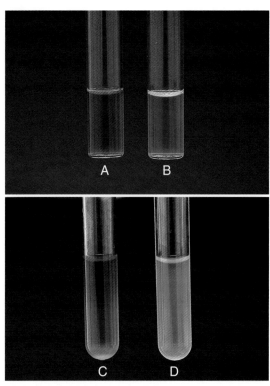

**Figure 13-26** Methyl red/Voges-Proskauer (MRVP) tests. **A,** Positive methyl red. **B,** Negative methyl red. **C,** Positive Voges-Proskauer. **D,** Negative Voges-Proskauer.

## Microdase Test (Modified Oxidase)

### Purpose
This test is used to differentiate gram-positive, catalase-positive cocci (micrococci from staphylococci).

### Principle
The microdase test is a rapid method to differentiate *Staphylococcus* from *Micrococcus* spp. by detection of the enzyme oxidase. In the presence of atmospheric oxygen, the oxidase enzyme reacts with the oxidase reagent and cytochrome C to form the colored compound, indophenol.

### Method
1. Using a wooden applicator stick, rub a small amount of several colonies of an 18- to 24-hour pure culture grown on blood agar onto a small area of the microdase disk. *Note:* Do not rehydrate the disk before use.
2. Incubate at room temperature for 2 minutes.

### Expected Results
Positive: Development of blue to purple-blue color (Figure 13-27, *A*).
Negative: No color change (Figure 13-27, *B*).

### Limitations
Staphylococci should yield a negative color change, except for *S. sciuri, S. lentus,* and *S. vitulus.*

### Quality Control
Positive: *Micrococcus luteus* (ATCC10240)
Negative: *Staphylococcus aureus* (ATCC25923)

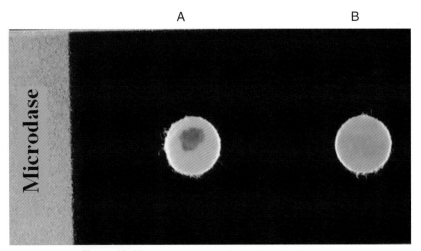

**Figure 13-27** Microdase test. **A,** Positive. **B,** Negative.

## Motility Testing

### Purpose

These tests are used to determine whether an enteric organism is motile. An organism must have flagella to be motile.

### Principle

The inoculum is stabbed into the center of a semisolid agar deep. Bacterial motility is evident by a diffuse zone of growth extending out from the line of inoculation. Some organisms grow throughout the entire medium, whereas others show small areas or nodules that grow out from the line of inoculation.

Media: Enzymatic digest of gelatin (10 g), beef extract (3 g), NaCl (5 g), agar (4 g), per 1000 mL, pH 7.3.

### Method

1. Touch a straight needle to a colony of a young (18- to 24-hour) culture growing on agar medium.
2. Stab once to a depth of only $\frac{1}{3}$ to $\frac{1}{2}$ inch in the middle of the tube.
3. Incubate at 35°-37°C and examine daily for up to 7 days.

### Expected Results

Positive: Motile organisms will spread out into the medium from the site of inoculation (Figure 13-28, *A*).

Negative: Nonmotile organisms remain at the site of inoculation (Figure 13-28, *B*).

### Limitations

Some organisms will not display sufficient growth in this medium to make an accurate determination, and additional follow-up testing is required.

### Quality Control

Positive: *Escherichia coli* (ATCC25922)
Negative: *Staphylococcus aureus* (ATCC25923)

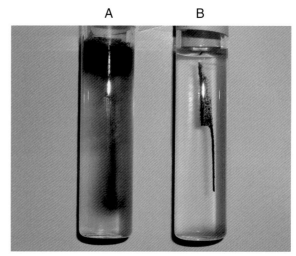

**Figure 13-28** Motility test. **A,** Positive. **B,** Negative.

## MRS Broth

### Purpose
This test is used to determine whether an organism forms gas during glucose fermentation. Some *Lactobacillus* spp. and *Leuconostoc* sp. produce gas.

### Principle
The MRS broth contains sources of carbon, nitrogen, and vitamins to support the growth of lactobacilli and other organisms. It is a selective medium that uses sodium acetate and ammonium citrate to prevent overgrowth by contaminating organisms. Growth is considered a positive result. A Durham tube may be added to differentiate *Lactobacillus* spp. from Leuconostoc *sp.*

Media: Enzymatic digest of animal tissue (10 g), beef extract (10 g), yeast extract (5 g), dextrose (20 g), $NaC_2H_3O_2$ (5 g), polysorbate 80 (1 g), $KH_2PO_4$ (2 g), ammonium citrate (2 g), $MgSO_4$ (0.1 g), $MnSO_4$ (0.05 g), per 1000 mL, pH 6.5.

### Method
1. Inoculate MRS broth with an 18- to 24-hour culture from agar or broth.

2. Incubate 24 to 48 hours at 35°-37°C in ambient air.

### Expected Results
Positive: *Leuconostoc* sp.—Growth, gas production indicated by a bubble in the Durham tube, (Figure 13-29, *A*).

Positive: *Lactobacillus* spp.—Growth, no gas production (Figure 13-29, *B*).
Negative: No growth (not shown).

### Quality Control
Positive: *Lactobacillus lactis* (ATCC19435)
Negative: *Escherichia coli* (ATCC25922)

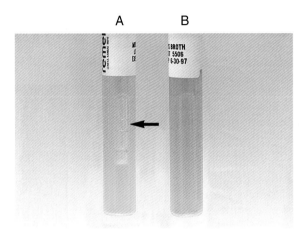

**Figure 13-29** MRS broth. **A,** Positive; gas production by *Leuconostoc* sp. *(arrow).* **B,** Positive: growth, no gas production by *Lactobacillus* sp.

## 4-Methylumbelliferyl-β-D-Glucuronide (MUG) Test

### Purpose
This test is used to presumptively identify various genera of Enterobacteriaceae and verotoxin-producing *Escherichia coli*.

### Principle
*E. coli* and other Enterobacteriaceae produce the enzyme β-d-glucuronidase, which hydrolyzes β-d-glucopyranosid-uronic derivatives to aglycons and d-glucuronic acid. The substrate 4-methylumbelliferyl-β-d-glucuronide is impregnated into the disk and is hydrolyzed by the enzyme to yield the 4-methylumbelliferyl moiety, which fluoresces blue under long wavelength ultraviolet light. However, verotoxin-producing strains of *E. coli* do not produce MUG, and a negative test result may indicate the presence of a clinically important strain.

### Method
1. Wet the disk with 1 drop of water.
2. Using a wooden applicator stick, rub a portion of a colony from an 18- to 24-hour-old pure culture onto the disk.
3. Incubate at 35°-37°C in a closed container for up to 2 hours.
4. Observe disk using a 366-nm ultraviolet light.

### Expected Results
Positive: Electric blue fluorescence (Figure 13-30, *A*).
Negative: Lack of fluorescence (Figure 13-30, *B*).

### Limitations
Do not test colonies isolated from medias containing dyes (EMB, MAC), because it may make the interpretation difficult.
Only test on oxidase-positive organisms, because some oxidase-negative organisms naturally fluoresce.

### Quality Control
Positive: *Escherichia coli* (ATCC25922)
Negative: *Klebsiella pneumoniae* (ATC13883)

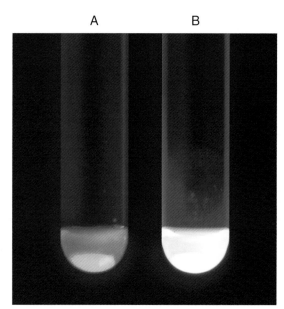

**Figure 13-30** MUG test. **A,** Positive. **B,** Negative.

# Nitrate Reduction

## Purpose
This test is used to determine the ability of an organism to reduce nitrate to nitrite. All members of the Enterobacteriaceae family reduce nitrate, but some members further metabolize nitrite to other compounds.

## Principle
Anaerobic metabolism requires an electron acceptor other than atmospheric oxygen ($O_2$). Many gram-negative bacteria use nitrate as the final electron acceptor. The organisms produce nitrate reductase, which converts the nitrate ($NO_3$) to nitrite ($NO_2$). The reduction of nitrate to nitrite is determined by adding sulfanilic acid and alpha-naphthylamine. The sulfanilic acid and nitrite react to form a diazonium salt. The diazonium salt then couples with the alpha-naphthylamine to produce a red, water-soluble azo dye. If no color change occurs, the organism did not reduce nitrate or reduced it further to $NH_3$, NO, or $N_2O_2$. Zinc is added at this point; if nitrate remains, the zinc will reduce the compound to nitrite and the reaction will turn positive, indicating a negative test result for nitrate reduction by the organism. If no color change occurs after the addition of zinc, this indicates that the organism reduced nitrate to one of the other nitrogen compounds previously described. A Durham tube is placed in the broth for two reasons: (1) to detect deterioration of the broth before inoculation, as evidenced by gas formation in the tube; and (2) to identify denitrification by organisms that produce gas by alternate pathways; if gas is formed in the tube before the addition of the color indicator, the test result is negative for nitrate reduction by this method.

Media: Pancreatic digest of gelatin (20 g), $KNO_3$ (2 g), per 1000 mL.

## Method
1. Inoculate nitrate broth (Figure 13-31, *D*) with 1 to 2 drops from a young broth culture of the test organism.
2. Incubate for 48 hours at 35°-37°C in ambient air (some organisms may require longer incubation for adequate growth). Test these cultures 24 hours after obvious growth is detected or after a maximum of 7 days.
3. After a suitable incubation period, test the nitrate broth culture for the presence of gas, reduction of nitrate, and reduction of nitrite according to the following steps:

a. Observe the inverted Durham tube for the presence of gas, indicated by bubbles inside the tube.
b. Add 5 drops each of nitrate reagent solution A (sulfanilic acid) and B (alpha-naphthylamine). Observe for at least 3 minutes for a red color to develop.
c. If no color develops, test further with zinc powder. Dip a wooden applicator stick into zinc powder and transfer only the amount that adheres to the stick to the nitrate broth culture to which solutions A and B have been added. Observe for at least 3 minutes for a red color to develop. Breaking the stick into the tube after the addition of the zinc provides a useful marker for the stage of testing.

## Expected Results
The nitrate reduction test is read for the presence or absence of three metabolic products: gas, nitrate ($NO_3$), and nitrite ($NO_2$). The expected results can be summarized as follows:

| Reaction | Gas | Color after Addition of Solutions A and B | Color after Addition of Zinc | Interpretation |
|---|---|---|---|---|
| $NO_3 \rightarrow NO_2$ (Figure 13-31, *A*) | None | Red | — | $NO_3$+, no gas |
| $NO_3 \rightarrow NO_2$, gas partial nongaseous end products | None | Red | — | $NO_3$+, no |
| $NO_3 \rightarrow NO_2$, gaseous end products (Figure 13-31, *B*) | Yes | Red | — | $NO_3$+, gas+ |
| $NO_3 \rightarrow$ gaseous end product (Figure 13-31, *C*) | Yes | None | None | $NO_3$+, $NO_2$+, gas+ *C*) |
| $NO_3 \rightarrow$ nongaseous end products | None | None | None | $NO_3$+, $NO_2$+, no gas |
| $NO_3 \rightarrow$ no reaction | None | None | Red | Negative |

## Limitations
Nitrate reduction is a supportive test for identification of Enterobacteriaceae to the genus level; however, additional follow-up, confirmatory testing is required for final identification.

## Quality Control
Positive: $NO_3$+, no gas: *Escherichia coli* (ATCC25922)
Positive: $NO_3$+, gas: *Pseudomonas aeruginosa* (ATCC17588)
Negative: *Acinetobacter baumannii* (ATCC19606)

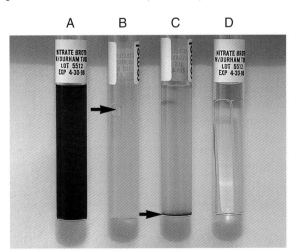

**Figure 13-31** Nitrate reduction. **A,** Positive, no gas. **B,** Positive, gas *(arrow)*. **C,** Positive, no color after addition of zinc *(arrow)*. **D,** Uninoculated tube.

## Nitrite Reduction

### Purpose
This test is used to determine whether an organism can reduce nitrites to gaseous nitrogen or to other compounds containing nitrogen.

### Principle
Microorganisms capable of reducing nitrite to nitrogen do not turn color and do produce gas in the nitrate reduction test (see Procedure 13-29). The test does not require the addition of zinc dust.

Media: Brain-heart infusion broth (2 g), pancreatic digest of casein (10 g), peptic digest of animal tissue (5 g), yeast extract (3 g), NaCl (5 g), $NaNO_2$ (0.1 g), per 1000 mL, pH 6.9.

### Method
1. Inoculate nitrite broth with 1 drop from a 24-hour broth culture.
2. Incubate for 48 hours at 35°-37°C.
3. Examine 48-hour nitrite broth cultures for nitrogen gas in the inverted Durham tube and add 5 drops each of the nitrate reagents A and B to determine whether nitrite is still present in the medium (reagents A and B are described under the nitrate reduction test in Procedure 13-29).

### Expected Results
Positive: No color change to red 2 minutes after the addition of the reagents; gas production observed in the Durham tube (Figure 13-32, A).

Negative: The broth becomes red after the addition of the reagents. No gas production is observed (Figure 13-32, B).

### Limitations
If the broth does not become red and no gas production is observed, zinc dust is added to determine if the nitrite has not been oxidized to nitrate (thus invalidating the test). If oxidation has occurred, the mixture turns red after the addition of zinc.

### Quality Control
Positive: *Proteus mirabilis* (ATCC12453)—colorless, gas production
Negative: *Acinetobacter baumannii* (ATCC19606)—red, no gas production

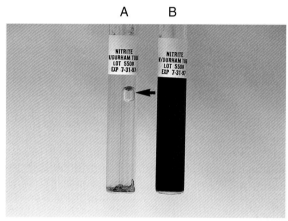

**Figure 13-32** Nitrite reduction. **A,** Positive, no color change after addition of zinc dust and gas in Durham tube *(arrow).* **B,** Negative.

**PROCEDURE 13-31**

## o-Nitrophenyl-β-D-Galactopyranoside (ONPG) Test

### Purpose
This test is used to determine the ability of an organism to produce β-galactosidase, an enzyme that hydrolyzes the substrate ONPG to form a visible (yellow) product, orthonitrophenol. The test distinguishes late lactose fermenters from non–lactose fermenters of Enterobacteriaceae.

### Principle
Lactose fermenters must be able to transport the carbohydrate (β-galactoside permease) and hydrolyze (β-galactosidase) the lactose to glucose and galactose. Organisms unable to produce β-galactosidase may become genetically altered through a variety of mechanisms and be identified as late-lactose fermenters. ONPG enters the cells of organisms that do not produce the permease but are capable of hydrolyzing the ONPG to galactose and a yellow compound, o-nitrophenol, indicating the presence of β-galactosidase.

Media (tube method): $Na_2HPO_4$ (9.46 g), phenylalanine (4 g), ONPG (2 g), $KH_2PO_4$ (0.907 g), per 1000 mL, pH 8.0.

### Method
1. Aseptically suspend a loop full of organism in 0.85% saline.
2. Place an ONPG disk in the tube.
3. Incubate for 4 hours at 37°C in ambient air.
4. Examine tubes for a color change.

### Expected Results
Positive: Yellow (presence of β-galactosidase) (Figure 13-33, *A*).
Negative: Colorless (absence of enzyme) (Figure 13-33, *B*).

### Quality Control
Positive: *Shigella sonnei* (ATCC9290)
Negative: *Salmonella typhimurium* (ATCC14028)

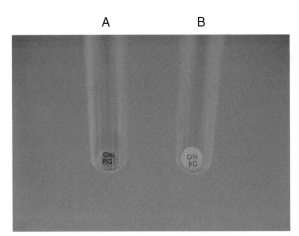

**Figure 13-33** OPNG test. **A,** Positive. **B,** Negative.

## Optochin (P disk) Susceptibility Test

### Purpose
This test is used to determine the effect of Optochin (ethyl hydrocupreine hydrochloride) on an organism. Optochin lyses pneumococci (positive test), but alpha-streptococci are resistant (negative test).

### Principle
Optochin is an antibiotic that interferes with the ATPase and production of adenosine triphosphate (ATP) in microorganisms. The Optochin-impregnated disk (TaxoP) is placed on a lawn of organism on a sheep blood agar plate, allowing the antibiotic to diffuse into the medium. The antibiotic inhibits the growth of a susceptible organism, creating a clearing, or zone of inhibition, around the disk. A zone of 14 to 16 mm is considered susceptible and presumptive identification for *Streptococcus pneumoniae*.

### Method
1. Using an inoculating loop, streak two or three suspect colonies of a pure culture onto half of a 5% sheep blood agar plate.
2. Using heated forceps, place an Optochin disk in the upper third of the streaked area. Gently tap the disk to ensure adequate contact with the agar surface.
3. Incubate the plate for 18 to 24 hours at 35°C in 5% $CO_2$. *Note:* Cultures do not grow as well in ambient air, and larger zones of inhibition occur.

4. Measure the zone of inhibition in millimeters, including the diameter of the disk.

### Expected Results
Positive: Zone of inhibition $\geq$ 14 mm in diameter, with 6-mm disk (Figure 13-34, *A*).
Negative: No zone of inhibition (Figure 13-34, *B*).

### Limitations
Equivocal: Any zone of inhibition less than 14 mm is questionable for pneumococci; the strain is identified as a pneumococcus with confirmation by a positive bile-solubility test.

### Quality Control
Positive: *Streptococcus pneumoniae* (ATCC6305)
Negative: *Streptococcus pyogenes* (ATCC12384)

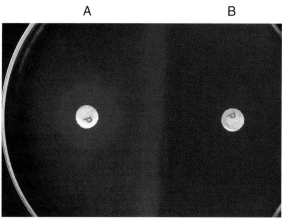

**Figure 13-34** Optochin (TaxoP disk) test. **A,** *Streptococcus pneumoniae* showing zone of inhibition greater than 14 mm. **B,** Alpha-hemolytic *Streptococcus* sp. growing up to the disk.

## Oxidase Test (Kovac's Method)

### Purpose
This test determines the presence of cytochrome oxidase activity in microorganisms for the identification of oxidase-negative Enterobacteriaceae, differentiating them from other gram-negative bacilli.

### Principle
To determine the presence of bacterial cytochrome oxidase using the oxidation of the substrate tetramethyl-p-phenylenediamine dihydrochloride to indophenol, a dark purple-colored end product. A positive test (presence of oxidase) is indicated by the development of a dark purple color. No color development indicates a negative test and the absence of the enzyme.

### Method
1. Moisten filter paper with the substrate (1% tetramethyl-p-phenylenediamine dihydrochloride) or select a commercially available paper disk that has been impregnated with the substrate.
2. Use a platinum wire or wooden stick to remove a small portion of a bacterial colony (preferably not more than 24 hours old) from the agar surface and rub the sample on the filter paper or commercial disk.
3. Observe the inoculated area of paper or disk for a color change to deep blue or purple (Figure 13-35) within 10 seconds (timing is critical).

### Expected Results
Positive: Development of a dark purple color within 10 seconds (Figure 13-35, *A*).
Negative: Absence of color (Figure 13-35, *B*).

### Limitations
Using nickel-base alloy wires containing chromium and iron (nichrome) to rub the colony paste onto the filter paper may cause false-positive results.

### Quality Control
Positive: *Pseudomonas aeruginosa* (ATCC27853)
Negative: *Escherichia coli* (ATCC25922)

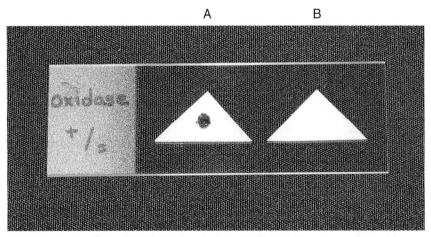

**Figure 13-35** Oxidase test. **A,** Positive. **B,** Negative.

## Oxidation/Fermentation (of) Medium (CDC Method)

### Purpose
This test is used to differentiate microorganisms based on the ability to oxidize or ferment specific carbohydrates.

### Principle
This test is used to determine whether an organism uses carbohydrate substrates to produce acid byproducts. Nonfermentative bacteria are routinely tested for their ability to produce acid from six carbohydrates (glucose, xylose, mannitol, lactose, sucrose, and maltose). In addition to the six tubes containing carbohydrates, a control tube containing the OF base without carbohydrate is also inoculated. Triple sugar iron agar (TSI) (see Procedure 13-40) is also used to determine whether an organism can ferment glucose. OF glucose is used to determine whether an organism ferments (Figure 13-36, *A*) or oxidizes (Figure 13-36, *B*) glucose. If no reaction occurs in either the TSI or OF glucose, the organism is considered a non-glucose utilizer (Figure 13-36, *C*). Hugh and Leifson's formula uses a low peptone-to-carbohydrate ratio and a limiting amount of carbohydrate. The reduced peptone limits the formation of alkaline amines that may mask acid production resulting from oxidative metabolism. Two tubes are required for interpretation of the OF test. Both are inoculated, and one tube is overlaid with mineral oil, producing an anaerobic environment. Production of acid in the overlaid tube results in a color change and is an indication of fermentation. Acid production in the open tube and color change is the result of oxidation. Media: Pancreatic digest of casein (2 g), glycerol (10.0 mL), phenol red (King method) (0.03 g), agar (3 g), per 1000 mL, pH 7.3.

### Method
1. To determine whether acid is produced from carbohydrates, inoculate agar deeps, each containing a single carbohydrate, with bacterial growth from an 18- to 24-hour culture by stabbing a needle 4 to 5 times into the medium to a depth of 1 cm. *Note:* Two tubes of OF dextrose are usually inoculated; one is overlaid with either sterile melted petrolatum or sterile paraffin oil to detect fermentation.

2. Incubate the tubes at 35°-37°C in ambient air for up to 7 days. *Note:* If screwcap tubes are used, loosen the caps during incubation to allow for air exchange. Otherwise, the control tube and tubes containing carbohydrates that are not oxidized might not become alkaline.

### Expected Results
Positive: Acid production (A) is indicated by the color indicator changing to yellow in the carbohydrate-containing deep.
Weak-positive (Aw): Weak acid formation can be detected by comparing the tube containing the medium with carbohydrate with the inoculated tube containing medium with no carbohydrate. Most bacteria that can grow in the OF base produce an alkaline reaction in the control tube. If the color of the medium in a tube containing carbohydrate remains about the same as it was before the medium was inoculated and if the inoculated medium in the control tube becomes a deeper red (i.e., becomes alkaline), the culture being tested is considered weakly positive, assuming the amount of growth is about the same in both tubes.

Negative: Red or alkaline (K) color in the deep with carbohydrate equal to the color of the inoculated control tube.
No change (NC) or neutral (N): There is growth in the media, but neither the carbohydrate-containing medium nor the control base turns alkaline (red).
*Note:* If the organism does not grow at all in the OF medium, mark the reaction as no growth (NG).

### Limitations
Slow-growing organisms may not produce results for several days.

### Quality Control
*Note:* Appropriate organisms depend on which carbohydrate has been added to the basal medium. Glucose is used as an example.
Fermenter: *Escherichia coli* (ATCC25922)
Oxidizer: *Pseudomonas aeruginosa* (ATCC27853)

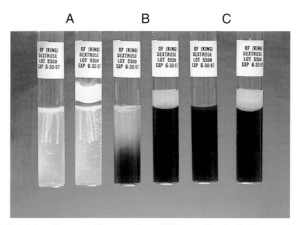

**Figure 13-36** Oxidation/fermentation medium (CDC method). **A,** Fermenter. **B,** Oxidizer. **C,** Nonutilizer.

## Phenylalanine Deaminase Agar

### Purpose
This test is used to determine the ability of an organism to oxidatively deaminate phenylalanine to phenylpyruvic acid. The genera *Morganella, Proteus,* and *Providencia* can be differentiated from other members of the Enterobacteriaceae family.

### Principle
Microorganisms that produce phenylalanine deaminase remove the amine ($NH_2$) from phenylalanine. The reaction results in the production of ammonia ($NH_3$) and phenylpyruvic acid. The phenylpyruvic acid is detected by adding a few drops of 10% ferric chloride; a green-colored complex is formed between these two compounds.

Media: Phenylalanine (2 g), yeast extract (3 g), NaCl (5 g), $Na_3PO_4$ (1 g), agar (12 g), per 1000 mL, pH 7.3.

### Method
1. Inoculate phenylalanine slant with 1 drop of a 24-hour brain-heart infusion broth.
2. Incubate 18 to 24 hours (or until good growth is apparent) at 35°-37°C in ambient air with cap loose.
3. After incubation, add 4 to 5 drops of 10% aqueous ferric chloride to the slant.

### Expected Results
Positive: Green color develops on slant after ferric chloride is added (Figure 13-37, *A*).
Negative: Slant remains original color after the addition of ferric chloride (Figure 13-37, *B*).

### Quality Control
Positive: *Proteus mirabilis* (ATCC12453)
Negative: *Escherichia coli* (ATCC25922)

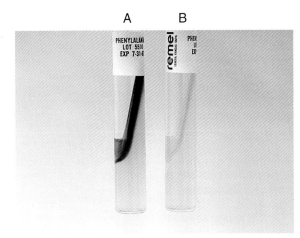

**Figure 13-37** Phenylalanine deaminase. **A,** Positive. **B,** Negative.

## L-Pyrrolidonyl Arylamidase (PYR) Test

### Purpose
This test is used for the presumptive identification of group A streptococci *(Streptococcus pyogenes)* and enterococci by the presence of the enzyme L-pyrrolidonyl arylamidase.

### Principle
The enzyme *L*-pyrrolidonyl arylamidase hydrolyzes the L-pyrrolidonyl- β-naphthylamide substrate to produce a β-naphthylamine. The β-naphthylamine can be detected in the presence of N,N-methylaminocinnamaldehyde reagent by the production of a bright red precipitate.

### Method
1. Before inoculation, moisten the disk slightly with reagent-grade water. Do not flood the disk.
2. Using a wooden applicator stick, rub a small amount of several colonies of an 18- to 24-hour pure culture onto a small area of the PYR disk.
3. Incubate at room temperature for 2 minutes.
4. Add a drop of detector reagent, N,N-dimethylaminocinnamaldehyde, and observe for a red color within 1 minute.

### Expected Results
Positive: Bright red color within 5 minutes (Figure 13-38, *A*).
Negative: No color change or an orange color (Figure 13-38, *B*).

### Quality Control
Positive: *Enterococcus faecalis* (ATCC29212)
*Streptococcus pyogenes* (ATCC19615)
Negative: *Streptococcus agalactiae* (ATCC10386)

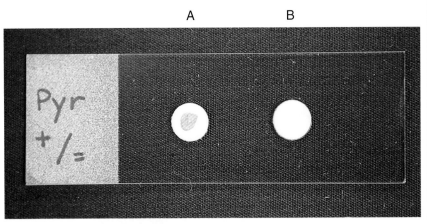

**Figure 13-38** PYR test. **A,** Positive. **B,** Negative.

## Pyruvate Broth

### Purpose
This test is used to determine the ability of an organism to utilize pyruvate. This aids in the differentiation between *Enterococcus faecalis* (positive) and *Enterococcus faecium* (negative).

### Principle
Pyruvate broth is a carbohydrate-free, nutrient-limited medium. Pyruvic acid is added to the broth to determine whether the microorganism is able to use pyruvate, resulting in the formation of metabolic acids. Bromthymol blue indicator changes from blue to yellow in the presence of acid as a result of the decrease in pH.

Media: Pancreatic digest of casein (10 g), pyruvic acid, sodium (10 g), yeast extract (5 g), $K_2HPO_4$ (5 g), NaCl (5 g), bromthymol blue (40 g), per 1000 mL, pH 7.3.

### Method
1. Lightly inoculate the pyruvate broth with an 18- to 24-hour culture of the organism from 5% sheep blood agar.
2. Incubate at 35°-37°C in ambient air for 24 to 48 hours.

### Expected Results
Positive: Indicator changes from green to yellow (Figure 13-39, *A*).
Negative: No color change; yellow-green indicates a weak reaction and should be regarded as negative (Figure 13-39, *B*).

### Quality Control
Positive: *Enterococcus faecalis* (ATCC29212)
Negative: *Streptococcus bovis* (ATCC9809)

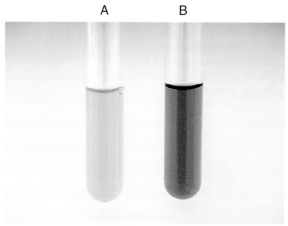

**Figure 13-39** Pyruvate broth. **A,** Positive. **B,** Negative.

## Salt Tolerance Test

### Purpose
This test is used to determine the ability of an organism to grow in high concentrations of salt. It is used to differentiate enterococci (positive) from nonenterococci (negative).

### Principle
The salt tolerance test is a selective and differential medium. Enterococci are resistant to high salt concentration. A heart infusion broth containing 6.5% NaCl is used as the test medium. This broth also contains a small amount of glucose and bromcresol purple as the indicator for acid production.

Media: Brain-heart infusion broth (BHI) may be used in place of the individual components with the addition of NaCl and indicator dye. Components: Heart digest (10 g), enzymatic digest of animal tissue (10 g), NaCl (65 g), dextrose (1 g), bromocresol purple (0.016 g), per 1000 mL.

### Method
1. Inoculate one or two colonies from an 18- to 24-hour culture into 6.5% NaCl broth.
2. Incubate the tube at 35°-37°C in ambient air for 48 hours.
3. Check daily for growth.

### Expected Results
Positive: Visible turbidity in the broth, with or without a color change from purple to yellow (Figure 13-40, *A*).
Negative: No turbidity and no color change (Figure 13-40, *B*).

### Quality Control
Positive: *Enterococcus faecalis* (ATCC29212)—growth, color change to yellow
Negative: *Streptococcus bovis* (ATCC9809)—inhibition, as demonstrated by little to no growth, no color change

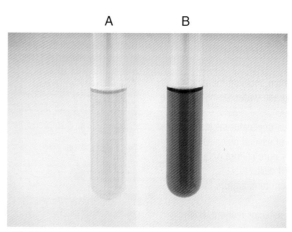

**Figure 13-40** Salt tolerance (6.5% NaCl) test. **A,** Positive. **B,** Negative.

## Spot Indole Test

### Purpose

This test is used to determine the presence of the enzyme tryptophanase. It is a rapid method that can be used in lieu of the tube test described in Procedure 13-20.

### Principle

Tryptophanase breaks down tryptophan to release indole, which is detected by its ability to combine with certain aldehydes to form a colored compound. For indole-positive bacteria, the blue-green compound formed by the reaction of indole with cinnamaldehyde is easily visualized. The absence of enzyme results in no color production (indole negative).

### Method

1. Saturate a piece of filter paper with the 1% paradimethylaminocinnamaldehyde reagent.
2. Use a wooden stick or bacteriologic loop to remove a small portion of a bacterial colony from the agar surface and rub the sample on the filter paper. Rapid development of a blue color indicates a positive test result. Most indole-positive organisms turn blue within 30 seconds.

### Expected Results

Positive: Development of a blue color within 20 seconds (Figure 13-41, *A*).

Negative: No color development or slightly pink color (Figure 13-41, *B*).

### Limitations

The bacterial inoculum should not be selected from MacConkey agar, because the color of lactose-fermenting colonies on this medium can interfere with test interpretation.

### Quality Control

Positive: *Escherichia coli* (ATCC25922)

Negative: *Klebsiella pneumoniae* (ATCC13883)

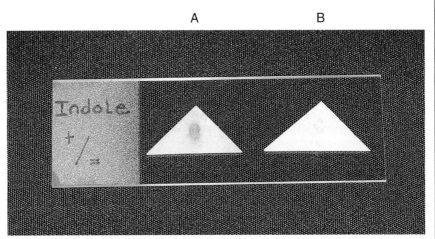

**Figure 13-41** Spot indole test. **A,** Positive. **B,** Negative.

## Triple Sugar Iron Agar (TSI)

### Purpose

TSI is used to determine whether a gram-negative rod ferments glucose and lactose or sucrose and forms hydrogen sulfide ($H_2S$). The test is used primarily to differentiate members of the Enterobacteriaceae family from other gram-negative rods.

### Principle

The composition of TSI is 10 parts lactose:10 parts sucrose:1 part glucose and peptone. Phenol red and ferrous sulfate serve as indicators of acidification and $H_2S$ formation, respectively. A glucose-fermenting organism turns the entire medium acidic (yellow) in 8 to 12 hours. The butt remains acidic after the recommended 18- to 24-hour incubation period because of the presence of organic acids resulting from the fermentation of glucose under anaerobic conditions in the butt of the tube. The slant, however, reverts to the alkaline (red) state because of oxidation of the fermentation products under aerobic conditions on the slant. This change is a result of the formation of $CO_2$ and $H_2O$ and the oxidation of peptones in the medium to alkaline amines. When, in addition to glucose, lactose and/or sucrose are fermented, the large amount of fermentation products formed on the slant neutralizes the alkaline amines and renders the slant acidic (yellow), provided the reaction is read in 18 to 24 hours. Reactions in TSI should not be read beyond 24 hours of incubation, because aerobic oxidation of the fermentation products from lactose and/or sucrose proceeds, and the slant eventually reverts to the alkaline state. The formation of $CO_2$ and hydrogen gas ($H_2$) is indicated by the presence of bubbles or cracks in the agar or by separation of the agar from the sides or bottom of the tube. The production of $H_2S$ (sodium thiosulfate reduced to $H_2S$) requires an acidic environment, and reaction with the ferric ammonium citrate produces a blackening of the agar butt in the tube.

Media: Enzymatic digest of casein (5 g), enzymatic digest of animal tissue (5 g), yeast-enriched peptone (10 g), dextrose (1 g), lactose (10 g) sucrose (10 g), ferric ammonium citrate (0.2 g), NaCl (5 g), sodium thiosulfate (0.3 g), phenol red (0.025 g), agar (13.5 g), per 1000 mL, pH 7.3.

### Method

1. With a straight inoculation needle, touch the top of a well-isolated colony.
2. Inoculate TSI (Figure 13-42, *D*) by first stabbing through the center of the medium to the bottom of the tube and then streaking the surface of the agar slant.
3. Leave the cap on loosely and incubate the tube at 35°-37°C in ambient air for 18 to 24 hours.

### Expected Results

Alkaline slant/no change in the butt (K/NC): glucose, lactose, and sucrose nonutilizer; this may also be recorded as K/K (alkaline slant/ alkaline butt) (Figure 13-42, *C*).

Alkaline slant/acid butt (K/A): glucose fermentation only.

Acid slant/acid butt (A/A): glucose, sucrose, and/or lactose fermenter (Figure 13-42, *A*)

*Note:* A black precipitate in the butt indicates production of ferrous sulfide and $H_2S$ gas ($H_2S+$) (Figure 13-42, *B*). Bubbles or cracks in the tube indicate the production of $CO_2$ or $H_2$. Drawing a circle around the A for the acid butt; that is, Ⓐ, usually indicates this means the organism ferments glucose and sucrose, glucose and lactose, or glucose, sucrose, and lactose, with the production of gas.

### Quality Control

Ⓐ, gas production: *Escherichia coli* (ATCC25922)

K/A, +/− gas production, $H_2S+$: *Salmonella typhimurium* (ATCC14028)

K/K: *Pseudomonas aeruginosa* (ATCC27853)

K/A, $H_2S+$: *Proteus mirabilis* (ATCC12453)

K/A: *Shigella flexneri* (ATCC12022)

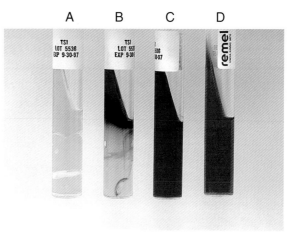

**Figure 13-42** Triple sugar iron agar. **A,** Acid slant/acid butt with gas, no $H_2S$ (A/A). **B,** Alkaline slant/acid butt, no gas, $H_2S$-positive (K/A $H_2S+$). **C,** Alkaline slant/alkaline butt, no gas, no $H_2S$ (K/K). **D,** Uninoculated tube.

## PROCEDURE 13-41

## Urease Test (Christensen's Method)

### Purpose
This test is used to determine an organism's ability to produce the enzyme urease, which hydrolyzes urea. *Proteus* sp. may be presumptively identified by the ability to rapidly hydrolyze urea.

### Principle
Urea is the product of decarboxylation of amino acids. Hydrolysis of urea produces ammonia and $CO_2$. The formation of ammonia alkalinizes the medium, and the pH shift is detected by the color change of phenol red from light orange at pH 6.8 to magenta (pink) at pH 8.1. Rapid urease-positive organisms turn the entire medium pink within 24 hours. Weakly positive organisms may take several days, and negative organisms produce no color change or yellow as a result of acid production.

Media: Enzymatic digest of gelatin (1 g), dextrose (1 g), NaCl (5 g), $KH_2PO_4$ (2 g), urea (20 g), phenol red (0.012 g), per 1000 mL, pH 6.8.

### Method
1. Streak the surface of a urea agar slant with a portion of a well-isolated colony or inoculate slant with 1 to 2 drops from an overnight brain-heart infusion broth culture.
2. Leave the cap on loosely and incubate the tube at 35°-37°C in ambient air for 48 hours to 7 days.

### Expected Results
Positive: Change in color of slant from light orange to magenta (Figure 13-43, *A*).
Negative: No color change (agar slant and butt remain light orange) (Figure 13-43, *B*).

### Limitations
Alkaline reactions may appear after prolonged incubation and may be the result of peptone or other protein utilization raising the pH. To eliminate false-positive reactions, perform a control test with the base medium without urea.

### Quality Control
Positive: *Proteus vulgaris* (ATCC13315)
Weak positive: *Klebsiella pneumoniae* (ATCC13883)
Negative: *Escherichia coli* (ATCC25922)

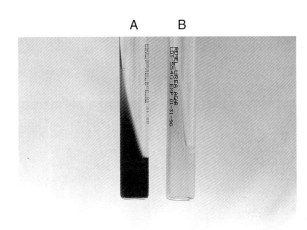

**Figure 13-43** Urea hydrolysis (Christensen's method). **A,** Positive. **B,** Negative.

## X and V Factor Test

### Purpose
The X and V factor test is used to differentiation *Haemophilus* species. Members of the genus *Haemophilus* require accessory growth factors in vitro. Some *Haemophilus* spp. require X factor (hemin) alone, V factor (nicotinamide adenine dinucleotide [NAD]) alone, or a combination of the two.

### Principle
A lawn of the test organism is streaked onto heart infusion agar, tryptic soy agar, *Haemophilus* agar, or nutrient agar. The impregnated disks or strips (X, V, or XV) are placed directly on the confluent inoculation, allowing diffusion of the accessory growth factor into the medium. The organisms will grow only around the disk that provides the appropriate factor for growth of the organism.

### Method
1. Make a very light suspension (MacFarland 0.5) of the organism in sterile saline. *Note:* It is important not to carry over any X factor in the medium from which the organism is taken. Therefore, a loop, not a swab, should be used to make the suspension.
2. Dip a sterile swab into the organism suspension. Roll the swab over the entire surface of a trypticase soy agar plate.
3. Place the X, V, and XV factor disks on the agar surface. If using separate disks, place them at least 4 to 5 cm apart.
4. Incubate overnight at 35°-37°C in ambient air.

### Expected Results
Positive: Growth around the XV disk only shows a requirement for both factors (Figure 13-44, *A*). Growth around the V disk, no growth around the X disk, and light growth around the XV disk shows a V factor requirement (Figure 13-44, *B*).
Negative: Growth over the entire surface of the agar indicates no requirement for either X or V factor (Figure 13-44, *C*).

### Quality Control
Positive:
*Haemophilus influenza* (ATCC35056): halo of growth around the XV disk, no growth on the rest of the agar surface
*Haemophilus parainfluenzae* (ATCC7901): halo of growth around the XV and V disks
*Haemophilus ducreyi* (ATCC27722): halo of growth around the XV and X disks

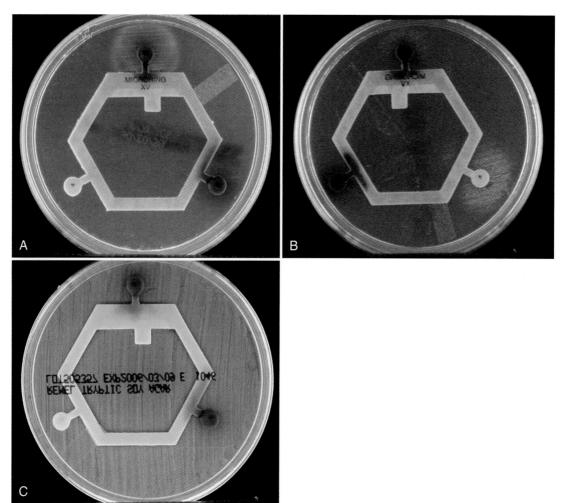

**Figure 13-44** X (hemin) and V (nicotinamide adenine dinucleotide [NAD]) factor test. **A,** Positive: growth around XV disk only. **B,** Positive: growth around V disk. **C,** Negative: growth over entire plate.

# BIBLIOGRAPHY

Alatoom AA, Cunningham SA, Ihde SM et al: Comparison of direct colony method versus extraction method for identification of gram-positive cocci by use of Bruker Biotype matrix-assisted laser desorption/ionization time-of-flight mass spectrometry, *J Clin Microbiol* 49:2868, 2011.

American Type Culture Collection, P.O. Box 1549, Manassas, Va 20108.

Baker JS, Hackett MF, Simard DJ: Variations in bacitracin susceptibility observed in *Staphylococcus* and *Micrococcus* species, *J Clin Microbiol* 23:963, 1986.

Becton, Dickinson & Co: Quality control technical bulletins, BD Company, 7 Loveton Circle, Sparks, Md 21152.

Chauard C, Reller LB: Bile-Esculin test for presumptive identification of enterococci and streptococci: effects of bile concentration, inoculation technique, and incubation time, *J Clin Microbiol* 36:1135, 1998.

Darling CL: Standardization and evaluation of the CAMP reaction for the prompt, presumptive identification of *Streptococcus agalactiae* (Lancefield group B) in clinical material, *J Clin Microbiol* 1:171, 1975.

Hawn CVZ, Beebe E: Rapid method for demonstrating bile solubility of *Diplococcus pneumoniae*, *J Bacteriol* 90:549, 1965.

Heimbrook ME, Wang WL, Campbell G: Staining bacterial flagella easily, *J Clin Microbiol* 26:2612, 1989.

HiMedia Laboratories: Technical data, Bhaveshwar Plaza, Marg, Mumbai, India.

McDade JJ, Weaver RH: Rapid methods for the detection of gelatin hydrolysis, *Reprint J Bacteriol* 1977.

National Committee for Clinical Laboratory Standards: *Abbreviated identification of bacteria and yeast: approved guideline M35-A*, Wayne, Pa, 2002, NCCLS.

Neogen Corp: Acumedia, 620 Lesher Place, Lansing, Mich, 48912.

Oberhofer TR: Characteristics of human isolates of unidentified pseudomonads capable of growth at 42°C, *J Clin Microbiol* 14:492, 1981.

Perez JL, Pulido A, Pantozzi F, Martin R: Butyrate esterase (4-methylumbelliferyl butyrate) spot test: a simple method for immediate identification of *Moraxella (Branhamella) catarrhalis*, *J Clin Microbiol* 28:2347, 1990.

Pilsucki RW, Clayton NW, Cabelli VJ et al: Limitations of the Moeller lysine and ornithine decarboxylase tests, *Appl Environ Microbiol* 37:254, 1979.

Qadri SMH, DeSilva MI, Zubairi S: Rapid test for determination of esculin hydrolysis, *J Clin Microbiol* 12:472, 1980.

Saffert RT, Cunningham SA, Ihde SM et al: Comparison of Bruker Biotyper matrix-assisted laser desorption/ionization time-of-flight mass spectrometer to BD Phoenix automated microbiology system for identification of gram-negative bacilli, *J Clin Microbiol* 49:887, 2011.

Westly JW, Anderson PJ, Close VA et al: Aminopeptidase profiles of various bacteria, *Appl Microbiol* 15:822, 1967.

York MK, Traylor MM, Hardy J et al: Biochemical tests for the identification of aerobic bacteria. In Isenberg HD, editor: *Clinical microbiology procedures handbook*, ed 2, Washington, DC, 2004, ASM Press.

# Catalase-Positive, Gram-Positive Cocci

# Staphylococcus, Micrococcus, and Similar Organisms

## OBJECTIVES

1. Describe the general characteristics of *Staphylococcus* spp. and *Micrococcus* spp., including oxygenation, microscopic gram staining characteristics, and macroscopic appearance on blood agar.
2. Describe the chemical principle of the media used for the isolation and differentiation of staphylococci, including 5% sheep blood agar, mannitol salt, phenyl-ethyl alcohol, and colistin nalidixic acid agars.
3. Explain the principle of the coagulase test, including the different principles associated with the slide versus the tube test and the clinical significance.
4. List the various types of diseases specifically associated with *Micrococcus* spp., *S. aureus*, *S. saprophyticus*, and *S. epidermidis*.
5. Outline the basic biochemical testing procedure to differentiate *Staphylococcus* spp. from *Micrococcus* spp., including coagulase negative and coagulase positive staphylococci.
6. Identify key biochemical reactions to identify the clinically significant *Staphylococcus* spp., and explain the chemical principle associated with each test.
7. Define methicillin-resistant *staphylococcus aureus* (MRSA) as it relates to antibiotic susceptibility.
8. Explain the D Zone test principle and clinical significance in the treatment of *S. aureus*.
9. Describe methods utilized to control the transmission of multiple drug resistant organisms such as MRSA within the community and health care settings.

### GENERA AND SPECIES TO BE CONSIDERED

*Staphylococcus aureus*
Coagulase-negative staphylococci (most commonly encountered)
- *Staphylococcus epidermidis*
- *Staphylococcus haemolyticus*
- *Staphylococcus saprophyticus*
- *Staphylococcus lugdunensis*
- *Staphylococcus schleiferi*
Coagulase-negative staphylococci
- *Staphylococcus capitis*
- *Staphylococcus caprae*
- *Staphylococcus warneri*
- *Staphylococcus hominis*
- *Staphylococcus auricularis*
- *Staphylococcus cohnii*
- *Staphylococcus xylosus*
- *Staphylococcus simulans*
*Micrococcus* spp. and related genera
*Alloiococcus*

## GENERAL CHARACTERISTICS

The gram-positive cocci are a very heterogenous group. Historically, the genus *Staphylococcus* was included with the genus *Micrococcus* in the family Micrococcaceae. However, molecular phylogenetic and chemical analysis has indicated that these two genera are not closely related. The *Staphylococcus* spp. has now been combined with the Bacillaceae, Planococcaceae, and Listeriaceae into the order Bacillales. There are approximately 39 species and 21 subspecies within the genus *Staphylococcus*. Several of the *Micrococcus* species are now reclassified into the genera *Kocuria, Nesterenkonia, Kytococcus*, and *Dermacoccus*. These genera have now been reorganized into two families, the Micrococcaceae and the Dermacoccaceae. The only other organism, *Alloiococcus otitidis*, that biochemically reacts similar to the families included in this chapter belongs to the family Carnobacteriaceae. The species described in this chapter are all catalase-positive, gram-positive cocci. The organisms are aerobic or facultative anaerobic with the exception of *S. aureus* subsp. *anaerobius* and *S. saccharolyticus*, obligate anaerobes, and may be catalase negative. However, only those belonging to the genus *Staphylococcus* are of primary clinical significance. *Staphylococcus* are nonmotile and non-spore forming. Several of the coagulase-negative staphylococci (CoNS or non–*Staphylococcus aureus*) species listed may be encountered in clinical specimens. The CoNS have been subdivided into two groups based on their novobiocin susceptibility pattern. The CoNS group that demonstrates novobiocin susceptibility includes *S. epidermidis, S. capitis, S. haemolyticus, S. hominis* subsp. *hominis, S. lugdunensis, S. saccharolyticus, S. warneri*, and other species. The novobiocin resistant group consists of such species as *S. cohnii, S. kloosii, S. saprophyticus*, and *S. xylosus*. The skin colonizers *Micrococcus* sp., *Kocuria* sp. and *Kytococcus* sp. are easily confused with staphylococci. Occasionally, these genera will be associated with skin lesions and are more commonly isolated form immunocompromised patients.

## EPIDEMIOLOGY

As outlined in Table 14-1, the staphylococci associated with infections in humans are colonizers of various skin and mucosal surfaces. There are three types of nasal

**TABLE 14-1** Epidemiology

| Organism | Habitat (Reservoir) | Mode of Transmission |
| --- | --- | --- |
| *Staphylococcus aureus* | Normal flora:<br>Anterior nares<br>Nasopharynx<br>Perineal area<br>Skin<br>Colonizer of mucosa | Endogenous strain: sterile site by traumatic introduction (e.g., surgical wound or microabrasions)<br>Direct contact: person-to-person, fomites<br>Indirect contact: aerosolized |
| *Staphylococcus epidermidis* | Normal flora:<br>Skin<br>Mucous membranes | Endogenous strain: sterile site, by implantation of medical devices (e.g., shunts, prosthetic devices)<br>Direct contact: person-to-person |
| *Staphylococcus haemolyticus*<br>*Staphylococcus lugdunensis* | Normal flora:<br>Skin<br>Mucous membranes (low numbers) | Same as previously indicated for *S. epidermidis* |
| *Staphylococcus saprophyticus* | Normal flora:<br>Skin<br>Genitourinary tract<br>Mucosa | Endogenous strain: sterile urinary tract, notably in young, sexually active females |
| *Micrococcus* spp.<br>*Kocuria* spp.<br>*Kytococcus* spp. | Normal flora:<br>Skin<br>Mucosa<br>Oropharynx | Endogenous strain: uncertain<br>Rarely implicated in infections<br>Immunocompromised hosts: brain abscess, meningitis, pneumonia, endocarditis |

carrier states associated with *S. aureus*: persistent carriers that harbor a single strain for an extended period of time, intermittent carriers that will harbor different strains over time, and then individuals that do not harbor any organisms or non-carriers. Because the carrier state is common among the human population, infections are frequently acquired when the colonizing strain gains entrance to a normally sterile site as a result of trauma or abrasion to the skin or mucosal surface. However, the traumatic event often may be so minor that it goes unnoticed. Health care workers have a high incidence of carrier state along with immunocompromised individuals, including those with insulin-dependent diabetes mellitus, long-term hemodialysis patients, and IV drug users. Vaginal carriage may be seen in premenopausal women.

Staphylococci are also transmitted from person to person. Upon transmission, the organisms may become established as part of the recipient's normal flora and later introduced to sterile sites by trauma or invasive medical procedures, such as surgery. Person-to-person spread of staphylococci, particularly antimicrobial-resistant strains, occurs in hospitals and presents substantial infection control problems. However, more recently serious *S. aureus* infections have been encountered in the community setting as well.

# PATHOGENESIS AND SPECTRUM OF DISEASE

Without question, *S. aureus* is the most virulent species of staphylococci encountered. A wide spectrum of factors, not all of which are completely understood, contribute to this organism's ability to cause infections and disease.

*S. aureus* and *S. epidermidis* produce a polysaccharide capsule that inhibits phagocytosis. The capsule, which is produced in various amounts by individual clinical isolates, may appear as a slime layer or biofilm, allowing the organisms to adhere to inorganic surfaces and circumventing the actions of antibiotics. The gram-positive cell wall chemical composition is also implicated in the mediation of pathogenesis. The peptidoglycan resembles the endotoxin effect of gram negatives by activating complement, interleukin 1 (IL-1), and acting as a chemotactic factor for the recruitment of PMNs. This cascade of events causes swelling and may lead to the exacerbation of tissue damage because of the additional virulent factors produced by the organisms. *S. aureus* produces a surface protein, known as protein A. This protein is bound to the cytoplasmic membrane of the organism and has a high affinity for the Fc receptor on IgG molecules as well as complement. This provides a mechanism for the organisms to bind the immune active molecules, decreasing the ability for clearance of the organism from the site of infection. Several toxins and enzymes mediate tissue invasion and survival at the infection site (Table 14-2). Cytotoxins alpha, beta, delta, and gamma are produced by a variety of species. Most strains of *S. aureus* produce alpha toxin, which disrupts the smooth muscle in blood vessels and is toxic to erythrocytes, leukocytes, hepatocytes, and platelets. Beta toxin, believed to work in conjunction with the alpha toxin, is a heat-labile sphingomyelinase, which catalyzes the hydrolysis of membrane phospholipids resulting in cell lysis. *S. aureus, S. epidermidis,* and *S. haemolyticus* have been identified as capable of producing Delta toxin, which is cytolytic to erythrocytes and demonstrates nonspecific membrane toxicity to other mammalian cells. Gamma toxin is produced by all strains of *S. aureus* and may actually function in

**TABLE 14-2** Pathogenesis and Spectrum of Diseases

| Organism | Virulence Factors | Spectrum of Diseases and Infections |
|---|---|---|
| *Staphylococcus aureus* | Polysaccharide capsule: Inhibits phagocytosis (slime layer or biofilm) <br> Peptidoglycan: activates complement, IL-1, chemotactic to PMNs <br> Teichoic acids: species specific, mediate binding to fibronectin <br> Protein A: affinity for Fc receptor of IgG and complement. <br> Exotoxins: <br> Cytotoxins (alpha, beta, delta and gamma) <br> Leukocidins, PVL <br> Exfoliative toxins <br> Enterotoxins: A-E, G-I heat stable <br> Toxic Shock Syndrome Toxin I (TSST-1); pyrogenic exotoxin C <br> Enzymes: <br> Coagulase, clumping factor <br> Catalase <br> Hyaluronidase <br> Fibrinolysin: staphylokinase <br> Lipases <br> Nucleases <br> Penicillinase | Carriers: Persistent in older children and adults, nasopharynx <br> Toxin mediated: <br> Scalded skin syndrome: Ritter's disease involves ≥90% of the body, pemphigus neonatorum is the localized form evident by a few blisters; both are exfoliative dermatitis caused by toxins A and B <br> Toxic shock syndrome <br> Food poisoning; preformed enterotoxins, resulting in gastrointestinal symptoms within 2-6 hours of consumption of contaminated food <br> Localized skin infections: folliculitis <br> Furuncles and carbuncles <br> Impetigo <br> Tissue and systemic: <br> Wounds <br> Bacteremia; any localized infection can become invasive and lead to bacteremia <br> Endocarditis <br> Osteomyelitis <br> Cerebritis <br> Pyelonephritis |
| *Staphylococcus epidermidis* | Exopolysaccharide "slime" or biofilm; antiphagocytic. <br> Exotoxins: delta toxin | Normal flora: nosocomial Infections: bacteremia associated with indwelling vascular catheters; endocarditis involving prosthetic cardiac valves (rarely involves native valves); infection at intravascular catheter sites, frequently leading to bacteremia; and other infections associated with CSF shunts, prosthetic joints, vascular grafts, postsurgical ocular infections, and bacteremia in neonates under intensive care |
| *S. haemolyticus* and *S. lugdunensis* | Uncertain; probably similar to those described for *S. epidermidis* | *S. haemolyticus* <br> Endocarditis <br> Bacteremia <br> Peritonitis <br> Urinary tract <br> Wound, bone, and joint infections <br> *S. lugdunensis* <br> Bacteremia <br> Wound infections <br> Endocarditis <br> Endophthalmitis <br> Septic arthritis <br> Vascular catheter infections <br> Urinary tract infections |
| *S. saprophyticus* | Uncertain | Urinary tract infections in sexually active, young females; infections in sites outside urinary tract are not common |
| *S. schleiferi* | Uncertain | Endocarditis <br> Septicemia <br> Osteomyelitis <br> Joint infections <br> Wounds |
| *Micrococcus* spp., *Kocuria* spp. *Kytococcus* spp. | Unknown; probably of extremely low virulence | Usually considered contaminants of clinical specimens; rarely implicated as cause of infections in humans |

association with the Panton-Valentine leukocidin (PVL). Elaboration of these factors is chiefly responsible for the various skin, wound, and deep tissue infections commonly caused by *S. aureus*. Many of these infections can rapidly become life threatening if not treated and managed appropriately.

Thirty to fifty percent of all *S. aureus* strains are capable of producing one of eight distinct serologic types of a heat-stable enterotoxin. The enterotoxins are resistant to hydrolysis by the gastric and intestinal enzymes. The toxins, which are often found in milk products, are associated with pseudomembranous enterocolitis and toxic shock syndrome, and they may exacerbate the normal immune response, resulting in further tissue damage and systemic pathology.

Localized skin or soft tissue infections (SSTIs) may involve hair follicles (i.e., folliculitis) and spread into the tissue causing boils (i.e., furuncles). More serious, deeper infections result when the furuncles coalesce to form carbuncles. Impetigo, the *S. aureus* skin infection involving the epidermis, is typified by the production of vesicles that rupture and crust over. Regardless of the initial site of infection, the invasive nature of this organism always presents a threat for deeper tissue invasion, bacteremia, and spread to one or more internal organs including the respiratory tract. Furthermore, these serious infections have emerged more frequently among the general population and are associated with strains that produce the PVL toxin. PVL is toxic to white blood cells, preventing clearance of the organism by the immune system. These serious soft tissue "community-associated" infections are frequently mediated by methicillin-resistant *S. aureus* (community-acquired MRSA or CA-MRSA).

*S. aureus* also produces toxin-mediated diseases, such as scalded skin syndrome and toxic shock syndrome. In these cases, the organisms may remain relatively localized, but production of potent toxins causes systemic or widespread effects. With scalded skin syndrome (Ritter's disease), which usually afflicts neonates, the exfoliative toxin is a serine protease that splits the intracellular bridges of the epidermidis, resulting in extensive sloughing of epidermis to produce a burnlike effect on the patient. The toxic shock syndrome toxin (TSST-1), also referred to as pyrogenic exotoxin C, has several systemic effects, including fever, desquamation, and hypotension potentially leading to shock and death.

Other coagulase-positive or variable staphylococci are normal flora of a variety of animal species including dogs. These species include *S. intermedius, S. pseudointermedius,* and *S. delphini.* These organisms may be associated with skin infections in dogs, as well as invasive infections in immunocompromised humans or a result of a bite or scratch wound.

The coagulase-negative staphylococci, among which *S. epidermidis* is the most commonly encountered, are substantially less virulent than *S. aureus* and are opportunistic pathogens. Their prevalence as nosocomial pathogens is as much, if not more, related to medical procedures and practices than to the organism's capacity to establish an infection. Infections with *S. epidermidis* and, less commonly, *S. haemolyticus* and *S. lugdunensis* usually involve implantation of medical devices (see Table 14-2). This kind of medical intervention allows invasion by these normally noninvasive organisms. Two organism characteristics that do enhance the likelihood of infection include production of a slime layer or biofilm-facilitating attachment to implanted medical devices and the ability to acquire resistance to most of the antimicrobial agents used in hospital environments. *S. lugdunensis* infections resemble *S. aureus* infections.

Although most coagulase-negative staphylococci are primarily associated with nosocomial infections, urinary tract infections caused by *S. saprophyticus* are clear exceptions. This organism is most frequently associated with community-acquired urinary tract infections in young, sexually active females but is not commonly associated with hospital-acquired infections or any infections at non–urinary tract sites. It is the second most common (following *Escherichia coli*) as the cause of urinary tract infections in young women.

Because coagulase-negative staphylococci are ubiquitous colonizers, they are frequently found as contaminants in clinical specimens. This fact, coupled with the emergence of these organisms as nosocomial pathogens, complicates laboratory interpretation of their clinical significance. When these organisms are isolated from clinical specimens, every effort should be made to substantiate their clinical relevance in a particular patient.

The Micrococcaceae and Dermacoccaceae are generally normal flora of the skin, some of the genera including *Micrococcus, Kocuria,* and *Kytococcus* spp. have been associated with infections such as endocarditis, pneumonia, sepsis, and skin infections in immunocompromised patients. What, if any, virulence factors are produced by the remaining genera within this group is not known. Because these organisms are rarely associated with infections in healthy individuals, they are probably of low virulence.

# LABORATORY DIAGNOSIS

## SPECIMEN COLLECTION AND TRANSPORT

No special considerations are required for specimen collection and transport of the organisms discussed in this chapter. Refer to Table 5-1 for general information on specimen collection and transport.

## SPECIMEN PROCESSING

No special considerations are required for processing of the organisms discussed in this chapter. Refer to Table 5-1 for general information on specimen processing.

## DIRECT DETECTION METHODS
### Microscopy

The majority of the genera included within this chapter produce spherical, gram-positive cells. However, some of the species within the Micrococcaceae or Dermacoccaceae exhibit rod-shaped cells and are motile. During cell division, the organisms divide along both longitudinal and horizontal planes, forming pairs, tetrads, and, ultimately, irregular clusters (Figure 14-1). Gram stains should be performed on young cultures, because very old cells may lose their ability to retain crystal violet and may appear gram variable or gram negative. Staphylococci appear as gram-positive cocci, usually in clusters. Micrococci typically appear as gram-positive cocci in tetrads, rather than large clusters. The additional related genera (i.e., *Kytococcus, Nesterenkonia, Dermacoccus, Arthrobacter,* and *Kocuria*) resemble the staphylococci microscopically.

### Nucleic Acid Testing

Several rapid nucleic acid amplification methods have been developed including the Staphylo Resist (plus) (Amplex Diagnostics, Gars-Bahnhof, Germany) and StaphPlex Panel (Qiagen). These methods are PCR amplification approaches capable of detecting methicillin-resistant staphylococci from clinical swabs. The assays detect the *mecA* gene (which encodes the methicillin resistance) in conjunction with a species-specific target gene. Caution should be used in the interpretation of these results, as several species of staphylococci may reside in the normal flora including methicillin-resistant CoNS causing false positives.

Single-locus amplification is available in several test systems, including the BD Gene OHM MRSA assay (BD, Franklin Lakes, New Jersey), Genotype MRSA Direct and

Geno-Quick MRSA (Hain Lifescience, Xpert MRSA (Cepheid, Sunnyvale, California), and the Roche Light-Cycler MRSA (Roche, Basel, Switzerland). These methods utilize a set of oligonucleotide primers that bind to the downstream sequence of the staphylococcal cassette chromosome region encoding the mec region (*SCCmec*) and the flanking open reading frame (*orfX*). This allows for amplification of the nucleic acid region that indicates antibiotic resistance coupled with a species-specific marker. However, presence of the amplicon does not ensure the presence of or the absence of methicillin-resistant *S. aureus*. This is due to the variability associated with chromosomal recombination within the cassette region that may include partial or full deletion or exchange of antibiotic genes within the cassette. For this reason, it is recommended that positive nucleic acid–based testing be utilized as a preliminary result and confirmatory culture and antimicrobial sensitivity testing is recommended.

## CULTIVATION

### Media of Choice

The organisms will grow on 5% sheep blood and chocolate agars. They also grow well in broth-blood culture systems and common nutrient broths, such as thioglycollate, dextrose broth, and brain-heart infusion.

Selective media can also be used to isolate staphylococci from clinical material. Phenylethyl alcohol (PEA) or Columbia colistin-nalidixic acid (CNA) agars may be used to eliminate contamination by gram-negative organisms in heavily contaminated specimens such as feces. In addition, mannitol salt agar may be used for this purpose. This agar contains a high concentration of salt (10%), the sugar mannitol, and phenol red as the pH indicator. *S. aureus* ferments mannitol and produces a yellow halo on this media as a result of acid production altering the pH (Figure 14-2). CHROMagar (originally invented by Alain Rambach) is a selective and differential media for the identification of methicillin-resistant *Staphylococcus aureus*. The media are now available from a variety of manufacturers. These media are becoming more widely used for the direct detection of nasal colonization. The medium is selective

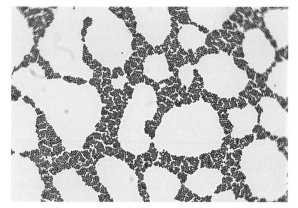

**Figure 14-1** Gram stain of *Staphylococcus aureus* from blood agar.

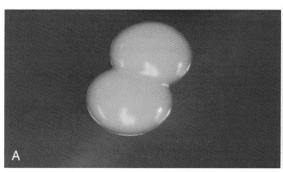
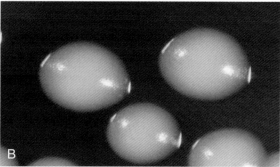

**Figure 14-2 A,** Yellow colonies of *S. aureus* fermenting mannitol as evident by the yellow color of the agar. **B,** White colonies of *S. epidermidis,* no-mannitol fermenting, as evident by the original pink color of the agar. (Photos courtesy of Malissa Tille, Sioux Falls, South Dakota.)

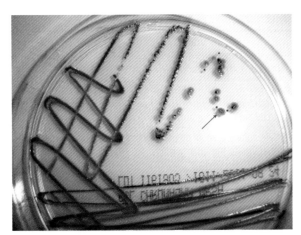

**Figure 14-3** CHROMagar for the identification of MRSA isolates through the selective and differential formation of mauve-colored colonies. (Photo courtesy of Stacie Lansink, Sioux Falls, South Dakota.)

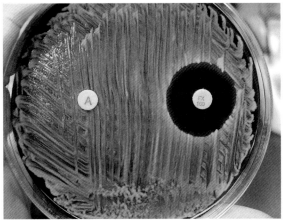

**Figure 14-4** *Staphylococcus epidermis* screening plate showing resistance to bacitracin (taxo A disk) and susceptible to furazolidone (FX disk).

because it contains cefoxitin, and MRSA is resistant to this antibiotic. The addition of chromogenic substrates hydrolyzed by the organisms produce a mauve-colored colony, allowing for the identification of the organisms. Other organisms will hydrolyze various chromogenic substances within the media, resulting in a variety of colored colonies from white to blue to green (Figure 14-3).

### Incubation Conditions and Duration

Visible growth on 5% sheep blood and chocolate agars incubated at 35° C in carbon dioxide ($CO_2$) or ambient air usually occurs within 24 hours of inoculation. Mannitol salt agar and other selective media may require incubation for at least 48 to 72 hours before growth is detected.

### Colonial Appearance

Table 14-3 describes the colonial appearance and other distinguishing characteristics (e.g., hemolysis) of each genus and various staphylococcal species on 5% sheep blood agar. Growth on chocolate agar is similar. *S. aureus* yields colonies surrounded by a yellow halo on mannitol salt agar. In addition, small colony variants of *S. aureus* appear as small pinpoint, nonhemolytic and nonpigmented colonies on blood agar. Small colony variants (SCVs) may result from limited nutrients or other selective pressures and may revert to the normal *S. aureus* phenotype following subculture. However, other staphylococci (particularly *S. saprophyticus*) may also ferment mannitol and thus resemble *S. aureus* on this medium.

## APPROACH TO IDENTIFICATION

The commercial systems for identification of *Staphylococcus* spp. and *Micrococcus* spp. are discussed in Chapter 13. Most commercial systems are successful in the identification of *S. aureus*, *S epidermidis*, and *S. saprophyticus*. The identification of the other species varies from system to system. In addition, automated systems may not correctly identify nutritionally variant forms such as small colony variants and other unusual isolates.

Gram stains are used in the clinical laboratory as the initial presumptive identification method for all gram-positive cocci. Microscopic along with macroscopic colonial morphology (see Table 14-3) provides a presumptive identification. The *Staphylococci* spp. and *Micrococci* spp. are distinguishable from the related family Streptococcaceae (see Chapter 15) by the catalase test. Table 14-4 shows how the catalase-positive, gram-positive cocci can be differentiated. Because they may show a pseudocatalase reaction—that is, they may appear to be catalase-positive—*Aerococcus* and *Enterococcus* are included in Table 14-4; *Rothia* (formerly *Stomatococcus*) is included for the same reason. Once an organism has been characterized as a gram-positive, catalase-positive, coccoid bacterium, complete identification may involve a series of tests, including (1) atmospheric requirements, (2) resistance to 0.04 U of bacitracin (Taxo A disk) and furazolidone, and (3) possession of cytochrome C as determined by the microdase (modified oxidase) test. However, in the busy setting of many clinical laboratories, microbiologists proceed immediately to a coagulase test based on recognition of a staphylococcal-like colony and a positive catalase test.

Microdase disks, a modified oxidase test, are available commercially (Remel, Inc., Lenexa, Kansas). The test is used for differentiating *Micrococcus* spp. from *Staphylococcus* spp. A visible amount of growth from an 18- to 24-hour-old culture is smeared on the disk; *Micrococcus* spp. turn blue within 2 minutes (see Figure 13-27). A variety of tests including the formation of acid from carbohydrates followed by tests for glycosidases, hydrolases, and peptidases are used for species identification and are included in a variety of identification panels.

Both for bacitracin and for furazolidone resistance, disk tests are used (Figure 14-4). A 0.04-U bacitracin-impregnated disk and a 100-µg furazolidone-impregnated disk, both available from Becton Dickinson and Company, are placed on the surface of a 5% sheep blood agar streaked in three directions with a cotton-tipped swab that has been dipped in a bacterial suspension prepared to match the turbidity of the 0.5 McFarland

**TABLE 14-3** Colonial Appearance and Characteristics on 5% Sheep Blood Agar

| Organism | Appearance |
|---|---|
| *Micrococcus* spp. and related organisms* | Small to medium (1-2 μm); opaque, convex; nonhemolytic; wide variety of pigments (white, tan, yellow, orange, pink) |
| *Staphylococcus aureus* | Medium to large (0.5-1.5 μm); smooth, entire, slightly raised, low convex, opaque; most colonies pigmented creamy yellow; most colonies beta-hemolytic |
| *S. epidermidis* | Small to medium; opaque, gray-white colonies; most colonies nonhemolytic; slime-producing strains are extremely sticky and adhere to the agar surface |
| *S. haemolyticus* | Medium; smooth, butyrous, and opaque; beta-hemolytic |
| *S. hominis* | Medium to large; smooth, butyrous, and opaque; may be unpigmented or cream-yellow-orange |
| *S. lugdunensis* | Medium to large; smooth, glossy, entire edge with slightly domed center; unpigmented or cream to yellow-orange, may be β-hemolytic |
| *S. warneri* | Resembles *S. lugdunensis* |
| *S. saprophyticus* | Large; entire, very glossy, smooth, opaque, butyrous, convex; usually white but colonies can be yellow or orange |
| *S. schleiferi* | Medium to large; smooth, glossy, slightly convex with entire edges; unpigmented |
| *S. intermedius* | Large; slightly convex, entire, smooth, glossy, translucent; usually nonpigmented |
| *S. hyicus* | Large; slightly convex, entire, smooth, glossy, opaque; usually nonpigmented |
| *S. capitis* | Small to medium; smooth, slightly convex, glistening, entire, opaque; *S. capitis* subsp. *urealyticus* usually pigmented (yellow or yellow-orange); *S. capitis* subsp. capitis is nonpigmented |
| *S. cohnii* | Medium to large; convex, entire, circular, smooth, glistening, opaque; *S. cohnii* subsp. urealyticum usually pigmented (yellow or yellow-orange); *S. cohnii* subsp. cohnii is nonpigmented |
| *S. simulans* | Large; raised, circular, nonpigmented, entire, smooth, slightly glistening |
| *S. auricularis* | Small to medium; smooth, butyrous, convex, opaque, entire, slightly glistening; nonpigmented |
| *S. xylosus* | Large; raised to slightly convex, circular, smooth to rough, opaque, dull to glistening; some colonies pigmented yellow or yellow-orange |
| *S. sciuri* | Medium to large; raised, smooth, glistening, circular, opaque; most strains pigmented yellow in center of colonies |
| *S. caprae* | Small to medium; circular, entire, convex, opaque, glistening; nonpigmented |

*Includes Kytococcus, Nesterenkonia, Dermacoccus, Kocuria, and Arthrobacter.

standard (i.e., the same as that used in preparing inoculum for disk diffusion susceptibility tests as described in Chapter 12). The tests are then interpreted based on the inhibition or sensitivity of the bacteria by measuring the zone of inhibition present around the disk.

Additional rapid identification systems are available for presumptive screening for the detection of clumping factor A, a cell wall-associated adhesin for fibrinogen and protein A.

### Comments Regarding Specific Organisms

*Micrococcus* spp. and related genera are (1) not lysed with lysostaphin, (2) resistant to the antibiotic furazolidone, (3) susceptible to 0.04 U of bacitracin, and (4) microdase-positive; they usually will only grow aerobically. In contrast, staphylococci are (1) lysed with lysostaphin, (2) resistant to 0.04 U of bacitracin, (3) susceptible to furazolidone, (4) microdase-negative, and (5) facultatively anaerobic.

Once an isolate is identified as, or strongly suspected to be, a species of staphylococci, a test for coagulase production is performed to separate *S. aureus* from the other species collectively referred to as coagulase-negative staphylococci (Figure 14-5).

The enzyme coagulase produced by *S. aureus* binds plasma fibrinogen and activates a cascade of reactions causing plasma to clot. An organism can produce two types of coagulase, referred to as bound and free (see Procedure 13-13 for further information on coagulase tests). Bound coagulase, or clumping factor, is detected using a rapid slide test (i.e., the slide coagulase test), in which a positive test is indicated when the organisms agglutinate on a glass slide when mixed with plasma (see Figure 13-13, *A*). Most, but not all, strains of *S. aureus* produce clumping factor and thus are readily detected by this slide test. Approximately 10% to 15% of strains may give a negative slide coagulase test as a result of the masking by capsular polysaccharides. In addition, false positives may occur as a result of auto agglutination

**TABLE 14-4** Differentiation among Gram-Positive, Catalase-Positive Cocci

| Organism | Catalase | Microdase (modified oxidase) | Aerotolerance | RESISTANCE TO: Bacitracin (0.04 U)[a] | RESISTANCE TO: Furazolidone (100 µg)[a] | RESISTANCE TO: Lysostaphin (200 µg/µL) |
|---|---|---|---|---|---|---|
| *Staphylococcus* | +[b] | −[c] | FA | R | S | S |
| *Micrococcus* (and related organisms) | + | + | A[d] | S | R | R[e] |
| Macrococcus | + | + | ± | + | S | S |
| *Rothia* | ± | − | FA | R or S | R or S | R |
| *Aerococcus* | −[f] | − | FA[g] | S | S | R |
| *Alloiococcus* | ± | − | A | ND | ND | ND |
| *Enterococcus* | −[f] | − | FA | R | S | R |
| *Streptococcus* | − | − | FA | +[d] | − | + |

[a]For bacitracin, susceptible ≥10 mm; for furazolidone, susceptible ≥15 mm.
[b]*S. aureus subsp. anaerobius* and *S. saccharolyticus* are catalase-negative and only grow anaerobically.
[c]*S. sciuri, Macrococcus caseolyticus, S. lentus,* and *S. vitulus* are microdase-positive.
[d]*Kocuria (Micrococcus) kristinae* is facultatively anaerobic.
[e]Some strains of *Micrococcus, Arthrobacter (Micrococcus) agilis,* and *Kocuria* are susceptible to lysostaphin.
[f]Some strains may show a pseudocatalase reaction.
[g]Grows best at reduced oxygen tension and may not grow anaerobically.
[h]Eleven percent to 89% of species or strains are positive.
+, ≥90% of species or strains positive; ±, ≥90% of species or strains weakly positive; −,≥90% of species or strains negative; A, strict aerobe; FA, facultative anaerobe or microaerophile; R, resistant; S, sensitive; ND, no data available.
Data compiled from Schumann P, Spröer C, Burghardt J, et al: Reclassification of the species *Kocuria erythromyxa* (Brooks and Murray, 1981) as *Kocuria rosea* (Flügge, 1886), *Int J Syst Bacteriol* 49:393, 1999; Stackerbrandt E, Koch C, Gvozdiak O, et al: Taxonomic dissection of the genus Micrococcus: Kocuria gen nov Nesterenkonia gen nov, Kytococcus gen nov, Dermacoccus gen nov, and Micrococcus (Cohn, 1872) gen emend, *Int J Syst Bacteriol* 45:682, 1995; and Versalovic J: *Manual of clinical microbiology,* ed 10, Washington, DC, 2011, ASM Press.

when colonies are grown on media with high salt concentrations.

Isolates suspected of being *S. aureus* but failing to produce bound coagulase must be tested for production of extracellular (i.e., free) coagulase because S. *lugdunensis* and *S. schleiferi* may give a positive slide coagulase test. This test, referred to as the tube coagulase test, is performed by inoculation of a tube containing plasma and incubating at 35° C. Production of the enzyme results in a clot formation within 1 to 4 hours of inoculation (see Figure 13-13, *B*). Some strains produce fibrinolysin, dissolve the clot after 4 hours of incubation at 35° C, and may appear to be negative if allowed to incubate longer than 4 hours. Because citrate-utilizing organisms may yield false-positive results, plasma containing ethylenediaminetetraacetic (EDTA) rather than citrate should be used.

Various commercial systems are available that substitute for the conventional coagulase tests previously described. Latex agglutination procedures that detect clumping factor and protein A and passive hemagglutination tests capable detecting clumping factor are no longer used as extensively because they often fail to detect methicillin-resistant *S. aureus* strains, which are being isolated from an increasing number of community-acquired infections. In addition, the recent third-generation assays that include monoclonal antibodies to the capsular polysaccharide serotypes 5 and 8 or other molecules have a higher sensitivity but are not as specific.

False-positive reactions occur in the presence of some CoNS species such as *S. haemolyticus, S. hominis,* and *S. saprophyticus.*

In addition to the screening tests previously described, a variety molecular testing methodologies have been developed for the rapid identification of staphylococci. Accuprobe is a commercially available DNA probe assay available for the confirmation of an identification of *S. aureus* (Gen-Probe, Inc., San Diego, California). *S. aureus* may also be identified by amplification of the *nuc* gene, which encodes a thermostable nuclease. The amplified DNA product is approximately a 270 bp fragment. The detection limit for successful isolation and amplification is less than 10 colony-forming units or 0.69 pg of DNA. This method is highly specific. Additional amplification assays have been developed that detect species-specific genes or chromosomal sequences including 16S and 23SrRNA genes and spacer regions, elongation factor (*tuf*), DNA gyrase (*gyrA*), superoxide dismutase (*sodA*), glyceraldehyde-3-phosphate dehydrogenase gene (gap), and a heat shock protein (*HSP60/GroE*). MRSA has been identified using the staphylococcal insertion sequence *IS431.*

A qualitative nucleic acid hybridization assay that targets rRNA sequences in *S. aureus* and CoNS has been developed by bioMerieux. The hybridization assay is based on the binding of a peptide nucleic acid (PNA) labeled with a fluorescent dye to *S. aureus* in a blood smear prepared from a positive blood culture bottle.

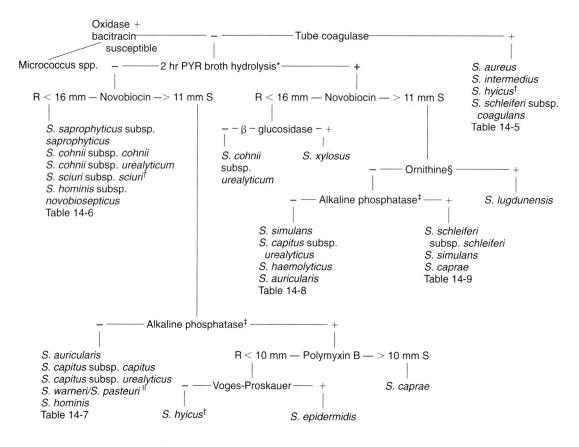

*Available commercially from Remel, Inc., Lenexa, Kan.
†Rarely involved in infections in humans.
‡Alkaline phosphatase available as a disk (Becton Dickinson and Company, Sparks, Md.) or a tablet (KEY Scientific Products, Round Rock, Texas).
§Moeller's decarboxylase medium.
‖rRNA gene restriction site polymorphism with pBA2 as a probe may be required to separate these species.

**Figure 14-5** Staphylococcal identification to species. (Based on the methods in Hébert GA, Crowder CG, Hancock GA, et al: Characteristics of coagulase-negative Staphylococci that help differentiate these species and other members of the family Micrococcaceae, *J Clin Microbiol* 26:1939, 1988.)

Table 14-5 provides the results for various tests used to differentiate the coagulase-positive staphylococci; *S. intermedius* is an important agent isolated from dog bite wound infections and may be misidentified as *S. aureus* if only coagulase testing is performed. Microbiologists should perform additional confirmatory tests in cases in which coagulase-positive staphylococci are isolated from dog bite infections. Otherwise, catalase-positive, gram-positive cocci in clusters from a white to yellow, creamy, opaque colony on blood agar that is slide coagulase-positive and tube coagulase-positive in 4 hours may be presumptively identified as *S. aureus*.

Most laboratories do not identify the coagulase-negative staphylococci to species. However, exceptions may include isolates from normally sterile sites (blood, joint fluid, or cerebrospinal fluid [CSF]), isolates from prosthetic devices, catheters, and shunts; and isolates from urinary tract infections that may be *S. saprophyticus*.

The coagulase-negative staphylococci may be identified based on the criteria shown in Figure 14-5 and Tables 14-5 through 14-9. Isolates not identified to species are reported as "coagulase-negative staphylococci."

It is particularly important to differentiate *S. lugdunensis* from other coagulase-negative staphylococci from sterile sites because there are different interpretive criteria for susceptibility to oxacillin for this organism. *S. lugdunensis* is positive for both the 2-hour PYR and ornithine decarboxylase tests.

## SERODIAGNOSIS

Serologic testing for antibodies associated with infections with Staphylococcal organisms is not clinically relevant due to low specificity and cross-reacting antibodies. Antibodies to teichoic acid, a major cell wall component of gram-positive bacteria, are usually produced in long-standing or deep-seated staphylococcal infections, such as osteomyelitis. This procedure is usually performed in reference laboratories. However, the clinical utility of performing this assay is, at best, uncertain. The identification of protective antibodies in toxin-mediated

**TABLE 14-5** Differentiation among the Most Clinically Significant Coagulase-Positive Staphylococci

| Organism | Clumping Factor | Tube Coagulase | Heat Stable Nuclease | Alkaline Phosphatase | Ornithine Decarboxylase | Acetoin Production | Novobiocin Resistance | Polymyxin B Resistance | β-galactosidase | PYR* | D-trehalose | D-Mannitol | Maltose | Sucrose | D. Mannose |
|---|---|---|---|---|---|---|---|---|---|---|---|---|---|---|---|
| S. aureus subsp. aureus | + | + | + | + | − | + | − | + | − | − | + | + | + | + | + |
| S. lugdunensis | + | v | − | − | + | + | − | v | − | + | + | − | + | + | + |
| S. intermedius† | v | v | + | + | − | − | − | − | + | + | + | v | v | + | + |
| S. pseudintermedius† | − | + | ND | v | ND | + | − | + | + | + | + | v | + | + | + |
| S. hyicus†‡ | − | v | + | + | − | − | − | + | − | − | + | − | − | + | + |

*Performed from disk (Becton Dickinson and Company, Sparks, Maryland) or tablet (KEY Scientific Products, Round Rock, Texas).
†Primarily isolated from animals.
‡Rarely a cause of infections in humans.
+, >90% of strains positive; −, >90% of strains negative; PYR, pyrrolidonyl aminopeptidase; v, variable; ND, no data available.
Data compiled from Behme RJ, Shuttleworth R, McNabb A, et al: Identification of staphylococci with a self-educating system using fatty acid analysis and biochemical tests (published erratum appears in *J Clin Microbiol* 35:1043, 1997), *J Clin Microbiol* 34:2267, 1996; Hébert GA: Hemolysin and other characteristics that help differentiate and biotype *Staphylococcus lugdunensis* and *Staphylococcus schleiferi*, *J Clin Microbiol* 28:2425, 1990; Kloos WE, Wolfshohl JF: Identification of *Staphylococcus* species with API STAPH-IDENT System, *J Clin Microbiol* 16:509, 1982; Roberson JR, Fox LK, Hancock DD, et al: Evaluation of methods for differentiation of coagulase-positive staphylococci, *J Clin Microbiol* 30:3217, 1992; and Versalovic J: *Manual of clinical microbiology*, ed 10, Washington, DC, 2011, ASM Press.


**TABLE 14-6** Differentiation among Coagulase-Negative, PYR-Negative, Novobiocin-Resistant Staphylococci

| Organism | Urease | Oxidase | Alkaline Phosphatase* | Acid from D-Trehalose† | D-Mannitol | Maltose | Sucrose | D-Mannose |
|---|---|---|---|---|---|---|---|---|
| S. saprophyticus subsp. saprophyticus | + | − | − | + | v | + | + | − |
| S. cohnii subsp. cohnii | − | − | − | + | v | − | − | v |
| S. cohnii subsp. urealyticus | + | − | v | + | + | + | − | + |
| S. sciuri subsp. sciuri‡ | − | + | + | (+) | + | v | + | v |
| S. hominis subsp. novobiosepticus | + | − | − | − | − | + | + | − |

*Performed from disk (Becton Dickinson and Company, Sparks, Mdaryland) or tablet (KEY Scientific Products, Round Rock, Texas).
†Performed by the method of Kloos and Schleifer. Results obtained by other methods may vary.
‡Primarily isolated from animals; rarely a cause of infections in humans.
+, >90% of strains positive; −, >90% of strains negative; (+), delayed positive; v, variable.
Data compiled from Kloos WE, Ballard DN, Webster JA, et al: Ribotype delineation and description of *Staphylococcus sciuri* subspecies and their potential as reservoirs of methicillin resistance and staphylolytic enzyme genes, *Int J Syst Bacteriol* 47:313, 1997; Kloos WE, George CG, Olgiate JS, et al: *Staphylococcus hominis* subsp novobiosepticus subsp nov, a novel trehalose- and N-acetyl-d-glucosamine-negative, novobiocin- and multiple-antibiotic-resistant subspecies isolated from human blood cultures, *Int J Syst Bacteriol* 48:799, 1998; and Versalovic J. *Manual of clinical microbiology*, ed 10, Washington, DC, 2011, ASM Press.


**TABLE 14-7** Differentiation among Coagulase-Negative, PYR-Negative, Novobiocin-Susceptible, Alkaline Phosphatase-Negative Staphylococci

| Organism | Urease | β-Glucosidase* | Anaerobic Growth | Acid from D-Trehalose† | D-Mannitol | Maltose | Sucrose | D-Mannose |
|---|---|---|---|---|---|---|---|---|
| S. auricularis | − | − | (±) | (+) | − | (+) | v | − |
| S. capitis subsp. capitis | − | − | (+) | − | + | − | (+) | + |
| S. capitis subsp. urealyticus | + | − | (+) | − | + | + | + | + |
| S. warneri | + | + | + | + | v | (+) | + | − |
| S. hominis subsp. hominis | + | − | − | v | − | v | v | − |

*Performed from disk (Becton Dickinson and Company, Sparks, Maryland) or tablet (KEY Scientific Products, Round Rock, Texas).
†Performed by the method of Kloos and Schleifer. Results obtained by other methods may vary.
+, >90% of strains positive; (+), >90% of strains delayed positive; −, >90% of strains negative; ±, 90% or more strains are weakly positive; ( ), reaction may be delayed; v, variable results.
Data compiled from Versalovic J: *Manual of clinical microbiology*, ed 10, Washington, DC, 2011, ASM Press.

**TABLE 14-8** Differentiation of Coagulase-Negative, PYR-Positive, Novobiocin-Susceptible, Alkaline Phosphatase-Negative Staphylococci

| Organism | Urease | β-Glucuronidase* | β-Galactosidase* | Acid from Mannitol† |
|---|---|---|---|---|
| S. simulans | + | v | + | + |
| S. capitis subsp. urealyticus | + | – | – | + |
| S. haemolyticus‡ | – | v | – | v |
| S. auricularis‡ | – | – | (v) | – |

*Performed from disk (Becton Dickinson Microbiology Systems, Sparks, Maryland) or tablet (KEY Scientific Products, Round Rock, Texas).
†Performed by the method of Kloos and Schliefer. Results obtained by other methods may vary.
‡S. haemolyticus and S. auricularis are very difficult to separate; even fatty acid analysis does not work well.
+, >90% of strains positive; –, >90% of strains negative; (v), variable, positive reactions may be delayed.
Data compiled from Kloos WE, Schleifer KH: Simplified scheme for routine identification of human Staphylococcus species, *J Clin Microbiol* 1:82, 1975; and Roberson JR, Fox LK, Hancock DD, et al: Evaluation of methods for differentiation of coagulase-positive staphylococci, *J Clin Microbiol* 30:3217, 1992.

**TABLE 14-9** Differentiation of Coagulase-Negative, PYR-Positive, Novobiocin-Susceptible, Alkaline Phosphatase–Positive Staphylococci

| Organism | β-Galactosidase* | Urease |
|---|---|---|
| S. schleiferi subsp. schleiferi | (+) | – |
| S. simulans | + | + |
| S. caprae | – | + |

*Performed from disk (Becton Dickinson Microbiology Systems, Sparks, Md) or tablet (KEY Scientific Products, Round Rock, Texas).
+, >90% of strains positive; (+), >90% of strains delayed positive; –, >90% of strains negative.
Data compiled from references Kloos WE, Schleifer KH: Simplified scheme for routine identification of human Staphylococcus species, *J Clin Microbiol* 1:82, 1975; and Roberson JR, Fox LK, Hancock DD, et al: Evaluation of methods for differentiation of coagulase-positive staphylococci, *J Clin Microbiol* 30:3217, 1992.

syndromes such as toxic shock syndrome and staphylococcal scalded skin syndrome may be absent or present at very low levels. However, seroconversion following the onset of symptoms and during convalescence may be observed. Various kits are available for the detection of staphylococcal toxins in foods or patient specimens that may be helpful in clinical diagnosis. Additional assays for the detection of other staphylococcal proteins are being examined for their clinical utility in identifying staphylococcal infections.

# ANTIMICROBIAL SUSCEPTIBILITY TESTING AND THERAPY

Identification of species using susceptibility testing is still useful in the differentiation of *S. saprophyticus* (novobiocin resistant) from other CoNS species (novobiocin sensitive). In addition, polymyxin B resistance is common in clinical isolates of *S. aureus*, *S. epidermidis*, *S. hyicus*, *S. chromogenes*, and some strains of *S. lugdunensis*. Resistance is indicated by an inhibition zone diameter of < 10 mm.

Antimicrobial therapy is vital to the management of patients suffering from staphylococcal infections (Table 14-10). Although a broad spectrum of agents may be used for therapy (see Table 12-6 for a detailed listing), most staphylococci are capable of acquiring and using one or more of the resistance mechanisms presented in Chapter 11. The unpredictable nature of any clinical isolate's antimicrobial susceptibility requires testing as a guide to therapy. As discussed in Chapter 12, several standard methods and commercial systems have been developed for testing staphylococci.

Although penicillinase-resistant penicillins, such as methicillin, nafcillin, or oxacillin, are the mainstay of antistaphylococcal therapy, resistance is common. The primary mechanism for this resistance is production of an altered penicillin-binding protein (i.e., PBP 2a), which renders all currently available β-lactams essentially ineffective. Strains that carry the *mecA* gene, which encodes for PBP 2a, are referred to as methicillin resistant *Staphylococcus aureus* (MRSA). The *mecA* gene is carried on a mobile DNA element (SSS*mec*) that mediates wide dissemination of the antibiotic resistance. The prevalence of hospital-acquired, methicillin-resistant staphylococcus (HA-MRSA) has increased to >50% in some areas within the United States. In addition an increasing prevalence of community-acquired (CA-MRSA) and livestock-associated methicillin-resistant *S. aureus* has been associated with clinical infections. In addition, β-lactamase–producing strains should be considered resistant to all penicillins. Some strains have been identified that overproduce β-lactamase and may appear resistant to oxacillin on routine disk diffusion sensitivity testing but do not possess the *mecA* gene. HA-MRSA are often resistant to aminoglycosides, fosfomycin, fusidic acid, glycopeptides, ketolides, lincosamides, macrolides, quinolones, rifampin, tetracyclines, and trimethoprimsulfamethoxazole. Additional reports have identified isolates of *S. aureus* and CoNS resistant to linezolid, daptomycin, and tigecycline. CA-MRSA isolates are typically more susceptible to non-β-lactam antibiotics.

MRSA isolates can also contain two subpopulations within a single culture, one that is oxacillin sensitive and one that is resistant. The resistant population grows much more slowly and is undetectable by routine susceptibility methods. MRSA Screen agar may be used to clarify and interpret the oxacillin sensitivity pattern for

**TABLE 14-10** Antimicrobial Therapy and Susceptibility Testing

| Organism | Therapeutic Options | Potential Resistance to Therapeutic Options | Validated Testing Methods* | Comments |
|---|---|---|---|---|
| *Staphylococcus* spp. | Several agents from each major class of antimicrobials, including aminoglycosides, beta-lactams, quinolones, and vancomycin; new agent available for use against MRSA includes linezolid, tigecycline daptomycin; see Table 12-6 for listing of specific agents that could be selected for testing and use; for many isolates, a penicillinase-resistant penicillin (e.g., nafcillin, oxacillin, methicillin) is used; vancomycin is used when isolates resistant to these penicillin derivatives are encountered | Yes; resistance to every therapeutically useful antimicrobial has been described | As documented in Chapter 12: disk diffusion, broth dilution, agar dilution, and commercial systems | In vitro susceptibility testing results are important for guiding therapy; for species other than *S. aureus*, clinical significance should be established before testing is done |
| *Micrococcus* spp. and *Kocuria* spp. | No specific guidelines, because these species are rarely implicated in infections; potentially susceptible to β-lactams, macrolides, tetracycline, linezolid, rifampin, and glycopeptides | Unknown Strains have also been identified that are resistant to these agents | †Note | |
| *Kytococcus* spp. | Often susceptible to carbapenems, gentamicin, ciprofloxacin, tetracycline, rifampin, and glycopeptides; recommended treatment includes vancomycin, rifampin, and gentamicin combination | Typically resistant to penicillin G, cephalosporins, and oxacillin | †Note | |
| *Alloiococcus* spp. | May be susceptible to ampicillin, cefotaxime, tetracycline, and vancomycin | Resistant to macrolides, azithromycin, and co-trimoxazole | †Note | |

*Validated testing methods include those standard methods recommended by the Clinical and Laboratory Standards Institute (CLSI) and those commercial methods approved by the Food and Drug Administration (FDA).
†Note: There are no currently recommended Clinical and Laboratory Standards methods for susceptibility testing.

such isolates. The MRSA Screen agar uses oxacillin and promotes the growth of the resistant population by the addition of 2% to 4% NaCl. This medium is then incubated at 35° C for a full 24 hours in order to determine the oxacillin-resistance pattern. Any growth on the MRSA screen agar indicates oxacillin resistance. Current recommendations indicate that successful detection of mixed populations may be enhanced by incubation at a lower temperature, 30° to 35° C for up to 48 hours. Alternatively, cefoxitin (30 μg) disk diffusion can be used to detect methicillin resistance in *S. aureus* and *S. lugdunensis*. An inhibition zone of ≤ 21 mm is reported as resistant and ≥ 20 mm is reported as sensitive. Other coagulase negative *Staphylococcus* spp. should be reported as resistance with a zone diameter of ≤ 24 mm. If microdilution testing is used to detect *mecA* resistance using either oxacillin or cefoxitin, *S. aureus* and *S. lugdunensis* should be reported as follows: resistant to cefoxitin (minimal inhibitory concentrations [MIC] ≥ 8 ug/uL) and oxacillin (MIC ≥ 4 ug/uL) with CoNS resistant to oxacillin at an MIC ≥ 0.5ug/uL. Susceptibility testing with cefoxitin is the recommended method for the detection of the susceptibility or resistance to penicillinase-resistant penicillins.

In addition to the increased penicillin resistance in *S. aureus*, many coagulase negative staphylococcal species within the health care settings are now becoming resistant because of the production of β-lactamase. Many isolates are resistant to methicillin and other antibiotics.

Interpretive guidelines for *S. aureus* with penicillin MICs of ≤ 12 μg/mL or zones of ≥ 29 using screen tests should be retested using disk diffusion. The same interpretive guidelines as indicated here for *S. aureus* are recommended for use with *S. lugdunensis*. However, it is important to use nitrocefin-based testing in place of penicillin for reliable results. Isolates that test beta-lactamase-positive should demonstrate a disk diffusion zone with a clear, sharp zone at the edge of the disk or "cliff." If the isolates demonstrate a fuzzy zone or "beach" edge, the isolate should be considered beta-lactamase-negative. In addition, any isolates that demonstrate a high level of mupirocin resistance should be retested using disk diffusion (200-μg mupirocin disk) or by broth microdilution using a single mupirocin 256 μg/mL well.

The increasing incidence of methicillin-resistant *Staphylococcus* spp. isolated from infections has resulted in an increase in the use of macrolide antibiotics for treatment. Lincomycin antibiotics such as clindamycin are hydrophobic and capable of diffusing into the tissues, providing a means for killing deep infections with *Staphylococci* spp. However, macrolide resistance may be expressed as a constitutive mechanism or an inducible mechanism that is activated by the presence of erythromycin. This is typically identified in erythromycin-resistant strains of *S. aureus*. Although erythromycin and clindamycin are different classes of antibiotics, their resistance mechanisms are similar. Resistance is mediated by either an efflux pump, *msrA*, resulting in macrolide resistance or the activity of a methylase enzyme that alters the ribosomal binding site, *erm*, which confers resistance to macrolides-lincosamide-streptogramin B and is referred to as MLS$_B$ resistant. The MLS$_B$ resistance phenotype is the macrolide resistance that may be expressed as a constitutive or inducible mechanism. To determine the organism's susceptibility to clindamycin, a modified Kirby Bauer test, known as the D zone, has been used in microbiology laboratories. Two antibiotic disks are used: a clindamycin (2 µg) disk is placed 15 mm from an erythromycin disk (15 µg) on a Mueller Hinton agar plate streaked with confluent growth of the isolate. If the organism is able to express inducible clindamycin resistance in the presence of erythromycin, the cells will demonstrate a resistance in the zone of inhibition nearest the erythromycin disk demonstrating a characteristic D zone pattern. If this occurs, an alternate therapy is required for successful treatment of the infection.

Vancomycin is the most commonly used cell wall–active agent that retains activity and is an alternative drug of choice for the treatment of infections with resistant strains. High-level resistance to vancomycin (MIC >8 µg/mL) has been described in several clinical *S. aureus* isolates, and strains with MIC in the intermediate range have been encountered. These reduced intermediate susceptible *S. aureus* (VISAs, MIC 4 to 8 µg/mL) are believed to have structural alterations within the organism's cell wall. VISAs are also often resistant to teicoplanin. Vancomycin-resistant *S. aureus* are currently defined by the identification of an MIC ≥ 16 µg/mL and are readily detected using standard microdilution techniques. Intermediate vancomycin-resistant CoNS are currently defined as having an MIC 8 to 16 µg/mL. However, as resistance patterns increase, the detection of VISA has proved to be unreliable and probably underreported. Two relatively newer agents available for use against such resistant strains are linezolid and daptomycin. Because of the substantial clinical and public health impact of vancomycin resistance emerging among staphylococci, laboratories should have a heightened awareness of this resistance pattern.

*Staphylococci* spp. that demonstrate no intrinsic antibiotic resistance include *S. aureus*, *S. lugdunensis*, *S. epidermidis*, and *S. haemolyticus*. Intrinsic resistance has been reported in *S. saprophyticus* (novobiocin, fosfomycin, and fusidic acid), *S. capitis* (fosfomycin), *S. cohnii* (novobiocin), and *S. xylosus* (novobiocin). In addition, gram-positive bacteria are intrinsically resistant to polymyxin B/colistin, nalidixic acid, and aztreonam. Any clinical isolates that are identified as oxacillin-resistant *S. aureus*, or coagulase-negative staphylococci should be considered resistant to all other beta-lactam antibiotics.

Because *Micrococcus* spp. are rarely encountered in infections in humans, therapeutic guidelines and standardized testing methods do not exist (see Table 14-10). However, in vitro results indicate that these organisms generally appear to be susceptible to most β-lactam antimicrobials.

# PREVENTION

There are no approved antistaphylococcal vaccines. Health care workers identified as intranasal carriers of an epidemic strain of *S. aureus* are treated with topical mupirocin and, in some cases, with rifampin. Some physicians advocate the use of antibacterial substances such as gentian violet, acriflavine, chlorhexidine, or bacitracin to the umbilical cord stump to prevent staphylococcal disease in hospital nurseries. During epidemics, it is recommended that all full-term infants be bathed with 3% hexachlorophene as soon after birth as possible and daily thereafter until discharge.

The Centers for Disease Control and Prevention recommend a concerted effort to battle multiple drug-resistant organisms identified in health care settings. Current recommended strategies for the control of spread and prevention of infection within health care settings include the screening of patients for MRSA prior to admission along with a variety of contact isolation procedures. Guidelines for the prevention and control of such organisms are included in the Campaign to Reduce Antimicrobial Resistance in Healthcare Settings (www.cdc.gov/drugresistance/healthcare/default.htm).

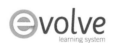 *Visit the Evolve site to complete the review questions.*

## CASE STUDY 14-1

A teenage male had a history of colitis, most likely Crohn's disease. He had difficulty controlling his disease with medical management and had been treated with parenteral nutrition and pain medication. He attends high school and is socially adjusted, even though his illness has caused him to be small in stature. He lives with his mother, who works for a veterinarian. The reason for this admission was abdominal discomfort and erythema at the exit site and along the tunnel of his central line. Blood cultures were collected, and both the blood cultures and his catheter tip cultures grew catalase-positive, gram-positive cocci (Figure 14-6). The coagulase tube test was positive, but the slide and latex test for coagulase were negative (see Procedure 13-13, Coagulase Test).

### QUESTIONS

1. What further biochemical testing should be performed?
2. What additional test should always be performed from staphylococci that are PYR-positive from blood cultures?
3. Susceptibility testing for the penicillinase-resistant penicillins is problematic for coagulase-negative staphylococci, because they can be heteroresistant and express resistance poorly in vitro. This characteristic makes testing in the laboratory difficult, leading to reports of false susceptibility. What is the only reported mechanism of resistance to these agents?

4. Because of the difficulties in expression of the *mecA* gene product in staphylococci, studies have been done to determine which antimicrobial agent best induces the microorganism to produce PBP2a. After extensive studies with many challenge strains, which antimicrobial agent was found to best predict the susceptibility or resistance to the penicillinase-resistant penicillins?

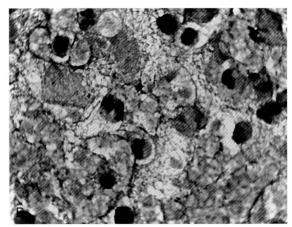

**Figure 14-6** Gram stain clinical specimen demonstrating the presence of gram-positive cocci in clusters and infiltrated with white blood cells.

## CASE STUDY 14-2

An 81-year-old female was admitted to the hospital for a total knee arthroplasty. Following the surgical procedure she had no postoperative complications and a successful recovery. Two years later, while living independently at home, she began to experience chronic, daily pain in the knee and joint. To control the pain, she would take acetaminophen every several hours as directed. She finally presented to her orthopedic surgeon following a 2-month history of the pain. She could not recall any injury or change in activity that may have initiated the pain. Physical examination of the knee and joint demonstrated moderate swelling and mile erythema of the artificial joint. She experienced increased pain with weight bearing and passive range of motion. A new x-ray revealed no acute fractures or deformities but did point out that there was a small effusion, indicating the need for an arthrocentesis. Joint fluid revealed no crystals, 110,000 white blood cells, and 25,000 red blood cells.

### QUESTIONS

1. Describe the proper interpretation for the Gram stain depicted in Figure 14-7.
2. What additional laboratory tests would assist in the diagnosis of the patient's condition?
3. Review the laboratory tests in the following table:

| Laboratory Test | Patient Results | Normal Range |
| --- | --- | --- |
| WBC | 16 | $5\text{-}10 \times 10^9$/L |
| RBC | 4.3 | $4\text{-}5 \times 10^{12}$/L |
| Hgb | 13.5 | 12-16 |
| Hct | 0.40 | 0.36-0.46 L/L |
| MCV | 94 | 80-100 fL |
| MCH | 31 | 26-34 pg |

| Laboratory Test | Patient Results | Normal Range |
| --- | --- | --- |
| MCHC | 33 | 30%-37% |
| Platelets | 156 | $150\text{-}400 \times 10^9$/L |
| Neutrophils | 85 | 25%-60% |
| Lymphocytes | 12 | 20%-50% |
| ESR | 72 | 0-15 mm/h |
| CRP | 15.5 | <1 mg/dL |

Identify the abnormal results. What is the possible diagnosis based on the woman's history and laboratory results?

4. What follow-up treatment would be indicated in this case?

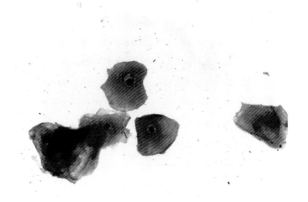

**Figure 14-7** Single microscopic field of vision of the Gram stain of the patient's synovial fluid.

# BIBLIOGRAPHY

Barker KF, O'Driscoll JC, Bhargava A: Staphylococcus ludgdunensis, *J Clin Pathol* 44:873-874, 1991.

Behme RJ, Shuttleworth R, McNabb A, et al: Identification of staphylococci with a self-educating system using fatty acid analysis and biochemical tests (published erratum appears in J *Clin Microbiol* 35:1043, 1997), *J Clin Microbiol* 34:2267, 1996.

Brakstad OG, Aasbakk K, Maeland JA: *Detection of Staphylococcus aures by polymerase chain reaction amplification of the nuc gene.* Clinical and Laboratory Standards Institute, 2009. Methods for Dilution Antimicrobial Susceptibility Testing for Bacteria That Grow Aerobically; Approved Standard-Eight ed. CLSI document M07-A8. Clinical and Laboratory Science Institute, Wayne, PA.

Clinical and Laboratory Standards Institute: Performance standards for antimicrobial susceptibility testing; M100-S23, Wayne, Pa., 2013, CLSI.

Hébert GA: Hemolysin and other characteristics that help differentiate and biotype *Staphylococcus lugdunensis* and *Staphylococcus schleiferi*, *J Clin Microbiol* 28:2425, 1990.

Hébert GA, Crowder CG, Hancock GA, et al: Characteristics of coagulase-negative staphylococci that help differentiate these species and other members of the family Micrococcaceae, *J Clin Microbiol* 26:1939, 1988.

Isaac DW, Pearson TA, Hurwitz CA, et al: Clinical and microbiologic aspects of *Staphylococcus haemolyticus* infections, *Pediatr Infect J* 12:1018, 1993.

Kloos WE, Ballard DN, Webster JA, et al: Ribotype delineation and description of *Staphylococcus sciuri* subspecies and their potential as reservoirs of methicillin resistance and staphylolytic enzyme genes, *Int J Syst Bacteriol* 47:313, 1997.

Kloos WE, Bannerman TL: Update on clinical significance of coagulase-negative staphylococci, *Clin Microbiol Rev* 7:117, 1994.

Kloos WE, George CG, Olgiate JS, et al: *Staphylococcus hominis* subsp novobiosepticus subsp nov, a novel trehalose- and N-acetyl-d-glucosamine-negative, novobiocin- and multiple-antibiotic-resistant subspecies isolated from human blood cultures, *Int J Syst Bacteriol* 48:799, 1998

Kloos WE, Schleifer KH: Simplified scheme for routine identification of human Staphylococcus species, *J Clin Microbiol* 1:82, 1975.

Koontz F: Is there a clinical necessity to identify coagulase-negative staphylococci to the species level? "Okay, so I was wrong!" *Clin Microbiol Newsletter* 20:78, 1998.

LeLoir Y, Baron F, Gautier M: *Staphylococcus aureus* food poisoning, *Genet Mol Res* 2:63, 2003.

Lyytikainen O, Vaara M, Jaarviluoma E, et al: Increased resistance among *Staphylococcus epidermidis* isolates in a large teaching hospital over a 12-year period, *Eur J Clin Microbiol Infect Dis* 15:133, 1996.

Mulligan ME, Murray-Leisure KA, Ribner BS, et al: Methicillin-resistant *Staphylococcus aureus:* a consensus review of the microbiology, pathogenesis, and epidemiology with implications for prevention and management, *Am J Med* 94:313, 1993.

Roberson JR, Fox LK, Hancock DD, et al: Evaluation of methods for differentiation of coagulase-positive staphylococci, *J Clin Microbiol* 30:3217, 1992.

Shantala GB, Shetty AD, Rahul RK, et al: Detection of inducible clindamycin clinical isolates of *Staphylococcus aureus* by the Disc Diffusion Induction Test, *J Clin Diag Res* 5:35-37, 2011.

Stackerbrandt E, Koch C, Gvozdiak O, et al: Taxonomic dissection of the genus Micrococcus: Kocuria gen nov Nesterenkonia gen nov, Kytococcus gen nov, Dermacoccus gen nov, and Micrococcus (Cohn, 1872) gen emend, *Int J Syst Bacteriol* 45:682, 1995.

Vandenesch F, Etienne J, Reverdy ME, et al: Endocarditis due to *Staphylococcus lugdunensis:* report of 11 cases and review, *Clin Infect Dis* 17:871, 1993.

Versalovic J: *Manual of clinical microbiology*, ed 10, Washington, DC, 2011, ASM Press.

Woolford N, Johnson AP, Morrison D, et al: Current perspectives on glycopeptide resistance, *Clin Microbiol Rev* 8:585, 1995.

# Streptococcus, Enterococcus, and Similar Organisms

## OBJECTIVES

1. Describe the general characteristics of *Streptococcus* spp. and *Enterococcus* spp., including oxygenation, microscopic Gram-staining characteristics, and macroscopic appearance on blood agar.
2. Explain the Lancefield classification system for *Streptococcus* spp.
3. Identify the clinical infections associated with *Streptococcus* spp., *Enterococcus* spp., and related gram-positive cocci.
4. Describe the patterns of hemolysis for clinically significant species of Streptococci and Enterococci.
5. Explain the chemical principles for isolation of *Streptococcus* spp. and *Enterococcus* spp. on selective and differential media; include 5% sheep blood agar and Enterococcosel agar.
6. Compare and contrast streptolysin O and streptolysin S, including oxygen stability, immunogenicity, and appearance on blood agar.
7. Describe the major significance of serologic testing procedures for Anti streptolysin O and Anti streptolysin S, in combination with anti-DNase for diagnosis of poststreptococcal sequelae.
8. Explain the activity for the virulence factors of *Streptococcus pyogenes* and the pathogenic effects of each including M protein, hyaluronic acid capsule, streptokinase, F protein, hylauronidase, and the streptococcal pyrogenic exotoxins.
9. Explain the significance of *S. agalactiae* (group B) in perinatal infections.
10. Identify the two major virulence factors associated with *S. pneumoniae,* and describe their effect on the pathogenesis of the infection.
11. Describe the colony morphology, clinical significance, and laboratory techniques for the identification and recovery of the nutritionally variant streptococci.
12. List the appropriate clinical specimens for isolation of the individual *Streptococcus* spp., *Enterococcus* and *Aerococcus viridans*, *Alloiococcus otitidis*, *Gemella*, *Leuconostoc*, and *Pediococcus*.
13. Identify a clinical isolate based on the results from standard laboratory diagnostic procedures.

- *Streptococcus mitis* group
- *Streptococcus bovis* group
- *Streptococcus urinalis*
- *Streptococcus anginosus* group (also called *Streptococcus milleri* group)

Nutritionally variant streptococci
- *Abiotrophia defectiva*
- *Granulicatella adiacens*
- *Granulicatella balaenopterae*
- *Granulicatella elegans*

Enterococci (most commonly isolated)
- *Enterococcus faecalis*
- *Enterococcus faecium*
- Other *Enterococcus* spp. isolated from humans
  - *E. durans*
  - *E. mundtii*
  - *E. dispar*
  - *E. gallinarum*
  - *E. avium*
  - *E. hirae*
  - *E. raffinosus*
  - *E. casseliflavus*

*Leuconostoc* spp.
*Lactococcus* spp.
*Globicatella* sp.
*Pediococcus* spp.
*Aerococcus* spp.
*Gemella* spp.
*Helcococcus* sp.
*Alloiococcus otitidis*
*Dolosicoccus paucivorans*
*Facklamia*
*Dolosigranulum pigrum*
*Ignavigranum ruoffiae*
*Tetragenococcus*

## GENERA AND SPECIES TO BE CONSIDERED

Beta-hemolytic streptococci
- *Streptococcus pyogenes* (group A beta-hemolytic streptococci)
- *Streptococcus agalactiae* (group B beta-hemolytic streptococci)
Groups C, F, and G beta-hemolytic streptococci
*Streptococcus pneumoniae*
Viridans (alpha-hemolytic) *streptococci*
- *Streptococcus mutans* group
- *Streptococcus salivarius* group

## GENERAL CHARACTERISTICS

The organisms discussed in this chapter are all catalase-negative, gram-positive cocci. The Streptococcaceae consist of a large family of medically important species including *Streptococcus* spp. and *Enterococcus* spp. *Alloiococcus*, which is catalase negative only when tested on media devoid of whole blood (e.g., chocolate agar), is included here because it morphologically resembles the viridans streptococci. Some strains of *Enterococcus faecalis* produce a pseudocatalase when grown on blood-containing media and may appear weakly catalase positive. Organisms included in this chapter are differentiated based on cell wall structure, hemolytic patterns on blood agar, physiologic characteristics, the Lancefield Classification scheme, and biochemical identification. This traditional system of classification is still useful within the clinical laboratory, although it differs in some cases with the molecular analysis of the 16srRNA sequences. Of the organisms considered in this chapter, those that are most commonly encountered in infections in humans include *Streptococcus pyogenes*, *S. agalactiae*, *S. pneumoniae*, viridans streptococci, and enterococci, usually *E. faecalis* or *E. faecium*. The other species listed in the tables either are rarely found in clinically relevant settings or are usually considered contaminants that can be mistaken for viridans streptococci or enterococci.

# EPIDEMIOLOGY

Many of these organisms are commonly found as part of normal human flora and are encountered in clinical specimens as contaminants or as components of mixed cultures with minimal or unknown clinical significance (Table 15-1). However, when these organisms gain access to normally sterile sites, they can cause life-threatening infections. Other organisms, most notably *Streptococcus pneumoniae* and *Streptococcus pyogenes*, are notorious pathogens. Although *S. pneumoniae* can be found as part of the normal upper respiratory flora, this organism is also the leading cause of bacterial pneumonia and meningitis. Similarly, although *S. pyogenes* may be carried in the upper respiratory tract of humans, it is rarely considered to be normal flora and should be deemed clinically important whenever it is encountered. At the other extreme, organisms such as *Leuconostoc* spp. and *Pediococcus* spp. usually are only capable of causing infections in severely compromised patients.

Many of the organisms listed in Table 15-1 are spread person to person by various means and subsequently establish a state of colonization or carriage; infections may then develop when colonizing strains gain entrance to normally sterile sites. In some instances, this may involve trauma (medically or non-medically induced) to skin or mucosal surfaces or, as in the case of *S. pneumoniae* pneumonia, may result from aspiration into the lungs of organisms colonizing the upper respiratory tract.

# PATHOGENESIS AND SPECTRUM OF DISEASE

The capacity of the organisms listed in Table 15-2 to produce disease and the spectrum of infections they cause vary widely with the different genera and species.

## BETA-HEMOLYTIC STREPTOCOCCI

*S. pyogenes,* the most clinically important Lancefield group A, produces several factors that contribute to its virulence; it is one of the most aggressive pathogens encountered in clinical microbiology laboratories. Among these factors are streptolysin O and S, which not only contribute to virulence but are also responsible for the beta-hemolytic pattern on blood agar plates used as a guide to identify this species. Streptolysin S is an oxygen stable, nonimmunogenic hemolysin capable of lysing erythrocytes, leukocytes, and platelets in the presence of room air. Streptolysin O is immunogenic, capable of lysing the same cells and cultured cells, is broken down by oxygen, and will produce hemolysis only in the absence of room air. Streptolysin O is also inhibited by the cholesterol in skin lipids resulting in the absence of the development of protective antibodies associated with skin infection. The infections caused by *S. pyogenes* may be localized or systemic; other problems may arise as a result of the host's antibody response to the infections caused by these organisms. Localized infections include acute pharyngitis, for which *S. pyogenes* is the most common bacterial etiology, and skin infections, such as impetigo and erysipelas (see Chapter 76 for more information on skin and soft tissue infections).

*S. pyogenes* infections are prone to progression with involvement of deeper tissues and organs, a characteristic that has earned the designation in general publications as the "flesh-eating bacteria." Such systemic infections are life threatening. Additionally, even when infections remain localized, streptococcal pyrogenic exotoxins (SPEs) may be released and produce scarlet fever, which occurs in association with streptococcal pharyngitis and is manifested by a rash of the face and upper trunk. The SPEs are erythrogenic toxins produced by lysogenic strains. They are heat labile and rarely found in group C and G streptococci. The SPEs act as superantigens activating macrophages and T-helper cells inducing the release of powerful immune mediators including IL-1, IL-2, IL-6, TNF-alpha, TNF-beta, interferons, and cytokines, which induce shock and organ failure. Streptococcal toxic shock syndrome, typified by multisystem involvement including renal and respiratory failure, rash, and diarrhea, is a serious disease mediated by production of potent SPE.

Other complications that result from *S. pyogenes* infections are the poststreptococcal diseases rheumatic fever and acute glomerulonephritis. The poststreptococcal diseases are mediated by the presence of the M protein, not present in any other Lancefield groups. The M protein consists of two alpha helical polypeptides anchored in the cytoplasmic membrane of the organism and extending through the cell wall to the outer surface. The outer amino terminus of the protein is highly variable, consisting of greater than 100 serotypes. Class 1 M protein is associated with rheumatic fever, and class I or II is typically associated with glomerulonephritis. Rheumatic fever, which is manifested by fever, endocarditis (inflammation of heart muscle), subcutaneous nodules, and polyarthritis, usually follows respiratory tract infections and is thought to be mediated by antibodies produced against *S. pyogenes* M protein that cross-react with human heart tissue. Acute glomerulonephritis, characterized by edema, hypertension, hematuria, and proteinuria, can follow respiratory or cutaneous infections and is

**TABLE 15-1** Epidemiology

| Organism | Habitat (reservoir) | Mode of Transmission |
|---|---|---|
| *Streptococcus pyogenes* (group A) | Normal flora: Not considered normal flora Inhabits skin and upper respiratory tract of humans, carried on nasal, pharyngeal, and, sometimes, anal mucosa; presence in specimens is almost always considered clinically significant | Direct contact: person to person Indirect contact: aerosolized droplets from coughs or sneezes |
| *Streptococcus agalactiae* (group B) | Normal flora: female genital tract and lower gastrointestinal tract Occasional colonizer of upper respiratory tract | Endogenous strain: gaining access to sterile site(s) probable Direct contact: person to person from mother in utero or during delivery; or nosocomial transmission by unwashed hands of mother or health care personnel |
| Groups C, F, and G beta-hemolytic streptococci | Normal flora: Skin Nasopharynx Gastrointestinal tract Genital tract | Endogenous strain: gain access to sterile site Direct contact: person to person |
| *Streptococcus pneumoniae* | Colonizer of nasopharynx | Direct contact: person to person with contaminated respiratory secretions |
| Viridans streptococci | Normal flora: Oral cavity Gastrointestinal tract Female genital tract | Endogenous strain: gain access to sterile site; most notably results from dental manipulations |
| *Enterococcus* spp. | Normal flora: Humans, animals, and birds *E. faecalis* and *E. faecium*) are normal flora of the human gastrointestinal tract and female genitourinary tract Colonizers | Endogenous strain: gain access to sterile sites Direct contact: person to person Contaminated medical equipment; immunocompromised patients are at risk of developing infections with antibiotic resistant strains |
| *Abiotrophia* spp. (nutritionally variant streptococci) | Normal flora: Oral cavity | Endogenous strains: gain access to normally sterile sites |
| *Leuconostoc* spp. | Plants, vegetables, dairy products | Mode of transmission for the miscellaneous gram-positive cocci listed is unknown; most are likely to transiently colonize the gastrointestinal tract after ingestion; from that site they gain access to sterile sites, usually in compromised patients; all are rarely associated with human infections |
| *Lactococcus* spp. (group N) | Foods and vegetation | |
| *Globicatella* sp. | Uncertain | |
| *Pediococcus* spp. | Foods and vegetation | |
| *Aerococcus* spp. | Environmental; occasionally found on skin | |
| *Gemella* spp. | Normal flora of human oral cavity and upper respiratory tract | |
| *Helcococcus* sp. | Uncertain | |
| *Alloiococcus otitidis* | Occasionally isolated from human sources, but natural habitat is unknown | Uncertain; rarely implicated in infections |

**TABLE 15-2** Pathogenesis and Spectrum of Disease

| Organism | Virulence Factors | Spectrum of Diseases and Infections |
|---|---|---|
| *Streptococcus pyogenes* | Protein F mediates epithelial cell attachment (fibronectin binding); hyaluronic acid capsule inhibits phagocytosis; M protein is antiphagocytic (> 100 serotypes); produces several enzymes and hemolysins that contribute to tissue invasion and destruction, including streptolysin O, streptolysin S, streptokinase, DNase, and hyaluronidase. Streptococcal pyrogenic exotoxins (Spes) mediate production of rash (i.e., scarlet fever) or multisystem effects that may result in death; C5a Peptidase-destroying complement chemotactic factors. | Acute pharyngitis, impetigo, cellulitis, erysipelas, necrotizing fasciitis and myositis, bacteremia with potential for infection in any of several organs, pneumonia, scarlet fever, streptococcal toxic shock syndrome |
| | Cross-reactions of antibodies produced against streptococcal antigens and human heart tissue | Rheumatic fever |
| | Deposition of antibody-streptococcal antigen complexes in kidney results in damage to glomeruli | Acute, poststreptococcal glomerulonephritis |
| *Streptococcus agalactiae* | Uncertain; capsular material interferes with phagocytic activity and complement cascade activation | Infections most commonly involve neonates and infants, often preceded by premature rupture of mother's membranes; transient vaginal carriage in 10%-30% of females; infections often present as multisystem problems, including sepsis, fever, meningitis, respiratory distress, lethargy, and hypotension; infections may be classified as early onset (occur within first 5 days of life) or late onset (occur 7 days to 3 months after birth); infections in adults usually involve postpartum infections such as endometritis, which can lead to pelvic abscesses and septic shock; infections in other adults usually reflect compromised state of the patient and include bacteremia, pneumonia, endocarditis, arthritis, osteomyelitis, and skin and soft tissue infections |
| Groups C, F, and G beta-hemolytic streptococci | None have been definitively identified, but likely include factors similar to those produced by *S. pyogenes* and *S. agalactiae* | Cause similar types of acute infections in adults as described for *S. pyogenes* and *S. agalactiae*, but usually involve compromised patients; a notable proportion of infections caused by group G streptococci occur in patients with underlying malignancies; group C organisms occasionally have been associated with acute pharyngitis |
| *Streptococcus pneumoniae* | Polysaccharide capsule that inhibits phagocytosis is primary virulence factor; pneumolysin has various effects on host cells, and several other factors likely are involved in eliciting a strong cellular response by the host; secretory IgA protease | A leading cause of meningitis and pneumonia with or without bacteremia; also causes sinusitis and otitis media |
| Viridans streptococci | Generally considered to be of low virulence; production of extracellular complex polysaccharides (e.g., glucans and dextrans) enhance attachment to host cell surfaces, such as cardiac endothelial cells or tooth surfaces in the case of dental caries | Slowly evolving (subacute) endocarditis, particularly in patients with previously damaged heart valves; bacteremia and infections of other sterile sites do occur in immunocompromised patients; meningitis can develop in patients suffering trauma or defects that allow upper respiratory flora to gain access to the central nervous system; *S. mutans* plays a key role in the development of dental caries |

**TABLE 15-2** Pathogenesis and Spectrum of Disease—cont'd

| Organism | Virulence Factors | Spectrum of Diseases and Infections |
|---|---|---|
| *Enterococcus* spp. | Little is known about virulence; adhesions, cytolysins, and other metabolic capabilities may allow these organisms to proliferate as nosocomial pathogens; multidrug resistance also contributes to proliferation | Most infections are nosocomial and include urinary tract infections, bacteremia, endocarditis, mixed infections of abdomen and pelvis, wounds, and occasionally, ocular infections; CNS and respiratory infections are rare |
| *Abiotrophia* spp. (nutritionally variant streptococci) | Unknown | Endocarditis; rarely encountered in infections of other sterile sites |
| *Leuconostoc* spp., *Lactococcus* spp., *Globicatella* sp., *Pediococcus* spp., *Aerococcus* spp., *Gemella* spp., *Helcococcus* sp. *Facklamia* spp. *Ignavigranum ruoffiae* *Dolosigranulum pigrum* *Dolosicoccus paucivorans* | Unknown; probably of low virulence; opportunistic organisms that require impaired host defenses to establish infection; intrinsic resistance to certain antimicrobial agents (e.g., *Leuconostoc* spp. and *Pediococcus* spp. resistant to vancomycin) may enhance survival of some species in the hospital setting | Whenever encountered in clinical specimens, these organisms should first be considered as probable contaminants; *Aerococcus urinae* is notably associated with urinary tract infections |
| *Alloiococcus* sp. | Unknown | Chronic otitis media in children |

mediated by antigen-antibody complexes that deposit in glomeruli, where they initiate damage.

The organism adheres and invades the epithelial cells through the mediation of various proteins and enzymes. Internalization of the organism is believed to be important for persistent and deep tissue infections. Additional virulence factors are included in Table 15-2.

*S. pyogenes* is also a powerful modulator of the host immune system, preventing clearance of the infection. The M protein is able to bind beta globulin factor H, a regulatory protein of the alternate complement pathway involved in the degradation of C3b. The M protein also binds to fibrinogen blocking complement alternate pathway activation. In addition, all strains produce a C5a peptidase, which is a serine protease capable of inactivating the chemotactic factor for neutrophils and monocytes (C5a).

*S. agalactiae*, group B, infections usually are associated with neonates and are acquired before or during the birthing process (see Table 15-2). The organism is known to cause septicemia, pneumonia, and meningitis in newborns. Although the virulence factors associated with the other beta-hemolytic streptococci have not been definitively identified, groups C, G, and F streptococci cause infections similar to those associated with *S. pyogenes* (i.e., skin and soft tissue infections and bacteremia) but are less commonly encountered, often involve compromised patients, and do not produce postinfection sequelae.

## STREPTOCOCCUS PNEUMONIAE AND VIRIDANS STREPTOCOCCI

*S. pneumoniae* contains the C polysaccharide unrelated to the Lancefield grouping and is still one of the leading causes of morbidity and mortality. The organism is the primary cause of bacterial pneumonia, meningitis, and otitis media. The antiphagocytic property of the

polysaccharide capsule is associated with the organism's virulence. There are more than 90 different serotypes of encapsulated strains of *S. pneumoniae.* Nonencapsulated strains are avirulent. The organism may harmlessly inhabit the upper respiratory tract with a 5% to 75% carriage rate in humans. *S. pneumoniae* is capable of spreading to the lungs, paranasal sinuses, and middle ear. In addition, this organism accesses the bloodstream and the meninges to cause acute, purulent, and often life-threatening infections.

*S. pneumoniae* is capable of mobilizing inflammatory cells mediated by its cell wall structure, including peptidoglycan, teichoic acids, and a pneumolysin. The pneumolysis activates the classical complement pathway. The pneumolysin mediates suppression of the oxidative burst in phagocytes providing for effective evasion of immune clearance. In addition, the organism contains phosphorylcholine within the cell wall, which binds receptors for platele- activating factor in endothelia cells, leukocytes, platelets, and tissue cells of the lungs and meninges providing for entry and spread of the organism.

The viridans (greening) streptococci and *Abiotrophia* spp. (formally known as nutritionally variant streptococci) are a heterogenous group consisting of alpha hemolytic and nonhemolytic species generally considered to be opportunistic pathogens of low virulence. The organisms colonize the gastrointestinal and genitourinary tract. These organisms are not known to produce any factors that facilitate invasion of the host. However, when access is gained, a transient bacteremia occurs and endocarditis and infections at other sites in compromised patients may result.

## ENTEROCOCCI

Enterococci, previously classified as group D streptococci, commonly colonizes the gastrointestinal tract.

Greater than 29 species exist, including commensals that lack potent toxins and other well-defined virulence factors. Although virulence factors associated with enterococci are a topic of increasing research interest, little is known about the characteristics that have allowed these organisms to become a prominent cause of nosocomial infections. Enterococci are one of the most feared nosocomial pathogens isolated from the urinary tract, peritoneum, heart tissue, bacteremia, endocarditis, and intra-abdominal infections.

Compared with other clinically important gram-positive cocci, this genus is intrinsically more resistant to the antimicrobial agents commonly used in hospitals and is especially resistant to all currently available cephalosporins and aminoglycosides. In addition, these organisms are capable of acquiring and exchanging genes encoding resistance to antimicrobial agents. This genus is the first clinically relevant group of gram-positive cocci to acquire and disseminate resistance to vancomycin, the single cell–wall active agent available for use against gram-positive organisms resistant to beta-lactams (e.g., methicillin-resistant staphylococci). Spread of this troublesome resistance marker from enterococci to other clinically relevant organisms is a serious public health concern and appears to have occurred with the emergence of vancomycin-resistant *S. aureus*.

A wide variety of enterococcal species have been isolated from human infections, but *E. faecalis* and *E. faecium* still clearly predominate as the species most commonly encountered. *E. faecalis* and *E. faecium* have been isolated from the respiratory tract and the myocardium. Between these two species, *E. faecalis* is the most commonly encountered, but the incidence of *E. faecium* infections is on the rise in many hospitals, which is probably related in some way to the acquisition of resistance to vancomycin and other antimicrobial agents. Two additional species, *E. gallinarum* and *E. casseliflavus*, have been associated with intestinal infections.

## MISCELLANEOUS OTHER GRAM-POSITIVE COCCI

The other genera listed in Table 15-2 are of low virulence and are almost exclusively associated with infections involving compromised hosts. A possible exception is the association of *Alloiococcus otitidis* with chronic otitis media in children. Certain intrinsic features, such as resistance to vancomycin among *Leuconostoc* spp. and *Pediococcus* spp., may contribute to the ability of these organisms to survive in the hospital environment. However, whenever they are encountered, strong consideration must be given to their clinical relevance and potential as contaminants. These organisms can also challenge many identification schemes used for gram-positive cocci, and they may be readily misidentified as viridans streptococci.

# LABORATORY DIAGNOSIS

## SPECIMEN COLLECTION AND TRANSPORT

No special considerations are required for specimen collection and transport of the organisms discussed in this chapter. Refer to Table 5-1 for general information on specimen collection and transport.

## SPECIMEN PROCESSING

No special considerations are required for processing of the organisms discussed in this chapter. Refer to Table 5-1 for general information on specimen processing.

## DIRECT DETECTION METHODS

### Antigen Detection

Antigen detection screening methods are available for several streptococcal antigens. Detection of antigens is possible using latex agglutination or enzyme-linked immunosorbent assay (ELISA) technologies. These commercial kits have been reported to be very specific, but false-negative results may occur if specimens contain low numbers of *S. pyogenes*. Sensitivity has ranged from approximately 60% to greater than 95% depending on the methodology and other variables. Therefore, many microbiologists recommend collecting two throat swabs from each patient. If the first swab yields a positive result by a direct antigen method, the second swab can be discarded. However, for those specimens in which the rapid antigen test yielded a negative result, a blood agar plate or selective streptococcal blood agar plate should be inoculated with the second swab.

Several commercial antigen detection kits are available for diagnosis of neonatal sepsis and meningitis caused by group B streptococci. Developed for use with serum, urine, or cerebrospinal fluid (CSF), the best results have been achieved with CSF; false-positive results have been a problem using urine. Because neonates acquire *S. agalactiae* infection during passage through the colonized birth canal, direct detection of group B streptococcal antigen from vaginal swabs has also been attempted. However, direct extraction and latex particle agglutination have not been sensitive enough for use alone as a screening test.

Latex agglutination kits to detect the capsular polysaccharide antigen of the pneumococcus have also been developed for use with urine, serum, and CSF, although they are no longer commonly used in clinical microbiology laboratories.

### Molecular Diagnostic Testing

Nucleic acid based testing is available and offers a rapid and increased specificity as compared to traditional identification schemes. Polymerase chain reaction is available for the detection of an internal sequence of the CAMP-factor (*cfb gene*) for group B streptococci. Analyte-specific reagents are available from Roche Applied Science (Indianapolis, Indiana) for the detection of the *ptsI* gene of group B and group A streptococci. The two groups are differentiated based on specificity of the sequences within the primer pairs for the assay. Gen-Probe Incorporated (San Diego, California) has developed several DNA probe assays for the differentiation of streptococci. The GASDirect test is a DNA probe hybridization assay for the detection of group streptococcal RNA from throat swabs. The ACCUPROBE group B Streptococcus assay is a hybridization protection assay that utilizes a DNA probe for the detection of 16 s ribosomal RNA sequences unique to *Streptococcus agalactiae*.

A fully integrated automated real-time PCR-based GeneXpert system has been developed by Cepheid (Sunnyvale, California). The system completely automates the sample preparation, DNA extraction, amplification, and detection of the target sequence within a closed system. The GeneXpert platform offers a qualitative assay for the detection of group B Streptococcus DNA directly from a swab.

## Gram Stain

All the genera described in this chapter are gram-positive cocci. Microscopically, streptococci are round or oval-shaped, occasionally forming elongated cells that resemble pleomorphic corynebacteria or lactobacilli. They may appear gram-negative if cultures are old or if the patient has been treated with antibiotics. *Gemella haemolysans* is easily decolorized. *S. pneumoniae* is typically lancet-shaped and occurs singly, in pairs, or in short chains (Figure 15-1).

Growth in broth should be used for determination of cellular morphology if there is a question regarding staining characteristics from solid media. In fact, the genera described in this chapter are subdivided based on whether they have a "strep"-like Gram stain or a "staph"-like Gram stain. For example, *Streptococcus* and *Abiotrophia* growing in broth form long chains of cocci (Figure 15-2), whereas *Aerococcus*, *Gemella*, and *Pediococcus* grow as large, spherical cocci arranged in tetrads or pairs or as individual cells. *Leuconostoc* may elongate to form coccobacilli, although cocci are the primary morphology. The cellular arrangements of the genera in this chapter are noted in Tables 15-3 and 15-4.

## CULTIVATION

### Media of Choice

Except for *Abiotrophia* and *Granulicatella*, the organisms discussed in this chapter will grow on standard laboratory media such as 5% sheep blood and chocolate agars. They will not grow on MacConkey agar but will grow on gram-positive selective media such as CNA (Columbia agar with colistin and nalidixic acid) and PEA (phenylethyl alcohol agar).

*Abiotrophia* and *Granulicatella* will not grow on blood or chocolate agars unless pyridoxal (vitamin $B_6$) is supplied either by placement of a pyridoxal disk, by cross-streaking with *Staphylococcus*, or by inoculation of vitamin $B_6$–supplemented culture media.

Blood culture media support the growth of all of these organisms, as do common nutrient broths, such as thioglycollate or brain-heart infusion. Blood cultures that appear positive and show chaining gram-positive cocci on Gram stain but do not grow on subculture should be resubcultured with a pyridoxal disk to consider the possibility of *Abiotrophia* or *Granulicatella* bacteremia.

Other selective media are available for isolating certain species from clinical specimens. For isolating group A streptococci from throat swabs, the most common medium is 5% sheep blood agar supplemented with trimethoprim-sulfamethoxazole (SXT) to suppress the growth of normal flora. However, this medium also inhibits growth of groups C, F, and G beta-hemolytic streptococci.

To detect genital carriage of group B streptococci during pregnancy, Todd-Hewitt broth with antimicrobials (gentamicin, nalidixic acid, or colistin and nalidixic acid) is used to suppress the growth of vaginal flora and allow growth of *S. agalactiae* following subculture to blood agar. LIM broth is one medium formulation used for this purpose (see Chapter 7).

Differentiation of Enterococci and group D streptococci is traditionally based on the ability of the organisms to hydrolyze the glycoside esculin to esculetin and dextrose. The Esculetin reacts with an iron salt to form a dark brown precipitate surrounding the colonies. Entero-

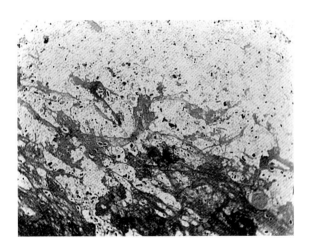

**Figure 15-1** *S. pneumoniae* lancet-shaped diplococci in Gram stain; note the encapsulated organisms as evident by the clear "halo."

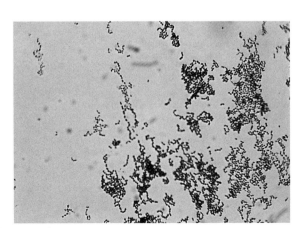

**Figure 15-2** Chains of streptococci seen in Gram stain prepared from broth culture.

**TABLE 15-3** Differentiation of Catalase-Negative, Gram-Positive Coccoid Organisms Primarily in Chains

| Organisms | Gram Stain from Thio Broth | Hemolysis α, β, or non[a] | Cytochrome[b]/ Catalase | Van | LAP | PVR | Gas in MRS Broth | Motility | on BE | in 6.5% NaCl Broth | GROWTH At 10°C | At 45°C | Comments |
|---|---|---|---|---|---|---|---|---|---|---|---|---|---|
| *Leuconostoc* | cb, pr, ch | α, non | –/– | R | V | – | + | – | V | V | V | V | |
| *Enterococcus* Vancomycin R | c, ch | α, β, or non | –/–[c] | R | + | + | – | – | + | + | + | + | |
| *Streptococcus* (all) | c, ch | α, β, or non | –/– | S | +[e] | V[f] | – | – | V[d] | V[h] | – | V | |
| *S. agalactiae* | c, ch | β, non | –/– | S | + | – | NT | – | – | V | NT | NT | |
| *S. bovis* | c, ch | α, non | –/– | S | + | – | – | – | + | – | – | + | |
| Viridans streptococci | c, ch | α, non | –/– | S | + | – | – | – | – | – | – | V | |
| *S. urinalis* | c, pr, ch | non | –/– | S | + | + | – | – | + | + | – | + | |
| *Abiotrophia* | c, ch | α, non | –/– | S | V | V | – | – | – | – | – | V | Satellitism around *S. aureus* |
| *Granulicatella* | c, pr, ch | α | –/– | S | + | + | – | – | NT | – | – | V | Satellitism around *S. aureus* |
| *Lactococcus* | cb, ch | α, non | –/– | S | + | V | – | – | + | V | + | V[i] | |
| *Dolosicoccus paucivorans* | c, pr, ch | α | –/– | S | – | + | – | – | – | – | – | – | |
| *Globicatella sanguinis* | c, ch, pr | α, non | –/– | S | – | V | – | – | + | + | + | V | |
| *Vagococcus* | c, ch | α, non | –/– | S | + | + | – | + | + | V | + | V | |
| *Lactobacillus* | cb, ch | α, non | –/– | V | V | – | V | – | V | V | + | V | |
| *Weissella confusa* | Elongated bacilli[k] | α | –/– | R | – | NT | + | V | + | V | NT | + | Arginine positive |

[a]Hemolysis tested on TSA with 5% sheep blood.
[b]Cytochrome enzymes as detected by the porphyrin broth test.
[c]Enterococci may produce a positive "pseudocatalase" effervescence. This occurs when *E. faecalis* strains grown on a blood-containing medium are tested for catalase production.
[d]*Vagococcus fluvialis* is negative for l-arabinose and raffinose, but the motile *Enterococcus gallinarum* is positive for both.
[e]The most common isolates are positive.
[f]*S. pyogenes, S. pneumoniae*, and *S. urinalis* are PYR positive.
[g]Five percent to 10% of viridans streptococci and *S. bovis* are bile esculin positive.
[h]Some beta streptococci grow in 6.5% salt broth.
[i]Occasional isolates are positive or give weakly positive reactions that are difficult to interpret.
[j]Majority of strains will not grow at 45° C in less than or equal to 48 hours.
[k]From blood agar, the organism resembles a gram-positive coccobacillus.
α, alpha-hemolytic; β, beta-hemolytic; BE, bile esculin hydrolysis; c, cocci; cb, coccobacilli; ch, chaining; pr, pairs; LAP, leucine aminopeptidase; MRS, gas from glucose in Mann, Rogosa, Sharp Lactobacillus broth; NT, not tested; PYR, pyrrolidonyl arylamidase; THIO, thioglycollate broth; Van, vancomycin (30 µg) susceptible (S) or resistant (R); +, 90% or more of species or strains are positive; –, 90% or more of species or strains negative; V, variable reactions.

Data compiled from Collins MD, Lawson PA: The genus *Abiotrophia* (Kawamura et al) is not monophyletic: proposal of Granulicatella gen nov, *Granulicatella adiacens* comb nov, *Granulicatella elegans* comb nov and *Granulicatella balaenopterae* comb nov, *Int J Syst Evol Microbiol* 50:365, 2000; Collins MD, Rodriguez Jovita M, Hutson RA, et al: *Dolosicoccus paucivorans* gen nov, sp nov, isolated from human blood, *Int J Syst Bacteriol* 49:1439, 1999; Facklam RR: Newly described, difficult-to-identify, catalase-negative, gram-positive cocci, *Clin Microbiol Newsl* 23:1, 2001; Schlegel L, Grimont F, Collins MD, et al: *Streptococcus infantarius* sp nov, *Streptococcus infantarius* subsp infantarius subsp nov, and *Streptococcus infantarius* subsp coli subsp nov, isolated from humans and food, *Int J Syst Evol Microbiol* 50:1425, 2000; Schlegel L, Grimont F, Ageron E, et al: Reappraisal of the taxonomy of the *Streptococcus bovis/Streptococcus equinus* complex and related species: description of *Streptococcus gallolyticus* subsp. gallolyticus subsp. nov, *S. gallolyticus* subsp. macedonicus subsp. nov and *S. gallolyticus* subsp. pasteurians subsp. nov, *Int J Syst Evol Microbiol* 53: 631, 2003; and Versalovic J: *Manual of Clinical Microbiology,* ed 10, Washington, DC, 2011, ASM Press.

coccosel agar is a selective differential medium based on the esculin hydrolysis and is also selective by incorporation of inhibitory oxgall (bile salts) for other grampositive organisms and sodium azide for gram-negative organisms.

### Incubation Conditions and Duration

Most of the organisms within this group are facultative anaerobes with some preferring a $CO_2$-enriched environment. Laboratories typically incubate blood or chocolate agar plates in 5% to 10% carbon dioxide. This is the preferred atmosphere for *S. pneumoniae* and is acceptable for all other genera discussed in this chapter. However, visualization of beta-hemolysis is enhanced by anaerobic conditions. Therefore, the blood agar plates should be inoculated by stabbing the inoculating loop into the agar several times (Figure 15-3, *A*). Colonies can then grow throughout the depth of the agar, producing subsurface oxygen-sensitive hemolysins (i.e., streptolysin O) (Figure 15-3, *B*). Most organisms will grow on agar media within 48 hours of inoculation.

### Colonial Appearance

Table 15-5 describes the colonial appearance and other distinguishing characteristics (e.g., hemolysis) of each genus on 5% sheep blood agar. The beta-hemolytic streptococci may have a distinctive buttery odor.

## APPROACH TO IDENTIFICATION

None of the commercial identification systems has been found to accurately identify all species of viridans streptococci or enterococci.

### Comments Regarding Specific Organisms

Useful characteristics for differentiation among catalasenegative, gram-positive cocci are shown in Tables 15-3 and 15-4. Organisms that may be weakly catalase positive, such as *Rothia mucilaginosa* (formerly *Stomatococcus mucilaginosus*), or coccobacillary, such as *Lactobacillus*, are included in these tables.

The cellular arrangement and the type of hemolysis are important considerations in identification (Figure 15-4). If the presence of hemolysis is uncertain, the colony should be moved aside with a loop and the medium directly beneath the original colony should be examined by holding the plate in front of a light source.

A screening test for vancomycin susceptibility is often useful for differentiating among many alpha-hemolytic cocci. All streptococci, aerococci, gemellas, lactococci,

**TABLE 15-4** Differentiation of Catalase-Negative, Gram-Positive, Coccoid Organisms Primarily in Clusters or Tetrads

| Organisms | Gram Stain from Thio Broth[a] | Hemolysis α, β, or non[β] | Cytochrome[c]/ Catalase | Van | LAP | PYR | Gas in MRS Broth | Motility | on BE | in 6.5% NaCl Broth | GROWTH At 10° C | At 45° C | Comments |
|---|---|---|---|---|---|---|---|---|---|---|---|---|---|
| *Alloiococcus* | c, pr, tet | non | –/+[k] | S | + | + | – | – | – | +[e] | – | – | Chronic otitis, no growth anaerobically at 72 hrs |
| *Facklamia* | c, pr, ch, cl | α, non | –/– | S | + | + | – | – | NT | +[f] | – | – | |
| *Dolosigranulum pigrum* | c, cl | non | – | S | + | +wk | – | – | – | + | – | – | |
| *Ignavigranum ruoffiae* | c, pr, cl | α | –/– | S | + | + | – | – | – | + | – | –[g] | Enhanced growth around *S. aureus;* sauerkraut odor on SBA |
| *Rothia* (formerly *Stomatococcus mucilaginosa*) | c, pr, cl | non | +/– or +[wk] | S | + | +[h] | – | – | NT | – | – | – | Strong adherence to agar surface |
| *Gemella* | c, pr, ch, cl, tet[i] | α, non | –/– | Sj | V[k] | V[l] | – | – | – | – | – | – | |
| *Pediococcusm* | c, pr, tet, cl | α, non | –/– | R | + | – | – | – | + | V | – | V | |
| *Tetragenococcusn* | c, tet, cl | α | –/– | S | + | – | – | – | + | + | – | + | Rarely found in humans |

*Continued*

**TABLE 15-4** Differentiation of Catalase-Negative, Gram-Positive, Coccoid Organisms Primarily in Clusters or Tetrads—cont'd

| Organisms | Gram Stain from Thio Broth[a] | Hemolysis α, β, or non[β] | Cytochrome[c]/ Catalase | Van | LAP | PYR | Gas in MRS Broth | Motility | on BE | in 6.5% NaCl Broth | GROWTH At 10° C | At 45° C | Comments |
|---|---|---|---|---|---|---|---|---|---|---|---|---|---|
| *Aerococcus* | c, pr, tet, cl | α | −/− | S | + | − | − | − | − | + | − | V[o] | |
| *Aerococcus urinae* | | | | | | | | | | | | | |
| *A. viridans* | c, pr, tet, cl | α | −/+[wk] | S | − | + | − | − | V | + | V | V | |
| *Helcococcus kunzii*[p] | c, pr, ch, cl | non | −/− | S | − | + | − | − | − | +[q] | − | − | Lipophilic |

[a]*Alloiococcus* will not grow in thioglycollate broth; Gram stain must be done from a solid medium. *D. pigrum* grows poorly in thioglycollate broth.
[b]Hemolysis tested on TSA with 5% sheep blood.
[c]Cytochrome enzymes as detected by the porphyrin broth test.
[d]No growth anaerobically. May be catalase negative when grown on non–blood-containing media.
[e]May take 2 to 7 days.
[f]*Facklamia hominis, F. ignava,* and *F. languida* are positive and *F. sourekii* is negative.
[g]Positive after 7 days.
[h]Most are positive.
[i]*G. haemolysans* easily decolorizes when Gram stained. They resemble *Neisseria* with adjacent flattened sides of pairs of cells.
[j]There is one literature report of a vancomycin-resistant *Gemella haemolysans*.
[k]*G. haemolysans* and G. sanguinis are LAP negative, and *G. morbillorum* and *G. bergeri* are positive.
[l]Weakly positive. Use a large inoculum.
[m]The most commonly isolated pediococci are arginine deaminase positive.
[n]Reactions are based on one isolate only.
[o]If inoculated too heavily, the organism will grow at 45° C.
[p]Lipophilic-growth stimulated on HIA (heart infusion agar) with 1% horse serum or 0.1% Tween.
[q]Because *Helcococcus* is lipophilic, the salt broth may appear to be negative unless supplemented with 1% horse serum or 0.1% Tween 80.
α, alpha-hemolytic; β, beta-hemolytic; BE, bile esculin hydrolysis; c, cocci; cb, coccobacilli; ch, chaining; cl, clusters; pr, pairs; tet, tetrads; LAP, leucine aminopeptidase; MRS, gas from glucose in Mann, Rogosa, Sharp Lactobacillus broth; NT, not tested; PYR, pyrrolidonyl arylamidase; SBA, 5% sheep blood agar; THIO, thioglycollate broth; Van, vancomycin (30 μg) susceptible reactions. (S) or resistant (R); +, 90% or more of species or strains are positive; +wk, strains or species may be weakly positive; −, 90% or more of species or strains negative; V, variable.
Data compiled from Arbique JC, Poyart C, Trieu-Cuot P, et al: Accuracy of phenotypic and genotypic testing for identification of *Streptococcus pneumoniae* and description of *Streptococcus pseudopneumoniae* sp. nov, *J Clin Microbiol* 42:4686, 2004; Christensen JJ, Vibits H, Ursing J, et al: Aerococcus-like organism: a newly recognized potential urinary tract pathogen, *J Clin Microbiol* 29:1049, 1991; Collins MD, Falsen E, Lemozy J, et al: Phenotypic and phylogenetic characterization of some Globicatella-like organisms from human sources: description of *Facklamia hominis* gen nov, sp nov, *Int J Syst Bacteriol* 47:880, 1997; Collins MD, Hutson RA, Falsen E, et al: An unusual Streptococcus from human urine, *Streptococcus urinalis* sp nov, *Int J Syst Evol Microbiol* 50:1173, 2000; Collins MD, Hutson RA, Falsen E, et al: Description of *Gemella sanguinis* sp nov, isolated from human clinical specimen, *J Clin Microbiol* 36:3090, 1998; Collins MD, Hutson RA, Falsen E, et al: *Facklamia sourekii* sp nov, isolated from human sources, *Int J Syst Bacteriol* 49:635, 1999; Collins MD, Hutson RA, Falsen E, et al: *Gemella bergeriae* sp nov, isolated from human clinical specimens, *J Clin Microbiol* 36:1290, 1998; Collins MD, Lawson PA, Monasterio R, et al: *Facklamia ignava* sp nov, isolated from human clinical specimens, *J Clin Microbiol* 36:2146, 1998; Collins MD, Lawson PA, Monasterio R, et al: *Ignavigranum ruoffiae* sp nov, isolated from human clinical specimens, *Int J Syst Bacteriol* 49:97, 1999; Collins MD, Williams AM, Wallbanks S: The phylogeny of Aerococcus and Pediococcus as determined by 16S rRNA sequence analysis: description of Tetragenococcus gen nov, *FEMS Microbiol Lett* 70:255, 1990; Facklam RR: Newly described, difficult-to-identify, catalase-negative, gram-positive cocci, *Clin Microbiol Newsl* 23:1, 2001; LaClaire L, Facklam R: Antimicrobial susceptibility and clinical sources of *Dolosigranulum pigrum* cultures, *Antimicrob Agents Chemother* 44:2001, 2000; and Lawson PA, Collins MD, Falsen E, et al: *Facklamia languida* sp nov, isolated from human clinical specimen, *J Clin Microbiol* 37:1161, 1999.

and most enterococci are susceptible to vancomycin (any zone of inhibition), whereas pediococci, leuconostocs, and many lactobacilli are typically resistant (growth up to the disk). Other useful tests listed in Tables 15-3 and 15-4 includes leucine aminopeptidase (LAP) and pyrrolidonyl arylamidase (PYR), which are commercially available as disks (see Chapter 13).

*Leuconostoc* produces gas from glucose in MRS broth; this distinguishes it from all other genera, except the lactobacilli. However, unlike *Leuconostoc* spp., lactobacilli appear as elongated bacilli when Gram stained from thioglycollate broth. Several organisms (e.g., *Leuconostoc, Pediococcus, Lactococcus, Helcococcus, Globicatella, Tetragenococcus, Streptococcus urinalis,* and *Aerococcus viridans*) will show growth on bile-esculin agar and in 6.5% salt broth;

this is the reason these two tests no longer solely can be used to identify enterococci.

Serologic grouping of cell wall carbohydrates (Lancefield classifications) has classically been used to identify species of beta-hemolytic streptococci. The original Lancefield precipitin test is now rarely performed in clinical laboratories. It has been replaced by either latex agglutination or coagglutination procedures available as commercial kits. Serologic tests have the advantage of being rapid, confirmatory, and easily performed on one or two colonies. However, they are more expensive than biochemical screening tests.

The PYR and hippurate or CAMP tests can be used to identify groups A and B streptococci, respectively. However, use of the 0.04-U bacitracin disk is no longer

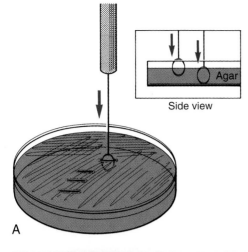

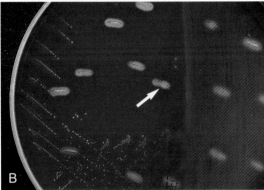

**Figure 15-3** Stabbing the inoculating loop vertically into the agar after streaking the blood agar plate (A) allows subsurface colonies to display hemolysis caused by streptolysin O (B).
*Based on the reactions of only one isolate.
†*S. bovis* variant includes *S. infantarius* subsp. *infantarius, S. lutetiensis,* and *S. gallolyticus* subsp. *pasteurianus.* Most *S. bovis* variant strains will be positive for α-galactosidase and *S. salivarius* will be negative.
‡Optochin test must be performed in $CO_2$ to avoid misidentification with *S. pseudopneumoniae.*

recommended for *S. pyogenes,* because groups C and G streptococci are also susceptible to this agent. *S. pyogenes* is the only species of beta-hemolytic streptococci that will give a positive PYR reaction.

   *S. agalactiae* is able to hydrolyze hippurate and is positive in the CAMP test. The CAMP test detects production of a diffusible, extracellular protein that enhances the hemolysis of sheep erythrocytes by *Staphylococcus aureus.* A positive test is recognized by the appearance of an arrowhead shape at the juncture of the *S. agalactiae* and *S. aureus* streaks (Figure 15-5). Occasionally, non–beta-hemolytic strains of Streptococcus agalactiae may be encountered, but identification of such isolates can be accomplished using the serologic agglutination approach. Enterococci can also be hippurate hydrolysis positive.

   Table 15-6 shows the differentiation of the clinically relevant beta-hemolytic streptococci. Minute beta-hemolytic streptococci are all likely to be of the *S. anginosus* group; a positive Voges-Proskauer test and negative

**TABLE 15-5** Colonial Appearance and Characteristics on 5% Sheep Blood Agar

| Organism | Appearance |
|---|---|
| Group A beta-hemolytic streptococci[a] | Grayish white, transparent to translucent, matte or glossy; large zone of beta hemolysis |
| Group B beta-hemolytic streptococci[b] | Larger than group A streptococci; translucent to opaque; flat, glossy; narrow zone of beta hemolysis; some strains nonhemolytic |
| Group C beta-hemolytic streptococci[c] | Grayish white, glistening; wide zone of beta hemolysis |
| Group F beta-hemolytic streptococci[d] | Grayish white, small, matte; narrow to wide zone of beta hemolysis |
| Group G beta-hemolytic streptococci[e] | Grayish white, matte; wide zone of beta hemolysis |
| *S. pneumoniae* | Small, gray, glistening; colonies tend to dip down in the center and resemble a doughnut (umbilicated) as they age; if organism has a polysaccharide capsule, colony may be mucoid; alpha-hemolytic |
| Viridans streptococci[f] | Minute to small, gray, domed, smooth or matte; alpha-hemolytic or nonhemolytic |
| *Abiotrophia* spp. and *Granulicatella* spp.[g] | Resemble viridans streptococci |
| *Enterococcus* spp. | Small, cream or white, smooth, entire; alpha-, beta-, or nonhemolytic |
| *Leuconostoc, Aerococcus, Pediococcus, Gemella, Lactococcus, Globicatella, Helcococcus, Alloiococcus, Tetragenococcus, Dolosigranulum, Facklamia, Ignavigranum, Dolosicoccus, Vagococcus,* and *Weissella* | Resemble viridans streptococci; see Tables 15-3 and 15-4 for hemolytic reactions |

[a]Two colony sizes, that is, small (called large-colony and named *S. pyogenes*) and minute (called small-colony and named *S. anginosus* group).
[b]*S. agalactiae.*
[c]Two colony sizes, that is, small (called large-colony and named *S. dysgalactiae* subsp. *equisimilis*) and minute (called small-colony and named *S. anginosus* group).
[d]*S. anginosus* group.
[e]Two colony sizes—that is, small (called large-colony and named *S. dysgalactiae* subsp. *equisimilis*) and minute (called small-colony and named *S. anginosus* group).
[f]Includes *S. mutans* group, *S. salivarius* group, *S. anginosus* group, *S. bovis* and variants, and *S. urinalis* and *S. mitis* group.
[g]May satellite around staphylococcal colonies on 5% sheep blood or chocolate agars.

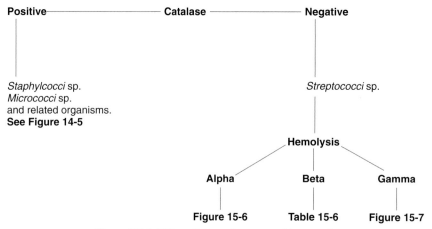

Positive ─────────── Catalase ─────────── Negative

Staphylcocci sp.
Micrococci sp.
and related organisms.
**See Figure 14-5**

Streptococci sp.

Hemolysis

Alpha                    Beta                    Gamma

Figure 15-6            Table 15-6            Figure 15-7

**Figure 15-4** Differentiation of gram-positive cocci.

**TABLE 15-6** Differentiation of the Clinically Relevant Beta-Hemolytic Streptococci

| Species | Colony Size | Lancefield Group | Pyr | Vp | Hipp | Camp Test |
|---|---|---|---|---|---|---|
| S. pyogenes | Large | A | + | − | − | − |
| S. anginosus group[a] | Small | A | − | + | − | − |
| S. agalactiae | Medium | B | − | −[b] | + | + |
| S. dysgalactiae subsp. equisimilis | Large | C and G | − | − | − | − |
| S. anginosus group[a] | Small | C and G | − | + | − | − |
| S. anginosus group[a] | Small | F | − | + | − | − |
| S. anginosus group[a] | Small | Non-groupable | − | + | − | − |

[a]Also called S. milleri group.
[b]Mixed reports of this result in the literature.
Hipp, Hydrolysis of hippurate; PYR, pyrrolidonyl arylamidase; VP, Voges-Proskauer test; +, >90% of strains positive; −, >90% of strains negative.
Data compiled from Vandamme P, Pot B, Falsen E, et al: Taxonomic study of Lancefield streptococcal groups C, G, and L (Streptococcus dysgalactiae) and proposal of S. dysgalactiae subsp equisimilis subsp nov, Int J Syst Bacteriol 46:774, 1996; Whiley RA, Hall LM, Hardie JM, et al: A study of small-colony, β-hemolytic, Lancefield group C streptococci within the anginosus group: description of Streptococcus constellatus subsp pharyngis subsp nov, associated with the human throat and pharyngitis, Int J Syst Bacteriol 49:1443, 1999; and Versalovic J: Manual of clinical microbiology, ed 10, Washington, DC, 2011, ASM Press.

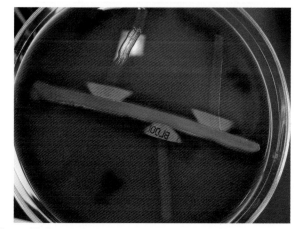

**Figure 15-5** Positive CAMP reaction as indicated by enlarged zone of hemolysis shaped like a tip of the arrow, S. agalactiae intersecting with S. aureus streak line.

PYR test identify a beta-hemolytic streptococcal isolate as such.

Suspicious colonies thought to be S. pneumoniae must be tested for either bile solubility or susceptibility to optochin (ethylhydrocupreine hydrochloride). The bile solubility test is confirmatory and is based on the ability of bile salts to induce lysis of S. pneumoniae. In the optochin test, which is presumptive, a filter paper disk ("P" disk) impregnated with optochin is placed on a blood agar plate previously streaked with a lawn of the suspect organism. The plate is incubated at 35° C for 18 to 24 hours and read for inhibition. S. pneumoniae produce a zone of inhibition, whereas viridans streptococci grow up to the disk. A newly discovered organism, Streptococcus pseudopneumoniae, may interfere with appropriate interpretation of the optochin disk test. S. pseudopneumoniae are resistant to optochin (zone ≤14 mm) when they are incubated under increased $CO_2$, but are susceptible to optochin (zone >14 mm) when they are incubated in ambient atmosphere. Therefore, optochin disk tests should be incubated under 5% $CO_2$ and all tests should be confirmed by a bile solubility test. Unfortunately, the commercial molecular probe for S. pneumoniae, AccuProbe Pneumococcus (Gen-Probe, San Diego,

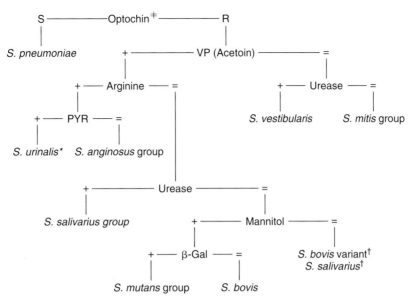

*Based on the reactions of only one isolate.
†*S. bovis* variant includes *S. infantarius* subsp. infantarius, *S. lutetiensis*, and *S. gallolyticus* subsp. *pasteurianus.* Most *S. bovis* variant strains will be positive for α-galactosidase and *S. salivarius* will be negative.
‡Optochin test must be performed in $CO_2$ to avoid misidentification with *S. pseudopneumoniae.*

**Figure 15-6** Differentiation of clinically relevant viridans streptococcal groups. *S. mitis* group includes *S. mitis, S. sanguinis, S. parasanguinis, S. gordonii, S. oralis,* and *S. cristatus. S. mutans* group includes *S. mutans* and *S. sobrinus. S. anginosus* group includes *S. anginosus, S. constellatus subsp. constellatus,* and *S. intermedius. S. salivarius* group includes *S. salivarius* and *S. vestibularis.* β-gal, Beta-galactosidase; *PYR,* pyrrolidonyl arylamidase; *R,* resistant; *S,* sensitive; +, positive; =, negative. (Compiled from Collins MD, Hutson RA, Falsen E, et al: An unusual Streptococcus from human urine, Streptococcus urinalis sp nov, *Int J Syst Evol Microbiol* 50:1173, 2000; Poyart C, Quesne G, Trieu-Cuot P: Taxonomic dissection of the Streptococcus bovis group by analysis of manganese-dependent superoxide dismutase gene (sodA) sequences: reclassification of "Streptococcus infantarius subsp. coli" as *Streptococcus lutetiensis* sp. nov. and of Streptococcus bovis biotype II.2 as *Streptococcus pasteurianus* sp. nov, *Int J Syst Evol Microbiol* 52:1247, 2002; and Schlegel L, Grimont F, Collins MD, et al: Streptococcus infantarius sp nov, Streptococcus infantarius subsp infantarius subsp nov, and Streptococcus infantarius subsp coli subsp nov, isolated from humans and food, *Int J Syst Evol Microbiol* 50:1425, 2000.)

California), does not discriminate between *S. pneumoniae* and *S. pseudopneumoniae.* Because the pathogenic potential of *S. pseudopneumoniae* is currently unknown, it is important to differentiate it from *S. pneumoniae,* a known pathogen. Serologic identification of *S. pneumoniae* is also possible using coagglutination or latex agglutination test kits.

Once *S. pneumoniae* has been ruled out as a possibility for an alpha-hemolytic isolate, viridans streptococci and enterococci must be considered. Figure 15-6 outlines the key tests for differentiating among the viridans streptococci. Carbohydrate fermentation tests are performed in heart infusion broth with bromcresol purple indicator. Although alpha-hemolytic streptococci are not often identified to species, there are cases (i.e., endocarditis, isolation from multiple blood cultures) in which full identification is indicated. This is particularly true for blood culture isolates of *S. bovis* that have been associated with gastrointestinal malignancy and may be an early indicator of gastrointestinal cancer. *S. bovis* possesses group D antigen that may be detected using commercially available typing sera. However, this is not a definitive test, because other organisms (e.g., *Leuconostoc*) may also produce a positive result.

Except for species not usually isolated from humans (*E. saccharolyticus, E. cecorum, E. columbae,* and *E. pallens*),

all enterococci hydrolyze PYR and possess group D antigen. A flowchart that may be used to identify enterococcal species is shown in Figure 15-7. Identifying the species of enterococcal isolates is important for understanding the epidemiology of antimicrobial resistance among isolates of this genus and for managing patients with enterococcal infections. Most clinical laboratories identify *Enterococcus* spp. presumptively by demonstrating that the isolate is PYR and LAP positive and that it grows at 45° C and in 6.5% NaCl. However, the recent discovery of *Streptococcus urinalis* presents a problem in this regard. *S. urinalis* and the commonly isolated Enterococcus spp. exhibit identical reactions in the four tests listed here and only differ in the ability to grow at 10° C (*S. urinalis* cannot).

## SERODIAGNOSIS

Individuals with disease caused by *S. pyogenes* produce antibodies against various antigens. The most common are antistreptolysin O (ASO), anti-DNase B, antistreptokinase, and antihyaluronidase. Pharyngitis seems to be followed by rises in antibody titers against all antigens, whereas patients with pyoderma, an infection of the skin, only show a significant response to anti-DNase B. Use of serodiagnostic tests is most useful to demonstrate prior

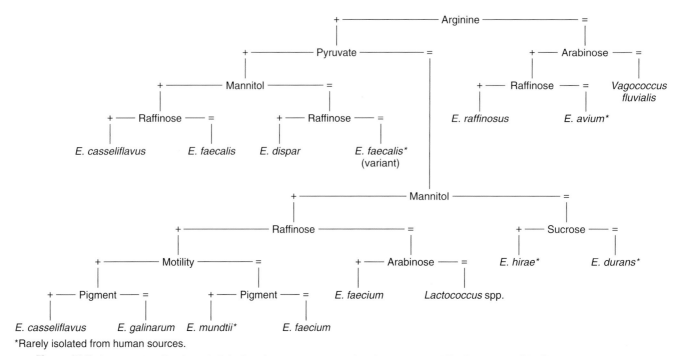

**Figure 15-7** Species identification of clinically relevant enterococcal and enterococcal-like isolates. =, Signifies a negative result.

streptococcal infection in patients from whom group A *Streptococcus* has not been cultured but who present with sequelae suggestive of rheumatic fever or acute glomerulonephritis. Serum obtained as long as 2 months after infection usually demonstrates increased antibodies. As with other serologic tests, an increasing titer over time is most useful for diagnosing previous streptococcal infection.

Commercial products are available for detection of anti-streptococcal antibodies. Streptozyme (Alere Inc., Waltham, MA), which detects a mixture of antibodies, is a commonly used test. Unfortunately, no commercial system has been shown to accurately detect all streptococcal antibodies.

# ANTIMICROBIAL SUSCEPTIBILITY TESTING AND THERAPY

For *S. pyogenes* and the other beta-hemolytic streptococci, penicillin is the drug of choice (Table 15-7). Because penicillin resistance has not been encountered among these organisms, susceptibility testing of clinical isolates for reasons other than resistance surveillance is not necessary. However, if a macrolide such as erythromycin is being considered for use, as is the case with patients who are allergic to penicillin, testing is needed to detect resistance that has emerged among these organisms. For serious infections caused by *S. agalactiae*, an aminoglycoside may be added to supplement β-lactam therapy and enhance bacterial killing.

In contrast to beta-hemolytic streptococci, the emergence of resistance to a variety of different antimicrobial classes in *S. pneumoniae* and viridans streptococci dictates that clinically relevant isolates be subjected to in vitro

susceptibility testing. When testing is performed, methods that produce minimal inhibitory concentration (MIC) data for β-lactams are preferred. The level of resistance (i.e., MIC in μg/mL) can provide important information regarding therapeutic management of the patient, particularly in cases of pneumococcal meningitis in which relatively slight increases in MIC can have substantial impact on the clinical efficacy of penicillins and cephalosporins. Vancomycin resistance has not been described in either *S. pneumoniae* or viridans streptococci.

*S. pneumoniae* or other beta-hemolytic *Streptococcus* spp. that demonstrate resistance to erythromycin and susceptible or intermediate to clindamycin should be examined for inducible clindamycin resistance as previously described for *Staphylococcus* spp. in Chapter 14. Disk diffusion using Mueller Hinton or Tryptic soy agar supplemented with 5% sheep blood may be used. Place a 15-μg erythromycin disk and a 2-μg disk 12 mm apart. If inducible resistance is present, the clindamycin zone adjacent to the erythromycin disk will demonstrate the classic flattening or D-zone appearance. Alternately, a broth microdilution using Mueller Hinton containing lysed horse blood (2.5% to 5%) may be used by adding 1 μg/mL erythromycin and 0.5 μg/mL clindamycin within a single well. Any visible growth within the well would indicate inducible clindamycin resistance.

Enterococci are intrinsically resistant to a wide array of antimicrobial agents, and they generally are resistant to killing by any of the single agents (e.g., ampicillin or vancomycin) that are bactericidal for most other gram-positive cocci. Therefore, effective bactericidal activity can only be achieved with the combination of a cell wall–active agent, such as ampicillin or vancomycin, and an aminoglycoside, such as gentamicin or streptomycin.

Unfortunately, many *E. faecalis* and *E. faecium* isolates have acquired resistance to one or more of these

**TABLE 15-7** Antimicrobial Therapy and Susceptibility Testing

| Organism | Therapeutic Options | Resistance to Therapeutic Options | Validated Testing Methods* | Comments |
|---|---|---|---|---|
| *Streptococcus pyogenes* | Penicillin is drug of choice; alternatives may include macrolides (e.g., azithromycin, clarithromycin, or erythromycin), telithromycin, and certain cephalosporins; vancomycin for penicillin-allergic patients with serious infections | No resistance to penicillin, cephalosporins, vancomycin known; resistance to macrolides does occur | As documented in Chapter 12: disk diffusion, broth dilution, and agar dilution | Testing to guide therapy is not routinely needed, unless a macrolide is being considered |
| *Streptococcus agalactiae* | Penicillin, with or without an aminoglycoside; ceftriaxone or cefotaxime may be used instead of penicillin; vancomycin is used for penicillin-allergic patients | No resistance to penicillins, cephalosporins, or vancomycin known | As documented in Chapter 12: disk diffusion, broth dilution, agar dilution, and some commercial methods | Testing to guide therapy is not routinely needed |
| Groups C, F, and G beta-hemolytic streptococci | Penicillin; vancomycin for penicillin-allergic patients | No resistance known to penicillin or vancomycin | Same as used for *S. pyogenes* and *S. agalactiae* | Testing to guide therapy is not routinely needed |
| *Streptococcus pneumoniae* | Penicillin, ceftriaxone, or cefotaxime; telithromycin; macrolides, trimethoprim-sulfamethoxazole, and certain quinolones (levofloxacin, moxifloxacin, gemifloxacin) | Yes. Resistance to penicillin, cephalosporins, and macrolides is frequently encountered; vancomycin resistance has not been encountered. Fluoroquinolone resistance is rare | As documented in Chapter 12; disk diffusion, broth dilution, and certain commercial methods | In vitro susceptibility testing results are important for guiding therapy |
| Viridans streptococci | Penicillin or ceftriaxone, with or without an aminoglycoside; vancomycin is used in cases of penicillin allergies and beta-lactam resistance | Resistance to penicillin and cephalosporins is frequently encountered; vancomycin resistance has not been encountered | As documented in Chapter 12: disk diffusion, broth dilution, agar dilution, and some commercial methods | In vitro susceptibility testing results are important for guiding therapy |
| *Abiotrophia* spp. (nutritionally variant streptococci) | Penicillin, or vancomycin, plus an aminoglycoside | Resistance to penicillin in known, but impact on efficacy of combined penicillin and aminoglycoside therapy is not known | See CLSI document M45: methods for antimicrobial dilution and disk susceptibility testing of infrequently isolated or fastidious bacteria | Testing to guide therapy is not necessary |
| *Enterococcus* spp. | For systemic, life-threatening infections a cell wall–active agent (i.e. penicillin, ampicillin, or vancomycin) plus an aminoglycoside (gentamicin or streptomycin); newer agents such as linezolid and daptomycin may also be effective; occasionally, other agents such as chloramphenicol may be used when multidrug-resistant strains are encountered. For urinary tract isolates, ampicillin, nitrofurantoin, tetracycline, or quinolones may be effective | Resistance to every therapeutically useful antimicrobial agent, including vancomycin, linezolid, and daptomycin has been described | As documented in Chapter 12: disk diffusion, broth dilution, various screens, agar dilution, and commercial systems | In vitro susceptibility testing results are important for guiding therapy |

*Continued*

**TABLE 15-7** Antimicrobial Therapy and Susceptibility Testing—cont'd

| Organism | Therapeutic Options | Resistance to Therapeutic Options | Validated Testing Methods* | Comments |
|---|---|---|---|---|
| *Leuconostoc* spp., *Lactococcus* spp., *Globicatella* sp., *Pediococcus* spp., *Aerococcus* spp., *Gemella* spp., *Helcococcus* sp., and *Alloiococcus otitidis* and other miscellaneous opportunistic cocci | Frequently susceptible to penicillins and aminoglycosides | Unknown. *Leuconostoc* and pediococci are intrinsically resistant to vancomycin | See CLSI document M45: Methods for Antimicrobial Dilution and Disk Susceptibility Testing of Infrequently Isolated or Fastidious Bacteria | Whenever isolated from clinical specimens, the potential of the isolate being a contaminant should be strongly considered |

*Validated testing methods include those standard methods recommended by the Clinical and Laboratory Standards Institute (CLSI) and those commercial methods approved by the Food and Drug Administration (FDA).

components of combination therapy. This resistance generally eliminates any contribution that the target antimicrobial agent could make to the synergistic killing of the organism. Therefore, performance of in vitro susceptibility testing with clinical isolates from systemic infections is critical for determining which combination of agents may still be effective therapeutic choices.

For uncomplicated urinary tract infections, bactericidal activity is usually not required for clinical efficacy, so that single agents such as ampicillin, nitrofurantoin, or a quinolone are often sufficient.

All gram-positive bacteria demonstrate intrinsic antibiotic resistance to polymyxin B/colistin, nalidixic acid, and axtreonam. In addition, several species of enterococci are intrinsically resistant to additional antibiotics, including the following: *E. faecalis* (cephalosporins, aminoglycosides, clindamycin, quinpristin-dalfopristin, trimethoprim, trimethoprim/sulfamethoxazole, and fusidic acid), *E. facieum* (all of these included for *E. faecalis* except quinupristin-dalfopristin), *E. gallinarum*, and *E. casseliflavus* (all of those included for *E. faecalis* and, in addition, vancolycin). Careful consideration should be taken when reporting susceptibilities, cephalosporins, aminoglycosides (except for high-level resistance screening), clindamycin, and trimethoprim-sulfamethoxazole may appear to be effective in the laboratory using in vitro methods, but they are not clinically effective and should not be reported as susceptible.

infection by the most common serotypes of *S. pneumoniae* is available in the United States. Vaccination is recommended for children 2 years and older with medical conditions such as sickle cell disease, diabetes, cochlear implants, damaged spleen, diseases that affect the immune system, chronic heart or lung failure, and for individuals older than 65. The vaccine is not effective in children younger than 2 years of age. Vaccination with PCV13 is recommended for children and infants who may be at risk for infection. PCV13 is a pneumococcal conjugate vaccine that protects against 13 types of *Streptococcus pneumoniae*. The serotypes included in this vaccine account for the majority of cases of bacteremia, meningitis, and otitis media in children younger than 6 years of age.

Lifetime chemoprophylaxis with penicillin, given either monthly (intramuscular administration) or daily (oral administration), is recommended for patients with rheumatic heart disease to prevent development of bacterial endocarditis on a damaged heart valve. Likewise, penicillin may be indicated to control outbreaks of *S. pyogenes* in individuals in close physical contact, such as in households, military populations, or newborn nurseries.

# PREVENTION

A single-dose, 23-valent vaccine (Pneumovax, Merck & Co., Inc., West Point, Pennsylvania) to prevent

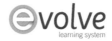 *Visit the Evolve site to complete the review questions.*

# CASE STUDY 15-1

A 76-year-old man with atherosclerosis was previously admitted for abdominal aneurysm and resection of the perirenal aorta. He had several follow-up admissions over the next year for postoperative wound infections, with accompanying bacteremia, alternating between *Pseudomonas aeruginosa,* vancomycin-resistant *Enterococcus faecium,* and *Candida glabrata.* On his final admission, blood cultures were positive, with numerous gram-positive cocci in pairs and chains in the smear, but subculture of the bottle showed no growth aerobically with increased $CO_2$ on blood agar or chocolate agar or anaerobically on Brucella agar.

## QUESTIONS

1. What is this organism, and what media should be used for culture?
2. To control infection, screening for vancomycin resistance in enterococci on selected hospitalized patients is important. What is a cost-effective screening method?
3. Many genera of gram-positive cocci are catalase negative, but only a few are vancomycin resistant. Name these genera, and indicate how they can be differentiated from vancomycin-resistant enterococci.

# CASE STUDY 15-2

A 75-year-old man lives at home with his wife and is in relatively good health aside from hypertension and mild diabetes mellitus type 2. Through medications and lifestyle, the man is able to keep both of his medical conditions under control. He has never used tobacco, but his wife was a smoker for 35 years. She quit approximately 20 years ago. She always smoked in the house and in the car with other family members present, including her husband.

The man presented with a 3-day history of fatigue, chills, and lack of appetite. He has no acute respiratory complaints other than mild dyspnea and a fever of 101. On an almost daily basis he coughs up yellow sputum (Figure 15-8) in the morning and has for several years. He has attributed this to his "old age" and has never discussed this with his physician.

## LABORATORY RESULTS

Patient was found to have an elevated white blood count of 16,000 with >10 bands per hpf.

| Chemistry Panel | Patient | Reference Range |
|---|---|---|
| Sodium | 146 | 136-145 meq/L |
| Potassium | 3.9 | 3.6-5.0 meq/L |
| Chloride | 111 | 101-111 meq/L |
| $HCO_3^-$ | 27 | 24-34 meq/L |
| Glucose | 120 | 80-120 mg/dL |
| Bilirubin, total | 1.0 | 0.2-1.2 mg/dL |
| AST | 28 | 5-40 IU/L |
| ALP | 56 | 30-157 IU/L |
| Total protein | 7.1 | 6.0-8.4 g/dL |
| BUN | 91.2 | 7-24 mg/dL |
| Creatinine | 2.4 | 0.5-1.2 mg/dL |

Bun/Creatinine ration = 38

| Arterial Blood Gases | Patient | Reference Range |
|---|---|---|
| $PCO_2$ | 47 | 35-45 mm Hg |
| $PO_2$ | 75 | 83-108 mmHg |
| $HCO_3^-$ | 29 | 22-28 mEq/L |
| pH | 7.34 | 7.35-7.45 |
| $SaO_2$ | 88 | 95%-98% |

$PCO_2$, partial pressure of carbon dioxide; $PO_2$, partial pressure of oxygen, $SaO_2$, oxygen saturation.

## QUESTIONS

1. What risk factors are associated with this individual's condition that predispose him to bacterial infections?
2. Review the laboratory results provided. Identify the abnormal results, and provide an explanation for recommended follow-up laboratory tests and any other recommended diagnostics.
3. Review the Gram stain provided from the patient's sputum. Is it stain consistent with the patient's condition? What, if any, additional tests would be recommended?

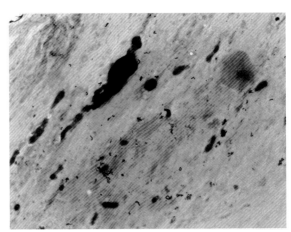

**Figure 15-8** Patient's sputum Gram stain.

# BIBLIOGRAPHY

Arbique JC, Poyart C, Trieu-Cuot P, et al: Accuracy of phenotypic and genotypic testing for identification of *Streptococcus pneumoniae* and description of *Streptococcus pseudopneumoniae* sp. nov, *J Clin Microbiol* 42:4686, 2004.

Bosley GS, Whitney AM, Prucker JM, et al: Characterization of ear fluid isolates of Alloiococcus otitidis from patients with recurrent otitis media, *J Clin Microbiol* 33:2876, 1995.

Bouvet A: Human endocarditis due to nutritionally variant streptococci: *Streptococcus adjacens* and *Streptococcus defectivus*, *Eur Heart J* 16(suppl B):24, 1995.

Carratala J, Alcaide F, Fernandez-Sevilla A, et al: Bacteremia due to viridans streptococci that are highly resistant to penicillin: increase among neutropenic patients with cancer, *Clin Infect Dis* 20:1169, 1995.

Chapin, KC, Blake P, Wilson CD: Performance characteristics and utilization of rapid antigen test, DNA probe, and culture for detection in an acute care clinic, *J Clin Microbiol* 40:4207-4210, 2002.

Christensen JJ, Vibits H, Ursing J, et al: Aerococcus-like organism: a newly recognized potential urinary tract pathogen, *J Clin Microbiol* 29:1049, 1991.

Clinical and Laboratory Standards Institute: Performance standards for antimicrobial susceptibility testing; M100-S23, Wayne, Pa., 2013, CLSI.

Collins MD, Falsen E, Lemozy J, et al: Phenotypic and phylogenetic characterization of some Globicatella-like organisms from human sources: description of *Facklamia hominis* gen nov, sp nov, *Int J Syst Bacteriol* 47:880, 1997.

Collins MD, Hutson RA, Falsen E, et al: An unusual Streptococcus from human urine, Streptococcus urinalis sp nov, *Int J Syst Evol Microbiol* 50:1173, 2000.

Collins MD, Hutson RA, Falsen E, et al: Description of *Gemella sanguinis* sp nov, isolated from human clinical specimen, *J Clin Microbiol* 36:3090, 1998.

Collins MD, Hutson RA, Falsen E, et al: *Facklamia sourekii* sp nov, isolated from human sources, *Int J Syst Bacteriol* 49:635, 1999.

Collins MD, Hutson RA, Falsen E, et al: *Gemella bergeriae* sp nov, isolated from human clinical specimens, *J Clin Microbiol* 36:1290, 1998.

Collins MD, Lawson PA: The genus Abiotrophia (Kawamura et al) is not monophyletic: proposal of Granulicatella gen nov, Granulicatella adiacens comb nov, Granulicatella elegans comb nov and Granulicatella balaenopterae comb nov, *Int J Syst Evol Microbiol* 50:365, 2000.

Collins MD, Lawson PA, Monasterio R, et al: *Facklamia ignava* sp nov, isolated from human clinical specimens, *J Clin Microbiol* 36:2146, 1998.

Collins MD, Lawson PA, Monasterio R, et al: *Ignavigranum ruoffiae* sp nov, isolated from human clinical specimens, *Int J Syst Bacteriol* 49:97, 1999.

Collins MD, Rodriguez Jovita M, Hutson RA, et al: Dolosicoccus paucivorans gen nov, sp nov, isolated from human blood, *Int J Syst Bacteriol* 49:1439, 1999.

Collins MD, Williams AM, Wallbanks S: The phylogeny of Aerococcus and Pediococcus as determined by 16S rRNA sequence analysis: description of Tetragenococcus gen nov, *FEMS Microbiol Lett* 70:255, 1990.

Facklam RR: Newly described, difficult-to-identify, catalase-negative, gram-positive cocci, *Clin Microbiol Newsl* 23:1, 2001.

Gerber MA: Antibiotic resistance in group A streptococci, *Pediatr Clin North Am* 42:539, 1995.

Hassan, AA, Abdulmawjood A, Yildirim AO, et al: Identification of streptococci isolated from various sources by determination of cfb gene and other CAMP-factor genes, *Can J Microbiol* 46: 946-951, 2000.

Jett BD, Huycke MM, Gilmore MS: Virulence of enterococci, *Clin Microbiol Rev* 7:462, 1994.

Johnson AP: The pathogenicity of enterococci, *J Antimicrob Chemother* 33:1083, 1994.

LaClaire L, Facklam R: Antimicrobial susceptibility and clinical sources of Dolosigranulum pigrum cultures, *Antimicrob Agents Chemother* 44:2001, 2000.

Lawson PA, Collins MD, Falsen E, et al: *Facklamia languida* sp nov, isolated from human clinical specimen, *J Clin Microbiol* 37:1161, 1999.

Leclercq R: Epidemiology and control of multiresistant enterococci, *Drugs* 2:47, 1996.

Poyart C, Quesne G, Trieu-Cuot P: Taxonomic dissection of the *Streptococcus bovis* group by analysis of manganese-dependent superoxide dismutase gene (sodA) sequences: reclassification of "Streptococcus infantarius subsp. coli" as *Streptococcus lutetiensis* sp. nov. and of *Streptococcus bovis* biotype II.2 as *Streptococcus pasteurianus* sp. nov, *Int J Syst Evol Microbiol* 52:1247, 2002.

Schlegel L, Grimont F, Collins MD, et al: *Streptococcus infantarius* sp nov, Streptococcus infantarius subsp infantarius subsp nov, and *Streptococcus infantarius* subsp coli subsp nov, isolated from humans and food, *Int J Syst Evol Microbiol* 50:1425, 2000.

Schlegel L, Grimont F, Ageron E, et al: Reappraisal of the taxonomy of the *Streptococcus bovis/Streptococcus equinus* complex and related species: description of *Streptococcus gallolyticus* subsp. gallolyticus subsp. nov, S. gallolyticus subsp. macedonicus subsp. nov and S. gallolyticus subsp. pasteurians subsp. nov, *Int J Syst Evol Microbiol* 53:631, 2003.

Vandamme P, Pot B, Falsen E, et al: Taxonomic study of Lancefield streptococcal groups C, G, and L (Streptococcus dysgalactiae) and proposal of S. dysgalactiae subsp equisimilis subsp nov, *Int J Syst Bacteriol* 46:774, 1996.

Whiley RA, Hall LM, Hardie JM, et al: A study of small-colony, β-hemolytic, Lancefield group C streptococci within the anginosus group: description of *Streptococcus constellatus* subsp pharyngis subsp nov, associated with the human throat and pharyngitis, *Int J Syst Bacteriol* 49:1443, 1999.

Versalovic J: *Manual of clinical microbiology*, ed 10, Washington, DC, 2011, ASM Press.

# Non-Branching, Catalase-Positive, Gram-Positive Bacilli

## *Bacillus* and Similar Organisms

## OBJECTIVES

1. Describe the general characteristics of *B. anthracis,* including colonial morphology and Gram stain appearance.
2. State the location of the organisms in the natural environment, and list the modes of transmission as they relate to human infections.
3. Describe the three forms of *B. anthracis* infection, including source, route of transmission, signs, and symptoms.
4. Summarize the types of infections associated with *B. cereus.*
5. Outline the laboratory tests utilized to differentiate *B. anthracis* from other *Bacillus* species.
6. State the culture media used to differentiate *Bacillus* spp., and include the chemical principle and interpretation.
7. Summarize the approach to species differentiation within the genera *Bacillus*, *Brevibacillus*, and *Paenibacillus*.
8. Indicate the appropriate therapy for *B. anthracis* infection.

---

### GENERA AND SPECIES TO BE CONSIDERED

- *Bacillus anthracis*
- *Bacillus cereus*
- *Bacillus mycoides*
- *Bacillus circulans*
- *Bacillus licheniformis*
- *Bacillus subtilis*
- *Bacillus megaterium*
- *Other Bacillus* spp.
- *Brevibacillus brevis*
- *Paenibacillus* spp.

---

## GENERAL CHARACTERISTICS

*Bacillus* species previously were phenotypically classified. With the development of rapid nucleic acid sequencing, the genus has been reorganized based on 16srRNA sequence analysis. The group now contains 53 genera. *Bacillus* remains the largest genus within this group and contains the most important medically relevant organisms. *Bacillus* spp. and related genera *Brevibacillus* and *Paenibacillus* are aerobic and facultative anaerobic, gram-positive, spore-forming rods. Only the species most commonly associated with human infections are discussed.

## BACILLUS ANTHRACIS

Clinical microbiologists are sentinels for recognition of a bioterrorist event, especially involving microorganisms such as *B. anthracis*. Even though this organism is rarely found, sentinel laboratory protocols require ruling out the possibility of anthrax before reporting any blood, CSF, or wound cultures in which a large gram-positive aerobic rod is isolated. During the 2001 terrorist attacks on the United States, the index case associated with the anthrax distribution was discovered by an astute clinical microbiologist who identified large gram-positive rods in a patient's cerebrospinal fluid. *B. anthracis* should be suspected if typical nonhemolytic "Medusa head" or ground glass colonies are observed on 5% sheep blood agar. The Red Line Alert Test (Tetracore, Inc., Gaithersburg, Maryland) is a Food and Drug Administration (FDA)-cleared immunochromatographic test that presumptively identifies *B. anthracis* from blood agar (Figure 16-1). The sentinel laboratory anthrax protocol was revised in 2005 and again in 2010 to use FDA-cleared tests in order to rule out nonhemolytic, nonmotile *Bacillus* spp. as potential isolates of *B. anthracis*.

### Epidemiology

Anthrax remains the most widely recognized bacillus in clinical microbiology laboratories. It is primarily a disease of wild and domestic animals including sheep, goats, horses, and cattle. The decline in animal and human infections is a result of the development of veterinary and human vaccines as well as improvements in industrial applications for handing and importing animal products. The organism is normally found in the soil and primarily causes disease in herbivores. Humans acquire infections when inoculated with the spores, either by traumatic introduction, ingestion, or inhalation during exposure to contaminated animal products, such as hides (Table 16-1). *Bacillus anthracis* produces endospores, which are highly resistant to heat and desiccation. The spores remain viable in a dormant state until they are deposited in a suitable environment for growth, including moisture, temperature, oxygenation, and nutrient availability. Because of the ability to survive harsh environments, infectiousness, ease of aerosol dissemination, and high mortality rate, the spores may be effectively used as an agent of biologic warfare (see Chapter 80 for additional information).

**TABLE 16-1** Epidemiology

| Species | Habitat (Reservoir) | Mode of Transmission |
| --- | --- | --- |
| *Bacillus anthracis* | Soil: contracted by various herbivores | Direct contact: animal tissue or products such as wool or hair (infecting organisms)<br>Trauma or insect bites: organisms or spores<br>Inhalation: spores; Woolsorters' disease<br>Ingestion: contaminated meat<br>Person-to-person transmission has not been documented |
| *Bacillus cereus, Bacillus circulans, Bacillus licheniformis, Bacillus subtilis,* other *Bacillus* spp., *Brevibacillus* sp., and *Paenibacillus* spp. | Vegetative cells and spores ubiquitous in nature; may transiently colonize skin or the gastrointestinal or respiratory tracts | Trauma<br>Associated with immunocompromised patients<br>Ingestion of food (rice) contaminated with *B. cereus* or toxins formed by this organism |

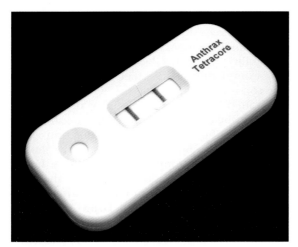

**Figure 16-1** Red Line Alert Test. A red line appears on the cassette if the culture isolate is presumptive *Bacillus anthracis*. (Courtesy Tetracore, Inc., Gaithersburg, Maryland.)

### Pathogenesis and Spectrum of Disease

*B. anthracis* is the most highly virulent species for humans and is the causative agent of anthrax. The three forms of disease are cutaneous, gastrointestinal (ingestion), and pulmonary (inhalation) or woolsorters' disease (Table 16-2). The cutaneous form accounts for most human infections and is associated with contact with infected animal products. Infection results from close contact and inoculation of endospores through a break in the skin. Following inoculation and incubation period of approximately 2 to 6 days in most cases, a small papule appears that progresses to a ring of vesicles. The vesicles then develop into an ulceration. The typical presentation is of a black, necrotic lesion known as an **eschar.** The mortality rate for untreated cutaneous anthrax is low, approximately 1%.

Ingestion anthrax results from ingestion of spores and is presented in two forms: oral or oropharyngeal with the lesion in the buccal cavity, on the tongue, tonsils, or pharyngeal mucosa and gastrointestinal anthrax with the lesions developing anywhere in the gastrointestinal tract. Oropharyngeal symptoms may include sore throat, lymphadenopathy, and edema of the throat and chest.

The initial symptoms on gastrointestinal anthrax may be nonspecific with progression to abdominal pain, bloody diarrhea, and hematemesis. The mortality rate is much higher than that of cutaneous anthrax and usually attributed to toxemia and sepsis.

Pulmonary (inhalation) anthrax is due to inhalation of the spores. The endospores are ingested by macrophages and taken to the lymph nodes where the infection develops into a systemic infection. The disease develops from flulike symptoms to respiratory distress, edema, cyanosis, shock, and death. Patients typically demonstrate abnormal chest x-rays with pleural effusion, infiltrates, and mediastinal widening. Woolsorters' disease and ragpickers' disease are used to describe respiratory infections that result from exposure to endospores during the handling of animal hides, hair, or fibers and other animal products.

Complications often follow all three forms of anthrax disease. Patients often develop meningitis within 6 days after exposure. Recovery results in long-term immunity to subsequent infections.

Virulence is attributed to the production of anthrax toxin. The toxin consists of three proteins. One of these proteins, protective antigen (PA), facilitates the transport of the other two proteins into the cell. Edema factor, EF, is responsible for edema, whereas lethal factor, LF, is primarily responsible for death.

## BACILLUS CEREUS

*B. cereus* is another clinically relevant species worthy of identification. It is penicillin resistant, beta-hemolytic, and motile, and it produces a wide zone of lecithinase on egg yolk agar (Figure 16-2).

### Epidemiology

*B. cereus,* a very close relative of *B. anthracis,* is also found within the soil. The organism is considered an opportunistic pathogen and is often associated with foodborne illness.

### Pathogenesis and Spectrum of Disease

*B. cereus* "food poisoning" is associated with the ingestion of a wide variety of foods including meats, vegetables,

**TABLE 16-2** Pathogenesis and Spectrum of Disease

| Species | Virulence Factors | Spectrum of Diseases and Infections |
|---|---|---|
| *Bacillus anthracis* | Capsule exotoxins (edema toxin and lethal toxin) swelling and tissue death | Causative agent of anthrax, of which there are three forms: <br> Cutaneous anthrax occurs at site of spore penetration 2 to 5 days after exposure and is manifested by progressive stages from an erythematous papule to ulceration and finally to formation of a black scar (i.e., eschar); may progress to toxemia and death <br> Pulmonary anthrax, also known as woolsorters' disease, follows inhalation of spores and progresses from malaise with mild fever and nonproductive cough to respiratory distress, massive chest edema, cyanosis, and death <br> Gastrointestinal anthrax may follow ingestion of spores and affects either the oropharyngeal or the abdominal area; most patients die from toxemia and overwhelming sepsis |
| *Bacillus cereus* | Enterotoxins and pyogenic toxin | Food poisoning of two types: diarrheal type, characterized by abdominal pain and watery diarrhea, and emetic type, which is manifested by profuse vomiting; *B. cereus* is the most commonly encountered species of *Bacillus* in opportunistic infections including posttraumatic eye infections, endocarditis, and bacteremia; infections of other sites are rare and usually involve intravenous drug abusers or immunocompromised patients |
| *Bacillus circulans, Bacillus licheniformis, Bacillus subtilis,* other *Bacillus* spp., *Brevibacillus* sp., and *Paenibacillus* spp. | Virulence factors unknown | Food poisoning has been associated with some species but is uncommon; these organisms may also be involved in opportunistic infections similar to those described for *B. cereus* |

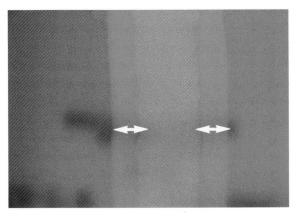

**Figure 16-2** Lecithinase production by *Bacillus cereus* on egg yolk agar. The organism has been streaked down the center of the plate. The positive test for lecithinase is indicated by the opaque zone of precipitation around the bacterial growth *(arrows)*.

deserts, sauces, and milk. A higher incidence is seen following the ingestion of rice dishes. Following ingestion patients present with one of two types of symptoms: diarrhea and abdominal pain within 8 to 16 hours or nausea and vomiting within 1 to 5 hours. *B. cereus* produces several toxins implicated in the diarrheal symptoms, including hemolysin BL (Hbl), nonhemolytic enterotoxin (Nhe), and cytotoxin K (CytK). The three toxins are believed to act synergistically, with Nhe responsible for the major symptoms in the diarrheal presentation of the infection. The emetic form of illness is associated with a heat-stable, proteolysis, and acid resistant toxin, cereulide, produced in food.

In addition to the food poisoning associated with *B. cereus*, it is a serious pathogen of the eye, causing progressive endophthalmitis. Identification of *B. cereus* from a patient's eye can cause permanent damage and should be reported to the physician immediately.

## BACILLUS THURINGIENSIS

*B. thurigiensis* has been identified harboring the genes of the *B. cereus*–associated enterotoxins. Occupational exposure with insecticides and pesticides containing the organism has resulted in the identification of the organism in feces without the presence of gastrointestinal symptoms. Additional rare cases of wound, burn, pulmonary, and ocular infections have been attributed to *B. thurigiensis*.

## BACILLUS SUBTILIS, BREVIBACILLUS SP., AND PAENIBACILLUS SPP.

*B. subtilis* has been identified in clinical specimens in a variety of cases including pneumonia, bacteremia, septicemia, surgical wounds, meningitis following head trauma, and other surgical infections. Rare human infections have been associated with a variety of *Bacillus* spp., including *B. clausii, B. licheniformis, B. circulans, B. coagulans, B. pumilus, Paenibacillus polymyxa,* and *Brevibacillus* sp. Many of these organisms are common environmental contaminants. Identification of these organisms is not recommended unless isolated from a sterile site (e.g., blood) or found in large numbers in pure culture. Therefore, identification and interpretation should be closely evaluated in conjunction with the patient's signs and symptoms and consultation with the attending physician.

### Epidemiology

Most other *Bacillus* spp. are generally considered to be opportunistic pathogens of low virulence and are associated with immunocompromised patients following exposure to contaminated materials.

### Pathogenesis and Spectrum of Disease

The spores of *Bacillus* spp. are ubiquitous in nature; and contamination of various clinical specimens may occur. Therefore, the clinical significance of the isolate should be carefully established during the identification of the microorganism.

# LABORATORY DIAGNOSIS

## SPECIMEN PROCESSING

With few exceptions, special processing considerations are not required. The organisms are capable of survival in fresh clinical specimens and standard transport medium. Refer to Table 5-1 for general information on specimen processing.

Specimens collected from patients suspected of having anthrax should be placed in leak-proof containers and placed in a secondary container. Cutaneous anthrax specimens should be collected from underneath the eschar. Two specimens of the vesicular fluid should be collected from underneath the lesion with a swab. For histochemical testing, the physician may collect a punch biopsy. Inhalation anthrax specimens should include blood cultures, pleural fluid, and a serum specimen for serology. Again, the physician may collect biopsy of bronchial or pleural tissue. Specimens required for inhalation anthrax include blood cultures, ascites fluid, and material from any lesions as well as serum for serologic testing. Preferred collection of specimens from patients suspected of infection with *B. anthracis* should be accumulated prior to antibiotic therapy.

Clinical specimens for the isolation of *Bacillus* species other than *B. anthracis* and *B. cereus* may be handled safely under normal standard laboratory practices. The exceptions are processing procedures for foods implicated in *B. cereus* food poisoning outbreaks and animal hides or products, and environmental samples, for the isolation of *B. anthracis*. These specimens may contain spores posing an aerosolization and inhalation risk to the laboratory professional and requiring the use of personal protective equipment including a proper respiratory mask.

Specimen processing may include heat or alcohol shock prior to plating on solid media. The pretreatment removes contaminating organisms, and only the spore-forming bacilli survive. This technique is considered an enrichment and selection procedure designed to increase the chance for laboratory isolation of the organisms.

Despite the publicity associated with *B. anthracis* as a potential agent of biologic warfare, the organism is not highly contagious. However, disinfection with formaldehyde, glutaraldehyde, or hydrogen peroxide and peracetic acid should be performed before the disposal of specimens suspected of containing a large number of spores. *B. anthracis* is classified by the Department of Health and Human Services/Centers for Disease Control and Prevention (CDC) and the U.S. Department of Agriculture/Animal and Plant Health Inspection Service (APHIS) as a select agent. Any laboratory in possession of the organism must register with one of these agencies and notify the organization within 7 days upon identification of the organism. If the organism is identified in an unregistered laboratory, the isolate must be shipped, using the request to transfer select agents and toxins approval from CDC or APHIS, to a registered laboratory for proper disposal.

## DIRECT DETECTION METHODS

The Gram stain is the only specific procedure for the direct detection of *Bacillus* spp. in clinical specimens. Microscopically the organisms appear as large gram-positive rods in singles, pairs, or serpentine changes (Figure 16-3).

*Bacillus* spp. are the only clinically relevant aerobic organisms capable of producing endospores in the presence of oxygen. Sporulation is inhibited by high concentrations of $CO_2$. The production of spores may be induced by growth in triple sugar iron (TSI), urea, or nutrient agar containing 5 mg/L manganese sulfate. Spores may appear as intra or extracellular clear oval structures upon Gram staining. Special staining is required in order to visualize endospores. The smear is covered with malachite green, and a piece of filter paper is placed over the stain. The microscope slide is then heated for several minutes to force the dye into the cell walls of the spore. During the heating process, it is important to keep the filter paper moist so that the stain is steamed rather than baked into the endospores. A safranin counterstain follows the primary stain. The endospores stain green and the vegetative cells will appear pink from the secondary stain, safranin (Figure 16-4).

The vegetative cell width of *B. anthracis*, *B. cereus*, *B. mycoides*, *B. thuringiensis*, and *B. megaterium* is usually greater than 1 µm, and the spores do not cause swelling of the cell. The vegetative cell width of *B. subtilis*, *B. pumilus*, and *B. licheniformis* is less than 1 µm, and the spores do not cause swelling of the cell. The cell width of *B. circulans*, *B. coagulans*, *B. sphaericus*, *B. brevis*,

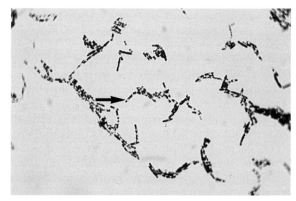

**Figure 16-3** Gram stain of *Bacillus cereus*. The arrow is pointed at a spore, the clear area inside the gram-positive vegetative cell.

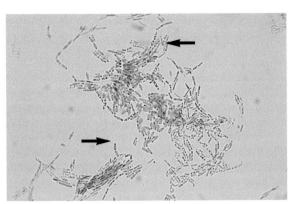

**Figure 16-4** Spore stain of *Bacillus cereus*. The arrows are pointed at green spores in a pink vegetative cell.

**TABLE 16-3** Colonial Appearance and Other Characteristics

| Organism | Appearance on 5% Sheep Blood Agar |
|---|---|
| *B. anthracis* | Medium-large, gray, flat, irregular with swirling projections ("Medusa head") or ground glass appearance; nonhemolytic |
| *B. cereus* and *B. thuringiensis* | Large, feathery, spreading; beta-hemolytic |
| *B. mycoides* | Rhizoid colony that resembles a fungus; weakly beta-hemolytic |
| *B. megaterium* | Large, convex, entire, moist; nonhemolytic |
| *B. licheniformis* | Large blister colony; becomes opaque with dull to rough surface with age; beta-hemolytic |
| *B. pumilus* | Large, moist, blister colony; may be beta-hemolytic |
| *B. subtilis* | Large, flat, dull, with ground-glass appearance; may be pigmented (pink, yellow, orange, or brown); may be beta-hemolytic |
| *B. circulans* | Large, entire, convex, butyrous; smooth, translucent surface; may be beta-hemolytic |
| *B. coagulans* | Medium-large, entire, raised, butyrous, creamy-buff; may be beta-hemolytic |
| *B. sphaericus* | Large, convex, smooth, opaque, butyrous; nonhemolytic |
| *Brevibacillus brevis* | Medium-large, convex, circular, granular; may be beta-hemolytic |
| *Paenibacillus macerans* | Large, convex, fine granular surface; nonhemolytic |
| *P. alvei* | Swarms over agar surface; discrete colonies are large, circular, convex, smooth, glistening, translucent or opaque; may be beta-hemolytic |
| *P. polymyxa* | Large, moist blister colony with "ameboid spreading" in young cultures; older colonies wrinkled; nonhemolytic |

*P. macerans, P. alvei*, and *P. polymyxa* is less than 1 μm, and the spores cause the cell to swell. When determining cell width, only the cells that stain gram-positive should be measured. Organisms that fail to retain the crystal violet appear narrower.

Direct detection of *B. anthracis* in clinical and environmental samples is also available using molecular and antigen-based methods. The immunohistochemical method available from the CDC uses antibodies specific to the organism's cell wall antigen or capsule for the detection of *B. anthracis*. A positive molecular amplification assay, PCR, from a normally sterile site is considered a presumptive diagnosis for anthrax infection.

## CULTIVATION

### Media of Choice

All *Bacillus* and related genera grow well on 5% sheep blood agar, chocolate agar, routine blood culture media, and nutrient broths. Isolates susceptible to nalidixic acid will not grow on Columbia agar with nalidixic acid and colistin (CNA), a selective and differential medium for gram-positive organisms. Phenylethyl alcohol agar (PEA), an additional selective agar for gram-positive organisms, is useful for the removal of contaminating organisms and the isolation of *Bacillus* spp. Polymyxin-lysozyme-EDTA-thallous acetate (PLET) can be used for selection and isolation from contaminated specimens. Colonies appear as creamy white, domed, circular colonies. Additionally, bicarbonate agar is used to induce *B. anthracis* capsule formation, providing a means for presumptive morphologic identification.

*B. cereus* media referred to as mannitol, egg yolk, and polymyxin B agar (MEYP or MYP); polymyxin B, egg yolk, mannitol, bromthymol blue (PEMBA); and *B. cereus* medium (BCM) have been developed for the specific isolation and identification of the organism. These media take advantage of the phospholipase C positive reaction on egg yolk agar, no production of acid from mannitol, and incorporation of pyruvate or polymyxin as the selective agents.

Heat shock treatment can be utilized for the growth and enhancement of endospores from clinical specimens. Heat treatment at 70° C for 30 minutes or 80° C for 10 minutes is effective for killing vegetative cells and retaining spores for most *Bacillus* spp. *B. anthracis* heat treatment is carried out at lower temperatures, 62° to 65° C for 15 to 20 minutes. Following heat treatment, samples are plated to culture medium along with a sample of untreated specimen to ensure maximal recovery of the isolate.

### Incubation Conditions and Duration

Most species will produce detectable growth within 24 hours following incubation on media incubated at 35° C, in ambient air, or in 5% carbon dioxide ($CO_2$). Bicarbonate agar requires incubation in $CO_2$.

### Colonial Appearance

Table 16-3 describes the colonial appearance on blood agar and other distinguishing characteristics (e.g., hemolysis) of each species of *Bacillus* or related genera.

Colonies of *B. anthracis* growing on bicarbonate agar appear large and mucoid.

## APPROACH TO IDENTIFICATION

Commercial biochemical identification systems or molecular techniques may be used in clinical laboratories for identification of *Bacillus* spp. Species differentiation within the genera *Bacillus*, *Brevibacillus*, and *Paenibacillus* is based on the size of the vegetative cell, sporulation resulting in swelling of the vegetative cell, and biochemical analysis (Table 16-4), including the production of the enzyme lecithinase (see Figure 16-2).

## SERODIAGNOSIS

Serologic methods are available for the detection of *B. cereus* toxin in food and feces, the Oxoid BCET-RPLA (Oxoid Ltd.), and the TECRA VIA (TECRA Diagnostics, New South Wales, Australia). Indirect hemagglutination and enzyme-linked immunosorbent assays are available to detect antibodies to *B. anthracis,* but serodiagnostic methods are not used to diagnose infections caused by other opportunistic *Bacillus* spp. Serodiagnosis of *B. anthracis* is typically available for the detection of the PA antigen or toxin protein, lethal factor (LF), and edema factor (EF).

## MOLECULAR DIAGNOSTICS

Various methods exist for the genetic analysis of *B. anthracis*. There are several sequence methods including multilocus sequence typing (MLST) and multiple-locus variable-number tandem-repeat analysis. MLST has also been used to discriminate between different isolates of *B. cereus*. Each of these assays examines a variety of genes and compares the genetic pattern between isolates. Additional genotyping techniques that examine single nucleotide polymorphisms and DNA microarrays are available for strain typing.

## ANTIMICROBIAL SUSCEPTIBILITY TESTING AND THERAPY

Although ciprofloxacin has been established as the preferred therapy for anthrax, the infrequent nature with which other species are encountered limits recommendations concerning therapy (Table 16-5). Nonetheless, the threat of bioterrorism has spawned interest in the development of in vitro testing of antimicrobial agents against *B. anthracis*. The Clinical and Laboratory Standards Institute (CLSI) document M100 addresses the technical issues required for antimicrobial sensitivity testing for *Bacillus* spp. Most other *Bacillus* spp. will grow on the media under the conditions recommended for testing the common organisms encountered in clinical specimens (see Chapter 12 for more information regarding validated testing methods), and technical information regarding the testing of the additional species is provided in CLSI document M45, "Methods for Antimicrobial Dilution and Disk Susceptibility Testing of Infrequently Isolated or Fastidious Bacteria." Careful evaluation of the organism's clinical significance must be established before extensive antimicrobial susceptibility testing efforts are undertaken.

## PREVENTION

A cell-free inactivated vaccine (BioThrax, Emergent Biodefense Operations, Lansing, Michigan) given in five doses (0 weeks, 4 weeks, 6 months, 12 months, and 18 months) with annual boosters thereafter is available for immunizing high-risk adults (i.e., public health laboratory workers, workers handling potentially contaminated industrial raw materials, and military personnel) against anthrax. Chemoprophylaxis with ciprofloxacin (or doxycycline) for a minimum of 4 weeks is recommended following aerosol exposure to *B. anthracis* such as may follow a bioterrorist event.

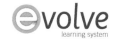 *Visit the Evolve site to complete the review questions.*

**TABLE 16-4** Differentiation of Clinically Relevant *Bacillus* spp., *Brevibacillus*, and *Paenibacillus*

| Organism | Bacillary Body Width >1 μm | Wide Zone Lecithinase | Spores Swell Sporangium | Voges Proskauer | Glucose with Gas | FERMENTATION OF: Mannitol | Xylose | Anaerobic Growth | Citrate | Indole | Motility | Parasporal Crystals |
|---|---|---|---|---|---|---|---|---|---|---|---|---|
| *Bacillus anthracis* | + | + | − | + | − | − | − | + | v | − | − | − |
| *B. cereus* | + | + | − | + | − | − | − | + | + | − | + | − |
| *B. thuringiensis* | + | + | − | + | − | − | − | + | + | − | + | + |
| *B. mycoides* | + | + | − | + | − | − | − | + | + | − | − | − |
| *B. megaterium* | + | − | − | − | − | + or (+) | v | − | + | − | + | − |
| *B. licheniformis* | − | − | − | + | − | + | + | + | + | − | + | − |
| *B. pumilus* | − | − | − | + | − | + | + | − | + | − | + | − |
| *B. subtilis* | − | − | − | + | − | + | + | − | + | − | + | − |
| *B. circulans* | − | − | + | − | − | + | + | v | + | − | + | − |
| *B. coagulans* | − | − | v | v | − | − | v | + | v | − | + | − |
| *Brevibacillus brevis* | − | − | + | − | − | + | − | − | v | − | + | v |
| *Paenibacillus macerans* | − | −* | + | − | + | + | + | + | − | − | + | − |
| *P. alvei* | − | − | + | + | − | − | − | + | − | + | + | − |
| *P. polymyxa* | − | −* | + | + | + | v | + | + | − | − | + | − |

*Weak lecithinase production only seen under the colonies.
+, 90% or more of species or strains are positive; −, 90% or more of species or strains are negative; v, variable reactions; ( ), reactions may be delayed.

Compiled from Drobniewski FA: *Bacillus cereus* and related species, *Clin Microbiol Rev* 6:324, 1993; Logan NA, Turnbull PC: Bacillus and other aerobic endospore-forming bacteria. In Murray PR, Baron EJ, Jorgensen JH, et al, editors: *Manual of clinical microbiology*, ed 10, Washington, DC, 2011, ASM Press; and Parry JM, Turnbull PC, Gibson JR: *A colour atlas of Bacillus species*, London, 1983, Wolf Medical Publications.

**TABLE 16-5** Antimicrobial Therapy and Susceptibility Testing

| Species | Therapeutic Options | Resistance to Therapeutic Options | Validated Testing Methods* | Comments |
|---------|--------------------|----------------------------------|---------------------------|----------|
| *Bacillus anthracis* | Ciprofloxacin or doxycycline plus one or two other antibiotics; other agents with in vitro activity include rifampin, vancomycin, penicillin, ampicillin, chloramphenicol, imipenem, clindamycin, and clarithromycin | Beta-lactamases | See CLSI document M100-S22; performed in approved reference laboratories only | |
| Other *Bacillus* spp., *Brevibacillus* sp., *Paenibacillus* spp. | No definitive guidelines; vancomycin, ciprofloxacin, imipenem, and aminoglycosides may be effective | *B. cereus* frequently produces beta-lactamase | See CLSI document M45; methods for antimicrobial dilution and disk susceptibility testing of infrequently isolated or fastidious bacteria | Whenever isolated from clinical specimens, the potential for the isolate to be a contaminant must be strongly considered |

*Validated testing methods include those standard methods recommended by the Clinical Laboratory Science Institute (CLSI) and those commercial methods approved by the Food and Drug Administration (FDA).

---

## CASE STUDY 16-1

A 46-year-old male welder from central Louisiana was healthy until 5 days before admission, when he experienced cough, congestion, chills, and fever. The symptoms had resolved, but he experienced a bout of hemoptysis and was referred to the emergency department by his local physician. His temperature was normal, pulse was 128 bpm, respiratory rate was 26, and blood pressure was 170/98. Chest radiograph was markedly abnormal with a confluent alveolar infiltrate in the right lung, with only a small amount of aeration in the apex. The left lung had a confluent density in the midline suggestive of a mass. Oxygen therapy was started, and the patient was placed on ciprofloxacin and cefotaxime. Shortly thereafter, the patient vomited coffee-colored emesis and had a cardiorespiratory arrest. Aerobic blood cultures were positive the next day for a large gram-positive rod with spores.

### QUESTIONS

1. The spore-forming bacteria grew well aerobically. What characteristics of the colony would be useful in identifying this bacterium to the species level?
2. What tests can you do to confirm the identification?
3. If you were to isolate a nonhemolytic, nonmotile, aerobic spore-forming bacterium from a clinical specimen, what should you do as quickly as possible?

---

## BIBLIOGRAPHY

Ash CF, Priest G, Collins MD: Molecular identification of rRNA group 3 bacilli (Ash, Farrow, Wallbanks, and Collins) using a PCR probe test, *Antonie van Leeuwenhoek* 64:253, 1993.

Claus D, Berkeley RC: Genus bacillus. In Vos P, Garrity G, Jones D, et al, editors: Bergey's manual of systematic bacteriology: Volume 3, New York, 2009, Springer.

Drobniewski FA: *Bacillus cereus* and related species, *Clin Microbiol Rev* 6:324, 1993.

Hollis DG, Weaver RE: Gram-positive organisms: a guide to identification, Atlanta, 1981, Centers for Disease Control.

Logan NA, Turnbull PC: Bacillus and other aerobic endospore-forming bacteria. In Murray PR, Baron EJ, Jorgensen JH, et al, editors: Manual of clinical microbiology, ed 9, Washington, DC, 2007, ASM Press.

Lucey D: *Bacillus anthracis* (anthrax). In Mandell GL, Bennett JE, Dolin R, editors: Principles and practice of infectious diseases, ed 7, Philadelphia, 2009, Elsevier Churchill.

Parry JM, Turnbull PC, Gibson JR: A colour atlas of Bacillus species, London, 1983, Wolf Medical Publications.

Shida O, Takagi H, Kadowaki K, et al: Proposal for two new genera, Brevibacillus gen nov and Aneurinibacillus gen nov, *Int J Syst Bacteriol* 46:939, 1996.

Turnbull P, Böhm R, Cosivi O, et al: Guidelines for the surveillance and control of anthrax in humans and animals, Geneva, Switzerland, 1998, World Health Organization.

# Listeria, Corynebacterium, and Similar Organisms

1. Describe the general characteristics of the *Corynebacterium* spp., including Gram stain morphology, culture media, and colonial appearance.
2. List two selective and differential media used for identification of *Corynebacterium diphtheriae* and describe the chemical principle for each.
3. Identify the clinically relevant indicators (e.g., signs, symptoms) associated with the need to identify *Corynebacterium* spp.
4. Describe four methods used to detect *C. diphtheriae* toxin, along with the chemical principle of each test.
5. Describe two methods used to observe motility in *Listeria monocytogenes*.
6. Explain how diphtheria is controlled by immunization and describe the course of treatment for individuals exposed to the disease.
7. Define "cold enrichment" and explain how it enhances the isolation of *L. monocytogenes*.
8. List the foods pregnant women and immunocompromised patients should avoid to reduce the risk of infection with *L. monocytogenes*.
9. Describe the clinical significance of identification of *Corynebacterium pseudotuberculosis*, *Corynebacterium ulcerans*, and *Rhodococcus* sp.

---

## GENERA AND SPECIES TO BE CONSIDERED

- *Arthrobacter* spp.
- *Brevibacterium* spp.
- *Cellulomonas* spp.
- *Cellulosimicrobium cellulans*
- *Corynebacterium amycolatum*
- *Corynebacterium auris*
- *Corynebacterium diphtheriae*
- *Corynebacterium jeikeium*
- *Corynebacterium minutissimum*
- *Corynebacterium pseudodiphtheriticum*
- *Corynebacterium pseudotuberculosis*
- *Corynebacterium striatum*
- *Corynebacterium ulcerans*
- *Corynebacterium urealyticum*
- *Corynebacterium xerosis*
- *Dermabacter hominis*
- *Exiguobacterium acetylicum*
- *Kurthia* spp.
- *Leifsonia aquatica* (formerly *Corynebacterium aquaticum*)
- *Listeria monocytogenes*
- *Microbacterium* spp. (includes former genus *Aureobacterium*)
- *Oerskovia* spp.
- Other *Corynebacterium* spp. and CDC Coryneform groups
- *Rothia* spp.
- *Turicella otitidis*

## GENERAL CHARACTERISTICS

The genera of bacteria described in this chapter are catalase-positive, gram-positive rods. They are non–acid-fast, non-spore-forming and mostly nonbranching rods. *Rothia* and *Oerskovia* spp. are included with the gram-positive rods because some species are rodlike. Furthermore, although *Oerskovia* spp. exhibit extensive branching and vegetative hyphae and penetrate into the agar surface, they do not display aerial hyphae, as do *Nocardia* spp. *Corynebacterium* spp. are aerobic or facultative anaerobic fastidious organisms that may demonstrate slow growth on an enriched medium.

## EPIDEMIOLOGY

Most of the organisms listed in Table 17-1 are part of the normal human flora and colonize various parts of the human body, are found in the environment, or are associated with various animals. The two most notable pathogens are *Listeria monocytogenes* and *Corynebacterium diphtheriae*. However, these two species differ markedly in epidemiology. *L. monocytogenes* is widely distributed in nature and occasionally colonizes the human gastrointestinal tract. Many foods are contaminated with *L. monocytogenes*, including milk, raw vegetables, cheese, and meats. *C. diphtheriae* is only carried by humans, but in rare cases it is isolated from healthy individuals. Primary transmission for *C. diphtheriae* is through respiratory secretions or exudates from skin lesions.

In contrast to these two organisms, *C. jeikeium* is commonly encountered in clinical specimens, mostly because it tends to proliferate as skin flora of hospitalized individuals. However, *C. jeikeium* is not considered to be highly virulent. The penetration of the patient's skin by intravascular devices is usually required for this organism to cause infection.

## PATHOGENESIS AND SPECTRUM OF DISEASE

*L. monocytogenes*, by virtue of its ability to survive within phagocytes, and *C. diphtheriae*, by production of an extremely potent cytotoxic exotoxin, are the most virulent species listed in Table 17-2. Not all strains of *C. diphtheriae* are toxin-producing strains. The toxin gene is present in strains that have acquired the gene by viral transduction. The result is the incorporation of the toxin gene into the organisms' genome. *C. diphtheriae* occurs in four biotypes: *gravis*, *intermedius*, *belfanti*, and *mitis*;

**TABLE 17-1** Epidemiology

| Organism | Habitat (Reservoir) | Mode of Transmission |
|---|---|---|
| *Listeria monocytogenes* | Colonizer:<br>Animals, soil, and vegetable matter; widespread in these environments<br>Human gastrointestinal tract | Direct contact:<br>Ingestion of contaminated food, such as meat and dairy products<br>Endogenous strain:<br>Colonized mothers may pass organism to fetus. Portal of entry is probably from gastrointestinal tract to blood and in some instances from blood to meninges. |
| *Corynebacterium diphtheriae* | Colonizer:<br>Human nasopharynx but only in carrier state; not considered part of normal flora<br>Isolation from healthy humans is not common. | Direct contact:<br>Person to person by exposure to contaminated respiratory droplets<br>Contact with exudate from cutaneous lesions<br>Exposure to contaminated objects |
| *Corynebacterium jeikeium* | Colonizer:<br>Skin flora of hospitalized patients, most commonly in the inguinal, axillary, and rectal sites | Uncertain<br>Direct contact:<br>May be person to person<br>Endogenous strain:<br>Selection during antimicrobial therapy<br>Introduction during placement or improper care of intravenous catheters |
| *Corynebacterium ulcerans* | Normal flora:<br>Humans and cattle | Uncertain<br>Zoonoses:<br>Close animal contact, especially during summer |
| *Corynebacterium pseudotuberculosis* | Normal flora:<br>Animals such as sheep, goats, and horses | Uncertain<br>Zoonoses:<br>Close animal contact, but infections in humans are rare |
| *Corynebacterium pseudodiphtheriticum* | Normal flora:<br>Human pharyngeal and occasionally skin flora | Uncertain<br>Endogenous strain:<br>Access to normally sterile site |
| *Corynebacterium minutissimum* | Normal flora:<br>Human skin | Uncertain<br>Endogenous strain:<br>Access to normally sterile site |
| *Corynebacterium urealyticum* | Normal flora:<br>Human skin | Uncertain<br>Endogenous strain:<br>Access to normally sterile site |
| *Leifsonia aquatica* (formerly *Corynebacterium aquaticum*) | Environment:<br>Fresh water | Uncertain |
| *Corynebacterium xerosis* | Normal flora:<br>Human conjunctiva<br>Skin<br>Nasopharynx | Uncertain<br>Endogenous strain:<br>Access to normally sterile site |
| *Corynebacterium striatum* | Normal flora:<br>Skin | Uncertain<br>Endogenous strain:<br>Access to normally sterile site |
| *Corynebacterium amycolatum* | Normal flora:<br>Human conjunctiva<br>Skin<br>Nasopharynx | Uncertain<br>Endogenous strain:<br>Access to normally sterile site |
| *Corynebacterium auris* | Uncertain:<br>Probably part of normal human flora | Uncertain<br>Rarely implicated in human infections |
| *Kurthia* spp. | Environment | Uncertain<br>Rarely implicated in human infections |
| *Brevibacterium* spp. | Normal flora:<br>Human<br>Various foods | Uncertain<br>Rarely implicated in human infections |

**TABLE 17-1** Epidemiology—cont'd

| Organism | Habitat (Reservoir) | Mode of Transmission |
|---|---|---|
| *Dermabacter hominis* | Normal flora:<br>Human skin | Uncertain<br>Rarely implicated in human infections |
| *Turicella otitidis* | Uncertain:<br>Probably part of normal human flora | Uncertain<br>Rarely implicated in human infections |
| *Arthrobacter* spp.,<br>  *Microbacterium* spp.,<br>  *Cellulomonas* spp., and<br>  *Exiguobacterium* sp. | Uncertain<br>Probably environmental | Uncertain<br>Rarely implicated in human infections |

**TABLE 17-2** Pathogenesis and Spectrum of Diseases

| Organism | Virulence Factors | Spectrum of Diseases and Infections |
|---|---|---|
| *Listeria monocytogenes* | Listeriolysin O:<br>A hemolytic and cytotoxic toxin that allows for survival within phagocytes<br>Internalin: Cell surface protein that induces phagocytosis<br>Act A:<br>Induces actin polymerization on the surface of host cells, producing cellular extensions and facilitating cell-to-cell spread.<br>Siderophores:<br>Organisms capable of scavenging iron from human transferrin and of enhanced growth of organism.* | Systemic:<br>Bacteremia, without any other known site of infection<br>CNS infections: Meningitis, encephalitis, bran abscess, spinal cord infections<br>Neonatal:<br>Early onset: Granulomatosis infantisepticum—in utero infection disseminated systemically that causes stillbirth<br>Late onset: Bacterial meningitis<br>Immunosuppressed patients |
| *Corynebacterium diphtheriae* | Diphtheria toxin:<br>A potent exotoxin that destroys host cells by inhibiting protein synthesis. | Respiratory diphtheria is a pharyngitis characterized by the development of an exudative membrane that covers the tonsils, uvula, palate, and pharyngeal wall; if untreated, life-threatening cardiac toxicity, neurologic toxicity, and other complications occur. Respiratory obstruction develops and release of toxin into the blood can damage various organs, including the heart. |
|  | Nontoxigenic strains:<br>Uncertain | Cutaneous diphtheria is characterized by nonhealing ulcers and membrane formation.<br>Immunocompromised patients, drug addicts, and alcoholics.<br>Invasive endocarditis, mycotic aneurysms, osteomyelitis, and septic arthritis* |
| *Corynebacterium jeikeium* | Unknown:<br>Multiple antibiotic resistance allows survival in hospital setting | Systemic:<br>Septicemia<br>Skin infections:<br>Wounds, rashes and nodules<br>Immunocompromised:<br>Malignancies, neutropenia, AIDS patients.<br>Associated with indwelling devices such as catheters, prosthetic valves, and CSF shunts* |
| *Corynebacterium ulcerans* | Unknown | Zoonoses:<br>Bovine mastitis<br>Has been associated with diphtheria-like sore throat, indistinguishable from *C. diphtheriae*<br>Skin infections<br>Pneumonia |
| *Corynebacterium pseudotuberculosis* | Unknown | Zoonoses:<br>Suppurative granulomatous lymphadenitis |

*Continued*

**TABLE 17-2** Pathogenesis and Spectrum of Diseases—cont'd

| Organism | Virulence Factors | Spectrum of Diseases and Infections |
|---|---|---|
| *Corynebacterium pseudodiphtheriticum* | Unknown<br>Some stains have been identified that are resistant to macrolides* | Systemic:<br>Septicemia<br>Endocarditis<br>Pneumonia and lung abscesses; primarily in immunocompromised |
| *Corynebacterium minutissimum* | Unknown<br>Probably of low virulence | Superficial, pruritic skin infections known as erythrasma<br>Immunocompromised:<br>Septicemia<br>Endocarditis<br>Abscess formation |
| *Corynebacterium urealyticum* | Unknown<br>Multiple antibiotic resistance allows survival in hospital setting. | Immunocompromised and elderly:<br>Urinary tract infections<br>Wound infections<br>Rarely: endocarditis, septicemia, osteomyelitis, and tissue infections |
| *Leifsonia aquatica (* formerly *Corynebacterium aquaticum)* | Unknown | Immunocompromised:<br>Bacteremia<br>Septicemia |
| *Corynebacterium xerosis* | Unknown | Immunocompromised:<br>Endocarditis<br>Septicemia |
| *Corynebacterium striatum* | Unknown | Immunocompromised:<br>Bacteremia<br>Pneumonia and lung abscesses<br>Osteomyelitis<br>Meningitis |
| *Corynebacterium amycolatum* | Unknown<br>Multiple antibiotic resistance patterns | Immunocompromised:<br>Endocarditis<br>Septicemia<br>Pneumonia<br>Neonatal sepsis |
| *Corynebacterium auris* | Unknown<br>Multiple antibiotic resistance patterns | Uncertain disease association but has been linked to otitis media |
| *Kurthia* spp., *Brevibacterium* and *Dermabacter* sp. | Unknown | Immunocompromised:<br>Rarely causes infections in humans<br>Bacteremia in association with indwelling catheters or penetrating injuries |
| *Turicella otitidis* | Unknown | Uncertain disease association but has been linked to otitis media |
| *Arthrobacter* spp., *Microbacterium* spp., *Aureobacterium* spp., *Cellulomonas* spp., and *Exiguobacterium* sp. | Unknown | Uncertain disease association |

*AIDS,* Acquired immunodeficiency syndrome; *CSF,* cerebrospinal fluid; *CNS,* central nervous system.

*C. gravis* causes the most severe form of disease. The biotypes can be differentiated based on colonial morphology, biochemical reactions, and hemolytic patterns on blood agar.

*L. monocytogenes* is ingested through contaminated food. Once the organism has been phagocytized by white blood cells, it produces listeriolysin O, the major virulence factor. Listeriolysin O in combination with phospholipases enables the organism to escape from the white blood cells and spread to the bloodstream, eventually reaching the central nervous system and the placenta.

Most of the remaining organisms in Table 17-2 are opportunistic, and infections are associated with immunocompromised patients. For this reason, whenever *Corynebacterium* spp. or the other genera of gram-positive rods are encountered, careful consideration must be given to their role as infectious agents or contaminants. *Corynebacterium urealyticum* is an up-and-coming cause of cystitis in hospitalized patients, in those who have undergone urologic manipulation, and in the elderly.

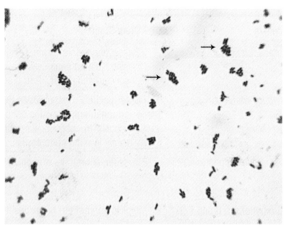

**Figure 17-1** Gram stain of *Corynebacterium diphtheriae.* Note palisading and arrangements of cells in formations that resemble Chinese letters *(arrows).*

# LABORATORY DIAGNOSIS

## SPECIMEN COLLECTION AND TRANSPORT

No special considerations are required for specimen collection and transport of the organisms discussed in this chapter. Refer to Table 5-1 for general information on specimen collection and transport.

## SPECIMEN PROCESSING

No special considerations are required for processing of most of the organisms discussed in this chapter. (Refer to Table 5-1 for general information on specimen processing.) One exception is the isolation of *L. monocytogenes* from placental and other tissue. Because isolating *Listeria* organisms from these sources may be difficult, cold enrichment may be used to enhance the recovery of the organism. The specimen is inoculated into a nutrient broth and incubated at 4°C for several weeks to months. The broth is subcultured at frequent intervals to enhance recovery.

## DIRECT DETECTION METHODS

Gram stain of clinical specimens is the only procedure used for the direct detection of these organisms. Most of the genera in this chapter (except *Listeria, Rothia,* and *Oerskovia* spp.) are classified as coryneform bacteria; that is, they are gram-positive, short or slightly curved rods with rounded ends; some have rudimentary branching. Cells are arranged singly, in "palisades" of parallel cells, or in pairs of cells connected after cell division to form V or L shapes. Groups of these morphologies seen together resemble and are often referred to as Chinese letters (Figure 17-1). The Gram stain morphologies of clinically relevant species are described in Table 17-3. *L. monocytogenes* is a short, gram-positive rod that may occur singly or in short chains, resembling streptococci.

## CULTIVATION

### Media of Choice

*Corynebacterium* spp. usually grow on 5% sheep blood and chocolate agars. Some coryneform bacteria do not grow on chocolate agar, and the lipophilic (lipid loving) species (e.g., *C. jeikeium, C. urealyticum, C. afermentans* subsp. *lipophilum, C. accolens,* and *C. macginleyi*) produce much larger colonies when cultured on 5% sheep blood agar supplemented with 1% Tween 80 (Figure 17-3).

Selective and differential media for *C. diphtheriae* should be used if diphtheria is suspected. The two media commonly used for this purpose are cystine-tellurite blood agar and modified Tinsdale agar (TIN). Tellurite

blood agar maybe used with or without cystine. Cystine enhances the growth of fastidious organisms, including *C. diphtheriae.* Both media contain a high concentration of potassium tellurite that is inhibitory to normal flora. Organisms capable of growing on Tinsdale agar are differentiated based on the conversion of the tellurite to tellurium. This conversion results in color variations of grey to black colonies on the two media. *C. diphtheriae* also produces a halo on both media. *C. diphtheriae* can be presumptively identified by observing brown-black colonies with a gray-brown halo on Tinsdale agar (Figure 17-4). The brown halo is produced when the organism uses tellurite to produce hydrogen sulfide. The halo produced on cystine-tellurite blood agar appears brown as a result of the organism breaking down the cystine. In addition, Loeffler medium, which contains serum and egg, stimulates the growth of *C. diphtheriae* and the production of metachromatic granules in the cells. *C. diphtheriae* grows rapidly on the highly enriched agar and produces gray to white, translucent colonies within 12 to 18 hours. Primary inoculation of throat swabs to Loeffler serum slants is no longer recommended because of the inevitable overgrowth of normal oral flora.

*Corynebacterium* spp. are unable grow on MacConkey agar. They all are capable of growth in routine blood culture broth and nutrient broths, such as thioglycollate or brain-heart infusion. Lipophilic coryneform bacteria demonstrate better growth in broths supplemented with rabbit serum.

### Incubation Conditions and Duration

Detectable growth of corynebacterium on 5% sheep blood and chocolate agars, incubated at 35°C in either ambient air or in 5% to 10% carbon dioxide, should occur within 48 to 72 hours after inoculation. The lipophilic organisms grow more slowly; it takes 3 days or longer to identify visible growth on routine media. For growth of *C. diphtheriae,* cystine-tellurite blood agar and modified Tinsdale agar should be incubated for at least 48 hours in ambient air. Five percent to 10% carbon

**TABLE 17-3** Gram Stain Morphology, Colonial Appearance, and Other Distinguishing Characteristics

| Organism | Gram Stain | Appearance on 5% Sheep Blood Agar |
|---|---|---|
| *Arthrobacter* spp. | Typical coryneform gram-positive rods after 24 hr, with "jointed ends" giving L and V forms, and coccoid cells after 72 hr (i.e., rod-coccus cycle*) | Large colony; resembles *Brevibacterium* spp. |
| *Brevibacterium* spp. | Gram-positive rods; produce typical coryneform arrangements in young cultures (<24 hr) and coccoid-to-coccobacillary forms that decolorize easily in older cultures (i.e., rod-coccus cycle*) | Medium to large; gray to white, convex, opaque, smooth, shiny; nonhemolytic; cheeselike odor |
| *Cellulomonas* spp. | Irregular, short, thin, branching gram-positive rods | Small to medium; two colony types, one starts out white and turns yellow within 3 days and the other starts out yellow |
| CDC coryneform group F-1 | Typical coryneform gram-positive rods | Small, gray to white |
| CDC coryneform group G† | Typical coryneform gram-positive rods | Small, gray to white; nonhemolytic |
| *Corynebacterium accolens* | Resembles *C. jeikeium* | Resembles *C. jeikeium* |
| *C. afermentans* subsp. *afermentans* | Typical coryneform gram-positive rods | Medium; white; nonhemolytic; nonadherent |
| *C. afermentans* subsp. *lipophilum* | Typical coryneform gram-positive rods | Small; gray, glassy |
| *C. amycolatum* | Pleomorphic gram-positive rods with single cells, V forms, or Chinese letters | Small; white to gray, dry |
| *C. argentoratense* | Typical coryneform gram-positive rods | Medium; cream-colored; nonhemolytic |
| *C. aurimucosum* | Typical coryneform gram-positive rods | Slightly yellowish sticky colonies; some strains black-pigmented |
| *C. auris* | Typical coryneform gram-positive rods | Small to medium; dry, slightly adherent, become yellowish with time; nonhemolytic |
| *C. coyleae* | Typical coryneform gram-positive rods | Small, whitish and slightly glistening with entire edges; either creamy or sticky |
| *C. diphtheriae* group‡ | Irregularly staining, pleomorphic gram-positive rods | Various biotypes of *C. diphtheriae* produce colonies ranging from small, gray, and translucent (biotype *intermedius*) to medium, white, and opaque (biotypes *mitis, belfanti,* and *gravis*); *C. diphtheriae* biotype *mitis* may be beta-hemolytic; *C. ulcerans* and *C. pseudotuberculosis* resemble *C. diphtheriae* |
| *C. falsenii* | Typical coryneform gram-positive rods | Small; whitish, circular with entire edges, convex, glistening, creamy; yellow pigment after 72 hr |
| *C. freneyi* | Typical coryneform gram-positive rods | Whitish; dry; rough |
| *C. glucuronolyticum* | Typical coryneform gram-positive rods | Small; white to yellow, convex; nonhemolytic |
| *C. jeikeium* | Pleomorphic; occasionally, club-shaped gram-positive rods arranged in V forms or palisades | Small; gray to white, entire, convex; nonhemolytic |
| *C. imitans* | Typical coryneform gram-positive rods | Small, white to gray, glistening, circular, convex; creamy; entire edges |
| *C. macginleyi* | Typical coryneform gram-positive rods | Tiny colonies after 48 hr; nonhemolytic |
| *C. matruchotii* | Gram-positive rods with whip-handle shape and branching filaments | Small; opaque, adherent |
| *C. minutissimum* | Typical coryneform gram-positive rods with single cells, V forms, palisading and Chinese letters | Small; convex, circular, shiny, and moist |
| *C. mucifaciens* | Typical coryneform gram-positive rods | Small, slightly yellow and mucoid; circular, convex, glistening |
| *C. propinquum* | Typical coryneform gram-positive rods | Small to medium with matted surface; nonhemolytic |
| *C. pseudodiphtheriticum* | Typical coryneform gram-positive rods | Small to medium; slightly dry |

**TABLE 17-3** Gram Stain Morphology, Colonial Appearance, and Other Distinguishing Characteristics—cont'd

| Organism | Gram Stain | Appearance on 5% Sheep Blood Agar |
|---|---|---|
| *C. pseudotuberculosis* | Typical coryneform gram-positive rods | Small, yellowish white, opaque, convex; matted surface |
| *C. riegelii* | Typical coryneform gram-positive rods | Small, whitish, glistening, convex with entire edges; either creamy or sticky |
| *C. simulans* | Typical coryneform gram-positive rods | Grayish white; glistening; creamy |
| *C. singulare* | Typical coryneform gram-positive rods | Circular; slightly convex with entire margins; creamy |
| *C. striatum* | Regular medium to large gram-positive rods; can show banding | Small to medium; white, moist and smooth (resembles colonies of coagulase-negative staphylococci) |
| *C. sundsvallense* | Gram-positive rods, some with terminal bulges or knobs; some branching | Buff to slight yellow, sticky, adherent to agar |
| *C. thomssenii* | Typical coryneform gram-positive rods | Tiny after 24 hr; whitish, circular, mucoid and sticky |
| *C. ulcerans* | Typical coryneform gram-positive rods | Small, dry, waxy, gray to white |
| *C. urealyticum* | Gram-positive coccobacilli arranged in V forms and palisades | Pinpoint (after 48 hr); white, smooth, convex; nonhemolytic |
| *C. xerosis* | Regular medium to large gram-positive rods can show banding; | Small to medium; dry, yellowish, granular |
| *Dermabacter hominis* | Coccoid to short gram-positive rods | Small; gray to white, convex; distinctive pungent odor |
| *Exiguobacterium acetylicum* | Irregular, short, gram-positive rods arranged singly, in pairs, or short chains; (i.e., rod-coccus cycle*) | Golden yellow |
| *Kurthia* spp. | Regular gram-positive rods with parallel sides; coccoid cells in cultures >3 days old | Large, creamy or tan-yellow; nonhemolytic |
| *Leifsonia aquatica* | Irregular, slender, short gram-positive rods | Yellow |
| *Listeria monocytogenes* | Regular, short, gram-positive rods or coccobacilli occurring in pairs (resembles streptococci) | Small; white, smooth, translucent, moist; beta-hemolytic |
| *Microbacterium* spp. | Irregular, short, thin, gram-positive rods | Small to medium; yellow |
| *Oerskovia* spp. | Extensive branching; hyphae break up into coccoid to rod-shaped elements | Yellow-pigmented; convex; creamy colony grows into the agar; dense centers |
| *Rothia* spp. | Extremely pleomorphic; predominately coccoid and bacillary (broth, Figure 17-2, *A*) to branched filaments (solid media, Figure 17-2, *B*) | Small, smooth to rough colonies; dry; whitish; raised |
| *Turicella otitidis* | Irregular, long, gram-positive rods | Small to medium; white to cream, circular, convex |

*Rod-coccus cycle means rods are apparent in young cultures; cocci are apparent in cultures greater than 3 days old.
†Includes strains G-1 and G-2.
‡Includes *C. diphtheriae, C. ulcerans,* and *C. pseudotuberculosis.*

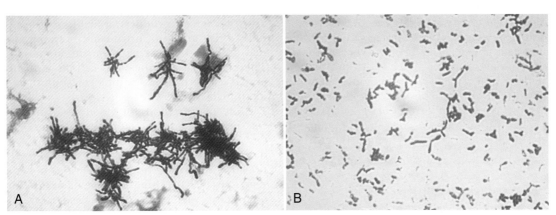

**Figure 17-2 A,** *Rothia dentocariosa* from broth. **B,** *R. dentocariosa* from solid media. (Courtesy Deanna Kiska, SUNY Upstate Medical University, Syracuse, NY.)

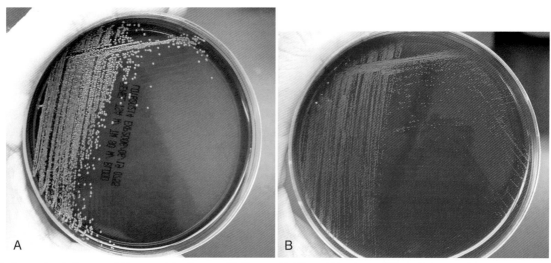

**Figure 17-3** *Corynebacterium urealyticum* on blood agar with Tween 80 **(A)** and blood agar **(B)** at 48 hours. This organism is lipophilic and grows much better on the lipid-containing medium.

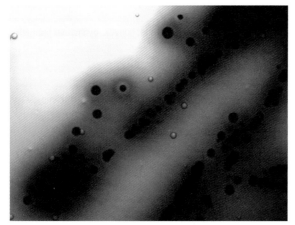

**Figure 17-4** Colony of *Corynebacterium diphtheriae* on Tinsdale agar. Note black colonies with brown halo.

dioxide ($CO_2$) retards the formation of halos on TIN agar.

### Colonial Appearance

Table 17-3 describes the colonial appearance and other distinguishing characteristics (e.g., hemolysis and odor) of each clinically relevant genus or species of corynebacteria on blood agar. Colonies of *C. diphtheriae* on cystine-tellurite blood agar appear black or gray, whereas those on modified Tinsdale agar are black with dark brown halos (see Figure 17-4). *C. diphtheriae* colonies may be recognized by one of four varieties of colony morphologies. These colony types are referred to as *gravis, intermedius, belfanti,* and *mitis,* based on the phenotypic characteristics of size, texture, color, hemolysis, and the presence of metachromatic granules.

### APPROACH TO IDENTIFICATION

Except for *L. monocytogenes* and a few *Corynebacterium* spp., identification of the organisms in this chapter generally

is complex and problematic. A multiphasic approach is required for definitive identification. This often requires biochemical testing, whole-cell fatty acid analysis, cell wall diamino acid analysis, or 16S rRNA gene sequencing. The last three methods are usually not available in routine clinical laboratories, so identification of isolates requires expertise available in reference laboratories. Further complicating the situation is the fact that coryneforms are present as normal flora throughout the body. Thus, only clinically relevant isolates should be identified fully. Indicators of clinical relevance include (1) isolation from normally sterile sites or multiple blood culture bottles; (2) isolation in pure culture or as the predominant organism from symptomatic patients who have not yielded any other known etiologic agent; and (3) isolation from urine if present as a pure culture at greater than 10,000 colony-forming units per milliliter (CFU/mL) or the predominant organism at greater than 100,000 CFU/mL. Coryneforms are more likely to be the cause of a urinary tract infection if the pH of the urine is alkaline or if struvite crystals composed of phosphate, magnesium, and ammonia are present in the sediment.

The API Coryne strip (bioMérieux, St. Louis, Missouri) and the RapID CB Plus (Remel, Lenexa, Kansas) are commercial products available for rapid identification of this group of organisms; however, the databases may not be current with recent taxonomic changes. Therefore, misidentifications can occur if the code generated using these kits is the exclusive criterion used for identification.

Molecular methods for the identification of *C. diphtheriae,* including ribotyping, pulsed-field gel electrophoresis, and multilocus sequence typing, have been demonstrated to be more sensitive and effective for identification during an outbreak. Various polymerase chain reaction (PCR) techniques have been developed for the quantitative detection of *L. monocytogenes* in food products. *L. monocytogenes* DNA in cerebrospinal fluid (CSF) and tissue (fresh or paraffin blocks) can be detected by molecular assays, although these are not available in most clinical laboratories.

Table 17-4 shows the key tests needed to separate the genera discussed in this chapter. In addition to the features shown, the Gram stain and colonial morphology should be carefully noted.

### Comments on Specific Organisms

Two tests (halo on Tinsdale agar and urea hydrolysis) can be used to separate *C. diphtheriae* from other corynebacteria. Definitive identification of a *C. diphtheriae* as a true pathogen requires demonstration of toxin production by the isolate in question. A patient may be infected with several strains at once, so testing is performed using a pooled inoculum of at least 10 colonies. Several toxin detection methods are available:

- Guinea pig lethality test to ascertain whether diphtheria antitoxin neutralizes the lethal effect of a cell-free suspension of the suspect organism
- Immunodiffusion test originally described by Elek (Figure 17-5)
- Tissue culture cell test to demonstrate toxicity of a cell-free suspension of the suspect organism in tissue culture cells and the neutralization of the cytopathic effect by diphtheria antitoxin
- PCR to detect the toxin gene

Because the incidence of diphtheria in the United States is so low (fewer than 5 cases/year), it is not practical to perform these tests in routine clinical laboratories. Toxin testing is usually performed in reference laboratories.

Identification criteria for *Corynebacterium* spp. (including *C. diphtheriae*) are shown in Tables 17-5 through 17-9. Most clinically relevant strains are catalase positive, nonmotile, nonpigmented, and esculin and gelatin negative. Therefore, isolation of an organism failing to demonstrate any of these characteristics provides a significant clue that another genus shown in Table 17-4 should be considered. In addition, an irregular, gram-positive rod isolate that is strictly aerobic, nonlipophilic and oxidizes or does not utilize glucose, will likely be *Leifsonia aquatica,* or *Arthrobacter, Brevibacterium,* or *Microbacterium* spp.

The enhancement of growth by lipids (e.g., Tween 80 or serum) of certain coryneform bacteria (e.g., *C. jeikeium* and *C. urealyticum*) is useful for preliminary identification. These two species are also resistant to several antibiotics commonly tested against gram-positive bacteria.

*L. monocytogenes* can be presumptively identified by observation of motility by direct wet mount. The organism exhibits characteristic end-over-end tumbling motility when incubated in nutrient broth at room temperature for 1 to 2 hours. Alternatively, characteristic motility can be seen by an umbrella-shaped pattern (Figure 17-6) that develops after overnight incubation at room temperature of a culture stabbed into a tube of semisolid agar. *L. monocytogenes* ferments glucose and is Voges-Proskauer positive and esculin positive. Isolation of a small, gram-positive, catalase-positive rod with a narrow zone of beta-hemolysis from blood or CSF should be considered strong presumptive evidence for listeriosis. *L. monocytogenes* can be differentiated from other *Listeria* spp. by a positive result on the Christie, Atkins, Munch-Petersen (CAMP) test, as described in Chapter 15 for the identification of *Streptococcus agalactiae*. A reverse CAMP reaction (i.e., an arrow of no hemolysis formed at the junction of the test organism with the staphylococci) is used to identify *C. pseudotuberculosis* and *C. ulcerans*. *C. urealyticum* is rapidly urea positive.

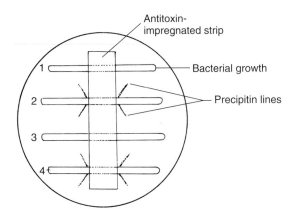

**Figure 17-5** Diagram of an Elek plate for demonstration of toxin production by *Corynebacterium diphtheriae*. A filter paper strip impregnated with diphtheria antitoxin is buried just beneath the surface of a special agar plate before the agar hardens. Strains to be tested and known positive and negative toxigenic strains are streaked on the agar's surface in a line across the plate and at a right angle to the antitoxin paper strip. After 24 hours of incubation at 37°C, the plates are examined with transmitted light for the presence of fine precipitin lines at a 45-degree angle to the streaks. The presence of precipitin lines indicates that the strain produced toxin that reacted with the homologous antitoxin. Line 1 is the negative control. Line 2 is the positive control. Line 3 is an unknown organism that is a nontoxigenic strain. Line 4 is an unknown organism that is a toxigenic strain.

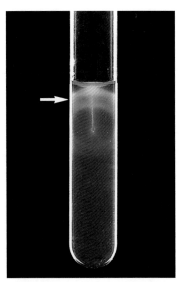

**Figure 17-6** Umbrella motility of *Listeria monocytogenes* grown at room temperature.

**TABLE 17-4** Catalase-Positive, Non–Acid-Fast, Gram-Positive Rods[a]

| Organism | Metabolism[b] | Motility | Pigment[c] | Nitrate Reduction | Esculin | Glucose Fermentation | CAMP[d] | Mycolic Acid[e] | Cell Wall Diamino Acids[f] | Other Comments |
|---|---|---|---|---|---|---|---|---|---|---|
| *Corynebacterium* | F/O | – | n, w, y, bl | v | –[g] | v | v | +[h] | meso-DAP | |
| *Arthrobacter* | O | v[i] | w, g | v | v | –[j] | – | – | L-lys | Gelatin-positive |
| *Brevibacterium* | O | – | w, g, sl y, t | v | – | –[j] | – | – | meso-DAP | Gelatin- and casein-positive; cheese odor |
| *Microbacterium*[k] | F/O[m] | v[n] | y, o, y-o | v | v[o] | v | –[p] | – | L-lys, D-orn | Gelatin and casein variable |
| *Turicella otitidis* | O | – | w | – | – | – | + | – | meso-DAP | Isolated from ears |
| *Dermabacter hominis* | F | – | n, w | – | + | + | – | – | meso-DAP | Pungent odor; decarboxylates lysine and ornithine; gelatin positive |
| *Cellulomonas* | F[l] | v | sl y, y | + | + | + | – | – | L-orn | Gelatin-positive; casein-negative |
| *Leifsonia aquatica* | O | + | y | v | v | –[q] | – | – | DAB | Gelatin- and casein-negative |
| *Rhodococcus equi* | O | – | p | v | – | – | + | + | meso-DAP | Usually mucoid; can be acid-fast; urease-positive |
| *Cellulosimicrobium cellulans* (formerly *Oerskovia xanthineolytica*) | F | – | y | + | + | + | NT | – | L-lys | Hydrolyzes xanthine; colonies pit agar |
| *Oerskovia turbata* | F | v | y | + | + | + | NT | – | L-lys | Does not hydrolyze xanthine |
| *Listeria monocytogenes* | F | +[r] | w | – | + | + | + | – | meso-DAP | Narrow zone of beta hemolysis on sheep blood agar; hippurate-positive |
| *Kurthia* | O | +[r] | n, c | – | – | – | NT | – | L-lys | Large, "Medusa-head" colony with rhizoid growth on yeast nutrient agar; may be $H_2S$-positive in TSI butt; gelatin-negative |

**TABLE 17-4** Catalase-Positive, Non–Acid-Fast, Gram-Positive Rods—cont'd

| Organism | Metabolism[b] | Motility | Pigment[c] | Nitrate Reduction | Esculin | Glucose Fermentation | CAMP[d] | Mycolic Acid[e] | Cell Wall Diamino Acids[f] | Other Comments |
|---|---|---|---|---|---|---|---|---|---|---|
| *Exiguobacterium acetylicum* | F | + | Golden | v | + | + | NT | – | L-lys | Most are oxidase positive; casein and gelatin positive |
| *Rothia dentocariosa* | F | – | w | + | + | + | – | – | L-lys | If sticky, probably *R. mucilaginosa;* some strains are black pigmented |
| *Actinomyces neuii* | F | – | n | v | – | + | + | – | NT | Nonhemolytic |
| *Actinomyces viscosus* | F | – | n | + | – | + | – | – | NT | |
| *Propionibacterium avidum/granulosum* | F | – | w, n | – | v | v | + | – | NT | Beta-hemolytic, branching |

[a]The aerotolerant catalase-positive *Propionibacterium* spp. and *Actinomyces* spp. are also included in Table 23-4.
[b]F, Fermentative; O, oxidative.
[c]c, Cream; g, gray; n, nonpigmented; o, orange; sl, slightly; t, tan; w, white; y, yellow; y-o, yellowish-orange; p, pink; bl, black.
[d]CAMP test using a beta-lysin–producing strain of *Staphylococcus aureus.*
[e]Mycolic acids of various lengths are also present in the partially acid-fast *Nocardia, Gordona, Rhodococcus,* and *Tsukamurella* and the completely acid-fast *Mycobacterium* genera.
[f]*DAB,* diaminobutyric acid; *D-orn,* d-ornithine; *L-lys,* L-lysine; *L-orn,* L-ornithine; *meso-DAP,* meso-diaminopimelic acid.
[g]Of the significant clinical *Corynebacterium* isolates, only *C. matruchotii* and *C. glucuronolyticum* are esculin-positive.
[h]Of the significant *Corynebacterium* isolates, *Corynebacterium amycolatum* does not have mycolic acid as a lipid in the cell wall, as determined by high-performance liquid chromatography (HPLC) profiling methods.
[i]Rod forms of some species are motile.
[j]Glucose may be variably oxidized, but it is not fermented.
[k]*Microbacterium* spp. now include the former *Aureobacterium* spp.
[l]Some grow poorly anaerobically.
[m]Slow and weak oxidative production of acid from some carbohydrates.
[n]Only the orange-pigmented species *M. imperiale* and *M. arborescens* are motile at 28°C.
[o]Positive reaction may be delayed.
[p]Some strains of *M. arborescens* are CAMP-positive.
[q]Glucose is usually oxidized, but it is not fermented.
[r]Motile at 20° to 25°C.

*NT,* Not tested; *TSI,* triple sugar iron agar; *v,* variable reactions; +, ≥90% of species or strains positive; –, ≥90% of species or strains negative.

**TABLE 17-5** Fermentative, Nonlipophilic, Tinsdale-Positive *Corynebacterium* spp.*

| Organism | Urease[†] | Nitrate Reduction[†] | Esculin Hydrolysis[†] | Fermentation of Glycogen[†] | Lipophilic |
|---|---|---|---|---|---|
| *C. diphtheriae* subsp. *gravis* | − | + | − | + | − |
| *C. diphtheriae* subsp. *mitis* | − | + | − | − | − |
| *C. diphtheriae* subsp. *belfanti* | − | − | − | − | − |
| *C. diphtheriae* subsp. *intermedius* | − | + | − | − | + |
| *C. ulcerans*[‡§] | + | − | − | + | − |
| *C. pseudotuberculosis*[‡§] | + | v | − | − | − |

*Separation of lipophilic and nonlipophilic species can be determined by comparing growth on sheep blood agar and sheep blood agar with 1% Tween 80 or growth in brain-heart infusion broth with and without 1 drop of Tween 80 or rabbit serum.
[†]Reactions from API Coryne.
[‡]Propionic acid produced as a product of glucose metabolism.
[§]Reverse CAMP positive.
+, ≥90% of species or strains positive; −, ≥90% of species or strains are negative; v, variable reactions.
Data compiled from Coyle MB, Lipsky BA: Coryneform bacteria in infectious diseases: clinical and laboratory aspects, *Clin Microbiol* Rev 3:227, 1990; Funke G, Carlotti A: Differentiation of *Brevibacterium* spp. encountered in clinical specimens, *J Clin Microbiol* 32:1729, 1994; and Gruner E, Steigerwalt AG, Hollis DG et al: Human infections caused by *Brevibacterium casei,* formerly CDC groups B-1 and B-3, *J Clin Microbiol* 32:1511, 1994.

**TABLE 17-6** Fermentative, Nonlipophilic, Tinsdale-Negative Clinically Relevant *Corynebacterium* spp.*[†]

| Organism | Urea[‡] | Nitrate Reduction[‡] | Propionic Acid[§] | Motility | Esculin Hydrolysis[‡] | Fermentation of Glucose[‡] | Maltose[‡] | Sucrose[‡] | Xylose[‡] | CAMP[¶] |
|---|---|---|---|---|---|---|---|---|---|---|
| *C. amycolatum*[a] | v | v | + | − | − | + | v | v | − | − |
| *C. argentoratense* | − | − | + | − | − | + | − | − | − | − |
| *C. aurimucosum*[b,c] | − | − | − | − | − | + | + | + | − | − |
| *C. coyleae* | − | − | ND | − | − | (+) | − | − | − | + |
| *C. falsenii*[d] | (+) | v | ND | − | v | (+) | v | − | − | − |
| *C. freneyi*[b] | − | v | − | − | − | + | + | + | − | ND |
| *C. glucuronolyticum* | v | v | + | − | v | + | v | + | v | + |
| *C. imitans* | − | v | ND | − | − | + | + | (+) | − | + |
| *C. matruchotii* | − | + | + | − | v + | + | + | + | − | − |
| *C. minutissimum*[f] | − | − | − | − | − | + | + | v | − | − |
| *C. riegelii* | + | − | ND | − | − | − | (+) | − | − | − |
| *C. simulans*[g] | − | + | − | − | − | + | − | + | − | − |
| *C. singulare* | + | − | − | − | − | + | + | + | − | − |
| *C. striatum* | − | + | − | − | − | + | − | v | − | v |
| *C. sundsvallense*[b] | + | − | ND | − | − | (+) | + | + | − | − |
| *C. thomssenii*[b] | + | − | ND | − | − | (+) | + | + | − | − |
| *C. xerosis* | − | v | − | − | − | + | + | + | − | − |

*Consider also *Dermabacter, Cellulomonas, Exiguobacterium,* and *Microbacterium* spp. if the isolate is pigmented, motile, or esculin or gelatin positive (see Table 17-4). The aerotolerant catalase-positive *Propionibacterium* spp. and *Actinomyces* spp. (see Table 18-4) should also be considered in the differential with the organisms in this table.
[†]Separation of lipophilic and nonlipophilic species can be determined by comparing growth on sheep blood agar and sheep blood agar with 1% Tween 80 or growth in brain-heart infusion broth with and without 1 drop of Tween 80 or rabbit serum.
[‡]Reactions from API Coryne.
[§]Propionic acid as an end-product of glucose metabolism.
[¶]CAMP data using a beta-lysin-producing strain of *Staphylococcus aureus.*
[a]Most frequently encountered species in human clinical material; frequently misidentified as *C. xerosis.*
[b]Sticky colonies.
[c]Yellow or black-pigmented; black-pigmented strains have been previously listed as *C. nigricans;* may be pathogenic from female genital tract.
[d]Yellow after 72 hours.
[e]Grows at 42°C; frequently misidentified as *C. xerosis.*
[f]DNase positive.
[g]Nitrite reduced.
*ND,* No data; *v,* variable reactions; +, ≥90% of species or strains are positive; +[W], (+), delayed positive reaction; −, ≥90% of species or strains are negative.

**TABLE 17-7** Strictly Aerobic, Nonlipophilic, Nonfermentative, Clinically Relevant *Corynebacterium* spp.[a,b]

| Organism | Oxidation of Glucose | Nitrate Reduction[c] | Urease[c] | Esculin Hydrolysis[c,d] | Gelatin[c,d] | Camp[e] | Other Comments |
|---|---|---|---|---|---|---|---|
| *C. afermentans* subsp. *afermentans* | − | − | − | − | − | v | Isolated from blood; nonadherent colony |
| *C. auris*[f] | − | − | − | − | − | + | Isolated from ears; dry, usually adherent colony |
| *C. mucifaciens* | + | − | − | − | NT | − | Slightly yellow, mucoid colonies |
| *C. pseudodiphtheriticum* | − | + | + | − | − | − | |
| *C. propinquum* | − | + | − | − | − | − | |

[a]*Kurthia* sp. is also a strictly aerobic, nonlipophilic, nonfermentative organism. However, as described in Table 17-3, the colonial and cellular morphology of *Kurthia* organisms should easily distinguish it from the organisms in this table.
[b]Separation of lipophilic and nonlipophilic species can be determined by comparing growth on sheep blood agar and sheep blood agar with 1% Tween 80 or growth in brain-heart infusion broth with and without 1 drop of Tween 80 or rabbit serum.
[c]Reactions from API Coryne.
[d]Consider also *Brevibacterium* and *Microbacterium* spp., *Leifsonia aquatica,* and *Arthrobacter* sp. in the differential if the isolate is gelatin or esculin positive (see Table 17-4).
[e]CAMP test using a beta-lysin–producing strain of Staphylococcus aureus.
[f]For isolates from the ear, also consider *Turicella otitidis,* which is nitrate and urease positive, in the differential (see Table 17-4).
*NT,* Not tested; *v,* variable reactions; +, ≥90% of species or strains are positive; −, ≥90% of species or strains are negative.
Data compiled from Coyle MB, Lipsky BA: Coryneform bacteria in infectious diseases: clinical and laboratory aspects, *Clin Microbiol Rev* 3:227, 1990; Funke G, Carlotti A: Differentiation of *Brevibacterium* spp. encountered in clinical specimens, *J Clin Microbiol* 32:1729, 1994; and Mandell GL, Bennett JE, Dolin R: *Principles and practices of infectious diseases,* 2010, Churchill Stone and Livingston, Elsevier.

**TABLE 17-8** Strictly Aerobic, Lipophilic, Nonfermentative, Clinically Relevant Corynebacterium spp.*

| Organism | OXIDATION OF | | | | |
|---|---|---|---|---|---|
| | Nitrate Reduction[†] | Urease[†] | Esculin Hydrolysis[†] | Glucose | Maltose |
| *C. lipophiloflavum*[‡] | − | − | − | − | − |
| *C. jeikeium*[§] | − | − | − | + | v |
| *C. afermentens* subsp. *lipophilum* | − | − | − | − | − |
| *C. urealyticum*[§] | − | + | − | − | − |

*Separation of lipophilic and nonlipophilic species can be determined by comparing growth on sheep blood agar and sheep blood agar with 1% Tween 80 or growth in brain-heart infusion broth with and without one drop of Tween 80 or rabbit serum.
[†]Reactions from API Coryne.
[‡]Yellow.
[§]Isolates are usually multiply antimicrobial resistant.
+, ≥90% of species or strains positive; −, ≥90% of species or strains negative; *v,* variable reactions.
Data compiled from Coyle MB, Lipsky BA: Coryneform bacteria in infectious diseases: clinical and laboratory aspects, *Clin Microbiol Rev* 3:227, 1990; Funke G, Carlotti A: Differentiation of *Brevibacterium* spp. encountered in clinical specimens, *J Clin Microbiol* 32:1729, 1994; Mandell GL, Bennett JE, Dolin R: *Principles and practices of infectious diseases,* 2010, Churchill Stone and Livingston, Elsevier; and Riegel P, de Briel D, Prévost G et al: Genomic diversity among *Corynebacterium jeikeium* strains and comparison with biochemical characteristics, *J Clin Microbiol* 32:1860, 1994.

**TABLE 17-9** Lipophilic, Fermentative, Clinically Relevant *Corynebacterium* spp.*

| Organism | Urease[†] | Esculin Hydrolysis[†] | Alkaline Phosphatase[†] | Pyrazinamidase[†] |
|---|---|---|---|---|
| *C. kroppenstedtii*[‡] | − | + | − | + |
| *C. bovis* | − | − | + | − |
| *C. accolens*[§] | − | − | − | v |
| *C. macginleyi*[§] | − | − | + | − |
| CDC coryneform group F-1 | + | − | − | + |
| CDC coryneform group G | − | − | + | + |

*Separation of lipophilic and nonlipophilic species can be determined by comparing growth on sheep blood agar and sheep blood agar with 1% Tween 80 or growth in brain-heart infusion broth with and without one drop of Tween 80 or rabbit serum.
[†]Reactions from API Coryne.
[‡]Propionic acid produced as a product of glucose metabolism.
[§]Nitrate reduced.
+, ≥90% of species or strains positive; −, ≥90% of species or strains negative; v, variable reactions.
Data compiled from Coyle MB, Lipsky BA: Coryneform bacteria in infectious diseases: clinical and laboratory aspects, *Clin Microbiol Rev* 3:227, 1990; Funke G, Carlotti A: Differentiation of *Brevibacterium* spp. encountered in clinical specimens, *J Clin Microbiol* 32:1729, 1994; Mandell GL, Bennett JE, Dolin R: *Principles and practices of infectious diseases*, 2010, Churchill Stone and Livingston, Elsevier; and Riegel P, Ruimy R, de Briel D et al: Genomic diversity and phylogenetic relationships among lipid-requiring diphtheroids from humans and characterization of *Corynebacterium macginleyi* sp nov, *Int J Syst Bacteriol* 45:128, 1995.

**TABLE 17-10** Antimicrobial Therapy and Susceptibility Testing

| Organism | Therapeutic Options | Resistance to Therapeutic Options | Validated Testing Methods* |
|---|---|---|---|
| *Listeria monocytogenes* | Ampicillin, or penicillin (MIC ≤2 µg/mL), with or without an aminoglycoside | Occasional resistance to tetracyclines | Yes, but testing is rarely needed to guide therapy; typically treated empirically. |
| *Corynebacterium diphtheriae* | Antitoxin to neutralize diphtheria toxin plus penicillin or erythromycin to eradicate organism | Not to recommended agents; rare instances of penicillin or macrolide resistance | See CLSI document M45-A: Methods for Antimicrobial Dilution and Disk Susceptibility Testing of Infrequently Isolated or Fastidious Bacteria. |
| Other *Corynebacterium* spp. | No definitive guidelines. All are susceptible to vancomycin and teicoplanin. | Multiple resistance to penicillins, macrolides, aminoglycosides, fluoroquinolones, tetracyclines, clindamycin and cephalosporins | See CLSI document M45-A: Methods for Antimicrobial Dilution and Disk Susceptibility Testing of Infrequently Isolated or Fastidious Bacteria. |
| *Kurthia* spp., *Brevibacterium* spp., *Dermabacter* sp., *Arthrobacter* spp., *Microbacterium* spp., *Cellulomonas* spp., and *Exiguobacterium* sp. | No definitive guidelines | Unknown | Not available |

*Validated testing methods include the standard methods recommended by CLSI and commercial methods approved by the U.S. Food and Drug Administration (FDA).
*CLISI,* Clinical and Laboratory Standards Institute; *MIC,* minimum inhibitory concentration.

## SERODIAGNOSIS

Serodiagnostic techniques are not generally used for the laboratory diagnosis of infections caused by the organisms discussed in this chapter. Anti–listeriolysin O antibodies (IgG) can be detected in cases of listeriosis, although IgM antibodies are undetectable. However, these tests are not commonly used for the clinical diagnosis.

## ANTIMICROBIAL SUSCEPTIBILITY TESTING AND THERAPY

Definitive guidelines have been established for antimicrobial therapy for *L. monocytogenes* against certain antimicrobial agents. Because there is no resistance to the therapeutic agents of choice, antimicrobial susceptibility testing is not routinely necessary (Table 17-10).

As shown in Table 17-10, Clinical and Laboratory Standards Institute (CLSI) document M45 provides some guidelines for testing of *Corynebacterium* spp. Chapter 12 should be reviewed for strategies that can be used to provide susceptibility information and data when warranted. It is important to note that some strains of *Corynebacterium* spp. may require 48 hours of incubation for growth. If growth is insufficient or if the isolate appears susceptible to β-lactams at 24 hours, the medium should be incubated for a total of 48 hours before the result is reported.

# PREVENTION

The only effective control of diphtheria is through immunization with a multidose diphtheria toxoid prepared by inactivation of the toxin with formaldehyde. Immunization is usually initiated in infancy as part of a triple antigen vaccine (DTaP— previously referred to as DPT) containing diphtheria toxoid, pertussis, and tetanus toxoid. Boosters are recommended every 10 years to maintain active protection and are given as part of a double-antigen vaccine with tetanus toxoid.

A single dose of intramuscular penicillin or a 7- to 10-day course of oral erythromycin is recommended for all individuals exposed to diphtheria, regardless of their immunization status. Follow-up throat cultures from individuals taking prophylaxis should be obtained at least 2 weeks after therapy. If the patient still harbors *C. diphtheriae,* an additional 10-day course of oral erythromycin should be given. Previously immunized contacts should receive a booster dose of diphtheria toxoid; nonimmunized contacts should begin the primary series of immunizations.

The general population should always properly wash raw vegetables and thoroughly cook vegetables and meat to prevent listerosis. Patients who are immunocompromised and pregnant women should avoid eating soft cheeses (e.g., Mexican-style cheese, feta, brie, Camembert, and blue-veined cheese) to prevent food-borne listeriosis. Additionally, leftover or ready-to-eat foods such as hot dogs or cold cuts should be thoroughly heated before consumption and stored for only a short period before disposal, because *L. monocytogenes* is able to replicate during refrigeration at 4°C.

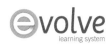

***Visit the Evolve site to complete the review questions.***

---

## CASE STUDY 17-1

A 27-year-old man received a pancreas and kidney transplant. The patient was readmitted 3 months later for possible rejection of the organs. Five days earlier, he had developed fever, nausea, and dizziness. His creatinine was elevated, and he had white blood cells in his urine. All other laboratory findings were normal. A biopsy did not demonstrate rejection. At this point, the laboratory reported greater than 100,000 gram-positive rods in the urine. The colonies were catalase positive and beta-hemolytic. The next day, blood cultures were positive with the same organism.

**QUESTIONS**

1. A simple laboratory test indicated that the isolate was not a *Corynebacterium* sp. What was that test?
2. Which method is used for routine susceptibility testing for *Listeria* sp.?
3. List the *Corynebacterium* spp. that are considered urinary tract pathogens. What test is helpful to screen for these pathogens?

---

# BIBLIOGRAPHY

Barreau C, Bimet F, Kiredjian M, et al: Comparative chemotaxonomic studies of mycolic acid–free coryneform bacteria of human origin, *J Clin Microbiol* 31:2085, 1993.

Bernard K, Bellefeuille M, Hollis DG, et al: Cellular fatty acid composition and phenotypic and cultural characterization of CDC fermentative coryneform groups 3 and 5, *J Clin Microbiol* 32:1217, 1994.

Collins MD, Bernard KA, Hutson RA, et al: *Corynebacterium sundsvallense* sp nov, from human clinical specimens, *Int J Syst Bacteriol* 49:361, 1999.

Coyle MB, Lipsky BA: Coryneform bacteria in infectious diseases: clinical and laboratory aspects, *Clin Microbiol Rev* 3:227, 1990.

Daneshvar MI, Hollis DG, Weyant RS, et al: Identification of some charcoal black–pigmented CDC fermentative coryneform group 4 isolates as *Rothia dentocariosa* and some as *Corynebacterium aurimucosum*: proposal of *Rothia dentocariosa* (emend Georg and Brown, 1967), *Corynebacterium aurimucosum* (emend Yassin, et al, 2002), and *Corynebacterium nigricans* (Shukla et al, 2003) pro synon. *Corynebacterium aurimucosum, J Clin Microbiol* 42:4189, 2004.

Evtushenko LI, Dorofeeva LV, Subbotin SA, et al: *Leifsonia poae* gen nov, sp nov, isolated from nematode galls on *Poa annua,* and reclassification of "*Corynebacterium aquaticum*" (Leifson, 1962) as *Leifsonia aquatica* (ex Leifson, 1962) gen nov, nom rev, comb nov and *Clavibacter xyli* (Davis et al, 1984) with two subspecies as *Leifsonia xyli* (Davis et al, 1984) gen nov, comb nov, *Int J Syst Evol Microbiol* 50:371, 2000.

Funke G, Carlotti A: Differentiation of *Brevibacterium* spp encountered in clinical specimens, *J Clin Microbiol* 32:1729, 1994.

Funke G, Efstratiou A, Kuklinska D, et al: *Corynebacterium imitans* sp nov isolated from patients with suspected diphtheria, *J Clin Microbiol* 35:1978, 1997.

Funke G, Falsen E, Barreau C: Primary identification of *Microbacterium* spp encountered in clinical specimens as CDC coryneform group A-4 and A-5 bacteria, *J Clin Microbiol* 33:188, 1995.

Funke G, Hutson RA, Bernard KA, et al: Isolation of *Arthrobacter* spp. from clinical specimens and description of *Arthrobacter cumminsii* sp nov and *Arthrobacter woluwensis* sp nov, *J Clin Microbiol* 34:2356, 1996.

Funke G, Lawson PA, Collins MD: *Corynebacterium mucifaciens* sp nov, and unusual species from human clinical material, *Int J Syst Bacteriol* 47:952, 1997.

Funke G, Lawson PA, Collins MD: *Corynebacterium riegelii* sp nov: an unusual species isolated from female patients with urinary tract infections, *J Clin Microbiol* 36:624, 1998.

Funke G, Lawson PA, Collins MD: Heterogeneity within Centers for Disease Control and Prevention coryneform group ANF-1-like bacteria and description of *Corynebacterium auris* sp nov, *Int J Syst Bacteriol* 45:735, 1995.

Funke G, Lawson PA, Bernard KA, et al: Most *Corynebacterium xerosis* strains identified in the routine clinical laboratory correspond to *Corynebacterium amycolatum*, *J Clin Microbiol* 34:1124, 1996.

Funke G, von Graevenitz A, Clarridge JE, et al: Clinical microbiology of coryneform bacteria, *Clin Microbiol Rev* 10:125, 1997.

Gruner E, Steigerwalt AG, Hollis DG, et al: Human infections caused by *Brevibacterium casei*, formerly CDC groups B-1 and B-3, *J Clin Microbiol* 32:1511, 1994.

Mandell GL, Bennett JE, Dolin R: *Principles and practices of infectious diseases*, 2010, Churchill Stone Livingston/Elsevier.

McNeil MM, Brown JM: The medically important aerobic actinomycetes: epidemiology and microbiology, *Clin Microbiol Rev* 7:357, 1994.

Riegel P, de Briel D, Prévost G, et al: Genomic diversity among *Corynebacterium jeikeium* strains and comparison with biochemical characteristics, *J Clin Microbiol* 32:1860, 1994.

Riegel P, Ruimy R, de Briel D, et al: Genomic diversity and phylogenetic relationships among lipid-requiring diphtheroids from humans and characterization of *Corynebacterium macginleyi* sp nov, *Int J Syst Bacteriol* 45:128, 1995.

Shukla SK, Bernard KA, Harney M, et al: *Corynebacterium nigricans* sp. nov.: proposed name for a black-pigmented *Corynebacterium* species recovered from the human female urogenital tract, *J Clin Microbiol* 41:4353, 2003.

Versalovic J: *Manual of clinical microbiology*, ed 10, 2011, Washington, DC, ASM Press.

Zimmermann O, Spröer C, Kroppenstedt RM, et al: *Corynebacterium thomssenii* sp nov: a *Corynebacterium* with N-acetyl-β-glucosaminidase activity from human clinical specimens, *Int J Syst Bacteriol* 48:489, 1998.

# Non-Branching, Catalase-Negative, Gram-Positive Bacilli

# *Erysipelothrix, Lactobacillus,* and Similar Organisms

## OBJECTIVES

1. Describe the Gram stain morphology of *Arcanobacterium, Lactobacillus, Erysipelothrix,* and *Gardnerella* spp.
2. Identify the media of choice and morphologic appearance of *Gardnerella* sp. and describe its incubation conditions, including time, oxygen requirements, and temperature.
3. List the disease states associated with *Erysipelothrix, Gardnerella,* and *Lactobacillus* spp.
4. Identify the correct specimens for the isolation of *Erysipelothrix, Gardnerella,* and *Lactobacillus* spp.
5. Explain why in vitro susceptibility testing is usually not necessary to guide therapy of *Erysipelothrix* or *Gardnerella* spp.

---

### GENERA AND SPECIES TO BE CONSIDERED

- *Erysipelothrix rhusiopathiae*
- *Arcanobacterium* spp.
- *Gardnerella vaginalis*
- *Lactobacillus* spp.
- *Weissella confusa*

---

## GENERAL CHARACTERISTICS

The genera described in this chapter are all catalase-negative, non-spore-forming, gram-positive rods; some may exhibit rudimentary branching. *Erysipelothrix rhusiopathiae* is one of three species in the genus, but it is considered the only human pathogen. *E. rhusiopathiae* consists of several serovars based on peptidoglycan structure. The serovars most commonly associated with human infection include serovars 1 and 2. *Arcanobacterium* spp. demonstrate irregular, gram-positive rods on Gram stain. *Gardnerella* sp. fermentation byproducts include acetic and lactic acid. The cell wall of *Gardnerella* sp. is significantly thinner and contains less peptidoglycan than the typically gram-positive bacteria. *Weissella confusa,* formerly classified as *Lactobacillus confusus,* is included in Tables 18-3 and 18-4 because it is easily confused on culture media with the organisms included in this chapter, and in rare cases it has been isolated associated with bacteremia and endocarditis.

## EPIDEMIOLOGY

*Erysipelothrix* spp. are found worldwide in a variety of vertebrate and invertebrate animals, including mammals, birds, and fish. Other domestic animals that may be infected include sheep, rabbits, cattle, and turkeys. The organism may be transmitted through direct contact or ingestion of contaminated water or meat. *Arcanobacterium* spp. are normal inhabitants of the mucosal membranes of cattle, sheep, dogs, cats, and pigs. The organisms listed in Table 18-1 include those that are closely associated with animals and are contracted by humans through animal exposure (e.g., *E. rhusiopathiae* and *Arcanobacterium pyogenes*) and those that are part of the normal human flora (e.g., *Lactobacillus* spp. and *Gardnerella vaginalis*).

## PATHOGENESIS AND SPECTRUM OF DISEASE

*G. vaginalis* and *Lactobacillus* spp. (Table 18-2) are natural inhabitants of the human vagina. Vaginal infections with *G. vaginalis* are often found in association with a variety of mixed anaerobic flora. Extravaginal infections are uncommon but have been identified associated with postpartum endometritis, septic abortion, and cesarean birth.

*Lactobacillus* spp. are important for maintaining the proper pH balance in vaginal secretions. The organisms metabolize glucose to lactic acid, producing an acidic vaginal pH and resulting in an environment that is not conducive to the growth of pathogenic bacteria. *W. confusa* is a *Lactobacillus*-like organism that has been recovered in blood cultures from patients with clinical symptoms of endocarditis.

*Erysipelothrix* infections are associated with individuals employed in occupations such as fish handlers, farmers, slaughterhouse workers, food preparation workers, and veterinarians. Infections are typically a result of a puncture wound or skin abrasion. Three categories of human disease have been characterized, including localized skin lesions (erysipeloid), diffuse cutaneous infection with systemic symptoms, and bacteremia. Bacteremia results in dissemination of the organism and can manifest as endocarditis.

*Arcanobacterium* spp. are primarily an animal pathogen, but they have been associated with pharyngitis septicemia, tissue abscesses, and ulcers in immunocompromised patients.

Often the primary challenge is to determine the clinical relevance of these organisms when they are found in specimens from normally sterile sites.

**TABLE 18-1**  Epidemiology

| Species | Habitat (Reservoir) | Mode of Transmission |
|---|---|---|
| *Erysipelothrix rhusiopathiae* | Normal flora; carried by and causes disease in animals | Zoonoses; abrasion or puncture wound of skin with animal exposure |
| *Arcanobacterium haemolyticum* | Normal flora of human skin and pharynx | Uncertain; infections probably caused by person's endogenous strains |
| *Arcanobacterium pyogenes* | Normal flora; carried by and causes disease in animals. | Uncertain: Abrasion or undetected wound during exposure to animals |
| *Gardnerella vaginalis* | Normal flora: Human vaginal tissue Colonizers: Distal urethra of males | Endogenous strain |
| *Lactobacillus* spp. | Environmental: Widely distributed in foods and nature Normal flora: Human mouth, gastrointestinal tract, and female genital tract | Endogenous strain Infections are rare. |

# LABORATORY DIAGNOSIS

## SPECIMEN COLLECTION AND TRANSPORT

Generally, no special considerations are required for specimen collection and transport of the organisms discussed in this chapter. Of note, skin lesions for *Erysipelothrix* should be collected by biopsy of the full thickness of skin at the leading edge of the discolored area. Refer to Table 5-1 for other general information on specimen collection and transport.

## SPECIMEN PROCESSING

No special considerations are required for processing of the organisms discussed in this chapter. Refer to Table 5-1 for general information on specimen processing.

## DIRECT DETECTION METHODS

Gram staining of *Arcanobacterium* spp. demonstrates delicate, curved, gram-positive rods with pointed ends and occasional rudimentary branching. This branching is more pronounced after these organisms have been cultured anaerobically. *Arcanobacterium* spp. stain unevenly after 48 hours of growth on solid media and also exhibit coccal forms.

*Lactobacillus* is highly pleomorphic, occurring in long chaining rods and in coccobacilli and spiral forms (Figure 18-1).

*E. rhusiopathiae* stains as both short rods and long filaments. These morphologies correspond to two colonial types: (1) rough colonies that contain slender, filamentous, gram-positive rods with a tendency to overdecolorize and appear gram negative and (2) smooth colonies that contain small, slender rods. This variability in staining and colonial morphology may be mistaken for a polymicrobial infection both on direct examination and culture.

**TABLE 18-2**  Pathogenesis and Spectrum of Disease

| Organisms | Virulence Factors | Spectrum of Diseases and Infections |
|---|---|---|
| *Erysipelothrix rhusiopathiae* | Capsule Neuraminidase Hyaluronidase Surface proteins | Localized: Erysipeloid, a skin infection that is painful and may spread slowly Systemic: Erysipeloid may cause diffuse skin infection with systemic symptoms. Bacteremia Endocarditis is rare. |
| *Arcanobacterium haemolyticum* | Unknown | Systemic: Pharyngitis Cellulitis, and other skin infections |
| *Arcanobacterium pyogenes* | Unknown | Rarely associated with human infection. When infections occur, they generally are cutaneous and may be complicated by or lead to bacteremia. |
| *Gardnerella vaginalis* | Uncertain Produces cell adherence factors and cytotoxin | Bacterial vaginosis; less commonly associated with urinary tract infections; bacteremia is extremely rare. |
| *Lactobacillus* spp. | Uncertain | Most frequently encountered as a contaminant. Immunocompromised: Bacteremia |

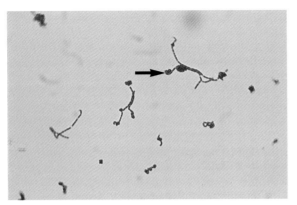

**Figure 18-1** Gram stain of *Lactobacillus* spp. Note spiral forms *(arrow).*

**TABLE 18-3** Colonial Appearance on 5% Sheep Blood Agar and Other Characteristics

| Organism | Appearance |
|---|---|
| *Arcanobacterium* spp. | Small to large colonies with various appearances, including smooth, mucoid, and white and dry, friable, and gray; may be surrounded by narrow zone of beta-hemolysis |
| *Erysipelothrix rhusiopathiae* | Two colony types: large and rough or small, smooth, and translucent; shows alpha-hemolysis after prolonged incubation |
| *Gardnerella vaginalis* | Pinpoint; nonhemolytic |
| *Lactobacillus* spp. | Multiple colonial morphologies, ranging from pinpoint, alpha-hemolytic colonies resembling streptococci to rough, gray colonies |
| *Weissella confusa* | Pinpoint; alpha-hemolytic and may be confused with organisms presented in this chapter |

*Gardnerella* organisms are small, pleomorphic gram-variable or gram-negative coccobacilli and short rods. Wet mount and Gram staining of vaginal secretions are key tests for diagnosing bacterial vaginosis caused by *G. vaginalis.* A wet mount prepared in saline reveals the characteristic "clue cells," which are large, squamous epithelial cells with numerous attached small rods. A Gram-stained smear of the discharge shows the attached organisms to be gram-variable coccobacilli. In bacterial vaginosis, clue cells are typically present, and large numbers of other gram-positive rods (i.e., lactobacilli), representing normal vaginal flora, are absent or few in number. In addition, the BDaffirm vaginal DNA probe (VDP) may be used for direct detection from genital specimens. Special vials containing transport reagent are used to stabilize the organism's nucleic acids prior to testing (Becton, Dickinson and Company Franklin Lakes, NJ).

## Cultivation

**Media of Choice.** All the genera described in this chapter grow on 5% sheep blood and chocolate agars. They do not grow on MacConkey agar but do grow on Columbia colistin-nalidixic acid (CNA) agar. CNA agar is a nutritional base that may include 5% sheep blood to enhance the growth of fastidious organisms. The antibiotics colistin and nalidixic acid prevent the overgrowth of gram-negative organisms. All genera except *Gardnerella* sp. grow in commercially available blood culture broths. *Gardnerella* organisms are inhibited by sodium polyanetholsulfonate (SPS), which currently is used as an anticoagulant in most commercial blood culture media. An SPS-free medium or a medium with SPS that is supplemented with gelatin should be used when *G. vaginalis* sepsis is suspected.

Isolation of *G. vaginalis* from female genital tract specimens is best accomplished using the selective medium human blood bilayer Tween agar (HBT). HBT is CNA agar with amphotericin B added to prevent the growth of yeasts and filamentous fungi. Human blood is layered over the top to enhance the beta-hemolytic pattern of *G. vaginalis.*

## Incubation Conditions and Duration

Detectable growth of these organisms should occur on 5% sheep blood and chocolate agars, CNA, and HBT

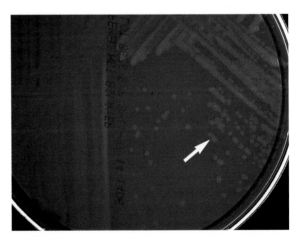

**Figure 18-2** *Gardnerella vaginalis* on human blood bilayer Tween (HBT) agar. Note small colonies with diffuse zone of beta-hemolysis *(arrow).*

incubated at 35°C in 5% to 10% carbon dioxide ($CO_2$) within 48 hours of inoculation.

## Colonial Appearance

Table 18-3 describes the colonial appearance and other distinguishing characteristics (e.g., hemolysis) of each genus on sheep blood agar. *G. vaginalis* produces small, gray, opaque colonies surrounded by a diffuse zone of beta-hemolysis on HBT agar (Figure 18-2).

## APPROACH TO IDENTIFICATION

The identification of the four genera described in this chapter must be considered along with that of *Actinomyces, Bifidobacterium,* and *Propionibacterium* spp., which are discussed in Chapter 42. Although the latter genera are usually considered with the anaerobic bacteria, they grow on routine laboratory media in 5% to 10% $CO_2$. Some

**TABLE 18-4** Biochemical and Physiologic Characteristics of Catalase-Negative, Gram-Positive, Aerotolerant, Non–Spore-Forming Rods

| | Urease | Nitrate Reduction | Beta-Hemolysis[b] | FERMENTATION[a] OF: Glucose | Maltose | Mannitol | Sucrose | Xylose | CAMP[c] | GLC[d] | Other Comments |
|---|---|---|---|---|---|---|---|---|---|---|---|
| *Actinomyces israelii* | − | v | − | + | + | v | + | + | − | A, L, S | |
| *A. odontolyticus* | − | + | −[e] | + | v | − | + | v | − | A, S | Red pigment produced after 1 week on SBA |
| *A. naeslundii* | + | + | −[w] | + | + | v | + | v | − | A, L, S | |
| *A. radingae* | − | − | −[w] | + | + | − | + | + | − | S? | Pyrazinamidase, beta-galactosidase–positive and esculin-positive |
| *A. turicensis* | − | − | −[w] | + | v | − | + | + | − | NT | Pyrazinamidase, beta-galactosidase–negative and esculin-negative |
| *A. graevenitzii* | − | − | − | + | + | + | + | − | ND | L > S | |
| *Actinobaculum schaalii* | − | − | − | + | + | − | v | + | +[w] | A, s | Beta-galactosidase–negative |
| *Arcanobacterium haemolyticum* | − | − | + | + | + | − | v | − | Reverse +[f] | A, L, S | Gelatin-negative at 48 hr; beta-hemolysis is stronger on agar containing human or rabbit blood |
| *A. pyogenes* | − | − | +[g] | + | v | v | v | + | − | A, L, S | Gelatin-positive at 48 hr; casein-positive |
| *A. bernardiae* | − | − | − | + | + | − | − | − | − | A, L, S | |
| *Bifidobacterium adolescentis* | − | − | − | + | + | − | + | + | ND | A > L (s) | |
| *Erysipelothrix* sp. | − | − | − | +[h] | − | − | − | − | | A, L, S | H$_2$S-positive in TSI butt; vancomycin-resistant; alpha-hemolytic |
| *Lactobacillus* spp. | − | − | − | + | + | v | + | ND | ND | L (a s) | Some strains vancomycin-resistant; alpha-hemolytic |
| *Propionibacterium acnes* | − | + | − | + | − | − | − | − | + | A, P (iv L s) | Indole-positive; may show beta-hemolysis on rabbit blood agar |
| *P. propionicum[j]* | − | + | − | + | + | + | + | − | ND | A, P, S, (L) | Colony may show red fluorescence under long-wavelength UV light |
| *Gardnerella vaginalis* | − | − | − | + | + | − | v | −[k] | ND | A (l s) | Beta-hemolysis on HBT; usually hydrolyses hippurate |
| *Weissella* spp. | NT | − | − | + | + | − | + | v | NT | L (as) | Vancomycin-resistant, small, short rods; produces gas from MRS broth; alpha-hemolytic; esculin-positive; arginine–positive |

*HBT,* Human blood bilayer Tween agar; *iv,* isovaleric acid; *ND,* not done; *NT,* not tested; *SBA,* 5% sheep blood agar; *TSI,* triple sugar iron agar; *v,* variable; *w,* weak; +, ≥90% of strains positive; −, ≥90% of strains negative.

[a]Fermentation is detected in peptone base with Andrade's indicator.

[b]On sheep blood agar.

[c]CAMP test using a beta-lysin–producing strain of *Staphylococcus aureus.*

[d]End products of glucose metabolism: *A,* Acetic acid; *L,* lactic acid; *P,* propionic acid; *S,* succinic acid; (), may or may not produce acid end product.

[e]May show beta-hemolysis on brain-heart infusion agar with sheep or human blood.

[f]Reverse CAMP test; *Staphylococcus aureus* beta-lysins are inhibited by a diffusible substance produced by *A. haemolyticum* (Figure 18-3).

[g]May also show beta-hemolysis on brain-heart infusion agar with human blood.

[h]Reaction may be weak or delayed.

[i]Some strains are catalase negative.

[j]Formerly *Arachnia propionica.*

[k]*Gardnerella vaginalis*–like organisms ferment xylose.

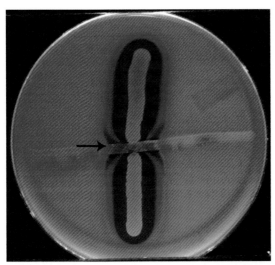

**Figure 18-3** Reverse Christie, Atkins, Munch-Petersen (CAMP) test. *Arcanobacterium haemolyticum* is streaked on a blood agar plate. *Staphylococcus aureus* is then streaked perpendicular to the *Arcanobacterium* path. A positive reverse CAMP test result is indicated *(arrow)*.

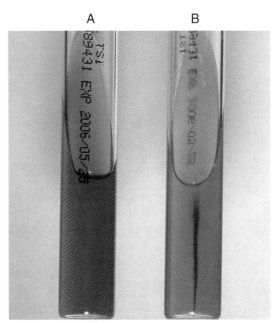

**Figure 18-4** $H_2S$ production by *Erysipelothrix rhusiopathiae* in TSI **(B)**. A negative TSI **(A)** is included for comparison.

are catalase negative. Therefore, as shown in Table 18-4, these organisms must be considered together when a laboratory encounters catalase-negative, gram-positive, non-spore-forming rods.

Several commercial systems for fastidious gram-negative bacterial identifications will adequately identify *Gardnerella.* The HNID panel (*Haemophilus-Neisseria* identification panel, Dade MicroScan, West Sacramento, California) works particularly well. However, rapid identification panels usually are used for isolates from extragenital sources (e.g., blood).

### Comments Regarding Specific Organisms

A presumptive identification of *G. vaginalis* is sufficient for genital isolates, based on typical appearance on Gram stain, beta-hemolysis on HBT agar, and negative tests for oxidase and catalase. *Corynebacterium lipophiloflavum,* a bacteria isolated from females with bacterial vaginosis, is catalase positive.

The beta-hemolytic *Arcanobacterium* spp. resemble the beta-hemolytic streptococci but can be differentiated from them by Gram stain morphology. *A. haemolyticum* and *A. pyogenes* can be differentiated based on liquefaction of gelatin; *A. pyogenes* is positive and *A. haemolyticum* is negative. *A. bernardiae* is nonhemolytic.

*Erysipelothrix* sp. is the only catalase-negative, gram-positive non-spore-forming rod that produces hydrogen sulfide ($H_2S$) when inoculated into triple sugar iron (TSI) agar (Figure 18-4). Some *Bacillus* spp. also blacken the butt of TSI, but they are catalase positive and produce spores. Automated identification with the Vitek2 and Phoenix systems and the API ID system is reliable for identification.

*Lactobacillus* spp. are usually identified based on colony and Gram stain morphologies and catalase reaction (negative). Differentiation from viridans streptococci may be difficult, but the formation of rods in chains rather than cocci in thioglycollate broth is helpful. Alternatively, a Gram stain of growth just outside the zone of inhibition surrounding the 10-U penicillin disk placed on a blood agar plate inoculated with a lawn of the organism should show long bacilli rather than coccoid forms if the organism is *Lactobacillus* spp.

## SERODIAGNOSIS

Serodiagnostic techniques are not generally used for the laboratory diagnosis of infections caused by the organisms discussed in this chapter.

## ANTIMICROBIAL SUSCEPTIBILITY TESTING AND THERAPY

The rarity with which most of these organisms are encountered as the cause of infection has made the development of validated in vitro susceptibility testing methods difficult (Table 18-5). However, most of the organisms are susceptible to the agents used to eradicate them, therefore in vitro testing is not usually necessary to guide therapy. *Lactobacillus* spp. can be resistant to various antimicrobial agents. Fortunately, these organisms are rarely implicated in infections. When they are encountered in specimens from normally sterile sites, careful evaluation of their clinical significance is warranted before any attempt is made at performing a non-standardized susceptibility test.

Although some of these organisms may grow on the media and under the conditions recommended for testing other bacteria (see Chapter 12 for more information regarding validated testing methods), this does not necessarily mean that interpretable and reliable results

**TABLE 18-5** Antimicrobial Therapy and Susceptibility Testing

| Organism | Therapeutic Options | Resistance to Therapeutic Options | Validated Testing Methods* | Comments |
|---|---|---|---|---|
| *Erysipelothrix rhusiopathiae* | Susceptible to penicillins, cephalosporins, erythromycin, clindamycin, tetracycline, and ciprofloxacin | Not common | See CLSI document M45 (Methods for Antimicrobial Dilution and Disk Susceptibility Testing of Infrequently Isolated or Fastidious Bacteria) | Susceptibility testing not needed to guide therapy |
| *Arcanobacterium haemolyticum* | No definitive guidelines. Usually susceptible to penicillin, erythromycin, and clindamycin | Not known | Not available | Susceptibility testing not needed to guide therapy |
| *Arcanobacterium pyogenes* | No definitive guidelines. Usually susceptible to cephalosporins, penicillins, ciprofloxacin, and chloramphenicol | Not known | Not available | Susceptibility testing not needed to guide therapy |
| *Gardnerella vaginalis* | Metronidazole is the drug of choice; also susceptible to ampicillin | Not known | Not available | Susceptibility testing not needed to guide therapy |
| *Lactobacillus* spp. | No definitive guidelines. Systemic infections may require the use of a penicillin with an aminoglycoside | Frequently resistant to cephalosporins; not killed by penicillin alone; frequently highly resistant to vancomycin | See CLSI document M45 (Methods for Antimicrobial Dilution and Disk Susceptibility Testing of Infrequently Isolated or Fastidious Bacteria) | Confirm that the isolate is clinically relevant and not a contaminant |

*Validated testing methods include standard methods recommended by the Clinical and Laboratory Standards Institute (CLSI) and commercial methods approved by the U.S. Food and Drug Administration (FDA).

will be produced. Chapter 12 should be reviewed for preferable strategies that can be used to provide susceptibility information when validated testing methods do not exist for a clinically important bacterial isolate.

# PREVENTION

Many of these organisms are ubiquitous in nature, and many are part of the normal human flora commonly encountered without deleterious effects on healthy human hosts. Currently, there are no recommended vaccination or prophylaxis protocols for prevention and treatment of diseases caused by these organisms.

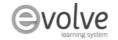 *Visit the Evolve site to complete the review questions.*

---

## CASE STUDY 18-1

Police found an elderly, intoxicated man unconscious near his fishing gear. He was taken to the hospital, and samples for blood cultures were collected. However, despite their efforts, the emergency department staff was unable to revive him. At autopsy, several vegetations were seen on both his aortic and mitral valves, and both valves were perforated. Blood cultures were reported positive with a gram-positive rod.

### QUESTIONS

1. What test should the laboratory perform to confirm the genus of this gram-positive, catalase-negative rod, growing both aerobically and anaerobically?

2. Although susceptibility testing for this organism is not generally performed, what important information about the organisms susceptibility is important to communicate to those caring for the patient?

3. What is the likely source of this patient's infection with *Erysipelothrix* sp.?

# BIBLIOGRAPHY

Carlson P, Kontiainen S, Renkonen O: Antimicrobial susceptibility of *Arcanobacterium haemolyticum, Antimicrob Agents Chemother* 38:142, 1994.

Coyle MB, Lipsky BA: Coryneform bacteria in infectious disease: clinical and laboratory aspects, *Clin Microbiol Rev* 3:227, 1990.

Drancourt M, Oules O, Bouche V et al: Two cases of *Actinomyces pyogenes* infections in humans, *Eur J Clin Microbiol Infect Dis* 12:55, 1993.

Flaherty JD, Levett PN, Dewhirst FE et al: Fatal case of endocarditis due to *Weissella confusa, J Clin Microbiol* 41:2237, 2003.

Funke G, Martinett Lucchini G, Pfyffer GE et al: Characteristics of CDC group 1 and group 1-like coryneform bacteria isolated from clinical specimens, *J Clin Microbiol* 31:2907, 1993.

Funke G, von Graevenitz A, Clarridge JE et al: Clinical microbiology of coryneform bacteria, *Clin Microbiol Rev* 10:125, 1997.

Kharsany AB, Hoosen AA, Van den Ende J: Antimicrobial susceptibilities of *Gardnerella vaginalis, Antimicrob Agents Chemother* 37:2733, 1993.

Lidbeck A, Nord CE: Lactobacilli and the normal human anaerobic microflora, *Clin Infect Dis* 16(suppl 4):S181, 1993.

Mackenzie A, Fuite LA, Chan TH et al: Incidence and pathogenicity of *Arcanobacterium haemolyticum* during a 2-year study in Ottawa, *Clin Infect Dis* 21:177, 1995.

Pascual Ramos C, Foster G, Collins MD: Phylogenetic analysis of the genus *Actinomyces* based on 16S rRNA gene sequences: description of *Arcanobacterium phocae* sp nov, *Arcanobacterium bernardiae* comb nov, and *Arcanobacterium pyogenes* comb nov, *Int J Syst Bacteriol* 47:46, 1997.

Patel R, Cockerill FR, Porayko MK, et al: Lactobacillemia in liver transplant patients, *Clin Infect Dis* 18:207, 1994.

Schuster MG, Brennan PJ, Edelstein P: Persistent bacteremia with *Erysipelothrix rhusiopathiae* in a hospitalized patient, *Clin Infect Dis* 17:783, 1993.

Spiegel CA: Bacterial vaginosis, *Clin Microbiology Rev* 4:485, 1991.

Vandamme P, Falsen E, Vancanneyt M et al: Characterization of *Actinomyces turicensis* and *Actinomyces radingae* strains from human clinical samples, *Int J Syst Bacteriol* 48:503, 1998.

Versalovic J: Manual of clinical microbiology, ed 10, Washington, DC, 2011, ASM Press.

# Branching or Partially Acid-Fast, Gram-Positive Bacilli

# *Nocardia, Streptomyces, Rhodococcus,* and Similar Organisms

## OBJECTIVES

1. Describe the general characteristics of the aerobic actinomycetes, including their Gram stain morphology, microscopic morphology, colonial morphology, and biochemical reactions.
2. Describe the habitats of actinomycetes and the routes of transmission.
3. Describe the three types of skin infections caused by *Nocardia* spp. in immunocompromised individuals.
4. List the laboratory tests used to differentiate the clinically relevant aerobic actinomycetes.
5. List the laboratory tests used to differentiate the pathogenic *Nocardia* spp.
6. Describe the chemical structures required for an organism to be classified as acid-fast.
7. List the virulence factors associated with *Nocardia asteroides.*
8. Define mycetoma and actinomycetoma.
9. List the various selective media used to isolate aerobic actinomycetes and describe their usefulness in achieving optimal recovery.

### GENERA AND SPECIES TO BE CONSIDERED

- *Actinomadura madurae*
- *Actinomadura pelletieri*
- *Dermatophilus congolensis*
- *Gordonia* spp.
- *Nocardia asteroides*
- *Nocardia brasiliensis*
- *Nocardia farcinica*
- *Nocardia nova*
- *Nocardia otitidiscaviarum*
- *Nocardia pseudobrasiliensis*
- *Nocardiopsis dassonvillei*
- *Rhodococcus* spp.
- *Streptomyces anulatus*
- *Streptomyces paraguayensis*
- *Streptomyces somaliensis*
- *Thermophilic actinomycetes*
- *Tsukamurella* spp.

The actinomycetes are a large and diverse group of gram-positive bacilli. For the most part, cells of all actinomycetes elongate to form branching, filamentous forms. The rate and extent of filament elongation with lateral branching depends on the strain of actinomycetes, the growth medium, and the temperature

of incubation. Some organisms form filaments, or hyphae, on the agar surface or into the agar, whereas others produce hyphae that extend into the air.

These organisms are aerobic, facultatively anaerobic, or obligately anaerobic; only the aerobic actinomycetes are discussed in this chapter. Aerobic actinomycetes belong to the order Actinomycetales. Actinomycetes comprise more than 40 genera, but only the clinically relevant aerobic actinomycetes genera are considered here (Table 19-1). In this chapter, only aerobic actinomycetes that exhibit branching and/or partial acid-fastness are addressed. Although both the *Corynebacterium* and *Mycobacterium* genera belong to the order Actinomycetales, *Corynebacterium* spp. do not usually exhibit branching filaments or partial acid-fastness, and *Mycobacterium* spp. do not exhibit branching and are strongly (acid-alcohol) acid-fast; for these reasons, the Corynebacteriaceae and Mycobacteriaceae are addressed in Chapters 17 and 43, respectively. Another clinically significant aerobic actinomycete is *Tropheryma whipplei;* because this organism has not been cultured on artificial media, it is reviewed in Chapter 44. For purposes of discussion, the remaining genera of aerobic actinomycetes are divided into the two large groups: those with cell walls that contain mycolic acid and are therefore partially acid-fast and those with cell envelopes that do not contain mycolic acid and therefore are non–acid-fast.

In general, the aerobic actinomycetes are not frequently isolated in the clinical laboratory; nevertheless, these organisms are causes of serious human disease. Not only are infections caused by these organisms difficult to recognize in the clinical laboratory, the organisms are also difficult to isolate. Further complications include difficulty classifying, identifying, and performing antibiotic susceptibilities on aerobic actinomycetes isolated from clinical specimens. At the time of this writing, the taxonomy of the aerobic actinomycetes is complex and continues to evolve. New and reliable methods that can identify cell wall amino acids and sugars and characterize mycolic acid, menaquinones, and phospholipids in conjunction with nucleic acid phylogenetic studies are proving extremely useful for resolving the taxonomy of the actinomycetes.

## GENERAL CHARACTERISTICS

The genera *Nocardia, Rhodococcus, Gordonia,* and *Tsukamurella* are partially acid-fast aerobic actinomycetes.

**TABLE 19-1**  Clinically Relevant Aerobic Actinomycetes*

| Cell Wall Containing Mycolic Acid | Genus |
| --- | --- |
| Present | *Nocardia*<br>*Rhodococcus*<br>*Gordonia*<br>*Tsukamurella*<br>*Corynebacterium* |
| Absent | *Streptomyces*<br>*Actinomadura*<br>*Dermatophilus*<br>*Nocardiopsis*<br>*Oerskovia* |

*The genera *Williamsia, Skermania,* and *Dietzia* are also aerobic actinomycetes but to date are not clinically relevant.

**BOX 19-1**  *Nocardia* spp. Considered Human Pathogens or Have Been Implicated in Human Disease

- *Nocardia asteroides sensu stricto* type VI
- *N. nova*
- *N. farcinica*
- *N. brasiliensis*
- *N. otitidiscaviarum*
- *N. pseudobrasiliensis*

**Less Common or Prevalence Not Established**
- *N. transvalensis*
- *N. brevicatena*
- *N. carnea*
- *N. abscessus*
- *N. africana*
- *N. paucivorans*
- *N. veterana*

*Nocardia* and *Rhodococcus* belong to the family Nocardiaceae, and *Gordonia* and *Tsukamurella* are in the Gordoniaceae and Tsukamurellaceae families, respectively. However, the variability associated with the classification of an organism as partially acid-fast depends on the particular strain and culture conditions. Therefore, this characteristic should be interpreted with caution. The genus *Actinomadura* includes approximately 67 species and subspecies, with significant variation. The cell walls of this group contain the sugar madurose, a characteristic shared with the genus *Dermatophilus.*

## PARTIALLY ACID-FAST AEROBIC ACTINOMYCETES

### *Nocardia* spp.

Organisms belonging to the genus *Nocardia* are gram positive (often with a beaded appearance), variably acid-fast, catalase positive, and strictly aerobic. As they grow, *Nocardia* spp. form branched filaments that extend along the agar surface (substrate hyphae) and into the air (aerial hyphae). As the organisms age, nocardiae fragment into pleomorphic rods or coccoid elements. Nocardiae also are characterized by the presence of mesodiaminopimelic acid (DAP) and the sugars arabinose and galactose in peptidoglycan in the cell wall.

Currently, the taxonomy in the genus *Nocardia* is changing rapidly. Recognition and description of new species continue and remain controversial regarding the number of validly described species; recent publications cite 22 to 30 valid species. Of significance, Cloud et al.[1] reported that the most commonly identified species was *Nocardia cyriacigeorgica,* not *N. asteroides,* as determined by partial 16S rRNA DNA sequencing, followed by *N. farcinica, N. nova, N. africana,* and *N. veterana.* The species considered human pathogens or that have been implicated as human pathogens are listed in Box 19-1. *N. asteroides, N. nova, N. farcinica, N. brasiliensis, N. otitidiscaviarum* (formerly *N. caviae*), *N. pseudobrasiliensis,* and *N. transvalensis* account for most of the diseases in humans caused by *Nocardia* spp.

**TABLE 19-2**  Species Included in the Genera *Rhodococcus, Gordonia,* and *Tsukamurella*

| Genus | Species |
| --- | --- |
| *Rhodococcus* | *equi, erythropolis, rhodnii, rhodochrous* (other species of unknown significance include *globerulus, marinonascens,* and *ruber*) |
| *Gordonia* | *aichiensis, bronchialis, polyisoprenivorans, rubripertincta, sputi, terrae* (remaining species isolated from environmental sources) |
| *Tsukamurella* | *paurometabola, pulmonis, tyrosinosolvens, strandjordae* (*T. ichonensis, T. wratislaviensis* isolated from nature) |

Data compiled from Brown JM et al: In Murray PR, Baron EJ, Pfaller MA et al, editors: *Manual of clinical microbiology,* ed 10, Washington, DC, 2003, American Society for Microbiology; Goodfellow M, Chun J, Stubbs S et al: *Lett Appl Microbiol* 19:401, 1994; Klatte S, Rainey FA, Kroppenstedt RM: *Int J Syst Bacteriol* 44:769, 1994; Lasker BA, Brown JM, McNeil MM: *Clin Infect Dis* 15:233, 1992; Maertens J et al: *Clin Microbiol Infect* 4:51, 1998; Riegel P et al: *J Clin Microbiol* 34:2045, 1996; Yassin AF, Rainey FA, Burrghardt J et al: *Int J Syst Bacteriol* 47:607, 1997; Arenskötter M et al: *Appl Environ Microbiol* 70:3195, 2004

### *Rhodococcus, Gordonia, Tsukamurella* spp.

Organisms belonging to the *Rhodococcus, Gordonia,* and *Tsukamurella* genera are similar to *Nocardia* spp. in that they are gram-positive, aerobic, catalase-positive, partially acid-fast, branching, filamentous bacteria that can fragment into rods and cocci. The extent of acid-fastness depends on the amount and complexity of mycolic acids in the organism's cell envelope and on culture conditions. The differentiation of these three genera, as well as species identification, is difficult. In particular, the genus *Rhodococcus* consists of a very diverse group of organisms in terms of morphology, biochemical characteristics, and ability to cause disease. As previously mentioned, the taxonomy of these organisms continues to evolve; species included in these three genera, as of this writing, are summarized in Table 19-2.

**TABLE 19-3** Non–Acid-Fast Aerobic Actinomycetes Associated with Human Disease

| Genus | Number of Species | Species Associated with Human Disease |
|---|---|---|
| Streptomyces | >3000 | S. somaliensis<br>S. paraguayensis<br>S. anulatus |
| Actinomadura | 27 | A. madurae<br>A. pelletieri<br>A. latina |
| Dermatophilus | 2 | D. congolensis |
| Nocardiopsis | 8 | N. dassonvillei<br>N. synnemataformans |

## NON–ACID-FAST AEROBIC ACTINOMYCETES: *STREPTOMYCES, ACTINOMADURA, DERMATOPHILUS, NOCARDIOPSIS,* AND THE THERMOPHILIC ACTINOMYCETES

The non–acid-fast aerobic actinomycetes (i.e., *Streptomyces, Actinomadura, Dermatophilus, Nocardiopsis,* and the thermophilic actinomycetes) are gram-positive, branching filaments that do not contain mycolic acids in their cell envelopes and are therefore non–acid-fast. This group of actinomycetes is heterogeneous and is encountered infrequently in the clinical laboratory. Only the non–acid-fast actinomycetes associated with human disease are addressed (Table 19-3).

Another group of non–acid-fast actinomycetes, the thermophilic actinomycetes, are associated with infections in humans and include the medically relevant genera *Thermoactinomyces, Saccharomonospora,* and *Saccharopolyspora.*

## ▪ EPIDEMIOLOGY AND PATHOGENESIS

### PARTIALLY ACID-FAST AEROBIC ACTINOMYCETES

*Nocardia* spp.

*Nocardia* organisms are normal inhabitants of soil and water and are primarily responsible for the decomposition of plant material. Infections caused by *Nocardia* spp. are found worldwide. Because they are ubiquitous, isolation of these organisms from clinical specimens does not always indicate infection. Rather, isolation may indicate colonization of the skin and upper respiratory tract or laboratory contamination, although the latter is rare. *Nocardia* infections can be acquired either by traumatic inoculation or inhalation. *N. asteroides sensu stricto* type VI is evenly distributed throughout the United States, as is *N. farcinica.* The prevalence of other species varies regionally; *N. brasiliensis* is associated with tropical climates and has a higher prevalence in the southwestern and southeastern United States.

*Nocardia* spp., particularly *N. asteroides,* are facultative intracellular pathogens capable of growth in various human cells. The mechanisms of pathogenesis are complex and not completely understood. However, the virulence of *N. asteroides* appears to be associated with several factors, such as stage of growth at the time of infection, resistance to intracellular killing, tropism for neuronal tissue, and ability to inhibit phagosome-lysosome fusion; other characteristics, such as production of large amounts of catalase and hemolysins, may also be associated with virulence.

### *Rhodococcus, Gordonia, Tsukamurella* spp.

*Rhodococcus, Gordonia,* and *Tsukamurella* spp. can be isolated from several environmental sources, especially soil and farm animals, as well as from fresh water and salt water. The organisms are believed to be acquired primarily by inhalation. For the most part, these aerobic actinomycetes are infrequently isolated from clinical specimens.

To date, *Rhodococcus equi* has been the organism most commonly associated with human disease, particularly in immunocompromised patients, such as those infected with the human immunodeficiency virus (HIV). *R. equi* is a facultative intracellular organism that can persist and replicate within macrophages. Determinants of the virulence of *R. equi* are under investigation and may involve cell wall mycolic acids that may play a role in intracellular survival, production of interleukin-4, and granuloma formation. Although *Gordonia* spp. and *Tsukamurella* are able to cause opportunistic infections in humans, little is known about their pathogenic mechanisms.

## NON–ACID-FAST AEROBIC ACTINOMYCETES: *STREPTOMYCES, ACTINOMADURA, DERMATOPHILUS, NOCARDIOPSIS,* AND THE THERMOPHILIC ACTINOMYCETES

Aspects of the epidemiology of the non–acid-fast aerobic actinomycetes are summarized in Table 19-4. Little is known about how these agents cause infection.

## ▪ SPECTRUM OF DISEASE

### PARTIALLY ACID-FAST AEROBIC ACTINOMYCETES

The partially acid-fast actinomycetes cause various infections in humans.

*Nocardia* spp.

Infections caused by *Nocardia* spp. can occur in immunocompetent and immunocompromised individuals. *N. asteroides, N. brasiliensis,* and *N. otitidiscaviarum* are the major causes of these infections, with *N. asteroides* causing greater than 80% of infections.

*Nocardia* spp. cause three types of skin infections in immunocompetent individuals:

- Mycetoma, a chronic, localized, painless, subcutaneous infection

**TABLE 19-4** Epidemiology of the Non–Acid-Fast Aerobic Actinomycetes

| Organism | Habitat (Reservoir) | Distribution | Routes of Primary Transmission |
|---|---|---|---|
| *Streptomyces somaliensis* | Sandy soil | Africa, Saudi Arabia, Mexico, South America | Penetrating wound/abrasions in the skin |
| *S. anulatus* | Soil | Most common isolate in United States | Penetrating wound/abrasions in the skin |
| *Actinomadura madurae* | Soil | Tropical and subtropical countries | Penetrating wound/abrasions in the skin |
| *A. pelletieri, A. latina* | Unknown, possibly soil | Tropical and subtropical countries | Penetrating wound/abrasions in the skin |
| *Dermatophilus congolensis* | Unknown; skin commensal or saprophyte in soil(?) | Worldwide, but more prevalent in humid, tropical, and subtropical regions | Trauma to the epidermis caused by insect bites and thorns; contact with tissues of infected animals through abrasions in the skin |
| *Nocardiopsis dassonvillei\** | Unknown | Unknown | Unknown |
| *Thermophilic actinomycetes* | Ubiquitous; water, air, soil, compost piles, dust, hay | Worldwide | Inhalation |

*Only a few cases of infection identified in the literature.

- Lymphocutaneous infections
- Skin abscesses or cellulites

Of note, *N. brasiliensis* is the predominant cause of these skin infections.

In immunocompromised individuals, *Nocardia* spp. can cause invasive pulmonary infections and disseminated infections. Patients receiving systemic immunosuppression, such as transplant recipients, individuals with impaired pulmonary immune defenses, and intravenous drug abusers, are examples of immunosuppressed patients at risk for these infections. Patients with pulmonary infections caused by *Nocardia* spp. can exhibit a wide range of symptoms, from an acute to a more chronic presentation. Unfortunately, no specific signs indicate pulmonary nocardiosis. Patients usually appear systemically ill, with fever, night sweats, weight loss, and a productive cough that may be bloody. Pulmonary infection can lead to complications such as pleural effusions, empyema, mediastinitis, and soft tissue infection. An acute inflammatory response follows infection, resulting in necrosis and abscess formation; granulomas are not usually formed.

*Nocardia* spp. can often spread hematogenously throughout the body from a primary pulmonary infection. Disseminated infection can result in lesions in the brain and skin; hematogenous dissemination involving the central nervous system is particularly common, occurring in about 30% of patients. Disseminated nocardiosis has a very poor prognosis.

### *Rhodococcus, Gordonia, Tsukamurella* spp.

The types of infections caused by *Rhodococcus, Gordonia,* and *Tsukamurella* spp. are listed in Table 19-5. For the most part, these organisms are considered opportunistic pathogens, because most infections occur in immunocompromised individuals.

**TABLE 19-5** Infections Caused by *Rhodococcus, Gordonia,* and *Tsukamurella* spp.

| Organism | Clinical Manifestations |
|---|---|
| *Rhodococcus* spp. | Pulmonary infections (pneumonia, lung abscess, pulmonary nodules)<br>Bacteremia<br>Skin, urinary tract, and wound infections<br>Endophthalmitis<br>Peritonitis<br>Catheter-associates sepsis<br>Abscesses: prostatic/splenic, thyroid, renal, brain, subcutaneous<br>Osteomyelitis |
| *Gordonia* spp. | Skin infections<br>Chronic pulmonary disease<br>Catheter-associated sepsis<br>Wound infection: sterna<br>Bacteremia |
| *Tsukamurella* spp. | Peritonitis<br>Catheter-associated sepsis<br>Skin infection |

## NON–ACID-FAST AEROBIC ACTINOMYCETES: *STREPTOMYCES, ACTINOMADURA, DERMATOPHILUS, NOCARDIOPSIS,* AND THE THERMOPHILIC ACTINOMYCETES

Infection caused by the non–acid-fast aerobic actinomycetes is usually associated with chronic, granulomatous lesions of the skin referred to as **mycetomas.** Mycetoma is an infection of subcutaneous tissues that results in tissue swelling and drainage of the sinus tracts. These infections are acquired by traumatic inoculation of organisms (usually in the lower limbs) and are usually caused by fungi. If mycetoma is caused by an actinomycete, the infection is called **actinomycetoma.**

Except for the thermophilic actinomycetes, most of these agents have rarely been associated with other types of infections (Table 19-6). These nonmycetomic infections have occurred in immunosuppressed patients, such as those infected with HIV.

The thermophilic actinomycetes are responsible for hypersensitivity pneumonitis, an allergic reaction to these agents. This is an occupational disease that occurs in farmers, factory workers, and others who are repeatedly exposed to these agents. The disease has acute and chronic forms. Patients with acute hypersensitivity pneumonitis experience malaise, sweats, chills, loss of appetite, chest tightness, cough, and fever within 4 to 6 hours after exposure; typically symptoms resolve within a day. Under some circumstances involving continued exposure to the organisms, patients suffer from a chronic form of disease in which symptoms progressively worsen with subsequent development of irreversible lung fibrosis.

**TABLE 19-6** Clinical Manifestations of Infections Caused by Non–Acid-Fast Aerobic Actinomycetes

| Organism | Clinical Manifestations |
|---|---|
| *Streptomyces* spp. (*S. somaliensis* and other species such as *S. anulatus* and *S. albus*) | Actinomycetoma Other (rare): pericarditis, bacteremia, and brain abscess |
| *Actinomadura* spp. (*A. madurae, A. pelletieri,* and *A. latina*) | Actinomycetoma Other (rare): peritonitis, wound infection, pneumonia, and bacteremia |
| *Dermatophilus congolensis* | Exudative dermatitis with scab formation (dermatophilosis) |
| *Nocardiopsis dassonvillei* | Actinomycetoma and other skin infections |

# LABORATORY DIAGNOSIS

## SPECIMEN COLLECTION, TRANSPORT, AND PROCESSING

Appropriate specimens should be collected aseptically from affected areas. For the most part, no special requirements are needed for specimen collection, transport, or processing of the organisms discussed in this chapter (refer to Table 5-1 for general information). When nocardiosis is clinically suspected, multiple specimens should be submitted for culture, because smears and cultures are simultaneously positive in only a third of the cases. The significance of random isolation of *Nocardia* spp. from the respiratory tract is questionable, because these organisms are so widely distributed in nature. Some of the actinomycetes tend to grow as a microcolony in tissues, leading to the formation of granules. Most commonly, these granules are formed in actinomycetomas, such as those caused by *Nocardia, Streptomyces, Nocardiopsis,* and *Actinomadura* spp. Therefore, material from draining sinus tracts is an excellent specimen for direct examination and culture.

## DIRECT DETECTION METHODS

Direct microscopic examination of Gram-stained preparations of clinical specimens is of utmost importance in the diagnosis of infections caused by the aerobic actinomycetes. Often, the demonstration of gram-positive, branching or partially branching beaded filaments provides the first clue to the presence of an aerobic actinomycete (Figure 19-1). Unfortunately, the actinomycetes do not always exhibit such characteristic morphology; many times these organisms are not seen at all or appear as gram-positive cocci, rods, or short filaments. Nevertheless, if gram-positive, branching or partially branching organisms are observed, a modified acid-fast stain should be performed (i.e., 1% sulfuric acid rather than 3% hydrochloric acid as the decolorizing agent) (see Procedure 19-1 on the Evolve site). The modified acid-fast stain is positive in only about half of these smears showing gram-positive beaded, branching filaments subsequently

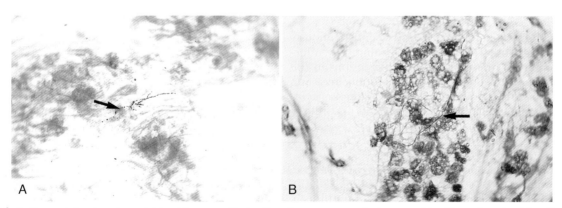

**Figure 19-1 A,** Gram stain of sputum obtained from a patient with pulmonary nocardiosis caused by *Nocardia asteroides.* **B,** The same sputum stained with a modified acid-fast stain. The organism is indicated by the arrow.

confirmed as *Nocardia* sp. Histopathologic examination of tissue specimens using various histologic stains, such as Gomori's methenamine-silver (GMS) stain, can also detect the presence of actinomycetes.

It is important to examine any biopsy or drainage material from actinomycetomas for the presence of granules. If observed, the granules are washed in saline, emulsified in 10% potassium hydroxide or crushed between two slides, Gram stained, and examined microscopically for the presence of filaments.

## MOLECULAR DIAGNOSTICS

Amplification techniques (i.e., polymerase chain reaction [PCR]) involving the 16srRNA sequence have been used to examine the relatedness among the genera and species within the non–acid-fast aerobic actinomycetes and thermophilic actinomycetes. When the MicroSeq System was used for identification (see Chapter 8), almost 15% of isolates were identified as *Nocardia* spp., but no definitive species were given. PCR paired with restriction endonuclease analysis has been used to identify commonly isolated *Nocardia* spp. Housekeeping heat shock protein genes coupled with the 16srRNA sequence are used in this assay. DNA sequencing of several genes, including the 16srRNA, a heat shock protein gene, and a housekeeping gene are referred to as *secA1*. These methods currently are not available in the clinical laboratory; they are predominantly used for taxonomic, epidemiologic, and research studies.

## CULTIVATION

Many of the aerobic actinomycetes do not have complex growth requirements; they are able to grow on routine laboratory media, such as sheep blood, chocolate, Sabouraud dextrose, and brain-heart infusion agar. However, because many of the aerobic actinomycetes grow slowly, they may be overgrown by other normal flora present in contaminated specimens. This is particularly true for the nocardiae that require a minimum of 48 to 72 hours of incubation before colonies become visible. Because of their slow growth and the possibility of being overgrown with contaminating flora, various selective media have been used to recover nocardiae. A solid medium using paraffin as the sole source of carbon has been effective for isolating *Nocardia* spp. and rapidly growing mycobacteria from contaminated clinical specimens. Selective media formulated for the isolation of *Legionella* spp. from contaminated specimens, such as buffered charcoal-yeast extract medium with polymyxin, anisomycin, and vancomycin, have been successful in the recovery of nocardiae from contaminated specimens. Martin Lewis and colistin-nalidixic acid media also have been used. *Nocardia* spp. grow well on Sabouraud dextrose agar and on fungal media containing cycloheximide, such as Mycosel. Because *Nocardia* organisms are able to withstand the decontamination procedures used to isolate mycobacteria, isolates may be identified on mycobacterial culture media.

If other aerobic actinomycetes are considered, a selective medium, such as brain-heart infusion agar with chloramphenicol and cycloheximide, is recommended in addition to routine agar to enhance isolation from contaminated specimens. Although most aerobic actinomycetes grow at 35°C, recovery is increased at 30°C. Therefore, selective and nonselective agars should be incubated at 35°C and 30°C. Plates should be incubated for 2 to 3 weeks. The typical Gram-stain morphology and colonial appearance of the aerobic actinomycetes are summarized in Table 19-7. Examples of Gram stains and cultures of different aerobic actinomycetes are shown in Figures 19-2 and 19-3.

Clinical laboratories are rarely asked to diagnose hypersensitivity pneumonitis caused by the thermophilic actinomycetes. These organisms grow rapidly on trypticase soy agar with 1% yeast extract. The ability to grow at temperatures of 50°C or greater is a characteristic of all thermophilic actinomycetes. Differentiation of the various agents is based on microscopic and macroscopic morphologies.

## APPROACH TO IDENTIFICATION

If Gram-stain morphology or colonial morphology suggests a possible actinomycetes (see Table 19-7), an acid-fast stain should be performed first to rule out rapidly growing mycobacteria (see Chapter 43), followed by a modified acid-fast stain (see Procedure 19-1). If the modified acid-fast stain results are positive, the isolate is a probable partially acid-fast aerobic actinomycete (i.e., *Nocardia*, *Rhodococcus*, *Tsukamurella*, or *Gordonia* sp). If the acid-fast stain result is negative, these organisms still are not completely ruled out because of the variability of acid-fastness among isolates belonging to this group. Aerobic actinomycetes can be initially placed into major groupings by considering the following:

- Gram-stain morphology (see Figures 19-1 and Figure 19-2)
- Modified acid-fast stain results
- Presence or absence of aerial hyphae when grown on tap water agar
- Growth or no growth in nutrient broth containing lysozyme (250 µg/mL (Figure 19-4) (see Procedure 19-2 on the Evolve site)
- Other tests: urea hydrolysis, nitrate reduction, and ability to grow anaerobically

Table 19-8 summarizes the key characteristics of aerobic actinomycetes.

Accurate identification of *Nocardia* to the species level is important, because differences among the species have emerged in terms of virulence, antibiotic susceptibility, and epidemiology. However, identification of the pathogenic nocardiae to the species level can be problematic, because no single method can identify all *Nocardia* isolates, and the methods used are time-consuming, often requiring 2 weeks. Useful phenotypic tests include the use of casein, xanthine, and tyrosine hydrolysis; growth at 45°C; acid production from rhamnose; gelatin hydrolysis; opacification of Middlebrook agar; and antimicrobial susceptibility patterns. Some of these reactions with the nocardial pathogens are summarized in Table 19-9.

**TABLE 19-7** Typical Gram-Stain Morphology and Colonial Appearance

| Organism | Gram Stain* | Colonial Appearance on Routine Agar |
|---|---|---|
| *Nocardia* spp. | Branching, fine, delicate filaments with fragmentation | Extremely variable; adherent; some isolates are beta-hemolytic on sheep blood agar; wrinkled; often dry, chalky-white appearance to orange-tan pigment; crumbly |
| *Rhodococcus* spp. | Diphtheroid-like with minimal branching or coccobacillary; colonial growth appears as coccobacilli in zigzag configuration | Nonhemolytic; round; often mucoid with orange to red, salmon-pink pigment developing within 4 to 7 days (pigment may vary widely) |
| *Gordonia* spp. | Nonmotile, short rods | Somewhat pigmented; *G. sputi:* smooth, mucoid and adherent to media; *G. bronchialis:* dry and raised |
| *Tsukamurella* spp. | Mostly long rods that fragment, no spores or aerial hyphae | May have rhizoid edges, dry, white to creamy to orange |
| *Streptomyces* spp. | Extensive branching with chains and spores; does not fragment easily | Glabrous or waxy heaped colonies; variable morphology |
| *Actinomadura* spp. | Moderate, fine, intertwining branching with short chains of spores, fragmentation | White-to-pink pigment, mucoid, molar tooth appearance after 2 weeks' incubation |
| *Dermatophilus* sp. | Branched filaments divided in transverse and longitudinal planes; fine, tapered filaments | Round, adherent, gray-white colonies that later develop orange pigments; often beta-hemolytic |
| *Nocardiopsis* sp. | Branching with internal spores | Coarsely wrinkled and folded with well-developed aerial mycelium |

Data compiled from Brown JH, Mcneil MM: In Murray PR, Baron EJ, Pfaller MA et al, editors: *Manual of clinical microbiology,* ed 10, Washington, DC, American Society for Microbiology, 2003; McNeil MM, Brown JM: *Clin Microbiol Rev* 7:357, 1994.
*Aerobic actinomycetes are gram-positive organisms that are often beaded in appearance.

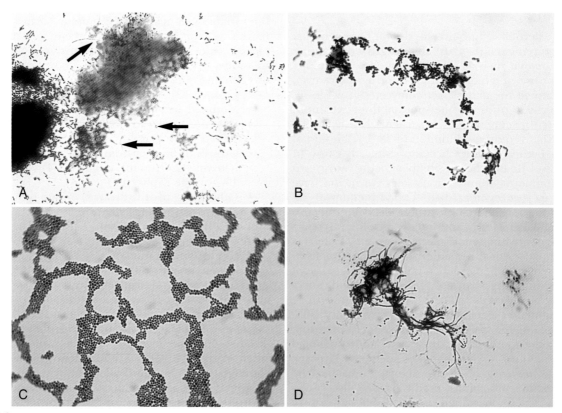

**Figure 19-2** Gram stains of different aerobic actinomycetes. **A,** *Nocardia asteroides* grown on Löwenstein-Jensen medium. The arrows indicate branching rods. **B,** *Rhodococcus equi* from broth. **C,** *R. equi* grown on chocolate agar. **D,** *Streptomyces* spp. grown on Sabouraud dextrose agar.

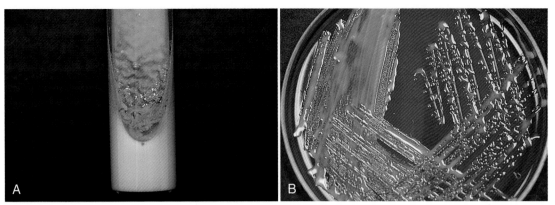

**Figure 19-3** Aerobic actinomycetes grown on solid media. **A,** *Nocardia asteroides* grown on Löwenstein-Jensen medium. **B,** *Rhodococcus equi* grown on chocolate agar.

**TABLE 19-8** Preliminary Grouping of the Clinically Relevant Aerobic Actinomycetes

| Characteristics | *Nocardia* spp. | *Rhodococcus* spp. | *Gordonia* spp. | *Tsukamurella* spp. | *Streptomyces* spp. | *Actinomadura* spp. | *Dermatophilus* sp. | *Nocardiopsis* spp. |
|---|---|---|---|---|---|---|---|---|
| Partially acid-fast | + | ± | ± | ± | − | − | − | − |
| Appearance on tap water agar*: branching/aerial hyphae | Extensive/+ | Minimal/− | Minimal/− | Minimal/− | Extensive/+ | Variable/ sparse | Branching | Extensive/+ |
| Lysozyme resistance | + | ± | − | + | − | − | − | − |
| Urea hydrolysis | + | ± | + | + | ± | − | + | + |
| Nitrate reduction | ± | ± | + | − | ± | + | − | + |
| Growth anaerobically | − | − | − | − | − | − | − | − |

Modified from Brown JM, McNeil MM: In Murray PR, Baron EJ, Pfaller MA et al, editors: *Manual of clinical microbiology,* ed 10, Washington, DC, 2003, American Society for Microbiology.

+, predominantly positive; −, predominantly negative; ±, mostly positive with some negative isolates.

*Tap water agar: Bacto agar (Difco Laboratories, Detroit, Mich.) is added to 100 mL of tap water, sterilized, and then poured into plates. Two plates are lightly inoculated using a single streak and incubated at 30°C for up to 7 days and examined daily.

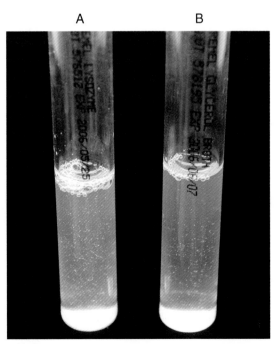

**Figure 19-4** Lysozyme **(A)** and glycerol **(B)** broths. The lysozyme broth demonstrates enhanced growth, which is typical of *Nocardia asteroides.*

**TABLE 19-9** Key Tests for Differentiation of the Pathogenic Nocardia spp.

| Test | N. asteroides sensu stricto | N. farcinica* | N. nova | N. travalensis (N. asteroides type IV) | N. transvalensis sensu stricto | N. brasiliensis | N. otitidiscaviarum | N. pseudobrasiliensis |
|---|---|---|---|---|---|---|---|---|
| Hydrolysis of: | | | | | | | | |
| Casein | − | − | − | − | −/+ | + | − | + |
| Xanthine | − | − | − | − | −/+ | − | − | − |
| Tyrosine | − | − | − | − | −/+ | + | −/+ | + |
| Growth at 42°C after 3 days | ± | + | − | − | − | − | ± | − |
| 14-day arylsulfatase | − | − | + | NT | − | − | − | − |
| Acid from rhamnose | ± | ± | − | − | − | − | − | − |
| Gelatin hydrolysis | − | − | − | − | − | + | − | − |
| Opacification of Middlebrook agar 4 | − | + | − | − | − | − | −/+ | − |
| Api 20C assimilation: | | | | | | | | |
| Galactose | − | − | − | + | + | + | − | + |
| Glycerol | + | + | − | + | + | + | + | + |
| Trehalose | − | − | − | + | + | + | + | + |
| Adonitol | − | − | − | − | + | − | − | − |
| Sensitivity by Kirby Bauer disk diffusion†: | | | | | | | | |
| Gentamicin | S | R | S/R | R/S | R/S | S | S | S |
| Tobramycin | S/R | R | S/R | R | R | S | S/R | S |
| Amikacin | S | S | S | S/R | R | S | S | S |
| Erythromycin | R | S/R | S | R | R | R | R | R |

*NT*, Not tested; +, predominantly positive; −, predominantly negative; ±, mostly positive with some negative isolates; −/+, mostly negative with some positive isolates.
*Cefotaxime resistant.
†Sensitive (S) or resistant (R) as determined by Kirby Bauer disk diffusion.

Many tests are needed to confirm the identification of the other actinomycetes at the level of speciation; these are beyond the capabilities of the routine clinical microbiology laboratory, and such cases therefore should be referred to a reference laboratory.

## SERODIAGNOSIS

Currently, no reliable serodiagnostic tests are available to help identify patients with active nocardiosis; such tests are used only to augment culture results. Infections caused by other aerobic actinomycetes currently cannot be diagnosed serologically.

# ANTIMICROBIAL SUSCEPTIBILITY TESTING AND THERAPY

A standard for susceptibility testing by broth microdilution and with cation-supplemented Mueller-Hinton broth has been approved by the Clinical and Laboratory Standards Institute (CLISI; formerly the National Committee for Clinical and Laboratory Standards), along with interpretive guidelines. Other methods, including modified disk diffusion, agar dilution, broth microdilution, E-test, and radiometric growth index have been used for antimicrobial susceptibility testing of *Nocardia* spp. However,

**TABLE 19-10** Primary Drugs of Choice for Infections Caused by Aerobic Actinomycetes

| Organisms | Primary Drugs of Choice |
| --- | --- |
| *Nocardia* spp. | Sulfonamides<br>Trimethoprim-sulfamethoxazole<br>Other primary agents: amikacin, ceftriaxone, cefotaxime, linezolid, or imipenem<br>Minocycline<br>Combination of sulfa-containing agent and one of the primary agents is recommended for serious systemic disease. |
| *Rhodococcus, Gordonia, Tsukamurella* spp. | Erythromycin and rifampin<br>Gentamicin, tobramycin, or ciprofloxacin<br>Vancomycin and imipenem |
| *Streptomyces* spp. | Streptomycin and trimethoprim-sulfamethoxazole or dapsone |
| *Actinomadura* spp. | Streptomycin and trimethoprim-sulfamethoxazole or dapsone Amikacin and imipenem |
| *Nocardiopsis dassonvillei* | Trimethoprim-sulfamethoxazole |
| *Dermatophilus congolensis* | Highly variable susceptibilities; no specific drugs of choice |

although these methods demonstrate good interlaboratory and intralaboratory agreement and reproducibility, correlation of in vitro susceptibility testing results with clinical outcome has not been systematically performed at the time of this writing. Nevertheless, antimicrobial susceptibility testing should be performed on clinically significant isolates of *Nocardia* spp. If required, the isolate should be sent to a reference laboratory. For all other actinomycetes, no standardized methods currently are available. In some instances, susceptibility studies of *Rhodococcus* and *Gordonia* spp. can be used as a guide for directing therapy.

The primary drugs of choice against the aerobic actinomycetes are shown in Table 19-10; no effective antimicrobial therapy is available for hypersensitivity pneumonitis caused by the thermophilic actinomycetes.

# PREVENTION

No vaccines are available for the prevention of infection with aerobic actinomycetes; some have been developed, but with little success. With respect to hypersensitivity pneumonitis caused by the thermophilic actinomycetes, patients must prevent the disease by avoiding exposure to these sensitizing microorganisms.

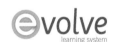 *Visit the Evolve site to complete the review questions.*

# CASE STUDY 19-1

A 60-year-old woman with a history of steroid-treated rheumatoid arthritis presented to the emergency department with increasing confusion, lethargy, and fever, which began approximately 2 weeks before admission. She had an elevated white blood cell (WBC) count. A spinal tap was performed, which showed elevated protein, low glucose, and a WBC count of 200 mm³. The cerebrospinal fluid was cultured, and two colonies of nonhemolytic, catalase-positive, gram-positive rods grew on the second quadrant of the blood agar plate after 48 hours. The chocolate plate had no growth.

## QUESTIONS

1. Because the colonies were nonhemolytic, *Listeria* sp. was not in the differential. Before these colonies are dismissed as plate contaminants, what testing should be performed?

2. Identification and susceptibility testing for such isolates are important but are usually left to reference laboratories. However, a simple disk test using an inoculum equivalent to a 0.5 McFarland standard showed that the isolate was resistant to gentamicin, erythromycin, and cefotaxime. Which species is characteristically resistant to these antimicrobial agents?

3. If the isolate was mucoid and salmon pink in color, what testing would be helpful for identification?

# REFERENCE

1. Cloud JL, Conville PS, Croft A et al: Evaluation of partial 16S ribosomal DNA sequencing for identification of *Nocardia* species by using the MicroSeq 500 system with an expanded database, *J Clin Microbiol* 42:578, 2004.

# BIBLIOGRAPHY

Beaman BL, Beaman L: *Nocardia* species: host-parasite relationships, *Clin Microbiol Rev* 7:213, 1994.
Chun J, Goodfellow M: A phylogenetic analysis of the genus *Nocardia* with 16S rRNA gene sequences, *Int J Syst Bacteriol* 45:240, 1995.

Flores M, Desmond E: Opacification of Middlebrook agar as an aid in identification of *Nocardia farcinica*, *J Clin Microbiol* 31:3040, 1993.

Garrett MA, Holmes HT, Nolte FS: Selective buffered charcoal-yeast extract medium for isolation of nocardiae from mixed cultures, *J Clin Microbiol* 30:1891, 1992.

Kiska DL, Hicks K, Pettit DJ: Identification of medically relevant *Nocardia* species with an abbreviated battery of tests, *J Clin Microbiol* 40:1346, 2002.

Klatte S, Rainey FA, Kroppenstedt RM: Transfer of *Rhodococcus aichensis* (Tsukamura, 1982) and *Nocardia amarae* (Lechevalier and Lechevalier, 1974) to the genus *Gordonia* as *Gordonia aichiensis* comb nov and *Gordonia amarae* comb nov, *Int J Syst Bacteriol* 44: 769, 1994.

Roth A, Andrees S, Kroppenstedt RM et al: Phylogeny of the genus *Nocardia* based on reassessed 16S rRNA gene sequences reveals underspeciation and division of strains classified as *Nocardia asteroides* into three established species and two unnamed taxons, *J Clin Microbiol* 41:851, 2003.

Saubolle MA, Sussland D: Nocardiosis: review of clinical laboratory experience, *J Clin Microbiol* 41:4497, 2003.

Versalovic J. *Manual of clinical microbiology*, ed 10, Washington, DC, 2011, ASM Press.

Vickers RM, Rihs JD, Yu VL: Clinical demonstration of isolation of *Nocardia asteroides* on buffered charcoal-yeast extract media, *J Clin Microbiol* 30:227, 1992.

Weinstock DM, Brown AE: *Rhodococcus equi:* an emerging pathogen, *Clin Infect Dis* 34:1379, 2002.

Woods GL, Brown-Elliott BA, Desmond EP et al: *Susceptibility testing of Mycobacteria, Nocardia, and other actinomycetes: approved standard M24-A*, vol 23, no. 18 NCCLS, Wayne, Pa, 2003.

# Enterobacteriaceae

## OBJECTIVES

1. Describe the general characteristics of the Enterobacteriaceae, including oxygenation, microscopic Gram staining characteristics, and macroscopic appearance on blood and MacConkey agar.
2. Describe the chemical principle of the media used for the isolation and differentiation of Enterobacteriaceae, including xylose-lysine-deoxycholate agar (XLD), Salmonella-Shigella agar (SS), Hektoen enteric agar (HE), MacConkey agar (MAC), eosin methylene blue agar (EMB), cefsulodin-irgasan-novobiocin agar (CIN), Simmons citrate agar (CIT), gram-negative broth (GN), MacConkey agar with sorbitol (MAC-SOR), lysine iron agar (LIA), and triple sugar iron agar (TSI).
3. Describe the antigens used for serotyping in Enterobacteriaceae, including bacterial location, chemical structure, heat stability, and nomenclature.
4. List the members of the Enterobacteriaceae that are considered intestinal pathogens (rather than extraintestinal pathogens).
5. Compare and contrast infections with the various pathotypes of Escherichia coli (i.e., uropathogenic E. coli [UPEC], meningitis/sepsis–associated E. coli [MNEC], enterotoxigenic E. coli [ETEC], enteroinvasive E. coli [EIEC], enteroaggregative E. coli [EAEC], enteropathogenic E. coli [EPEC], and enterohemorrhagic E. coli [EHEC]), including the route of transmission, types of infection, and pathogenesis.
6. Explain the clinical significance of E. coli O157:H7 and the recommended diagnostic testing for confirmation of infection.
7. Outline the basic biochemical testing procedure to differentiate Enterobacteriaceae from other gram-negative rods.
8. Define ESBL and interpret an antibiotic profile as either positive, negative for ESBL, including corrections required before reporting results.
9. Define MDRTF and the antibiotic susceptibility recommendations associated with identification of an MDRTF isolate.
10. Define an extended spectrum cephalosporin resistance and explain the clinical significance and identification in the clinical laboratory.
11. Describe the modified Hodge test (MHT) procedure, including the chemical principle and clinical significance of the test with regard to carbapenemase resistance.
12. Differentiate Salmonella spp. and Shigella spp. based on biochemical testing.
13. Differentiate Yersinia spp. from the major pathogens among the Enterobacteriaceae.
14. Correlate signs and symptoms of infection with the results of laboratory diagnostic procedures for the identification of a clinical isolate in the Enterobacteriaceae family.

## GENERA AND SPECIES TO BE CONSIDERED

### Opportunistic Pathogens

*Citrobacter freundii*
*Citrobacter (diversus) koseri*
*Citrobacter braakii*
*Cronobacter sakazakii* (previously *Enterobacter sakazakii*)
*Edwardsiella tarda*
*Enterobacter aerogenes*
*Enterobacter cloacae*
*Enterobacter gergoviae*
*Enterobacter amnigenus*
*Enterobacter (cancerogenous) taylorae*
*Escherichia coli* (including extraintestinal)
*Ewingella americana*
*Hafnia alvei*
*Klebsiella pneumoniae*
*Klebsiella oxytoca*
*Morganella morganii* subsp. *morganii*
*Morganella psychrotolerans*
*Pantoea agglomerans* (previously *Enterobacter agglomerans*)
*Proteus mirabilis*
*Proteus vulgaris*
*Proteus penneri*
*Providencia alcalifaciens*
*Providencia heimbachae*
*Providencia rettgeri*
*Providencia stuartii*
*Serratia marcescens*
*Serratia liquefaciens* group
*Serratia odorifera*

### Pathogenic Organisms
#### *Primary Intestinal Pathogens*

*E. coli* (diarrheagenic)
*Plesiomonas shigelloides*
**Salmonella, all serotypes**
*Shigella dysenteriae* (group A)
*Shigella flexneri* (group B)
*Shigella boydii* (group C)
*Shigella sonnei* (group D)

### Pathogenic *Yersinia* spp.

*Yersinia pestis*
*Yersinia enterocolitica* subsp. *enterocolitica*
*Yersinia frederiksenii*

Because of the large number and diversity of genera included in the Enterobacteriaceae, it is helpful to consider the bacteria of this family as belonging to one of two major groups. The first group comprises species that either commonly colonize the human gastrointestinal tract or are most notably associated with human infections. Although many Enterobacteriaceae that cause human infections are part of our normal gastrointestinal flora, there are exceptions, such as *Yersinia pestis*. The second group consists of genera capable of colonizing humans but rarely associated with human infection and commonly recognized as environmental inhabitants or colonizers of other animals. For this reason, the discovery of these species in clinical specimens should alert laboratorians to possible identification errors; careful confirmation of both the laboratory results and the clinical significance of such isolates is warranted.

## GENERAL CHARACTERISTICS

Molecular analysis has not proven effective for definitively characterizing all the organisms and genera included within the Enterobacteriaceae family. Therefore, species names and reclassification of organisms continually evolve. In general, the Enterobacteriaceae consist of a diverse group of gram-negative bacilli or coccobacilli; they are non–spore forming, facultative anaerobes capable of fermenting glucose; they are oxidase negative (except for *Plesiomonas* sp.); and, with rare exception (*Photorhabdus* and *Xenorhabdus* spp.), they reduce nitrates to nitrites. Furthermore, except for *Shigella dysenteriae* type 1, all commonly isolated Enterobacteriaceae are catalase positive.

## EPIDEMIOLOGY

Enterobacteriaceae inhabit a wide variety of niches, including the human gastrointestinal tract, the gastrointestinal tract of other animals, and various environmental sites. Some are agents of zoonoses, causing infections in animal populations (Table 20-1). Just as the reservoirs for

these organisms vary, so do their modes of transmission to humans.

For species capable of colonizing humans, infection may result when a patient's own bacterial strains (i.e., endogenous strains) establish infection in a normally sterile body site. These organisms can also be passed from one patient to another. Such infections often depend on the debilitated state of a hospitalized patient and are acquired during the patient's hospitalization (nosocomial). However, this is not always the case. For example, although *E. coli* is the most common cause of nosocomial infections, it is also the leading cause of community-acquired urinary tract infections.

Other species, such as *Salmonella* spp., *Shigella* spp., and *Yersinia enterocolitica*, inhabit the bowel during infection and are acquired by ingestion of contaminated food or water. This is also the mode of transmission for the various types of *E. coli* known to cause gastrointestinal infections. In contrast, *Yersinia pestis* is unique among the Enterobacteriaceae that infect humans. This is the only species transmitted from animals by an insect vector (i.e., flea bite).

## PATHOGENESIS AND SPECTRUM OF DISEASES

The clinically relevant members of the Enterobacteriaceae can be considered as two groups: the opportunistic pathogens and the intestinal pathogens. Typhi and Shigella spp. are among the latter group and are causative agents of typhoid fever and dysentery, respectively. *Yersinia pestis* is not an intestinal pathogen, but it is the causative agent of plague. The identification of these organisms in clinical material is serious and always significant. These organisms, in addition to others, produce various potent virulence factors and can cause life-threatening infections (Table 20-2).

The opportunistic pathogens most commonly include *Citrobacter* spp., *Enterobacter* spp., *Klebsiella* spp., *Proteus* spp., *Serratia* spp., and a variety of other organisms. Although considered opportunistic pathogens, these organisms produce significant virulence factors, such as endotoxins capable of mediating fatal infections. However, because they generally do not initiate disease in healthy, uncompromised human hosts, they are considered opportunistic.

Although *E. coli* is a normal bowel inhabitant, its pathogenic classification is somewhere between that of the overt pathogens and the opportunistic organisms. Diuretic strains of this species, such as enterotoxigenic *E. coli* (ETEC), enteroinvasive *E. coli* (EIEC), and enteroaggregative *E. coli* (EAEC), express potent toxins and cause serious gastrointestinal infections. Additionally, in the case of enterohemorrhagic *E. coli* (EHEC) also referred to as verocytotoxin producing *E. coli* (VTEC) or Shiga-like toxin producing *E. coli* (STEC), the organism may produce life-threatening systemic illness. Furthermore, as the leading cause of Enterobacteriaceae nosocomial infection, *E. coli* is likely to have greater virulence

**TABLE 20-1** Epidemiology of Clinically Relevant Enterobacteriaceae

| Organism | Habitat (Reservoir) | Mode of Transmission |
|---|---|---|
| *Escherichia coli* | Normal bowel flora of humans and other animals; may also inhabit female genital tract | Varies with the type of infection. For nongastrointestinal infections, organisms may be endogenous or spread person to person, especially in the hospital setting. For gastrointestinal infections, the transmission mode varies with the strain of *E. coli* (see Table 20-2); it may involve fecal-oral spread between humans in contaminated food or water or consumption of undercooked beef or unpasteurized milk from colonized cattle |
| *Shigella* spp. | Only found in humans at times of infection; not part of normal bowel flora | Person-to-person spread by fecal-oral route, especially in overcrowded areas, group settings (e.g., daycare) and areas with poor sanitary conditions |
| *Salmonella* serotype Typhi *Salmonella* serotypes Paratyphi A, B, C | Only found in humans but not part of normal bowel flora | Person-to-person spread by fecal-oral route by ingestion of food or water contaminated with human excreta |
| Other *Salmonella* spp. | Widely disseminated in nature and associated with various animals | Ingestion of contaminated food products processed from animals, frequently of poultry or dairy origin. Direct person-to-person transmission by fecal-oral route can occur in health care settings when hand-washing guidelines are not followed |
| *Edwardsiella tarda* | Gastrointestinal tract of cold-blooded animals, such as reptiles | Uncertain; probably by ingestion of contaminated water or close contact with carrier animal |
| *Yersinia pestis* | Carried by urban and domestic rats and wild rodents, such as the ground squirrel, rock squirrel, and prairie dog | From rodents to humans by the bite of flea vectors or by ingestion of contaminated animal tissues; during human epidemics of pneumonic (i.e., respiratory) disease, the organism can be spread directly from human to human by inhalation of contaminated airborne droplets; rarely transmitted by handling or inhalation of infected animal tissues or fluids |
| *Yersinia enterocolitica* | Dogs, cats, rodents, rabbits, pigs, sheep, and cattle; not part of normal human microbiota | Consumption of incompletely cooked food products (especially pork), dairy products such as milk, and, less commonly, by ingestion of contaminated water or by contact with infected animals |
| *Yersinia pseudotuberculosis* | Rodents, rabbits, deer, and birds; not part of normal human microbiota | Ingestion of organism during contact with infected animal or from contaminated food or water |
| *Citrobacter* spp., *Enterobacter* spp., *Klebsiella* spp., *Morganella* spp., *Proteus* spp., *Providencia* spp., and *Serratia* spp. | Normal human gastrointestinal microbiota | Endogenous or person-to-person spread, especially in hospitalized patients |

capabilities than the other species categorized as "opportunistic" Enterobacteriaceae.

# SPECIFIC ORGANISMS

## OPPORTUNISTIC HUMAN PATHOGENS

### *Citrobacter* spp. *(C. freundii, C. koseri, C. braakii)*

*Citrobacter* organisms are inhabitants of the intestinal tract. The most common clinical manifestation in patients as a result of infection occurs in the urinary tract. However, additional infections, including septicemias, meningitis, brain abscesses, and neurologic complications, have been associated with *Citrobacter* spp. Transmission is typically person to person. Table 20-3 provides an outline of the biochemical differentiation of the most common clinically isolated *Citrobacter* species. *C. freundii* may harbor inducible *AmpC* genes that encode resistance to ampicillin and first-generation cephalosporins.

### *Cronobacter sakazakii*

*Cronobacter sakazakii*, formerly *Enterobacter sakazakii*, is a pathogen associated with bacteremia, meningitis, and necrotizing colitis in neonates. The organism produces a yellow pigment that is enhanced by incubation at 25°C. *C. sakazakii* may be differentiated from *Enterobacter* spp. as Voges-Proskauer, arginine dihydrolase, ornithine decarboxylase positive. In addition, the organism displays the following fermentation reactions: D-sorbitol negative, raffinose positive, L-rhamnose positive, melibiose positive,

**TABLE 20-2** Pathogenesis and Spectrum of Disease for Clinically Relevant Enterobacteriaceae

| Organism | Virulence Factors | Spectrum of Disease and Infections |
|---|---|---|
| *Escherichia coli* (as a cause of extraintestinal infections) | Several, including endotoxin, capsule production pili that mediate attachment to host cells | Urinary tract infections, bacteremia, neonatal meningitis, and nosocomial infections of other various body sites. Most common cause of gram-negative nosocomial infections. |
| Enterotoxigenic *E. coli* (ETEC) | Pili that permit gastrointestinal colonization. Heat-labile (LT) and heat-stable (ST) enterotoxins that mediate secretion of water and electrolytes into the bowel lumen | Traveler's and childhood diarrhea, characterized by profuse, watery stools. Transmitted by contaminated food and water. |
| Enteroinvasive *E. coli* (EIEC) | Virulence factors uncertain, but organism invades enterocytes lining the large intestine in a manner nearly identical to *Shigella* | Dysentery (i.e., necrosis, ulceration, and inflammation of the large bowel); usually seen in young children living in areas of poor sanitation. |
| Enteropathogenic *E. coli* (EPEC) | Bundle-forming pilus, intimin, and other factors that mediate organism attachment to mucosal cells of the small bowel, resulting in changes in cell surface (i.e., loss of microvilli) | Diarrhea in infants in developing, low-income nations; can cause a chronic diarrhea. |
| Enterohemorrhagic *E. coli* (EHEC, VTEC, or STEC) | Toxin similar to Shiga toxin produced by *Shigella dysenteriae*. Most frequently associated with certain serotypes, such as *E. coli* O157:H7 | Inflammation and bleeding of the mucosa of the large intestine (i.e., hemorrhagic colitis); can also lead to hemolytic-uremic syndrome, resulting from toxin-mediated damage to kidneys. Transmitted by ingestion of undercooked ground beef or raw milk. |
| Enteroaggregative *E. coli* (EAEC) | Probably involves binding by pili, ST-like, and hemolysin-like toxins; actual pathogenic mechanism is unknown | Watery diarrhea that in some cases can be prolonged. Mode of transmission is not well understood. |
| *Shigella* spp. | Several factors involved to mediate adherence and invasion of mucosal cells, escape from phagocytic vesicles, intercellular spread, and inflammation. Shiga toxin role in disease is uncertain, but it does have various effects on host cells. | Dysentery defined as acute inflammatory colitis and bloody diarrhea characterized by cramps, tenesmus, and bloody, mucoid stools. Infections with *S. sonnei* may produce only watery diarrhea. |
| *Salmonella* serotypes | Several factors help protect organisms from stomach acids, promote attachment and phagocytosis by intestinal mucosal cells, allow survival in and destruction of phagocytes, and facilitate dissemination to other tissues. | Three general categories of infection are seen:<br><br>• Gastroenteritis and diarrhea caused by a wide variety of serotypes that produce infections limited to the mucosa and submucosa of the gastrointestinal tract. *S.* serotype Typhimurium and *S.* serotype Enteritidis are the serotypes most commonly associated with *Salmonella* gastroenteritis in the United States.<br>• Bacteremia and extraintestinal infections occur by spread from the gastrointestinal tract. These infections usually involve *S.* Choleraesuis or *S.* dublin, although any serotype may cause these infections.<br>• Enteric fever (typhoid fever, or typhoid) is characterized by prolonged fever and multisystem involvement, including blood, lymph nodes, liver, and spleen. This life-threatening infection is most frequently caused by *S.* serotype Typhi; more rarely, *S.* serotypes Paratyphi A, B or C. |
| *Yersinia pestis* | Multiple factors play a role in the pathogenesis of this highly virulent organism. These include the ability to adapt for intracellular survival and production of an antiphagocytic capsule, exotoxins, endotoxins, coagulase, and fibrinolysin. | Two major forms of infection are bubonic plague and pneumonic plague. Bubonic plague is characterized by high fever and painful inflammatory swelling of axilla and groin lymph nodes (i.e., the characteristic buboes); infection rapidly progresses to fulminant bacteremia that is frequently fatal if untreated. Pneumonic plague involves the lungs and is characterized by malaise and pulmonary signs; the respiratory infection can occur as a consequence of bacteremic spread associated with bubonic plague or can be acquired by the airborne route during close contact with other pneumonic plague victims; this form of plague is also rapidly fatal. |

**TABLE 20-2** Pathogenesis and Spectrum of Disease for Clinically Relevant Enterobacteriaceae—cont'd

| Organism | Virulence Factors | Spectrum of Disease and Infections |
|---|---|---|
| *Yersinia enterocolitica* subsp. *enterocolitica* | Various factors encoded on a virulence plasmid allow the organism to attach to and invade the intestinal mucosa and spread to lymphatic tissue. | Enterocolitis characterized by fever, diarrhea, and abdominal pain; also can cause acute mesenteric lymphadenitis, which may present clinically as appendicitis (i.e., pseudoappendicular syndrome). Bacteremia can occur with this organism but is uncommon. |
| *Yersinia pseudotuberculosis* | Similar to those of *Y. enterocolitica* | Causes infections similar to those described for *Y. enterocolitica* but is much less common. |
| *Citrobacter* spp., *Enterobacter* spp., *Klebsiella* spp., *Morganella* spp., *Proteus* spp., *Providencia* spp., and *Serratia* spp. | Several factors, including endotoxins, capsules, adhesion proteins, and resistance to multiple antimicrobial agents | Wide variety of nosocomial infections of the respiratory tract, urinary tract, blood, and several other normally sterile sites; most frequently infect hospitalized and seriously debilitated patients. |

**TABLE 20-3** Biochemical Differentiation of *Citrobacter* Species

| Species | Indole | ODC | Malonate | ACID FERMENTATION | | | |
|---|---|---|---|---|---|---|---|
| | | | | Adonitol | Dulcitol | Melibiose | Sucrose |
| *C. braakii* | V | pos | neg | neg | V | V | neg |
| *C. freundii* | V | neg | neg | neg | neg | pos | V |
| *C. koseri* | pos | pos | pos | pos | V | neg | V |

From Versalovic J: *Manual of clinical microbiology,* ed 10, 2011, Washington, DC, ASM Press. *neg,* Negative < 15%; *ODC,* ornithine decarboxylase; *pos,* positive ≥ 85%; *V,* variable 15% to 84%.

D-arabitol negative, and sucrose positive. *C. sakazakii* is intrinsically resistant to ampicillin and first- and second-generation cephalosporins as a result of an inducible *AmpC* chromosomal β-lactamase. Mutations to the *AmpC* gene may result in overproduction of β-lactamase, conferring resistance to third-generation cephalosporins.

### Edwardsiella tarda

*Edwardsiella tarda* is infrequently encountered in the clinical laboratory as a cause of gastroenteritis. The organism is typically associated with water harboring fish or turtles. Immunocompromised individuals are particularly susceptible and may develop serious wound infections and myonecrosis. Systemic infections occur in patients with underlying liver disease or conditions resulting in iron overload.

### Enterobacter spp. (E. aerogenes, E. cloacae, E. gergoviae, E. amnigenus, E. taylorae)

*Enterobacter* spp. are motile lactose fermenters that produce mucoid colonies. *Enterobacter* spp. are reported as one of the genera listed in the top 10 most frequently isolated health care–associated infections by the National Healthcare Safety Network. The infections are typically associated with contaminated medical devices, such as respirators and other medical instrumentation. The organism has a capsule that provides resistance to phagocytosis. *Enterobacter* spp. may harbor plasmids that encode multiple antibiotic resistance genes, requiring antibiotic susceptibility testing to identify appropriate therapeutic options.

### Escherichia coli (UPEC, MNEC, ETEC, EIEC, EAEC, EPEC and EHEC)

Molecular analysis of *E. coli* has resulted in the classification of several pathotypes as well as commensal strains. The genus consists of facultative anaerobic, glucose-fermenting, gram-negative, oxidase-negative rods capable of growth on MacConkey agar. The genus contains motile (peritrichous flagella) and nonmotile bacteria. Most *E. coli* strains are lactose fermenting, but this function may be delayed or absent in other *Escherichia* spp.

Isolates of extraintestinal *E. coli* strains have been grouped into two categories: uropathogenic *E. coli* (UPEC) and meningitis/sepsis–associated *E. coli* (MNEC). UPEC strains are the major cause of *E. coli*–associated urinary tract infections. These strains contain a variety of pathogenicity islands that code for specific adhesions and toxins capable of causing disease, including cystitis and acute pyelonephritis. MNEC causes neonatal meningitis that results in high morbidity and mortality. Eighty percent of MNEC strains test positive for the K1 antigen. The organisms are spread to the meninges from a blood infection and gain access to the central nervous system via membrane-bound vacuoles in microvascular endothelial cells.

As mentioned, intestinal *E. coli* may be classified as enterohemorrhagic (or serotoxigenic [STEC], or verotoxigenic [VTEC]), enterotoxigenic, enteropathogenic, enteroinvasive, or enteroaggregative. EHEC is recognized as the cause of hemorrhagic diarrhea, colitis, and hemolytic uremic syndrome (HUS). HUS, which is characterized by a hemolytic anemia and low platelet count, often results in kidney failure and death. Unlike in dysentery, no white blood cells are found in the stool. Although more than 150 non-O157 serotypes have been associated with diarrhea or HUS, the two most common are O157:H7 and O157:NM (nonmotile). The O antigen is a component of the lipopolysaccharide of the outer membrane, and the H antigen is the specific flagellin associated with the organism. ETEC produces a heat-labile enterotoxin (LT) and a heat-stable enterotoxin (ST) capable of causing mild watery diarrhea. ETEC is uncommon in the United States but is an important pathogen in young children in developing countries. EIEC may produce a watery to bloody diarrhea as a result of direct invasion of the epithelial cells of the colon. Cases are rare in the United States. EPEC typically does not produce exotoxins. The pathogenesis of these strains is associated with attachment and effacement of the intestinal cell wall through specialized adherence factors. Symptoms of infection include prolonged, nonbloody diarrhea; vomiting; and fever, typically in infants or children. EAEC has been isolated from a variety of clinical cases of diarrhea. The classification as aggregative results from the control of virulence genes associated with a global aggregative regulator gene, *AggR*, responsible for cellular adherence. EAEC-associated stool specimens typically are not bloody and do not contain white blood cells. Inflammation is accompanied by fever and abdominal pain.

### *Ewingella americana*

*Ewingella americana* has been identified from blood and wound isolates. The organism is biochemically inactive, and currently no recommended identification scheme has been identified.

### *Hafnia alvei*

*Hafnia alvei* (formerly *Enterobacter hafniae*) has been associated with gastrointestinal infections. The organism, resides in the gastrointestinal tract of humans and many animals It is a motile non–lactose fermenter and is often isolated with other pathogens. Most infections with *H. alvei* are indentified in patients with severe underlying disease (e.g., malignancies) or after surgery or trauma. However, a distinct correlation with clinical signs and symptoms has not been clearly developed, probably because of the lack of identified clinical cases. Treatment is based on antimicrobial susceptibility testing.

### *Klebsiella* spp. (*K. pneumoniae, K. oxytoca*)

*Klebsiella* spp. are inhabitants of the nasopharynx and gastrointestinal tract. Isolates have been identified in association with a variety of infections, including liver abscesses, pneumonia, septicemia, and urinary tract infections. Some strains of *K. oxytoca* carry a heat-labile cytotoxin, which has been isolated from patients who have developed a self-limiting antibiotic-associated hemorrhagic colitis. K1 capsular–containing *K. pneumoniae* organisms are increasingly isolated from community-acquired pyogenic liver abscess worldwide. All strains of *K. pneumoniae* are resistant to ampicillin. In addition, they may demonstrate multiple antibiotic resistance patterns from the acquisition of multidrug-resistant plasmids, with enzymes such as carbapenemase.

### *Morganella* spp. (*M. morganii, M. psychrotolerans*)

*Morganella* spp. are found ubiquitously throughout the environment and are often associated with stool specimens collected from patients with symptoms of diarrhea. They are normal inhabitants of the gastrointestinal tract. *M. morganii* is commonly isolated in the clinical laboratory; however, its clinical significance has not been clearly defined. *Morganella* spp. are deaminase positive and urease positive.

### *Pantoea agglomerans*

*Pantoea agglomerans* appears as a yellow-pigmented colony and is lysine, arginine, and ornithine negative. In addition, the organism is indole positive and mannitol, raffinose, salicin, sucrose, maltose, and xylose negative. The organism is difficult to identify using commercial or traditional biochemical methods due to the high variability of expression in the key reactions. Sporadic infections can occur due to trauma from objects contaminated with soil or from contaminated fluids (i.e., IV fluids).

### *Plesiomonas shigelloides*

*Plesiomonas shigelloides* is a fresh water inhabitant that is transmitted to humans by ingestion of contaminated water or by exposure of disrupted skin and mucosal surfaces. *P. shigelloides* can cause gastroenteritis, most frequently in children, but its role in intestinal infections is still unclear.

*P. shigelloides* is unusual in that it is among the few species of clinically relevant bacteria that decarboxylate lysine, ornithine, and arginine. It is important to distinguish *Aeromonas* spp. from *P. shigelloides*., since both are oxidase positive. This is accomplished by using the string test described in Chapter 26. The DNase test may also be used to differentiate these organisms. *Aeromonas* spp. are DNase positive and *Plesiomonas* organisms are DNase negative.

### *Proteus* spp. (*P. mirabilis, P. vulgaris, P. penneri*) and *Providencia* spp. (*P. alcalifaciens, P. heimbachae, P. rettgeri, P. stuartii, P. rustigianii*)

The genera *Proteus* and *Providencia* are normal inhabitants of the gastrointestinal tract. They are motile, non–lactose fermenters capable of deaminating phenylalanine. *Proteus* spp. are easily identified by their classic "swarming" appearance on culture media. However, some strains lack the swarming phenotype. *Proteus* has a distinct odor that is often referred to as a "chocolate cake" or "burnt chocolate" smell. For safety reasons, smelling plates is strongly discouraged in the clinical laboratory. Because of its motility, the organism is often associated with urinary tract infections; however, it also has been isolated from wounds and ears. The organism has also been associated with diarrhea and sepsis.

*Providencia* spp. are most commonly associated with urinary tract infections and the feces of children with diarrhea. These organisms may be associated with nosocomial outbreaks. No clear clinical association exists when these organisms are isolated.

### Serratia spp. (S. marcescens, S. liquefaciens group)

*Serratia* spp. are known for colonization and the cause of pathagenic infections in health care settings. *Serratia* spp. are motile, slow lactose fermenters, DNAse, and orthonitrophenyl galactoside (ONPG) positive. *Serratia* spp. are ranked the twelfth most commonly isolated organism from pediatric patients in North America, Latin America, and Europe. Transmission may be person to person but is often associated with medical devices such as urinary catheters, respirators intravenous fluids, and other medical solutions. *Serratia* spp. have also been isolated from the respiratory tract and wounds. The organism is capable of survival under very harsh environmental conditions and is resistant to many disinfectants. The red pigment (prodogiosin) produced by *S. marcescens* typically is the key to identification among laboratorians, although pigment-producing strains tend to be of lower virulence. Other species have also been isolated from human infections. *Serratia* spp. are resistant to ampicillin and first-generation cephalosporins because of the presence of an inducible, chromosomal *AmpC* β-lactamase. In addition, many strains have plasmid-encoded antimicrobial resistance to other cephalosporins, penicillins, carbapenems, and aminoglycosides.

## PRIMARY INTESTINAL PATHOGENS

### Salmonella (All Serotypes)

*Salmonella* are facultative anaerobic, motile gram-negative rods commonly isolated from the intestines of humans and animals. Identification is primarily based on the ability of the organism to use citrate as the sole carbon source and lysine as a nitrogen source in combination with hydrogen sulfide ($H_2S$) production. The genus is comprised of two primary species, *S. enterica* (human pathogen) and *S. bongori* (animal pathogen). *S. enterica* is subdivided into six subspecies: subsp. *enterica*, subsp. *salamae*, subsp. *arizonae*, subsp. *diarizonae*, subsp. *houtenae*, and subsp. *indica*. *S. enterica* subsp. *enterica* can be further divided into serotypes with unique virulence properties. Serotypes are differentiated based on the characterization of the heat-stable O antigen, included in the LPS, the heat-labile H antigen flagellar protein, and the heat-labile Vi antigen, capsular polysaccharide. A DNA sequence–based method has been developed for molecular identification of DNA motifs in the flagella and O antigens.

### Shigella spp. (S. dysenteriae, S. flexneri, S. boydii, S. sonnei)

*Shigella* spp. are nonmotile; lysine decarboxylase–negative; citrate-, malonate-, and $H_2S$-negative; non–lactose fermenting; gram-negative rods that grow well on MacConkey agar. The four subgroups of *Shigella* spp. are: *S. dysenteriae* (group A), *S. flexneri* (group B), *S. boydii*(group C), and *S. sonnei* (group D). Each subgroup has several serotypes. Serotyping is based on the somatic LPS O antigen. After presumptive identification of a suspected *Shigella* species based on traditional biochemical methods, serotyping should be completed, especially in the case of

*S. dysenteriae.* Suspected strains of *Shigella* sp. that cannot be typed by serologic methods should be referred to a reference laboratory for further testing.

### Yersinia spp. (Y. pestis, Y. enterocolitica, Y. frederiksenii, Y. intermedia, Y. pseudotuberculosis)

*Yersinia* spp. are gram-negative; catalase-, oxidase-, and indole-positive, non–lactose fermenting; facultative anaerobes capable of growth at temperatures ranging from 4° to 43°C. The gram-negative rods exhibit an unusual bipolar staining. Based on the composition of the LPS in the outer membrane, colonies may present with either a rough form lacking the O-specific polysaccharide chain (*Y. pestis*) or a smooth form containing the lipid A-oligosaccharide core and the complete O-polysaccharide (*Y. pseudotuberculosis* and *Y. enterocolitica*). Complex typing systems exist to differentiate the various *Yersinia* spp., including standard biochemical methods coupled with biotyping, serotyping, bacteriophage typing, and antibiogram analysis. In addition, epidemiologic studies often include pulsed-field gel electrophoresis (PFGE) studies.

## RARE HUMAN PATHOGENS

A variety of additional Enterobacteriaceae may be isolated from human specimens, such as *Cedecea* spp., *Kluyvera* spp., *Leclercia adecarboxylata, Moellerella wisconsensis, Rahnella aquatilis, Tatumella ptyseos,* and *Yokenella regensburgei.* These organisms are typically opportunistic pathogens found in environmental sources.

# LABORATORY DIAGNOSIS

## SPECIMEN COLLECTION AND TRANSPORT

Enterobacteriaceae are typically isolated from a variety of sources in combination with other more fastidious organisms. No special considerations are required for specimen collection and transport of the organisms discussed in this chapter. (See Table 5-1 for general information on specimen collection and transport.)

## SPECIMEN PROCESSING

No special considerations are required for processing of the great majority of organisms discussed in this chapter. The one exception is *Yersinia pestis.* This organism is a select agent. Manipulation of specimens suspected of containing this organism would generate aerosols and should be handled using Biosafety Level 3 (BSL-3) conditions. Refer to Table 5-1 for general information on specimen processing.

## DIRECT DETECTION METHODS

All Enterobacteriaceae have similar microscopic morphology; therefore, Gram staining is not significant for the presumptive identification of Enterobacteriaceae. Generally isolation of gram-negative organisms from a sterile site, including cerebrospinal fluid (CSF), blood, and other body fluids, is critical and may assist the physician in prescribing appropriate therapy.

Direct detection of Enterobacteriaceae in stool by Gram staining is insignificant because of the presence of a large number of normal gram-negative microbiota. The presence of increased white blood cells may indicate an enteric infection; however, the absence is not sufficient to rule out a toxin-mediated enteric disease.

Other than Gram staining of patient specimens, specific procedures are required for direct detection of most Enterobacteriaceae. Microscopically the cells of these organisms generally appear as coccobacilli, or straight rods with rounded ends. *Y. pestis* resembles a closed safety pin when it is stained with methylene blue or Wayson stain; this is a key characteristic for rapid diagnosis of plague.

*Klebsiella granulomatis* can be visualized in scrapings of lesions stained with Wright's or Giemsa stain. Cultivation in vitro is very difficult, so direct examination is important diagnostically. Groups of organisms are seen in mononuclear endothelial cells; this pathognomonic entity is known as a *Donovan body,* named after the physician who first visualized the organism in such a lesion. The organism stains as a blue rod with prominent polar granules, giving rise to the safety-pin appearance, surrounded by a large, pink capsule. Subsurface infected cells must be present; surface epithelium is not an adequate specimen.

*P. shigelloides* tend to be pleomorphic gram-negative rods that occur singly, in pairs, in short chains, or even as long, filamentous forms.

## CULTIVATION

### Media of Choice

Most Enterobacteriaceae grow well on routine laboratory media, such as 5% sheep blood, chocolate, and MacConkey agars. In addition to these media, selective agars, such as Hektoen enteric (HE) agar, xylose-lysine-deoxycholate (XLD) agar, and *Salmonella-Shigella* (SS) agar, are commonly used to cultivate enteric pathogens from gastrointestinal specimens (see Chapter 59 for more information about laboratory procedures for the diagnosis of bacterial gastrointestinal infections). The broths used in blood culture systems, as well as thioglycollate and brain-heart infusion broths, all support the growth of Enterobacteriaceae.

Cefsulodin-irgasan-novobiocin (CIN) agar is a selective medium specifically used for the isolation of *Y. enterocolitica* from gastrointestinal specimens. Similarly, MacConkey-sorbitol agar (MAC-SOR) is used to differentiate sorbitol-negative *E. coli* O157:H7 from other strains of *E. coli* that are capable of fermenting this sugar alcohol.

*Klebsiella granulomatis* will not grow on routine agar media. Recently, the organism was cultured in human monocytes from biopsy specimens of genital ulcers of patients with donovanosis. Historically, the organism has also been cultivated on a special medium described by Dienst that contains growth factors found in egg yolk. In clinical practice, however, the diagnosis of granuloma inguinale is made solely on the basis of direct examination.

Table 20-4 presents a complete description of the laboratory media used to isolate Enterobacteriaceae.

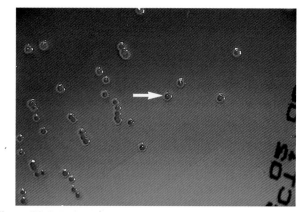

**Figure 20-1** Bull's-eye colony of *Yersinia enterocolitica (arrow)* on cefsulodin-irgasan-novobiocin (CIN) agar.

### Incubation Conditions and Duration

Under normal circumstances, most Enterobacteriaceae produce detectable growth in commonly used broth and agar media within 24 hours of inoculation. For isolation, 5% sheep blood and chocolate agars may be incubated at 35°C in carbon dioxide or ambient air. However, MacConkey agar and other selective agars (e.g., SS, HE, XLD) should be incubated only in ambient air. Unlike most other Enterobacteriaceae, *Y. pestis* grows best at 25° to 30°C. Colonies of *Y. pestis* are pinpoint at 24 hours but resemble those of other Enterobacteriaceae after 48 hours. CIN agar, used for the isolation of *Y. enterocolitica,* should be incubated 48 hours at room temperature to allow for the development of typical "bull's-eye" colonies (Figure 20-1).

### Colonial Appearance

Table 20-5 presents the colonial appearance and other distinguishing characteristics (pigment and odor) of the most commonly isolated Enterobacteriaceae on MacConkey, HE, and XLD agars (see Figures 7-4, 7-6, and 7-8 for examples). All Enterobacteriaceae produce similar growth on blood and chocolate agars; colonies are large, gray, and smooth. Colonies of *Klebsiella* or *Enterobacter* may be mucoid because of their polysaccharide capsule. *E. coli* is often beta-hemolytic on blood agar, but most other genera are nonhemolytic. As a result of motility, *Proteus mirabilis, P. penneri,* and *P. vulgaris* "swarm" on blood and chocolate agars. Swarming results in the production of a thin film of growth on the agar surface (Figure 20-3) as the motile organisms spread from the original site of inoculation.

Colonies of *Y. pestis* on 5% sheep blood agar are pinpoint at 24 hours but exhibit a rough, cauliflower appearance at 48 hours. Broth cultures of *Y. pestis* exhibit a characteristic "stalactite pattern" in which clumps of cells adhere to one side of the tube.

*Y. enterocolitica* produces bull's-eye colonies (dark red or burgundy centers surrounded by a translucent border; see Figure 20-1) on CIN agar at 48 hours. However, because most *Aeromonas* spp. produce similar colonies on CIN agar, it is important to perform an oxidase test to verify that the organisms are *Yersinia* spp. (oxidase negative). The oxidase test should be performed on suspect

**TABLE 20-4** Biochemical Media used in the Differentiation and Isolation of Enterobacteriaceae

| Media | Selective | Differential | Nutritional | Purpose |
|---|---|---|---|---|
| Blood agar (sheep) (SBA, BAP) | | Hemolysis of RBCs: Beta: Complete lysis Alpha: Partial, greening Gamma: Nonhemolytic | Routinely used to cultivate moderately fastidious organisms; TSA with 5% to 10% defibrinated blood. | Screening colonies for the oxidase enzyme |
| Cefsulodin-irgasan-novobiocin agar (CIN) | Selective inhibition of gram-negative and gram-positive organisms | Fermentation of mannitol in the presence of neutral red. Macroscopic colonial appearance: colorless or pink colonies with red center. | | Isolation of *Yersinia enterocolitica* |
| Citrate agar, Simmons (CIT) | | Citrate as the sole carbon source, ammonium salt as nitrate. Ammonium salt alteration changes pH to alkaline, bromthymol blue shifts from green to blue. | | Detect organisms capable of citrate utilization |
| Decarboxylases (ornithine, arginine, lysine) | | Incorporate amino acid as differential media (e.g., lysine, arginine, or ornithine). Decarboxylation yields alkaline, pH-sensitive bromcresol purple dye. Basal medium serves as a control. Incubate for up to 4 days. Fermentative organisms turn media yellow, using glucose. [H+] increases, making optimal conditions for decarboxylation. Conversion of the aa to amines raises the pH, reversing the yellow to purple. Nonfermenters turn the purple a deeper color. | | Differentiate fermentative and nonfermentative gram-negative bacteria. |
| Eosin/ methylene blue agar (EMB) | Eosin Y and methylene blue dyes inhibit the growth of gram-positive bacteria. | Lactose and sucrose for differentiation based on fermentation. Sucrose is an alternate energy source for slow lactose fermenters, allowing quick differentiation from pathogens. | | Identification of gram-negative bacteria. *E coli:* Lactose fermenter, forms blue-black with a metallic green sheen. Other coliform fermenters form pink colonies. Nonfermenters: Translucent, either amber or colorless. |
| Gram-negative broth (GN) | Deoxycholate and citrate salts inhibit gram-positive bacteria. | | Increasing mannitol, which temporarily favors the growth of mannitol-fermenting, gram-negative rods (e.g., *Salmonella* and *Shigella* spp.) | Enhances the recovery of enteric pathogens from fecal specimens |
| Hektoen enteric agar (HEK) | Bile salts inhibit gram-positive and many gram-negative normal intestinal flora. | Differential lactose, salicin, and sucrose with a pH indicator bromthymol blue and ferric salts to detect hydrogen sulfide ($H_2S$). Most pathogens ferment one or both sugars and appear bright orange to salmon pink because of the pH interaction with the dye. Nonfermenters appear green to blue green. $H_2S$ production produces a black precipitate in the colonies. | | Detection of enteric pathogens from feces or from selective enrichment broth |

*Continued*

**TABLE 20-4** Biochemical Media used in the Differentiation and Isolation of Enterobacteriaceae—cont'd

| Media | Selective | Differential | Nutritional | Purpose |
|---|---|---|---|---|
| Lysine iron agar (LIA) | | Contains lysine, glucose, and protein, bromocresol purple (pH indicator) and sodium thiosulfate/ferric ammonium citrate. Purple denotes alkaline (K), red color (R), acid (A). <br><br> K/K: Organism decarboxylates but cannot deaminate, ferments glucose, first butt is yellow. Decarboxylates lysine producing alkaline; changes back to purple. <br><br> K/A: Organism fermented glucose but was unable to deaminate or decarboxylate lysine. <br> Bordeaux red and yellow butt. <br><br> R/A: Organism deaminated lysine but could not decarboxylate it. The lysine deamination combines with the ferric ammonium citrate, forming a burgundy color. <br> Blackening of the butt indicates production of $H_2S$. | | Measures three parameters that are useful for identifying Enterobacteriaceae (lysine decarboxylation, lysine deamination, and $H_2S$ production) |
| MacConkey agar (MAC) | Bile salts and crystal violet inhibit most gram-positive organisms and permit growth of gram-negative rods. | Lactose serves as the sole carbohydrate. Lactose fermenters produce pink or red colonies, may be precipitated bile salts may surround colonies. Non–lactose fermenters appear colorless or transparent. | | Selection for gram-negative organisms and differentiating Enterobacteriaceae |
| MacConkey-sorbitol (MAC-SOR) | | Same as regular MacConkey except D-sorbitol is substituted for lactose. Sorbitol-negative organisms are clear and may indicate E. coli O157:H7. | | Used to isolate *Escherichia coli* O157:H7 |
| Motility test medium | | Nonmotile organisms grow clearly only on stab line, and the surrounding medium remains clear. Motile organisms move out of the stab line and make the medium appear diffusely cloudy. | | Determine motility for an organism. Identification and differentiation of Enterobacteriaceae. *Shigella* and *Klebsiella* spp. are nonmotile; *Yersinia* sp. are motile at room temperature. *Listeria monocytogenes* (not an Enterobacteriaceae) has umbrella-shaped motility. |
| *Salmonella-Shigella* agar (SS) | Bile salts, sodium citrate, and brilliant green, which inhibit gram-positive organisms and some lactose-fermenting, gram-negative rods normally found in the stool. | Lactose is the sole carbohydrate, and neutral red is the pH indicator. Fermenters produce acid and change the indicator to pink-red. Sodium thiosulfate is added as a source of sulfur for the production of hydrogen sulfide. Also includes ferric ammonium citrate to react with $H_2S$ and produce a black precipitate in the center of the colony. *Shigella* spp. appear colorless. *Salmonella* spp. are colorless with a black center. | | Select for *Salmonella* spp. and some strains of *Shigella* from stool specimens. |

**TABLE 20-4** Biochemical Media used in the Differentiation and Isolation of Enterobacteriaceae—cont'd

| Media | Selective | Differential | Nutritional | Purpose |
|---|---|---|---|---|
| Triple sugar iron agar (TSI) | | Contains glucose, sucrose, and lactose. Sucrose and lactose are present in 10 times the quantity of the glucose; phenol red is the pH indicator. Turns to yellow when sugars are fermented because of drop in pH. Sodium thiosulfate plus ferric ammonium sulfate as $H_2S$ indicator.<br>Acid/acid (A/A): Glucose and lactose and/or sucrose (or both) fermentation.<br>Gas bubbles: Production of gas.<br>Visible air breaks or pockets in agar.<br>Black precipitate: $H_2S$.<br>Alkaline/acid (K/A): Glucose fermentation but not lactose or sucrose.<br>Alkaline/alkaline (K/K): No fermentation of dextrose, lactose, or sucrose. | | Differentiates glucose fermenters from non–glucose fermenters; also contains tests for sucrose and/or lactose fermentation, as well as gas production during glucose fermentation and $H_2S$ production. |
| Urea agar | | Urea is hydrolyzed to form carbon dioxide, water, and ammonia. Ammonia reacts with components of the medium to form ammonium carbonate, raising the pH, which changes the pH indicator, phenol red, to pink. Limited protein in the medium prevents protein metabolism from causing a false-positive reaction. | | Identification of Enterobacteriaceae species capable of producing urease. (*Citrobacter, Klebsiella, Proteus, Providencia,* and *Yersinia* spp.) |
| Xylose-lysine-deoxycholate agar (XLD) | Sodium deoxycholate inhibits gram-positive cocci and some gram-negative rods. Contains less bile salts than other formulations of enteric media (e.g., SS, HEK) and therefore permits better recovery. | Sucrose and lactose in excess concentrations and xylose in lower amounts. Phenol red is the pH indicator.<br>Lysine is included to detect decarboxylation. Sodium thiosulfate/ferric ammonium citrate allows the production of $H_2S$.<br>The following types of colonies may be seen:<br>*Yellow:* Fermentation of the excess carbohydrates to produce acid; because of the carbohydrate use, the organisms do not decarboxylate lysine, even though they may have the enzyme.<br>*Colorless or red:* Produced by organisms that do not ferment any of the sugars.<br>*Yellow to red:* Fermentation of xylose (yellow), but because it is in small amounts, it is used up quickly, and the organisms switch to decarboxylation of lysine, turning the medium back to red.<br>Black precipitate is formed from the production of $H_2S$. | | Selective media used to isolate *Salmonella* and *Shigella* spp. from stool and other specimens containing mixed flora |

colonies that have been subcultured to sheep blood agar (Table 20-4). Pigments present in the CIN agar will interfere with correct interpretation of the oxidase test results.

## APPROACH TO IDENTIFICATION

In the early decades of the twentieth century, Enterobacteriaceae were identified using more than 50 biochemical tests in tubes; this method is still used today in reference and public health laboratories. Certain key tests such as indole, methyl red, Voges-Proskauer, and citrate, known by the acronym IMViC, were routinely performed to group the most commonly isolated pathogens. Today, this type of conventional biochemical

identification of enterics has become a historical footnote in most clinical and hospital laboratories in the United States.

In the latter part of the twentieth century, manufacturers began to produce panels of miniaturized tests for identification, first of enteric gram-negative rods and later of other groups of bacteria and yeast. Original panels were inoculated manually; these were followed by semiautomated and automated systems, the most sophisticated of which inoculate, incubate, read, and discard the panels. Practically any commercial identification system can be used to reliably identify the commonly isolated Enterobacteriaceae. Depending on the system, results are available within 4 hours or after overnight

**TABLE 20-5** Colonial Appearance and Characteristics of the Most Commonly Isolated Enterobacteriaceae*

| Organism | Medium | Appearance |
|---|---|---|
| *Citrobacter* spp. | MAC | Late LF; therefore, NLF after 24 hr; LF after 48 hr; colonies are light pink after 48 hr |
| | HE | Colorless |
| | XLD | Red, yellow, or colorless colonies, with or without black centers ($H_2S$) |
| *Edwardsiella* spp. | MAC | NLF |
| | HE | Colorless |
| | XLD | Red, yellow, or colorless colonies, with or without black centers ($H_2S$) |
| *Enterobacter* spp. | MAC | LF; may be mucoid |
| | HE | Yellow |
| | XLD | Yellow |
| *Escherichia coli* | MAC | Most LF, some NLF (some isolates may demonstrate slow or late fermentation); and generally flat, dry, pink colonies with a surrounding darker pink area of precipitated bile salts[†] |
| | HE | Yellow |
| | XLD | Yellow |
| *Hafnia alvei* | MAC | NLF |
| | HE | Colorless |
| | XLD | Red or yellow |
| *Klebsiella* spp. | MAC | LF; mucoid |
| | HE | Yellow |
| | XLD | Yellow |
| *Morganella* spp. | MAC | NLF |
| | HE | Colorless |
| | XLD | Red or colorless |
| *Plesiomonas shigelloides* | BAP | Shiny, opaque, smooth, nonhemolytic |
| | MAC | Can be NLF or LF |
| *Proteus* spp. | MAC | NLF; may swarm, depending on the amount of agar in the medium; characteristic foul smell |
| | HE | Colorless |
| | XLD | Yellow or colorless, with or without black centers |
| *Providencia* spp. | MAC | NLF |
| | HE | Colorless |
| | XLD | Yellow or colorless |
| *Salmonella* spp. | MAC | NLF |
| | HE | Green, black center as a result of $H_2S$ production |
| | XLD | Red with black center |
| *Serratia* spp. | MAC | Late LF; *S. marcescens* may be red pigmented, especially if plate is left at 25°C (Figure 20-2) |
| | HE | Colorless |
| | XLD | Yellow or colorless |
| *Shigella* spp. | MAC | NLF; *S. sonnei* produces flat colonies with jagged edges |
| | HE | Green |
| | XLD | Colorless |
| *Yersinia* spp. | MAC | NLF; may be colorless to peach |
| | HE | Salmon |
| | XLD | Yellow or colorless |

*HE,* Hektoen enteric agar; *LF,* lactose fermenter, pink colony; *MAC,* MacConkey agar; *NLF,* non–lactose fermenter, colorless colony; *XLD,* xylose-lysine-deoxycholate agar.

*Most Enterobacteriaceae are indistinguishable on blood agar; see text for colonial description.

[†]Pink colonies on MacConkey agar with sorbitol are sorbitol fermenters; colorless colonies are non–sorbitol fermenters.

incubation. The extensive computer databases used by these systems include information on unusual biotypes. The number of organisms used to define individual databases is important; in rare cases, isolated organisms or new microorganisms may be misidentified or not identified at all.

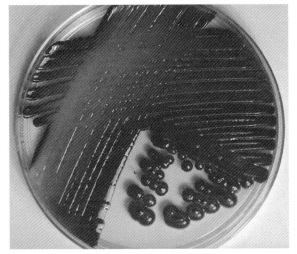

**Figure 20-2** Red-pigmented *Serratia marcescens* on MacConkey agar.

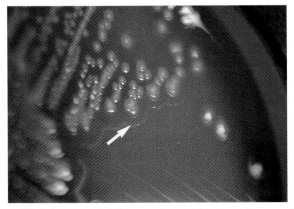

**Figure 20-3** *Proteus mirabilis* swarming on blood agar (arrow points to swarming edge).

The definitive identification of enterics can be enhanced based on molecular methods, especially 16S ribosomal RNA (rRNA) sequencing and DNA-DNA hybridization. Through the use of molecular methods, the genus *Plesiomonas*, composed of one species of oxidase-positive, gram-negative rods, now has been included in the family Enterobacteriaceae. *Plesiomonas* sp. clusters with the genus *Proteus* in the Enterobacteriaceae by 16S rRNA sequencing. However, like all other Enterobacteriaceae, *Proteus* organisms are oxidase-negative. The clustering together of an oxidase-positive genus and an oxidase-negative genus is a revolutionary concept in microbial taxonomy.

In the interests of cost containment, many clinical laboratories use an abbreviated scheme to identify commonly isolated enterics. *E. coli*, for example, the most commonly isolated enteric organism, may be identified by a positive spot indole test (see Procedure 13-41). For presumptive identification of an organism as *E. coli*, the characteristic colonial appearance on MacConkey agar, as described in Table 20-5, is documented along with positive spot indole test result. A spot indole test can also be used to quickly separate swarming Proteae, such as *P. mirabilis* and *P. penneri*, which are negative, from the indole-positive *P. vulgaris*.

Table 20-6 provides an overview of common reactions for identifying biochemically unusual enteric pathogens. Figure 20-4 depicts the biochemical reactions typically used to differentiate some of the representative enteric pathogens. To aid the development of an understanding of the separation of common enteric pathogens based on groupings, Figure 20-5 provides a systematic algorithm for grouping pathogens into a working identification scheme.

### Specific Considerations for Identifying Enteric Pathogens

The common biochemical tests used to differentiate the species in the genus *Citrobacter* are illustrated in Table 20-3.

Table 20-7 illustrates the use of biochemical profiles obtained with triple sugar iron (TSI) agar and lysine iron agar (LIA) to presumptively identify enteric pathogens (see Chapter 13 for information on the principles,

**TABLE 20-6** Biochemical Differentiation of Unusual LDC-, ODC- and ADH-negative Enterobacteriaceae

| Genus | Gas from Glucose | Motility | KCN | VP | ACID FERMENTATION | | |
|---|---|---|---|---|---|---|---|
| | | | | | L-Arabitol | Sucrose | Trehalose |
| *Budvicia* | | | neg | | | | |
| *Ewingella* | neg | V | neg | pos | neg | neg | pos |
| *Leclercia* | pos | pos | pos | neg | pos | pos | pos |
| *Moellerella* | pos | pos | V | neg | pos | neg | pos |
| *Rahnella* | pos | neg | neg | neg | neg | pos | pos |
| *Tatumella* | neg | neg | neg | neg | neg | pos | pos |
| *Photorhabdus* | neg | pos | neg | neg | neg | neg | neg |

*ADH,* Arginine dihydrolase; *KCN,* potassium cyanide; *LDC,* lysine decarboxylase; *ODC,* ornithine decarboxylase; *neg,* negative 10%. *pos,* positive 90%; *V,* variable 11% to 89%; *VP,* Voges-Proskauer test.

| Test | Yersinia enterocolitica | Providencia P. stuartii | Providencia P. rettgeri | Morganella morganii | Proteus P. mirabilis | Proteus P. vulgaris | Serratia S. odorifera biotype 2 | Serratia S. marcescens | Pantoea agglomerans (was Enterobacter) | Cronobacter sakazakii | Enterobacter E. aerogenes | Enterobacter E. cloacae | Klebsiella K. oxytoxa | Klebsiella K. pneumoniae | Citrobacter C. koseri (formerly diversus) | Citrobacter C. braakii | Citrobacter C. freundii | Edwardsiella tarda | S. typhi | S. enteritidis | Other Shigella | Shigella sonnei | Plesiomonas shigelloides (oxidase +)* | H. alvei | Ewingella americana | Escherichia coli |
|---|---|---|---|---|---|---|---|---|---|---|---|---|---|---|---|---|---|---|---|---|---|---|---|---|---|---|
| Indole | V | + | + | + | − | + | V | − | −(v) | − | − | − | + | − | + | −(v) | − | + | − | − | V | − | + | − | − | + |
| Methyl red | + | + | + | + | + | + | +(v) | V | V | − | − | − | −(v) | V | + | + | + | + | + | + | + | + | V | −(v) | + | + |
| Voges Proskauer | − | − | − | − | V | − | + | + | +(v) | + | + | + | + | + | − | − | − | − | − | − | − | − | − | +(v) | + | − |
| Simmons' citrate | − | + | + | − | V | −(v) | + | + | V | + | + | + | + | + | + | +(v) | + | − | − | +(v) | − | − | − | + | + | − |
| Hydrogen Sulfide (TSI) | − | + | + | − | +(v) | + | − | − | − | − | − | − | − | − | − | +(v) | + | + | +w | +(v) | − | − | − | − | − | − |
| Urea | + | −(v) | + | + | + | + | + | −(v) | −(v) | +(v) | − | +(v) | + | + | +(v) | −(v) | −(v) | − | − | − | − | − | − | − | − | − |
| Motility | − | +(v) | + | V | + | + | + | + | + | + | + | + | − | − | + | + | + | + | + | + | − | − | + | + | − | V |
| Lysine decarboxylase | − | − | − | + | − | − | + | + | − | − | + | − | + | + | − | − | − | + | + | + | − | − | + | + | − | +(v) |
| Arginine dihydrolase | + | − | − | + | − | − | + | − | + | + | − | + | − | − | + | + | +(v) | − | − | +(v) | V | − | + | − | − | −(v) |
| Ornithine decarboxylase | + | − | − | + | + | − | + | + | − | + | + | + | − | − | + | + | − | + | − | + | − | + | + | + | − | +(v) |
| Phenylalinine deaminase | − | + | + | + | + | + | − | − | −(v) | +(v) | − | − | − | − | − | − | − | − | − | − | − | − | − | − | − | − |
| Gas from D-glucose | − | −(v) | − | + | + | + | + | + | −(v) | + | + | + | + | + | + | + | + | + | − | + | − | − | − | + | − | + |
| Lactose | − | − | − | − | − | − | + | −(v) | −(v) | + | + | + | + | + | V | + | +(v) | − | − | − | − | − | V | + | +(v) | + |
| Sucrose | + | V | − | − | − | + | + | + | +(v) | + | + | + | + | + | −(v) | − | +(v) | − | − | − | − | − | − | − | − | V |
| D-Mannitol | + | −(v) | + | − | − | − | + | + | + | + | + | + | + | + | + | + | + | − | + | + | + | + | − | + | + | + |
| Adonitol | − | − | + | − | − | − | +(v) | −(v) | − | − | + | −(v) | + | + | + | − | − | − | − | − | − | − | + | − | − | − |
| Inositol | − | + | + | − | − | − | + | V | − | + | + | −(v) | + | + | − | − | − | − | − | − | − | − | + | − | − | − |
| D-Sorbitol | + | − | − | − | − | − | + | + | + | − | + | + | + | + | + | + | + | − | + | + | V | − | + | − | − | +(v) |
| L-Arabinose | + | − | − | − | − | − | + | − | + | + | + | + | + | + | + | + | + | − | + | + | V | + | − | + | − | + |
| Raffinose | + | − | − | − | − | − | + | − | −(v) | + | + | + | + | + | + | − | −(v) | − | − | − | V | − | − | − | − | V |
| L-Rhamnose | − | −(v) | +(v) | − | − | − | + | −(v) | + | + | + | + | + | + | + | + | + | − | − | + | −(v) | +(v) | − | + | − | − |
| KCN, growth in | − | + | + | + | + | + | − | + | + | + | + | + | − | − | − | + | + | − | − | − | − | − | − | + | − | − |
| Gelatin (22°C) | − | − | − | − | + | + | + | −(v) | − | − | − | − | − | − | − | − | − | − | − | − | − | − | − | − | − | − |
| DNase | − | − | − | − | − | − | − | + | − | − | − | − | − | − | − | − | − | − | − | − | − | − | − | − | − | − |

**Figure 20-4** Biochemical differentiation of representative Enterobacteriaceae. *V*, Variability can be equally either positive or negative; +(v), greater probability for positive reaction >50%; −(v), greater probability for negative reaction >50%; (+), positive > 80%; (−), negative > 80%. The pink squares indicate a pattern useful for preliminary recognition. The green squares indicate a key characteristic for biochemical identification.

**Lactose Fermenters:** *E. coli, K. pneumoniae. *C. freundii (LF), *C. koseri (LF), Other *Citrobacter species (LF), E. aerogenes, E. cloacae*

**Non-lactose Fermenters:** *\*C. freundii, \*C. koseri, \*Other Citrobacter species, E. tarda, H. alvei, E. coli (inactive), M. morganii, P. mirabilis, P. penneri, P. vulgaris, P rettgeri, P. stuartii, Salmonella spp., Shigella spp., Serratia marcencens.*

ONPG +
**S. serotype Typhi**
C–
**S. serotype Paratyphi B**
C+
**S. serotype Typhimurium**
C+
LD positive

**H₂S Negative**

**Citrobacter spp.** [other than C. freundii]
I–U+C+
K/A with gas (KI)
Motile
**C. koseri**
I+U–C+
K/A with gas (KI)
Motile
**E. coli** [inactive]
I+/–U–C–
K/A no gas (KI)
**Hafnia spp.**
I–U–C–
K/A with gas (KI)
Motile
AD positive
**S. paratyphi A**
I–U–C–
K/A with gas (KI)
Motile
**S. marscecens**
I–U–C+
K/A 55% no gas (KI)
Motile
**Shigella spp.**
I–U–C–
K/A no gas (KI)
Non Motile

---

| Indole Positive | Indole Negative | PPA Positive | PPA Negative |
|---|---|---|---|
| E.coli, Citrobacter species other than C. freundii K. oxytoxa | C.freundii K. pneumoniae Enterobacter spp. | Proteus spp. Providencia spp. Morganella morganii | Citrobacter spp. Edwardsiella tarda E. coli [inactive] Hafnia spp. Salmonella spp. Shigella spp. S. marcescens |

**Indole Positive → Biochemical Division**
**E. coli** I+U–C–
**C. koseri** I+U+/–C+ (motile) MR positive
**K. oxytoca** I+U+C+ (nonmotile) MR negative

**Indole Negative:**
**C. freundii** I–/+U–/+C+/– H₂S+ (KI)
**E. aerogenes** I–U–C+ A/A with gas (KI); OD positive
**E. cloacae** I–U+/–C+ A/A with gas (KI); AD positive
**K. pneumoniae** I–U+C+ A/A with gas (KI); gas (KI)

**PPA Positive:**

| H₂S Positive | H₂S Negative |
|---|---|
| P. mirabilis P. vulgaris P. penneri (30%) M. morganii (20%) | P. rettgeri P. stuartii P. penneri (70%) M. morganii (80%) |

| Biochemical | Biochemical |
|---|---|
| **P. mirabilis** I–U+C+/– **P. vulgaris** I+U+C–/+ **P. penneri** I–U+C– **M. morganii** I+U+C– | **P. rettgeri** M+ no gas I+C+C+ K/A(KI) **P. stuartii** M– no gas I+C+U–/+ K/A (KI) **P. penneri** M– with gas I–C–U+ K/A (KI) **M. morganii** M– with gas I+C–U+ K/A (KI) |

**PPA Negative:**

| Mannitol Positive | Mannitol Negative |
|---|---|
| **Citrobacter spp.** **E. coli** [inactive] **Hafnia spp.** **Salmonella spp.** **Shigella spp.** [other than S. dysenteriae] **S. marscecens** | **Edwardsiella tarda** isolated from a variety of body sites I+H₂S+ (KI) **S. dysenteriae** usually isolated from stool I-H₂S - (KI) |

**H₂S Positive**

**C. freundii**

**Figure 20-5** Algorithm for the identification of Enterobacteriaceae. * Denotes variability in lactose fermentation reactions. *LF,* Late fermenter; *C,* indicates growth on Simmons citrate agar; *U,* indicates urease reaction; *I,* indicates indole reaction; *MR,* methyl red; +, positive > 90%; – indicates ≤ 10% negative; +/–, > 50%; +, –/+, indicates less than 5% positive]; *KI,* Kligler iron agar; *OD,* ornithine decarboxylase positive; *AD,* arginine decarboxylase positive; *LD,* lysine decarboxylase positive; *PPA,* phenylalanine deamination to phenylpyruvic acid; *M,* mannitol fermentation; *ONPG,* ortho-nitrophenyl-beta-galactoside test. (Algorithm modified from Gould LH et al: Recommendations for diagnosis of Shiga toxin–producing *Escherichia coli* in clinical laboratories, *MMR* 58(RR12):1, 2009.)

**TABLE 20-7** TSI and LIA Reactions Used to Screen for Enteropathogenic Enterobacteriaceae and *Aeromonas/Vibrio* spp.*†

| TSI Reactions‡ | LIA Reactions‡ | Possible Identification |
|---|---|---|
| K/Ⓐ or K/A H₂S + | K/K or K/NC H₂S+ | *Salmonella* serotypes *Edwardsiella* spp. |
| K/A H₂S+ | K/K or K/NC H₂S+ | *Salmonella* serotypes (rare) |
| K/Ⓐ | K/K or K/NC | *Salmonella* serotypes (rare) |
| K/A, H₂S | K/K or K/NC H₂S+ | *Salmonella typhi* (rare) |
| K/Ⓐ | K/A H₂S+ | *Salmonella paratyphi* A (usually H₂S−) |
| K/Ⓐ | K/A or A/A | *Escherichia coli* *Salmonella paratyphi* A *Shigella flexneri* 6 (uncommon) *Aeromonas* spp. (oxidase positive) |
| K/A | K/K or K/NC | *Plesiomonas* sp. (oxidase positive) *Salmonella typhi* (rare) *Vibrio* spp. (oxidase positive) |
| K/A | K/A or A/A | *Escherichia coli* *Shigella* groups A-D *Yersinia* spp. |
| A/Ⓐ H₂S+ | K/K or K/NC H₂S+ | *Salmonella* serotypes (rare) |
| A/A | K/A or A/A | *Escherichia coli* *Yersinia* spp. *Aeromonas* spp. (oxidase positive) *Vibrio cholerae* (rare, oxidase positive) |
| A/A | K/K or K/NC | *Vibrio* spp. (oxidase positive) |

*A*, Acid; Ⓐ, acid and gas production; *H₂S*, hydrogen sulfide; *K*, alkaline; *LIA*, lysine iron agar; *NC*, no change; *TSI*, triple sugar iron agar.

*Vibrio* spp. and *Aeromonas* spp. are included in this table because they grow on the same media as the Enterobacteriaceae and may be enteric pathogens; identification of these organisms is discussed in Chapter 28.

†TSI and LIA reactions described in this table are only screening tests. The identity of possible enteric pathogens must be confirmed by specific biochemical and serologic testing.

‡Details regarding the TSI and LIA procedures can be found in Chapter 13.

performance, and interpretation of these tests). Organisms that exhibit the profiles shown in Table 20-7 require further biochemical profiling and, in the case of *Salmonella* spp. and *Shigella* spp., serotyping to establish a definitive identification. Bacterial species not considered capable of causing gastrointestinal infections give profiles other than those shown, but further testing may be required.

In most clinical laboratories, serotyping of Enterobacteriaceae is limited to the preliminary grouping of *Salmonella* spp., *Shigella* spp., and *E. coli* O157:H7. Typing should be performed from a non–sugar-containing medium, such as 5% sheep blood agar or LIA. Use of sugar-containing media, such as MacConkey or TSI agars, can cause the organisms to autoagglutinate.

Commercially available polyvalent antisera designated A, B, C₁, C₂, D, E, and Vi are commonly used to preliminarily group *Salmonella* spp. because 95% of isolates belong to groups A through E. The antisera A through E contain antibodies against somatic ("O") antigens, and the Vi antiserum is prepared against the capsular ("K") antigen of *S.* serotype Typhi. Typing is performed using a slide agglutination test. If an isolate agglutinates with the Vi antiserum and does not react with any of the "O" groups, then a saline suspension of the organism should be prepared and heated to 100°C for 10 minutes to inactivate the Vi antigen. The organism should then be retested. *S. typhi* is positive with Vi and group D. Complete typing of *Salmonella* spp., including the use of antisera against the flagellar ("H") antigens, is performed at reference laboratories.

Preliminary serologic grouping of *Shigella* spp. is also performed using commercially available polyvalent somatic ("O") antisera designated A, B, C, and D. As with *Salmonella* spp., *Shigella* spp. may produce a capsule and therefore heating may be required before typing is successful. Subtyping of *Shigella* spp. beyond the groups A, B, and C (*Shigella* group D only has one serotype) is typically performed in reference laboratories.

*P. shigelloides*, a new member of the Enterobacteriaceae that can cause gastrointestinal infections (see Chapter 26), might cross-react with *Shigella* grouping antisera, particularly group D, and lead to misidentification. This mistake can be avoided by performing an oxidase test.

Sorbitol-negative *E. coli* can be serotyped using commercially available antisera to determine whether the somatic "O" antigen 157 and the flagellar "H" antigen 7 are present. Latex reagents and antisera are now also available for detecting some non-O157, sorbitol-fermenting, Shiga toxin–producing strains of *E. coli* (Meridian Diagnostics, Cincinnati, Ohio; Oxoid, Ogdensburg, New York). Some national reference laboratories therefore are simply performing tests for Shiga toxin rather than searching for O157 or non-O157 strains by culture. Unfortunately, isolates are not available then for strain typing for epidemiologic purposes. Laboratory tests to identify enteropathogenic, enterotoxigenic, enteroinvasive, and enteroaggregative *E. coli* that cause gastrointestinal infections usually involve animal, tissue culture, or molecular studies performed in reference laboratories.

The current recommendation for the diagnosis of Shiga toxin–producing *E. coli* includes testing all stools submitted from patients with acute community-acquired diarrhea to detect enteric pathogens (*Salmonella*, *Shigella*, and *Campylobacter* spp.) should be cultured for O157 STEC on selective and differential agar. In addition, these stools should be tested using either a Shiga toxin detection assay or a molecular assay to simultaneously determine whether the sample contains a non-O157 STEC. To save media, some laboratories may elect to perform the assay first, then attempt to grow organisms from broths with an assay-positive result on selective media. In any case, any isolate or broth positive for O157STEC, non-O157STEC, or shiga toxin should be forwarded to the public health laboratory for confirmation and direct immunoassay testing. Any isolate positive for O157 STEC should be forwarded to the public health laboratory for additional epidemiologic analysis. Any specimens or enrichment broths that are positive for Shiga toxin or STEC but negative for O157 STEC should also be forward to the public health laboratory for further testing.

Most commercial systems can identify *Y. pestis* if a heavy inoculum is used. All isolates biochemically grouped as a *Yersinia* sp. should be reported to the public health laboratory. *Y. pestis* should always be reported and confirmed.

## SERODIAGNOSIS

Serodiagnostic techniques are used for only two members of the family Enterobacteriaceae; that is, *S. typhi* and *Y. pestis*. Agglutinating antibodies can be measured in the diagnosis of typhoid fever; a serologic test for *S. typhi* is part of the "febrile agglutinins" panel and is individually known as the Widal test. Because results obtained by using the Widal test are somewhat unreliable, this method is no longer widely used.

Serologic diagnosis of plague is possible using either a passive hemagglutination test or enzyme-linked immunosorbent assay; these tests are usually performed in reference laboratories.

## ANTIMICROBIAL SUSCEPTIBILITY TESTING AND THERAPY

For many of the gastrointestinal infections caused by Enterobacteriaceae, inclusion of antimicrobial agents as part of the therapeutic strategy is controversial or at least uncertain (Table 20-8).

For extraintestinal infections, antimicrobial therapy is a vital component of patient management (Table 20-9). Although a broad spectrum of agents may be used for therapy against Enterobacteriaceae (see Table 12-6 for a detailed list), every clinically relevant species is capable of acquiring and using one or more of the resistance mechanisms discussed in Chapter 14. The unpredictable nature of any clinical isolate's antimicrobial susceptibility requires that testing be done as a guide to therapy. As discussed in Chapter 12, several standard methods and commercial systems have been developed for this purpose. Table 20-10 presents intrinsic patterns of resistance identified in Enterobacteriaceae.

## EXTENDED SPECTRUM β-LACTAMASE (ESBL)–PRODUCING ENTEROBACTERIACEAE

Enterobacteriaceae are capable of producing β-lactamases that hydrolyze penicillins and cephalosporins, including the extended spectrum cephalosporins (cefoxime, ceftriazone, ceftizoxime, and ceftazidime). These enzymes are referred to as *ESBLs*. A chromogenic agar has been developed for the detection of ESBLs. The agar chrom ID ESBL (bioMerieux, Marcy l'Etolle, France) uses cefpodoxime as a substrate to increase the recovery and sensitivity of CTX-M type ESBL isolates. Some limitations must be considered in the use of this medium, including hyperproducing *AmpC* (*Enterobacter* and *Citrobacter* spp.) and hyperproducing penicillinase (*K. oxytoca*) false positives. In addition, both Vitek 2 (bioMerieux, Durham, North Carolina) and Phoenix (Becton Dickinson, Sparks, Maryland) have ESBL panels, with expert interpretation

**TABLE 20-8** Therapy for Gastrointestinal Infections Caused by Enterobacteriaceae

| Organisms | Therapeutic Strategies |
|---|---|
| Enterotoxigenic *Escherichia coli* (ETEC)<br>    Enteroinvasive *E. coli* (EIEC)<br>    Enteropathogenic *E. coli* (EPEC)<br>    Enterohemorrhagic *E. coli* (EHEC)<br>    Enteroaggregative *E. coli* (EAEC) | Supportive therapy, such as oral rehydration, is indicated in cases of severe diarrhea; for life-threatening infections, such as hemolytic-uremic syndrome associated with EHEC, transfusion and hemodialysis may be necessary. Antimicrobial therapy may shorten the duration of gastrointestinal illness, but many of these infections resolve without such therapy. Because these organisms may develop resistance (see Table 20-7), antimicrobial drug therapy for non–life-threatening infections may be contraindicated |
| *Shigella* spp. | Oral rehydration; antimicrobial drug therapy may be used to shorten the period of fecal excretion and perhaps limit the clinical course of the infection. However, because of the risk of resistance, using antimicrobial drug therapy for less serious infections may be questioned. |
| *Salmonella* serotypes | For enteric fevers (e.g., typhoid fever) and extraintestinal infections (e.g., bacteremia), antimicrobial agents play an important role in therapy. Potentially effective agents for typhoid include quinolones, chloramphenicol, trimethoprim/sulfamethoxazole, and advanced-generation cephalosporins, such as ceftriaxone; however, first- and second-generation cephalosporins and aminoglycosides are not effective. For nontyphoidal *Salmonella* bacteremia, a third-generation cephalosporin (e.g., ceftriaxone) is frequently used. For gastroenteritis, replacement of fluids is most important. Antimicrobial therapy generally is not recommended either for treatment of the clinical infection or for shortening the amount of time a patient excretes the organism. |
| *Yersinia enterocolitica* and *Yersinia pseudotuberculosis* | The need for antimicrobial therapy for enterocolitis and mesenteric lymphadenitis is not clear. In cases of bacteremia, pseudotuberculosis piperacillin, third-generation cephalosporins, aminoglycosides, and trimethoprim/sulfamethoxazole are potentially effective agents. *Y. enterocolitica* is frequently resistant to ampicillin and first-generation cephalosporins, whereas *Y. pseudotuberculosis* isolates are generally susceptible |

**TABLE 20-9** Antimicrobial Therapy and Susceptibility Testing of Clinically Relevant Enterobacteriaceae

| Organism | Therapeutic Options | Potential Resistance to Therapeutic Options | Testing Methods* | Comments |
|---|---|---|---|---|
| *Escherichia coli, Citrobacter* spp., *Enterobacter* spp., *Morganella* spp., *Proteus* spp., *Providencia* spp., *Serratia* spp. | Several agents from each major class of antimicrobials, including aminoglycosides, beta-lactams, and quinolones, have activity. See Table 12-7 for a list of specific agents that should be selected for in vitro testing. For urinary tract infections, single agents may be used; for systemic infections, potent beta-lactams are used, frequently in combination with an aminoglycoside. | Yes; every species is capable of expressing resistance to one or more antimicrobials belonging to each drug class. | As documented in Chapter 12; disk diffusion agar dilution and commercial systems | In vitro susceptibility testing results are important for guiding broth dilution and therapy. |
| *Yersinia pestis* | Streptomycin is the therapy of choice; tetracycline and chloramphenicol are effective alternatives. | Yes, but rare | See CLSI document M100-515; testing must be performed only in a licensed reference laboratory. | Manipulation of cultures for susceptibility testing is dangerous for laboratory personnel and is not necessary. |

*Validated testing methods include standard methods recommended by the Clinical and Laboratory Standards Institute (CLSI) and commercial methods approved by the U.S. Food and Drug Administration (FDA).

available for clinical diagnostic use. Table 20-11 presents an example of an ESBL pattern from a clinical isolate that may require technical interpretation and correction before the results are reported.

ESBLs can occur in bacteria other than *Klebsiella* spp., *E. coli*, and *Proteus mirabilis*. The Clinical and Laboratory Standards Institute and (CLSI) has created guidelines (CLISI document M-100 and M100-S23) for the minimum inhibitory concentration (MIC) and disk diffusion breakpoints for aztreonam, cefotaxime, cefpodoxime, ceftazidime, and ceftriaxone for *E. coli*, *Proteus*, and *Klebsiella* spp., as well as for cefpodoxime, ceftazidime, and cefotaxime for *P. mirabilis*. The sensitivity of the screening increases with the use of more than a single drug. ESBLs are inhibited by clavulanic acid; therefore, this property can be used as a confirmatory test in the identification process. In addition, with regard to cases in which moxalactam, cefonicid, cefamandole, or cefoperazone is being considered to treat infection caused by *E. coli*, *Klebsiella* spp., or *Proteus* spp., it is important to note that interpretive guidelines have not been evaluated, and ESBL testing should be performed. If isolates test ESBL positive, the results of the antibiotics listed should be reported as resistant.

CLSI has revised the interpretive criteria for cephalosporins (cefazolin, cefotaxime, ceftazidime, ceftizoxime, and ceftriaxone) and aztreonam. Using the new interpretive guidelines, routine ESBL testing is no longer necessary, and it is no longer necessary to edit results for cephalosporins, aztreonam, or penicillins from susceptible to resistant. ESBL testing will remain useful for epidemiologic and infection control purposes.

# EXPANDED-SPECTRUM CEPHALOSPORIN RESISTANCE AND CARBAPENEMASE RESISTANCE

The explosion of molecular biology in the past two decades has provided alternatives to phenotypic strategies for the identification of organisms and the genotyping of drug resistance. The bacterial chromosome represents the majority of the genetic make-up or genome within a single organism. However, many genes may be located on extra-chromosomal elements, including transposons and plasmids that are capable of independent replication and movement between organisms. Plasmids exist as double-stranded, closed, circular miniature chromosomes. A single bacterial cell may contain several plasmids. Transposable elements are pieces of DNA that move from one genetic element to another, such as from the plasmid to the chromosome or vice versa (see Chapter 2). Multi-drug resistant organisms are increasing in frequency on a worldwide basis due to the presence of these mobile genetic elements. In addition, these elements may have a complex structure, including the presence of integrans, which are genetic elements specifically designed to take up and incorporate or integrate genes such as those that encode antibiotic resistance.

In the last decade, a very serious emerging mechanism of resistance referred to as carbapenemase resistance has developed in the Enterobacteriaceae family in both hospital and community-acquired infections. Carbapenemase is currently the last treatment option for infections caused by multi-drug resistant bacteria. The various

**TABLE 20-10** Intrinsic Antibiotic Resistance in Enterobacteriaceae*

| | Escherichia hermannii | Hafnia alvei | Serratia marcescens | Yersinia enterocolitica | K. pneumoniae | CITROBACTER | | ENTEROBACTER | | PROTEUS | | | PROVIDENCIA | |
| --- | --- | --- | --- | --- | --- | --- | --- | --- | --- | --- | --- | --- | --- | --- |
| | | | | | | C. freundii | C. koseri | E. cloacae | E. aerogenes | P. vulgaris | P. mirabilis | P. penneri | P. rettgeri | P. stuartii |
| Ampicillin | R | R | R | R | R | R | R | R | R | R | | R | R | R |
| Amoxicillin/ clavulanate | R | R | R | R | | R | R | R | R | | | | R | R |
| Ampicillin/ sulbactam | R | R | R | | | R | R | R | R | | | | | |
| Piperacillin | | | | | | | R | | | | | | | |
| Ticarcillin | R | | | R | R | | R | | | R | | R | R | R |
| Cephalosporins I: cefazolin and cephalothin | | R | R | R | | R | | R | R | R | | R | R | |
| Cephamycins cefoxitin, and cefotetan | | R | R | | | R | | R | R | | | | | |
| Cephalosporins II: cefuroxime | | | R | | | R | | R | R | R | | R | | |
| Tetracyclines | | | | | | | | | | R | R | R | R | R |
| Nitrofurantoin | | | R | | | | | | | R | R | R | R | R |
| Polymyxin B Colistin | | | R | | | | | | | R | R | R | R | R |

Modified from Clinical and Laboratory Standards Institute (CLSI): *Performance standards for antimicrobial susceptibility testing—nineteenth informational supplement*, CLS Document M100-S21, Wayne, Pa, 2011.

*Cephalosporins III, cefepime, aztreonam, ticarcillin/clavulanate, piperacillin/tazobactam, and the carbapenems are not listed because the Enterobacteriaceae have no intrinsic resistance in to these antibiotics.

**TABLE 20-11** Extended Beta-Lactamase Antibiotic Resistance Pattern Based on Vitek 2 Gram-Negative Susceptibility AST-GN24 of an *E. coli* Isolate

| Antibiotic | Vitek 2 | | Expert* | | Final† | |
|---|---|---|---|---|---|---|
| Amikacin | 16 | S | 16 | S | 16 | S |
| Ampicillin | ≥32 | R | ≥32 | R | ≥32 | R |
| Ampicillin/sulbactam | ≥32 | R | ≥32 | R | ≥32 | R |
| Cefazolin | ≥64 | R | ≥64 | R | >-64 | R |
| Cefepime | 2 | S | 2 | R | 2 | R |
| Cefoxitin | ≥64 | R | ≥64 | R | ≥64 | R |
| Ceftazidime | ≥64 | R | ≥64 | R | ≥64 | R |
| Ceftriaxone | ≥64 | R | ≥64 | R | ≥64 | R |
| Ciprofloxacin | ≥4 | R | ≥4 | R | ≥4 | R |
| Ertapenem | ≤0.5 | S | ≤0.5 | S | ≤0.5 | S |
| ESBL | Pos | + | Pos | + | Pos | + |
| Gentamicin | ≤1 | S | ≤1 | S | ≤1 | S |
| Imipenem | ≤1 | S | ≤1 | S | ≤1 | S |
| Levofloxacin | ≥8 | R | ≥8 | R | ≥8 | R |
| Nitrofurantoin | ≤16 | S | ≤16 | S | ≤16 | S |
| Piperacillin/tazobactam | 16 | S | 16 | S | 16 | S |
| Tobramycin | ≥16 | R | ≥16 | R | ≥16 | R |
| Trimethoprim/sulfamethoxazole | ≤20 | S | ≤20 | S | ≤20 | S |

Suggested antibiogram correction: Therapeutic interpretations suggest corrections to cefepime; all other cephalosporins were already resistant.
*Note:* All the cephalosporins except cefepime display a resistance pattern.
*Expert findings indicate that susceptibility results are fully consistent with the organism identification.
†Final column indicates that the laboratory technologist corrected the interpretation as indicated before reporting the results to the physician.

classes of carbapenemases include KPC (Class A) VIM, IMP, NDM (Class B), and OXA-48 (Class D). Class A, C, and D β-lactamases are the enzymes that contain serine at the active site. The metallo-β-lactamases (Class B) require a zinc ion for hydrolysis. Genes encoding the β-lactamase enzymes mutate continuously in response to the heavy pressure exerted by antibiotic use. Amp-C class (Class C) genes that were originally carried on chromosomes are now found on plasmids. The last class of β-lactamases is referred to as oxacillanses (Class D) and contains a higher hydrolysis rate for oxacillin than penicillin.

The resistant mechanism is typically plasmid-borne, and the gene product is capable of hydrolyzing almost all known β-lactam antibiotics. The plasmids that harbor these mobile genetic elements include the various classes of non-typeable plasmids (using current PCR-based replicon typing) and the IncHI family of plasmids. These plasmids demonstrate conjugative transfer (movement between individual bacterial cells) at a higher frequency at 30 °C than at 37 °C. The carbapenemase resistance gene within these plasmids may also be included in a cassette of genes that are flanked by insertion sequences or small transposons that facilitate the movement of the gene between genetic elements. In addition, many of these genes in particular the NDM (Class B) are neither species- nor plasmid-specific, therefore indicating a limitless boundary for spread of this resistance. OXA-48 is carried on a composite transposon known as TN1999 or variants of the transposon known as TN1999.2 and TN1999.3. The metallo-β lactamases are also transferable via a plasmid, and in addition to β-lactamase resistance, the strains are frequently resistant to aminoglycosides and fluorquinolones while remaining susceptible to polymixins.

It appears that these resistant determinants are capable of existing in a very diverse genetic background and able to move from one genetic element to another, one organism to another, and across genus and species lines in an unlimited capacity. It is therefore important for practitioners and laboratorians to not overlook or ignore any new emerging antibiotic patterns of resistance where they least expect them to occur. On February 14, 2013 the Center for Disease Control distributed an official CDC Health Alert through their Health Alert Network indicating that new carbapenem-resistant Enterobacteriaceae warrant additional action by healthcare providers. This alert was based on four key points:

1. While carbapenemase resistance may still be uncommon in some areas, at least 15 unusual biochemical resistance forms have been reported in the United States since July, 2012.

2. This increases the need for healthcare providers to work to aggressively prevent the emergence of CRE.

3. Guidelines are currently available from CDC to prevent CRE (e.g., contact precautions). Guidelines are available at http://www.cdc.gov/hai/organisms/cre/cre-toolkit/index.html.

4. Many of these organisms have been identified in patients within the United States following previous treatment and/or medication outside of the United States. These isolates should be referred to a reference laboratory for confirmatory susceptibility testing that should minimally include an evaluation for KPC and NDM carbapenemases.

## MULTIDRUG-RESISTANT TYPHOID FEVER (MDRTF)

Multidrug-resistant typhoid fever is caused by *S.* serotype Typhi strains resistant to chloramphenicol, ampicillin, and cotrimoxazole. Isolates classified as MDRTF have been indentified since the early 1990s in patients of all ages. The risk for the development of MDRTF is associated with the overuse, misuse and inappropriate use of antibiotic therapy. Susceptibility tests should be performed using the typical first-line antibiotics, including chloramphenicol, ampicillin, and trimethoprim-sulfamethoxazole, along with a fluoroquinolone and a nalidixic acid (to detect reduced susceptibility to fluoroquinolones), a third-generation cephalosporin, and any other antibiotic currently used for treatment.

## PREVENTION

Vaccines are available for typhoid fever and bubonic plague; however, neither is routinely recommended in the United States. An oral, multiple-dose vaccine prepared against *S.* serotype Typhi strain Ty2la or a parenteral single-dose vaccine containing Vi antigen is available for people traveling to an endemic area or for household contacts of a documented *S.* serotype Typhi carrier.

An inactivated multiple-dose, whole-cell bacterial vaccine is available for bubonic plague for people traveling to an endemic area. However, this vaccine does not provide protection against pneumonic plague. Individuals exposed to pneumonic plague should be given chemoprophylaxis with doxycycline (adults) or trimethoprim/sulfamethoxazole (children younger than 8 years of age).

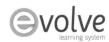 *Visit the Evolve site to complete the review questions.*

---

## CASE STUDY 20-1

A 47-year-old woman who had undergone kidney transplantation 2 years earlier presented to the hospital with fever and confusion. Blood cultures obtained on admission were positive with a gram-negative rod. A direct identification strip was inoculated from the blood culture that keyed out as *Shigella* spp., with very few positive reactions. It did not type with *Shigella* antisera. The test was repeated from a colony the next day, with the same low number of positive reactions. However, the technologist noticed that the original strip had been incubating on the counter and was now positive for urease and a number of sugar fermentation reactions. A new code was determined adding the additional reactions, and the organism keyed out as *Yersinia pseudotuberculosis*. When the patient was questioned, she admitted that she had been eating unpasteurized imported goat cheese.

### QUESTIONS

1. What tests would you do to confirm the identification of *Y. pseudotuberculosis*?

2. Why did the reactions change in the second incubation period?

3. Had this organism been *Yersinia pestis,* which causes plague and is included on the list of potential agents for biologic warfare, what reactions would have been different?

4. If the isolate had been urease negative and nonmotile, what be the next step in the diagnostic process?

---

## CASE STUDY 20-2

An 84-year-old rancher presents to the outpatient clinic with a chief complaint of abdominal cramps and diarrhea for 2 days. He is diagnosed with viral gastroenteritis and sent home on antidiarrheal medication.

Three days later he returns, complaining of several bloody, liquid stools per day with associated severe abdominal cramping. He has associated weakness, dizziness on standing, and dyspnea.

He has a past history of renal insufficiency, congestive heart failure (CHF), coronary artery disease (CAD), peripheral artery disease (PAD), and chronic obstructive pulmonary disease (COPD). In addition to several other prescription medications, he takes 40 mg of prednisone daily, because he was diagnosed with polymyalgia rheumatica 1 month ago.

He denies any travel history or known ill contacts. He continues to operate his own ranch and often butchers his cattle for his own use. He has not eaten at any restaurants; however, when asked about his eating habits, he admits to eating raw hamburger almost daily. He explains that he prepares it according to his native Lebanese custom, and he believes that it is safe to do this because the meat comes from his own ranch and therefore is not "contaminated" in a packing plant.

He is found to be febrile and dehydrated and is admitted to the hospital for intravenous (IV) hydration and further investiga-

## CASE STUDY 20-2—cont'd

tion. Empirically, he is started on IV tigecycline. Given his previous vascular disease history, ischemic colitis is suspected.

### PATIENT VITAL SIGNS

WEIGHT IS DOWN 8 LB FROM PRIOR VISIT, temperature 101.0, pulse 110, respirations 20, blood pressure 100/59

### INITIAL EVALUATION

CT scan of the abdomen revealed bowel wall thickening consistent with colitis.

BUN 59, creatinine (CR) 1.6, K (potassium) 3.0, Na (sodium) 138, Cl (chloride)100

Liver function tests (LFTs) were normal.

Amylase and lipase were normal.

Complete blood count: WBC 16K, HGB 15.5, HCT 47, PLTS 242

Stool for *Clostridium difficile* testing and culture was obtained. Three consecutive stools were all negative for *C. diff.* Two days later stool culture was negative for *Salmonella, Shigella* and *Campylobacter* spp.

After 3 days of hospitalization, subsequent evaluation revealed:

WBC 11K, HGB 12, HCT 36

BUN 30, CR 1.6

Peripheral smear was positive for a few schistocytes.

LFTs revealed slightly elevated bilirubin (BILI) of 3.0

The patient received aggressive hydration therapy. His infection proved self-limited, resolving by day 4 of hospitalization. He was when discharged.

### QUESTIONS

1. What is the most likely route of transmission or source of the patient's infection?
2. What is *the most likely* etiologic agent of this infection?
3. Describe the spectrum of disease possible with this type of infection.

## BIBLIOGRAPHY

Bear N, Klugman KP, Tobiansky L et al: Wound colonization by *Ewingella americana, J Clin Microbiol* 23:650, 1986.

Clinical and Laboratory Standards Institute (CLISI): *Performance standards for antimicrobial susceptibility testing—nineteenth informational supplement,* CLS Document M100-S21, Wayne, Pa, 2011, the Institute.

CLSI Supplement: *Performance Standards for Antimicrobial Susceptibility Testing; twenty third informational supplement,* Wayne, Pa., M100-S23, 2013, CLSI.

Committee on Infectious Diseases: *2006 Red book: report of the Committee on Infectious Diseases,* ed 27, Elk Grove, Ill, 2006, American Academy of Pediatrics.

Devreese K, Claeys, G, Verschraegen G: Septicemia with *Ewingella americana, J Clin Microbiol* 30:2746, 1992.

Difco Laboratories: *Differentiation of Enterobacteriaceae by biochemical tests,* Detroit, 1980, Difco Laboratories.

Dolejska M, Villa L, Poirel L, et al: Complete sequencing of an IncHI1 plasmid encoding the carbapenemase NDM-1, the ARMA 16S RNA methylase and a resistance-nodulation-cell division/multidrug efflux pum, *J Antimicrob Ther* 68(1): 34-39, 2013.

Gould LH et al: Recommendations for diagnosis of Shiga toxin-producing *Escherichia coli* in clinical laboratories, *MMR* 58(RR12):1, 2009.

Holt JG, Krieg NR, Sneath PH et al, editors: *Bergey's manual of determinative bacteriology,* ed 9, Baltimore, 1994, Williams & Wilkins.

Khan R, Rizvi M, Shukia I, Malik A: A novel approach for identification of members of Enterobacteriaceae isolated from clinical samples, *Biol Med* 3:313, 2011.

Mandell GL, Bennett JE, Dolin R: *Principles and practices of infectious diseases,* ed 7, Philadelphia, 2010, Churchill Livingstone/Elsevier.

Mortimer CKB, Peters TM, Bharbia SE et al: Towards the development of a DNA sequence– based approach to serotyping of *Salmonella enterica, BMC Microbiol* 4:31, 2004.

National Committee for Clinical Laboratory Standards (NCCLS): *Abbreviated identification of bacteria and yeast: approved guideline M35-A,* Wayne, Pa, 2002, NCCLS.

Noyal MJS, Menezes GA, Harish BN, et al: Simple screening for detection of carbapenemases in clinical isolates of nonfermenting Gram-negative bacteria, *Indian J Med Res* 129, 2009.

Oteo J, Hernandez JM, Espasa M, et al: Emergence of OXA-48 producing *Klebsiella pneumoniae* and the novel cabapenemeases OXA-244 and OXA-245 in Spain, *J Antimicrob Chemo* 68:317-321, 2013.

Schultsz C, Geerlings S: Plasmid-mediated resistance in Enterobacteriaceae, changing landscape and implications for therapy, *Drugs* 72(1):1-16, 2012.

Stiles ME, Ng LK: Biochemical characteristics and identification of Enterobacteriaceae isolated from meats, *Apply Environ Microbiol* 41:639, 1981.

Versalovic J: *Manual of clinical microbiology,* ed 10, Washington, DC, 2011, ASM Press.

Zaki SA, Karande S: Multidrug-resistant typhoid fever: a review, *J Infect Dev Ctries* 5:324, 2011.

Yong DCT, Thompson JS, Prytula A: Rapid microbiochemical method for presumptive identification of gastroenteritis-associated members of the family Enterobacteriaceae, *J Clin Microbiol* 21:914, 1985.

# Acinetobacter, Stenotrophomonas, and Similar Organisms

1. List the most common gram-negative organisms discussed in this chapter that are encountered in clinical specimens.
2. Explain where *Acinetobacter* spp. are found and the patients most at risk of infection.
3. Describe the Gram stain morphology of *Acinetobacter, Bordetella,* and *Stenotrophomonas* spp.
4. Describe the appearance and odor of *Stenotrophomonas maltophilia* when grown on blood agar.
5. Differentiate between the two groups of *Acinetobacter* organisms and identify the most dependable test to distinguish between the groups.

## GENERA AND SPECIES TO BE CONSIDERED

| Current Name | Previous Name |
|---|---|
| *Acinetobacter* spp.; saccharolytic, nonhemolytic | *Acinetobacter baumannii, A. calcoaceticus, A. anitratus, A. calcoaceticus* subsp. *anitratus* |
| *Acinetobacter* spp.; saccharolytic, hemolytic | *Acinetobacter alcaligenes, A. anitratus, A. haemolyticus* |
| *Acinetobacter* spp.; asaccharolytic, nonhemolytic | *Acinetobacter calcoaceticus* subsp *lwoffi, A. johnsonii, A. junii, A. lwoffi* |
| *Acinetobacter* spp.; asaccharolytic, hemolytic | |
| *Bordetella holmesii* | CDC group NO-2 |
| *Bordetella parapertussis* | |
| *Bordetella trematum* | |
| *Burkholderia gladioli* | *Pseudomonas gladioli, P. marginata* |
| **CDC group NO-1** | |
| *Pseudomonas luteola* | *Chrysemonas luteola,* CDC Group Ve-1 |
| *Pseudomonas oryzihabitans* | *Flavimonas oryzihabitans,* CDC Group Ve-2 |
| *Stenotrophomonas maltophilia* | *Xanthomonas maltophilia, Pseudomonas maltophilia* |

## GENERAL CHARACTERISTICS

The organisms discussed in this chapter are considered together because, except for CDC group NO-1, they are all oxidase negative and grow on MacConkey agar, as do the Enterobacteriaceae. However, unlike the Enterobacteriaceae, which ferment glucose, these organisms either oxidize glucose (i.e., they are saccharolytic), or they do not utilize glucose (i.e., they are nonoxidizers, or asaccharolytic). Although CDC group NO-1 is oxidase negative and does not usually grow on MacConkey agar, it is included here because it must be distinguished from the asaccharolytic *Acinetobacter* spp. Based on molecular studies, approximately 21 species and/or strains of

*Acinetobacter* spp. have been identified. The specific morphologic and physiologic features of the organisms are considered later in this chapter in the discussion of laboratory diagnosis. Of note, only *Acinetobacter* and *Stenotrophomonas* spp. are routinely found in clinical specimens. *Bordetella parapertussis* is included in Table 21-4 in this chapter but is discussed in Chapter 37.

## EPIDEMIOLOGY

The organisms discussed in this chapter inhabit environmental niches. *Acinetobacter* spp. and *Stenotrophomonas maltophilia* are widely distributed in moist natural and hospital environments (Table 21-1). *Acinetobacter* spp. can be found on fomites and in soil, water, and animal food products. These organisms are capable of survival on inanimate objects for extended periods. *Acinetobacter* spp. is a human skin colonizer in 0.5% to 3% of the general population and has been identified from a number of human sources, including sputum, urine, feces, and vaginal secretions. *S. maltophilia* may be found in tap water and salads. Although none of these organisms are considered normal human flora, the relatively high prevalence of *Acinetobacter* spp. and *S. maltophilia* in hospitals frequently results in colonization of the skin and respiratory tract of patients. The prevalence of these organisms is evidenced by the fact that, excluding the Enterobacteriaceae, *Acinetobacter* spp. and *S. maltophilia* are the second and third most common gram-negative bacilli, respectively, encountered in clinical specimens. In contrast, *Pseudomonas luteola, Pseudomonas oryzihabitans,* and CDC group NO-1 are not commonly found in clinical specimens but have been isolated from wounds, blood cultures, and dialysis fluids.

## PATHOGENESIS AND SPECTRUM OF DISEASE

All of the organisms listed in Table 21-2 are opportunistic pathogens for which no definitive virulence factors are known. Because *Acinetobacter* spp. and *S. maltophilia* are relatively common colonizers of hospitalized patients, their clinical significance when found in patient specimens can be difficult to establish. In fact, these organisms are more frequently isolated as colonizers than as infecting agents. When infection does occur, it usually is seen in debilitated patients, such as those in burn or intensive care units and those who have undergone medical instrumentation and/or have received multiple antimicrobial agents. *Acinetobacter baumannii* is typically the species identified in hospital-acquired infections. Infections caused by *Acinetobacter* spp. and *S. maltophilia* usually

**TABLE 21-1** Epidemiology

| Species | Habitat (Reservoir) | Mode of Transmission |
|---|---|---|
| *Acinetobacter* spp. | Widely distributed in nature, including the hospital environment. May become established as part of skin and respiratory flora of patients hospitalized for prolonged periods | Colonization of hospitalized patients from environmental factors; medical instrumentation (e.g., intravenous or urinary catheters) introduces organism to normally sterile sites |
| *Stenotrophomonas maltophilia* | Widely distributed in nature, including moist hospital environments. May become established as part of respiratory flora of patients hospitalized for prolonged periods | Colonization of hospitalized patients from environmental factors; medical instrumentation introduces organism to normally sterile sites (similar to transmission of *Acinetobacter* spp.) |
| CDC group NO-1 | Oropharynx of animals. Not part of human flora | Animal bite or scratch |
| *Burkholderia gladioli* | Environmental pathogen of plants; occasionally found in respiratory tract of patients with cystic fibrosis but not part of normal flora | Transmission to humans uncommon, mode of transmission not known |
| *Pseudomonas luteola* *Pseudomonas oryzihabitans* | Environmental, including moist hospital environments (e.g., respiratory therapy equipment). Not part of normal human flora | Uncertain; probably involves exposure of debilitated hospital patients to contaminated fluids and medical equipment |
| *Bordetella holmesii* *B. trematum* | Unknown or part of normal human flora | Unknown; rarely found in humans |

**TABLE 21-2** Pathogenesis and Spectrum of Diseases

| Species | Virulence Factors | Spectrum of Disease and Infections |
|---|---|---|
| *Acinetobacter* spp. | Unknown | Clinical isolates are often colonizers. True infections are usually nosocomial, occur during warm seasons, and most commonly involve the genitourinary tract, respiratory tract, wounds, soft tissues, and bacteremia |
| *Bordetella holmesii* *Bordetella trematum* | Unknown | Bacteremia is the only type of infection described. |
| *Burkholderia gladioli* | Unknown | Role in human disease is uncertain; occasionally found in sputa of patients with cystic fibrosis, but clinical significance in this setting is uncertain. |
| *Pseudomonas luteola,* *P. oryzihabitans* | Unknown | Catheter-related infections, septicemia, and peritonitis, usually associated with continuous ambulatory peritoneal dialysis, and miscellaneous mixed infections of other body sites. |
| *Stenotrophomonas maltophilia* | Unknown. Intrinsic resistance to almost every commonly used antibacterial agent supports the survival of this organism in the hospital environment. | Most infections are nosocomial and include catheter-related infections, bacteremia, wound infections, pneumonia, urinary tract infections, and miscellaneous infections of other body sites. |
| CDC group NO-1 | Unknown | Animal bite wound infections |

involve the respiratory or genitourinary tract, bacteremia and, occasionally, wound infections, although infections involving several other body sites have been described. Community-acquired infections with these organisms can occur, but the vast majority of infections are nosocomial.

# LABORATORY DIAGNOSIS

## SPECIMEN COLLECTION AND TRANSPORT

No special considerations are required for specimen collection and transport of the organisms discussed in this chapter. Refer to Table 5-1 for general information on specimen collection and transport.

## SPECIMEN PROCESSING

No special considerations are required for processing of the organisms discussed in this chapter. Refer to Table 5-1 for general information on specimen processing.

## DIRECT DETECTION METHODS

Other than Gram stain of patient specimens, there are no specific procedures for the direct detection of these organisms in clinical material. *Acinetobacter* spp. are plump coccobacilli that tend to resist alcohol decolorization; they may be mistaken for *Neisseria* spp. The *Bordetella* spp. are coccobacilli or short rods. *S. maltophilia, P. oryzihabitans,* and *P. luteola* are short to medium-size straight rods. CDC group NO-1 are coccoid to medium-size bacilli.

## CULTIVATION

### Media of Choice

In addition to their ability to grow on MacConkey agar, all of the genera described in this chapter, except CDC group NO-1, grow well on 5% sheep blood and chocolate agars. These organisms also grow well in the broth of blood culture systems and in common nutrient broths, such as thioglycollate and brain-heart infusion.

### Incubation Conditions and Duration

These organisms generally produce detectable growth on 5% sheep blood and chocolate agars when incubated at 35°C in carbon dioxide or ambient air for a minimum of 24 hours. MacConkey agar should be incubated only in ambient air.

### Colonial Appearance

Table 21-3 describes the colonial appearance and other distinguishing characteristics (e.g., hemolysis and odor)

of each genus when grown on 5% sheep blood and MacConkey agars.

## APPROACH TO IDENTIFICATION

*Acinetobacter* spp. and *S. maltophilia* are reliably identified by the API 20E system (bioMérieux, St. Louis, Missouri), although other commercial systems may not perform as well. Automated identification systems typically identify the organisms in this chapter to the genus level. Additional testing may be required to speciate the organisms using conventional biochemical and physiologic characteristics, such as those outlined in Table 21-4.

Molecular methods are invaluable for the speciation of *Acinetobacter* spp. Sequence-based methods, including amplification of the ribosomal RNA (rRNA) sequence, genomic fingerprinting, and restriction endonuclease analysis, have been used to identify *Acinetobacter* spp.

### Comments Regarding Specific Organisms

The genus *Acinetobacter* has 21 genospecies or genomospecies. Each genospecies comprises a distinct DNA hybridization group and is given a numeric designation, which has replaced previous species names. *Acinetobacter* species are oxidase negative, catalase positive and nonmotile. The genus also is divided into two groups: the saccharolytic (glucose oxidizing) species and the asaccharolytic (non–glucose utilizing) species.

**TABLE 21-3** Colonial Appearance and Characteristics

| Organism | Medium | Appearance |
|---|---|---|
| *Stenotrophomonas maltophilia* | BA | Large, smooth, glistening colonies with uneven edges and lavender-green to light purple pigment; greenish discoloration underneath growth; ammonia smell |
| | Mac | NLF |
| *Acinetobacter* spp. | BA | Smooth, opaque, raised, creamy, and smaller than Enterobacteriaceae; some genospecies are beta-hemolytic |
| | Mac | NLF, but colonies exhibit a purplish hue that may cause the organism to be mistaken for LF (Figure 21-1) |
| *Burkholderia gladioli* | BA | Yellow |
| | Mac | NLF |
| *Bordetella parapertussis* | BA | Smooth, opaque, beta-hemolytic |
| | Mac | NLF, delayed growth |
| *Bordetella holmesii* | BA | Punctate, semiopaque, convex, round, with greening of blood usually accompanied by lysis |
| | Mac | NLF, delayed growth |
| *Bordetella trematum* | BA | Convex, circular, grayish cream to white |
| | Mac | NLF |
| *Pseudomonas oryzihabitans* | BA | Wrinkled, rough or smooth, transparent, yellow |
| | Mac | NLF |
| *Pseudomonas luteola* | BA | Maybe rough and smooth, opaque, yellow |
| | Mac | NLF |
| CDC group NO-1 | BA | Small colonies that can be transferred intact with an inoculating needle |
| | Mac | NLF, but only 20% of strains grow |

*BA,* 5% Sheep blood agar; *LF,* lactose fermenter; *Mac,* MacConkey agar; *NLF,* non–lactose fermenter.

Most glucose-oxidizing, nonhemolytic strains were previously identified as *Acinetobacter baumannii,* and most non–glucose utilizing, nonhemolytic strains were designated as *Acinetobacter lwoffi.* The majority of beta-hemolytic organisms previously were called *Acinetobacter*

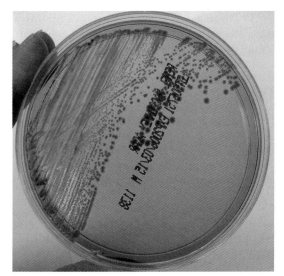

**Figure 21-1** Colony of *Acinetobacter* spp. on MacConkey agar. Note purple color.

*haemolyticus.* Nitrate-reducing strains of asaccharolytic *Acinetobacter* spp. are difficult to differentiate from CDC group NO-1. The *Acinetobacter* transformation test provides the most dependable criterion for this purpose, but this test is not commonly performed in clinical microbiology laboratories.

*S. maltophilia* is an oxidase-negative, nonfermentative, gram-negative bacillus that can produce biochemical profiles similar to those of *Burkholderia cepacia.* A negative oxidase test result most often rules out the latter. *S. maltophilia* also oxidizes maltose faster than glucose (hence the species name, *maltophilia,* or "maltose loving"), and it produces a brown pigment on heart infusion agar that contains tyrosine.

*Pseudomonas* spp. (*Chrysemonas* and *Flavimonas* spp.) are gram-negative, nonfermentative, oxidase-negative, catalase-positive bacilli. The organisms characteristically produce rough colonies that are often yellow pigmented on sheep blood agar.

## SERODIAGNOSIS

Serodiagnostic techniques are not generally used for the laboratory diagnosis of infections caused by the organisms discussed in this chapter.

**TABLE 21-4** Key Biochemical and Physiologic Characteristics

| Organism | Growth on MacConkey | Motile | Oxidizes Glucose | Oxidizes Maltose | Esculin Hydrolysis | Lysine Decarboxylase | Nitrate Reduction | Urea Christensen's |
|---|---|---|---|---|---|---|---|---|
| *Stenotrophomonas maltophilia* | + | + | + | + | V | + | V | – |
| Saccharolytic *Acinetobacter* | + | – | + | – | – | – | – | V |
| Asaccharolytic *Acinetobacter* | + | – | – | V | – | – | – | V |
| *Burkholderia gladioli** | + | + | + | – | – | – | V | V |
| *Bordetella parapertussis* | + | – | – | – | – | ND | – | + |
| *Bordetella holmesii*[†] | + or (+) | – | – | – | – | – | – | – |
| *Bordetella trematum* | + | + | – | – | – | – | V | – |
| *Pseudomonas oryzihabitans* | + | + p, 1-2 | + | + | – | – | – | V |
| *Pseudomonas luteola* | + | + p, >2 | + | + | + | – | V | V |
| CDC group NO-1 | V | – | – | – | – | – | + | – |

Compiled from Reed RP: *Flavimonas oryzihabitans* sepsis in children, *Clin Infect Dis* 22:733, 1996; Seifert H, Strate A, Pulverer G: Nosocomial bacteremia due to *Acinetobacter baumannii:* clinical features, epidemiology, and predictors of mortality, *Medicine* 74:340, 1995; and Weyant RS, Hollis DG, Weaver RE et al: *Bordetella holmesii* sp nov: a new gram-negative species associated with septicemia, *J Clin Microbiol* 33:1, 1995.
*V,* Variable; +, > 90% of strains are positive; –, > 90% of strains are negative; ( ), delayed; *ND,* no data; *p,* polar flagella.
**B. gladioli* is included with the oxidase-negative organisms because oxidase reactions are frequently weak and may only be positive with Kovacs method.
[†]Brown, soluble pigment.

**TABLE 21-5** Antimicrobial Therapy and Susceptibility Testing

| Species | Therapeutic Options | Potential Resistance to Therapeutic Options | Validated Testing Methods* | Comments |
|---|---|---|---|---|
| *Acinetobacter* spp. | No definitive guidelines. Potentially active agents include β-lactam, β-lactam inhibitor, combinations, ceftazidime, imipenem, ciprofloxacin, tigecycline, and aminoglycosides | Yes; resistance to β-lactams, carbapenems, aminoglycosides, and quinolones | Disk diffusion, broth dilution, and agar dilution | In vitro susceptibility testing results are important for guiding therapy. |
| *Bordetella holmesii* | No definitive guidelines. Potentially active agents include penicillins, cephalosporins, and quinolones | Unknown | Not available | |
| *Burkholderia. gladioli* | No definitive guidelines. Potentially active agents include imipenem, piperacillin, and. ciprofloxacin | Yes | See CLSI document M100, Performance Standards for Antimicrobial Susceptibility Testing | Rarely involved in human infections. Reliable therapeutic data are limited. |
| *Pseudomonas luteola* *P. oryzihabitans* | No definitive guidelines. Potentially active agents include cefotaxime, ceftriaxone, ceftazidime, imipenem, quinolones, and aminoglycosides | Yes | See CLSI document M100. | Rarely involved in human infection. |
| *Stenotrophomonas maltophilia* | Multiple resistance leaves few therapeutic choices; therapy of choice is trimethoprim-sulfamethoxazole. Potential alternatives include minocycline, ticarcillin/clavulanic acid, and chloramphenicol | Yes; intrinsically resistant to most beta-lactams and aminoglycosides; frequently resistant to quinolones | See CLSI document M100. | May be tested by various methods, but profiles obtained with beta-lactams can be seriously misleading. |
| CDC group NO-1 | No definitive guidelines. Appear susceptible to beta-lactam antibiotics | Unknown | Not available | |

*Validated testing methods include standard methods recommended by the Clinical and Laboratory Standards Institute (CLSI) and commercial methods approved by the U.S. Food and Drug Administration (FDA).

# ANTIMICROBIAL SUSCEPTIBILITY TESTING AND THERAPY

*Acinetobacter* spp. and *S. maltophilia* can exhibit resistance to a wide array of antimicrobial agents, making the selection of agents for optimal therapy difficult (Table 21-5). In addition, automated methods for determining the minimum inhibitory concentration (MIC) for *Acinetobacter* spp. does not correlate with disk diffusion methods. This underscores the importance of establishing the clinical significance of individual isolates before antimicrobial testing is performed and results are reported (see Chapter 12 for a discussion of criteria used to establish significance). Failure to do so could lead to inappropriate treatment of patients with expensive and potentially toxic agents. If susceptibility testing must be performed, it is recommended that an overnight MIC method be used.

For urinary tract infections caused by *Acinetobacter* spp., single-drug therapy is usually sufficient. In contrast,

more serious infections, such as pneumonia or bacteremia, may require the use of a β-lactam in combination with an aminoglycoside. Tigecycline also has potent activity against these organisms. Because this genus is able to acquire and express resistance to most antimicrobial agents, including imipenem, in vitro testing is recommended for clinically relevant isolates. Methods outlined by the Clinical and Laboratory Standards Institute (CLSI) appear to be suitable for testing *Acinetobacter* spp., *S. maltophilia,* and other organisms listed in Table 21-5.

*S. maltophilia* is notoriously resistant to most currently available antimicrobial agents, leaving trimethoprim-sulfamethoxazole as the primary drug of choice for infections caused by this species. Although a few other agents, such as minocycline, ticarcillin/clavulanic acid, and chloramphenicol, often exhibit in vitro activity, clinical experience with these agents is not extensive. Therefore, trimethoprim-sulfamethoxazole remains the drug of choice.

The other agents should be considered only when trimethoprim-sulfamethoxazole–resistant strains are encountered. Even then, the potential efficacy of these other agents is suspect because of the ability of *S. malto-philia* to rapidly develop resistance. As indicated in Table 21-5, CLSI guidelines are available for the testing of several of the organisms listed in this chapter.

# PREVENTION

Because these organisms are ubiquitous in nature and are not generally a threat to human health, there are no recommended vaccination or prophylaxis protocols. Hospital-acquired infections are best controlled by following appropriate sterile techniques and infection control guidelines and by implementing effective protocols for the sterilization and decontamination of medical supplies.

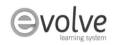 *Visit the Evolve site to complete the review questions.*

---

## CASE STUDY 21-1

A 3-month-old boy who has been hospitalized in the intensive care nursery since birth is recovering from corrective congenital heart surgery. The infant develops signs of sepsis. It is noted that a central line has been in place for some time, through which heparin has been given to reduce clot formation. A blood culture specimen drawn through the line tests positive. Subsequently, a second culture specimen is collected from a peripheral stick. Both specimens grow a gram-negative rod. The child is diagnosed with catheter-related bacteremia; antibiotics and removal of the catheter succeed in clearing the infection.

#### QUESTIONS

1. A commercial system identified the gram-negative bacilli as *Acinetobacter* sp.; however, it indicated that all the biochemical tests in the system, including utilization of glucose, were negative and the identification should be confirmed. What rapid biochemical tests should be used to confirm the identification?
2. The isolate did not grow on MacConkey agar. Which test is needed to separate this genus from NO-1?
3. How did the patient acquire the infection with this microorganism?
4. What is the meaning of a glucose-oxidizing, gram-negative rod?
5. What is the best method of distinguishing an asaccharolytic microorganism from a fastidious gram-negative rod that is unable to grow in of media?

---

# BIBLIOGRAPHY

Bergogne-Berezin E, Towner KJ: *Acinetobacter* spp. as nosocomial pathogens: microbiological, clinical, and epidemiological features, *Clin Microbiol Rev* 9:148, 1996.

Clinical and Laboratory Standards Institute: *Methods for dilution antimicrobial tests for bacteria that grow aerobically, M7-A6,* Villanova, Pa, 2005, CLSI.

Clinical and Laboratory Standards Institute: *Performance standards for antimicrobial disk susceptibility tests, M2-A8,* Villanova, Pa, 2005, CLSI.

CLSI Supplement: Performance standards for antimicrobial susceptibility testing: 23rd informational supplement, Wayne, Pa., 2013, CLSI, M100-S23.

Esteban J, Valero-Moratalla ML, Alcazar R et al: Infections due to *Flavimonas oryzihabitans*: case report and literature review, *Eur J Clin Microbiol Infect Dis* 12:797, 1993.

Garrison MW, Anderson DE, Campbell DM et al: *Stenotrophomonas maltophilia:* emergence of multidrug-resistant strains during therapy and in an in vitro pharmacodynamic chamber model, *Antimicrob Agents Chemother* 40:2859, 1996.

Mandell GL, Bennett JE, Dolin R: *Principles and practices of infectious diseases,* ed 7, Philadelphia, 2010, Churchill Livingstone/Elsevier.

Rahav G, Simhon A, Mattan Y et al: Infections with *Chrysemonas luteola* (CDC group Ve-1) and *Flavimonas oryzihabitans* (CDC group Ve-2), *Medicine* 74:83, 1995.

Reed RP: *Flavimonas oryzihabitans* sepsis in children, *Clin Infect Dis* 22:733, 1996.

Seifert H, Strate A, Pulverer G: Nosocomial bacteremia due to *Acinetobacter baumannii:* clinical features, epidemiology, and predictors of mortality, *Medicine* 74:340, 1995.

Versalovic J: *Manual of clinical microbiology,* ed 10, Washington, DC, 2011, ASM Press.

Weyant RS, Hollis DG, Weaver RE et al: *Bordetella holmesii* sp nov: a new gram-negative species associated with septicemia, *J Clin Microbiol* 33:1, 1995.

# *Pseudomonas, Burkholderia,* and Similar Organisms

## OBJECTIVES

1. Describe the normal sources (habitat) for *Pseudomonas aeruginosa, Burkholderia cepacia, Burkholderia pseudomallei,* and *Burkholderia mallei,* including the routes of transmission.
2. Identify the factors that contribute to the pathogenicity of *P. aeruginosa* and explain the physiologic mechanism for each.
3. List the various disease states associated with *P. aeruginosa* and *Burkholderia* spp.
4. Compare and contrast the Gram stain appearance of the gram-negative bacilli discussed in this chapter.
5. List the appropriate scheme for identifying *P. aeruginosa.*
6. Describe the media and chemical principle of each used, including differential and selective agars that aid the cultivation of *Pseudomonas, Brevundimonas,* and *Ralstonia* spp.
7. Describe the potential therapies for *B. cepacia* and *B. pseudomallei* and the concerns about optimal therapy.
8. Describe and identify the patterns of antibiotic resistance in *P. aeruginosa.*

### GENERA AND SPECIES TO BE CONSIDERED

| Current Name | Previous Name |
|---|---|
| *Acidovorax delafieldii* | *Pseudomonas delafieldii* |
| *Acidovorax facilis* | |
| *Acidovorax temperans* | |
| *Brevundimonas diminuta* | *Pseudomonas diminuta* |
| *Brevundimonas vesicularis* | *Pseudomonas vesicularis* |
| *Burkholderia cepacia* complex | *Pseudomonas cepacia* |
| *Burkholderia pseudomallei* | *Pseudomonas pseudomallei* |
| *Burkholderia mallei* | *Pseudomonas mallei* |
| *Pandoraea* spp. | CDC group WO-2 (five distinct species) |
| *Pseudomonas aeruginosa* | |
| *Pseudomonas fluorescens* | |
| *Pseudomonas mendocina* | |
| *Pseudomonas monteilii* | |
| *Pseudomonas putida* | |
| *Pseudomonas stutzeri* (includes CDC group Vb-3) | CDC group IVd |
| *Pseudomonas veronii* | |
| *Pseudomonas*-like group 2 | |
| **CDC group Ic** | |
| *Ralstonia mannitolilytica* | "*Pseudomonas thomasii,*" *Ralstonia pickettii* biovar 3 |
| *Ralstonia insidiosa* | CDC group IVc-2 |
| *Ralstonia pickettii* | *Pseudomonas pickettii, Burkholderia pickettii,* Va-1, Va-2 |

## GENERAL CHARACTERISTICS

At one time, most of the species belonging to the genera *Brevundimonas, Burkholderia, Ralstonia,* and *Acidovorax* were members of the genus *Pseudomonas.* Organisms in these genera have many similar characteristics. They are aerobic, non–spore-forming, straight, slender, gram-negative bacilli with cells that range from 1 to 5 $\mu$m long and 0.5 to 1 $\mu$m wide. All species except *B. mallei* are motile, having one or several polar flagella. Members of these genera use a variety of carbohydrate, alcohol, and amino acid substrates as carbon and energy sources. Although they are able to survive and possibly grow at relatively low temperatures (i.e., as low as 4°C), the optimum temperature range for growth of most species is 30° to 37°C; that is, they are mesophilic. *Burkholderia gladioli, Pseudomonas luteola,* and *Pseudomonas oryzihabitans* are oxidase negative and are discussed in Chapter 21. *Pseudomonas alcaligenes, Pseudomonas pseudoalcaligenes, Ralstonia paucula, Ralstonia gilardii, Comamonas* spp. (including the former *Pseudomonas testosteroni*), and *Delftia acidovorans* (formerly *Pseudomonas acidovorans*) are not able to utilize glucose and are discussed in Chapter 25. *Acidovorax facilis* is MacConkey negative. *Pseudomonas* spp. are catalase positive. The organisms in this chapter are all oxidase-positive, grow on MacConkey agar, and oxidize glucose.

## EPIDEMIOLOGY

### *BURKHOLDERIA* SPP. AND *RALSTONIA PICKETTII*

*Burkholderia* spp. and *Ralstonia pickettii* are inhabitants of the environment and are not considered part of the normal human flora (Table 22-1). As such, their transmission usually involves human contact with heavily contaminated medical devices or substances encountered in the hospital setting.

*B. cepacia,* which is among the *Burkholderia* spp. found in the United States, is a complex of 10 distinct genomic species (genomovars) isolated from clinical specimens. Plants, soil, and water serve as reservoirs. These organisms are able to survive on or in medical devices and disinfectants. Intrinsic resistance to multiple antimicrobial agents contributes to the organism's survival in

**TABLE 22-1** Epidemiology

| Species | Habitat (Reservoir) | Mode of Transmission |
|---|---|---|
| *Burkholderia cepacia* | Environmental (soil, water, plants); survives well in hospital environment; not part of normal human flora; may colonize respiratory tract of patients with cystic fibrosis | Exposure of medical devices and solutions contaminated from the environment; person-to-person transmission also documented |
| *B. pseudomallei* | Environmental (soil, streams, surface water, such as rice paddies); limited to tropical and subtropical areas, notably Southeast Asia; not part of human flora | Inhalation or direct inoculation from environment through disrupted epithelial or mucosal surfaces |
| *B. mallei* | Causative agent of glanders in horses, mules, and donkeys; not part of human flora | Transmission to humans is extremely rare; associated with close animal contact and introduced through mucous membranes or broken skin. |
| *Ralstonia pickettii* | Environmental (multiple sources); found in variety of clinical specimens; not part of human flora | Mode of transmission is not known; likely involves exposure to contaminated medical devices and solutions |
| *Pseudomonas aeruginosa* | Environmental (soil, water, plants); survives well in domestic environments (e.g., hot tubs, whirlpools, contact lens solutions) and hospital environments (e.g., sinks, showers, respiratory equipment); rarely part of normal flora of healthy humans | Ingestion of contaminated food or water; exposure to contaminated medical devices and solutions; introduction by penetrating wounds; person-to-person transmission is assumed to occur |
| *P. alcaligenes, P. pseudoalcaligenes, Pseudomonas* sp. CDC group 1, "*P. denitrificans,*" *Pseudomonas*-like group 2, and CDC group Ic | Environmental; not part of normal human flora | Uncertain. Rarely encountered in clinical specimens |
| *P. fluorescens, P. putida, P. stutzeri,* (including Vb-3), *P. luteola,* and *P. mendocina* | Environmental (soil and water); not part of normal human flora | Exposure to contaminated medical devices and solutions |
| *Brevundimonas vesicularis* and *B. diminuta* | Environmental; not part of normal human flora | Uncertain. Rarely encountered in clinical specimens |
| *Acidovorax* spp. | Environmental, soil; not part of human flora | Unknown. Rarely found in humans |

hospitals. Human acquisition of *B. cepacia* that results in colonization or infection usually involves direct contact with contaminated foods, devices such as respiratory equipment, or medical solutions, including disinfectants. Person-to-person transmission also has been documented.

*B. pseudomallei* is another environmental inhabitant of niches similar to those described for *B. cepacia;* however, it is geographically restricted to tropical and subtropical areas of Australia and Southeast Asia. The organism is widely disseminated in soil, streams, ponds, and rice paddies. Human acquisition occurs through inhalation of contaminated debris or by direct inoculation through damaged skin or mucous membranes.

Although *B. mallei* causes severe infections in horses and related animals, it has been identified in rare human localized suppurative or acute pulmonary infections. When transmission has occurred, it has been associated with close animal contact. *B. gladioli* is a plant pathogen that is only rarely found in the sputa of patients with cystic fibrosis or associated with chronic granulomatous

disease; the mode of transmission to humans and its clinical significance are unknown.

*R. pickettii* is another environmental organism that is occasionally found in a variety of clinical specimens, such as blood, the sputa of patients with cystic fibrosis, and urine. The mode of transmission is uncertain, but isolates have been found in contaminated sterile hospital fluids.

## PSEUDOMONAS SPP. AND BREVUNDIMONAS SPP.

The genera *Pseudomonas* and *Brevundimonas* comprise several environmental species that rarely inhabit human skin or mucosal surfaces. In the clinical setting, *P. aeruginosa* is the most commonly encountered gram-negative species that is not a member of the family Enterobacteriaceae and is an uncommon member of the normal human flora. The organism survives in various environments in nature and in homes and hospitals (see Table 22-1). *Brevundimonas* spp. are environmental and are

**TABLE 22-2** Pathogenesis and Spectrum of Disease

| Species | Virulence Factors | Spectrum of Disease and Infections |
|---|---|---|
| *Burkholderia cepacia* | Unknown. Binding of mucin from patients with cystic fibrosis may be involved. Intrinsic resistance to multiple antibiotics complicates therapy and may promote organism survival in hospital | Nonpathogenic to healthy human hosts; able to colonize and cause life-threatening infections in patients with cystic fibrosis or chronic granulomatous disease; other patients may suffer nonfatal infections of the urinary tract, respiratory tract, and other sterile body sites |
| *B. pseudomallei* | Unknown. Bacilli can survive within phagocytes | Wide spectrum from asymptomatic infection to melioidosis, of which there are several forms, including infections of the skin and respiratory tract, multisystem abscess formation, and bacteremia with septic shock |
| *B. mallei* | Unknown for human infections | Human disease is extremely rare. Infections range from localized acute or chronic suppurative infections of skin at site of inoculation to acute pulmonary infections and septicemia |
| *Ralstonia pickettii* | Unknown | Rarely encountered as cause of disease; nonpathogenic to healthy human host, but may be isolated from a variety of clinical specimens, including blood, sputum, and urine; when encountered environmental contamination should be suspected |
| *Pseudomonas aeruginosa* | Exotoxin A, endotoxins, proteolytic enzymes, alginate, and pili; intrinsic resistance to many antimicrobial agents | Opportunistic pathogen that can cause community- or hospital-acquired infections<br>Community-acquired infections: skin (folliculitis); external ear canal (otitis externa); eye, following trauma; bone (osteomyelitis), following trauma; heart (endocarditis) in IV drug abusers; and respiratory tract (patients with cystic fibrosis)<br>Hospital acquired infections: respiratory tract, urinary tract, wounds, bloodstream (bacteremia), and central nervous system<br>Key pathogen that infects lungs of cystic fibrosis patients |
| *P. fluorescens, P. putida,* and *P. stutzeri* (includes Vb-3) | Unknown. Infection usually requires patient with underlying disease to be exposed to contaminated medical devices or solutions | Uncommon cause of infection; have been associated with bacteremia, urinary tract infections, wound infections, and respiratory tract infections; when found in clinical specimen, significance should always be questioned |
| *P. mendocina, P. alcaligenes, P. pseudoalcaligenes, Pseudomonas* sp. CDC group 1, "*P. denitrificans,*" *Pseudomonas*-like group 2, and CDC group Ic | Unknown | Not typically known to cause human infections. *P. mendocina* has been isolated from a patient with endocarditis (R) |
| *Brevundimonas vesicularis* and *B. diminuta* | Unknown | Rarely associated with human infections. *B. vesicularis* is rare cause and of bacteremia in patients suffering underlying disease |
| *Acidovorax* spp. | Unknown | Rarely isolated from clinical specimens. Not implicated in human infections |

encountered primarily in nature in water, soil, and on plants, including fruits and vegetables. Because of the ubiquitous nature of *P. aeruginosa* and *Brevundimonas* spp., the transmission of to humans can occur in a variety of ways.

*P. fluorescens, P. putida,* and *P. stutzeri* are environmental inhabitants, but they are much less commonly found in clinical specimens than is *P. aeruginosa.* The other pseudomonads and *Brevundimonas* spp. listed in Table 22-1 are also environmental organisms. Because they are rarely encountered in patient specimens, the mode of transmission to humans remains uncertain.

# PATHOGENESIS AND SPECTRUM OF DISEASE

## BURKHOLDERIA SPP. AND RALSTONIA PICKETTII

Because *Burkholderia* spp. and *R. pickettii* are uncommon causes of infection in humans, very little is known about what, if any, virulence factors they exhibit. Except for *B. pseudomallei,* the species listed in Table 22-2 generally are nonpathogenic for healthy human hosts.

The capacity of *B. cepacia* to survive in the hospital environment, which may be linked to the organism's intrinsic resistance to many antibiotics, provides the opportunity for this species to occasionally colonize and infect hospitalized patients. In patients with cystic fibrosis or chronic granulomatous disease, the organism can cause fulminant lung infections and bacteremia, resulting in death. In other types of patients, infections of the blood, urinary tract, and respiratory tract usually result from exposure to contaminated medical solutions or devices but are rarely fatal.

Infections caused by *B. pseudomallei* (capable of survival in human macrophages) can range from asymptomatic to severe. The disease is referred to as *melioidosis;* it has several forms, including the formation of skin abscesses, sepsis and septic shock, abscess formation in several internal organs, and acute pulmonary disease.

The remaining species listed in Table 22-2 are rarely encountered in human disease, and their clinical significance should be questioned when they are found in clinical specimens.

## *PSEUDOMONAS* SPP. AND *BREVUNDIMONAS* SPP.

Of the species in the *Pseudomonas* and *Brevundimonas* genera, *P. aeruginosa* is the most thoroughly studied with regard to infections in humans. *Brevundimonas* spp. are rarely associated with human infection. *B. vesicularis* has been isolated in clinical cases of bacteremia and from cervical specimens. *B. diminuta* has been recovered from cancer patients in blood, urine and pleural fluid. Although *P. aeruginosa* is an environmental inhabitant, it is also a very successful opportunistic pathogen. Factors that contribute to the organism's pathogenicity include production of exotoxin A, which kills host cells by inhibiting protein synthesis, and production of several proteolytic enzymes and hemolysins capable of destroying cells and tissue. On the bacterial cell surface, pili mediate attachment to host cells. Some strains produce alginate, a polysaccharide polymer that inhibits phagocytosis and contributes to the infection potential in patients with cystic fibrosis. Pyocyanin, the blue phenazine pigment that contributes to the characteristic green color of *P. aeruginosa*, damages cells by producing reactive oxygen species. The reactive oxygen species are also bacteriocidal to the organism. In order to protect itself from destruction, the organism must produce catalase enzymes.

*P. aeruginosa* also contains several genes involved in quorum sensing, a mechanism for detecting bacterial products in the immediate environment. When the growth of the organism or neighboring bacteria reaches a critical mass, the concentration of these "inducing" molecules reaches a level that activates transcription of virulence factors, including genes related to metabolic processes, enzyme production, and the formation of biofilm. Although many in vitro studies have examined biofilm formation, no clear evidence exists that demonstrates a clear role for biofilm in the organism's pathogenesis. Although biofilm studies have been examined in the laboratory, it is evident that *P. aeruginosa* does not form the same type of biofilm in vivo as is seen on artificial surfaces. Biofilm production related to the overproduction of alginate and the mucoid phenotype isolated from patients with cystic fibrosis is associated with serious infections. *P. aeruginosa* forms microcolonies in tissue that are associated with quorum-sensing, biofilm-producing strains, which indicates that the quorum sensing is also linked to the formation of microcolonies. These microcolonies contain DNA, mucus, actin, and other products from dying bacterial and host cells. Additionally, *P. aeruginosa* can survive harsh environmental conditions and displays intrinsic resistance to a wide variety of antimicrobial agents, two factors that facilitate the organism's ability to survive in the hospital setting (see Table 22-2).

Even with the variety of potential virulence factors discussed, *P. aeruginosa* remains an opportunistic pathogen that requires compromised host defenses to establish infection. In normal, healthy hosts, infection is usually associated with events that disrupt or bypass protection provided by the epidermis (e.g., burns, puncture wounds, use of contaminated needles by intravenous drug abusers, eye trauma with contaminated contact lenses). The result is infections of the skin, bone, heart, or eye (see Table 22-2).

In patients with cystic fibrosis, *P. aeruginosa* has a predilection for infecting the respiratory tract. Although organisms rarely invade through respiratory tissue and into the bloodstream of these patients, the consequences of respiratory involvement alone are serious and life-threatening. In other patients, *P. aeruginosa* is a notable cause of nosocomial infections of the respiratory and urinary tracts, wounds, bloodstream, and even the central nervous system. For immunocompromised patients, such infections are often severe and frequently life-threatening. In some cases of bacteremia, the organism may invade and destroy the walls of subcutaneous blood vessels, resulting in the formation of cutaneous papules that become black and necrotic. This condition is known as *ecthyma gangrenosum*. Similarly, patients with diabetes may suffer a severe infection of the external ear canal (malignant otitis externa), which can progress to involve the underlying nerves and bones of the skull.

No known virulence factors have been associated with *P. fluorescens*, *P. putida*, or *P. stutzeri*. When infections caused by these organisms occur, they usually involve a compromised patient exposed to contaminated medical materials. Such exposure has been known to result in infections of the respiratory and urinary tracts, wounds, and bacteremia (see Table 22-2). However, because of their low virulence, whenever these species are encountered in clinical specimens, their significance should be highly suspect. Similar caution should be applied whenever the other *Pseudomonas* spp. or *Brevundimonas* spp. listed in Table 22-2 are encountered.

# LABORATORY DIAGNOSIS

## SPECIMEN COLLECTION AND TRANSPORT

No special considerations are required for specimen collection and transport of organisms discussed in this chapter. Refer to Table 5-1 for general information on specimen collection and transport.

## SPECIMEN PROCESSING

No special considerations are required for processing of the organisms discussed in this chapter. Refer to Table 5-1 for general information on specimen processing.

## DIRECT DETECTION METHODS

Other than Gram staining, no specific procedures have been established for the direct detection within clinical samples of the organisms discussed in this chapter. These organisms usually appear as medium-size, straight rods on Gram staining. Exceptions are *B. diminuta,* which is a long, straight rod; *B. mallei,* which is a coccobacillus; *P. pseudomallei,* which is a small, gram-negative rod with bipolar staining; and CDC group Ic, which is a thin, pleomorphic rod.

## NUCLEIC ACID DETECTION

Culture remains the standard approach for organism identification. However, rapid screening may be useful when evaluating a large outbreak or during environmental epidemiologic studies. Polymerase chain reaction (PCR) assays have been developed for various genes, including 16s rRNA, heat shock protein, and exotoxin A. Undoubtedly, with further development and expansion in molecular diagnostics, useful clinical assays related to rapid diagnosis for respiratory infections and other serious infections will continue to emerge.

Several genotyping methods have been developed to examine the heterogeneity and diversity of the pseudomonads, including restriction fragment length polymorphism (RFLP); pulsed-field gel electrophoresis (PFGE); additional PCR-based typing methods, such as rapid amplification of polymorphic DNA (RAPD); and multilocus sequence typing (MLST). Discriminatory techniques are typically limited to specialized reference laboratories and are not considered routine laboratory testing.

## CULTIVATION

### Media of Choice

*Pseudomonas* spp., *Brevundimonas* spp., *Burkholderia* spp., *R. pickettii,* and CDC group Ic grow well on routine laboratory media, such as 5% sheep blood agar and chocolate agar (Figure 22-1). Except for *B. vesicularis,* all usually grow on MacConkey agar. All four genera also grow well in broth-blood culture systems and common nutrient broths, such as thioglycollate and brain-heart infusion. Specific selective media, such as *Pseudomonas cepacia* (PC) agar or oxidative–fermentative base–polymyxin B–bacitracin–lactose (OFPBL) agar may be used to isolate *B. cepacia* from the respiratory secretions of patients with cystic fibrosis (Table 22-3). PC agar contains crystal violet, bile salts, polymyxin B, and ticarcillin to inhibit grampositive and rapid-growing, gram-negative organisms. Inorganic and organic components, including pyruvate

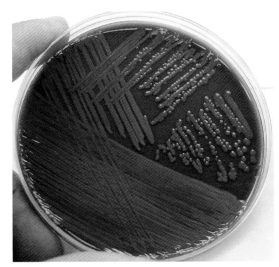

**Figure 22-1** *Burkholderia cepacia* on chocolate agar. Note green pigment.

and phenol red, also are added. *B. cepacia* breaks down the pyruvate, creating an alkaline pH and resulting in a color change of the pH indicator (phenol red) from yellow to pink. OFPBL incorporates bacitracin as an added selective agent and uses lactose fermentation to differentiate isolates. *B. cepacia* ferments lactose and appears yellow, whereas nonfermenters appear green. Ashdown medium is used to isolate *B. pseudomallei* when an infection caused by this species is suspected. The medium contains crystal violet and gentamicin as selective agents to suppress the growth of contaminating organisms. Neutral red is incorporated into the medium and is taken up by the organism, making it distinguishable from other bacteria.

### Incubation Conditions and Duration

Detectable growth on 5% sheep blood and chocolate agars, incubated at 35°C in carbon dioxide or ambient air, generally occurs in 24 to 48 hours after inoculation. Growth on MacConkey agar incubated in ambient air at 35°C is detectable within this same time frame. Selective media used for patients with cystic fibrosis (e.g., PC or OFPBL) may require incubation at 35°C in ambient air for up to 72 hours before growth is detected.

### Colonial Appearance

Table 22-3 describes the colonial appearance and other distinguishing characteristics (e.g., hemolysis and odor) of each genus on common laboratory media.

## APPROACH TO IDENTIFICATION

Most of the commercial systems available for identification of these organisms reliably identify *Pseudomonas aeruginosa* and *Burkholderia cepacia* complex, but their reliability for identification of other species is less certain.

Table 22-4 provides the key phenotypic characteristics for identifying the species discussed in this chapter. These tests provide useful information for presumptive organism identification, but definitive identification

**TABLE 22-3** Colonial Appearance and Other Characteristics of *Pseudomonas, Brevundimonas, Burkholderia, Ralstonia,* and Other Organisms

| Organism | Medium | Appearance |
|---|---|---|
| *Acidovorax delafieldii* | BA | No distinctive appearance |
| | Mac | NLF |
| *Acidovorax facilis* | BA | No distinctive appearance |
| | Mac | Unable to grow |
| *A. temperans* | BA | No distinctive appearance |
| | Mac | NLF |
| *Brevundimonas diminuta* | BA | Chalk white |
| | Mac | NLF |
| *B. vesicularis* | BA | Orange pigment |
| | Mac | NLF, but only 66% grow |
| *Burkholderia cepacia complex* | BA | Smooth and slightly raised; dirtlike odor |
| | Mac | NLF; colonies become dark pink to red due to oxidation of lactose after 4-7 days |
| | PC or OFPBL | Smooth |
| *B. pseudomallei* | BA | Smooth and mucoid to dry and wrinkled (may resemble *P. stutzeri*) |
| | Mac | |
| | Ashdown | NLF |
| | | Dry, wrinkled, violet-purple |
| *B. mallei* | BA | No distinctive appearance |
| | Mac | NLF |
| *Pandoraea* spp. | BA | No distinctive appearance |
| | Mac | NLF |
| *Pseudomonas aeruginosa* | BA | Spreading and flat, serrated edges; confluent growth; often shows metallic sheen; bluish green, red, or brown pigmentation; colonies often beta–hemolytic; grapelike or corn tortilla–like odor; mucoid colonies commonly seen in patients with cystic fibrosis |
| | Mac | NFL |
| *P. fluorescens* | BA | No distinctive appearance |
| | Mac | NLF |
| *P. mendocina* | BA | Smooth, nonwrinkled, flat, brownish–yellow pigment |
| | Mac | NLF |
| *P. monteilii* | BA | No distinctive appearance |
| | Mac | NLF |
| *P. mosselii* | BA | No distinctive appearance |
| | Mac | NLF |
| | | No acid production from xylose |
| *P. putida* | BA | No distinctive appearance |
| | Mac | NLF |
| *P. stutzeri* and CDC group Vb–3 | BA | Dry, wrinkled, adherent, buff to brown |
| | Mac | NLF |
| *P. veronii* | BA | No distinctive appearance |
| | Mac | NLF |

**TABLE 22-3** Colonial Appearance and Other Characteristics of *Pseudomonas, Brevundimonas, Burkholderia, Ralstonia,* and Other Organisms—cont'd

| Organism | Medium | Appearance |
|---|---|---|
| *Pseudomonas*–like group 2 | BAP | No distinctive appearance but colonies tend to stick to agar |
| | Mac | NLF |
| CDC group Ic | BAP | No distinctive appearance |
| | Mac | NLF |
| *Ralstonia mannitolilytica* | BAP | No distinctive appearance |
| | Mac | NLF |
| *R. pickettii* | BAP | No distinctive appearance but may take 72 hr to produce visible colonies |
| | Mac | NLF |

*BAP,* 5% sheep blood agar; *Mac,* MacConkey agar; *NLF,* non–lactose-fermenter; *OFPBL,* oxidative–fermentative base–polymyxin B–bacitracin–lactose; *PC, Pseudomonas cepacia* agar.

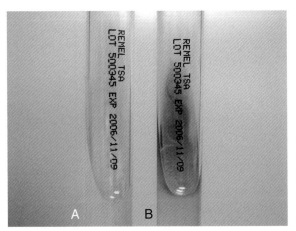

**Figure 22-2** *Pseudomonas aeruginosa* on tryptic soy agar **(B).** Note bluish-green color. Uninoculated tube **(A)** is shown for comparison.

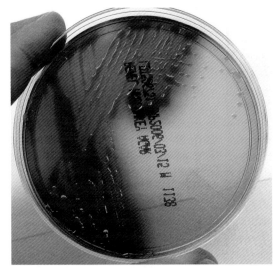

**Figure 22-3** *Pseudomonas aeruginosa* on MacConkey agar.

often requires the use of a more extensive battery of tests performed by reference laboratories.

### Comments Regarding Specific Organisms

A convenient and reliable identification scheme for *P. aeruginosa* involves the following conventional tests and characteristics:

- Oxidase-positive
- Triple sugar iron slant with an alkaline/no change (K/NC) reaction
- Production of bright bluish (pyocyanin) green (pyoverdin), red (pyorubin), or brown (pyomelanin) diffusible pigment on Mueller-Hinton agar or trypticase soy agar (Figures 22-2 and 22-3)

*P. aeruginosa, P. fluorescens, P. putida, P. veronii,* and *P. monteilii* comprise the group known as the fluorescent pseudomonads. *P. aeruginosa* can be distinguished from the others in this group by its ability to grow at 42°C. Mucoid strains of *P. aeruginosa* from patients with cystic fibrosis may not exhibit the characteristic pigment and may react more slowly in biochemical tests than nonmucoid strains. The organisms may undergo several phenotypic changes, including slow growth, changes in pigment production, and altered biochemical activity. Therefore, standard biochemicals should be held for the complete 7 days before being recorded as negative. This slow biochemical activity is often what prevents the identification of mucoid *P. aeruginosa* by commercial systems. *P. monteilii* can be distinguished from *P. putida* by its inability to oxidize xylose. Both can be distinguished from *P. fluorescens* by their inability to liquefy gelatin.

*B. cepacia* should be suspected whenever a nonfermentative organism that decarboxylates lysine is encountered. Lysine decarboxylation is positive in 80% of strains. Correct identification of the occasional lysine-negative (20%), or oxidase-negative (14%) strains requires full biochemical profiling. *Pandoraea* spp. may be differentiated from *B. cepacia* by their failure to decarboxylate lysine and their inability to liquefy gelatin. Unlike *R. paucula,* they do not hydrolyze Tween 80,

The presumptive identification of other species in this chapter is fairly straightforward using the key

**TABLE 22-4** Biochemical and Physiologic Characteristics

| Organisms | Growth at 42°C | Nitrate Reduction | Gas from Nitrate | Gelatin Liquefied | Arginine Dihydrolase | Lysine Decarboxylase | Urea Hydrolysis | Oxidizes Glucose | Oxidizes Lactose | Oxidizes Mannitol | Oxidizes Xylose |
|---|---|---|---|---|---|---|---|---|---|---|---|
| Acidovorax delafieldii | v | + | - | - | + | - | + | + | - | v | v |
| Acidovorax facilis | - | + | - | + | + | - | + | + | - | + | + |
| Acidovorax temperans | + | + | - | - | - | - | v | + | - | v | - |
| Brevundimonas diminuta | v | - | - | v | - | - | - | v | - | - | - |
| B. vesicularis | v | - | - | v | - | - | - | v | - | - | v |
| Burkholderia cepacia complex | v | v | - | v | + | v | v | + | v | + | v |
| B. pseudomallei | + | + | + | v | + | - | v | + | + | + | + |
| B. mallei | - | + | - | - | + | - | v | + | v | - | v |
| Pandoraea spp. | v | v | - | - | - | - | v | +w | - | - | - |
| Pseudomonas aeruginosa | + | + | + | v | + | - | v | + | - | v | + |
| P. fluorescens | - | - | - | + | + | - | v | + | v | v | + |
| P. mendocina | + | + | + | - | + | - | v | + | - | - | + |
| P. monteilii | - | - | - | - | + | - | v | + | - | - | - |
| P. mosselii | - | - | - | + | + | - | ND | + | - | v | - |
| P. putida | - | - | - | - | + | - | v | + | v | v | + |
| P. stutzeri | v | + | + | - | - | - | v | + | - | + | + |
| Pseudomonas veronii | - | + | + | v | + | ND | v | + | ND | + | + |
| Pseudomonas–like group 2 | v | v | - | - | v | - | + | + | + | + | + |
| CDC group Ic | + | + | - | - | + | - | v | + | - | - | - |
| Ralstonia insidiosa | + | + | ND | ND | N | - | v | - | v | ND | ND |
| Ralstonia mannitolilytica | + | - | - | v | - | - | + | + | + | + | + |
| R. pickettii | v | + | v | v | - | - | + | + | v | - | + |

*ND*, No data; *v*, variable; +, >90% of strains are positive; -, >90% of strains are negative; *w*, weak.
*Arginine-positive strains of *P. stutzeri* formerly classified as CDC group Vb-3.

characteristics given in Table 22-4. However, a few notable exceptions exist. First, when *B. cepacia* complex is identified by a commercial system in a patient with cystic fibrosis, species confirmation should be completed by a combination of phenotypic and genotypic methods. This is also true if a rapid system identifies an organism as *B. gladioli* or *R. pickettii*. The *B. cepacia* complex has 10 genomovars, and appropriate speciation is crucial.

## SERODIAGNOSIS

Serodiagnostic techniques are not generally used for laboratory diagnosis of infections caused by the organisms discussed in this chapter. An indirect hemagglutination assay is available in endemic areas in the Far East to diagnose infections caused by *P. pseudomallei;* acute and convalescent sera are required. Cross-reactions with other organisms (e.g., *B. cepacia* complex) occur, and interpretation of any serology must include compatible clinical symptoms.

An indirect hemagglutination assay has been used in the diagnosis of *B. pseudomallei* infections. The serologic test is not available commercially and has limited value in endemic areas. No current validated method exists; therefore, results should be interpreted carefully.

## ANTIMICROBIAL SUSCEPTIBILITY TESTING AND THERAPY

Many of these organisms grow on the media and under the conditions recommended for testing of the more commonly encountered bacteria (see Chapter 12 for more information about validated testing methods); however, the ability to grow under test conditions does not guarantee reliable detection of important antimicrobial resistance. Therefore, even though testing can provide an answer, it poses a substantial risk of erroneous interpretations. Validated susceptibility testing methods are available for a limited number of antibiotics.

*Burkholderia* spp. and *R. pickettii* are infrequently encountered in human infections. Potential therapies for *B. cepacia* and *B. pseudomallei* are provided, but antimicrobial therapy rarely eradicates *B. cepacia*, especially from the respiratory tract of patients with cystic fibrosis, and the optimum therapy for melioidosis remains controversial. *Burkholderia* spp. are capable of expressing resistance to various antibiotics, so devising effective treatment options can be problematic. Establishing the clinical significance of these species is important in the care of the patient.

Among *Pseudomonas* spp. and *Brevundimonas* spp., *P. aeruginosa* is the only species for which valid in vitro susceptibility testing methods exist and for which extensive therapeutic evidence exists (see Table 22-5; also see Chapter 12 for a discussion of available testing methods). Therapy usually involves the use of a beta-lactam developed for antipseudomonal activity and an aminoglycoside. The particular therapy used depends on several clinical factors and on the laboratory antimicrobial resistance profile for the *P. aeruginosa* isolate. *P. aeruginosa* isolated from patients with cystic fibrosis may require extended incubation for up to 24 hours before obtaining a reliable susceptibility pattern. In addition, the organism may develop resistance during prolonged therapy with any antimicrobial agent within 3 to 4 days requiring repeat susceptibility testing.

*P. aeruginosa* is intrinsically resistant to various antimicrobial agents; only those with potential activity are shown in Table 22-5. However, *P. aeruginosa* also readily acquires resistance to the potentially active agents listed, necessitating susceptibility testing for each clinically relevant isolate.

Although antimicrobial resistance is also characteristic of the other *Pseudomonas* spp. and *Brevundimonas* spp., the fact that these organisms are rarely clinically significant and the lack of validated testing methods prohibit the provision of specific guidelines (see Table 22-5). Antimicrobial agents used for *P. aeruginosa* infections are often considered for use against the other species; however, before proceeding with the development of treatment strategies, the first critical step should be to establish the clinical significance of the organism.

## PREVENTION

Because these organisms are ubiquitous in nature and many are commonly encountered without deleterious effects on healthy human hosts, there are no recommended vaccination or prophylaxis protocols. Hospital-acquired infections can be minimized by ensuring that appropriate infection control guidelines are followed and protocols for the sterilization and decontamination of medical supplies are implemented.

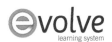 *Visit the Evolve site to complete the review questions.*

**TABLE 22-5** Antimicrobial Therapy and Susceptibility Testing

| Species | Therapeutic Options | Potential Resistance to Therapeutic Options | Validated Testing Methods* | Comments |
|---|---|---|---|---|
| *Burkholderia cepacia* | Potentially active agents include piperacillin, ceftazidime imipenem, ciprofloxacin, chloramphenicol, and trimethoprim/sulfamethoxazole | Yes | Disk diffusion, broth dilution, and E-tests | Antimicrobial therapy rarely eradicates organism. Development of resistance during therapy may warrant additional susceptibility testing. |
| *B. pseudomallei* | Potentially active agents include ceftazidime, piperacillin/ tazobactam, ticarcillin/clavulanate, amoxicillin/clavulanate, imipenem, trimethoprim/sulfamethoxazole, and chloramphenicol | Yes | Disk diffusion, broth dilution, agar dilution, and E-tests | Disk diffusion testing for TMP-SMX is unreliable |
| *B. mallei* | No definitive guidelines Potentially active agents. may include those listed for *B. pseudomallei* | Yes | Disk diffusion, broth dilution, agar dilution, and E-tests | Relapses may occur following therapy |
| *Ralstonia pickettii* | No definitive guidelines. Potentially active agents include those listed for *B. cepacia* | Yes | Not available | Rarely involved in human infections, so reliable therapeutic data are limited |
| *Pseudomonas aeruginosa* | An antipseudomonal beta-lactam (listed below) with or without an aminoglycoside; certain quinolones may also be used. Specific agents include piperacillin/tazobactam, ceftazidime, cefepime, aztreonam, imipenem, meropenem, gentamicin, tobramycin, amikacin, netilmicin, ciprofloxacin, and levofloxacin | Yes | Disk diffusion, broth dilution, agar dilution, and commercial systems | In vitro susceptibility testing results important for guiding therapy |
| *P. fluorescens, P. putida, P. stutzeri* (includes Vb-3), *P. mendocina, P. alcaligenes, P. pseudoalcaligenes, Pseudomonas* sp. CDC group 1, "*P. denitrificans,*" *Pseudomonas*-like group 2, and CDC group Ic | Because rarely implicated in human infections, there are no definitive guidelines; agents used for *P. aeruginosa* may be effective for these species | Yes | Not available | Most will grow on susceptibility testing media, but standards for interpretation of results do not exist |
| *Pseudomonas luteola P. oryzihabitans* | No definitive guidelines. Potentially active agents include cefotaxime, ceftriaxone, ceftazidime, imipenem, quinolones, and aminoglycosides | Yes, activity of penicillins is variable; commonly resistant to first- and second-generation cephalosporins | Not available | |
| *Brevundimonas vesicularis B. diminuta* | Because rarely implicated in human infections, there are no definitive guidelines | Unknown | Not available | Rarely involved in human infection |
| *Acidovorax* spp. | No definitive guidelines | Unknown | Not available | No clinical experience |

*Validated testing methods include standard methods recommended by the Clinical and Laboratory Standards Institute (CLSI) and commercial methods approved by the U.S. Food and Drug Administration (FDA).
TMP-SMX – Trimethoprim-Sulfamethoxazole.

# CASE STUDY 22-1

A 31-year-old man presents to his physician with a low-grade fever and chronic cough with purulent sputum production. A radiograph shows diffuse shadowing of the upper lungs. These chronic respiratory symptoms have been present since youth, when the patient was diagnosed with cystic fibrosis (CF). A sputum is sent for culture for CF pathogens, and the patient is admitted for antimicrobial therapy and supportive care. A smear of the sputum is not performed. However, several mucoid and nonmucoid morphologies of oxidase-positive, gram-negative, non–glucose-fermenting rods are isolated. The mucoid organism (Figure 22-4) has a grapelike odor but does not produce blue-green or fluorescent pigment (see Figure 22-2). The disk method is used, and the isolates are found to be resistant to aminoglycosides and fluoroquinolone antibiotics. Growth is seen around the colistin disk on the plate only from the nonmucoid strain.

## QUESTIONS

1. What are the likely gram-negative agents found in cultures from patients with CF?
2. What is the likely identification of the mucoid gram-negative rod? Why did the organism produce atypical reactions?
3. The Cystic Fibrosis Foundation recommends against using rapid methods to perform susceptibility testing on isolates from patients with CF. What is the reason for this recommendation?
4. Give the reasons the disk method is useful for testing for pathogens in patients with CF.

5. What is the likely identification of the colistin-resistant gram-negative rod? This organism might be confused with what other nonfermenting, gram-negative rods?
6. Why was the smear not useful for evaluation of the patient's infection?

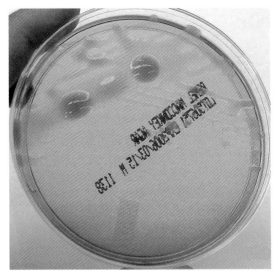

**Figure 22-4** *Pseudomonas aeruginosa* on MacConkey Agar.

# CASE STUDY 22-2

A 50-year-old male presents to the hospital emergency department (ED) intoxicated and febrile. The man has a significant history of alcoholism. Because he is unable to provide a coherent history related to his condition, it is unclear how long he has been ill. The patient was found unconscious on the sidewalk by law enforcement officers.

The patient has come to the ED frequently. He is well known to be a noncompliant diabetic with neuropathy.

Upon presentation to the ED, the patient's blood sugar is 310 mg/dL (normal range, 80-120 mg/dL). Among other laboratory abnormalities, he is found to have a WBC of 14,000 (normal, $5\text{-}10 \times 10^9$/L) with 6% bands.

Additional physical evaluation reveals a 2-cm ulcer on the plantar surface of his left foot. A bright green purulent exudate is expressed from the wound. The resulting Gram stain is shown in Figure 22-5. Radiographs of the patient's food reveal evidence of bone infection. His laboratory results are shown in the following table.

*Continued*

# CASE STUDY 22-2—cont'd

| Value | Patient | Reference Range |
|---|---|---|
| Sodium | 135 | 135-145 mEq/L |
| Potassium | 3.2 | 3.6-5.0 mEq/L |
| Chloride | 99 | 98-107 mEq/L |
| $CO_2$ | 24.0 | 24.0-34.0 mEq/L |
| Glucose | 310 | 80-120 mg/dL |
| Bilirubin, total | 3.0 | 0.2-1.9 mg/dL |
| AST | 100 | 5-40 IU/L |
| ALT | 90 | 5-40 IU/L |
| ALP | 40 | 30-157 IU/L |
| Protein | 7.0 | 6.0-8.4 g/dL |
| BUN | 45 | 7-24 mg/dL |
| Creatinine | 2.4 | 0.5-1.2 mg/dL |
| Hgb $A_1C$ | 11.3 | 4%-5.9% |
| pH | 7.34 | 7.35-7.45 |
| $PCO_2$ | 33 | 35-45 mm Hg |
| $PO_2$ | 83.5 | 83-108 mm Hg |
| $HCO_3^-$ | 18 | 22-28 mEq/L |
| $SaO_2$ | 96 | 95%-98% |

## QUESTIONS

1. Review the laboratory results provided and identify all abnormal values. Are the results consistent with the patient's present condition?
2. Based on the patient's presentation and the Gram stain result in Figure 22-5, what, if any, additional tests should be performed?
3. What is the likely agent of infection in this case? What treatment would be recommended?

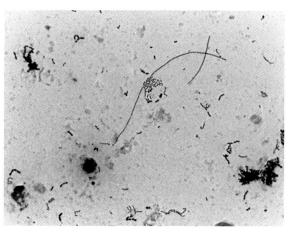

**Figure 22-5** Gram stain result for the wound specimen obtained from the patient in Case Study 22-2. Note the cluster of organisms in the center of the photograph.

# ▓ BIBLIOGRAPHY

Anzai Y, Kudo Y, Oyaizu H: The phylogeny of the genera *Chryseomonas, Flavimonas* and *Pseudomonas* supports synonymy of these three genera, *Int J Syst Bacteriol* 47:249, 1997.

Balows A, Truper HG, Dworkin M et al, editors: *The prokaryotes: a handbook on the biology of bacteria—ecophysiology, isolation, identification, applications,* ed 2, New York, 1981, Springer-Verlag.

Christenson JC, Welch DF, Mukwaya G et al: Recovery of *Pseudomonas gladioli* from respiratory tract specimens of patients with cystic fibrosis, *J Clin Microbiol* 27:270, 1989.

CLSI Supplement: Performance standards for antimicrobial susceptibility testing: 23rd informational supplement, Wayne, Pa., 2013, CLSI, M100-S23.

Coenye T, Falsen E, Hoste B et al: Description of *Pandoraea* gen nov with *Pandoraea apista* sp nov, *Pandoraea pulmonicola* sp nov, *Pandoraea pnomenusa* sp nov, *Pandoraea sputorum* sp nov and *Pandoraea norimbergensis* comb nov, *Int J Syst Evol Microbiol* 50:887, 2000.

Dance DA: Melioidosis: the tip of the iceberg? *Clin Microbiol Rev* 4:52, 1991.

Daneshvar MI, Hollis DG, Steigerwalt AG et al: Assignment of CDC weak oxidizer group 2 (WO-2) to the genus *Pandoraea* and characterization of three new *Pandoraea* genomospecies, *J Clin Microbiol* 39:1819, 2001.

De Baere T, Steyaert S, Wauters G, Des Vos P et al: Classification of *Ralstonia pickettii* biovar 3/"thomasii' strains (Pickett 1994) and of new isolates related to nosocomial recurrent meningitis as *Ralstonia mannitolytica* sp nov, *J Syst Evol Microbiol* 51(pt 2):547, 2001.

Elomari M, Caroler L, Verhille S: *Pseudomonas monteilii* sp nov, isolated from clinical specimens, *Int J Syst Bacteriol* 47:846, 1997.

Fick RB Jr: *Pseudomonas aeruginosa: the opportunist,* Boca Raton, Fla, 1993, CRC Press.

Gilligan PH: Microbiology of airway disease in patients with cystic fibrosis, *Clin Microbiol Rev* 4:35, 1991.

Godfrey AJ, Wong S, Dance DA et al: *Pseudomonas pseudomallei* resistance to β-lactam antibiotics due to alterations in the chromosomally encoded β-lactamase, *Antimicrob Agent Chemother* 35:1635, 1991.

Gold R, Jin E, Levison H et al: Ceftazidime alone and in combination in patients with cystic fibrosis: lack of efficacy in treatment of severe respiratory infections caused by *Pseudomonas cepacia, J Antimicrob Chemother* 12(suppl A):331, 1983.

Lewin C, Doherty C, Govan J: In vitro activities of meropenem, PD12731, PD 131628, ceftazidime, chloramphenicol, co-trimoxazole, and ciprofloxacin against *Pseudomonas cepacia, Antimicrob Agents Chemother* 37:123, 1993.

Livermore D: β-lactamases in laboratory and clinical resistance, *Clin Microbiol Rev* 8:557, 1995.

Mandell GL, Bennett JE, Dolin R, editors: *Principles and practice of infectious diseases,* ed 7, New York, 2010, Churchill Livingstone.

Nelson JW, Butler SL, Krieg D, et al: Virulence factors of *Burkholderia cepacia,* FEMS Immunol Med Microbiol 8:89, 1994.

Noble RC, Overman SB: *Pseudomonas stutzeri* infection: a review of hospital isolates and a review of the literature, *Diagn Microbiol Infect Dis* 19:51, 1994.

Oberhelman RA, Humbert JR, Santorelli FW: *Pseudomonas vesicularis* causing bacteremia in a child with sickle cell anemia, *South Med J* 87:821, 1994.

O'Neil KM, Herman JH, Modlin JF et al: *Pseudomonas cepacia:* an emerging pathogen in chronic granulomatous disease, *J Pediatr* 108:940, 1986.

Pallent LJ, Hugo WB, Grant DJ et al: *Pseudomonas cepacia* as a contaminant and infective agent, *J Hosp Infect* 4:9, 1983.

Papapetropoulou M, Iliopoulou J, Rodopoulou G et al: Occurrence and antibiotic resistance of *Pseudomonas* species isolated from drinking water in southern Greece, *J Chemother* 6:111, 1994.

Pegues DA, Carson LA, Anderson RL et al: Outbreak of *Pseudomonas cepacia* bacteremia in oncology patients, *Clin Infect Dis* 16: 407, 1993.

Pruksachartvuthi S, Aswapokee N, Thankerngpol K: Survival of *Pseudomonas pseudomallei* in human phagocytes, *J Med Microbiol* 31:109, 1990.

Segers P, Vancanneyt M, Pot B et al: Classification of *Pseudomonas diminuta* (Leifson and Hugh, 1954) and *Pseudomonas vesicularis* (Basing, Dîll, and Freytag, 1953) in *Brevundimonas* gen nov as *Brevundimonas diminuta* comb nov and *Brevundimonas vesicularis* comb nov, respectively, *Int J Syst Bacteriol* 44:499, 1994.

Simpson IN, Finlay J, Winstanleyet DJ et al: Multi-resistance isolates possessing characteristics of both *Burkholderia (Pseudomonas) cepacia* and *Burkholderia gladioli* from patients with cystic fibrosis, *J Antimicrob Chemother* 34:353, 1994.

Smith MD, Wuthiekanum V, Walsh AL et al: Susceptibility of *Pseudomonas pseudomallei* to some newer β-lactam antibiotics and antibiotic combinations using time-kill studies, *J Antimicrob Chemother* 33:145, 1994.

Sookpranee M, Boonma P, Susaengrat M et al: Multicenter prospective randomized trial comparing ceftazidime plus co-trimoxazole with chloramphenicol plus doxycycline and co-trimoxazole for treatment of severe melioidosis, *Antimicrob Agents Chemother* 36:158, 1992.

Sokpranee T, Sookpranee M, Mellencamp MA et al: *Pseudomonas pseudomallei:* a common pathogen in Thailand that is resistant to the bactericidal effects of many antibiotics, *Antimicrob Agents Chemother* 35:484, 1991.

Stryjewski ME, LiPuma JJ, Messier RH Jr et al: Sepsis: multiple organ failure, and death due to *Pandoraea pnomenusa* infection after lung transplantation, *J Clin Microbiol* 41:2255, 2003.

Vandamme P, Goris J, Coenye T: Assessment of Centers for Disease Control group IVc-2 to the genus *Ralstonia* as *Ralstonia paucula* sp nov, *Int J Syst Bacteriol* 49:663, 1999.

Versalovic J. *Manual of clinical microbiology,* ed 10, Washington, DC, 2011, ASM Press.

Weyant RS, Moss CW, Weaver RE et al, editors: *Identification of unusual pathogenic gram-negative aerobic and facultatively anaerobic bacteria,* ed 2, Baltimore, 1996, Williams & Wilkins.

Yabuuchi E, Kosako Y, Yano H et al: Transfer of two *Burkholderia* and an *Alcaligenes* species to *Ralstonia* gen nov: proposal of *Ralstonia pickettii* (Ralston, Palleroni, and Doudoroff, 1973) comb nov, *Ralstonia solanacearum* (Smith, 1896) comb nov and *Ralstonia eutropha* (Davis, 1969) comb nov, *Microbiol Immunol* 39:897, 1995.

# Rhizobium, Ochrobactrum, and Similar Organisms

## OBJECTIVES

1. Describe the general characteristics of the organisms discussed in this chapter, including their normal habitat, Gram stain characteristics, and morphology.
2. List the types of diseases associated with each organism.
3. Compare and contrast the Gram stain appearance of the various species.
4. Create an algorithm that outlines the major tests used to differentiate *Achromobacter* spp., *Alcaligenes xylosoxidans*, *Ochrobactrum anthropi*, and *Rhizobium radiobacter*.

---

### GENERA AND SPECIES TO BE CONSIDERED

| Current Name | Previous Name |
|---|---|
| CDC group EF-4b | CDC group EF-4 |
| CDC group Ic | |
| CDC group O-3 | |
| CDC group OFBA-1 | |
| *Ochrobactrum anthropi* | CDC group Vd1 -2 |
| *Ochrobactrum intermedium* | |
| *Paracoccus yeei* | CDC group EO-2 |
| *Psychrobacter immobilis* (saccharolytic strains) | Part of CDC group EO-2 |
| *Rhizobium radiobacter* | *Agrobacterium radiobacter,* CDC group Vd-3 |
| *Shewanella putrefaciens* | *Alteromonas putrefaciens,* |
| *Shewanella algae* | *Achromobacter putrefaciens,* CDC group Ib |

*Quotation marks indicate a proposed organism name.

---

## GENERAL CHARACTERISTICS

Most of the organisms discussed in this chapter exist in the environment. CDC group EF-4b inhabits the upper respiratory tract of certain animals. *Ochrobactrum anthropi* may occasionally inhabit the human gastrointestinal tract. All are nonpigmented, oxidase positive, and oxidize glucose; most grow on MacConkey agar. However, their specific morphologic and physiologic features are somewhat diverse; these are considered later in this chapter in the discussion of laboratory diagnosis.

## EPIDEMIOLOGY

As environmental organisms, these bacteria are rarely encountered in human specimens or infections. When they are encountered, they are found on contaminated medical devices or are isolated from immunocompromised or debilitated patients. Of the organisms listed in Table 23-1, *Rhizobium radiobacter,* and *O. anthropi* are the species most commonly encountered in the clinical setting. *Ochrobactrum intermedium* is phenotypically indistinguishable from *O. anthropi.* The other bacteria have rarely been discovered in clinical material, and several have never been established as the cause of human infection.

*R. radiobacter* inhabits the soil, and human infections occur by exposure to contaminated medical devices.

The specific environmental niche of *O. anthropi* is unknown, but this organism is capable of survival in water, including moist areas in the hospital environment. The organism may also be a transient colonizer of the human gastrointestinal tract. Similar to *R. radiobacter,* human infections caused by *O. anthropi* are associated with implantation of intravenous catheters or other foreign bodies in patients with a debilitating illness. Acquisition by contaminated pharmaceuticals and by puncture wounds has also been documented.

The epidemiology of CDC group EF-4b is unlike that of the other bacteria discussed in this chapter. Animals, rather than the environment, are the reservoir, and transmission to humans occurs by dog or cat bites and scratches.

## PATHOGENESIS AND SPECTRUM OF DISEASE

Because these organisms rarely cause human infections, little is known about what, if any, virulence factors they may produce to facilitate infectivity (Table 23-2). The fact that *R. radiobacter* and *O. anthropi* infections frequently involve contaminated medical materials and immunocompromised patients, and rarely, if ever, occur in healthy hosts, suggests that these bacteria have relatively low virulence. One report suggests that *R. radiobacter* is capable of capsule production. The ability of *O. anthropi* to adhere to the silicone material of catheters may contribute to this organism's propensity to cause catheter-related infections. No known virulence factors have been described for CDC group EF-4b. Infection appears to require traumatic introduction by a puncture wound, bite, or scratch, which indicates that the organism itself does not express any invasive properties.

For both *R. radiobacter* and *O. anthropi,* bacteremia is the most common type of infection (see Table 23-2); peritonitis, endocarditis, meningitis, urinary tract, and pyogenic infections are much less commonly encountered. *R. radiobacter* is frequently isolated from blood, peritoneal dialysate, urine, and ascitic fluid. Cellulitis and abscess formation typify the infections resulting from

**TABLE 23-1** Epidemiology

| Species | Habitat (Reservoir) | Mode of Transmission |
|---|---|---|
| *"Achromobacter"* group | Uncertain, probably environmental; may be part of endogenous flora of the ear and gastrointestinal tract | Unknown<br>Nosocomial infections related to contaminated disinfectants, dialysis fluids, saline solution, and water |
| *Rhizobium radiobacter* | Environmental, soil and plants; not part of human flora | Contaminated medical devices, such as intravenous and peritoneal catheters |
| CDC group EF-4b | Animal oral and respiratory flora; not part of human flora | Animal contact, particularly bites or scratches from dogs and cats |
| *Paracoccus yeei* | Environmental; not part of human flora | Identified in human peritonitis |
| *Psychrobacter immobilis* | Environmental, particularly cold climates such as the Antarctic; not part of human flora | Unknown. Rarely found in humans. Has been found in fish, poultry, and meat products |
| CDC group OFBA-1 | Uncertain, probably environmental; not part of human flora | Unknown. Rarely found in humans |
| *Ochrobactrum anthropi* | Uncertain, probably environmental; found in water and hospital environments; may also be part of human flora | Uncertain. Most likely involves contaminated medical devices, such as catheters or other foreign bodies, or contaminated pharmaceuticals. Also can be acquired in community by puncture wounds |
| *Shewanella putrefaciens*<br>*Shewanella algae* | Environmental and foods; not part of human flora | Unknown, rarely found in humans<br>Isolated from abscesses and wounds |

**TABLE 23-2** Pathogenesis and Spectrum of Disease

| Species | Virulence Factors | Spectrum of Disease and Infections |
|---|---|---|
| *"Achromobacter"* group | Unknown | Rarely isolated from humans.<br>Isolates have been recovered from wounds, blood, respiratory and gastrointestinal tract. |
| *Rhizobium radiobacter* | Unknown. One blood isolate described as mucoid, suggestive of exopolysaccharide capsule production. | Exposure of immunocompromised or debilitated patient to contaminated medical devices resulting in bacteremia and, less commonly, peritonitis, endocarditis, or urinary tract infection. |
| CDC group EF-4b | Unknown | Infected bite wounds of fingers, hands, or arm leading to cellulitis or abscess formation. Systemic infections are rare. |
| Paracoccus yeei | Unknown | No infections described in humans. Rarely encountered in clinical specimens. |
| *Psychrobacter immobilis* | Unknown | Rare cause of infection in humans. Has been described in wound and catheter site infections, meningitis, and eye infections. |
| CDC group OFBA-1 | Unknown | Rarely isolated from clinical specimens; found in blood, respiratory, wound, and catheter specimens. |
| *Ochrobactrum anthropi* | Unknown. Exhibits ability to adhere to silicone catheter material in a manner similar to staphylococci. | Catheter- and foreign body–associated bacteremia. May also cause pyogenic infections, community-acquired wound infections, and meningitis in tissue graft recipients. Patients are usually immunocompromised or otherwise debilitated. |
| *Shewanella putrefaciens* | Unknown | Clinical significance uncertain; often found in mixed cultures. Has been implicated in cellulites, otitis media, and septicemia; also may be found in respiratory tract, urine, feces and pleural fluid |

the traumatic introduction of CDC group EF-4b into the skin and subcutaneous tissue.

Although other species listed in Table 23-2 may be encountered in clinical specimens, their association with human infection is rare, and their clinical significance in such encounters should be carefully analyzed.

## ■ LABORATORY DIAGNOSIS

### SPECIMEN COLLECTION AND TRANSPORT

No special considerations are required for specimen collection and transport of the organisms discussed in this chapter. Refer to Table 5-1 for general information on specimen collection and transport.

### SPECIMEN PROCESSING

No special considerations are required for processing the organisms discussed in this chapter. Refer to Table 5-1 for general information on specimen processing.

### DIRECT DETECTION METHODS

Other than Gram staining, no specific procedures are required for direct detection of these organisms in clinical material. *Ochrobactrum* spp., CDC group OFBA-1, and CDC group Ic are slender, short to long rods, and CDC group O-3 are thin, medium to slightly long, curved rods with tapered ends, resembling a sickle. *R. radiobacter* is a short, pleomorphic rod. *Psychrobacter immobilis*, CDC group EF-4b, and *Paracoccus yeei* are coccobacilli. *P. yeei* has a characteristic O appearance on Gram staining (Figure 23-1). *Shewanella putrefaciens* organisms are long, short, or filamentous rods.

### CULTIVATION

#### Media of Choice

*Rhizobium* sp., *P. yeei*, CDC group Ic, CDC group O-3, *S. putrefaciens*, CDC group EF-4b, *Ochrobactrum* spp., CDC group OFBA-1, and *Psychrobacter* spp. grow well on routine laboratory media such as 5% sheep blood, chocolate, and MacConkey agars. These organisms also grow well in the broth of blood culture systems and in common nutrient broths such as thioglycollate and brain-heart infusion.

#### Incubation Conditions and Duration

These organisms produce detectable growth on 5% sheep blood and chocolate agars in 5% carbon dioxide ($CO_2$) and on MacConkey agar in ambient air when incubated at 35°C for a minimum of 24 hours. *Psychrobacter* spp. are an exception in that they usually grow poorly at 35°C and grow best at 20° to 25°C. *R. radiobacter* optimally grows at 25° to 28°C but is also capable of growth at 35°C.

#### Colonial Appearance

Table 23-3 presents descriptions of the colonial appearance and other distinguishing characteristics (e.g., hemolysis and odor) of each genus when grown on 5% sheep blood or MacConkey agar.

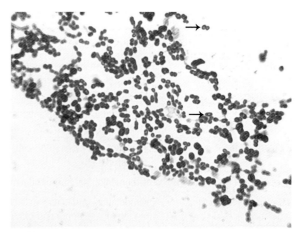

**Figure 23-1** *Paracoccus yeei;* note doughnut-shaped organism on Gram stain *(arrows).*

### APPROACH TO IDENTIFICATION

The ability of most commercial identification systems to accurately identify the organisms discussed in this chapter is limited or uncertain. Identification often requires the use of conventional biochemical profiles.

The key biochemical reactions used to presumptively differentiate among the genera discussed in this chapter are provided in Table 23-4. However, definitive identification of these organisms often requires performing an extensive battery of biochemical tests not commonly available in many clinical microbiology laboratories. Therefore, full identification of clinically relevant isolates may require identification by a reference laboratory.

#### Comments Regarding Specific Organisms

Although the EF portion of the CDC group EF-4b designation stands for eugonic fermenter (an organism that grows well on common laboratory media), most CDC group EF-4b strains oxidize glucose, so the designation as a eugonic fermenter is a misnomer. *P. yeei*, formerly CDC group EO-2 (a eugonic oxidizer), has a biochemical profile very similar to that of the saccharolytic, nonhemolytic *Acinetobacter* spp., except that the latter are oxidase negative (see Chapter 21 for more information about this genus).

The notable characteristic of CDC group OFBA-1 is that it produces an acidlike reaction in the OF medium tube, even though no carbohydrates are present. In contrast, *R. radiobacter* produces acid from various carbohydrates, but it does not acidify the OF tube.

*R. radiobacter* may be differentiated from *Ochrobactrum* spp. by a positive β-galactosidase test result. *O. anthropi* often requires cellular fatty acid analysis for differentiation. *Psychrobacter* spp. can be either saccharolytic or asaccharolytic, although all members of this genus have an optimal growth temperature of less than 35°C.

CDC group O-3 is often misidentified as *Campylobacter* spp. because of its curved shape on Gram stain.

*Shewanella* spp. are notable for the production of hydrogen sulfide ($H_2S$) in the butt of triple sugar iron

**TABLE 23-3** Colonial Appearance and Characteristics

| Organism | Medium | Appearance |
|---|---|---|
| *"Achromobacter"* group | BA | Flat, spreading and rough colonies |
| | Mac | NLF; biovar F does not grow |
| CDC group EF-4b | BA | No distinctive appearance, but cultures smell like popcorn |
| | Mac | NLF |
| CDC group Ic | BA | No distinctive appearance |
| | Mac | NLF |
| CDC group O-3 | BA | Circular, entire, translucent, very punctate |
| | Mac | NLF, may grow poorly or not at all |
| CDC group OFBA-1 | BA | Beta-hemolytic |
| | Mac | NLF |
| *Ochrobactrum anthropi* | BA | Resembles colonies of Enterobacteriaceae, only smaller |
| | Mac | NLF |
| *Paracoccus yeei* | BA | Growth frequently mucoid |
| | Mac | NLF |
| *Psychrobacter immobilis* | BA | No distinctive appearance but usually does not grow well at 35°C; grows best at 20°C; cultures (saccharolytic strains) smell like roses |
| | Mac | NLF |
| *Rhizobium radiobacter* | BA | No distinctive appearance |
| | Mac | NLF (mucoid pink after extended incubation [>48 hr]) |
| *Shewanella putrefaciens* | BA | Convex, circular, smooth; occasionally mucoid; lavender greening of blood agar; soluble brown to tan pigment |
| | Mac | NLF |

*BA,* 5% sheep blood agar; *Mac,* MacConkey agar; *NLF,* non–lactose fermenter.

**TABLE 23-4** Key Biochemical and Physiologic Characteristics

| Organism | Oxidizes Glucose | Oxidizes Xylose | Oxidizes Mannitol | Nitrate Reduction | Gas from Nitrate | Arginine Dihydrolase | Esculin Hydrolyzed | Growth on Cetrimide |
|---|---|---|---|---|---|---|---|---|
| *"Achromobacter"* group[a,b] | + | + | v | + | + | + | + | v |
| CDC group EF–4b | + | − | − | + | − | − | − | ND |
| CDC group Ic | + | − | − | + | − | + | − | + |
| CDC group O–3 | + | + | − | − | − | − | + | ND |
| CDC group OFBA–1[c] | + | + | (+) | + | + | + | − | + |
| *Ochrobactrum anthropi*[b] | + | + | v | v | v | v | v | − |
| *Paracoccus yeei* | + | + | − | + | v | v | − | − |
| *Psychrobacter immobilis*[d] | (+) | (+) | − | v | − | v | − | − |
| *Rhizobium radiobacter* | + | + | + | v | − | − | + | − |
| *Shewanella putrefaciens*[e] | v | − | − | + | − | − | − | − |

Compiled from data in Weyant RS, Moss CW, Weaver RE et al, editors: *Identification of unusual pathogenic gram-negative aerobic and facultatively anaerobic bacteria,* ed 2, Baltimore, 1996, Williams & Wilkins; and Young JM, Kuykendall LD, Martínez-Romero E et al: A revision of *Rhizobium Frank, 1889,* with an emended description of the genus, and the inclusion of all species of *Agrobacterium Conn, 1942* and *Allorhizobium undicola de Lajudie et al, 1998* as new combinations: *Rhizobium radiobacter, R. rhizogenes, R. rubi, R. undicola* and *R. vitis, Int J Syst Evol Microbiol* 51:89, 2001.
*ND,* No data available; *v,* variable; +, >90% of strains are positive; −, >90% of strains are negative; (+), delayed.
[a]Includes biovars B, E, and F; F does not grow on MacConkey agar.
[b]Usually motile by peritrichous flagella.
[c]Oxidizes base.
[d]Saccharolytic variety; prefers growth at 25°C.
[e]$H_2S$ in butt of triple sugar iron (TSI) agar.

(TSI) agar; this characteristic is rare among the nonfermentive gram-negative rods. *S. algae* is halophilic.

## SERODIAGNOSIS

Serodiagnostic techniques are not generally used in the laboratory diagnosis of infections caused by the organisms discussed in this chapter.

## ANTIMICROBIAL SUSCEPTIBILITY TESTING AND THERAPY

No validated susceptibility testing methods are available for the organisms discussed in this chapter. Although many of these organisms grow on the media and under the conditions recommended for testing of more commonly encountered bacteria (see Chapter 12 for more information on validated testing methods), no standardized reference exists for antimicrobial resistance for these organisms. The lack of validated in vitro susceptibility testing methods does not allow definitive treatment and testing guidelines to be given for the organisms listed in Table 23-5. Although susceptibility data for some of these bacteria can be found in the literature, the lack of understanding of potential underlying resistance mechanisms prohibits the validation of the data. Review Chapter 12 for preferable strategies used to provide susceptibility information and data when validated testing methods do not exist for a clinically relevant bacterial isolate.

Because *R. radiobacter* and *O. anthropi* infections are frequently associated with implanted medical devices, therapeutic management of the patient often involves removal of the contaminated material. Although definitive antimicrobial therapies for these infections have not been established, in vitro data suggest that certain agents could be more effective than others (see Table 23-5). Most strains of *R. radiobacter* are susceptible to cephalosporins, carbapenems, tetracyclines, and gentamicin.

*O. anthropi* is commonly resistant to all currently available penicillins, cephalosporins, aztreonam, and

**TABLE 23-5** Antimicrobial Therapy and Susceptibility Testing

| Species | Therapeutic Options | Potential Resistance to Therapeutic Options | Validated Testing Methods* | Comments |
|---|---|---|---|---|
| "Achromobacter" group | No definitive guidelines. Human infections are rare. | Resistant to narrow-spectrum penicillins, other cephalosporins, and aminoglycosides. | Methods are not standardized. Methods used may include broth macrodilution and microdilution, agar dilution, breakpoint, and Etest. | |
| Rhizobium radiobacter | Optimal therapy uncertain. Treatment involves removal of foreign body. Potentially active agents include ceftriaxone, cefotaxime imipenem, gentamicin, and ciprofloxacin | Yes | Not available | Grows on susceptibility testing media, but standards for interpretation of results do not exist. |
| CDC group EF-4b | No definitive guidelines. Potentially active agents include penicillin, ampicillin, ciprofloxacin, and ofloxacin | Unknown; some cephalosporins may be less active than the penicillins. | Not available | Limited clinical data |
| Paracoccus yeei | No definitive guidelines | Unknown | Not available | No clinical data |
| Psychrobacter immobilis | No definitive guidelines. Usually penicillin susceptible. | Unknown | Not available | Limited clinical data |
| CDC group OFBA-1 | No definitive guidelines | Unknown | Not available | No clinical data |
| Ochrobactrum anthropi | Optimal therapy uncertain. Treatment involves removal of foreign body. Potentially active agents include trimethoprim-sulfamethoxazole, ciprofloxacin, and imipenem; aminoglycoside activity variable | Commonly resistant to all penicillins and cephalosporins. | Not available | Grows on susceptibility testing media, but standards for interpretation of results do not exist. |
| Shewanella putrefaciens | No definitive guidelines. Generally susceptible to various antimicrobial agents | Often resistant to ampicillin and cephalothin | Not available | |

*Validated testing methods include standard methods recommended by the Clinical and Laboratory Standards Institute (CLSI) and commercial methods approved by the U.S. Food and Drug Administration (FDA).

amoxicillin-clavulanate but usually is susceptible to aminoglycosides, fluoroquinolones, imipenem, tetracycline, and trimethoprim-sulfamethoxazole. *O. anthropi* (colistin susceptible) may be differentiated from *O. intermedium* by colistin resistance. This resistance profile is sufficiently consistent with the species, making it potentially useful for confirming the organism's identification. The organism may also appear susceptible to trimethoprim-sulfamethoxazole and ciprofloxacin, but antimicrobial therapy without removal of the contaminated medical device may not successfully eradicate the organism.

## PREVENTION

Because these organisms are ubiquitous in nature and are not generally a threat to human health, no recommended vaccination or prophylaxis protocols have been established. Hospital-acquired infections are controlled by following appropriate sterile techniques, infection control guidelines and by implementing effective protocols for the sterilization and decontamination of medical supplies.

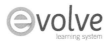

*Visit the Evolve site to complete the review questions.*

---

## CASE STUDY 23-1

A 31-year-old female bartender, who is right-hand dominant, presents with a dog bite on her right second finger. She is treated at the emergency department for pain and swelling of the finger. Flexor tenosynovitis and tendon laceration are diagnosed. She has surgery the next day, and culture samples are obtained. The patient does well following surgery, and the physicians want to send her home on ampicillin/sulbactam. However, the laboratory isolates an unidentified gram-negative coccobacilli from the bite wound. Although the organism does not grow on MacConkey agar, it is an oxidase- and catalase-positive glucose oxidizer without any pigment production. It emits the distinct odor of popcorn.

### QUESTIONS

1. What is the most likely identity of this bacterium, and how would the laboratory definitively identify it?
2. List the other common microorganisms that would be expected to be isolated from dog and cat bites.
3. This isolate had an unusual reaction in nitrate medium, which is characteristic of EF-4b and a very few other microorganisms. No gas was present in the Durham tube; no red color was detected with the addition of the reagents; and no pink color was present after the addition of zinc. (See Procedure 13-29, Nitrate Reduction.) If no pink color is present after the addition of zinc, is the microorganism positive for nitrate reduction?

---

## BIBLIOGRAPHY

Alnor D, Frimodt-Moller N, Espersen F et al: Infections with the unusual human pathogens *Agrobacterium* species and *Ochrobactrum anthropi, Clin Infect Dis* 18:914, 1994.

Chang HJ, Christenson JC, Pavia AT et al: *Ochrobactrum anthropi* meningitis in pediatric pericardial allograft transplant recipients, *J Infect Dis* 173:656, 1996.

Cieslak TJ, Drabick CJ, Robb ML: Pyogenic infections due to *Ochrobactrum anthropi, Clin Infect Dis* 22:845, 1996.

Cieslak TJ, Robb ML, Drabick CJ et al: Catheter-associated sepsis caused by *Ochrobactrum anthropi:* report of a case and review of related nonfermentative bacteria, *Clin Infect Dis* 14:902, 1992.

Dunne WM, Tillman J, Murray JC: Recovery of a strain of *Agrobacterium radiobacter* with a mucoid phenotype from an immunocompromised child with bacteremia, *J Clin Microbiol* 31:2541, 1993.

Lloyd-Puryear M, Wallace D, Baldwin T et al: Meningitis caused by *Psychrobacter immobilis* in an infant, *J Clin Microbiol* 29:2041, 1991.

Lozano F, Florez C, Recio FJ et al: Fatal *Psychrobacter immobilis* infection in a patient with AIDS, *AIDS* 8:1189, 1994.

Nozue H, Hayashi T, Hashimoto Y: Isolation and characterization of *Shewanella algae* from human clinical specimens and emendation of the description of *S. algae* (*Simidu et al, 1990, 335*), *Int J Syst Bacteriol* 42:628, 1992.

Shideh K, Janda JM: Biochemical and pathogenic properties of *Shewanella alga* and *Shewanella putrefaciens, J Clin Microbiol* 36:783, 1998.

Validation of publication of new names and new combinations previously effectively published outside the IJSEM, *Int J Syst Evol Microbiol* 53:935, 2003.

Versalovic J: *Manual of clinical microbiology,* ed 10, Washington, DC, 2011, ASM Press.

Weyant RS, Moss CW, Weaver RE et al, editors: *Identification of unusual pathogenic gram-negative aerobic and facultatively anaerobic bacteria,* ed 2, Baltimore, 1996, Williams & Wilkins.

Young JM, Kuykendall LD, Martínez-Romero E et al: A revision of *Rhizobium Frank, 1889,* with an emended description of the genus, and the inclusion of all species of *Agrobacterium conn, 1942,* and *Allorhizobium undicola de Lajudie et al, 1998,* as new combinations: *Rhizobium radiobacter, R. rhizogenes, R. rubi, R. undicola* and *R. vitis, Int J Syst Evol Microbiol* 51:89, 2001.

## OBJECTIVES

1. Describe the general characteristics of the organisms discussed in this chapter.
2. Identify the normal habitat and the routes of transmission for the organisms.
3. List the appropriate media for cultivation of the organisms listed, particularly *E. meningoseptica*.
4. Describe the colonial appearance of *E. meningoseptica*.
5. Outline the tests used to differentiate the major genera in this group, including *Elizabethkingia* sp., *Myoides* spp., *Sphingobacterium* spp., and *Bergeyella zoohelicum*.

### GENERA AND SPECIES TO BE CONSIDERED

| Current Name | Previous Name |
|---|---|
| *Rhizobium radiobacter* | |
| *Bergeyella zoohelicum* | *Weeksella zoohelicum,* CDC group IIj |
| CDC group IIb* | *Flavobacterium* spp. (IIb) |
| CDC group EO-3 | |
| CDC group EO-4 | |
| CDC group 0-1, 0-2, and 0-3 | |
| *Chryseobacterium* spp.† | *Flavobacterium gleum* and |
| | *Flavobacterium indologenes* |
| *Elizabethkingia meningoseptica* | *Chryseobacterium meningosepticum,* |
| | *Flavobacterium meningosepticum,* |
| | and CDC group IIa |
| *Empedobacter brevis* | *Flavobacterium breve* |
| *Myoides odoratus* | *Flavobacterium* spp. |
| *Myoides odoratimimus* | *Flavobacterium* spp. |
| *Sphingobacterium multivorum* | *Flavobacterium multivorum* and CDC |
| | group IIK-2 |
| *Sphingobacterium spiritivorum* | *Flavobacterium spiritivorum* and |
| | CDC group IIK-3 |
| *Sphingobacterium thalpophilum* | |
| *Weeksella virosa* | CDC group IIf |

*Includes clinical strains of *C. gleum* and *C. indologenes* other than the type strains.
†Includes type strain of *C. gleum* and *C. indologenes* (formerly *Flavobacterium gleum* and *F. indologenes*).

## GENERAL CHARACTERISTICS

The organisms discussed in this chapter are environmental inhabitants that are occasionally encountered in human specimens. Most of the organisms originated in the heterogenous group *Flavobacterium*. However, when subjected to molecular analysis, they did not prove to be closely related and therefore have been reclassified. They are considered together here because they share similar physiologic and morphologic characteristics. Most are yellow-pigmented, oxidase-positive, glucose oxidizers that grow on MacConkey agar. *Sphingobacterium* spp. have an unusually large amount of sphingophospholipid compounds in their cell membranes. *Sphingobacterium mizutaii,* which does not grow on MacConkey agar, is discussed in Chapter 27.

## EPIDEMIOLOGY

As environmental inhabitants, these organisms may be found in various niches (Table 24-1). Most notable in terms of clinical relevance is their ability to survive in hospital environments, especially in moist areas. Although they are not considered part of normal human flora, these species can colonize a patient's respiratory tract during hospitalization. This results from exposure to contaminated water or medical devices. Transmission also may occur directly from contaminated pharmaceutical solutions and, in the case of *E. meningoseptica,* from person to person.

Because of their ability to survive well in hospital environments, these organisms have the potential to contaminate laboratory culture media and blood culture systems. Whenever these species are encountered, their clinical significance and the potential for contamination should be seriously considered.

## PATHOGENESIS AND SPECTRUM OF DISEASE

As environmental organisms, no specific virulence factors have been identified for these species. However, the ability to survive in chlorinated tap water may give these organisms an edge in their ability to thrive in hospital water systems.

The development of infection basically requires exposure of debilitated patients to a contaminated source, resulting in respiratory colonization (Table 24-2). Depending on the patient's health, subsequent infections, such as bacteremia and pneumonia, may develop. These infections are most frequently caused by *Elizabethkingia meningoseptica* or *Myoides odoratus.* Infections of several other body sites, which may or may not be preceded by respiratory colonization, have been associated with the other species.

Meningitis caused by *E. meningoseptica* is the most notable infection associated with the organisms listed in Table 24-2. This life-threatening infection, which may be accompanied by bacteremia, originally gained attention because it occurred in neonates. However, *E. meningoseptica* meningitis can also occur in compromised adults.

TABLE 24-1 Epidemiology

| Species | Habitat (Reservoir) | Mode of Transmission |
|---|---|---|
| *Elizabethkingia meningoseptica, Chryseobacterium* spp., *Empedobacter brevis, Sphingobacterium* spp. | Soil, plants, water, food, and hospital water sources, including incubators, sinks, faucets, tap water, hemodialysis systems, saline solutions, and other pharmaceuticals Not part of human flora | Exposure of patients to contaminated medical devices or solutions, but source is not always known. May colonize upper respiratory tract. *E. meningoseptica* occasionally may be transmitted from birth canal to neonate. |
| *Chryseobacterium indologenes* | | Catheter-related infections |
| *Bergeyella zoohelicum* | Normal oral flora of dogs and other animals | Dog and cat bites |

TABLE 24-2 Pathogenesis and Spectrum of Diseases

| Species | Virulence Factors | Spectrum of Disease and Infections |
|---|---|---|
| *Elizabethkingia meningoseptica, Chryseobacterium* spp., *Empedobacter brevis, Sphingobacterium* spp. | Specific virulence factors are unknown. Able to survive chlorinated tap water. *E. meningoseptica,* the species most often associated with human infections, can be encapsulated or produce proteases and gelatinases that destroy host cells and tissues. | Bacteremia (often associated with implanted devices, such as catheters, or contaminated medical solutions). *E. meningoseptica* is particularly associated with meningitis in neonates and less commonly in adults. Other organisms are associated with pneumonia, mixed infections of wounds, ocular and urinary tract infections, and occasionally sinusitis, endocarditis, peritonitis, and fasciitis. |
| *Chryseobacterium indologenes* | | Catheter-related bacteremia Bacteremia associated with malignancies and neutropenia |
| *Bergeyella zoohelicum* | | Dog and cat bite wounds Rarely meningitis and bacteremia |
| *Myroides odoratus, Myroides odoratimimus* | Pathogenesis unknown | Rarely isolated from humans. Associated with urine, blood, wounds, and respiratory specimens. |
| *Weeksella virosa* | Pathogenesis unknown | Genitourinary isolation, most often in women. |

The organism has been implicated in hospital-based outbreaks of both meningitis and pneumonia.

# LABORATORY DIAGNOSIS

## SPECIMEN COLLECTION AND TRANSPORT

No special considerations are required for specimen collection and transport of the organisms discussed in this chapter. Refer to Table 5-1 for general information on specimen collection and transport.

## SPECIMEN PROCESSING

No special considerations are required for processing the organisms discussed in this chapter. Refer to Table 5-1 for general specimen processing information.

## DIRECT DETECTION METHODS

Gram staining is used to detect these organisms in clinical material. The *Chryseobacterium* spp., *E. meningoseptica,*

and CDC group IIb are medium to long straight rods that often appear as "II-forms" (i.e., cells that appear thin in the center and thicker at the ends). *Empedobacter brevis* varies in being short to long rods. *Sphingobacterium* spp. are short straight rods, *S. thalpophilum* may exhibit II-forms. *Rhizobium radiobacter* yellow group are slender, medium to long, gram-negative rods. CDC groups EO-3 and EO-4 are coccobacilli, and CDC groups O-1, O-2, and O-3 are short, gram-negative, curved rods.

## CULTIVATION

### Media of Choice

All genera and CDC groups in this chapter grow well on routine laboratory media such as 5% sheep blood and chocolate agars. They also grow well in the broth of blood culture systems and in common nutrient broths such as thioglycollate and brain-heart infusion.

### Incubation Conditions and Duration

These organisms will produce detectable growth on blood and chocolate agars when incubated at 35°C in

**TABLE 24-3** Colonial Appearance and Characteristics

| Organism | Medium | Appearance |
|---|---|---|
| *Rhizobium radiobacter* | BAP<br>MAC | Yellow<br>NLF |
| *Bergeyella zoohelicum* | BAP | Nonmucoid<br>Sticky, nonpigmented |
| CDC group IIb | BAP<br>MAC | Yellow to orange pigment<br>NLF, growth variable |
| CDC group EO-3 | BAP<br>MAC | Yellow<br>NLF |
| CDC group EO-4 | BAP<br>MAC | Most strains yellow<br>NLF |
| CDC group O-1 | BAP<br>MAC | Yellow<br>NLF, growth variable |
| *Chryseobacterium* spp.;<br>*C. indologenes* | BAP<br>Choc | Circular, smooth, shiny with entire edge; light yellow to orange.<br>Dark yellow pigment* (flexirubin) |
| *Elizabethkingia meningoseptica* | BAP<br>Choc<br>MAC | Usually nonpigmented, although may exhibit a slight yellow pigment;<br>smooth, circular, large, shiny with entire edge<br>NLF |
| *Empedobacter brevis* | BAP<br>MAC | Circular, smooth, shiny with entire edge; light yellow<br>NLF, if growth |
| *Myroides odoratus, Myroides odoratimimus* | BAP<br>MAC | Yellow pigmented, fruity odor<br>NLF |
| *Sphingobacterium multivorum* | BAP<br>MAC | Small, circular, convex, smooth, opaque with light yellow pigment after<br>overnight incubation at room temperature<br>NLF |
| *Sphingobacterium spiritivorum* | BAP<br>MAC | Small, circular, convex, smooth with pale yellow pigment<br>NLF, if growth |
| *Sphingobacterium thalpophilum* | BAP<br>MAC | Pale yellow<br>NLF |
| *Weeksella virosa* | BAP | Mucoid, slimy<br>Yellow-green pigment |

*BA,* 5% sheep blood agar; *Mac,* MacConkey agar; *Choc,* chocolate agar; *NLF,* non–lactose fermenter.
*\*Chryseobacterium* spp. produce a yellow pigment that turns red upon the addition of 20% KOH.

either carbon dioxide or ambient air for a minimum of 24 hours. Growth on MacConkey agar is usually detectable within 24 hours of inoculation.

Colonial Appearance

Table 24-3 presents descriptions of the colonial appearance and other distinguishing characteristics of each genus on 5% sheep blood and MacConkey agars.

## APPROACH TO IDENTIFICATION

The ability of most commercial identification systems to accurately identify the organisms discussed in this chapter is limited or uncertain. The key biochemical reactions used to presumptively differentiate among the genera discussed in this chapter are provided in Table 24-4. However, definitive identification of these organisms often requires a battery of biochemical tests not commonly available in many clinical microbiology

laboratories. Therefore, full identification of clinically relevant isolates may require that they be sent to a reference laboratory.

Comments Regarding Specific Organisms

The growth of *Sphingobacterium spiritivorum* and *Chryseobacterium* spp. is variable on MacConkey agar. Therefore, these organisms often need to be differentiated from the yellow-pigmented, MacConkey-negative, oxidase-positive genera considered in Chapters 27 and 31.

Indole and urea hydrolysis are key biochemical tests for distinguishing *E. brevis, E. meningoseptica,* and *Chryseobacterium* spp. from *Sphingobacterium* spp.

## SERODIAGNOSIS

Serodiagnostic techniques are not generally used for the laboratory diagnosis of infections caused by the organisms discussed in this chapter.

**TABLE 24-4** Key Biochemical and Physiologic Characteristics

| Organism | Oxidizes Mannitol | Indole | Gelatin | Urea | Nitrate Reduction | Esculin Hydrolysis | Motility |
|---|---|---|---|---|---|---|---|
| *Agrobacterium* yellow group[a] | – | – | – | + | – | (+) | p,1-2 |
| CDC group EO–3 | (+) | – | – | (+) | – | – | nm |
| CDC group EO–4 | – | – | – | + | – | – | nm |
| CDC group 0–1 | – | – | v | – | – | + | p, 1-2 |
| *Chryseobacterium* spp.[b,d] | – | + | v | v | v | v | nm |
| *Elizabethkingia meningoseptica*[b,c] | + | + | + | – | – | + | nm |
| *Empedobacter brevis*[b,c] | – | + | + | – | – | – | nm |
| *Myoides* spp. | ND | – | + | + | + | ND | nm |
| *Sphingobacterium multivorum* | – | – | – | + | – | + | nm |
| *Sphingobacterium spiritivorum* | + | – | v | + or (+) | – | + | nm |
| *Sphingobacterium thalpophilum* | – | – | v | + | + | + | nm |

*ND,* No data; *nm,* nonmotile; *p,* polar flagella; *v,* variable; +, >90% of strains are positive; –, >90% of strains are negative; (+), reaction may be delayed.
[a]Only a positive 3-ketolactonate test differentiates this group from *Sphingomonas paucimobilis.*
[b]Colonial pigmentation is critical to separate *Chryseobacterium* spp. and *Empedobacter brevis.*
[c]DNase positive.
[d]Includes *Chryseobacterium gleum, C. indologenes,* and CDC group IIb.

**TABLE 24-5** Antimicrobial Therapy and Susceptibility Testing

| Species | Therapeutic Options | Potential Resistance to Therapeutic Options | Validated Testing Methods* | Comments |
|---|---|---|---|---|
| *Bergeyella zoohelicum* | Susceptible to penicillin | | Not available | |
| *Chryseobacterium indologenes, Elizabethkingia meningoseptica, Empedobacter brevis, Sphingobacterium* spp. | No definitive guidelines. Potentially active agents include ciprofloxacin rifampin, clindamycin, trimethoprim/ sulfamethoxazole, and vancomycin | Produce β-lactamases and are frequently resistant to aminoglycosides | Not available | In vitro susceptibility results with disk diffusion may be seriously misleading |

*Validated testing methods include standard methods recommended by the Clinical and Laboratory Standards Institute (CLSI) and commercial methods approved by the U.S. Food and Drug Administration (FDA).

# ANTIMICROBIAL SUSCEPTIBILITY TESTING AND THERAPY

Validated susceptibility testing methods do not exist for these organisms. Although they grow on the media and under the conditions recommended for testing (see Chapter 12 for more information about validated testing methods), the ability to grow and the ability to detect important antimicrobial resistances are not the same. Therefore, the lack of validated in vitro susceptibility testing methods does not allow definitive treatment and testing guidelines to be given for any of the organisms listed in Table 24-5.

Although susceptibility data for some of these bacteria can be found in the literature, the lack of understanding of potential underlying resistance mechanisms prohibits the validation of such data. Review Chapter 12 for preferable strategies that can be used to provide susceptibility information and data when validated testing

methods do not exist for a clinically important bacterial isolate.

In general, the species considered in this chapter are frequently resistant to β-lactams (including penicillins, cephalosporins, and carbapenems) and aminoglycosides commonly used to treat infections caused by other gram-negative bacilli. However, the susceptibility data can vary substantially with the type of testing method used. An unusual feature of many of these species is that they often appear susceptible to, and may be treated with, antimicrobial agents that are usually considered effective against gram-positive bacteria; clindamycin, rifampin, and vancomycin are notable examples.

# PREVENTION

Because these organisms are ubiquitous in nature and are not generally a threat to human health, no recommended vaccination or prophylaxis protocols have been established. Hospital-acquired infections are controlled through the use of appropriate sterile technique, infection control, and implementation of effective protocols for sterilization and decontamination of medical supplies.

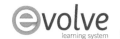 **Visit the Evolve site to complete the review questions.**

---

## CASE STUDY 24-1

A 48-year-old male with underlying acute myelogenous leukemia develops fever during a hospitalization for induction chemotherapy. At the time of infection, the patient is severely neutropenic. Blood drawn through an indwelling venous catheter tests positive for an indole- and oxidase-positive yellow bacterium. Subsequent blood cultures are negative on therapy. Fourteen days into treatment, the patient develops progressive dyspnea (difficulty breathing), fever, and a pulmonary infiltrate. A subsequent sputum specimen grows the same yellow bacteria, now resistant to therapy. The patient is treated with minocycline, and the pneumonia resolves.

### QUESTIONS

1. List the bacteria that would be in the differential for indole-positive, glucose-nonfermenting, gram-negative rods.

2. *E. meningoseptica* is the most significant pathogen in this group. How can this species be distinguished from the other indole-positive bacteria?

3. Although *E. meningoseptica* is a ubiquitous inhabitant of the aqueous environment, disease is rare. However, it can be present in the hospital environment, resulting in serious disease in the neonate. Ninety percent of cases of meningitis caused by *E. meningoseptica* occur in neonates, predominantly in premature infants. The mortality rate is high; more than half of the infants succumb to the disease. Because of this bacterium's importance and rarity, which method should be used to perform susceptibility testing for it?

---

## BIBLIOGRAPHY

Blahovea J, Hupkova M, Krcmery V et al: Resistance to and hydrolysis of imipenem in nosocomial strains of *Flavobacterium meningosepticum*, *Eur J Clin Microbiol Infect Dis* 13:833, 1994.

Fass RJ, Barnishan J: In vitro susceptibilities of nonfermentative gram-negative bacilli other than *Pseudomonas aeruginosa* to 32 antimicrobial agents, *Rev Infect Dis* 2:841, 1980.

Ferrer C, Jakob E, Pastorino G et al: Right-sided bacterial endocarditis due to *Flavobacterium odoratum* in a patient on chronic hemodialysis, *Am J Nephrol* 15:82, 1995.

Hsueh P, Wu J, Hsiue T et al: Bacteremic necrotizing fasciitis due to *Flavobacterium odoratum*, *Clin Infect Dis* 21:1337, 1995.

Jorgensen JH, Maher LA, Howell AW: Activity of meropenem against antibiotic-resistant or infrequently encountered gram-negative bacilli, *Antimicrob Agents Chemother* 35:2410, 1991.

Kim KK, Kim MK, Lim JH et al: Transfer of *Chryseobacterium meningosepticum* and *Chryseobacterium miricola* to *Elizabethkingia meningoseptica* comb nov and *Elizabethkingia miricola* comb nov, *Int J Syst Evol Microbiol* 55:1287, 2005.

Mandell GL, Bennett JE, Dolin R: *Principles and practices of infectious diseases*, ed 7, Philadelphia, 2010, Churchill Livingstone/Elsevier.

Marnejon T, Watanakunakorn C: *Flavobacterium meningosepticum* septicemia and peritonitis complicating CAPD, *Clin Nephrol* 38:176, 1992.

Pokrywka M, Viazanko K, Medvick J et al: A *Flavobacterium meningosepticum* outbreak among intensive care patients, *Am J Infect Control* 21:139, 1993.

Reina J, Borrell N, Figuerola J: *Sphingobacterium multivorum* isolated from a patient with cystic fibrosis, *Eur J Clin Microbiol Infect Dis* 11:81, 1992.

Sader HS, Jones RN, Pfaller MA: Relapse of catheter-related *Flavobacterium meningosepticum* bacteremia demonstrated by DNA macrorestriction analysis, *Clin Infect Dis* 21:997, 1995.

Schreckenberger PG, Daneshvar MI, Weyant RS, et al: *Acinetobacter, Achromobacter, Chryseobacterium, Moraxella,* and other nonfermentative gram-negative bacteria. In Murray PR, Baron EJ, Jorgensen JH, et al, editors: *Manual of clinical microbiology*, ed 8, Washington, DC, 2003, ASM Press.

Skapek SX, Jones WS, Hoffman KM et al: Sinusitis and bacteremia caused by *Flavobacterium meningosepticum* in a sixteen-year-old with Shwachman Diamond syndrome, *Pediatr Infect Dis J* 11:411, 1992.

Tizer KB, Cervia JS, Dunn A et al: Successful combination of vancomycin and rifampin therapy in a newborn with community acquired *Flavobacterium meningosepticum* neonatal meningitis, *Pediatr Infect Dis J* 14:916, 1995.

Vandamme P et al: New perspectives in the classification of the flavobacteria: description of *Chryseobacterium* gen nov, *Bergeyella* gen nov, and *Empedobacter* nov rev, *Int J Syst Bacteriol* 44:827, 1994.

Versalovic J: *Manual of clinical microbiology*, ed 10, Washington, DC, 2011, ASM Press.

Weyant RS, Moss CW, Weaver RE et al, editors: *Identification of unusual pathogenic gram-negative aerobic and facultatively anaerobic bacteria*, ed 2, Baltimore, 1996, Williams & Wilkins.

# Alcaligenes, Bordetella (Non-pertussis), Comamonas, and Similar Organisms

## OBJECTIVES

1. Describe the normal habitat of the organisms discussed in this chapter and the means of transmission for human infection.
2. List the general characteristics of the bacteria discussed in this chapter.
3. Identify unusual biochemical reactions and incubation conditions required of organisms discussed in this chapter.
4. Outline the major tests used to identify the organisms in these groups.
5. Compare the appearance of the different genera in Gram stain preparations.
6. Describe the colonial appearance of the clinically significant species.

## GENERA AND SPECIES TO BE CONSIDERED

| Current Name | Previous Name |
|---|---|
| Achromobacter denitrificans | Alcaligenes denitrificans, Achromobacter xylosoxidans subsp. denitrificans |
| Achromobacter piechaudii | Alcaligenes piechaudii |
| Achromobacter xylosoxidans | Achromobacter xylosoxidans subsp. xylosoxidans |
| Alcaligenes faecalis type species | Pseudomonas or Alcaligenes odorans |
| A. faecalis subsp. faecalis | |
| A. faecalis subsp. parafaecalis | |
| A. faecalis subsp. phenolicus | |
| Bordetella bronchiseptica | CDC group IVa |
| CDC Alcaligenes-like group 1 | |
| CDC group IIg | |
| Comamonas spp. | |
| Cupriavidus pauculus | CDC group IVc-2, Wautersia paucula, Ralstonia paucula |
| Delftia acidovorans | Comamonas acidovorans, Pseudomonas acidovorans |
| Ignatzchineria spp. | Ciliari rod group 1 |
| Myroides spp. | Flavobacterium odoratum |
| Oligella ureolytica | CDC group IVe |
| Oligella urethralis | Moraxella urethralis, CDC group M-4 |
| Pseudomonas alcaligenes | |
| Pseudomonas pseudoalcaligenes | |
| Psychrobacter spp. (asaccharolytic strains) | Moraxella phenylpyruvia |
| Psychrobacter phenylpyruvicus | Moraxella phenylpyruvica |
| Roseomonas spp. | |

## GENERAL CHARACTERISTICS

The genera discussed in this chapter are considered together because most of them are usually oxidase-positive, non–glucose utilizers capable of growth on MacConkey agar. They are a diverse group of organisms.

The organism's specific morphologic and physiologic features are presented later in this chapter in the discussion of laboratory diagnosis.

*Achromobacter* species are gram-negative, nonsporulating, motile rods with 1 to 20 peritrichous flagella. They are strictly aerobic and nonfermentative. However, some strains are capable of anaerobic growth. The genus *Alcaligenes* is limited to the pathogenic type species *A. faecalis,* with two subspecies that are limited to environmental isolates: *A. faecalis* subsp. *parafaecalis* and *A. faecalis* subsp. *phenolicus.* *Alcaligenes* species are gram-negative, strict aerobic rods or coccobacilli that are oxidase and catalase positive. They are motile and have 1 to 12 peritrichous flagella. *Comamonas* spp. are typically environmental species that may be problematic opportunistic nosocomial pathogens. *Comamonas* and *Delftia* spp. are aerobic, non–spore forming, straight or slightly curved, gram-negative rods with one or more polar flagella. The genus *Oligella* comprises two asaccharolytic coccobacilli species, *O. ureolytica* and *O. urethralis. O. ureolytica* are motile by peritrichous flagella, and *O. urethralis* are nonmotile. *Roseomonas* spp. are coccoid, plump rods in pairs or short chains. They are typically motile by one or two polar flagella.

## EPIDEMIOLOGY

The habitats of the species listed in Table 25-1 vary from soil and water environments to the upper respiratory tract of various mammals. Certain species have been exclusively found in humans, whereas the natural habitat for other organisms remains unknown.

The diversity of the organisms' habitats is reflected in the various ways they are transmitted. For example, transmission of environmental isolates such as *Achromobacter denitrificans* frequently involves exposure of debilitated patients to contaminated fluids or medical solutions. In contrast, *Bordetella bronchiseptica* transmission primarily occurs by close contact with animals, whereas *Bordetella holmesii* has been detected only in human blood, and no niche or mode of transmission is known.

## PATHOGENESIS AND SPECTRUM OF DISEASE

Identifiable virulence factors are not known for most of the organisms listed in Table 25-2. However, because infections usually involve exposure of compromised patients to contaminated materials, most of these species are probably of low virulence. Among the environmental organisms listed, *Achromobacter* spp. are most frequently associated with various infections, including bacteremia, meningitis, pneumonia, and peritonitis. They also have

**TABLE 25-1** Epidemiology

| Species | Habitat (Reservoir) | Mode of Transmission |
|---|---|---|
| *Achromobacter xylosoxidans* | Environment, including moist areas of hospital. Transient colonizer of human gastrointestinal or respiratory tract in patients with cystic fibrosis | Not often known. Usually involves exposure to contaminated fluids (e.g., intravenous fluids, hemodialysis fluids, irrigation fluids), soaps, and disinfectants |
| *Achromobacter piechaudii* | Environment | Unknown. Rarely found in humans |
| *Alcaligenes faecalis* | Environment; soil and water, including moist hospital environments. May transiently colonize the skin | Exposure to contaminated medical devices and solutions |
| *Bordetella bronchiseptica* | Normal respiratory flora of several mammals, including dogs, cats, and rabbits. Not part of human flora | Probably by exposure to contaminated respiratory droplets during close contact with animals |
| *Comamonas* spp. | Environment, soil and water; can be found in hospital environment. Not part of human flora | Nosocomial opportunistic pathogens because of their ability to survive in aqueous environments |
| CDC group IVc-2 | Uncertain. Probably water sources, including those in the hospital setting. Not part of human flora | Usually involves contaminated dialysis systems or exposure of wounds to contaminated water |
| *Delftia acidovorans* | Environment, soil and water; can be found in hospital environment. Not part of human flora | Uncertain. Rarely found in humans. Probably involves exposure to contaminated solutions or devices |
| Ignatzchineria spp. | Unknown. Probably environmental. Not part of human flora | Unknown. Rarely found in humans |
| *Oligella urethralis* *Oligella ureolytica* | Unknown. May colonize distal urethra | Manipulation (e.g., catheterization) of urinary tract |
| *Psychrobacter* spp. | Unknown | Unknown |
| *Roseomonas* spp. | Unknown | Unknown. Rarely found in humans |

been implicated in outbreaks of nosocomial infections. *Achromobacter piechaudii* has been isolated from pharyngeal swabs, wounds, blood, and ear discharge. *Achromobacter xylosoxidans* increasingly has been recovered from patients with cystic fibrosis. However, it is unclear whether the organism is implicated in causing clinical disease in patients with cystic fibrosis or whether it simply colonizes the respiratory tract. *A. denitrificans* has been recovered from urine, prostrate secretions, the buccal cavity, pleural fluid, and eye secretions. *A. faecalis* has been isolated from a wide range of clinical specimens and has been identified in bacteremia, ocular infections, pancreatic abscesses, bone infections, urine, and ear discharge. *Comamonas* spp. have been identified in cases of endocarditis, meningitis, and catheter-associated bacteremia. They have also been recovered from sputum in patients with cystic fibrosis. Other organisms, such as *O. urethralis* and *O. ureolytica* have been isolated predominantly from the human urinary tract. *Pseudomonas alcaligenes* and *Pseudomonas pseudoalcaligenes* rarely have been identified in clinical samples.

# LABORATORY DIAGNOSIS

## SPECIMEN COLLECTION AND TRANSPORT

No special considerations are required for collection and transport of the organisms discussed in this chapter.

Refer to Table 5-1 for general information on specimen collection and transport.

## SPECIMEN PROCESSING

No special considerations are required for processing of the organisms discussed in this chapter. Refer to Table 5-1 for general information on specimen processing.

## DIRECT DETECTION METHODS

Other than Gram staining of patient specimens, there are no specific procedures for the direct detection of these organisms in clinical material. *B. bronchiseptica* is a medium-sized straight rod, whereas *O. urethralis*, *Psychrobacter* spp., *Roseomonas* spp., and *Moraxella* spp. are all coccobacilli, although *Psychrobacter phenylpyruvicus* may appear as a broad rod, and some *Roseomonas* spp. may appear as short, straight rods. *O. ureolytica* is a short, straight rod; *Myroides* spp. are pleomorphic rods and are either short or long and straight to slightly curved.

*Alcaligenes* and *Achromobacter* spp. are medium to long straight rods, as are CDC *Alcaligenes*-like group 1, *Cupriavidus pauculus*, *Delftia acidovorans*, *P. alcaligenes*, and *P. pseudoalcaligenes*. The *Comamonas* spp. are pleomorphic and may appear as long, paired, curved rods or filaments. The cells of CDC group IIg appear as small, coccoid-to-rod forms or occasionally as rods with long filaments.

**TABLE 25-2** Pathogenesis and Spectrum of Disease

| Species | Virulence Factors | Spectrum of Disease and Infections |
|---|---|---|
| *Achromobacter dentrificans* | Unknown. Survival in hospital the result of inherent resistance to disinfectants and antimicrobial agents | Infections usually involve compromised patients and include bacteremia, urinary tract infections, meningitis, wound infections, pneumonia, and peritonitis; occur in various body sites; can be involved in nosocomial outbreaks. |
| *Achromobacter xylosoxidans* | Unknown. Survival in hospital the result of inherent resistance to disinfectants and antimicrobial agents | Infections usually involve compromised patients and include meningitis, pneumonia, otitis media, urinary tract infections, surgical wound infections, and bacteremia. |
| *Alcaligenes faecalis* | Unknown | Infections usually involve compromised patients. Often a contaminant; clinical significance of isolates should be interpreted with caution. Has been isolated from blood, respiratory specimens, and urine. |
| *Alcaligenes piechaudii* | Unknown | Rare cause of human infection. |
| *Bordetella bronchiseptica* | Unknown for humans. Has several factors similar to *B. parapertussis* | Opportunistic infection in compromised patients with history of close animal contact. Infections are uncommon and include pneumonia, bacteremia, urinary tract infections, meningitis, and endocarditis. |
| CDC group IVc-2 | Unknown | Rare cause of human infection. Infections in compromised patients include bacteremia and peritonitis. |
| *Comamonas testosteroni Comamonas* spp. | Unknown | Isolated from respiratory tract, eye, and blood but rarely implicated as being clinically significant. |
| *Cupriavidus* spp. | Unknown | Recovered from cystic fibrosis patients. Additional infections include bacteremia, peritonitis and tenosynovitis. |
| *Delftia acidovorans* | Unknown | Isolated from respiratory tract, eye, and blood but rarely implicated as being clinically significant. |
| Ignatzchineria spp. | Unknown | Clinical significance uncertain, has been isolated from wounds, urine, and blood. |
| *Oligella urethralis* | Unknown | Urinary tract infections, particularly in females. |
| *Oligella ureolytica* | Unknown | Also isolated from kidney, joint, and peritoneal fluid. |
| *P. alcaligenes P. pseudoalcaligenes* | Unknown; low virulence associated with administration of contaminated solutions and medicines | Recovered from the respiratory secretions of patients with cystic fibrosis. |
| *Psychrobacter* spp. | Unknown | Rare cause of human infection |
| *Roseomonas* spp. | Unknown; uncommon isolates from humans | Clinical significance uncertain. Typically opportunistic infections. Most isolated from blood, wounds, exudates, abscesses, or genitourinary tract of immunocompromised or debilitated patients. |

## CULTIVATION

### Media of Choice

*B. bronchiseptica* grows on 5% sheep blood, chocolate, and MacConkey agars, usually within 1 to 2 days after inoculation. It should also grow in thioglycollate broth. *Psychrobacter* spp., *Myroides* spp., *Oligella* spp., *Achromobacter* spp., *D. acidovorans,* *Alcaligenes* spp., CDC *Alcaligenes*-like group 1, *Comamonas* spp., *Roseomonas* spp., *P. alcaligenes, P. pseudoalcaligenes, C. pauculus,* and CDC group IIg all grow well on 5% sheep blood, chocolate, and MacConkey agars. Most of these genera should also grow well in the broth of blood culture systems, as well as in common nutrient broths such as thioglycollate and brain-heart infusion.

### Incubation Conditions and Duration

Most of the organisms produce detectable growth on media incubated at 35°C in ambient air or 5% carbon dioxide ($CO_2$). *Psychrobacter* spp. usually grow better at 25°C than at 35°C.

### Colonial Appearance

Table 25-3 describes the colonial appearance and other distinguishing characteristics (e.g., pigment and odor) of each genus on 5% sheep blood and MacConkey agars.

## APPROACH TO IDENTIFICATION

The ability of most commercial identification systems to accurately identify the organisms discussed in this chapter is limited or uncertain. Strategies for identification of these genera therefore are based on the use of conventional biochemical tests and special staining for flagella. Although most clinical microbiology laboratories do not routinely perform flagella stains, motility and flagella

**TABLE 25-3** Colonial Appearance and Characteristics

| Organism | Medium | Appearance |
|---|---|---|
| *Achromobacter denitrificans* | BAP MAC | Small, convex, and glistening NLF |
| *Achromobacter xylosoxidans* | BAP MAC | Small, convex, and glistening NLF |
| *Achromobacter piechaudii* | BAP MAC | Nonpigmented, glistening, convex colonies surrounded by zone of greenish brown discoloration NLF |
| *Alcaligenes faecalis* | BAP MAC | Feather-edged colonies usually surrounded by zone of green discoloration; produces a highly characteristic, fruity odor resembling apples or strawberries NLF |
| *Bordetella bronchiseptica* | BAP MAC | Small, convex, round NLF |
| CDC *Alcaligenes*-like group 1 | BAP MAC | Resembles *A. denitrificans* NLF |
| CDC group IIg | BAP MAC | No distinctive appearance NLF |
| *Comamonas* spp. | BAP MAC | No distinctive appearance NLF |
| *Cupriavidus* sp. | BAP MAC | Small, yellow NLF |
| *Delftia acidovorans* | BAP MAC | No distinctive appearance NLF |
| Ignatzchineria spp. | BAP MAC | No distinctive appearance NLF |
| *Myroides* spp. | BAP MAC | Most colonies are yellow, have a characteristic fruity odor, and tend to spread NLF |
| *Oligella* spp. | BAP MAC | Small, opaque, whitish NLF |
| *Pseudomonas alcaligenes* | BAP MAC | No distinctive appearance NLF |
| *Pseudomonas pseudoalcaligenes* | BAP MAC | No distinctive appearance NLF |
| *Psychrobacter* spp. (asaccharolytic strains) | BAP MAC | Smooth, small, translucent to semiopaque NLF |
| *Roseomonas* spp. | BAP MAC | Pink-pigmented; some colonies may be mucoid NLF |

*BA,* 5% sheep blood agar; *Mac,* MacConkey agar; *NLF,* non–lactose fermenter.

placement are the easiest ways to differentiate among these organisms.

Many microbiologists groan at the mere mention of having to perform a flagella stain, but the method described in Procedure 13-16 is a wet mount that is easy to perform. At the very least, a simple wet mount to observe cells for motility helps distinguish between the motile and nonmotile genera. The pseudomonads and *Brevundimonas, Burkholderia,* and *Ralstonia* species described in Chapter 22 are motile by means of single or multiple polar flagella; the motile organisms described in this chapter have peritrichous flagella (e.g., *B.*

*bronchiseptica, Alcaligenes* spp., and *Achromobacter* spp.), or polar flagella (e.g., *Delftia, Comamonas* spp.).

Organisms are first categorized on the basis of Gram stain morphology (i.e., coccoid [Table 25-4] or rod shaped [Tables 25-5 through 25-7]). They are then further characterized based on whether the organisms are non-motile (see Table 25-5), peritrichously flagellated (see Table 25-6), or flagellated by polar tufts (see Table 25-7).

## Comments Regarding Specific Organisms

*B. bronchiseptica* is oxidase-positive, motile, and rapidly urease positive, sometimes in as little as 4 hours. This

**TABLE 25-4** Key Biochemical and Physiologic Characteristics for Coccoid Species

| Organisms | Motility | Urea Hydrolysis | Nitrate Reduction | Nitrite Reduction |
|---|---|---|---|---|
| *Oligella ureolytica* | + or (+)* | + | + | + |
| *Oligella urethralis* | nm | − | − | + |
| *Psychrobacter phenylpyruvicus*[†] | nm | + | v | − |
| *Psychrobacter immobilis*[‡] (asaccharolytic strains) | nm | v | v | ND |

Data compiled from Holt JG, Krieg NR, Sneath PH et al, editors: *Bergey's manual of determinatative bacteriology,* ed 9, Baltimore, 1994, Williams & Wilkins; and Versalovic J: *Manual of clinical microbiology,* ed 10, Washington, DC, 2011, ASM Press.
*ND,* No data available; *nm,* nonmotile; *v,* variable; +, >90% of strains are positive; −, >90% of strains are negative; (+), positive delayed.
*Petrichous flagella but motility may be delayed or difficult to demonstrate,
[†]Deaminates phenylalanine.
[‡]Best growth at 25°C.

**TABLE 25-5** Key Biochemical and Physiologic Characteristics for Rod-Shaped Nonmotile Species

| Organisms | Insoluble Pigment | Indole | Urea Hydrolysis | Nitrite Reduction |
|---|---|---|---|---|
| CDC group IIg | v, tan or salmon | + | − | + |
| *Myroides* spp. | v, yellow | − | + | v |

Data compiled from Holt JG, Krieg NR, Sneath PH et al, editors: *Bergey's manual of determinatative bacteriology,* ed 9, Baltimore, 1994, Williams & Wilkins; and Versalovic J: *Manual of clinical microbiology,* ed 10, Washington, DC, 2011, ASM Press.
*v,* Variable; +, >90% of strains are positive; −, >90% of strains are negative

organism must be differentiated from *C. pauculus* and *O. ureolytica.*

Urea hydrolysis is a key test for *Myroides* spp., which is also distinguished by production of a characteristic fruity odor. CDC group IIg is the only indole-positive, nonmotile species included in this chapter.

The genus *Oligella* includes one nonmotile species (*O. urethralis*) and one motile species (*O. ureolytica*). Urease hydrolysis is a key test for differentiating between these species; *O. ureolytica* often turns positive within minutes. *O. urethralis* is urease and nitrate reductase negative. *P. phenylpyruvicus* is nonmotile and urease positive, arginine dihydrolase positive and phenylalanine deaminase positive.

*Achromobacter denitrificans* and *Alcaligenes piechaudii* reduce nitrate to nitrite, but only the former reduces nitrite to gas. *Achromobacter* species are oxidase and catalase positive and negative for urease, DNase, lysine decarboxylase, ornithine decarboxylase, arginine dihydrolase, and gelatinase. *A. faecalis* has a fruity odor and also reduces nitrite to gas. CDC *Alcaligenes*-like group 1 is similar to *Achromobacter denitrificans* but is usually urea positive.

*Delftia acidovorans* is unique in producing an orange color when Kovac's reagent is added to tryptone broth (indole test).

*Roseomonas* spp. must be separated from other pink-pigmented, gram-negative (e.g., *Methylobacterium* spp.) and gram-positive (e.g., certain *Rhodococcus* spp. or *Bacillus* spp.) organisms. *Roseomonas* spp. differ from *Rhodococcus* and *Bacillus* spp. by being resistant to vancomycin, as determined by using a 30-μg vancomycin disk on an inoculated 5% blood agar plate. Unlike *Methylobacterium* spp., *Roseomonas* spp. grow on MacConkey agar and at 42°C. All *Roseomonas* species strongly hydrolyze urea but not esculin and are β-galactosidase negative.

*P. alcaligenes* is differentiated from *P. pseudoalcaligenes* by its inability to oxidize fructose. These two species are often referred to as "*Pseudomonas* spp., not *aeruginosa*" in clinical situations.

## SERODIAGNOSIS

Serodiagnostic techniques are not generally used for the laboratory diagnosis of infections caused by the organisms discussed in this chapter.

## ANTIMICROBIAL SUSCEPTIBILITY TESTINGAND THERAPY

Validated susceptibility testing methods do not exist for these organisms. Although they will grow on the media and under the conditions recommended for testing the more commonly encountered bacteria (see Chapter 12 for more information regarding validated testing methods), this does not necessarily mean that interpretable and reliable results will be produced. Chapter 12 should be reviewed for preferable strategies that can be used to provide susceptibility information when validated testing methods do not exist for a clinically important bacterial isolate.

The lack of validated in vitro susceptibility testing methods does not allow definitive treatment and testing guidelines to be given for most organisms listed in Table 25-8. If antimicrobial sensitivity testing is required for *Achromobacter* and *Alcaligenes* spp., methods include broth macrodilution and microdilution, agar dilution, breakpoint methods, and Etest. *Bordetella parapertussis* is an

**TABLE 25-6** Key Biochemical and Physiologic Characteristics for Rod-Shaped Motile Species with Polar Flagella

| Organism | Number of Flagella | Oxidizes Mannitol | Insoluble Pigment | Growth at 42°C | Nitrate Reduction |
|---|---|---|---|---|---|
| *Delftia acidovorans* | >2 | + | – | v | + |
| *Comamonas* spp. | >2 | – | – | v | + |
| *Pseudomonas alcaligenes* | 1-2 | – | v[a] | v | v |
| *Pseudomonas pseudoalcaligenes*[b] | 1-2 | – | – | + | + |
| *Roseomonas* spp.[c] | 1-2[d] | v | pink | v | v |

Data compiled from Holt JG, Krieg NR, Sneath PH, et al, editors: *Bergey's manual of determinatative bacteriology,* ed 9, Baltimore, 1994, Williams & Wilkins; and Versalovic J: *Manual of clinical microbiology,* ed 10, 2011, Washington, DC, ASM Press.
*v,* Variable; +, >90% of strains are positive; –, >90% of strains are negative.
[a]Some strains have a yellow-orange insoluble pigment.
[b]Oxidizes fructose.
[c]Represents composite of several species and genomospecies.
[d]Genomospecies 5 is nonmotile.

**TABLE 25-7** Key Biochemical and Physiologic Characteristics for Rod-Shaped Motile Species with Peritrichous Flagella

| Organism | Urea Hydrolysis | Nitrate Reduction | Gas from Nitrate | Growth on Cetrimide | Jordan's Tartrate* |
|---|---|---|---|---|---|
| *Achromobacter denitrificans* | – | + | + | v | + |
| *Achromobacter xylosoxidans* | | + | + | + | |
| *Achromobacter piechaudii* | – | + | – | + | + |
| *Alcaligenes faecalis*[†] | – | – | – | v | – |
| CDC *Alcaligenes*-like group 1 | v | + | + | – | – |
| *Bordetella bronchiseptica* | + | + | – | – | – |
| *Cupriavidus pauculus* | + | v | – | – | + |

Data compiled from Holt JG, Krieg NR, Sneath PH et al, editors: *Bergey's manual of determinatative bacteriology,* ed 9, Baltimore, 1994, Williams & Wilkins; and Versalovic J: *Manual of clinical microbiology,* ed 10, 2011, Washington, DC, ASM Press.
*v,* Variable; +, >90% of strains are positive; –, >90% of strains are negative.
*Jordan's tartrate agar deeps is a medium used to differentiate gram-negative enteric microorganisms based on the utilization of tartrate.
[†]Reduces nitrite.

**TABLE 25-8** Antimicrobial Therapy and Susceptibility Testing

| Species | Therapeutic Options | Potential Resistance to Therapeutic Options | Validated Testing Methods* | Comments |
|---|---|---|---|---|
| *Achromobacter denitrificans* | No definitive guidelines. Potentially active agents include mezlocillin, piperacillin, ticarcillin/clavulanic acid, ceftazidime, imipenem, trimethoprim/sulfamethoxazole, and quinolones | Capable of beta-lactamase production | Not available | |
| *Achromobacter xylosoxidans* | No definitive guidelines. Potentially active agents include imipenem, piperacillin, ticarcillin/ clavulanic acid, ceftazidime, and trimethoprim-sulfamethoxazole | Aminoglycosides, expanded spectrum cephalosporins other than ceftazidime, and quinolones demonstrated no activity. Resistant to tobramycin, azithromycin, and clarithromycin | Not available | |
| *Achromobacter piechaudii* | No definitive guidelines. | Resistant to ampicillin, cefpodoxime, and gentamicin | Not available | |

**TABLE 25-8** Antimicrobial Therapy and Susceptibility Testing—cont'd

| Species | Therapeutic Options | Potential Resistance to Therapeutic Options | Validated Testing Methods* | Comments |
|---|---|---|---|---|
| *Alcaligenes faecalis* | No definitive guidelines. Potentially active agents include combinations of amoxicillin or ticarcillin with clavulanic acid, various cephalosporins, and ciprofloxacin | Capable of beta-lactamase production. Commonly resistant to ampicillin, amoxicillin, ticarcillin, aztreonam, kanamycin, gentamicin, and nalidixic acid. | Not available | |
| *Bordetella bronchiseptica* | No definitive guidelines. May be sensitive to amoxicillin-clavulanic acid, tetracycline, gentamicin or quinolones. | Possesses a ß-lactamase. Commonly resistant to many penicillins and cephalosporins and mostly resistant to trimethoprim-sulfamethoxazole. | Not available | |
| CDC group IVc-2 | No definitive guidelines. Potentially active agents include cefotaxime ceftazidime, ceftriaxone, and imipenem | Often resistant to penicillins, even with beta-lactamase inhibitor, and aminoglycosides | Not available | |
| *Comamonas acidovorans, Comamonas testosteroni, Comamonas* spp. | No definitive guidelines. Potentially active agents include extended- to broad-spectrum cephalosporins, carbapenems, quinolones and trimethoprim-sulfamethoxazole | Unknown | Not available | *C. acidovorans* tends to be more resistant than the other two species, especially to aminoglycosides. |
| *Delftia acidovorans* | No definitive guidelines | Frequently resistant to aminoglycosides | Not available | |
| Ignatzchineria spp. | No definitive guidelines | Unknown | Not available | Generally susceptible to various antimicrobial agents |
| *Oligella urethralis* *Oligella ureolytica* | No definitive guidelines. Potentially active agents include several penicillins, cephalosporins, and quinolones | Produces beta-lactamases; may develop resistance to quinolones | Not available | |
| *Roseomonas* spp. | No definitive guidelines. Potentially active agents include aminoglycosides, imipenem, and quinolones. | Generally resistant to cephalosporins and penicillins | Not available | |

*Validated testing methods include standard methods recommended by the Clinical and Laboratory Standards Institute (CLSI) and commercial methods approved by the U.S. Food and Drug Administration (FDA).

exception; significant clinical experience indicates that erythromycin is the antimicrobial agent of choice for whooping cough caused by this organism (see Chapter 37 for more information on therapy for *Bordetella pertussis* and *B. parapertussis* infections). Standardized testing methods do not exist for this species, but the recent recognition of erythromycin resistance in *B. pertussis* indicates that development of such testing may be warranted for the causative agents of whooping cough.

Even though standardized methods have not been established for the other species discussed in this chapter, in vitro susceptibility studies have been published, and antimicrobial agents that have potential activity are noted, where appropriate, in Table 25-8. *A. xylosoxidans* demonstrates variable susceptibility to β-lactams, ureidopenicillins, and carbapenems; the organism is resistant to narrow-spectrum penicillins and cephalosporins, including cefotaxime.

# PREVENTION

Because the organisms may be encountered throughout nature and do not generally pose a threat to human health, there are no recommended vaccination or prophylaxis protocols. For those organisms occasionally associated with nosocomial infections, prevention of infection is best accomplished by following appropriate sterile techniques and infection control guidelines.

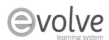 **Visit the Evolve site to complete the review questions.**

## CASE STUDY 25-1

A patient who has tested positive for the human immunodeficiency virus (HIV) develops pneumonia while traveling in Europe. His cultures are reported as negative for pathogens, and he does not respond to the usual treatment with cephalosporin therapy. The patient returns home and submits a sputum culture to the local laboratory. The smear shows white blood cells but low numbers of bacteria. No pathogens are detected within 24 hours, but after 48 hours, heavy growth of a gram-negative coccobacilli is observed. After the cause of the patient's pneumonia is identified, he is successfully treated with ciprofloxacin. Later it comes to light that he has a pet dog.

### QUESTIONS

1. The organism is able to grow on MacConkey agar. but the colonies are small and colorless. The organism tests oxidase and catalase positive. Colonies on blood agar are without pigment. What rapid tests can be done to identify this bacterium?
2. In this case, indole and PDA are negative, but motility and urease are positive. Which genera are in the differential for the pathogen?
3. Had the organism been nonmotile, which serious pathogen should have been considered?
4. The patient was not diagnosed at another hospital. What do you suspect as the reason for the inability to detect the organism?

## BIBLIOGRAPHY

Balows A, Truper HG, Dworkin M, et al, editors: *The prokaryotes: a handbook on the biology of bacteria—ecophysiology, isolation, identification, applications*, ed 2, New York, 1981, Springer-Verlag.

Bowman JP, Cavanagh J, Austin JJ, et al: Novel *Psychrobacter* species from Antarctic ornithogenic soils, *Int J Syst Bacteriol* 46:841, 1996.

Castagnola E, Tasso L, Conte M, et al: Central venous catheter–related infection due to *Comamonas acidovorans* in a child with non-Hodgkin's lymphoma, *Clin Infect Dis* 19:559, 1994.

Dunne WM, Maisch S: Epidemiological investigation of infections due to *Alcaligenes* species in children and patients with cystic fibrosis: use of repetitive-element–sequence polymerase chain reaction, *Clin Infect Dis* 20:836, 1995.

Holt JG, Krieg NR, Sneath PH, et al, editors: *Bergey's manual of determinative bacteriology*, ed 9, Baltimore, 1994, Williams & Wilkins.

Hoppe JE, Tschirner T: Comparison of media for agar dilution susceptibility testing of *Bordetella pertussis* and *Bordetella parapertussis*, *Eur J Clin Microbiol Infect Dis* 14:775, 1995.

Lindquist SW, Weber DJ, Mangum ME, et al: *Bordetella holmesii* sepsis in an asplenic adolescent, *Pediatr Infect Dis J* 14:813, 1995.

Mandell GL, Bennett JE, Dolin R, editors: *Principles and practice of infectious diseases*, ed 7, Philadelphia, 2010, Churchill Livingstone/Elsevier.

Moss CW, Daneshvar MI, Hollis DG: Biochemical characteristics and fatty acid composition of *Gilardi* rod group 1 bacteria, *J Clin Microbiol* 31:689, 1993.

Pugliese A, Pacris B, Schoch PE, et al: *Oligella urethralis* urosepsis, *Clin Infect Dis* 17:1069, 1993.

Rihs JD, Brenner DJ, Weaver RE, et al: *Roseomonas*: a new genus associated with bacteremia and other human infections, *J Clin Microbiol* 31:3275, 1993.

Riley UBG, Bignardi G, Goldberg L, et al: Quinolone resistance in *Oligella urethralis*–associated chronic ambulatory peritoneal dialysis peritonitis, *J Infect* 32:155, 1996.

Saiman L, Chen Y, Tabibi S, et al: Identification and antimicrobial susceptibility of *Alcaligenes xylosoxidans* isolated from patients with cystic fibrosis, *J Clin Microbiol* 39:3942, 2001.

Validation of the publication of new names and new combinations previously effectively published outside the IJSB, Validation List No 65, *Int J Syst Bacteriol* 48:627, 1998.

Vancanneyt M, Segers P, Torck U, et al: Reclassification of *Flavobacterium odoratum (Stutzer 1929)* strains to a new genus, *Myroides*, as *Myroides odoratus* comb nov and *Myroides odoratimimus* sp nov, *Int J Syst Bacteriol* 46:926, 1996.

Vandamme P, Heyndrickx M, Vancanneyt M, et al: *Bordetella trematum* sp nov, isolated from wounds and ear infections in humans, and reassessment of *Alcaligenes denitrificans (Rüger and Tan, 1983)*, *Int J Syst Bacteriol* 46:849, 1996.

Versalovic J: *Manual of clinical microbiology*, ed 10, Washington, DC, 2011, ASM Press.

Wen A, Fegan M, Hayward C, et al: Phylogenetic relationships among members of the Comamonadaceae, and description of *Delftia acidovorans (den Dooren de Jong, 1926 and Tamaoka et al, 1987)* gen nov, comb nov, *Int J Syst Bacteriol* 49:567, 1999.

Yabuuchi E, Kawamura Y, Kosako Y, et al: Emendation of the genus *Achromobacter* and *Achromobacter xylosoxidans* (Yabuuchi and Yano) and proposal of *Achromobacter ruhlandii* (Packer and Vishniac) comb nov, *Achromobacter piechaudii* (Kiredjian et al) comb nov, and *Achromobacter xylosoxidans* subsp *denitrificans* (Rüger and Tan) comb nov, *Microbiol Immunol* 42:429, 1998.

Yohei D, Poirel L, Paterson DL, Nordmann P: Characterization of a naturally occurring class D beta-lactamase from *Achromobacter xylosoxidans*, *Antimicrob Agents Chemother* 52:1952, 2008.

# Vibrio, Aeromonas, Chromobacterium, and Related Organisms

## OBJECTIVES

1. Describe the general characteristics of the organisms discussed in this chapter, including natural habitat, route of transmission, Gram stain reactions, and cellular morphology.
2. Describe the media used to isolate *Vibrio* spp. and the organisms' colonial appearance.
3. Explain the physiologic activity of the cholera toxin and its relationship to the pathogenesis of the organism.
4. Describe the clinical significance of *Aeromonas* spp., *Chromobacterium* sp., and *Vibrio* spp. other than *Vibrio cholerae.*
5. Correlate the patient's signs and symptoms and laboratory data to identify an infectious agent.

### GENERA AND SPECIES TO BE CONSIDERED

| Current Name | Previous Name |
|---|---|
| *Aeromonas caviae* complex | |
| *A. caviae* | |
| *A. media* | |
| *Aeromonas hydrophila* complex | |
| *A. hydrophila* subsp. *hydrophila* | |
|    *A. hydrophila* subsp. *dhakensis* | |
|    *A. bestiarum* | |
| *A. salmonicida* | |
| *Aeromonas veronii* complex | |
| *A. veronii* biovar *sobria* | |
|    *A. veronii* biovar *veronii* | |
|    *A. jandaei* | |
| *A. schubertii* | |
| *Chromobacterium violaceum* | |
| *Photobacterium damselae* | *Vibrio damsela* |
| *Grimontia hollisae* | CDC group EF-13; *Vibrio hollisae* |
| *Vibrio alginolyticus* | *Vibrio parahaemolyticus* biotype 2 |
| *Vibrio cholerae* | |
| *Vibrio cincinnatiensis* | |
| *Vibrio fluvialis* | CDC group EF-6 |
| *Vibrio furnissii* | |
| *Vibrio harveyi* | *Vibrio carchariae* |
| *Vibrio metschnikovii* | CDC enteric group 16 |
| *Vibrio mimicus* | *Vibrio cholerae* (sucrose negative) |
| *Vibrio parahaemolyticus* | *Pasteurella parahaemolyticus* |
| *Vibrio vulnificus* | CDC group EF-3 |

## GENERAL CHARACTERISTICS

The organisms discussed in this chapter are considered together because they are all oxidase-positive, glucose-fermenting, gram-negative bacilli capable of growth on MacConkey agar. Their individual morphologic and physiologic features are presented later in this chapter

in the discussion of laboratory diagnosis. Other halophilic organisms, such as *Halomonas venusta* and *Shewanella algae*, require salt but do not ferment glucose, as do the halophilic *Vibrio* spp.

*Aeromonas* spp. are gram-negative straight rods with rounded ends or coccobacillary facultative anaerobes that occur singly, in pairs, or in short chains. They are typically oxidase and catalase positive and produce acid from oxidative and fermentative metabolism. *Chromobacterium violaceum* is a facultative anaerobic, motile, gram-negative rod or cocci.

The family Vibrionaceae includes six genera, three of which are discussed in this chapter. The *Photobacterium* and *Grimontia* each include a single species. The genus *Vibrio* consists of 10 species of gram-negative, facultative anaerobic, curved or comma-shaped rods. Most species are motile and are catalase and oxidase positive except *Vibrio metschnikovii*. All *Vibrio* spp. require sodium for growth and ferment glucose.

## EPIDEMIOLOGY

Many aspects of the epidemiology of *Vibrio* spp., *Aeromonas* spp., and *C. violaceum* are similar (Table 26-1). The primary habitat for most of these organisms is water; generally, brackish or marine water for *Vibrio* spp., freshwater for *Aeromonas* spp., and soil or water for *C. violaceum*. *Aeromonas* spp. may also be found in brackish water or marine water with a low salt content. None of these organisms are considered part of the normal human flora. Transmission to humans is by ingestion of contaminated water, fresh produce, meat, dairy products, or seafood or by exposure of disrupted skin and mucosal surfaces to contaminated water.

The epidemiology of the most notable human pathogen in this chapter, *Vibrio cholerae*, is far from being fully understood. This organism causes epidemics and pandemics (i.e., worldwide epidemics) of the diarrheal disease cholera. Since 1817 the world has witnessed seven cholera pandemics. During these outbreaks the organism is spread among people by the fecal-oral route, usually in environments with poor sanitation.

The niche that *V. cholerae* inhabits between epidemics is uncertain. The form of the organism shed from infected humans is somewhat fragile and cannot survive long in the environment. However, evidence suggests that the bacillus has survival, or dormant, stages that allow its long-term survival in brackish water or saltwater environments during interepidemic periods. These dormant stages are considered viable but nonculturable. Asymptomatic carriers of *V. cholerae* have been documented, but they are not thought to be a significant reservoir for maintaining the organism between outbreaks.

**TABLE 26-1** Epidemiology

| Species | Habitat (Reservoir) | Mode of Transmission |
|---|---|---|
| Vibrio cholerae | Niche outside of human gastrointestinal tract between occurrence of epidemics and pandemics is uncertain; may survive in a dormant state in brackish or saltwater; human carriers also are known but are uncommon | Fecal-oral route, by ingestion of contaminated washing, swimming, cooking, or drinking water; also by ingestion of contaminated shellfish or other seafood |
| V. alginolyticus | Brackish or saltwater | Exposure to contaminated water |
| V. cincinnatiensis | Unknown | Unknown |
| Photobacterium damsela | Brackish or saltwater | Exposure of wound to contaminated water |
| V. fluvialis | Brackish or saltwater | Ingestion of contaminated water or seafood |
| V. furnissii | Brackish or saltwater | Ingestion of contaminated water or seafood |
| Grimontia hollisae | Brackish or saltwater | Ingestion of contaminated water or seafood |
| V. metschnikovii | Brackish, salt and freshwater | Unknown |
| V. mimicus | Brackish or saltwater | Ingestion of contaminated water or seafood |
| V. parahaemolyticus | Brackish or saltwater | Ingestion of contaminated water or seafood |
| V. vulnificus | Brackish or saltwater | Ingestion of contaminated water or seafood |
| Aeromonas spp. | Aquatic environments around the world, including freshwater, polluted or chlorinated water, brackish water and, occasionally, marine water; may transiently colonize gastrointestinal tract; often infect various warm- and cold-blooded animal species | Ingestion of contaminated food (e.g., dairy, meat, produce) or, water; exposure of disrupted skin or mucosal surfaces to contaminated water or soil; traumatic inoculation of fish fins and or fishing hooks |
| Chromobacterium violaceum | Environmental, soil and water of tropical and subtropical regions. Not part of human flora | Exposure of disrupted skin to contaminated soil or water |

# PATHOGENESIS AND SPECTRUM OF DISEASE

As a notorious pathogen, *V. cholerae* elaborates several toxins and factors that play important roles in the organism's virulence. Cholera toxin (CT) is primarily responsible for the key features of cholera (Table 26-2). Release of this toxin causes mucosal cells to hypersecrete water and electrolytes into the lumen of the gastrointestinal tract. The result is profuse, watery diarrhea, leading to dramatic fluid loss. The fluid loss results in severe dehydration and hypotension that, without medical intervention, frequently lead to death. This toxin-mediated disease does not require the organism to penetrate the mucosal barrier. Therefore, blood and the inflammatory cells typical of dysenteric stools are notably absent in cholera. Instead, "rice water stools," composed of fluids and mucous flecks, are the hallmark of cholera toxin activity.

*V. cholerae* is divided into three major subgroups; *V. cholerae* O1, *V. cholerae* O129, and *V. cholerae* non-O1. The somatic antigens O1 and O139 associated with the *V. cholerae* cell envelope are positive markers for strains capable of epidemic and pandemic spread of the disease. Strains carrying these markers almost always produce cholera toxin, whereas non-O1/non-O139 strains do not produce the toxin and hence do not produce cholera. Therefore, although these somatic antigens are not virulence factors per se, they are important virulence and epidemiologic markers that provide important information about *V. cholerae* isolates. The non-O1/non-O139 strains are associated with nonepidemic diarrhea and extraintestinal infections.

*V. cholerae* produces several other toxins and factors, but the exact role of these in disease is still uncertain (see Table 26-2). To effectively release toxin, the organism first must infiltrate and distribute itself along the cells lining the mucosal surface of the gastrointestinal tract. Motility and chemotaxis mediate the distribution of organisms, and mucinase production allows penetration of the mucous layer. Toxin coregulated pili (TCP) provide the means by which bacilli attach to mucosal cells for release of cholera toxin.

Depending on the species, other vibrios are variably involved in three types of infection: gastroenteritis, wound infections, and bacteremia. Although some of these organisms have not been definitively associated with human infections, others, such as *Vibrio vulnificus*, are known to cause fatal septicemia, especially in patients suffering from an underlying liver disease.

*Aeromonas* spp. are similar to *Vibrio* spp. in terms of the types of infections they cause. Although these organisms can cause gastroenteritis, most frequently in children, their role in intestinal infections is not always clear. Therefore, the significance of their isolation in stool specimens should be interpreted with caution. Severe watery diarrhea has been associated with *Aeromonas* strains that produce a heat-labile enterotoxin and a heat-stable enterotoxin. In addition to diarrhea, complications of

**TABLE 26-2** Pathogenesis and Spectrum of Diseases

| Species | Virulence Factors | Spectrum of Disease and Infections |
|---------|-------------------|-----------------------------------|
| *Vibrio cholerae* | Cholera toxin; zonula occludens (Zot) toxin (enterotoxin); accessory cholera enterotoxin (Ace) toxin; O1 and O139 somatic antigens, hemolysin/cytotoxins, motility, chemotaxis, mucinase, and toxin coregulated pili (TCP) pili. | Cholera: profuse, watery diarrhea leading to dehydration, hypotension, and often death; occurs in epidemics and pandemics that span the globe. May also cause nonepidemic diarrhea and, occasionally, extra intestinal infections of wounds, respiratory tract, urinary tract, and central nervous system |
| *V. alginolyticus* | Specific virulence factors for the non–*V. cholerae* species are uncertain. | Ear infections, wound infections; rare cause of septicemia; involvement in gastroenteritis is uncertain |
| *V. cincinnatiensis* | | Rare cause of septicemia |
| *P. damsela* | | Wound infections and rare cause of septicemia |
| *V. fluvialis* | | Gastroenteritis |
| *V. furnissii* | | Rarely associated with human infections |
| *Grimontia hollisae* | | Gastroenteritis; rare cause of septicemia |
| *V. metschnikovii* | | Rare cause of septicemia; involvement in gastroenteritis is uncertain |
| *V. mimicus* | | Gastroenteritis; rare cause of ear infection |
| *V. vulnificus* | | Wound infections and septicemia; involvement in gastroenteritis is uncertain |
| *Aeromonas* spp. | *Aeromonas* spp. produce various toxins and factors, but their specific role in virulence is uncertain. | Gastroenteritis, wound infections, bacteremia, and miscellaneous other infections, including endocarditis, meningitis, pneumonia, conjunctivitis, and osteomyelitis |
| *Chromobacterium violaceum* | Endotoxin, adhesins, invasins and cytolytic proteins have been described. | Rare but dangerous infection. Begins with cellulitis or lymphadenitis and can rapidly progress to systemic infection with abscess formation in various organs and septic shock |

infection with *Aeromonas* spp. include hemolytic-uremic syndrome and kidney disease.

*C. violaceum* is not associated with gastrointestinal infections, but acquisition of this organism by contamination of wounds can lead to fulminant, life-threatening systemic infections.

# LABORATORY DIAGNOSIS

## SPECIMEN COLLECTION AND TRANSPORT

Because no special considerations are required for isolation of these genera from extraintestinal sources, the general specimen collection and transport information provided in Table 5-1 is applicable. However, stool specimens suspected of containing *Vibrio* spp. should be collected and transported only in Cary-Blair medium. Buffered glycerol saline is not acceptable, because glycerol is toxic for vibrios. Feces is preferable, but rectal swabs are acceptable during the acute phase of diarrheal illness.

## SPECIMEN PROCESSING

No special considerations are required for processing of the organisms discussed in this chapter. Refer to Table 5-1 for general information on specimen processing.

**Figure 26-1** Gram stain of *Vibrio parahaemolyticus.*

## DIRECT DETECTION METHODS

*V. cholerae* toxin can be detected in stool using an enzyme-linked immunosorbent assay (ELISA) or a commercially available latex agglutination test (Oxoid, Inc., Odgensburg, New York), but these tests are not widely used in the United States.

Microscopically, vibrios are gram-negative, straight or slightly curved rods (Figure 26-1). When stool specimens from patients with cholera are examined using dark-field microscopy, the bacilli exhibit characteristic rapid darting or shooting-star motility. However, direct microscopic examination of stools by any method is not commonly used for laboratory diagnosis of enteric bacterial infections.

*Aeromonas* spp. are gram-negative, straight rods with rounded ends or coccobacilli. No molecular or serologic methods are available for direct detection of *Aeromonas* spp. Cells of *C. violaceum* are slightly curved, medium to long, gram-negative rods with rounded ends. A polymerase chain reaction (PCR) amplification assay has been developed for identification of *C. violaceum*.

## CULTIVATION

### Media of Choice

Stool cultures for *Vibrio* spp. are plated on the selective medium thiosulfate citrate bile salts sucrose (TCBS) agar. TCBS contains 1% sodium chloride, bile salts that inhibit the growth of gram-positive organisms, and sucrose for the differentiation of the various *Vibrio* spp. Bromothymol blue and thymol blue pH indicators are added to the medium. The high pH of the medium (8.6) inhibits the growth of other intestinal flora. Although some *Vibrio* spp. grow very poorly on this medium, those that grow well produce either yellow or green colonies, depending on whether they are able to ferment sucrose (which produces yellow colonies). Alkaline peptone water (pH 8.4) may be used as an enrichment broth for obtaining growth of vibrios from stool. After inoculation, the broth is incubated for 5 to 8 hours at 35°C and then subcultured to TCBS.

Chromogenic *Vibrio* agar, which was developed for the recovery of *Vibrio parahaemolyticus* from seafood, supports the growth of other *Vibrio* spp. Colonies on this agar range from white to pale blue and violet.

*Aeromonas* spp. are indistinguishable from *Yersinia enterocolitica* on modified cefsulodin-irgasan-novobiocin (CIN) agar (4 µg/mL of cefsulodin); therefore, it is important to perform an oxidase test to differentiate the two genera. *Aeromonas* agar is a relatively new alternative medium that uses D-xylose as a differential characteristic. These organisms typically grow on a variety of differential and selective agars used for the identification of enteric pathogens. They are also beta-hemolytic on blood agar.

*C. violaceum* grows on most routine laboratory media. The colonies may be beta-hemolytic and have an almond-like odor. Most strains produce violacein, an ethanol-soluble violet pigment.

All of the genera considered in this chapter grow well on 5% sheep blood, chocolate, and MacConkey agars. They also grow well in the broth of blood culture systems and in thioglycollate or brain-heart infusion broths.

### Incubation Conditions and Duration

These organisms produce detectable growth on 5% sheep blood and chocolate agars when incubated at 35°C in carbon dioxide or ambient air for a minimum of 24 hours. MacConkey and TCBS agars only should be incubated at 35°C in ambient air. The typical violet pigment of *C. violaceum* colonies (Figure 26-2) is optimally produced when cultures are incubated at room temperature (22°C).

### Colonial Appearance

Table 26-3 describes the colonial appearance and other distinguishing characteristics (e.g., hemolysis and odor)

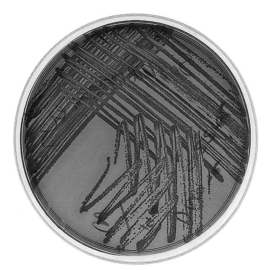

**Figure 26-2** Colonies of *Chromobacterium violaceum* on DNase agar. Note violet pigment.

**TABLE 26-3** Colonial Appearance and Characteristics

| Organism | Medium | Appearance |
|---|---|---|
| *Aeromonas* spp. | BA Mac | Large, round, raised, opaque; most pathogenic strains are beta-hemolytic except *A. caviae*, which is usually nonhemolytic Both NLF and LF |
| *Chromobacterium violaceum* | BA Mac | Round, smooth, convex, some strains are beta-hemolytic; most colonies appear black or very dark purple; cultures smell of ammonium cyanide (almond-like) NLF |
| *Vibrio* spp. and *Grimontia hollisae* | BA Mac | Medium to large, smooth, opaque, iridescent with a greenish hue; *V. cholerae*, *V. fluvialis*, and *V. mimicus* can be beta-hemolytic NLF except *V. vulnificus*, which may be LF |
| *P. damsela* | BA Mac | Medium to large, smooth, opaque, iridescent with a greenish hue; may be beta-hemolytic NLF |

*BA*, 5% sheep blood agar; *Mac*, MacConkey agar; *LF*, lactose fermenter, *NLF*, non–lactose fermenter.

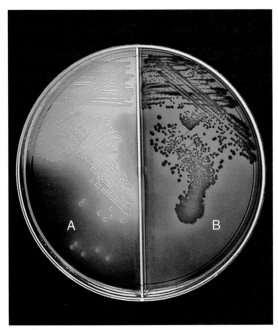

**Figure 26-3** Colonies of *Vibrio cholerae* **(A)** and *V. parahaemolyticus* **(B)** on TCBS agar.

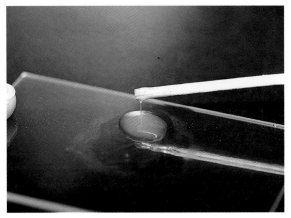

**Figure 26-4** String test used to differentiate *Vibrio* spp. (positive) from *Aeromonas* spp. and *P. shigelloides* (negative).

of each genus on 5% sheep blood and MacConkey agars. The appearance of *Vibrio* spp. on TCBS is described in Table 26-4 and shown in Figure 26-3.

## APPROACH TO IDENTIFICATION

The colonies of these genera resemble those of the family Enterobacteriaceae but can be distinguished notably by their positive oxidase test result (except for *V. metschnikovii,* which is oxidase negative). The oxidase test must be performed from 5% sheep blood or another medium without a fermentable sugar (e.g., lactose in MacConkey agar or sucrose in TCBS), because fermentation of a carbohydrate results in acidification of the medium, and a false-negative result may occur if the surrounding pH is below 5.1. Likewise, if the violet pigment of a suspected *C. violaceum* isolate interferes with performance of the oxidase test, the organism should be grown under anaerobic conditions (where it cannot produce pigment) and retested.

The reliability of commercial identification systems has not been widely validated for identification of these organisms, although most are listed in the databases of several systems. The API 20E system (bioMérieux, St. Louis, Missouri) is one of the best for vibrios. Because the inoculum is prepared in 0.85% saline, the amount of salt often is enough to allow growth of the halophilic (salt-loving) organism.

The ability of most commercial identification systems to accurately identify *Aeromonas* organisms to the species level is limited and uncertain, and with some kits, difficulty arises in separating *Aeromonas* spp. from *Vibrio* spp. Therefore, identification of potential pathogens should be confirmed using conventional biochemical tests or serotyping. Tables 26-4 and 26-5 show several

characteristics that can be used to presumptively group *Vibrio* spp., *Aeromonas* spp., and *C. violaceum.*

### Comments Regarding Specific Organisms

*V. cholerae* and *Vibrio mimicus* are the only *Vibrio* spp. that do not require salt for growth. Therefore, a key test for distinguishing the halophilic species from *V. cholerae, V. mimicus,* and *Aeromonas* spp. is growth in nutrient broth with 6% salt. Furthermore, the addition of 1% NaCl to conventional biochemical tests is recommended to allow growth of halophilic species.

The string test can be used to differentiate *Vibrio* spp. from *Aeromonas* spp. In this test, organisms are emulsified in 0.5% sodium deoxycholate, which lyses *Vibrio* cells, but not those of *Aeromonas* spp. Cell lysis releases DNA, which can be pulled up into a string with an inoculating loop (Figure 26-4).

A *Vibrio* static test using 0/129 (2,4-diamino-6, 7-diisopropylpteridine)–impregnated disks also has been used to separate vibrios (susceptible) from other oxidase-positive glucose fermenters (resistant) and to differentiate *V. cholerae* O1 and non-O1 (susceptible) from other *Vibrio* spp. (resistant). However, recent strains of *V. cholerae* O139 have demonstrated resistance, so the dependability of this test is questionable.

Serotyping should be performed immediately to further characterize *V. cholerae* isolates. Toxigenic strains of serogroup O1 and O139 can be involved in cholera epidemics. Strains that do not type in either antiserum are identified as non-O1. Although typing sera are commercially available, isolates of *V. cholerae* are usually sent to a reference laboratory for serotyping.

Identification of *V. cholerae* or *V. vulnificus* should be reported immediately because of the life-threatening nature of these organisms.

*Aeromonas* spp. and *C. violaceum* can be identified using the characteristics shown in Table 26-5. *Aeromonas* spp. identified in clinical specimens should be identified as *A. hydrophilia, A. caviae* complex, or *A. veronii* complex.

Pigmented strains of *C. violaceum* are so distinctive that a presumptive identification can be made based on colonial appearance, oxidase, and Gram staining. Nonpigmented strains (approximately 9% of isolates) may be

TABLE 26-4　Key Biochemical and Physiologic Characteristics of *Vibrio* spp. and *Grimontia hollisae*

| Species | Oxidase | Indole | Gas from Glucose | FERMENTATION OF Lactose | FERMENTATION OF Sucrose | Lysine Decarboxylase[a] | Arginine Dihydrolase[a] | Ornithine Decarboxylase[a] | Growth in 0% NaCl[b] | Growth in 6% NaCl[b] | TCBS[c] Growth | Colony on TCBS[c] |
|---|---|---|---|---|---|---|---|---|---|---|---|---|
| *Grimonti hollisae* | + | + | − | − | − | − | − | − | − | + | Very poor | Green |
| *Vibrio alginolyticus* | + | v | − | − | + | + | − | v | − | + | Good | Yellow |
| *Vibrio cholerae* | + | + | − | v | + | + | − | + | + | v | Good | Yellow |
| *Vibrio cincinnatiensis*[d] | + | v | − | − | + | v | − | − | − | + | Very poor | Yellow |
| *P. damsela* | + | − | − | − | − | v | + | − | − | + | Reduced at 36°C | Green[e] |
| *Vibrio fluvialis* | + | v | − | − | + | − | + | − | − | + | Good | Yellow |
| *Vibrio furnissi* | + | v | + | − | + | − | + | − | − | + | Good | Yellow |
| *Vibrio harveyi* | + | + | − | − | v | + | − | − | − | + | Good | Yellow |
| *Vibrio metschnikovii* | − | v | − | v | + | v | v | − | − | v | May be reduced | Yellow |
| *Vibrio mimicus* | + | + | − | v | − | + | − | + | + | v | Good | Green |
| *Vibrio parahaemolyticus* | + | + | − | − | − | + | − | + | − | + | Good | Green[f] |
| *Vibrio vulnificus* | + | + | − | (+) | − | + | − | + | − | + | Good | Green[g] |

*V*, Variable; +, >90% of strains are positive; −, >90% of strains are negative; (+), delayed.
[a]1% NaCl added to enhance growth.
[b]Nutrient broth with 0% or 6% NaCl added.
[c]Thiosulfate citrate bile salts sucrose agar.
[e]5% yellow.
[f]1% yellow.
[g]0% yellow.
[d]Ferments myoinositol.

**TABLE 26-5** Key Biochemical and Physiologic Characteristics of *Aeromonas* spp., *P. shigelloides*, and *C. violaceum*

| Species | Oxidase | Indole | Gas from Glucose | Esculin Hydrolysis | Fermentation of Sucrose | Lysine Decarboxylase | Arginine Dihydrolase | Ornithine Decarboxylase | Growth in 0% NaCl[a] | Growth in 6% NaCl[a] | TCBS[b] Growth |
|---|---|---|---|---|---|---|---|---|---|---|---|
| *Aeromonas caviae* complex | + | V | − | + | + | − | + | − | + | − | − |
| *Aeromonas hydrophila* complex | + | + | V | V | V | V | + | − | + | V | − |
| *Aeromonas jandaei* (*A. veronii* complex) | + | + | + | − | − | + | + | − | + | − | − |
| *Aeromonas schubertii* (*A. veronii* complex) | + | V | − | − | − | + | + | − | + | − | − |
| *Aeromonas veronii* biovar *sobria* | + | + | + | − | + | + | + | − | + | − | − |
| *Aeromonas veronii* biovar *veronii* | + | + | + | + | + | + | − | + | + | − | − |
| *Chromobacterium violaceum*[c] | V | V | −[d] | − | V | − | + | − | + | − | ND |

*ND,* No data; *V,* variable; +, >90% of strains are positive; −, >90% of strains are negative.
[a]Nutrient agar with 0% or 6% NaCl added.
[b]Thiosulfate citrate bile salts sucrose agar.
[c]91% produce an insoluble violet pigment; often, nonpigmented strains are indole positive.
[d]Gas-producing strains have been described.

differentiated from *Pseudomonas, Burkholderia, Brevundimonas,* and *Ralstonia* organisms based on glucose fermentation and a positive test result for indole. Negative lysine and ornithine reactions are useful criteria for distinguishing *C. violaceum* from *Plesiomonas shigelloides.* In addition to the characteristics listed in Table 26-5, failure to ferment either maltose or mannitol also differentiates *C. violaceum* from *Aeromonas* spp.

## SERODIAGNOSIS

Agglutination, vibriocidal, or antitoxin tests are available for diagnosing cholera using acute and convalescent sera. However, these methods are most commonly used for epidemiologic purposes. Serodiagnostic techniques are not generally used for laboratory diagnosis of infections caused by the other organisms discussed in this chapter.

## ANTIMICROBIAL SUSCEPTIBILITY TESTING AND THERAPY

Two components of the management of patients with cholera are rehydration and antimicrobial therapy (Table 26-6). Antimicrobials reduce the severity of the illness and shorten the duration of organism shedding. The drug of choice for cholera is tetracycline or doxycycline; however, resistance to these agents is known, and the use of other agents, such as chloramphenicol, ampicillin, or trimethoprim-sulfamethoxazole, may be necessary. The Clinical and Laboratory Standards Institute (CLSI) has established methods for testing for *V. cholerae,* and the CLSI document should be consulted for this purpose.

The need for antimicrobial intervention for gastrointestinal infections caused by other *Vibrio* spp. and *Aeromonas* spp. is less clear. However, extraintestinal infections with these organisms and with *C. violaceum* can be life-threatening, and directed therapy is required. *C. violaceum* is often resistant to β-lactams and colistin.

Antimicrobial agents with potential activity are listed, where appropriate, in Table 26-6. It is important to note these organisms' ability to show resistance to therapeutic agents; especially noteworthy is the ability of *Aeromonas* spp. to produce various beta-lactamases.

## PREVENTION

No cholera vaccine is available in the United States. Two oral vaccines are available outside the United States,

**TABLE 26-6** Antimicrobial Therapy and Susceptibility Testing

| Species | Therapeutic Options | Potential Resistance to Therapeutic Options | Validated Testing Methods* | Comments |
|---|---|---|---|---|
| *Vibrio cholerae* | Adequate rehydration plus antibiotics. Recommended agents include tetracycline or doxycycline; alternatives include trimethoprim-sulfamethoxazole, erythromycin, chloramphenicol, and quinolones | Resistance to tetracycline, chloramphenicol, and trimethoprim-sulfamethoxazole is known | See Clinical and Laboratory Standards Institute (CLSI) standards | |
| Other *Vibrio* spp. | No definitive guidelines. For gastroenteritis, therapy may not be needed; for wound infections and septicemia, potentially active agents include tetracycline, chloramphenicol, nalidixic acid, most cephalosporins, and quinolones | Similar to resistance reported for *V. cholerae* | See CLSI standards | |
| *Aeromonas* spp. | No definitive guidelines. For gastroenteritis, therapy may not be needed; for soft tissue infections and septicemia, potentially active agents include ceftriaxone, cefotaxime, ceftazidime, imipenem, aztreonam, amoxicillin-clavulanate, quinolones, and trimethoprim-sulfamethoxazole | Capable of producing various beta-lactamases that mediate resistance to penicillins and certain cephalosporins | See CLSI standards | |
| *Chromobacterium violaceum* | No definitive guidelines. Potentially active agents include cefotaxime, ceftazidime, imipenem, and aminoglycosides | Activity of penicillins is variable; activity of first- and second-generation cephalosporins is poor | Not available | Grows on Mueller-Hinton agar, but interpretive standards do not exist |

*Validated testing methods include standard methods recommended by the Clinical and Laboratory Standards Institute (CLSI) and commercial methods approved by the U.S. Food and Drug Administration (FDA).

although the World Health Organization no longer recommends immunization for travel to or from cholera-infected areas. Individuals who have recently shared food and drink with a patient with cholera (e.g., household contacts) should be given chemoprophylaxis with tetracycline, doxycycline, or trimethoprim-sulfamethoxazole. However, mass chemoprophylaxis during epidemics is not indicated. No approved vaccines or chemoprophylaxis exists for the other organisms discussed in this chapter.

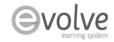 *Visit the Evolve site to complete the review questions.*

---

## CASE STUDY 26-1

After vacationing in San Diego, a 21-year-old male surfer sees his physician complaining of severe left ear pain. He is afebrile, but the auditory canal and tympanic membrane are erythematous. Amoxicillin is prescribed for presumed otitis media. Over the next 4 days, the symptoms persist and a bloody discharge develops. The patient returns to his physician, who cultures the drainage and prescribes gentamicin eardrops. The patient's symptoms improve over the next 7 days. On culture, a non–lactose fermenter was isolated from MacConkey agar.

QUESTIONS

1. The isolate is indole and oxidase positive. A biochemical identification system had positive reactions for lysine and ornithine but not arginine. What genus and species of bacteria are in the differential and how would you identify this microorganism?
2. How do you think the patient acquired this infection?
3. Commercial systems are known to misidentify the *Vibrio* spp. as *Aeromonas* spp. and vice versa. What is the reason for such a critical error?
4. Susceptibility testing using the disk method is not problematic for *Vibrio* spp. as long as which extra step is taken with testing?

# BIBLIOGRAPHY

Clark RB, Lister PD, Arneson-Rotert L, et al: In vitro susceptibilities of *Plesiomonas shigelloides* to 24 antibiotics and antibiotic-β-lactamase-inhibitor combinations, *Antimicrob Agents Chemother* 34:159, 1990.

Colwell RR: Global climate and infectious disease: the cholera paradigm, *Science* 274:2025, 1996.

Committee on Infectious Diseases: *2006 Red book: report of the Committee on Infectious Diseases,* ed 27, Elk Grove, Ill, 2006, American Academy of Pediatrics.

Jones BL, Wilcox MH: *Aeromonas* infections and their treatment, *J Antimicrob Chemother* 35:453, 1995.

Kimura B, Hokimoto S, Takahasi H: *Photobacterium histaminum* (Okuzumi et al, 1994) is a later subjective synonym for *Photobacterium damselae* subsp *damselae* (Love et al, 1981; Smith et al, 1991), *Int J Syst Evol Microbiol* 50:1339, 2000.

Mandell GL, Bennett JR, Dolin R: *Principles and practices of infectious diseases,* ed 7, Philadelphia, 2010, Churchill Livingstone/Elsevier.

Thompson FL, Hoste B, Vandemeulebroecke K et al: Reclassification of *Vibrio hollisae* as *Grimontia hollisae* gen nov, comb nov, *Int J Syst Evol Microbiol* 53:1615, 2003.

Ti TY, Tan CW, Chong AP et al: Nonfatal and fatal infections caused by *Chromobacterium violaceum, Clin Infect Dis* 17:505, 1993.

von Graevenitz A, Zbinden R, Mutters R: *Actinobacillus, Capnocytophaga, Eikenella, Kingella, Pasteurella,* and other fastidious or rarely encountered gram-negative rods. In Murray PR, Baron EJ, Jorgensen JH, et al, editors: *Manual of clinical microbiology,* ed 8, Washington, DC, 2003, ASM Press.

Versalovic J: Manual of Clinical Microbiology, ed 10, 2011, Washington, DC, ASM Press.

# Gram-Negative Bacilli and Coccobacilli (MacConkey-Negative, Oxidase-Positive)

# *Sphingomonas paucimobilis* and Similar Organisms

## OBJECTIVES

1. Identify cultivation methods and colonial characteristics for *Sphingomonas paucimobilis* and similar organisms.
2. State the initial clues that alert the CL to the presence of this group of organisms for clinical laboratorians.
3. Select identification approaches for this group of organisms.
4. Identify susceptibility testing methods appropriate for this group of organisms.
5. Recognize the pathogenicity of organisms in this group.

### ORGANISMS TO BE CONSIDERED

| Current Name | Previous Name |
|---|---|
| *Acidovorax facilis* | *Pseudomonas facilis* |
| CDC group IIc | |
| CDC group IIe | |
| CDC group IIh | |
| CDC group IIi | |
| CDC group O-1 | |
| CDC group O-2 | |
| CDC group O-3 | |
| *Sphingobacterium mizutaii* | *Flavobacterium mizutaii* |
| *Sphingobacterium multivorum* | *Flavobacterium multivorum*, CDC IIk-2 |
| *Sphingobacterium spiritivorum* | *Flavobacterium spiritivorum, Flavobacterium yabuuchiae, Sphingobacterium versatilis,* CDC IIk-3 |
| *Sphingomonas parapaucimobilis* | |
| *Sphingomonas paucimobilis* | *Pseudomonas paucimobilis,* CDC IIk-1 |

## GENERAL CONSIDERATIONS

The organisms discussed in this chapter are considered together because they usually fail to grow on MacConkey agar, are oxidase positive, and oxidatively utilize glucose.

## EPIDEMIOLOGY, SPECTRUM OF DISEASE, AND ANTIMICROBIAL THERAPY

As demonstrated in Table 27-1, these organisms are rarely or only occasionally isolated from human materials and

have limited roles as agents of infection. Because they are infrequently encountered in the clinical setting, little information is available on their epidemiology, ability to cause human infections, and potential for antimicrobial resistance. For example, even though O-1 and O-2 organisms have been submitted to the Centers for Disease Control and Prevention (CDC) after being isolated from clinical materials such as blood, cerebrospinal fluid (CSF), wounds, and pleural fluid, their natural habitat is unknown. The genus *Sphingobacterium* is ubiquitous in nature, and *Sphingomonas* spp. are known for their waterborne nature. Some of these groups are present in hospital settings, such as hospital water supplies. When the organisms discussed in this chapter are encountered in clinical specimens, their clinical significance and potential as contaminants should be considered; human infections have been documented, so care must be taken to determine whether these organisms are infectious agents or contaminants.

## LABORATORY DIAGNOSIS

### SPECIMEN COLLECTION AND TRANSPORT

No special considerations are required for specimen collection and transport of the organisms discussed in this chapter. Refer to Table 5-1 for general information on specimen collection and transport.

### SPECIMEN PROCESSING

No special considerations are required for processing of the organisms discussed in this chapter. Refer to Table 5-1 for general information on specimen processing.

### DIRECT DETECTION METHODS

No specific procedures other than microscopy are required for direct detection of these organisms in clinical material.

### CULTIVATION

Media of Choice

*Sphingomonas* spp., *Sphingobacterium* spp., *Acidovorax facilis,* and all CDC groups considered in this chapter grow well on routine laboratory media, such as 5% sheep

**TABLE 27-1** Epidemiology, Spectrum of Disease, and Antimicrobial Therapy

| Organism | Epidemiology | Disease Spectrum | Antimicrobial Therapy |
|---|---|---|---|
| *Acidovorax facilis* | *A. facilis* is found in soil and has been used as a soil additive to improve plant growth in areas of agriculture and horticulture. | Commonly found in soil. Rarely found in clinical material and not substantiated as a cause of human infections. | No guidelines; little is known about antimicrobial resistance potential. Disk diffusion testing cannot be performed. |
| CDC group IIc CDC group IIe CDC group IIh CDC group IIi | CDC groups IIc, IIe, IIh, and IIi are found in soil, plants, foodstuffs, and water, including moist areas in hospitals. Not part of human flora. | Rarely found in clinical material and rarely substantiated as a cause of human infections; have been isolated from blood, eyes, and wounds. | No guidelines; little is known about antimicrobial resistance potential |
| CDC group O-1 CDC group O-2 CDC group O-3 | Epidemiology is unknown. | Rarely found in clinical material and rarely implicated as a cause of human infections. CDC group O-3 has been isolated from bone, blood, lung, and lymph node tissue. | No guidelines; one report indicates susceptibility of CDC group O-3 to aminoglycosides, imipenem, trimethoprim-sulfamethoxazole, and chloramphenicol (however, the breakpoints used were based on those for the Enterobacteriaceae family). |
| *Sphingobacterium mizutaii* *S. multivorum* *S. spiritivorum* | Sphingobacteria are ubiquitous in nature. | Rarely involved in human infections. *S. mizutaii* has been associated with blood, cerebrospinal fluid, and wound infections; *S. multivorum* with blood and wound infections; and *S. spiritivorum* with blood and urine infections. | Literature references report the following susceptibilities: *S. mizutaii*—erythromycin, trimethoprim-sulfamethoxazole, and pefloxacin. *S. multivorum*—amikacin, gentamicin, aztreonam, cefepime, cefotaxime, ceftazidime, meropenem, piperacillin, piperacillin/tazobactam, and chloramphenicol. *S. spiritivorum*—amikacin, gentamicin, aztreonam, cefepime, cefotaxime, chloramphenicol. |
| *Sphingomonas paucimobilis* *S. parapaucimobilis* | *S. paucimobilis* inhabits environmental niches and is known especially as a waterborne organism that can exist in hospital water systems. Not part of human flora. Mode of transmission is uncertain but probably involves patient exposure to contaminated medical devices or solutions. | *S. paucimobilis* virulence factors are unknown. It has been implicated in community- and hospital-acquired infections, specifically in blood and urine infections. | No definitive guidelines; potentially active agents include trimethoprim-sulfamethoxazole, chloramphenicol, ciprofloxacin, and aminoglycosides; resistance to beta-lactams is known, but validated susceptibility testing methods do not exist. |

blood and chocolate agars; however, most fail to grow on MacConkey agar. They usually grow well in thioglycollate and brain-heart infusion broths and in broths used in blood culture systems.

### Incubation Conditions and Duration

Within 24 to 48 hours of inoculation and incubation, most of these organisms produce detectable growth on media incubated at 35° to 37°C in 5% carbon dioxide ($CO_2$) or ambient air.

### Colonial Appearance

Table 27-2 describes the colonial appearance and distinguishing characteristics (e.g., pigment) of each organism on 5% sheep blood agar. When these organisms do grow on MacConkey agar, they appear as lactose nonfermenters.

## APPROACH TO IDENTIFICATION

The ability of many commercial identification systems to identify accurately the organisms discussed in this chapter may be limited or uncertain. Tables 27-3 through 27-6 show some biochemical tests that are helpful for presumptive differentiation among the various organisms in this group.

### Comments Regarding Specific Organisms

***Acidovorax facilis.*** *A. facilis* is a straight to slightly curved, gram-negative rod that occurs singly or in short chains. It is aerobic and has a single polar flagellum, which makes it motile. On nutrient agar, it forms unpigmented colonies, and 30°C is its optimum temperature. *A. facilis* is oxidase positive and urease variable (some grow on Christensen urea agar but lack urease activity). Key characteristics are shown in Table 27-3. *A. facilis* is commonly found in soil, and no evidence of pathogenicity in healthy humans has been identified. A role for *A. facilis* as an opportunistic pathogen has not been proven or rejected.

**CDC groups IIc, IIe, IIh, IIi, 0-1, 0-2, and 0-3.** CDC groups IIc, IIe, IIh, IIi, 0-1, and 0-2 are short, straight rods that may appear as "II-forms" (i.e., bacteria with thickened ends and thin centers). The phenotypic characteristics of CDC group IIc are most similar to those of CDC groups IIe and IIh, the major difference being that CDC group IIc produces acid from sucrose, hydrolyzes esculin, and usually reduces nitrate. Strains of CDC groups IIe and IIh are similar to *Empedobacter brevis* (see Chapter 26) in that they oxidize glucose and maltose and produce indole. CDC group IIi resembles *S. multivorum* but produces indole. *S. parapaucimobilis* resembles CDC group O-1 in that both are motile, esculin positive, and positive for hydrogen sulfide ($H_2S$) in lead acetate; however, *S. parapaucimobilis* oxidizes more carbohydrates (CDC O-1 is weakly positive in OF glucose and negative in OF xylose, maltose, and mannitol).

CDC groups O-1 and O-2 are similar in that they are motile, oxidase-positive, esculin-positive, gram-negative rods that grow with yellow pigment and do not grow on MacConkey agar. CDC groups O-1 and O-2 have been isolated from clinical sources; antimicrobial susceptibility testing on these organisms has not been reported. CDC group O-2 does not oxidize xylose, mannitol, or lactose; this can help distinguish it from the other yellow-pigmented organisms growing on blood agar discussed in this chapter.

CDC O-3 bacteria, which are predominantly curved rods, do not produce yellow pigment. They are motile by a single polar flagellum. They grow well on a *Campylobacter*-selective medium and may be misidentified as a *Campylobacter* sp. CDC group O-3 are aerobic, glucose-oxidizing organisms that utilize xylose, sucrose, and maltose. They do not grow on MacConkey agar. They are oxidase positive, hydrolyze esculin, and are negative for urease, indole, nitrate, and gelatin. Key characteristics of the CDC groups are shown in Tables 27-3 and 27-4. CDC O-3 has been reported as susceptible to aminoglycosides, imipenem, chloramphenicol, and trimethoprim-sulfamethoxazole and resistant to beta-lactam antimicrobials.

*Sphingobacterium mizutaii.* *S. mizutaii* exhibits II-forms. It can produce a yellow pigment, and it does not grow on MacConkey agar. Although aflagellate and therefore frequently classified as nonmotile, it can be motile by gliding movement. It is able to grow in the presence of 40% bile; it also is oxidase positive, catalase positive, esculin positive, indole negative, and urease negative (although a report exists that 20% are positive for Christensen urease). Key characteristics are shown in Tables

**TABLE 27-2** Colonial Appearance and Characteristics

| Organism | Medium | Appearance |
|---|---|---|
| *Acidovorax facilis* | BA | No distinctive appearance |
| CDC group IIc | BA | No distinctive appearance but colonies sticky |
| CDC group IIe | BA | No distinctive appearance |
| CDC group IIh | BA | No distinctive appearance |
| CDC group IIi | BA | No distinctive appearance |
| CDC group 0-1, 0-2, 0-3 | BA | Yellow pigment present in 0-1 and 0-2 but not in 0-3 |
| Sphingobacterium spp. | BA | Yellow pigment present in *S. mizutaii* |
| *Sphingomonas paucimobilis* *S. parapaucimobilis* | BA | Small, circular, smooth, convex; bright yellow growth pigment |

*BA,* 5% sheep blood agar.

**TABLE 27-3** Key Biochemical and Physiologic Characteristics

| Organism | Insoluble Pigment | Glucose Oxidized | Xylose Oxidized | Sucrose Oxidized | Esculin Hydrolysis | Motility |
|---|---|---|---|---|---|---|
| *Acidovorax facilis* | − | + | (+) | − | − | + |
| CDC group IIc | Tan or buff | + | − | + | + | nm |
| CDC group IIe | − | + | − | − | − | nm |
| CDC group IIh | − | + | − | − | + | nm |
| CDC group IIi | Yellow | + | + | + | + | nm |
| CDC group 0-2 | Yellow to orange | v | − | + | v | v* |
| *Sphingobacterium mizutaii* | v[†] | + | (+) | + | + | nm |
| *Sphingomonas* spp.[‡] | Yellow | + | + | + | + | +[§] |

Data compiled from Daneshvar MI, Hill B, Hollis DG et al: CDC group O-3: phenotypic characteristics, fatty acid composition, isoprenoid quinone content, and in vitro antimicrobic susceptibilities of an unusual gram-negative bacterium isolated from clinical specimens, *J Clin Microbiol* 36:1674, 1998; Hollis DG, Moss CW, Daneshvar MI, Wallace-Shewmaker PL: CDC group IIc phenotypic characteristics, fatty acid composition, and isoprenoid quinone content, *J Clin Microbiol* 34:2322, 1996; and Weyant RS, Moss CW, Weaver RE et al, editors: *Identification of unusual pathogenic gram-negative aerobic and facultatively anaerobic bacteria,* ed 2, Baltimore, 1996, Williams & Wilkins.

*nm,* Nonmotile; *v,* variable; +, >90% strains positive; −, >90% strains negative; (+), delayed.
*Only 20% are motile; motility is only apparent upon wet mount or flagellar staining.
[†]Yellow pigment production may be enhanced by incubation at room temperature.
[‡]Includes *S. paucimobilis* and *S. parapaucimobilis.*
[§]Usually nonmotile in motility medium, but motility is present on wet mount.

**TABLE 27-4** Specific Biochemical Characteristics for Differentiation of CDC groups IIc, IIe, and IIh*

| Biochemical Test | CDC Group IIc (n = 20) | CDC Group IIe (n = 18) | CDC Group IIh (n = 21) |
|---|---|---|---|
| Growth on MacConkey agar | 0 | 7 | 0 |
| Oxidase | 100 | 88 | 100 |
| Acid from OF glucose | 100 | 100 | 100 |
| Acid from OF xylose | 0 | 0 | 0 |
| Acid from OF mannitol | 0 | 0 | 0 |
| Acid from OF lactose | 0 | 0 | 0 |
| Acid from OF sucrose | 100 | 0 | 0 |
| Acid from OF maltose | 100 | 100 | 100 |
| Catalase | 100 | 88 | 100 |
| Christensen urea | 0 | 0 | 0 |
| Nitrate reduction | 90 | 0 | 0 |
| Indole | 100 | 100 | 100 |
| Simmons citrate | 0 | 0 | 0 |
| Motility | 0 | 0 | 0 |
| Gelatin hydrolysis | 20 | 0 | 7 |
| Esculin hydrolysis | 100 | 0 | 100 |
| Growth at 25°C | 100 | 100 | 100 |
| Growth at 35°C | 100 | 100 | 100 |
| Growth at 42°C | 5 | 0 | 5 |

Data compiled from Hollis DG, Moss CW, Daneshvar MI, Wallace-Shewmaker PL: CDC group IIc phenotypic characteristics, fatty acid composition, and isoprenoid quinone content, *J Clin Microbiol* 34:2322, 1996.
*Results indicate percent positive after 48 hours.

**TABLE 27-5** Specific Biochemical Characteristics for Differentiation of the *Sphingobacterium* spp.

| Biochemical Test | *S. multivorum* | *S. spiritivorum* | *S. mizutaii* |
|---|---|---|---|
| Oxidation of ethanol | Negative | Positive | Negative |
| Oxidation of mannitol | Negative | Positive | Negative |
| Oxidation of rhamnose | Negative | Positive | Positive |
| Christensen urease | Positive | Positive | Negative* |
| DNase | Negative† | Positive | ND‡ |
| Susceptibility to polymyxin B | Resistant | Resistant | Resistant |
| Indole | Negative | Negative | Negative |

Data compiled from Freney J, Hansen W, Ploton C et al: Septicemia caused by *Sphingobacterium multivorum. J Clin Microbiol* 25:1126, 1987.
*Reported positive: 20%.
†Reported positive: 40%.
‡Not determined. Some microbiology texts classify *S. mizutaii* as DNase positive, and some major literature references identify it as DNase negative.

**TABLE 27-6** Specific Biochemical Characteristics for Differentiation of the *Sphingomonas* spp.

| Biochemical Test | *S. paucimobilis* | *S. parapaucimobilis* |
|---|---|---|
| Oxidation of glucose | Positive | Positive |
| Oxidation of xylose | Positive | Positive |
| Oxidation of maltose | Positive | Positive |
| Esculin hydrolysis | Positive | Positive |
| Motility | Positive* | Positive |
| Indole | Negative | Negative |
| Susceptibility to polymyxin B | Susceptible | Variable |
| Hydrogen sulfide ($H_2S$) (lead acetate paper suspended over KIA) | Negative | Positive |
| Citrate | Negative | Positive |
| DNase | Positive | Negative |

Data compiled from Winn WC, Allen SD, Janda WM et al: *Koneman's color atlas and textbook of diagnostic microbiology,* ed 6, Philadelphia, 2006, Lippincott Williams & Wilkins.
$H_2S$, Hydrogen sulfide; *KIA,* Kligler iron agar.
*Motility positive by wet mount or in motility medium incubated at 18° to 22°C, but organism is nonmotile when incubated at 37°C.

27-3 and 27-5. Reported infections in humans have included septicemia (blood culture), meningitis (CSF specimen), and cellulitis (wound source). This bacterium has been reported to be susceptible to erythromycin, trimethoprim-sulfamethoxazole, and pefloxacin.

**Sphingobacterium multivorum.** *S. multivorum* is yellow pigmented, oxidase positive, and esculin positive. It is OF glucose positive; it does not produce acid from mannitol, ethanol, or rhamnose; and it is Christensen urease positive. This bacterium grows on blood agar plate (BAP), Mueller-Hinton agar, *Burkholderia cepacia*–selective agar (BCSA), and MacConkey agar. Key characteristics are shown in Table 27-5. These organisms are ubiquitous in nature and rarely associated with serious infection; however, cases of septicemia and peritonitis have been reported. This bacterium is nonmotile and resistant to

polymyxin B, characteristics that distinguish it from *S. paucimobilis*. Susceptibility to amikacin, gentamicin, aztreonam, cefepime, cefotaxime, ceftazidime, meropenem, piperacillin, and chloramphenicol has been reported in a small study of eight isolates.

**Sphingobacterium spiritivorum.** *S. spiritivorum* is yellow pigmented and positive for oxidase and esculin. It does not grow on MacConkey agar but does grow on BAP,

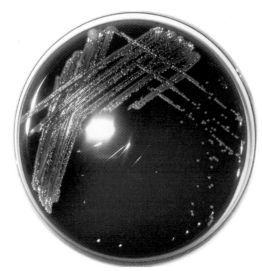

**Figure 27-1** *Sphingomonas paucimobilis* growth on BAP. (From Seo SW, Chung IY, Kim E, Park JM: A case of postoperative *Sphingomonas paucimobilis* endophthalmitis after cataract extraction, *Kor J Ophthalmol* 22:63, 2008.)

Mueller-Hinton agar, and BCSA. It produces acid in OF glucose and in mannitol, ethanol, and rhamnose. Like *S. multivorum*, this bacterium is ubiquitous in nature but rarely pathogenic for humans. It can be distinguished from *S. paucimobilis* by the fact that it is nonmotile and resistant to polymyxin B. Key characteristics are shown in Table 27-5. *S. spiritivorum* has been isolated environmentally from hospitals, most commonly from blood and urine. Susceptibility testing by Kirby-Bauer (KB) disk diffusion on 13 isolates showed susceptibility to amikacin, gentamicin, aztreonam, cefepime, cefotaxime, and chloramphenicol.

*Sphingomonas paucimobilis.* *S. paucimobilis* is a medium-size, straight, gram-negative rod with a single polar flagellum; growth requires at least 48 hours' incubation on sheep blood agar (Figure 27-1). Optimal growth occurs at 30°C in 5% $CO_2$ or ambient air; it does grow at 37°C but not at 42°C. It grows as a deep yellow colony on tryptic soy and blood agars. It is obligately aerobic, grows in broth (e.g., brain-heart infusion, thioglycollate, blood culture media), and does not grow on MacConkey agar (90% do not grow; 10% grow as lactose nonfermenters). *S. paucimobilis* oxidatively utilizes glucose, xylose, and sucrose. Biochemical test results of interest include the following: esculin hydrolysis positive; motile by wet mount or in motility medium when incubated at 18° to 22°C (nonmotile when incubated at 37°C); oxidase positive (90% to 94% positive); catalase positive; urease negative; and indole negative. *S. paucimobilis* is susceptible to polymyxin B, a trait that distinguishes it from *Sphingobacterium* spp. Key characteristics are shown in Table 27-6.

Antimicrobial susceptibility testing indicates that *S. paucimobilis* is susceptible to tetracycline, chloramphenicol, trimethoprim-sulfamethoxazole, and aminoglycosides. Susceptibility to vancomycin has been noted when the organism is grown on sheep blood agar with a vancomycin disk (30 μg). *S. paucimobilis* is ubiquitous in soil and water and has been isolated environmentally from swimming pools, hospital equipment, and water and laboratory supplies. It has been associated with human infections and found in a variety of clinical specimens, specifically, peritonitis associated with wound infections (chronic ambulatory peritoneal dialysis, leg ulcer, empyema, splenic abscess, brain abscess), blood cultures, and CSF, urine, vaginal, and cervical samples. Recent literature indicates that *S. paucimobilis* is usually regarded as having minor clinical significance; however, community-acquired infection, diabetes mellitus, and alcoholism have been identified as significant risk factors for primary bacteremia. A retrospective study suggests that the prevalence of *S. paucimobilis* infection in humans seems to have increased in recent times, and although it has low virulence, infection can lead to septic shock, particularly in immunocompromised patients. Another report indicates that although this bacterium has low mortality associated with infection, it frequently causes complications in hospitalized patients.

*Sphingomonas parapaucimobilis.* *S. parapaucimobilis* is similar to *S. paucimobilis* in many ways. It is a medium-size, straight, gram-negative rod that grows with a deep yellow pigment. It is obligately aerobic, motile, and does not grow on MacConkey agar. *S. parapaucimobilis* can be distinguished from *S. paucimobilis* by several characteristics. *S. parapaucimobilis* is $H_2S$ positive, as indicated by blackening of lead acetate paper suspended over Kligler iron agar (KIA); it is Simmons citrate positive (*S. paucimobilis* is negative); and it is negative for extracellular DNAse (*S. paucimobilis* is positive). Like *S. paucimobilis*, *S. parapaucimobilis* is acid in OF glucose, OF xylose, and OF maltose but negative in OF mannitol. It has been distinguished from *Sphingobacterium* spp. by its susceptibility to polymyxin B; however, *S. parapaucimobilis* is sometimes variable to polymyxin B. Key characteristics are shown in Table 27-6. Antimicrobial susceptibility testing indicates that *S. parapaucimobilis* displays variable resistance but is usually susceptible to tetracycline, chloramphenicol, sulfamethoxazole, aminoglycosides, third-generation cephalosporins, and fluoroquinolone. *S. parapaucimobilis* has been associated with human infections; specifically, it has been isolated from sputum, urine, and the vagina.

## ANTIMICROBIAL SUSCEPTIBILITY

Antimicrobial susceptibility for this group of bacteria ranges from variable resistance to identifiable patterns of susceptibility. Standardized guidelines are not available. However, when clinically necessary, susceptibility testing should be completed using an overnight MIC or E-test method.

## SERODIAGNOSIS

Serodiagnostic techniques are not generally used for the laboratory diagnosis of infections caused by the organisms discussed in this chapter.

## PREVENTION

Because these organisms are rarely implicated or only recently have been identified in human infections, no vaccines or prophylactic measures are available.

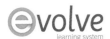

*Visit the Evolve site to complete the review questions.*

## CASE STUDY 27-1

A 16-year-old patient with acute lymphoblastic leukemia presents to his oncologist with pain and swelling of the left knee. He recently received a course of chemotherapy and radiotherapy, and he is taking oral steroids. Straw-colored fluid with 2+ WBC is aspirated from his knee. No microorganisms are seen on the smear, and none grow in culture. Unfortunately, only a few drops of the fluid are cultured on plate media. Over the next 6 months, the patient is in and out of the hospital, receiving antibiotics and having more cultures done, with no positive findings to explain his pain and swelling. He is admitted to the hospital, where an arthroscopic procedure is performed to evaluate the problem. Widespread synovitis is seen. Culture samples obtained from the surgery grow a yellow-pigmented, gram-negative rod on blood agar, but no growth is observed on MacConkey agar. Indole and urease testing are negative, but the oxidase test and wet mount motility are positive. The bacterium is identified as *Sphingomonas paucimobilis*. The patient is treated with a 6-week course of intravenous amikacin and ceftazidime. Despite the effectiveness of treatment, the patient is left with residual knee pain and stiffness because of articular cartilage destruction.

### QUESTIONS

1. Which microorganisms are in the differential diagnosis for the patient?
2. What tests can be done to provide differential evidence for bacterial identification?
3. What method or methods should be used to test for susceptibility of the pathogens identified in this case?

From Charity R, Foukas A: Osteomyelitis and secondary septic arthritis caused by *Sphingomonas paucimobilis*, *Infection* 33:93, 2005.

## CASE STUDY 27-2

A 20-month-old girl is diagnosed with cystic fibrosis at the age of 6 months. She is taken to the hospital on her second day of respiratory difficulty and presents with cough, abundant mucus expectoration, and a temperature of 37.9°C. Because she has a history of *Pseudomonas aeruginosa* infections, treatment is started with ceftazidime and amikacin. Bronchial aspirates are obtained for culture, plated on blood, chocolate, and MacConkey agars, and incubated (37°C, 48 hours). A medium specific for isolation of slow-growing *Burkholderia* organisms also is inoculated and incubated appropriately. Abundant growth of oxidase-positive colonies that are nonmotile, catalase-positive, gram-negative rods is identified as *Sphingobacterium multivorum* by means of a Vitek GNI card and API 20NE.

Definitive identification is provided by biochemical tests that show the following positive results: growth on MacConkey agar; urease; esculin hydrolysis; beta-D-galactosidase production; assimilation of glucose, arabinose, mannose, N-acetyl-glucosamine, and maltose; and acidification of glucose, lactose, maltose, sucrose, and xylose. Negative results are identified for the following: motility at 23°C (room temperature), 37°C, and 42°C; nitrate and nitrite reduction; indole production; arginine dihydrolase; lysine and ornithine decarboxylase; gelatin hydrolysis; hydrogen sulfide production; and assimilation of mannitol, gluconate, malate, and citrate.

Antimicrobial susceptibility testing identifies susceptibility to carbenicillin, ceftazidime, ceftriaxone, cefuroxime, chloramphenicol, azlocillin, cefotaxime, ticarcillin, ciprofloxacin, imipenem, piperacillin, and amikacin. Resistance to aztreonam, mezlocillin, gentamicin, tobramycin, and cotrimoxazole also is identified. A *Burkholderia*-specific medium shows no growth. The patient responds well to fluid and antimicrobial therapy and is discharged from the hospital.

### QUESTIONS

1. Which microorganisms are in the differential diagnosis for this patient?
2. What tests can be done to provide differential evidence for bacterial identification?
3. What method or methods should be used to test for susceptibility of the pathogens identified in this case?

From Reina J, Borrell N, Figuerola J: *Sphingobacterium multivorum* isolated from a patient with cystic fibrosis, *Eur J Clin Microbiol Infect Dis* 11:81, 1992.

## ▤ BIBLIOGRAPHY

Boken DJ, Romero JR, Cavalieri SJ: *Sphingomonas paucimobilis* bacteremia: four cases and review of the literature, *Infect Dis Clin Pract* 7:286, 1998.

Charity RM, Foukas AF: Osteomyelitis and secondary septic arthritis caused by *Sphingomonas paucimobilis*, *Infection* 33:93, 2005.

Daneshvar MI, Hill B, Hollis DG et al: CDC group O-3: phenotypic characteristics, fatty acid composition, isoprenoid quinone content, and in vitro antimicrobic susceptibilities of an unusual Gramnegative bacterium isolated from clinical specimens, *J Clin Microbiol* 36:1674, 1998.

Freney J, Hansen W, Ploton C et al: Septicemia caused by *Sphingobacterium multivorum*, *J Clin Microbiol* 25:1126, 1987.

Hollis DG, Moss CW, Daneshvar MI et al: CDC group IIc phenotypic characteristics, fatty acid composition, and isoprenoid quinone content, *J Clin Microbiol* 34:2322, 1996.

Lambiase A, Rossano F, Del Pezzo M et al: *Sphingobacterium* respiratory tract infection in patients with cystic fibrosis, *BMC Res Notes* 2:262, 2009.

Lemaitre D, Elaichouni A, Hundhausen M et al: Tracheal colonization with *Sphingomonas paucimobilis* in mechanically ventilated neonates due to contaminated ventilator temperature probes, *J Hosp Infect* 32:199, 1996.

Lin JN, Lai CH, Chen YH et al: *Sphingomonas paucimobilis* bacteremia in humans: 16 case reports and a literature review, *J Microbiol Immunol Infect* 43:35, 2010.

Reina J, Bassa A, Llompart I et al: Infections with *Pseudomonas paucimobilis:* report of four cases and review, *Rev Infect Dis* 13:1072, 1991.

Salazar R, Martino R, Suredo A et al: Catheter-related bacteremia due to *Pseudomonas paucimobilis* in neutropenic cancer patients: report of two cases, *Clin Infect Dis* 20:1573, 1995.

Toh HS, Tay HT, Kuar WK et al: Risk factors associated with *Sphingomonas paucimobilis* infection, *J Microbiol Immunol Infect* 44(4):2289-95 2011.

Weyant RS, Moss CW, Weaver RE et al, editors: *Identification of unusual pathogenic gram-negative aerobic and facultatively anaerobic bacteria*, ed 2, Baltimore, 1996, Williams & Wilkins.

Willems A, Falsen E, Pot B et al: *Acidovorax,* a new genus for *Pseudomonas facilis, Pseudomonas delafieldii*, E. Falsen (EF) group 13, EF group 16, and several clinical isolates, with the species *Acidovorax facilis* comb nov, *Acidovorax delafieldii* comb nov, and *Acidovorax temperans* sp nov, *Intl J System Bacteriol* 40:384, 1990.

Winn WC, Allen SD, Janda WM et al: *Koneman's color atlas and textbook of diagnostic microbiology*, ed 6, Philadelphia, 2006, Lippincott Williams & Wilkins.

# Moraxella and Related Organisms

## CHAPTER 28

## OBJECTIVES

1. Identify the distinguishing characteristics of the species within the genera *Moraxella* and *Neisseria*.
2. Identify what species within this group of bacteria that are frequently isolated as pathogens and which are considered potential contaminants.
3. Explain the procedure the microbiologist can use to determine whether the bacteria in this grouping exist as true cocci and name these organisms.
4. Identify the species of *Moraxella* and *Neisseria* that may be isolated from human wounds resulting from a dog or cat bite.
5. Identify the species of *Moraxella* frequently isolated from cases of human conjunctivitis.
6. Explain the media used for culture for this group of organisms, including the chemical principle and composition.
7. List some of the conventional biochemical tests that can be used to distinguish these organisms from other bacteria, and explain the principle for each.
8. Correlate patient signs and symptoms with laboratory data, and identify the most likely etiologic agent.

## GENERA AND SPECIES TO BE CONSIDERED

| Current Name | Previous Name |
|---|---|
| *Moraxella atlantae* | |
| *Moraxella canis* | |
| *Moraxella lacunata* | |
| *Moraxella lincolnii* | |
| *Moraxella nonliquefaciens* | |
| *Moraxella osloensis* | |
| *Neisseria elongata* subspecies *elongata* | CDC group M6 |
| *Neisseria elongata* subspecies *glycolytica* | |
| *Neisseria elongata* subspecies *nitroreducens* | |
| *Neisseria weaverii* | CDC group M5 |

## GENERAL CHARACTERISTICS

The organisms discussed in this chapter are either coccobacilli or short to medium-sized, gram-negative rods. This group of bacteria consists of several species within the genera *Moraxella* and *Neisseria*, other than the three frequently isolated pathogens, *Moraxella catarrhalis*, *Neisseria. gonorrhoeae*, and *Neisseria meningitidis*. Most of these organisms rarely cause infection and should be considered as potential contaminants. Many *Moraxella* spp. are considered to be normal mucosal flora with low virulence. Two of these species, *N. weaverii* and *M. canis*, are oropharyngeal flora in dogs and cats and are sometimes seen in humans as a result of a bite wound. Subinhibitory concentrations of penicillin, such as occurs in the presence of a 10-unit penicillin disk, cause the coccoid forms of these bacteria to elongate to bacilli morphology. In contrast, true cocci, such as most *Neisseria* spp. and *Moraxella (Branhamella) catarrhalis*, with which these organisms may be confused, maintain their original cocci shape in the presence of penicillin. In addition, the organisms discussed in this chapter do not use glucose and most do not grow on MacConkey agar but will grow well on blood and chocolate agar, as well as in commercial blood culture systems. Specific morphologic and physiologic features are presented later in this chapter in the discussion of laboratory diagnosis.

## EPIDEMIOLOGY, SPECTRUM OF DISEASE, AND ANTIMICROBIAL THERAPY

Infections caused by *Moraxella* spp. and *Neisseria elongata* most likely result when a breakdown of the patient's mucosal or epidermal defensive barriers allows subsequent invasion of sterile sites by an organism that is part of the patient's normal flora (i.e., an endogenous strain; Table 28-1). The fact that these organisms rarely cause infection indicates that they have low virulence. Whenever these organisms are encountered in clinical specimens, the possibility that they are contaminants should be seriously considered. This is especially the case when the specimen source may have come in contact with a mucosal surface.

*Moraxella catarrhalis* is the species most commonly associated with human infections, primarily of the respiratory tract. However, because the cellular morphology of this species is more similar to that of *Neisseria* spp. than that of the other *Moraxella* spp., details of this organism's characteristics are discussed in Chapter 40.

Data collected from the Centers for Disease Control and Prevention (CDC) show that these rare isolates may also be a cause of infection. In a study of the bacteria, *Neisseria elongate* subsp. *nitroreducens*, one fourth of the isolates received at the CDC for analysis were from cases of bacterial endocarditis. Data collected during a 16-year period found that most of these isolates were from blood, but they were also recovered from wounds, respiratory secretions, and peritoneal fluid. Individuals at risk had preexisting heart damage or had undergone dental manipulations.

The rarity with which these organisms are encountered as the cause of infection and the lack of validated in vitro susceptibility testing methods does not allow definitive treatment guidelines to be given (Table 28-2). Although many of these organisms may grow on the media and under the conditions recommended for

**TABLE 28-1** Epidemiology, Pathogenesis, and Spectrum of Disease

| Organism | Habitat (Reservoir) | Mode of Transmission | Virulence Factors | Spectrum of Disease and Infections |
|---|---|---|---|---|
| *Moraxella nonliquefaciens, Moraxella lacunata, Moraxella osloensis, Moraxella lincolnii, Moraxella canis,* and *Moraxella atlantae* | Normal human flora that inhabit mucous membranes covering the nose, throat, other parts of the upper respiratory tract, conjunctiva, and, for some species (i.e., *M. osloensis*), the urogenital tract; may also colonize the skin | Infections are rare; when they occur, they are probably caused by the patient's endogenous strains; person-to-person transmission may be possible, but this has not been documented | Unknown; because they are rarely associated with infections, they are considered opportunistic organisms of low virulence | *M. lacunata* has historically been associated with eye infections, but these infections also may be caused by other *Moraxella* spp.; other infections include bacteremia, endocarditis, septic arthritis, and, possibly, respiratory infections |
| *Neisseria elongate* | Normal flora of upper respiratory tract | When infections occur, they are probably caused by the patient's endogenous strains | Unknown; an opportunistic organism of low virulence | Rarely implicated in infections; has been documented as a cause of bacteremia, endocarditis, and osteomyelitis |
| *Neisseria weaverii* | Oral flora of dogs | Dog bite | Unknown | Infections of dog bite wounds |

**TABLE 28-2** Antimicrobial Therapy and Susceptibility Testing

| Organism | Therapeutic Options | Potential Resistance to Therapeutic Options | Validated Testing Methods* |
|---|---|---|---|
| *Moraxella* spp. | No definitive guidelines; generally susceptible to penicillins and cephalosporins | β-lactamase–mediated resistance to penicillins common | Not available Exception: See CLSI document M45 for testing guidelines for *M. catarrhalis* (see Chapter 40) |
| *Neisseria elongata* and *Neisseria weaverii* | No definitive guidelines; generally susceptible to penicillins and cephalosporins | None known | Not available |

*Validated testing methods include those standard methods recommended by the Clinical and Laboratory Standards Institute (CLSI) and those commercial methods approved by the Food and Drug Administration (FDA).

testing other bacteria, this does not necessarily mean that interpretable and reliable results will be produced. Chapter 12 should be reviewed for preferable strategies that can be used to provide susceptibility information when validated testing methods do not exist for a clinically important bacterial isolate.

In general, β-lactam antibiotics are thought to be effective against these species. However, some evidence suggests that β-lactamase–mediated resistance may be capable of spreading among *Moraxella* spp.

# LABORATORY DIAGNOSIS

## SPECIMEN COLLECTION AND TRANSPORT

No special considerations are required for specimen collection and transport of the organisms discussed in this chapter. Refer to Table 5-1 for general information on specimen collection and transport.

# SPECIMEN PROCESSING

No special considerations are required for processing of the organisms discussed in this chapter. Refer to Table 5-1 for general information on specimen processing.

## DIRECT DETECTION METHODS

Other than a Gram stain of patient specimens, there are no specific procedures for the direct detection of these organisms in clinical material. *M. atlantae, M. nonliquefaciens,* and *M. osloensis* may appear as either coccobacilli or as short, broad rods that tend to resist decolorization and may appear gram-variable. This is also true for *M. canis*, which appears as cocci in pairs or short chains. *M. lacunata* is a coccobacilli or medium-sized rod, and *M. lincolnii* is a coccobacilli that may appear in chains. All subspecies of *Neisseria elong*ata are either coccobacilli or short, straight rods, and *N. weaverii* is a medium-length, straight bacillus.

## CULTIVATION

### Media of Choice

*Moraxella* spp. and the elongated *Neisseria* spp. grow well on 5% sheep blood and chocolate agars. Most strains grow slowly on MacConkey agar and resemble the non-lactose-fermenting *Enterobacteriaceae*. Both genera also grow well in the broth of commercial blood culture systems and in common nutrient broths, such as thioglycollate and brain-heart infusion.

### Incubation Conditions and Duration

Five percent sheep blood and chocolate agars should be incubated at 35° C in carbon dioxide or ambient air for a minimum of 48 hours. For those species that may grow on MacConkey agar, the medium should be incubated at 35° C in ambient air.

### Colonial Appearance

Table 28-3 describes the colonial appearance and other distinguishing characteristics (e.g., pitting) of each species on 5% sheep blood and MacConkey agars. The ability of most commercial identification systems to accurately identify the organisms discussed in this chapter is limited or uncertain. Table 28-4 lists some conventional biochemical tests that can be used to presumptively differentiate the species in this chapter. This is a simplified scheme; clinically important isolates should be sent to a reference laboratory for definitive identification.

## APPROACH TO IDENTIFICATION

As previously mentioned, these organisms can be difficult to differentiate from gram-negative diplococci (see Chapter 40 for more information about gram-negative diplococci). In addition, these organisms are relatively biochemically inert. Elongation in the presence of penicillin is a useful criterion for differentiating them from true cocci. The effect of penicillin is determined by streaking a blood agar plate, placing a 10-unit penicillin disk in the first quadrant and overnight incubation at 35° C. A Gram stain of the growth taken from around the edge of the zone of inhibition readily demonstrates whether the isolate in question is a true cocci or has elongated.

### Comments Regarding Specific Organisms

*M. nonliquefaciens* and *M. osloensis*, the two most frequently isolated species, can be differentiated by the ability of *M. osloensis* to utilize acetate. *M. lacunata* is able to liquefy serum, so depressions are formed on the surface of Loeffler's serum agar slants. Most of the species considered in this chapter do not utilize glucose; *Neisseria*

**TABLE 28-3** Colonial Appearance and Characteristics

| Organism | Medium | Appearance |
|---|---|---|
| *Moraxella atlantae* | BAP | Small, pitting and spreading |
| | Mac | NLF |
| *M. lacunata* | BAP | Small colonies that pit the agar |
| | Mac | No growth |
| *M. lincolnii* | BAP | Smooth, translucent to semiopaque |
| | Mac | No growth |
| *M. nonliquefaciens* | BAP | Smooth, translucent to semiopaque; occasionally, colonies spread and pit agar |
| | Mac | NLF, if growth |
| *M. osloensis* | BAP | Smooth, translucent to semiopaque |
| | Mac | NLF, if growth |
| *M. canis* | BAP | Resemble colonies of Enterobacteriaceae |
| | Mac | NLF |
| *Neisseria elongata* (all subspecies) | BAP | Gray, translucent, smooth, glistening; may have dry, claylike consistency |
| | Mac | NLF, if growth |
| *N. weaverii* | BAP | Small, smooth, semiopaque |
| | Mac | NLF, if growth |

*BAP,* 5% sheep blood agar; *Mac,* MacConkey agar; *NLF,* non-lactose-fermenter.

*elongata* subsp. *glycolytica,* which produces acid from glucose in the rapid sugar test used for *Neisseria* spp., is the only exception. Unlike *Oligella* spp. (see Chapter 25 for more information regarding this genus), none of the organisms considered here are motile.

## SERODIAGNOSIS

Serodiagnostic techniques are not generally used for the laboratory diagnosis of infections caused by the organisms discussed in this chapter.

## PREVENTION

Because these organisms do not generally pose a threat to human health, there are no recommended vaccination or prophylaxis protocols.

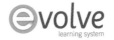 *Visit the Evolve site to complete the review questions.*

**TABLE 28-4** Key Biochemical and Physiologic Characteristics

| Organism | Growth on MacConkey | Catalase | Nitrate Reduction | Nitrite Reduction | DNase | Digests Loeffler's Slant | Sodium Acetate Utilization | Growth in Nutrient Broth |
|---|---|---|---|---|---|---|---|---|
| *Moraxella atlantae* | + | + | – | – | – | – | ND | – |
| *M. lacunata* | – | + | + | – | – | + | – | – |
| *M. lincolnii* | – | + | – | –* | – | – | – | – |
| *M. nonliquefaciens* | – | + | + | – | – | – | – | v |
| *M. osloensis* | v | + | v | – | – | – | + | + |
| *M. canis* | + | + | + | v | + | – | + | + |
| *Neisseria elongata* subsp. *elongata* | v | – | | + | ND | ND | v | + |
| *Neisseria elongata* subsp. *glycolytica* | + | + | – | v | ND | ND | + | + |
| *Neisseria elongata* subsp. *nitroreducens* | v | – | + | + | ND | ND | v | v |
| *N. weaverii* | v | + | – | + | ND | ND | – | v |

*Nitrite-positive strains have been reported.
*ND*, No data; *v*, variable; +, >90% of strains positive; –, >90% of strains negative.
Note: Organisms listed are generally indole-negative.

---

## CASE STUDY 28-1

A 44-year-old woman was rehospitalized following a gastroje-junostomy. She had increased white blood cells (21,000/μL) and was thought to have a postsurgical infection. X-rays showed a leakage from the gastrojejunostomy site into the left upper abdomen and communication with the large cavity. Aspiration of the fluid found by radiologic examination contained small, gram-variable bacilli. Tiny, yellowish nonhemolytic colonies grew on blood agar that slightly pitted the agar. They were cata-lase negative and oxidase positive, but they failed to grow on MacConkey.

### QUESTIONS

1. Both rapid indole and hanging drop motility tests were negative for this bacillus. What microorganisms are in the differential, and how would you approach this identification?

2. The nitrate test was negative and the organism did not ferment glucose. The oxidative-fermentation (OF) glucose test was also negative, meaning that the organism was a glucose nonoxidizer. What is the most likely identification, and how would you confirm it?

3. How is the nitrite reduction test performed when the nitrate test is negative?

---

## BIBLIOGRAPHY

Grant PE, Brenner DJ, Steigerwalt AG, et al: *Neisseria elongata* subsp *nitroreducens* subsp *nov*, formerly CDC group M-6, a gram-negative bacterium associated with endocarditis, *J Clin Microbiol* 28:2591, 1990.

Jannes G, Vaneechoutte M, Lannoo M, et al: Polyphasic taxonomy leading to the proposal of *Moraxella canis* sp *nov* for *Moraxella catarrhalis*–like strains, *Int J Syst Bacteriol* 43:438, 1993.

Kodjo A, Richard Y, Tønjum T: *Moraxella boevrei* sp *nov*, a new *Moraxella* species found in goats, *Int J Syst Bacteriol* 47:115, 1997.

Mandell GL, Bennett JE, Dolin R: *Principles and practices of infectious Diseases*, ed 7, Philadelphia, 2010, Churchill Livingstone Elsevier.

Montejo M, Ruiz-Irastorza G, Aguirrebengoa K, et al: Endocarditis due to *Neisseria elongata* subspecies *nitroreducens*, *Clin Infect Dis* 20:1431, 1995.

Mueleman P, Erard K, Herregods MC, et al: Bioprosthetic valve endo-carditis caused by *Neisseria elongata* subspecies *nitroreducens*, *Infection* 24:258, 1996.

Nagano N, Sato J, Cordevant C, et al: Presumed endocarditis caused by BRO B-lactamase-producing *Moraxella lacunata* in an infant with Fallot's tetrad, *J Clin Microbiol* 41:5310, 2003

Struillou L, Raffi F, Barrier JH: Endocarditis caused by *Neisseria elongata* subspecies *nitroreducens:* case report and literature review, *Eur J Clin Microbiol Infect Dis* 12:625, 1993.

Vandamme P, Gillis M, Vancanneyt M, et al: *Moraxella lincolnii* sp *nov*, isolated from the human respiratory tract, and reevaluation of the taxonomic position of *Moraxella osloensis*, *Int J Syst Bacteriol* 43:474, 1993.

Versalovic J: *Manual of clinical microbiology*, ed 10, Washington, DC, 2011, ASM Press.

Wallace RJ, Steingrube DR, Nash DR, et al: BRO β-lactamases of *Branhamella catarrhalis* and *Moraxella* subgenus *Moraxella*, including evidence for chromosomal β-lactamase transfer by conjugation in *B. catarrhalis, M. nonliquefaciens*, and *M. lacunata*, *Antimicrob Agent Chemother* 30:1845, 1989.

Wong JD, Janda JM: Association of an important *Neisseria* species, *Neisseria elongate* subsp. *nitroreducens*, with bacteremia, endocarditis, and osteomyelitis, *J Clin Microbiol* 30:719, 1992.

# Eikenella and Similar Organisms

## OBJECTIVES

1. Identify and explain the key morphologic and biochemical characteristics for *Eikenella corrodens*.
2. Describe the normal habitat for *Eikenella* spp. and situations that provide optimal conditions for the opportunistic bacteria to become a pathogen.
3. Define the acronym HACEK; what organisms does this acronym refer to, and what medical conditions are associated with these organisms?
4. Define the general characteristics for *Eikenella corrodens*, *Methylobacterium* spp., *Weeksella virosa*, and *Bergeyella zoohelcum*, and explain how the organisms are distinguished from one another.
5. Describe the Gram stain characteristics for each type of bacteria listed in objective 4.
6. Identify the normal habitat for *Methylobacterium* and explain why the organism is frequently isolated from water distribution systems.
7. Explain how the pink colonies produced in culture by *Methylobacterium* spp. are differentiated from other species of bacteria capable of producing pink colonies.
8. Describe the culture techniques used to isolate *Eikenella corrodens* and *Methyolobacterium* spp.
9. Correlate patient signs, symptoms, and laboratory results to identify the most probable etiologic agent associated with the data.

### GENERA AND SPECIES TO BE CONSIDERED

| Current Name | Previous Name |
|---|---|
| *Eikenella corrodens* | |
| *Methylobacterium* spp. | *Pseudomonas mesophilica, Pseudomonas extorquens, Vibrio extorquens* |
| *Weeksella virosa* | CDC group IIf |
| *Bergeyella zoohelcum* | *Weeksella zoohelcum,* CDC group IIj |

## GENERAL CHARACTERISTICS

The organisms discussed in this chapter are considered together because they are all asaccharolytic, oxidase-positive bacilli that fail to grow on MacConkey agar. Their individual morphologic and physiologic features are presented later in this chapter.

## EPIDEMIOLOGY, SPECTRUM OF DISEASE, AND ANTIMICROBIAL THERAPY

The organisms listed in Table 29-1 are not commonly associated with human infections, but they are occasionally encountered in clinical specimens. *Eikenella corrodens* is normal flora of the human oral cavity. The organism is a facultative anaerobe, nonmotile, gram-negative rod. Among the organisms considered in this chapter, it is the organism most frequently isolated and is usually found in mixed infections resulting from human bites or clenched-fist wounds. The organism can be isolated from dental plaque and has been implicated in periodontitis, osteomyelitis, bite wound infections, bacteremia, and endocarditis. It is an opportunistic pathogen predominantly in immunocompromised patients, causing abscesses and infections, and may lead to death. Patients with diabetes are often at risk for Eikenella infections as a result of the daily microtrauma to their skin via glucose monitoring, insulin injections, and the potential for introduction of the organism from oral secretions by licking or biting their skin. The organism is often the cause of soft tissue infections in intravenous drug abusers who lick the injection site.

This organism also is the "E," for Eikenella, in the HACEK group of bacteria known to cause subacute bacterial endocarditis (see Chapter 68 for more information regarding endocarditis and bloodstream infections). HACEK is an acronym used to represent the slow-growing gram-negative bacilli associated with endocarditis. The additional members of the HACEK group of bacteria include *Aggregatibacter aphrophilus, Actinobacillus actinomycetemcometans, Cardiobacterium hominis,* and *Kingella kingae.*

*Methylobacterium* sp. bacteria are gram-negative bacilli predominantly found in water and soil. There are currently 20 recognized species. They can be opportunistic pathogens but are considered to be of low virulence as most human infections are associated with immunocompromised patients. *M. mesophilicum* and *M. zatmanii* are the two species most commonly isolated from clinical samples. *Methylobacterium* spp. are chlorine resistant and have been isolated from water-distribution systems.

The rarity with which these organisms are encountered in the clinical laboratory and the lack of validated in vitro susceptibility testing methods do not provide enough data to recommend definitive treatment guidelines (Table 29-2). Although ß-lactamase production has been described in *E. corrodens,* this species is usually susceptible to penicillin and other ß-lactam antimicrobials. Penicillin-resistant strains of *E. corrodens* have been identified.

## LABORATORY DIAGNOSIS

### SPECIMEN COLLECTION AND TRANSPORT

No special considerations are required for specimen collection and transport for the organisms discussed in this

**TABLE 29-1** Epidemiology, Pathogenesis, and Spectrum of Disease

| Organism | Habitat (Reservoir) | Mode of Transmission | Virulence Factors | Spectrum of Disease and Infections |
|---|---|---|---|---|
| *Eikenella corrodens* | Normal human flora of mouth and gastrointestinal tract | Person to person involving trauma associated with human teeth incurred during bites or clenched-fist wounds incurred as a result of facial punches; infection may be a result of the patient's endogenous strains (e.g., endocarditis) | Unknown; opportunistic organism usually requires trauma for introduction into normally sterile sites; also may enter bloodstream to cause transient bacteremia or be introduced by intravenous drug abuse | Human bite wound infections, head and neck infections, and aspiration pneumonias as part of mixed infection; can also cause endocarditis that is slow to develop and indolent (i.e., sub acute); less commonly associated with brain and intra-abdominal abscesses |
| *Methylobacterium* spp. | Found on vegetation and occasionally in the hospital environment; not considered normal human flora | Uncertain; probably involves contaminated medical devices such as catheters | Unknown; an opportunistic organism probably of low virulence Uncommon cause of infection | Bacteremia and peritonitis in patients undergoing chronic ambulatory peritoneal dialysis (CAPD) |
| *Weeksella virosa* | Uncertain; probably environmental; not considered normal human flora | Uncertain; rarely found in clinical material | Unknown; role in human disease is uncertain | Asymptomatic bacteriuria; also isolated from female genital tract |
| *Bergeyella zoohelcum* | Normal oral flora of dogs and other animals; not considered normal human flora | Bite or scratch of dog or cat | Unknown; an opportunistic organism that requires traumatic introduction to normally sterile site | Dog and cat bite wound infections |

chapter. Refer to Table 5-1 for general information on specimen collection and transport.

## SPECIMEN PROCESSING

No special considerations are required for processing of the organisms discussed in this chapter. Refer to Table 5-1 for general information on specimen processing.

## DIRECT DETECTION METHODS

Other than Gram stain and microscopic examination, there are no specific procedures for the direct detection of these organisms in clinical material. *E. corrodens* is a slender, medium-length gram-negative, straight rod with rounded ends. *Methylobacterium* is a vacuolated, pale-staining, short to medium-length gram-negative bacillus that may resist decolorization. *Weeksella virosa* and *Bergeyella zoohelcum* are medium to long gram-negative rods with parallel sides and rounded ends that may form "II-forms" (parallel sides) similar to the *Sphingobacterium* (see Chapter 24 for more information regarding this genus).

## CULTIVATION

### Media of Choice

Because it is a facultative anaerobe, *Eikenella corrodens* grows slowly on blood and chocolate agar with small colonies developing within 48 hours. The organism will not grow on MacConkey agar. The organism also displays limited growth in blood culture broth media, thioglycollate broth, and brain-heart infusion broth. The hallmark characteristics for the presence of *E. corrodens* in culture include the organism's tendency to pit or corrode the agar, demonstrate a slightly yellow hue after several days, and exude a chlorine bleach odor. Most strains require hemin for growth unless incubated in 5% to 10% $CO_2$. Detection may be improved using selective media containing clindamycin.

*Methylobacterium* is also difficult to grow on routine laboratory media producing small colonies in 4 to 5 days on sheep blood agar, modified Thayer-Martin, buffered charcoal-yeast extract, and Middlebrook 7H11 agar. Reports have indicated that improved growth may be

**TABLE 29-2** Antimicrobial Therapy and Susceptibility Testing

| Organism | Potential Resistance to Therapeutic Options | Therapeutic Options | Validated Testing Methods* |
|---|---|---|---|
| *Eikenella corrodens* | Often susceptible to penicillins, quinolones, cephalosporins, and trimethoprim-sulfamethoxazole | May produce beta-lactamases; usually resistant to clindamycin, metronidazole, and aminoglycosides | See CLSI document M45, section on "HACEK" organisms |
| *Methylobacterium* spp. | No guidelines | Unknown | Not available |
| *Weeksella virosa* and *Bergeyella zoohelcum* | No guidelines; potentially active agents include beta-lactams and quinolones | Susceptibility to tetracycline, aminoglycosides, and trimethoprim-sulfamethoxazole | Not available |

*Validated testing methods include those standard methods recommended by the Clinical and Laboratory Standards Institute (CLSI) and those commercial methods approved by the Food and Drug Administration (FDA).

achieved using BYCE agar and Sabouraud agar. As previously indicated, the organism is not capable of growth on MacConkey agar. Optimal growth occurs at 15° to 30° C. *Methylobacterium* produce small, dry, coral pink-pigmented colonies. Pink colonies are also produced by *Roseomonas*. The two genera can be differentiated by incubation at 42° C. *Roseomonas* is capable of growth at 42° C, whereas *Methylobacterium* is temperature sensitive and incapable of growth in increased temperatures. In addition, *Methylobacterium* can metabolize acetate, and *Roseomonas* cannot.

### Incubation Conditions and Duration

To detect growth on 5% sheep blood and chocolate agars, incubation at 35° to 37° C in carbon dioxide for a minimum of 48 hours is required. In contrast to the other genera, *Methylobacterium* grows at lower temperatures, as previously indicated.

### Colonial Appearance

Table 29-3 describes the colonial appearance and other distinguishing characteristics (e.g., odor and pigment) of each genus on 5% sheep blood agar.

**TABLE 29-3** Colonial Appearance and Characteristics

| Organism | Medium* | Appearance |
|---|---|---|
| *Bergeyella zoohelcum* | BA | Colonies may be sticky; tan to yellow in color |
| *Eikenella corrodens* | BA | Colonies are tiny at 24 hours; mature colonies have moist, clear centers surrounded by flat, spreading growth; colonies may pit or corrode the agar surface; slight yellow pigmentation in older cultures; sharp odor of bleach |
| *Methylobacterium* spp. | BA | Pink to coral pigment; does not grow well on blood agar |
| *Weeksella virosa* | BA | Small colonies at 24 hours; mature colonies mucoid and adherent with a tan to brown pigment |

*These organisms usually do not grow on MacConkey agar; if breakthrough growth occurs, the organisms appear as non-lactose-fermenters.
BA, 5% sheep blood agar.

## APPROACH TO IDENTIFICATION

The ability of most commercial identification systems to accurately identify the organisms discussed in this chapter is limited or, at best, uncertain. Therefore, strategies for identification of these genera are based on the use of conventional biochemical tests. Table 29-4 outlines basic criteria useful for differentiating the genera discussed in this chapter.

### Comments Regarding Specific Organisms

As previously indicated, *Methylobacterium* may be differentiated from other pink-pigmented, gram-negative rods by its ability to utilize acetate and its inability to grow at 42° C. Some strains of *Methylobacterium* weakly oxidize glucose and oxidize xylose.

The most recognizable feature of *E. corrodens* in culture is the distinctive bleachlike odor. The organism is asaccharolytic (does not utilize glucose or other carbohydrates). The organism is oxidase positive, catalase negative, reduces nitrate to nitrite, and hydrolyzes both ornithine and lysine.

*Weeksella* and *Bergeyella* are oxidase and catalase positive. A distinguishing feature of the two bacteria is that they are indole positive, an unusual characteristic for most nonfermentative bacteria. *W. virosa* is urease-negative and *B. zoohelcum* is urease-positive, pyrrolidonyl aminopeptidase negative, and resistant to colistin. *W. virosa* will grow on selective media such as modified Thayer martin (MTM) for *Neisseria gonorrhoeae* but can differentiated from the gonococci using indole and Gram-stain morphology.

## SERODIAGNOSIS

Serodiagnostic techniques are not generally used for the laboratory diagnosis of infections caused by the organisms discussed in this chapter.

**TABLE 29-4** Key Biochemical and Physiologic Characteristics

| Organism | Catalase | Oxidizes Xylose | Indole | Arginine Dihydrolase |
|---|---|---|---|---|
| *Eikenella corrodens* | – | – | – | – |
| *Methylobacterium* spp.* | + | + | – | ND |
| *Weeksella virosa* | + | – | + | – |
| *Bergeyella zoohelcum* | + | – | + | + |

*Colonies are pigmented pink and must be differentiated from *Roseomonas* spp.; *Roseomonas* spp. usually grow on MacConkey agar and will grow at 42° C.
*ND,* No data; +, >90% of strains positive; –, >90% of strains negative.
Data compiled from Weyant RS, Moss CW, Weaver RE, et al, editors: *Identification of unusual pathogenic gram-negative aerobic and facultatively anaerobic bacteria,* ed 2, Baltimore, 1997, Williams & Wilkins.

# PREVENTION

Because these organisms do not generally pose a threat to human health, there are no recommended vaccination or prophylaxis protocols.

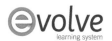 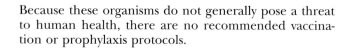

*Visit the Evolve site to complete the review questions.*

---

## CASE STUDY 29-1

A 64-year-old Indonesian man was in good health until 3 months ago when he awoke with back pain localized to the upper thoracic area. His symptoms were not improved with physical therapy or acupuncture. A bone scan was positive for inflammation at C5 and C6, and he was treated with antibiotics for 2 weeks. His symptoms returned when antibiotics were discontinued. A vertebrectomy of C5 and C6 was performed, and bone tissue was sent for culture. A nonhemolytic gram-negative rod was isolated that was catalase negative and oxidase positive, but did not grow on MacConkey. Colonies showed pits in the agar and exuded an odor of bleach. When questioned, the patient indicated that he had no dental procedures prior to the illness but indicated he had previously sought medical attention for a swallowed fishbone that was not successfully removed. Review of the radiology films indicated a dense area that could have been the foreign body.

### QUESTIONS

1. Because the bacterium is catalase negative, it needs to be separated from the genera described in Chapters 28, 30, and 31. However, one unique positive biochemical reaction will definitively identify the organism. What is that test?
2. Why was the physician interested in whether dental work had been performed prior to the onset of symptoms?
3. Explain why this bacterium is included in the HACEK group?

---

# BIBLIOGRAPHY

Cercenado E, Cercenado S, Bouza E: In vitro activities of tigecycline (GAR-936) and 12 other antimicrobial agents against 90 *Eikenella corrodens* clinical isolates, *Antimicrob Agents Chemother* 47:2644, 2003

Chen CK, Wilson ME: Eikenella corrodens in human oral and non-oral infections: a review, *J Periodontol* 63:941, 1992.

Fass RJ, Barnishan J, Solomon MC, et al: In vitro activities of quinolones, β-lactams, tobramycin, and trimethoprim-sulfamethoxazole, against nonfermentative gram-negative bacilli, *Antimicrob Agents Chemother* 40:1412, 1996.

Goldstein EJ, Tarenzi LA, Agyare EO et al: Prevalence of *Eikenella corrodens* in dental plaque, *J Clin Microbiol* 17:363, 1983

Hornei B, Lüneberg E, Schmidt-Rotte H, et al: Systemic infection of an immunocompromised patient with *Methylobacterium zatmanii, J Clin Microbiol* 37:248, 1999

Kay KM, Macone S, Kazanjian PH: Catheter infections caused by Methylobacterium in immunocompromised hosts: report of three cases and review of the literature, *Clin Infect Dis* 14:1010, 1992.

Lacroix JM, Walker CB: Identification of a streptomycin resistance gene and a partial Tn3 transposon coding for a β-lactamase in a periodontal strain of Eikenella corrodens, *Antimicrob Agents Chemother* 36:740, 1992.

Newfield RS, Vargas I, Huma Z: Eikenella corrodens infections: case report in two adolescent females with IDDM, *Diabetes Care* 19:1011-1013, 1996

Reina J, Borell N: Leg abscess caused by *Weeksella zoohelcum* following a dog bite, *Clin Infect Dis* 14:1162, 1992.

Reina J, Gil J, Alomar P: Isolation of *Weeksella virosa* (formally CDC group IIf) from a vaginal sample, *Eur J Clin Microbiol Infect Dis* 8:569, 1989.

Versalovic J: *Manual of clinical microbiology,* ed 10, Washington, DC, 2011, ASM Press.

Weyant RS, Moss CW, Weaver RE, et al, editors: Identification of unusual pathogenic gram-negative aerobic and facultatively anaerobic bacteria, ed 2, Baltimore, 1997, Williams & Wilkins.

# Pasteurella and Similar Organisms

## OBJECTIVES

1. Describe the general characteristics of *Pasteurella* spp. and the additional organisms included in this chapter.
2. Describe the epidemiology associated with human infections caused by *Pasteurella* spp. and similar organisms, including the normal habitat and route of transmission.
3. Compare the Gram-stain appearance of the organisms included in this chapter.
4. Explain the limitations of antimicrobial susceptibility testing with respect to *Pasteurella* spp. and similar organisms.
5. Identify limitations associated with identification of *Pasteurella* spp. and similar organisms.

---

### GENERA AND SPECIES TO BE CONSIDERED

| Current Name | Previous Name |
|---|---|
| *Mannheimia haemolytica* | *Pasteurella haemolytica* |
| *Pasteurella aerogenes*\* | |
| *Pasteurella bettyae*\* | CDC group HB-5 |
| *Pasteurella caballi*\* | |
| *Pasteurella canis* | |
| *Pasteurella dagmatis* | |
| *Pasteurella multocida* subspecies *multocida* | *Pasteurella multocida* |
| *Pasteurella multocida* subspecies *gallicida* | *Pasteurella multocida* |
| *Pasteurella multocida* subspecies *septica* | *Pasteurella multocida* |
| *Pasteurella pneumotropica*\* | |
| *Pasteurella stomatis* | |
| *Suttonella indologenes* | *Kingella indologenes* |

\*Pending potential classification changes based on DNA sequencing.

---

## GENERAL CHARACTERISTICS AND TAXONOMY

The organisms discussed in this chapter are small, gram-negative, non-motile, oxidase-positive bacilli that ferment glucose. The majority of the organisms discussed in this chapter will not grow on MacConkey agar. Their individual morphologic and physiologic features are presented later in this chapter in the discussion of laboratory diagnosis.

Taxonomy of *Pasteurella* spp. and similar organisms has significantly changed since the early 2000s and may be subject to additional revision. Genera now classified into the Pasteurellaceae family include *Actinobacillus*, *Aggregatibacter* (aggregation of the former *Actinobacillus actinomycetemcomitans*, *Haemophilus aphrophilus*, *H. paraphrophilus*, and *H. segnis*), *Haemophilus*, and *Pasteurella*.

## EPIDEMIOLOGY, SPECTRUM OF DISEASE, AND ANTIMICROBIAL THERAPY

Most of the organisms presented in this chapter constitute portions of both domestic and wild animal flora and are transmitted to humans during close animal contact, including bites. For most of these species, virulence factors are not recognized. As a result, the organisms may be considered opportunistic pathogens that require mechanical disruption of host anatomic barriers (i.e., bite-induced wounds; Table 30-1). Of the organisms listed in Table 30-2, *P. multocida* subsp. *multocida* is most commonly encountered in clinical specimens. Reported virulence factors for this subspecies include lipopolysaccharide, cytotoxin, six serotypes of the antiphagocytic capsule, surface adhesins, and iron-acquisition proteins. Other manifestations of infection by *P. multocida* subsp. *multocida* can include respiratory disease and systemic disease such as endocarditis and septicemia. Liver cirrhosis is viewed as a risk factor for systemic disease. Other *Pasteurella* spp. can be agents of systemic infection (*P. pneumotropica*) and genital tract-associated disease (*P. bettyae*).

An unusual feature of the organisms considered in this chapter is that most are susceptible to penicillin. Although most other clinically relevant Gram-negative bacilli are intrinsically resistant to penicillin, it is the drug of choice for infections involving *P. multocida* and several other species listed in Table 30-3. The general therapeutic effectiveness of penicillin and the lack of resistance to this agent among *Pasteurella* spp. suggest that in vitro susceptibility testing is typically not indicated. This is especially true with isolates emanating from bite wounds. Moreover, bite wounds can be complicated by polymicrobial infection. In this case, the empiric therapy directed toward multiple agents is generally also effective against *Pasteurella* spp. As a result, antimicrobial susceptibility testing for *Pasteurella* spp. may have greater utility for isolates recovered from sterile sources (blood, deep tissue) and from respiratory specimens obtained from immunocompromised patients.

Clinical and Laboratory Standards Institute (CLSI) document M45-A2, published in 2010, provides guidelines for broth microdilution (cation-adjusted Mueller Hinton broth medium supplemented with 2.5% to 5% lysed horse blood) and disk diffusion (Mueller Hinton agar medium supplemented with 5% sheep blood) susceptibility testing of *Pasteurella* spp. Both formats are incubated in 35° C ambient air. Interpretation of disk diffusion and broth microdilution formats occurs at 16 to 18 hours and 18 to 24 hours of incubation, respectively. Antimicrobial agents to consider for testing

**TABLE 30-1** Epidemiology of Selected *Pasteurella* spp. and Similar Organisms

| Organism | Habitat (Reservoir) | Mode of Transmission |
|---|---|---|
| *P. multocida*, other *Pasteurella* spp. | Commensal found in nasopharynx and gastrointestinal tract of wild and domestic animals; potential upper respiratory commensal in humans having extensive occupational exposure to animals | Bite or scratch from variety of veterinary hosts (usually feline or canine); infections may be associated with non-bite exposure to animals; less commonly, infections may occur without history of animal exposure |
| *S. indologenes* | Unknown; rarely encountered in clinical specimens but may be part of human flora | Unknown |

**TABLE 30-2** Pathogenesis and Spectrum of Disease of Selected *Pasteurella* spp. and Similar Organisms

| Organism | Virulence Factors | Spectrum of Disease and Infections |
|---|---|---|
| *P. bettyae* | Unknown | Genital tract infection; neonatal infection |
| *P. multocida* subsp. *multocida* | Endotoxin, cytotoxin, surface adhesins, capsule associated with *P. multocida* | Focal soft tissue infection; chronic respiratory infection, usually in patients with preexisting chronic lung disease and heavy exposure to animals; systemic disease (hematogenous dissemination) such as meningitis, endocarditis, osteomyelitis, dialysis-associated peritonitis, septicemia |
| *P. multocida* subsp. *septica* | Unknown | Focal soft tissue infection |
| *P. pneumotropica* | Unknown | Rare systemic infection |
| *S. indologenes* | Unknown | Rare ocular infection |

include penicillin, ampicillin, amoxicillin, amoxicillin-clavulanate, ceftriaxone, moxifloxacin, levofloxacin, tetracycline, doxycycline, erythromycin, azithromycin, chloramphenicol, and trimethoprim-sulfamethoxazole. Of these agents, breakpoints for categorical interpretation of resistance or intermediate susceptibility have only been established for erythromycin.

# LABORATORY DIAGNOSIS

## SPECIMEN COLLECTION AND TRANSPORT

No special considerations are required for specimen collection and transport of the organisms discussed in this chapter. Refer to Table 5-1 for general information on specimen collection and transport.

## SPECIMEN PROCESSING

No special considerations are required for processing of the organisms discussed in this chapter. Refer to Table 5-1 for general information on specimen processing.

## DIRECT DETECTION METHODS

Other than Gram staining, there are no commonly employed procedures for the direct detection of these organisms from primary clinical material. *Pasteurella* spp. are typically short, straight bacilli, although *P. aerogenes* may also present as coccobacilli. Bipolar staining is frequent. The bacillus of *P. bettyae* is usually thinner than those of the other species. *M. haemolytica* is a small bacillus or coccobacillus. *S. indologenes* is a broad bacillus of variable length.

## CULTIVATION

### Media of Choice

The bacteria described in this chapter grow well on routine laboratory media such as tryptic soy agar supplemented with 5% sheep blood (blood agar) and chocolate agar. With the exception of *P. aerogenes* and some strains of *P. bettyae* and *P. pneumotropica*, most species do not grow on MacConkey agar. *M. haemolytica*, *Pasteurella* spp., and *S. indologenes* also grow well in broth blood culture systems and common nutrient broths such as thioglycollate and brain-heart infusion. *Pasteurella* spp. may

**TABLE 30-3** Antimicrobial Therapy and Susceptibility Testing for *Pasteurella* spp. and Similar Organisms

| Organism | Therapeutic Options | Potential Resistance to Therapeutic Options | Validated Testing Methods |
|---|---|---|---|
| *Pasteurella* spp. | Penicillin, ampicillin, amoxicillin are recommended agents; doxycycline, amoxicillin-clavulanate are alternative agents; ceftriaxone, fluoroquinolones may be effective | Clindamycin, cephalexin, nafcillin, erythromycin (deduced from susceptibility testing) | CLSI document M45-A2 |
| *S. indologenes* | Not well characterized; purported susceptibility to penicillins, chloramphenicol, tetracycline | Unknown | Not available |

be differentiated from *Haemophilus* spp. via $CO_2$-independence and growth on media containing sheep blood.

### Incubation Conditions and Duration

Inoculated blood and chocolate agar are incubated at 35° C in ambient air or an environment enriched with 5% $CO_2$ for a minimum of 24 hours. *S. indologenes* may grow especially slowly on primary media.

### Colonial Appearance

Table 30-4 describes the colonial appearance and other distinguishing characteristics (e.g., hemolysis and odor) of these genera on blood agar.

## APPROACH TO IDENTIFICATION

The accuracy of commercial biochemical identification systems has been called into question for the definitive identification of *Pasteurella* spp. and similar organisms. Table 30-5 summarizes conventional biochemical tests that can assist in the presumptive differentiation or species confirmation of organisms discussed in this chapter. These organisms closely resemble those described in Chapter 31. Therefore, data discussed in both Chapters 30 and 31 can be considered when evaluating an isolate in the clinical laboratory. A more complete conventional biochemical battery, offered as part of a reference laboratory workup, may be required for

**TABLE 30-4** Colonial Appearance and Characteristics of Selected *Pasteurella* spp. and Similar Organisms on Sheep Blood Agar

| Organism | Appearance |
|---|---|
| *M. haemolytica** | Convex, smooth, grayish, beta-hemolytic (feature may be lost on subculture) |
| *P. aerogenes** | Convex, smooth, translucent, nonhemolytic[†] |
| *P. bettyae*[‡] | Convex, smooth, nonhemolytic |
| *P. caballi* | Convex, smooth, nonhemolytic |
| *P. canis* | Convex, smooth, nonhemolytic |
| *P. dagmatis* | Convex, smooth, nonhemolytic |
| *P. multocida* | Convex, smooth, gray, nonhemolytic; rough and mucoid variants can occur; may have a musty or mushroom odor |
| *P. pneumotropica** | Smooth, convex, nonhemolytic |
| *P. stomatis* | Smooth, convex, nonhemolytic |
| *S. indologenes* | Resembles *Kingella* spp. (see Chapter 31); may spread or pit the surface of blood agar |

*Breakthrough growth may occur on MacConkey agar; will appear as lactose fermenter.
[†]After 48 hours, colonies may be surrounded by a narrow green to brown halo.
[‡]Breakthrough growth may occur on MacConkey agar; will appear as non-lactose fermenter.

**TABLE 30-5** Key Biochemical Characteristics of Selected *Pasteurella* spp. and Similar Organisms

| Organism | PHENOTYPE | | | | | | | |
|---|---|---|---|---|---|---|---|---|
| | Indole | Urea | Nitrate Reduction | Catalase | ODC[†] | Mannitol | Sucrose | Maltose |
| *M. haemolytica* | − | − | + | + | − | (+) | + | + |
| *P. aerogenes* | − | (+) | (+) | + | v | − | + | + |
| *P. bettyae* | (+) | − | (+) | − | − | − | − | − |
| *P. caballi* | − | − | (+) | − | (+) | (+) | (+) | (+) |
| *P. canis* | + | − | + | + | (+) | − | (+) | − |
| *P. dagmatis* | (+) | (+) | (+) | + | − | − | + | (+) |
| *P. multocida* | (+) | − | (+) | + | (+) | + | + | − |
| *P. pneumotropica* | (+) | (+)* | (+) | + | (+) | − | + | + |
| *P. stomatis* | (+) | − | + | + | − | − | (+) | − |
| *S. indologenes* | (+) | − | − | v | − | − | (+) | (+) |

Data compiled from Angen O, Mutters R, Caugant DA, et al: Taxonomic relationships of the [*Pasteurella*] *haemolytica* complex as evaluated by DNA-DNA hybridization and 16S rRNA sequencing with proposal of *Mannheimia haemolytica* gen. nov., comb. nov., *Mannheimia granulomatis* comb. nov., *Mannheimia glucosida* sp. nov., *Mannheimia ruminalis* sp. nov. and *Mannheimia varigena* sp. nov., *Int J Syst Bacteriol* 49:67, 1999; Versalovic J, Carroll KC, Funke G, et al, editors: *Manual of clinical microbiology,* ed 10, Washington, DC, 2011, ASM Press; and Weyant RS, Moss CW, Weaver RE, et al, editors: *Identification of unusual pathogenic gram-negative aerobic and facultatively anaerobic bacteria,* ed 2, Baltimore, 1996, Williams & Wilkins.
*May require a drop of rabbit serum on the slant or a heavy inoculum.
[†]Ornithine decarboxylase
+, >90% of strains positive; (+), >90% of strains positive but reaction may be delayed (i.e., 2 to 7 days); −, >90% of strains negative; *v,* variable.

definitive identification of the isolates. Alternatively, past attempts to definitively identify *Pasteurella* spp. on the basis of cellular fatty acid analysis have been replaced by 16S rDNA gene sequencing and *sodA* gene sequencing. Matrix-assisted laser desorption ionization-time of flight (MALDI-TOF) mass spectrometry may provide future utility.

### Comments Regarding Specific Organisms

*Pasteurella* spp. typically yield a positive tetramethyl-p-phenylenediamine dihydrochloride-based oxidase result. With the exception of *P. bettyae* and *P. caballi*, these organisms are catalase positive; all *Pasteurella* spp. reduce nitrates to nitrites. *P. aerogenes* and some strains of *P. dagmatis* ferment glucose with the production of gas. *P. multocida* can be differentiated from other *Pasteurella* spp. on the basis of positive reactions for ornithine decarboxylase and indole, with a negative reaction for urease. Within *P. multocida*, subsp. *multocida* ferments sorbitol and fails to ferment dulcitol, subsp. *gallicida* ferments dulcitol but not sorbitol, and subsp. *septica* ferments neither carbohydrate.

*M. haemolytica* may be differentiated from members of the *Pasteurella* genus by its inability to produce indole or ferment mannose. *S. indologenes* can be separated from *Pasteurella* spp. with a negative nitrate test and is further delineated from *Kingella* spp. (discussed in Chapter 31) by indole production and sucrose fermentation.

## SERODIAGNOSIS

Serodiagnostic techniques are of little utility for the laboratory diagnosis of infections caused by the organisms discussed in this chapter.

## PREVENTION

Because these organisms do not generally pose a threat to human health, there are no recommended vaccination or prophylaxis protocols.

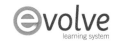 *Visit the Evolve site to complete the review questions.*

---

## CASE STUDY 30-1

A 55-year-old woman sustained a bite from the family cat on the left ring finger and the palm of the right hand. Within the next 12 to 18 hours, the patient noted increased redness, pain, and swelling (particularly in the left hand) and presented to the emergency department. Physical examination was significant for a puncture wound on the proximal phalanx of the left ring finger, with erythema extending from the midphalanx to the midmetacarpal area. Tendon sheaths were nontender, and proximal interphalangeal (PIP) joints had full range of motion. The right hand exhibited a small puncture wound and 1 to 2 cm of surrounding erythema. Minimal drainage emanated from each wound.

The patient was afebrile upon presentation, but slightly tachycardic and tachypneic (pulse 78; respiratory rate 20). Blood pressure was 100/65 and pO$_2$ was 95% on room air. Significant laboratory data included a C-reactive protein level of 30 mg/L (reference range, 0 to 8 mg/L), a peripheral leukocyte count of 12,100/μL (77.8% segmented neutrophils; 15.6% lymphocytes), and further indicated renal dysfunction (blood urea nitrogen and serum creatinine values elevated 35% to 45%

above the upper end of respective reference ranges). Liver function testing was within normal limits. Radiology revealed moderate soft tissue swelling about the PIP joint of the left ring finger.

An initial diagnosis of cellulitis was made, and the patient was admitted for intravenous empiric ampicillin-sulbactam therapy and fluid replacement. Within 24 hours, improvement of the cellulitis and acute renal failure was observed. A gram-negative bacillus was isolated in the microbiology laboratory on blood agar and chocolate agar (no growth on a selective enteric medium). Antimicrobial susceptibility testing of this isolate demonstrated resistance only to erythromycin and allowed clinicians to convert the patient to a 10-day regimen of oral penicillin. The patient was discharged on hospital day 3.

### QUESTIONS

1. What is the likely identification of this organism?
2. Describe the value of empiric ampicillin-sulbactam therapy in this case study.
3. Discuss the potential significance of acute renal failure in this case study.

---

## BIBLIOGRAPHY

Angen O, Mutters R, Caugant DA, et al: Taxonomic relationships of the [*Pasteurella*] *haemolytica* complex as evaluated by DNA-DNA hybridization and 16S rRNA sequencing with proposal of *Mannheimia haemolytica* gen. nov., comb. nov., *Mannheimia granulomatis* comb. nov., *Mannheimia glucosida* sp. nov., *Mannheimia ruminalis* sp. nov. and *Mannheimia varigena* sp. nov., *Int J Syst Bacteriol* 49:67, 1999.

Clinical and Laboratory Standards Institute: *Methods for antimicrobial dilution and disk susceptibility testing of infrequently isolated or fastidious bacteria; M45-A2*, Wayne, Pa, 2010, CLSI.

Cuadrado-Gómez LM, Arranz-Caso JA, Cuadros-González J, Albarrán-Hernández F: *Pasteurella pneumotropica* pneumonia in a patient with AIDS, *Clin Infect Dis* 21:445, 1995.

Donnio P-Y, Lerestif-Gautier A-L, Avril J-L: Characterization of *Pasteurella* spp. strains isolated from human infections, *J Comp Pathol* 130:137, 2004.

Gautier A-L, Dubois D, Escande F, et al: Rapid and accurate identification of human isolates of *Pasteurella* and related species by sequencing of the *sodA* gene, *J Clin Microbiol* 43:2307, 2005.

Gregersen RH, Neubauer C, Christensen H, et al: Characterization of Pasteurellaceae-like bacteria isolated from clinically affected psittacine birds, *J Appl Microbiol* 108:1235, 2010.

Guillard T, Duval V, Jobart R, et al: Dog bite wound infection by *Pasteurella dagmatis* misidentified as *Pasteurella pneumotropica* by automated system Vitek 2, *Diagn Microbiol Infect Dis* 65:347, 2009.

Harper M, Boyce JD, Adler B: *Pasteurella multocida* pathogenesis: 125 years after Pasteur, *FEMS Microbiol Lett* 265:1, 2006.

Hayashimoto N, Takakura A, Itoh T: Genetic diversity of 16S rDNA sequence and phylogenetic tree analysis in *Pasteurella pneumotropica* strains isolated from laboratory animals, *Curr Microbiol* 51:239, 2005.

Holst E, Roloff J, Larsson L, Nielsen JP: Characterization and distribution of *Pasteurella* species recovered from infected humans, *J Clin Microbiol* 30:2984, 1992.

Korczak B, Christensen H, Emler S, et al: Phylogeny of the family *Pasteurellaceae* based on *rpoB* sequences, *Int J Syst Evol Microbiol* 54:1393, 2004.

Mandell GL, Bennett JE, Dolin R, editors: *Principles and practice of infectious diseases*, ed 7, Philadelphia, 2010, Elsevier Churchill Livingstone.

Norskov-Lauritsen N, Kilian M: Reclassification of *Actinobacillus actinomycetemcomitans, Haemophilus aphrophilus, Haemophilus paraphrophilus,* and *Haemophilus segnis* as *Aggregatibacter actinomycetemcomitans* gen. nov., comb. nov., *Aggregatibacter aphrophilus*, comb. nov., and *Aggregatibacter segnis* comb. nov., and emended description of *Aggregatibacter aphrophilus* to include V factor-dependent and V factor-independent isolates, *Int J Syst Evol Microbiol* 56:2135, 2006.

Shapiro DS, Brooks PE, Coffey DM, Browne KF: Peripartum bacteremia with CDC group HB-5 (*Pasteurella bettyae*), *Clin Infect Dis* 22:1125, 1996.

Versalovic J, Carroll KC, Funke G, et al, editors: *Manual of clinical microbiology*, ed 10, Washington, DC, 2011, ASM Press.

Weber DJ, Wolfson JS, Swartz MN, Hooper DC: *Pasteurella multocida* infections. Report of 34 cases and review of the literature, *Medicine* 63:133, 1984.

Weyant RS, Moss CW, Weaver RE, et al, editors: *Identification of unusual pathogenic gram-negative aerobic and facultatively anaerobic bacteria*, ed 2, Baltimore, 1996, Williams & Wilkins.

# Actinobacillus, Aggregatibacter, Kingella, Cardiobacterium, Capnocytophaga, and Similar Organisms

## OBJECTIVES

1. Describe the general characteristics of the bacteria included in this chapter.
2. Describe the normal habitat and the routes of transmission for the organisms included in this chapter.
3. Identify the major clinical diseases associated with *Actinobacillus, Aggregatibacter, Kingella, Cardiobacterium,* and *Capnocytophaga* spp.
4. Explain the incubation conditions for the bacteria discussed in this chapter including oxygenation, time, and temperature.
5. Define *dysgonic*.
6. List the media used to cultivate the organisms discussed in this chapter.
7. Discuss the unique colonial presentation of the various genera of the clinically significant species.

### GENERA AND SPECIES TO BE CONSIDERED

| Current Name | Previous Name |
|---|---|
| *Actinobacillus* spp., including | |
| *A. suis* (pigs) | |
| *A. lignieresii* (sheep and cattle) | |
| *A. hominis* | |
| *A. equuli* (horses and pigs) | |
| *A. ureae* | |
| *Aggregatibacter* sp. (newly proposed) | |
| *A. actinomycetemcomitans* | Formerly *Actinobacillus actinomycetemcomitans* |
| *A. aphrophilus* | Formerly *Haemophilus aphrophilus, H. paraphrophilus* |
| *A. segnis* | Formerly *Haemophilus segnis* |
| *Capnocytophaga canimorsus* (dogs and cats) | CDC group DF-2 |
| *Capnocytophaga cynodegmi* (dogs and cats) | CDC group DF-2 |
| *Capnocytophaga haemolytica* | |
| *Capnocytophaga granulosa* | |
| *Capnocytophaga leadbetteri* | |
| *Capnocytophaga* genospecies AHN8471 | |
| *Cardiobacterium hominis* | |
| *Cardiobacterium valvarum* | |
| *Dysgonomonas gadei* | |
| *Dysgonomonas mossii* | |
| *Dysgonomonas hofstadii* | |
| *Dysgonomonas capnocytophagoides* | CDC group DF-3 |
| *Kingella denitrificans* | |
| *Kingella kingae* | |
| *Kingella oralis* | |
| *Kingella potus* | |

## GENERAL CHARACTERISTICS

The organisms discussed in this chapter are dysgonic—that is, they grow slowly (48 hours at 35° to 37° C) or poorly. Although they all ferment glucose, their fastidious nature requires that serum be added to the basal fermentation medium to enhance growth and detect fermentation byproducts. These bacteria are capnophiles—that is, they require additional carbon dioxide (5% to 10% $CO_2$) for growth, and most species will not grow on MacConkey agar. *Actinobacillus actinomycetemcomitans* has been reclassified to be included in the *Aggregatibacter* genus based on 16sRRNA sequencing. *Haemophilus aphrophilus* and *Haemophilus paraphrophilus* have been reclassified as a single species based on multilocus sequence analysis. *Aggregatibacter aphrophilus* now includes both the hemin-dependent and hemin-independent isolates. *Haemophilus segnis* has been reclassified as *Aggregatibacter segnis*. *A. segnis* requires V-factor, but does not require X-factor.

## EPIDEMIOLOGY, PATHOGENESIS, AND SPECTRUM OF DISEASE, AND ANTIMICROBIAL THERAPY

The organisms listed in Table 31-1 are part of the normal flora of the nasopharynx or oral cavity of humans and other animals and are parasitic. Species associated with animals are specifically indicated in the table at the beginning of the chapter. As such, they generally are of low virulence and, except for those species associated with periodontal infections, usually only cause infections in humans after introduction into sterile sites following trauma such as bites, droplet transmission from human to human, sharing paraphernalia, or manipulations in the oral cavity. *Cardiobacterium* spp. are not only associated with the human oropharynx and oral cavity, but they may also be identified in the gastrointestinal and urogenital tract. The natural habitat for *Dysgonomonas* is unknown. Rare isolates have been identified in the feces of immunocompromised patients.

The types of infections caused by these bacteria vary from periodontitis to endocarditis (Table 31-2). *Actinobacillus* spp. cause granulomatous disease in animals and have been associated with soft tissue infection in humans following animal bites. Additionally, *A. equuli* and *A. suis* have been isolated from the human respiratory tract. Additional species have been isolated from patients that have developed meningitis following trauma or surgery. *Actinobacillus* spp. may harbor a pore-forming protein toxin known as an RTX toxin that is cytotoxic and

**TABLE 31-1** Epidemiology

| Organism | Habitat (Reservoir) | Mode of Transmission |
|---|---|---|
| *Aggregatibacter actinomycetemcomitans* | Normal flora of human oral cavity | Endogenous; enters deeper tissues by minor trauma to mouth, such as during dental procedures |
| *Actinobacillus* spp. | Normal oral flora of animals such as cows, sheep, and pigs; not part of human flora | Rarely associated with human infection; transmitted by bite wounds or contamination of preexisting wounds during exposure to animals |
| *Kingella* spp. | Normal flora of human upper respiratory and genitourinary tracts | Infections probably caused by patient's endogenous strains |
| *Cardiobacterium hominis* and *Cardiobacterium valvarum* | Normal flora of human upper respiratory tract | Infections probably caused by patient's endogenous strains |
| *Capnocytophaga gingivalis, Capnocytophaga ochracea, Capnocytophaga sputigena,* and other species | Subgingival surfaces and other areas of human oral cavity | Infections probably caused by patient's endogenous strains |
| *Capnocytophaga canimorsus* and *Capnocytophaga cynodegmi* | Oral flora of dogs | Dog bite or wound (scratch), long exposure to dogs *Capnocytophaga cynodegmi* |
| *Dysgonomonas capnocytophagoides* and other species | Uncertain; possibly part of human gastrointestinal flora | Uncertain; possibly endogenous |

**TABLE 31-2** Pathogenesis and Spectrum of Diseases

| Organism | Virulence Factors | Spectrum of Diseases and Infections |
|---|---|---|
| *Aggregatibacter* spp. | Unknown; probably of low virulence; an opportunistic pathogen | *A. actinomycetemcomitans* has been associated with destructive periodontitis that may cause bone loss or endocarditis; endocarditis, often following dental manipulations; soft tissue and human bite infections, often mixed with anaerobic bacteria and *Actinomyces* spp.; *A. aphrophilus* is an uncommon cause of endocarditis and is the H member of the HACEK group of bacteria associated with slowly progressive (subacute) bacterial endocarditis |
| *Actinobacillus* spp. | Unknown for human disease; probably of low virulence | Rarely cause infection in humans but may be found in animal bite wounds, such as meningitis or bacteremia; association with other infections, such as meningitis or bacteremia, is extremely rare and involves compromised patients |
| *Kingella* spp. | Unknown; probably of low virulence; opportunistic pathogens | Endocarditis and infections in various other sites, especially in immunocompromised patients; *K. kingae* associated with blood, bone, and joint infections of young children; periodontitis and wound infections |
| *Cardiobacterium hominis* | Unknown; probably of low virulence | Infections in humans are rare; most commonly associated with endocarditis, especially in persons with anatomic heart defects |
| *Capnocytophaga gingivalis, Capnocytophaga ochracea,* and *Capnocytophaga sputigena* | Unknown; produce wide variety of enzymes that may mediate tissue destruction | Most commonly associated with periodontitis and other types of periodontal disease; less commonly associated with bacteremia in immunocompromised patients |
| *Capnocytophaga canimorsus* and *Capnocytophaga cynodegmi* | Unknown | Range from mild, local infection at bite site to bacteremia culminating in shock and disseminated intravascular coagulation; most severe in splenectomized or otherwise debilitated (e.g., alcoholism) patients but can occur in healthy people; miscellaneous other infections such as pneumonia, endocarditis, and meningitis may also occur |
| *Dysgonomonas capnocytophagoides* and other species | Unknown; probably of low virulence | Role in disease is uncertain; may be associated with diarrheal disease in immunocompromised patients; rarely isolated from other clinical specimens, such as urine, blood, and wounds |

**TABLE 31-3** Antimicrobial Therapy and Susceptibility Testing

| Organism | Therapeutic Options | Potential Resistance to Therapeutic Options | Validated Testing Methods* |
|---|---|---|---|
| *Aggregatibacter actinomycetemcomitans* | No definitive guidelines; for periodontitis, debridement of affected area; potential agents include ceftriaxone, ampicillin, amoxicillin-clavulanic acid, fluoroquinolone, or trimethoprim-sulfamethoxazole; for endocarditis, penicillin, ampicillin, or a cephalosporin (perhaps with an aminoglycoside) may be used | Some strains appear resistant to penicillin and ampicillin, but clinical relevance of resistance is unclear | See CLSI document M45 |
| *Actinobacillus* spp. | No guidelines (susceptible to extended-spectrum cephalosporins and fluoroquinolones) | Unknown (same as Aggregatibacter) | Not available |
| *Kingella denitrificans, Kingella kingae* | A beta-lactam with or without an aminoglycoside; other active agents include erythromycin, trimethoprim/ sulfamethoxazole, and ciprofloxacin | Some strains produce beta-lactamase that mediates resistance to penicillin, ampicillin, ticarcillin, and cefazolin | See CLSI document M45 |
| Cardiobacterium hominis | For endocarditis, penicillin with or without an aminoglycoside; usually susceptible to other β-lactams, chloramphenicol, and tetracycline | Unknown (same as Aggregatibacter) | See CLSI document M45 |
| *Capnocytophaga gingivalis, Capnocytophaga ochracea, Capnocytophaga sputigena* | No definitive guidelines; generally susceptible to clindamycin, erythromycin, tetracyclines, chloramphenicol, imipenem, and other beta-lactams | β-lactamase–mediated resistance to penicillin | Not available |
| *Capnocytophaga canimorsus, Capnocytophaga cynodegmi* | Penicillin is drug of choice; also susceptible to penicillin derivatives, imipenem, and third-generation cephalosporins | Unknown | Not available |
| *Dysgonomonas capnocytophagoides* | No guidelines; potentially effective agents include chloramphenicol, trimethoprim/ sulfamethoxazole, tetracycline, and clindamycin | Often resistance to β-lactams and ciprofloxacin | Not available |

*Validated testing methods include those standard methods recommended by the Clinical and Laboratory Standards Institute (CLSI) and those commercial methods approved by the Food and Drug Administration (FDA).

hemolytic. *A. actinomycetemcomitans* is often associated with periodontitis. Virulence factors include the RTX leukotoxin, cytotoxic distending toxin, and the EmaA adhesin. Three of these organisms, *Aggregatibacter actinomycetemcomitans*, *Cardiobacterium hominis*, and *Kingella* spp., are the A, C, and K, respectively, of the HACEK group of organisms that cause slowly progressive (i.e., subacute) bacterial endocarditis, soft tissue infections, and other infections. *Capnocytophaga* are associated with septicemia and endogenous infections in immunocompromised patients. Infections with *C. canimorsus* and *C. cynodegmi* following a dog or cat bat can result in serious illness including disseminated intravascular coagulation, renal failure, shock, and hemolytic-uremic syndrome. *Kingella* spp. can also be involved in other serious infections involving children, especially osteoarthritic infections. The pathogenic mechanisms are unknown, and disease associated with *Dysgonomonas* spp. is quite variable and includes diarrhea, bacteremia, blood, and wound infections.

Infections are frequently treated using β-lactam antibiotics, occasionally in combination with an aminoglycoside (Table 31-3). β-lactamase production has been described in *Kingella* spp., but the impact of this resistance mechanism on the clinical efficacy of beta-lactams is uncertain. When in vitro susceptibility testing is required, Clinical and Laboratory Standards Institute (CLSI) document M45 does provide guidelines for testing *A. actinomycetemcomitans*, *Cardiobacterium* spp., and *Kingella* spp.

# LABORATORY DIAGNOSIS

## SPECIMEN COLLECTION AND TRANSPORT

No special considerations are required for specimen collection and transport of the organisms discussed in this chapter. Refer to Table 5-1 for general information on specimen collection and transport.

## SPECIMEN PROCESSING

No special considerations are required for processing of the organisms discussed in this chapter. Refer to Table 5-1 for general information on specimen processing.

# DIRECT DETECTION METHODS

Other than Gram stain of patient specimens, there are no specific procedures for the direct detection of these organisms in clinical material. *Actinobacillus* spp. are short to very short gram-negative bacilli. They occur singly, in pairs, and in chains, and they tend to exhibit bipolar staining. This staining morphology gives the overall appearance of the dots and dashes of Morse code. *Aggregatibacter aphrophilus* are very short bacilli but occasionally are seen as filamentous forms. *Aggregatibacter segnis* are pleomorphic rods.

*Kingella* spp. stain as short, plump coccobacilli with squared-off ends that may form chains. *Cardiobacterium hominis* is a pleomorphic gram-negative rod with one rounded end and one tapered end, giving the cells a teardrop appearance. *C. hominis* tends to form clusters, or rosettes, when Gram stains are prepared from 5% sheep blood agar.

*Capnocytophaga* spp. are gram-negative, fusiform-shaped bacilli with one rounded end and one tapered end and occasional filamentous forms; *C. cynodegmi* and *C. canimorsus* may be curved. *Dysgonomonas capnocytophagoides* stains as short gram-negative rods or coccobacilli.

Amplification methods (PCR) have been developed for the identification of some of the organisms discussed in this chapter. However, these tests are not routinely available in the clinical laboratory and are predominantly used in reference or research laboratories.

# CULTIVATION

## Media of Choice

All genera described in this chapter grow on 5% sheep blood and chocolate agars. *Dysgonomonas capnocytophagoides* can be recovered from stool on CVA (cefoperazone-vancomycin-amphotericin B) agar. For recovery of *D. capnocytophagoides*, this medium, a *Campylobacter* selective agar, is incubated at 35° C instead of 42° C.

These genera grow in the broths of commercial blood culture systems and in common nutrient broths such as thioglycollate and brain-heart infusion. Growth of Aggregatibacter in broth media is often barely visible, with no turbidity produced. Microcolonies may be seen as tiny puffballs growing on the blood cell layer in blood culture bottles or as a film or tiny granules on the sides of a tube.

## Incubation Conditions and Duration

The growth of all genera discussed in this chapter occurs best at 35° C and in the presence of increased $CO_2$. Therefore, 5% sheep blood and chocolate agars should be incubated in a $CO_2$ incubator or candle jar. In addition, *Actinobacillus, Aggregatibacter,* and *Cardiobacterium* grow best in conditions of elevated moisture; a candle jar with a sterile gauze pad moistened with sterile water is ideal for this purpose. *Capnocytophaga* requires $CO_2$ and enriched media. The organism is inhibited by sodium polyanethole sulfonate (SPS). Selective media containing bacitracin, polymyxin B, vancomycin, and trimethoprim, or Thayer-Martin and Martin Lewis agars have been used to isolate species of *Capnocytophaga*. Selective media containing cefoperazone, vancomycin, and amphotericin B has been used to isolate *Dysgonomonas* spp. from stool specimens.

Even when optimum growth conditions are met, the organisms discussed here are all slow growing; therefore, inoculated plates should be held 2 to 7 days for colonies to achieve maximal growth.

## Colonial Appearance

Table 31-4 describes the colonial appearance and other distinguishing characteristics (e.g., hemolysis and pigment) of each genus on 5% sheep blood agar. Most species will not grow on MacConkey agar; exceptions are noted in Table 31-4.

# APPROACH TO IDENTIFICATION

Table 31-5 outlines some conventional biochemical tests that are useful for differentiating among *Actinobacillus, Aggregatibacter, Cardiobacterium,* and *Kingella*; these are four of the five HACEK bacteria that cause subacute bacterial endocarditis. *A. aphrophilus* does not require either X or V factors for growth. However, it is catalase negative and ferments lactose or sucrose. *A. actinomycetemcomitans* yields the opposite reactions in these tests.

Table 31-6 shows key conventional biochemicals that can be used to differentiate *Capnocytophaga* spp., *Dysgonomonas capnocytophagoides,* and aerotolerant *Leptotrichia buccalis*.

## Comments Regarding Specific Organisms

*Actinobacillus* spp. are facultative anaerobic, nonmotile, gram-negative rods. The genus *Actinobacillus* is similar to *Aggregatibacter* and *Pasteurella* (see Chapter 30), which must also be considered when a fastidious gram-negative rod requiring rabbit serum is isolated. *A. actinomycetemcomitans,* the most frequently isolated of the aggregatibacters, can be distinguished from *A. aphrophilus* by its positive test for catalase and negative test for lactose fermentation.

*A. actinomycetemcomitans* differs from *C. hominis* in being indole-negative and catalase positive; catalase is also an important test for differentiating *Kingella* spp., which are catalase negative, from *A. actinomycetemcomitans. C. hominis* is indole positive following extraction with xylene and addition of Ehrlich's reagent; this is a key feature in differentiating it from *A. aphrophilus, A. actinomycetemcomitans,* and CDC group EF-4a. *C. hominis* is similar to *Suttonella indologenes* but can be distinguished by its ability to ferment mannitol and sorbitol.

*Kingella* spp. are catalase negative, which helps to separate them from *Neisseria* spp. (see Chapter 40), with which they are sometimes confused. *K. denitrificans* may be mistaken for *Neisseria gonorrhoeae* when isolated from modified Thayer-Martin agar. Nitrate reduction is a key test in differentiating *K. denitrificans* from *N. gonorrhoeae,* which is nitrate negative.

The species in the former CDC group DF-1—that is, *C. ochracea, C. sputigena,* and *C. gingivalis*—are catalase and oxidase negative; however, members of CDC group DF-1 cannot be separated by conventional biochemical tests. *C. canimorsus* and *C. cynodegmi* are catalase and oxidase positive; these species are also difficult to

**TABLE 31-4** Colonial Appearance and Characteristics on 5% Sheep Blood Agar

| Organism | Appearance |
|---|---|
| *Aggregatibacter actinomycetemcomitans* | Pinpoint colonies after 24 hours; rough, sticky, adherent colonies surrounded by a slight greenish tinge after 48 hours; characteristic finding is presence of a four- to six-pointed star-like configuration in the center of a mature colony growing on a clear medium (e.g., brain-heart infusion agar) resembling crossed cigars, which can be visualized by examining the colony under low power (100×) of a standard light microscope |
| *Aggregatibacter aphrophilus* | Round; convex with opaque zone near center on chocolate agar |
| *Aggregatibacter segnis* | Convex, grayish white, smooth or granular at 48 hours on chocolate agar |
| *Actinobacillus equuli** | Small colonies at 24 hours that are sticky, adherent, smooth or rough, and nonhemolytic |
| *A. lignieresii** | Resembles *A. equuli* |
| *A. suis** | Beta-hemolytic but otherwise resembles *A. equuli* and *A. lignieresii* |
| *A. ureae* | Resembles the pasteurellae (see Chapter 32) |
| *Cardiobacterium hominis* | After 48 hours, colonies are small, slightly alpha-hemolytic, smooth, round, glistening and opaque; pitting may be produced |
| *Capnocytophaga* spp. | After 48 to 74 hours, colonies are small- to medium-size, opaque, shiny; nonhemolytic; pale beige or yellowish color may not be apparent unless growth is scraped from the surface with a cotton swab; gliding motility may be observed as outgrowths from the colonies or as a haze on the surface of the agar, similar to swarming of Proteus |
| *Dysgonomonas capnocytophagoides* | Pinpoint colonies after 24 hours; small, wet, gray-white colonies at 48 to 72 hours; usually nonhemolytic, although some strains may produce a small zone of beta-hemolysis; characteristic odor alternately described as fruity strawberry-like odor or bitter |
| *Kingella denitrificans* | Small, nonhemolytic; frequently pits agar; can grow on *Neisseria gonorrhoeae* selective agar (e.g., Thayer-Martin agar) |
| *K. kingae* | Small, with a small zone of beta-hemolysis; may pit agar |

*May grow on MacConkey agar as tiny lactose fermenters.

**TABLE 31-5** Biochemical and Physiologic Characteristics of *Actinobacillus* spp. and Related Organisms

| Organism | Oxidase | Catalase | Nitrate Reduction | Indole | Urea | Esculin Hydrolysis | FERMENTATION OF:[†] Xylose | Lactose | Trehalose |
|---|---|---|---|---|---|---|---|---|---|
| *Aggregatibacter actinomycetemcomitans* | −** | + | + | − | − | − | v | − | − |
| *Aggregatibacter aphrophilus* | − | − | + | − | − | − | − | (+) | (+) |
| *Actinobacillus equuli* | + | v | + | − | (+)* | − | + | + | (+) |
| *Actinobacillus lignieresii* | + | v | + | − | (+)* | − | + or (+) | v | − |
| *Actinobacillus suis* | + | v | + | − | (+)* | + | + | + or (+) | + |
| *Actinobacillus ureae* | + | v | + | − | (+)* | − | − | − | − |
| *Cardiobacterium hominis* | + | − | − | + | − | − | − | − | ND |
| *Kingella denitrificans* | + | − | (+)[‡] | − | − | − | − | − | ND |
| *K. kingae* | + | − | − | − | − | − | − | − | ND |

Data compiled from Weyant RS, Moss CW, Weaver RE, et al, editors: *Identification of unusual pathogenic gram-negative aerobic and facultatively anaerobic bacteria,* ed 2, Baltimore, 1996, Williams & Wilkins.
*ND,* No data; *v,* variable; +, >90% of strains positive; (+), >90% of strains positive but reaction may be delayed (i.e., 2 to 7 days); −, >90% of strains negative.
*May require a drop of rabbit serum on the slant or a heavy inoculum.
[†]May require the addition of 1 to 2 drops rabbit serum per 3 mL of fermentation broth to stimulate growth.
[‡]Nitrate is usually reduced to gas.
**Occassional strain is oxidase positive.

**TABLE 31-6** Biochemical and Physiologic Characteristics of *Capnocytophaga* spp., Dysgonomonas spp., and Similar Organisms

| Organism | Oxidase | Catalase | Esculin Hydrolysis | Indole | Nitrate Reduction | Xylose Fermentation |
|---|---|---|---|---|---|---|
| *Capnocytophaga* spp. (CDC group DF-1)* | – | – | (v) | – | v | – |
| *C. canimorsus* (CDC group DF-2)† | (+) | (+) | v | – | – | –‡ |
| *C. cynodegmi* (CDC group DF-2-like)† | (+) | (+) | + or (+) | – | – | – |
| *Leptotrichia buccalis** | – | – | v | – | – | –‡ |
| *Dysgonomonas capnocytophagoides** | – | – | (+) | (v) | – | + or (+)‡ |
| CDC group DF-3-like | – | v | v | (+) | – | –‡ |

Data compiled from Jensen KT, Schonheyder H, Thomsen VF: In-vitro activity of β-lactam and other antimicrobial agents against *Kingella kingae,* J Antimicrob Chemother 33:635, 1994; and Weyant RS, Moss CW, Weaver RE, et al, editors: *Identification of unusual pathogenic gram-negative aerobic and facultatively anaerobic bacteria,* ed 2, Baltimore, 1996, Williams & Wilkins.
*Lactic acid is the major fermentation end product of glucose fermentation for *Leptotrichia buccalis,* and succinic acid and propionic is the major fermentation end product of glucose fermentation for *Capnocytophaga* spp. (CDC group DF-1) and *Dysgonomonas capnocytophagoides.*
†*C. canimorsus* does not ferment the sugars inulin, sucrose, or raffinose; *C. cynodegmi* will usually ferment one or all of these sugars.
‡May require the addition of 1 to 2 drops of rabbit serum per 3 mL of fermentation broth to stimulate growth.
+, >90% of strains positive; (+), >90% of strains positive, but reaction may be delayed (i.e., 2 to 7 days); –, >90% of strains negative; v, variable; (v), positive reactions may be delayed.

differentiate from each other. However, for most clinical purposes, a presumptive identification to genus—that is, *Capnocytophaga*—is sufficiently informative and precludes the need to identify an isolate to the species level. Presumptive identification of an organism as *Capnocytophaga* spp. can be made when a yellow-pigmented, thin, gram-negative rod with tapered ends that exhibits gliding motility (see Table 31-4) and does not grow in ambient air is isolated.

*Dysgonomonas capnocytophagoides,* although similar to the other organisms in this chapter, are oxidase negative. They are nonmotile, unlike the *Capnocytophaga,* which exhibit gliding motility. Gas-liquid chromatography is useful in separating *D. capnocytophagoides* and *Capnocytophaga* spp., but this technology is not commonly available in most clinical laboratories. *D. capnocytophagoides* produces succinic and propionic acid, whereas *Capnocytophaga* produces only succinic acid. Cellular fatty acid analysis can provide information necessary to distinguish *Capnocytophaga, D. capnocytophagoides,* and the aerotolerant strains of *Leptotrichia buccalis.*

## SERODIAGNOSIS

Serodiagnostic techniques are not generally used for the laboratory diagnosis of infections caused by the organisms discussed in this chapter.

## PREVENTION

Because the organisms discussed in this chapter do not generally pose a threat to human health, there are no recommended vaccination or prophylaxis protocols.

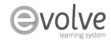 *Visit the Evolve site to complete the review questions.*

---

## CASE STUDY 31-1

A 71-year-old woman with acute myeloid leukemia was being treated with immunosuppressive therapy and was neutropenic with 100 white blood cells per microliter. She had a low-grade fever and was not responding to treatment with a third-generation cephalosporin. Severe periodontal disease was noted. Her blood cultures became positive after 48 hours with a gram-negative fusiform rod that did not grow on MacConkey and was neither oxidase nor catalase positive. On blood agar, the organism was nonhemolytic but spread out from the initial colony, producing a haze on the agar. The laboratory reported that the organism was resistant to beta-lactam drugs. The

patient's therapy was changed to ciprofloxacin, and she became afebrile within 24 hours.

### QUESTIONS

1. What is the likely organism isolated from the blood culture, and what is the likely source of the organism?
2. Which tests will confirm the identification?
3. The patient was not responding to cephalosporin antimicrobial agents. What rapid testing can the laboratory perform to aid in the appropriate treatment of this organism?

# BIBLIOGRAPHY

Clinical and Laboratory Standards Institute: *Methods for antimicrobial dilution and disk susceptibility testing of infrequently isolated or fastidious bacteria; M45*, Villanova, PA, 2007, CLSI.

Gordillo EM, Rendel M, Sood R, et al: Septicemia due to β-lactamase–Kingella kingae, *Clin Infect Dis* 17:818, 1993.

Hassan IJ, Hayek L: Endocarditis caused by *Kingella denitrificans, J Infect* 27:291, 1993.

Hofstad T, Olsen I, Eribe ER: *Dysgonomonas* gen nov to accommodate *Dysgonomonas gadei* sp nov, an organism isolated from human gall bladder, and *Dysgonomonas capnocytophagoides* (formerly CDC group DF-3), *Int J Syst Evol Microbiol* 50:2189, 2000.

Jensen KT, Schonheyder H, Thomsen VF: In-vitro activity of β-lactam and other antimicrobial agents against Kingella kingae, *J Antimicrob Chemother* 33:635, 1994.

Norskov-Lauritsen N, Kilian M: Reclassification of *Actinobacillus actinomycetemcomitans, Haemophilus aphrophilus, Haemophilus paraphrophilus* and *Haemophilus segnis* as Aggregatibacter actinomycetemcomitans gen. nov., comb. nov., *Aggregatibacter aphrophilus* comb. nov. and *Aggregatibacter segnis* comb. nov., and emended description of *Aggregatibacter aphrophilus* to include V factor-dependent and V factor-independent isolates. *Int J Syst Evol Microbiol* 56:2135-2146, 2006.

Pers C, Gahrn-Hansen B, Frederiksen W: Capnocytophaga canimorsus septicemia in Denmark, 1982-1995: review of 39 cases, *Clin Infect Dis* 23:71, 1996.

Versalovic J: *Manual of clinical microbiology*, ed 10, 2011, Washington, DC, ASM Press.

Weyant RS, Moss CW, Weaver RE, et al, editors: *Identification of unusual pathogenic gram-negative aerobic and facultatively anaerobic bacteria*, ed 2, Baltimore, 1996, Williams & Wilkins.

Yagupsky P, Dagan R: Kingella kingae bacteremia in children, *Pediatr Infect Dis J* 13:1148, 1994.

# Gram-Negative Bacilli and Coccobacilli (MacConkey-Negative, Oxidase-Variable)

# Haemophilus

## OBJECTIVES

1. List the general characteristics within the genus *Haemophilus*, including general habitat, atmosphere, and temperature requirements.
2. Describe the infections caused by *Haemophilus influenzae* and *Haemophilus ducreyi*.
3. Describe the difference in the typeable and nontypeable categories of *Haemophilus*, their virulence factors, and the disease they cause.
4. Describe the Gram stain and colonial morphology of the various *Haemophilus* species.
5. Describe the isolation requirements necessary for optimal recovery of *Haemophilus*, including any special specimen processing or transport requirements.
6. Explain the satellite phenomenon and the chemical basis for the phenomenon.
7. List the X and V factor requirements for *H. influenzae, H. parainfluenzae,* and *H. ducreyi.*
8. Explain the principle of the porphyrin test.
9. Explain why routine susceptibility testing of clinical isolates for *H. influenzae* is only necessary on strains of clinical significance (i.e., sterile sites).
10. Correlate patient signs, symptoms, and laboratory data to identify the most probable etiologic agent associated with an infection.

### ORGANISMS TO BE CONSIDERED

| Current Name | Previous Name |
|---|---|
| *Haemophilus influenzae* | |
| *Haemophilus aegyptius* | *Haemophilus* biogroup aegyptius |
| *Haemophilus ducreyi* | |
| *H. parainfluenzae* | |
| *H. parahaemolyticus* | |
| *H. paraphrohaemolyticus* | |
| *H. pittmaniae* | |
| *H. haemolyticus* | |

## GENERAL CHARACTERISTICS

The genus *Haemophilus* contains significant genetic diversity. Members of the genus are small, nontile, pleomorphic gram-negative bacilli. The cells are typically coccobacilli or short rods. Species of the genus *Haemophilus* require protoporphyrin IX (a metabolic intermediate of the hemin biosynthetic pathway) referred to as X factor

and the V factor, nicotine adenine dinucleotide (NAD) or NADP for in vitro growth. *Haemophilus* are facultative anaerobes enhanced in a 5% to 7% $CO_2$-enriched atmosphere. The morphologic and physiologic features of individual species are presented in the discussion of laboratory diagnosis. *Aggregatibacter aphrophilus* and *Aggregatibacter paraphrophilus* have been reclassified as a single species based on their multilocus sequence analysis (*A. aphrophilus*).

## EPIDEMIOLOGY

As presented in Table 32-1, except for *Haemophilus ducreyi, Haemophilus* spp. normally inhabit the upper respiratory tract of humans. Asymptomatic colonization with *H. influenzae* type b is rare. Although *H. ducreyi* is only found in humans, the organism is not part of our normal flora, and its presence in clinical specimens indicates infection.

Among *H. influenzae* strains, there are two broad categories: typeable and nontypeable (NTHi). Strains are typed based on capsular characteristics. The capsule is composed of a sugar-alcohol phosphate (i.e., polyribitol phosphate) complex. Differences in this complex are the basis for separating encapsulated strains into one of six groups: type a, b, c, d, e, or f. *H. influenzae* type b (Hib) is most commonly encountered in serious infections in humans. Nontypeable strains do not produce a capsule and are most commonly encountered as normal inhabitants of the upper respiratory tract.

Although person-to-person transmission plays a key role in infections caused by *Haemophilus influenzae* and *H. ducreyi,* infections caused by other *Haemophilus* strains and species likely arise endogenously as a person's own flora gains access to a normally sterile site. The colonizing organism invades the mucosa and enters the patient's bloodstream. Encapsulated strains are protected from clearance from host phagocytes. Once in the circulation, the organism is able to spread to additional sites and tissues including the lungs, pericardium, pleura, and meninges.

## PATHOGENESIS AND SPECTRUM OF DISEASE

Production of a capsule and factors that mediate bacterial attachment to human epithelial cells are the primary virulence factors associated with *Haemophilus* spp. In general, infections caused by *Haemophilus influenzae* are often systemic and life threatening, whereas infections caused by nontypeable (do not have a capsule) strains are usually localized (Table 32-2). The majority of serious infections caused by *H. influenzae* type b are typically biotypes I and II. The development and use of the conjugate vaccine in children since 1993 has reduced the infection rate by 95% in children younger than 5 years old in the United States.

The majority of *H. influenzae* infections are now caused by nontypeable strains (NTHi). Transmission is often via respiratory secretions. The organism is able to gain access to sterile sites from colonization in the upper respiratory tract. Clinical infections include otitis media (ear infection), sinusitis, bronchitis, pneumonia, and conjunctivitis. Immunodeficiencies and chronic respiratory problems such as chronic obstructive pulmonary disease may predispose an individual to infection with NTHi.

Chancroid is the sexually transmitted disease caused by *H. ducreyi* (see Table 32-2). The initial symptom is the development of a painful genital ulcer and inguinal lymphadenopathy. Although small outbreaks of this disease have occurred in the United States, this disease is more common among socioeconomically disadvantaged populations inhabiting tropical environments. Epidemics of disease are associated with poor hygiene, prostitution, drug abuse, and poor socioeconomic conditions.

# LABORATORY DIAGNOSIS

## SPECIMEN COLLECTION AND TRANSPORT

*Haemophilus* spp. can be isolated from most clinical specimens. The collection and transport of these specimens are outlined in Table 5-1, with emphasis on the following points. First, *Haemophilus* spp. are susceptible to drying

**TABLE 32-1** Epidemiology

| Organism | Habitat (Reservoir) | Mode of Transmission |
|---|---|---|
| *Haemophilus influenzae* | Normal flora: upper respiratory tract | Person-to-person: respiratory droplets Endogenous strains |
| *Haemophilus ducreyi* | Not part of normal human flora; only found in humans during infection | Person-to-person: sexual contact |
| Other *Haemophilus* spp. *H. parainfluenzae* *H. parahaemolyticus* | Normal flora: upper respiratory tract | Endogenous strains |

**TABLE 32-2** Pathogenesis and Spectrum of Diseases

| Organism | Virulence Factors | Spectrum of Disease and Infections |
|---|---|---|
| *Haemophilus influenzae* | Capsule: Antiphagocytic, type b most common Additional cell envelope factors Mediate attachment to host cells Unencapsulated strains: pili and other cell surface factors mediate attachment | Encapsulated strains: Meningitis Epiglottitis Cellulitis with bacteremia Septic arthritis Pneumonia Nonencapsulated strains: Localized infections Otitis media Sinusitis Conjunctivitis Immunocompromised patients: Chronic bronchitis Pneumonia Bacteremia |
| *Haemophilus influenzae* | Uncertain; probably similar to those of other *H. influenzae* | Purulent conjunctivitis single strain identified as the Brazilian purpuric fever, high mortality in children between ages 1 and 4; infection includes purulent meningitis, bacteremia, high fever, vomiting, purpura (i.e., rash), and vascular collapse |
| *Haemophilus ducreyi* | Uncertain, but capsular factors, pili, and certain toxins are probably involved in attachment and penetration of host epithelial cells | Chancroid; genital lesions progress from tender papules (i.e., small bumps) to painful ulcers with several satellite lesions; regional lymphadenitis is common |
| Other *Haemophilus* spp. and *Aggregatibacter* spp. | Uncertain; probably of low virulence. Opportunistic pathogens | Associated with wide variety of infections similar to *H. influenzae*; *A. aphrophilus* is an uncommon cause of endocarditis and is the H member of the HACEK group of bacteria associated with slowly progressive (subacute) bacterial endocarditis |

and temperature extremes. Therefore, specimens suspected of containing these organisms should be inoculated to the appropriate media immediately. Specimens susceptible to contamination with normal flora such as a lower respiratory specimen should be collected by bronchioalveolar lavage. In cases of pneumonia or cerebrospinal fluid (CSF) infection or suspected infection of any other normally sterile body fluid, blood cultures should also be collected.

Second, the recovery of *H. ducreyi* from genital ulcers requires special processing. The ulcer should be cleaned with sterile gauze moistened with sterile saline. A cotton swab moistened with phosphate-buffered saline is then used to collect material from the base of the ulcer. To maximize the chance for recovering the organism, the swab must be plated to special selective media within 10 minutes of collection.

## SPECIMEN PROCESSING

Other than the precautions required for the collection of *H. ducreyi*, no special considerations are required for specimen processing of *Haemophilus* spp. Refer to Table 5-1 for general information on specimen processing.

## DIRECT DETECTION METHODS

### Direct Observation

Gram stain is generally used for the direct detection of *Haemophilus* in clinical material (Figure 32-1). However, in some instances the acridine orange stain (AO; see Chapter 6 for more information on this technique) is used to detect smaller numbers of organisms that may be undetectable by gram staining.

To increase the sensitivity of direct Gram stain examination of body fluid specimens, especially CSF, specimens may be centrifuged (2000 rpm for 10 minutes) and the smear is prepared from the pellet deposited in the bottom of the tube. Most laboratories are now equipped with a cytocentrifuge (10,000 × g for 10 minutes) used for concentration of specimens. This is highly recommended over traditional centrifugation for non-turbid specimens. This concentration step can increase the sensitivity of direct microscopic examination from five to tenfold. Moreover, cytocentrifugation of the specimen, in which clinical material is concentrated by centrifugation directly onto microscope slides, reportedly increases sensitivity of the Gram stain by as much as 100-fold (see Chapter 71 for information on infections of the central nervous system).

Gram stains of the smears from clinical specimens must be examined carefully. *Haemophilus* spp. stain a pale pink and may be difficult to detect in the pink background of proteinaceous material often found in clinical specimens. Underdecolorization may result in misidentification of *H. influenzae* as either *Streptococcus* spp. or *Listeria monocytogenes*.

*H. influenzae* appears as pleomorphic coccobacilli or small rods, whereas the cells usually appear as long, slender rods. *H. haemolyticus* are small coccobacilli or short rods with occasional cells appearing as tangled filaments.

*H. parainfluenzae* produce either small pleomorphic rods or long filamentous forms, whereas *H. parahaemolyticus* usually are short to medium-length bacilli. *Aggregatibacter aphrophilus* is a very short bacillum but occasionally are seen as filamentous forms. *H. ducreyi* may be either slender or coccobacillary. Traditionally, *H. ducreyi* cells are described as appearing as "schools of fish." However, this morphology is rarely seen in clinical specimens.

Table 32-3 presents *Haemophilus influenzae* and *H. parainfluenzae* biotypes.

**TABLE 32-3** Differentiation of *Haemophilus influenzae* and *H. parainfluenzae* Biotypes

| Organism and Biotype | Indole | Ornithine Decarboxylase | Urease |
|---|---|---|---|
| ***H. influenzae*** | | | |
| I | pos | pos | pos |
| II | pos | pos | neg |
| III | neg | pos | neg |
| IV | neg | pos | pos |
| V | pos | neg | pos |
| VI | neg | pos | neg |
| VII | pos | neg | neg |
| VIII | neg | neg | neg |
| ***H. parainfluenzae*** | | | |
| I | neg | neg | pos |
| II | neg | pos | pos |
| III | neg | pos | neg |
| IV | pos | pos | pos |
| V | neg | neg | neg |
| VI | pos | neg | pos |
| VII | pos | pos | neg |
| VIII | pos | neg | neg |

Modified from Versalovic J: *Manual of clinical microbiology,* ed 10, Washington, DC, 2011, ASM Press.

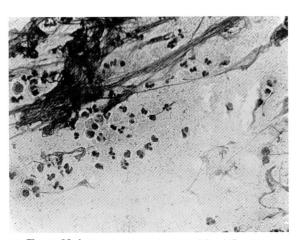

**Figure 32-1** Gram stain of *Haemophilus influenzae.*

### Antigen Detection

*Haemophilus influenzae* type b capsular polysaccharide in clinical specimens, such as CSF and urine, can be detected directly using commercially available particle agglutination assays (see Chapter 9). Organisms in clinical infections are usually present at a sufficiently high concentration to be visualized by Gram stain. Therefore, most clinical laboratories no longer perform the latex test for the identification of *Haemophilus* spp. Latex tests are sensitive and specific for detection of *H. influenzae* type b, especially in patients treated with antimicrobial therapy prior to specimen collection. However, false positives have been reported in CSF and urine of patients who have recently immunized with the Hib vaccine.

### Molecular Testing

Rapid screening procedures are very useful for patient therapy and evaluating outbreaks and have been developed for detection from CSF, plasma, serum, and whole blood. A PCR method for *Haemophilus influenzae* capsular types a and f has been developed. PCR product was amplified for the specific capsular type for which the primer was designed. PCR has its advantages over serotyping in that problems of cross-reaction and autoagglutination are gone. Detection from some clinical samples has been problematic based on the presence of small numbers of organisms in the sample increasing the need for large samples and concentration procedures.

Diagnosis of chancroid and the identification of *H. ducreyi* have been successfully completed using a variety of molecular targets. Amplification of the 16SrRNA, the *rrs* (16S)-*rri* (23S) spacer region, or the heat shock protein gene *groEL* has been used in molecular assays. Molecular methods have demonstrated improved sensitivity over traditional methods.

In addition to molecular methods for the identification, pulsed-field gel electrophoresis is considered the gold standard for typing *Haemophilus* isolates. Additional amplification methods such as repetitive-element sequence-based PCR, ribotyping, restriction fragment length polymorphism (RFLP), multilocus enzyme electrophoresis, and rapidly amplified polymorphic DNA (RAPD) have also been used.

## CULTIVATION

### Media of Choice

*Haemophilus* spp. typically grows on chocolate agar as smooth, flat or convex buff, or slightly yellow colonies. Chocolate agar provides hemin (X factor) and NAD (V factor), necessary for the growth of *Haemophilus* spp. Most strains will not grow on 5% sheep blood agar, which contains protoporphyrin IX but not NAD. Several bacterial species, including *Staphylococcus aureus*, produce NAD as a metabolic byproduct. Therefore, tiny colonies of *Haemophilus* spp. may be seen growing on sheep blood agar very close to colonies of bacteria capable of producing V factor; this is known as the satellite phenomenon (Figure 32-2). The satellite phenomenon has become important in this era of needing to rapidly identify potential agents of a bioterrorist attack. To examine an isolate for the satellite phenomenon, place a single streak of a hemolysin-producing strain of *Staphylococcus* spp. on a

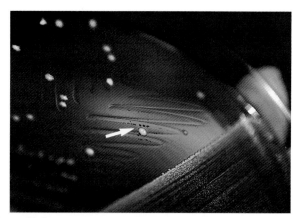

**Figure 32-2** *Haemophilus influenzae* satellite phenomenon *(arrow)* around colonies of *Staphylococcus aureus.*

sheep blood agar plate that has been inoculated with a suspected *Haemophilus* spp. The Staphylococcus lyses the red blood cells adjacent to the streak line, releasing hemin (x factor) and NAD (v factor), providing the necessary components for growth of *Haemophilus* spp. *Haemophilus* spp. will grow adjacent to the streak line where the nutrients are available.

A selective medium, such as horse blood–bacitracin agar, may be used for isolation of *H. influenzae* from respiratory secretions of patients with cystic fibrosis. This medium is designed to prevent overgrowth of *H. influenzae* by mucoid *Pseudomonas aeruginosa*. *Haemophilus* spp. are unable to grow on MacConkey agar.

*H. ducreyi* requires additional growth factors and special media for cultivation in the laboratory. Two types of media utilized within the laboratory include (1) Mueller-Hinton–based chocolate agar supplemented with 1% IsoVitaleX and 3 μg/mL vancomycin and (2) heart infusion–based agar supplemented with 10% fetal bovine serum and 3 μg/mL vancomycin. The vancomycin inhibits gram-positive colonizing organisms of the genital tract.

*Haemophilus* spp. will grow in commercial blood culture broth systems and in common nutrient broths such as thioglycollate and brain-heart infusion. However, the growth is often slower, produces weakly turbid suspensions, and may not be readily visible in broth cultures. For this reason, blind subcultures to chocolate agar or examination of smears by AO or Gram stain have been used to enhance detection. Subcultures have not demonstrated a clinically significant effect on the isolation and detection of *Haemophilus* spp. from blood culture systems.

Rabbit or horse blood agars are commonly used for detecting hemolysis by hemolysin-producing strains of *Haemophilus* strains unable to grow on 5% sheep blood.

### Incubation Conditions and Duration

Most strains of *Haemophilus* spp. are able to grow aerobically and anaerobically (facultative anaerobes). Growth is stimulated by 5% to 10% carbon dioxide ($CO_2$). It is recommended that cultures be incubated in a candle extinction jar, $CO_2$ pouch, or $CO_2$ incubator. These organisms usually grow within 24 hours, but cultures are routinely held 72 hours before being discarded as

**TABLE 32-4** Colonial Appearance and Characteristics

| Organism | Medium | Appearance |
|---|---|---|
| *Aggregatibacter aphrophilus* | CHOC | Round; convex with opaque zone near center |
| *H. ducreyi* | Selective medium | Small, flat, smooth, and translucent to opaque at 48-72 hours; colonies can be pushed intact across agar surface |
| *H. haemolyticus* | CHOC | Resembles *H. influenzae* except beta-hemolytic on rabbit or horse blood agar |
| *H. influenzae* | CHOC | Unencapsulated strains are small, smooth, and translucent at 24 hours; encapsulated strains form larger, more mucoid colonies; mouse nest odor; nonhemolytic on rabbit or horse blood agar |
| *H. influenzae* biotype aegyptius | CHOC | Resembles *H. influenzae* except colonies are smaller at 48 hours |
| *H. parahaemolyticus* | CHOC | Resembles *H. parainfluenzae* beta-hemolytic on rabbit or horse blood agar |
| *H. parainfluenzae* | CHOC | Medium to large, smooth, and translucent; nonhemolytic on rabbit or horse blood agar |
| *Aggregatibacter segnis* | CHOC | Convex, grayish white, smooth or granular at 48 hours |

*CHOC*, Chocolate agar.

negative. An exception is *H. ducreyi*, which may require as long as 7 days to grow.

Optimal growth of all *Haemophilus* spp., except *H. ducreyi*, occurs at 35° to 37° C. Cultures for *H. ducreyi* should be incubated at 33° C. In addition, *H. ducreyi* requires high humidity, which may be established by placing a sterile gauze pad moistened with sterile water inside the candle jar or $CO_2$ pouch.

### Colonial Appearance

Table 32-4 describes the colonial appearance and other distinguishing characteristics (e.g., odor and hemolysis) of each species.

## APPROACH TO IDENTIFICATION

Commercial identification systems for *Haemophilus* spp. are available. All of the systems incorporate several rapid enzymatic tests and generally work well for identifying these organisms.

Traditional identification criteria include hemolysis on horse or rabbit blood and the requirement for X and V factors for growth. To establish X and V factor require-

ments, disks impregnated with each factor are placed on unsupplemented media, usually Mueller-Hinton agar or trypticase soy agar, inoculated with a light suspension of the organism (see Figure 13-42). After overnight incubation at 35° C in ambient air, the plate is examined for growth around each disk. Many X factor–requiring organisms are able to carry over enough factor from the primary medium to give false-negative results (i.e., growth occurs at such a distance from the X disk as to falsely indicate that the organism does not require the X factor).

The porphyrin test is another means for establishing an organism's X-factor requirements and eliminates the potential problem of carryover. This test detects the presence of enzymes that convert δ-aminolevulinic acid (ALA) into porphyrins or protoporphyrins. The porphyrin test may be performed in broth, in agar, or on a disk.

Isolates from CSF or respiratory tract specimens that (1) are gram-negative rods or gram-negative coccobacilli, (2) grow on chocolate agar in $CO_2$ but not blood agar or satellite around other colonies on blood agar, and (3) are porphyrin negative and nonhemolytic on rabbit or horse blood may be identified as *H. influenzae*. *Haemophilus* isolates may also be identified to species using rapid sugar fermentation tests; an abbreviated identification scheme for the X- and V-requiring organisms is shown in Table 32-5.

## SEROTYPING

Although serologic typing of *H. influenzae* may be used to establish an isolate as being any one of the six serotypes (i.e., a, b, c, d, e, and f), it is used primarily to identify type b strains. All *H. influenzae* from cases of invasive infections should be serotyped to determine whether or not *H. influenzae* type b is the cause of the infection. Testing can be performed using a slide agglutination test (see Chapter 9); a saline control without the reagent antibodies should always be tested simultaneously alongside the patient's specimen in order to detect auto agglutination (i.e., the nonspecific agglutination of the test organism without homologous antiserum).

## SERODIAGNOSIS

An enzyme-linked immunosorbent assay (ELISA) has been developed to detect antibodies to *H. ducreyi*. ELISA has been used to show seroconversion following Hib vaccination. None of these assays are commonly used for diagnostic purposes.

## ANTIMICROBIAL SUSCEPTIBILITY TESTING AND THERAPY

Standard methods have been established for performing in vitro susceptibility testing with clinically relevant isolates of *Haemophilus* spp. (see Chapter 12 for details on these methods). In addition, various agents may be considered for testing and therapeutic use (Table 32-6). Although widespread *H. influenzae* is capable of producing beta-lactamase (penicillin resistance), third-generation cephalosporins are not notably affected by the enzyme (i.e., ceftriaxone and cefotaxime) and

**TABLE 32-5** Key Biochemical and Physiologic Characteristics of *Haemophilus* spp.

| Organism | X Factor | V Factor | Beta-Hemolytic on Rabbit Blood Agar | Catalase | Lactose | Glucose | Xylose | Sucrose | Mannose | β-galactosidase |
|---|---|---|---|---|---|---|---|---|---|---|
| *Haemophilus influenzae* | pos | pos | neg | pos | neg | pos | pos | neg | neg | neg |
| *H. aegyptius* | pos | pos | pos | pos | neg | pos* | neg | neg | neg | neg |
| *H. haemolyticus* | pos | pos | pos | pos | neg | pos | V | neg | neg | neg |
| *H. parahaemolyticus* | neg | pos | pos | V | neg | pos | neg | pos | neg | V |
| *H. parainfluenzae* | neg | pos | V | V | neg | pos | neg | pos | pos | V |
| *H. pittmaniae* | neg | pos | pos | pos^w | neg | pos | neg | pos | pos | pos |
| *H. paraphrohaemolyticus* | neg | pos | pos | pos | neg | pos | neg | pos | neg | V |
| *H. ducreyi* | pos | neg | neg* | neg | neg | V | neg | neg | neg | neg |

Data compiled from Versalovic J: *Manual of clinical microbiology,* ed 10, Washington, DC, 2011, ASM Press; and Weyant RS, Moss CW, Weaver RE, et al, editors: *Identification of unusual pathogenic gram-negative aerobic and facultatively anaerobic bacteria,* ed 2, Baltimore, 1996, Williams & Wilkins.
+, >90% of strains positive; –, >90% of strains negative; *w,* indicates a weak reaction; *v,* indicates a variable reaction.
*Delayed reactions in some strains.

**TABLE 32-6** Antimicrobial Therapy and Susceptibility Testing

| Organism | Therapeutic Options | Potential Resistance to Therapeutic Options | Validated Testing Methods* | Comments |
|---|---|---|---|---|
| *Haemophilus influenzae* | Usually ceftriaxone or cefotaxime for life-threatening infections; for localized infections several cephalosporins, β-lactam/β-lactamase inhibitor combinations, macrolides, trimethoprim-sulfamethoxazole, and certain fluoroquinolones are effective | β-Lactamase–mediated resistance to ampicillin is common; β-lactam resistance by altered PBP target is rare (≤1% of strains) | As documented in Chapter 12: disk diffusion, broth dilution, and certain commercial systems | Resistance to third-generation cephalosporins has not been documented; testing to guide therapy is not routinely needed |
| *Haemophilus ducreyi* | Erythromycin is the drug of choice; other potentially active agents include ceftriaxone and ciprofloxacin | Resistance to trimethoprim-sulfamethoxazole and tetracycline has emerged; β-lactamase–mediated resistance to ampicillin and amoxicillin is also known | Not available | |
| Other *Haemophilus* spp. | Guidelines the same as for *H. influenzae* | β-Lactamase–mediated resistance to ampicillin is known | As documented in Chapter 12: disk diffusion, broth dilution, and certain commercial systems. Also see CLSI document M45 | Resistance to third-generation cephalosporins has not been documented; testing to guide therapy is not routinely needed |

*Validated testing methods include standard methods recommended by the Clinical and Laboratory Standards Institute (CLSI) and commercial methods approved by the Food and Drug Administration (FDA).

may be effective therapeutic agents. Therefore, routine susceptibility testing of clinical isolates as a guide to therapy may not be necessary. Care should be taken when preparing inoculum concentrations (0.5 McFarland) for Haemophilus spp.; in particular, beta-lactamase-producing strains of *H. influenzae*, as higher suspensions may lead to false-resistant results.

# PREVENTION

Several multiple-dose protein-polysaccharide conjugate vaccines are licensed in the United States for *H. influenzae* type b. These vaccines have substantially reduced the incidence of severe invasive infections caused by type b organisms, and vaccination of children starting at 2 months of age is strongly recommended.

Antibody to the Hib capsule and activation of the complement pathway within the host play a primary role in clearance and protection from infection. Newborns are protected for a short period following birth due to the presence of maternal antibodies.

Rifampin chemoprophylaxis is recommended for all household contacts of index cases of Hib meningitis in which there is at least one unvaccinated household member younger than 4 years of age. Children and staff of daycare centers should also receive rifampin prophylaxis if at least two cases have occurred among the children.

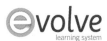 *Visit the Evolve site to complete the review questions.*

---

## CASE STUDY 32-1

A 20-year-old man presented to the emergency department with a history of temperature up to 103° F and mild respiratory distress. He reported that he had the worst sore throat of his life and was having difficulty swallowing. On physical examination, the patient was found to have a "cherry-red" epiglottis. Blood and throat cultures were obtained, and the patient was treated with cefotaxime. An endotracheal tube was placed for 48 hours until the inflammation of the epiglottis subsided. The throat culture grew normal respiratory microbiota, but a gram-negative rod was isolated from the blood culture in 24 hours only on chocolate agar.

### QUESTIONS

1. What is the genus of the organism that was isolated from this patient's blood?
2. The organism grew on blood agar only around a colony of Staphylococcus (see Figure 32-2) but produced porphyrins from delta-aminolevulinic acid and fermented lactose. What is the species of this organism?
3. What is the importance of identification of *Haemophilus* to the species level from specimens isolated from sterile sites?

---

# BIBLIOGRAPHY

Centers for Disease Control and Prevention (CDC): Progress toward eliminating *Haemophilus influenza* type b disease among infants and children—United States, 1987-1997, *MMWR* 47:993, 1998.

Chadwick PR, Malnick H, Ebizie AO: *Haemophilus paraphrophilus* infection: a pitfall in laboratory diagnosis, *J Infect* 30:67, 1995.

Clinical and Laboratory Standards Institute: *Methods for antimicrobial dilution and disk susceptibility testing of infrequently isolated or fastidious bacteria; M45*, Villanova, Pa, 2007, CLSI.

CLSI Supplement: Performance standards for antimicrobial susceptibility testing: 23rd informational supplement, Wayne, Pa., 2013, CLSI, M100-S23.

Coll-Vinent B, Suris X, Lopez-Soto A, et al: *Haemophilus paraphrophilus* endocarditis: case report and review, *Clin Infect Dis* 20:1381, 1995.

Committee on Infectious Diseases: *2006 Red book: report of the Committee on Infectious Diseases*, ed 27, Elk Grove, Ill, 2006, American Academy of Pediatrics.

Darville T, Jacobs RF, Lucas RA, et al: Detection of *Haemophilus influenzae* type b antigen in cerebrospinal fluid after immunization, *Pediatr Infect Dis J* 11:243, 1992.

Falla TJ, Crook DW, Broply LN, et al: PCR for capsular typing of Haemophilus influenza, *J Clin Microbiol* 32:2382, 1994.

Foweraker JE, Cooke NJ, Hawkey PM: Ecology of *Haemophilus influenzae* and *Haemophilus parainfluenzae* in sputum and saliva and effects of antibiotics on their distribution in patients with lower respiratory tract infections, *Antimicrob Agents Chemother* 37: 804, 1993.

Jones RG, Bass JW, Weisse ME, et al: Antigenuria after immunization with *Haemophilus influenzae* oligosaccharide CRM197 conjugate (H6OC) vaccine, *Pediatr Infect Dis J* 10:557, 1991.

Lageragard T: *Haemophilus ducreyi:* pathogenesis and protective immunity, *Trends Microbiol* 3:87, 1995.

Merino D, Saavedra J, Pujol E, et al: *Haemophilus aphrophilus* as a rare cause of arthritis, *Clin Infect Dis* 19:320, 1994.

National Committee for Clinical Laboratory Standards: *Abbreviated identification of bacteria and yeast; M35-A*, Wayne, Pa, 2002, NCCLS.

Shanholtzer CJ, Schaper PJ, Peterson LR: Concentrated Gram-stained smears prepared with a cytospin centrifuge, *J Clin Microbiol* 16:1052, 1982.

St Geme JW III: Nontypeable *Haemophilus influenzae* disease: epidemiology, pathogenesis, and prospects for prevention, *Infect Agents Dis* 2:1, 1993.

Van Dyck E, Bogaerts J, Smet H, et al: Emergence of *Haemophilus ducreyi* resistance to trimethoprim-sulfamethoxazole in Rwanda, *Antimicrob Agents Chemother* 38:1647, 1994.

Versalovic J: *Manual of clinical microbiology*, ed 10, Washington, DC, 2011, ASM Press.

Weyant RS, Moss CW, Weaver RE, et al, editors: *Identification of unusual pathogenic gram-negative aerobic and facultatively anaerobic bacteria*, ed 2, Baltimore, 1996, Williams & Wilkins.

# Gram-Negative Bacilli that Are Optimally Recovered on Special Media

CHAPTER

# 33 | Bartonella and Afipia

## OBJECTIVES

1. Explain the routes of transmission for *Bartonella* infections, and describe the organism's interaction with the host.
2. Discuss the clinical manifestations of Trench fever, including signs, symptoms, and individuals at risk of acquiring the disease.
3. Explain the criteria used to diagnose *Bartonella henselae*.
4. Describe the two methods for culturing *Bartonella,* including growth rates, media, incubation temperature, and other relevant conditions.
5. Explain why the sensitivity and specificity has been questioned with indirect fluorescent antibody and enzyme-linked immunoassay testing.
6. Describe the strategies to prevent exposure and infection by these organisms in immunocompromised individuals.

---

### GENERA AND SPECIES TO BE CONSIDERED

*Bartonella bacilliformis*
Other *Bartonella* spp., including
   *B. quintana*
   *B. henselae*
   *B. elizabethae*
   *B. clarridgeiae*
*Afipia felis*

---

The two genera, *Bartonella* and *Afipia*, are able to grow on chocolate agar and, albeit very slowly, on routine blood (trypticase soy agar with 5% sheep blood agar), typically appearing after 12 to 14 days and sometimes requiring as long as 45 days; neither organism grows on MacConkey agar. Presently, there is no optimal procedure for the isolation of these organisms from clinical specimens. Because of these similarities and because two organisms, *Bartonella henselae* and *Afipia felis*, cause cat-scratch disease (CSD), these genera are addressed together in this chapter.

## BARTONELLA

### GENERAL CHARACTERISTICS

*Bartonella* spp. were previously grouped with members of the family Rickettsiales. However, because of extensive differences, the family Bartonellaceae was removed from this order. As a result of phylogenetic studies using molecular biologic techniques, the genus *Bartonella* currently includes 22 species and subspecies, most of which were reclassified from the genus *Rochalimeae* and from the genus *Grahamella.* Only five species are currently recognized as major causes of disease in humans (Table 33-1), but other members of the genus have been found in animal reservoirs such as rodents, ruminants, and moles. *Bartonella* spp. are most closely related to *Brucella abortus* and *Agrobacterium tumefaciens* and are short, gram-negative, rod-shaped, facultative intracellular, fastidious organisms that are oxidase negative and grow best on blood-enriched media or cell co-culture systems.

## EPIDEMIOLOGY AND PATHOGENESIS

Organisms belonging to the genus *Bartonella* cause numerous infections in humans; most of these infections are thought to be zoonoses. Interest in these organisms has increased because of their recognition as causes of an expanding array of clinical syndromes in immunocompromised and immunocompetent patients. For example, *Bartonella* species have been recognized with increasing frequency since the early 2000s as a cause of culture-negative endocarditis. Humans acquire infection either naturally (infections caused by *Bartonella quintana* or *Bartonella bacilliformis*) or incidentally (other *Bartonella* species) via arthropod-borne transmission. Nevertheless, questions remain regarding the epidemiology of these infections; some epidemiologic information is summarized in Table 33-1.

*Bartonella* is a facultative intracellular bacterium that closely interacts with the host cells and has unique abilities to cause either acute or chronic infection as well as the proliferation of microvascular endothelial cells and angiogenesis (forming new capillaries from preexisting ones) or suppurative manifestations. Three *Bartonella* species (*B. quintana, B. bacilliformis,* and *B. henselae*) are capable of causing angiogenic lesions. Research has demonstrated that some species are capable of interacting with host red blood cells, endothelial cells, and possibly bone marrow progenitor cells. Colonization of vascular endothelium is considered a crucial step in the establishment and maintenance of *Bartonella*-triggered angioproliferative lesions. Within several hours following infection of cultured human umbilical vein endothelial cells,

**TABLE 33-1** Organisms Belonging to the Genus *Bartonella* and Recognized to Cause Disease in Humans*

| Organism | Habitat (Reservoir) | Mode of Transmission | Clinical Manifestation(s) |
|---|---|---|---|
| *Bartonella alsatica* | Rabbits | Unknown; fleas or ticks suspected | Humans accidental hosts |
| *B. bacilliformis* | Uncertain; humans; possibly cats and dogs | Fleas and sandflies | Carrión's disease* |
| *B. quintana* | Uncertain; small rodents, gerbils, humans | Human body louse and fleas | Trench fever<br>Chronic bacteremia<br>Endocarditis<br>Bacillary angiomatosis<br>Chronic lymphadenopathy<br>Pericarditis |
| *B. henselae* | Domestic cats | Domestic cats and dogs; bites or scratches, fleas | Bacteremia<br>Endocarditis<br>Cat-scratch disease<br>Bacillary angiomatosis<br>Peliosis hepatitis<br>Neuroretinitis |
| *B. clarridgeiae* | Domestic cats | Domestic cat; bites or scratches and fleas | Bacteremia<br>Cat-scratch disease |
| *B. elizabethae* | Rats | Fleas | Endocarditis |

Note: Other *Bartonella* species have caused incidental infections in humans, but only one or a few cases have been documented.
*Disease confined to a small endemic area in South America; characterized by a septicemic phase with anemia, malaise, fever, and enlarged lymph nodes in the liver and spleen, followed by a cutaneous phase with bright red cutaneous nodules, usually self-limited.

*Bartonella* species adhere to and enter these cells by an actin-dependent process resembling other bacterial-directed phagocytosis or uptake into host cells. Recent studies have also shown that *B. henselae* possess nine outer membrane proteins (OMP), one of which is able to bind to endothelial cells.

Typically, *Bartonella* species multiply and persist in the red blood cells in the reservoir host and share common persistence and dissemination strategies. In addition to angioproliferation, recent data indicate bartonellae can inhibit endothelial cell apoptosis (programmed cell death); these organisms also activate monocyte and macrophage cells capable of producing potent angiogenic factors. Although more research is needed regarding the pathogenesis of infections caused by *Bartonella*, it is evident these organisms possess unique pathogenic strategies to expand their bacterial niche in order to sustain survival within the human host. It is evident that the pathologic response to these infections varies substantially with the status of the host immune system. For example, infection with the same *Bartonella* species, such as *B. henselae*, can cause a focal suppurative reaction (i.e., CSD) in immunocompetent patients or a multifocal angioproliferative lesion (i.e., bacillary angiomatosis) in immunocompromised patients. *B. quintana*, the etiologic agent for trench fever, also causes bacillary angiomatosis in immunocompromised patients.

## SPECTRUM OF DISEASE

The diseases caused by *Bartonella* species are listed in Table 33-1. Because *B. quintana* and *B. henselae* are more

common causes of infections in humans, these agents are addressed in greater depth.

Trench fever, caused by *B. quintana*, was largely considered a disease of the past. Clinical manifestations of trench fever range from a mild influenza-like headache and bone pain to splenomegaly (enlarged spleen) and a short-lived maculopapular rash. During the febrile stages of trench fever, infection may persist long after the disappearance of all clinical signs; some patients may have six or more recurrences. *B. quintana* has reemerged and has been reported in cases of bacteremia, endocarditis, chronic lymphadenopathy, and bacillary angiomatosis primarily in low socioeconomic groups in Europe and the United States, as well as in patients infected with the human immunodeficiency virus (HIV). Bacillary angiomatosis is a vascular proliferative disease involving the skin (other organs such as the liver, spleen, and lymph nodes may also be involved) and occurs in immunocompromised individuals such as organ transplant recipients and HIV-positive individuals. Prolonged bacteremia with *B. quintana* infections may be associated with the development of endocarditis and bacillary angiomatosis.

*B. henselae* is associated with bacteremia, endocarditis, and bacillary angiomatosis. Of note, recent observations indicate that *B. henselae* infections appear to be subclinical and are markedly underreported, as problems with current diagnostic approaches are recognized (see Laboratory Diagnosis). In addition, *B. henselae* causes CSD and peliosis hepatitis. About 24,000 cases of CSD occur annually in the United States; about 80% of these occur in children. The infection begins as a papule or pustule at the primary inoculation site; regional tender lymphade-nopathy develops in 1 to 7 weeks. The spectrum of disease ranges from chronic, self-limited adenopathy to a severe systemic illness affecting multiple body organs. Although complications such as a suppurative (draining) lymph node or encephalitis are reported, fatalities are rare. Diagnosis of CSD requires three of the four following criteria:

- History of animal contact plus site of primary inoculation (e.g., a scratch)
- Negative laboratory studies for other causes of lymphadenopathy
- Characteristic histopathology of the lesion
- A positive skin test using antigen prepared from heat-treated pus collected from another patient's lesion

*Bartonella clarridgeiae* is a newly described species capable of causing CSD and bacteremia.

Peliosis hepatitis caused by *B. henselae* may occur independently or in conjunction with cutaneous bacillary angiomatosis or bacteremia. Patients with peliosis hepatitis demonstrate gastrointestinal symptoms. Symptoms include fever, chills, and an enlarged liver and spleen that contain blood filled cavities. This systemic disease develops in patients infected with HIV and other immunocompromised individuals.

## LABORATORY DIAGNOSIS

### Specimen Collection, Transport, and Processing

Clinical specimens submitted to the laboratory for direct examination and culture include blood, which has been collected in a lysis-centrifugation blood culture tube (Isolator; Wampole Laboratories, Cranbury, New Jersey), as well as aspirates and tissue specimens (e.g., lymph node, spleen, or cutaneous biopsies). There are no special requirements for specimen collection, transport, or processing that enhances organism recovery. Refer to Table 5-1 for general information on specimen collection, transport, and processing.

### Direct Detection Methods

Detection of *Bartonella* spp. during the histopathologic examination of tissue biopsies is enhanced with staining using the Warthin-Starry silver stain orimmunofluorescence and immunohistochemical techniques. Because of the fastidious nature of the organisms and slow growth, molecular methods to identify *Bartonella* spp. directly in clinical specimens allows earlier detection. Polymerase chain reaction (PCR) targeting the 16S-23S rRNA gene intergenic transcribed spacer region has been proposed as a reliable method for the detection of *Bartonella* DNA in clinical samples. However, a recent study revealed some potential limitations based on insufficient primer specificity. As the number of species included in the genus expand, PCR and restriction fragment length polymorphism (RFLP) (see Chapter 8) as well as sequencing may require targeting several genes and subsequent sequencing for accurate species identification.

### Cultivation

The optimum conditions required for recovery of bartonellae from clinical specimens has yet to be fully defined. Currently, two methods are recommended including direct inoculation onto fresh chocolate agar plates (less than 2 weeks old) and co-cultivation in cell culture. Fresh agar helps supply moisture necessary for growth. Lysed, centrifuged sediment of blood collected in an isolator tube or minced tissue is directly inoculated onto fresh chocolate agar plates and incubated at 35° C in a very humid atmosphere containing 5% to 10% carbon dioxide ($CO_2$), examined daily for 3 days, and examined again after 2 weeks of incubation. One study indicated that collection of blood in EDTA and subsequent freezing may improve the sensitivity of recovering *B. henselae*. Biopsy material is co-cultivated with an endothelial cell culture system; co-cultures are incubated at 35° C in 5% to 10% $CO_2$ for 15 to 20 days. Blood-enriched agar, such as Columbia or heart infusion agar base with 5% sheep blood, has been used, but horse or rabbit blood has been reported to be a more effective supplement for recovery of organisms. Lymph node tissue, aspirates, or swabs can be inoculated onto laked horse blood agar slopes supplemented with hemin; plates are sealed and incubated in 5% $CO_2$ up to 6 weeks at 37° C with 85% humidity.

### Approach to Identification

*Bartonella* spp. should be suspected when colonies of small, gram-negative bacilli are recovered after prolonged incubation (Figure 33-1). Organisms are all oxidase, urease, nitrate reductase, and catalase negative.

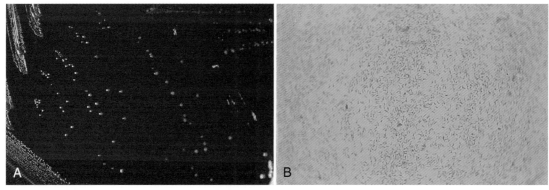

**Figure 33-1 A,** Colonies of *Bartonella henselae* on blood agar. **B,** Gram stain of a colony of *B. henselae* from blood agar.

Various methods may be used for confirmation and identification of *Bartonella* spp. Species identification is possible by adding 100 µg/mL of hemin to the test medium, as well as biochemical profiling using the MicroScan rapid or Rapid ANAII system (Innovative Diagnostic Systems, Norcross, Georgia) anaerobe panels, polyvalent antisera, or a variety of molecular methods.

### Serodiagnosis

Several serologic methods for detecting antibodies to *Bartonella* spp. have been developed. An indirect fluorescent antibody has been developed using antigen prepared from *Bartonella* spp. co-cultivated with Vero cells and enzyme-linked immunoassays. However, the sensitivity and specificity of these assays have been questioned. Cross-reactivity between *Bartonella*, *Chlamydia* spp. and *Coxiella burnettii* has been reported. Serology testing is not recommended in HIV-positive or immunocompromised patients because of a decreased antibody response to infection.

A 5-year study by LaScola and colleagues of various samples obtained for culture for *Bartonella* species demonstrated that successful recovery or detection of *B. henselae* or *B. quintana* was dependent on several factors. These factors include the clinical form of the disease (i.e., endocarditis, bacteremia, bacillary angiomatosis, or CSD), previous antibiotic therapy, the type of clinical specimen (e.g., blood, heart valve, skin, or lymph node), and the type of laboratory diagnostic method employed (serology, PCR, shell vial cultures with human endothelial cell monolayers, direct plating of blood onto agar or broth blood cultures). In other words, the organisms are not unlike other microorganisms cultured and identified in the microbiology laboratory. The knowledge required for sufficient recovery and appropriate methods is yet to be established.

## ANTIMICROBIAL SUSCEPTIBILITY TESTING AND THERAPY

Treatment recommendations for *Bartonella* diseases, including CSD, depend on the specific disease presentation. The efficacy of various antibiotics for CSD is difficult to assess as a result of the self-limiting nature of the disease and the decrease in symptoms in the absence of therapy. In addition to the clinical presentation, the treatment must be specifically adapted to the correct *Bartonella* sp. Antimicrobial susceptibilities have been determined in the presence of eucaryotic cells or without cells (i.e., axenic media). However, these conditions have not been standardized and interpretive criteria have not been determined, according to Clinical and Laboratory Standards Institute (CLSI). Moreover, results of in vitro

testing may not correlate with clinical efficacy; for example, the administration of penicillin is not effective therapy despite susceptibility in vitro. Recent treatments with azithromycin indicate successful, more rapid resolution of adenopathy of CSD; however, it is presently unclear if antibiotic therapy is effective in immunocompetent patients. For patients with severe CSD (about 5% to 14% of cases), other successful antibiotic regimens have included rifampin, doxycycline, erythromycin, and azithromycin or doxycycline in combination with rifampin. For bacillary angiomatosis and peliosis, doxycycline and erythromycin are considered the drugs of choice. Suggested therapy for endocarditis, suspected or documented, is gentamicin with or without doxycycline, respectively.

## PREVENTION

There are no vaccines available to prevent infections caused by *Bartonella* spp. Exposure to cats or cat fleas has been implicated in the transmission of *B. henselae* to humans. Therefore, it is recommended that immunocompromised individuals avoid contact with cats, especially kittens, and control flea infestation.

## AFIPIA FELIS

CSD was first reported in 1931; however, the causative agent was unknown for several decades. Finally a bacterial agent was isolated and characterized and given the name *Afipia felis*. However, the role of *A. felis* in the etiology of CSD was subsequently questioned because patients with CSD failed to mount an immune response to *A. felis* antigen. In addition, and the organism was unsuccessfully isolated from culture or detected by PCR. Subsequently, additional data demonstrated that patients with CSD mounted an immune response to *B. henselae* and the organism was isolated in culture as well as detected using PCR and immunocytochemistry. The organism *B. henselae* was also detected in CSD skin test antigens, from cats, and cat fleas. In light of all the data, *B. henselae* is now recognized as the primary causative agent of CSD, and *A. felis* is loosely implicated in the disease. Despite its rare isolation, indirect evidence suggests *A. felis* may be commonly linked to CSD; however, it is impossible to determine at this time because current laboratory methods are insufficient.

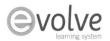 *Visit the Evolve site to complete the review questions.*

## CASE STUDY 33-1

A 52-year-old male with a 25-year smoking history had been living on the street for an unknown period of time. He sought medical attention because of overall poor health and was found to be anemic with weight loss. A spiculated mass was observed in his left middle lung lobe on chest film, and a lobectomy was performed with the possible diagnosis of carcinoma. The pathology department reported numerous necrotizing granulomas and chronic inflammation, but no carcinoma was observed in the lung tissue. Gram staining demonstrated "dark-staining gram-variable debris" but no definitive organisms. The patient had an uneventful recovery without anti-infective therapy. Routine bacterial and fungal cultures of the lung tissue were negative, but the broth mycobacterial culture grew a gram-negative rod. The rod only grew on charcoal yeast extract agar (CYE), but not on blood or chocolate agars. It was oxidase and urease positive, motile, and beta-lactamase positive. The catalase reaction was weak; nitrate was negative. It did not react with *Legionella* antiserum.

### QUESTIONS

1. The significant characteristics of this bacterium include growth in broth and on CYE plates. Most laboratories typically do not have CYE available for routine culture. What would be the recommended procedure following isolation of a gram-negative rod from a normally sterile specimen with an original order for mycobacterium testing?

2. The isolate was identified as *Afipia broomeae* using DNA homology testing. According to Weyant and colleagues, this bacterium is characterized for its growth on CYE and in broth, but not on other laboratory media. The species identification is based on a positive oxidase, catalase, urease, and xylose and a negative nitrate reduction. *A. felis* is identical except it is nitrate positive. Although the CDC collection of *A. felis* is mostly from lymph nodes, most of the *A. broomeae* were from respiratory specimens. What is the likely route of transmission, or how was the individual exposed to the organism resulting in the infection?

3. Because both *Afipia* and *Bartonella* are difficult to grow, should the laboratory attempt to provide culture services?

## ▄ BIBLIOGRAPHY

Avidor B, Graidy M, Efrat G, et al: *Bartonella* koehlerae, a new cat-associated agent of culture-negative human endocarditis, *J Clin Microbiol* 42:3462, 2004.

Berger P, Papazian L, Drancourt M, et al: Ameba-associated microorganisms and diagnosis of nosocomial pneumonia, *Emerg Infect Dis* 12:248, 2006.

Breitschwerdt EB, Kordick DL: *Bartonella* infections in animals: carriership, reservoir potential, and zoonotic potential for human infection, *Clin Microbiol Rev* 13:428, 2000.

Brenner SA, Rooney JA, Manzewitsch P, et al: Isolation of *Bartonella* (*Rochalimaea*) henselae: effects of methods of blood collection and handling, *J Clin Microbiol* 35:544, 1997.

Dehio C: Recent progress in understanding *Bartonella*-induced vascular proliferation, *Curr Opin Microbiol* 6:61, 2003.

Drancourt M, Raoult D: Proposed tests for the routine identification of *Rochalimaea* species, *Eur J Clin Microbiol Infect Dis* 12:710, 1993.

Fournier PE, Robson J, Zeaiter Z, et al: Improved culture from lymph nodes of patients with cat scratch disease and genotypic characterization of *Bartonella henselae* isolates in Australia, *J Clin Microbiol* 40:3620, 2002.

Garcia-Caceres U, Garcia FU: Bartonellosis: an immunosuppressive disease and the life of Daniel Alcides Carrión, *Am J Clin Pathol* 95(suppl 1):S58, 1991.

Giladi M, Avidor B, Kletter Y, et al: Cat scratch disease: the rare role of *Afipia felis*, *J Clin Microbiol* 36:2499, 1998.

Greub G, Raoult D: *Bartonella*: new explanations for old diseases, *J Med Microbiol* 51:915, 2002.

Jacomo V, Raoult D: Human infections caused by *Bartonella* spp. Parts 1 and 2, *Clin Microbiol Newsletter* 22:1-5, 9-13, 2000.

Jacomo V, Raoult D: Natural history of *Bartonella* infections (an exception to Koch's postulates), *Clin Diagn Lab Immunol* 9:8, 2002.

Kordick DL, Hilyard EJ, Hadfield TL, et al: *Bartonella clarridgeiae*: a newly recognized zoonotic pathogen causing inoculation papules, fever, and lymphadenopathy (cat-scratch disease), *J Clin Microbiol* 35:1813, 1997.

LaScola B, Raoult D: Culture of *Bartonella quintana* and *Bartonella henselae* from human samples: a 5-year experience (1993-1998), *J Clin Microbiol* 37:1899, 1999.

Lawson PA, Collins MD: Description of *Bartonella clarridgeiae* sp nov isolated from the cat of a patient with *Bartonella henselae* septicemia, *Med Microbiol Lett* 5:640, 1996.

Maggie RG, Breitschwerdt EB: Potential limitations of the 16S-23S rRNA intergenic region for molecular detection of *Bartonella* species, *J Clin Microbiol* 43:1171, 2005.

Manfredi R, Sabbatini S, Chiodo F: Bartonellosis: light and shadows in diagnostic and therapeutic issues, *Clin Microbiol Infect* 11:167, 2004.

Maurin M, Raoult D: *Bartonella* (*Rochalimaea*) quintana infections, *Clin Microbiol Rev* 9:273, 1996.

Midani S, Ayoub EM, Anderson B: Cat scratch disease, *Adv Pediatr* 43:397, 1996.

Rolain JM, Brouqui P, Koehler JE, et al: Recommendations for treatment of human infections caused by *Bartonella* species, *Antimicrob Agents Chemother* 48:1921, 2004.

Versalovic J: *Manual of clinical microbiology*, ed 10, Washington, DC, 2011, ASM Press.

Weisburg WG, Woese CR, Dobson ME, et al: A common origin of rickettsiae and certain plant pathogens, *Science* 230:556, 1985.

Weyant, RS, Moss CW, Weaver RE, et al, editors: *Identification of unusual pathogenic gram-negative aerobic and facultatively anaerobic bacteria*, ed 2, Baltimore, 1996, Williams & Wilkins.

# Campylobacter, Arcobacter, and Helicobacter

## OBJECTIVES

1. List the *Campylobacter* species most often associated with infections in humans, and explain how they are transmitted.
2. Identify the culture methods for optimum recovery of *Campylobacter jejuni* and *Campylobacter coli,* including agar, temperatures, oxygenation, and length of incubation.
3. Describe how to isolate *Campylobacter* from blood, including special stains, atmospheric conditions, and length of incubation.
4. List the colonial morphology, microscopic, and biochemical reactions of *Campylobacter* and *Helicobacter.*
5. List the key biochemical test to identify *Helicobacter pylori* in specimens.
6. Describe how *H. pylori* colonize in the stomach and how motility plays an important role in the pathogenesis of the organism.
7. Describe why therapy is often problematic for *H. pylori.*

---

### GENERA AND SPECIES TO BE CONSIDERED

*Campylobacter coli*
*Campylobacter concisus*
*Campylobacter curvus*
*Campylobacter fetus* subsp. *fetus*
*Campylobacter fetus* subsp. *venerealis*
*Campylobacter gracilis*
*Campylobacter hyointestinalis* subsp. *hyointestinalis*
*Campylobacter jejuni* subsp. *doylei*
*Campylobacter jejuni* subsp. *jejuni*
*Campylobacter lari*
*Campylobacter rectus*
*Campylobacter showae*
*Campylobacter sputorum* biovar. *sputorum*
*Campylobacter upsaliensis*
*Arcobacter cryaerophilus*
*Arcobacter butzleri*
*Helicobacter pylori*
*Helicobacter cinaedi*
*Helicobacter fennelliae*

---

Because of morphologic similarities and an inability to recover these organisms using routine laboratory media for primary isolation, the genera *Campylobacter, Arcobacter,* and *Helicobacter* are considered in this chapter (Figure 34-1). All organisms belonging to these genera are small, curved, motile, gram-negative bacilli. With few exceptions, most of these bacteria also have a requirement for a microaerobic (5% to 10% $O_2$) atmosphere.

## CAMPYLOBACTER AND ARCOBACTER

### GENERAL CHARACTERISTICS

*Campylobacter* and *Arcobacter* spp. are relatively slow growing, fastidious, and, in general, asaccharolytic; organisms known to cause disease in humans and are listed in Table 34-1.

### EPIDEMIOLOGY AND PATHOGENESIS

The majority of *Campylobacter* species are pathogenic and associated with a wide variety of diseases in humans and other animals. These organisms demonstrate considerable ecologic diversity. *Campylobacter* spp. are microaerobic (5% to 10% $O_2$) inhabitants of the gastrointestinal tracts of various animals, including poultry, dogs, cats, sheep, and cattle, as well as the reproductive organs of several species. When random fecal samples from chicken carcasses from butcher shops in the New York City area were tested for *Campylobacter,* 83% of the samples yielded more than 10 colony-forming units per gram of feces. In general, *Campylobacter* spp. produce three syndromes in humans: febrile systemic disease, periodontal disease, and, most commonly, gastroenteritis. *Arcobacter* species appear to be associated with gastroenteritis. Studies have indicated that *A. butzleri* was the fourth most common *Campylobacter*-like organism isolated from stool and was associated with a persistent, watery diarrhea. In addition, more recent data indicate that *Arcobacter* is underreported in gastrointestinal infections and diarrhea throughout many European countries. The organism is found in the environment and in untreated water. It is also prevalent in commercially prepared meats including chicken, beef, pork, lamb, and poultry.

Within the genus *Campylobacter, C. jejuni* and *C. coli* are commonly associated with infections in humans and are transmitted via contaminated food, milk, or water. Outbreaks have been associated with contaminated drinking water and improperly pasteurized milk, among other sources. In contrast to other agents of foodborne gastroenteritis, including *Salmonella* and staphylococci, *Campylobacter* spp. does not multiply in food. Other campylobacters have been isolated from patients as a result of consumption of untreated water as well as from immunocompromised

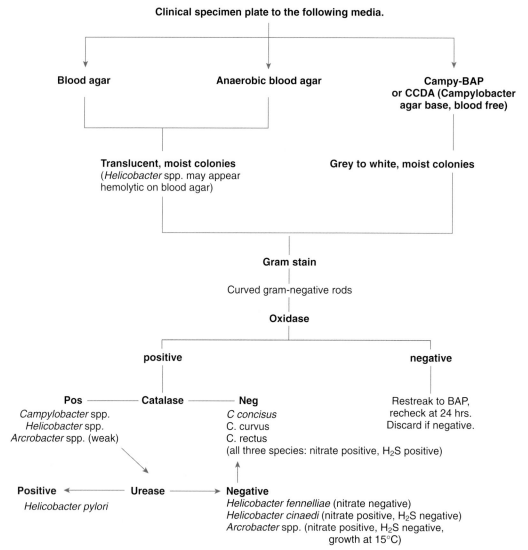

**Figure 34-1** Identification scheme for the differentiation of the genera *Helicobacter, Campylobacter,* and *Arcobacter. BAP,* Blood agar plate.

patients, or patients recently returned from international travel. *C. jejuni* subsp. *doylei* has been isolated from children with diarrhea and from gastric biopsies in adults. In developed countries, the majority of *C. jejuni* infections are transmitted by direct contact during the preparation and eating of chicken. Person-to-person transmission of *Campylobacter* infections plays only a minor role in the transmission of disease. There is a marked seasonality with the rates of *C. jejuni* infection in the United States; the highest rates of infection occur in late summer and early fall. *Campylobacter* spp. has been recognized as the most common etiologic agent of gastroenteritis in the United States.

Although infections with *C. jejuni* are evident as a result of acute inflammatory enteritis of the small intestine and colon, the pathogenesis remains unclear. However, multiplication of organisms in the intestine leads to cell damage and an inflammatory response. Blood and polymorphonuclear neutrophils are often observed in patient stool specimens. Most strains of *C. jejuni* are susceptible to the nonspecific bactericidal

activity of normal human serum; this susceptibility probably explains why *C. jejuni* bacteremia is uncommon.

## SPECTRUM OF DISEASE

As previously mentioned, *Campylobacter* species are the causative agent of gastrointestinal or extraintestinal infections. An increase in extraintestinal disease, including meningitis, endocarditis, and septic arthritis has been reported in patients with acquired immunodeficiency syndrome (AIDS) and other immunocompromised individuals. The different campylobacters and the associated diseases are summarized in Table 34-1. Gastroenteritis associated with *Campylobacter* spp. is usually a self-limiting illness and does not require antibiotic therapy. Most recently, postinfectious complications with *C. jejuni* have been recognized and include reactive arthritis and Guillain-Barré syndrome, an acute demyelination (removal of the myelin sheath from a nerve) of the peripheral nerves. Studies indicate that 20% to 40% of patients with this syndrome are infected

**TABLE 34-1** *Campylobacter* and *Arcobacter* spp., Their Source, and Spectrum of Disease in Humans

| Organism | Source | Spectrum of Disease in Humans |
|---|---|---|
| C. concisus, C. curvus, C. rectus, C. showae | Humans | Periodontal disease; gastroenteritis (?) |
| C. gracilis | Humans | Deep-tissue infections: head, neck, and viscera; gingival crevices |
| C. coli | Pigs, poultry, sheep, bulls, birds | Gastroenteritis* Septicemia |
| C. jejuni subsp. jejuni | Poultry, pigs, bulls, dogs, cats, birds, and other animals | Gastroenteritis* Septicemia Meningitis Proctitis |
| C. jejuni subsp. doylei | Humans | Gastroenteritis* Gastritis Septicemia |
| C. lari | Birds, poultry, other animals; river and seawater | Gastroenteritis* Septicemia Prosthetic joint infection |
| C. hyointestinalis subsp. hyointestinalis | Pigs, cattle, hamsters, deer | Gastroenteritis |
| C. upsaliensis | Dogs, cats | Gastroenteritis Septicemia abscesses |
| C. fetus subsp. fetus | Cattle, sheep | Septicemia Gastroenteritis Abortion Meningitis |
| C. fetus subsp. venerealis | Cattle | Septicemia |
| C. sputorum biovar sputorum | Humans, cattle, pigs | Abscesses Gastroenteritis |
| Arcobacter cryaerophilus | Pigs, bulls, and other animals | Gastroenteritis* Septicemia |
| A. butzleri | Pigs, bulls, humans, other animals; water | Gastroenteritis* Septicemia |

*Most common clinical presentation.

with *C. jejuni* 1 to 3 weeks prior to the onset of neurologic symptoms.

## LABORATORY DIAGNOSIS

### Specimen Collection, Transport, and Processing

There are no special requirements for the collection, transport, and processing of clinical specimens for the detection of campylobacters; the two most common clinical specimens submitted to the laboratory are feces (rectal swabs are also acceptable for culture) and blood. Specimens should be processed as soon as possible. Delays of more than 2 hours require the stool specimen to be placed either in Cary-Blair transport medium or in campy thio, a thioglycollate broth base with 0.16% agar and vancomycin (10 mg/L), trimethoprim (5 mg/L), cephalothin (15 mg/L), polymyxin B (2500 U/L), and amphotericin B (2 mg/L). Cary-Blair transport medium is suitable for other enteric pathogens; specimens received in transport medium should be processed immediately or stored at 4° C until processed.

### Direct Detection

Upon gram staining, *Campylobacter* spp. display a characteristic microscopic morphology as small, curved or seagull-winged, faintly staining, gram-negative rods (Figure 34-2). Polymerase chain reaction (PCR) amplification may provide an alternative to culture methods for the detection of *Campylobacter* spp. from clinical specimens. The detection of *Campylobacter* DNA in stools from a large number of patients with diarrhea suggests that *Campylobacter* spp. other than *C. jejuni* and *C. coli* may account for a proportion of cases of acute gastroenteritis in which no etiologic agent is identified.

### Antigen Detection

Several commercial antigen detection systems are available for the direct detection of Campylobacter in stool specimens. These enzyme immunoassays (EIA) can be used to detect antigens in stool samples for several days if stored at 4° C.

### Media

Campy-BAP is an enriched selective blood agar plate used to isolate *C. jejuni*. The medium is composed of a Brucella agar base, sheep red blood cells and vancomycin, trimethoprim, polymyxin B, amphotericin B, and cephalothin. Campy medium (CVA) contains cefoperazone, vancomycin, and amphotericin B. The antibiotics in both media suppress the growth of normal fecal flora. *Campylobacter* agar base blood free (CCDA) is a modified agar that does not include blood. The blood is replaced with charcoal, sodium pyruvate, and ferrous sulfate. The medium supports growth of most *Campylobacter* spp.

### Cultivation

**Stool.** Successful isolation of *Campylobacter* spp. from stool requires selective media and optimum incubation conditions. Recommended inoculation of two selective agars is associated with increased recovery of the organisms. Because *Campylobacter* and *Arcobacter* spp. have different optimum temperatures, two sets of selective plates should be incubated, one at 42° C and one at 37° C. Extended incubation may be required, 48 to 72 hours, before there is evidence of visible growth. Table 34-2 describes the selective plating media and incubation conditions required for the recovery of *Campylobacter* spp. from stool specimens.

A filtration method can also be used in conjunction with a nonselective medium to enhance recovery of *Campylobacter* and *Arcobacter* spp. A filter (0.65-µm pore-size

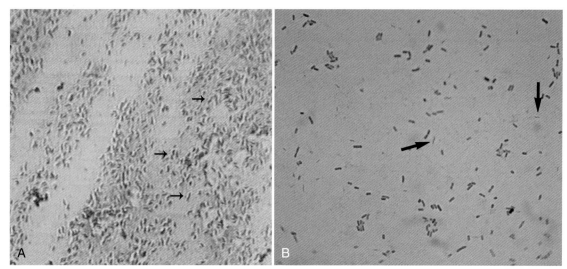

**Figure 34-2 A,** Gram stain appearance of *Campylobacter jejuni* subsp. *jejuni* from a colony on a primary isolation plate. Note seagull and curved forms *(arrows).* **B,** Appearance of *Campylobacter jejuni* subsp. *jejuni* in a direct Gram stain of stool obtained from a patient with campylobacteriosis. *Arrows* point to the seagull form.

**TABLE 34-2** Selective Media and Incubation Conditions to Recover *Campylobacter* and *Arcobacter* spp. from Stool Specimens

| Organism | Primary Plating Media | Incubation Conditions |
|---|---|---|
| *C. jejuni*<br>*C. coli* | Modified Skirrow's medium: Columbia blood agar base, 7% horse-lysed blood, and antibiotics (vancomycin, trimethoprim, and polymyxin B)<br>Campy-BAP: *Brucella* agar base with antibiotics (trimethoprim, polymyxin B, cephalothin, vancomycin, and amphotericin B) and 10% sheep blood<br>Blood-free, charcoal-based selective medium: Columbia base with charcoal, hemin, sodium pyruvate, and antibiotics (vancomycin, cefoperazone, and cycloheximide)<br>Modified charcoal cefoperazone deoxycholate agar (CCDA)<br>Semisolid motility agar: Mueller-Hinton broth II, agar, cefoperazone, and trimethoprim lactate<br>Campy-CVA: *Brucella* agar base with antibiotics (cefoperazone, vancomycin, and amphotericin B) and 5% sheep blood | 42° C microaerobic conditions* for 72 hours |
| *C. fetus* subsp. *fetus*[†]<br>*C. jejuni* subsp. *doylei*<br>*C. upsaliensis*<br>*C. lari*<br>*C. hyointestinalis* | Modified Skirrow's medium<br>Blood-free charcoal-based selective media<br>Campy-CVA<br>CCDA<br>Semisolid motility agar | 37° C under microaerobic conditions for at least 72 hours up to 7 days[‡] |
| *A. cryaerophilus, A. butzleri* | Campy-CVA | 37° C under microaerobic conditions[§] for 72 hours |

*Atmosphere can be generated in several ways, including commercially produced, gas-generating envelopes to be used with plastic bags or jars. Evacuation and replacement in plastic bags or anaerobic jars with an atmosphere of 10% $CO_2$, 5% $O_2$, and the balance of nitrogen ($N_2$) is the most cost-effective method, although it is labor intensive.
[†]All these organisms are susceptible to cephalothin.
[‡]*C. upsaliensis* will grow at 42° C but not on cephalothin-containing selective agar.
[§]*A. cryaerophilus* does not require microaerobic conditions.

cellulose acetate) is placed on the agar surface, and a drop of stool is placed on the filter. The plate is incubated upright. After 60 minutes at 37° C, the filter is removed and the plates are reincubated in a microaerobic atmosphere. The organisms are motile and capable of migrating through the filter, producing isolated colonies on the agar surface and effectively removing contaminating stool flora. *C. concisus, A. butzleri, A. cryaerophilus,* and *H. cinaedi* have been isolated following

5 to 6 days of incubation using the filter technique. An enrichment broth may also be used for the recovery of *Arcobacter* or *Campylobacter* species from stool.

**Blood.** *Campylobacter* spp. are capable of growth in less than 5 days in most blood culture media, although they may require extended incubation periods of up to 2 weeks for detection. Subcultures should be incubated in 5% to 10% $O_2$ (microaerobic) environment. Turbidity may not be visible in blood culture media; therefore,

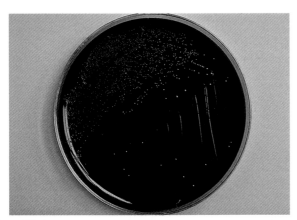

**Figure 34-3** Colonies of *Campylobacter jejuni* following 48 hours of incubation on a selective medium in a microaerobic atmosphere.

blind subcultures or microscopic examination using acridine orange stain may be necessary. The presence of *Campylobacter* spp. in blood cultures is effectively detected through carbon dioxide ($CO_2$) monitoring. Isolation from sources other than blood or feces is extremely rare. Recovery of the organisms is enhanced by inoculation (minced tissue, wound exudate) to a nonselective blood or chocolate agar plate and incubation at 37° C in a $CO_2$-enriched, microaerobic atmosphere. (Selective agars containing a cephalosporin, rifampin, and polymyxin B may inhibit growth of some strains and should not be used for isolation from sterile sites.)

### Approach to Identification

Plates should be examined for characteristic colonies, which are gray to pinkish or yellowish gray and slightly mucoid looking; some colonies may exhibit a tailing effect along the streak line (Figure 34-3). Colony morphology varies with the type of medium used for isolation. Suspicious-looking colonies observed on selective media incubated at 42° C may be presumptively identified as *Campylobacter* spp., usually *C. jejuni* or *C. coli*, with a few basic tests. A wet preparation of the organism in broth may be examined for characteristic darting motility and curved morphology on Gram stain. Both organisms are cephalothin resistant, nalidixic acid sensitive, and sensitive to lysis by complement. *C. fetus* is incapable of growth at 42°, and optimal growth is 37°; it is cephalothin sensitive, nalidixic acid resistant, and resistant to complement lysis.

Almost all the pathogenic *Campylobacter* spp. are oxidase positive and catalase positive. Frequently laboratories will report stool isolates as "*Campylobacter* spp."

Most *Campylobacter* spp. are asaccharolytic, unable to grow in 3.5% NaCl, although strains of *Arcobacter* appear more resistant to salt and, except for *Arcobacter cryaerophilus*, unable to grow in ambient air. Growth in 1% glycine is variable. Susceptibility to nalidixic acid and cephalothin, as previously described (Table 34-3), is determined by inoculating a 5% sheep blood or Mueller-Hinton agar plate with a McFarland 0.5 turbidity suspension of the organism, placing 30-mg disks on the agar surface and incubating in 5% to 10% $CO_2$ at 37° C. Other tests useful for identifying these species are the rapid hippurate

hydrolysis test, production of hydrogen sulfide ($H_2S$) in triple sugar iron agar slants, nitrate reduction, and hydrolysis of indoxyl acetate. Indoxyl acetate disks are available commercially. Cellular fatty acid analysis is useful for species identification. This method is not available in routine clinical microbiology laboratories. Several commercial products are available for species identification, including particle agglutination methods and nucleic acid probes.

Molecular assays based on PCR amplification of the 16S rRNA gene and direct sequencing of the PCR product have successfully been used to identify the majority of *Campylobacter* species. The assays accurately discriminate related taxa including *Campylobacter*, *Arcobacter*, or *Helicobacter* species. Finally, another approach using 16S-23S PCR-based amplification with a DNA probe colorimetric membrane assay proved to rapidly detect and identify *Campylobacter* in stool specimens.

### Serodiagnosis

Serodiagnosis is not widely applicable for the diagnosis of infections caused by these organisms.

## ANTIMICROBIAL SUSCEPTIBILITY TESTING AND THERAPY

Susceptibility tests for *Campylobacter* spp. are not standardized, and therefore testing of isolates is not routinely performed. *C. jejuni* and *C. coli* are susceptible to many antimicrobial agents, including macrolides, tetracyclines, aminoglycosides, and quinolones. Erythromycin is the drug of choice for patients with severe gastroenteritis (severe dehydration, bacteremia), with ciprofloxacin as an alternative therapeutic option. Previously, fluoroquinolones were the antibiotic therapy most frequently prescribed for *Campylobacter* infection; however, a rapidly increasing proportion of *Campylobacter* strains worldwide have been identified as fluoroquinolone resistant. Parenteral therapy (not taken through the alimentary canal but by an alternate route such as intravenous) is used to treat systemic infections.

## PREVENTION

No vaccines are available for *Campylobacter* spp. Infections caused by *Campylobacter* spp. are acquired by ingesting contaminated foodstuffs or water. Proper preparation and cooking of all foods derived from animal sources, particularly poultry, will decrease the risk of transmission. All milk should be pasteurized and drinking water chlorinated. Care must be taken during food preparation to prevent cross-contamination from raw poultry to other food items.

# HELICOBACTER

## GENERAL CHARACTERISTICS

In 1983, spiral-shaped organisms resembling *Campylobacter* spp. were isolated from the human stomach; these organisms were named *Campylobacter pylori*. Based on

**TABLE 34-3** Differential Characteristics of Clinically Relevant *Campylobacter, Arcobacter,* and *Helicobacter* spp.

| Genus and Species | Growth at 25° C | Growth at 42° C | Hippurate Hydrolysis | Catalase | H₂S in Triple Sugar Iron Agar | Indoxyl Acetate Hydrolysis | Nitrate to Nitrite | Susceptible to 30-μg Disk Cephalothin | Nalidixic Acid (30 μg) |
|---|---|---|---|---|---|---|---|---|---|
| *C. coli* | − | + | − | + | − | + | + | − | + |
| *C. concisus* | − | + | − | − | + | − | + | − | − |
| *C. curvus** | − | + | − | − | + | + | + | ND | + |
| *C. fetus* subsp. *fetus* | + | −/+ | − | + | − | + | + | + | − |
| *C. hyointestinalis* | +/− | − | − | + | + | − | + | + | − |
| *C. jejuni* subsp. *jejuni* | − | + | + | + | − | + | + | − | + |
| *C. jejuni* subsp. *doylei* | − | +/− | + | +/− or weak + | − | + | − | + | + |
| *C. lari* | − | + | − | + | − | − | + | − | − |
| *C. rectus** | − | Slight + | − | − | + | + | + | ND | + |
| *C. sputorum* | − | + | − | −/+ | + | − | + | + | −/+ |
| *C. upsaliensis* | − | + | − | −/weak + | − | + | + | + | + |
| *A. butzleri*† | + | − | − | −/weak + | − | + | + | −/+ | +/− |
| *A. cryaerophilus*‡ | + | − | − | +/− | − | + | + | −/+ | +/− |
| *H. cinaedi* | − | −/+ | − | + | − | −/+ | + | +/− | + |
| *H. fennelliae* | − | − | − | + | − | + | − | + | + |
| *H. pylori*§ | − | + | − | + | − | − | +/− | + | − |

*Anaerobic, not microaerobic.
†Grows at 40° C.
‡Aerotolerant, not microaerobic; except for a few strains, *A. cryaerophilus* cannot grow on MacConkey agar, whereas *A. butzleri* grows on MacConkey agar.
§Strong and rapid positive urease.
*ND*, Test not done; +, most strains positive; −, most strains negative; +/−, variable (more often positive); −/+, variable (more often negative).

many studies, the genus *Helicobacter* was established in 1989 and *C. pylori* was renamed *Helicobacter pylori*. Approximately 32 species are included in this genus, the majority of which colonize mammalian stomachs or intestines. The genus *Helicobacter* consists of curved, microaerophilic, gram-negative rods, the majority of species exhibiting urease activity. Human isolates include *H. pylori, H. cinaedi, H. fennelliae, H. heilmannii* (formerly known as *Gastrospirillum hominis*), *H. westmeadii, H. canis, H. canadensis* sp. nov., *H. pullorum,* and "*H. rappini*" (formerly known as "*Flexispira rappini*"). Human pathogens discussed here include *H. pylori, H. cinaedi,* and *H. fennelliae.*

## EPIDEMIOLOGY AND PATHOGENESIS

*Helicobacter pylori*'s primary habitat is the human gastric mucosa. The organism is distributed worldwide. Although acquired early in life in underdeveloped countries, the exact mode of transmission is unknown. An oral-oral, fecal-oral, and a common environmental source have been proposed as possible routes of transmission, with familial transmission associated with *H. pylori* infections. Research studies suggest mother-to-child transmission as the most probable cause of intrafamilial spread. In industrialized nations, antibody surveys indicate that approximately 50% of adults >60 years of age are infected by *H. pylori*. Gastritis incidence increases with age. *H. pylori* has occasionally been cultured from feces and dental plaque, thereby suggesting a fecal-oral or oral-oral transmission.

The habitat *for H. cinaedi* and *H. fennelliae* appears to be the human gastrointestinal tract, and the organisms may be normal flora; hamsters have also been proposed as a reservoir for *H. cinaedi.* Although the epidemiology of these organisms is not clearly delineated, these two bacterial agents have been associated with sexual transmission among homosexual men.

*H. pylori* is capable of colonizing the mucous layer of the antrum and fundus of the stomach but fails to invade the epithelium. Motility allows *H. pylori* to escape the acidity of the stomach and burrow through and colonize the gastric mucosa in close association with the epithelium. In addition, the organism produces urease that hydrolyzes urea-forming ammonia ($NH_3$) significantly increasing the pH around the site of infection. The change in pH protects the organism from the acidic environment produced by gastric secretions. *H. pylori* also produces a protein called CagA and injects the protein into the gastric epithelial cells. The protein subsequently affects host cell gene expression inducing cytokine release and altering cell structure, and interactions with neighboring cells enabling *H. pylori* to successfully

**TABLE 34-4** Genes and Their Possible Role in Enhancing Virulence of *H. pylori*

| Gene | Possible Role |
|------|---------------|
| VacA | Exotoxin (VacA)<br>Creates vacuoles in epithelial cells, decreases apoptosis, and loosens cell junctions |
| CagA | Pathogenicity island<br>Encodes a type IV secretion system for transferring CagA proteins into host cells |
| BabA | Encodes outer membrane protein: mediates adherence to blood group antigens on the surface of gastric epithelial cells |
| IceA | Presence associated with peptic ulcer disease in some populations |

invade the gastric epithelium. Individuals who demonstrate positive antibody response to cag protein are at increased risk of developing both peptic ulcer disease and gastric carcinoma. Other possible virulence factors include adhesins for colonization of mucosal surfaces, mediators of inflammation, and a cytotoxin capable of causing damage to host cells (Table 34-4). Although *H. pylori* is noninvasive, untreated colonization persists despite the host's immune response.

# SPECTRUM OF DISEASE

*H. cinaedi* and *H. fennelliae* cause proctitis, enteritis, and sepsis in homosexual men. Septic shock caused by *H. fennelliae* was reported in a non-HIV-infected heterosexual immunocompromised patient. *H. cinaedi* has also been reported to cause septicemia, cellulitis, and meningitis in immunocompromised patients. *H. pylori* causes gastritis, peptic ulcer disease, and gastric cancer. However, most individuals tolerate the presence of *H. pylori* for decades with few, if any, symptoms.

## LABORATORY DIAGNOSIS

### Specimen Collection, Transport, and Processing
There are no special requirements for the collection, transport, or processing of stool or blood specimens for *H. cinaedi* and *H. fennelliae*. Tissue biopsy material of the stomach for detection of *H. pylori* should be placed directly into transport media such as Stuart's transport medium to prevent drying. Specimens for biopsy may be refrigerated up to 24 hours before processing; tissues should be minced and gently homogenized.

### Direct Detection
Pathologists use the Warthin-Starry or other silver stains and Giemsa stains to examine biopsy specimens. Squash preparations of biopsy material can be Gram-stained with good results; the 0.1% basic fuchsin counterstain enhances recognition of the bacteria's typical morphology. Sampling error may occur during processing, therefore resulting in no identification of the organisms.

Presumptive evidence of the presence of *H. pylori* in biopsy material may be obtained by placing a portion of crushed tissue biopsy material directly into urease broth or onto commercially available urease agar kits. A positive test is considered indicative of the organism's presence. Another noninvasive indirect test to detect *H. pylori* is the urea breath test. This test relies on the presence of *H. pylori* urease. The patient ingests radioactively labeled ($13°$ C) urea, and if the organism is present, the urease produced by *H. pylori* hydrolyzes the urea to form ammonia and labeled bicarbonate that is exhaled as $CO_2$; the labeled $CO_2$ is detected by either a scintillation counter or a special spectrometer. This test has excellent sensitivity and specificity. Two enzyme immunoassays *H. pylori* stool antigen tests (Premier Platinum HpSA, Meridian Diagnostics, Inc., Cincinnati, Ohio; FemtoLab *H. pylori*, Connex, Martinsried, Germany) and a one-step immunochromatographic assay using monoclonal antibodies (Immunocard STAT! HpSA, Meridian Bioscience Europe) have been introduced to directly detect *H. pylori*. Finally, a variety of molecular methods have been developed to directly detect *H. pylori* in clinical specimens and to identify bacterial strains and host genotype characteristics, bacterial density in the stomach, as well as antimicrobial resistance patterns.

### Cultivation
Stool specimens submitted for culture of *H. cinaedi* and *H. fennelliae* are inoculated onto selective media used for *Campylobacter* isolation but without cephalothin such as Campy-CVA. For the recovery of *H. pylori* from tissue biopsy specimens including gastric antral biopsies, nonselective agar media, including chocolate agar and Brucella agar with 5% sheep blood, have resulted in successful recovery of the organisms. Selective agar such as Skirrow's and modified Thayer-Martin agar also support growth. Recently, the combination of a selective agar (Columbia agar with an egg yolk emulsion, supplements, and antibiotics) and a nonselective agar (modified chocolate agar with Columbia agar, 1% Vitox, and 5% sheep blood) was reported as the optimal combination for recovering *H. pylori* from antral biopsies. Incubation up to 1 week in a humidified, 5% to 10% $O_2$ environment, at 35° to 37° C may be required before growth is visible.

### Approach to Identification
Colonies of *Helicobacter* spp. may require 4 to 7 days of incubation before small, translucent, circular colonies are observed. Organisms are identified presumptively as *Helicobacter pylori* by the typical cellular morphology and positive results for oxidase, catalase, and rapid urease tests. *H. pylori*, *H. cinaedi*, and *H. fennelliae* are definitively identified by using a similar approach to *Campylobacter* spp. (see Table 34-3).

### Serodiagnosis
Serologic diagnosis is also available for *H. pylori*. Numerous serologic enzyme-linked immunoassays (EIAs) designed to detect immunoglobulin G (IgG) and immunoglobulin A (IgA) antibodies to *H. pylori* are commercially available. Reported performance of these assays varies as a result of the reference method used to confirm

*H. pylori* infection, antigen source for the assay, and the population studied. In addition to variability in assay performance, the clinical utility of these assays has not been determined. It is uncertain as to whether or not these assays are capable of differentiation of active versus past *H. pylori* infections. However, a single study has confirmed the role of seroconversion in determining a cure of *H. pylori* infection.

## ANTIMICROBIAL SUSCEPTIBILITY TESTING AND THERAPY

Except for metronidazole and clarithromycin, most laboratory susceptibility assays are unsuccessful in predicting clinical outcome. Routine testing of *H. pylori* isolates' susceptibility to metronidazole is recommended using the E-test and agar or broth dilution methods.

Therapy for *H. pylori* infection is problematic. *H. pylori* readily becomes resistant when metronidazole, clarithromycin, azithromycin, rifampin, or ciprofloxacin is prescribed as a single agent. Current regimens recommend triple-drug therapy including metronidazole, a bismuth salt, and either amoxicillin or tetracycline. An alternative and simple regimen for patients with metronidazole-resistant strains includes omeprazole or lansoprazole (proton pump inhibitors cause rapid symptom relief while working synergistically with the antibiotics) and amoxicillin or clarithromycin. Relapses occur often. *Helicobacter* spp. associated with enteritis and proctitis may respond to quinolones; however, appropriate therapy has not been established.

## PREVENTION

No vaccines are available for *H. pylori*. However, several vaccines are under development.

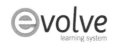 *Visit the Evolve site to complete the review questions.*

---

## CASE STUDY 34-1

A 10-year-old boy became ill a few days after a Fourth of July picnic where fried chicken was served. He complained of diarrhea, abdominal pain, and fever. Symptoms continued over the next week and he was seen at the local clinic. Blood was found in his stool and cultures were ordered. He was treated with ampicillin but switched to azithromycin (a macrolide similar to erythromycin) for 5 days when the culture results were reported.

**QUESTIONS**

1. At 42° C in a microaerobic environment, water droplet–type oxidase and catalase-positive colonies were isolated. A Gram stain showed gram-negative rods with seagull-shaped morphology. What rapid test is used to confirm the identity of this bacterium?
2. What follow-up testing would be required if the hippurate hydrolysis is negative?
3. What is the most likely route of transmission to the patient in this incident?
4. Why is the nalidixic acid disk not required for the identification of *C. jejuni/coli*?

---

## BIBLIOGRAPHY

Allos BM: *Campylobacter jejuni* infections: update on emerging issues and trends, *Clin Infect Dis* 32:1201, 2001.

Blaser MJ: The biology of cag in the *Helicobacter pylori*-human interaction, *Gastroenterology* 128:1512, 2005.

Butzler JP: *Campylobacter*, from obscurity to celebrity, *J Clin Microbiol Infect* 10:868, 2004.

Crowe SE: *Helicobacter* infection, chronic inflammation, and the development of malignancy, *Curr Opin Gastroenterol* 21:32, 2005.

Day AS, Jones NL, Lynetl JT, et al: cagE is a virulence factor associated with *Helicobacter pylori*-induced duodenal ulceration in children, *J Infect Dis* 181:1370, 2000.

Dunn BE, Cohen H, Blaser MJ: Helicobacter pylori, *Clin Microbiol Rev* 10:720, 1997.

Endtz HP, Ruijs GJ, van Klingeren B, et al: Comparison of six media, including a semisolid agar, for the isolation of various *Campylobacter* species from stool specimens, *J Clin Microbiol* 29:1007, 1991.

Engberg J, On SL, Harrington CS, et al: Prevalence of *Campylobacter, Arcobacter, Helicobacter* and *Sutterella* spp. in human fecal samples as estimated by a reevaluation of isolation methods for campylobacters, *J Clin Microbiol* 38:286, 2000.

Feldman M, Cryer B, Lee E, et al: Role of seroconversion in confirming cure of *Helicobacter pylori* infection, *JAMA* 280:363, 1998.

Goodwin CS: Antimicrobial treatment of *Helicobacter pylori* infection, *Clin Infect Dis* 25:1023, 1997.

Gorkiewicz G, Feierl G, Schober C, et al: Species-specific identification of campylobacters by partial 16S rRNA gene sequencing, *J Clin Microbiol* 41:2537, 2003.

Han S, Zschausch H, Meyer HW, et al: *Helicobacter pylori*: clonal population structure and restricted transmission within families revealed by molecular typing, *J Clin Microbiol* 38:3646, 2000.

Henriksen TH, Brorson Ö, Schöyen R, et al: A simple method for determining metronidazole resistance of *Helicobacter pylori*, *J Clin Microbiol* 35:1424, 1997.

Konno M, Fujii N, Yakota S, et al: Five year follow-up study of mother-to-child transmission of *Helicobacter pylori* infection detected by a random amplified polymorphic DNA fingerprinting method, *J Clin Microbiol* 43:2246, 2005.

Maher M, Finnegan C, Collins E, et al: Evaluation of culture methods and a DNA probe-based PCR assay for detection of *Campylobacter* species in clinical specimens of feces, *J Clin Microbiol* 41:2980, 2003.

Marchildon PA, Ciota LM, Zamaniyan FZ, et al: Evaluation of three commercial enzyme immunoassays compared with the C urea breath test for detection of *Helicobacter pylori* infection, *J Clin Microbiol* 34:1147, 1996.

On SL: Identification methods for campylobacters, helicobacters, and related organisms, *Clin Microbiol* 9:405, 1996.

Pavicic MJ, Namavar F, Verboom T, et al: In vitro susceptibility of *Helicobacter pylori* to several antimicrobial combinations, *Antimicrob Agents Chemother* 37:1184, 1993.

Piccolomini R, Di Bonaventura G, Catamo G, et al: Optimal combination of media for primary isolation of *Helicobacter pylori* from gastric biopsy specimens, *J Clin Microbiol* 35:1541, 1997.

Rieder G, Fischer W, Haas R: Interaction of *Helicobacter pylori* with host cells: function of secreted and translocated molecules, *Curr Opin Microbiol* 8:67, 2005.

Simala-Grant J, Taylor DE: Molecular biology methods for the characterization of *Helicobacter pylori* infections and their diagnosis, *APMIS* 112:886, 2004.

Tajada P, Gomez-Graces JL, Alos JI, et al: Antimicrobial susceptibilities of *Campylobacter jejuni* and *Campylobacter coli* to 12 β-lactam agents and combinations with β-lactamase inhibitors, *Antimicrob Agents Chemother* 40:1924, 1996.

Vandenberg O, Dediste A, Houf K, et al: *Arcobacter* species in humans, *Emerg Infect Dis* 10:1863, 2004.

Versalovic J: *Manual of clinical microbiology*, ed 10, Washington, DC, 2011, ASM Press.

## OBJECTIVES

1. Identify the causative agent of Legionnaires' disease.
2. List sources for *Legionella* in the environment, including those that are both man-made and naturally occurring.
3. Describe how *Legionella* infections are acquired.
4. Describe how *Legionella* avoids destruction by the host, including where the organisms survive and replicate.
5. Compare and contrast the three primary clinical manifestations of *Legionella,* including signs and symptoms.
6. List the specimens acceptable for *Legionella* testing, including storage and transportation of specimens.
7. Describe the different types of testing for *Legionella*, including sensitivity and specificity.
8. Explain the chemical principle for buffered charcoal-yeast extract (BCYE) with and without inhibitory agents and the proper use for each.
9. Describe the morphology of the *Legionella* when grown under optimal growth conditions, including oxygenation, temperature, and length of incubation.
10. State the drugs of choice for effective therapy.

---

### GENUS AND SPECIES TO BE CONSIDERED

*Legionella pneumophila*

*Legionella* spp.

---

This chapter addresses organisms that will not grow on routine primary plating media and belong to the genus *Legionella*. *Legionella* belongs to the family Legionellaceae and includes a single genus, *Legionella*, comprising approximately 52 species. *Legionella pneumophila* is the causative agent of Legionnaires' disease, a febrile and pneumonic illness with numerous clinical presentations. *Legionella* was discovered in 1976 by scientists at the Centers for Disease Control and Prevention (CDC) who were investigating an epidemic of pneumonia among Pennsylvania State American Legion members attending a convention in Philadelphia. There is retrospective serologic evidence of *Legionella* infection as far back as 1947. Bacteria resembling *Legionella* that are capable of living in amoebae have been designated as *Legionella*-like amoebal pathogens (LLAPs).

## GENERAL CHARACTERISTICS

All *Legionella* spp. are mesophilic (20° to 45° C), obligately aerobic, faintly staining, thin, gram-negative fastidious bacilli that require a medium supplemented with iron and L-cysteine, and buffered to pH 6.9 for optimum growth. The organisms utilize protein for energy generation rather than carbohydrates. The overwhelming majority of *Legionella* spp. are motile. As of this writing, more than 52 species belong to this genus. Nevertheless, the organism *Legionella pneumophila* predominates as a human pathogen within the genus and consists of 16 serotypes. In approximately decreasing order of clinical importance are *L. pneumophila* serotype 1 (about 70% to 90% of the cases of Legionnaires' disease), *L. pneumophila* serotype 6, *L. micdadei, L. dumoffii, L. anisa,* and *L. feeleii*. Of note, many species of *Legionella* have only been isolated from the environment or recorded as individual cases. To date, 20 species of *Legionella* are documented as human pathogens in addition to *L. pneumophila*. Box 35-1 is an abbreviated list of some of the species of *Legionella*.

## EPIDEMIOLOGY

*Legionellae* are ubiquitous and widely distributed in the environment. As a result, most individuals are exposed to *Legionella* spp.; however, few develop symptoms. In nature, *legionellae* are found primarily in aquatic habitats and thrive at warmer temperatures; these bacteria are capable of surviving extreme ranges of environmental conditions for long periods; studies have shown that *L. pneumophila* can survive for up to 14 months in water with only a slight loss in viability. *Legionella* spp. have been isolated from the majority of natural water sources investigated, including lakes, rivers, and marine waters, as well as moist soil. Organisms are also widely distributed in man-made facilities, including air-conditioning ducts and cooling towers; potable water; large, warm-water plumbing systems; humidifiers; whirlpools; and technical-medical equipment in hospitals.

*Legionella* infections are acquired exclusively from environmental sources; no person-to-person spread has been documented. Inhalation of infectious aerosols (1 to 5 μm in diameter) is considered the primary means of transmission. Exposure to these aerosols can occur in the workplace or in industrial or nosocomial settings; for example, nebulizer's filled with tap water and showers have been implicated. Infection is acquired through the inhalation of aerosols or microaspiration. Legionnaires' disease occurs in sporadic, endemic, and epidemic forms. The incidence of disease varies greatly and appears to depend on the geographic area, but it is estimated that *Legionella* spp. cause less than 1% to 5% of cases of pneumonia.

## PATHOGENESIS AND SPECTRUM OF DISEASE

*Legionella* spp. can infect and multiply within some species of free-living amoebae (*Hartmannella, Acanthamoeba,* and

*Naegleria* spp.), as well as within *Tetrahymena* spp., a ciliated protozoa, or within biofilms (well-organized microcolonies of bacteria usually enclosed in polymer matrices that are separated by water channels that remove wastes and deliver nutrients). This contributes to the organism's survival in the environment. In addition, *L. pneumophila* exists in two well-defined, morphologically distinct forms in Hela cells: (1) a highly differentiated, cystlike form that is highly infectious, metabolically dormant, and resistant to antibiotics and detergent-mediated lysis and (2) a replicative intracellular form that is ultrastructurally similar to agar-grown bacteria. The existence of this cystlike form may account for the ability of *L. pneumophila* to survive for long periods between hosts (amoebae or humans).

---

**BOX 35-1** Some *Legionella* spp. Isolated from Humans and Environmental Sources

**Species Isolated From Humans**
*L. pneumophila,* serotypes 1-16
*L. micdadei*
*L. bozemanii*
*L. dumoffii*
*L. feelei*
*L. gormanii*
*L. hackeliae*
*L. longbeachae*
*L. oakridgensis*
*L. wadsworthii*

**Species Isolated From the Environment Only**
*L. cherrii*
*L. erythra*
*L. gratiana*
*L. jamestowniensis*
*L. brunensis*
*L. fairfieldensis*
*L. santicrucis*

---

Although the exact mechanisms by which *L. pneumophila* causes disease are not totally delineated, its ability to avoid destruction by the host's phagocytic cells plays a significant role in the disease process. *L. pneumophila* is considered a facultative intracellular pathogen. Following infection, organisms are taken up by phagocytosis primarily in alveolar macrophages, where they survive and replicate within a specialized, membrane-bound vacuole by resisting acidification and evading fusion with lysosomes; it is still unknown how *Legionella* prevent vacuole acidification. Following replication, the organisms will kill the phagocyte releasing them into the lungs and will again be phagocytized by a mononuclear cell, and multiplication of the organism will increase.

The sequestering of *legionellae* within macrophages also makes it difficult to deliver and accumulate effective antimicrobials. Of significance, studies have shown that although certain antimicrobials can penetrate the macrophage and inhibit bacterial multiplication, *L. pneumophila* is not killed and, when drugs are removed, the organism resumes replicating. Therefore, a competent cell-mediated immune response is also important for recovery from *Legionella* infections. Humoral immunity appears to play an insignificant role in the defense against this organism.

In eukaryotic cells, most proteins secreted or transported inside vesicles to other cellular compartments are synthesized at the endoplasmic reticulum (ER) (Figure 35-1). Many bacterial pathogens use secretion systems as a part of how they cause disease. *L. pneumophila* possesses genes that are able to "trick" eukaryotic cells into transporting them to the endoplasmic reticulum; these virulence genes are called dot (defective organelle trafficking) or icm (intracellular multiplication). This dot/icm secretion system in *L. pneumophila* consists of 23 genes and is a type IV secretion system. Bacterial type IV secretion systems are bacterial devices that deliver macromolecules such as proteins across and into cells. After entry but before bacterial replication, *L. pneumophila,* residing in a membrane-bound vacuole, is surrounded

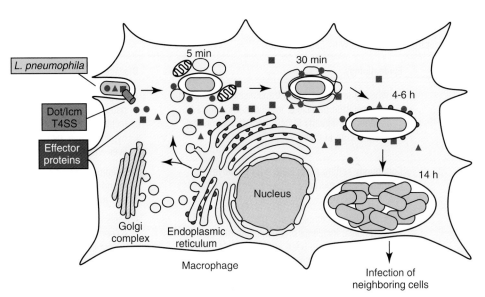

**Figure 35-1** (Modified from 2009annualreport.nichd.nih.gov/ump.html.)

by a ribosome-studded membrane derived from the host cell's ER and mitochondria. Thus, by exploiting host cell functions, *L. pneumophila* is able to gain access to the lumen of the ER, which supports its survival and replication where the environment is rich in peptides. A second type II secretion system has also been implicated in the virulence of some strains of *Legionella*. The type II secretion system carries numerous genes for enzymatic degradation including lipases, proteinases, and a number of novel proteins. Mutations within the type II secretion system results in decreased infectivity of the organism. A number of additional bacterial factors have also been identified as crucial for intracellular infection; some of these are listed in Box 35-2.

Finally, several cellular components and extracellular products of *L. pneumophila,* such as an extracellular cytotoxin that impairs the ability of phagocytic cells to use oxygen and various enzymes (e.g., phospholipase C), have been purified and proposed as virulence factors. However, their exact role in the pathogenesis of *Legionella* infections is not completely clear.

*Legionella* spp. are associated with a spectrum of clinical presentations, ranging from asymptomatic infection to severe, life-threatening diseases. Serologic evidence exists for the presence of asymptomatic disease, because many healthy people surveyed possess antibodies to *Legionella* spp. Table 35-1 provides a more detailed description of the following three primary clinical manifestations:

- Pneumonia with a case fatality rate of 10% to 20% (referred to as Legionnaires' disease)
- Pontiac fever, which is a self-limited, nonfatal, influenza-like respiratory infection
- Other rare extrapulmonary sites, such as wound abscesses, encephalitis, or endocarditis.

Individuals at risk for pneumonia are those who are immunocompromised, older than age 60, or heavy smokers. The clinical manifestations following infection with a particular species are primarily caused by differences in the host's immune response and perhaps by inoculum size; the same *Legionella* sp. gives rise to different expressions of disease in different individuals.

There are a number of bacteria that grow only within amoebae and are closely related phylogenetically based on 16S rRNA gene sequencing to *Legionella* species; these organisms are referred to as "*Legionella*-like amoeba pathogens" (LLAPs). Several LLAPs have been assigned to the *Legionella* genus. One LLAP has been isolated from the sputum of a patient with pneumonia after the specimen was incubated with the amoeba *Acanthamoeba polyphaga.* Serologic surveys of patients with community-acquired pneumonia suggest LLAPs may be occasional human pathogens.

---

**BOX 35-2** Examples of *L. pneumophila* Factors Crucial for Intracellular Infection

- Heat shock protein 60
- Outer membrane protein
- Macrophage infectivity potentiator
- Genes encoding for the type II secretion systems required for intracellular growth
- Type IV pili
- Flagella
- Dot/icm type IV secretion system

---

# LABORATORY DIAGNOSIS

## SPECIMEN COLLECTION AND TRANSPORT

Specimens from which *Legionella* can be isolated include respiratory tract secretions of all types, including expectorated sputum, additional lower respiratory specimens, and pleural fluid; other sterile body fluids, such as blood; and lung, transbronchial, or other biopsy material. Because sputum from patients with Legionnaires' disease is usually nonpurulent and may appear bloody or watery, the grading system used for screening sputum for routine cultures is not applicable. Patients with Legionnaires'

---

**TABLE 35-1** Disease Spectrum Associated with *Legionella* sp.

| | Epidemiology | Disease |
|---|---|---|
| **Pneumonia (Legionnaires' Disease)** | Community and nosocomial transmission (inhalation of aerosolized particles); immunocompromised patients, particularly in cell-mediated immunity; rarely occurs in children | Acute pneumonia indistinguishable from other bacterial pneumonias; clinical syndrome may include nonproductive cough, myalgia, diarrhea, hyponatremia, hypophosphatemia, and elevated liver enzymes |
| **Pontiac Fever** | Community setting associated with employment (industrial or recreational) or other group | Self-limiting, febrile illness; symptoms may include cough, dyspnea, abdominal pain, fever, and myalgia; pneumonia does not occur |
| **Extrapulmonary** | Rare, metastatic complications from underlying pneumonia; incidents of inoculation into sites via punctures have been identified or therapeutic bathing; highly associated with immunocompromised patients | Abscesses have been identified in the brain, spleen, lymph nodes, muscles, surgical wounds, and a variety of tissues and organs |

From Mandell GL, Bennett JE, Dolin R: *Principles and practices of infectious diseases,* ed 7, Philadelphia, 2010, Elsevier.

disease usually have detectable numbers of organisms in their respiratory secretions, even for some time after antibiotic therapy has been initiated. If the disease is present, the initial specimen is often likely to be positive. However, additional specimens should be processed if the first specimen is negative and suspicion of the disease persists. Pleural fluid has not yielded many positive cultures in studies performed in several laboratories, but it may contain organisms. Urine for antigen collection should be collected in a sterile container. The sample should be transported to the laboratory and refrigerated if a delay in processing occurs. Specimens should be transported without holding media, buffers, or saline, which may inhibit the growth of *Legionella*. The organisms are hardy and are best preserved by maintaining specimens in a small, tightly closed container to prevent desiccation and transporting them to the laboratory within 30 minutes of collection. If a longer delay is anticipated, specimens should be refrigerated. If one cannot ensure that specimens will remain moist, 1 mL of sterile broth may be added.

## SPECIMEN PROCESSING

All specimens for *Legionella* culture should be handled and processed in a class II biologic safety cabinet (BSC). When specimens from nonsterile body sites are submitted for culture, selective media or treatment of the specimen to reduce the numbers of contaminating organisms is proposed. Brief treatment of sputum specimens with hydrochloric acid before culture has been shown to enhance the recovery of *legionellae*. However, this technique is time consuming and is only recommended on specimens from patients with cystic fibrosis. Respiratory secretions may be held for up to 48 hours at 5° C before culture; if culturing is delayed longer, then the specimen may be frozen.

Tissues are homogenized before smears and cultures are performed, and clear, sterile body fluids are centrifuged for 30 minutes at 4000× g. The sediment is then vortexed and used for culture and smear preparation. Blood for culture of *Legionella* may be processed with the lysis-centrifugation tube system (Isolator; Wampole Laboratories, Cranbury, New Jersey) and plated directly to buffered charcoal-yeast extract (BCYE) agar. Specimens collected by bronchoalveolar lavage are quite dilute and therefore should be concentrated at least tenfold by centrifugation before culturing.

## DIRECT DETECTION METHODS

Several laboratory methods are used to detect *Legionella* spp. directly in clinical specimens.

### Stains

The cellular morphology of the organism differs from primary isolated colonies on media, long, filamentous bacilli, and lung or sputum specimens that appear as small coccobacilli or rods. Because of their faint staining, *Legionella* spp. are not usually detectable directly in clinical material by Gram stain. The use of 0.1% fuchsin substituted for safranin in the Gram-stain procedure may

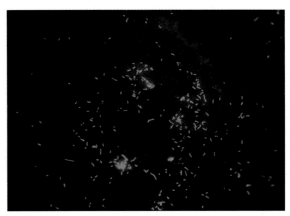

**Figure 35-2** Fluorescent antibody-stained *Legionella pneumophila*.

enhance the visibility of the organisms. Organisms can be observed on histologic examination of tissue sections using silver or Giemsa stains.

### Antigens

One approach to direct detection of *legionellae* in clinical specimens is the direct immunofluorescent antibody (DFA) test of respiratory secretions. Polyclonal and monoclonal antisera conjugated with fluorescein are available from several commercial suppliers. Specimens are first tested with pools of antisera containing antibodies to several serotypes of *L. pneumophila* or several *Legionella* spp. Those that exhibit positive results are then reexamined with specific conjugated antisera. One reagent made by Genetic Systems Corporation (Seattle, Washington) is a monoclonal antibody directed against a cell wall protein common to *L. pneumophila*. The manufacturer's directions should be followed explicitly, and material from commercial systems should never be divided and used separately. Laboratories should decide which serotypes to test for routinely based on the prevalence of isolates in their geographic area. The sensitivity of the DFA test ranges from 25% to 75%, and its specificity is greater than 95%. If positive, organisms appear as brightly fluorescent rods (Figure 35-2). Of importance, cultures always must be performed, because *Legionella* spp. or serotypes not included in the antisera pool can be recovered. In addition, even in the hands of an experienced microbiologist, false positives may occur. The high complexity of the test and lack of high reproducible sensitivity has reduced the number of laboratories offering DFA testing for *Legionella* sp.

Rapid detection of *Legionella* antigen in urine and other body fluids has been accomplished by enzyme immunoassay (EIA) and immunochromatography. Antigen may be present in the prodromal period and by 3 days after the onset of symptoms. Urine should be tested for *L. pneumophila*, although a drawback of the immunochromatographic urine antigen assay is that it only detects the presence of antigen of *L. pneumophila* serogroup 1, which constitutes 80% to 90% of all *Legionella* infections. In addition, false positives may occur in urine in the presence of rheumatoid-like factors, urinary sediment, and freeze-thawing of urine. All positive urine antigen tests should be confirmed. The urine sample should be clarified by brief centrifugation and boiled for 5-15 minutes (dependent on protocol) to remove rheumatoid-like factors. One *Legionella* EIA (Biotest, Dreieich, Germany) that utilizes a broadly cross-reactive antibody is available for the detection of all serotypes of *L. pneumophila*. The relative sensitivity of urine antigen tests in detecting infections ranges from 5% for some serogroups and up to 90% for *L. pneumophila* serogroup 1. Of note, a comparison of two EIAs demonstrated that the clinical utility for the diagnosis of Legionnaires' disease differed depending on the category of infection being investigated. Sensitivity (about 45%) for both EIAs was significantly lower for nosocomial cases than for either community-acquired or travel-associated ones. These assays have a sensitivity of 80% in their ability to detect infection caused by *L. pneumophila* serogroup 1 and are highly specific, although nonspecific false-positive results do occur as a result of excessive urinary sediment and rheumatoid-like factors. Boiling urine for 5-15 minutes (dependent on protocol) and concentrating urine by centrifugation help increase assay specificity and sensitivity, respectively. Of importance, because bacterial antigen may persist in urine for days to weeks after initiation of antibiotic therapy, these assays may be positive when other diagnostic tests are negative.

### Nucleic Acid Amplification

Although a single commercial assay was approved by the Food and Drug Administration (FDA) in the United States in 2004 (Becton Dickinson BD ProbeTec), molecular methods are predominantly research based and are becoming increasingly available in reference and public health laboratories. The BD Probe Tec assay is only available for sputum specimens and detects serotypes 1 through 14. The direct detection of *Legionella* nucleic acid by conventional and real-time polymerase chain reaction (PCR) has the potential to offer rapid results and increased sensitivity on respiratory and urine samples over current methods; of significance, PCR assays can detect all *Legionella* spp., not just *L. pneumophila*.

### CULTIVATION

Specimens for culture should be inoculated to two agar plates for recovery of *Legionella*, at least one of which is BCYE without inhibitory agents. This medium contains charcoal to detoxify the medium, remove carbon dioxide ($CO_2$), and modify the surface tension to allow the organisms to proliferate more easily. BCYE is also prepared with ACES buffer (N-(2-Acetoamido)-2-aminoethanesulfonic acid) and the growth supplements cysteine (required by *Legionella*), yeast extract, α-ketoglutarate, and iron. A second medium, BCYE base with polymyxin B, anisomycin (to inhibit fungi), and cefamandole, is recommended for specimens, such as sputum, that are likely to be contaminated with other flora. These media are commercially available. Several other media, including a selective agar containing vancomycin and a differential agar containing bromthymol blue and bromcresol purple, are also available from Remel (Lenexa, Kansas) and others.

Specimens obtained from sterile body sites may be plated to two media without selective agents and may also be inoculated into special blood culture broth without SPS. (Specimens should always be plated to standard media for recovery of pathogens other than *Legionella* that may be responsible for the disease.)

*L. pneumophila* grows at a temperature range from approximately 20° to 42° C. Plates are typically incubated in a candle jar at the optimal temperature of 35° to 37° C in a humid atmosphere. Some *Legionella* spp. may be stimulated by increased 2% to 5% concentration of $CO_2$, including *L. sainthelensi* and *L. oakridgensis*. The low level of $CO_2$ will not prevent the growth of *L. pneumophila*. If this concentration is not possible, incubation in air is preferable to 5% to 10% $CO_2$, which may inhibit some *legionellae*, specifically *L. pneumophila*. Within 3 to 4 days, colonies should be visible. Plates are held for a maximum of 2 weeks before they are discarded. Blood cultures in biphasic media should be held for 1 month. At 5 days, colonies are 3 to 4 mm in diameter, gray-white to blue-green, glistening, convex, and circular and may exhibit a cut-glass type of internal granular speckling (Figure 35-3). A Gram stain yields thin, gram-negative bacilli (Figure 35-4).

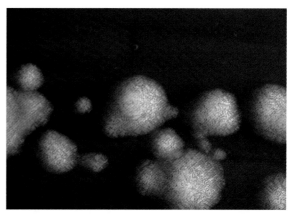

**Figure 35-3** Colonies of *Legionella pneumophila* on buffered charcoal-yeast extract agar.

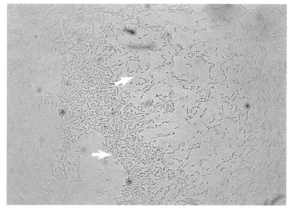

**Figure 35-4** Gram stain of a colony of *Legionella pneumophila* showing thin, gram-negative bacilli (*arrows*).

## APPROACH TO IDENTIFICATION

Because *Legionella* spp. are biochemically inert and many tests produce equivocal results, extensive biochemical testing is of little use. Definitive identification requires the facilities of a specialized reference laboratory. Suspect colonies should be Gram stained to determine if bacteria are small to filamentous, gram-negative rods. Colonies should be plated to two media, including a BYCE plate containing L-cysteine and one made without. *L. pneumophila* will only grow on the BYCE L-cysteine media, providing a more definitive identification. In addition, if only a small amount of growth is present on the primary medium, the growth may be emulsified in sterile water and used for subculturing, staining, and serologic identification. Once the isolate has been determined to be L-cysteine dependent, further identification is completed using serotyping. *L. pneumophila* spp. can be identified using a monoclonal immunofluorescent stain (Genetic Systems Corporation). Emulsions of organisms from isolated colonies are made in 10% neutral formalin, diluted 1:100 (to produce a very thin suspension), and placed on slides for fluorescent antibody staining. Clinical laboratories probably perform sufficient service to clinicians by indicating the presence of *Legionella* spp. in a specimen. Serologic typing is a simple method and should provide sufficient characterization. If further identification is necessary, the isolate should be forwarded to an appropriate reference laboratory.

## SERODIAGNOSIS

Most patients with legionellosis have been diagnosed retrospectively by detection of a fourfold rise in anti-*Legionella* antibody with an indirect fluorescent antibody (IFA) test. Serum specimens should be tested no closer than 2 weeks apart. Diagnostic efficacy associated with serologic testing increases with the collection and testing of acute and convalescent paired sera. Convalescent sera should be collected at 4, 6, and 12 weeks following the appearance of the disease. Disease is confirmed by a fourfold rise in titer to more than 128. A single serum with a titer of more than 256 and a characteristic clinical picture may be presumptive for legionellosis; however, because as many as 12% of healthy persons yield titers as high as 1:256, this practice is strongly discouraged.

Unfortunately, individuals with Legionnaires' disease may not exhibit an increase in serologic titers until as long as 10 weeks after the primary illness or they may never display significant antibody titer increases. It is essential to correlate serologic findings with the patient's clinical presentation because of the variation in antibody response associated with legionellosis. Most patients will develop a classic IgM, IgG, and IgA response. However, some patients may only develop antibodies for a single class (in other words, IgG, IgM, or IgA only). Commercially prepared antigen-impregnated slides for IFA testing are available from numerous suppliers.

## ANTIMICROBIAL SUSCEPTIBILITY TESTING AND THERAPY

In vitro susceptibility studies are not predictive of clinical response and should not be performed for individual isolates of *legionellae*. Because newer agents such as fluoroquinolones and the newer macrolides (e.g., clarithromycin and azithromycin) are more active against *L. pneumophila*, erythromycin has been replaced. Alternative regimens include doxycycline and the combination of erythromycin and rifampin. Clinical response usually follows within 48 hours after the introduction of effective therapy. Penicillins, cephalosporins of all generations, and aminoglycosides are not effective and should not be used.

## PREVENTION

Although under development, a vaccine against *Legionella* infections is not currently available. The effectiveness of other approaches to the prevention of *Legionella* infections, such as the elimination of its presence from cooling towers and potable water, is uncertain.

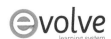 *Visit the Evolve site to complete the review questions.*

---

**CASE STUDY** 35-1

A 6-month-old infant was diagnosed clinically with pneumonia. She was treated with intramuscular ceftriaxone followed by an oral cephalosporin for 3 days. The next day she was found to be unresponsive and rushed to the hospital. She was afebrile but tachypneic (increased breathing) and tachycardic (increased heart rate); she had an increased white blood cell (WBC) count predominated with lymphocytes. A bronchoalveolar lavage was collected and was positive for *Legionella* by direct fluorescent antibody. A culture grew *Legionella pneumophila* serogroup 6 after 8 days. Despite appropriate therapy with erythromycin and rifampin, the infant's pulmonary disease was fatal. No underlying disease was found in the baby.

**QUESTIONS**

1. The *Legionella* urine antigen test was negative in this baby. What is the explanation for this finding?
2. The baby appeared to be a normal infant. List as many risk factors as possible for acquiring *Legionella* pneumonia.
3. List the factors that hamper the laboratory diagnosis of *Legionella*.
4. In general, sputum sent to the laboratory to diagnosis pneumonia will be purulent with mucus and increased polymorphonuclear WBCs. Describe the type of sputum observed with *Legionella* infection.

## ADVANCED CASE STUDY 35-2

A 78-year-old male retired executive presented to the clinic with a 3- to 5-day illness that consisted of headache and diarrhea. Over-the-counter remedies and hydration were recommended as empiric therapy for viral gastroenteritis. Two days later his wife drove him to the clinic, as the man was too weak to drive. She reported that her husband had become confused and had a high fever for the past 24 hours. In addition, he had developed a dry cough and was complaining of feeling short of breath. The patient has a previous medical history of hypertension and dyslipidemia. He is a former smoker but has no structural lung disease and no history of heart failure.

Physical examination revealed a temperature of 102.5° F, blood pressure of 110/65, a pulse of 110 bpm, a respiratory rate of 26 breaths per minute, and an oxygen saturation of 86%. A lung exam revealed crackles bilaterally in both left and right lungs. There were no signs of heart murmur or cyanosis. The patient had no other significant physical findings. Chest x-ray revealed diffuse pulmonary infiltrates bilaterally. The patient was admitted to the hospital with a provisional diagnosis of pneumonia and potentially H1N1 influenza. The following laboratory results were obtained:

### Laboratory Results

| Chemistry | Patient | Reference Range |
|---|---|---|
| Arterial pH | 7.35 | 7.35-7.45 |
| $PCO_2$ | 40 | 35-45 mmHg |
| $PO_2$ | 60 | 75-85 mmHg |
| $HCO_3^-$ | 24 | 20-25 mmol/L |
| CRP (C reactive protein) | 12 | <1 mg/dL |
| BNP (B type natriuretic peptide) | 100 | 9-86 pg/mL (male 75-83 years) |
| **Hematology** | | |
| WBC | 14 | $5-10 \times 10^9$/L |
| RBC | 5.11 | $5-6 \times 10^{12}$/L |
| Hgb | 15.5 | 13.5-17.5 |
| Hct | 0.46 | 0.41-0.53 L/L |

| Chemistry | Patient | Reference Range |
|---|---|---|
| Platelets | 120 | $150-400 \times 10^9$/L |
| Segmented neutrophils | 85% | 25%-60% |
| Lymphocytes | 13% | 20%-50% |
| Monocytes | 2% | 2%-11% |
| Eosinophils | 0% | 0%-8% |
| Basophils | 0% | 0%-2% |

### QUESTIONS

1. Evaluate the laboratory results as presented. Are there any unusual indicators here or in the patient's history that would signify a predisposition for unusual respiratory infections?
2. What additional laboratory tests would be indicated at this time?
3. Following hospitalization, the patient continued to demonstrate a low sodium level of 120 to 123 (reference range 135-145 mEq/L) despite rehydration efforts. His diarrhea and headache resolved by day 6 of his hospitalization, but his hypoxia increased. He was subsequently intubated and placed on mechanical ventilation for respiratory failure and continued to have a markedly elevated temperature of up to 104.3° F despite antibiotic treatment with cefotaxime and azithromycin. Repeat chest x-ray indicated an increase in infiltrates. His antibiotic treatment was broadened to include fungal and anaerobic antimicrobial agents, and the patient was placed in respiratory isolation. The following serologic test results were obtained: Influenza Rapid Antigen Test—negative; TB skin test—negative, sputum by endotracheal suction for acid-fast bacteria—negative; Mycoplasma IgM <1:16 (negative); *Legionella* Urine Antigen Test—positive.

A diagnosis of *Legionella* pneumonia was made. The azithromycin was maximized to optimal dosing of 500 mg per day, and the additional antibiotic treatment was discontinued.

Eventually the patient was extubated and made a full recovery from the pneumonia.

What are the major factors in the patient's clinical history that would point to an atypical pneumonia related to *Legionella pneumophila* infection?

# BIBLIOGRAPHY

Barker J, Brown MRW: Speculations on the influence of infecting phenotype on virulence and antibiotic susceptibility of *Legionella pneumophila*, *J Antimicrob Chemother* 36:7, 1995.

Becton, Dickenson and Company: *BD ProbeTec ET Legionella pneumophila (LP) Amplified DNA Assay, Package Insert*, Sparks, Md, 2006, Becton, Dickenson & Company.

Breiman RF: Modes of transmission in epidemic and non-epidemic *Legionella* infections: directions of further study. In Barbaree JM, Breiman RF, and Dufour AP, editors: *Legionella: current status and emerging perspectives*, Washington, DC, 1993, American Society for Microbiology.

Buesching WJ, Brust RA, Ayers LW: Enhanced primary isolation of *Legionella pneumophila* from clinical specimens by low pH treatment, *J Clin Microbiol* 17:1153, 1983.

Garduño RA, Garduño E, Hiltz M et al: Intracellular growth of *Legionella pneumophila* gives rise to a differentiated form dissimilar to stationary-phase forms, *Infect Immun* 70:6273, 2002.

Harb OS, Kwaik YA: Interaction of *Legionella pneumophila* with protozoa provides lessons, *ASM News* 66:609, 2000.

Helbig JH, Uldum SA, Bernander S, et al: Clinical utility of urinary antigen detection for diagnosis of community-acquired, travel-associated, and nosocomial Legionnaires' disease, *J Clin Microbiol* 41:838, 2003.

Mandell GL, Bennett JE, Dolin R: *Principles and practices of infectious diseases*, ed 7, Philadelphia, 2010, Churchill-Livingstone Elsevier.

Marrie TJ, Raoult D, LaScola B, et al: *Legionella*-like and other amoebal pathogens as agents of community-acquired pneumonia, *Emerg Infect Dis* 7:1026, 2001.

Muder RR, Yu VL: Infection due to *Legionella* species other than *Legionella pneumophila*, *Clin Infect Dis* 35:990, 2002.

Murdock DR: Diagnosis of *Legionella* infection, *Clin Infect Dis* 36:64, 2003.

Pasculle W: Update on *Legionella*, *Clin Microbiol Newsletter* 22:97, 2000.

Roy CR, Tilney LG: The road less traveled: transport of *Legionella* to the endoplasmic reticulum, *J Cell Biol* 158:415, 2002.

Salcedo SP, Holden DW: Bacterial interactions with the eukaryotic secretory pathway, *Curr Opin Microbiol* 8:92, 2005.

Shelhamer JH, Gill VJ, Quinn TC, et al: The laboratory evaluation of opportunistic pulmonary infections, *Ann Intern Med* 124:585, 1996.

Versalovic J: *Manual of clinical microbiology*, ed 10, Washington, DC, 2011, ASM Press.

Winn WC: *Legionella* and the clinical microbiologist, *Infect Dis Clin North Am* 7:377, 1993.

# *Brucella*

## OBJECTIVES

1. Identify the primary routes of transmission for *Brucella* spp.
2. Name the populations at risk for developing brucellosis.
3. Identify the signs and symptoms associated with brucellosis.
4. State two reasons the microbiology laboratory should be notified when *Brucella* infection is suspected.
5. Describe the principle and procedure for the rapid test for presumptive identification of *Brucella* spp.
6. Describe the differential characteristics of *Brucella abortus*, *Brucella melitensis*, *Brucella suis*, and *Brucella canis*.

---

### GENERA AND SPECIES TO BE CONSIDERED

*Brucella abortus*
*Brucella melitensis*
*Brucella suis*
*Brucella canis*

---

The family Brucellaceae comprises three genera: *Ochrobactrum*, *Mycoplana*, and *Brucella*. *Brucella* spp. are discussed in this chapter. Brucellae are free-living organisms that are subcategorized into nine recognized species. Six of the species are terrestrial, and four of those have been associated with human disease: *B. abortus* (seven biovars), *B. melitensis* (three biovars), *B. suis* (five biovars), and *B. canis*. Of the four species capable of causing human infection, all but *B. canis* are considered potential agents of bioterrorism.

## GENERAL CHARACTERISTICS

Brucellae are small, facultative, intracellular, nonmotile, aerobic, gram-negative coccobacilli or short rods that stain poorly by conventional Gram stain. Many isolates require supplementary carbon dioxide ($CO_2$) for growth, especially on primary isolation. *Brucella* spp. are closely related to *Bartonella*, *Rhizobium*, and *Agrobacterium* spp.

## EPIDEMIOLOGY AND PATHOGENESIS

The disease brucellosis occurs worldwide, especially in Mediterranean and Persian Gulf countries, India, and parts of Mexico and Central and South America. The organisms are capable of survival for extended periods (e.g., soil, 10 weeks; aborted fetuses, 11 weeks; bovine stool, 17 weeks, milk and ice cream, 3 weeks); they can survive in fresh cheese for several months. Brucellosis is

a zoonosis and is recognized as a cause of devastating economic loss among domestic livestock.

Each of the four *Brucella* spp. that are pathogenic for humans has a limited number of preferred animal hosts (Table 36-1). In the host, *Brucella* tend to localize in tissues rich in erythritol (e.g., placental tissue), a four-carbon alcohol that enhances their growth. Humans become infected by four primary routes:

- Ingestion of infected unpasteurized animal milk products (most common means of transmission)
- Inhalation of infected aerosolized particles (laboratory-acquired infection is the most important source of transmission)
- Direct contact with infected animal parts through ruptures of skin and mucous membranes
- Accidental inoculation of mucous membranes by aerosolization

Rare cases of transmission by blood and bone marrow transplantation and by sexual intercourse, in addition to neonatal brucellosis, have been reported. Individuals considered at risk for contracting brucellosis include dairy farmers, livestock handlers, slaughterhouse employees, veterinarians, and laboratory personnel. The organism has a very low infectious dose (100 organisms or fewer). Mishandling and misidentification of the organism is often associated with laboratory transmission of the organism.

*Brucella* spp. are facultative, intracellular parasites that are able to exist in both intracellular and extracellular environments. Other bacteria classified as facultative intracellular infectious agents include *Salmonella*, *Shigella*, *Yersinia*, *Listeria*, and *Francisella* spp. After infecting a host, brucellae are ingested by neutrophils, within which they replicate, causing cell lysis. Neutrophils containing viable organisms circulate in the bloodstream and are subsequently phagocytized by reticuloendothelial cells in the spleen, liver, and bone marrow. If the infection goes untreated, granulomas develop in these organs, and the brucellae survive in monocytes and macrophages. Brucellae tend to show a tendency to invade and persist in the human host by inhibiting apoptosis (programmed cell death). Resolution of the infection depends on the host's nutritional and immune status, the size of the inoculum and route of infection, and the *Brucella* species causing the infection; in general, *B. melitensis* and *B. abortus* are more virulent for humans.

Survival and multiplication of *Brucella* organisms in phagocytic cells are features essential to the establishment, development, and chronicity of the disease. The mechanisms by which brucellae avoid intracellular killing are not completely understood. *Brucella* spp. can change from a smooth to a rough colonial morphology based on the composition of their cell wall lipopolysaccharide O-side chain (LPS); those with a smooth LPS are more resistant to intracellular killing by neutrophils than those

**TABLE 36-1** *Brucella* spp. and Their Respective Natural Animal Hosts

| Organism | Preferred Animal Host |
|----------|----------------------|
| *B. abortus* | Cattle |
| *B. melitensis* | Sheep or goats |
| *B. suis* | Swine |
| *B. canis* | Dogs |
| *B. ovis* | Rams (not associated with human infection) |
| *B. neotomae* | Desert and wood rats (not associated with human infection) |

with a rough LPS. The smooth phenotype has been identified in *B. abortus* and *B. melitensis*. Brucellae ensure intracellular survival by interfering with the phagosome-lysosome fusion in macrophages and epithelial cells. In addition, as do *Legionella* spp. (see Chapter 35), brucellae use a type IV secretion system, VirB, for intracellular survival and replication. Unlike *Legionella* spp., however, brucellae modulate phagosome transport to avoid being delivered to lysosomes. Essentially, VirB is involved in controlling the maturation of the *Brucella* vacuole into an organelle that allows replication. In the mouse model, if mutations occur in this gene region, *B. abortus* is unable to establish chronic infections. In addition, *Brucella* spp. produce urease, which provides protection during passage through the digestive system when the organism is ingested in food products. Urease breaks down urea, producing ammonia, and neutralizes the gastric pH. Despite our current knowledge, many questions remain about the pathogenesis of disease caused by *Brucella* spp.

# SPECTRUM OF DISEASE

The clinical manifestations of brucellosis vary greatly, ranging from asymptomatic infection to serious, debilitating disease. For the most part, brucellosis is a systemic infection that can involve any organ of the body. Symptoms, which are nonspecific, include fever, chills, weight loss, sweats, headache, muscle aches, fatigue, and depression. Lymphadenopathy and splenomegaly are common physical findings. After an incubation period of about 2 to 4 weeks, the onset of disease is commonly insidious. Complications can occur, such as arthritis; spondylitis (inflammation of the spinal cord); genital, pulmonary, and renal complications; and endocarditis. Relapse is considered an important feature of brucellosis; it is associated with delayed initiation of treatment, ineffective antibiotic therapy, and positive blood culture findings during the initial presentation.

# LABORATORY DIAGNOSIS

## SPECIMEN COLLECTION, TRANSPORT, AND PROCESSING

A definitive diagnosis of brucellosis requires isolation of the organisms in cultures of blood, bone marrow,

cerebrospinal fluid (CSF), pleural and synovial fluids, urine, abscesses, or other tissues. If processing will be delayed, the specimen may be held in the refrigerator.

It is essential that the clinical microbiology laboratory be notified whenever brucellosis is suspected:

- To ensure that specimens are cultivated in an appropriate manner for optimum recovery from clinical specimens
- To avoid accidental exposure of laboratory personnel handling the specimens, because *Brucella* spp. are considered class III pathogens (specimen labels should indicate that *Brucella* spp. are a potential pathogen)

Blood for culture can be collected routinely (see Chapter 68) into most commercially available blood culture bottles and the lysis-centrifugation system (Isolator; Alere, Waltham, MA). For other clinical specimens, no special requirements must be met for collection, transport, or processing.

## DIRECT DETECTION METHODS

Direct stains of clinical specimens are not particularly useful for the diagnosis of brucellosis. Conventional and real-time polymerase chain reaction (PCR) assays are reliable and specific means of directly detecting *Brucella* organisms in clinical specimens. Sensitivity varies among assays, ranging from 50% to 100%. Several gene targets have been used, including a cell surface protein (BCS P31), a periplasmic protein (BP26), 16S rRNA, and transposon insertion sequence 711(IS711). Molecular assays currently are not available in routine laboratory testing; therefore, use of a reference laboratory may be required.

## CULTIVATION

Although most isolates of *Brucella* spp. grow on blood and chocolate agars (some isolates are also able to grow on MacConkey agar), more enriched agars and special incubation conditions generally are needed to achieve optimal recovery of these fastidious organisms from clinical specimens. *Brucella* agar or infusion base is recommended for specimen types other than blood. The addition of 5% heated horse or rabbit serum enhances growth on all media. Cultures should be incubated in 5% to 10% $CO_2$ in a humidified atmosphere; inoculated plates are incubated for up to 3 weeks before they are considered negative and discarded.

Commercial blood culture systems (e.g., BacT/Alert, BACTEC, and lysis-centrifugation systems) all have successfully detected brucellae in blood. Other blood culture bottles, such as those with brain-heart infusion and trypticase soy broth, also support the growth of brucellae if the bottles are continuously vented and placed in a $CO_2$ incubator. Most isolates can be detected within 5 to 7 days using commercial systems. Bottles need not be incubated longer than 10 to 14 days. Culture bottles may not become turbid. All subculture plates should be held for a minimum of 7 days.

On culture, colonies appear small, convex, smooth, translucent, nonhemolytic, and slightly yellow and opalescent after at least 48 hours of incubation (Figure 36-1).

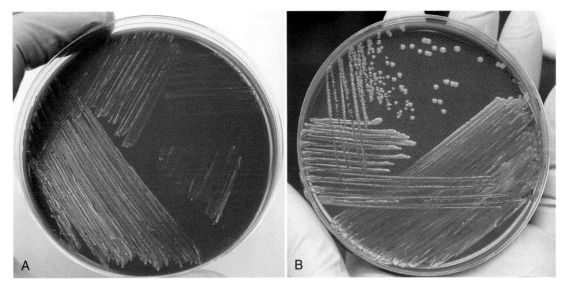

**Figure 36-1** Growth of *Brucella* spp. on chocolate agar after incubation for 2 days **(A)** and 4 days **(B)**.

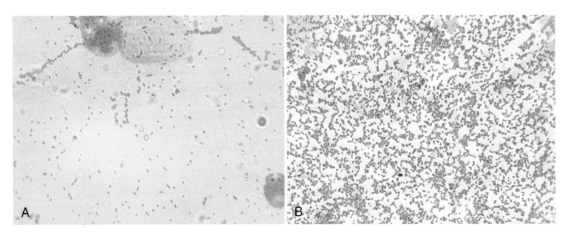

**Figure 36-2** *Brucella melitensis* with traditional Gram stain **(A)** and Gram stain with 2-minute safranin counterstain **(B)** to allow easier visualization of the organism.

Rough variants may be seen with *B. canis*. The colonies may become brownish with age.

## APPROACH TO IDENTIFICATION

Because brucellosis is the most commonly reported laboratory-acquired bacterial infection, all handling and manipulations of suspected *Brucella* spp. should be performed in a class II or higher biologic safety cabinet. On Gram stain, the organisms are small coccobacilli that resemble fine grains of sand (Figure 36-2). *Brucella* spp. are catalase and urease positive, and most strains are oxidase positive. Other nonfermentative gram-negative coccobacilli that may be confused with brucellae are *Bordetella*, *Moraxella*, *Kingella*, and *Acinetobacter* spp. *Brucella* spp., however, are nonmotile, urease and nitrate positive, and strictly aerobic. The most rapid test for presumptive identification of *Brucella* spp. is the particle agglutination test with anti–smooth *Brucella* serum (Difco Laboratories, Detroit, Michigan).

*Brucella* spp. are differentiated by the rapidity with which an organism hydrolyzes urea, its relative ability to produce hydrogen sulfide ($H_2S$), its requirements for $CO_2$, and its susceptibility to the aniline dyes thionine and basic fuchsin (Table 36-2). For determination of the $CO_2$ requirement, identical plates of Brucella agar or brain-heart infusion agar should be given equal inocula (e.g., with a calibrated loop) of a broth suspension of the organism to be tested. One plate should be incubated in a candle jar and the other plate in air in the same incubator. Most strains of *B. abortus* do not grow in air but show growth in the candle jar. Presumptive identification can be reported based on the colony's morphology and a positive catalase, oxidase, urease, and slide agglutination reaction (see next section). *Brucella* isolates should be sent to state or other reference laboratories for confirmation or definitive identification, because most clinical laboratories lack the necessary media and containment facilities.

Subtyping of biovars may be performed using a variety of molecular techniques, including pulsed-field electrophoresis, random amplification of polymorphic DNA, amplified fragment length polymorphism, various PCR techniques, and multilocus sequence typing.

**TABLE 36-2** Characteristics of *Brucella* spp. That Are Pathogenic for Humans

| Species | CO₂ Required for Growth | Time to Positive Urease | H₂S Produced | INHIBITION BY DYE Thionine* | Fuchsin* |
|---|---|---|---|---|---|
| *B. abortus* | ± | 2 hr (rare 24 hr) | + (most strains) | + | – |
| *B. melitensis* | – | 2 hr (rare 24 hr) | + | – | – |
| *B. suis* | – | 15 min | ± | – | + (most) |
| *B. canis* | – | 15 min | – | – | + |

+, >90% of strains positive; –, >90% of strains negative; ±, variable results.
*Dye tablets (Key Scientific Products, Round Rock, Texas).

## SERODIAGNOSIS

Because isolating brucellae is difficult, a serologic test is widely used (e.g., serum agglutination test [SAT] or microplate agglutination [MAT]). This technique detects antibodies to *B. abortus*, *B. melitensis*, and *B. suis*; however, the SAT does not detect *B. canis* antibodies. An indirect Coombs' test is performed after the SAT. This test detects nonagglutinating or incomplete antibodies in complicated and chronic cases of brucellosis.

The serology associated with *Brucella* infection follows the classic antibody response: IgM appears initially, followed by IgG. A titer of 1:160 or greater in the SAT is considered diagnostic if this result fits the clinical and epidemiologic findings. The SAT can cross-react with class M immunoglobulins with a variety of bacteria, such as *Francisella tularensis* and *Vibrio cholerae*. Enzyme-linked immunosorbent assays (ELISAs) also have been developed. Purified LPS or protein extracts are primarily used in ELISAs. However, currently no reference antigen exists; therefore, it is important to identify the antigen in the commercial antigen when evaluating test results. In patients with neurobrucellosis, ELISA offers significant diagnostic advantages over conventional agglutination methods.

Additional serologic assays are commercially available, including a lateral flow dipstick for screening outbreaks and an immunocapture agglutination method. The immunocapture assay demonstrates sensitivity and specificity similar to a Coombs' test and is less cumbersome to perform. The dipstick test has a high degree of sensitivity (greater than 90%).

## ANTIMICROBIAL SUSCEPTIBILITY TESTING AND THERAPY

Because of the fastidious nature of the brucellae and their intracellular localization, in vitro susceptibility testing is not reliable. To prevent relapse of infection, patients with brucellosis undergo prolonged treatment (6 weeks) with antibiotics that can penetrate macrophages and act in the acidic intracellular environment. For initial therapy, doxycycline or tetracycline in combination with streptomycin or rifampin is recommended. In some cases surgical drainage is also required to treat localized foci of infection.

## PREVENTION

Successful vaccines against *Brucella* infection have been developed for livestock. However, the development of human vaccines has met with serious medical contraindications and low efficacy. The prevention of brucellosis in humans depends on elimination of the disease in domestic livestock.

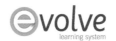 *Visit the Evolve site to complete the review questions.*

---

## CASE STUDY 36-1

A 67-year-old woman from the Middle East has total arthroplasty of the right knee, and 3 years later the same procedure is performed in the left knee. She seeks medical attention because of pain in her left knee. Her knee is aspirated, and a finding of 3600 WBCs/µL is reported, but no organisms are seen on Gram stain. Coagulase-negative staphylococci are grown from joint fluid cultured in blood culture bottles after 3 days of incubation. A few tiny, poorly staining gram-negative rods are present on the direct blood and chocolate agar plates after 5 days of incubation, but not in the blood culture. The rods are oxidase and catalase positive. A repeat culture 2 weeks later grows only the gram-negative rods. Surgical debridement with appropriate antimicrobial therapy results in control of the infection.

### QUESTIONS

1. When a fastidious, gram-negative coccobacilli is isolated from a normally sterile site, what is the first step that should be taken in the laboratory?
2. What rapid test can expedite the identification of this fastidious coccobacillus? Describe the limitations associated with this method.
3. How did this woman acquire the infection with this organism?
4. How is the diagnosis confirmed?

# BIBLIOGRAPHY

Boschiroli ML, Ouahrani-Betlache S, Foulongne V et al: Type IV secretion and *Brucella* virulence, *Vet Microbiol* 90:341, 2002.

Fortier AH, Green SJ, Polsinelli T et al: Life and death of an intracellular pathogen: *Francisella tularensis* and the macrophage, *Immunol Series* 60:349, 1994.

Hall WH: Modern chemotherapy for brucellosis in humans, *Rev Infect Dis* 12:1060, 1990.

Maria-Pilar J, Dudal S, Jacques D et al: Cellular bioterrorism: how *Brucella* corrupts macrophage physiology to promote invasion and proliferation, *Clin Immunol* 114:227, 2004.

Pappas G, Akritidis N, Bosilkovski M et al: Brucellosis, *N Engl J Med* 352:2325, 2005.

Radolf JD: Brucellosis: don't let it get your goat! *Am J Med Sci* 307:64, 1994.

Roy CR: Exploitation of the endoplasmic reticulum by bacterial pathogens, *Trends Microbiol* 10:418, 2002.

Smith LD, Ficht TA: Pathogenesis of *Brucella*, *Crit Rev Microbiol* 17:209, 1990.

Versalovic J: *Manual of clinical microbiology*, ed 10, Washington, DC, 2011, ASM Press.

Yagupsky P: Detection of *Brucella* in blood cultures, *J Clin Microbiol* 37:3437, 1999.

Yagupsky P: Detection of *Brucella melitensis* by BACTEC NR660 blood culture system, *J Clin Microbiol* 32:1899, 1994.

# Bordetella pertussis, Bordetella parapertussis, and Related Species

## OBJECTIVES

1. Describe the general characteristics of the *Bordetella* spp.
2. State the normal habitat and routes of transmission for *Bordetella pertussis* and *Bordetella parapertussis*.
3. Describe the three stages of pertussis, including the duration and symptoms.
4. Describe the proper collection and transport of specimens for the detection of *B. pertussis* and *B. parapertussis*.
5. Explain the limitations of direct fluorescent antibody (DFA) and polymerase chain reaction (PCR) methods for detecting *B. pertussis*, including assay specificity and sensitivity.
6. Describe the optimum condition for culturing *B. pertussis*, including specimens of choice for optimal recovery.
7. Outline the major tests used to identify and differentiate *B. pertussis* and *B. parapertussis*.
8. Correlate the patient's signs and symptoms and laboratory results to identify the etiologic agent associated with infection.

---

### GENERA AND SPECIES TO BE CONSIDERED

*Bordetella avium*
*Bordetella ansorpii*
*Bordetella bronchiseptica* (Chapter 25)
*Bordetella hinzii*
*Bordetella holmesii* (Chapter 21)
*Bordetella pertussis*
*Bordetella parapertussis* (Chapter 21)
*Bordetella petrii*
*Bordetella trematum* (Chapter 21)

---

The genus *Bordetella* includes three primary human pathogens: *Bordetella bronchiseptica*, *B. pertussis*, and *B. parapertussis*. *B. bronchiseptica* is reviewed in Chapter 25 because it grows on MacConkey agar. Although *B. parapertussis* also can grow on MacConkey agar, it is discussed with *B. pertussis* in this chapter for two reasons: *B. pertussis* and *B. parapertussis* both cause human upper respiratory tract infections, with almost identical symptoms, epidemiology, and therapeutic management; and optimal recovery of both organisms from respiratory specimens requires the addition of blood and/or other suitable factors to culture media. Additional *Bordetella* species may cause rare asymptomatic infections in immunocompromised patients; these include *B. hinzii*, *B. holmesii*, *B. petrii*, and *B. trematum*. (See the chapter cross-references in the preceding table for information on organisms not discussed in this chapter.)

## GENERAL CHARACTERISTICS

General features of *Bordetella* spp. other than *B. pertussis* and *B. parapertussis* are summarized in Chapter 25. In contrast to *B. bronchiseptica*, *B. pertussis* and *B. parapertussis* are nonmotile and infect only humans. In the evolutionary process, these exclusive human pathogens have a close genetic relationship. They remain separate species based on their differences in pathogenesis and host range.

### EPIDEMIOLOGY AND PATHOGENESIS

#### Epidemiology

Before the introduction of the vaccine (and currently in nonimmunized populations), pertussis (whooping cough) periodically became an epidemic disease that cycled approximately every 2 to 5 years. Transmission occurs person to person through inhalation of respiratory droplets. Humans are the only known reservoir.

Pertussis is a highly contagious, acute infection of the upper respiratory tract caused primarily by *B. pertussis* and less commonly by *B. parapertussis*. The latter agent generally has a less severe clinical presentation both in duration of symptoms and in the percentage of identified cases. Recently, *B. holmesii* was reported to cause a pertussis-like illness, but little is known about the biology, virulence mechanisms, and pathogenic significance. Pertussis was first described in the sixteenth century and occurs worldwide, totaling about 48.5 million cases annually. Although the incidence has decreased significantly since vaccination became widespread, outbreaks of pertussis occur periodically. *B. pertussis* infections appear to be endemic in adults and adolescents, most likely because of waning vaccine-induced immunity; these infections may serve as the source of the epidemic cycles involving unvaccinated or partially immunized infants and children.

#### Pathogenesis

*B. pertussis*, the primary pathogen of whooping cough, uses several mechanisms to overcome the immune defenses of healthy individuals. The mechanisms are complex and involve the interplay of several virulence factors (Table 37-1). Some factors help establish infection; others are toxigenic to the host; and still others override specific components of the host's mucosal defense system. For example, when *B. pertussis* reaches the host's respiratory tract, its surface adhesins attach to respiratory ciliated epithelial cells and paralyze the

**TABLE 37-1** Major Virulence Determinants of *Bordetella pertussis*

| Function | Factor/Structure |
|---|---|
| Adhesion (auto transporters) | Fimbriae (FIM), types 2 and 3: Serotype-specific agglutinins for colonization of respiratory mucosa.<br>Filamentous hemagglutinin (FHA): Mediates adhesion to the ciliated upper respiratory tract<br>Pertactin (PRN): Mediates eukaryotic cell binding and is highly immunogenic.<br>Tracheal colonization factor<br>Brk A* |
| Toxicity | Pertussis toxin (encoded by the *ptx* gene, an A/B toxin related to cholera toxin): Induces lymphocytosis and suppresses chemotaxis and oxidative responses in neutrophils and macrophages<br>Adenylate cyclase toxin: Hemolyzes red cells and activates cyclic adenosine monophosphate, thereby inactivating several types of host immune cells<br>Dermonecrotic toxin (exact role unknown)<br>Tracheal cytotoxin (ciliary dysfunction and damage)<br>Endotoxin (lipopolysaccharide)<br>Type III secretion† |
| Overcome host defenses | Outer membrane: Inhibits host lysozyme<br>Siderophore production: Prevents host lactoferrin and transferrin from limiting iron |

*Plays a role in pathogenesis by conferring serum resistance.
†This type of secretion allows *Bordetella* organisms to transport proteins directly into host cells; it is required for persistent tracheal colonization.

beating cilia by producing a tracheal cytotoxin. A major virulence factor, pertussis toxin (PT), is produced by the attached organism. PT enters the bloodstream, subsequently binding to specific receptors on host cells. After binding, PT disrupts several host cell functions, such as initiation of host cell translation; inability of host cells to receive signals from the environment causes a generalized toxicity. The center membrane of *B. pertussis* blocks access of the host's lysozyme to the bacterial cell wall via its outer membrane. *B. pertussis* and *B. parapertussis* share a nearly identical virulence control system encoded by the bvgAS locus that is responsive to variation in environmental conditions. Because of this very complex system, *Bordetella* organisms appear to be able to alter phenotypic expression, enhancing transmission, colonization, and survival.

# SPECTRUM OF DISEASE

Several factors influence the clinical manifestations of *B. pertussis* (Box 37-1). Classic pertussis is usually a disease of children and can be divided into three symptomatic stages: catarrhal, paroxysmal, and convalescent. During the catarrhal stage, symptoms are the same as for a mild cold with a runny nose and mild cough; this stage may last several weeks. Episodes of severe and violent coughing increase in number, marking the beginning of the paroxysmal stage. As many as 15 to 25 paroxysmal coughing episodes can occur in 24 hours; these are associated with vomiting and with "whooping," the result of air rapidly inspired into the lungs past the swollen glottis. Lymphocytosis occurs, although typically the patient has no fever and no signs and symptoms of systemic illness. This stage may last 1 to 4 weeks.

In addition to classic pertussis, *B. pertussis* can cause mild illness and asymptomatic infection, primarily in household contacts and in a number of unvaccinated and previously vaccinated children. Since the 1990s, a shift in the age distribution of pertussis cases to adolescence and adults has been observed in highly vaccinated populations. Adults and adolescents are now recognized as a reservoir for transmitting infection to vulnerable infants. Among these immunized individuals, a prolonged cough may be the only manifestation of pertussis; a scratchy throat, other pharyngeal symptoms, and episodes of sweating commonly occur in adults with pertussis. A number of studies have documented that 13% to 32% of adolescents and adults with an illness involving a cough of 6 days' duration or longer have serologic and/or culture evidence of *B. pertussis* infection.

Other *Bordetella* species have been associated with infection in immunocompromised patients. *B. bronchiseptica, B. holmesii,* and *B. hinzii* produce a pertussis-like respiratory illness. *B. trematum* has been isolated from individuals working with poultry, and *B. ansorpii* has been associated with septicemia.

# LABORATORY DIAGNOSIS

## SPECIMEN COLLECTION, TRANSPORT, AND PROCESSING

Confirming the diagnosis of pertussis is challenging. Culture, which is most sensitive early in the illness, has been the traditional diagnostic standard for pertussis and shows nearly 100% specificity but varied sensitivity. Organisms may become undetectable by culture 2 weeks after the start of paroxysms. Nasopharyngeal aspirates or a nasopharyngeal swab (calcium-alginate or Dacron on a wire handle) are acceptable specimens, because *B. pertussis* colonizes the ciliated epithelial cells of upper respiratory tract. Calcium-alginate swabs with aluminum shafts are not recommended for PCR, because they may inhibit the polymerase enzyme in PCR detection. In addition,

**TABLE 37-2** Examples of Selective Media for Primary Isolation of *B. pertussis* and *B. parapertussis*

| Agar Media | Description |
|---|---|
| Bordet-Gengou | Potato infusion agar with glycerol and sheep blood with methicillin or cephalexin* (short shelf-life) |
| Modified Jones-Kendrick charcoal | Charcoal agar with yeast extract, starch, and 40 μg cephalexin (2- to 3-month shelf-life but inferior to Regan-Lowe agar) |
| Regan-Lowe† | Charcoal agar with 10% horse blood and cephalexin (4- to 8-week shelf-life) |
| Stainer-Scholte | Synthetic agar lacking blood products |

*Cephalexin is superior to methicillin and penicillin for inhibiting normal respiratory flora.
†Regan-Lowe agar has been found to work best for recovery of *B. pertussis* from nasopharyngeal swabs.

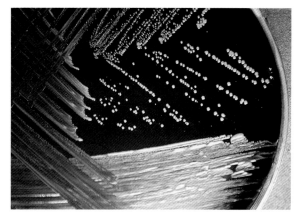

**Figure 37-1** Growth of *Bordetella pertussis* on Regan-Lowe agar.

cotton swabs may be inhibitory to specimen growth and are not recommended. Specimens obtained from the throat, sputum, or anterior nose are unacceptable, because these sites are not lined with ciliated epithelium. For collection, the swab is bent to conform to the nasal passage and held against the posterior aspect of the nasopharynx. If coughing does not occur, another swab is inserted into the other nostril to initiate the cough. The swab is left in place during the entire cough, removed, and immediately inoculated onto a selective medium at the bedside (Table 37-2).

Transport time is critical. A fluid transport medium may be used for swabs but must be held for less than 2 hours. Half-strength Regan-Lowe agar enhances recovery when used as a transport and enrichment medium. Cold casein hydrolysate medium and casamino acid broth (available commercially) have proved to be effective transport media, particularly for preparation of slides for direct fluorescent antibody staining. Dry swabs may be transported in ambient air for PCR testing.

## DIRECT DETECTION METHODS

A DFA stain using polyclonal antibodies against *B. pertussis* and *B. parapertussis* is commercially available for detection of *B. pertussis* in smears made from nasopharyngeal (NP) material (Becton Dickinson, Sparks, Maryland); an NP specimen that is DFA positive for *B. pertussis* is shown in Figure 6-15, *B*. Although rapid, this DFA stain has limited sensitivity and variable specificity; therefore, the DFA test should always be used in conjunction with culture. DFA monoclonal reagent is also commercially available with two antisera with different fluorophores to detect *B. pertussis* and *B. parapertussis* (Accu-Mab, Altachem Pharma, Edmonton, Canada).

Because of the limitations associated with culture and serologic diagnostic methods, significant effort has been put into developing nucleic acid amplification methods. Most diagnostic studies use direct detection of *B. pertussis*

and *B. parapertussis* by various PCR procedures, including real-time PCR. These assays have a diagnostic sensitivity at least comparable (and in most cases superior) to that of culture. A word of caution: Positive results have been obtained with samples containing *B. holmesii* and *B. bronchiseptica* (see Chapter 25) depending on the sequence targeted in conventional and real-time PCR assays. Most laboratories use transposon insertion sequences IS481 for *B. pertussis* and IS1001 for *B. parapertussis*. However, strains of *B. holmesii*, *B. parapertussis*, and *B. bronchiseptica* that carry IS481 have been identified; therefore, careful interpretation of results and correlation with the clinical presentation are required. Additional PCR assays are available for the detection of the pertussis toxin, fimbriae, pertactin and a porin gene. However, because these are single-copy genes and not multicopy insertion sequences, assay sensitivity is reduced. Nasopharyngeal swabs (rayon or Dacron swabs on plastic shafts) and aspirates are the two types of samples primarily used for pertussis PCR; calcium-alginate swabs are unacceptable, as previously mentioned, because these inhibit PCR-based detection.

## CULTIVATION

Plates are incubated at 35°C in a humidified atmosphere without elevated carbon dioxide for up to 12 days. Most isolates are detected in 3 to 7 days; *B. parapertussis* appears in 2 to 3 days. Colony morphology is not distinct for the identification of other *Bordetella* spp.

Regan-Lowe agar, Bordet-Gengou agar, and Stainer-Scholte synthetic medium are suitable culture media. Regan-Lowe agar contains beef extract, starch, casein digest, and charcoal supplemented with horse blood. Bordet-Gengou agar is a potato fusion base containing glycerol and either sheep or horse blood. Most media contain cephalexin as an additive for suppression of contaminating organisms. Young colonies of *B. pertussis* and *B. parapertussis* are small and shiny, resembling mercury drops; colonies become whitish gray with age (Figure 37-1).

Sensitivity of culture approaches 100% in the best of hands and depends on the stage of illness at the time of

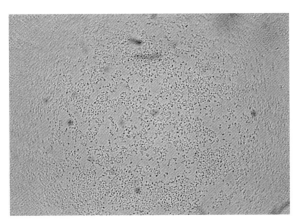

**Figure 37-2** Typical Gram stain appearance of *Bordetella pertussis.*

**TABLE 37-3** Characteristics That Differentiate *Bordetella* spp.

| Characteristic | B. pertussis | B. parapertussis | B. bronchiseptica |
|---|---|---|---|
| Catalase | + | + | + |
| Oxidase | + | − | + |
| Motility | − | − | + |
| Nitrate | − | − | + |
| Urease | − | + (24 hours) | + (4 hours) |
| **Growth** Regan-Lowe agar | 3-6 days | 2-3 days | 1-2 days |
| Blood agar | − | + | + |
| MacConkey agar | − | +/− | + |

specimen collection, the technique used for specimen collection, specimen adequacy and transport, and culture conditions.

## APPROACH TO IDENTIFICATION

A Gram stain of the organism reveals minute, faintly staining coccobacilli singly or in pairs (Figure 37-2). Use of a 2-minute safranin "O" counterstain or a 0.2% aqueous basic fuchsin counterstain enhances their visibility. *Bordetella* spp. characteristics are presented in Table 37-3. The DFA reagent is used to presumptively identify organisms. Whole-cell agglutination reactions in specific antiserum can be used for species identification.

## SERODIAGNOSIS

Although several serologic tests are available for the diagnosis of pertussis, including agglutination, complement fixation, and enzyme immunoassay, no single method can be recommended for serologic diagnosis at this time.

The current most reliable serologic test available for diagnosis is an anti-PT (antibody to pertussis toxin) enzyme-linked immunosorbent assay (ELISA) that has been used with acute and paired convalescent sera successfully in older children, adolescents, and adults. A titer greater than 100 to 125 IU/mL has been reported as a reliable indicator of exposure of patients to PT-producing bacteria.

## ANTIMICROBIAL SUSCEPTIBILITY TESTING AND THERAPY

Laboratories currently do not perform routine susceptibility testing of *B. pertussis* and *B. parapertussis,* because the organisms remain susceptible to erythromycin or the newer macrolides (clarithromycin, azithromycin), ketolides, quinolones, and other antibiotics, such as tetracyclines, chloramphenicol, and trimethoprim-sulfamethoxazole. However, three erythromycin-resistant isolates of *B. pertussis* have been discovered; therefore, continued surveillance of *B. pertussis* is advised. Both *B. pertussis* and *B. parapertussis* are resistant to most oral cephalosporins. Caution is recommended when antimicrobial susceptibility testing for *Bordetella* spp. is considered, because no standardized procedure currently exists.

## PREVENTION

Whole-cell vaccines to prevent pertussis, made from various *B. pertussis* preparations, are manufactured in many countries and are efficacious in controlling epidemic pertussis. However, because of reactions to these vaccines and an apparent lack of long-term immunity, new acellular vaccines have replaced whole-cell vaccines in the United States and elsewhere. In addition, some countries, such as Germany, France, and Canada, now recommend routine vaccination of adolescents. The United States uses three different formulas for diphtheria, tetanus, and pertussis vaccines. Children should receive five doses of DTaP vaccine before they are 6 years of age. Adolescents between 11 and 18 years of age and adults 19 to 64 years of age should receive a single dose of Tdap. Td vaccine can be given as a booster for adults every 10 years. Prompt recognition of clinical cases and treatment of contacts and cases also are very important in preventing the transmission of *B. pertussis* and *B. parapertussis;* viable organisms can be recovered from untreated patients for 3 weeks after the onset of cough. To prevent nosocomial outbreaks, patients with suspected or confirmed pertussis should be placed on droplet precautions.

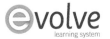 *Visit the Evolve site to complete the review questions.*

## CASE STUDY 37-1

A 36-year-old female surgeon is discharged from the hospital after an uncomplicated delivery of a healthy second child. Three days after arriving home, she awakes with a fever, malaise, and nonproductive cough. An induced sputum specimen grows *Pseudomonas aeruginosa*. She is admitted to the hospital and treated with ceftazidime and tobramycin. Her white blood cell count on admission is 13,500/mm$^3$, and scattered, coarse rhonchi are heard on deep inspiration. The rest of the family is in good health. The Infectious Disease Service (IDS) does not believe that the patient has *Pseudomonas* pneumonia and suggests that a nasopharyngeal aspirate be collected for *Bordetella pertussis* PCR, even though the patient is feeling better. The laboratory performs the test, and the result is positive. Subsequent culture on Regan-Lowe medium is positive for the organism (see Figure 37-1).

### QUESTIONS

1. Why was the IDS so interested in having the diagnosis correct in a patient whose disease was improving?
2. Pertussis in young and older adults is underdiagnosed. What are some of the reasons?
3. Why is the pertussis PCR assay so sensitive?
4. What biochemical tests uniquely identify *B. pertussis*?

## ≡ BIBLIOGRAPHY

Cattaneo LA, Reed GW, Haase DH et al: The seroepidemiology of *Bordetella pertussis* infections: a study of persons ages 1 to 65 years, *J Infect Dis* 173:1257, 1996.

Cherry JD: Historical review of pertussis and the classical vaccine, *J Infect Dis* 174(suppl 3):S259, 1996.

Fernandez RC, Weiss AA: Cloning and sequencing of a *Bordetella pertussis* serum resistance locus, *Infect Immunol* 62:4727, 1994.

Gordon KA, Fusco J, Biedenback DJ et al: Antimicrobial susceptibility testing of clinical isolates of *Bordetella pertussis* from Northern California: report from the SENTRY antimicrobial surveillance program, *Antimicrob Agents Chemother* 45:3599, 2001.

Guris D, Strebel PM, Bardenheier B et al: Changing epidemiology of pertussis in the United States: increasing reported incidence among adolescents and adults, 1990-1996, *Clin Infect Dis* 28:1230, 1999.

Hewlett EL, Edwards KM: Pertussis: not just for kids, *N Engl J Med* 352:1215, 2005.

Hoppe JE, Vogl R: Comparison of three media for cultures of *Bordetella pertussis*, *Eur J Clin Microbiol* 5:361, 1986.

Katzko C, Hofmeister M, Church D: Extended incubation of culture plates improves recovery of *Bordetella* spp., *J Clin Microbiol* 34:1563, 1996.

Mastrantonio P, Stefanelli P, Giuliano M et al: *Bordetella parapertussis* infection in children: epidemiology, clinical symptoms, and molecular characteristics of isolates, *J Clin Microbiol* 36:999, 1998.

Mattoo S, Cherry JD: Molecular pathogenesis, epidemiology, and clinical manifestations of respiratory infections due to *Bordetella pertussis* and other *Bordetella* species, *Clin Microbiol Rev* 18: 326, 2005.

Rappuoli R: Pathogenicity mechanisms of *Bordetella*, *Curr Top Microbiol Immunol* 192:319, 1994.

Stauffer LR, Brown DR, Sandstrom RE: Cephalexin-supplemented Jones-Kendrick charcoal agar for selective isolation of *Bordetella pertussis*: comparison with previously described media, *J Clin Microbiol* 17:60, 1983.

Versalovic J: *Manual of clinical microbiology*, ed 10, 2011, Washington, DC, ASM Press.

Weiss A: Mucosal immune defenses and the response of *Bordetella pertussis*, *ASM News* 63:22, 1997.

Yih WK, Silva EA, Ida JH et al: *Bordetella holmesii*–like organisms isolated from Massachusetts patients with pertussis-like symptoms, *Emerg Infect Dis* 5:441, 1999.

# Francisella

## OBJECTIVES

1. List the media of choice for optimal recovery and cultivation of *Francisella tularensis*.
2. Describe the optimal incubation conditions for *F. tularensis*.
3. Describe the normal habitat and means of transmission of *Francisella* spp.
4. Describe the symptoms of tularemia and differentiate the various clinical presentations, including ulceroglandular, glandular, oculoglandular, oropharyngeal, systemic (typhoidal), and pneumonic tularemia.

---

**GENERA AND SPECIES TO BE CONSIDERED**

*Francisella tularensis*
   subsp. *tularensis* (type A): includes three subclades (A1a, A1b, A2)
   subsp. *holartica* (type B): includes 10 different subclades
   subsp. *mediasiatica*
*Francisella noatunensis* (formerly *F. philomiragia* subsp. *noatunensis*)
*Francisella novicida*
*Francisella philomiragia*

---

Blood, chocolate, and Thayer-Martin agars can be used for the primary isolation of organisms belonging to the genus *Francisella*. *Francisella* organisms are facultative, intracellular pathogens that require cysteine, cystine, or another sulfhydryl and a source of iron for enhanced growth. They thus require a complex medium for isolation and growth.

## GENERAL CHARACTERISTICS

Organisms belonging to the genus *Francisella* are faintly staining, tiny, gram-negative coccobacilli that are oxidase and urease negative, catalase-positive, nonmotile, non–spore forming, strict aerobes. The taxonomy of this genus continues to be in flux. Current members of the genus share greater than 97% identity based on 16SrRNA sequence analysis. The most current proposed taxonomy is summarized in Table 38-1. For the most part, different subspecies are associated with different geographic regions.

## EPIDEMIOLOGY AND PATHOGENESIS

Francisellaceae are widely distributed throughout the environment. *F. tularensis* is the agent of human and animal tularemia. *F. novicida* and *F. philomiragia* are present in the environment and are opportunistic human pathogens. Worldwide in distribution, *F. tularensis* is carried by many species of wild rodents, rabbits, beavers, and muskrats in North America. Humans become infected by handling the carcasses or skin of infected animals; by inhaling infective aerosols or ingesting contaminated water; through insect vectors (primarily deerflies and ticks in the United States); and by being bitten by carnivores that have themselves eaten infected animals. Some evidence indicates that francisellae can persist in waterways, possibly in association with amebae.

Most cases in the United States are sporadic, occurring during the summer months, and most cases are seen in the states of South Dakota, Arkansas, Missouri, and Oklahoma.

The capsule of *F. tularensis* appears to be a necessary component for expression of full virulence, allowing the organism to avoid immediate destruction by polymorphonuclear neutrophils. In addition to being extremely invasive, *F. tularensis* is an intracellular parasite that can survive in the cells of the reticuloendothelial system, where it resides after a bacteremic phase. Granulomatous lesions may develop in various organs. Humans are infected by fewer than 50 organisms by either aerosol or cutaneous routes. *F. tularensis* subsp. *tularensis* is the most virulent for humans, with an infectious dose of less than 10 colony forming units. *F. philomiragia* has been isolated from several patients, many of whom were immunocompromised or victims of near-drowning incidents. The organism is present in animals and ground water.

## SPECTRUM OF DISEASE

The disease associated with *F. tularensis*, known as *tularemia*, is recognized worldwide. In the United States the clinical manifestations have been referred to as rabbit fever, deer fly fever, and market men's disease. The clinical manifestation depends on the mode of transmission, the virulence of the infecting organism, the immune status of the host, and the length of time from infection to diagnosis and treatment. The typical clinical presentation after inoculation of *F. tularensis* through abrasions in the skin or by arthropod bites includes the development of a lesion at the site and progresses to an ulcer; lymph nodes adjacent to the site of inoculation become enlarged and often necrotic. Once the organism enters the bloodstream, patients become systemically ill with high temperature, chills, headache, and generalized aching. Clinical manifestations of infection with *F. tularensis* range from mild and self-limiting to fatal; they include glandular, ulceroglandular, oculoglandular, oropharyngeal, systemic, and pneumonic forms. These clinical presentations are briefly summarized in Table 38-2.

**TABLE 38-1** Most Recent Taxonomy of the Genus *Francisella* and Key Characteristics

| Organism | Primary Region | Disease in Humans | Requires Cystine/Cysteine |
|---|---|---|---|
| *F. tularensis* subsp. *tularensis* | North America (United States and Canada) | Most severe: Tularemia (all forms, see Table 38-2) | + |
| *F. tularensis* subsp. *holartica* | Europe, former Soviet Union, Japan, North America | Least severe: Tularemia (all forms) | + |
| *F. tularensis* subsp. *mediasiatica* | Kazakhstan, Uzbekistan | Severe: Tularemia | + |
| *F. noatunensis* (formerly *F. philomiragia* subsp. *noatunensis*) | North and South America | Emerging pathogen of fish; no human infections identified | − |
| *F. novicida* | North America | Mild illness; virulent in immunocompromised patients | − |
| *F. philomiragia* (formerly *Yersinia philomiragia*) | North America | Mild illness; virulent only in immunocompromised individuals and near-drowning victims | − |

**TABLE 38-2** Clinical Manifestations of *Francisella tularensis* Infection

| Types of Infection | Clinical Manifestations and Description |
|---|---|
| Ulceroglandular | Common; ulcer and lymphadenopathy; rarely fatal |
| Glandular | Common; lymphadenopathy; rarely fatal |
| Oculoglandular | Conjunctivitis, lymphadenopathy |
| Oropharyngeal | Ulceration in the oropharynx |
| Systemic (typhoidal) tularemia | Acute illness with septicemia; 30% to 60% mortality rate; no ulcer or lymphadenopathy |
| Pneumonic tularemia | Acquired by inhalation of infectious aerosols or by dissemination from the bloodstream; pneumonia; most serious form of tularemia |

# LABORATORY DIAGNOSIS

*F. tularensis* is a Biosafety Level 2 pathogen, a designation that requires technologists to wear gloves and to work in a biologic safety cabinet (BSC) when handling clinical material that potentially harbors this agent. The organism is designated Biosafety Level 3 when the laboratorian is working with cultures; therefore, a mask is recommended for the handling of all clinical specimens and is very important for preventing aerosol acquisition of *F. tularensis*. Because tularemia is one of the most common laboratory-acquired infections, most microbiologists do not attempt to work with infectious material from suspected patients. It is recommended that specimens be sent to reference laboratories or state or other public health laboratories that are equipped to handle *Francisella* spp.

## SPECIMEN COLLECTION, TRANSPORT, AND PROCESSING

The most common specimens submitted to the laboratory are scrapings from infected ulcers, lymph node biopsies, and sputum. Whole blood is an acceptable specimen for all types of tularemia; however, false-negative results may occur during early stages of disease. Serum is generally collected from all patients early in disease and during convalescence. The blood should be separated from the serum as soon as possible, preferably within 24 hours, and may be stored at 2° to 8°C for up to 10 days. If long-term storage is required, the serum may be frozen. To minimize the loss of viable organisms, samples should be transported to the laboratory within 24 hours. If specimens are to be held longer than 24 hours, specimens should be refrigerated in Amie's transport medium. *F. tularensis* should remain viable for up to 7 days stored at ambient temperature in Amie's medium. Swab specimens should be placed in Amie's transport media containing charcoal. Specimens for molecular testing should be placed in guanidine isothiocyanate buffer for up to 1 month.

Specimen collection for the identification of *F. tularensis* is highly dependent on the type of clinical manifestation. A detailed description of the recommended type of specimen associated with the patient's clinical presentation is presented in Table 38-3. In light of recent events and concerns about bioterrorism, laboratories must keep in mind that isolation of *F. tularensis* from blood cultures might be considered a potential bioterrorist attack; *F. tularensis* is considered one of the Select Biological Agents of Human Disease (see Chapter 80).

## DIRECT DETECTION METHODS

Gram staining of clinical material is of little use with primary specimens unless the concentration of organisms is high, as in swabs from wounds or ulcers, tissues, and respiratory aspirates. The organisms tend to counterstain poorly with safranin. Replacing safranin with basic fuchsin may enhance identification. Fluorescent

**TABLE 38-3** Recommended Specimen Type Based on Clinical Manifestation

| | CLINICAL MANIFESTATION | | | | | |
|---|---|---|---|---|---|---|
| | Ulceroglandular | Glandular | Oculoglandular | Oropharyngeal | Typhoidal | Pneumonic |
| Whole blood | X | X | X | X | X | X |
| Serum | X | X | X | X | X | X |
| Pharyngeal swabs, bronchial/tracheal washes or aspirates, sputum, transthoracic lung aspirates, and pleural fluid | | | | X | X | X |
| Swabs from visible lesions | X | | X | | | |
| Aspirates from lymph nodes or lesions | X | X | X | | | |

antibody stains and immunohistochemical stains are commercially available for direct detection of the organism in lesion smears and tissues and are typically available in reference laboratories. Conventional and real-time polymerase chain reaction (PCR) assays have been developed to detect *F. tularensis* directly in clinical specimens. Of significance, several patients with clinically suspected tularemia with negative serology and culture had detectable DNA by PCR. Currently most PCR-based assays are unable to discriminate *F. tularensis* from *F. novicida*, which limits the value of the epidemiologic data.

## CULTIVATION

Isolation of *F. tularensis* is difficult. The organism is strictly aerobic and is enhanced by enriched media containing sulfhydryl compounds (cysteine, cystine, thiosulfate or IsoVitaleX) for primary isolation. Two commercial media for cultivation of the organism are available: glucose cystine agar (BBL; Microbiology Systems, Sparks, Maryland) and cystine-heart agar (Difco Laboratories, Detroit, Michigan); both require the addition of 5% sheep or rabbit blood. *F. tularensis* also may grow on chocolate agar supplemented with IsoVitaleX, the nonselective buffered charcoal-yeast extract agar (BCYE) used for isolation of legionellae, or modified Mueller-Hinton broth and tryptic soy broth supplemented with 1% to 2% IsoVitaleX. Growth is not enhanced by carbon dioxide.

These slow-growing organisms require 2 to 4 days for maximal colony formation; they are weakly catalase positive and oxidase negative. Some strains may require up to 2 weeks to develop visible colonies. *F. philomiragia* is less fastidious than *F. tularensis*. Although *F. philomiragia* does not require cysteine or cystine for isolation, it is similar to *F. tularensis* in that it is a small, coccobacillary rod that grows poorly or not at all on MacConkey agar. This organism grows well on heart infusion agar with 5% rabbit blood or BCYE agar with or without cysteine. *F. tularensis* can be detected in commercial blood culture systems in 2 to 5 days; because these organisms Gram stain poorly, an acridine orange stain may be required to visualize the organisms in a positive blood culture bottle.

**BOX 38-1** Indications of a Possible *Francisella* Species

- Unusual Gram stain: small, poorly staining gram-negative rods seen mostly as single cells or amorphous gram-negative mass without distinct cell forms *(F. philomiragia)*
- Subcultures yield primarily pinpoint colonies on chocolate agar
- Oxidase-negative; weak or negative catalase test
- Negative satellite or X and V tests
- Small, gram-negative coccobacillus observed in a Gram-stained smear of a positive blood culture in which time to detection is longer than 24 hours
- Organism requires prolonged incubation on chocolate agar

## APPROACH TO IDENTIFICATION

Colonies are transparent, mucoid, and easily emulsified. Although carbohydrates are fermented, isolates should be identified serologically (by agglutination) or by a fluorescent antibody stain. Ideally, isolates should be sent to a reference laboratory for characterization.

*F. philomiragia* differs from *F. tularensis* biochemically; *F. philomiragia* is oxidase-positive by Kovac's modification, and most strains produce hydrogen sulfide in triple sugar iron agar medium, hydrolyze gelatin, and grow in 6% sodium chloride (no strains of *F. tularensis* share these characteristics).

In previous reports, problems have been identified in association with *Francisella* species isolated from clinical specimens. Twelve microbiology employees were exposed to *F. tularensis* even though bioterrorism procedures were in place; the organism had been isolated from blood, respiratory, and autopsy specimens and grew on chocolate agar. In this situation, multiple cultures were worked up on open benches without any additional personal protective equipment for what had been thought to be most consistent with a *Haemophilus* species. As a result of this report, microbiologists must be aware of not only the key characteristics of this group of organisms (Box 38-1), but also the possible pitfalls in their identification (e.g., some strains grow well on sheep blood agar;

identification kits may incorrectly suggest an identification of *Actinobacillus actinomycetemcomitans*). If *F. tularensis* is suspected, all culture Petri dishes should be taped from the top to the bottom in two places to keep them together for safety purposes.

## SERODIAGNOSIS

Because of the risk of infection to laboratory personnel and other inherent difficulties with culture, diagnosis of tularemia is usually accomplished serologically by whole-cell agglutination (febrile agglutinins or newer enzyme-linked immunosorbent assay techniques). Serum antibody detection is useful for all forms of tularemia. After the initial specimen, a convalescent sample should be collected at 14 days and preferable up to 3 to 4 weeks after the appearance of symptoms. A fourfold difference in titers in acute versus convalescent phase serum samples, in conjunction with one additional positive diagnostic test, such as culture or molecular tests, is considered a presumptive diagnosis for tularemia.

## ANTIMICROBIAL SUSCEPTIBILITY TESTING AND THERAPY

No standardized antimicrobial susceptibility test exists for *Francisella* spp. The organism is susceptible to aminoglycosides, and streptomycin is the drug of choice. Gentamicin is a possible alternative; doxycycline and chloramphenicol also have been used, although these two agents have been associated with a higher rate of relapse after treatment. Fluoroquinolones appear promising for treatment of even severe tularemia.

## PREVENTION

The primary means of preventing tularemia is to reduce the possibility of exposure to the etiologic agent in nature, such as by wearing protective clothing to prevent insect bites and by refraining from handling dead animals. An investigative live-attenuated vaccine is available.

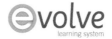 *Visit the Evolve site to complete the review questions.*

---

## CASE STUDY 38-1

A 36-year-old man with human immunodeficiency virus (HIV) infection had been doing well on a prophylactic regimen. After camping in Yosemite National Yosemite Park, he presents to his physician for a nonhealing, erythematous, 3-mm "cyst" on his neck. He had been treated with ampicillin-sulbactam without resolution, so a biopsy is performed. No organisms are seen on Gram staining, but the culture grows a tiny, gram-negative rod only on chocolate agar after 3 days of incubation (Figure 38-1). The microbiologist finds the organism to be oxidase and urease negative but weakly catalase positive. It does not satellite around a staphylococcal dot on blood agar. A beta-lactamase test result is positive. The patient is treated with a 4-week course of ciprofloxacin, and the lesion resolves.

### QUESTIONS

1. The local health department identifies the isolate as *Francisella tularensis* by PCR and by fluorescent stain. What do you think is the most commonly misidentified genus and species submitted as *F. tularensis?* What test differentiates these two organisms?
2. The isolate is oxidase and urease negative but weakly catalase positive. After it is determined to be negative for satelliting around a staphylococcal dot on blood agar, what precautions should be taken when working with the culture?
3. Why is a beta-lactamase test performed?

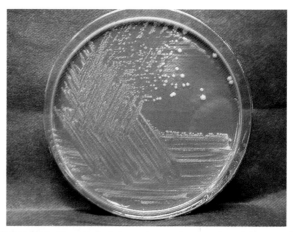

**Figure 38-1** *Francisella tularensis* growing on chocolate agar after 72 hours of incubation. (Courtesy Mary K. York.)

# BIBLIOGRAPHY

Craven R, Barnes AM: Plague and tularemia, *Infect Dis Clin North Am* 5:165, 1991.

Ellis J, Oyston PC, Green M et al: Tularemia, *Clin Microbiol Rev* 15:631, 2002.

Enderlin G, Morales L, Jacobs RF et al: Streptomycin and alternative agents for the treatment of tularemia: review of the literature, *Clin Infect Dis* 19:42, 1994.

Fortier AH, Green SJ, Polsinelli T et al: Life and death of an intracellular pathogen: *Francisella tularensis* and the macrophage, *Immunol Series* 60:349, 1994.

Friis-Møller A, Lemming LE, Valerius NH et al: Problems in identification of *Francisella philomiragia* associated with fatal bacteremia in a patient with chronic granulomatous disease, *J Clin Microbiol* 42:1840, 2004.

Hollis DG, Weaver RE, Steigerwalt AG et al: *Francisella philomiragia* comb nov (formerly *Yersinia philomiragia*) and *Francisella tularensis* biogroup *novicida* (formerly *Francisella novicida*) associated with human disease, *J Clin Microbiol* 27:1601, 1989.

Limaye AP, Hooper CJ: Treatment of tularemia with fluoroquines: two cases and review, *Clin Infect Dis* 29:922, 1999.

Mandell GL, Bennett JE, Dolin R, editors: *Principles and practice of infectious diseases*, ed 7, Philadelphia, 2010, Churchill Livingstone/Elsevier.

Shapiro DS, Schwartz DR: Exposure of laboratory workers to *Francisella tularensis* despite a bioterrorism procedure, *J Clin Microbiol* 40:2278, 2002.

Sjöstedt A: Virulence determinants and protective antigens of *Francisella tularensis*, *Curr Opin Microbiol* 6:66, 2003.

Versalovic J: *Manual of clinical microbiology*, ed 10, Washington, DC, 2011, ASM Press.

# *Streptobacillus moniliformis* and *Spirillum minus*

## OBJECTIVES

1. Describe the natural habitats of *Streptobacillus moniliformis* and *Spirillum minus*.
2. List the two ways in which *S. moniliformis* is transmitted to humans.
3. Define Haverhill fever, rat-bite fever, and sodoku.
4. List the symptoms of rat-bite fever.
5. Describe the optimal conditions for culturing *S. moniliformis*, including media, supplements, atmospheric conditions, and length of incubation.
6. Describe the different appearances of *S. moniliformis* colonial morphology when grown on various media.
7. Describe how *S. minus* is detected in the laboratory.
8. Compare and contrast the microscopic appearance of *S. minus* and *S. moniliformis* in Gram-stained or other smears.

---

### GENERA AND SPECIES TO BE CONSIDERED

*Streptobacillus moniliformis*
*Spirillum minus*

---

*S*treptobacillus moniliformis is a gram-negative bacillus that requires media containing blood, serum, or ascites fluid as well as incubation under carbon dioxide ($CO_2$) for isolation from clinical specimens. This organism causes rat-bite fever and Haverhill fever in humans. *Spirillum minus* has never been grown in culture but, because both are causative agents of rat-bite fever, these organisms are considered in this chapter.

## STREPTOBACILLUS MONILIFORMIS

### GENERAL CHARACTERISTICS

The genus *Streptobacillus* is a member of the Fusobacteriaceae family. The *Streptobacillus* genus has only one species, *S. moniliformis*, a facultative, nonmotile anaerobe that tends to be highly pleomorphic.

### EPIDEMIOLOGY AND PATHOGENESIS

The natural habitat of *S. moniliformis* is the upper respiratory tract (nasopharynx, larynx, upper trachea, and middle ear) of wild and laboratory rats (mice, gerbils, squirrels, ferrets, weasels); in addition, this organism occasionally has been isolated from other animals, such as cats and dogs that have fed on rodents. *S. moniliformis* is pathogenic for humans and is transmitted by two routes:

- Rat bite, or possibly through direct contact with rat feces or saliva
- Ingestion of contaminated food, such as unpasteurized milk or milk products and, less frequently, water

The incidence of *S. moniliformis* infections is unknown, but human infections appear to occur worldwide.

The pathogenic mechanisms of *S. moniliformis* are unknown. The organism is known to spontaneously develop L forms (bacteria without cell walls), which may allow its persistence in some sites.

### SPECTRUM OF DISEASE

Despite the different modes of transmission, the clinical manifestations of *S. moniliformis* infection are similar. When *S. moniliformis* is acquired by ingestion, the disease is called *Haverhill fever*.

Patients with rat-bite or Haverhill fever develop acute onset of chills, fever, headache, vomiting, and often severe joint pains. Febrile episodes may persist for weeks or months. In the first few days of illness, patients develop a rash on the palms, soles of the feet, and other extremities. Complications can occur, including endocarditis, septic arthritis, pneumonia, pericarditis, brain abscess, amnionitis, prostatitis, and pancreatitis.

### LABORATORY DIAGNOSIS

#### Specimen Collection, Transport, and Processing

Unfortunately, the diagnosis of rat-bite fever caused by *S. moniliformis* is often delayed because of lack of exposure history, an atypical clinical presentation, and the unusual microbiologic characteristics of the organism. Organisms may be cultured from blood or aspirates from infected joints, lymph nodes, or lesions. No special requirements have been established for the collection, transport, and processing of these specimens except for blood. Because recovering *S. moniliformis* from blood cultures is impeded by concentrations of sodium polyanethol sulfonate (SPS) used in blood culture bottles, an alternative to most commercially available bottles must be used. After collection by routine procedures (described in Chapter 68), blood and joint fluids are mixed with equal volumes of 2.5% citrate to prevent clotting and are then inoculated to brain-heart infusion cysteine broth supplemented with heated horse serum and yeast extract, commercially available fastidious anaerobe broth without SPS, or thiol broth.

#### Direct Detection Methods

Pus or exudates should be smeared, stained with Gram or Giemsa stain, and examined microscopically (Figure 39-1). *S. moniliformis* is a pleomorphic, gram-negative rod.

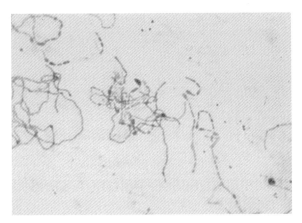

**Figure 39-1** Gram stain of *Streptobacillus moniliformis* from growth in thioglycollate broth with 20% serum. (Courtesy Robert E. Weaver, Centers for Disease Control and Prevention, Atlanta, Ga.)

Cells may appear straight of variable size or as long tangled chains and filaments with bulbar swellings. The cells may also appear spiral shaped and resemble a string of pearls. Direct detection of the 16sRNA gene sequence for *S. moniliformis* using polymerase chain reaction (PCF) analysis has been described.

### Cultivation

As previously mentioned, *S. moniliformis* requires the presence of blood, ascitic fluid, or serum for growth. Growth occurs on blood agar, incubated in a very moist environment with 5% to 10% carbon dioxide ($CO_2$), usually after 48 hours of incubation at 37°C. Colonies are nonhemolytic. The addition of 10% to 30% ascitic fluid (available commercially from some media suppliers) or 20% horse serum should facilitate recovery of the organism. In broth cultures, the organism grows as "fluff balls" or "bread crumbs" near the bottom of the tube of broth or on the surface of the sedimented red blood cell layer in blood culture media. Colonies grown on brain-heart infusion agar supplemented with 20% horse serum are small, smooth, glistening, colorless or grayish and have irregular edges.

Colonies are embedded in the agar and may also have a "fried egg" appearance, with a dark center and a flattened, lacy edge. These colonies are also referred to as *L-phase colonies* because they have undergone spontaneous transformation to the L form. Staining of L-form colonies yields coccobacillary or bipolar-staining coccoid forms (usually a special stain, such as the Dienes stain performed by pathologists), is required. Acridine orange stain also reveals the bacteria when Gram stain fails because of lack of cell wall constituents.

As previously stated, Gram-stained organisms from standard colonies show extreme pleomorphism, with long, looped, filamentous forms, chains, and swollen cells. The club-shaped cells can be 2 to 5 times the diameter of the filament. Carbolfuchsin counterstain or Giemsa stain may be necessary for visualization (see Figure 39-1).

### Approach to Identification

*S. moniliformis* does not produce indole and is catalase, oxidase, and nitrate negative, in contrast to organisms with which the *Streptobacillus* sp. may be confused, such as *Actinobacillus* spp., *Haemophilus aphrophilus*, and *Cardiobacterium* spp. In addition, *S. moniliformis* is nonmotile and urea and lysine decarboxylase negative; hydrogen sulfide ($H_2S$) is not produced in triple sugar iron agar but can be detected using lead acetate paper.

### Serodiagnosis

Serologic diagnosis of rat-bite fever is also useful; most patients develop agglutinating titers to the causative organism. The specialized serologic tests are performed only at national reference laboratories, because the disease is extremely rare in the United States. A titer of 1:80 is considered diagnostic unless a fourfold rise in titer is demonstrated.

## ANTIMICROBIAL SUSCEPTIBILITY TESTING AND THERAPY

No standardized methods have been established for determining *S. moniliformis* susceptibility to various antimicrobials. Different in vitro techniques, such as agar dilution and disk diffusion, have had similar results. Although *S. moniliformis* is susceptible to a broad spectrum of antibiotics, penicillin is regarded as the drug of choice for human rat-bite fever. An aminoglycoside or tetracycline can be used to eliminate L forms or for patients allergic to penicillin.

## PREVENTION

There are no vaccines available to prevent rat-bite fever. Disease is best prevented by avoiding contact with animals known to harbor the organism. Individuals with frequent animal contact should wear gloves, practice regular handwashing and avoid hand-to-mouth contact when handling rats or cleaning rat cages.

## *SPIRILLUM MINUS*

### GENERAL CHARACTERISTICS

*Spirillum minus* is a gram-negative, helical, strictly aerobic organism.

### EPIDEMIOLOGY AND PATHOGENESIS

Little information is available regarding the epidemiology or pathogenesis of *S. minus*, but it is supposed to be similar in some regards to that of *S. moniliformis*. The mode of transmission of infection is by a rat bite.

### SPECTRUM OF DISEASE

*S. minus* also causes rat-bite fever in humans and is referred to as sodoku. The clinical signs and symptoms are similar to those caused by *S. moniliformis*, except that arthritis is rarely seen in patients with sodoku and swollen lymph nodes are prominent; febrile episodes are also more predictable in sodoku. The bite wound heals spontaneously, but 1 to 4 weeks later, it reulcerates to form a granulomatous lesion; at the same time, the patient develops constitutional symptoms of fever, headache, and a generalized, blotchy, purplish, maculopapular rash. Differentiation between rat-bite fever caused by *S. minus* and that caused by *S. moniliformis* is usually accomplished based on the clinical presentation of the two infections and isolation of the latter organism in culture. The incubation period for *S. minus* is much longer than that for streptobacillary rat-bite fever, which has occurred within 12 hours of the initial bite.

## LABORATORY DIAGNOSIS

### Specimen Collection, Transport, and Processing

Specimens commonly submitted for diagnosis of sodoku include blood, exudate, or lymph node tissues. There are no requirements for specimen collection, transport, or processing of the organisms discussed in this chapter. Refer to Table 5-1 for general information on this subject.

### Direction Detection Methods

Because *S. minus* cannot be grown on synthetic media, diagnosis relies on direct visualization of characteristic spirochetes in clinical specimens using Giemsa or Wright stains, or dark-field microscopy. *S. minus* appears as a thick, spiral, gram-negative organism with two or three coils and polytrichous polar flagella. Diagnosis is definitively made by injection of lesion material or blood into experimental white mice or guinea pigs and subsequent recovery 1 to 3 weeks after inoculation.

### Serodiagnosis

There is no specific serologic test available for *S. minus* infection.

## ANTIMICROBIAL SUSCEPTIBILITY TESTING AND THERAPY

Because this spirochete is nonculturable, routine antimicrobial susceptibility testing is not performed.

## PREVENTION

No vaccines are available to prevent rat-bite fever. Disease is best prevented by avoiding contact with animals known to harbor the organism.

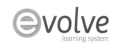 *Visit the Evolve site to complete the review questions.*

---

## CASE STUDY 39-1

An 8-year-old girl presented with a 7-day history of worsening flulike illness with fever, cough, and arthralgias. By admission, the arthralgia was so severe that she refused to walk. A rash was noted on the dorsal surface of her hands and feet. The pediatrician suspected *Streptobacillus moniliformis* because the child had a pet rat that slept with her. The rat had never bitten her, but she did carry it around her neck. A routine blood culture was drawn. A second blood culture was collected in a tube and plated to blood and chocolate agars. A third culture was collected. Doxycycline was then started and over the next few days the patient did well. The first and second cultures remained negative, but the third culture attempt was positive in less than 24 hours with a gram-negative rod. Subcultures of the bottle to blood, chocolate, *Brucella* (aerobic and anaerobic), and *Legionella* selective agars incubated in $CO_2$ were negative at 48 hours.

### QUESTIONS

1. Why did the laboratory set up a culture with more blood than recommended by the manufacturer?
2. Because *S. moniliformis* was suspected and there was no growth on any of the subcultures at 48 hours, what can the laboratory do to grow the organism on a plated medium to identify it?
3. How is the organism definitively identified?

---

## BIBLIOGRAPHY

Buranakitjaroen P, Nilganuwong S, Gherunpong V: Rat bite fever caused by *Streptobacillus moniliformis*, *Southeast Asian J Trop Med Public Health* 25:778, 1994.

Freundt EA: Experimental investigations into the pathogenicity of the L-phase variant of *Streptobacillus moniliformis*, *Acta Pathol Microbiol Scand* 38:246, 1956.

Lambe DW Jr, McPhedran AM, Mertz JA et al: *Streptobacillus moniliformis* isolated from a case of Haverhill fever: biochemical characterization and inhibitory effect of sodium polyanethol sulfonate, *Am J Clin Pathol* 60:854, 1973.

McEvoy MB, Noah ND, Pilsworth R: Outbreak of fever caused by *Streptobacillus moniliformis*, *Lancet* ii:1361, 1987.

Rupp ME: *Streptobacillus moniliformis* endocarditis: case report and review, *Clin Infect Dis* 14:769, 1992.

Shanson D, Pratt J, Green P: Comparison of media with and without "Panmede" for the isolation of *Streptobacillus moniliformis* from blood cultures and observations on the inhibitory effect of sodium polyanethol sulfonate, *J Med Microbiol* 19:181, 1985.

Versalovic J: *Manual of clinical microbiology*, ed 10, Washington, DC, 2011, ASM Press.

Wullenweber M: *Streptobacillus moniliformis*: a zoonotic pathogen—taxonomic considerations, host species, diagnosis, therapy, geographical distribution, *Lab Anim* 29:1, 1985.

# *Neisseria* and *Moraxella catarrhalis*

## OBJECTIVES

1. Identify the clinical specimens or sources for the isolation of pathogenic *Neisseria* spp.
2. List the *Neisseria* species considered normal flora and the sites where they colonize the human body.
3. Explain the routes of transmission for the organisms discussed in this chapter; include the clinical relevance of asymptomatic carriers.
4. Define and describe the diseases associated with *Moraxella catarrhalis* and the pathogenic *Neisseria* spp., *Neisseria gonorrhoeae* and *Neisseria meningitidis* (i.e., pelvic inflammatory disease, disseminated gonococcal infection, ophthalmia neonatorum, pharyngitis, meningitis, and septicemia); include the signs and symptoms, treatments, and prognosis.
5. Describe the method of transport that yields optimal recovery of *N. gonorrhoeae*, including transport media, growth temperatures, and atmospheric conditions.
6. Describe the benefits of amplified testing for *N. gonorrhoeae* over nonamplified testing as it relates to financial, diagnostic and clinical efficacy, and control measures.
7. Identify the optimal growth conditions for the *Neisseria* species.
8. Name the appropriate biochemical tests for differentiating the *Neisseria* species and explain the chemical principle for each test.
9. Biochemically differentiate the organisms in this chapter using carbohydrate utilization (cysteine trypticase agar [CTA]) and orthonitrophenyl galactoside (ONPG).
10. Describe the appropriate therapeutic agents for *N. gonorrhoeae*.
11. Compare and contrast the laboratory identification of *M. catarrhalis* and *Neisseria* spp.
12. Analyze laboratory data and disease signs and symptoms for correlation and identification of the etiologic agents discussed in this chapter.

---

### GENERA AND SPECIES TO BE CONSIDERED

| Current Name | Previous Name |
|---|---|
| *Moraxella catarrhalis* | *Branhamella catarrhalis, Neisseria catarrhalis* |
| *Neisseria gonorrhoeae* | |
| *Neisseria meningitidis* | |
| **Other *Neisseria* spp.** | |
| *N. animaloris* | CDC group EF-4a |
| *N. cinerea* | |
| *N. lactamica* | |
| *N. polysaccharea* | |
| *N. subflava* | *N. subflava, N. flava,* and *N. perflava* |
| *N. sicca* | |
| *N. mucosa* | |
| *N. flavescens* | |

## GENERAL CHARACTERISTICS

Species of the family Neisseriaceae, genus *Neisseria*, are discussed in this chapter, along with family Moraxellaceae, species *Moraxella catarrhalis*, because of their biochemical and morphologic similarities. The organisms are all oxidase-positive, gram-negative diplococci that do not elongate when exposed to subinhibitory concentrations of penicillin. The rodlike *Neisseria* spp. are described in Chapter 28.

## EPIDEMIOLOGY

Except for *Neisseria gonorrhoeae*, the organisms considered in Table 40-1 are normal inhabitants of the upper respiratory tract of humans. Humans are the only natural host for *N. gonorrhoeae*, primarily a clinically significant pathogen found in the urogenital tract and never considered normal flora. Asymptomatic carriers of gonorrhea are the primary reservoir for dissemination in the human population. The number of reported and identified cases of infection with *N. gonorrhoeae* is probably significantly higher than statistical data indicate because of the number of unreported cases.

The two pathogenic species of *Neisseria*, *N. gonorrhoeae* and *N. meningitidis*, are transmitted person to person. *N. gonorrhoeae* is sexually transmitted, and *N. meningitidis* is spread via contaminated respiratory droplets. Infections caused by *M. catarrhalis* and the other *Neisseria* spp. usually involve a patient's endogenous strain.

## PATHOGENESIS AND SPECTRUM OF DISEASE

As noted in Table 40-2, infections caused by *M. catarrhalis* are usually localized to the respiratory tract and rarely disseminate.

*N. gonorrhoeae* is a leading cause of sexually transmitted disease, and infections caused by this organism usually are localized to the mucosal surfaces where the host is initially exposed to the organism (e.g., cervix, conjunctiva, pharyngeal surface, anorectal area, or urethra of males). Localized infections may be asymptomatic or acute with a pronounced purulent response. Not all infections remain localized, and dissemination from the

**TABLE 40-1** Epidemiology

| Organism | Habitat (Reservoir) | Mode of Transmission |
|---|---|---|
| *Moraxella catarrhalis* | Normal human flora of upper respiratory tract; occasionally colonizes female genital tract | Spread of patient's endogenous strain to normally sterile sites. Person-to-person nosocomial spread by contaminated respiratory droplets also can occur |
| *Neisseria gonorrhoeae* | Not part of normal human flora. Only found on mucous membranes of genitalia, anorectal area, oropharynx, or conjunctiva at time of infection | Person-to-person spread by sexual contact, including rectal intercourse and orogenital sex. May also be spread from infected mother to newborn during birth. Asymptomatic carriers are a significant reservoir for increased disease transmission. |
| *Neisseria meningitidis* | Colonizes oropharyngeal and nasopharyngeal mucous membranes of humans. Humans commonly carry the organism without symptoms | Person-to-person spread by contaminated respiratory droplets, usually in settings of close contact |
| Other *Neisseria* spp. | Normal human flora of the upper respiratory tract | Spread of patient's endogenous strain to normally sterile sites. Person-to-person spread may also be possible, but these species are not common causes of human infections |
| *Neisseria animaloris* | Not part of normal human flora. Animal oral and respiratory commensal organism | Animal contact, particularly bites or scratches from dogs and cats |

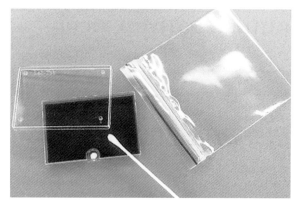

**Figure 40-1** JEMBEC system. Plate contains modified Thayer-Martin medium. The $CO_2$-generating tablet is composed of sodium bicarbonate and citric acid. After inoculation the tablet is placed in the well, and the plate is closed and placed in the zip-lock plastic pouch. The moisture in the agar activates the tablet, generating a $CO_2$ atmosphere in the pouch.

The other *Neisseria* spp. are not considered pathogens and are often referred to as the *saprophytic Neisseria*. Although they are most commonly encountered as contaminants in clinical specimens, they may occasionally be identified in bacteremia and endocarditis.

# LABORATORY DIAGNOSIS

## SPECIMEN COLLECTION AND TRANSPORT

The pathogenic *Neisseria* spp. described in this chapter are very sensitive to drying and temperature extremes. In addition to general information on specimen collection and transport provided in Table 5-1, there are some special requirements for isolation of *N. gonorrhoeae* and *N. meningitidis*.

Swabs are acceptable for *N. gonorrhoeae* testing if the specimen will be plated within 6 hours; however, reduced recovery may result within 30 minutes of collection. If cotton swabs are used, the transport medium should contain charcoal (Ames medium) to inhibit toxic fatty acids present in the fibers. Calcium alginate has also been found to be inhibitory. Dacron or rayon fibers are recommended. *N. gonorrhoeae* should be inoculated to growth media immediately after specimen collection. The sample should then be placed in a container able to sustain an atmosphere of increased carbon dioxide ($CO_2$) during transport. Specially packaged media consisting of selective agar in plastic trays that contain a $CO_2$-generating system are commercially available (JEMBEC plates). The JEMBEC system (Figure 40-1) is transported to the laboratory at room temperature. Upon receipt in the laboratory, the agar surface is cross-streaked to obtain isolated colonies, and the plate is incubated at 35°C in 3% to 5% $CO_2$. Additional commercial transport systems that may be useful, particularly when the collection site is separate from the diagnostic laboratory, are the Bio-Bag, Gono-Pak, and Transgrow.

initial infection site can lead to severe disseminated disease (see Table 40-2). Isolates with nutritional requirements for arginine, hypoxanthine, and uracil (AHU strains) are often isolated from disseminated infections, most often from women although also from asymptomatic males.

*N. meningitidis* is a leading cause of fatal bacterial meningitis. However, the virulence factors responsible for the spread of this organism from a patient's upper respiratory tract to the bloodstream and meninges, causing life-threatening infections, are not fully understood (see Table 40-2).

**TABLE 40-2** Pathogenesis and Spectrum of Disease

| Organism | Virulence Factors | Spectrum of Disease and Infections |
|---|---|---|
| *Moraxella catarrhalis* | Uncertain; factors associated with cell envelope probably facilitate attachment to respiratory epithelial cells | Most infections are localized to sites associated with the respiratory tract and include otitis media, sinusitis, and pneumonia. Lower respiratory tract infections often target elderly patients and those with chronic obstructive pulmonary disease. Rarely causes disseminated infections such as bacteremia or meningitis. |
| *Neisseria gonorrhoeae* | Several surface factors, such as pili (types T1-T2 virulent and T3-T5 avirulent), mediate the exchange of genetic material between strains and attachment to human mucosal cell surface, invasion of host cells, and survival through the inhibition of phagocytosis in the presence neutrophils.<br>Genetic-phase variation of pilus structure between types T1 through T5 allows the organism to vary its antigenic structure, preventing recognition by host immune cells.<br>Capsule, lipooligosaccharide (endotoxin), and outer cell membrane proteins I-III are important in antigenic variation and for eliciting an inflammatory response.<br>Protein II (Opa) facilitates adherence to phagocytic and epithelial cells.<br>Protein II (RMP) blocks the bactericidal effect of host IgG.<br>Outer membrane porin (PorB) provides protection from the host's immune response, including serum complement–mediated cell death. | A leading cause of sexually transmitted diseases. Genital infections include acute purulent urethritis, prostatitis, and epididymitis in males and acute cervicitis in females. These infections also may be asymptomatic in females.<br>Other localized infections include pharyngitis, anorectal infections, and conjunctivitis (e.g., ophthalmia neonatorum of newborns acquired during birth from an infected mother).<br>Disseminated infections result when the organism spreads from a local infection to cause pelvic inflammatory disease or disseminated gonococcal infection that includes bacteremia, arthritis, and metastatic infection at other body sites.<br>Pelvic inflammatory disease (PID) may cause sterility, ectopic pregnancy or perihepatitis also referred to as Fitz-Hugh–Curtis syndrome. |
| *Neisseria meningitidis* | Surface structures, perhaps pili, facilitate attachment to mucosal epithelial cells and invasion to the submucosa. Once in the blood, survival is mediated by production of a polysaccharide capsule. Endotoxin release mediates many of the systemic manifestations of infection, such as shock.<br>Cellular proteins are similar to those described for *N. gonorrhoeae*, including Por and Opa. Two porin proteins are produced (PorA and PorB).<br>IgA protease degrades membrane-associated IgA, increasing the host's susceptibility to invasion. | Life-threatening, acute, purulent meningitis. Meningitis may be accompanied by appearance of petechiae (i.e., rash) that is associated with meningococcal bacteremia (i.e., meningococcemia). Bacteremia leads to thrombocytopenia, disseminated intravascular coagulation, and shock. Disseminated disease is often fatal. Less common infections include conjunctivitis, pneumonia, and sinusitis. |
| Other *Neisseria* spp. | Unknown; probably of low virulence | Rarely involved in human infections. When infections occur, they can include bacteremia, endocarditis, and meningitis. |
| *Neisseria animaloris* | Unknown | Cellulitis or abscess formation secondary to infected bite wounds; systemic infection (rare). |

Recovery of *N. gonorrhoeae* or *N. meningitidis* from normally sterile body fluids requires no special methods, except for blood cultures. Both organisms are sensitive to sodium polyanethol sulfonate (SPS), the preservative typically found in blood culture broths. If a blood culture broth is inoculated, the SPS content should not exceed 0.025%. In addition, if blood is first collected in Vacutainer tubes containing SPS (Becton Dickinson, Sparks, Maryland), the specimen must be transferred to the broth culture system within 1 hour of collection.

Nasopharyngeal swabs collected to detect *N. meningitidis* carriers should be plated immediately to the JEMBEC system, or they should be submitted on swabs placed in charcoal transport media.

## SPECIMEN PROCESSING

The JEMBEC system should be incubated at 35° to 37°C as soon as the plate is received in the laboratory. Body fluids (e.g., joint or cerebrospinal fluid [CSF]) should be stored until cultured at 37°C, because both gonococci and meningococci are sensitive to cold.

Any volume of clear fluid greater than 1 mL suspected of containing either of these pathogens should be centrifuged at room temperature at 1500× g for 15 minutes. The supernatant fluid should then be removed and the sediment should be vortexed and inoculated onto the appropriate media (described later).

Any specimens or cultures in which *N. meningitidis* is a consideration should be handled in a biological safety cabinet to avoid laboratory-acquired infections.

## DIRECT DETECTION METHODS

### Gram Stain

The members of the genus *Neisseria* discussed in this chapter and *M. catarrhalis* appear as gram-negative diplococci (Figure 40-2) with adjacent sides flattened. They

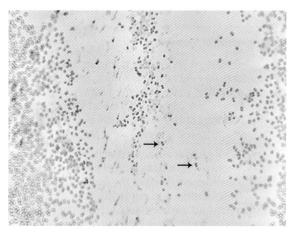

**Figure 40-2** Gram stain of *Neisseria gonorrhoeae* showing gram-negative diplococci *(arrows)*.

are often referred to as "kidney bean"–shaped diplococci. Direct Gram staining of urethral discharge from symptomatic males with urethritis is an important test for gonococcal disease. The appearance of gram-negative diplococci inside polymorphonuclear leukocytes is diagnostic in this situation. However, because the normal vaginal and rectal flora are composed of gram-negative coccobacilli, which can resemble *Neisseria* spp., direct examination of endocervical secretions in symptomatic women is only presumptive evidence of gonorrhea, and the diagnosis must be confirmed by culture. In addition, avirulent strains (i.e., pili types 3 to 5) may be present as extracellular diplococci; these are not pathogenic. Pharyngeal specimens should not be Gram stained, because nonpathogenic, commensal *Neisseria* spp. may be present, and these are not diagnostic of infection.

The direct Gram stain of body fluids for either *N. gonorrhoeae* or *N. meningitidis* is best accomplished using a cytocentrifuge, which can concentrate small numbers of organisms 100-fold.

### Commercial Molecular Assays

Molecular assays have replaced old enzyme-linked immunosorbent assay systems for rapid diagnosis of *N. gonorrhoeae*. The U.S. Food and Drug Administration (FDA) has cleared a number of amplified and nonamplified tests. (For a discussion of molecular technology, see Chapter 8.) The nonamplified DNA probe assay, PACE 2 (Hologic, Inc., Bedford, MA), has a chemiluminescent detection system for direct detection of gonococcal ribosomal RNA (rRNA) in genital and conjunctival specimens. This test performs well in high-risk patients, is rapid (results are available in 2 hours), and is suitable for screening many patients simultaneously. The Gen-Probe Accuprobe test targets rRNA after lysis of bacteria; the rRNA is detected using a single-strand chemiluminescent DNA probe. The hybrids are then detected in a luminometer. In addition, the Digene CT/GC Dual ID HC2 (HC2; Qiagen) detects RNA-DNA hybrids using antibody-mediated recognition of the hybrids and visualization of a chemiluminescent substrate.

Amplified assays, which are more sensitive than the nonamplified assay, are commercially available from

Roche Diagnostic Systems. They include the AMPLICOR and COBAS AMPLICOR PCR (Branchburg, New Jersey) and the Hologic Gen-Probe Aptima Combo 2 transcription-mediated amplification (Bedford, MA) and other tests produced by other manufacturers. The ProbeTec ET (Becton Dickinson, Sparks, Maryland) also is available. These tests are suitable for large-scale screening programs, but none are admissible as evidence in medicolegal cases. An advantage of all molecular assays is the ability to test for *Chlamydia trachomatis* from the same specimen at the same time. *N. gonorrhoeae* DNA can be found in a specimen for up to 3 weeks after successful treatment, so amplified molecular assays should not be used to assess cure.

Molecular assays have also been developed to detect *N. meningitidis*. Sequence-based typing methods combined with serologic typing are currently recommended. Molecular targets for identification include PCR and sequencing of a variety of genes, including PorA, PorB, FetA (associated with PorA), global housekeeping genes, penA (penicillin susceptibility) and Factor H binding protein.

Following the manufacturer's recommendations is important in evaluating molecular diagnostic tests to identify *Neisseria* spp. Some of the assays have limitations with regard to the type of specimen that may be used, cross-reactivity with nonpathogenic species, and assay inhibition and false-negative results caused by substances present in patient samples.

### Antigen Detection

The detection of *Neisseria meningitidis* capsular polysaccharide antigen in body fluids (e.g., urine, serum, CSF) is no longer recommended in the United States.

## CULTIVATION

### Media of Choice

*N. meningitidis*, *M. catarrhalis*, and saprophytic *Neisseria* spp. grow well on 5% sheep blood and chocolate agars. *N. gonorrhoeae* is more fastidious and requires an enriched chocolate agar for growth on primary culture. Because gonococci and sometimes meningococci must be isolated from sites that contain large numbers of normal flora (e.g., genital tract or upper respiratory tract), selective media have been developed to facilitate their recovery. The first of these was Thayer-Martin medium, a chocolate agar with an enrichment supplement (IsoVitaleX) and the antimicrobials colistin (to inhibit gram-negative bacilli), nystatin (to inhibit yeast), and vancomycin (to inhibit gram-positive bacteria). This original medium was subsequently modified to include trimethoprim (to inhibit swarming *Proteus* spp.), and its name was changed to modified Thayer-Martin medium (MTM). Martin-Lewis (ML) medium is similar to MTM except that anisomycin, an antifungal agent, is substituted for nystatin and the concentration of vancomycin is increased. GC-LECT agar is a selective medium that contains additional antimicrobials to inhibit bacteria found in oropharyngeal specimens; it includes vancomycin and lincomycin (to inhibit gram-positive bacteria), colistin (to inhibit gram-negative bacteria), amphotericin B (to

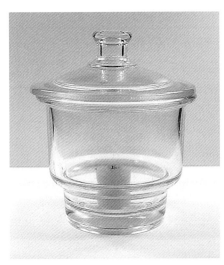

**Figure 40-3** Candle jar.

**TABLE 40-3** Colonial Appearance and Other Characteristics on Chocolate Agar*

| Organism | Appearance |
| --- | --- |
| *Moraxella catarrhalis* | Large, nonpigmented or gray, opaque, smooth; friable "hockey puck" consistency; colony may be moved intact over surface of agar |
| *Neisseria gonorrhoeae* | Small, grayish white, convex, translucent, shiny colonies with either smooth or irregular margins; may be up to five different colony types on primary plates |
| *N. meningitidis* | Medium, smooth, round, moist, gray to white; encapsulated strains are mucoid; may be greenish cast in agar underneath colonies |
| *N. animaloris* | Some strains exhibit yellow to tan pigment; odor resembles popcorn |
| *N. cinerea* | Small, grayish white; translucent; slightly granular |
| *N. flavescens* | Medium, yellow, opaque, smooth |
| *N. lactamica* | Small, nonpigmented or yellowish, smooth, transparent |
| *N. mucosa* | Large, grayish white to light yellow, translucent; mucoid because of capsule |
| *N. polysaccharea* | Small, grayish white to light yellow, translucent, raised |
| *N. sicca* | Large, nonpigmented, wrinkled, coarse and dry, adherent |
| *N. subflava* | Medium, greenish yellow to yellow, smooth, entire edge |

*Appearance on blood agar is the same as on chocolate agar except for pigmentation; colonies are less opaque on blood agar.

inhibit yeast), and trimethoprim (to inhibit swarming *Proteus* spp. and *Capnocytophaga* spp.).

New York City (NYC) medium, a transparent medium containing lysed horse blood, horse plasma, yeast dialysate, and the same antibiotics as MTM, also has been used. The advantage of NYC medium is that genital mycoplasmas (*Mycoplasma hominis* and *Ureaplasma urealyticum;* see Chapter 45) also grow on this agar. Some strains of *N. gonorrhoeae* are inhibited by the concentration of vancomycin in the selective media, so the addition of nonselective chocolate agar is recommended, especially in suspect cases that are culture negative or for sterile specimens (e.g., joint fluid).

Unlike the pathogenic species, some of the saprophytic *Neisseria* spp. (*N. flavescens, N. mucosa, N. sicca,* and *N. subflava*) may grow on MacConkey agar, although poorly. *N. gonorrhoeae* and *N. meningitidis* will grow in most broth blood culture media but grow poorly in common nutrient broths such as thioglycollate and brain-heart infusion. *M. catarrhalis* and the other *Neisseria* spp. grow well in almost any broth medium.

### Incubation Conditions and Duration

Agar plates should be incubated at 35° to 37°C for 72 hours in a $CO_2$-enriched, humid atmosphere. *N. gonorrhoeae, N. meningitidis,* and *M. catarrhalis* grow best under conditions of increased $CO_2$ (3% to 7%). This atmosphere can be achieved using a candle jar, $CO_2$-generating pouch, or $CO_2$ incubator. Only white, unscented candles should be used in candle jars, because other types may be toxic to *N. gonorrhoeae* and *N. meningitidis.*

Humidity can be provided by placing a pan with water in the bottom of a $CO_2$ incubator or by placing a sterile gauze pad soaked with sterile water in the bottom of a candle jar (Figure 40-3).

### Colonial Appearance

Table 40-3 describes the colonial appearance and other distinguishing characteristics (e.g., pigment) of *M. catarrhalis* and the *Neisseria* spp. on chocolate agar.

## APPROACH TO IDENTIFICATION

Various commercial systems are available for the rapid identification of the coccoid *Neisseria* spp. and *M. catarrhalis.* Some of these systems are described briefly in Table 13-1. These systems employ biochemical or enzymatic substrates and work very well for the pathogenic species (*N. gonorrhoeae, N. meningitidis,* and *M. catarrhalis*). A heavy inoculum of the organism is required, but because these systems detect the activity of preformed enzymes, viability of the organisms in the inoculum is not essential. Manufacturers' instructions should be followed exactly; several systems have been developed only for strains isolated on selective media and should not be used to test other gram-negative diplococci.

### Biochemical Identification

Table 40-4 presents some conventional biochemical tests that traditionally have been used to identify these organisms definitively. The extent to which identification of isolates is carried out depends on the source of the specimen and the suspected species of the organism involved.

An isolate from a child or a person involved in a case of sexual abuse must be identified unequivocally because

**TABLE 40-4** Biochemical and Physiologic Characteristics of *Moraxella catarrhalis* and Coccoid *Neisseria* spp.

| | GROWTH ON: | | | RAPID FERMENTATION SUGARS | | | | | |
|---|---|---|---|---|---|---|---|---|---|
| Organism | Modified Thayer-Martin* | Nutrient Agar at 35°C | Blood or Chocolate Agar at 25°C | Glucose | Maltose | Lactose | Nitrate Reduction | Gas from Nitrate Reduction | 0.1% Nitrite Reduction |
| *Moraxella catarrhalis*[†] | v | + | + | − | − | − | + | − | v |
| *Neisseria cinerea*[‡] | v | + | − | −[§] | − | − | − | − | + |
| *N. flavescens* | − | + | + | − | − | − | − | − | +[‖] |
| *N. gonorrhoeae*[¶] | + | − | − | + | − | − | − | − | − |
| *N. lactamica* | + | v | v | + | + | + | − | − | + |
| *N. meningitidis* | + | − | − | + | + | − | − | − | v |
| *N. mucosa* | − | + | + | + or (+) | + | − | + | + | + |
| *N. sicca*[#] | − | + | + | + or (+) | + | − | − | − | + |
| *N. subflava*[#] | − | + | + | v | + | − | − | − | + |

Data compiled from Janda WM, Knapp JS: *Neisseria* and *Moraxella catarrhalis.* In Murray PR, Baron EJ, Jorgensen JH et al, editors: *Manual of clinical microbiology,* ed 8, Washington, DC, 2003, ASM Press; and Weyant RS, Moss CW, Weaver RE et al, editors: *Identification of unusual pathogenic gram-negative aerobic and facultatively anaerobic bacteria,* ed 2, Baltimore, 1996, Williams & Wilkins.

+, >90% of strains positive; (+), >90% of strains positive but reaction may be delayed (i.e., 2 to 7 days); −, >90% of strains negative; *v,* variable.
*Growth defined as >10 colonies.
[†]Butyrate and DNase positive.
[‡]*Neisseria cinerea* may be differentiated from *N. flavescens* by a positive reaction with the amylosucrase test.
[§]Some strains of *N. cinerea* may appear glucose-positive in some rapid systems and be mistaken for *N. gonorrhoeae.* However, *N. cinerea* grows on nutrient agar at 35°C and reduces nitrite, unlike the gonococcus.
[‖]Only 2 of 10 strains were tested.
[¶]*Kingella denitrificans* may grow on modified Thayer-Martin agar and be mistaken for *N. gonorrhoeae* on microscopic examination. However, *K. denitrificans* can reduce nitrate and is catalase-negative, unlike the gonococcus.
[#]*Neisseria subflava* produces a yellow pigment on Loeffler's agar; *N. sicca* does not.

of the medicolegal ramifications of these results. It is recommended that these organisms be identified using at least two different types of tests; that is, biochemical, immunologic, enzymatic, or the nonamplified DNA probe previously discussed. Isolates from normally sterile body fluids should also be completely identified. However, isolates from genital sites in adults at risk of sexually transmitted disease (STD) can be identified presumptively; that is, oxidase-positive, gram-negative diplococci that grow on gonococcal selective agar. Likewise, an oxidase-positive, gram-negative diplococcus that hydrolyzes tributyrin from an eye or ear culture can be identified as *M. catarrhalis* (see Figure 13-8).

### Comments About Specific Organisms

Determination of carbohydrate utilization patterns historically has been performed in cysteine trypticase soy agar (CTA) with 1% dextrose, maltose, lactose, and sucrose (see Procedure 40-1 on the Evolve site). This medium is no longer widely used, because it does not work well for oxidative *Neisseria* spp., specifically *N. gonorrhoeae* and *N. meningitidis.* Therefore, carbohydrate utilization patterns are currently determined by inoculating an extremely heavy suspension of the organism to be tested in a small volume of buffered, low-peptone substrate with the appropriate carbohydrate. These methods do not require subculture or growth, and results are available in approximately 4 hours. Commercially available methods include the Rim-*Neisseria* Test (Rapid Identification Method–*Neisseria*) (Remel Laboratories), the

*Neisseria* Kwik Test (Micro-Biologics) and the Gonobio Test (I.A.F Production).

The saprophytic *Neisseria* spp. are not routinely identified in the clinical laboratory. *N. cinerea* may be misidentified as *N. gonorrhoeae* if the isolate produces a weak positive glucose reaction. However, it grows on nutrient agar at 35°C, whereas the gonococcus does not. Moreover, *N. cinerea* is inhibited by colistin, whereas *N. gonorrhoeae* is not.

*M. catarrhalis* can be differentiated from the gonococci and meningococci based on its growth on blood agar at 22°C and on nutrient agar at 35°C, the reduction of nitrate to nitrite, its inability to utilize carbohydrates, and its production of DNase. *M. catarrhalis* is the only member of this group of organisms that hydrolyzes DNA.

Chromogenic substrate enzyme tests for beta-galactosidase, gamma-glutamyl aminopeptidase, and prolyl-hydroxylprolyl aminopeptidase are available for the differentiation of *N. gonorrhoeae,* *N. meningitidis,* *N. lactamica,* and *M. catarrhalis. M. catarrhalis* lacks all three of these enzymes. The presence of prolyl-hydroxylprolyl aminopeptidase alone identifies an organism as *N. gonorrhoeae.* The presence of beta-galactosidase and gamma-glutamyl aminopeptidase indicates *N. meningitidis.* Two commercial chromogenic substrate kits are the Gonocheck II (EY Laboratories, San Mateo, California) and BactiCard *Neisseria* (Remel Laboratories, Lenexa, Kansas). A limitation of these methods is misidentification of various nonpathogenic strains of *Neisseria* spp. In addition, isolate colonies on selective media should be used to avoid misidentification of contaminants as a *Neisseria* spp. Modified chromogenic substrate kits, such as the Bacti-Card *Neisseria,* can be used to identify and speciate *Neisseria* and *Haemophilus* organisms from selective and nonselective media. These modified tests use a combination of enzyme substrate tests and additional biochemical tests.

*N. lactamica* may grow on selective media and may be confused with *N. meningitidis.* The ONPG test (Procedure 13-33) is used to determine an organism's ability to produce beta-galactosidase, which is an indicator of lactose utilization. *N. lactamica* is ONPG positive, and *N. gonorrhoeae* is ONPG negative.

The eugonic fermenter *N. animaloris* propagates well on routine laboratory media and ferments glucose; this distinguishes it from dysgonic fermenters that grow poorly on blood and chocolate agars (see Chapter 31). *N. animaloris* ferments no carbohydrates other than glucose and is indole negative and arginine dihydrolase positive.

### Immunoserologic Identification

Particle agglutination methods are available for immunoserologic identification of *N. gonorrhoeae.* They include the Phadebact GC OMNI test (Karo Bio Diagnostics AB, Huddinge, Sweden), the MicroTrak Culture Confirmation test (Trinity Biotech, Bray, Ireland), and the GonoGen II test (Becton Dickinson, Sparks, Maryland). These tests can be performed from colonies growing on primary plates; isolates are typed with specific monoclonal antibodies. The Phadebact GC OMNI test is a coagglutination assay that contains inactivated *Staphylococcus aureus* cells coated with antibodies to staphylococcal protein A via the Fc region. The GonoGen II is a colorimetric test using antibodies adsorbed to metal sol particles. The MicroTrak assay uses fluorescein isothiocyanate-labeled antibodies (FITC) for confirmation of *N. gonorrhoeae* using a fluorescent microscope.

### Serotyping

Twelve different serogroups are distinguishable for *N. meningitidis.* Antisera are commercially available for identifying *N. meningitidis* serogroups A, B, C, H, I , K, L, X, Y, Z, W135, and 29E. Serologic identification is usually performed by slide agglutination. A, B, C, Y, and W135 are the serotypes that most frequently cause systemic disease in the United States. Serotyping has been replaced in many laboratories by DNA sequence typing methods related to the hypervariable outer membrane proteins. Information is available at http://neisseria.org.

## SERODIAGNOSIS

Serodiagnostic techniques are not generally used for the laboratory diagnosis of infections caused by the organisms discussed in this chapter.

## ■ ANTIMICROBIAL SUSCEPTIBILITY TESTING AND THERAPY

Although beta-lactamase production is common among *M. catarrhalis* isolates, many beta-lactam antibiotics maintain activity. Because several other agents are also effective, susceptibility testing to guide therapy is not routinely required (Table 40-5).

Standard methods have been established for performing in vitro susceptibility testing with *N. gonorrhoeae* and *N. meningitidis* (see Chapter 12). The Clinical and Laboratory Standards Institute (CLSI) recommends the use of agar dilution for minimum inhibitory concentration (MIC) measurements and GC agar containing 1% growth supplement for *N. gonorrhoeae* disk diffusion methods.

In addition, various agents can be considered for testing and therapeutic use. Quinolones were widely used to treat gonorrhea; however, resistance to these agents has emerged (i.e., quinolone-resistant *N. gonorrhoeae* [QRNG]), and they are no longer recommended for treatment of gonorrhea.

The Gonococcal Isolate Surveillance Project (GISP) has identified six categories of antibiotic susceptibility patterns for the characterization of isolates: PPNG (plasmid-mediated beta-lactamase positive); TRNG (plasmid-mediated tetracycline resistance, MIC ≥ 16 µg/mL); PPNG-TRNG; Penr; Tetr (MIC = 2-8 µg/mL) (chromosomal-mediated resistance patterns); and CMRNG (Penr combined with Tetr).

Because of the increase in QRNG and PPNG isolates, broad-spectrum cephalosporins have become the treatment of choice for *N. gonorrhoeae.* However, treatment failures have been associated with the use of broad-spectrum cephalosporins. Oral and intravenous regimens are recommended, depending on the severity and location of the infection.

Beta-lactamase production in *N. meningitidis* is extremely rare, although decreased susceptibility to penicillin, mediated by altered penicillin-binding proteins, is emerging. Optimum laboratory methods for detecting this relatively low level of resistance have not yet been established, and the impact of this resistance on the clinical efficacy of penicillin is not known. The CLSI recommends that susceptibility testing be performed by disk diffusion on Mueller-Hinton agar or using cation-adjusted Mueller-Hinton broth in microdilution.

## ■ PREVENTION

Two types of single-dose vaccine to the polysaccharide capsulare antigens of *N. meningitidis* groups A, C, Y, and W135 are available in the United States. MCV4 vaccine is a conjugated vaccine for individuals 55 years of age and younger. MPSV4 (meningococcal polysaccharide vaccine) is licensed for use in immunization for individuals older than 55 years of age. Chemoprophylaxis with rifampin or ciprofloxacin (orally) or ceftriaxone (intramuscularly) is indicated for close contacts of patients with meningococcal meningitis. Household contacts, day care contacts, and health care workers who have given mouth-to-mouth resuscitation are at risk and should be treated within 24 hours. No chemoprophylaxis is necessary for asymptomatic carriers.

A single application of either a 2.5% solution of povidone-iodine, 1% tetracycline eye ointment, 0.5% erythromycin eye ointment, or 1% silver nitrate eye drops is instilled in newborns within 1 hour of delivery to prevent gonococcal ophthalmia neonatorum.

**TABLE 40-5** Antimicrobial Therapy and Susceptibility Testing

| Species | Therapeutic Options | Potential Resistance to Therapeutic Options | Validated Testing Methods* | Comments |
|---------|---------------------|---------------------------------------------|----------------------------|----------|
| Moraxella catarrhalis | Several beta-lactams are effective, including beta-lactam/beta-lactamase–inhibitor combinations, cephalosporins, macrolides, quinolones, and trimethoprim-sulfamethoxazole | Commonly produce beta-lactamases that mediate resistance to ampicillin. Although not common, resistance to erythromycin and trimethoprim-sulfamethoxazole may occur | See CLSI document M45 methods | Testing to guide therapy is not routinely needed |
| Neisseria gonorrhoeae | Recommended therapy includes ceftriaxone and other broad-spectrum cephalosporins. Macrolides also may be used | Penicillin resistance by beta-lactamase production is common | As documented in Chapter 12: disk diffusion, agar dilution, limited commercial methods | Testing by disk diffusion may not detect decrease in quinolone activity. No ceftriaxone resistance has been documented |
| Neisseria meningitidis | Supportive therapy for shock and antimicrobial therapy using penicillin, ceftriaxone, cefotaxime, or chloramphenicol | Subtle increases in beta-lactam resistance have been described, but clinical relevance is uncertain. Beta-lactamase production is extremely rare. Reduced fluoroquinolone susceptibility possible | As documented in Chapter 12: broth dilution, agar dilution and CLSI guidelines | Testing to guide therapy is not routinely needed |
| Other Neisseria spp. | Usually susceptible to penicillin and other beta-lactams | Uncertain; potential for beta-lactamase production | Not available | |
| Neisseria animaloris | Not well characterized; purported susceptibility to penicillin, ampicillin, ciprofloxacin, and ofloxacin | Unknown; first-generation cephems appear less active than penicillins | Not available | |

*Validated testing methods include standard methods recommended by the Clinical and Laboratory Standards Institute (CLSI) and commercial methods approved by the U.S. Food and Drug Administration (FDA).

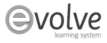 **Visit the Evolve site to complete the review questions.**

## CASE STUDY 40-1

An elderly man has a history of chronic obstructive pulmonary disease (COPD) after 20 years of heavy smoking. He presents to the emergency department with shortness of breath, severe cough, and profuse, yellow sputum production. Crackles and wheezing can be heard on chest examination. A sputum culture is positive for many intracellular gram-positive, lancet-shaped diplococci. Gram-negative diplococci are also observed in the smear. The patient is placed on amoxicillin/clavulanic acid, and other supportive measures are provided.

QUESTIONS

1. List the pathogenic agents most often found to be involved in acute infections of patients with COPD.

2. List the tests required to identify *Moraxella catarrhalis* definitively and rapidly.

3. The culture from this patient grows *Streptococcus pneumoniae* and *Moraxella catarrhalis*. The *S. pneumoniae* was susceptible to penicillin, but the organism was still present in the sputum, even though the patient was being treated with amoxicillin before the acute episode that brought him to the emergency department. Can you explain this observation?

# BIBLIOGRAPHY

Abadi FJ, Yakubu DE, Pennington TH: Antimicrobial susceptibility of penicillin-sensitive and penicillin-resistant meningococci, *J Antimicrob Chemother* 35:687, 1995.

Blondeau JM, Ashton FE, Isaacson M, et al: *Neisseria meningitidis* with decreased susceptibility to penicillin in Saskatchewan, Canada, *J Clin Microbiol* 33:1784, 1995.

CLSI Supplement: Performance standards for antimicrobial susceptibility testing: 23rd informational supplement, Wayne, Pa., 2013, CLSI, M100-S23.

Committee on Infectious Diseases: *2006 Red book: report of the Committee on Infectious Diseases*, ed 27, Elk Grove, Ill, 2006, American Academy of Pediatrics.

Heiddal S, Sverrisson JT, Yngvason FE, et al: Native valve endocarditis due to *Neisseria sicca*: case report and review, *Clin Infect Dis* 16:667, 1993.

Kam KM, Wong PW, Cheung MM, et al: Detection of quinolone-resistant *Neisseria gonorrhoeae*, *J Clin Microbiol* 34:1462, 1996.

Myer GA, Shope TR, Waeker NJ, et al: *Moraxella (Branhamella) catarrhalis* bacteremia in children, *Clin Pediatr* 34:146, 1995.

National Committee for Clinical Laboratory Standards (NCCLS): *Abbreviated identification of bacteria and yeast*, M35-A, ed 2, Wayne, Pa, 2008, NCCLS.

Riedo FX, Plikaytis BD, Broome CV: Epidemiology and prevention of meningococcal disease, *Pediatr Infect Dis J* 14:643, 1995.

Tanaka M, Matsumoto T, Kobayashi I, et al: Emergence of in vitro resistance to fluoroquinolones in Neisseria gonorrhoeae isolated in Japan, *Antimicrob Agents Chemother* 39:2367, 1995.

Vandamme P, Holmes B, Bercovier H, Coenye T: Classification of Centers for Disease Control group eugonic fermenter (EF)-4a and EF-4b as *Neisseria animaloris* sp nov and *Neisseria zoodegmatis* sp nov, respectively, *Int J Syst Evol Microbiol* 56:1801, 2006.

Verghese A, Berk SL: Moraxella (Branhamella) catarrhalis, *Infect Dis Clin North Am* 5:523, 1991.

Versalovic J: *Manual of clinical microbiology*, ed 10, Washington, DC, 2011, ASM Press.

Weyant RS, Moss CW, Weaver RE, et al, editors: *Identification of unusual pathogenic gram-negative aerobic and facultatively anaerobic bacteria*, ed 2, Baltimore, 1996, Williams & Wilkins.

Woods CR, Smith AL, Wasilauskas BL, et al: Invasive disease caused by *Neisseria meningitidis* relatively resistant to penicillin in North Carolina, *J Infect Dis* 170:453, 1994.

# Overview and General Considerations

## OBJECTIVES

*This chapter provides an overview of the methods used to identify anaerobic microorganisms. The detailed technical procedures discussed should be used in conjunction with specifics provided in Chapter 42 to develop a clear understanding of the full process, from specimen collection to identification. However, readers should consider the following general objectives for the information and methods provided.*

1. State the specific diagnostic purpose for the test methodology.
2. Briefly describe the test principle associated with the test methodology.
3. Outline limitations and describe a process for trouble-shooting or reporting results if a test result is equivocal or indistinguishable.
4. State the appropriate quality control organisms and results used with each testing procedure.
5. Define and differentiate obligate (strict), moderate, facultative, and aerotolerant anaerobes.
6. List suitable specimens for isolation of anaerobic bacteria and characteristics of these specimens that might suggest the presence of an anaerobic infection.
7. Explain the proper techniques for collecting, transporting, and processing clinical specimens for anaerobic bacteriology.
8. Explain the use of antigen detection methodologies in the diagnosis of anaerobic infections.
9. List the media used for cultivation of anaerobic bacteria.
10. Describe the appropriate incubation conditions for cultivation of anaerobic bacteria.
11. Describe the procedures for the identification of and antibiotic susceptibility testing for anaerobic bacteria.

## GENERAL CHARACTERISTICS

The organisms described in this chapter and in Chapter 42 usually do not grow in the presence of oxygen ($O_2$); they are obligate, or strict, anaerobes (0% $O_2$). Obligate anaerobes are killed upon brief exposure (less than a few minutes) to atmospheric oxygen. Obligate anaerobes include *Prevotella* sp., *Fusobacterium* sp., and *Bacteroides* spp. These chapters also include some aerotolerant organisms (5% $O_2$), such as *Actinomyces* spp., *Bifidobacterium* spp., and *Clostridium* spp., which are capable of growth in the presence of either reduced or atmospheric oxygen but grow best under anaerobic conditions. Finally, facultative anaerobes do not require atmospheric oxygen

but are capable of growth in oxygen and anaerobic environments.

Anaerobic organisms lack superoxide dismutase and catalase, the enzymes required to breakdown reactive oxygen species produced during respiration or aerobic metabolism. In addition, oxygen has a high affinity for organic compounds containing nitrogen, hydrogen, carbon, and sulfur, which interferes with normal biologic activity. Because they are unable to protect themselves against the action of oxygen, anaerobes require an environment free of oxygen to survive and grow.

## SPECIMEN COLLECTION AND TRANSPORT

The importance of proper collection and transport of specimens for anaerobic culture cannot be overemphasized. Because indigenous anaerobes are often present in large numbers as normal flora on mucosal surfaces, even minimal contamination of a specimen can produce misleading results. Box 41-1 shows the specimens acceptable for anaerobic culture; Box 41-2 presents specimens that are likely to be contaminated and therefore are unacceptable for anaerobic culture. In general, material for anaerobic culture is best obtained by tissue biopsy or by aspiration using a needle and syringe. Use of swabs is a poor alternative because of excessive exposure of the specimen to the deleterious effects of drying, the possibility of contamination during collection, and the easy retention of microorganisms in the fibers of the swab. If a swab must be used, it should be from an oxygen-free transport system.

A crucial factor in obtaining valid results with anaerobic cultures is the transport of the specimen; the lethal effect of atmospheric oxygen must be nullified until the specimen can be processed in the laboratory. Recapping a syringe and transporting the needle and syringe to the laboratory is no longer acceptable because of safety concerns involving needle stick injuries. Therefore, even aspirates must be injected into an oxygen-free transport tube or vial.

Three kinds of anaerobic transport systems are shown in Figures 41-1 to 41-3. Figure 41-1 shows is a rubber-stoppered collection vial containing an agar indicator system. The vial is gassed out with oxygen-free carbon dioxide ($CO_2$) or nitrogen. The specimen (pus, body

---

**BOX 41-1** Clinical Specimens Suitable for Anaerobic Culture

Bile
Biopsy of endometrial tissue obtained with an endometrial
   suction curette (Pipelle; Unimar, Wilton, Connecticut)
Blood
Bone marrow
Bronchial washings obtained with a double-lumen plugged
   catheter
Cerebrospinal fluid
Culdocentesis aspirate
Decubitus ulcer (if obtained from base of the lesion after
   thorough debridement of the ulcer's surface)
Fluid from normally sterile site (e.g., joint)
Material aspirated from abscesses (the best specimens are
   from loculated or walled-off lesions)
Percutaneous (direct) lung aspirate or biopsy
Peritoneal (ascitic) fluid
Sulfur granules from a draining fistula
Suprapubic bladder aspirate
Thoracentesis (pleural) fluid
Tissue obtained at biopsy or autopsy
Transtracheal aspirate
Uterine contents (if collected using a protected swab)

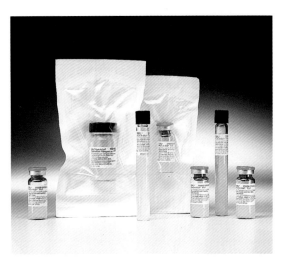

**Figure 41-1** Anaerobic transport system for liquid specimens. The specimen is injected into the tube through the rubber septum. Agar at the bottom contains an oxygen tension indicator. (Courtesy BD Diagnostic Systems, Sparks, Md.)

---

**BOX 41-2** Clinical Specimens Unsuitable for
Anaerobic Culture

Bronchial washing or brush (unless collected with a double-
   lumen plugged catheter)
Coughed (expectorated) sputum
Feces (except for *Clostridium difficile*)
Gastric or small-bowel contents (except in blind loop
   syndrome)
Ileostomy or colostomy drainage
Nasopharyngeal swab
Rectal swab
Secretions obtained by nasotracheal or orotracheal suction
Swab of superficial (open) skin lesion
Throat swab
Urethral swab
Vaginal or cervical swab
Voided or catheterized urine

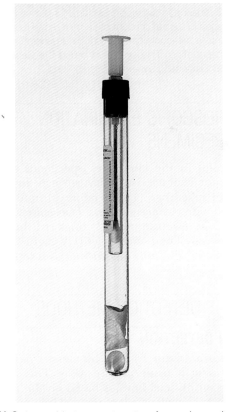

**Figure 41-2** Anaerobic transport system for swab specimens: Vacutainer Anaerobic Specimen Collector (BD Diagnostic Systems, Sparks, Md.). The sterile pack contains a sterile swab and an oxygen-free inner tube. After the specimen has been collected, the swab is inserted back into the inner tube. Agar on the bottom of the outer tube contains an oxygen tension indicator.

fluid, or other liquid material) is injected through the rubber stopper after all air has been expelled from the syringe and needle. If only a swab specimen can be obtained, a special collection device with an oxygen-free atmosphere is required (see Figure 41-2). When the swab is reinserted, care must be taken not to tip the container, which would cause the oxygen-free $CO_2$ or nitrogen to spill out and be displaced by ambient air. A tissue specimen can be immersed in a small amount of liquid to prevent it from drying and then placed in an anaerobic pouch (see Figure 41-3). All specimens should be held at room temperature pending processing in the laboratory, because refrigeration can oxygenate the specimen.

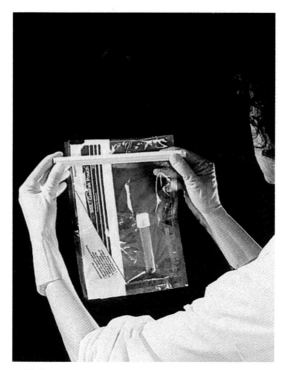

**Figure 41-3** Anaerobic transport system for tissue specimens. Tissue is placed in a small amount of saline to keep it moist. It then is inserted into a self-contained, atmosphere-generating anaerobic bag for transportation. This system is called the GasPak Pouch. (Courtesy BD Diagnostic Systems, Sparks, Md.)

# MACROSCOPIC EXAMINATION OF SPECIMENS

Upon receipt in the laboratory, specimens should be inspected for characteristics that strongly indicate the presence of anaerobes: (1) foul odor; (2) sulfur granules (associated with *Actinomyces* spp., *Propionibacterium* spp., or *Eubacterium nodatum*); and (3) brick red fluorescence under long wavelength ultraviolet (UV) light (associated with pigmented *Prevotella* or *Porphyromonas* spp).

# DIRECT DETECTION METHODS

## ANTIGEN DETECTION

The cytotoxin (toxin B) of *Clostridium difficile* can be detected using a tissue culture assay. This assay, performed in various cell lines, is based on the neutralization of cytopathic effect when the cell-free fecal extract is adsorbed using either *Clostridium sordellii* or *C. difficile* antitoxins. Latex particle agglutination tests or enzyme-linked immunosorbent assays (ELISA) to detect toxin A or toxin B (or both) are also available.

Screening of stool samples for the production of glutamate dehydrogenase (GDH) using enzyme immunoassays is commonly used. GDH-positive samples should be examined for production of toxin A and B. Commercially available DNA-based methods are available. However, *C. difficile* colonization occurs, and therefore molecular testing does not indicate *C. difficile* enteric disease.

# GRAM STAINING

The Gram stain is an important rapid tool for anaerobic bacteriology. Not only does it reveal the types and relative numbers of microorganisms and host cells present, it also serves as a quality control measure for the adequacy of anaerobic techniques. The absence of leukocytes does not rule out the presence of a serious anaerobic infection, however, because certain organisms, such as clostridia, produce necrotizing toxins that destroy white blood cells. A positive Gram stain with a negative culture may indicate (1) poor transport methods, (2) excessive exposure to air during specimen processing, (3) failure of the system (jar, pouch, or chamber) to achieve an anaerobic atmosphere, (4) inadequate types of media or old media, or (5) killing of microorganisms by antimicrobial therapy.

Standard Gram stain procedures and reagents are used, except that the safranin counterstain is left on for 3 to 5 minutes. Gram-negative anaerobes often stain poorly with safranin, resulting in failure to visualize pathogenic organisms. As an alternative, 0.5% aqueous basic fuchsin can be used as the counterstain to improve identification of gram-negative anaerobes. In addition, some gram-positive anaerobes (e.g., *Clostridium* spp.) stain pink. Enhanced Gram stain reagents are available that contain different concentrations in the reagents, in addition to a Gram Enhancer, which is applied after decolorization to suppress the red color in the background, aiding the differentiation of gram-negative anaerobes.

Table 41-1 presents the cellular morphology seen with Gram staining of common anaerobes.

# SPECIMEN PROCESSING

Specimens for anaerobic culture may be processed in the biologic safety cabinet, after which they are incubated in anaerobic jars or pouches or in an anaerobic chamber. The roll tube method developed at Virginia Polytechnic Institute is no longer widely used and is not discussed here.

## ANAEROBE JARS OR POUCHES

The most frequently used system for creating an anaerobic atmosphere is the anaerobe jar. Anaerobe jars are available commercially from several companies. For example, the GasPak (Figure 41-4) is made by Becton Dickinson (Sparks, Maryland); other companies that produce these devices include EM Diagnostic Systems (Gibbstown, New Jersey) and Oxoid U.S.A. (Columbus, Maryland). All of these systems use a clear, heavy plastic jar with a lid that is clamped down to make it airtight. Anaerobic conditions can be set up by two methods. The easiest method uses a commercially available envelope containing a hydrogen and $CO_2$ generator that is activated either by adding water (GasPak) or by the moisture on the agar plates (EM Diagnostic Systems and Oxoid USA). The production of heat within a few minutes (detected by touching the top of the jar) and subsequent development of moisture on the walls of the jar are

**TABLE 41-1** Gram Stain Morphology, Colonial Appearance, and Other Distinguishing Features of Common Anaerobic Bacteria

| Organism | Gram Stain* | Media | Appearance |
|---|---|---|---|
| *Actinomyces* spp. | Gram-positive, branching, beaded or banded, thin, filamentous rods | Ana BAP | Colonies of most species are small, smooth, flat, convex, gray-white, translucent, with entire margins; colonies of *A. israelii* and *A. gerencseriae* are white, opaque, and may resemble a "molar tooth"; *A. odontolyticus* turns red after several days in ambient air and may be beta-hemolytic |
| *Anaerococcus* spp. | Gram-positive cocci arranged in short chains or tetrads | Ana BAP | Small, white, translucent, smooth |
| *Atopobium* spp. | Elongated gram-positive cocci; occur singly, in pairs, or in short chains | Ana BAP | Resemble lactobacilli |
| *Bacteroides distasonis* | Gram-negative, straight rods with rounded ends; occur singly or in pairs | Ana BAP | Gray-white, circular, entire, convex, smooth, translucent to opaque; nonhemolytic |
| | | BBE | At 48 hr, colonies are >1 mm, circular, entire, raised, and either (1) low convex, dark gray, friable, and surrounded by a dark gray zone (esculin hydrolysis) and sometimes a precipitate (bile) or (2) glistening, convex, light to dark gray, and surrounded by a gray zone |
| *B. fragilis* | Gram-negative, pale-staining, pleomorphic rods with rounded ends; occur singly or in pairs; cells often described as resembling a safety pin (see Figure 42-4) | Ana BAP | White to gray, circular, entire, convex, translucent to semiopaque; nonhemolytic (see Figure 42-5) |
| | | BBE | At 48 hr, colonies are >1 mm, circular, entire, raised, and either (1) low convex, dark gray, friable, and surrounded by a dark gray zone (esculin hydrolysis) and sometimes a precipitate (bile) or (2) glistening, convex, light to dark gray, and surrounded by a gray zone (see Figure 42-6) |
| *B. ovatus* | Gram-negative, ovoid rods with rounded ends; occur singly or in pairs | Ana BAP | Pale buff, circular, entire, convex, semiopaque; often mucoid; nonhemolytic |
| | | BBE | At 48 hr, colonies are >1 mm, circular, entire, raised, and either (1) low convex, dark gray, friable, and surrounded by a dark gray zone (esculin hydrolysis) and sometimes a precipitate (bile) or (2) glistening, convex, light to dark gray, and surrounded by a gray zone |
| *B. thetaiotaomicron* | Gram-negative, irregularly staining, pleomorphic rods with rounded ends; occur singly or in pairs | Ana BAP | White, circular, entire, convex, semiopaque, shiny, punctiform; nonhemolytic |
| | | BBE | At 48 hr, colonies are >1 mm, circular, entire, raised, and either (1) low convex, dark gray, friable, and surrounded by a dark gray zone (esculin hydrolysis) and sometimes a precipitate (bile) or (2) glistening, convex, light to dark gray, and surrounded by a gray zone |
| *B. ureolyticus* | Gram-negative, pale-staining, thin, delicate rods with rounded ends; some curved | Ana BAP | Small, translucent or transparent; may produce greening of agar on exposure to air; colonies corrode (pit) the agar (see Figure 42-9) or may be smooth and convex or spreading |
| *B. vulgatus* | Gram-negative, pleomorphic rods with rounded ends; occur singly, in pairs, or in short chains; swellings or vacuoles may be seen | Ana BAP | Gray, circular, entire, convex, semiopaque; nonhemolytic |
| | | BBE | At 48 hr, colonies are >1 mm, circular, entire, raised, glistening, convex, light to dark gray but with no gray zone (esculin not hydrolyzed) |

*Continued*

**TABLE 41-1** Gram Stain Morphology, Colonial Appearance, and Other Distinguishing Features of Common Anaerobic Bacteria—cont'd

| Organism | Gram Stain* | Media | Appearance |
|---|---|---|---|
| *Bifidobacterium* spp. | Gram-positive diphtheroid; coccoid or thin, pointed shape; or larger, highly irregular, curved rods with branching; rods terminate in clubs or thick, bifurcated (forked) ends ("dog bones") | Ana BAP | Small, white, convex, shiny, with irregular edge |
| *Bilophila wadsworthia* | Gram-negative, pale-staining, delicate rods | Ana BAP | Small, translucent |
|  |  | BBE | Grows at 3-5 days; colonies are usually gray with a black center because of production of hydrogen sulfide ($H_2S$); black center may disappear after exposure to air |
| *Clostridium botulinum* | Gram-positive, straight rods; occur singly or in pairs; spores usually subterminal and resemble a tennis racket | Ana BAP | Gray-white; circular to irregular; usually beta-hemolytic |
| *C. clostridioforme* | Gram-positive rod that stains gram negative; long, thin rods; spores usually not seen; elongated football shape with cells often in pairs | Ana BAP | Small, convex, entire edge; nonhemolytic |
| *C. difficile* | Gram-positive straight rods; may produce chains of up to six cells aligned end to end; spores oval and subterminal | Ana BAP | Large, white, circular, matte to glossy, convex, opaque; nonhemolytic; horse stable odor; fluoresces yellow-green |
|  |  | CCFA | Yellow, ground-glass colony (see Figure 42-2) |
| *C. perfringens* | Gram-variable straight rods with blunt ends; occur singly or in pairs; spores seldom seen but if present are large and central to subterminal, oval, and swell cell; large boxcar shapes (see Figure 44-6) | Ana BAP | Gray to grayish yellow; circular, glossy, dome shaped, entire, translucent; double zone of beta-hemolysis (see Figure 42-3) |
| *C. ramosum* | Gram-variable straight or curved rods; spores rarely seen but are round and terminal; more slender and longer than *C. perfringens* | Ana BAP | Small, gray-white to colorless; circular to slightly irregular, smooth, translucent or semiopaque; nonhemolytic |
| *C. septicum* | Gram positive in young cultures but becomes gram negative with age; stains unevenly; straight or curved rods; occur singly or in pairs; spores subterminal, and oval and swell cells | Ana BAP | Gray; circular, glossy, translucent; markedly irregular to rhizoid margins resembling a "Medusa head"; beta-hemolytic; swarms over entire agar surface in less than 24 hr |
| *C. sordellii* | Gram-positive rods; subterminal spores | Ana BAP | Large colony with irregular edge |
| *C. sporogenes* | Gram-positive rods; subterminal spores | Ana BAP | Colonies firmly adhere to agar; may swarm over agar surface |
| *C. tertium* | Gram-variable rods; terminal spores | Ana BAP | Resembles *Lactobacillus* spp. |
| *C. tetani* | Gram positive, becoming gram negative after 24-hr incubation; occur singly or in pairs; spores oval and terminal or subterminal with drumstick or tennis racket appearance | Ana BAP | Gray; matte surface, irregular to rhizoid margin, translucent, flat; narrow zone of beta-hemolysis; may swarm over agar surface |
| *Collinsella aerofaciens* | Gram-positive chains of coccoid cells | Ana BAP | Circular, entire, white center with translucent edge |
| *Eggerthella lenta* | Gram-positive, small, straight rod with rounded ends | Ana BAP | Small, gray, translucent, circular, entire, convex |
| *Eubacterium* spp. | Gram-positive pleomorphic rods or coccobacilli; occur in pairs or short chains; *E. alactolyticum* has a seagull-wing shape similar to *Campylobacter* spp.; *E. nodatum* is similar to Actinomyces spp. with beading, filaments, and branching | Ana BAP | Small, gray, transparent to translucent, raised to convex; colonies of *E. nodatum* may resemble *A. israelii* |

**TABLE 41-1** Gram Stain Morphology, Colonial Appearance, and Other Distinguishing Features of Common Anaerobic Bacteria—cont'd

| Organism | Gram Stain* | Media | Appearance |
|---|---|---|---|
| *Finegoldia magna* | Gram-positive cocci with cells > 0.6 μm in diameter; in pairs and clusters; resemble staphylococci | Ana BAP | Tiny, gray, translucent; nonhemolytic |
| *Fusobacterium mortiferum* | Gram-negative, pale-staining, irregularly stained, highly pleomorphic rods with swollen areas, filaments, and large, bizarre, round bodies | Ana BAP | Circular; entire or irregular edge, convex or slightly umbonate, smooth, translucent; nonhemolytic |
| | | BBE | >1 mm in diameter, flat and irregular |
| *F. necrophorum* subsp. *necrophorum* | Gram-negative, pleomorphic rods with round to tapered ends; may be filamentous or contain round bodies; becomes more pleomorphic with age | Ana BAP | Circular, umbonate, ridged surface, translucent to opaque; fluoresces chartreuse; greening of agar on exposure to air; some strains beta-hemolytic |
| *F. nucleatum* subsp. *nucleatum* | Gram negative; pale staining; long, slender, spindle-shaped with sharply pointed or tapered ends; occasionally cells occur in pairs end to end; resembles *Capnocytophaga* spp. (see Figure 42-11) | Ana BAP | Three colony types: bread crumb–like (white; see Figure 42-10), speckled, and smooth (gray to gray-white); greening of agar on exposure to air; fluoresces chartreuse; usually nonhemolytic |
| *F. varium* | Gram negative, unevenly staining, pleomorphic; coccoid and rod shapes; occurs singly or in pairs | Ana BAP | Gray-white center with colorless edge resembling a fried egg; circular, entire, convex, translucent; nonhemolytic |
| | | BBE | >1 mm in diameter, flat and irregular |
| *Lactobacillus* spp. | Gram-variable pleomorphic rods or coccobacilli; straight, uniform rods have rounded ends; short coccobacilli resemble streptococci | Ana BAP | Resemble *Lactobacillus* spp. colonies on aerobic blood or chocolate agar, except colonies are usually larger when incubated anaerobically |
| *Leptotrichia* spp. | Gram-negative, large, fusiform rods with one pointed end and one blunt end | Ana BAP | Large, raspberry-like colonies |
| *Parvimonas micra* | Gram-positive cocci with cells < 0.7 μm in diameter; occur in packets and short chains | Ana BAP | Tiny, white, opaque; nonhemolytic |
| *Mobiluncus* spp. | Gram-variable, small, thin, curved rods; the two species can be divided based on cell length | Ana BAP | Tiny colonies after 48 hr-incubation; after 3-5 days, colonies are small, low convex, and translucent |
| *Peptococcus niger* | Gram-positive, spherical cells; occur singly or in pairs, tetrads, and irregular masses | Ana BAP | Tiny, black, convex, shiny, smooth, circular, entire edge; becomes light gray when exposed to air |
| *Peptostreptococcus anaerobius* | Gram-positive, large coccobacillus; often in chains | Ana BAP | Medium, gray-white, opaque; sweet, fetid odor; colonies usually larger than most anaerobic cocci |
| *Porphyromonas* spp. | Gram-negative coccobacilli | Ana BAP | Dark brown to black; more mucoid than *Prevotella* spp.; except for *P. gingivalis*, fluoresces brick red |
| *Prevotella disiens* | Gram-negative rods; occur in pairs or short chains | Ana BAP | White, circular, entire, convex, translucent to opaque, smooth, shiny; nonhemolytic; fluoresces brick red |
| | | LKV | Black pigment |
| *P. melaninogenica* | Gram-negative coccobacilli | Ana BAP | Dark center with gray to light brown edges; circular, entire, convex, smooth, shiny; nonhemolytic; fluoresces brick red |
| | | LKV | Black pigment |
| *Propionibacterium* spp. | Gram-positive, pleomorphic, diphtheroid-like rod; club-shaped to palisade arrangements; called *anaerobic diphtheroids* | Ana BAP | Young colonies are small and white to gray-white and become larger and more yellowish tan with age; *P. avidum* is beta-hemolytic |
| *Veillonella parvula* | Gram-negative, tiny diplococci in clusters, pairs, and short chains; unusually large cocci, especially in clusters, suggests *Megasphaera* or *Acidaminococcus* spp. | Ana BAP | Small, almost transparent; grayish white; smooth, entire, opaque, butyrous; may show red fluorescence under UV light (360 nm) |

*Ana BAP,* Anaerobic blood agar plate; *BBE, Bacteroides* bile esculin agar; *CCFA,* cycloserine cefoxitin fructose agar; *LKV,* laked kanamycin-vancomycin blood agar; *UV,* ultraviolet.
*Typical Gram stain appearance is seen from broth (thioglycollate or peptone-yeast-glucose).

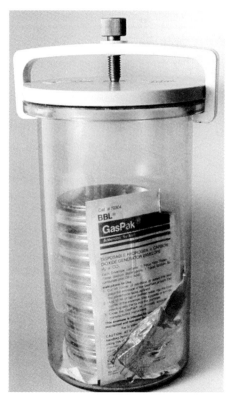

**Figure 41-4** GasPak anaerobe jar (BD Diagnostic Systems, Sparks, Md.). Inside the jar are inoculated plates, an activated gas-generating envelope, and an indicator strip. A wire-mesh basket attached to the lid of the jar contains palladium-coated alumina pellets that catalyze the reaction to remove oxygen. Newer models of the GasPak jar use reagent packs that simply require the addition of water to catalyze a reaction (see chapter text).

indications that the catalyst and generator envelope are functioning properly. Reduced conditions are achieved in 1 to 2 hours, although the methylene blue or resazurin indicators take longer to decolorize. Alternatively, the "evacuation-replacement" method can be used. Air is removed from the sealed jar by drawing a vacuum of 25 inches (62.5 cm) of mercury. This process is repeated two times, with the jar being filled with an oxygen-free gas, such as nitrogen, between evacuations. The final fill of the jar is made with a gas mixture containing 80% to 90% nitrogen, 5% to 10% hydrogen, and 5% to 10% $CO_2$. Many anaerobes require $CO_2$ for maximal growth.

The atmosphere in the jars is monitored using an indicator to check anaerobiosis. Anaerobe bags or pouches are useful for laboratories processing small numbers of anaerobic specimens. A widely used anaerobic pouch, the GasPak Pouch, is shown in Figure 41-3. Besides specimen transport, the pouch also can be used to incubate one or two agar plates.

## HOLDING JARS

If anaerobic jars or pouches are used for incubation, holding jars should be used during specimen processing and examination of cultures. Holding jars are anaerobic jars with loosely fitted lids attached by rubber tubing to nitrogen gas. Uninoculated plates are kept in holding jars pending use for culture setup, and inoculated plates are kept in holding jars pending incubation or examination; this minimizes exposure to oxygen.

## ANAEROBE CHAMBER

Anaerobic chambers, or glove boxes, are made of molded or flexible clear plastic. The flexible clear plastic chambers are the most widely used type. Specimens and other materials are placed in the chamber through an air lock. The technologist uses gloves (Forma Scientific, Marietta, Ohio) or sleeves (Sheldon Manufacturing, Cornelius, Oregon), to form airtight seals around the arms (Figure 41-5). Media stored in the chamber are kept oxygen free, and all work on a specimen, from inoculation through workup, is performed under anaerobic conditions. A gas mixture of 5% $CO_2$, 10% hydrogen, and 85% nitrogen, plus a palladium catalyst, maintain the anaerobic environment inside the chamber.

## ANAEROBIC MEDIA

Initial processing of anaerobic specimens involves inoculation of appropriate media. Table 41-2 lists commonly used anaerobic media. Primary plates should be freshly prepared or used within 2 weeks of preparation. Plates stored for longer periods accumulate peroxides and become dehydrated; this results in growth inhibition. Reduction of media in an anaerobic environment eliminates dissolved oxygen but has no effect on the peroxides. Prereduced, anaerobically sterilized (PRAS) media are produced, packaged, shipped, and stored under anaerobic conditions. They are commercially available from Anaerobe Systems (Morgan Hill, California) (Figure 41-6) and have an extended shelf life of up to 6 months.

In general, anaerobic media should include a nonselective anaerobic blood agar and one or all of the following selective media: *Bacteroides* bile esculin agar (BBE), laked kanamycin-vancomycin blood agar (LKV), and anaerobic phenylethyl alcohol agar (PEA). In addition, aerobic 5% sheep blood agar, chocolate agar, and MacConkey agar are set up because most anaerobic infections are polymicrobic and may include aerobic or facultative anaerobic bacteria. A backup broth, usually thioglycollate, is inoculated to enrich small numbers of anaerobes in tissues and other sterile specimens. Most anaerobes grow well on any of the foregoing media.

Cultures for *C. difficile* are plated on a special selective medium, cycloserine cefoxitin fructose agar (CCFA) or egg yolk agar (EYA). There are also selective media for certain groups of anaerobes, such as *Actinomyces* spp., although they are rarely used in the clinical laboratory.

Special anaerobic blood culture systems containing various media, including thioglycollate broth, thiol broth, and Schaedler's broth, are commercially available. Although many anaerobes will grow in the aerobic blood culture bottle, it is better to use an unvented anaerobic broth when attempting to isolate these organisms from blood or bone marrow.

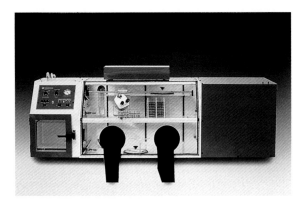

**Figure 41-5** Gloveless anaerobe chamber. Anaerobic chambers were developed more than 40 years ago, and a variety of new models are being used in cutting-edge research. (Courtesy Anaerobe Systems, Morgan Hill, Calif.)

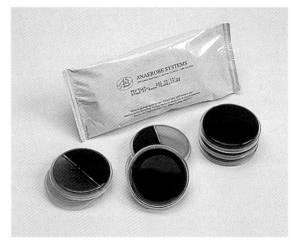

**Figure 41-6** Prereduced, anaerobically sterilized (PRAS) plated media. (Courtesy Anaerobe Systems, Morgan Hill, Calif.)

**TABLE 41-2** Common Anaerobic Media

| Medium | Components/Comments | Primary Purpose |
|---|---|---|
| Anaerobic blood agar | May be prepared with Columbia, Schaedler, CDC, *Brucella*, or brain-heart infusion base supplemented with 5% sheep blood, 0.5% yeast extract, hemin, L-cystine, and vitamin $K_1$ | Nonselective medium for isolation of anaerobes and facultative anaerobes |
| *Bacteroides* bile esculin agar (BBE) | Trypticase soy agar base with ferric ammonium citrate and hemin; bile salts and gentamicin act as inhibitors | Selective and differential for *Bacteroides fragilis* group; good for presumptive identification |
| Laked kanamycin-vancomycin (LKV) | *Brucella* agar base with kanamycin (75 $\mu$g/ mL), vancomycin (7.5 $\mu$g/mL), vitamin $K_1$ (10 $\mu$g/mL), and 5% laked blood | Selective for isolation of *Prevotella* and *Bacteroides* spp. |
| Anaerobic phenylethyl alcohol agar (PEA) | Nutrient agar base, 5% blood, phenylethyl alcohol | Selective for inhibition of enteric gram-negative rods and swarming by some clostridia |
| Egg yolk agar (EYA) | Egg yolk base | Nonselective for determination of lecithinase and lipase production by clostridia and fusobacteria |
| Cycloserine cefoxitin fructose agar (CCFA) | Egg yolk base with fructose, cycloserine (500 mg/L), and cefoxitin (16 mg/L); neutral red indicator | Selective for *Clostridium difficile* |
| Cooked meat (also called chopped meat) broth | Solid meat particles initiate growth of bacteria; reducing substances lower oxidation-reduction potential (Eh) | Nonselective for cultivation of anaerobic organisms; with addition of glucose, can be used for gas-liquid chromatography |
| Peptone–yeast extract–glucose broth (PYG) | Peptone base, yeast extract, glucose, cysteine (reducing agent), resazurin (oxygen tension indicator), salts | Nonselective for cultivation of anaerobic bacteria for gas-liquid chromatography |
| Thioglycollate broth | Pancreatic digest of casein, soy broth, and glucose to enrich growth of most bacteria. Thioglycollate and agar reduce Eh. May be supplemented with hemin and vitamin $K_1$ | Nonselective for cultivation of anaerobes, facultative anaerobes, and aerobes |

## INCUBATION CONDITIONS AND DURATION

Inoculated plates should be immediately incubated under anaerobic conditions at 35° to 37°C for 48 hours. In general, cultures should not be exposed to oxygen until after 48 hours' incubation, because anaerobes are most sensitive to oxygen during their log phase of growth. Plates may be removed from the anaerobic environment at 24 hours, briefly evaluated, and returned to the anaerobic environment. Plates incubated in an anaerobe chamber or bag can be examined at 24 hours without oxygen exposure for typical colonies of *B. fragilis* group or *Clostridium perfringens*. Plates that show no growth at 48 hours should be incubated for at least 5 days before being discarded.

Thioglycollate broth can be incubated anaerobically with the cap loose or anaerobically with the cap tight. Broths should be inspected daily for 7 days.

# APPROACH TO IDENTIFICATION

Complete identification of anaerobes can be costly, often requiring various biochemical tests, gas-liquid chromatography to analyze the metabolic end products of glucose fermentation, and/or gas chromatography for whole-cell long chain fatty acid methyl ester (FAME) analysis. Most clinical laboratories no longer perform complete identification of anaerobes, because presumptive identification is just as useful in assisting the physician in determining appropriate therapy. Therefore, the approach to identification taken in this chapter emphasizes simple, rapid methods to identify commonly isolated anaerobic bacteria. Identification should proceed in a stepwise fashion, beginning with examination of the primary plates.

## EXAMINATION OF PRIMARY PLATES

Anaerobes are usually present in mixed culture with other anaerobes and facultative bacteria. The combination of selective and differential agar plates yields information that suggests the presence and perhaps the types of one or more anaerobes. Primary anaerobic plates should be examined with a hand lens (×8) or, preferably, a stereoscopic microscope. Colonies should be described from the various media and semiquantitated.

All colony morphotypes from the nonselective anaerobic blood agar should be characterized and subcultured to purity plates, because facultative and obligate anaerobic bacteria frequently have similar colonial appearances.

Colonies on PEA are processed further if they are different from colonies growing on the anaerobic blood agar or if colonies on the anaerobic blood agar are impossible to subculture because of overgrowth by swarming clostridia, *Proteus*, or other organisms.

The backup broth (e.g., thioglycollate) should be Gram stained; if cellular types are seen that were not present on the primary plates, the broth should be subcultured. In addition, if no growth is seen on the primary plates, the backup broth should be subcultured to the battery of anaerobic media included in the primary plating setup.

## SUBCULTURE OF ISOLATES

A single colony of each distinct morphotype is examined microscopically using a Gram stain and is subcultured for aerotolerance testing. Figure 41-7 presents a basic algorithm for processing isolated colonies. A sterile wooden stick or platinum loop should be used to subculture colonies to:

- A chocolate agar plate (CHOC) to be incubated in carbon dioxide ($CO_2$) for aerotolerance
- An anaerobic blood agar plate (BAP) and a chocolate plate to be incubated anaerobically (purity plate)

The chocolate agar plate should be inoculated first, so that if only the anaerobic blood agar plate grows, there is no question of not having enough organisms to initiate growth. The following antibiotic identification disks are placed on the first quadrant of the purity plate (see Procedure 41-1 on the Evolve site):

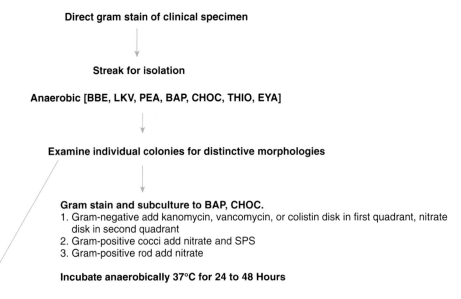

Direct gram stain of clinical specimen

↓

Streak for isolation

Anaerobic [BBE, LKV, PEA, BAP, CHOC, THIO, EYA]

↓

Examine individual colonies for distinctive morphologies

↓

**Gram stain and subculture to BAP, CHOC.**
1. Gram-negative add kanomycin, vancomycin, or colistin disk in first quadrant, nitrate disk in second quadrant
2. Gram-positive cocci add nitrate and SPS
3. Gram-positive rod add nitrate

**Incubate anaerobically 37°C for 24 to 48 Hours**

Aerotolerance Test: Subculture organisms to a CHOC plate, incubate 37°C for 24 to 48 hours in 5% $CO_2$ to detect slow growing aerobes such as *Capnocytophaga*, *Eikenella* and *Actinobacillus* spp.

**Figure 41-7** Algorithm for isolation and identification of anaerobic bacteria. *BAP*, Sheep blood agar; *CHOC*, chocolate agar; *BBE*, *Bacteroides* bile esculin agar; *LKV*, laked kanamycin-vancomycin agar; *PEA*, phenylethyl agar; *EYA*, egg yolk agar (for suspected *Clostridium* spp.), *THIO*, thioglycollate enrichment broth (should be examined daily and incubated for up to 7 days if no growth is identified on primary media; subculture to anaerobic media if growth is detected in broth culture).

- Kanamycin, 1 mg
- Colistin, 10 µg
- Vancomycin, 5 µg

These disks aid preliminary grouping of anaerobes and verify the Gram stain results, but they do not imply susceptibility of an organism for antibiotic therapy.

Three other disks may be added to the anaerobic blood agar plate at this time. A nitrate disk may be placed on the second quadrant for subsequent determination of nitrate reduction; a sodium polyanethol sulfonate (SPS) disk can be placed near the colistin disk for rapid presumptive identification of *Peptostreptococcus anaerobius* if gram-positive cocci are seen on Gram staining; and a bile disk may be added to the second quadrant to detect bile inhibition if gram-negative rods are seen on Gram staining.

If processing is performed on the open bench, all plates should promptly be incubated anaerobically, because some clinical isolates (e.g., *Fusobacterium necrophorum* subsp. *necrophorum* and some *Prevotella* spp.) may die after relatively short exposure to oxygen. The primary plates are reincubated, along with the purity plates, for an additional 48 to 72 hours and are again inspected for slowly growing or pigmenting strains.

## PRESUMPTIVE IDENTIFICATION OF ISOLATES

Information from the primary plates in conjunction with the atmospheric requirements, Gram stain results, and colony morphology of a pure isolate provides preliminary differentiation of many anaerobic organisms. Table 41-3 summarizes the extent to which isolates can be identified using this information. Considering the specimen source and expected organisms from the site can be a useful aid in this process.

Presumptive identification of many clinically relevant anaerobic bacteria can be accomplished using a few simple tests (Tables 41-4 and 41-5).

## DEFINITIVE IDENTIFICATION

Various techniques can be used for definitive identification of anaerobic bacteria. Such methods may include the following:

- PRAS biochemicals
- Miniaturized biochemical systems (e.g., API 20A [bioMérieux, St. Louis, Missouri])
- Rapid, preformed enzyme detection panels (e.g., AnIdent [bioMérieux]; RapID-ANA II [Remel, Lenexa, Kansas]; BBL Brand Crystal Anaerobe ID

**TABLE 41-3** Preliminary Grouping of Anaerobic Bacteria Based on Minimal Criteria

| Organism | Gram Stain Reaction | Cell Shape | Gram Stain Morphology | Aerotolerance | Distinguishing Characteristics |
|---|---|---|---|---|---|
| *Bacteroides fragilis* group | – | B | Can be pleomorphic with safety pin appearance | – | Grows on BBE; >1 mm in diameter; some strains hydrolyze esculin |
| Pigmented gram-negative bacilli | – | B, CB | Can be very coccoid or *Haemophilus*-like | – | Foul odor; black or brown pigment; some fluoresce brick red |
| *Bacteroides ureolyticus* | – | B | Thin; some curved | – | May pit agar or spread; transparent colony |
| *Fusobacterium nucleatum* | – | B | Slender cells with pointed ends | – | Foul odor; three colony types; bread crumb–like, speckled, and smooth |
| Gram-negative bacillus | – | B | | – | |
| Gram-negative coccus | – | C | *Veillonella* cells are tiny | – | |
| Gram-positive coccus | + | C, CB | Variable size | – | |
| *Clostridium perfringens* (presumptive) | + | B | Large; boxcar shape; no spores observed; may appear gram negative | – | Double-zone beta-hemolysis |
| *Clostridium* spp. | + | B | Spores usually observed; may appear gram negative | –* | |
| Gram-positive bacillus | + | B, CB | No spores observed; no boxcar-shaped cells | –* | |
| *Actinomyces*-like | + | B | Branching cells | –* | Sulfur granules on direct examination; "molar tooth" colony |

*B,* Bacillus; *BBE, Bacteroides* bile esculin agar; *C,* coccus; *CB,* coccobacillus; –, negative; + positive.
*Some strains are aerotolerant; these include *Clostridium tertium, C. histolyticum,* some bifidobacteria, some propionibacteria, and most *Actinomyces* spp.

**TABLE 41-4** Abbreviated Identification of Gram-Negative Anaerobes

| | Cell Shape | Slender Cells with Pointed Ends | Kanamycin (1 mg) | Vancomycin (5 μg) | Colistin (10 mg) | Growth in Bile | Spot Indole | Catalase | Pigmented Colony | Brick Red Fluorescence | Lipase | Pits the Agar | Requires Formate/Fumarate | Nitrate Reduction | Urease | Motile |
|---|---|---|---|---|---|---|---|---|---|---|---|---|---|---|---|---|
| **Gram-Negative Rods** | | | | | | | | | | | | | | | | |
| *Bacteroides fragilis* group | B | − | R | R | R | + | V | V | − | − | − | − | − | − | − | − |
| *Bacteroides ureolyticus* | B | − | S | R | S | − | − | − | − | − | − | +⁻ | + | + | + | − |
| Pigmented spp. | B, CB | − | R | R | V | − | V | − | +* | V | V | − | − | − | − | − |
| *Prevotella intermedia* | B, CB | − | R | R | S | − | + | − | + | + | + | − | − | − | − | − |
| *Prevotella loescheii* | B, CB | − | R | R | ˢRˢ | − | − | − | +* | + | −† | − | − | − | − | − |
| **Other** | | | | | | | | | | | | | | | | |
| *Prevotella* spp. | B, CB | − | R | R | V | − | V | − | −† | − | − | − | − | − | − | − |
| *Porphyromonas* s spp. | B, CB | − | R | ‡**S**‡ | R | − | + | − | + | +ˢ | − | − | − | − | − | − |
| *Bilophila* sp. | B | − | S | R | S | + | − | + | − | − | − | − | − | + | +⁻ | − |
| *Fusobacterium* spp. | Bǁ | V | **S** | **R** | **S** | V | V | − | − | − | V | − | − | − | − | − |
| *F. nucleatum* subsp. *nucleatum* | B | + | S | R | S | − | + | − | − | − | − | − | − | − | − | − |
| *F. necrophorum* subsp. *necrophorum* | B | − | S | R | S | −⁺ | + | − | − | − | +⁻ | − | − | − | − | − |
| *F. mortiferum varium* | B | − | S | R | S | + | V | − | − | − | − | − | − | − | − | − |
| *Leptotrichia* spp. | B | +¶ | S | R | S | V | − | − | − | − | − | − | − | − | − | − |
| **Gram-Negative Cocci** | | | | | | | | | | | | | | | | |
| *Veillonella* spp. | C | − | S | R | S | − | − | V | − | −† | − | − | − | + | − | − |

Reactions in **bold type** are key tests; superscripts indicate reactions of occasional strains.
B, Bacillus; C, coccus; CB, coccobacillus; R, resistant; S, sensitive; V, variable; +, positive; −, negative.
*P. melaninogenica group often requires prolonged incubation before pigment is observed.
†P. bivia produces pigment on prolonged incubation.
‡Will not grow on laked kanamycin-vancomycin (LKV) because of susceptibility to vancomycin.
§P. gingivalis does not fluoresce.
ǁThin, pointed fusiform cells.
¶One pointed end, one blunt end.

**TABLE 41-5** Abbreviated Identification of Gram-Positive Anaerobes

| | Cell Shape | Spores Observed | Boxcar-Shaped Cells | Double-Zone Beta Hemolysis | Kanamycin (1 mg) | Vancomycin (5 mg) | Colistin (10 mg) | Spot Indole | Sodium Polyanethol Sulfonate | Catalase | Survives Ethanol Spore Test | Lecithinase | Nagler Test | Strong Reverse-Camp Test | Arginine Stimulation | Urease | Nitrate Reduction | Ground-Glass, Yellow Colonies on CCFA* Medium | Comment |
|---|---|---|---|---|---|---|---|---|---|---|---|---|---|---|---|---|---|---|---|
| **Gram-Positive Cocci** | C, CB | – | – | – | V | S | R | V | V | V | – | – | – | | – | | $-^+$ | – | |
| *Peptostreptococcus anaerobius* | C, CB | – | – | – | $\mathbf{R^s}$ | S | R | – | S | $-^+$ | – | – | – | | – | | – | – | Sweet, putrid odor; may chain |
| *Finegoldia magna* | C† | – | – | – | S | S | R | – | R | V | – | – | – | | – | – | – | – | |
| *Parvimonas micros* | C‡ | – | – | – | S | S | R | – | $V^\S$ | – | – | – | – | | – | – | – | – | |
| *Peptococcus niger* | C | – | – | – | S | S | R | – | R | – | – | – | – | | – | – | – | – | Black to olive green colonies |
| **Gram-Positive, Spore-Forming Rods** *Clostridium* spp. | B | $-^+$ | $-^+$ | – | V | S | R | V | | $-^+$ | $+^-$ | V | – | | – | V | $-^+$ | V | |
| NAGLER POSITIVE *C. perfringens* | B | – | + | $-^+$ | S | S | R | – | | $-^+$ | $-^+$ | + | + | + | – | – | $+^-$ | – | |
| *C. baratii* | B | + | – | – | S | S | R | – | | – | + | + | $+^w$ | – | – | – | V | – | |
| *C. sordellii* | B | + | – | – | S | S | R | + | | $-^+$ | + | + | $+^w$ | – | $+^-$ | – | – | – | Swarming with serpentine-edged colonies |
| *C. bifermentans* | B | + | – | – | S | S | R | + | | $-^+$ | + | + | $+^w$ | – | – | – | – | – | |
| NAGLER NEGATIVE *C. difficile* | B | $+^-$ | – | – | S | S | R | – | | $-^+$ | + | – | – | – | – | | – | + | Horse stable odor; fluoresces chartreuse |
| *C. septicum* | B | + | – | – | S | S | R | – | | $-^+$ | $+^-$ | – | – | – | – | – | V | – | Smoothly swarming over agar surface |
| **Non–Spore Forming** | B, CB | – | – | – | V | S | R | V | | $V^+$ | – | V | – | | V | V | V | – | |
| *Propionibacterium acnes* | B, CB | – | – | – | S | S | R | $+^-$ | | $+^+$ | – | – | – | – | – | – | + | – | May branch; diphtheroid |
| *Eggerthella lenta* | B | – | – | – | S | S | R | – | | $-^+$ | – | – | – | – | + | – | + | – | Small rod |
| *Bifidobacterium* spp. | B‖ | – | – | – | S | S | R | V | | – | | | | | | – | | | Some strains are aerotolerant (e.g., *B. adolescentis*) |
| *Eubacterium* spp. | B | – | – | – | S | S | R | V | | – | | | | | | – | | | |

Reactions in **bold type** are key tests; superscripts indicate reactions of occasional strains.

*B*, Bacillus; *C*, coccus; *CB*, coccobacillus; *R*, resistant; *S*, sensitive; *V*, variable; *w*, weak; +, positive; –, negative.

*Cycloserine cefoxitin fructose agar.

†Cell size > 0.6 μm.

‡Cell size < 0.6 μm.

§Some strains inhibited but zone usually < 12 mm.

‖Rods with or without one bifurcated end.

See Procedure 41-2.

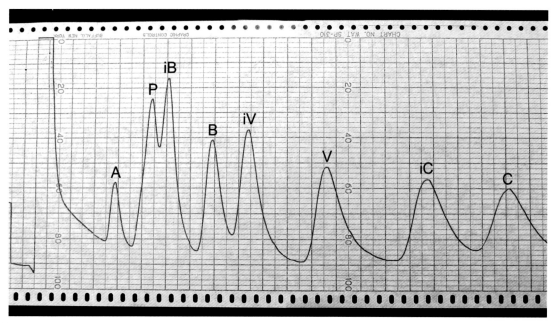

**Figure 41-8** Actual chromatogram of volatile acid standard. *A,* Acetic acid; *P,* propionic acid; *iB,* isobutyric acid; *B,* butyric acid; *iV,* isovaleric acid; *V,* valeric acid; *iC,* isocaproic acid; *C,* caproic acid.

[Becton Dickinson]; Rapid Anaerobe Identification Panel [Dade MicroScan, West Sacramento, California]; Vitek ANI card [bioMérieux]).

- Gas-liquid chromatography (GLC) for end products of glucose fermentation (Supelco, Bellefonte, Pennsylvania). GLC is used to separate and identify anaerobic metabolic end products (i.e., volatile fatty acids [Figure 41-8] and nonvolatile organic acids) of carbohydrate fermentation and amino acid degradation. Chromatograms produced with anaerobic bacteria can greatly facilitate identification of certain genera and species not readily identified based on other phenotypic characteristics.
- High-resolution GLC for cellular fatty acid analysis. GLC application has been expanded for the analysis of longer chain fatty acids (i.e., 9 to 20 carbons in length) to produce chromatograms for identifying organisms often without the need for other phenotypic information (e.g., Gram stain morphology). One such commercial system (MIDI Microbial Identification System, Inc.; Newark, Del.) has more than 600 bacteria in the chromatographic database. Although this approach may not be practical for identification of many commonly encountered bacterial species, it has great potential for use as a reference method for organisms that are difficult to identify by conventional methods.

For commonly isolated anaerobic bacteria, the commercial identification systems and biochemical kits reliably identify the anaerobic bacteria. However, caution must be used in interpretation, and the results must be correlated with other clinical information, including the site of infection, Gram staining results, and colonial morphology. The high cost of some methods alone does not justify their use in most clinical laboratories. To ensure accurate identification, reference or research laboratories use a combination of PRAS biochemicals and GLC or high-resolution GLC.

# ANTIMICROBIAL SUSCEPTIBILITY TESTING AND THERAPY

When mixed infections are encountered, definitive information about the identification of each species present usually does not affect therapeutic management. Because most clinically relevant anaerobes are susceptible to first-line antimicrobials (Table 41-6), knowledge of their presence and Gram stain morphologies in mixed cultures is usually sufficient for guiding therapy. Therefore, definitive identification methods that follow the schemes outlined should be judiciously applied to clinical situations in which an anaerobic organism is isolated in pure culture from a normally sterile site (e.g., clostridial myonecrosis).

The therapeutic options listed in Table 41-6 for each of the major groups of anaerobic bacteria are rapidly changing; therefore, therapeutic use of the antimicrobial agents listed generally requires the performance of antimicrobial susceptibility testing with anaerobic isolates. Although standard susceptibility testing methods have been established for testing anaerobic bacteria against various antimicrobial agents (Table 41-7), the fastidious nature of many species and the labor intensity involved in using these methods indicate that testing should be done only under recommended circumstances (Box 41-3).

Although certain commercial methods (e.g., Etest, Spiral Gradient; see Chapter 12) may facilitate anaerobic

**TABLE 41-6** Antimicrobial Therapy and Susceptibility Testing of Anaerobic Bacteria

| Organism Group | Therapeutic Options | Potential Resistance to Therapeutic Options | Validated Testing Methods* |
|---|---|---|---|
| *Bacteroides fragilis* group, other *Bacteroides* spp., *Porphyromonas* spp., *Prevotella* spp., and *Fusobacterium* spp. | Highly effective agents include most beta-lactam/beta-lactamase–inhibitor combinations, imipenem, metronidazole, and chloramphenicol<br>Cefoxitin (cephalosporin)<br>Moxifloxacin (fluoroquinolone) | Beta-lactamase production does occur but generally does not significantly affect imipenem or beta-lactamase–inhibitor combinations. However, isolates of *B. fragilis* are known to produce beta-lactamases capable of hydrolyzing imipenem. Metronidazole resistance has been reported; resistance to various cephalosporins or clindamycin does occur, and susceptibility to these agents cannot be assumed. Decreasing susceptibility to ampicillin-sulbactam and amoxicillin-clavulanate has been reported. | Yes; see Table 41-7 |
| *Clostridium* spp. | Penicillins, with or without beta-lactamase–inhibitor combinations and imipenem; metronidazole or vancomycin for *C. difficile*–induced gastrointestinal disease; antimicrobial therapy is not indicated for botulism and *C. perfringens* food poisoning | Resistance to therapeutic options is not common, but cephalosporins and clindamycin show uncertain clinical efficacy | Yes; see Table 41-7 |
| *Actinomyces* spp., *Propionibacterium* spp., *Bifidobacterium* spp., *Eubacterium* spp. | Penicillins, with or without beta-lactamase–inhibitor combinations, imipenem, cefotaxime, and ceftizoxime | Resistance to therapeutic options not common; generally resistant to many cephalosporins and metronidazole | Yes; see Table 41-7 |
| *Peptostreptococcus* spp., and *Peptococcus niger* | Penicillins, most cephalosporins, imipenem, vancomycin, clindamycin, and chloramphenicol | Resistance to therapeutic options is not common | Yes; see Table 41-7 |

Data from the Clinical Laboratory Science Institute (CLSI): *Abbreviated identification of bacteria and yeast,* Approved guideline, M35-A2, Wayne, Pa, 2002, CLSI; and Versalovic J: *Manual of clinical microbiology,* ed 10, Washington, DC, 2011, ASM Press.
*Validated testing methods include standard methods recommended by the Clinical and Laboratory Standards Institute (CLSI) and commercial methods approved by the U.S. Food and Drug Administration (FDA).

**TABLE 41-7** Summary of Antimicrobial Susceptibility Testing Methods for Anaerobic Bacteria

| Test Conditions | TEST METHODS | | |
|---|---|---|---|
| | Agar Dilution | Broth Microdilution | Etest |
| Medium | *Brucella* agar supplemented with hemin (5 $\mu$g/mL), vitamin K (1 $\mu$g/mL), and 5% (V/V) laked sheep blood | *Brucella* broth supplemented with hemin (5 $\mu$g/mL), vitamin K (1 $\mu$g/mL), and lysed horse blood (5%) | *Brucella* blood agar |
| Inoculum size | $1 \times 10^5$ CFU/spot | $1 \times 10^6$ CFU/mL | 0.1-1 McFarland standard, swab plate |
| Incubation conditions | Anaerobic, 35°-37° C | Anaerobic, 35°-37° C | Anaerobic, 35°-37° C |
| Incubation duration | 48 hr | 48 hr | 24-48 hr |

Data from the National Committee for Clinical Laboratory Standards (NCCLS): *Abbreviated identification of bacteria and yeast,* Approved guideline, M35-A2, Wayne, Pa, 2002, NCCLS; and Versalovic J: *Manual of clinical microbiology,* ed 10, Washington, DC, 2011, ASM Press.
*CFU,* Colony forming units; *V/V,* volume/volume.

---

**BOX 41-3** Indications for Performing Antimicrobial Susceptibility Testing with Anaerobic Bacteria

- To establish patterns of susceptibility of anaerobes to new antimicrobial agents
- To periodically monitor susceptibility patterns of anaerobic bacteria collected in and among specific geographic areas or particular health care institutions
- To assist in the therapeutic management of patients, when such information may be critical because of the following:
  - Known resistance of a particular species to commonly used agents
  - Therapeutic failures and/or persistence of an organism at a site of infection
  - Lack of a precedence for therapeutic management of a particular infection
  - Severity of an infection (e.g., brain abscess, osteomyelitis, infections of prosthetic devices, and refractory or recurrent bacteremia)

Modified from Clinical and Laboratory Standards Institute (CLSI): Document M11-A8.

---

susceptibility testing in some way, the difficulty of assigning clinical significance to many anaerobic isolates and the availability of several highly effective empiric therapeutic choices significantly challenge a laboratory policy of routinely performing susceptibility testing with these organisms.

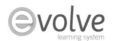 *Visit the Evolve site to complete the review questions.*

---

# BIBLIOGRAPHY

Committee on Infectious Diseases: *2006 Red book: report of the Committee on Infectious Diseases,* ed 27, Elk Grove, Ill, 2006, American Academy of Pediatrics.

Coy B: The role of the anaerobic chamber in microbiology today, *American Laboratory,* 2010.

Johnson CC: Susceptibility of anaerobic bacteria to β-lactam antibiotics in the United States, *Clin Infect Dis* 16(suppl 4):S371, 1993.

Knoop FC, Owens M, Crocker IC: *Clostridium difficile:* clinical disease and diagnosis, *Clin Microbiol Rev* 6:251, 1993.

Microlog Minutes: Biolog, Inc.: Gram-negative and Gram-positive bacteria, Hayward, Calif, Volume 1, Issue 1, 2003.

National Committee for Clinical Laboratory Standards (NCCLS): *Abbreviated identification of bacteria and yeast,* Approved guideline, M35-A2, Wayne, Pa, 2008, NCCLS.

Versalovic J: *Manual of clinical microbiology,* ed 10, Washington, DC, 2011, ASM Press.

# Overview of Anaerobic Organisms

## OBJECTIVES

1. For each group of organisms listed, provide the general characteristics, including Gram stain reactions, colonial morphology, growth requirements (media, oxygen requirement, temperature), laboratory identification, and clinical significance.
2. Differentiate normal anaerobic bacteria from pathogenic bacteria isolated from clinical specimens.
3. Describe the pathogenesis and virulence factors associated with the *Clostridium* species *C. perfringens, C. botulinum, C. difficile,* and *C. septicum.*
4. Define and discuss the pathogenesis for anaerobic cellulitis, gas gangrene, clostridial gastroenteritis, pseudomembranous enterocolitis, botulism, actinomycosis, bacterial vaginosis, and enteritis necroticans.
5. Differentiate the three forms of botulism (food poisoning, wound botulism, and infant botulism).
6. Compare paralysis associated with botulism with tetanus.
7. Explain the procedure for spore isolation and growth using the ethyl alcohol shock procedure.
8. List the appropriate specimen collection, transport, and storage conditions for the recovery of anaerobic organisms.
9. Explain aerotolerance testing, including how to perform the test, what media is used, and the reason or reasons the media is important.
10. Identify the special potency antibiotics and explain the typical resistance patterns used to identify the various anaerobic groups (e.g., gram-positive cocci, gram-negative cocci).
11. Correlate disease signs and symptoms with laboratory data to identify the etiologic agent of infection.

### GENERA AND SPECIES TO BE CONSIDERED

| Current Name | Previous Name |
|---|---|
| **Gram-Positive, Spore-Forming Bacilli** | |
| *Clostridium botulinum* | |
| *Clostridium difficile* | |
| *Clostridium perfringens* | |
| *Clostridium septicum* | |
| *Clostridium sordellii* | |
| *Clostridium tetani* | |
| Other *Clostridium* spp. | |
| **Gram-Positive, Non–Spore-Forming Bacilli** | |
| *Actinomyces israelii* | |
| *Actinomyces naeslundii* | |
| *Actinomyces odontolyticus* | |
| Other *Actinomyces* spp. | |
| *Atopobium minutum* | *Lactobacillus minutum* |
| *Atopobium parvulum* | *Streptococcus parvulum* |
| *Bifidobacterium* spp. | |
| *Collinsella aerofaciens* | *Eubacterium aerofaciens* |
| *Eggerthella lenta* | *Eubacterium lentum* |
| *Eubacterium* spp. | |

### GENERA AND SPECIES TO BE CONSIDERED—cont'd

| Current Name | Previous Name |
|---|---|
| *Lactobacillus* spp. | |
| *Mobiluncus* spp. | |
| *Propionibacterium* spp. | |
| **Gram-Positive Cocci** | |
| *Anaerococcus prevotii* | *Peptostreptococcus prevotii* |
| *Anaerococcus tetradius* | *Peptostreptococcus tetradius* |
| *Finegoldia magna* | *Peptostreptococcus magnus* |
| *Gallicola barnesae* | *Peptostreptococcus barnesae* |
| *Parvimonas micra* | *Micromonas micros, Peptostreptococcus micros* |
| *Peptococcus niger* | |
| *Peptoniphilus* spp. | |
| *Peptostreptococcus anaerobius* | |
| *Staphylococcus saccharolyticus* | *Peptostreptococcus saccharolyticus* |
| **Gram-Negative Bacilli** | |
| *Bacteroides fragilis* group | |
| Other *Bacteroides* spp. | |
| *Bacteroides ureolyticus* | |
| *Bilophila wadsworthia* | |
| *Fusobacterium* spp. | |
| *Leptotrichia* spp. | |
| *Porphyromonas* spp. | |
| *Prevotella* spp. | |
| *Sutterella wadsworthensis* | |
| **Gram-Negative Cocci** | |
| *Acidaminococcus* | |
| *Megasphaera* | |
| *Veillonella* spp. | |

As previously described in Chapter 41, the organisms in this chapter predominantly do not grow in the presence of oxygen.

## EPIDEMIOLOGY

Most of the anaerobic bacteria that cause infections in humans are also part of our normal flora. The ecology of these organisms is such that various species and genera exhibit preferences for the body sites they inhabit (endogenous anaerobes) (Table 42-1). Other pathogenic anaerobes (e.g., *Clostridium botulinum* and *Clostridium tetani*) are soil and environmental inhabitants (exogenous anaerobes) and are not considered part of the normal human flora.

The ways in which anaerobic infections are acquired are summarized in Table 42-2. Person-to-person nosocomial spread of *Clostridium difficile* among hospitalized patients presents an enormous clinical and infection control dilemma; however, most anaerobic infections

TABLE 42-1 Incidence of Anaerobes as Normal Flora of Humans

| Genus | Skin | Upper Respiratory Tract* | Intestine | External Genitalia | Urethra | Vagina |
|---|---|---|---|---|---|---|
| **Gram-Negative Bacteria** | | | | | | |
| *Bacteroides* | 0 | ± | 2 | ± | ± | ± |
| *Prevotella* | 0 | 2 | 2 | 1 | ± | 1 |
| *Porphyromonas* | 0 | 1 | 1 | U | U | ± |
| *Fusobacterium* | 0 | 2 | 1 | U | U | ± |
| *Veillonella* | 0 | 2 | 1 | 0 | U | 1 |
| **Gram-Positive Bacteria** | | | | | | |
| *Finegoldia* | 1 | 2 | 2 | 1 | ± | 1 |
| *Parvimonas* | 1 | 2 | 2 | 1 | ± | 1 |
| *Clostridium* | ± | ± | 2 | ± | ± | ± |
| *Actinomyces* | 0 | 1 | 1 | 0 | 0 | ± |
| *Bifidobacterium* | 0 | 1 | 2 | 0 | 0 | ± |
| *Eubacterium* | 0 | 1 | 2 | U | U | 1 |
| *Lactobacillus* | 0 | 1 | 1 | 0 | ± | 2 |
| *Propionibacterium* | 2 | 1 | ± | ± | ± | 1 |

Modified from Summanen PE, Baron EJ, Citron DM et al: *Wadsworth anaerobic bacteriology manual,* ed 5, Belmont, Calif, 1993, Star.
*U,* Unknown; *0,* not found or rare; ±, irregular; *1,* usually present; *2,* present in large numbers.
*Includes nasal passages, nasopharynx, oropharynx, and tonsils.

TABLE 42-2 Acquisition of Anaerobic Infections and Diseases

| Mode of Acquisition | Examples |
|---|---|
| Endogenous strains of normal flora gain access to normally sterile sites, usually as result of one or more predisposing factors that compromise normal anatomic barriers (e.g., surgery or accidental trauma) or alter other host defense mechanisms (e.g., malignancy, diabetes, burns, immunosuppressive therapy, aspiration) | Wide variety of infections involving several anatomic locations, including bacteremia, head and neck infections, dental and orofacial infections, pneumonia and other infections of the thoracic cavity, intraabdominal and obstetric and gynecologic infections, bite wound and other soft tissue infections, and gangrene (i.e., clostridial myonecrosis). Organisms most commonly encountered in these infections include *Bacteroides fragilis* group, *Prevotella* spp., *Porphyromonas* spp., *Fusobacterium nucleatum*, *Peptostreptococcus* spp., and *Clostridium perfringens*. |
| Contamination of existing wound or puncture by objects contaminated with toxigenic *Clostridium* spp. | Tetanus (*Clostridium tetani*), gas gangrene (*Clostridium perfringens* and, less commonly, *C. septicum, C. novyi,* and others) |
| Ingestion of preformed toxins in vegetable- or meat-based foods | Botulism (*Clostridium botulinum*) and other clostridial food poisonings (*C. perfringens*) |
| Colonization of gastrointestinal tract with potent toxin-producing organism | Infant botulism (*C. botulinum*) |
| Person-to-person spread | Nosocomial spread of *Clostridium difficile*–induced diarrhea and pseudomembranous colitis; bite wound infections caused by a variety of anaerobic species |

occur when a patient's normal flora gains access to a sterile site as a result of disruption of some anatomic barrier.

# PATHOGENESIS AND SPECTRUM OF DISEASE

The types of infections and diseases in humans caused by anaerobic bacteria span a wide spectrum. Certain species, such as *C. botulinum* and *C. tetani*, produce some of the most potent toxins known. In contrast, specific virulence factors for the organisms commonly encountered in infections (e.g., *B. fragilis* group, *C. difficile*) are not well understood (Table 42-3).

Most anaerobic infections involve a mixture of anaerobic and facultative anaerobic organisms (e.g., Enterobacteriaceae), which creates problems in identification and diagnosis to establish the extent to which a particular anaerobic species contributes to infection. In addition,

**TABLE 42-3** Pathogenesis and Spectrum of Disease for Anaerobic Bacteria

| Organism | Virulence Factors | Spectrum of Disease and Infections |
| --- | --- | --- |
| *Clostridium perfringens* | Produces several exotoxins; alpha-toxin, the most important, mediates destruction of host cell membranes; enterotoxin inserts and disrupts membranes of mucosal cells<br>Beta-toxin—cytotoxin | Gas gangrene (myonecrosis): Life-threatening, toxin-mediated destruction of muscle and other tissues after traumatic introduction of the organism.<br>Food poisoning: Caused by release of the toxin after ingestion of large numbers of the organism. Usually self-limiting and benign; manifested by abdominal cramps, diarrhea, and vomiting.<br>Enteritis necroticans (necrotizing enteritis; NEC): Life-threatening infection that causes ischemic necrosis of the jejunum. Often associated with immunocompromised patients (e.g., those with diabetes, alcohol-induced liver disease, or neutropenia). NEC, a gastrointestinal disease that causes bowel necrosis and inflammation, affects low-birth-weight, premature infants. |
| *Clostridium sordellii* | Produces a variety of bacterial proteases, phospholipases<br>Produces up to seven exotoxins, including lethal toxin (LT), hemorrhagic toxin (HT), and enterotoxins A, B, and C | Gas gangrene of the uterus as a result of abortion, normal delivery, or cesarean section.<br>Patient presents with little or no fever, lack of purulent discharge, hypotension, peripheral edema, and an increased white blood cell (WBC) count. Infection is typically fatal, and death is rapid. |
| *Clostridium tetani* | Produces tetanospasmin (TeNT), a neurotoxic exotoxin that disrupts nerve impulses to muscles | Tetanus (commonly known as lockjaw). Organism establishes a wound infection and elaborates TeNT, a potent toxin that mediates generalized muscle spasms. If the disease goes untreated, spasms continue to be triggered by even minor stimuli, leading to exhaustion and, eventually, respiratory failure. |
| *Clostridium botulinum* | Produces an extremely potent neurotoxin (BoNT) | Foodborne botulism: Results from ingestion of preformed toxin in nonacidic vegetable or mushroom foodstuffs. Absorption of the toxin leads to nearly complete flaccid (rag doll) paralysis of respiratory and other essential muscle groups.<br>Infant botulism: Occurs when the organism elaborates the toxin after it has colonized the gastrointestinal tract of infants (i.e., infant botulism).<br>Wound botulism: Occurs when *C. botulinum* produces the toxin from an infected wound site |
| *Clostridium difficile* | Produces toxin A (TcdA), an enterotoxin, and toxin B (TcdB), a cytotoxin<br>Both toxin A and toxin B are classified as large clostridial cytotoxins<br>The toxins glycosylate guanosine triphosphate (GTP) signaling proteins, leading to a breakdown of the cellular cytotoxin and cell death | Organism requires diminution of normal gut flora by the activity of various antimicrobial agents to become established in the gut of hospitalized patients. Once established, elaboration of one or more toxins results in antibiotic-associated diarrhea or potentially life-threatening inflammation of the colon. When the surface of the inflamed bowel is overlaid with a "pseudomembrane" composed of necrotic debris, white blood cells, and fibrin, the disease is referred to as *pseudomembranous colitis.*<br>Only strains producing toxin A or toxin B (or both) cause infections. |
| *Actinomyces* spp., including *A. israelii, A. meyeri, A. naeslundii,* and *A. odontolyticus* | No well-characterized virulence factors. Infections usually require disruption of protective mucosal surface of the oral cavity, respiratory tract, gastrointestinal tract, and/or female genitourinary tract | Usually involved in mixed oral or cervicofacial, thoracic, pelvic, and abdominal infections caused by patient's endogenous strains.<br>Certain species (*A. viscosus* and *A. naeslundii*) also involved in periodontal disease and dental caries.<br>Identified in a variety of soft tissue infections, including perianal, groin, ancillary, breast, and periaural abscesses. |
| *Propionibacterium* spp. | No definitive virulence factors known | Associated with inflammatory process in acne.<br>Identified in systemic opportunistic infections, including endocarditis, central nervous system (CNS) infections, osteomyelitis, and arthritis.<br>As part of normal skin flora, the organism is considered the most common anaerobic contaminant of blood cultures and is often ignored. |
| *Atopobium* spp. | No definitive virulence factors known | Isolated from various infections in the genital tract, including bacterial vaginosis.<br>Considered normal flora of the female genital tract. |

*Continued*

**TABLE 42-3** Pathogenesis and Spectrum of Disease for Anaerobic Bacteria—cont'd

| Organism | Virulence Factors | Spectrum of Disease and Infections |
|---|---|---|
| *Bifidobacterium* spp. | No definitive virulence factors known | Not commonly found in clinical specimens. Usually encountered in mixed infections of the pelvis or abdomen. |
| *Eggerthella* spp. | No definitive virulence factors known | Recovered from a variety of infections including intraabdominal and periabdominal infections. |
| *Eubacterium* spp. | No definitive virulence factors known | Usually associated with mixed infections of the oral cavity, abdomen, pelvis, or genitourinary tract. |
| *Lactobacillus* spp. | No definitive virulence factors known | Associated with advanced dental caries. Organism has also been identified in endocarditis and bacteremia. |
| *Mobiluncus* spp. | No definitive virulence factors known | Organisms are found in the vagina and have been associated with bacterial vaginosis, but their precise role in gynecologic infections is unclear. Rarely encountered in infections outside the female genital tract. |
| *Bacteroides fragilis* group, other *Bacteroides* spp., including *B. gracilis* and *B. ureolyticus* *Prevotella* spp. *Porphyromonas* spp. *Fusobacterium nucleatum* and other *Fusobacterium* spp. | Anaerobic, gram-negative bacilli that produce capsules, endotoxin, and succinic acid, which inhibit phagocytosis, and various enzymes that mediate tissue damage. Most infections still require some breach of mucosal integrity that allows the organisms to gain access to deeper tissues | Organisms most commonly encountered in anaerobic infections. Infections are often mixed with infections caused by other anaerobic and facultative anaerobic organisms. Infections occur throughout the body, usually as localized or enclosed abscesses, and may involve the cranium, periodontium, thorax, peritoneum, liver, and female genital tract. May also cause bacteremia, aspiration pneumonia, septic arthritis, chronic sinusitis, decubitus ulcers, and other soft tissue infections. The hallmark of most but not all infections is the production of a foul odor. In general, infections caused by *B. fragilis* group occur below the diaphragm; pigmented *Prevotella* spp., *Porphyromonas* spp., and *F. nucleatum* generally are involved in head and neck and pleuropulmonary infections. |
| *Finegoldia magna* *Parvimonas micra* | No definitive virulence factors known *P. micra* has been shown to produce a variety of enzymes capable of tissue destruction, including collagenase, hemolysin, and elastase. | Most often found mixed with other anaerobic and facultatively anaerobic bacteria in cutaneous, respiratory, oral, or female pelvic infections. |
| *Peptostreptococcus anaerobius* | No definitive virulence factors known | Most often isolated from polymicrobic infections, including abscesses. |
| *Veillonella* spp. | No definitive virulence factors known | May be involved in mixed infections. Organisms have been isolated in increasingly serious infections, including meningitis, osteomyelitis, endocarditis, bacteremia, and prosthetic infections. |

as ubiquitous members of our normal flora, anaerobic organisms frequently contaminate clinical materials. For these reasons, assigning clinical significance to anaerobic bacteria isolated in the laboratory is important, although often difficult.

## GRAM-POSITIVE, SPORE-FORMING BACILLI

The clostridia are the endospore-forming, obligately anaerobic (or aerotolerant), catalase-negative, gram-positive bacilli (Figure 42-1). The rods are pleomorphic and may be arranged in pairs or short chains. If spores are not present on Gram stain, the ethanol shock spore or heat shock spore test can separate this group from the non–spore-forming anaerobic bacilli (see Procedure 42-1

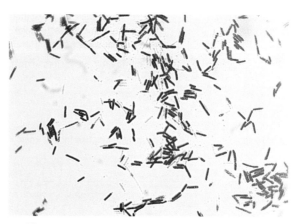

**Figure 42-1** Gram stain of *Clostridium perfringens*.

on the Evolve site). Some strains of *C. perfringens, C. ramosum,* and *C. clostridioforme* may not produce spores or survive a spore test, so it is important to recognize these organisms using other characteristics. Some clostridia typically stain gram negative, although they are susceptible to vancomycin on the disk test. Several species of clostridia grow aerobically (*C. tertium, C. carnis, C. histolyticum,* and occasional strains of *C. perfringens*), but they produce spores only under anaerobic conditions. *C. perfringens* may appear weakly catalase positive.

*Clostridium* species are widespread in nature because of their ability to form spores, referred to as *endospores,* in the mother cell (Table 42-4). In addition, they are present in large numbers as normal flora in the gastrointestinal tract of humans and animals, the female genital tract, and the oral mucosa.

**TABLE 42-4** Characteristics of Clinically Significant *Clostridium* species

| Species | Spore Location | Gelatin | Lecithinase | Lipase | Indole | Esculin | Nitrate |
|---|---|---|---|---|---|---|---|
| *C. argentinense* | ST | + | − | − | − | − | − |
| *C. baratii* | ST | − | + | − | − | + | V |
| *C. bifermentans* | ST | + | + | − | + | V | − |
| *C. bolteae* | ST | − | − | − | − | V | − |
| *C. botulinum* Types A,B, and F | ST | + | − | + | − | + | − |
| Types B, E, and F-nonproteolytic | ST | + | − | + | − | − | − |
| Types C and D | T | + | V | + | V | − | − |
| *C. butyricum* | ST | − | − | − | − | + | − |
| *C. cadaveris* | T | + | - | - | + | − | − |
| *C. canis* | ST | − | − | − | − | + | − |
| *C. clostridioforme* | ST | − | − | − | − | + | − |
| *C. difficile* | ST⁽ᵀ⁾ | + | − | − | − | + | − |
| *C. glycolicum* | ST | − | − | − | − | V | − |
| *C. hastiforme* | T | + | − | − | − | − | V |
| *C. hathewayi* | ST | − | − | − | − | + | − |
| *C. histolyticum* | ST | + | − | − | − | − | − |
| *C. indolis* | T | − | − | − | + | + | V |
| *C. innocuum* | T | − | − | − | − | + | − |
| *C. limosum* | ST | + | + | − | − | − | − |
| *C. novyi A* | ST | + | + | + | − | − | − |
| *C. paraputrificum* | T⁽ˢᵀ⁾ | − | − | − | − | + | V |
| *C. perfringens* | ST | + | + | − | − | V | V |
| *C. putrificum* | T⁽ˢᵀ⁾ | + | − | − | − | V | − |
| *C. ramosum* | T | − | − | − | − | + | − |
| *C. septicum* | ST | + | − | − | − | + | V |
| *C. sordelli* | ST | + | + | − | + | V | − |
| *C. sphenoides* | ST⁽ᵀ⁾ | − | − | − | + | + | V |
| *C. sporogenes* | ST | + | − | + | − | + | − |
| *C. subterminale* | ST | + | V | − | − | V | − |
| *C. symbiosum* | ST | − | − | − | − | − | − |
| *C. tertium* | T | − | − | − | − | + | V |
| *C. tetani* | T | + | − | − | V | − | − |

Modified from Versalovic J: *Manual of clinical microbiology,* ed 10, 2011, Washington, DC, ASM Press.
+, Positive reaction; −negative reaction; *V,* variable reaction; *ST,* subterminal; *T,* terminal; superscript indicates variability.

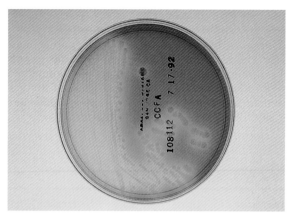

**Figure 42-2** *Clostridium difficile* on cycloserine cefoxitin fructose agar (CCFA). (Courtesy Anaerobe Systems, Morgan Hill, Calif.)

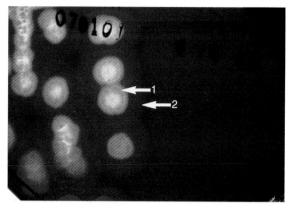

**Figure 42-3** *Clostridium perfringens* on anaerobic blood agar. Note double zone of beta-hemolysis. *1,* First zone; *2,* second zone. (Courtesy Anaerobe Systems, Morgan Hill, Calif.)

*C. botulinum* is listed by the Centers for Disease Control and Prevention (CDC) as a potential agent of bioterrorism (see Chapter 80). A diagnosis of botulism is made by the demonstration of botulinum neurotoxin in serum, feces, gastric contents, vomitus, or suspect food (food poisoning) or environmental specimen (potential bioterrorism incident). This means that most hospital laboratories must know how to package and ship such a specimen to the State Health Department or CDC. Isolation of *C. botulinum* is rarely seen in the clinical microbiology laboratory. Table 42-3 describes the pathogenesis of the frequently encountered *Clostridium* spp.

## Laboratory Diagnosis and Specimen Collection

As stated in Chapter 41, the proper collection and transport of specimens for anaerobic culture cannot be overemphasized. General considerations are included in the discussion in Chapter 41. However, special collection instructions must be followed for some clostridial illnesses, specifically foodborne *C. perfringens* and *C. botulinum*, *C. difficile* pseudomembranous enterocolitis, and *C. septicum* neutropenic enterocolitis (NEC). Food and freshly passed fecal specimens must be sent to a public health laboratory for confirmation of *C. perfringens* food poisoning; these should be transported at 4° C. The specimens should be processed within 24 hours of collection. The clinical diagnosis of botulism is confirmed by demonstration of botulinum toxin in serum, feces, vomitus, or gastric contents, as well as by recovery of the organism from the stool of patients (Figure 42-2). Several methods are available, including cell culture assays, enzyme-linked immunosorbent assay (ELISA), and latex agglutination.

*C. perfringens*–associated enteritis necroticans infection requires the collection of three blood cultures, stool and bowel contents, or bowel tissue. Specimens should be Gram-stained and cultured. Follow-up tests to identify the organism are determined by the interpretation of the initial Gram stain. The isolate should be serologically typed. In addition, polymerase chain reaction (PCR) testing is available for *C. perfringens*.

Suspected *C. difficile* infection (CDI) indicates collection of a freshly passed stool specimen for culture and toxin assays for both toxin A and toxin B. Only liquid or unformed stools should be processed for CDI to prevent the treatment of patients colonized with the bacterium. Formed stools or rectal swabs are adequate to detect carriers. Specimens should be cultured within 2 hours after collection. Figure 42-3 demonstrates the isolation of *C. difficile* on cycloserine cefoxitin fructose agar (CCFA) and on anaerobic blood agar. Specimens may be stored in anaerobic transport bags at 4° C for up to 48 hours; however, this reduces the recovery rate of viable organisms in culture. Specimens for toxin assays may be stored at 4° for 72 hours or frozen at −70° C if a longer delay is expected.

A variety of immunoassays are commercially available for the identification of *C. difficile* enterotoxin. In addition, a variety of molecular-based assays have been developed for the amplification of the toxin A (tcdA) and toxin B (tcdB) genes. Stool samples may be submitted for PCR amplification. The assays include amplification of the glutamate dehydrogenase (GDH) gene or 16srRNA as internal control housekeeping genes. Detection of the GDH and 16s rRNA genes without the presence of a toxin gene would indicate a nonpathogenic strain or carrier state. A new molecular assay is currently available: Illumigene *C. difficile*, (Meridian Bioscience, Inc., Memphis, TN), using LAMP isothermal amplification. See Chapter 8 for information on LAMP methodology. Cell culture cultivation is still recommended for molecular stain typing and epidemiologic studies.

The CDC maintains a 24-hour/day, 365-day/year hotline to provide emergency assistance in cases of botulism. Botulinum toxin is a potential bioweapon. Acceptable specimens for the diagnosis of *C. botulinum* or *C. tetani* infection include feces, enema fluid, gastric aspirates, vomitus, tissue, exudates, or postmortem specimens. Specimens for infant botulism should include serum and stool; those for wound botulism should include serum, stool, and tissue biopsy. Serum specimens should be collected immediately after the onset of symptoms. All specimens should be stored and shipped at 4° C. Detection of the toxin BoNT is diagnostic for *C. botulinum* infection. The mouse bioassay remains the recommended method of analysis for the identification of BoNT. The bioassay requires that the specimen be split

**TABLE 42-5** Differentiation of Representative Gram-Negative Bacilli and Gram-Positive Cocci

| | GRAM-NEGATIVE BACILLI | | |
| | B. fragilis | B. thetaiotaomicron | F. nucleatum |
|---|---|---|---|
| **Test Method** | | | |
| Arabinose | Neg | Pos | Neg |
| Bile 20%, growth | Pos | Pos | Neg |
| Catalase | Pos | Pos | Neg |
| Colistin (Col) | R | R | S |
| Esculin hydrolysis | Pos | Pos | Neg |
| Gelatinase | 0 | 0 | 0 |
| Indole | Neg | Pos | Pos |
| Kanamycin (Km) | R | R | S |
| Nitrate | Neg | Neg | Neg |
| Vancomycin (Van) | R | R | R |
| | GRAM-POSITIVE BACILLI | | |
| | P. anaerobius | P. asaccharolyticus | F. magna |
| **Test Method** | | | |
| Indole | Neg | Pos | Neg |
| Nitrate | Neg | Neg | Neg |
| Sodium polyanethol sulfonate (SPS) | S | R | R |

From Versalovic J: *Manual of clinical microbiology,* ed 10, Washington, DC, 2011, ASM Press.*Neg,* Negative reaction; *Pos,* positive reaction; *R,* resistant; *S,* sensitive; *V,* variable.
>10 mm = sensitive for Km, Van, Col; >12 mm = sensitive for SPS.

into two samples. One sample is boiled at 80° C for 10 minutes, inactivating the toxins. The two samples are each injected intraperitoneally into a mouse. One mouse serves as the negative control (inactivated specimen), and the other serves as the "test" sample. The mice are then observed for neurologic symptoms. The presence of toxin is presumptively indicated with the development of symptoms and death in the test animal but not the control animal. The toxins associated with *C. botulinum* and *C. tetani* (BoNT and tetanus neurotoxin) are considered extremely dangerous. The CDC recommends the use of Biosafety Level 3 practices and precautions, including immunization for the toxins.

The specimens of choice for neutropenic enterocolitis involving *C. septicum* are three different blood cultures, stool, and lumen contents or tissue from the involved ileocecal area; a muscle biopsy sample should also be collected if myonecrosis (death of muscle tissue) is suspected. Table 42-5 provides an identification scheme for representative anaerobic organisms.

## GRAM-POSITIVE, NON–SPORE-FORMING BACILLI

The genera *Actinomyces, Bifidobacterium, Eubacterium, Eggerthella, Collinsella,* anaerobic *Lactobacillus, Mobiluncus, Atopobium,* and *Propionibacterium* are among the anaerobic, gram-positive, non–spore-forming bacilli. These organisms are typically found as normal flora on the mucosal surfaces of the human digestive tract and urogenital tract and on the skin. These organisms rarely cause infections independently. They typically are identified in a polymicrobic infection of a mucosal surface, such as the oral or vaginal cavity or the urogenital tract.

The genera *Actinomyces* (anaerobic and aerotolerant) and *Mobiluncus* (strictly anaerobic) include species that show non–acid-fast, gram-positive, pleomorphic branching rods or coccobacilli. Direct examination and the macroscopic presence in purulent exudate of "sulfur granules," which reveal gram-positive filaments when crushed, is diagnostic for an infection with *Actinomyces* spp. *Mobiluncus* spp., a cause of bacterial vaginosis, usually is diagnosed on Gram staining of vaginal secretions by observation of gram-variable, curved rods with tapered ends. It is rarely isolated in the clinical laboratory, because vaginal secretions are not acceptable specimens for anaerobic culture. *Propionibacterium* spp. are anaerobic and aerotolerant, pleomorphic, gram-positives rods. The bacterium produces propionic acid from glucose. *Bifidobacterium* spp. are strictly anaerobic or microaerophilic, gram-positive, pleomorphic rods that appear as rods or as branched or club shaped. *Lactobacillus* spp. contain microaerophilic, catalase-negative, gram-positive rods capable of producing lactic acid from glucose fermentation. The genus *Eubacterium* remains poorly characterized, although its species are commonly isolated from oral infections. The pathogenic mechanisms and the spectrum of diseases associated with these organisms are included in Table 42-3.

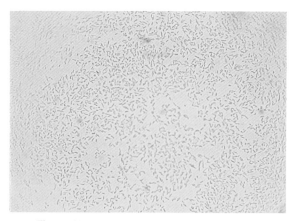

**Figure 42-4** Gram stain of *Bacteroides fragilis*.

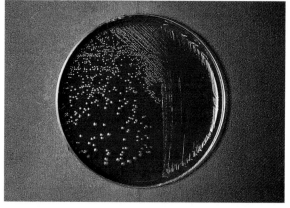

**Figure 42-5** *Bacteroides fragilis* on anaerobic blood agar.

## Laboratory Diagnosis

Differentiation of the gram-positive, non–spore forming anaerobes is based on colony and Gram stain morphology. Follow-up tests to identify the organism are determined by the interpretation of the initial Gram stain results. Additional tests include an aerotolerance test (see Procedure 42-2 on the Evolve site) or growth in 5% $CO_2$, followed by routine screening of special-potency antibiotic susceptibility patterns. The gram-positive organisms typically are resistant to colistin (10 μg), susceptible to vancomycin (5 μg), and have variable sensitivity to kanamycin (1 mg). Additional rapid testing includes a 15% catalase test, production of indole, and nitrate reduction. Although currently no rapid molecular amplification tests are available in the clinical laboratory, isolates can be submitted to reference laboratories for 16s RNA sequence analysis. Table 42-5 provides an identification scheme for representative anaerobic organisms.

## GRAM-NEGATIVE RODS

### Bacteroides Fragilis Group

The anaerobic gram-negative rods typically are isolated from the mucosal surfaces of the human oral cavity and gastrointestinal tract (Figure 42-4). (Table 42-3 presents an overview of the pathogenesis and infections associated with these organisms.) The Bacteroidaceae family consists of the saccharolytic, bile-resistant, nonpigmented *Bacteroides fragilis* group. *B. fragilis* is the most common organism isolated from clinical specimens, followed by *B. thetaiotaomicron* and *B. ovatus*. These organisms have been associated with a variety of infections.

The gram-negative *Bacteroides fragilis* group grows in 20% bile, and the organisms are almost always resistant to all three special-potency antibiotic disks (Figures 42-5 and 42-6). Rare strains of *B. fragilis* are susceptible to colistin.

### Nonpigmented *Prevotella* spp.

*Prevotella* spp. are ubiquitous in the oral cavity and are an important component of dental biofilms. *Prevotella* organisms have also been identified in the esophagus and stomach. Most are bile-sensitive, kanamycin-resistant,

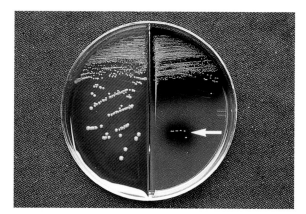

**Figure 42-6** *Bacteroides fragilis* on a biplate containing anaerobic blood agar and *Bacteroides* bile esculin agar (BBE) *(arrow)*. (Courtesy Anaerobe Systems, Morgan Hill, Calif.)

gram-negative rods. Colistin susceptibility is variable, and almost all strains are catalase and indole negative.

### Pigmented *Porphyromonas* and *Prevotella* spp.

The Porphyromonadaceae family comprises five genera, including the genera, *Parabacteroides*, *Porphyromonas*, *Tannerella*, *Odoribacter*, and *Barnesiella*. *Porphyromonas* generally is considered the pathogenic genus in the Porphyromonadaceae family. Most *Porphyromonas* spp. are asaccharolytic and pigmented. The Prevotellaceae includes saccharolytic organisms that have been isolated from a variety of body sites, including the oral cavity and feces. Colonies that fluoresce brick red or produce brown to black pigment are placed among the pigmented *Prevotella* (Figure 42-7) and *Porphyromonas* spp. (Figure 42-8). Some species appear coccobacillary on Gram staining.

### Bacteroides ureolyticus

*Bacteroides ureolyticus* is asaccharolytic, reduces nitrate, and requires formate and fumarate for growth in broth culture. Its disk pattern is the same as for the fusobacteria; however, the colony morphology is different. *B. ureolyticus* forms small, translucent to transparent colonies

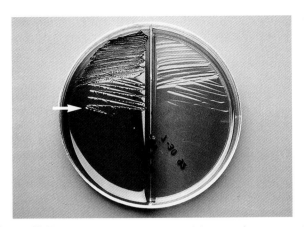

**Figure 42-7** *Prevotella disiens* on laked kanamycin-vancomycin blood agar. Note black pigment *(arrow)*.

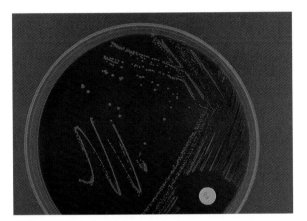

**Figure 42-8** *Porphyromonas* spp. on anaerobic blood agar. Red fluorescence is seen under ultraviolet light (365 nm). (Courtesy Anaerobe Systems, Morgan Hill, Calif.)

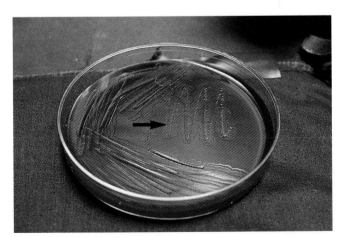

**Figure 42-9** *Bacteroides ureolyticus* on anaerobic blood agar. Note pitting of agar *(arrow)*. (Courtesy Anaerobe Systems, Morgan Hill, Calif.)

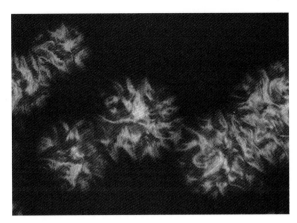

**Figure 42-10** *Fusobacterium nucleatum* subsp. *nucleatum* on anaerobic blood agar. Note bread crumb–like colonies and greening of agar.

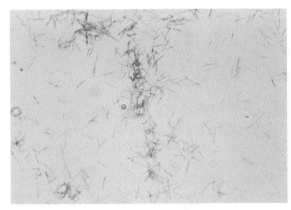

**Figure 42-11** Gram stain of *Fusobacterium nucleatum* subsp. nucleatum. Note pointed ends.

that may corrode the agar (Figure 42-9), whereas the *Fusobacterium* colony generally is larger and more opaque (Figure 42-10). *B. ureolyticus* formerly was grouped with organisms that have been transferred to the genus *Campylobacter* (*C. gracilis, C. concisus, C. recta,* and *C. curva*).

The campylobacters are all microaerophiles, not anaerobes, and are discussed in Chapter 34. Curved or motile organisms that grow anaerobically but not in 5% $CO_2$ should be retested in a microaerophilic atmosphere with approximately 6% oxygen.

### Fusobacteriaceae

The Fusobacteriaceae family includes the genera *Fusobacterium, Leptotrichia,* and *Sneathia*. These organisms typically are isolated from the oral cavity as integral components of dental biofilms (Figure 42-11). The gram-negative *Fusobacterium* spp. are sensitive to kanamycin, and most strains fluoresce chartreuse. Different species have characteristic cell and colony morphologies (Figure 42-12).

*Leptotrichia* spp. are very large, fusiform rods with one pointed end and one blunt end. Colonies are large, gray, and convoluted. They are most often isolated from the oral cavity or urogenital tract.

### Protobacteria

The phylum Protobacteria contains a variety of clinically significant organisms, including *Bilophila wadsworthia*

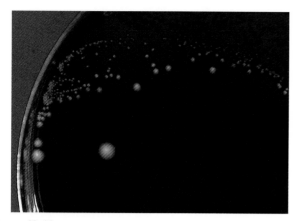

**Figure 42-12** *Peptostreptococcus anaerobius* on anaerobic blood agar.

and *Sutterella wadsworthensis*. *B. wadsworthia* is an anaerobic, asaccharolytic, bile-resistant, gram-negative rod. *S. wadsworthensis* is an asaccharolytic, bile-resistant, short, gram-negative rod. *B. wadsworthia* phenotypically resembles *B. ureolyticus* but is resistant to bile and is strongly catalase positive.

## ANAEROBIC GRAM-POSITIVE AND GRAM-NEGATIVE COCCI

As stated earlier in this chapter and in Chapter 41, the proper collection and transport of specimens for anaerobic culture cannot be overemphasized. General considerations are included in the discussion in Chapter 41. The gram-positive anaerobic cocci typically are found as part of the normal flora of the oral cavity, upper respiratory tract, gastrointestinal tract, female genitourinary tract, and the skin. The anaerobic cocci are non-spore forming and may appear slightly elongated. The cells vary in size and may be arranged in tetrads, chains, clusters, pairs, or clumps. Carbohydrate utilization varies among the genera. In addition, organisms typically classified as aerobic, such as *Staphylococcus epidermidis*, include strictly anaerobic strains. *Staphylococcus saccharolyticus* and *Staphylococcus aureus* subsp. *anaerobius* grow under anaerobic conditions, although after subculture they may develop aerotolerance. If a gram-positive coccus demonstrates resistance to metronidazole (5 µg) after 48 hours of incubation, it is likely a *Streptococcus* species.

The gram-negative anaerobic cocci are part of the normal flora of the oral cavity and the gastrointestinal, genitourinary, and respiratory tracts of humans. Among anaerobic gram-positive cocci, the genera of clinical importance are *Peptostreptococcus*, *Finegoldia*, *Gallicola*, *Parvimonas* (previously *Micromonas*), *Peptoniphilus*, *Murdochiella*, *Staphylococcus*, and *Anaerococcus*.

The category of anaerobic gram-negative cocci is based on Gram stain morphology. This category includes the genera *Veillonella*, *Megasphaera*, *Anaeroglobus*, *Negativicoccus*, and *Acidaminococcus*. The genus *Veillonella* is

ubiquitous as part of the normal flora of the human oral cavity and the genitourinary, respiratory, and gastrointestinal tracts.

### Laboratory Diagnosis

Direct examination of clinical specimens reveals grampositive or gram-negative cocci in chains, pairs, or singly. Follow-up tests to identify the organism are determined by interpretation of the initial Gram stain results. Organisms typically are isolated on anaerobic blood agar, and they can be differentiated using the special-potency antibiotic disks previously described in this chapter. Grampositive cocci are sensitive to vancomycin and resistant to colistin. Gram-negative cocci typically are resistant to vancomycin. *Peptostreptococcus anaerobius* and *Parvimonas micra* demonstrate sensitivity to sodium polyanethol sulfonate (SPS). *P. micra* also produces a milky halo around the colonies on blood agar. Interpretation and identification of either gram-positive or gram-negative cocci from a clinical specimen should be reported with caution and should correlate with the patient's signs and symptoms. Table 42-5 provides an identification scheme for representative anaerobic organisms.

## PREVENTION

A multiple-dose vaccine is available for the prevention of tetanus. The immunogen, which is adsorbed tetanus toxoid (inactivated toxin), generally is administered with diphtheria toxoid and pertussis vaccine as a triple antigen called *Tdap* or *DTP*. Single boosters of diphtheria and tetanus (Td or DT) or tetanus alone are recommended every 10 years. These vaccines can be used to catch-up individuals who did not complete their full childhood vaccinations of DTap or DTP as children.

Immunoprophylaxis in wound management is based on the type of wound. Completely immunized individuals with minor and/or uncontaminated wounds do not require specific treatment. However, completely immunized individuals with major and/or contaminated wounds should get a booster of tetanus toxoid if they have not had one in the previous 5 years. Finally, a partially immunized individual or one who has never been immunized should receive a dose of tetanus toxoid immediately. In addition, passive immunization with human tetanus immune globulin (TIG) should be given if the individual has a major wound or a wound contaminated with soil that contains animal feces.

Individuals who have eaten food suspected of containing botulinum toxin should be purged with cathartics (laxatives), have their stomach pumped, and be given high enemas.

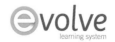 *Visit the Evolve site to complete the review questions.*

# BIBLIOGRAPHY

Dowell VR, Hawkins TM: *Laboratory methods in anaerobic bacteriology: CDC laboratory manual*, Centers for Disease Control, DHHS Pub No (CDC) 81-8272, Atlanta, 1981, US Department of Health & Human Services.

Dzink JL, Sheenan MT, Socransky SS: Proposal of three subspecies of *Fusobacterium nucleatum* Knorr, 1922: *Fusobacterium nucleatum* subsp nov, comb nov; *Fusobacterium nucleatum* subsp *polymorphum* subsp nov, nom rev, comb nov; and *Fusobacterium nucleatum* subsp *vincentii* subsp nov, nom rev, comb nov, *Int J Syst Bacteriol* 40:74, 1990.

Holdeman LV, Cato EP, Moore WEC, editors: *Anaerobic laboratory manual*, ed 4, Blacksburg, Va, 1977, Virginia Polytechnic Institute and State University.

Holdeman LV, Cato EP, Moore WEC, editors: *Anaerobic laboratory manual: update*, ed 4, Blacksburg, Va, 1987, Virginia Polytechnic Institute and State University.

Jousimies-Somer HR, Summanen P, Citron DM et al: *Wadsworth anaerobic bacteriology manual*, ed 6, Belmont, Calif, 2002, Star.

Johnson CC: Susceptibility of anaerobic bacteria to β-lactam antibiotics in the United States, *Clin Infect Dis* 16(suppl 4):S371, 1993.

Kageyama A, Benno Y, Nakase T: Phylogenetic and phenotypic evidence for the transfer of *Eubacterium aerofaciens* to the genus *Collinsella* as *Collinsella aerofaciens* gen nov, comb nov, *Int J Syst Bacteriol* 49:557, 1999.

Kageyama A, Benno Y, Nakase T: Phylogenetic evidence for the transfer of *Eubacterium lentum* to the genus *Eggerthella* as *Eggerthella lenta* gen nov, comb nov, *Int J Syst Bacteriol* 49:1725, 1999.

Koransky JR, Allen SD, Dowell VR: Use of ethanol for selective isolation of spore forming microorganisms, *Appl Environ Microbiol* 35:762, 1978.

Murdoch DA, Shah HN: Reclassification of *Peptostreptococcus magnus* (Prevot, 1933) Holdeman and Moore, 1972 as *Finegoldia magna* comb nov and *Peptostreptococcus micros* (Prevot, 1933) Smith, 1957 as *Micromonas micros* comb nov, *Anaerobe* 5:553, 1999.

National Committee for Clinical Laboratory Standards (NCCLS): *Abbreviated identification of bacteria and yeast; approved guideline*, M35-A, Wayne, Pa, 2002, NCCLS.

Shinjo T, Fujisawa T, Mitsuoka T: Proposal of two subspecies of *Fusobacterium necrophorum* (Flügge) Moore and Holdeman: *Fusobacterium necrophorum* subsp *necrophorum* subsp nov, nom rev (ex Flügge, 1886), and *Fusobacterium necrophorum* subsp *funduliforme* subsp nov, nom rev (ex Halle, 1898), *Int J Syst Bacteriol* 41:395, 1991.

Versalovic J: *Manual of clinical microbiology*, ed 10, Washington, DC, 2011, ASM Press.

## OBJECTIVES

1. Describe the general characteristics of the *Mycobacterium* spp., including oxygen requirements, staining patterns and cell morphology, artificial media required for cultivation and growth, and pigmentation.
2. Explain the chemical composition of the bacterial cell wall.
3. Explain the microscopic staining characteristics of *Mycobacterium* spp. using the Gram stain and acid-fast staining methods.
4. List the most common pathogenic species in the *Mycobacterium* genus and state the natural habitat, mode of transmission, and reservoir for each.
5. Differentiate *M. tuberculosis* clinical infections based on the signs and symptoms of the following: primary infection, latent infection, disseminated infection, and reactivation.
6. Compare the current safety and containment methods recommended for handling mycobacterial infectious materials and routine bacteriology in a diagnostic laboratory.
7. Describe the purified protein derivative (PPD; also referred to as the tuberculin skin test). What is the significance of a positive result?
8. List the clinical specimens acceptable for recovery of mycobacteria and describe the limitations of recovery from each type of specimen.
9. Justify the use of DNA probes and molecular sequencing or amplification methods to identify *Mycobacterium* spp.
10. Evaluate the effectiveness of the staining procedures—Kinyoun, Ziehl-Neelsen, and fluorescent staining (auramine-rhodamine or acridine orange)—for identifying mycobacteria.
11. Describe the requirements for using digestion and decontamination procedures to improve the recovery of *Mycobacterium* spp.
12. Explain the limitations of digestion and decontamination procedures.
13. Explain the methods commonly used for biochemical identification of *Mycobacterium* spp. (i.e., niacin, nitrate, urease, modified catalase, Tween 80, tellurite, arylsulfatase, thiophene-2-carboxylic acid hydrazide [TCH], and 5% NaCl tests), including the purpose, principle, and control organisms used for each.
14. Describe the role of the human immunodeficiency virus (HIV) and acquired immunodeficiency syndrome (AIDS) in the dissemination and/or pathogenesis of infections with *Mycobacterium* spp.
15. Explain the recommended susceptibility testing methods and state when susceptibility testing is required or recommended for *Mycobacterium* spp.

---

### MAJOR GENERA AND SPECIES TO BE CONSIDERED

**Mycobacterium tuberculosis Complex**

Mycobacterium tuberculosis
Mycobacterium bovis
Mycobacterium bovis BCG
Mycobacterium africanum
Mycobacterium caprae
Mycobacterium canettii
Mycobacterium microti
Mycobacterium pinnipedii

**Nontuberculous Mycobacteria**
**Early-Pigmented, Rapid-Growing Mycobacterium spp.**

M. canariasense
M. cosmeticum
M. monacense
M. neoaurum
Mycobacterium chelonae and M. abscessus group
    M. abscessus subsp. abscessus
    M. abscessus subsp. bolletii
    M. chelonae
    M. immunogenum
    M. salmoniphilum
Mycobacterium fortuitum group
    M. boenickei
    M. brisbanense
    M. fortuitum
    M. houstonense
    M. neworleansense
    M. peregrinum
    M. porcinum
    M. senegalense
    M. septicum
    M. setense
Mycobacterium mageritense and M. wolinskyi group
    M. mageritense
    M. wolinskyi
Mycobacterium mucogenicum group
    M. aubagnense
    M. mucogenicum
    M. phocaicum
Mycobacterium smegmatis group
    M. goodii
    M. smegmatis
(see Box 43-1 for an extensive listing.)

---

Traditionally, *Mycobacterium* spp. have been classified according to phenotypic characteristics. However, since the late 1980s, molecular diagnostics have been used to shift the characterization of these organisms to genotypic studies. This chapter discusses both the phenotypic characterization and the new taxonomy based on molecular genetic data.

The organisms that belong to the genus *Mycobacterium* are aerobic (although some may grow in reduced oxygen concentrations), non–spore forming (except for *M. marinum*), nonmotile, very thin, slightly curved or straight rods (0.2 to 0.6 × 1 to 10 $\mu$m). Some species may display a branching morphology. *Mycobacterium* is the only genus in the Mycobacteriaceae family (Actinomycetales order, Actinomycetes class). Genera that are closely related to *Mycobacterium* include *Nocardia*, *Rhodococcus*, *Tsukamurella* and *Gordonia*.

*Mycobacterium* spp. have an unusual cell wall structure. The cell wall contains N-glycolylmuramic acid instead of N-acetylmuramic acid, and it has a very high lipid content, which creates a hydrophobic permeability barrier. Because of this cell wall structure, mycobacteria are difficult to stain with commonly used basic aniline dyes, such as those used in Gram staining. Although these organisms cannot be readily Gram stained, they generally are considered gram positive. However, they resist decolorization with acidified alcohol (3% hydrochloric acid) after prolonged application of a basic fuchsin dye or with heating of this dye after its application. This important property of mycobacteria, which derives from their cell wall structure, is referred to as *acid fastness;* this characteristic distinguishes mycobacteria from other genera. Rapid-growing mycobacteria (RGMs) may partially or completely lose this characteristic as a result of their growth characteristics.

Another important feature of many species is that they grow more slowly than most other human pathogenic bacteria because of their hydrophobic cell surface. Because of this hydrophobicity, organisms tend to clump, so that nutrients are not easily allowed into the cell. A single cell's *generation time* (the time required for a cell to divide into two independent cells) may range from approximately 20 hours to 36 hours for *Mycobacterium ulcerans*. This slow growth results in the formation of visible colonies in 2 to 60 days at optimum temperature.

Currently, the genus *Mycobacterium* includes more than 100 recognized or proposed species. These organisms produce a spectrum of infections in humans and animals ranging from localized lesions to disseminated disease. Some species cause only human infections, and others have been isolated from a wide variety of animals. Many species are also found in water and soil.

For the most part, mycobacteria can be divided into two major groups, based on fundamental differences in epidemiology and association with disease: those belonging to the *Mycobacterium tuberculosis* complex and those referred to as *nontuberculous mycobacteria (NTM)* (Box 43-1).

# MYCOBACTERIUM TUBERCULOSIS COMPLEX

Tuberculosis was endemic in animals in the Paleolithic period, long before it ever affected humans. This disease

---

**BOX 43-1** Major Groupings of Organisms Belonging to the Genus *Mycobacterium**

**Mycobacterium tuberculosis Complex**
M. tuberculosis
M. bovis
M. bovis BCG
M. africanum
M. caprae
M. canettii
M. microti
M. pinnipedii

**Nontuberculous Mycobacteria**
*Slow-Growing Nonphotochromogens*
M. avium complex
M. avium
   subsp. avium
   subsp. silvaticum
   subsp. paratuberculosis
M. intracellulare
M. celatum
M. ulcerans
M. gastri
M. genavense
M. haemophilum
M. malmoense
M. shimoidei
M. xenopi
M. heidelbergense
M. branderi
M. simiae
M. triplex
M. conspicuum

*Photochromogens*
M. kansasii
M. asiaticum
M. marinum

*Scotochromogens*
M. szulgai
M. scrofulaceum
M. interjectum
M. gordonae
M. cookii
M. hiberniae
M. lentiflavum
M. conspicuum
M. heckeshornense
M. tusciae
M. kubicae
M. ulcerans
M. bohemicum

*Noncultivatable*
M. leprae

*Rapid-Growing, Potentially Pathogenic*
M. fortuitum
M. chelonae
M. abscessus subsp. abscessus
M. abscessus subsp. bolletii
M. smegmatis
M. peregrinum
M. immunogenum

*Continued*

**BOX 43-1** Major Groupings of Organisms Belonging to the Genus *Mycobacterium*—cont'd

*M. mucogenicum*
*M. neworleansense*
*M. brisbanense*
*M. senegalense*
*M. porcinum*
*M. houstonense*
*M. boenickei*
*M. wolinskyi*
*M. goodii*
*M. septicum*
*M. mageritense*
*M. canariasense*
*M. alvei*
*M. novocastrense*
*M. cosmeticum*
*M. boenickei*
*M. canariasense*
*M. setense*

**Rarely Pathogenic or Not Yet Associated with Infection**
*M. agri, M. aichiense, M. austroafricanum, M. aurum,*
*M. brumae, M. chitae, M. chubuense, M. diernhoferi,*
*M. duvalii, M. fallax, M. flavescens, M. gadium,*
*M. gilvum, M. hassiacum, M. komossense, M. moriokaense,*
*M. murale, M. neoaurum, M. obuense, M. parafortuitum,*
*M. phlei, M. pulveris, M. rhodesiae, M. senegalense,*
*M. sphagni, M. thermoresistibile, M. tokaiense, M. vaccae*
*M. elephantis, M. lacticola, M. mageritense, M. phocaicum*

---

*This box is not inclusive; rather, it lists only the prominent mycobacteria isolated from humans.

(also called *consumption*) has been known in all ages and climates. For example, tuberculosis was the subject of a hymn in a sacred text from India dating from 2500 BC, and DNA unique to *Mycobacterium tuberculosis* was identified in lesions from the lung in 1000-year-old human remains found in Peru.

## GENERAL CHARACTERISTICS

In the clinical microbiology laboratory, the term *complex* frequently is used to describe two or more species for which distinction is complicated and has little or no medical importance. The mycobacterial species that occur in humans and belong to the *M. tuberculosis* complex include *M. tuberculosis, M. bovis, M. bovis* BCG, *M. africanum, M. caprae, M. microti, M. canettii,* and *M. pinnipedii*. All of these species are capable of causing tuberculosis. It should be noted that species identification might be required for epidemiologic and public health reasons. The organisms that belong to the *M. tuberculosis* complex are considered slow growers, and colonies are nonpigmented.

## EPIDEMIOLOGY AND PATHOGENESIS

### Epidemiology

*M. tuberculosis* is the cause of most cases of human tuberculosis, particularly in developed countries. An estimated

1.7 billion people, or one third of the world's population, are infected with *M. tuberculosis*. This reservoir of infected individuals results in 8 million new cases of tuberculosis and 2.9 million deaths annually. Tuberculosis continues to be a public health problem in the United States. An additional complicating factor in the management of tuberculosis is the increasing incidence of co-infection with the human immunodeficiency virus (HIV). HIV-associated tuberculosis remains a significant challenge to world health, with an estimated 1.1 million individuals living with HIV-associated tuberculosis. In the United States, tuberculosis typically is found among the poor, homeless, intravenous (IV) drug users, alcoholics, the elderly, or medically underserved populations. Although the organisms belonging to the *M. tuberculosis* complex have numerous characteristics in common, including extreme genetic homogeneity, they differ in certain epidemiologic aspects (Table 43-1).

### Pathogenesis

The pathogenesis of tuberculosis caused by organisms of the *M. tuberculosis* complex is discussed in Chapter 69. Inhalation of a single viable organism has been shown to lead to infection, although close contact is usually necessary. Of those who become infected with *M. tuberculosis*, 15% to 20% develop disease. The disease usually occurs some years after the initial infection, when the patient's immune system breaks down for some reason other than the presence of tuberculosis bacilli in the lung. In a small percentage of infected hosts, the disease becomes systemic, affecting a variety of organs.

After ingestion of milk from infected cows, *Mycobacterium bovis* may penetrate the gastrointestinal mucosa or invade the lymphatic tissue of the oropharynx. An attenuated strain of *M. bovis*, bacillus Calmette-Guérin (BCG), has been used extensively in many parts of the world to immunize susceptible individuals against tuberculosis. Because mycobacteria are the classic examples of intracellular pathogens and the body's response to BCG hinges on cell-mediated immunoreactivity, immunized individuals are expected to react more aggressively against all antigens that elicit cell-mediated immunity. In rare cases, an unfortunate individual's immune system is so compromised that it cannot handle the BCG, and systemic BCG infection may develop.

## SPECTRUM OF DISEASE

Tuberculosis may mimic other diseases, such as pneumonia, neoplasm, or fungal infections. In addition, clinical manifestations in patients infected with *M. tuberculosis* complex may range from asymptomatic to acutely symptomatic. Patients who are symptomatic can have systemic symptoms, pulmonary signs and symptoms, signs and symptoms related to other organ involvement (e.g., the kidneys), or a combination of these features. Cases of pulmonary disease caused by *M. tuberculosis* complex organisms are clinically, radiologically, and pathologically indistinguishable.

Primary tuberculosis typically is considered a disease of the respiratory tract. Common presenting symptoms include low-grade fever, night sweats, fatigue, anorexia

**TABLE 43-1** Epidemiology of Organisms Belonging to *M. tuberculosis* Complex That Cause Human Infections

| Organism | Habitat | Primary Route of Transmission | Distribution |
|---|---|---|---|
| *M. tuberculosis* | Patients with cavitary disease are primary reservoir | Person to person by inhalation of droplet nuclei: droplet nuclei containing the organism (infectious aerosols, 1 to 5 μm) are produced when people with pulmonary tuberculosis cough, sneeze, speak, or sing; infectious aerosols may also be produced by manipulation of lesions or processing of clinical specimens in the laboratory. Droplets are so small that air currents keep them airborne for long periods; once inhaled, they are small enough to reach the lungs' alveoli* | Worldwide |
| *M. bovis* | Humans and a wide range of host animals, such as cattle, nonhuman primates, goats, cats, buffalo, badgers, possums, dogs, pigs, and deer | Ingestion of contaminated milk from infected cows[†]; airborne transmission[‡] | Worldwide |
| *M. africanum* | Humans[§] | Inhalation of droplet nuclei | East and West tropical Africa; some cases have been identified in the United States |
| *M. caprae* | Humans rarely; predominately infects a wide range of animals | Inhalation of droplet nuclei | Europe |
| *M. microti* | Humans rarely; small animals (e.g., voles and other wild rodents) | Inhalation of droplet nuclei | Europe; Great Britain, Netherlands |
| *M. canettii* | Natural reservoir has not been clearly defined. Rarely infects humans. | Unclear | Africa |
| *M. pinnipedii* | Humans rarely; predominantly infects a wide range of animals | Unclear | Europe |

*Infection occasionally can occur through the gastrointestinal tract or skin.
[†]The incidence has decreased significantly in developed countries since the introduction of universal pasteurization of milk and milk products and the institution of effective control programs for cattle.
[‡]Can be transmitted human to human, animal to human, and human to animal.
[§]Infections in animals have not been totally excluded.

(loss of appetite), and weight loss. A patient who presents with pulmonary tuberculosis usually has a productive cough, along with low-grade fever, chills, myalgias (aches), and sweating; however, these signs and symptoms are similar for influenza, acute bronchitis, and pneumonia.

Upon respiratory infection with *M. tuberculosis* complex organisms, the cellular immune system T cells and macrophages migrate to the lungs, and the organisms are phagocytized by the macrophages. However, these organisms are capable of intracellular multiplication in the macrophages. Often the host is unable to eliminate the organisms, and the result is a systemic hypersensitivity to *Mycobacterium* antigens. Granulomas or a hard tubercle forms in the lung from the lymphocytes, macrophages, and cellular pathology, including giant cell formation (cellular fusion displaying multiple nuclei). If the *Mycobacterium* antigen concentration is high, the hypersensitivity reaction may result in tissue necrosis, caused by

enzymes released from the macrophages. In this case no granuloma forms, and a solid or semisolid, caseous material is left at the primary lesion site.

In some patients infected with primary active tuberculosis, the disease may spread via the lymph system or hematogenously, leading to meningeal or miliary (disseminated) tuberculosis. This most often occurs in patients with depressed or ineffective cellular immunity.

As previously mentioned, in a small percentage of patients, organs besides the lungs can become involved after infection with *M. tuberculosis* complex organisms. These organs include the following:

- Genitourinary tract
- Lymph nodes (cervical lymphadenitis)
- Central nervous system (meningitis)
- Bone and joint (arthritis and osteomyelitis)
- Peritoneum
- Pericardium

- Larynx
- Pleural lining (pleuritis)

Disseminated tuberculosis may be diagnosed by a positive tuberculin skin test (described later in the chapter).

Patients also may have latent disease (i.e., they have no apparent signs, symptoms, or pathologic condition). A patient with latent tuberculosis is not infectious and does not have active disease, although the organism is present in granulomas. Patients with latent tuberculosis may progress to active disease (also referred to as *reactivation of tuberculosis*) at any time. Reactivation tuberculosis typically occurs after an incident in which cellular immunity is suppressed or damaged as a result of a change in life style or other health condition.

Individuals infected with HIV are particularly susceptible to developing active tuberculosis. These patients are likely to have rapidly progressive primary disease instead of a subclinical infection.

Diagnosing tuberculosis is more difficult in people infected with HIV, because chest radiographs of the pulmonary disease often lack specificity, and patients frequently are anergic (lack a biologic response) to tuberculin skin testing, a primary means of identifying individuals infected with *M. tuberculosis*. The tuberculin skin test, or purified protein derivative (PPD) test, is based on the premise that after infection with *M. tuberculosis*, an individual develops a delayed hypersensitivity cell-mediated immunity to certain antigenic components of the organism. To determine whether a person has been infected with *M. tuberculosis*, a culture extract of *M. tuberculosis* (i.e., PPD of tuberculin) is injected intracutaneously. After 48 to 72 hours, an infected individual shows a delayed hypersensitivity reaction to the PPD, characterized by erythema (redness) and, most important, induration (firmness as a result of influx of immune cells). The diameter of induration is measured and then interpreted as to whether the patient has been infected with *M. tuberculosis;* different interpretative criteria are used for different patient populations (e.g., immunosuppressed individuals, such as those infected with HIV). More recently, the T-Spot TB test (Oxford, Immunotec, United Kingdom) offers next-day results and does not require a follow-up visit with a physician. The assay measures T cells that have been activated by *Mycobacterium tuberculosis* antigens. Peripheral blood mononuclear cells are incubated with *M. tuberculosis*-specific antigens stimulating any sensitized T cells in the patient sample. T cell cytokines released in the sample are measured using antibody to capture them and then detected with a secondary antibody conjugated to alkaline phosphatase. This assay should be interpreted in correlation with the patient's signs and symptoms.

The PPD test is not 100% sensitive or specific, and a positive reaction to the skin test does not necessarily signify the presence of disease. Because of these issues, a new test approved by the U.S. Food and Drug Administration (FDA) has become available. It is an enzyme-linked immunosorbent assay (ELISA) called QuantiFERON-TB Gold (Cellestis Limited, Carnegie, Victoria, Australia). The assay measures a component of the cell-mediated immune response to *M. tuberculosis* to diagnose latent tuberculosis infection and tuberculosis disease. It is based on the quantification of interferon-gamma released from sensitized lymphocytes in heparinized whole blood that has been incubated overnight with a mixture of synthetic peptides simulating two proteins in *M. tuberculosis*. The test assesses responses to multiple antigens; it can be performed in a single patient visit; and it is less subject to reader bias and error. An important feature is that the results of the assay are unaffected by previous BCG vaccination. Guidelines published by the Centers for Disease Control and Prevention (CDC) recommend the use of this assay in all circumstances in which the tuberculin skin test currently is used (e.g., contact investigations and evaluation of recent immigrants). The guidelines also provide specific cautions for interpreting negative results in individuals from selected populations.

# NONTUBERCULOUS MYCOBACTERIA

The NTM include all mycobacterial species that do not belong to *M. tuberculosis* complex. Currently, approximately 130 species of nontuberculous mycobacteria have been recognized. The members of this large group of mycobacteria have been known by several names (Box 43-2). Significant geographic variability is seen both in the prevalence of and the species responsible for NTM disease. As previously mentioned, NTM are present everywhere in the environment and sometimes colonize the skin and respiratory and gastrointestinal tracts of healthy individuals. Little is known about how infection is acquired, but some mechanisms appear to be trauma, inhalation of infectious aerosols, and ingestion; a few diseases are nosocomial or are acquired as an iatrogenic infection. In contrast to *M. tuberculosis* complex, NTM are not usually transmitted from person to person, nor does isolation of these organisms necessarily mean they are associated with a disease process. Interpretation of a positive NTM culture is complicated, because these organisms are widely distributed in nature, their pathogenic potential varies greatly from one species to another, and humans can be colonized by these mycobacteria without necessarily developing infection or disease. With few exceptions, little is known about the pathogenesis of infections caused by these bacterial agents.

---

**BOX 43-2** Other Names That Have Been Used to Designate the Nontuberculous Mycobacteria

Anonymous
Atypical
Unclassified
Unknown
Tuberculoid
Environmental
Opportunistic
Mycobacteria other than tubercle bacilli (MOTT)

From Debrunner M et al: Epidemiology and clinical significance of nontuberculous mycobacteria in patients negative for human immunodeficiency virus in Switzerland, *Clin Infect Dis* 15:330, 1992.

In 1959 Runyon[1] classified NTM into four groups (Runyon groups I to IV) based on the phenotypic characteristics of the various species, most notably the growth rate and colonial pigmentation (Table 43-2). Runyon's system first categorizes the slow-growing NTM (Runyon groups I to III) and then the rapid-growers (Runyon group IV). One other NTM, *M. leprae,* which cannot be cultivated on artificial media, is also reviewed. (As with many classification schemes, the Runyon classification does not always hold true. For example, some NTM can be either a photochromogen or a nonphotochromogen.)

Because determining the clinical significance of isolating NTM from a clinical sample is difficult, several clinical classification schemes also have been proposed. One such scheme classifies NTM recovered from humans into four major groups (pulmonary, lymphadenitis, cutaneous, or disseminated) based on the clinical disease they cause. Other NTM classifications are based on the pathogenic potential of a species.

## SLOW-GROWING NONTUBERCULOUS MYCOBACTERIA

The slow-growing NTM can be subdivided into three groups based on the phenotypic characteristics of the species. *Mycobacterium* spp. synthesize carotenoids (a group of yellow to red pigments) in varying amounts and thus can be categorized into three groups based on the production of these pigments: photochromogens, scotochromogens, and nonphotochromogens. Some of these NTM are considered potentially pathogenic for humans, whereas others are rarely associated with disease.

### Photochromogens

The photochromogens (Table 43-3) are slow-growing NTM that produce colonies that require light to form pigment.

### Scotochromogens

The scotochromogens (Table 43-4) are slow-growing NTM that produce pigmented colonies whether grown in the dark or the light. The epidemiology of the potentially pathogenic scotochromogens has not been definitively described. In contrast to potentially pathogenic nonphotochromogens, these agents are rarely recovered in the clinical laboratory.

### Nonphotochromogens

The nonphotochromogens (Table 43-5) are slow-growing NTM that produce unpigmented colonies whether grown in the dark or the light. Of the organisms in this group,

**TABLE 43-2** Runyon Classification of Nontuberculous Mycobacteria (NTM)

| Runyon Group Number | Group Name | Description |
|---|---|---|
| I | Photochromogens | NTM colonies that develop pigment on exposure to light after being grown in the dark and take longer than 7 days to appear on solid media |
| II | Scotochromogens | NTM colonies that develop pigment in the dark or light and take longer than 7 days to appear on solid media |
| III | Nonphotochromogens | NTM colonies that are nonpigmented regardless of whether they are grown in the dark or light and take longer than 7 days to appear on solid media |
| IV | Rapid growers | NTM colonies that grow on solid media and take fewer than 7 days to appear |

**TABLE 43-3** Characteristics of Nontuberculous Mycobacteria—Photochromogens

| Organism | Epidemiology | Pathogenicity | Type of Infection |
|---|---|---|---|
| *M. kansasii* | Infection more common in white males; natural reservoir is tap water; aerosols are involved in transmission | Potentially pathogenic | Chronic pulmonary disease; extrapulmonary diseases, such as cervical lymphadenitis and cutaneous disease |
| *M. asiaticum* | Not commonly encountered (primarily seen in Australia) | Potentially pathogenic | Pulmonary disease |
| *M. marinum* | Natural reservoirs are freshwater and saltwater as a result of contamination from infected fish and other marine life. Transmission is by contact with contaminated water and organism entry by means of trauma or small breaks in the skin; associated with aquatic activity usually involving fish | Potentially pathogenic | Cutaneous disease; bacteremia |
| *M. intermedium* | Unknown | Potentially pathogenic | Pulmonary disease |
| *M. novocastrense* | Unknown | Potentially pathogenic | Cutaneous disease |

**TABLE 43-4** Characteristics of Nontuberculous Mycobacteria—Scotochromogens

| Organism | Epidemiology/Habitat | Pathogenicity | Type of Infection |
|---|---|---|---|
| *M. szulgai* | Water and soil | Potentially pathogenic | Pulmonary disease, predominantly in middle-aged men; cervical adenitis; bursitis |
| *M. scrofulaceum* | Raw milk, soil, water, dairy products | Potentially pathogenic | Cervical adenitis in children, bacteremia, pulmonary disease, skin infections |
| *M. interjectum* | Unknown | Potentially pathogenic | Chronic lymphadenitis, pulmonary disease |
| *M. heckeshornense* | Unknown | Potentially pathogenic | Pulmonary disease (rare) |
| *M. tusciae* | Unknown—isolated from tap water | Potentially pathogenic | Cervical lymphadenitis (rare) |
| *M. kubicae* | Unknown | Potentially pathogenic | Pulmonary disease |
| *M. gordonae* | Tap water, water, soil | Nonpathogenic* | NA |
| *M. cookie* | Sphagnum moss, surface waters in New Zealand | Nonpathogenic* | NA |
| *M. hiberniae* | Sphagnum moss, soil in Ireland | Nonpathogenic* | NA |

*NA,* Not applicable.*Rarely, if ever, causes disease.

**TABLE 43-5** Characteristics of the Nontuberculous Mycobacteria—Nonphotochromogens and Species Considered Potential Pathogens

| Organism | Epidemiology | Type of Infection |
|---|---|---|
| *M. avium* complex | Environmental sources, including natural waters, and soil | Patients without AIDS: Pulmonary infections in patients with preexisting pulmonary disease; cervical lymphadenitis; and disseminated disease* in immunocompromised patients who are HIV negative<br>Patients with AIDS: Disseminated disease |
| *M. xenopi*[†] | Water, especially hot water taps in hospitals; believed to be transmitted in aerosols | Primarily pulmonary infections in adults; less common, extrapulmonary infections (bone, lymph nodes, sinus tract) and disseminated disease |
| *M. ulcerans* | Stagnant tropical waters; also harbored in an aquatic insect's salivary glands; infections occur in tropical or temperate climates | Indolent cutaneous and subcutaneous infections (African Buruli ulcer or Australian Bairnsdale ulcer) |
| *M. malmoense* | Most cases from England, Wales, and Sweden. Rarely isolated from patients infected with HIV. Little is known about epidemiology; to date, isolated only from humans and captured armadillos | Chronic pulmonary infections, primarily in patients with preexisting disease; cervical lymphadenitis in children; less common, infections of the skin or bursae |
| *M. genovense* | Isolated from pet birds and dogs. Mode of acquisition unknown | Disseminated disease in patients with AIDS (wasting disease characterized by fever, weight loss, hepatosplenomegaly, anemia) |
| *M. haemophilum* | Unknown | Disseminated disease; cutaneous infections in immunosuppressed adults; mild and limited skin infections in preadolescence or early adolescence; cervical lymphadenitis in children |
| *M. heidelbergense* | Unknown | Lymphadenitis in children; also isolated from sputum, urine, and gastric aspirate |
| *M. shimoidei* | To date has not been isolated from environmental sources; few case reports, but widespread geographically | Tuberculosis-like pulmonary infection; disseminated disease |
| *M. simiae* | Tap water and hospital water tanks; rarely isolated | Tuberculosis-like pulmonary infection |

*AIDS,* Acquired immunodeficiency syndrome; *HIV,* human immunodeficiency virus.
*Disseminated disease can involve multiple sites, such as bone marrow, lungs, liver, lymph nodes.
[†]Can be either nonphotochromogenic or scotochromogenic.

*M. terrae* complex (*M. terrae, M. triviale,* and *M. nonchromogenicum*) and *M. gastri* are considered nonpathogenic for humans. The other nonphotochromogens are considered potentially pathogenic, and many are frequently recovered in the clinical laboratory. The nonphotochromogens belonging to *Mycobacterium avium* complex are frequently isolated in the clinical laboratory and are able to cause infection in the human host.

**Mycobacterium avium Complex (MAC).** Largely because of the increasing populations of immunosuppressed patients, the incidence of infection caused by *M. avium* complex spp., as well as these organisms' clinical significance, has changed significantly since they were first recognized as human pathogens in the 1950s. The introduction of highly active antiretroviral therapy (HAART) has dramatically reduced the infections caused by these organisms in patients with acquired immunodeficiency syndrome (AIDS).

**General Characteristics.** Taxonomically, *M. avium* complex comprises *M. avium, M. intracellulare, M. avium* subsp. *avium, M. avium* subsp. *paratuberculosis, M. avium* subsp. *silvaticum* (wood pigeon bacillus), *M. vulneris, M. marseillense, M. bouchedurhonense,* and *M. timonense.* The name *M. avium* subsp. *hominissuis* has been proposed for another subspecies capable of infecting humans. Unfortunately, the nomenclature is somewhat confusing. Although *M. avium* and *M. intracellulare* are clearly different organisms, they so closely resemble each other that the distinction cannot be made by routine laboratory determinations or on clinical grounds. As a result, these organisms sometimes are referred to as *M. avium-intracellulare.* Furthermore, because isolation of *M. avium* subsp. *paratuberculosis* in a routine laboratory setting is exceedingly rare, the term *M. avium* complex is most commonly used to report the isolation of *M. avium-intracellulare.*

**Epidemiology and Pathogenesis.** MAC is an important pathogen in both immunocompromised and immunocompetent populations. These are among the most commonly isolated NTM species in the United States. MAC is particularly noteworthy for its potentially pathogenic role in pulmonary infections in patients with AIDS and also in patients who are not infected with HIV. The organisms are ubiquitous in the environment and have been isolated from natural water, soil, dairy products, pigs, chickens, cats, and dogs. As a result of extensive studies, it is generally accepted that natural waters serve as the major reservoir for most human infections.

Infections caused by MAC are acquired by inhalation or ingestion. The pathogenesis of MAC infections is not clearly understood. The organisms are commonly associated with respiratory disease clinically similar to tuberculosis in adults, lymphadenitis in children, and disseminated infection in patients with HIV. However, these organisms and other environmental NTM have extraordinary starvation survival. They can persist well over a year in tap water, and MAC tolerates temperature extremes. In addition, similar to legionellae, *M. avium* can infect and replicate in protozoa. *Amoebae*-grown *M. avium* is more invasive toward human epithelial and macrophage cells.

MAC cultures can have an opaque, a translucent, or a transparent colony morphology. Studies suggest that transparent colonies are more virulent because they are more drug resistant, are isolated more frequently from the blood of patients with AIDS, and appear more virulent in macrophage and animal models.

*M. avium* subsp. *paratuberculosis* is known to cause an inflammatory bowel disease (known as *Johne's disease*) in cattle, sheep, and goats. It also has been isolated from the bowel mucosa of patients with Crohn's disease, a chronic inflammatory bowel disease of humans. The organism is extremely fastidious, seems to require a growth factor (mycobactin, produced by other species of mycobacteria, such as *M. phlei,* a saprophytic strain) and may take as long as 6 to 18 months for primary isolation. Whether these and other mycobacteria actually contribute to development of Crohn's disease or are simply colonizing an environmental niche in the bowel of these patients remains to be elucidated.

**Clinical Spectrum of Disease.** The clinical manifestations of *M. avium* complex infections are summarized in Table 43-5.

**Other Nonphotochromogens.** Several other mycobacterial species that are considered nonphotochromogens are potentially pathogenic in humans. The epidemiology and spectrum of disease for these organisms are summarized in Table 43-5. In addition to the species in this table, other, newer species of mycobacteria that are nonphotochromogens have been described, such as *M. celatum* and *M. conspicuum.* These newer agents appear to be potentially pathogenic in humans.

# RAPIDLY GROWING NONTUBERCULOUS MYCOBACTERIA (RGM)

Mycobacteria that produce colonies on solid media in 7 days or earlier constitute the second major group of NTM. Currently, approximately 70 species have been classified into this group.

## General Characteristics

The large group of organisms that constitute the RGM is divided into six major groups of potentially pathogenic species, based on pigmentation and molecular studies (see Box 43-1). Unlike the majority of other mycobacteria, most rapid-growers can grow on routine bacteriologic media and on media specific for cultivation of mycobacteria. On Gram staining, these organisms appear as weakly gram-positive rods resembling diphtheroids.

## Epidemiology and Pathogenesis

The rapidly growing mycobacteria considered potentially pathogenic can cause disease in either healthy or immunocompromised patients. Like many other NTM, these organisms are ubiquitous in the environment and are present worldwide. They have been found in soil, marshes, rivers, and municipal water supplies (tap water) and in marine and terrestrial life forms. Infections caused by rapidly growing mycobacteria can be acquired in the community from environmental sources. They also can be nosocomial infections, resulting from medical interventions (including bone marrow transplantation), wound infections, and catheter sepsis. These organisms

**TABLE 43-6** Common Types of Infections Caused by Rapidly Growing Mycobacteria

| Organism | Common Types of Infection |
|---|---|
| *M. abscessus* subsp. *abscessus* | Disseminated disease, primarily in immunocompromised individuals; skin and soft tissue infections; pulmonary infections; postoperative infections |
| *M. fortuitum* | Postoperative infections in breast augmentation and median sternotomy; skin and soft tissue infections; pulmonary infections, usually single. localized lesions. Central nervous system (CNS) disease is rare but has high morbidity and mortality |
| *M. chelonae* | Skin and soft tissue infections, postoperative wound infections, keratitis |
| **Less Common Types of Infection (More Than 10 Cases)** *M. peregrinum* | Skin and soft tissue infections; bacteremia |
| *M. mucogenicum* | Posttraumatic wound infections, catheter-related sepsis, health care associated |
| *M. smegmatis* | Skin or soft tissue infections; less frequently, pulmonary infections |
| *M. abscessus* subsp. *bolletii* | Health care–associated infections, skin and soft tissue infections, pulmonary infections |
| *M. boenickei* | Bone and joint infections |
| *M. canariasense* | Bacteremia |
| *M. cosmeticum* | Pulmonary and urosepsis |
| *M. goodii* | Bone and joint infections, osteomyelitis |
| *M. houstonense* | Bone and joint infections |
| *M. immunogenum* | Hypersensitivity pneumonitis |
| *M. neoaurum* (closely related to *M. lacticola*) | Catheter-related sepsis |
| *M. porcinum* | Surgical site infection |
| *M. senegalense* | Catheter-related sepsis |
| **Rare Infections (Fewer Than 10 Cases)** *M. aubagnense* | Various opportunistic health care–associated infections |
| *M. brisbanense* | Various opportunistic health care–associated infections |
| *M. brumae* | Various opportunistic health care–associated infections |
| *M. elephantis* | Various opportunistic health care–associated infections |
| *M. mageritense* | Skin and soft tissue infections |
| *M. monacense* | Various opportunistic health care–associated infections |
| *M. moriokaense* | Various opportunistic health care–associated infections |
| *M. neworleansense* | Various opportunistic health care–associated infections |
| *M. novocastrense* | Various types of opportunistic health care–associated infections |
| *M. phocaicum* | Catheter-related sepsis |
| *M. septicum* | Various opportunistic health care–associated infections |
| *M. setense* | Bone and joint infections |
| *M. wolinskyi* | Skin and soft tissue infections, bone infection, osteomyelitis |

may be commensals on the skin. They gain entry into the host by inoculation into the skin and subcutaneous tissues as a result of trauma, injections, or surgery, or through animal contact.

The RGM also can cause disseminated cutaneous infections. The description of chronic pulmonary infections caused by rapidly growing mycobacteria suggests a possible respiratory route for acquisition of organisms present in the environment. Of the potentially pathogenic, rapidly growing NTM, *M. fortuitum, M. chelonae,* and *M. abscessus* are commonly encountered; these three species account for approximately 90% of clinical disease. Little is known about the pathogenesis of these organisms.

### Spectrum of Disease

The spectrum of disease caused by the most commonly encountered rapid-growers is summarized in Table 43-6. The most common infection associated with RGM is posttraumatic wound infection. An increase in wound infections has been associated with planktonic *M. abscessus,* which can be identified as a rough colonial phenotype on artificial media; these organisms are capable of infecting macrophages. The smooth colonial phenotype typically is identified in biofilms and lacks infectivity.

## NONCULTIVATABLE NONTUBERCULOUS MYCOBACTERIA—*MYCOBACTERIUM LEPRAE*

The nontuberculous mycobacterium *M. leprae* is a close relative of *M. tuberculosis*. This organism causes leprosy (also called *Hansen's disease*). Leprosy is a chronic disease of the skin, mucous membranes, and nerve tissue. Leprosy remains a worldwide public health concern as a result of the development of drug-resistant isolates.

### General Characteristics

*M. leprae* has not yet been cultivated in vitro, although it can be cultivated in the armadillo and in the footpads of mice. Molecular biologic techniques have provided most of the information about this organism's genomic structure and its various genes and their products. Although polymerase chain reaction (PCR) assays have been used to detect and identify *M. leprae* in infected tissues, the technique thus far has not proved as effective diagnostically as anticipated in indeterminate or paucibacillary (few organisms present) disease. Therefore, diagnosis of leprosy is based on distinct clinical manifestations, such as hypopigmented skin lesions and peripheral nerve involvement, in conjunction with a skin smear that tests positive for acid-fast bacilli.

### Epidemiology and Pathogenesis

Understanding of the epidemiology and pathogenesis of leprosy is hampered by the inability to grow the organism in culture. In tropical countries, where the disease is most prevalent, it may be acquired from infected humans; however, infectivity is very low. Prolonged close contact and the host's immunologic status play roles in infectivity.

**Epidemiology.** The primary reservoir for *M. leprae* is infected humans. The disease is transmitted person to person through inhalation or contact with infected skin. The more important mode of transmission appears to be inhalation of *M. leprae* discharged in the nasal secretions of an infected individual.

**Pathogenesis.** Although the host's immune response to *M. leprae* plays a key role in control of infection, the immune response is also responsible for the damage to skin and nerves; in other words, leprosy is both a bacterial and an immunologic disease. After acquisition of *M. leprae*, the infection passes through many stages, which are characterized by their histopathologic and clinical features. Although the infection has many intermediate stages, the two primary phases are a silent phase, during which the leprosy bacilli multiply in the skin in macrophages, and an intermediate phase, in which the bacilli multiply in peripheral nerves and begin to cause sensory impairment. More severe disease states may follow. A patient may recover spontaneously at any stage.

### Spectrum of Disease

Based on the host's response, the spectrum of disease caused by *M. leprae* ranges from subclinical infection to intermediate stages of disease to full-blown and serious clinical manifestations involving the skin, upper respiratory system, testes, and peripheral nerves. The two major forms of the disease are a localized form, called *tuberculoid leprosy*, and a more disseminated form, called *lepromatous leprosy*. Patients with lepromatous leprosy are anergic to *M. leprae* because of a defect in their cell-mediated immunity. Because the organisms' growth is unimpeded, these individuals develop extensive skin lesions containing numerous acid-fast bacilli; the organisms can spill over into the blood and disseminate. In contrast, individuals with tuberculoid leprosy do not have an immune defect, so the disease is localized to the skin and nerves; few organisms are observed in skin lesions. Most of the serious sequelae associated with leprosy are the result of this organism's tropism for peripheral nerves.

## LABORATORY DIAGNOSIS OF MYCOBACTERIAL INFECTIONS

Specimens received by the laboratory for mycobacterial smear and culture must be handled in a safe manner. Tuberculosis ranks high among laboratory-acquired infections; therefore, laboratory and hospital administrators must provide laboratory personnel with facilities, equipment, and supplies that reduce this risk to a minimum. *M. tuberculosis* has a very low infective dose for humans (i.e., an infection rate of approximately 50% with exposure to fewer than 10 acid-fast bacilli). All tuberculin-negative personnel should have a skin test at least annually. The CDC recommends Biosafety Level 2 practices, containment equipment, and facilities for preparing acid-fast smears and culture for nonaerosolizing manipulations. If *M. tuberculosis* is grown and then propagated and manipulated, biologic safety cabinet (BSC) class II safety precautions are required; however, Biosafety Level 3 practices are recommended. BSC Level 3 practices are recommended for opening centrifuge vials, adding reagents to biochemical testing medias, and sonication; these practices include restricted laboratory access, negative pressure airflow, and special personal protective equipment (e.g., certified respirators). Respiratory devices should be certified through the National Institute for Occupational Safety and Health (NIOSH).

### SPECIMEN COLLECTION AND TRANSPORT

Acid-fast bacilli can infect almost any tissue or organ of the body. Successful isolation of these organisms depends on the quality of the specimen obtained and the use of appropriate processing and culture techniques by the mycobacteriology laboratory. In suspected mycobacterial disease, as in all other infectious diseases, the diagnostic procedure begins at the patient's bedside. Collection of proper clinical specimens requires careful attention to detail by health care professionals. Most specimens are respiratory samples, such as sputum, tracheal or bronchial aspirates, and specimens obtained by bronchial alveolar lavage. Other samples may include urine, gastric aspirates, tissue (biopsy) specimens, cerebrospinal fluid (CSF), and pleural and pericardial fluid. Blood or fecal specimens may be collected from immunocompromised patients. Specimens should be collected in sterile, leak-proof, disposable, and appropriately labeled containers without fixatives and placed in bags to contain leakage. If transport and processing will be delayed longer than 1 hour, all specimens except blood should be refrigerated at 4° C until processed.

### Pulmonary Specimens

Pulmonary secretions may be obtained by any of the following methods: spontaneously produced or induced sputum, gastric lavage, transtracheal aspiration, bronchoscopy, and laryngeal swabbing. Most specimens submitted for examination are sputum, aerosol-induced sputum, bronchoscopic aspirations, or gastric lavage samples. Spontaneously produced sputum is the specimen of choice. To raise sputum, patients must be instructed to take a deep breath, hold it momentarily, and then cough deeply and vigorously. Patients must also be instructed to cover the mouth carefully while coughing and to discard tissues in an appropriate receptacle. Saliva and nasal secretions should not be collected, nor should the patient use oral antiseptics during the collection period. Sputum specimens must be free of food particles, residues, and other extraneous matter.

The aerosol (saline) induction procedure can best be done on ambulatory patients who are able to follow instructions. Aerosol-induced sputum specimens have been collected from children as young as 5 years of age. This procedure should be performed in an enclosed area with appropriate airflow. Operators should wear particulate respirators and take appropriate safety measures to prevent exposure. The patient is told that the procedure is being performed to induce coughing to raise sputum that the patient cannot raise spontaneously and that the salt solution is irritating. The patient is instructed to inhale slowly and deeply through the mouth and to cough at will, vigorously and deeply, coughing and expectorating into a collection tube. The procedure is discontinued if the patient fails to raise sputum after 10 minutes or feels any discomfort. Ten milliliters of sputum should be collected; if the patient continues to raise sputum, a second specimen should be collected and submitted. Specimens should be delivered promptly to the laboratory and refrigerated if processing is delayed.

Sputum collection guidelines recommend collection of an early morning specimen for 3 consecutive days. In many cases the third specimen demonstrates minimal recovery of organisms, and this collection may not be recommended in some laboratories. Pooled specimens are unacceptable because of an increased risk of contamination.

### Gastric Lavage Specimens

Gastric lavage is used to collect sputum from patients who may have swallowed sputum during the night. The procedure is limited to senile, nonambulatory patients; children younger than 3 years of age (specimen of choice); and patients who fail to produce sputum by aerosol induction. The most desirable gastric lavage is collected at the patient's bedside before the patient arises and before exertion empties the stomach. Gastric lavage cannot be performed as an office or clinic procedure.

The collector should wear a cap, gown, and particulate respirator mask and should stand beside (not in front of) the patient, who should sit up on the edge of the bed or in a chair, if possible. The Levine collection tube is inserted through a nostril, and the patient is instructed to swallow the tube. When the tube has been fully inserted, a syringe is attached to the end of the tube and filtered distilled water is injected into the tube. The syringe is then used to withdraw 5 to 10 mL of gastric secretions, which is expelled slowly down the sides of the 50-mL conical collecting tube. Samples should be adjusted to a neutral pH. The laboratory may choose to provide sterile receptacles containing 100 mg of sodium carbonate to reduce the acidity; this improves the recovery of organisms. The top of the collection tube is screwed on tightly, and the tube is held upright during prompt delivery to the laboratory. Three specimens should be collected over a period of consecutive days. Specimens should be processed within 4 hours.

Bronchial lavages, washings, and brushings are collected and submitted by medical personnel. These are the specimens of choice for detecting nontuberculous mycobacteria and other opportunistic pathogens in patients with immune dysfunction.

### Urine Specimens

The incidence of urogenital infections shows little evidence of decreasing. About 2% to 3% of patients with pulmonary tuberculosis show urinary tract involvement, but 30% to 40% of patients with genitourinary disease have tuberculosis at some other site. The clinical manifestations of urinary tuberculosis, which are variable, include frequency of urination (most common), dysuria, hematuria, and flank pain. Definitive diagnosis requires recovery of acid-fast bacilli from the urine.

Early morning voided urine specimens (40 mL minimum) in sterile containers should be submitted daily for at least 3 days. The collection procedure is the same as for collecting a clean-catch midstream urine specimen (see Chapter 73). The 24-hour urine specimen is undesirable because of excessive dilution, higher contamination, and difficulty in concentrating. Catheterization should be used only if a midstream voided specimen cannot be collected.

### Fecal Specimens

Acid-fast staining or culture of stool (or both) from patients with AIDS has been used to identify patients who may be at risk for developing disseminated *M. avium* complex disease. The clinical utility of this practice remains controversial; however, if screening stains and/or cultures are positive, dissemination often follows. Feces should be submitted in a clean, dry, wax-free container without preservative or diluent. Contamination with urine should be avoided.

### Tissue and Body Fluid Specimens

Tuberculous meningitis is uncommon but occurs in both immunocompetent and immunosuppressed patients. A sufficient quantity of specimen is crucial for isolation of acid-fast bacilli from CSF. Very few organisms may be present in the spinal fluid, which makes their detection difficult. At least 10 mL of CSF is recommended for recovery of mycobacteria. Similarly, as much as possible of other body fluids (10 to 15 mL minimum), such as pleural, peritoneal, and pericardial fluids, should be collected in a sterile container or syringe with a Luer-tip cap. Tissues may be immersed in saline or wrapped in gauze. Swabs are discouraged, because the recovery of organisms is decreased.

### Blood Specimens

Immunocompromised patients, particularly those infected with HIV, can have disseminated mycobacterial infection; most of these infections are caused by *M. avium* complex. A blood culture positive for MAC is always associated with clinical evidence of disease. Recovery of mycobacteria is improved with blood collection in either a broth or the Isolator lysis-centrifugation system (see Chapter 68). Some studies have indicated that the lysis-centrifugation system is advantageous, because quantitative data can be obtained with each blood culture; in patients with AIDS, quantitation of such organisms can be used to monitor therapy and determine the prognosis. However, the necessity of quantitative blood cultures remains unclear.

Blood for culture of mycobacteria should be collected as for routine blood cultures. Blood collected in regular phlebotomy procedures in anticoagulants such as sodium polyanethol sulfonate (SPS), heparin, and citrate may be used to inoculate cultures for the recovery of *Mycobacterium* species. Conventional blood culture collection systems are unacceptable for the isolation of *Mycobacterium* spp. However, specialized automated systems are available for growth of Mycobacterium spp., including the Bactec MGIT 960 system (Becton-Dickinson, Franklin Lakes, N.J.), and the BacT/ALERT 3D (Biomerieux, Durham, N.C.).

### Wounds, Skin Lesions, and Aspirates

An aspirate is the best type of specimen for culturing of a skin lesion or wound. The skin should be cleansed with alcohol before aspiration of the material into a syringe. If the volume is insufficient for aspiration, pus and exudates may be obtained on a swab and then placed in a transport medium, such as Amie's or Stuart's medium (dry swabs are unacceptable). However, a negative culture of a specimen obtained on a swab is not considered reliable, and this should be noted in the culture report.

## SPECIMEN PROCESSING

Processing to recover acid-fast bacilli from clinical specimens involves several complex steps, each of which must be carried out with precision. Specimens from sterile sites can be inoculated directly to media (small volume) or concentrated to reduce volume. Other specimens require decontamination and concentration. A processing scheme is shown in Figure 43-1, and the procedures are explored in detail in the following discussions.

### Contaminated Specimens

Most specimens submitted for mycobacterial culture consist of organic debris, such as mucin, tissue, serum, and other proteinaceous material contaminated with organisms. A typical example of such a specimen is sputum. Laboratories must process these specimens to kill or reduce contaminating bacteria that can rapidly outgrow mycobacteria, and mycobacteria are released from mucin and/or cells. After decontamination, mycobacteria are concentrated, usually by centrifugation, to enhance their detection by acid-fast stain and culture. Unfortunately, there is no single ideal method for decontaminating and digesting clinical specimens. Although continuously faced with the inherent limitations of various methods, laboratories must strive to maximize the survival and detection of mycobacteria while maximizing the elimination of contaminating organisms. Rapidly growing mycobacteria are especially susceptible to high or prolonged exposure to greater than or equal to 2% sodium hydroxide (NaOH). Digestion-decontamination procedures should be as gentle as possible.

### Inadequate Specimens and Rejection Criteria

Identification and detection of *Mycobacterium* spp. is costly and time consuming. It is essential that the laboratory have a detailed policy regarding the rejection of inadequate specimens for the identification of these organisms. Specimens should be rejected according to the following guidelines: (1) insufficient volume, (2) contamination with saliva, (3) dried swabs, (4) pooled sputum or urine, (5) container has been compromised, broken or leaking, and (6) length of time from collection to processing is too long.

**Overview.** Commonly used digestion-decontamination methods are the NaOH method, the Zephiran-trisodium phosphate method, and the N-acetyl-L-cysteine (NALC)–2% NaOH method. The NALC-NaOH method is presented in detail in Procedure 43-1, which can be found on the Evolve site. Another decontaminating procedure that uses oxalic acid is very useful for treating specimens known to harbor gram-negative rods, particularly *Pseudomonas* and *Proteus* spp., which are extremely troublesome contaminants. It is important to note that oxalic acid, NaOH, and mild hydrogen chloride (HCl) may reduce the recovery of *M. ulcerans*.

NaOH, a commonly used decontaminant that is also mucolytic, should be used with caution. It not only reduces contamination, but also reduces recovery of *Mycobacterium* spp. as alkalinity increases, temperature rises, and exposure time increases. The sample should be homogenized by centrifugal swirling, minimizing physical agitation. The container then should be allowed to sit for 15 minutes so that aerosolized droplets can fall to the bottom, thus reducing the risk of infection for the laboratory professional.

Several agents can be used to liquefy a clinical specimen, including NALC, dithiothreitol (sputolysin), and enzymes. None of these agents are inhibitory to bacterial cells. In most procedures, liquefaction (release of the organisms from mucin or cells) is enhanced by vigorous mixing with a vortex-type mixer in a closed container. After mixing as previously described, the container

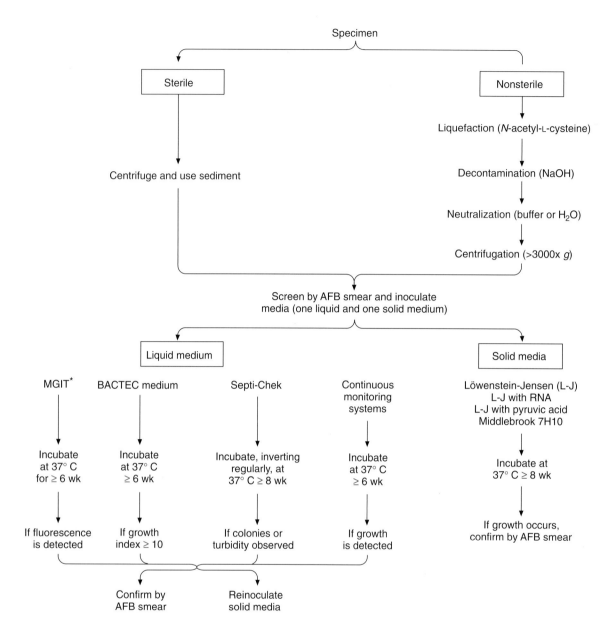

**Figure 43-1** Flowchart for specimen processing to isolate mycobacteria.

should be allowed to stand for 15 minutes before opening, to prevent the dispersion of fine aerosols generated during mixing. Of utmost importance during processing is strict adherence to processing and laboratory safety protocols. All of these procedures should be carried out in a biologic safety cabinet (BSC).

After digestion and decontamination, specimens are concentrated by centrifugation at greater than or equal to 3000× *g*.

**Special Considerations.** Many specimen types besides respiratory samples contain normal flora and require decontamination and concentration.

Aerosol-induced sputum should be treated as sputum. Gastric lavages should be processed within 4 hours of collection or neutralized with 10% sodium carbonate (check with pH paper to make sure the specimen is at

neutral pH) and refrigerated until processed as for sputum. If more than 10 mL of watery-appearing aspirate was obtained, the specimen can be centrifuged at 3600× *g* for 30 minutes, the supernatant decanted, and the sediment processed as for sputum.

Urine specimens should be divided into a maximum of four 50-mL centrifuge tubes and centrifuged at 3600× *g* for 30 minutes. The supernatant should be decanted, leaving approximately 2 mL of sediment in each tube. The tubes are vortexed to suspend the sediments, and sediments are combined. If necessary, distilled water can be added to a total volume of 10 mL. This urine concentrate is treated as for sputum or with the sputolysin–oxalic acid method.

For fecal specimens, approximately 0.2 g of stool (a portion about the size of a pea) is emulsified in 11 mL of sterile, filtered, distilled water. The suspension is vortexed thoroughly, and particulate matter is allowed to settle for 15 minutes. Ten milliliters of the supernatant is then transferred to a 50-mL conical centrifuge tube and decontaminated using the oxalic acid or NALC-NaOH method.

Swabs and wound aspirates should be transferred to a sterile, 50-mL conical centrifuge tube containing a liquid medium (Middlebrook 7H9, Dubos Tween albumin broth) at a ratio of 1 part specimen to 5 to 10 parts liquid medium. The specimen is vortexed vigorously and allowed to stand for 20 minutes. The swab is removed, and the resulting suspension is processed as for sputum.

Large pieces of tissue should be finely minced with a sterile scalpel and scissors. This material is homogenized in a sterile tissue grinder with a small amount of sterile saline (0.85%) or sterile 0.2% bovine albumin; the suspension then is processed as for sputum. If the tissue is not known to be sterile, it is homogenized, and half is directly inoculated to solid and liquid media. The other half is processed as for sputum. If the tissue is collected aseptically (i.e., it is sterile), it may be processed without being treated with NALC-NaOH.

### Specimens Not Requiring Decontamination

Tissues or body fluids collected aseptically usually do not require the digestion and decontamination methods used with contaminated specimens. The processing of clinical specimens that do not routinely require decontamination for acid-fast culture is described here. If such a specimen appears contaminated because of color, cloudiness, or foul odor, Gram staining is performed to detect bacteria other than acid-fast bacilli. Specimens found to be contaminated should be processed as described in the preceding section.

CSF should be handled aseptically and centrifuged for 30 minutes at 3600× *g* to concentrate the bacteria. The supernatant is decanted, and the sediment is vortexed thoroughly before the smear is prepared and the media inoculated. If insufficient quantity of spinal fluid is received, the specimen should be used directly for smear and culture. Recovery of acid-fast bacilli from CSF is difficult, and additional solid or liquid media should be inoculated if material is available.

Pleural fluid should be collected in sterile anticoagulant (1 mg/mL ethylenediaminetetraacetic acid [EDTA] or 0.1 mg/mL heparin). If the fluid becomes clotted, it should be liquefied with an equal volume of sputolysin and vigorously mixed. To lower the specific gravity and density of pleural fluid, 20 mL is transferred to a sterile, 50-mL centrifuge tube, and the specimen is diluted by filling the tube with distilled water. The tube is inverted several times to mix the suspension and then centrifuged at 3600× *g* for 30 minutes. The supernatant should be removed, and the sediment should be suspended for smear and culture.

Joint fluid and other sterile exudates can be handled aseptically and inoculated directly to media. Bone marrow aspirates may be injected into Pediatric Isolator tubes (Alere, Waltham, MA), which help prevent clotting; the specimen can be removed with a needle and syringe for preparation of smears and cultures. As an

alternative, these specimens are either inoculated directly to media or, if clotted, treated with sputolysin or glass beads and distilled water before concentration.

## DIRECT DETECTION METHODS

### Microscopy

Microscopy is considered a reasonably sensitive and rapid procedure for the presumptive identification of *Mycobacterium* spp. in clinical specimens.

### Acid-Fast Stains

The cell walls of mycobacteria contain long-chain, multiply cross-linked fatty acids, called *mycolic acids*. Mycolic acids probably complex basic dyes, contributing to the characteristic of acid-fastness that distinguishes mycobacteria from other bacteria. Mycobacteria are not the only group with this unique feature. Species of *Nocardia* and *Rhodococcus* are also partially acid-fast; *Legionella micdadei*, a causative agent in pneumonia, is partially acid-fast in tissue. Cysts of the genera *Cryptosporidium* and *Isospora* are distinctly acid-fast. The mycolic acids and lipids in the mycobacterial cell wall probably account for the unusual resistance of these organisms to the effects of drying and harsh decontaminating agents in addition to the property of acid-fastness.

When Gram stained, mycobacteria usually appear as slender, poorly stained, beaded, gram-positive bacilli (Figure 43-2); sometimes they appear as "gram neutral," or "gram-ghosts," by failing to take up either crystal violet or safranin. Acid-fastness is affected by the age of colonies, the medium on which growth occurs, and exposure to ultraviolet light. Rapidly growing species appear to be acid-fast variable.

Three types of staining procedures are used in the laboratory for rapid detection and confirmation of acid-fast bacilli: fluorochrome, Ziehl-Neelsen, and Kinyoun. Smears for all methods are prepared in the same way (see Procedure 43-2 on the Evolve site).

Visualization of acid-fast bacilli in sputum or other clinical material should be considered only presumptive

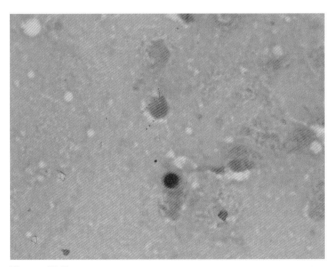

**Figure 43-2** Gram staining of *M. marinum* demonstrates beaded appearance. (Courtesy Stacie Lansink, Sioux Falls, S.D.)

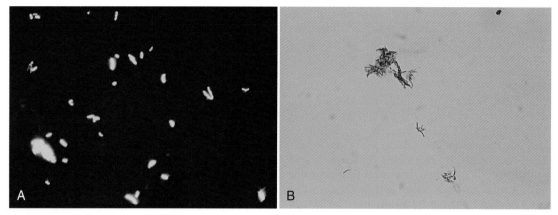

**Figure 43-3** *M. tuberculosis* stained with **(A)** fluorochrome stain (×400) and **(B)** Kinyoun acid-fast stain (×1000).

evidence of tuberculosis, because staining does not specifically identify *M. tuberculosis*. The report form should indicate this. For example, *M. gordonae*, a nonpathogenic scotochromogen commonly found in tap water, has been a problem when tap water or deionized water has been used in the preparation of smears or even when patients have rinsed their mouths with tap water before using an aerosolized saline solution to induce sputum. However, the incidence of false-positive smears is very low when good quality control is maintained. Conversely, acid-fast–stained smears of clinical specimens require at least $10^4$ acid-fast bacilli per milliliter for detection from concentrated specimens.

**Methods** *Fluorochrome Stain.* Fluorochrome staining is the screening procedure recommended for laboratories that have a fluorescent (ultraviolet) microscope (see Procedure 43-3 on the Evolve site). Fluorochrome stain is more sensitive than the conventional carbolfuchsin stains, because the fluorescent bacilli stand out brightly against the background (Figure 43-3). Because the smear can be examined initially at lower magnifications (×250 to ×400), more fields can be visualized in a short period. In addition, a positive fluorescent smear may be restained using the conventional Ziehl-Neelsen or Kinyoun procedure, thereby saving the time needed to make a fresh smear. Screening of specimens with rhodamine or rhodamine-auramine results in a higher yield of positive smears and substantially reduces the time needed to examine smears.

One drawback of the fluorochrome stains is that many rapid-growers may not appear fluorescent with these reagents. All positive fluorescent smears should be confirmed with a Ziehl-Neelsen stain or by examination by another technologist. It is important to wipe the immersion oil from the objective lens after examining a positive smear, because stained bacilli can float off the slide into the oil, possibly contributing to a false-positive reading for the next smear examined.

**Fuchsin Acid-Fast Stains.** The classic carbolfuchsin stain (Ziehl-Neelsen) requires heating of the slide for better penetration of the stain into the mycobacterial cell wall; hence, it is also known as the *hot stain procedure* (see Procedure 6-3 on the Evolve site). With Ziehl-Neelsen staining, *Mycobacterium* spp. appear red or have a red-blue, beaded appearance, whereas nonmycobacteria appear blue.

Procedure 6-4, which can be found on the Evolve site, describes the Kinyoun acid-fast stain. The method is similar to Ziehl-Neelsen staining, but no heat is used (see Figure 43-3); this technique is known as the *cold stain procedure*. If present, typical acid-fast bacilli appear as purple to red, slightly curved, short or long rods (2 to 8 μm); they also may appear beaded or banded (*M. kansasii*). For some nontuberculous species, such as *M. avium* complex, they appear pleomorphic, usually coccoid.

**Examination, Interpretation, and Reporting of Smears.** Before a smear is reported as negative, it should be examined carefully by scanning at least 300 oil immersion fields (magnification ×1000), equivalent to three full horizontal sweeps of a smear that is 2 cm long and 1 cm wide. Because the fluorescent stain can be examined using a lower magnification (×250 or ×450) than that required for a fuchsin-stained smear, the equivalent number of fields (30) can be examined in less time, which makes the fluorochrome stain the preferred method.

When acid-fast organisms are observed on a smear, the report should include information about the type of staining method used and the quantity of organisms. The recommended interpretations and ways to report smear results are shown in Table 43-7.

The overall sensitivity of an acid-fast smear ranges from 20% to 80%. Factors such as specimen type, staining method, and culture method can influence the acid-fast smear sensitivity. In general, specificity of acid-fast smear examination is very high. However, cross-contamination of slides during the staining process and use of water contaminated with saprophytic mycobacteria can lead to false-positive results. Staining receptacles should not be used; acid-fast bacilli can also be transferred from one slide to another in immersion oil. For these reasons, the best course is to confirm a positive result.

Although not without some limitations, because of its simplicity and speed, the stained smear is an important and useful test, particularly for detection of smear-positive patients ("infectious reservoirs"), who pose the greatest risk to others in their environment.

**TABLE 43-7** Acid-Fast Smear Reporting

| Number of AFB Seen Fuchsin Stain (1000× Magnification) | Number of AFB Seen Fluorochrome Stain (450× Magnification) | Number of AFB Seen Fluorochrome Stain (250× Magnification) | Report |
|---|---|---|---|
| 0 | 0 | 0 | No AFB seen |
| 1-2/300 fields | 1-2/70 fields | 1-2/30 fields | Doubtful; request another specimen |
| 1-9/100 fields | 2-18/50 fields | 1-9/10 fields | 1+ |
| 1-9/10 fields | 4-36/10 fields | 1-9/field | 2+ |
| 1-9/field | 4-36/field | 10-90/field | 3+ |
| >9/field | >36/field | >90/field | 4+ |

Modified from Kent PT, Kubica GP: *Public health mycobacteriology: a guide for the level III laboratory,* US Department of Health and Human Service, Public Health Service, Washington, DC, 1985, Centers for Disease Control and Prevention; and Versalovic J: *Manual of clinical microbiology,* ed 10, 2011, Washington, DC, ASM Press.
*AFB,* Acid-fast bacilli.

## Antigen-Protein Detection

The detection of microbial products or components has been used in recent years to diagnose infections caused by *M. tuberculosis.* For example, tuberculostearic acid is a fatty acid that can be extracted from the cell wall of mycobacteria and detected by gas chromatography or mass spectrometry in clinical samples containing few mycobacteria. Because of the limited number of species that can cause meningitis and because *M. tuberculosis* appears to be the only one of these species that releases tuberculostearic acid into the surrounding environment, the presence of this substance in CSF is thought to be diagnostic of tuberculous meningitis. Performance of this assay is limited to a few laboratories. Various immunoassays for antigen detection directly in clinical specimens, including sputum and CSF, have been evaluated and show some promise.

Production of adenosine deaminase, a host enzyme, is increased in certain infections caused by *M. tuberculosis.* For example, elevated levels of this enzyme were found in most patients with tuberculous pleural effusions (98% sensitive); the test for the enzyme also was determined to be highly specific (96% specificity).

## Immunodiagnostic Testing

As previously discussed, interferon-gamma release assays have become more widely used for the diagnosis of tuberculosis. The available test systems, T-SPOT-TB (Oxford Immunotec, Oxford, United Kingdom) and Quanti*F-ERON* Gold In-Tube (QFNG-IT; Cellestis, Chadstone, Victoria, Australia), do not typically cross react with nontuberculous mycobacterium, are not affected by the BCG vaccine, and are not as variable as the historical serologic tuberculin skin tests. The T-SPOT-TB assay is an enzyme-linked immunospot assay that requires isolation and incubation of peripheral blood mononuclear cells (PBMCs). It takes approximately 2 days and is technically complicated. The QFNG-IT assay measures the stimulation of T-cell interferon-gamma in whole blood in a tube precoated with *M. tuberculosis* antigens. It yields results in approximately 8 hours. Neither assay distinguishes between latent and active infections. In addition, specificity and sensitivity vary in the population tested, including immunocompromised patients and children. Variation is associated with the patient's CD4 cell count; therefore, interpretations and results should be evaluated with caution.

## Genetic Sequencing and Nucleic Acid Amplification

Subsequent to the introduction of commercially available hybridization assays, commercially available and in-house–developed nucleic acid amplification tests were used successfully for early identification of *M. tuberculosis* complex grown in liquid cultures. Currently, PCR-based sequencing for mycobacterial identification consists of PCR amplification of mycobacterial DNA with genus-specific primers and sequencing of the amplicons. The organism is identified by comparison of the nucleotide sequence with reference sequences. The most reliable sequence for identification of mycobacteria is the approximately 1500 bp 16S rRNA gene. However, only a 600 bp sequence at the 5′ end is required for identification. The sequence homogeneity in the *M. tuberculosis* complex prevents the use of this sequence to differentiate these species. This region contains both conserved and variable regions, which makes it an ideal target for identification purposes.

Despite the accuracy of PCR-based sequencing to identify mycobacteria, problems remain: the sequences in some databases are not accurate; no present consensus exists as to the quantitative definition of a genus or species based on 16S rRNA gene sequence data; and procedures are not standardized. In addition, the 16S rRNA 5′ region contains two hypervariable regions, A and B. The A region provides the signature sequences for species identification. However, *M. chelonae* and *M. abscessus* both require additional sequencing, because the A and B regions are identical and the 3′ end of the 16srRNA contains a 4-bp sequence difference.

Several other genes have also been used to identify mycobacterial species, including the 23S rRNA, ITS 1, *hsp65, rpoB,* and *gyrB* gene. The 23S rRNA sequence is 3100 bp in length, which limits accurate sequencing. ITS 1 is a spacer sequence located between the 16S and 23S rRNA genes. This sequence, which is only 200 to 330 bp, is more easily analyzed. The limitation of this sequence is that it is not a genus-specific sequence; therefore, results may be affected by contaminating bacteria. The 65 kDa heat shock protein, also referred to as the *groEL2* gene, is a 440-bp fragment that can be amplified and analyzed with restriction digestion, followed by agarose electrophoresis. The *hsp65* is highly conserved but contains a greater variation in polymorphisms than the 16S RNA, particularly in a 441-bp region referred to as the "Telanti fragment." This allows for differentiation of *Mycobacterium* species based on the variation in restriction fragment length polymorphisms (RFLPs). Repetitive sequence–based PCR, Diversilab (Biomérieux, Durham, N.C.), demonstrates better species discrimination than RFLP. In addition, a commercially available system in which the 16S to 23S rRNA spacer region of mycobacterial species (INNO-LiPA Mycobacteria; Innogenetics, Ghent, Belgium) has been successfully used to directly detect and identify several of the most clinically relevant mycobacterial species in aliquots of positive liquid culture. However, caution should be used in interpretation of results, because some cross reactivity has occurred with closely related species.

Another commercial system, GenoType Mycobacterium (Hain Lifescience GmbH, Nehrin, Germany), which uses a similar format, has additional probes from *M. celatum, M. malmoense, M. peregrinum, M. phlei,* and two subgroups of *M. fortuitum,* in addition to a supplemental kit that allows for 16 additional mycobacterial species. Yet another commercial system, MicroSeq500 16S rRNA (Applied Biosystems, Foster City, California), sequences a 500-bp region and uses a comparative database for species identification.

The *rpoB* gene encodes the beta-subunit in the organism's RNA polymerase. Mutations in this gene confer rifampin resistance to *M. tuberculosis.* Different regions in this gene have been used to identify rapid-growing isolates, but little data are available for the slow-growing species. Finally, the *gyrB* gene encodes the beta-subunit in the organism's topoisomerase II. Several single nucleotide polymorphisms have been identified in this gene that are useful in distinguishing species in the *M. tuberculosis* complex. After amplification, identification and differentiation of species requires restriction analysis and gel electrophoresis.

Additional molecular techniques, such as conventional and real-time PCR, have been used to detect *M. tuberculosis* directly in clinical specimens. For example, the Amplicor *Mycobacterium tuberculosis* test (Roche Diagnostic Systems, Branchburg, New Jersey) uses PCR to detect *M. tuberculosis* directly in respiratory specimens. The Amplified *Mycobacterium tuberculosis* Direct Test (AMTD; Gen-Probe, San Diego, California) is based on ribosomal RNA amplification. The Roche assay currently is approved by the FDA for use only on acid-fast, smear-positive specimens, because numerous studies have demonstrated less than optimum sensitivity on smear-negative specimens. Because of subsequent kit modifications that improved sensitivity, Gen-Probe's assay is approved on both smear-positive and smear-negative specimens. Ribosomal RNA is released from the mycobacteria by means of a lysing agent, sonication, and heat. The specific DNA probe is allowed to react with the extracted rRNA to form a stable DNA-RNA hybrid. Any nonhybridized DNA–acridinium ester probes are chemically degraded. When an alkaline hydrogen peroxide solution is added to elicit chemiluminescence, only the hybrid-bound acridinium ester is available to emit light; the amount of light emitted is directly related to the amount of hybridized probe. The light produced is measured on a chemiluminometer. Numerous laboratories have incorporated these tests into their routine procedures.

The Amplicor test (Roche Diagnostic Systems), which uses TaqMan technology and is a real-time PCR test, has received FDA approval for smear-positive respiratory specimens from patients suspected of having tuberculosis. These tests are limited in the number of species they are able to identify. Clinical laboratories have developed their own PCR assays to detect *M. tuberculosis* directly in clinical specimens.

Line probe assays (DNA strip assays) involve PCR amplification coupled with a reverse hybridization step. The target sequence is amplified using biotinylated primers. The amplicon is then hybridized to membrane-immobilized, sequence-specific probes for each species. The membrane is developed using an enzyme-mediated reaction and color indicator to analyze the banding pattern. Banding patterns are species specific based on the immobilized probe map on the membrane. A commercially available line probe assay (GenoType MTBC; Hain Lifescience, Nehren, Germany) enables the identification of *M. tuberculosis* complex organisms at the species level using the 23S rRNA.

In addition to assays developed in-house and the Genotype MTBC, five non-FDA-approved commercial amplification tests are widely used outside the United States. The Artus *M. tuberculosis* PCR kit (Qiagen GmbH, Hilden/Hamburg, Germany) assay uses real-time PCR for amplification of the 16S rRNA gene; the ProbeTec Direct TB energy transfer system (Becton Dickinson, Sparks, Maryland) uses strand displacement amplification technology; the RealArt *M. tuberculosis* TM PCR reagents (Abbott Laboratories, Abbott Park, Illinois) is a real-time PCR assay using the ABI Prism 7000 system; and the Loop-mediated isothermal amplification test (Eiken Chemical, Tokyo) uses isothermal amplification and UV light detection. These systems have sensitivities and specificities comparable to those of the FDA-approved amplification assays. The GeneXpert system (Cepheid, Sunnyvale, California), which is used for real-time PCR detection of *M. tuberculosis* complex and resistance to rifampin, uses amplification of the *rpoB* gene previously discussed in this section.

Currently no molecular assays are available for direct detection of nontuberculous mycobacteria. In 2004, the Centers for Disease Control established a national tuberculosis genotyping system. Details and updates are available at http://www.cdc.gov/tb/programs/default.htm.

**DNA Microarrays.** DNA microarrays are also attractive for rapid examination of large numbers of DNA sequences by a single hybridization step. This approach has been used to simultaneously identify mycobacterial species and detect mutations that confer rifampin resistance in mycobacteria. Fluorescent-labeled PCR amplicons generated from bacterial colonies are hybridized to a DNA array containing nucleotide probes. The bound amplicons emit a fluorescent signal that is detected with a scanner. With this approach, 82 unique 16S rRNA sequences allow for differentiation of 54 mycobacterial species and 51 sequences that contain unique *rpoB* gene mutations (mutations that confer resistance to rifampin).

### Chromatographic Analysis

Analysis of mycobacterial lipids by chromatographic methods, including thin-layer chromatography, gas-liquid

**BOX 43-3** Suggested Media for Cultivation of Mycobacteria from Clinical Specimens*

| Media | Comments | Media | Comments |
|---|---|---|---|
| **Solid** | | **Liquid†** | |
| ***AGAR BASED—GROWTH WITHIN 10 TO 12 DAYS*** | | BACTEC 12B medium | Used in the MGIT960 system; PANTA is added before incubation; $^{14}$C-labeled palmitic acid is metabolized to produce $^{14}CO_2$, which is detected by the instrument |
| Middlebrook | Contains 2% glycerol, which enhances the growth of *Mycobacterium avium* complex (MAC). | | |
| Middlebrook 7H10 | Supplemented with carbenicillin (for inhibition | Middlebrook 7H9 broth Dubos Tween albumin | |
| Middlebrook 7H10 selective | of pseudomonads), polymyxin B, trimethoprim lactate, and amphotericin B | Septi-Chek AFB | 20 mL of Middlebrook 7H9 broth is incubated in 20% $CO_2$; solid phase contains three media: modified L-J, Middlebrook 7H11, and a chocolate agar slab |
| Middlebrook 7H11 | Contains 0.1% enzymatic hydrolysate of | | |
| Middlebrook 7H11 selective | casein, which improves recovery of isoniazid-resistant *M. tuberculosis*) | | |
| Middlebrook 7H11 | Supplemented with mycobactin J, which provides for growth of *M. genovense* | | |
| Middlebrook 7H11 thin pour plates, 10 × 90 mm (Remel, Lenexa, Kansas) | Enhances visibility of colonies within 11 days | **Media Used in Commercially Supplied Growth and Semiautomated or Fully Automated Systems** | |
| Middlebrook biplate (7H10/7H11S agar) | | Mycobacteria Growth Indicator Tube [MGIT] (Becton Dickinson Microbiology Systems, Cockeysville, Md.) | MGIT 460TB (semiautomated system) or MGIT 960 (fully automated system); MGIT is a modified Middlebrook 7H9 broth that incorporates a fluorescence-quenching–based oxygen sensor for detection |
| ***EGG BASED—GROWTH WITHIN 18 TO 24 DAYS*** | | | |
| Löwenstein-Jensen (L-J) | Commonly used medium; good recovery of *M. tuberculosis* but poor recovery of many other species; *M. genovense* fails to grow | MB Redox (Heipha Diagnostica Biotest, Eppelheim, Germany) | Nonradiometric medium; a modified Kirchner medium, enriched with additives and antibiotics, that uses tetrazolium salt as the redox indicator |
| L-J Gruft | Supplemented with penicillin and nalidixic acid | ESP Culture System II and versa TREK Culture System II (Trek Diagnostic Systems, Cleveland, Ohio) | Modified Middlebrook 7H9 broth |
| L-J Mycobactosel | Supplemented with cycloheximide, lincomycin, and nalidixic acid | | |
| L-J with pyruvic acid | Enhances recovery of *M. bovis* | MB/BacT Alert 3D (bioMérieux, Durham, N.C.) | Uses Middlebrook 7H9 broth |
| L-J with glycerol | Enhances recovery of *M. ulcerans* | | |
| Petragnani medium | Contains twice the concentration of malachite than Lowenstein-Jensen green (an inhibitor of contaminating organisms); improves recovery from heavily contaminated specimens | BACTEC 9000 MB (Becton Dickinson); recently discontinued by manufacturer | Used Middlebrook 7H9 broth |
| Heme-supplemented media (egg or agar based) | Supplemented with hemin, hemoglobin or ferric ammonium citrate increases recovery of *M. haemophilum*. | | |

*For optimal recovery of mycobacteria, a minimum combination of liquid medium and solid media is recommended.
†Tween 80 added to liquid media acts as a surfactant, breaking up clumps of organisms and increasing recovery rates.

chromatography (GLC), capillary gas chromographic methods, and reverse-phase high-performance liquid chromatography (HPLC), has been used to identify mycobacteria. In HPLC, a liquid mobile phase is combined with various technical advances to separate large cellular metabolites and components. HPLC of extracted mycobacteria is a specific and rapid method for identifying species. Many state health departments and the CDC now use this method routinely. The long-chain mycolic acids are separated better by HPLC than by GLC, because they do not withstand the high temperatures needed for GLC. The patterns produced by different species are very easily reproducible, and a typical identification requires only a few hours.

## Cultivation

A combination of different culture media is required to optimize recovery of mycobacteria from culture; at least one solid medium in addition to a liquid medium should be used. The ideal media combination should be economical and should support the most rapid and abundant growth of mycobacteria, allow for the study of colony morphology and pigment production, inhibit the growth of contaminants.

### Solid Media

Solid media, such as those listed in Box 43-3, are recommended because of the development of characteristic, reproducible colonial morphology, good growth from small inocula, and a low rate of contamination. Optimally, at least two solid media (a serum [albumin] agar base medium, [e.g., Middlebrook 7H10] and an egg-potato base medium [e.g., Löwenstein-Jensen, or L-J]) should be used for each specimen (these media are available from commercial sources). All specimens must be processed appropriately before inoculation. It is imperative to inoculate test organisms to commercially available products for quality control (see Procedure 43-4 on the Evolve site).

Cultures are incubated at 35° C in the dark in an atmosphere of 5% to 10% carbon dioxide ($CO_2$) and high humidity. Tube media are incubated in a slanted position with screw caps loose for at least 1 week to allow for evaporation of excess fluid and the entry of $CO_2$; plated media are either placed in a $CO_2$-permeable plastic bag or wrapped with $CO_2$-permeable tape. If specimens obtained from the skin or superficial lesions are suspected to contain *M. marinum* or *M. ulcerans*, an additional set of solid media should be inoculated and incubated at 25° to 30° C. In addition, a chocolate agar plate (or placement of an X-factor [hemin] disk on conventional media) and incubation at 25° to 33° C is needed for recovery of *M. haemophilum* from these specimens. RGM optimally require incubation at 28° to 30° C.

Cultures are examined weekly for growth. Contaminated cultures are discarded and reported as "contaminated, unable to detect presence of mycobacteria"; additional specimens are also requested. If available, sediment may be recultured after enhanced decontamination or by inoculating the sediment to a more selective medium. Most isolates appear between 3 and 6 weeks; a few isolates appear after 7 or 8 weeks of incubation. When growth appears, the rate of growth, pigmentation, and colonial morphology are recorded. The typical colonial appearance of *M. tuberculosis* and other mycobacteria is shown in Figure 43-4. After 8 weeks of incubation, negative cultures (those showing no growth) are reported, and the cultures are discarded.

Because of the resurgence of tuberculosis in the United States in the late 1980s and early 1990s, significant effort has been put into developing methods to provide more rapid diagnosis of tuberculosis. Welch et al.[2] refined a method that reduced the time to detection of mycobacterial growth by half or more, compared with conventional culture methods, by using a thinly poured Middlebrook 7H11 plate. These plates are inoculated in a routine manner, sealed, incubated, and examined microscopically (×40) at regular intervals for the appearance of microcolonies. Presumptive identification of *M. tuberculosis* or *M. avium* complex could be made for about 83% of the isolates within 10 and 11 days after inoculation, respectively.

### Liquid Media

In general, use of a liquid media system reduces the turnaround time for isolation of acid-fast bacilli to approximately 10 days, compared with 17 days or longer for conventional solid media. Several different systems are available for culturing and detecting the growth of mycobacteria in liquid media. The most commonly used systems are summarized in Table 43-8. Growth of mycobacteria in liquid media, regardless of the type, requires 5% to 10% $CO_2$; $CO_2$ is either already provided in the culture vials or is added according to the manufacturer's instructions. When growth is detected in a liquid medium, acid-fast staining of a culture aliquot is performed to confirm the presence of acid-fast bacilli, and the material

is subcultured to solid agar. Gram staining can also be performed if contamination is suspected.

### Interpretation

Although isolation of MAC organisms indicates infection, the clinician must determine the clinical significance of isolating NTM in most cases; in other words, does the organism represent mere colonization or significant infection? Because these organisms vary greatly in their pathogenic potential, can colonize an individual without causing infection, and are ubiquitous in the environment, interpretation of a positive NTM culture is complicated. Therefore, the American Thoracic Society has recommended diagnostic criteria for NTM disease to help physicians interpret culture results.

## APPROACH TO IDENTIFICATION

Regardless of the identification methods used, the first test always performed on organisms growing on solid or liquid mycobacterial media is acid-fast staining, to confirm that the organisms are indeed mycobacteria. Identification of species other than MAC and the more frequently isolated NTM (MAC, *M. avium*, *M. intracellulare*, *M. gordonae*, and *M. kansasii*) has become challenging for routine clinical microbiology laboratories, particularly in light of the ever-increasing number of new mycobacterial species. Traditional methods (i.e., phenotypic methods) for identifying mycobacteria, particularly the NTM, are based on growth parameters, biochemical characteristics, and analysis of cell wall lipids, all of which are slow, cumbersome, and often inconclusive procedures. Over the past decade, the rate of non-AIDS–associated infections has been increasing, and many of the newly identified NTM species have been associated with various diseases. As a result, identification of species is vital to selecting effective antimicrobial therapy and to deciding whether to perform susceptibility testing on accurately speciated NTM. Most of the newer species have been identified using nucleic acid sequencing with limited published phenotypic characteristics. Because of these issues and limitations with conventional phenotypic methods for identification, molecular and genetic investigations are becoming indispensable to identify the NTM accurately. Therefore, for timely and accurate identification of mycobacteria, molecular approaches in conjunction with some phenotypic characteristics should be used.

Regardless of whether molecular or phenotypic methods are used, when growth is detected, broth subcultures of colonies growing in liquid media or on solid media (several colonies inoculated to Middlebrook 7H9 broth [5 mL] and incubated at 35° C for 5 to 7 days with daily agitation to enhance growth) are then used to determine pigmentation and growth rate and to inoculate all test media for biochemical tests, if performed. Additional cultures may be inoculated and then incubated at different temperatures when more definitive identification is needed.

### Conventional Phenotypic Tests

**Growth Characteristics.** Preliminary identification of mycobacterial isolates depends on the organisms' rate of

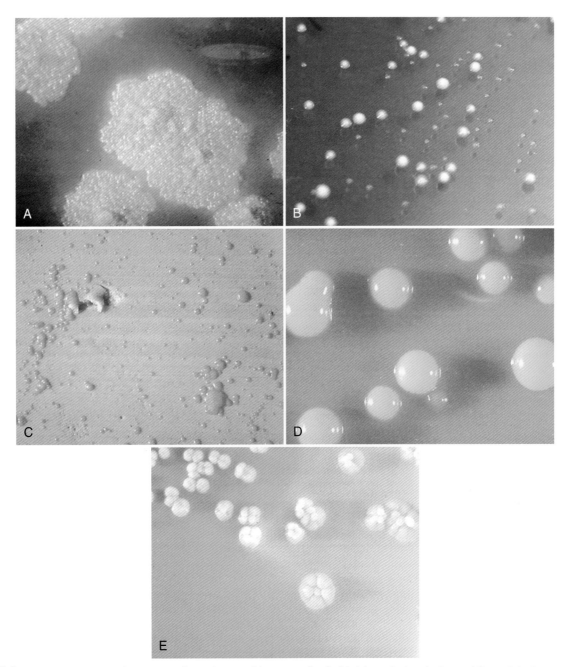

**Figure 43-4** Typical appearance of some mycobacteria on solid agar media. **A,** *M. tuberculosis* colonies on Löwenstein-Jensen agar after 8 weeks of incubation. **B,** A different colonial morphology is seen on culture of one strain of *M. avium* complex. **C,** *M. kansasii* colonies exposed to light. **D,** Scotochromogen *M. gordonae* showing yellow colonies. **E,** Smooth, multilobate colonies of *M. fortuitum* on Löwenstein-Jensen medium.

growth, colonial morphology (see Figure 43-4), colonial texture, pigmentation and, in some instances, the permissive incubation temperatures of mycobacteria. Despite the limitations of phenotypic tests, the mycobacterial growth characteristics are helpful for determining a preliminary identification (e.g., an isolate appears as rapidly growing mycobacteria). To perform identification procedures, quality control organisms should be tested along with unknowns (Table 43-9). The commonly used quality control organisms can be maintained in broth at room temperature and transferred monthly. In this way

they are always be available for inoculation to test media along with suspensions of the unknown mycobacteria being tested.

***Growth Rate.*** The rate of growth is an important criterion for determining the initial category of an isolate. Rapid-growers usually produce colonies within 3 to 4 days after subculture. However, even a rapid-grower may take longer than 7 days to initially produce colonies because of inhibition by a harsh decontaminating procedure. Therefore, the growth rate (and pigment production) must be determined by subculture (see Procedure 43-5

**TABLE 43-8** Liquid Media Systems Commonly Used to Culture and Detect the Growth of Mycobacteria

| System | Basic Principles of Detection |
|---|---|
| BACTEC 460 TB (Becton Dickinson Diagnostic Systems, Cockeysville, Md.) | Culture medium contains $^{14}$C-labeled palmitic acid. If present in the broth, mycobacteria metabolize the $^{14}$C-labeled substrates and release radioactively labeled $^{14}CO_2$ in the atmosphere, which collects above the broth in the bottle. The instrument withdraws this carbon dioxide ($CO_2$)-containing atmosphere and measures the amount of radioactivity present. Bottles that yield a radioactive index, called a *growth index,* greater than or equal to 10 are considered positive. |
| Septi-Chek AFB System (Becton Dickinson) | Biphasic culture system made up of a modified Middlebrook 7H9 broth with a three-sided paddle containing chocolate, egg-based, and modified 7H11 solid agars. After inoculation, a supplement is added to the liquid that includes glucose, glycerol, oleic acid, pyridoxal HCl, catalase, albumin, and antibiotics (PANTA). The bottle is inverted regularly to inoculate the solid media. Growth is detected by observing the three-sided paddle. |
| Mycobacteria Growth Indicator Tube (MGIT) (Becton Dickinson) | A culture tube contains Middlebrook 7H9 broth and a fluorescent compound embedded in a silicone sensor. Growth is detected visually using an ultraviolet light. Oxygen ($O_2$) diminishes the fluorescent output of the sensor; therefore, $O_2$ consumption by organisms present in the medium is detected as an increase in fluorescence under ultraviolet (UV) light at 365 nm. The MGIT medium is supplemented with oleic acid-albumin-dextrose and PANTA before incubation. |
| **Continuous Growth Monitoring Systems** Versa TREK (TREK Diagnostic Systems, Cleveland, Ohio) | Organisms are cultured in a modified Middlebrook 7H9 broth with enrichment and a cellulose sponge to increase the culture's surface area. The instrument detects growth by monitoring pressure changes that occur as a result of $O_2$ consumption or gas production by the organisms as they grow. |
| BacT/Alert System (bioMérieux, Durham, N.C.) | Organisms are cultured in modified Middlebrook 7H9 broth. The instrument detects growth by monitoring $CO_2$ production by means of a colorimetric $CO_2$ sensor in each bottle. |
| BACTEC 9000 MB (Becton Dickinson-recently discontinued) | Organisms are cultured in a modified Middlebrook 7H9 broth. The instrument detects growth by monitoring $O_2$ consumption by means of a fluorescent sensor. |
| BACTEC MGIT 960 (Becton Dickinson) | See above for basic principle (MGIT). The instrument detects growth by monitoring $O_2$ consumption by means of a fluorescent sensor. |
| MB Redox (Heipha Diagnostica Biotest, Eppelheim, Germany) | This is a nonradiometric medium. It is a modified Kirchner medium enriched with additives and antibiotics, and tetrazolium salt is the redox indicator. AFB are identified as pink to purple, pinhead-sized particles. |

on the Evolve site). The dilution of the organism used to assess the growth rate is critical. Even slow-growing mycobacteria appear to produce colonies in less than 7 days if the inoculum is too heavy. One organism particularly likely to exhibit false-positive rapid growth is *M. flavescens.* This species therefore serves as an excellent quality control organism for this procedure.

*Pigment Production.* As previously discussed, mycobacteria may be categorized into three groups based on pigment production. Procedure 43-5, which can be found on the Evolve site, describes how to determine pigment production. To achieve optimum photochromogenicity, colonies should be young, actively metabolizing, isolated, and well aerated. Although some species (e.g., *M. kansasii*) turn yellow after a few hours of light exposure, others (e.g., *M. simiae*) may take prolonged exposure to light. Scotochromogens produce pigmented colonies even in the absence of light, and colonies often become darker with prolonged exposure to light (Figure 43-5). One member of this group, *M. szulgai,* is peculiar in that it is a scotochromogen at 35° C and nonpigmented when grown at 25° to 30° C. For this reason, all pigmented colonies should be subcultured to test for

photoactivated pigment at both 35° C and 25° to 30° C. Nonchromogens are not affected by light.

*Biochemical Testing.* Once categorized into a preliminary subgroup based on its growth characteristics, an organism must be definitively identified to species or complex level. Although conventional biochemical tests can be used for this purpose, new methods (discussed later in this section) have replaced biochemical tests for identifying mycobacterial species because of the previously discussed limitations of phenotypic testing. Although key biochemical tests are still discussed in this edition, the reader must be aware that this approach to identification ultimately will be replaced by molecular methods. Table 43-10 summarizes distinctive properties of the more commonly cultivable mycobacteria isolated from clinical specimens; key biochemical tests for each of the major mycobacterial groupings, including *M. tuberculosis* complex, are listed in Table 43-11. The following sections address key biochemical tests.

*Niacin.* Niacin (nicotinic acid) plays an important role in the oxidation-reduction reactions that occur during mycobacterial metabolism. Although all species produce

**TABLE 43-9** Controls and Media Used for Biochemical Identification of Mycobacteria

| Biochemical Test | CONTROL ORGANISMS | | RESULT | | | | |
| | Positive | Negative | Positive | Negative | Medium Used | Duration | Incubation Conditions |
|---|---|---|---|---|---|---|---|
| Niacin | *M. tuberculosis* | *M. intracellulare* | Yellow | No color change | 0.5 mL DH₂O | 15-30 min | Room temperature |
| Nitrate | *M. tuberculosis* | *M. intracellulare* | Pink or red | No color change | 0.3 mL DH₂O | 2 hours | 37°C bath |
| Urease | *M. fortuitum* | *M. avium* | Pink or red | No color change | Urea broth for AFB | 1, 3, and 5 days | 37°C incubator (without CO₂) |
| 68°C Catalase | *M. fortuitum* or *M. gordonae* | *M. tuberculosis* | Bubbles | No bubbles | 0.5 mL phosphate buffer (pH, 7.0) | 20 min | 68°C bath |
| SQ Catalase | *M. kansasii* or *M. gordonae* | *M. avium* | >45 mm | <45 mm | Commercial medium | 14 days | 37°C incubator (with CO₂) |
| Tween 80 | *M. kansasii* | *M. intracellulare* | Pink or red | No color change | 1 mL DH₂O | 5 or 10 days | 37°C incubator (in the dark, without CO₂) |
| Tellurite | *M. avium* | *M. tuberculosis* | Smooth, fine, black precipitate (smokelike action) | Gray clumps (no smokelike action) | Middlebrook 7H9 broth | 7, then 3 additional days | 37°C incubator (with CO₂) |
| Arylsulfatase | *M. fortuitum* | *M. intracellulare* | Pink or red | No color change | Wayne's arylsulfatase medium | 3 days | 37°C incubator (without CO₂) |
| 5% NaCl | *M. fortuitum* | *M. gordonae* | Substantial growth | Little or no growth | Commercial slant with and without 5% NaCl | 28 days | 37°C incubator (with CO₂) |
| TCH | *M. bovis* | *M. tuberculosis* | No growth (i.e., susceptible) | Growth (i.e., resistant or ≥1% of colonies are resistant) | TCH slant | 3 weeks | 37°C incubator (with CO₂) |

*AFB,* Acid-fast bacilli; *CO₂,* carbon dioxide; *DH₂O,* distilled water; *NaCl,* sodium chloride; *SQ,* semiquantitative; *TCH,* thiophene-2-carboxylic acid hydrazide.

nicotinic acid, *M. tuberculosis* accumulates the largest amount. (*M. simiae* and some strains of *M. chelonae* also produce niacin.) Niacin therefore accumulates in the medium in which these organisms are growing. A positive niacin test (see Procedure 43-6 on the Evolve site) is preliminary evidence that an organism that exhibits a buff-colored, slow-growing, rough colony may be *M. tuberculosis* (Figure 43-6). However, this test is not sufficient to confirm identification. If sufficient growth is present on an initial L-J slant (the egg-base medium enhances accumulation of free niacin), a niacin test can be performed immediately. If growth on the initial culture is scant, the subculture used for growth rate determination can be used. If this culture yields only rare colonies, the colonies should be spread around with a sterile cotton swab (after the growth rate has been determined) to distribute the inoculum over the entire slant.

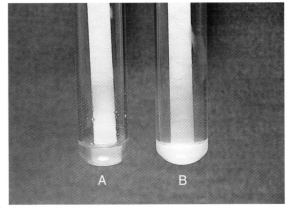

**Figure 43-6** Niacin test performed with filter paper strips. With a positive test result **(A),** the liquid turns yellow. With a negative result **(B),** the liquid remains milky white or clear.

**TABLE 43-10** Distinctive Properties of Commonly Cultivable Mycobacteria Encountered in Clinical Specimens

| Group/Complex | Species | Optimal Temp (°C) | Usual Colonial Morphology[a] | Niacin | Growth on TCH (10 mg/mL)[b] | Nitrate Reduction | Semi quantitative Catalase (>45 mm) | 68° C Catalase | Tween Hydrolysis, 5 Days | Tellurite Reduction | Tolerance to 5% NaCl | Arylsulfatase, 3 Days | Iron Uptake | Growth on MacConkey Agar | Urease | Pyrazinamidase, 4 Days |
|---|---|---|---|---|---|---|---|---|---|---|---|---|---|---|---|---|
| M. tuberculosis complex | M. tuberculosis | 37 | R | + | + | + | − | − | −[c] | ∓ | − | − | − | − | ± | + |
| | M. bovis | 37 | Rt | − | − | − | − | − | | ∓ | − | − | − | − | ± | − |
| | M. africanum | 37 | R | V | V | V | − | − | − | − | − | − | − | − | + | − |
| Photochromogens | M. marinum | 30 | S/SR | ∓ | + | − | − | − | + | ∓ | − | − | ∓[d] | − | −/+ | + |
| | M. kansasii | 35 | SR/S | − | + | + | + | + | + | ∓ | − | − | − | − | + | − |
| | M. simiae | 37 | S | ± | + | − | + | + | − | + | − | − | − | | ± | + |
| | M. asiaticum | 37 | S | − | + | − | + | + | + | − | − | − | − | | − | − |
| Scotochromogens | M. scrofulaceum | 37 | S | − | + | − | + | + | − | ∓ | − | − | V | − | V | ± |
| | M. szulgai | 37 | S or R | − | + | + | + | + | ∓[c] | ± | − | − | V | − | + | + |
| | M. gordonae | 37 | S | − | + | − | + | + | + | − | − | − | V | − | V | ± |
| Nonphotochromogens | M. avium complex | 35-37 | St/R | − | + | − | + | ± | − | + | − | − | − | ∓ | − | + |
| | M. genavense[e] | 37 | St | − | + | − | + | + | | | − | − | | | + | + |
| | M. gastri | 35 | S/SR/R | − | + | − | + | − | + | ∓ | − | − | − | − | ∓ | − |
| | M. malmoense | 30 | S | − | + | − | − | ± | + | + | − | − | − | | − | + |
| | M. haemophilum[f] | 30 | R | − | + | − | − | − | − | − | − | − | − | | − | + |
| | M. shimoidei | 37 | R | − | + | − | − | − | + | | | | − | | | + |
| | M. ulcerans | 30 | R | − | + | − | − | + | − | | | | − | | | − |
| | M. flavescens[g] | 37 | S | − | + | + | + | + | + | ∓ | + | − | − | − | + | + |
| | M. xenopi[h] | 42 | Sf | − | + | − | + | − | ∓ | − | − | ± | − | − | − | V |
| | M. terrae complex M. terrae M. triviale[i] M. nonchromogenicum | 35 | SR | − | − | + | + | + | + | − | − | − | − | V | − | V |
| Rapidly growing | M. fortuitum group | 28-30 | Sf/Rf | − | + | + | + | + | V | + | + | + | + | + | + | + |
| | M. chelonae | 28-30 | S/R | −/+ | + | − | + | V | V | + | − | − | + | + | + | + |
| | M. abscessus | 28-30 | S/R | − | | − | + | V | V | + | + | − | + | + | + | |
| | M. smegmatis | 28-30 | R/S | − | + | + | + | + | + | + | + | + | − | − | | |

Plus and minus signs indicate the presence or absence, respectively, of the feature; blank spaces indicate either that the information is not currently available or that the property is unimportant.

V, Variable; ±, usually present; ∓, usually absent.

See Versalovic J: *Manual of clinical microbiology*, ed 10, Washington, DC, 2011, ASM Press, for biochemical reactions of other mycobacterial species and for additional biochemical reactions on the mycobacteria included in this table.

[a]R, Rough; S, smooth; SR, intermediate in roughness; t, thin or transparent; f, filamentous extensions.

[b]TCH, Thiophene-2-carboxylic acid hydrazide.

[c]Tween hydrolysis may be positive at 10 days.

[d]Arylsulfatase, 14 days, is positive.

[e]Requires mycobactin for growth on solid media.

[f]Requires hemin as a growth factor.

[g]Young cultures may be nonchromogenic or have only pale pigment that may intensify with age.

[h]Strains of *M. xenopi* can be nonphotochromogenic or scotochromogenic.

[i]*M. triviale* is tolerant to 5% NaCl, and a rare isolate may grow on MacConkey agar.

**TABLE 43-11** Key Biochemical Reactions to Help Differentiate Organisms Belonging to the Same Mycobacterial Group

| Mycobacterial Group | Key Biochemical Tests |
|---|---|
| *M. tuberculosis* complex | Niacin, nitrate reduction; susceptibility to thiophene-2-carboxylic acid hydrazide (TCH) if *M. bovis* is suspected |
| Photochromogens | Tween 80 hydrolysis, nitrate reduction, pyrazinamidase, 14-day arylsulfatase, urease, niacin |
| Scotochromogens | Permissive growth temperature, Tween 80 hydrolysis, nitrate reduction, semiquantitative catalase, urease, 14-day arylsulfatase |
| Nonphotochromogens | Heat-resistant and semiquantitative catalase activity, nitrate reduction, Tween 80 hydrolysis, urease, 14-day arylsulfatase, tellurite reduction, acid phosphatase activity |
| Rapidly growing | Growth on MacConkey agar, nitrate reduction, Tween 80 hydrolysis, 3-day arylsulfatase, iron uptake |

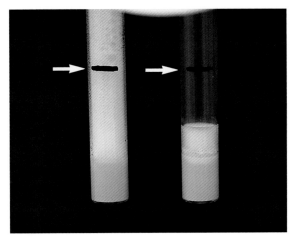

**Figure 43-7** Semiquantitative catalase test. The tube on the left contains a column of bubbles that has risen past the line (*arrow*), indicating 45-mm height (a positive test result). The tube on the right is the negative control.

The slant then is incubated until light growth over the surface of the medium is visible. For reliable results, the niacin test should be performed only from cultures on L-J medium that are at least 3 weeks old and show at least 50 colonies; otherwise, enough detectable niacin might not have been produced.

**Nitrate Reduction.** This test is valuable for identifying *M. tuberculosis, M. kansasii, M. szulgai,* and *M. fortuitum.* The ability of acid-fast bacilli to reduce nitrate is influenced by the age of the colonies, temperature, pH, and enzyme inhibitors. Although rapid-growers can be tested within 2 weeks, slow-growers should be tested after 3 to 4 weeks of luxuriant growth. Commercially available nitrate strips yield acceptable results only with strongly nitrate-positive organisms, such as *M. tuberculosis.* This test may be tried first because of its ease of performance. The *M. tuberculosis*–positive control must be strongly positive in the strip test, or the test results are unreliable. If the paper strip test is negative or if the control test result is not strongly positive, the chemical procedure (see Procedure 43-7 on the Evolve site) must be carried out using strong and weakly positive controls.

**Catalase.** Most species of mycobacteria, except for certain strains of *M. tuberculosis* complex (some isoniazid-resistant strains) and *M. gastri,* produce the intracellular enzyme catalase, which splits hydrogen peroxide into water and oxygen. Catalase can be assessed by using the semiquantitative catalase test or the heat-stable catalase test.

- The semiquantitative catalase test is based on the relative activity of the enzyme, as determined by the height of a column of bubbles of oxygen (Figure 43-7) formed by the action of untreated enzyme produced by the organism. Based on the

semiquantitative catalase test, mycobacteria are divided into two groups: those that produce less than 45 mm of bubbles and those that produce more than 45 mm of bubbles.

- The heat-stable catalase test is based on the ability of the catalase enzyme to remain active after heating (i.e., it is a measure of the enzyme's heat stability). When heated to 68° C for 20 minutes, the catalase of *M. tuberculosis, M. bovis, M. gastri,* and *M. haemophilum* becomes inactivated.

**Tween 80 Hydrolysis.** The commonly nonpathogenic, slow-growing scotochromogens and nonphotochromogens produce a lipase that can hydrolyze Tween 80 (the detergent polyoxyethylene sorbitan monooleate) into oleic acid and polyoxyethylated sorbitol, whereas pathogenic species do not. Tween 80 hydrolysis is useful for differentiating species of photochromogens, nonchromogens, and scotochromogens. Because laboratory-prepared media have a very short shelf life, the CDC recommends use of a commercial Tween 80 hydrolysis substrate (Becton-Dickinson, Franklin Lakes, N.J. or Remel Laboratories, Lenexa, Kansas) that is stable for up to 1 year.

**Tellurite Reduction.** Some species of mycobacteria reduce potassium tellurite at variable rates. The ability to reduce tellurite in 3 to 4 days distinguishes members of MAC from most other nonchromogenic species. All rapid-growers reduce tellurite in 3 days.

**Arylsulfatase.** The enzyme arylsulfatase is present in most mycobacteria. Test conditions can be varied to differentiate different forms of the enzyme. The rate at which this enzyme breaks down phenolphthalein disulfate into phenolphthalein (which forms a red color in the presence of sodium bicarbonate) and other salts helps to differentiate certain strains of mycobacteria. The 3-day test is particularly useful for identifying the potentially pathogenic rapid-growers *M. fortuitum* and *M. chelonae.* Slow-growing *M. marinum* and *M. szulgai* are positive in the 14-day test (Figure 43-8).

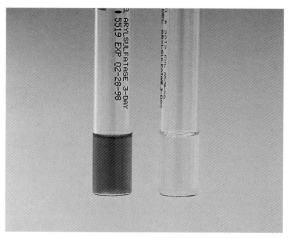

**Figure 43-8** A positive arylsulfatase test result is shown on the left; the tube containing the negative control is on the right.

***Growth Inhibition by Thiophene-2-Carboxylic Acid Hydrazide (TCH).*** This test is used to distinguish *M. bovis* from *M. tuberculosis*, because only *M. bovis* is unable to grow in the presence of 10 mg/mL of TCH.

***Other Tests.*** Other tests are often performed to make more subtle distinctions between species (see Table 43-11). However, performing all the procedures necessary for definitive identification of mycobacteria is not cost-effective for routine clinical microbiology laboratories; therefore, specimens that require further testing can be forwarded to regional laboratories.

# ANTIMICROBIAL SUSCEPTIBILITY TESTING AND THERAPY

Drug-resistant tuberculosis is a major health threat; more than 500,000 cases of multidrug-resistant (MDR) tuberculosis occur each year. Multidrug-resistant tuberculosis is resistant to rifampin and isoniazid, the two drugs most often used as effective treatment against tuberculosis. In addition, strains of extensively drug-resistant tuberculosis (XDR TB) are emerging that are resistant not only to rifampin and isoniazid, but also to quinolones and other drugs, such as aminoglycosides and capreomycin.

Standardized methods for susceptibility testing, including direct and indirect testing and new molecular tools, currently are available for susceptibility testing.

## M. TUBERCULOSIS COMPLEX

In vitro drug susceptibility testing should be performed on the first isolate of *M. tuberculosis* from all patients. Susceptibility testing of *M. tuberculosis* requires meticulous care in the preparation of the medium, selection of adequate samples of colonies, standardization of the inoculum, use of appropriate controls, and interpretation of results. Laboratories that see very few positive cultures should consider sending isolates to a reference laboratory for testing. Isolates must be saved in sterile 10% skim milk in distilled water at −70° C for possible future additional studies (e.g., susceptibilities if the patient does not respond well to treatment).

### Direct Versus Indirect Susceptibility Testing

Susceptibility tests may be performed by either the direct or indirect method. The direct method uses as the inoculum a smear-positive concentrate containing more than 50 acid-fast bacilli per 100 oil immersion fields; the indirect method uses a culture as the inoculum source. Although direct testing provides more rapid results, it is less standardized, and contamination may occur.

### Conventional Methods

The development of primary drug resistance in tuberculosis represents an increase in the proportion of resistant organisms. This increase in resistant organisms results from a spontaneous mutation and subsequent selection to predominance of these drug-resistant mutants by the action of a single or ineffective drug therapy. A poor clinical outcome is predicted with an agent when more than 1% of bacilli in the test population are resistant. If an isolate is reported as resistant to a drug, treatment failure is likely if this drug is used for therapy.

Drug resistance is defined for *M. tuberculosis* complex in terms of the critical concentration of the drug. The *critical concentration* of a drug is the amount of drug required to prevent growth above the 1% threshold of the test population of tubercle bacilli.

Four general methods are used throughout the world to determine the susceptibility of *M. tuberculosis* isolates to various antituberculous agents (Table 43-12). Initial isolates of *M. tuberculosis* are tested against five antimicrobials, which are referred to as prima*ry drugs* (Box 43-4.) If resistance to any of the primary drugs is detected, a second battery of agents is tested (Box 43-4).

### New Approaches

Several technologies recently introduced show promise of being faster, more reliable, and/or easier to perform

**TABLE 43-12** Overview of Conventional Methods to Determine Susceptibility of *M. tuberculosis* Isolates to Antimycobacterial Agents

| Method | Principle |
|---|---|
| Absolute concentration | For each drug tested, a standardized inoculum is inoculated to control (drug free) media and media containing several appropriately graded drug concentrations. Resistance is expressed as the lowest concentration of drug that inhibits all or almost all of the growth; that is, the minimum inhibitory concentration (MIC) |
| Resistance ratio | The resistance of the test organism is compared with that of a standard laboratory strain. The two strains are tested in parallel by inoculating a standard inoculum to media containing twofold serial dilutions of the drug. Resistance is expressed as the ratio of the MIC of the test strain divided by the MIC for the standard strain for each drug |
| Proportion | For each drug tested, several dilutions of standardized inoculum are inoculated onto control and drug-containing agar media. The extent of growth in the absence or presence of drug is compared and expressed as a percentage. If growth at the critical concentration of a drug is >1%, the isolate is considered clinically resistant. This is the standard method for all drugs except pyrazinamide. |
| Commercial systems approved for use by the FDA: BACTEC 460TB (Becton Dickinson, Sparks, Md.); BACTEC MGIT 960 (Becton Dickinson); VersaTREK (Trek Diagnostic Systems, Cleveland, Ohio); MB/BacT Alert 3D (bioMérieux, Durham, N.C.) | Using the principles of the agar proportion method, these methods use liquid media. Growth is indicated by the amount of $^{14}$C-labeled carbon dioxide ($CO_2$) released (as measured by the BACTEC 460 instrument) or the amount of fluorescence or gas produced (as measured by the MB/BacT Alert 3D and VersaTREK systems, respectively). For each drug tested, a standardized inoculum is inoculated into a drug-free and a drug-containing vial. The rate and amount of $CO_2$ produced in the absence or (with the BACTEC MGIT 960) presence of drug are then compared. The BACTEC 460TB is being replaced in many laboratories by the MGIT 960 to avoid hazardous waste disposal of radioactive materials, in addition to the cross-contamination that may occur with the 460TB. |
| Alternate methods and molecular methods | Several molecular methods have been developed that identify the mutations in the rifampin-resistant gene *(rpoB)*. Greater than 96% of rifampin resistance correlates to mutations in an 81 bp segment. Additional molecular methods have been developed for the identification of resistance to isoniazid, ethambutol, and pyrazinamide.<br>Molecular methods should be followed up with culture, especially for confirmation of second-line drug resistance and in XDR TB. |

*FDA,* U.S. Food and Drug Administration. *XDR TB,* extensively drug-resistant tuberculosis.

than most conventional methods of susceptibility testing. For example, mutations leading to rifampin resistance have been detected using molecular methods. One molecular method, the line probe assay (INNO-LiPA Rif TB; Innogenetics, Ghent, Belgium), is a commercially available, reverse hybridization–based probe assay for rapid detection of rifampin mutations leading to rifampin resistance in *M. tuberculosis*. Many different genotypic assays are currently available for drug susceptibility testing. Most are based on PCR amplification of a specific region of an *M. tuberculosis* gene, followed by analysis of the amplicon for specific mutations associated with resistance to a particular drug. The presence or absence of mutations can then be detected by several methods, such as automated sequencing.

As previously mentioned, high-density DNA probe assays (see Chapter 8) have been used to detect rifampin resistance and to identify mycobacterial species identification.

An innovative approach used by Jacobs et al.[3] to perform susceptibility testing involved the use of a luciferase-reporter mycobacteriophage (bacterial viruses). The basis for this assay is simple: viable mycobacteria can become infected with and replicate the mycobacteriophage; dead tubercle bacilli cannot. The mycobacteriophage was constructed to have the firefly luciferase gene next to a mycobacterial promoter; therefore, the presence and growth of the mycobacteriophage is detected by chemiluminescence. In brief, the isolate of *M. tuberculosis* to be tested is grown in the presence and absence of drug, and the specially constructed mycobacteriophage is added. After infection, luciferin, a substrate of luciferase, is added. If organisms are viable (i.e., thereby allowing infection of the bacteriophage and subsequent transcription and translation of the luciferase gene), the luciferin is broken down and light is emitted that can be measured; the amount of light emitted is directly proportional to the number of viable *M. tuberculosis* organisms. Therefore, if an organism is resistant to the drug, light is emitted; organisms susceptible to the drug do not emit light. Another commercially available assay that uses mycobacteriophages is the FAST Plaque TB–RIF test (Bio Tec Laboratories, Ipswich, UK).

Susceptibility testing should be repeated if the patient remains culture positive after 3 months following appropriate therapy or fails to respond clinically to therapy.

### Therapy

Therapy directed against *M. tuberculosis* depends on the susceptibility of the isolate to various antimicrobial agents. To prevent the selection of resistant mutants, treatment of tuberculosis requires four drugs: isoniazid, rifampin, ethambutol, and pyrazinamide. Initial therapy includes all four drugs for 8 weeks. However, if drug

**TABLE 43-13** CLSI Recommendations for Susceptibility Testing of Nontuberculous Mycobacteria

| Organism | Isolates to Be Tested | Recommended Method | Drugs to Be Tested |
|---|---|---|---|
| *M. avium* complex | • Clinically significant isolates from patients on previous macrolide therapy<br>• Isolates from patients who become bacteremic while on macrolide preventive therapy<br>• Isolates from patients who relapse while on macrolide therapy<br>• Initial isolates from blood or tissue of patients with disseminated disease or respiratory samples from patients with pulmonary disease<br>• Repeat testing after 3 months for patients with disseminated disease and after 6 months for patients with chronic pulmonary disease | Broth-based method; microdilution or BACTEC | Clarithromycin or azithromycin<br>Second line: Moxifloxacin or linezolid<br>Isolates typically are intrinsically resistant to isoniazid and pyrazinamide |
| *M. kansasii* | • All initial isolates<br>• Repeat testing if cultures remain positive after 3 months of appropriate therapy | Agar proportion<br>Broth based | Rifampin<br>If rifampin resistant, test rifabutin, ethambutol, isoniazid, linezolid, moxifloxacin, streptomycin, clarithromycin, amikacin, ciprofloxacin, and trimethoprim-sulfamethoxazole |
| *M. marinum* | Susceptibility testing not recommended; should be done only if patient fails to respond clinically after several months of therapy and remains culture positive | Agar proportion<br>Agar disk elution<br>Broth microdilution | Rifampin, ethambutol, clarithromycin, doxycycline, minocycline or trimethoprim-sulfamethoxazole |
| Rapidly growing mycobacteria | • Clinically significant isolates<br>• Isolates: M. fortuitum group, *M. chelonae, M. abscessus*<br>• Repeat testing if cultures remain positive after 6 months of appropriate therapy | Broth microdilution | Amikacin, cefoxitin, ciprofloxacin, clarithromycin, doxycycline, imipenem, linezolid, trimethoprim-sulfamethoxazole, tobramycin, moxifloxacin |

*CLSI,* Clinical and Laboratory Standards Institute.

susceptibility is determined for isoniazid, rifampin, and pyrazinamide, ethambutol may be discontinued. This is the preferred therapy for initial treatment, followed by isoniazid and rifampin for an additional 18 weeks. The most common two-drug regimen is isoniazid (INH, also known as isonicotinylhydrazine) and rifampin. The combination is administered for 9 months in cases of uncomplicated tuberculosis; if pyrazinamide is added to this regimen during the first 2 months, the total duration of therapy can be shortened to 6 months. Ethambutol may also be added to the regimen. INH prophylaxis is recommended for individuals with a recent skin test conversion who are disease free.

## NONTUBERCULOUS MYCOBACTERIA

In general, the treatment of patients infected with NTM requires more individualization of therapy than does the treatment of patients with tuberculosis. This individualization is based on the species of mycobacteria recovered, the site and severity of infection, antimicrobial drug susceptibility results, concurrent diseases, and the patient's general condition. Currently, sufficient data exist to allow general recommendations for susceptibility testing of MAC, *M. kansasii,* and *M. marinum.* Pulmonary infections with *M. avium* complex are often treated with clarithromycin, rifampin, and ethambutol (or streptomycin or amikacin for severe disease). If the infection is disseminated, clarithromycin, ethambutol, and rifabutin may be prescribed. Pulmonary infections with *M. kansasii* are treated with isoniazid, rifampin, and ethambutol. *M. marinum* skin and soft tissue infections may be treated with either clarithromycin and ethambutol, clarithromycin and rifampin, or rifampin and ethambutol.

Susceptibility testing should be performed on clinically significant, rapidly growing mycobacteria (Table 43-13). Skin and soft tissue infections, if susceptible, are treated with clarithromycin and at least one additional drug based on susceptibility testing. Pulmonary infections with *M. abscessus* should also be treated with a multidrug regimen that includes clarithromycin, if susceptible, and then additional drugs based on susceptibility testing.

## PREVENTION

As previously mentioned, prophylactic chemotherapy with INH is used when known or suspected primary tuberculous infection poses a risk of clinical disease. At present, the BCG vaccine is the only vaccine available against tuberculosis. The effectiveness of this live vaccine is controversial, because studies have demonstrated ineffectiveness to 80% protection. The greatest potential value for this vaccine is in developing countries with high prevalence rates for tuberculosis. At this time, at least four types of antituberculosis vaccines are currently being evaluated in experimental studies in animals.

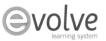

*Visit the Evolve site to complete the review questions.*

## CASE STUDY 43-1

A 40-year-old man who has tested positive for human immunodeficiency virus (HIV) infection and who is undergoing highly active antiretroviral therapy (HAART) presents with progressive encephalomyeloradiculopathy. He has severe headaches but no fever, cough, or weakness. Cerebrospinal fluid (CSF) is collected. The test results for the specimen are: 25 WBC/mm³ (25 white blood cells per cubic millimeter), low glucose, elevated protein, and no organisms on Gram stain or acid-fast stain. His studies are negative for cryptococcal antigen, *Toxoplasma* organisms (by serology), and herpes simplex virus (HSV) (by polymerase chain reaction [PCR]). Routine bacterial culture is negative. Despite therapy for HSV and routine aerobic bacterial causes of meningitis, over the next 4 days the patient spikes fevers. A second CSF specimen shows 415 WBC/mm³, with no diagnosis. A battery of viral encephalitis serology tests are done, and all are negative. In-house PCR testing on a third CSF specimen is positive for *Mycobacterium tuberculosis,* which grows in culture after 4 weeks.

### QUESTIONS

1. Why are the acid-fast smear results from all three of the specimens negative, but the second PCR result is positive?
2. How can *M. tuberculosis* be identified to the species level?
3. List the organisms present in the *Mycobacterium tuberculosis* complex.
4. Sometimes in processing for mycobacterial culture, an aerosol is created and one specimen splashes into another tube and contaminates it. If the physician states that the patient does not appear to have tuberculosis, how can the laboratory confirm that the positive culture does not represent contamination?

## ▤ BIBLIOGRAPHY

Badak FZ, Kiska DL, Setterquist S et al: Comparison of mycobacteria growth indicator tube with BACTEC 460 for detection and recovery of mycobacteria from clinical specimens, *J Clin Microbiol* 34:2236, 1996.

Banales JL, Pineda PR, Fitzgerald JM et al: Adenosine deaminase in the diagnosis of tuberculous pleural effusions: a report of 218 patients and review of the literature, *Chest* 99:355, 1991.

Brown-Elliott BA, Griffith DE, Wallace RJ: Newly described or emerging human species of nontuberculous mycobacteria, *Infect Dis Clin North Am* 16:187, 2002.

Brown-Elliott BA, Griffith DE, Wallace RJ: Diagnosis of nontuberculous mycobacterial infections, *Clin Lab Med* 22:911, 2002.

Colston MJ: The microbiology of *Mycobacterium leprae:* progress in the last 30 years, *Trans R Soc Trop Med Hyg* 87:508, 1993.

Greendyke R, Byrd TF: Differential antibiotic susceptibility of *Mycobacterium abscessus* variants in biofilms and macrophages compared to that of planktonic bacteria, *Antimicrob Agents Chemother* 52:2019, 2008.

Griffith DE, Girard WM, Wallace RJ: Clinical features of pulmonary disease caused by rapidly growing mycobacteria, *Am Rev Respir Dis* 147:1271, 1993.

Harries AD, Lawn SD, Getahun H, et al: HIV and tuberculosis–science and implementation to turn the tide and reduce deaths, *J Int AIDS Soc* 15(2):17396, 2012.

Havlik JA Jr, Metchock B, Thompson SE III et al: A prospective evaluation of *Mycobacterium avium* complex colonization of the respiratory and gastrointestinal tracts of persons with human immunodeficiency virus infection, *J Infect Dis* 168:1045, 1993.

Heifets L: Mycobacterial infections caused by nontuberculous mycobacteria, *Semin Respir Crit Care Med* 25:283, 2004.

Horsburgh C Jr, Metchock BG, McGowan JE Jr et al: Clinical implications of recovery of *Mycobacterium avium* complex from the stool or respiratory tract of HIV-infected individuals, *AIDS* 6:512, 1992.

Jacobs WR Jr, Barletta RG, Udani R et al: Rapid assessment of drug susceptibilities of *Mycobacterium tuberculosis* by means of luciferase reporter phages, *Science* 260:819, 1993.

Kent PT, Kubica GP: *Public health mycobacteriology: a guide for the level III laboratory,* US Department of Health and Human Services, Public Health Service, Atlanta, 1985, Centers for Disease Control and Prevention.

Lipsky BJ, Gates J, Tenover FC et al: Factors affecting the clinical value of microscopy for acid-fast bacilli, *Rev Infect Dis* 6:214, 1984.

Mazurek GH, Jereb J, LoBue P et al: Guidelines for using QuantiFERON-TB Gold Test for detecting *Mycobacterium tuberculosis* infection, *MMWR* 54:15, 2005.

Mijs W, de Haas P, Rossau R et al: Molecular evidence to support a proposal to reserve the designation *Mycobacterium avium* subsp. *avium* for bird-type isolates and *M. avium* subsp. *hominissuis* for the human/porcine type of *M. avium, Int J Syst Bacteriol* 52:1505, 2002.

Morris A, Reller LB, Salfinger M et al: Mycobacteria in stool specimens: the nonvalue of smears for predicting culture results, *J Clin Microbiol* 31:1385, 1993.

Moschella SL: An update on the diagnosis and treatment of leprosy, *J Am Acad Dermatol* 51:417, 2004.

O'Reilly LM, Daborn CJ: The epidemiology of *Mycobacterium bovis* infections in animals and man: a review, *Tubercle Lung Dis* 76(suppl 1):1, 1995.

Oxford Immunotec, Ltd: *T-spot TB, package insert. An aid in the diagnosis of toberculosis infection,* Oxfordshire, England, 2012.

Pfaller MF: Application of new technology to the detection, identification, and antimicrobial susceptibility testing of mycobacteria, *Am J Clin Pathol* 101:329, 1994.

Primm TP, Lucero CA, Falkinham JO: Health impacts of environmental mycobacteria, *Clin Microbiol Rev* 17: 98, 2004.

Runyon EH: Anonymous bacteria in pulmonary disease, *Med Clin North Am* 43:273, 1959.

Shinnick TM, Good RC: Mycobacterial taxonomy, *Eur J Clin Microbiol Infect Dis* 13:884, 1994.

Springer B, Tortoli E, Richter I et al: *Mycobacterium conspicuum* sp nov, a new species isolated from patients with disseminated infections, *J Clin Microbiol* 33:2805, 1995.

Steele JH, Ranney AF: Animal tuberculosis, *Am Rev Tuberculosis* 77:908, 1958.

Taylor Z, Nolan CM, Blumberg HM: Controlling tuberculosis in the United States: recommendations from the American Thoracic

Society, CDC, and the Infectious Diseases Society of America, *MMWR* 54:1, 2005.

Thibert L, Lapierre S: Routine application of high-performance liquid chromatography for identification of mycobacteria, *J Clin Microbiol* 31:1759, 1993.

Tortoli E: Impact of genotypic studies on mycobacterial taxonomy: the new mycobacteria of the 1990s, *Clin Microbiol Rev* 16:319, 2003.

Vernet G, Jay C, Rodrigue M et al: Species differentiation and antibiotic susceptibility testing with DNA microarrays, *J Appl Microbiol* 96:59, 2004.

Versalovic J: *Manual of Clinical Microbiology*, ed 10, Washington, DC, 2011, ASM Press.

Wallace RJ: Recent changes in taxonomy and disease manifestations of the rapidly growing mycobacteria, *Eur J Clin Microbiol Infect Dis* 13:953, 1994.

Wallace RJ et al: Diagnosis and treatment of disease caused by nontuberculous mycobacteria, *Am Rev Respir Dis* 142:940, 1990.

Wayne LG: The role of air in the photochromogenic behavior of *Mycobacterium kansasii*, *Am J Clin Pathol* 42:431, 1964.

Welch DF, Guruswamy AP, Sides SJ et al: Timely culture for mycobacteria which utilizes a microcolony method, *J Clin Microbiol* 31:2178, 1993.

Wolinsky E: Mycobacterial diseases other than tuberculosis, *Clin Infect Dis* 15:1, 1992.

Woods GL: Mycobacterial susceptibility testing and reporting: when, how, and what to test, *Clin Microbiol Newsl* 27:67, 2005.

Yajko DM, Nassos PS, Sanders CA et al: Comparison of four decontamination methods for recovery of *Mycobacterium avium* complex from stools, *J Clin Microbiol* 31:302, 1993.

# Obligate Intracellular and Nonculturable Bacterial Agents

## OBJECTIVES

1. Define the following: bubo, proctitis, bartholinitis, salpingitis, elementary body, reticulate body, Whipple's disease, morulae, and Donovan body.
2. Describe the general characteristics for the organisms included in this chapter including gram stain characteristics, cultivation methods (media and growth conditions), transmission and clinical significance.
3. Explain the mechanism and location for the replication of *Chlamydia* spp.
4. Compare the clinical manifestations and diagnosis of trachoma and other oculogenital infections associated with *Chlamydia* spp.
5. List the appropriate specimens used for the isolation of the organisms included in this chapter.
6. Describe the correct collection method for a specimen to be submitted for *C. trachomatis* screening from the female genital tract.
7. Explain the three stages associated with lymphogranuloma venereum, and compare the disease with other genital infections.
8. Describe the laboratory methods used for the diagnosis of *Chlamydia* infections, including sensitivity, limitations and appropriate use for culture, cytology, antigen (DFA), and nucleic acid testing (NAAT).
9. Compare hybridization and amplification nucleic acid–based testing for chlamydia.
10. Describe the triad of symptoms associated with *Rickettsia* spp.
11. Compare human monocytic ehrlichiosis (HME) and granulocytic anaplasmosis (HGA).
12. Distinguish and describe the three groups of *Rickettsia* based on mode of transmission, clinical manifestations, and intracellular growth characteristics.
13. Describe the Weil-Felix reaction, including chemical principle and limitations.
14. Describe the clinical significance for *Coxiella burnetii* phase I and phase II forms, including laboratory diagnosis.
15. Explain the limitations of the laboratory tests used to diagnose disease caused by the obligate intracellular and nonculturable bacteria.
16. Correlate signs, symptoms, and laboratory data for the identification of the organisms included in this chapter.

### GENERA AND SPECIES TO BE CONSIDERED

| Current Name | Previous Name |
| --- | --- |
| Chlamydia trachomatis | |
| Chlamydia psittaci | Chlamydophila psittaci |
| Chlamydia pneumoniae | Chlamydophila pneumoniae |
| Rickettsia rickettsii | |
| Rickettsia prowazekii | |
| Rickettsia typhi | |
| Orientia tsutsugamushi | |
| Ehrlichia chaffeensis | |

### GENERA AND SPECIES TO BE CONSIDERED—cont'd

| Current Name | Previous Name |
| --- | --- |
| Anaplasma phagocytophilum | Ehrlichia phagocytophila, Ehrlichia equi, and human granulocytic ehrlichiosis agent |
| Neorickettsia sennetsu | Ehrlichia sennetsu |
| Coxiella burnetii | |
| Tropheryma whipplei | T. whippelii |
| Klebsiella granulomatis | Calymmatobacterium granulomatis |

The organisms addressed in this chapter are obligate intracellular bacteria or are considered either extremely difficult to culture or unable to be cultured. Organisms of the genera *Chlamydia*, *Rickettsia*, *Orientia*, *Anaplasma*, and *Ehrlichia* are prokaryotes that differ from most other bacteria with respect to their very small size and obligate intracellular parasitism. Three other organisms, *Coxiella*, *Calymmatobacterium granulomatis*, and *Tropheryma whipplei*, are discussed in this chapter because they are also difficult to cultivate or are noncultivable.

## CHLAMYDIA

The *Chlamydia* spp. are members of the order Chlamydiales and the family Chlamydiaceae. The members of the family Chlamydiaceae had been regrouped in 1999 from one genus, *Chlamydia*, into two genera, *Chlamydia* and *Chlamydophila*, based on differences in phenotype, 16S rRNA, and 23S rRNA. This nomenclature change was controversial, however, and additional research led to the rejection of *Chlamydophila* as a separate genus in the family, thereby returning all species to the genus *Chlamydia*.

Members of the order Chlamydiales are obligate intracellular bacteria that were once regarded as viruses because, like viruses, the chlamydiae require the biochemical resources of the eukaryotic host cell to fuel their metabolism for growth and replication by providing high-energy compounds such as adenosine triphosphate. *Chlamydia* spp. are similar to the gram-negative bacilli in that they have lipopolysaccharide (LPS) as a component of the cell wall. The chlamydial LPS, however, has little endotoxic activity. The chlamydiae have a major outer membrane protein (MOMP) that is very diverse. The variation in MOMP in *C. trachomatis* is used to separate the species into 18 distinct serovars, yet highly conserved in *C. pneumoniae*.

Chlamydiae have a unique developmental life cycle reminiscent of parasites, with an intracellular, replicative form, the reticulate body (RB), and an extracellular, metabolically inert, infective form, the elementary body (EB). The EB cannot survive outside of a host cell for an extended period. Following infection of a host cell, the EB differentiates into a RB. The RB divides by binary fission within vacuoles. As the numbers of RB increase, the vacuole expands forming an intracytoplasmic inclusion. The RB then revert to EB, and 48 to 72 hours postinfection, the EB are released from the host cell (Figure 44-1). In addition to the replicative cycle associated with acute chlamydial infections, there is evidence that *Chlamydia* can persist in an aberrant form in vitro depending on the amount of interferon-gamma (IFN-γ) and tryptophan in the host cell as well as the function of the tryptophan synthase encoded by the organism. Removal of the IFN-γ or increase in tryptophan will result in the differentiation of the chlamydiae into an active EB infection. The therapeutic implications of this persistence in vivo has not yet been completely defined; however, evidence suggests that the activity of the tryptophan synthase gene in *C. trachomatis* differs between isolates recovered from the eye versus the genital tract.

*C. trachomatis*, *C. pneumoniae*, and *C. psittaci* are important causes of human infection; *C. psittaci* and *C. pecorum* are common pathogens among animals. The three species that infect humans differ with respect to their antigens, host cell preference, antibiotic susceptibility, EB morphology, and inclusion morphology (Table 44-1).

## CHLAMYDIA TRACHOMATIS

Over the past few decades, the importance of both acute and chronic infections caused by *Chlamydia trachomatis* has been recognized. Not only are *C. trachomatis* infections associated with infertility and ectopic pregnancy,

**TABLE 44-1** Differential Characteristics among Chlamydiae That Cause Human Disease

| Property | *C. trachomatis* | *C. psittaci* | *C. pneumoniae* |
|---|---|---|---|
| Host range | Humans (except one biovar that causes mouse pneumonitis) | Birds, lower mammals, humans (rare) | Humans |
| Elementary body morphology | Round | Round | Pear-shaped |
| Inclusion morphology | Round, vacuolar | Variable, dense | Round, dense |
| Glycogen-containing inclusions | Yes | No | No |
| Plasmid DNA | Yes | Yes | No |
| Susceptibility to sulfonamides | Yes | No | No |

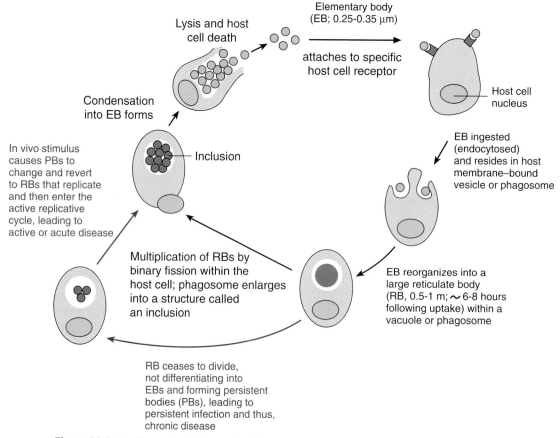

**Figure 44-1** The life cycle of chlamydiae. The entire cycle takes approximately 48 to 72 hours.

**TABLE 44-2** Primary Syndromes Caused by *C. trachomatis*

| Serovars | Clinical Syndrome | Route(s) of Transmission |
|---|---|---|
| A, B, Ba, C | Endemic trachoma (multiple or persistent infections that ultimately lead to blindness) | Hand to eye from fomites, flies |
| L1, L2, L2a, L3 | Lymphogranuloma venereum | Sexual |
| D-K | Urethritis, cervicitis, pelvic inflammatory disease, epididymitis, infant pneumonia, and conjunctivitis (does not lead to blindness) | Sexual, hand to eye by autoinoculation of genital secretions; eye to eye by infected secretions; neonatal |

but oftentimes *C. trachomatis* infections are asymptomatic, resulting in inadvertent transmission and high prevalence rates.

## General Characteristics

*C. trachomatis* infects humans almost exclusively and is responsible for various clinical syndromes. Based on MOMP antigenic differences, *C. trachomatis* is divided into 18 different serovars that are associated with different primary clinical syndromes (Table 44-2).

## Epidemiology and Pathogenesis

*C. trachomatis* causes significant infection and disease worldwide. In the United States, *C. trachomatis* is the most common sexually transmitted bacterial pathogen and a major cause of pelvic inflammatory disease (PID), ectopic pregnancy, and infertility (see Chapter 74 for more information on PID). An estimated 3 million cases of *C. trachomatis* infection occur annually in the United States. In 2010, more than 1.3 million cases of *C. trachomatis* infection were reported to the Centers for Disease Control and Prevention (CDC), corresponding to a rate of infection of 426 per 100,000 population and a 5.1% increase over the cases reported in 2009. In fact, of all the organisms causing sexually transmitted disease reported to the CDC, only *C. trachomatis* cases have increased every year. Genital tract infections caused by *C. trachomatis* were identified most frequently in women between the ages of 15 and 24 years. It is important to note, however, that data reported to the CDC, especially with regards to *Chlamydia*, come as a result of screening programs that primarily target women between the ages of 15 and 24 years.

Ocular trachoma, on the other hand, is a much more prevalent disease, affecting 84 million individuals worldwide, with 7 to 9 million infections resulting in blindness. Remote rural areas of Africa, Asia, Central and South America, Australia, and the Middle East are hyperendemic for trachoma, where the prevalence rate of *C. trachomatis* is 60% to 90% in preschool children. Trachoma is the cause for 3% of the cases of blindness in individuals around the world, with adult women more likely to be affected as a result of their exposure to children who serve as the major reservoir of the organism.

*C. trachomatis* infections are primarily transmitted from human to human by direct contact with infected secretions. Some infections, such as neonatal pneumonia or inclusion conjunctivitis, are transmitted from mother to infant during birth. The various routes of transmission for *C. trachomatis* infection are summarized in Table 44-2.

The natural habitat of *C. trachomatis* is humans. The mechanisms by which *C. trachomatis* cause inflammation and tissue destruction are not completely understood. The chlamydiae can infect a variety of different cells, including epithelial cells of the mucosa as well as blood vessels, smooth muscle cells, and monocytes. The chlamydial EB is phagocytosed into a host cell and resides in a vacuole that fails to fuse with a lysosome, leading to the intracellular persistence of the organism and escape from the host immune response. Chlamydiae are able to either turn on or turn off apoptosis (programmed cell death pathways) in infected host cells. By inducing host cell death, the organism facilitates its transmission to neighboring host cells and down-regulating inflammation in the acute disease process, whereas, by inhibiting apoptosis, the organism keeps the host cell alive, allowing for sustained survival in chronic infections.

The host's immune response accounts for the majority of the tissue destruction following infection with *C. trachomatis*. Infected epithelial cells secrete pro-inflammatory cytokines including Interleukin-1α (IL-1α), tumor necrosis factor (TNF) and IL-6. Quickly upon infection, neutrophils and monocytes migrate to the mucosa and eliminate exposed EB. Later CD4 T helper cells migrate to the site of infection. Responding neutrophils and T helper cells release cytokines, resulting in the influx of additional immune cells. The importance of multiple, recurrent infection with *C. trachomatis* is associated with the development of ocular trachoma. Immunity provides little protection from reinfection and appears to be short lived following infection with *C. trachomatis*.

## Spectrum of Disease

As previously mentioned, infection with different *C. trachomatis* serovars can lead to several clinical syndromes. These infections are summarized in Table 44-2.

**Trachoma.** Trachoma is manifested by a chronic inflammation of the conjunctiva and remains a major cause of preventable blindness worldwide. The organism is acquired as a result of contact with infected secretions on towels or fingers or by flies. Early symptoms of infection include mild irritation and itching of the eyes and eyelids. There may also be some discharge from the infected eye. The infection progresses slowly with increasing eye pain, blurred vision, and photophobia. Repeated infections result in scarring of the inner eyelid that may then turn the eyelid in toward the eye (entropion). As the inner eyelid continues to turn in, the eyelashes follow (trichiasis), resulting in rubbing and scratching of the cornea. The combined effects of the mechanical damage to the cornea and inflammation result in ulceration, scarring, and loss of vision.

**Lymphogranuloma Venereum.** Lymphogranuloma venereum (LGV) is a sexually transmitted disease rarely identified in North America but relatively frequent in Africa, Asia, and South America. It is reemerging in Europe, especially in homosexual males. *C. trachomatis* serovars L1, L2, L2b, and L3 are invasive causing LGV, in contrast to *C. trachomatis* serovars A-K, leaving the mucosa to spread to the regional lymph nodes. The disease is characterized by a brief appearance of a primary genital lesion at the initial infection site. This lesion is often small and may be unrecognized, especially by female patients. The second stage, acute lymphadenitis, often involves the inguinal lymph nodes, causing them to enlarge and become matted together, forming a large area of groin swelling, or bubo. During this stage, infection may become systemic and cause fever or may spread locally, causing granulomatous proctitis. In a few patients (more women than men), the disease progresses to a chronic third stage, causing the development of genital hyperplasia, rectal fistulas, rectal stricture, draining sinuses, and other manifestations.

**Oculogenital Infections.** *C. trachomatis* can cause acute inclusion conjunctivitis in adults and newborns. The organism is acquired when contaminated genital secretions get into the eyes via fingers or during passage of the neonate through the birth canal. Autoinfection rarely occurs. The organism can also be acquired from swimming pools, poorly chlorinated hot tubs, or by sharing eye makeup. Inclusion conjunctivitis is associated with swollen eyes and a purulent discharge. In contrast to trachoma, inclusion conjunctivitis does not lead to blindness in adults (or newborns).

Genital tract infections caused by *C. trachomatis* have surpassed gonococcal (*Neisseria gonorrhoeae*) infections as a cause of sexually transmitted disease in the United States. Similar to gonococci, *C. trachomatis* causes urethritis, cervicitis, bartholinitis (Bartholin glands or greater vestibular glands), proctitis, salpingitis (infection of the fallopian tubes), epididymitis, and acute urethral syndrome in women. In the United States, 60% of cases of nongonococcal urethritis are caused by chlamydiae. Both chlamydiae and gonococci are major causes of PID, contributing significantly to the rising rate of infertility and ectopic pregnancies in young women. Following a single episode of PID, as many as 10% of women may become infertile because of tubal occlusion. The risk increases dramatically with each additional episode.

Many genital chlamydial infections in both sexes are asymptomatic or not easily recognized by clinical criteria; asymptomatic carriage in both men and women may persist, often for months. As many as 50% of men and 70% to 80% of women identified as having chlamydial genital tract infections have no symptoms. Of significance, these asymptomatic infected individuals serve as a large reservoir to sustain transmission of the organism within a community.

When symptomatic, patients with a genital chlamydial infection will have an unusual discharge and pain or a burning sensation, symptoms similar to those for gonorrhea.

### Perinatal Infections

Approximately one fourth to half of infants born to women infected with *C. trachomatis* develop inclusion conjunctivitis. Usually, the incubation period is 5 to 12 days from birth, but it may be as long as 6 weeks. Although most develop inclusion conjunctivitis, about 10% to 20% of infants develop pneumonia. Perinatal acquired *C. trachomatis* infection may persist in the nasopharynx, urogenital tract, or rectum for more than 2 years.

### Laboratory Diagnosis

*C. trachomatis* can be diagnosed by cytology, culture, direct detection of antigen or nucleic acid, and serologic testing.

**Specimen Collection and Transport.** The organism can be recovered from or detected in infected cells of the urethra, cervix, conjunctiva, nasopharynx, rectum, and material aspirated from the fallopian tubes and epididymis. The endocervix is the preferred anatomic site to collect screening specimens from women. The specimen for *C. trachomatis* culture should be obtained following collection of all other specimens (e.g., those for Gram-stained smear, *Neisseria gonorrhoeae* culture, or Papanicolaou [Pap] smear). A large swab should first be used to remove all secretions from the cervix. The appropriate swab (for nonculture tests, use the swab supplied or specified by the manufacturer) or endocervical brush is inserted 1 to 2 cm into the endocervical canal, rotated against the wall for 10 to 30 seconds, withdrawn without touching any vaginal surfaces, and then placed in the appropriate transport medium or applied to a slide prepared for direct fluorescent antibody (DFA) testing.

Urethral specimens should not be collected until 2 hours after the patient has voided. A urogenital swab (or one provided or specified by the manufacturer) is gently inserted into the urethra (females, 1 to 2 cm; males, 2 to 4 cm), rotated at least once for 5 seconds, and then withdrawn. Again, swabs should be placed into the appropriate transport medium or onto a slide prepared for DFA testing. Screening of rectal or pharyngeal specimens for *C. trachomatis* by nucleic acid tests has proven useful in homosexual male patients. Urine specimens in appropriate transport media provided by manufacturers of nucleic acid testing methodologies are also available for both men and women. Because chlamydiae are relatively labile, viability can be maintained by keeping specimens cold and minimizing transport time to the laboratory. For successful culture, specimens should be submitted in a chlamydial transport medium such as 2SP (0.2 M sucrose-phosphate transport medium with antibiotics); a number of commercial transport media are available. Specimens should be refrigerated upon receipt, and if they cannot be processed for culture within 24 hours, they should be frozen at −70° C.

**Cultivation.** Cultivation of *C. trachomatis* is discussed before methods for direct detection and serodiagnosis because all nonculture methods for the diagnosis of *C. trachomatis* are compared with culture. Culture is being performed less often, however, with nucleic acid amplification tests (NAAT) being used almost exclusively for genital tract infections. For example, in a survey taken in 2007 of public health laboratories, 89.7% of tests for *Chlamydia* were NAAT.

Several different cell lines have been used to isolate *C. trachomatis* in cell culture, including McCoy, HeLa, and monkey kidney cells; cycloheximide-treated McCoy cells are commonly used. After shaking the clinical specimens with 5-mm glass beads, centrifugation of the specimen onto the cell monolayer (usually growing on a coverslip in the bottom of a vial, commonly called a "shell vial") presumably facilitates adherence of elementary bodies. After 48 to 72 hours of incubation, monolayers are stained with a fluorescein-labeled monoclonal antibody that is either species specific, targeting the MOMP of *C. trachomatis*, or genus specific, targeting the LPS. The monolayers are examined microscopically for inclusion. Use of iodine to detect inclusions is less specific and not recommended.

Although its specificity approaches 100%, the sensitivity of culture has been estimated at between 70% and 90% in experienced laboratories. Limitations of *Chlamydia* culture contributing to the lack of sensitivity include prerequisites to maintain viability of patient specimens by either rapid or frozen transport and to ensure the quality of the specimen submitted for testing (i.e., endocervical specimens devoid of mucus and containing endocervical epithelial or metaplastic cells or urethral epithelial cells). In addition, successful culture requires a sensitive cell culture system and a minimum of at least 2 days turnaround time between specimen receipt and the availability of results. Despite these limitations, culture is still recommended as the test of choice in some situations (Table 44-3). As of this writing, only chlamydia cultures should be used in situations with legal implications (e.g., sexual abuse) when the possibility of a false-positive test is unacceptable. Local and state requirements may vary.

### Direct Detection Methods

***Cytologic Examination.*** Cytologic examination of cell scrapings from the conjunctiva of newborns or persons with ocular trachoma can be used to detect *C. trachomatis* inclusions, usually after Giemsa staining. Cytology has also been used to evaluate endocervical and urethral scrapings, including those obtained for Pap smears. However, this method is insensitive compared with culture or other methods discussed in the following sections.

***Antigen Detection and Nucleic Acid Hybridization.*** To circumvent the shortcomings of cell culture, antigen detection methods are commercially available.

Direct fluorescent antibody (DFA) staining methods use fluorescein-isothiocyanate conjugated monoclonal antibodies to either MOMP or LPS of *C. trachomatis* to detect elementary bodies in smears of clinical material (Figure 44-2). The sensitivity and specificity of DFA are similar to those of culture. Chlamydial antigen can also be detected by enzyme immunoassays (EIA). Numerous U.S. Food and Drug Administration (FDA)-approved kits are commercially available. These assays use polyclonal or monoclonal antibodies that detect chlamydial LPS. These tests are not species-specific for *C. trachomatis* and may cross-react with LPS of other bacterial species present in the vagina or urinary tract and thereby produce a false-positive result.

Nucleic acid hybridization tests for *Chlamydia* were first available for the clinical microbiology laboratory in the late 1980s. Two hybridization tests are currently available, Gen-Probe PACE 2C (Hologic-Gen-Probe, San Diego, California) and Digene Hybrid Capture II assay (Digene, Silver Spring, Maryland). The Gen-Probe PACE

**TABLE 44-3** Use of Different Laboratory Tests to Diagnose *C. trachomatis* Infections

| Patient Population | Specimen Type | Acceptable Diagnostic Test |
|---|---|---|
| Prepubertal girls | Vaginal | Culture (if culture is unavailable, certain specialists accept NAAT) |
| Neonates and infants | Nasopharyngeal | Culture, DFA |
| | Rectal | Culture |
| | Conjunctiva | Culture, DFA, EIA, NAAT |
| Women | Cervical | NAAT*, culture, DFA, EIA, NAH, NAAT |
| | Vaginal | NAAT* |
| | Urethral | NAAT, culture, DFA, EIA, NAH |
| | Urine | NAAT* |
| Children, women and men | Rectal | Culture, DFA, NAAT* |
| Men | Urethral | NAAT* (DFA, EIA, NAH recommended when NAAT is unavailable) |
| | Urine† | NAAT* |

*Must be confirmed in a population with a low prevalence (<5%) of *C. trachomatis* infection.
†EIA can be used on urine from symptomatic men but not on urine from older men. Also, a positive result must be confirmed in a population with a low prevalence of *C. trachomatis* infection.
DFA, direct fluorescent antibody staining; EIA, enzyme immunoassay; NAH, nucleic acid hybridization; NAAT, nucleic acid amplification test.
Modified from Centers for Disease Control and Prevention: Recommendations for the prevention and management of *Chlamydia trachomatis* infections, *MMWR* 42(RR-12):1-39, 1993; Centers for Disease Control and Prevention: Screening tests to detect *Chlamydia trachomatis* and *Neisseria gonorrhoeae* infections, *MMWR* 51(RR-15):1-27, 2002; Centers for Disease Control and Prevention: Sexually transmitted diseases treatment guidelines, 2010, *MMWR* 59(RR-12):1, 2010.

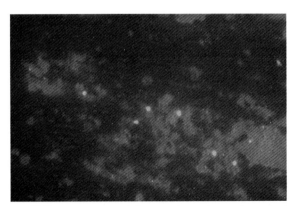

**Figure 44-2** Appearance of fluorescein-conjugated, monoclonal antibody–stained elementary bodies in direct smear of urethral cell scraping from a patient with chlamydial urethritis. (Courtesy Syva Co, San Jose, California)

2C assay uses a chemiluminescent-labeled DNA probe complementary to a sequence of ribosomal RNA (rRNA) in the chlamydial genome. If chlamydial rRNA is present in the sample, the labeled DNA probe will bind. In a unique hybridization protection assay, only bound label is detected by measuring chemiluminescence in a luminometer. The Digene Hybrid Capture II assay uses an RNA probe to detect chlamydial DNA in a sample. The DNA/RNA hybrids are captured using monoclonal antibodies imbedded on the side of the well that recognize the unique structure produced by the DNA/RNA hybrid. A second enzyme labeled anti-DNA/RNA hybrid antibody binds to captured hybrids, and enzyme activity is measured by chemiluminescence. Both assays are species specific for *C. trachomatis*.

Based on numerous studies, these nonculture tests are more reliable for the detection of infection in patients who are symptomatic and shedding large numbers of organisms than in those who are asymptomatic and most likely shedding fewer organisms. For the most part, these assays have sensitivities of greater than 70% and specificities of 97% to 99% in populations with a prevalence of *C. trachomatis* infection of 5% or more. In a low-prevalence population—that is, less than 5%—a significant proportion of positive tests will be falsely positive. Therefore, a positive result in a low-prevalence population should be handled with care, and a positive result should be verified. Positive results can be validated by the following methods:

- Culture
- Performing a second nonculture test that identifies a *C. trachomatis* antigen or nucleic acid sequence that is different from that used in the screening test
- Using a blocking antibody or competitive probe that verifies a positive test result by preventing attachment of a labeled antibody or probe used in the standard assay

***Nucleic Acid Amplification Tests.*** FDA-approved nucleic acid amplification tests (NAATs) for the laboratory diagnosis of *C. trachomatis* infection use three different formats: polymerase chain reaction (PCR), strand displacement amplification (SDA), and transcription-mediated amplification (TMA). The first two assay formats amplify DNA sequences present in the cryptic plasmid that is present in 7 to 10 copies in the chlamydial EB, whereas the last format amplifies 23S ribosomal RNA sequences. Studies clearly indicate that NAATs are more sensitive than culture and other non-nucleic acid amplification assays. Because of the increased sensitivity of detection, first-voided urine specimens from symptomatic and asymptomatic men and women are acceptable specimens to detect *C. trachomatis*, thereby affording a noninvasive means of chlamydia testing. NAATs are the preferred methodology for detecting *C. trachomatis* in most clinical situations because of increased sensitivity, ease of specimen collection, and the availability of automated high volume methods. Table 44-3 summarizes the possible uses of the different methodologies available for the detection of *C. trachomatis*; however, NAATs are used almost exclusively for the laboratory detection of *C. trachomatis*.

**Serodiagnosis.** Serologic testing has limited value for diagnosis of urogenital infections in adults. Most adults with chlamydial infection have had a previous exposure to *C. trachomatis* and are therefore seropositive. Serology can be used to diagnose LGV. Antibodies to a genus-specific antigen can be detected by complement fixation (CF), and a single-point titer greater than 1:64 is indicative of LGV. This test is not useful in diagnosing trachoma, inclusion conjunctivitis, or neonatal infections. The microimmunofluorescence assay (micro-IF), a tedious and difficult test, is used for type-specific antibodies of *C. trachomatis* and can also be used to diagnose LGV. A high titer of IgM (1:32) suggests a recent infection; however, not all patients produce IgM. In contrast to CF, micro-IF may be used to diagnose trachoma and inclusion conjunctivitis using acute and convalescent phase sera. Detection of *C. trachomatis*–specific IgM is useful in the diagnosis of neonatal infections. Negative serology can reliably exclude chlamydial infection.

### Antibiotic Susceptibility Testing and Therapy

Because *C. trachomatis* is an obligate intracellular bacterium, susceptibility testing is not practical in the routine clinical microbiology laboratory setting and is performed in only a few laboratories. In addition no standardized in vitro assay or an understanding of the relationship between in vitro test results and clinical outcome following treatment exist. Antibiotics typically used in infections with *C. trachomatis* include erythromycin and other macrolide antibiotics, tetracyclines, and fluoroquinolones.

### Prevention

Because no effective vaccines are available, strategies to prevent chlamydial urogenital infections focus on trying to manifest behavioral changes. By identifying and treating persons with genital chlamydia before infection is transmitted to sexual partners or from pregnant women to babies, the risk of acquiring or transmitting infection may be significantly decreased.

## CHLAMYDIA PSITTACI

Although members of this chlamydial species are common in birds and domestic animals, infections in humans are relatively uncommon.

### General Characteristics

*C. psittaci* differs from *C. trachomatis* in that it is sulfonamide resistant and in the morphology of its EB and inclusion bodies (see Table 44-1).

### Epidemiology and Pathogenesis

*C. psittaci* is an endemic pathogen of all bird species. Psittacine birds (e.g., parrots, parakeets) are a major reservoir for human disease, but outbreaks have occurred among turkey-processing workers and pigeon aficionados. The birds may show diarrheal illness or may be asymptomatic. Humans acquire the disease by inhalation of aerosols. The organisms are deposited in the alveoli; some are ingested by alveolar macrophages and then carried to regional lymph nodes. From there they are disseminated systemically, growing within cells of the reticuloendothelial system. Human-to-human transmission is rare, thus obviating the need for isolating patients if admitted to the hospital.

## Spectrum of Disease

Disease usually begins after an incubation period of 5 to 15 days. Onset may be insidious or abrupt. Clinical findings associated with this infection are diverse and include pneumonia, severe headache, mental status changes, and hepatosplenomegaly. The severity of infection ranges from unapparent or mild disease to a life-threatening systemic illness with significant respiratory problems.

## Laboratory Diagnosis

Diagnosis of psittacosis is almost always by serologic means. Because of hazards associated with working with the agent, only laboratories with Biosafety Level 3 biohazard containment facilities can culture *C. psittaci* safely. State health departments take an active role in consulting with clinicians about possible cases. Complement fixation and indirect microimmunofluorescence have been used to detect anti–*C. psittaci* antibodies in patients with suspected psittacosis infections. Either a fourfold rise in titer between acute and convalescent serum samples or a single IgM titer of 1:32 or greater in a patient with an appropriate illness is considered diagnostic of an infection.

Finally, amplification of rDNA sequences using a PCR assay followed by restriction fragment length polymorphism (RFLP) analysis was able to identify and distinguish all nine chlamydial species, including *C. psittaci*.

## Antibiotic Susceptibility Testing and Therapy

Because *C. psittaci* is an obligate intracellular pathogen and its incidence of infection is rare, susceptibility testing is not practical in the routine clinical microbiology laboratory. Tetracycline is the drug of choice for psittacosis. If left untreated, the fatality rate is about 20%.

## Prevention

Disease is prevented by treating infected birds or by quarantining imported birds for a month.

# CHLAMYDIA PNEUMONIAE

The TWAR strain of *C. pneumoniae* was first isolated from the conjunctiva of a child in Taiwan in 1965. It was initially considered to be a psittacosis strain, because the inclusions produced in cell culture resembled those of *C. psittaci*. The Taiwan isolate (TW-183) is serologically related to a pharyngeal isolate (AR-39) isolated from a college student in the United States, and thus the new strain was called "TWAR," an acronym for TW and AR (acute respiratory). Only one serotype of *C. pneumoniae* has been identified.

## General Characteristics

*C. pneumoniae* is considered more homogeneous than either *C. trachomatis* or *C. psittaci*, because all isolates tested are immunologically similar because of the homogeneity of the MOMP. One significant difference between *C. pneumoniae* and the other chlamydiae is the pear-shaped appearance of its EB (Figure 44-3).

## Epidemiology and Pathogenesis

*C. pneumoniae* appears to solely be a human pathogen; no bird or animal reservoirs have been identified. It is transmitted from person to person by aerosolized droplets via the respiratory route. The spread of infection is low. Antibody prevalence to *C. pneumoniae* starts to rise in school-aged children and reaches 30% to 45% in

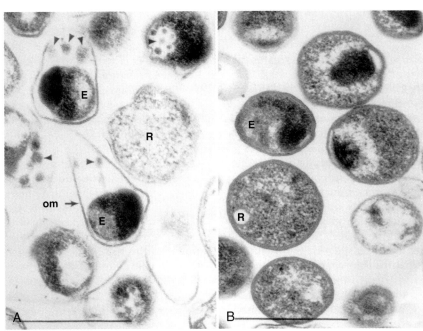

**Figure 44-3** Electron micrograph of *C. pneumoniae* (**A**) and *C. trachomatis* (**B**) (bar = 50.5 μm). *E*, Elementary body; *om*, outer membrane; *R*, reticulate body; arrowhead, small electron-dense bodies of undetermined function. (From Grayston JT, Kuo C-C, Campbell LA, and Wang S-P: *Chlamydia pneumonia* sp. nov. for *Chlamydia* sp. Strain TWAR. *Int J Syst Bacteriol* 39:88, 1989.)

adolescents; more than half of adults in the United States and in other countries have *C. pneumoniae* antibody. Of interest, *C. pneumoniae* infections are both endemic and epidemic. Unfortunately, little is known about the pathogenesis of *C. pneumoniae* infections, but it is similar to *C. trachomatis* in inducing inflammation that contributes to tissue damage.

### Spectrum of Disease

*C. pneumoniae* has been associated with pneumonia, bronchitis, pharyngitis, sinusitis, and a flulike illness. It causes 5% to 10% of cases of community-acquired pneumonia. Infection in young adults is usually mild to moderate; the microbiologic differential diagnosis primarily includes *Mycoplasma pneumoniae*. Severe pneumonia may occur in older or respiratory-compromised patients. Of note, asymptomatic infection or unrecognized, mildly symptomatic illnesses caused by *C. pneumoniae* are common. In addition, an association exists between *C. pneumoniae* infection and the development of asthmatic symptoms. Finally, an association between coronary artery disease and other atherosclerotic syndromes and *C. pneumoniae* infection has been suggested by seroepidemiologic studies and the demonstration of the organism in atheromatous plaques (yellow deposits within arteries containing cholesterol and other lipid material). Such an etiologic role by this organism is still under intense scrutiny. An excellent and comprehensive review of the literature related to whether *C. pneumoniae* is a cause of atherosclerosis was published in 2008 by Watson and Alp. Their research indicated that "it is difficult to attribute causality to a common infectious agent in a highly prevalent multifactorial disease." They also stated that "*C. pneumoniae* is neither alone sufficient nor is it necessary to cause atherosclerosis or its clinical consequences in humans," but they allowed for the possibility that treatment of *C. pneumoniae* may reduce the risk of atherosclerosis development.

### Laboratory Diagnosis

In the laboratory, *C. pneumoniae* infections are diagnosed by cell culture, serology, or NAATs.

**Direct Detection Methods.** To date, assays to directly detect *C. pneumoniae* antigens have poor sensitivity. A variety of NAAT, including conventional and real-time PCR assays, have been developed to detect *C. pneumoniae* nucleic acid sequences in clinical specimens. Several of these amplification assays are commercially available. Using these methods, the organism has been detected in throat swabs and other specimens, such as nasopharyngeal, bronchoalveolar lavage fluids, and sputum.

**Cultivation.** Specimens for isolation are usually swabs of the oropharynx; techniques for isolation of the organism from sputum are unsatisfactory. Swabs should be placed into chlamydial transport media, transported on ice, and stored at 4° C; organisms are rapidly inactivated at room temperature or by rapid freezing or thawing. A cell culture procedure similar to that used for *C. trachomatis* but using the more sensitive HL or Hep-2 cell lines must be substituted for McCoy cells. Multiple blind passages might be necessary to improve recovery rates. *C. pneumoniae* species-specific

monoclonal antibodies can detect the organism in cell culture.

**Serodiagnosis.** *C. pneumoniae* infection can also be diagnosed via serology. However, serologic testing has had variable success and questionable validity. Complement fixation using a genus-specific antigen has been used, but it is not specific for *C. pneumoniae*. A microimmunofluorescence test using *C. pneumoniae* elementary bodies as antigen is more reliable. However, availability is limited to specialized laboratories. A fourfold rise in either IgG or IgM is diagnostic, and a single IgM titer of 16 or greater or an IgG titer of 512 or greater suggests recent infection.

### Antibiotic Susceptibility Testing and Therapy

Methods for susceptibility testing of *C. pneumoniae* have been largely adapted from those used for *C. trachomatis*. Similar to *C. trachomatis*, susceptibility testing is not practical for the clinical microbiology laboratory and, because methods are not yet standardized, the results can be influenced by several variables. Treatment with tetracycline, doxycycline, macrolides, fluroquinolones, and erythromycin has been successful.

### Prevention

Little is known regarding effective ways to prevent *C. pneumoniae* infections beyond avoiding aerosolized droplets from infected people.

## RICKETTSIA, ORIENTIA, ANAPLASMA, AND EHRLICHIA

The rickettsias and rickettsia-like organisms are members of two families: the Rickettsiaceae (*Rickettsia* and *Orientia tsutsugamushi*) and the Anaplasmataceae (*Ehrlichia*, *Anaplasma*, and *Neorickettsia*). *Orientia tsutsugamushi* (formerly called *Rickettsia tsutsugamushi*) was placed into its own genus primarily based on the lack of LPS, the presence of a 54-58 kDa major surface protein, and the lack of a 17 kDa lipoprotein, all of which make it different from species of *Rickettsia*.

*Coxiella* and *Bartonella*, two other genera of intracellular bacteria causing human disease, were at one time included in the Rickettsiaceae family. However, based on phylogenetic differences, these two genera were removed from the Rickettsiaceae family and separated into two families, Coxiellaceae and Bartonellaceae. *Bartonella* spp. can be cultured on standard bacteriologic media; therefore, this group of organisms is addressed in Chapter 33. Because *Coxiella burnetii* can survive extracellularly, unlike the rickettsiae, yet requires cultivation in cell culture similar to the rickettsiae, this organism is discussed separately in this chapter.

## GENERAL CHARACTERISTICS

Rickettsiae are fastidious bacteria that are obligate, intracellular parasites. These bacterial agents survive only briefly outside of a host (reservoir or vector) and multiply only intracellularly. Organisms are small (0.3 μm × 1

**TABLE 44-4** Characteristics of Prominent *Rickettsia*\* *Orientia*, *Anaplasma*, and *Ehrlichia* spp.

| Agent | Disease | Vector | Distribution | Diagnostic Tests |
|---|---|---|---|---|
| **Spotted Fever Group**<br>*R. conorii* | Mediterranean and Israeli spotted fevers; Indian tick typhus; Kenya tick typhus | Ticks | Southern Europe, Middle East, Africa | Serology, immunohistology, PCR with sequencing |
| *R. rickettsii* | Rocky Mountain spotted fever | Ticks (*Dermacentor* spp.) | North and South America; particularly in southeastern states and Oklahoma in the United States | Serology, immunohistology, PCR with sequencing |
| **Typhus Group**<br>*R. prowazekii* | Epidemic typhus | Lice | Worldwide | Serology, PCR with sequencing |
| | Brill-Zinsser disease | None; recrudescent disease | Worldwide | Serology, PCR with sequencing |
| *R. typhi* | Murine typhus | Fleas | Worldwide | Serology, PCR with sequencing |
| **Scrub Typhus Group**<br>*O. tsutsugamushi* | Scrub typhus | Chiggers | South and Southeast Asia, South Pacific, | Serology, PCR with sequencing |
| **Ehrlichia/Anaplasma/ Neorickettsia**<br>*Ehrlichia chaffeensis* | Human monocytic ehrlichiosis | Ticks (*Amblyomma americanum*—Lone Star Tick) | Southeast, South Central, and mid-Atlantic United States | Serology, PCR, immunohistology, immunocytology |
| *E. ewingii* | | Ticks (Amblyomma americanum—Lone Star Tick) | United States (overlapping *with E. chaffeensis*) | PCR with species-specific primers or DNA sequencing of amplicons |
| *Anaplasma* | Human granulocytic anaplasmosis | Ticks (*Ixodes* spp.) | United States, Europe | Serology, PCR, immunohistology, phagocytophilum peripheral blood smear, immunocytology |
| *Neorickettsia sennetsu* | Sennetsu fever | Ticks | Southeast Asia (primarily Japan) | Serology |

\*Other *Rickettsia* species recognized as emerging human pathogens include *R. africae*, *R. sibirica*, *R. japonica*, *R. honei*, *R. australis*, *R. slovaca*, *R. aeschimannii*, *R. helvetica*, *R. heilongjiangensis*, and *R. parkeri*; all belong to the spotted fever group.

to 2 μm), pleomorphic, gram-negative bacilli that multiply by binary fission in the cytoplasm of host cells; the release of mature rickettsiae results in the lysis of the host cell.

## EPIDEMIOLOGY AND PATHOGENESIS

This group of organisms infects wild animals, with humans acting as accidental hosts in most cases. Most of these organisms are passed between animals by an insect vector. Similarly, humans become infected following the bite of an infected arthropod vector or by inhalation of infectious aerosols. Characteristics, including the respective arthropod vector of the prominent species of *Rickettsia*, *Orientia*, *Anaplasma*, and *Ehrlichia*, are summarized in Table 44-4.

Organisms belonging to the genus *Rickettsia* do not undergo any type of intracellular developmental cycle. Different species of *Rickettsia* share some antigenic properties, are genetically similar, and share a similar mechanism of pathogenesis. After being deposited directly into the bloodstream through the bite of an arthropod vector, these organisms induce the endothelial cells of the host's blood vessels to engulf them and are carried into the cell's cytoplasm within a vacuole. Following infection, organisms escape the vacuole, becoming free in the cytoplasm. *Rickettsia* spp. then multiply, causing cell injury and death. Subsequent vascular lesions caused by *Rickettsia*-induced damage to endothelial cells account for the changes that occur throughout the body, particularly in the skin, heart, brain, lung, and muscle. Rickettsiae also have numerous ways to evade human host defenses such as cell-to-cell spread, escaping from the phagosome, and entering into a latent state (primarily *R. prowazekii*).

In contrast to *Rickettsia* and *Orientia* spp., organisms belonging to the genus *Ehrlichia* undergo an intracellular developmental cycle following infection of circulating leukocytes. Similar to chlamydiae, *A. phagocytophilum*, *Ehrlichia* spp., and *N. sennetsu* cannot survive outside host cells and, once released, must rapidly induce signals for their own uptake into another host cell that is unique to each genus. How these organisms accomplish this entry, replicate in the host milieu and then exit is largely unknown. *E. chaffeensis* primarily infects monocytes and causes human monocytic ehrlichiosis (HME), whereas *A. phagocytophilum* infects bone marrow–derived cells, primarily infecting neutrophils, causing human granulocytic anaplasmosis (HGA).

## SPECTRUM OF DISEASE

Species in the genus *Rickettsia* are divided into three groups: the spotted fever group, the typhus group, and the scrub typhus group (*O. tsutsugamushi*), based on the arthropod mode of transmission, clinical manifestations, rate of intracellular growth, rate of intracellular burden, and extent of intracellular growth (see Table 44-4). Rickettsias are suspected when the triad of fever, headache, and rash is the primary clinical manifestation in patients with an exposure to insect vectors. Infections caused by these organisms may be severe and are sometimes fatal.

Although HME and HGA cause distinct infections, their clinical findings are similar. In general, patients with ehrlichial infections present with nonspecific symptoms such as fever, headache, and myalgias; rashes occur only rarely. The illness can range from asymptomatic to mild to severe.

## LABORATORY DIAGNOSIS

Because rickettsial and ehrlichial infections can be severe or even fatal, a timely diagnosis is essential.

### Direct Detection Methods

Immunohistology and conventional and real-time PCR have been used to diagnose rickettsial and ehrlichial infections. Biopsy of skin tissue from the rash caused by the spotted fever group rickettsiae is the preferred specimen. Organisms are identified using polyclonal antibodies and are detected with the use of fluorescein-labeled antibodies or enzyme-labeled indirect procedures. The sensitivity of these techniques is about 70% and depends on correct tissue sampling, examination of multiple tissue levels, and biopsy before or during the first 24 hours of therapy (see Table 44-4).

Direct detection of *Ehrlichia* and *Anaplasma* from peripheral blood or cerebrospinal fluid (CSF) includes PCR amplification, direct microscopic examination of Giemsa-stained or Wright's stained specimens, or immunocytologic or immunohistologic stains with *E. chaffeensis* or *Anaplasma* species antibodies. Direct microscopic examination of Giemsa-stained or Diff-Quik–stained peripheral blood buffy-coat smears can detect morulae (cytoplasmic vacuoles containing enriched organisms) during the febrile stage of infection in ehrlichiosis; morulae-like structures also can be observed in CSF cells and tissues. Finally, recent reports have described the development of rapid, species-specific real-time PCR assays to detect single or co-infections with *Anaplasma* species or *Ehrlichia* species in peripheral blood specimens.

### Cultivation

Although the rickettsiae can be cultured in embryonated eggs and in tissue culture, the risk of laboratory-acquired infection is extremely high, limiting the availability of culture to a few specialized laboratories. Blood should be collected as early as possible in the course of disease in a sterile, heparin-containing vial. Similarly, punch biopsies of skin or eschars (slough or dead skin) are also acceptable but must be collected early in the course of disease. These same specimens are also acceptable for PCR.

To date, culture of *Ehrlichia* and *Anaplasma* is limited and culture conditions are still being optimized. Currently, the preferred specimen for culture is peripheral blood obtained in a sterile, EDTA- or acid-citrate-dextrose-anti-coagulated blood tube; if specimens must be moved, they should be transported overnight at approximately 4° C.

### Serodiagnosis

Although it is not fast, the diagnosis of rickettsial disease and ehrlichiosis is primarily accomplished serologically. Serologic assays for the diagnosis of rickettsial infections include the indirect immunofluorescence assay (IFA), enzyme immunoassay (EIA), *Proteus vulgaris* OX-19 and OX-2 and *Proteus mirabilis* OX-K strain agglutination (the Weil-Felix reaction), line blot, and Western immunoblotting. The Weil-Felix reaction (see Procedure 44-1 on the Evolve site), the fortuitous agglutination of certain strains of *P. vulgaris* by serum from patients with rickettsial disease, may still be performed in developing countries, but because false-positive and false-negative tests are a continuing problem, these tests have been replaced by more accurate serologic methods such as IFA.

Except for latex agglutination, IFA, and DFA testing for diagnosing Rocky Mountain spotted fever, none of the serologic tests is useful for diagnosing disease in time to influence therapy. This lack of utility for serology is because antibodies to rickettsiae other than *R. rickettsii* cannot be reliably detected until at least 2 weeks after the patient has become ill. With newer immunologic recombinant reagents under development, the potential exists for new tests for all the rickettsial diseases.

To date, the sensitivity and specificity of serologic assays for ehrlichiosis is unknown but is presumed to be relatively high; indirect immunofluorescent antibody testing is available for *E. chaffeensis* or *A. phagocytophilum*. A fourfold or greater rise in antibody titer during the course of disease is considered significant.

## ANTIBIOTIC SUSCEPTIBILITY TESTING AND THERAPY

Tetracyclines, especially doxycycline, are the primary drugs of choice for treatment of most infections caused by *Rickettsia*, *Ehrlichia*, or *Anaplasma* species. Depending on the specific species of *Rickettsia*, some fluoroquinolones may be used, as may chloramphenicol.

## PREVENTION

The best means of preventing rickettsial and ehrlichial infection is to avoid contact with the respective vectors.

# COXIELLA

*Coxiella burnetii* is the causative agent of Q fever, an acute systemic infection that primarily affects the lungs.

## GENERAL CHARACTERISTICS

*C. burnetii* is smaller than *Rickettsia* spp. and is more resistant to various chemical and physical agents. Recent phylogenetic studies of this gram-negative coccobacillus have demonstrated that it is far removed from the rickettsiae and most closely related to *Legionella*. In contrast to the rickettsiae, *C. burnetii* can survive extracellularly; however, it can be grown only in lung cells. The organism has a sporelike life cycle and can exist in two antigenic states. When isolated from animals, *C. burnetii* is in phase I (large-cell variant form) and is highly infectious. In its phase II form (small-cell variant), *C. burnetii* has been grown in cultured cell lines and is not infectious, but it acts like a spore, assisting in extracellular survival of the organism.

## EPIDEMIOLOGY AND PATHOGENESIS

The most common animal reservoirs for the zoonotic disease caused by *C. burnetii* are cattle, sheep, and goats. In infected animals, organisms are shed in urine, feces, milk, and birth products. Usually, the infected animals are asymptomatic. Humans are infected by the inhalation of contaminated aerosols. Of significance, because of its resistance to desiccation and sunlight by virtue of forming spores, *C. burnetii* is able to withstand harsh environmental conditions. Q fever is endemic worldwide except in New Zealand.

Following infection, *C. burnetii* is passively phagocytized by host cells and multiplies within vacuoles. The incubation period is about 2 weeks to 1 month. After infection and proliferation in the lungs, organisms are picked up by macrophages and carried to the lymph nodes, from which they then reach the bloodstream.

## SPECTRUM OF DISEASE

After the incubation period, initial clinical manifestations of *C. burnetii* infections are systemic and nonspecific: headache, fever, chills, and myalgias. In contrast to rickettsial infections, a rash does not develop. Both acute and chronic forms of the disease are recognized. Possible clinical manifestations are listed in Box 44-1.

## LABORATORY DIAGNOSIS

Because laboratory-acquired infections caused by *C. burnetii* have occurred, cultivation of the organism must be done in a biosafety level 3 containment facility. However, the use of a shell vial assay with human lung fibroblasts to isolate the organism from buffy coat and biopsy

---

> **BOX 44-1** Clinical Manifestations of *C. burnetii* Infection
>
> Febrile, self-limited illness
> Atypical pneumonia
> Granulomatous hepatitis
> Endocarditis
> Neurologic manifestations (e.g., encephalitis, meningoencephalitis)
> Osteomyelitis

---

specimens has not resulted in any laboratory-acquired infections. Once inoculated, cultures are incubated for 6 to 14 days at 37° C in carbon dioxide. The organism is detected using a direct immunofluorescent assay.

Although organisms can be detected by nucleic acid amplification assays, serology is the most convenient and commonly used diagnostic tool. Three serologic techniques are available: IFA, complement fixation, and EIA. IFA is considered the reference method for both acute and chronic Q fever that is both highly specific and sensitive and is recommended for its reliability, cost effectiveness, and ease of performance. Many reference and state health laboratories perform phase I and phase II IgG and IgM serologic assays.

## ANTIBIOTIC SUSCEPTIBILITY TESTING AND THERAPY

Because *C. burnetii* does not multiply in bacteriologic culture media, susceptibility testing has been performed in only a limited number of laboratories. Tetracyclines are recommended for the treatment of acute and chronic Q fever.

## PREVENTION

The best way to prevent infection with *C. burnetii* is to avoid contact with infected animals. A vaccine is commercially available in Australia and Eastern European countries; a vaccine is being developed in the United States.

# *TROPHERYMA WHIPPLEI*

Although observed in diseased tissue, some organisms are nonculturable yet associated with specific disease processes, making the development of "traditional" diagnostic assays difficult (e.g., serology or antigen detection). With the ability to detect and classify bacteria using molecular techniques such as PCR to amplify ribosomal DNA sequences followed by sequencing and phylogenetic analysis, *Tropheryma whipplei* was identified as the causative agent of Whipple's disease.

## GENERAL CHARACTERISTICS

Phylogenetic analysis shows that this organism is a gram-positive actinomycete not closely related to any other genus known to cause infection.

## EPIDEMIOLOGY, PATHOGENESIS, AND SPECTRUM OF DISEASE

Whipple's disease, found primarily in middle-aged men, is characterized by the presence of periodic acid-Schiff (PAS)–staining macrophages (indicating mucopolysaccharide or glycoprotein) in almost every organ system. The bacillus is observed in macrophages and affected tissues, but it has never been cultured. Patients develop diarrhea, weight loss, arthralgia, lymphadenopathy, hyperpigmentation, often a long history of joint pain, and a distended and tender abdomen. Neurologic and sensory changes often occur. Although less common than intestinal or articular involvement, cardiac manifestations can also occur, including endocarditis. It has been suggested that a cellular immune defect is involved in the pathogenesis of this disease.

## LABORATORY DIAGNOSIS

Detection of *T. whipplei* is limited to only a few laboratories using conventional and real-time PCR.

## ANTIBIOTIC SUSCEPTIBILITY TESTING AND THERAPY

The organism is nonculturable, resulting in the inability to perform susceptibility testing. Patients usually respond well to long-term therapy with antibacterial agents, including trimethoprim/sulfamethoxazole, macrolides, aminoglycosides, tetracycline, and penicillin; tetracycline has been associated with serious relapses, however. Colchicine therapy appears to control symptoms. Without treatment the disease is uniformly fatal.

## PREVENTION

Little is known about the prevention of this disease.

# KLEBSIELLA GRANULOMATIS

*Klebsiella granulomatis* is the etiologic agent of granuloma inguinale, or donovanosis, a sexually transmitted disease.

## GENERAL CHARACTERISTICS

*K. granulomatis* is an encapsulated, pleomorphic, gram-negative bacillus that is usually observed in vacuoles in the cells of large mononuclear cells.

## EPIDEMIOLOGY AND PATHOGENESIS

Granuloma inguinale is uncommon in the United States but is recognized as a major cause of genital ulcers in India, Papua New Guinea, the Caribbean, Australia, and parts of South America. The causative agent is sexually transmitted, although there is a possibility that it may be nonsexually transmitted as well. Infectivity of this bacillus must be low, because sexual partners of infected patients often do not become infected or require repeated exposures to become infected.

## SPECTRUM OF DISEASE

Granuloma inguinale is characterized by the presence of enlarged subcutaneous nodules that evolve to form beefy, erythematous, granulomatous, painless lesions that bleed easily. The lesions, which usually occur on the genitalia, have been mistaken for neoplasms. Patients often have inguinal lymphadenopathy.

## LABORATORY DIAGNOSIS

The organism can be visualized in scrapings of lesions stained with Wright's or Giemsa stain. Subsurface infected cells must be present; surface epithelium is not an adequate specimen. Groups of organisms are seen within mononuclear endothelial cells; this pathognomonic entity is known as a Donovan body, named after the physician who first visualized the organism in such a lesion. The organism stains as a blue rod with prominent polar granules, giving rise to a "safety pin" appearance, surrounded by a large, pink capsule.

Cultivation in vitro is difficult, but it can be done using media containing some of the growth factors found in egg yolk. A medium described by Dienst has been used to culture *K. granulomatis* from aspirated bubo material. More recently, this agent was cultured in human monocytes from biopsies of genital ulcers of patients with donovanosis.

## ANTIBIOTIC SUSCEPTIBILITY TESTING AND THERAPY

No antibiotic susceptibility testing is performed. Trimethoprim/sulfamethoxazole and doxycycline are the most effective drugs for the therapy of granuloma inguinale. Ciprofloxacin, azithromycin, or erythromycin (in pregnancy) also provides effective treatment for granuloma inguinale.

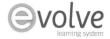 *Visit the Evolve site to complete the review questions.*

## CASE STUDY 44-1

A 13-year-old girl was well until 9 days before admission, when she developed headache, fever, and myalgias. Amoxicillin therapy was started 4 days before admission. Over the next few days, the symptoms continued and she developed abdominal pain and disorientation. Laboratory findings revealed neutropenia and elevated liver enzymes. On admission she presented with photophobia, nuchal rigidity (stiff neck), and disseminated intravascular coagulation. She had recently traveled to Arkansas where she stayed on a farm, rode horses, and removed multiple ticks from her legs. A bone marrow aspiration was performed, which yielded the diagnosis from the Wright's stain of the monocytes. After treatment with doxycycline, she had a complete recovery.

### QUESTIONS

1. What is the etiologic agent of this disease, and how was it detected?
2. Why is this disease called a zoonosis?
3. Diagnosis of this disease is difficult. What laboratory methods are available to the physician to diagnose a patient with this disease?

# BIBLIOGRAPHY

Bastian I, Bowden FJ: Amplification of *Klebsiella*-like sequences from biopsy samples from patients with donovanosis, *Clin Infect Dis* 23:1328, 1996.

Byrne GI, Ojcius DM: *Chlamydia* and apoptosis: life and death decisions of an intracellular pathogen, *Nat Rev* 2: 802, 2004.

Caldwell HD, Wood H, Crane D, et al: Polymorphisms in *Chlamydia trachomatis* tryptophan synthase genes differentiate between genital and ocular isolates, *J Clin Invest* 111: 1757, 2003.

Centers for Disease Control and Prevention: Sexually transmitted diseases treatment guidelines, 2010, *MMWR*, 59(RR-12):1, 2010.

Centers for Disease Control and Prevention: *2009 Sexually transmitted diseases surveillance, Chlamydia*, November 22, 2010, accessed from www.cdc.gov/std/stats09/chlamydia.htm, on September 7, 2011.

Centers for Disease Control and Prevention: *Volume and type of laboratory testing methods for sexually transmitted diseases in public health laboratories 2007.* Summary report published January 2011, accessed from www.cdc.gov/std/general/LabSurveyReport-2011.pdf on September 7, 2011.

Chapman AS: Diagnosis and management of tickborne rickettsial diseases: rocky mountain spotted fever, ehrlichiosis and anaplasmosis–United States, *MMWR*, 55(RR04):1, 2006.

Cook RL, Hutchison SL, Østergaard L, et al: Systematic review: noninvasive testing for *Chlamydia trachomatis* and *Neisseria gonorrhoeae*, *Ann Intern Med* 142:914, 2005.

Darville T, Hiltke TJ: Pathogenesis of genital tract disease due to *Chlamydia trachomatis*, *J Infect Dis* 201(S2): S114, 2010.

De Vries HJC, Morre SA, White JA: International union against sexually transmitted infections (IUSTI): 2010 European guideline on the management of lymphogranuloma venereum, *Int J STD AIDS* 21:533, 2010.

Dienst RB, Brownell GH: Genus *Calymmatobacterium* Aragao and Vianna 1913. In Krieg NR, Holt JG, editors: *Bergey's manual of systematic bacteriology*, vol 1, Baltimore, 1984, Williams & Wilkins.

Doyle CK, Labruna MB, Breitschwerdt EB, et al: Detection of medically important *Ehrlichia* by quantitative multicolor TaqMan real-time polymerase chain reaction of the dsb gene, *J Molec Diagn* 7:504, 2005.

Dumler JS, Bakken JS: Ehrlichial diseases of human: emerging tickborne infections, *Clin Infect Dis* 20:1102, 1994.

Dumler JS, Walker DH: Diagnostic tests for Rocky Mountain spotted fever and other rickettsial diseases, *Dermatol Clin* 12:25, 1994.

Everett KD, Andersen AA: Identification of nine species of the Chlamydiaceae using PCR-RFLP, *Int J Syst Bacteriol* 49:803, 1999.

Everett KD, Bush RM, Andersen AA: Emended description of the order Chlamydiales, proposal of Parachlamydiaceae fam nov and Simkaniaceae fam nov, each containing one monotypic genus, revised taxonomy of the family Chlamydiaceae, including a new genus and five new species, and standards for the identification of organisms, *Int J Syst Bacteriol* 49:415, 1999.

Falsey AR, Walsh EE: Transmission of *Chlamydia pneumoniae*, *J Infect Dis* 168:493, 1993.

Fournier PE, Raoult D: Suicide PCR on skin biopsy specimens for diagnosis of rickettsioses, *J Clin Microbiol* 42:3428, 2004.

Gaydos C, Essig A: Chlamydiaceae. In Versalovic J, editor: *Manual of clinical microbiology*, ed 10, Washington, DC, 2011, ASM Press.

Gaydos CA, Roblin PM, Hammerschlag MR, et al: Diagnostic utility of PCR-enzyme immunoassay, culture, and serology for detection of *Chlamydia pneumoniae* in symptomatic and asymptomatic patients, *J Clin Microbiol* 32:903, 1994.

Gaydos CA, Quinn TC: Urine nucleic acid amplification tests for the diagnosis of sexually transmitted infections in clinical practice, *Curr Opin Infect Dis* 18:55, 2005.

Goldberg J: Studies on granuloma inguinale. IV. Growth requirements of *Donovania granulomatis* and its relationship to the natural habitat of the organism, *Br J Ven Dis* 35:266, 1959.

Hackstadt T: The biology of rickettsiae, *Infect Agents Dis* 5:127, 1996.

Hammerschlag MR: Antimicrobial susceptibility and therapy of infections caused by *Chlamydia pneumoniae*, *Antimicrob Agents Chemother* 38:1873, 1994.

Hogan RJ, Mathews SA, Mukhopadhyay S, et al: Chlamydial persistence: beyond the biphasic paradigm, *Infect Immun* 72: 1843, 2004.

Jensenius M, Fournier PE, Raoult D: Rickettsioses and the international traveler, *Clin Infect Dis* 39:1493, 2004.

Johnson RE, Green TA, Schachter J, et al: Evaluation of nucleic acid amplification tests as reference tests for *Chlamydia trachomatis* infections in asymptomatic men, *J Clin Microbiol* 38:4382, 2000.

Kaplan JE, Schonberger LB: The sensitivity of various serologic tests in the diagnosis of Rocky Mountain Spotted Fever, *Am J Trop Med Hyg* 35:840, 1986.

Kellogg J: Impact of variation in endocervical specimen collection and testing techniques on frequency of false-positive and false-negative chlamydia detection results, *Am J Clin Pathol* 104:554, 1995.

Kharsany AB, Hoosen AA, Kiepiela P, et al: Culture of *Calymmatobacterium granulomatis*, *Clin Infect Dis* 22:391, 1996.

Kularatne SAM, Gawarammana IB: Validity of the Weil-Felix test in the diagnosis of acute rickettsial infections in Sri Lanka, *T Roy Soc Trop Med Hyg* 103:423, 2009.

Kuo CC, Jackson LA, Campbell LA, et al: *Chlamydia pneumoniae* (TWAR), *Clin Microbiol Rev* 8:451, 1995.

La Scola B, Raoult D: Laboratory diagnosis of rickettsioses: current approaches to diagnosis of old and new rickettsial diseases, *J Clin Microbiol* 35:2715, 1997.

Leber AL, Hall GS, LeBar WD: Nucleic acid amplification tests for detection of *Chlamydia trachomatis* and *Neisseria gonorrhoeae*. In Sharp SE, coordinating editor: *Cumitech 44*, Washington, DC, 2006, American Society for Microbiology.

Lepidi H, Fenollar F, Dumler JS, et al: Cardiac valves in patients with Whipple endocarditis: microbiological, molecular, quantitative histologic and immunohistochemical studies of 5 patients, *J Infect Dis* 190:935, 2004.

Mahajan SK, Kashyap R, Kanga A, et al: Relevance of Weil-Felix test in diagnosis of scrub typhus in India, *J Assoc Phys India* 54:619, 2006.

Martin DH: Chlamydial infections, *Med Clin North Am* 74:1367, 1990.

McMenemy A: Whipple's disease, a familial Mediterranean fever, adult-onset Still's disease, and enteropathic arthritis, *Curr Opin Rheumatol* 4:479, 1992.

Morrison RP: New insights into a persistent problem–chlamydial infections, *J Clin Invest* 111:1647, 2003.

Musso D, Raoult D: *Coxiella burnetii* blood cultures from acute and chronic Q-fever patients, *J Clin Microbiol* 33:3129, 1995.

Paddock CD, Childs JE: *Ehrlichia chaffeensis*: a prototypical emerging pathogen, *Clin Microbiol Rev* 16: 37, 2003.

Pariola P, Paddock C, Raoult D: Tick-borne rickettsioses around the world: emerging diseases challenging old concepts, *Clin Microbiol Rev* 18: 719, 2005.

Raoult D, Marrie T: Q fever, *Clin Infect Dis* 20:489, 1995.

Relman DA: The identification of uncultured microbial pathogens, *J Infect Dis* 168:1, 1983.

Relman DA, Schmidt TM, MacDermott RP, et al: Identification of the uncultured bacillus of Whipple's disease, *N Engl J Med* 327: 293, 1992.

Sirigireddy KR, Ganta RR: Multiplex detection of *Ehrlichia* and *Anaplasma* species pathogens in peripheral blood by real-time reverse transcriptase-polymerase chain reaction, *J Molec Diagn* 7:308, 2005.

Stephens RS, Myers G, Eppinger M, et al: Divergence without difference: phylogenetics and taxonomy of *Chlamydia* resolved, *FEMS Immunol Med Microbiol* 55:115, 2009.

Walker DH, Valbuena GA, Olano JP: Pathogenic mechanisms of diseases caused by *Rickettsia*, *Ann N Y Acad Sci* 990: 1, 2003.

Watson C, Alp NJ: Role of *Chlamydia pneumoniae* in atherosclerosis, *Clinical Science* 114:509, 2008.

Williams JC, Waag D: Antigens, virulence factors, and biological response modifiers of *Coxiella burnetii*: strategies for vaccine development. In Williams JC and Thompson HA, editors: *Q fever: the biology of Coxiella burnetii*, Boca Raton, Fla, 1991, CRC Press.

Williams KP, Sobral BW, Dickerman AW: A robust species tree for the Alphaproteobacteria, *J Bacti* 189:4578, 2007.

Wyrick PB: *Chlamydia trachomatis* persistence in vitro: an overview, *J Infect Dis* 201(S2):S88, 2010.

# Cell Wall–Deficient Bacteria: Mycoplasma and Ureaplasma

## OBJECTIVES

1. Describe the general characteristics of the Mycoplasmataceae, including microscopic and macroscopic appearance.
2. Identify key characteristic biochemical reactions for the differentiation of pathogenic *Mycoplasma* spp.
3. Explain the difficulties associated with isolation of these fastidious organisms, including nutritional requirements, immune response, cellular locations, and incubation requirements (length of time, temperature, and oxygenation requirements).
4. Compare the clinical presentation of *M. pneumoniae* to *S. pneumoniae*.
5. Describe the proper processing, collection, transport, and storage of specimens for the isolation of the organism discussed in this chapter.
6. State the site for colonization in the human host for *M. genitalium, M. hominis, M. pneumoniae,* and *U. urealyticum*.
7. Describe the clinical manifestations associated with each of the major species considered in this chapter.
8. Describe the complications of serologic diagnosis related to the variation in antibody formation in infection with *M. pneumoniae*.
9. Explain the current limitations and recommendations associated with susceptibility testing related to the Mycoplasmataceae.
10. Correlate signs and symptoms and evaluate laboratory data associated with the diagnosis of infections caused by the major pathogens discussed in this chapter.

---

### GENERA AND SPECIES TO BE CONSIDERED

*Mycoplasma fermentans*
*Mycoplasma genitalium*
*Mycoplasma hominis*
*Mycoplasma pneumoniae*
*Ureaplasma parvum*
*Ureaplasma urealyticum*

---

This chapter addresses a group of bacteria, the mycoplasmas, which are the smallest known free-living forms; unlike all other bacteria, these prokaryotes do not have a cell wall. Although mycoplasmas are ubiquitous in the plant and animal kingdoms (more than 200 different species exist within this class), this chapter predominantly addresses the most prominent varieties of *Mycoplasma* spp. and *Ureaplasma* spp. that colonize or infect humans and are not of animal origin.

## GENERAL CHARACTERISTICS

Organisms in this chapter belong to the class Mollicutes (Latin, meaning soft skin). This class comprises four orders, which, in turn, contain five families and eight genera (Figure 45-1). The mycoplasmas that colonize or infect humans belong to the family Mycoplasmataceae; this family comprises two genera, *Mycoplasma* and *Ureaplasma*. These organisms are highly fastidious, are slow growing, and most are facultative anaerobes that require nucleic acid precursor molecules, fatty acids, and sterols such as cholesterol for growth. These bacteria have a very small cell size ($0.3 \times 0.8 \ \mu m$) and small genome. The Mollicutes appear most closely related to the gram-positive bacterial subgroup that includes bacilli, streptococci, and lactobacteria that diverged from the Streptococcus branch of gram-positive bacteria.

## EPIDEMIOLOGY AND PATHOGENESIS

Mycoplasmas are part of the microbial flora of humans and are found mainly in the oropharynx, upper respiratory tract, and genitourinary tract. Besides those that are considered primarily as commensals, considerable evidence indicates the pathogenicity of some mycoplasmas; for others, a role in a particular disease is less clearly delineated.

### EPIDEMIOLOGY

The mycoplasmas usually considered as commensals are listed in Table 45-1, along with their respective sites of colonization. These organisms may be transmitted by direct sexual contact, transplanted tissue from donor to recipient, or from mother to fetus during childbirth or in utero. *M. pneumoniae* may be transmitted by respiratory secretions. One species of *Acholeplasma* (these organisms are widely disseminated in animals), *Acholeplasma laidlawii*, has been isolated from the oral cavity of humans a limited number of times; however, the significance of these mycoplasmas and their colonization of humans remains uncertain.

Of the other mycoplasmas that have been isolated from humans, the possible role that *M. pirum, M. amphoriforme, M. fermentans,* and *M. penetrans* might play in human disease is uncertain at this time. *M. pirum, M. fermentans,* and *M. penetrans* have been isolated from patients infected with the human immunodeficiency virus (HIV). It now appears that *M. genitalium* may account for as much as 15% to 20% of nongonococcal urethritis. *M. genitalium* is not associated with the presence of other mycoplasmas and ureaplasmas. In women, this organism may also cause cervicitis and endometritis. *M. fermentans* has been isolated from specimens such as bronchoalveolar lavage, bone marrow, peripheral blood, and the throats of children with pneumonia. The organism has been associated with infection in children and immunocompromised individuals. *M.*

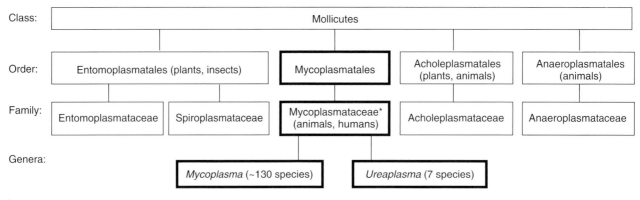

**Figure 45-1** Taxonomy of the class Mollicutes.

**TABLE 45-1** Mycoplasmas That Are Considered Normal Flora of the Oropharynx or Genital Tract

| Organism | Site of Colonization |
|---|---|
| *M. orale* | Oropharynx |
| *M. salivarium* | Oropharynx, gingiva |
| *M. amphoriforme* | Oropharynx, respiratory tract? |
| *M. buccale* | Oropharynx |
| *M. faucium* | Oropharynx |
| *M. fermentans* | Oropharynx |
| | Genital tract |
| *M. fermentans incognitus* strain | Oropharynx |
| *M. lipohilum* | Oropharynx |
| *M. penetrans* | Genital tract |
| *M. pirum* | Unknown |
| *M. primatum* | Genital tract, oropharynx |
| *M. spermatophilum* | Genital tract |
| *Acholeplasma laidlawii* | Oropharynx |

*amphoriforme* has been detected in the lower respiratory tract in patients with chronic respiratory disease and antibody deficiencies. The incidence of various *Mycoplasma* spp. infections in immunocompromised patients has been demonstrated following genital or respiratory tract colonization as well as medical procedures such as renal transplantation, genitourinary manipulations, or following trauma resulting in wound infections.

Finally, the remaining three species of mycoplasmas that have been isolated from humans—*M. pneumoniae, U. urealyticum,* and *M. hominis*—have well-established roles in human infections. Both *U. urealyticum* and *M. hominis* have been isolated from the genitourinary tract of humans, and *M. pneumoniae* has been isolated from the respiratory tract. Both *Ureaplasma* species have been isolated from the internal organs of stillborn, premature, and spontaneously aborted fetuses. However, the literature contains conflicting opinions as to the importance of *U. urealyticum* in comparison *to U. parvum.*

Infants are commonly colonized with *U. urealyticum* and *M. hominis.* Once an individual reaches puberty, colonization with these mycoplasmas can occur primarily as a result of sexual contact. In situations in which these agents cause disease in neonates, organisms are transmitted from a colonized mother to her newborn infant by an ascending route from colonization of the mother's urogenital tract, by crossing the placenta from the mother's blood, by delivery through a colonized birth canal, or postnatally from mother to infant.

*M. pneumoniae* is a cause of community-acquired atypical pneumonia, often referred to as walking pneumonia (see Chapter 69); infections caused by this agent are distributed worldwide, with an estimated 2 million cases per year in the United States. *M. pneumoniae* infection may also result in bronchitis or pharyngitis. *M. pneumoniae* may be transmitted person-to-person by respiratory secretions as previously stated or indirectly by inanimate objects contaminated with respiratory secretions (fomites). Infections can occur singly or as outbreaks in closed populations such as families and military recruit camps. Pneumonia caused by *M. pneumoniae* may present as asymptomatic to mild disease, with early nonspecific symptoms including malaise, fever, headache, sore throat, earache, and nonproductive cough. This differs significantly from the classic symptoms associated with pneumonia as a result of infection with *Streptococcus pneumoniae* (see Chapters 15 and 69). *M. pneumoniae* strongly attaches to the mucosal cells and may reside intracellularly within host cells, resulting in a chronic persistent infection that may last for months to years. The infections do not follow seasonal patterns as seen with influenzae and other respiratory pathogens. Besides respiratory infection, *M. pneumoniae* can cause extrapulmonary manifestations such as pericarditis, hemolytic anemia, arthritis, nephritis, Bell's palsy, and meningoencephalitis resulting in various additional forms of paralysis.

## PATHOGENESIS

In general, mycoplasmas colonize mucosal surfaces of the respiratory and urogenital tracts. Except for those mycoplasmas noted, most rarely produce invasive disease except in immunocompromised hosts or instrumentation. Of the mycoplasmas that are established as causes of human infections, these agents predominantly reside extracellularly, attaching with great affinity to ciliated and nonciliated epithelial cells. Recently, *M. fermentans*, *M. penetrans*, *M. genitalium*, and *M. pneumoniae* have been identified intracellularly. Intracellular invasion in bacterial infections is generally considered a means for immune evasion and may contribute to the persistent nature of infections and difficulties in cultivation or isolation of *Mycoplasma* spp. *M. pneumoniae* has a complex and specialized attachment organelle to accomplish this process that includes a P1 adhesin protein that primarily interacts with host cells. With respect to the mycoplasmas that are clearly able to cause disease, many of the disease processes are thought to be immunologically mediated. In addition to adherence properties and possibly immune-mediated injury, the ability to cause localized cell injury appears to contribute to their pathogenicity.

Of interest, the mycoplasmas associated with patients with HIV (*M. fermentans*, *M. penetrans*, and *M. pirum*) are all capable of invading human cells and modulating the immune system. Based on these findings, some investigators have proposed that these mycoplasmas might play a role in certain disease processes in these patients.

## SPECTRUM OF DISEASE

The clinical manifestations of infections caused by *M. pneumoniae* and the pathogenic genital mycoplasmas, *U. urealyticum*, *U. parvum*, *M. hominis*, and *M. genitalium* are summarized in Table 45-2.

## LABORATORY DIAGNOSIS

The laboratory diagnosis of mycoplasma infections is extremely challenging because of complex and time-consuming culture requirements and the lack of reliable, widely available rapid diagnostic tests. Accurate, rapid diagnosis for *M. pneumoniae* is highly desired, because penicillin and other β-lactam agents are ineffective treatments. The laboratory diagnosis of the mycoplasmas well recognized as able to cause human disease (i.e., *M.*

**TABLE 45-2** Clinical Manifestations of *Mycoplasma* Infections Caused by *Mycoplasma pneumoniae, Ureaplasma urealyticum, Ureaplasma parvum, M. hominis,* and *M. genitalium*

| Organism | Clinical Manifestations |
|---|---|
| *Mycoplasma pneumoniae* | Asymptomatic infection |
| | Upper respiratory tract infection in school-aged children: mild, nonspecific symptoms including runny nose, pharyngitis, coryza (symptoms of a head cold, stuffy or runny nose, cough, aches), and cough; most without fever |
| | Lower respiratory tract infection in adolescents or young adults: typically mild illness with nonproductive cough, fever, malaise, pharyngitis, myalgias; approximately 33% of patients develop pneumonia; complications include rash, arthritis, encephalitis, myocarditis, pericarditis, and hemolytic anemia |
| | Occasionally the organism has been associated with infection in children < 5 years of age and elderly patients |
| Genital mycoplasmas: *U. urealyticum* and *M. hominis* | Systemic infections in neonates as a result of vertical transmission from the mother to the fetus in 18%-55% when the mother is colonized: meningitis, abscess, bacteremia, and pneumonia; *U. urealyticum* is also associated with the development of chronic lung disease |
| | Invasive disease in immunosuppressed patients: bacteremia, arthritis (particularly in patients with agammaglobulinemia), abscesses and other wound infections, pneumonia, peritonitis |
| | Urogenital tract infections: prostatitis, pelvic inflammatory disease (PID), amnionitis, nongonococcal urethritis, acute polynephritis |
| | These organisms proliferate in the urogenital tract of patients suffering with bacterial vaginosis (BV) caused by other microorganisms; some studies link *M. hominis* to the development of BV and may be associated with the development of additional disease such as PID |
| *M. genitalium* | Nongonococcal urethritis in men; possible cause of cervicitis and endometritis in females |
| | Vertical transmission from mother to fetus has been identified; however, the clinical significance is currently unknown |
| *Ureaplasma* spp. | *Ureaplasma urealyticum* and less frequently *U. parvum* have been isolated from the tissues of spontaneously aborted fetuses, stillborns, and premature infants, as well as full-term infants; the organisms may infect the chorioamnion |

Data from Versalovic J: *Manual of clinical microbiology,* ed 10, Washington, DC, 2011, ASM Press.

*pneumoniae, U. urealyticum, M. hominis,* and *M. genitalium*) is addressed.

## SPECIMEN COLLECTION, TRANSPORT, AND PROCESSING

Various specimens are appropriate for the diagnosis of mycoplasma infections by culture or other means of detection. Acceptable specimens include body fluids (e.g., blood, joint fluid, amniotic fluid, urine, prostatic secretions, semen, pleural secretions, sputum, bronchoalveolar lavage specimens), tissues, wound aspirates and swabs of wounds, the throat, nasopharynx, urethra, cervix, or vagina. Blood for culture of genital mycoplasmas should be collected without anticoagulants and immediately inoculated into an appropriate broth culture medium. Mycoplasmas are inhibited by sodium polyanethol sulfonate (SPS), the anticoagulant typically found in commercial blood culture media. This may be overcome by the addition of 1% wt/vol of gelatin; however, commercial blood culture media and automated instruments are not adequate for the detection of *Mycoplasma* spp. Swab specimens should be obtained without the application of any disinfectants, analgesics, or lubricant; Dacron or polyester swabs on aluminum or plastic shafts should be used. Care must be taken to collect urine

samples to avoid contamination with lubricants and antiseptics used during gynecologic examination.

Because mycoplasmas have no cell wall, they are highly susceptible to drying; therefore, transport media are necessary, particularly when specimens are collected on swabs. Liquid specimens such as body fluids do not require transport media if inoculated to appropriate media within 1 hour of collection. Tissues should be kept moist; if a delay in processing is anticipated, they should also be placed in transport media. Specific media for the isolation of *Mycoplasma* spp. include those containing 10% heat-inactivated calf serum containing 0.2 M sucrose in a 0.02 M phosphate buffer, pH 7.2, such as SP4, Shepard's 10B broth or 2 SP. Additional commercial media available for cultivation of these organisms include Stuart's medium, trypticase soy broth supplemented with 0.5% bovine serum albumin, Mycotrans (Irvine Scientific, Irvine, California), and A3B broth (Remel, Inc.). Excessive delays in processing can result in decreased viability and recovery of organisms from clinical specimens. If the storage time is expected to exceed 24 hours prior to cultivation, the samples should be placed in transport media and frozen at −80°C. Frozen samples should be thawed in a hot water bath at 37°C. Transport and storage conditions of various types of specimens are summarized in Table 45-3.

**TABLE 45-3** Transport and Storage Conditions for *Mycoplasma pneumoniae, Ureaplasma urealyticum,* and *M. hominis*

| Specimen Type | Transport Conditions | Transport Media (examples)§ | Storage | Processing |
|---|---|---|---|---|
| Body fluid or liquid specimens* | Within 1 hr of collection on ice or at 4° C | Not required | 4° C up to 24 hr† | Concentrate by high-speed centrifugation and dilute (1:10 to 1:1000) in broth culture media to remove inhibitory substances and contaminating bacteria; urine should be filtered through a 0.45-μm pore size filter |
| Swabs | Place immediately into transport media | 0.5% albumin in trypticase soy broth modified Stuart's | 4°C up to 24 hr† | None |
| | | 2SP (sugar-phosphate medium with 10% heat-inactivated fetal calf serum) | | |
| | | Shepard's 10B broth for ureaplasmas | | |
| | | SP-4 broth for other mycoplasmas and *M. pneumoniae*‡ | | |
| | | *Mycoplasma* transport medium (trypticase phosphate broth, 10% bovine serum albumin, 100,000 U of penicillin/milliliter and universal transport media [Copan, Murrieta, CA]) | | |
| Tissue | Within 1 hr of collection on ice or at 4° C | Not required as long as prevented from drying out | 4° C up to 24 hr† | Mince (not ground) and dilute (1:10 and 1:100) in transport media |

*Except blood (see text).
†Can be stored indefinitely at -80° C if diluted in transport media following centrifugation.
‡SP-4 broth: sucrose phosphate buffer, 20% horse serum, *Mycoplasma* base, and neutral red.
§Not a complete list. A variety of commercial media is available.

**TABLE 45-4** Cultivation of *Mycoplasma pneumoniae, Ureaplasma* spp., and *M. hominis*

| Organism | Media (examples) | Incubation Conditions |
|---|---|---|
| *M. pneumoniae* | Biphasic SP-4 (pH 7.4)<br>Triphasic system (Mycotrim RS, Irvine Scientific, Irvine, California)<br>PPLO broth or agar with yeast extract and horse serum<br>Modified New York City medium | Broths: 37° C, ambient air for up to 4 wk<br>Agars: 37° C, ambient air supplemented with 5 to 10% $CO_2$ or anaerobically in 95% $N_2$ plus 5% $CO_2$.<br>All cultures should be retained for 4 weeks before reporting as negative. |
| *U. urealyticum/U. parvum*\*/M. hominis*† | A7 or A8 agar medium (Remel, Lenexa, Kansas); penicillin should be included to minimize bacterial overgrowth‡<br>New York City medium<br>Modified New York City medium<br>SP-4 glucose broth with arginine§<br>SP-4 glucose broth with urea‖<br>Triphasic system (Mycotrim GU, Irvine Scientific)<br>Shepard's 10B broth (or *Ureaplasma* 10C broth)‖ | Broths: 37° C, ambient air for up to 7 days<br>Agars: 37° C in 5 to 10% $CO_2$ or anaerobically in 95% $N_2$ plus 5% $CO_2$ for 2 to 5 days.<br>Genital cultures should be retained for 7 days before reporting as negative. |

\*Utilizes urea and requires acidic medium.
†Converts arginine to ornithine and grows over a broad pH range.
‡Commercially available.
§For *M. hominis* isolation.
‖For *U. urealyticum* isolation.

## DIRECT DETECTION METHODS

At present, no direct methods for identifying *M. pneumoniae, Ureaplasmas* spp., or other *Mycoplasma* spp. in clinical samples are recommended, although some methods have been described, such as immunoblotting and indirect immunofluorescence. Direct detection by gram staining may rule out the presence of other infectious organisms, but it will not stain cell wall-deficient mycoplasmas and ureaplasmas. Acridine orange or a fluorochrome stain may be useful to visualize organisms. However, these are nonspecific stains that will stain nucleic acids in bacteria as well as human cells.

### Molecular Diagnostics

Several amplification methods, such as polymerase chain reaction (PCR), have been developed for the detection of the clinically relevant *Mycoplasma* and *Ureaplasma* species. Various targets including 16srRNA sequences, insertion sequences, and organism specific genes have been used in the development of these assays. As a result of the fast turnaround time, specificity, and lack of need to cultivate fastidious organisms, PCR amplification for the diagnosis of these organisms is particularly attractive. When considering the use of molecular amplification methods for the detection of infectious diseases, it is important to note that although an organism is detectable, the patient's signs and symptoms must be correlated with the identified agent. It is possible to detect an organism by one method and not another—in other words, a patient may be PCR positive but culture negative or serologically negative for a *Mycoplasma* based on the patient's response to infection and current disease manifestation. Chapter 8 provides a more detailed description of the advantages, limitations, and methods used in the development of amplification assays. Multiplexed real-time PCR assays that detect *M. pneumoniae* as well as other atypical respiratory tract pathogens such as *Chlamydophila pneumoniae* and *Legionella pneumoniae* have been developed.

Because there is no reliable medium for its isolation, *M. genitalium* has been directly detected by PCR targeting its attachment protein in urine and urethral swabs in men. In women, vaginal or cervical swabs are used.

## CULTIVATION

In general, the medium for mycoplasma isolation contains a beef or soybean protein with serum, fresh yeast extract, and other factors. As a result of the slow growth of these organisms, the medium must be selective to prevent overgrowth of faster-growing organisms that may be present in a clinical sample. Culture media and incubation conditions for these organisms are summarized in Table 45-4. Culture methods for *M. pneumoniae, U. urealyticum,* and *M. hominis* are provided on the Evolve site in Procedures 45-1, 45-2, and 45-3, respectively. The quality control of the growth media with a fastidious isolate is of great importance.

For the most part, the different metabolic activity of the mycoplasmas for different substrates is used to detect their growth. Glucose (dextrose) is incorporated into media selective for *M. pneumoniae,* because this mycoplasma ferments glucose to lactic acid; the resulting pH change is then detected by a color change in a dye indicator. Similarly, urea or arginine can be incorporated into media to detect *U. urealyticum* and *M. hominis,* respectively (Table 45-5). If a color change—that is, a pH change—is detected, a 0.1- to 0.2-mL aliquot is immediately subcultured to fresh broth and agar media.

In some clinical situations, it may be necessary to provide quantitative information regarding the numbers of genital mycoplasmas in a clinical specimen. For example, quantitation of specimens taken at different stages during urination or after prostatic massage can help determine the location of mycoplasmal infection in the genitourinary tract.

**TABLE 45-5** Basic Biochemical Differentiation of the Major *Mycoplasma* spp. and *Ureaplasma urealyticum*

| Organism | Glucose Metabolism | Arginine Metabolism | Urease |
|---|---|---|---|
| *M. fermentans* | Positive | Positive | Negative |
| *M. genitalium* | Positive | Negative | Negative |
| *M. hominis* | Negative | Positive | Negative |
| *M. pneumoniae* | Positive | Negative | Negative |
| *U. urealyticum* | Negative | Negative | Positive |

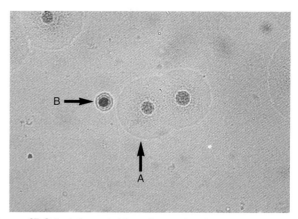

**Figure 45-3** Isolation of *Mycoplasma hominis* and *Ureaplasma urealyticum* (100× magnification). Note the "fried egg" appearance of the large *M. hominis* colony *(arrow A)* and the relatively small size of the *U. urealyticum* colony *(arrow B)*. (Courtesy Clinical Microbiology Laboratory, SUNY Upstate Medical University, Syracuse, NY.)

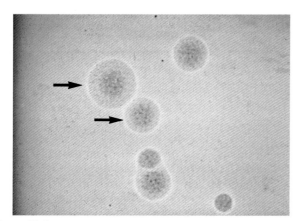

**Figure 45-2** Colonies of *Mycoplasma pneumoniae* visualized under 100× magnification. Note the variation in the size of the colonies *(arrows)*. (Courtesy Clinical Microbiology Laboratory, SUNY Upstate Medical University, Syracuse, NY.)

## APPROACH TO IDENTIFICATION

On agar, *M. pneumoniae* will appear as spherical, grainy, yellowish forms that are embedded in the agar, with a thin outer layer similar to those shown in Figure 45-2. The agar surface is examined under 20 to 60× magnification using a stereomicroscope daily for *Ureaplasma* spp., at 24 to 72 hours for *M. hominis*, and every 3 to 5 days for *M. pneumoniae* and other slow-growing species. Because only *M. pneumoniae* and one serovar of *U. urealyticum* hemadsorb, *M. pneumoniae* is definitively identified by overlaying suspicious colonies with 0.5% guinea pig erythrocytes in phosphate-buffered saline instead of water. After 20 to 30 minutes at room temperature, colonies are observed for adherence of red blood cells.

Cultures for the genital mycoplasmas are handled in a similar fashion, including culture examination and the requirement for subculturing. Colonies may be definitively identified on A8 agar as *U. urealyticum* by urease production in the presence of a calcium chloride indicator. *U. urealyticum* colonies (15 to 60 μm in diameter) will appear as dark brownish clumps. Colonies that are typical in appearance for *U. urealyticum* are shown in Figure 45-3. *M. hominis* are large (about 20 to 300 μm in diameter) and are urease negative (see Figure 45-3), with a characteristic "fried egg" appearance (Figure 45-4). On conventional blood agar, strains *of M. hominis*, but not of *U. urealyticum*, produce nonhemolytic, pinpoint colonies that do not stain with Gram stain. These colonies can

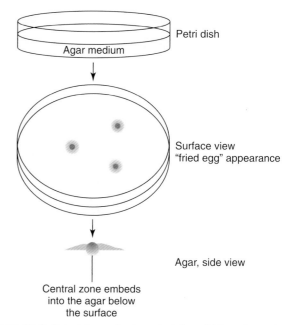

**Figure 45-4** Colonial growth characteristics of *Mycoplasma* in agar medium.

be stained with the Dienes or acridine orange stains. Numerous transport and growth media systems for the detection, quantitation, identification, and antimicrobial susceptibility testing of the genital mycoplasmas are commercially available in the United States and Europe.

## SERODIAGNOSIS

Laboratory diagnosis of *M. pneumoniae* is usually made serologically. Nonspecific production of cold agglutinins occurs in approximately half of patients with atypical pneumonia caused by this organism. Antibodies to *M. pneumoniae* are typically detectable following approximately 1 week of illness, peaking between 3 to 6 weeks, followed by a gradual decline. The antibody response to *M. pneumoniae* varies greatly from patient to patient. Some patients fail to produce a detectable IgM level, whereas in others the IgM level will persist for months. The variability associated with the antibody response necessitates the comparison of paired sera for proper diagnosis. In addition, cold agglutinins form in association with *M. pneumoniae* infection. The most widely used serologic tests today are enzyme-linked immunosorbent assay (ELISA) tests, although newly developed indirect fluorescent antibody tests are being used with some success. IgM-specific tests such as the Immuno Card (Meridian Diagnostics, Cincinnati, Ohio) are commercially available, and a single positive result in children, adolescents, and young adults may be considered diagnostic in some cases. In addition, there is a commercially available, membrane-based assay that simultaneously detects IgM and IgG against *M. pneumoniae* (Remel EIA, Lenexa, Kansas) with good sensitivity and specificity compared to other tests. Several additional commercial assays are available that include EIA microtiter assays.

Although serologic tests such as indirect hemagglutination and metabolism inhibition for genital mycoplasmas are available, they are rarely used. Because of the antigenic complexity of the mycoplasmas, the development of a specific and useful serologic assay is a challenge.

## SUSCEPTIBILITY TESTING AND THERAPY

Although agar and broth dilution methods may be used to determine antibiotic susceptibilities, the complex growth requirements of mycoplasmas have restricted their performance to a few laboratories. The Human Mycoplasma Susceptibility Testing Subcommittee of the Clinical and Laboratory Standards Institute has formulated agar and broth dilution methods. Most mycoplasmal infections are treated empirically.

Most *M. pneumoniae* infections are self-limited and usually do not require treatment. However, treatment can markedly shorten the illness, although complete eradication of the organism takes a long time, even after therapy. Because of the lack of a cell wall, *M. pneumoniae* as well as the other Mollicutes are innately resistant to all β-lactams. In addition they are resistant to sulfonamides, trimethoprim, and rifampin. Susceptibility patterns vary by species to macrolides and lincosamides. *M. pneumoniae* is usually susceptible to the macrolides, tetracycline, ketolides, and fluoroquinolones.

Unfortunately, the susceptibility of *M. hominis* and *U. urealyticum* to various agents is not as predictable. For the most part, the tetracyclines are the drugs of choice for these agents, although resistance has been reported.

Multidrug-resistant mycoplasmas and ureaplasmas have been identified in extragenital infections in immunocompromised patients. Treatment and clearance of these infections is extremely difficult and limited by the bacteriostatic concentrations of antimicrobials, as well as the slow growth and immune modulation associated with infections with these agents.

## PREVENTION

As of this writing, no vaccines have been developed for the mycoplasmas.

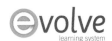 *Visit the Evolve site to complete the review questions.*

---

## CASE STUDY 45-1

A 29-year-old previously healthy female presented with a productive cough, fever to 102° F, and severe headache. She had cervical adenopathy (swollen glands), although she had a non-erythematous throat with no exudate. Chest examination showed crackles bilaterally at the lung base with decreased breath sounds diffusely. This finding was confirmed by chest film that showed bilateral multifocal areas of patchy consolidation. Her neck was not stiff, but because of the severity of the headache, she was admitted to the neurologic service. Spinal fluid was obtained and was negative for bacteria, *Cryptococcus*, and by acid-fast smear. No pathogens were isolated from blood and sputum cultures. The patient did not improve on ceftriaxone. On day 3 she was started on erythromycin. On day 4, cold agglutinins were done and were positive. The patient gradually improved, although the headache, photophobia, and cough continued for some time.

### QUESTIONS

1. What is the agent of this disease? Explain how the diagnosis was quickly made.
2. Can you explain why the bacterial cultures were negative?
3. Why is erythromycin an effective therapy for *M. pneumoniae,* but ceftriaxone is not?

---

## BIBLIOGRAPHY

Ainsworth JG, Katseni V, Hourshid S, et al: *Mycoplasma fermentans* and HIV-associated nephropathy, *J Infect* 29:323, 1994.

Bauer FA, Wear DJ, Angritt P, et al: *Mycoplasma fermentans* (incognitus strain) infection in the kidneys of patients with acquired immunodeficiency syndrome and associated nephropathy: a light microscopic, immunohistochemical and ultrastructural study, *Human Pathol* 22:63, 1991.

Goldenberg RL, Thompson BS: The infectious origins of stillbirth, *Am J Obstet Gynecol* 189:861-873, 2003.

Loens K, Ursi D, Goosens H, et al: Molecular diagnosis of *Mycoplasma pneumoniae* respiratory tract infections, *J Clin Microbiol* 4:4915, 2003.

Mandell GL, Bennett JE, Dolin R: *Principles and practices of infectious diseases*, ed 7, Philadelphia, 2010, Churchill-Livingston, Elsevier.

Mena L, Wang X, Mroczkowski TF, and Martin DH, et al: *Mycoplasma genitalium* infections in asymptomatic men and men with urethritis attending a sexually transmitted diseases clinic in New Orleans, *J Clin Infect Dis* 35:1167, 2001.

Montagnier L, Blanchard A: Mycoplasmas as cofactors in infection due to the human immunodeficiency virus, *Clin Infect Dis* 17 (suppl 1):S309, 1993.

Razin S, Yogev D, Naot V: Molecular biology and pathogenicity of mycoplasmas, *Microbiol Mol Biol Rev* 62:1094, 1998.

Sanchez P: Perinatal transmission of *Ureaplasma urealyticum:* current concepts based on review of the literature, *Clin Infect Dis* 17(suppl):S107, 1993.

Totten PA, Schwartz MA, Sjöström KE, et al: Association of *Mycoplasma genitalium* with nongonococcal urethritis in heterosexual men, *J Infect Dis* 183:269, 2001.

Versalovic J: *Manual of clinical microbiology,* ed 10, Washington, DC, 2011, ASM Press.

Waites KB, Bebear CM, Robertson JA, et al: Cumitech 34, Laboratory diagnosis of mycoplasmal infections. *Am Society Microbiology,* Washington, DC, 2001.

Waites KB, Talkington DF: *Mycoplasma pneumoniae* and its role as a human pathogen, *Clin Microbiol Rev* 17:697, 2004.

# The Spirochetes

## OBJECTIVES

1. Describe the bacterial agents discussed in this chapter in terms of morphology, taxonomy, and growth conditions.
2. Identify the four stages of syphilis (i.e., primary, secondary, latent, and tertiary) according to clinical symptoms, antibody production, transmission, and infectivity.
3. Explain congenital syphilis, including transmission and clinical manifestations.
4. Define reagin, cardiolipin, and biologic false positive.
5. Differentiate reagin and treponemal antibodies, including specificity and association with disease.
6. Identify the various serologic methods that utilize specific treponemal or nonspecific nontreponemal antigens.
7. Describe the basic principles for the RPR, VDRL, FTA-ABS, TP-PA, and MHA-TP assays.
8. Compare *Borrelia* spp. to the other spirochetes discussed in this chapter, including morphology and growth conditions.
9. Describe the pathogenesis for relapsing fever and Lyme disease, including the routes of transmission, vector, and disease presentation.
10. Explain the methodology and clinical significance for using a two-step diagnostic procedure for *Borrelia* spp. infections.
11. Describe the pathogenesis associated with leptospirosis, including the two major stages of the disease and the recommended clinical specimens.
12. Describe *Brachyspira* spp., including potential pathogenesis, appropriate specimen, transmission, and clinical significance.
13. Correlate patient signs and symptoms with laboratory data to identify the most likely etiologic agent.

---

### GENERA AND SPECIES TO BE CONSIDERED

*Treponema pallidum* subsp. *pallidum*
*Treponema pallidum* subsp. *pertenue*
*Treponema pallidum* subsp. *endemicum*
*Treponema carateum*
*Treponema denticola*
*Borrelia recurrentis*
*Borrelia burgdorferi sensu stricto*
*Borrelia garinii*
*Borrelia afzelii*
*Borrelia valaisiana*
*Brachyspira aalborgi*
*Brachyspira pilosicoli*
*Leptospira interrogans*

---

This chapter addresses the bacteria that belong in the order Spirochaetales. Although there are five genera in this family—the *Treponema, Borrelia, Brachyspira, Spirochaeta,* and *Leptospira*—only four are important in clinical diagnostics.

The spirochetes are all long, slender, helically curved, gram-negative bacilli, with the unusual morphologic features of axial fibrils and an outer sheath. These fibrils, or axial filaments, are flagella-like organelles that wrap around the bacteria's cell walls, are enclosed within the outer sheath, and facilitate motility of the organisms. The fibrils are attached within the cell wall by platelike structures, called *insertion disks,* located near the ends of the cells. The protoplasmic cylinder gyrates around the fibrils, causing bacterial movement to appear as a corkscrew-like winding. Differentiation of genera within the family Spirochaetaceae is based on the number of axial fibrils, the number of insertion disks present (Table 46-1), and biochemical and metabolic features. The spirochetes also fall into genera based loosely on their morphology (Figure 46-1): *Treponema* appear as slender with tight coils; *Borrelia* are somewhat thicker with fewer and looser coils; and *Leptospira* resemble *Borrelia* except for their hooked ends. *Brachyspira* are comma-shaped or helical, with tapered ends with four flagella at each end.

---

## TREPONEMA

### GENERAL CHARACTERISTICS

The major pathogens in the genus Treponema—*T. pallidum* subsp. *pallidum, T. pallidum* subsp. *pertenue, T. pallidum* subsp. *endemicum,* and *T. carateum*—infect humans and have not been cultivated for more than one passage in vitro. Most species stain poorly with Gram staining or Giemsa's methods and are best observed with the use of dark-field or phase-contrast microscopy. These organisms are considered to be microaerophilic.

Other treponemes such as *T. vincentii, T. denticola, T. refringens, T. socranskii,* and *T. pectinovorum* are normal inhabitants of the oral cavity or the human genital tract. These organisms are cultivable anaerobically on artificial media. Acute necrotizing ulcerative gingivitis, also known as Vincent's disease, is a destructive lesion of the gums. Methylene blue–stained material from the lesions of patients with Vincent's disease show certain morphologic types of bacteria. Observed morphologies include spirochetes and fusiforms; oral spirochetes, particularly an unusually large one, may be important in this disease, along with other anaerobes.

### EPIDEMIOLOGY AND PATHOGENESIS

Key features of the epidemiology of diseases caused by the pathogenic treponemes are summarized in Table 46-2. In general, these organisms enter the host by either penetrating intact mucous membranes (as is the case for *T. pallidum* subsp. *pallidum*—hereafter referred to as

**TABLE 46-1** Spirochetes Pathogenic for Humans

| Genus | Axial Filaments | Insertion Disks |
|---|---|---|
| Treponema | 6 to 10 | 1 |
| Borrelia | 30 to 40 | 2 |
| Leptospira | 2 | 3 to 5 |

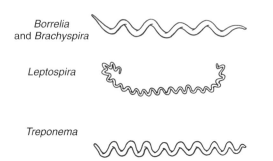

**Figure 46-1** Species designation of spirochetes based on morphology.

*T. pallidum*) or entering through breaks in the skin. *T. pallidum* is transmitted by sexual contact and vertically from mother to the unborn fetus. After penetration, *T. pallidum* subsequently invades the bloodstream and spreads to other body sites. Although the mechanisms by which damage is done to the host are unclear, *T. pallidum* has a remarkable tropism (attraction) to arterioles; infection ultimately leads to endarteritis (inflammation of the lining of arteries) and subsequent progressive tissue destruction.

## SPECTRUM OF DISEASE

*Treponema pallidum* causes venereal (transmitted through sexual contact) syphilis. The clinical presentation of venereal syphilis is varied and complex, often mimicking many other diseases. This disease is divided into stages: incubating, primary, secondary, early latent, latent, and tertiary. Primary syphilis is characterized by the appearance of a chancre (a painless ulcer) usually at the site of inoculation, most commonly the genitalia. Within 3 to 6 weeks, the chancre heals. Dissemination of the organism occurs during this primary stage; once the organism has reached a sufficient number (usually within 2 to 24 weeks), clinical manifestations of secondary syphilis become apparent. During this phase the patient is ill and seeks medical attention. Systemic symptoms such as fever, weight loss, malaise, and loss of appetite are present in about half of the patients. The skin is the organ most commonly affected in secondary syphilis, with patients having a widespread rash with generalized lymphadenopathy. Aseptic meningitis may also occur. After the secondary phase, the disease becomes subclinical but not necessarily dormant (inactive); during this *latent* period, diagnosis can be made using serologic methods. Relapses are common during early (≤ 1 year) latent syphilis. Late latent syphilis (≥ 1 year) is usually asymptomatic and

noninfectious. Tertiary syphilis is the tissue-destructive phase that appears 10 to 25 years after the initial infection in up to 35% of untreated patients. Complications of syphilis at this stage include central nervous disease (neurosyphilis), cardiovascular abnormalities, eye disease, and granuloma-like lesions, called *gummas*, found in the skin, bones, or visceral organs. Congenital syphilis is transmitted from mother to the unborn fetus during any stage of infection, but is most often associated with early syphilis. The unborn fetus may develop an asymptomatic infection or symptomatic infection with damage to the bone and teeth, deafness, neurosyphilis, or neonatal death.

The additional pathogenic treponemes are major health concerns in developing countries. Although morphologically and antigenically similar, these agents differ epidemiologically and with respect to their clinical presentation from *T. pallidum*. The diseases caused by these treponemes are summarized in Table 46-2.

## LABORATORY DIAGNOSIS

### Specimen Collection

Samples collected from ulcers and lesions should not be contaminated with blood, microorganisms, or tissue debris. The site should be cleansed with sterile gauze moistened with saline. The sample should be placed on a clean glass slide and cover slipped. Polymerase chain reaction (PCR) samples should be collected on a sterile Dacron or cotton swab and placed in a cryotube containing nucleic acid transport medium or universal transport medium. Tissue or needle aspirates of lymph nodes should be placed in 10% buffered formalin at room temperature. To test for congenital syphilis, a small section of the umbilical cord is collected and fixed in formalin or refrigerated until processed. Serum is the specimen of choice for serology; however, whole blood or plasma may be used in some assays.

### Direct Detection

Treponemes can be detected in material taken from skin lesions by dark-field examination or fluorescent antibody staining and microscopic examination. Material for microscopic examination is collected from suspicious lesions. The area around the lesion must first be cleansed with a sterile gauze pad moistened in saline. The surface of the ulcer is then abraded until some blood is expressed. After blotting the lesion until there is no further bleeding, the area is squeezed until serous fluid is expressed. The surface of a clean glass slide is touched to the exudate, allowed to air dry, and transported in a dust-free container for fluorescent antibody staining. A *T. pallidum* fluorescein-labeled antibody is commercially available for staining (Viro Stat, Portland, Maine). For dark-field examination, the expressed fluid is aspirated using a sterile pipette, dropped onto a clean glass slide, and cover slipped. The slide containing material for dark-field examination must be transported to the laboratory immediately. Because positive lesions may be teeming with viable spirochetes that are highly infectious, all supplies and patient specimens must be handled with

**TABLE 46-2** Epidemiology and Spectrum of Disease of the Treponemes Pathogenic for Humans

| Agent | Transmission | Geographic Location | Disease | Clinical Manifestations* | Age Group |
|---|---|---|---|---|---|
| *T. pallidum* subsp. *pallidum* | Sexual contact or congenital (mother to fetus) | Worldwide | Venereal syphilis[†] | Refer to text in this chapter | All ages |
| *T. pallidum* subsp. *pertenue* | Traumatized skin comes in contact with an infected lesion (person-to-person contact) | Humid, warm climates: Africa, South and Central America, Pacific Islands | Yaws | Skin—papules,[†] nodules, ulcers<br><br>Primary lesion (mother yaw), disseminated lesions (frambesia)<br><br>May progress to latent stage and late infection involving destructive lesions to bone and cartilage | Children |
| *T. pallidum* subsp. *endemicum* | Mouth to mouth by utensils, (person-to-person contact) | Arid, warm climates: North Africa, Southeast Asia, Middle East | Endemic nonvenereal syphilis | Skin/mucous patches, papules, macules, ulcers, scars[†]<br><br>May progress to disseminated oropharyngeal with generalized lymphadenopathy<br><br>May demonstrate a latent stage, and late syphilis destructive to skin, bone, and cartilage | Children or adults; rarely congenital |
| *T. carateum* | Traumatized skin comes in contact with an infected lesion (person-to-person contact) | Semiarid, warm climates: Central and South America, Mexico | Pinta | Skin papules, macules. Hyperkeratotic pigmented may lead to disseminated skin lesions and lymphadenopathy; late stage may result in pigmentary changes in skin (hyper- or hypopigmentation) | All ages but primarily children and adolescents |

*All diseases have a relapsing clinical course and prominent cutaneous manifestations.
[†]If untreated, organisms can disseminate to other parts of the body such as bone.

extreme caution and carefully discarded as required for contaminated materials. Gloves should always be worn.

Material for dark-field examination is examined immediately under 400× high-dry magnification for the presence of motile spirochetes. Treponemes are long (8 to 10 μm, slightly larger than a red blood cell) and consist of 8 to 14 tightly coiled, even spirals (Figure 46-2). Once seen, characteristic forms should be verified by examination under oil immersion magnification (1000×). Although the darkfield examination depends greatly on technical expertise and the numbers of organisms in the lesion, it can be highly specific when performed on genital lesions.

Lesion exudates or tissue samples may be used for direct fluorescent antibody detection for *T. pallidum* (DFA-TP). DFA-TP visualizes specimens on slides with fluorescein isothiocyanate (FITC) labeled antibodies. Polyclonal and monoclonal antibodies may be used; however, the Food and Drug Administration (FDA) in the United States has not approved this test.

## Molecular Diagnostics

Although molecular diagnostic assays are not currently available within many clinical laboratories, several methods have been developed using PCR for the detection of *T. pallidum*. These methods are primarily useful in the identification of organisms within exudate or lesions.

## Serodiagnosis

Serologic tests for treponematosis measure the presence of two types of antibodies: treponemal and nontreponemal. Treponemal antibodies are produced against antigens of the organisms themselves, whereas nontreponemal antibodies, often referred to as *reagin* antibodies, are produced in infected patients against components of mammalian cells. Reaginic antibodies, although almost always produced in patients with syphilis, are also produced in patients with other infectious diseases such as leprosy, tuberculosis, chancroid, leptospirosis, malaria, rickettsial disease, trypanosomiasis, lymphogranuloma venereum (LGV), measles, chickenpox, hepatitis, and infectious mononucleosis; noninfectious conditions such as drug addiction; autoimmune disorders, including rheumatoid disease and systemic lupus erythematosus; and in conjunction with increasing age, pregnancy, and recent immunization.

The two most widely used nontreponemal serologic tests are the Venereal Disease Research Laboratory (VDRL) and rapid plasma reagin (RPR) tests. Each of

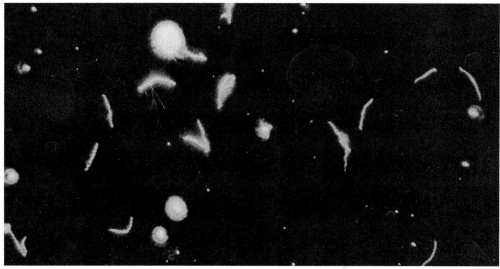

**Figure 46-2** Appearance of *Treponema pallidum* in dark-field preparation.

these tests is a flocculation (or agglutination) test, in which soluble antigen particles are coalesced to form larger particles that are visible as clumps when they are aggregated in the presence of antibody. The VDRL is used as a quantitative test and may be performed on serum or CSF in suspected cases of neurosyphilis. See Procedures 46-1 and 46-2 on the Evolve site for details and limitations for the VDRL and RPR.

Specific treponemal serologic tests include automated enzyme immunoassays (EIAs) and agglutination tests, such as the *T. pallidum* particle agglutination (TP-PA) test, the microhemagglutination assay (MHA-TP), *T. pallidum* indirect hemagglutination (TPHA), particle gel immunoassay (PaGIA), and the fluorescent treponemal antibody absorption (FTA-ABS) test. Once positive, their usefulness is limited because these tests tend to yield positive results throughout the patient's life. The FTA-ABS test is performed by overlaying whole treponemes fixed to a slide with serum from patients suspected of having syphilis. This test is typically performed following a positive VDRL or RPR screening test. The patient's serum is first absorbed with non–*T. pallidum* treponemal antigens (sorbent) to reduce nonspecific cross-reactivity. Fluorescein-conjugated antihuman antibody reagent is then applied as a marker for specific antitreponemal antibodies in the patient's serum. This test should not be used as a primary screening procedure. TP-PA (Fujirebio America, Fairfield, New Jersey) tests utilize gelatin particles sensitized with *T. pallidum* subsp. *pallidum* antigens. Serum samples are diluted in a microtiter plate and sensitized gelatin particles are added. The presence of specific antibody causes the gelatin particles to agglutinate and form a flat mat across the bottom of the microdilution well in which the test is performed. The MHA-TP is a passive hemagglutination assay of sensitized erythrocytes that are tested against the patient's serum. Agglutination indicates the presence of IgG or IgM antitreponemal antibodies in the patient's serum. TPHA is an indirect hemagglutination assay that uses sensitized red blood cells that aggregate when exposed to positive

patient serum. This test is similar to the MHA-TP. PaGIA test, which uses gel immunoassay technology, an established method in blood group serology. The assay contains recombinant antigens for the detection of *T. pallidum* antibodies in the patient's serum or plasma. The results are available in approximately 15 minutes. Several EIAs are available that utilize the direct, indirect sandwich, or competitive assay methodology. EIAs use recombinant antigens to detect IgM, IgG, or both. To date, no evidence indicates that these assays are more sensitive than the traditional treponeme tests. The Centers for Disease Control and Prevention (CDC) is currently evaluating rapid testing formats for syphilis that use lateral flow or flow through cassette methodology.

Several automated systems currently exist that use bead-capture technology. These assays use a capture antibody attached to a suspension of small micro polystyrene beads. The beads are dyed with fluorophores of differing intensity, giving each a unique fingerprint. The sandwich immunoassay uses a flow cytometry dual-laser system for detection. There are currently three Luminex commercial platforms that utilize this technology; Abbott Architect (Abbott Laboratories, Abbott Park, Illinois), Bio-Rad Bioplex (Bio-Rad Laboratories, Hercules, California), and Zeus AtheNA (Zeus Scientific, Branchburg, New Jersey). A fourth system, the DiaSorin Liaison (DiaSorin S.p.A., Vercelli, Italy) uses magnetic beads to capture patient antibodies with an isoluminol-antigen conjugate. Positive samples are then detected using a flash-chemiluminescent signal.

The nontreponemal serologic tests for syphilis can be used to determine antibody quantitative titers, which are useful to follow the patient's response to therapy. The relative sensitivity of each test is shown in Table 46-3 to confirm that a positive nontreponemal test result is due to syphilis rather than to one of the other infections or biologic false-positive conditions previously mentioned. Traditional diagnosis for syphilis is useful in active infections. However, early or treated infections may be incorrectly diagnosed. In addition, primary

**TABLE 46-3** Sensitivity of Commonly Used Serologic Tests for Syphilis

| METHOD | STAGE | | |
|---|---|---|---|
| | Primary | Secondary | Late |
| **Nontreponemal (Reaginic Tests)—Screening**<br>Venereal Disease Research Laboratory (reaginic) test (VDRL) | 70% | 99% | 60%-98% |
| Rapid plasma-reagin (RPR) card test and automated reagin test (ART) | 80% | 99% | 60%-98% |
| **Specific Treponemal Tests—Confirmatory**<br>Fluorescent treponemal antibody absorption test (FTA-ABS, TP-PA, TPHA, MHA-TP, EIA, PaGIA) | 85% | 100% | 98% |

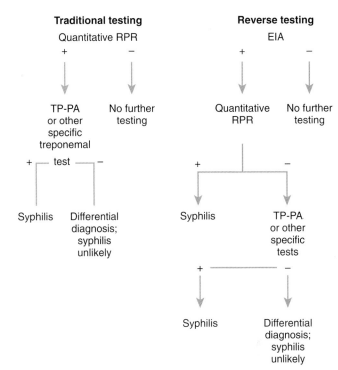

**Figure 46-3** Traditional testing versus reverse testing.

testing using RPR or VDRL may result in a high rate of false-positives. The Centers for Disease Control has recommended a reverse algorithm to detect early primary or treated infections that may be missed using traditional nonspecific screening methods. Reverse testing suggests the use of specific antibody testing for syphilis, using enzyme-linked immunoassay (EIA) for IgM and IgG or a similar technique. *T. pallidum* antibodies persist for many years following infection. Specific tests may then be followed by nonspecific screening tests, which become less reactive over time. However, reverse testing is not currently widely accepted, and more data are needed to resolve clinical diagnostic discrepancies (Figure 46-3).

## ANTIMICROBIAL SUSCEPTIBILITY TESTING AND THERAPY

Because the treponemes cannot be cultivated, susceptibility testing is not performed. For all treponemal infections, penicillin G is the drug of choice. Ceftriaxone is also highly active in most cases of syphilis other than early syphilis. Tetracycline or doxycycline is often the treatment of choice when patients are allergic to penicillin. Treatment varies depending on the stage of disease and the host (e.g., children or adults, HIV-infected or infected with congenital syphilis).

## PREVENTION

No vaccines are available for the treponematoses. Prevention is best accomplished by early and appropriate treatment, thereby preventing person-to-person spread.

# BORRELIA

## GENERAL CHARACTERISTICS

Borreliosis is considered a relapsing fever that is transmitted by a human-specific body louse or a tick. Organisms

belonging to the genus *Borrelia* are composed of 3 to 10 loose coils (see Figure 46-1) and are actively motile. They contain endoflagella located beneath the outer membrane. The cells contain a protoplasmic cylinder that is composed of a peptidoglycan layer and an inner membrane. In contrast to the treponemes, *Borrelia* spp. stain well with Giemsa's stain. Species that have been grown in vitro are microaerophilic or anaerobic.

## EPIDEMIOLOGY AND PATHOGENESIS

Although pathogens for mammals and birds, *Borrelia* are the causative agents of tickborne and louseborne relapsing fever and tickborne Lyme disease in humans.

### Relapsing Fever

Human relapsing fever is caused by more than 15 species of *Borrelia* and is transmitted to humans by the bite of a louse or tick. *B. recurrentis* is responsible for louseborne or epidemic relapsing fever. This spirochete is transmitted from the louse *Pediculus humanus* subsp. *humanus* and disease is found worldwide; humans are the only reservoir for *B. recurrentis*. All other borreliae that cause disease in the United States are transmitted via tick bites and are named after the species of tick, usually of the genus *Ornithodoros* (soft tick), from which they are recovered. Common species in the United States include *B. hermsii*, *B. turicatae*, *B. parkeri*, and *B. mazzottii*. Depending on the organisms and the disease, their reservoir is either humans or rodents in most cases. Although their pathogenic mechanisms are unclear, these spirochetes exhibit antigenic variability that may account for the cyclic fever patterns associated with this disease.

### Lyme Disease

Although there are currently at least 10 different *Borrelia* species within the *B. burgdorferi* sensu lato complex, only *Borrelia burgdorferi* sensu stricto (strict sense of *B. burgdorferi*) as well as *B. garinii*, *B. afzelii*, *B. spielmanii*, *B. lusitaniae*, and *B. valaisiana* are agents of Lyme disease and are transmitted by the bite of *Ixodes* ticks. Lyme disease is the most common vector-borne disease in North America and Europe and is an emerging problem in northern Asia. Hard ticks, belonging primarily to the genus *Ixodes*, act as vectors in the United States, including *Ixodes pacificus* in California and *I. scapularis* in other areas. The ticks' natural hosts are deer and rodents. However, the adult ticks will feed on a variety of mammals including raccoons, domestic and wild carnivores, and birds. The ticks will attach to pets as well as to humans; all stages of ticks—larva, nymph, and adult—can harbor the spirochete and transmit disease. The nymphal form of the tick is most likely to transmit disease because it is active in the spring and summer when people are dressed lightly and participating in outdoor activities in the woods. At this stage the tick is the size of a pinhead and the initial tick bite may be overlooked. Ticks require a period of attachment of at least 24 hours before they transmit disease. Endemic areas of disease have been identified in many states, including Massachusetts, Connecticut, Maryland, Minnesota, Oregon, and California, as well as in Europe, Russia, Japan, and Australia. Direct invasion of tissues by the organism is responsible for the clinical manifestations. However, IgM antibodies are produced continually months to years after initial infection as the spirochete changes its antigens. *B. burgdorferi*'s potential ability to induce an autoimmune process in the host because of cross-reactive antigens may contribute to the pathology associated with Lyme disease. Moreover, by virtue of its ability to vary its surface antigens (e.g., outer surface protein [Osp] A to G) as well as avoid complement attack, *B. burgdorferi* is able to avoid the human host response. The pathologic findings associated with Lyme disease are also believed to be due to the release of host cytokines initiated by the presence of the organism.

## SPECTRUM OF DISEASE

### Relapsing Fever

Two to 15 days following infection, patients have an abrupt onset of fever, headache, and myalgia that lasts for 4 to 10 days. Physical findings often include petechiae, diffuse abdominal tenderness, and conjunctival effusion. As the host produces specific antibody in response to the agent, organisms disappear from the bloodstream, becoming sequestered (hidden) in different organs during the afebrile period. Subsequently, organisms reemerge with newly modified antigens and multiply, resulting in another febrile period. Subsequent relapses are usually milder and of shorter duration. Generally, more relapses are associated with cases of untreated tickborne relapsing fever, but louseborne relapsing fevers tend to be more severe.

Treatment of relapsing fever with antibiotics may result in the formation of the Jarisch-Herxheimer

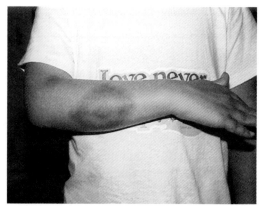

**Figure 46-4** Appearance of the classic erythema migrans lesion of acute Lyme disease.

reaction. This reaction is associated with the clearance of the organisms from the bloodstream and release of cytokines within hours of antibiotic treatment. The patient experiences tachycardia, chills, rigors, hypotension, fever, and diaphoresis. Death may be associated with the reaction. An acute respiratory distress syndrome has also been recognized in cases associated with tickborne relapsing fever.

### Lyme Disease

Lyme disease is characterized by three stages, not all of which occur in any given patient. The first stage, erythema migrans (EM), is the characteristic red, ring-shaped skin lesion with a central clearing that first appears at the site of the tick bite but may develop at distant sites as well (Figure 46-4). Patients may experience headache, fever, muscle and joint pain, and malaise during this stage. The second stage, beginning weeks to months after infection, may include arthritis, but the most important features are neurologic disorders (i.e., meningitis, neurologic deficits) and carditis. This is a result of the hematogenous spread of spirochetes to organs and tissues. In addition, neurologic symptoms and infection may occur in the meninges, spinal cord, peripheral nerves, and brain. The third stage is usually characterized by chronic arthritis or acrodermatitis chronica atrophicans (ACA), a diffuse skin rash, and may continue for years. There is an association between *Borrelia* species and distinct clinical manifestations. For example, *B. garinii* has been associated with up to 72% of European cases of neuroborreliosis.

## LABORATORY DIAGNOSIS

### Specimen Collection, Transport, and Processing

Peripheral blood is the specimen of choice for direct detection of borreliae that cause relapsing fever. *Borrelia burgdorferi* can be visualized and cultured, although serology is considered the best means to diagnose Lyme disease. Specimens submitted for stain or culture include blood, biopsy specimens, and body fluids including joint and cerebrospinal fluids. Body fluids should be transported without any preservatives. Tissue biopsy specimens should be placed in sterile saline to prevent drying.

## Direct Detection Methods

**Relapsing Fever.** Clinical laboratories rely on direct observation of the organism in peripheral blood from patients for diagnosis. Organisms can be found in 70% of cases when blood specimens from febrile patients are examined. The organisms can be seen directly in wet preparations of peripheral blood (mixed with equal parts of sterile, nonbacteriostatic saline) under dark- or bright-field illumination, in which the spirochetes move rapidly, often pushing the red blood cells around. The organisms may also be visualized by staining thick and thin films with Wright's or Giemsa stains using procedures similar to those used to detect malaria.

**Lyme Disease.** *B. burgdorferi* may be visualized in tissue sections stained with Warthin-Starry silver stain. In general, the number of spirochetes in blood of patients with Lyme borreliosis is below the lower limits of microscopic detection. Polymerase chain reaction (PCR) has become important in diagnosing Lyme disease. PCR has detected *B. burgdorferi* DNA in clinical specimens from patients with early and late clinical manifestations; optimal specimens include urine, synovial tissue, synovial fluid, and skin biopsies from patients with EM. Laboratories have used a variety of molecular methods to increase sensitivity and specificity and decrease turnaround time for diagnosing Lyme borreliosis. PCR has confirmed EM with an overall sensitivity and specificity of 68% and 100%, respectively. The ability to detect spirochetes in blood or plasma by PCR is dependent on the stage of illness (from 40% of patients with secondary EM to only 9.5% of patients with primary EM); PCR also does relatively well in detecting *B. burgdorferi* sensu lato in synovial fluids. In contrast, variable results using PCR have been achieved in cerebrospinal fluid (CSF) specimens obtained from patients with peripheral or central nervous system involvement with Lyme borreliosis; overall sensitivity is only in the range of 20%.

## Cultivation

Although the organisms that cause relapsing fever can be cultured in nutritionally rich media under microaerobic conditions, the procedures are cumbersome and unreliable and are used primarily as research tools. Similarly, the culture of *B. burgdorferi* may be attempted, although the yield is low. The best specimens for culture in untreated patients include the peripheral area of the EM ring lesion or synovial tissue. CSF and blood or plasma (greater than 9 mL) in general are of low diagnostic yield by culture or PCR. This seems to correlate with the duration of the neurologic disease—in other words, positive results decrease as the duration of the disease increases. To cultivate the organism, the plasma, spinal fluid sediment, or macerated tissue biopsy is inoculated into a tube of modified Kelly's medium (BSK II, BSK-H, or Preac-Mursic) and incubated at 30° to 34° C for up to 12 weeks under microaerophilic conditions. Blind subcultures (0.1 mL) are performed weekly from the lower portion of the broth to fresh media, and the cultures are examined by dark-field microscopy or by fluorescence microscopy after staining with acridine orange for the presence of spirochetes. Because of the long incubation time and low sensitivity associated with cultivation, cultivation is often confined to reference or research laboratories.

## Serodiagnosis

**Relapsing Fever.** Serologic tests for relapsing fever have not demonstrated reproducible or reliable data for diagnosis because of the many antigenic shifts *Borrelia* organisms undergo during the course of disease. Protein heterogeneity in strains of different species is quite variable. For example, the OspC protein has 21 major recognized antigenic types. In addition, patients may exhibit increased titers to Proteus OX K antigens (up to 1:80), but other cross-reacting antibodies are rare. Certain reference laboratories, such as those at the Centers for Disease Control and Prevention (CDC), may perform special serologic procedures on sera from selected patients.

**Lyme Disease.** Despite its inadequacies, serology continues to be the standard for the diagnosis of Lyme disease. *B. burgdorferi* has numerous immunogenic lipids, proteins, lipoproteins, and carbohydrate antigens on its surface and outer membrane. The earliest antibody response and development of IgM is in response to the OspC membrane protein, the flagellar antigens (FlaA and FlaB), or the fibronectin binding protein (BBK32). The IgM levels peak within several weeks but may be detectable for several months. The IgG response develops slowly during the first several weeks of disease and increases with antibody responses to Osp17 (decorin-binding protein) and additional proteins including p39 (BmpA) and p58. The late-stage infection demonstrates IgG antibodies to numerous antigens.

Numerous serologic tests are commercially available; however, these tests have not yet been standardized, and their performance characteristics vary greatly. The most common of these tests are the indirect immunofluorescence assay (IFA), the enzyme-linked immunosorbent assay (ELISA), and Western blot. Measuring antibody by enzyme-linked immunosorbent assay (ELISA) is the primary screening method because it is quick, reproducible, and relatively inexpensive. However, false-positive rates are high, mainly as a result of cross-reactivity. The specificity of IFA may be improved by adsorption of serum with *Treponema phagedenis* sonicate (IFA-ABS). Patients with syphilis, HIV infection, leptospirosis, mononucleosis, parvovirus infection, rheumatoid arthritis, and other autoimmune diseases commonly show positive results. Capture EIAs have been developed to avoid false positive reactions with rheumatoid factor. In addition, this may be overcome by pretreatment of the patient's sera with anti-IgG. For the United States, the CDC recommends a two-step approach to the serologic diagnosis of Lyme disease. The first step is to use a sensitive screening test such as an ELISA or IFA; if this test is positive or equivocal, the result must be confirmed by immunoblotting (Figure 46-5). In certain clinical situations, results of serologic tests must be interpreted with caution. For example, patients with Lyme arthritis frequently remain antibody-positive despite treatment but do not

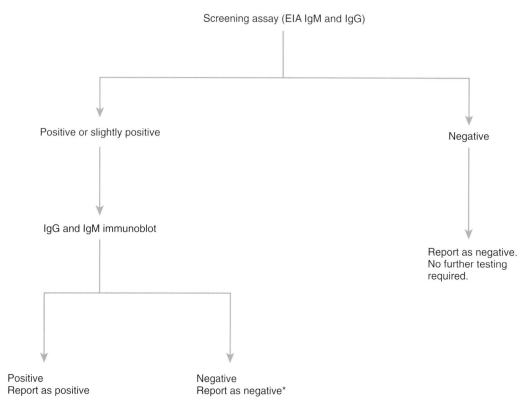

**Figure 46-5** Two-step serodiagnostic procedure. *Note: If neuroborreliosis is suspected, a paired sera and CSF specimen is recommended for testing. Any disease of short duration. For Lyme disease, it is recommended that a follow-up serologic test be performed at a later date. (Modified from Versalovic J: *Manual of clinical microbiology,* ed 10, Washington, DC, 2011, ASM Press.)

necessarily have persistent infection. Conversely, patients with a localized EM may be seronegative. Because of these limitations and others, the Food and Drug Administration (FDA) and the American College of Physicians have published guidelines regarding the use of laboratory tests for Lyme disease diagnosis. Of paramount importance is the clinician's determination before ordering serologic tests of the pretest probability of Lyme disease based on clinical symptoms and the incidence of Lyme disease in the population represented by the patient.

### Molecular Diagnostics

A variety of molecular methods have been developed for the diagnosis of borreliae infections. These methods have been used on blood, body fluids, and tissue specimens. Nucleic acid based methods are typically not available in routine clinical laboratories.

## ANTIBIOTIC SUSCEPTIBILITY TESTING AND THERAPY

Currently there are no standardized methods and borreliae are difficult to culture; therefore, antimicrobial susceptibility testing is not routinely performed.

Several antibiotics, including tetracycline, are effective in treating relapsing fever. Doxycycline, amoxicillin, or cefuroxime and parenteral cephalosporins are drugs of choice during the first stage of Lyme disease. Broad-spectrum cephalosporins, particularly ceftriaxone or cefotaxime, have been used successfully with patients who either fail initial treatment or present in later stages of the disease. Oral regimes are typically successful; however, in atrioventicular blocks, the patient may require IV therapy. Symptomatic treatment failures, particularly in patients with chronic Lyme disease, have been reported.

## PREVENTION

A recombinant outer surface protein A vaccine has been licensed for use in humans against Lyme disease caused by infection with organisms belonging to the *B. burgdorferi* complex. Although many issues surrounding vaccine use remain unsettled, the vaccine is expected to be in widespread use in endemic areas. Avoiding tick-infested areas; wearing protective clothing; checking your clothing, body, and pets for ticks; and removing them promptly will also assist in the prevention of infection. There are no vaccines against infections caused by other *Borrelia* spp.

# BRACHYSPIRA

## GENERAL CHARACTERISTICS

*Brachyspira aalborgi* requires anaerobic incubation and has not been isolated from animals, whereas *B. pilosicoli* colonizes the intestine of a variety of animal species. The organisms reside in the brush border within the intestine and appear as a "false brush border" upon histologic staining with hematoxylin and eosin.

## EPIDEMIOLOGY AND PATHOGENESIS

*B. aalborgi* is most likely transmitted via fecal-oral contamination. *B. pilosicoli* infection results from ingesting water contaminated with feces from infected animals. No pathogenic mechanisms have been identified; therefore, clinical significance must be carefully correlated with patient signs and symptoms.

## LABORATORY DIAGNOSIS

### Specimen Collection and Direct Detection

Fresh stool or rectal swabs may be collected and examined by dark-field microscopy. Additionally, tissue biopsy specimens may be submitted for histologic examination using periodic acid-Schiff (PAS) or hematoxylin and eosin staining. PCR amplification methods have been developed but are not available within the clinical laboratory.

### Cultivation

*Brachyspira* spp. can be grown in the laboratory on brain heart infusion (BHI) or tryptic soy agar containing 10% F bovine blood, 400 μg/mL of spectinomycin, and 5 μg/mL polymyxin in anaerobic conditions at 37° C. *B. aalborgi* is weakly beta-hemolytic on BHI medium.

### Approach to Identification

*B. aalborgi* can be differentiated from *B. pilosicoli* by a strong positive hippurate hydrolysis reaction and a weak indole reaction. *B. pilosicoli* is indole negative and has a weak hippurate hydrolysis reaction.

## ANTIBIOTIC SUSCEPTIBILITY AND THERAPY

Isolates of *B. pilosicoli* have demonstrated susceptibility to Augmentin (amoxicillin-clavulanic acid), ceftriaxone, chloramphenicol, meropenem, tetracycline, and metronidazole.

# LEPTOSPIRA

## GENERAL CHARACTERISTICS

The leptospires include both free-living and parasitic forms. The organisms are spiral-shaped, right-handed helices with hooked ends. The organisms contain two axial filaments and exhibit either a spinning motility or a rapid back-and-forth movement. *Leptospira* species are typically classified into two major groups, with *Leptospira interrogans* sensu stricto being the main species associated with human leptospirosis; in France, this organism is responsible for about 60% of human cases. *Leptospira biflexa* contains the saprophytic environmental strains. Molecular classification using 16srRNA sequencing currently separates the genus into three distinct groups of pathogens, environmental saprophytes, and other species of uncertain pathogenicity.

The pathogens include more than 260 serologically defined types that were formerly designated as species and are now referred to as serovars, or serotypes, of *L. interrogans* sensu stricto. Each serovar is usually associated with a particular animal host and therefore serovar identification is important for epidemiology studies and prevention strategies. The genotypic classification scheme now includes approximately 20 species, which incorporates all current serovars. Serovars cross species lines as a result of the horizontal transfer of genetic elements, making it difficult to fully classify species phenotypically.

## EPIDEMIOLOGY AND PATHOGENESIS

Leptospirosis, a zoonosis, has a worldwide distribution but is most common in developing countries and warm climates where contact with infected animals or water contaminated with urine is likely to occur. *L. interrogans* can infect most mammals throughout the world, as well as reptiles, amphibians, fish, birds, and invertebrates. The organism is maintained in nature by virtue of persistent colonization of renal tubules of carrier animals. Humans become infected through direct or indirect contact with the urine or blood of infected animals. Leptospires enter the human host through breaks in the skin, mucous membranes, or conjunctivae. Infection can be acquired in home and recreational settings (e.g., swimming, hunting, canoeing) or in people who work in certain occupational settings (e.g., farmers, ranchers, abattoir workers, trappers, veterinarians).

Pathogenic leptospires rapidly invade the bloodstream after entry and spread throughout all sites in the body such as the central nervous system and kidneys. Virulent strains show chemotaxis toward hemoglobin as well as the ability to migrate through host tissues. A number of potential virulence factors that might facilitate this process are shown in Box 46-1. Precisely how *L. interrogans* causes disease is not completely understood, but it appears that the presence of endotoxin and other toxins may play a role in which hemostasis pathways are activated as is an autoimmune response in the human host.

## SPECTRUM OF DISEASE

Symptoms begin abruptly 2 to 20 days after infection and include fever, headache, and myalgia. The most common

---

**BOX 46-1** Potential Virulence Factors of *Leptospira*

Hemolysins
Sphingomyelinases C and H
Fibronectin-binding protein for adhesion and invasion
Lipopolysaccharide and outer membrane proteins

clinical syndrome is anicteric leptospirosis, which is a self-limiting illness consisting of a septicemic stage, with high fever and severe headache that lasts 3 to 7 days, followed by the immune stage. Symptoms associated with the immune stage (onset coincides with the appearance of IgM) are varied but in general are milder than those associated with the septicemic stage. The hallmark of the immune stage is aseptic meningitis. Weil's disease, or icteric leptospirosis, is generally the most severe illness, with symptoms caused by liver, kidney, or vascular dysfunction with lethal pulmonary hemorrhage; death can occur in up to 10% of cases. Unfortunately, the clinical presentations of leptospirosis mimic those of many other diseases.

## LABORATORY DIAGNOSIS

### Specimen Collection, Transport, and Processing

During the first 10 days of illness, leptospires are present in the blood, CSF, and peritoneal dialysate. Urine specimens can be obtained beginning in the second week of illness and up to 30 days after the onset of symptoms. Specimens may be collected in citrate, heparin, or oxalate anticoagulants. There are no other special requirements for specimen collection, transport, or processing. Citrate or ethylenedaminetetraacetic acid (EDTA) is the preferred anticoagulant for molecular testing. Urine specimens should not be placed in preservatives and should be processed within 1 hour for optimal results. Specimens should be transported at room temperature and inoculated for culture within 24 hours.

### Direct Detection

Blood, CSF, and urine may be examined directly by dark-field microscopy examination. Detection of motile leptospires in these specimens is optimized following centrifuging at 1500× g for 30 minutes; sodium oxalate or heparin-treated blood is initially spun at 500× g for 15 minutes to remove blood cells. Other techniques, such as fluorescent antibody staining and hybridization techniques using leptospira-specific DNA probes, have also detected leptospires in clinical specimens. Conventional and real-time PCR assays have been used to detect leptospires in clinical and environmental samples.

### Molecular Diagnostics

Several nucleic acid–based amplification methods have been developed. Studies indicate that the sensitivity is comparable to paired sera testing using serologic methods. These methods are not readily available in routine clinical laboratories. However, PCR methodologies are not useful for the differentiation of serovars and therefore are of limited utility in epidemiologic studies. Highly complex and labor-intensive techniques such as pulsed field electrophoresis (PFGE) and restriction fragment length polymorphism (RFLP) are more useful for the identification of serovars.

### Cultivation

Albeit insensitive, the definitive method for laboratory diagnosis of leptospirosis is to culture the organisms from blood, CSF, or urine. A few drops of heparinized or sodium oxalate–anticoagulated blood are inoculated into tubes of semisolid media enriched with rabbit serum (Fletcher's or Stuart's) or bovine serum albumin. Urine should be inoculated soon after collection, because acidity (diluted out in the broth medium) may harm the spirochetes. One or 2 drops of undiluted urine and a 1:10 dilution of urine are added to 5 mL of medium. The addition of 200 µg/mL of 5-fluorouracil (an anticancer drug) may prevent contamination by other bacteria without harming the leptospires. Commercial media such as Ellinghausen-McCullough-Johnson-Harris (EMJH) or Fletcher's Medicum (Difco EMJH or Difco Fletcher's medium; BD Diagnostic Systems, Sparks, Maryland) are available that contain 5-fluorouracil for use at the patient's bedside. Tissue specimens, especially from the liver and kidney, may be aseptically macerated and inoculated in dilutions of 1:1, 1:10, and 1:100 as for urine cultures.

All cultures are incubated at room temperature or 30° C in the dark for up to 6 to 8 weeks. Because organisms grow below the surface, material collected from a few centimeters below the surface of broth cultures should be examined weekly for the presence of growth, using a direct wet preparation under dark-field illumination. Leptospires exhibit corkscrew-like motility.

### Approach to Identification

Based on the number of coils and hooked ends, leptospires can be distinguished from other spirochetes. Physiologically, the saprophytes can be differentiated from pathogens by their ability to grow to 10° C and lower, or at least 5° C lower than the growth temperature of pathogenic leptospires. Leptospires may also be visualized using dark-field or immunofluorescence.

### Serodiagnosis

Serodiagnosis of leptospirosis requires a fourfold or greater rise in titer of agglutinating antibodies. The microscopic agglutination (MA) test using live cells is the standard serologic procedure. Serologic diagnosis of leptospirosis is performed using pools of bacterial antigens containing many serotypes in each pool. Positive results are indicated by the presence of agglutination using dark-field microscopy. However, a macroscopic agglutination procedure is more readily accessible to routine clinical laboratories. Reagents are available commercially. Indirect hemagglutination and an ELISA test for IgM antibody are also available; IgM-detection assays are primarily used because IgM antibodies become detectable during the first week of illness.

### Molecular Testing

Recently several nucleic acid-based testing methods have been developed for detection of Leptospires. These techniques include traditional PCR, real-time PCR, and loop-mediated isothermal amplification. To date, no commercial molecular assays are available for diagnostic use.

## ANTIBIOTIC SUSCEPTIBILITY AND THERAPY

Treatment of leptospirosis is supportive management and the use of appropriate antibiotics. Ceftriaxone, penicillin, amoxicillin, doxycycline, and tetracycline are recommended for treatment of leptospirosis. Standardized procedures for antibiotic susceptibility are limited by the slow growth of the organisms and the need for serum during cultivation.

# PREVENTION

General preventive measures include the vaccination of domestic livestock and pet dogs. In addition, protective clothing, rodent control measures, and preventing recreational exposures, such as avoiding freshwater ponds, are indicated in preventing leptospirosis.

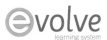 **Visit the Evolve site to complete the review questions.**

---

## CASE STUDY 46-1

A 43-year-old woman was referred to the infectious disease clinic for recurrent symptoms beginning about 4 months after she noticed a painful, swollen spot on her leg after removal of a tick. She had been treated with doxycycline for 14 days for presumed Lyme disease, documented by a positive IFA titer and presentation with migratory arthralgias, which were worse in the small joints of the hands. She also complained of fatigue, poor mentation, and occasional headaches. Because her symptoms recurred 2 months after treatment, she was unable to continue employment. Six months after a course of amoxicillin and later two courses of ceftriaxone, she again became symptomatic. A Western blot and PCR of her serum were ordered. The Western blot result was equivocal, but the PCR was positive for the agent of Lyme disease.

### QUESTIONS

1. How did this patient acquire Lyme disease?
2. Why did the physician order further testing to diagnose Lyme disease in this patient?
3. Our patient did not respond to therapy for *B. burgdorferi*. Can you explain why this can happen?

---

# BIBLIOGRAPHY

Aguero-Rosenfeld ME, Wang G, Schwartz I, et al: Diagnosis of Lyme borreliosis, *Clin Microbiol Rev* 18:484, 2005.

Bharti AR, Nally JE, Ricaldi JN, et al: Leptospirosis: a zoonotic disease of global importance, *Lancet Infect Dis* 3:757, 2003.

Centers for Disease Control: Discordant results from reverse sequence syphilis screening—five laboratories, United States, 2006-2010, *MMWR* 60(05):133-137, 2011.

Centers for Disease Control and Prevention: Sexually transmitted diseases treatment guidelines, *Morb Mortal Wkly Rep* 51:18, 2002.

Dummler JS: Molecular diagnosis of Lyme disease, *Mol Diagn* 6:1, 2001.

Erlandson KM, Klingler ET: Intestinal spirochetosis: epidemiology, microbiology and clinical significance, *Clin Microbiol Newsl* 27:91, 2005.

Li SJ, Zhang CC, Li XW et al: Molecular typing of Leptospira interrogans strains isolated from *Rattus tanezumi* in Guizhous province, southwest China, *Biomed Environ Sci* 25(5):542-548, 2012.

Mandell GL, Bennett JE, Dolin R, editors: *Principles and practice of infectious diseases*, ed 7, Philadelphia, 2010, Elsevier Churchill Livingstone.

Reed KD: Laboratory testing for Lyme disease: possibilities and practicalities, *J Clin Microbiol* 40:319, 2002.

Schmidt B: Evaluation of a new particle gel immunoassay for determination of antibodies against *Treponema pallidum, J Clin Microbiol* 42:2833, 2004.

Schmidt B, Muellegger RR, Stockenhuber C, et al: Detection of *Borrelia burgdorferi*-specific DNA in urine specimens from patients with erythema migrans before and after antibiotic therapy, *J Clin Microbiol* 34:1359, 1996.

Sonthayanon P, Chierakul W, Wuthiekanun V et al: Accuracy of loop-mediated isothermal amplification for diagnosis of human leptospirosis in Thailand, *Am J Trop Med Hyg* 84(4):614-620, 2011.

Versalovic J: *Manual of clinical microbiology*, ed 10, Washington, DC, 2011, ASM Press.

Wang G, van Dam A, Schwartz I, et al: Molecular typing of Borrelia burgdorferi sensu lato: taxonomic, epidemiological, and clinical manifestations, *Clin Microbiol Rev* 12:633, 1999.

Wilske B, Zöller L, Brade V, et al: MIQ 12, Lyme-Borreliose. In Mauch H, Lütticken R, editors: *Qualitätsstandards in der Mikrobiologisch-Infektiologischen Diagnostik.* Munich, Germany, 2000, Urban & Fischer Verlag, pp. 1-59.

Wilske B: Diagnosis of Lyme borreliosis in Europe, *Vector-Borne Zoonotic Dis* 3:215, 2003.

# Principles of Identification

# 47 Laboratory Methods for Diagnosis of Parasitic Infections: Overview

## OBJECTIVES

*This chapter provides an overview of the general epidemiology, pathogenesis, spectrum of disease, and approach to identification of parasites. The detailed technical procedures should be used in conjunction with additional specific chapters in this section to develop a clear understanding of the process, from specimen collection to identification. However, students should consider the following general objectives for the methods provided:*

1. State the specific diagnostic purpose for each test methodology.
2. Briefly describe the principle associated with the test method.
3. Determine specimen acceptability for parasite identification, including collection method, collection time/receipt time, number and/or quantity of specimen, and presence of interfering and contaminating substances.
4. Select appropriate preservatives for parasite specimens and explain the chemical principle and rationale for the preservative, including polyvinyl alcohol (PVA), formalin, and sodium acetate acetic acid formalin (SAF).
5. Select the appropriate method of detection and identification of parasites based on type of specimen.

The field of parasitology is often associated with tropical areas; however, many parasitic organisms that infect humans are worldwide in distribution and occur with some frequency in the temperate zones. Also, an increase in the number of compromised patients, particularly those who are immunodeficient or immunosuppressed, has led to increased interest in the field of parasitology. These individuals are greatly at risk for certain parasitic infections. Parasites of humans are classified into six major divisions:

- Protozoa (amebae, flagellates, ciliates, sporozoans, coccidia, microsporidia)
- Nematoda, or roundworms
- Platyhelminthes, or flatworms (cestodes, trematodes)
- Pentastomids, or tongue worms
- Acanthocephala, or thorny-headed worms
- Arthropoda (e.g., insects, spiders, mites, ticks)

Identification of parasitic organisms depends on morphologic criteria; accurate depiction of these criteria, in turn, depends on correct specimen collection and adequate fixation. Improperly submitted specimens may result in failure to detect or misidentification of the organisms. Tables 47-1 to 47-3 present information on the various groups of parasites, those that may be recovered from various body sites, the most frequently used specimen collection approaches, and appropriate processing methods.

## EPIDEMIOLOGY

Parasites usually are restricted to specialized environments inside and outside their hosts. A *zoonosis* is a disease of wild or domestic animals that occurs in humans as a result of parasitic infection. Animals that are potential sources of infection for humans are called *reservoir hosts*. The *host specificity* of any particular parasite influences factors associated with transmission and control. When humans are the only host for a parasite or a stage of its development, control options are relatively easy to define. However, if an infection is a zoonosis, control measures can become complex because of the existence of one or more reservoir animals. Some organisms are free-living during stages of their life cycles and do not depend on the human host for survival. In some cases, the human becomes an accidental host.

Parasites are transmitted from host to host through sexual means (venereal transmission) (*Trichomonas vaginalis*), from ingestion of infective forms in food or water (*Giardia lamblia, Cryptosporidium* spp., *Ascaris lumbricoides*), through skin penetration of infective larvae (*Strongyloides stercoralis*, hookworm), or through the bites of various arthropods (*Plasmodium, Trypanosoma, Leishmania*) (Table 47-4).

## PATHOGENESIS AND SPECTRUM OF DISEASE

Although a number of parasites can cause serious and life-threatening disease, particularly in the compromised patient, many organisms reach a "status quo" with the host and do no damage. Disease may not be the ultimate outcome of infection. Depending on the parasite, one or multiple body sites may be infected, resulting in no or few symptoms or, at the other extreme, death. Some parasites multiply in the human body, whereas others mature but do not increase in number. These life cycle

**TABLE 47-1** Description of the More Common Groups of Human Parasites

| Parasite Group | Description |
|---|---|
| **Protozoa, Intestinal**<br>Amebae | Single-celled organisms; pseudopodia (motility), trophozoite, and cyst stages in the life cycle.<br>Exceptions: Some have no identified cyst.<br>Fecal-oral transmission of the infective cyst.<br>*Entamoeba histolytica* causes amebiasis and is the most significant organism in this group. |
| Flagellates | Protozoa with characteristic flagella.<br>Fecal-oral transmission.<br>Exceptions: *Dientamoeba fragilis* (internal flagella) and the genus *Trichomonas* have a trophozoite and no cyst stage. Reproduction by longitudinal binary fission.<br>Examples: *Giardia lamblia* and *D. fragilis*. |
| Ciliates | Single-celled protozoa; cilia (motility), which beat in a coordinated, rhythmic pattern, moving the trophozoite in a spiral path.<br>Trophozoite and cyst stages in the life cycle; both stages show a large macronucleus and a micronucleus.<br>Fecal-oral transmission.<br>*Balantidium coli* is the single human pathogen in the group. |
| Coccidia | Protozoa; asexual and sexual life cycles.<br>Fecal-oral transmission via contaminated food and/or water. Infective stage (oocyst) containing sporocysts and/or sporozoites.<br>Examples: *Cryptosporidium* spp., *Cyclospora cayetanensis*, *Isospora belli*, and *Sarcocystis* spp. |
| Microsporidia | Small (1-2.5 $\mu$m) intestinal protozoa.<br>Transmission by ingestion, inhalation, or direct inoculation of spores.<br>Nine genera cause disease in humans; the two most important are *Encephalitozoon* and *Enterocytozoon*. |
| **Protozoa, Other Sites**<br>Amebae | Pathogenic, free-living organisms associated with warm freshwater environments.<br>Except for *Entamoeba gingivalis* (found in the mouth), they have been isolated from the central nervous system (CNS), eye, and other body sites.<br>Examples: *Naegleria fowleri*—acute CNS infection and death. Chronic CNS disease (*Acanthamoeba* spp., *Balamuthia mandrillaris*, and *Acanthamoeba* spp. can also cause keratitis). |
| Flagellates | Have flagella (long, proteinaceous organelles used for motility).<br>Sexual transmission.<br>Examples: *Trichomonas vaginalis* is located in the genitourinary system.<br>*Trichomonas tenax* can be identified in the mouth and is considered nonpathogenic. |
| Coccidia | Obligate intracellular, spore forming.<br>Transmission is typically fecal-oral through ingestion of contaminated materials or food.<br>Examples: *Cryptosporidium* spp. and *Toxoplasma gondii*. |
| Microsporidia | Small (1-2.5 $\mu$m) spore-forming protozoa.<br>Transmission is typically by ingestion of spores.<br>Life cycles vary considerably; some have an asexual life cycle, whereas others are complex and have both asexual and sexual life cycles and multiple hosts.<br>Examples: *Encephalitozoon*, *Pleistophora*, *Trachipleistophora*, and *Brachiola* spp. |
| **Protozoa, Blood and Tissue**<br>Malaria, babesiosis | Arthropod vector–borne protozoa.<br>Transmission via insect bite.<br>Examples: *Plasmodium* spp. includes parasites that undergo exoerythrocytic and pigment-producing erythrocytic schizogony in vertebrates and a sexual stage followed by sporogony in mosquitoes.<br>*Babesia* spp. are tick-borne and can cause severe disease in patients who have been splenectomized or otherwise immunologically compromised. |
| Flagellates<br>(leishmaniae) | Trypanosomatid protozoa; two morphologic forms—promastigotes (anterior flagellum) in the insect host and amastigote (no flagella) in the vertebrate host.<br>Transmission is through an insect vector.<br>Recovery and identification of the organisms are related to body site. Recovery of leishmanial amastigotes is limited to the site of the lesion in infections other than those caused by the *Leishmania donovani* complex (visceral leishmaniasis). |

*Continued*

**TABLE 47-1** Description of the More Common Groups of Human Parasites—cont'd

| Parasite Group | Description |
|---|---|
| Flagellates (trypanosomes) | Trypanosomatid protozoa; morphologic forms are identified based on the position, length, and attachment site of the flagella. At some time in their life cycle, these protozoa have the trypomastigote form with the typical undulating membrane and free flagellum at the anterior end. Transmission is typically through an insect vector. Some organisms cause African sleeping sickness (e.g., *Trypanosoma brucei gambiense, T. b. rhodesiense*). The etiologic agent of American trypanosomiasis is *T. cruzi*, which has amastigote and trypomastigote stages in the mammalian host and an epimastigote form in the arthropod host. |
| Nematodes, intestinal | Helminthic parasites; roundworms. Nematodes have separate sexes, are elongate-cylindrical and bilaterally symmetrical with a triradiate symmetry at the anterior end. Nematodes have an outer cuticle layer, no circular muscles, and a pseudocele that contains all systems (digestive, excretory, nervous, reproductive). Transmission is by ingestion of eggs or by skin penetration of larval forms from the soil. Examples: *Ascaris, Enterobius, Trichuris*, and *Strongyloides* spp. and hookworm. |
| Nematodes, tissue | Helminthic parasites; roundworms. Many of these organisms are rarely seen in the United States; however, some are important and are found worldwide. Diagnosis may be difficult if the only specimens are obtained through biopsy and/or autopsy, and interpretation must be based on examination of histologic preparations. Examples: *Trichinella* spp., visceral larva migrans (VLM), ocular larva migrans (OLM), cutaneous larva migrans (CLM). |
| Nematodes, filarial | Helminthic round worms. Transmission is via arthropods. Adult worms tend to live in the tissues or lymphatics of the vertebrate host. The diagnosis is made on the basis of recovery and identification of the larval worms (microfilariae) in the blood, other body fluids, or skin. Examples: *Wuchereria, Brugia, Loa*, and *Onchocerca* spp. |
| Cestodes, intestinal | Helminthic tapeworms. Adult tapeworm consists of a chain of egg-producing units called *proglottids*, which develop from the neck region of the attachment organ (scolex). Food is absorbed through the worm's integument. The intermediate host contains the larval forms that are acquired through ingestion of the adult tapeworm eggs. Transmission is through the ingestion of larval forms in poorly cooked or raw meat or freshwater fish. Examples: *Dipylidium caninum* (infection is acquired by accidental ingestion of dog fleas). *Hymenolepis nana* and *H. diminuta* are transmitted via ingestion of certain arthropods (fleas, beetles). Also, *H. nana* can be transmitted through egg ingestion (life cycle can bypass the intermediate beetle host). Humans can serve as both the intermediate and definitive hosts in *H. nana* and *Taenia solium* infections. |
| Cestodes, tissue | Tissue tapeworms. Transmission is through ingestion of certain tapeworm eggs or accidental contact with certain larval forms, leading to tissue infection. Humans serve as the accidental intermediate host. Examples: *Taenia solium, Echinococcus granulosus*, and several other species. |
| Trematodes, intestinal | Flatworms that are exclusively parasitic. Except for the schistosomes (blood flukes), flukes are hermaphroditic. They may be flattened; most have oral and ventral suckers. Transmission: Intestinal trematodes require a freshwater snail to serve as an intermediate host; these infections are food borne (freshwater fish, mollusks, or plants). Example: *Fasciolopsis buski*, the giant intestinal fluke. |
| Trematodes, liver, lung | Transmission: Liver and lung trematodes require a freshwater snail to serve as an intermediate host; these infections are food borne (freshwater fish, crayfish or crabs, or plants). Examples: Public health concerns include cholangiocarcinoma associated with *Clonorchis* and *Opisthorchis* infections, severe liver disease associated with *Fasciola* infections, and misdiagnosis of tuberculosis in individuals infected with *Paragonimus* spp. |
| Trematodes, blood | Schistosomes; sexes are separate. Males are characterized by an infolded body that forms the gynecophoral canal in which the female worm is held during copulation and oviposition. Transmission: Infection is acquired by skin penetration by the cercarial forms that are released from freshwater snails. The adult worms reside in the blood vessels over the small intestine, large intestine, or bladder. Examples: *Schistosoma mansoni, S. haematobium*, and *S. japonicum*. |

**TABLE 47-2** Body Sites and Parasite Recovery (Trophozoites, Cysts, Oocysts, Spores, Adults, Larvae, Eggs, Amastigotes, Trypomastigotes)

| Site | Parasites |
|---|---|
| **Blood**<br>Red cells | *Plasmodium* spp.<br>*Babesia* spp. |
| White cells | *Leishmania* spp.<br>*Toxoplasma gondii* |
| Whole blood/plasma | *Trypanosoma* spp.<br>Microfilariae |
| Bone marrow | *Leishmania* spp.<br>*Trypanosoma cruzi*<br>*Plasmodium* spp. |
| **Central Nervous System**<br>Cutaneous ulcers | *Taenia solium* (cysticerci)<br>*Echinococcus* spp.<br>*Naegleria fowleri*<br>*Acanthamoeba* spp.<br>*Balamuthia mandrillaris*<br>*Sappinia diploidea*<br>*Toxoplasma gondii*<br>Microsporidia<br>*Trypanosoma* spp. |
| Intestinal tract | *Leishmania* spp.<br>*Acanthamoeba* spp.<br>*Entamoeba histolytica*<br>*Entamoeba dispar*<br>*Entamoeba coli*<br>*Entamoeba hartmanni*<br>*Endolimax nana*<br>*Iodamoeba bütschlii*<br>*Blastocystis hominis*<br>*Giardia lamblia*<br>*Chilomastix mesnili*<br>*Dientamoeba fragilis*<br>*Pentatrichomonas hominis*<br>*Balantidium coli*<br>*Cryptosporidium* spp.<br>*Cyclospora cayetanensis*<br>*Isospora belli*<br>Microsporidia<br>*Ascaris lumbricoides*<br>*Enterobius vermicularis*<br>Hookworm<br>*Strongyloides stercoralis*<br>*Trichuris trichiura*<br>*Hymenolepis nana*<br>*Hymenolepis diminuta*<br>*Taenia saginata*<br>*Taenia solium*<br>*Diphyllobothrium latum*<br>*Clonorchis sinensis (Opisthorchis)*<br>*Paragonimus* spp.<br>*Schistosoma* spp.<br>*Fasciolopsis buski*<br>*Fasciola hepatica*<br>*Metagonimus yokogawai*<br>*Heterophyes heterophyes* |

**TABLE 47-2** Body Sites and Parasite Recovery (Trophozoites, Cysts, Oocysts, Spores, Adults, Larvae, Eggs, Amastigotes, Trypomastigotes)—cont'd

| Site | Parasites |
|---|---|
| Liver, spleen | *Echinococcus* spp.<br>*Entamoeba histolytica*<br>*Leishmania donovani*<br>Microsporidia |
| Lung | *Cryptosporidium* spp.*<br>*Echinococcus* spp.<br>*Paragonimus* spp.<br>Microsporidia |
| Muscle | *Taenia solium* (cysticerci)<br>*Trichinella* spp.<br>*Onchocerca volvulus* (nodules)<br>*Trypanosoma cruzi*<br>Microsporidia |
| Skin | *Leishmania* spp.<br>*Onchocerca volvulus*<br>Microfilariae |
| Urogenital system | *Trichomonas vaginalis*<br>*Schistosoma* spp.<br>Microsporidia<br>Microfilariae |
| Eye | *Acanthamoeba* spp.<br>*Toxoplasma gondii*<br>*Loa loa*<br>Microsporidia |

**NOTE:** This table does not include every possible parasite that can be found in a particular body site; the most likely organisms have been listed
*Disseminated in severely immunosuppressed individuals.

differences play important roles in pathogenicity and disease outcome. It is also important to remember that a patient who is debilitated or immunocompromised (including the very young and the very old) may react differently to a parasitic infection.

Certainly, it is not to the parasite's advantage to damage the host to the extent that severe illness or death occurs; this makes survival of the parasite difficult, at best, and transmission from host to host becomes a critical issue.

It is important to understand the life cycle of parasites, in terms both of potential control and prevention and of infectivity and disease outcomes in normal and immunosuppressed hosts (Table 47-5). Table 47-6 lists mechanisms of pathogenesis and the spectrum of parasitic diseases. Specific guidelines for physician requests are presented in Table 47-7.

# ■ LABORATORY DIAGNOSIS

The ability to detect and identify human parasites is directly linked to the quality of the clinical specimen, submission of the appropriate specimen or specimens, relevant diagnostic test orders, and the experience and

*Text continued on page 558*

**TABLE 47-3** Specimens and/or Body Site: Specimen Options, Collection and Transport Methods, and Processing

| Specimens and/ or Body Site | Specimen Options | Collection and Transport Methods | Specimen Processing | Comments |
|---|---|---|---|---|
| Stool for ova and parasite (O&P) examination | Fresh stool | ½ pint waxed container; 30 min if liquid, 60 min if semi formed, 24 h if formed; delivery to laboratory | Direct wet smear (not on formed specimen), concentration, permanent stained smear | Stool specimens containing barium are unacceptable; intestinal protozoa may be undetectable for 5 to 10 days after barium use. Certain substances and medications also impede detection of intestinal protozoa: mineral oil, bismuth, antibiotics, antimalarial agents, and nonabsorbable antidiarrheal preparations. After administration of any of these compounds, parasitic organisms may not be recovered for a week to several weeks. Specimen collection should be delayed after barium or antibiotics are administered for 5 to 10 days or at least 2 weeks, respectively. |
| | Preserved stool* | 5% or 10% formalin, MIF, SAF, Schaudinn's, PVA, modified PVA, single vial systems, universal fixative | Concentration, permanent stained smear Depending on specimen (fresh or preserved) and patient's clinical history, immunoassays may also be performed. | |
| Stool for culture of nematodes | Fresh stool, entire stool specimen | ½ pint waxed container; immediate delivery to laboratory | Filter paper strip, Petri dish, agar plate, charcoal cultures are all available. | Fresh stool (do not refrigerate) is required for these procedures. |
| Stool for recovery of tapeworm scolex | Preserved stool, entire stool specimen | 5% or 10% formalin (10% recommended) | The stool is filtered with a series of mesh screens and examined for the very small tapeworm scolex (proof of therapy efficacy) and/or proglottids (uncommon procedure but an option). | After treatment for tapeworm removal, the patient should be instructed to take a saline cathartic and to collect all stool material passed for the next 24 hr. The stool should be immediately placed in 10% formalin and thoroughly broken up and mixed with the preservative (1-gallon [3.8-liter] plastic jars are recommended, half full of 10% formalin). |
| | Adult worms, worm segments | Saline, 70% alcohol | | |
| Cellophane tape preparation for pinworms | Surface sample from perianal skin; anal impression smear | Cellulose (Scotch) tape preparation or commercial sampling paddle or swab | Tape is lifted from a slide, a drop of xylene substitute is added, the tape is replaced, and the specimen is ready for examination under the microscope. | Specimens should be collected late at night after the person has been asleep for several hours or first thing in the morning before going to the bathroom or taking a shower. At least 4 to 6 consecutive negative tapes are required to rule out the infection. |
| Sigmoid colon | Sigmoidoscopy material, prepared as smears | Fresh or PVA or Schaudinn's smears; specimen is taken with a spatula rather than cotton-tipped swabs; transported as smears in preservative | Direct wet smear, permanent stained smears | Material from the mucosal surface should be aspirated or scraped; it should not be obtained with cotton-tipped swabs. At least six representative areas of the mucosa should be sampled and examined (six samples, six slides). A parasitology specimen tray (containing Schaudinn's fixative, PVA, and 5% or 10% formalin) should be provided, or a trained technologist should be available at the time of sigmoidoscopy to prepare the slides. Examination of sigmoidoscopy specimens does not take the place of routine O&P examinations. If the amount of material is limited, use of a fixative containing PVA is highly recommended. |

| | | | |
|---|---|---|---|
| Duodenum | Duodenal contents | Entero-Test or aspirates; string in Petri dish or tube; immediate transport to laboratory | The specimen may be centrifuged (10 min at 500× *g*) and should be examined immediately as a wet mount for motile organisms. Iodine also can be used. Direct wet smear of mucus; permanent stained smears can also be prepared. | A fresh specimen is required; the amount may vary from < 0.5 mL to several milliliters of fluid. If the specimen cannot be completely examined within 2 hr after it is taken, any remaining material should be preserved in 5% to 10% formalin. |
| Entero-Test capsule (string) | Duodenal contents | Entero-Test (string test) in Petri dish (fresh) or preserved in PVA | Bile-stained mucus clinging to the yarn should be scraped off (mucus can also be removed by pulling the yarn between thumb and finger) and collected in a small Petri dish; disposable gloves are recommended. Usually 4 or 5 drops of material are obtained. The specimen should be examined immediately as a wet mount for motile organisms (iodine may be added later to facilitate identification of any organisms present). Organism motility is like that described previously for duodenal drainage. The pH of the terminal end of the yarn should be checked to ensure adequate passage into the duodenum (a very low pH means that it never left the stomach). The terminal end of the yarn should be yellow-green, indicating that it was in the duodenum (the bile duct drains into the intestine at this point). Permanent stained smears can also be prepared. | If the specimen cannot be completely examined within 1 hr after removal of the yarn, the material should be preserved in 5% to 10% formalin or PVA-mucus smears should be prepared. |
| Urogenital tract | Vaginal discharge Urethral discharge Prostatic secretions | Saline swab, transport swab (no charcoal), culture medium, plastic envelope culture, air-dried smear for FA | Direct wet smear; fluorescence; urine must be centrifuged before examination. | Fresh specimens are required; an air-dried smear may be an option for fluorescence. Do not refrigerate swabs and/or culture containers at any time, because motility and/or ability to grow will probably be lost. |
| | Urine | Single unpreserved specimen, 24-hr unpreserved specimen, early morning Nucleic acid-based testing media according to manufacturer's instructions | Examination of urinary sediment may be indicated in certain filarial infections. Administration of the drug diethylcarbamazine (Hetrazan) has been reported to enhance the recovery of microfilariae from the urine. The triple-concentration technique is recommended for the recovery of microfilariae. The membrane filtration technique can also be used with urine for the recovery of microfilariae. A membrane filter technique for the recovery of *Schistosoma haematobium* eggs has also been useful. | |

*Continued*

**TABLE 47-3** Specimens and/or Body Site: Specimen Options, Collection and Transport Methods, and Processing—cont'd

| Specimens and/or Body Site | Specimen Options | Collection and Transport Methods | Specimen Processing | Comments |
|---|---|---|---|---|
| Sputum | Sputum | True sputum (not saliva) | Direct wet smear; permanent stained smears; fluorescence also available (Calcofluor for microsporidia). Sputum is usually examined as a wet mount (saline or iodine), using low and high dry power (×100 and ×400). The specimen is not concentrated before preparation of the wet mount. If the sputum is thick, an equal amount of 3% sodium hydroxide (NaOH) (or undiluted chlorine bleach) can be added; the specimen is thoroughly mixed and then centrifuged. NaOH should not be used if the examiner is looking for *Entamoeba* spp. or *Trichomonas tenax*. After centrifugation, the supernatant fluid is discarded, and the sediment can be examined as a wet mount with saline or iodine. If examination must be delayed for any reason, the sputum should be fixed in 5% or 10% formalin to preserve helminth eggs or larvae or in PVA fixative to be stained later for protozoa. | True sputum is required; all specimens, especially induced specimens and BAL, should be delivered immediately to the laboratory (do not refrigerate). |
| | Induced sputum | No preservative (10% formalin if time delay) | | |
| | Bronchoalveolar lavage (BAL) | Sterile; immediate delivery to laboratory | | |
| Aspirates | Bone marrow | Sterile; immediate delivery to laboratory | Permanent stained smears; cultures can also be set (specifically designed for the recovery of blood parasites). | All aspirates for culture must be collected using sterile conditions and containers; this is mandatory for culture isolation of leishmaniae and trypanosomes. |
| | Cutaneous ulcers | Sterile plus air-dried smears | | |
| | Liver, spleen | Sterile, collected in 4 separate aliquots (liver) | | |
| | Lung | | | |
| | Transbronchial aspirate | Air-dried smears | | |
| | Tracheobronchial aspirate | Air-dried smears | | |
| Central nervous system | Cerebrospinal fluid (CSF) | Sterile | Direct wet smear, permanent stained smears; culture for free-living amebae (*Naegleria*, *Acanthamoeba* spp.). | All specimens must be transported immediately to the laboratory (STAT procedure). |

| Category | Specimen | Collection | Method | Comments |
|---|---|---|---|---|
| Biopsy | Intestinal tract | Routine histology | Direct wet smears, permanent stained smears; specimens to histology for routine processing. | The more material that is collected and tested, the more likely the organism is to be isolated and subsequently identified. Sterile collection is required for all specimens that will be cultured; bacterial and/or fungal contamination prevents isolation of parasites in culture. |
| | Cutaneous ulcers | Sterile, nonsterile to histopathology (formalin acceptable) | | |
| | Eye | Sterile (in saline), nonsterile to histopathology | | |
| | Scrapings | Sterile (in saline) | | |
| | Cornea (scrapings) | Collected by physician, placed directly on microscope slide | Fixed using methyl alcohol and stained using Calcofluor white | Helpful in diagnosis of *Acanthamoeba keratitis* |
| | Liver, spleen | Sterile, nonsterile to histopathology | | |
| | Lung | | | |
| | Brush biopsy | Air-dried smears | | |
| | Open lung biopsy | Air-dried smears | | |
| | Muscle | Fresh, squash preparation, nonsterile to histopathology | | |
| | Skin biopsy | Nonsterile to histopathology (formalin acceptable) | | |
| | Scrapings | Sterile (in saline), nonsterile to histopathology | | |
| | Skin snip | Aseptic, smear or vial No preservative | | |
| Blood | Smears of whole blood | Fresh (first choice) Thick and thin films; immediate delivery to laboratory | Thick and thin films, specialized concentrations and/or screening methods | Examination of blood films (particularly for malaria) is considered a STAT procedure; immediate delivery to the laboratory is mandatory. |

*Continued*

**TABLE 47-3** Specimens and/or Body Site: Specimen Options, Collection and Transport Methods, and Processing—cont'd

| Specimens and/ or Body Site | Specimen Options | Collection and Transport Methods | Specimen Processing | Comments |
|---|---|---|---|---|
| | Anticoagulated blood | Anticoagulant (second choice) EDTA* (first choice) Heparin (second choice) | Thick and thin films, specialized concentrations and/or rapid methods QBC Microhematocrit Centrifugation Method (Becton Dickinson, Tropical Disease Diagnostics, Sparks, Maryland) | Delivery to the laboratory within 30 min or less; if this time frame is not met, typical parasite morphology may not be seen in blood collected using anticoagulants. Knott concentration procedure: Used primarily to detect microfilariae in the blood, especially when a light infection is suspected. The disadvantage of the procedure is that the microfilariae are killed by the formalin and therefore are not seen as motile organisms. Membrane filtration technique: This technique, using Nuclepore filters, has proved highly efficient in demonstrating filarial infections when microfilaremias are of low density. It has also been successfully used in field surveys. |

Modified from Garcia LS: *Diagnostic medical parasitology*, ed 5, Washington, DC, 2007, ASM Press.

*A number of new stool fixatives are available; some use a zinc sulfate base rather than mercuric chloride. Some collection vials can be used as a single-vial system; both the concentration and permanent stained smear can be performed from the preserved stool. However, not all single-vial systems (proprietary formulas) provide material that can be used for fecal immunoassay procedures. A universal fixative is now available (TOTAL-FIX), which contains no formalin, no mercury, and no PVA.

†*EDTA*, Ethylenediaminetetraacetic acid; *FA*, fluorescent antibody; *MIF*, merthiolate-iodine-formalin; *PVA*, polyvinyl alcohol; *SAF*, sodium acetate–acetic acid–formalin.

**TABLE 47-4** Epidemiology of the More Common Groups of Human Parasites

| Parasite Group | Habitat (Reservoir) | Mode of Transmission | Prevention |
|---|---|---|---|
| **Protozoa, Intestinal**<br>Amebae | Single-celled organisms generally found in humans. Although certain animals harbor some of these organisms, they are not considered important reservoir hosts. | Humans acquire infections by ingesting food and water contaminated with fecal material containing the resistant, infective cyst stage of the protozoa. Various sexual practices have also been documented in transmission. | Preventive measures include increased attention to personal hygiene and sanitation measures; elimination of sexual activities that may involve fecal-oral contact. |
| Flagellates | The flagellates are generally found in humans. Although certain animals harbor some of these organisms, they are not considered important reservoir hosts; one exception may be animals, such as the beaver, that harbor *Giardia lamblia*. Contaminated water supplies are also a source. | Humans acquire infections by ingesting food and water contaminated with fecal material containing the resistant, infective cyst stage of the protozoa; in some cases (*Dientamoeba fragilis*), no cyst stage has been identified; the trophozoite forms may be transmitted from person to person in certain helminth eggs. | Preventive measures include increased attention to personal hygiene and sanitation measures; elimination of sexual activities that may involve fecal-oral contact; adequate water treatment (including filtration) is required; also awareness of environmental sources of infection. |
| Ciliates | *Balantidium coli* is generally found in humans, but it is also found in pigs. In some areas of the world, pigs are considered important reservoir hosts. | Humans acquire infections by ingesting food and water contaminated with fecal material containing the resistant, infective cyst stage of the protozoa. | Preventive measures include increased attention to personal hygiene and sanitation measures, as well as elimination of sexual activities that may involve fecal-oral contact. |
| Coccidia | Coccidia are found in humans. In some cases (e.g., cryptosporidiosis) animal reservoirs (cattle) can serve as important hosts. The muscle of various animals may contain sarcocysts that are infective for humans through the consumption of raw or poorly cooked meat. Numerous waterborne outbreaks with *Cryptosporidium* spp. have been reported throughout the world. Coccidian oocysts are extremely resistant to environmental conditions, particularly if they are kept moist. | These protozoa are acquired through ingestion of various meats or by fecal-oral transmission through contaminated food and/or water. The infective forms are called *oocysts* (*Cryptosporidium* spp., *Isospora* (*Cystoisospora*) *belli*, *Cyclospora cayetanensis*) or *sarcocysts* (*Sarcocystis* spp.), which are contained in infected meat. Cryptosporidia have also been implicated in nosocomial infections. | Preventive measures include increased attention to personal hygiene and sanitation measures; elimination of sexual activities that may involve fecal-oral contact. Adequate water treatment (including filtration) is mandatory; awareness of environmental sources of infection also is important. |
| Microsporidia | Microsporidia can infect every living animal, some of which probably serve as reservoir hosts for human infection. However, host specificity has not been well defined to date. The spores are environmentally resistant and can survive years if kept moist. | Infection with microsporidial spores usually occurs through ingestion; however, inhalation of spores and direct inoculation from the environment almost certainly occur. | Preventive measures include increased attention to personal hygiene and sanitation measures; increased awareness of environmental exposure possibilities; and adequate water treatment. |

*Continued*

**TABLE 47-4** Epidemiology of the More Common Groups of Human Parasites—cont'd

| Parasite Group | Habitat (Reservoir) | Mode of Transmission | Prevention |
|---|---|---|---|
| **Protozoa, Other Sites**<br>Amebae | Free-living amebae are associated with warm, freshwater environments; they are also found in soil. Although humans can harbor these organisms, person-to-person transfer is thought to be rare. Environmental sources are the primary link to human infection. Contaminated eye care solutions have been linked to organisms that cause keratitis. | Infection occurs through contact with contaminated water; organisms enter through the nasal mucosa and may travel via the olfactory nerve to the brain. Disease can be very severe and life-threatening; keratitis is also caused by these organisms, and infection can be linked to blindness or severe corneal damage. Eye infections can be linked to contaminated lens solutions or direct, accidental inoculation of the eye from environmental water and/or soil sources. | Avoidance of contaminated environmental water and soil sources; adequate care of contact lens systems. |
| Flagellates | *Trichomonas vaginalis* infection is found in a large percentage of humans; humans may present as symptomatic or asymptomatic. Person-to-person transfer is very common; reinfection is also common, particularly if sexual partners are not treated. | *T. vaginalis* is found in the genitourinary system and is usually acquired by sexual transmission. | Awareness of sexual transmission; treatment of all partners when infection is diagnosed in an individual patient. |
| **Protozoa, Blood and Tissue**<br>Malaria, babesiosis | Humans harbor the five species of malaria (*Plasmodium vivax, P. ovale, P. malariae, P. knowlesi,* and *P. falciparum*). Other animals can carry *Babesia* spp., and animal reservoir hosts play a large role in human transmission. | These organisms are arthropod-borne, *Plasmodium* spp. by the female anopheline mosquito and *Babesia* spp. by one or more genera of ticks. These infections can also be transmitted transplacentally, via shared needles, through blood transfusions, and from organ transplants. | Vector control; awareness of transmission through blood transfusions, shared drug needles, congenital infections, and organ transplants. Careful monitoring of the blood supply. Malaria prophylaxis if traveling to endemic areas. |
| Flagellates (leishmaniae) | Some strains of leishmaniae have reservoir hosts (e.g., dogs for the Mediterranean strain of *Leishmania donovani* and wild rodents for the African strains of *L. donovani*.) *L. tropica* also has been linked to the same two animal reservoirs. | Transmission is through the bite of infected sandflies. Infection can also occur from person to person (cutaneous lesions), from blood transfusion, shared needles, and organ transplants. | Vector control; avoiding environmental sources (e.g., dogs, wild rodents); careful handling of all clinical specimens from infected patients. |
| Flagellates (trypanosomes) | Humans are the only known hosts for *Trypanosoma brucei gambiense* (West African trypanosomiasis); *Trypanosoma brucei rhodesiense* (East African trypanosomiasis) infections are found in a number of antelope and other ungulates that act as reservoir hosts. Rodents and some mammals are reservoir hosts for *Trypanosoma cruzi*. | Transmission is through the bite of the infected tsetse fly and through blood transfusion, shared needles, and organ transplants.<br>Transmission of *T. cruzi* is through the infected feces of the triatomid bug; the bug takes a blood meal, immediately defecates, and the human host scratches the infected feces into the bite site; bug saliva contains an irritant that stimulates scratching. | Vector control; awareness of potential exposure/infection from blood sources (transfusions, shared needles, organ transplants). Laboratory accidents while handling infected blood have been reported. |

**TABLE 47-4** Epidemiology of the More Common Groups of Human Parasites—cont'd

| Parasite Group | Habitat (Reservoir) | Mode of Transmission | Prevention |
|---|---|---|---|
| Nematodes, intestinal | These roundworms generally do not have animal reservoirs relevant to human infection. One exception is the pig ascarid; human infections have been reported. These worms are found worldwide; *Ascaris lumbricoides* is probably the most common parasite of humans, although some would argue that *Enterobius vermicularis* is number one. *Strongyloides stercoralis* is particularly important as the causative agent of severe disease in the compromised host. | *A. lumbricoides* and *Trichuris trichiura* eggs must undergo development in the soil before they are infective; thus children who play in the dirt are a particularly high-risk group. Ingestion of food and water contaminated with infective eggs is the primary route of infection. Hookworm and *S. stercoralis* infections are initiated by larval penetration of the skin from contaminated soil. Pinworm infection (*E. vermicularis*) is acquired through ingestion of infective eggs from the environment (hand-to-mouth). | Avoiding ingestion of contaminated soil and/or avoiding frequenting soil contaminated with hookworm eggs (pets, soil, water, warmth, warm weather); treatment for pinworm is recommended, but reinfection is common. |
| Nematodes, tissue | *Trichinella* spp. have a number of animal reservoir hosts, including bears, walruses, pigs, rodents, and other animals. Dog and cat hookworms cause cutaneous larva migrans (CLM), and the dog and cat ascarid, *Toxocara* spp., causes visceral and ocular larva migrans (VLM, OLM). These infections can be serious and cause severe disease if not treated. | *Trichinella* organisms are acquired by ingestion of raw or poorly cooked infected meat. CLM is caused by skin penetration of infective larvae from the soil; children should avoid sandboxes where dogs and cats are known to defecate. Larval migration is limited to the skin. VLM and OLM are caused by accidental ingestion of *Toxocara* spp. eggs from contaminated soil; larval migration occurs throughout the body, including the eyes. | Adequate cooking of infected meat; awareness of possibility of contaminated soils for dog and cat hookworms and/or ascarids; covering of all sandboxes where pets have access to defecation and children play. |
| Nematodes, filarial | *Wuchereria bancrofti*, *Loa loa*, and *Onchocerca volvulus* have no animal reservoirs and are found only in humans, whereas *Brugia* spp. can also be found in cats and monkeys. *Dracunculus medinensis* can infect dogs, cats, and monkeys and also humans. | Filarial nematodes are transmitted through the bite of a blood-sucking arthropod (midges, mosquitoes, flies). *Dracunculus* infections are acquired through ingestion of water contaminated with small crustaceans, *Cyclops* spp., which contain infective larvae. | Vector control; protection of well-water sources. |
| Cestodes, intestinal | The human serves as the definitive host for beef (*Taenia saginata*) and pork (*Taenia solium*) tapeworms; cows/camels and pigs serve as intermediate hosts, respectively. Humans also serve as the intermediate host for *T. solium* (cysticercosis). *Diphyllobothrium latum* adult tapeworms can be found in a number of wild animals, the most important being dogs, bears, seals, and walruses, which serve as reservoir hosts; humans are the definitive host. *Hymenolepis nana* (dwarf tapeworm) can occur in rodents; humans can serve as both intermediate and definitive hosts, with development from the egg to adult worm occurring in the human intestine. | Human infection with the adult worm occurs through ingestion of raw or poorly cooked meat (beef, camel, pork) containing the intermediate forms, the cysticerci. Humans become the accidental intermediate host when eggs from an adult *T. solium* tapeworm are ingested. The cysticerci develop in the muscle and tissues of the human rather than the pig. Infection with the adult *D. latum* tapeworm occurs through ingestion of poorly cooked freshwater fish containing the sparganum or plerocercoid larval form. Infection with *H. nana* is primarily acquired through accidental ingestion of eggs from an adult tapeworm. | Adequate cooking of infected meat; treatment of patients harboring adult tapeworms (accidental ingestion of eggs can lead to infection). |

*Continued*

**TABLE 47-4** Epidemiology of the More Common Groups of Human Parasites—cont'd

| Parasite Group | Habitat (Reservoir) | Mode of Transmission | Prevention |
|---|---|---|---|
| Cestodes, tissue | Adult worms are found in a variety of animals; the human becomes the accidental intermediate host after ingestion of eggs from the adult worms. Reservoir hosts include dogs, cats, and rodents. | Ingestion of certain tapeworm eggs or accidental contact with certain larval forms can lead to tissue infection with *Taenia solium, Echinococcus* spp., and several others. | Preventive measures involve increased attention to personal hygiene and sanitation measures. |
| Trematodes, intestinal | Fish-eating wild and domestic animals serve as reservoir hosts. The definitive host of *Fasciolopsis buski* is the pig. | Ingestion of water chestnut and caltrop (raw, peeled with the teeth) is the source of infection; metacercariae are encysted on the plant material. Pig feces are used to fertilize various water plant crops. | Avoiding eating raw water plants that may contain encysted larval forms of the flukes; adequate waste disposal of farm animal feces (pigs). |
| Trematodes, liver, lung | Cats, dogs, and wild fish-eating mammals can serve as reservoir hosts for *Opisthorchis* spp., *Clonorchis sinensis*, and *Paragonimus* spp. *Fasciola hepatica* is normally a parasite of sheep, and *F. gigantica* is a parasite of cattle; humans are accidental hosts. | Infection occurs through ingestion of raw or poorly cooked fish, crabs, crayfish, and certain plants in or on which metacercariae are encysted. Infection with *Fasciola* spp. is not easily acquired (the parasite is not that well adapted to the human host). | Thorough cooking of potentially infected fish, crabs, crayfish; avoiding eating raw water plants that may contain encysted metacercariae. |
| Trematodes, blood | *Schistosoma mansoni* and *S. haematobium* appear to be restricted to the human host; *S. japonicum* can be found in cattle, deer, dogs, and rodents. The worms mature in the blood vessels, and eggs make their way outside the body in stool and/or urine. The freshwater snail is a mandatory part of the life cycle (contains developmental forms of schistosome). | Infection occurs through skin penetration by infected cercariae released from a freshwater snail containing the intermediate stages of the schistosome life cycle. Cercariae can be released from the snail intermediate host singly or in groups. | Protection from potentially contaminated water sources; awareness of mode of transmission; proper handling of human waste containing eggs (continued infection of snail intermediate hosts). |

training of laboratory personnel (Table 47-8). A summary of human parasites and applicable collection fixatives, clinical specimens, diagnostic tests, the elements of a positive finding, and comments are presented in Tables 47-9 and 47-10.

## SPECIMEN COLLECTION AND TRANSPORT

Depending on its stage of development in the clinical specimen (adult, larvae, eggs, trophozoites, cysts, oocysts, spores), a particular parasite may not be able to survive outside the host. For this reason, clinical specimens should be transported immediately to the laboratory to increase the likelihood of finding intact organisms. Because a lag time often occurs between collection of the specimen and its arrival in the laboratory, many facilities routinely use preservatives for collection and transport. This approach ensures that any parasites present maintain their morphology and can be identified after processing.

Correct processing depends on the use of appropriate fixatives, immediate fixation upon receipt of the specimen, and adequate mixing between the fixative and specimen (see Table 47-9). It is mandatory that specimen

collection guidelines are available for health care personnel and that all clients recognize the importance of following such guidelines. Specimen rejection criteria must be included as a part of the guidelines; guidelines must be followed and enforced to limit the possibility of reporting misleading or incorrect results. Detailed specimen descriptions and/or body sites, in addition to collection and transport information, are included in Table 47-3.

**NOTE:** Two ordering/collection/processing/examination situations are considered STAT orders (i.e., they require immediate attention for potentially life-threatening situations): central nervous system (CNS) specimens to be examined for free-living amebae and blood films in a potential malaria case.

## SPECIMEN PROCESSING

Diagnostic parasitology includes laboratory procedures designed to detect organisms in clinical specimens using morphologic criteria and visual identification (see Procedures 47-1 to 47-9 on the Evolve site). Many clinical specimens, such as those from the intestinal tract, contain numerous artifacts that complicate the differentiation of parasites from surrounding debris. Specimen

**TABLE 47-5** Parasitic Infections: Clinical Findings in Normal and Compromised Hosts

| Organism | Normal Host | Compromised Host |
|---|---|---|
| *Entamoeba histolytica* | Asymptomatic to chronic-acute colitis; extraintestinal disease may also occur (primary site: right upper lobe of liver). | Diminished immune capacity may lead to extraintestinal disease |
| Free-living amebae<br>*Naegleria fowleri*<br>*Acanthamoeba* spp.<br>*Balamuthia mandrillaris*<br>*Sappinia* spp. | Patients tend to have eye infections with *Acanthamoeba* spp. linked to poor lens care. | Primary amebic meningoencephalitis (PAM); granulomatous amebic encephalitis (GAE) |
| *Giardia lamblia* | Asymptomatic to malabsorption syndrome. | Certain immunodeficiencies tend to predispose an individual to infection. |
| *Toxoplasma gondii* | Approximately 50% of individuals have antibody and organisms in tissue but are asymptomatic. It is important to note that a developing fetus may be severally affected if the mother is infected; this is highly dependent on the time (trimester) when the infection occurs. | Disease in compromised hosts tends to involve the central nervous system (CNS), with various neurologic symptoms; it can mimic neurologic symptoms of infection with the human immunodeficiency virus (HIV). |
| *Cryptosporidium* spp.<br>*Cryptosporidium hominis* (humans)<br>*Cryptosporidium parvum* (humans and animals) | Self-limiting infection with diarrhea and abdominal pain. | Because of the autoinfective nature of the life cycle, infection is not self-limiting and may produce fluid loss of more than 10 L/day; multisystem involvement may occur. No totally effective therapy is known. |
| *Cyclospora cayetanensis* | Self-limiting infection with diarrhea (3-4 days); relapses common. | Diarrhea may persist for 12 weeks or longer; biliary disease has also been reported in this group, particularly those with acquired immunodeficiency syndrome (AIDS). |
| *Isospora (Cystoisospora) belli* | Self-limiting infection with mild diarrhea or no symptoms. | May lead to severe diarrhea, abdominal pain, and possibly death (rare case reports); diagnosis occasionally may be missed because of failure to recognize the oocyst stage; is not seen when concentrated from polyvinyl alcohol (PVA) fixative. |
| *Sarcocystis* spp. | Self-limiting infection with diarrhea or mild symptoms. | Symptoms may be more severe and last for a longer period. |
| Microsporidia<br>*Anncaliia*<br>*Nosema*<br>*Brachiola*<br>*Vittaforma*<br>*Encephalitozoon*<br>*Enterocytozoon*<br>*Pleistophora*<br>*Trachipleistophora*<br>*"Microsporidium"* | Little is known about these infections in the normal host. Most infections have been identified as causing intestinal symptoms (*Enterocytozoon, Encephalitozoon*) or eye infections (*Vittaforma, Encephalitozoon*). | Organisms infect various parts of the body; diagnosis often depends on histologic examination of tissues; routine examination of clinical specimens (e.g., stool, urine) is becoming more common; infection can probably cause death. |
| *Leishmania* spp. | Asymptomatic to mild disease. Depending on species, infection can result in cutaneous, diffuse cutaneous, or mucocutaneous disease. | More serious manifestations of visceral leishmaniasis; some cutaneous species manifest visceral disease; infection is difficult to treat and manage; definite co-infection with AIDS. |
| *Strongyloides stercoralis* | Asymptomatic to mild abdominal complaints; can remain latent for many years because of low-level infection maintained by internal autoinfective life cycle. | Can result in disseminated disease (hyperinfection syndrome resulting from autoinfective nature of life cycle); abdominal pain, pneumonitis, sepsis-meningitis with Gram-negative bacilli, eosinophilia; distinct link to certain leukemias or lymphomas; can be fatal. |
| Crusted (Norwegian) scabies | Infections can range from asymptomatic to moderate itching. | Severe infection with reduced itching response; hundreds of thousands of mites on the body; infection is very easily transferred to others; secondary infection is common. |

**TABLE 47-6** Pathogenesis and Spectrum of Parasitic Diseases

| Parasite Group | Pathogenesis | Spectrum of Disease |
|---|---|---|
| **Protozoa, Intestinal**<br>Amebae | Pathogens can cause severe disease; however, exposure does not always lead to disease; infection may be self-limiting; disease more likely in the compromised host. | Nonpathogens cause no disease, patients are asymptomatic; *Entamoeba histolytica* causes intestinal symptoms (bloody diarrhea) and the potential for amebic liver abscess; other tissues may be involved, especially in the immunocompromised patient. "*Blastocystis hominis*" comprises a number of strains, some considered pathogenic; patients' conditions range from asymptomatic to severe diarrhea. |
| Flagellates | Not all patients are infected upon exposure; disease spectrum varies; some patients may remain asymptomatic; if nonexposed patients become infected, symptoms are much more likely to occur. | Nonpathogens cause no disease, patients are asymptomatic; *Giardia lamblia* (malabsorption syndrome) and *Dientamoeba fragilis* cause intestinal symptoms ranging from "indigestion" to nonbloody diarrhea, cramping, gas, and so on. |
| Ciliates | *Balantidium coli* infection is rare in the United States; people who have regular contact with pigs are much more likely to become infected; wide range of symptoms. | *B. coli* causes intestinal symptoms, including severe watery diarrhea, similar to coccidial and microsporidial infections. |
| Coccidia | All coccidia infective to humans can cause severe disease, particularly in the immunocompromised patient; infections in the immunocompetent patient tend to be self-limiting; *Cryptosporidium* spp. can maintain the infective cycle in the patient as a result of the autoinfective portion of the life cycle (the immunocompromised patient cannot produce antibody to limit this autoinfective cycle); huge waterborne outbreaks have been documented for *Cryptosporidium* spp.; infecting dose is low for *Cryptosporidium* spp. | *Cryptosporidium* spp., *Cyclospora cayetanensis, and Isospora belli* cause intestinal symptoms, including severe watery diarrhea; infections are more severe in immunocompromised patients. Life-threatening infections can be seen with *Cryptosporidium* spp.; the organisms can disseminate to other tissues, primarily the lung. *Sarcocystis* can cause intestinal symptoms and/or muscle pain, depending on the mode of infection (ingestion of oocysts or infected meat). |
| Microsporidia | A number of genera are pathogenic for humans and for animals; wide range of body sites; disease varies, depending on patient's immune status; disease outcome is complicated by lack of treatment for some genera; albendazole is effective for *Encephalitozoon* spp. | Every human tissue may be infected; *Enterocytozoon bieneusi* and *Encephalitozoon (Septata) intestinalis* are the most common and are found in the intestinal tract; the latter can also disseminate to other tissues, including the kidneys. Eye infections have been seen in both healthy and compromised patients; severe corneal infections seen. |
| **Protozoa, Other Sites**<br>Amebae | Pathogenic for humans; disease ranging from acute meningoencephalitis to chronic encephalitis, cutaneous infections to keratitis, and the potential for other body sites; disease spectrum depends on patient's immune capacity and the organism involved; disease can be mild (*Acanthamoeba* spp.) to fatal (*Naegleria fowleri*). | Infection occurs through contact with contaminated water; organisms enter through the nasal mucosa and may travel via the olfactory nerve to the brain. Disease caused by *N. fowleri* can be severe and life-threatening (primary amebic meningoencephalitis [PAM]); chronic granulomatous amebic encephalitis (GAE) can be caused by *Acanthamoeba* spp. and *Balamuthia mandrillaris*; keratitis is also caused by these organisms, and infection can be linked to blindness or severe corneal damage. Eye infections can be linked to contaminated lens solutions or to direct, accidental inoculation of the eye from environmental water and/or soil sources. |
| Flagellates | *Trichomonas vaginalis* causes genitourinary disease, depending on vaginal pH, presence or absence of other organisms, sexual practices, and other factors. Disease can vary from mild to severe. | *T. vaginalis* is found in the genitourinary system and is usually acquired by sexual transmission. Disease can be asymptomatic in the male but can cause pain, itching, and discharge in females; some strains of drug-resistant *Trichomonas* have been documented. |

**TABLE 47-6** Pathogenesis and Spectrum of Parasitic Diseases—cont'd

| Parasite Group | Pathogenesis | Spectrum of Disease |
|---|---|---|
| **Protozoa, Blood and Tissue**<br>Malaria, babesiosis | *Plasmodium vivax, P. falciparum, P. ovale, P. knowlesi,* and *P. malariae* are pathogenic for humans; *P. falciparum* malaria is the leading cause of death in endemic areas; although the host can develop antibody, protection is strain specific and short-lived. | Malaria can cause a range of symptoms, with life-threatening illness caused by *P. falciparum;* symptoms include fever, chills, nausea, and central nervous system (CNS) symptoms; *Babesia* infections often mimic those seen with malaria but without the fever periodicity. |
| Flagellates (leishmaniae) | *Leishmania donovani* invades the spleen, liver, and bone marrow and can cause serious disease, particularly in compromised hosts. | Leishmaniasis can infect the skin and mucous membranes and the organs of the reticuloendothelial system; symptoms can be mild to life-threatening. |
| Flagellates (trypanosomes) | Humans are the only known hosts for *Trypanosoma brucei gambiense* (West African trypanosomiasis); *Trypanosoma brucei rhodesiense* (East African trypanosomiasis) infections are found in a number of antelope and other hoofed mammals that serve as reservoir hosts. *Trypanosoma cruzi* (American trypanosomiasis) can be found in rodents and chickens. | *T. b. gambiense* and *T.b. rhodesiense* cause African sleeping sickness, with eventual invasion of the CNS, leading to coma and death; Chagas disease *(T. cruzi)* causes acute to chronic problems, primarily linked to cardiac disease and diminished cardiac capacity; the muscles of the gastrointestinal (GI) tract are also infected, leading to loss of function in terms of movement of food through the GI tract. |
| Nematodes, intestinal | These worms can cause mild to severe disease, depending on the worm burden (original number of eggs ingested or infective larvae penetrating the skin); young children and debilitated patients are more likely to be symptomatic; severe infections are seen in hyperinfections caused by *Strongyloides stercoralis* (autoinfective life cycle and immunocompromised patients); outcome varies tremendously from patient to patient and depends on the original infective dose. | *Ascaris lumbricoides, Trichuris trichiura,* and hookworm symptoms range from none to diarrhea, pain, and so on, depending on the worm burden; anemia may be seen with severe hookworm infection; *S. stercoralis* infections can involve many body tissues (disseminated disease) in the immunocompromised patient and can cause death; pinworm infection (*Enterobius vermicularis*) symptoms range from none to anal itching, irritability, loss of sleep, and so on. |
| Nematodes, tissue | Depending on the infective dose, *Trichinella* spp. can cause mild to severe disease; both cutaneous larva migrans (CLM) (dog/cat hookworm larvae), and toxocariasis (visceral larva migrans [VLM], ocular larva migrans [OLM]) through ingestion of dog/cat ascarid eggs) cause serious disease if not treated; often CLM, VLM, and OLM are seen in children more than adults. | *Trichinella* spp. can cause eosinophilia, muscle aches and pains, and death, depending on the worm burden; CLM can cause severe itching and eosinophilia as a result of larval migration in the skin; VLM and OLM are caused by larval migration throughout the body, including the eyes (mimics retinoblastoma). |
| Nematodes, filarial | *Wuchereria bancrofti, Loa loa,* and *Onchocerca volvulus* cause human disease; however, some filarial infections are not well adapted to humans and require many years of exposure before disease is evident; some infections are not evident, some cause multiple disease manifestations. | Symptoms range from asymptomatic to elephantiasis, blindness, skin changes, lymphadenitis, lymphangitis; in some cases Loeffler's syndrome also may be seen. |
| Cestodes, intestinal | The beef *(Taenia saginata),* pork *(Taenia solium),* and freshwater fish *(Diphyllobothrium latum)* tapeworms infect humans and are generally found in the intestine as a single worm. In the case of cysticercosis; ingestion of *T. solium* eggs can cause mild to severe disease, depending on the infecting dose and body site (muscle, CNS). *Hymenolepis nana* (dwarf tapeworm) infection can lead to many worms in the intestinal tract (autoinfective cycle; the organism can go from egg to larval form to adult in the human host). | Human infection with the adult tapeworm can cause no symptoms, or mild intestinal symptoms may occur. When the human becomes the accidental intermediate host for *T. solium,* CNS symptoms may occur, including epileptic seizures. Infection with the adult *D. latum* tapeworm can also cause intestinal symptoms, such as pain, diarrhea, and so on, but the patient may also be asymptomatic; a vitamin $B_{12}$ deficiency may be seen. Infection with *H. nana* is primarily acquired from accidental ingestion of eggs from an adult tapeworm; symptoms may be absent, or diarrhea may be present. |

*Continued*

**TABLE 47-6** Pathogenesis and Spectrum of Parasitic Diseases—cont'd

| Parasite Group | Pathogenesis | Spectrum of Disease |
|---|---|---|
| Cestodes, tissue | *Echinococcus* spp. can cause severe disease, depending on the original infecting dose of tapeworm eggs; multiple organs can be involved, including brain, liver, lung, and bone; some cysts grow like a metastatic tumor; surgical removal can be very difficult, if not impossible. | Depending on the body site, hydatid cysts can cause pain, anaphylactic shock (fluid leakage), or CNS symptoms. The patient may be unaware of infection until a cyst begins to press on other body organs or a large fluid leak occurs. |
| Trematodes, intestinal | Many genera and species are pathogenic for humans; disease severity depends on the infective dose of metacercariae; some patients may be unaware of infection. | Intestinal trematodes can cause pain and diarrhea; intestinal toxicity can sometimes be seen in heavy infections with *Fasciolopsis buski*. |
| Trematodes, liver and lung | Many genera and species are pathogenic for humans; disease severity depends on the infective dose of metacercariae; some patients may be unaware of infection. | *Paragonimus* spp. infection in the lungs can be severe, resulting in coughing, shortness of breath, and other symptoms; liver fluke infection can involve the bile ducts and gallbladder; symptoms depend on worm burden. |
| Trematodes, blood | Schistosomes are pathogenic for humans; however, the loading dose of cercariae from infected water sources determines the outcome of disease; very light infections may not produce symptoms; heavy infections can lead to death. | Symptoms may range from asymptomatic in light infections to severe organ failure resulting from deposition of eggs and subsequent granuloma formation in the tissues; "pipe-stem" fibrosis is seen in blood vessels; collateral circulation may develop; severe disease can cause death. |

**TABLE 47-7** Recommendations for Stool Testing

| Patient and/or Situation | Test Ordered* | Follow-Up Test |
|---|---|---|
| Patient with diarrhea and acquired immunodeficiency syndrome (AIDS) or other cause of immune deficiency<br>Potential waterborne outbreak (municipal/city water supply) | *Cryptosporidium* or *Giardia/Cryptosporidium* immunoassay | If immunoassays are negative and symptoms continue, special tests for microsporidia (modified trichrome stain) and other coccidia (modified acid-fast stain), in addition to ova and parasite (O&P) exam, should be performed. |
| Patient with diarrhea (nursery school, day care center, camper, backpacker)<br>Patient with diarrhea and potential waterborne outbreak (resort setting)<br>Patient with diarrhea from areas where *Giardia* sp. is the most common parasite found | *Giardia* or *Giardia/Cryptosporidium* immunoassay (perform testing on two stools before reporting as negative)<br>**Particularly relevant for areas of the United States where *Giardia* sp. is the most common organism found.** | If immunoassays are negative and symptoms continue, special tests for microsporidia and other coccidia (see above) and O&P exam should be performed. |
| Patient with diarrhea and relevant travel history<br>Patient with diarrhea who is a past or present resident of a developing country<br>Patient in an area of the United States where parasites **other than** *Giardia* sp. are found | O&P examination, *Entamoeba histolytica/E. dispar* immunoassay; immunoassay for confirmation of *E. histolytica;* various tests for *Strongyloides* spp. may be relevant (even in the absence of eosinophilia). | If exams are negative and symptoms continue, special tests for coccidia and microsporidia should be performed. |
| Patient with unexplained eosinophilia and possible diarrhea; if chronic, patient may also have history of respiratory problems (larval migration) and/or sepsis or meningitis (hyperinfection) | Although the O&P exam is a possibility, the agar plate culture for *Strongyloides stercoralis* is recommended (it is more sensitive than the O&P exam). | If tests are negative and symptoms continue, additional O&P exams and special tests for microsporidia and other coccidia should be performed. |
| Patient with diarrhea (suspected food-borne outbreak) | Test for *Cyclospora cayetanensis* (modified acid-fast stain, autofluorescence) | If tests are negative and symptoms continue, special procedures for microsporidia and other coccidia and O&P exam should be performed. |

*Depending on the particular immunoassay kit used, various single or multiple organisms may be included. Selection of a particular kit depends on many variables, such as clinical relevance, cost, ease of performance, training, personnel availability, number of test orders, training of physician clients, sensitivity, specificity, equipment, and time to result. Very few laboratories handle this type of testing in exactly the same way. Many options are clinically relevant and acceptable for good patient care. It is critical that the laboratory report indicate specifically which organisms could be identified using the kit; a negative report should list the organisms relevant to that particular kit.

**TABLE 47-8** Stool Specimen Collection and Testing Options

| Option | Pros | Cons |
|---|---|---|
| Rejection of stools from inpatients who have been in-house for longer than 3 days | Data suggest that patients who begin to have diarrhea after they have been inpatients for a few days are not symptomatic from parasitic infections, but generally from other causes. | The chance always exists that the problem is related to a health care–associated (nosocomial) parasitic infection (rare); *Cryptosporidium* spp. and microsporidia may be possible considerations. |
| Examination of a single stool (ova and parasite [O&P]) Data suggest that 40% to 50% of organisms present are found with only a single stool exam. Two O&P exams (concentration, permanent stained smear) are acceptable but not always as good as three specimens (may be relatively cost-effective approach); any patient remaining symptomatic requires additional testing. | Some think that most intestinal parasitic infections can be diagnosed from examination of a single stool. If the patient becomes asymptomatic after collection of the first stool, subsequent specimens may not be necessary. | Diagnosis from a single stool examination depends on the experience of the microscopist, proper collection, and the parasite load in the specimen. In a series of three stool specimens, frequently not all three specimens are positive and/or may be positive for different organisms. |
| Examine a second stool only after the first is negative and the patient is still symptomatic. | With additional examinations, yield of protozoa increases (*Entamoeba histolytica*, 22.7%; *Giardia lamblia*, 11.3%; and *Dientamoeba fragilis*, 31.1%). | Assumes the second (or third) stool is collected within the recommended 10-day time frame for a series of stools; protozoa are shed periodically. May be inconvenient for patient. |
| Examination of a single stool and an immunoassay (enzyme immunoassay [EIA], fluorescent antibody [FA], lateral or vertical flow cartridge) This approach is a mix: one immunoassay may be acceptable; however, immunoassay testing of two separate specimens may be required to confirm the presence of *Giardia* antigen. One O&P exam is not the best approach (review last option below). | If the examinations are negative and the patient's symptoms subside, probably no further testing is required. | Patients may show symptoms (off and on), so ruling out parasitic infections with only a single stool and one fecal immunoassay may be difficult. If the patient remains symptomatic, then even if two *Giardia* immunoassays are negative, other protozoa may be missed (*Entamoeba histolytica/ E. dispar* group, *E. histolytica*, *Dientamoeba fragilis*, *Cryptosporidium* spp., microsporidia). Normally, there are specific situations in which fecal immunoassays OR O&P exams should be ordered. **It is not recommended to perform both the O&P and fecal immunoassay automatically as a stool exam for parasites.** |
| Pool three specimens for examination; perform one concentration and one permanent stain (the laboratory pools the specimens). | Three specimens are collected by the patient (three separate collection vials) over 7-10 days; pooling by the laboratory may save time and expense. | Organisms present in low numbers may be missed because of the dilution factor once the specimens have been pooled. |

preparation may require concentration, which is designed to increase the chance of finding the organism or organisms. Microscopic examination requires review of the prepared clinical specimen using multiple magnifications and different time frames; organism identification also depends on the skill of the microbiologist. Final identification is based on microscopic examination of stained preparations, often using high magnification, such as oil immersion (×1000). (See Table 47-3 for specific details on specimen processing.)

# APPROACH TO IDENTIFICATION

Protozoa are small, ranging from 1.5 μm (microsporidia) to approximately 80 μm (*Balantidium coli*, a ciliate). Some are intracellular and require multiple isolation and

staining methods for identification. Helminth infections usually are diagnosed by finding eggs, larvae, and/or adult worms in various clinical specimens, primarily from the intestinal tract. Identification to the species level may require microscopic examination of the specimen. Recovery and identification of blood parasites can require concentration, culture, and microscopy. Confirmation of suspected parasitic infections depends on proper collection, processing, and examination of clinical specimens; often, multiple specimens must be submitted and examined to find and confirm the suspected organism or organisms (see Table 47-10).

## MICROSCOPIC EXAMINATION

Good, clean microscopes and light sources are mandatory for examining specimens for parasites. Organism

**TABLE 47-9** Fecal Fixatives Used in Diagnostic Parasitology (Intestinal Tract Specimens)

| Fixative | Concentration | Permanent Stained Smear Trichrome, Iron-Hematoxylin, Special Stains/Coccidia and Microsporidia | Immunoassays: *Giardia lamblia* *Cryptosporidium* spp. | Comments |
|---|---|---|---|---|
| 5% or 10% Formalin | Yes | No | Yes | Concentrations and IAs (EIA, FA, Rapids) |
| 5% or 10% Buffered formalin | Yes | No | Yes | Concentrations and IAs (EIA, FA, Rapids) |
| MIF | Yes | Polychrome IV stain | ND | No published data |
| SAF | Yes | Iron-hematoxylin best | Yes | Concentrations, permanent stains, and IAs (EIA, FA, Rapids) |
| Schaudinn's (Hg base) no PVA* | Rare | Yes | No | Permanent stains; Hg interferes with IAs; primarily used with fresh stool specimens (no fixative collection vials) |
| Schaudinn's (Hg base) with PVA* | Rare | Yes | No | Permanent stains; Hg and PVA interfere with IAs; considered gold standard fixative for permanent stains |
| Schaudinn's (Cu base) with PVA[†] | Rare | Yes | No | Permanent stains; PVA interferes with IAs; stains not as good as with Schaudinn's fixative using Hg or Zn |
| Schaudinn's (Zn base) with PVA[‡] | Rare | Yes | No | Permanent stains; PVA interferes with IAs; the same fixative as TOTAL-FIX without PVA (see below) |
| Ecofriendly ECOFIX (PVA)[§] | Rare | Yes | No | Permanent stains; PVA interferes with IAs; works best with ECOSTAIN; Wheatley's trichrome second best |
| Universal fixative,[‖] ecofriendly TOTAL-FIX | Yes | Yes | Yes | No formalin, no mercury, no PVA; concentrations, permanent stains, special stains, fecal IAs |

*Cu,* Copper; *EIA,* enzyme immunoassay; *FA,* fluorescent antibody; *Hg,* mercury; *IA,* immunoassay; *MIF,* merthiolate-iodine-formalin fixative; *ND,* no data; *PVA,* polyvinyl alcohol; *Rapids,* cartridge-format, membrane-flow IAs; *SAF,* sodium acetate–acetic acid–formalin; *Zn,* zinc.
*These two fixatives use the mercuric chloride base in the Schaudinn's fixative; this formulation is still considered the gold standard against which all other fixatives are evaluated (organism morphology after permanent staining).
[†]This modification uses a copper sulfate base rather than mercuric chloride; the morphology of stained organisms is not as good as with Hg or Zn.
[‡]This modification (proprietary formula) uses a zinc base rather than mercuric chloride and works well with both trichrome and iron-hematoxylin.
[§]This fixative uses a combination of ingredients but is prepared from a proprietary formula (contains PVA).
[‖]This modification uses a combination of ingredients, including zinc, but is prepared from a proprietary formula. The aim is to provide a universal fixative that can be used for the fecal concentration, permanent stained smear, and available immunoassays for *Giardia lamblia*, *Cryptosporidium* spp., and *Entamoeba histolytica* (or the *Entamoeba histolytica/E. dispar* group). *However,* currently, fecal immunoassays for the *Entamoeba histolytica/E. dispar* group and *Entamoeba histolytica* (true pathogen) require fresh or frozen specimens; testing can also be performed from stool submitted in Cary-Blair transport medium.

**Commentary**
The most common collection option (original public health approach) is a two-vial system: one vial of 5% or 10% formalin or buffered formalin and one vial of fixative containing the plastic adhesive polyvinyl alcohol (PVA). The formalin vial is used for concentration and fecal immunoassays, and the PVA vial is used for the permanent stained smear. Regulations for formalin (see below) originally were developed for industry, not the clinical laboratory, where amounts of formalin tend to be quite low. However, a laboratory using any amount of formalin must be monitored (see below).

SEMIUNIVERSAL FIXATIVES
Examples of a semiuniversal fixative include sodium acetate–acetic acid–formalin (SAF) (no mercury or PVA; *contains formalin*) and ECOFIX (no mercury or formalin; *contains PVA*).

UNIVERSAL FIXATIVE
Currently, TOTAL-FIX is the only fixative that contains NO formalin, NO PVA, and NO mercury. **TOTAL-FIX can be used without adding PVA to the fixative; adequate drying time for smears before staining is the most important step (minimum of 1 hr in 37°C incubator; more time required for thicker fecal smears). This fixative can be used for concentration, permanent stained smear, special stains for coccidia or microsporidia, and fecal immunoassays for *Giardia* and *Cryptosporidium* spp.**

*Table 47-9 footnotes—cont'd*

FORMALIN FIXATIVE

Formalin has been used for many years as an all-purpose fixative that is appropriate for helminth eggs and larvae and for protozoan cysts, oocysts, and spores. Two concentrations are commonly used: 5%, which is recommended for preservation of protozoan cysts, and 10%, which is recommended for helminth eggs and larvae. Although 5% is often recommended for all-purpose use, most commercial manufacturers provide 10%, which is more likely to kill all helminth eggs. To help maintain organism morphology, the formalin can be buffered with sodium phosphate buffers (i.e., neutral formalin). Selection of specific formalin formulations is at the user's discretion. *Aqueous formalin permits examination of the specimen as a wet mount only, a much less accurate technique than a permanent stained smear for identifying intestinal protozoa.* However, the fecal immunoassays for *Giardia lamblia* and *Cryptosporidium* spp. can be performed from the aqueous formalin vial. Fecal immunoassays for the *Entamoeba histolytica/E. dispar* group and *E. histolytica* are limited to fresh or frozen fecal specimens or Cary-Blair transport medium. After centrifugation, special stains for the coccidia (modified acid-fast stains) and microsporidia (modified trichrome stains) can be performed from the concentrate sediment obtained from formalin-preserved stool material. Use of the sediment provides a more sensitive test.

OSHA REGULATIONS ON THE USE OF FORMALDEHYDE

Formaldehyde has been in use for more than a century as a disinfectant and preservative, and it is found in a number of industrial products. Disagreement exists about the carcinogenic potential of lower levels of exposure, and epidemiologic studies of the effects of formaldehyde exposure among humans have given inconsistent results. Studies of industry workers with known exposure to formaldehyde report little evidence of increased cancer risk. In addition, people with asthma appear to respond no differently than healthy individuals after exposure to concentrations of formaldehyde up to 3 ppm. The federal Occupational Safety and Health Administration (OSHA) requires all workers to be protected from dangerous levels of vapors and dust. Formaldehyde vapor is the most likely air contaminant to exceed the regulatory threshold in a laboratory, particularly in anatomic pathology. Current OSHA regulations require vapor levels not to exceed 0.75 ppm (measured as a time-weighted average [TWA]) and 2 ppm (measured as a 15-minute short-term exposure). *OSHA requires monitoring for formaldehyde vapor wherever formaldehyde is used in the work place. The laboratory must have evidence at the time of inspection that formaldehyde vapor levels have been measured, and both 8-hour and 15-minute exposures must have been determined.*

If each measurement is below the permissible exposure limit and the 8-hour measurement is below 0.5 ppm, no further monitoring is required as long as laboratory procedures remain constant. If the 0.5-ppm, 8-hour TWA or the 2-ppm, 15-minute level is exceeded, monitoring must be repeated semiannually. If either the 0.75-ppm, 8-hour TWA or the 2-ppm, 15-minute level is exceeded **(very unlikely in a routine microbiology laboratory setting)**, employees must be required to wear respirators. Accidental skin contact with aqueous formaldehyde must be prevented with the use of proper clothing and equipment (gloves, laboratory coats).

The amendments of 1992 add medical removal protection provisions to supplement the existing medical surveillance requirements for employees suffering significant eye, nose, or throat irritation and for those experiencing dermal irritation or sensitization from occupational exposure to formaldehyde. In addition, these amendments establish specific hazard-labeling requirements for all forms of formaldehyde, including mixtures and solutions composed of at least 0.1% formaldehyde in excess of 0.1 ppm. Additional hazard labeling, including a warning label that formaldehyde presents a potential cancer hazard, is required where formaldehyde levels, under reasonably foreseeable conditions of use, may potentially exceed 0.5 ppm. The final amendments also provide for annual training of all employees exposed to formaldehyde at levels of 0.1 ppm or higher.

**NOTE:** The use of monitoring badges may not be a sensitive enough method to correctly measure the 15-minute exposure level. Contact the OSHA office in your institution for monitoring options. Usually, the accepted method involves monitoring airflow in the specific area or areas in the laboratory where formaldehyde vapors are found.

POLYVINYL ALCOHOL (PVA) ADHESIVE (NOT A FIXATIVE)

Polyvinyl alcohol (PVA) is a water-soluble, synthetic polymer used as a viscosity-increasing agent in pharmaceuticals, as an adhesive in parasitology fecal fixatives, and as a lubricant and protectant in ophthalmic preparations. PVA is also defined as a water-soluble polymer made by hydrolysis of a polyvinyl ester (e.g., polyvinyl acetate); it is used in adhesives, a textile and paper sizer, and for emulsifying, suspending, and thickening solutions. **PVA is not a fixative, but rather an adhesive to help glue stool material onto the slide; this is the only purpose of PVA as an additive to parasitology fecal fixative formulations.**

PVA is a plastic resin that is normally incorporated into Schaudinn's fixative. Although some laboratories may perform a fecal concentration from a PVA-preserved specimen, some parasites do not concentrate well, and some do not exhibit the typical morphology that would be seen in concentration sediment from a formalin-based fixative. PVA fixative solution is highly recommended as a means of preserving cysts and trophozoites for later examination. Use of PVA fixative also allows specimens to be shipped (by regular mail service) from any location in the world to a laboratory for examination. PVA fixative is particularly useful for liquid specimens and should be used in the ratio of 3 parts PVA to 1 part fecal specimen.

**NOTE:** Very detailed information on all fixative options can be found in Garcia LS: *Diagnostic medical parasitology,* ed 5, Washington, DC, 2007, ASM Press,.

identification depends on morphologic differences, most of which must be seen using a stereoscopic microscope (magnification less than or equal to ×50) or a regular microscope at low (×100), high dry (×400), and oil immersion (×1000) magnifications. The use of a ×50 or ×60 oil immersion objective for scanning can be very helpful, particularly when the ×50 oil and ×100 oil immersion objectives are placed side by side.

A stereoscopic microscope is recommended for larger specimens (e.g., arthropods, tapeworm proglottids, various artifacts). The total magnification usually varies from approximately ×10 to ×45, either with a zoom capacity or with fixed objectives (×0.66, ×1.3, ×3) used with ×5 or ×10 oculars. Depending on the density of the specimen or object to be examined, the light source must be directed from under the stage or onto the top of the stage.

## Intestinal Tract

Stool specimens frequently are submitted to the diagnostic laboratory for parasite identification. The most commonly performed procedure in parasitology is the ova and parasite (O&P) examination, although use of the rapid fecal immunoassay tests has increased dramatically for the detection of Giardia and cryptosporidium. Several other diagnostic techniques are available for recovery and identification of parasitic organisms from the intestinal tract. Although most laboratories do not routinely offer all these relatively simple and inexpensive techniques, the clinician should be familiar with the relevance of information obtained from them. Examining stool specimens for scolices and proglottids of cestodes and adult nematodes and trematodes is rarely necessary to confirm the diagnosis or to identify the organism to the species level.

**TABLE 47-10** Common Human Parasites: Diagnostic Specimens, Tests, and Positive Findings

| Organism | Infection Acquired | Location in Host | Diagnostic Specimen | Diagnostic Test* | Positive Specimen | Comments |
|---|---|---|---|---|---|---|
| **Intestinal Amebae**<br>*Entamoeba histolytica*<br>*Entamoeba dispar*<br>*Entamoeba hartmanni*<br>*Entamoeba coli*<br>*Endolimax nana*<br>*Iodamoeba bütschlii*<br>*Blastocystis hominis* | Ingestion of food or water contaminated with infective cysts; fecal-oral transmission | Intestinal tract; *E. histolytica* infection may disseminate to the liver (extraintestinal amebiasis); *Blastocystis* strains are pathogenic or nonpathogenic; cannot differentiate on morphology | Stool; sigmoidoscopy specimens | O&P exam; stained sigmoidoscopy slides; stool immunoassays | Trophozoites and/or cysts | Many of the protozoa can look very much alike; see diagnostic tables for details; immunoassays for *E. histolytica/E. dispar* group and *E. histolytica* (fresh, frozen stool, Cary Blair required) |
| **Free-Living Amebae**<br>*Naegleria fowleri*<br>*Acanthamoeba* spp.<br>*Balamuthia mandrillaris*<br>*Sappinia* spp. | Contaminated water or soil; dust, contaminated eye solutions; organisms may enter through nasal mucosa, travel to brain via olfactory nerve | CNS (PAM, GAE); eye | CSF, corneal scrapings, biopsy, eye care solutions; CSF exam **STAT REQUEST** | Stains, culture, FA, biopsy; *B. mandrillaris* cannot be grown on agar culture, whereas *N. fowleri* and *Acanthamoeba* spp. can | Trophozoites or cysts | CNS disease life-threatening with *N. fowleri*; other CNS infections more chronic; keratitis can lead to blindness |
| **Intestinal Flagellates**<br>*Giardia lamblia*<br>*Dientamoeba fragilis*<br>*Chilomastix mesnili*<br>*Pentatrichomonas hominis* | Ingestion of food or water contaminated with infective cysts or trophozoites (*D. fragilis*, *T. hominis*); fecal-oral transmission | Intestinal tract | Stool; duodenal specimens or Entero-Test capsule (string test) for *Giardia lamblia* | O&P exam; wet preparations or stains of duodenal material; stool immunoassays (can use fresh or formalin fixed specimens; no PVA); need two specimens for IA for *G. lamblia* | Trophozoites or cysts | *G. lamblia* is very difficult to recover; stool immunoassays are more sensitive than routine O&P exams; *D. fragilis* requires permanent stain for identification |
| **Urogenital Flagellates**<br>*Trichomonas vaginalis* | Sexually transmitted; wet towels less likely but possible | Urinary tract; genital system; males may be asymptomatic | Vaginal secretions, prostatic fluid, often recovered in urine sediment | Wet preparations, culture, immunoassays; molecular testing | Trophozoites | Often diagnosed by motility in urine sediment or wet preparations |
| **Intestinal Ciliate**<br>*Balantidium coli* | Ingestion of food or water contaminated with infective cysts; fecal-oral transmission | Intestinal tract | Stool | O&P exam; wet preparations better than permanent stained smear | Trophozoites and/or cysts | Not common in the United States; associated with pigs; seen in proficiency testing specimens |
| **Intestinal Coccidia**<br>*Cryptosporidium* spp.<br>*Cyclospora cayetanensis*<br>*Isospora belli* | Ingestion of food or water contaminated with infective oocysts; fecal-oral transmission | Intestinal tract; *Cryptosporidium* can disseminate to other tissues in compromised host (lung, gallbladder) | Stool; biopsy; duodenal specimen; sputum | Modified acid-fast stains; stool immunoassays; concentration wet prep for *I. belli* | Oocysts in stool or scrapings; other developmental stages in tissues | *Cryptosporidium* spp. cause severe diarrhea in compromised patient; nosocomial transmission |

| Organism | Transmission | Body Site | Specimen | Diagnostic Methods | Positive Identification | Comments |
|---|---|---|---|---|---|---|
| **Intestinal Microsporidia†**<br>*Enterocytozoon bieneusi*<br>*Encephalitozoon (Septata) intestinalis* | Ingestion of food or water contaminated with infective spores; fecal-oral transmission | Intestinal tract; organisms can disseminate to other body sites (kidney) | Stool; biopsy | Modified trichrome stains; optical brightening agents; experimental immunoassays; biopsy and histology (tissue Gram stains) | Spores in stool; other developmental stages in tissues | Can cause serious diarrhea in compromised host; less known about infections in normal host |
| **Microsporidia, Other Body Sites**<br>*Encephalitozoon* spp.<br>*Brachiola vesicularum*<br>*Microsporidium*<br>*Anncalia*<br>*Pleistophora*<br>*Trachipleistophora*<br>*Vittaforma*<br>*Tubulinosema* | Ingestion of food or water contaminated with infective spores; fecal-oral transmission; inhalation; direct environmental contact to eyes; probably hands to eyes | All tissues | All body fluids and/or tissues relevant, depending on body site | Modified trichrome stains; optical brightening agents; experimental immunoassays; biopsy and histology (tissue Gram stains) | Spores in stool, urine, other body fluids; developmental stages in tissues | Can cause serious diarrhea in compromised host; less known about infections in normal host; a number of eye infections documented in immunocompetent patients |
| **Tissue Protozoa**<br>*Toxoplasma gondii* | *T. gondii:* ingestion of raw meat; ingestion of oocysts from cat feces | Eye, CNS in compromised patient (*T. gondii*) | Biopsies (any tissue), CSF | Serology, tissue culture; recovery from CSF | Positive serology; recovery of trophozoites in CSF | Many people have positive serologies for *T. gondii*; infections are serious in immunocompromised patients |
| **Intestinal Nematodes**<br>*Enterobius vermicularis*<br>*Trichuris trichiura*<br>*Ascaris lumbricoides*<br>Hookworm<br>*Strongyloides stercoralis* | Ingestion of food or water contaminated with infective eggs; penetration of skin by infective larvae in soil | Intestine; *S. stercoralis* may disseminate (hyperinfection), primarily in immunocompromised patients | Stool; duodenal contents (*S. stercoralis*); Scotch tape preps or paddles for *E. vermicularis* | O&P exam; special concentrates and cultures; examination of tapes for *E. vermicularis* | Adult worms, eggs and/or larvae, depending on the roundworm involved | Review direct and indirect life cycles (migration through heart, lung, trachea to intestine); 4 to 6 consecutive tapes required to rule out *Enterobius* infection |
| **Tissue Nematodes**<br>VLM, OLM (*Toxocara* spp.) | Ingestion of infective eggs | Migration through tissues | Serum | Serology | Positive serology | Human is accidental host for VLM, OLM, and CLM |
| CLM (dog/cat hookworm) | Skin penetration of larvae | Skin tracks, migration | Visual inspection | Presence of tracks/skin | Eosinophilia, visual tracks | |
| *Trichinella* spp. | Ingestion of raw pork | Muscle | Serum, muscle biopsy | Serology, squash prep | Positive serology, larvae | Outbreaks still occur |
| *Anisakis*, others | Ingestion of raw marine fish | Intestine | Submission of larvae | ID of larvae | Positive larval ID | Sometimes identified only after surgical removal |

*Continued*

**TABLE 47-10** Common Human Parasites: Diagnostic Specimens, Tests, and Positive Findings—cont'd

| Organism | Infection Acquired | Location in Host | Diagnostic Specimen | Diagnostic Test* | Positive Specimen | Comments |
|---|---|---|---|---|---|---|
| **Intestinal Cestodes** | | | | | | |
| *Taenia saginata* (beef) | Ingestion of: Raw beef | Intestine | Stool and/or proglottids | O&P, India ink proglottids | Eggs, proglottid branches | Eggs for the two *Taenia* spp. look alike; gravid proglottid or scolex is needed to make identification |
| *Taenia solium* (pork) | Raw pork | | Stool and/or proglottids | O&P, India ink proglottids | Eggs, proglottid branches | |
| *Diphyllobothrium latum* | Raw freshwater fish | | Stool and/or proglottids | O&P | Eggs, proglottid shape | |
| *Hymenolepis nana* | Tapeworm eggs | | Stool | O&P | Eggs | |
| *Hymenolepis diminuta* | Grain beetles | | Stool | O&P | Eggs | |
| *Dipylidium caninum* | Fleas from dogs/cats | | Stool and/or proglottids | O&P | Eggs, proglottid shape | |
| **Tissue Cestodes** | Ingestion of: | | | | | |
| *Echinococcus granulosus* | Eggs from dog tapeworm | Liver, lung, and so on | Serum, hydatid cyst aspirate; biopsy | Serology, centrifugation of fluid; histology | Positive serology; hydatid sand, tapeworm tissue | *E. granulosus* (enclosed cyst) |
| *E. multilocularis* | Eggs from fox tapeworm | | | | | *E. multilocularis* (cyst wanders through tissue) |
| *Taenia solium* (pork) | Eggs from human tapeworm | CNS, subcutaneous tissues | Serum, scans, biopsy | Serology, films, histology | Positive serology, positive scans, tapeworm tissue | Small, enclosed cysticerci (cysticercosis) |
| **Intestinal Trematodes** | Ingestion of metacercariae: | | | | | |
| *Fasciolopsis buski* | On water chestnuts | Intestine | Stool | O&P exam; M. *yokogawai*, H. *heterophyes* eggs very small; use high dry power | Eggs in stool | Eggs of *F. buski* look identical to those of the liver fluke, *Fasciola hepatica* |
| *Metagonimus yokogawai* | In raw fish | | | | | |
| *Heterophyes heterophyes* | | | | | | |
| **Liver and Lung Trematodes** | Ingestion of metacercariae: | | | | | |
| *Fasciola hepatica* | On watercress | Liver | Stool | O&P | Eggs in stool | Eggs of *F. hepatica* look almost identical to those of *F. buski*; lung fluke eggs in sputum resemble brown metal filings |
| *Clonorchis sinensis* | In raw fish | Liver, bile ducts | Stool, duodenal drainage | O&P | Eggs in stool, and so on | |
| *Paragonimus* spp. | In raw crabs | Lung | Stool, sputum | O&P | Eggs in stool and/or sputum | |

| Organism | Transmission | Location/Site | Specimen | Diagnostic Method | Finding | Comments |
|---|---|---|---|---|---|---|
| **Blood Trematodes** | | Veins over the: | | | | |
| *Schistosoma mansoni* | Skin penetration of cercariae released from the freshwater snail intermediate host | Large intestine | Because the adult worms may become located in the "incorrect" veins, both urine and stool (unpreserved) should be examined | O&P; hatching test for egg viability (all specimens collected with no preservatives); concentrates performed with saline, not water | Eggs in stool and/or urine | When schistosomiasis is suspected, stool, spot urines, and 24-hr urine specimen (collected with no preservatives) |
| *S. haematobium* | | Bladder | | | | |
| *S. japonicum* | | Small intestine | | | | |
| **Malaria** | | Preerythrocytic: | | | | |
| *Plasmodium vivax* | Infection through mosquito bite, blood transfusion, shared drug needles; transplacental | Liver | Drawn immediately: **STAT REQUEST** Blood; draw every 6 hr until confirmed as positive or negative | Thick, thin blood films; rapid immunoassay methods (not yet FDA approved in United States); concentration methods | Parasites present | *P. falciparum* and *P. knowlesi* infections are **medical** emergencies; complete patient history mandatory (travel, prophylaxis, prior history); Giemsa or other blood stain recommended |
| *P. ovale* | | Blood | | | | |
| *P. malariae* | | Blood | | | | |
| *P. knowlesi* | | Blood | | | | |
| *P. falciparum* | | Blood plus capillaries of deep tissues (spleen, liver, bone marrow) | | | | |
| **Babesiosis** *Babesia* spp. | Tick borne; transfusion; organ transplants | Blood | Blood | Thick, thin blood films | Parasites present | Can mimic ring forms of *P. falciparum*; patient will have no travel history outside of United States |
| **Trypanosomes** | | | | | | |
| *Trypanosoma brucei gambiense* | Bite of tsetse fly | Blood, lymph nodes, CNS | Blood, node aspirate, CSF | Thick, thin films | Trypomastigotes | African sleeping sickness more common with *T. b. gambiense* |
| *T. b. rhodesiense* | Bite of tsetse fly | Blood, lymph nodes, CNS | Blood, lymph nodes, CNS | Thick, thin films | Trypomastigotes | Chagas disease (American trypanosomiasis) |
| *Trypanosoma cruzi* | Feces of triatomid bug (kissing bug) (bug feces scratched into bite site) | Blood, striated muscle (e.g., heart, GI tract) | Blood, cardiac changes, muscle biopsy | Thick, thin films, histology; culture | Trypomastigotes in blood, amastigotes in tissue | (xenodiagnosis an option) |

*Continued*

**TABLE 47-10** Common Human Parasites: Diagnostic Specimens, Tests, and Positive Findings—cont'd

| Organism | Infection Acquired | Location in Host | Diagnostic Specimen | Diagnostic Test* | Positive Specimen | Comments |
|---|---|---|---|---|---|---|
| **Leishmaniae** | | Macrophages of: | | | | |
| Leishmania tropica complex (cutaneous) | Bite of sand fly | Skin | Skin biopsy | Stained smears, cultures | Amastigotes in clinical specimens indicated | Animal inoculation rarely used; some research labs now using PCR |
| L. braziliensis complex (mucocutaneous) | | Skin, mucous membranes | Skin, membrane biopsy | Stained smears, cultures | | |
| L. donovani complex (visceral) | | Spleen, liver, bone marrow (RE system) | Blood, bone marrow, liver/spleen biopsy | Thick, thin blood films; stained smears, cultures | | |
| **Filarial Nematodes** | Bite of: | | | | | |
| Wuchereria bancrofti (S) | Mosquito | Lymphatics (adults), blood (microfilariae) | Blood | Thick, thin films; various concentrations | Microfilariae | Elephantiasis possible; periodicity a factor in finding microfilariae; some microfilariae sheathed (S), some not (NS) |
| Onchocerca volvulus (NS) | Black fly | Nodules (adults), skin, eye (microfilariae) | Skin snips, blood; biopsy nodule | Biopsy, tease skin apart in water; thick, thin films | Microfilariae; adult in tissue nodules | |
| **Less Common** | | | | | | |
| Loa loa (S) | Black gnat | Eye (adults) | Blood | Thick, thin films; various concentrations | Microfilariae, adult worm | "African eye worm" |
| Brugia malayi (S) | Mosquito | Lymphatics (adults) blood (microfilariae) | | | Microfilariae | |
| Mansonella spp. (NS) | Mosquito | blood (microfilariae) for all three | | | Microfilariae | |

CLM, Cutaneous larva migrans; CSF, cerebrospinal fluid; CNS, central nervous system; FA, fluorescent antibody; GAE, granulomatous amebic encephalitis; IA, immunoassay; ID, identification; NS, not sheathed; OLM, ocular larva migrans; O&P, ova and parasite; PAM, primary amebic meningoencephalitis; PCR, polymerase chain reaction; RE, reticuloendothelium system; S, sheathed; VLM, visceral larva migrans.

*Although serologic tests are not always mentioned, they are available for a number of parasitic infections. Unfortunately, most are not routinely available. Contact your state Public Health Laboratory or the Centers for Disease Control and Prevention (CDC) in Atlanta, Georgia.

†The microsporidia are now classified with the fungi.

---

**BOX 47-1**  Direct Smear: Review

**Principle**

To assess the worm burden of the patient, to allow quick diagnosis of heavily infected specimens, to check organism motility (primarily protozoan trophozoites), and to diagnose organisms that cannot be identified from the permanent stain methods; visible organism motility is the primary objective.

**Specimen**

Any fresh liquid or soft stool specimen that has not been refrigerated or frozen.

**Reagents**

0.85% NaCl; Lugol's or D'Antoni's iodine

**Examination**

Low-power examination (×100) of entire 22 × 22 mm coverslip preparation (both saline and iodine); high dry power examination (×400) of at least one third of the coverslip area (both saline and iodine).

**Results**

Results from the direct smear examination often should be considered presumptive. However, some organisms can be identified definitively (*Giardia lamblia* cysts and *Entamoeba coli* cysts, helminth eggs and larvae, *Isospora belli* oocysts). These reports should be considered "preliminary"; the final report includes the results of the concentration and permanent stained smear procedures.

**Notes and Limitations**

When iodine is added to the preparation, the organisms are killed and motility is lost. Specimens submitted in stool preservatives and fresh, formed specimens should not be examined using this procedure; the concentration and permanent stained smear techniques should be performed instead. Oil immersion examination (×1000) is not recommended (the organism morphology is not that clear).

---

**BOX 47-2**  Concentration: Review

**Principle**

To concentrate the parasites present, either through sedimentation or by flotation. The concentration is specifically designed to allow recovery of protozoan cysts, coccidian oocysts, microsporidian spores, and helminth eggs and larvae.

**Specimen**

Any stool specimen that is fresh or preserved in formalin (most common), polyvinyl alcohol (PVA; mercury based or non–mercury based), sodium acetate–acetic acid–formalin (SAF), merthiolate-iodine-formalin (MIF), or the newer single vial–system fixatives Universal fixatives containing no mercury, formalin, or PVA.

**Reagents**

5% or 10% formalin, ethyl acetate, zinc sulfate (specific gravity, 1.18 for fresh stool and 1.20 for preserved stool); 0.85% sodium chloride (NaCl); Lugol's or D'Antoni's iodine.

**Examination**

Low-power examination (×100) of entire 22 × 22 mm coverslip preparation (iodine recommended but optional); high dry power examination (×400) of at least one third of the coverslip area (both saline and iodine).

**Results**

Often, results from the concentration examination should be considered presumptive. However, some organisms can be identified definitively (*Giardia lamblia* cysts and *Entamoeba coli* cysts, helminth eggs, and larvae, *Isospora belli* oocysts). These reports should be considered "preliminary"; the final report is produced after the results of the permanent stained smear become available.

**Notes and Limitations**

Formalin–ethyl acetate sedimentation concentration is most commonly used. Zinc sulfate flotation does not detect operculated or heavy eggs (*Clonorchis* eggs, unfertilized *Ascaris* eggs); both the surface film and sediment must be examined before a negative result is reported. Smears prepared from concentrated stool are normally examined at low power (×100) and high dry power (×400); oil immersion examination (×1000) is not recommended (the organism morphology is not that clear). The addition of too much iodine may obscure helminth eggs (i.e., it produces an effect that mimics debris).

---

Other specimens from the intestinal tract, such as duodenal aspirates or drainage, mucus from the Entero-Test Capsule technique, and sigmoidoscopy material, can also be examined as wet preparations and as permanent stained smears after processing with trichrome or iron-hematoxylin staining.

**O&P Examination.** The O&P examination comprises three separate protocols: the direct wet mount, the concentration, and the permanent stained smear.

The direct wet mount, which requires fresh stool, is designed to allow detection of motile protozoan trophozoites. The specimen is examined microscopically at low and high dry magnifications (×100, entire 22 × 22 mm coverslip; ×400, one third to one half of a 22 × 22 mm coverslip) (Box 47-1). However, because of potential problems resulting from the lag time between specimen passage and receipt in the laboratory, the direct wet examination has been eliminated from the routine O&P in many laboratories in favor of receipt of specimens collected in stool preservatives. The direct wet preparation is not performed for specimens received in the laboratory in stool collection preservatives. The various fixatives available are included in Table 47-9.

The second part of the O&P is the concentration, which is designed to facilitate recovery of protozoan cysts, coccidian oocysts, microsporidial spores, and helminth eggs and larvae (Box 47-2). Both flotation and sedimentation methods are available; the most common procedure is the formalin–ethyl acetate sedimentation method (formerly called the formalin-ether method). The concentrated specimen is examined as a wet preparation, with or without iodine, using low and high dry magnifications (×100, ×400) as indicated for the direct wet smear examination.

The third part of the O&P examination is the permanent stained smear, which is designed to facilitate identification of intestinal protozoa (Box 47-3). Several staining methods are available; the two most commonly used are the Wheatley modification of the Gomori tissue trichrome stain and the iron-hematoxylin stain (Figure 47-1). This part of the O&P examination is critical to confirmation of suspicious objects seen in the wet

## BOX 47-3 Permanent Stained Smear: Review

### Principle

To provide contrasting colors between the background debris and parasites present. This technique is designed to allow examination and recognition of detailed organism morphology under oil immersion examination (×100 objective, for a total magnification of ×1000), primarily allowing recovery and identification of intestinal protozoa.

### Specimen

Any stool specimen that is fresh or preserved in polyvinyl alcohol (PVA; mercury based or non–mercury based), sodium acetate–acetic acid–formalin (SAF), merthiolate-iodine-formalin (MIF), or the newer single vial–system fixatives (Universal fixatives).

### Reagents

Trichrome, iron-hematoxylin, modified iron-hematoxylin, polychrome IV, or chlorazol black E stains and their associated solutions; dehydrating solutions (alcohols and xylenes or xylene substitutes); mounting fluid (optional). Rather than the 95%/5% alcohol option for absolute alcohol, the use of true absolute alcohol (100% ethanol) is preferred.

### Examination

Oil immersion examination (×1000) of at least 300 fields; additional fields may be required if suspect organisms have been seen in the wet preparations from the concentrated specimen.

### Results

Most suspect protozoa and/or human cells can be confirmed by the permanent stained smear. These reports should be categorized as "final" and are reported as such (the direct wet smear and the concentration examination provide "preliminary" results).

### Notes and Limitations

The most commonly used stains are trichrome and iron-hematoxylin. Unfortunately, helminth eggs and larvae generally take up too much stain and may not be identified from the permanent stained smear. Coccidian oocysts and microsporidian spores also require other staining methods for identification.

Permanent stained smears are normally examined under oil immersion examination (×1000), and low and high dry power are not recommended. The slide may be screened using the ×50 or ×60 oil immersion objectives, but the results should not be reported until the examination has been completed using the ×100 oil immersion lens. Confirmation of intestinal protozoa (both trophozoites and cysts) is the primary purpose of this technique.

### Important Reminder

When nonmercury fixatives or one of the single-vial options (usually a zinc-based, proprietary formula or one of the Universal fixatives) is used, the iodine-alcohol step can be eliminated. After drying, the slides can be placed directly into the stain (trichrome or hematoxylin). However, if fecal specimens have been preserved with mercury-based fixatives, the iodine-alcohol step must be included in the routine staining protocol, as well as subsequent rinse steps to remove the mercury and iodine. Some laboratories leave the staining protocol as is; including the iodine-alcohol step does not harm smears preserved with non-mercury–based fixatives.

---

examination and to identification of protozoa that may not have been visible in the wet preparation. Permanent stained smears are examined using oil immersion objectives (×600 for screening, ×1000 for final review of 300 or more oil immersion fields).

The permanent stained smear is the most important procedure performed to confirm the diagnosis of intestinal protozoan infections.

Modified acid-fast stains are recommended for intestinal coccidia (Box 47-4), and modified trichrome stains are recommended for intestinal microsporidia (Box 47-5). These stains are specifically designed to allow identification of coccidian oocysts and microsporidian spores, respectively.

Figure 47-2 provides a diagrammatic overview for the processing of fecal specimens for parasite identification.

**Recovery of the Tapeworm Scolex.** The procedure for recovery of the tapeworm scolex is rarely requested and no longer clinically relevant because of the effective use of medication for treatment of tapeworm infections. However, stool specimens may be examined for scolices and gravid proglottids of cestodes for species identification. This procedure requires mixing a small amount of feces with water and straining the mixture through a series of wire screens (graduated from coarse to fine mesh) to look for scolices and proglottids. The appearance of scolices after therapy is an indication of successful treatment. If the scolex has not been passed, it may still be attached to the mucosa; the parasite is capable of producing more segments from the neck region of the scolex, and the infection continues. If this occurs, the patient can be retreated when proglottids begin to reappear in the stool.

**Examination for Pinworm.** *Enterobius vermicularis*, a roundworm parasite commonly found in children worldwide, is referred to as *pinworm* or *seatworm*. The adult female worm migrates out of the anus, usually at night, and deposits her eggs on the perianal area. The adult female (8 to 13 mm long) occasionally may be found on the surface of a stool specimen or on the perianal skin. Because the eggs usually are deposited around the anus, they are not commonly found in feces and must be detected by other diagnostic techniques. Diagnosis of pinworm infection is usually based on the recovery of typical eggs, which are described as thick-shelled, football-shaped eggs with one slightly flattened side. Often, each egg contains a fully developed embryo and is infective within a few hours after being deposited (Figure 47-3).

**Sigmoidoscopy Material.** Material obtained from sigmoidoscopy can be helpful in the diagnosis of amebiasis that has gone undetected by routine fecal examinations. However, a series of at least three routine stool examinations for parasites should be done before a sigmoidoscopy examination is performed. A sigmoidoscopy specimen should be processed immediately. Three methods of examination are recommended. However, depending on the availability of trained personnel, proper fixatives, or the amount of specimen obtained,

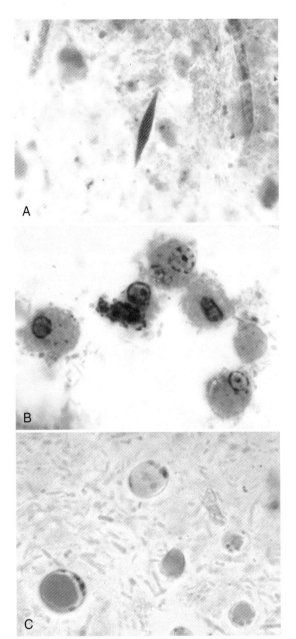

**Figure 47-1** Stool material stained with Wheatley's trichrome stain. **A,** Charcot-Leyden crystals. **B,** Polymorphonuclear leukocytes. **C,** *Blastocystis hominis* central body forms (larger objects) and yeast cells (smaller, more homogeneous objects).

one or two procedures may be used. It is important to note that even the most thorough examination will be meaningless if the specimen has been improperly collected, fixed, and transported.

**Duodenal Drainage.** In infections with *Giardia lamblia* or *Strongyloides stercoralis,* routine stool examinations may not be sufficient to identify the infecting organisms. Duodenal drainage material may increase the likelihood of identifying the parasites. However, the "falling leaf" motility often described for *Giardia* trophozoites is rarely seen in these preparations. The organisms may be caught in mucus strands, and the movement of the flagella on the *Giardia* trophozoites may be the only subtle motility

visible. *Strongyloides* larvae usually are very motile. It is important to keep the light intensity low for visualization of the moving parasites.

The duodenal fluid may contain mucus, and the organisms tend to be located in the mucus. Therefore, centrifugation of the specimen before examination is important. Fluorescent antibody or immunoassay detection kits (*Cryptosporidium* or *Giardia*) can also be used with fresh or formalinized material. It is important to check the package insert of each kit to see which specimen types are acceptable for that kit.

If a presumptive diagnosis of giardiasis is reached as a result of a wet prep examination, the coverslip can be removed and the specimen fixed with Schaudinn's fluid, other fixatives containing polyvinyl alcohol (PVA), or a "universal fixatives" (i.e., no formalin, no mercury, no PVA) for subsequent staining with trichrome or iron-hematoxylin. If the amount of duodenal material submitted is very small, permanent stains can be prepared in lieu of using a portion of the specimen for a wet prep. This approach provides a permanent record; it also may improve visualization of parasites using oil immersion examination of the stained specimen at ×1000 compared with examination of unstained organisms with minimal motility at a lower power.

**Duodenal Capsule Technique (Entero-Test).** The duodenal capsule technique is a simple, convenient method for collecting duodenal contents, eliminating the need for intestinal intubation. The technique involves the use of a length of nylon cord coiled inside a gelatin capsule. The cord protrudes through one end of the capsule and is taped to the side of the patient's face. The capsule is then swallowed. The gelatin dissolves in the stomach, and the weighted cord is carried by peristalsis into the duodenum. The cord is attached to the weight by a slipping mechanism; the weight is released and passes out in the stool when the cord is retrieved after 4 hours. The mucus collected on the cord is then examined for parasites, including *S. stercoralis, G. lamblia, Cryptosporidium* spp., microsporidia, and the eggs of *Clonorchis sinensis.*

### Urogenital Tract Specimens

*Trichomonas vaginalis* typically is identified by examination of wet preparations of vaginal and urethral discharges and prostatic secretions or urine sediment. Multiple specimens may be needed to detect the organisms. The specimens should be diluted with a drop of saline and examined for motile organisms under low power (×100) and reduced illumination; as the jerky motility begins to diminish, the undulating membrane may possibly be observed under high dry power (×400) (Figure 47-4). Unfortunately, the overall sensitivity of wet mount examinations is limited compared with culture and/or molecular testing, such as polymerase chain reaction (PCR) analysis. Stained smears usually are not necessary for identification of *T. vaginalis.* The number of false-positive and false-negative results reported from stained smears supports the value of confirmation by observation of motile organisms from the direct mount, culture media, or more sensitive direct antigen detection methods, such as the OSOM Trichomonas Rapid Test (Figure 47-5).

---

**BOX 47-4** Modified Acid-Fast Permanent Stained Smear: Review

**Principle**

To provide contrasting colors for background debris and parasites. This technique is designed to allow examination and recognition of acid-fast characteristic of organisms under high dry power (×40 objective, for a total magnification of ×400), primarily allowing recovery and identification of intestinal coccidian oocysts. The internal morphology (sporozoites) is seen in some *Cryptosporidium* oocysts under oil immersion (×1000); *Cyclospora* oocysts do not have a specific internal morphology.

**Specimen**

Any stool specimen that is fresh or preserved in formalin, sodium acetate–acetic acid–formalin (SAF), or the newer single vial–system fixatives (Universal fixatives).

**Reagents**

Kinyoun's acid-fast stain, modified Ziehl-Neelsen stain, and their associated solutions; dehydrating solutions (alcohols and xylenes or xylene substitutes); mounting fluid (optional). The decolorizing agents are less intense than the routine acid-alcohol used in routine acid-fast staining (this is what makes these "modified" acid-fast procedures). The recommended decolorizer is 1% to 3% sulfuric acid. Many laboratories use 1% so that the *Cyclospora* oocysts retain more color.

**Examination**

High dry examination (×400) of at least 300 fields; additional fields may be required if suspect organisms have been seen but are not clearly acid-fast.

**Results**

Identification of *Cryptosporidium* and *Isospora* oocysts should be possible. *Cyclospora* oocysts, which are twice the size of *Cryptosporidium* oocysts, should be visible but tend to be more acid-fast variable. Although microsporidia are acid-fast, their small size makes recognition very difficult. Final laboratory results depend heavily on the appearance of the quality control (QC) slides and comparison with positive patient specimens.

**Notes and Limitations**

Both the cold and hot modified acid-fast methods are excellent for staining coccidian oocysts. Some think that the hot method may result in better stain penetration, but the differences are probably minimal. Procedure limitations are related to specimen handling (proper centrifugation speeds and time, use of no more than two layers of wet gauze for filtration, and complete understanding of the difficulties in recognizing microsporidial spores). Also, some controversy exists over whether the organisms lose the ability to take up acid-fast stains after long-term storage in 10% formalin. The organisms are more difficult to find in specimens from patients who do not have the typical watery diarrhea (more formed stool contains more artifact material).

---

**BOX 47-5** Modified Trichrome Permanent Stained Smear: Review

**Principle**

To provide contrasting colors for the background debris and parasites present. This technique is designed to allow examination and recognition of organism morphology under oil immersion examination (×100 objective, for a total magnification of ×1000), primarily allowing recovery and identification of intestinal microsporidial spores. The internal morphology (horizontal or diagonal "stripes") may be seen in some spores under oil immersion.

**Specimen**

Any stool specimen that is fresh or preserved in formalin, sodium acetate–acetic acid–formalin (SAF), or the newer single vial–system fixatives (Universal fixatives).

**Reagents**

Modified trichrome stain (using high dye–content chromotrope 2R) and associated solutions; dehydrating solutions (alcohols, xylenes, or xylene substitutes); mounting fluid (optional).

**Examination**

Oil immersion examination (×1000) of at least 300 fields; additional fields may be required if suspect organisms have been seen but are not clearly identified.

**Results**

Identification of microsporidial spores may be possible; however, their small size makes recognition difficult. Final laboratory results depend heavily on the appearance of the quality control (QC) slides and comparison with positive patient specimens.

**Notes and Limitations**

Because of the difficulty in getting dye to penetrate the spore wall, this staining approach can be helpful. Procedure limitations are related to specimen handling (proper centrifugation speeds and time, use of no more than two layers of wet gauze for filtration, and complete understanding of the difficulties in recognizing microsporidial spores because of their small size [1 to 3 $\mu$m]).

**Commercial Suppliers**

Suppliers must be asked about specific fixatives and whether the fecal material can be stained with the modified trichrome stains and modified acid-fast stains. They also should be asked whether the fixatives prevent the use of any of the newer fecal immunoassay methods available for several of the intestinal amebae, flagellates, coccidia, and microsporidia.

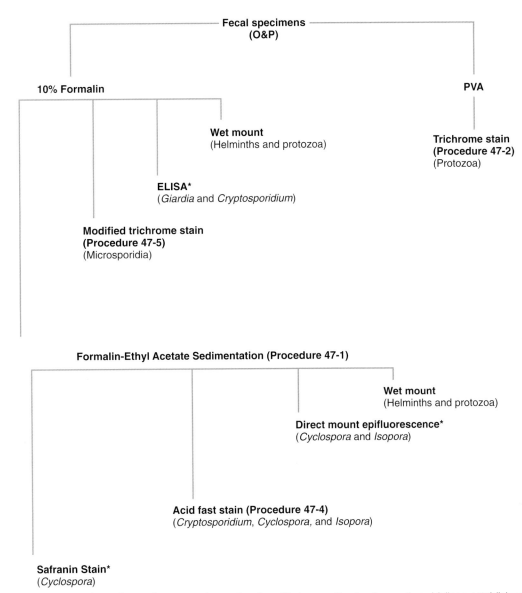

**Figure 47-2** Processing of fecal specimens for ova and parasites (modified according to diagnostic guidelines established by the Centers for Disease Control and Prevention). Asterisk (*) indicates a special test procedure.

## Sputum

Although not a common specimen, expectorated sputum may be submitted for parasitic examination. Organisms found in sputum that may cause pneumonia, pneumonitis, or Loeffler's syndrome include the migrating larval stages of *Ascaris lumbricoides, S. stercoralis,* and hookworm; the eggs of *Paragonimus* spp.; *Echinococcus granulosus* hooklets; and the protozoa *Entamoeba histolytica, Entamoeba gingivalis, Trichomonas tenax, Cryptosporidium* spp., and possibly the microsporidia. Some of the smaller organisms must be differentiated from fungi such as *Candida* spp. and *Histoplasma capsulatum.* In a *Paragonimus* infection, the sputum may be viscous, streaked with blood, and tinged with brownish flecks, which are clusters of eggs ("iron filings").

Induced sputa are collected after patients have used appropriate cleansing procedures to reduce oral contamination. The induction protocol is critical for the success of the procedure, and well-trained individuals are needed to recover the organisms.

## Aspirates

Examination of aspirated material for diagnosis of parasitic infections may be extremely valuable, particularly when routine testing methods have failed to demonstrate the presence of the organisms. These specimens should be transported to the laboratory immediately after collection. Aspirates include liquid specimens collected from a variety of sites. Aspirates most commonly processed in the parasitology laboratory include fine-needle aspirates and duodenal aspirates. Fluid specimens collected by bronchoscopy include bronchoalveolar lavages and bronchial washings.

Fine-needle aspirates may be submitted for slide preparation or culture, or both. Aspirates of cysts and abscesses for amebae may require concentration by centrifugation,

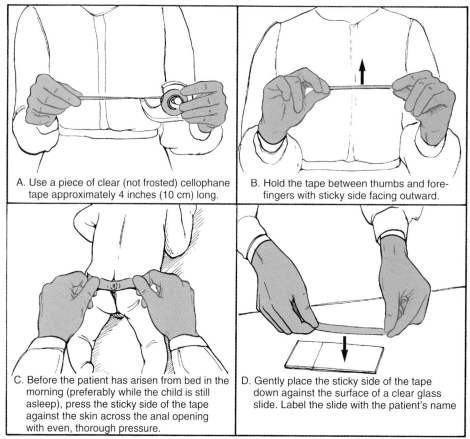

A. Use a piece of clear (not frosted) cellophane tape approximately 4 inches (10 cm) long.

B. Hold the tape between thumbs and fore-fingers with sticky side facing outward.

C. Before the patient has arisen from bed in the morning (preferably while the child is still asleep), press the sticky side of the tape against the skin across the anal opening with even, thorough pressure.

D. Gently place the sticky side of the tape down against the surface of a clear glass slide. Label the slide with the patient's name

**Figure 47-3** Method of collecting a cellophane (Scotch) tape preparation for pinworm diagnosis. This method dispenses with the tongue depressor, requiring only tape and a glass microscope slide. The tape must be pressed deep into the anal crack.

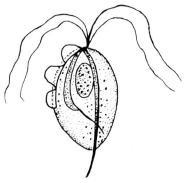

**Figure 47-4** *Trichomonas vaginalis* trophozoite. (Illustration by Nobuko Kitamura, Los Angeles.)

digestion, microscopic examination for motile organisms in direct preparations, cultures, and microscopic evaluation of stained preparations. Aspiration of cyst material (usually liver or lung) for diagnosis of hydatid disease usually is performed when surgical techniques are used for cyst removal. The aspirated fluid is submitted to the laboratory and examined for hydatid sand (scolices) or hooklets; absence of this material does not rule out the possibility of hydatid disease, because some cysts are sterile (Figure 47-6).

Bone marrow aspirates for *Leishmania* and *Trypanosoma cruzi* amastigotes or *Plasmodium* spp. require staining with any of the blood stains (Giemsa, Wright's,

Wright-Giemsa combination, rapid stains, or Field's stain). Examination of specimens may confirm an infection previously missed by examination of routine blood films.

Cases of primary amebic meningoencephalitis are rare, but examination of spinal fluid may reveal the causative agent, *Naegleria fowleri*, one of the free-living amebae (Figure 47-7).

### Biopsy Specimens

Biopsy specimens are recommended for diagnosis of tissue parasite infections. Impression smears and teased and squash preparations of biopsy tissue from skin, muscle, cornea, intestine, liver, lung, and brain can be used for this purpose, in addition to standard histologic preparations. An impression smear is a collection of cells, microorganisms, or fluids produced by pressing the surface of the specimen against a slide for review. Squash preparations are described in Chapter 6, and the tease mount preparation is outlined in Box 47-6. Tissue examined by permanent sections or electron microscopy should be fixed as specified by the processing laboratory. In certain cases, a biopsy may be the only means of confirming a suspected parasitic problem. Specimens examined as fresh material rather than as tissue sections should be kept moist in saline and submitted to the laboratory immediately.

Detection of parasites in tissue depends in part on specimen collection and adequate material to perform

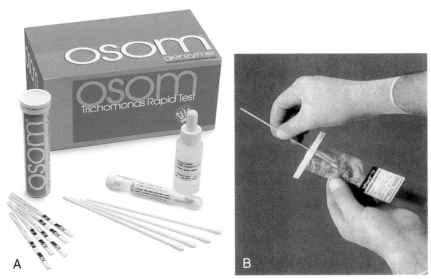

**Figure 47-5 A,** Rapid identification kit for *Trichomonas vaginalis.* **B,** Culture system for *T. vaginalis.* (**A** courtesy Sekisui Diagnostics, Farmingham, Mass.)

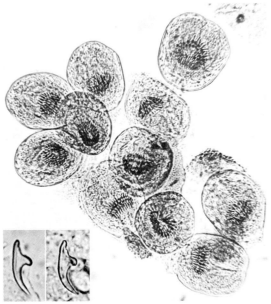

**Figure 47-6** *Echinococcus granulosus,* hydatid sand (×300). *Inset.* Two individual hooklets (×1000).

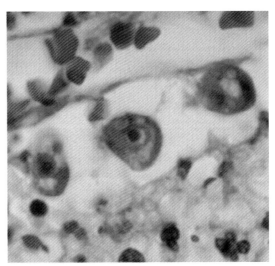

**Figure 47-7** *Naegleria fowleri* in brain tissue. (Hematoxylin and eosin stain.)

the recommended diagnostic procedures. Biopsy specimens are usually small and may not be representative of the diseased tissue. Multiple tissue samples often improve diagnostic results. To optimize the yield from any tissue specimen, all areas should be examined and as many procedures as possible performed. Tissues are obtained with invasive procedures, many of which are very expensive and lengthy; consequently, these specimens deserve the most comprehensive procedures possible. A muscle biopsy can be obtained for diagnosis of infection with *Trichinella* spp.; the specimen can be processed as a routine histology slide or can be examined as a squash preparation (Figure 47-8).

Tissue submitted in a sterile container on a sterile sponge dampened with saline may be used for cultures

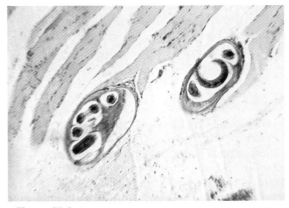

**Figure 47-8** *Trichinella* spp. larvae encysted in muscle.

## BOX 47-6 Thin Blood Films: Review

### Principle

To provide contrasting colors for background debris and parasites present, either outside or within the red blood cells (RBCs). This technique is designed to allow examination and recognition of detailed organism morphology under oil immersion examination (×100 objective, for a total magnification of ×1000), primarily allowing recovery and identification of *Plasmodium* spp., *Babesia* spp., *Trypanosoma* spp., *Leishmania donovani,* and filarial blood parasites. The thin blood film is routinely used for specific parasite identification, although the number of organisms per field is significantly reduced compared with the thick blood film. The primary purpose is to allow malarial parasites to be seen in the RBCs and to assess the size of infected RBCs compared with that of uninfected RBCs. RBC morphology is preserved using this method.

### Specimen

Finger-stick blood, whole blood, or anticoagulated blood (ethylenediaminetetraacetic acid [EDTA] recommended).

### Reagents

Giemsa stain (films must be prefixed with absolute methanol before staining), Wright's stain (the stain contains the fixative), or Wright-Giemsa stains and their associated solutions; mounting fluid (optional).

### Examination

Oil immersion examination (×1000) of at least 300 fields; additional fields may be required if suspect organisms have been seen in the thick blood film. The slide may be screened using the newer ×50 or ×60 oil immersion objectives, but the results should not be reported until the examination has been completed using the ×100 oil immersion lens. A blood film must be examined totally at a lower power to rule out the presence of microfilariae; this is particularly important for proficiency testing specimens.

### Results

The thin blood film is routinely used for parasite identification to the species level (*Plasmodium* spp.). Both the thick and thin films should be examined before the final result is reported.

### Notes and Limitations

The thin blood film is prepared exactly as one used for a differential count. A well-prepared film is thick at one end and thin at the other. The use of clean, grease-free slides is mandatory; long streamers of blood indicate that the slide used as a spreader was dirty or chipped. Streaks in the film usually are caused by dirt; holes in the film indicate grease on the slide. Although Giemsa stain is the stain of choice, blood parasites can be seen using other stains; however, the parasite morphology and color may not be consistent with that described for Giemsa-stained organisms. Giemsa stain does not stain the sheath of *Wuchereria bancrofti;* hematoxylin-based stains (e.g., Delafield's hematoxylin) are recommended for these organisms. The WBCs on the stained blood film serve as the quality control; if the WBC morphology and color are acceptable, then any parasites present will also appear normal and will be acceptable.

---

of protozoa after mounts for direct examination or impression smears for staining have been prepared. If cultures will be processed for parasites, sterile slides should be used for smear and mount preparation. Examination of tissue impression smears is detailed in Table 47-11.

### Blood

Depending on the life cycle, a number of parasites may be recovered in a blood specimen, including whole blood, buffy coat preparations, or various types of concentrations. Although organisms may be motile in fresh, whole blood, species identification is accomplished from examination of permanent stained thick and thin blood films. Blood films can be prepared from fresh, whole blood collected containing no anticoagulants, anticoagulated blood, or sediment from the various concentration procedures. In the past the stain of choice was Giemsa stain; however, parasites can also be seen on blood films stained with Wright's stain or other stains, including rapid staining options. Delafield's hematoxylin stain is often used to stain the microfilarial sheath; in some cases, Giemsa stain does not provide sufficient stain quality to allow differentiation of the microfilariae.

A request for examination of blood films for parasites is always a STAT request.

**Thin Blood Films.** In any examination of thin blood films for parasitic organisms, the initial screening should be done with the low-power microscope objective (×10). The entire film should be scanned to ensure that no microfilariae are missed. Microfilariae are rarely present in large numbers, and frequently only a few organisms are identified in each thin film preparation. Microfilariae are carried with the smear during preparation and typically are located at the edges or feathered end of the thin film. The feathered end of the film should be examined for intracellular and extracellular parasites. In these areas, the morphology and size of the infected red blood cells (RBCs) are more clearly visible (see Box 47-6).

Depending on the training and experience of the microscopist, examination of a thin film usually takes 15 to 20 minutes (300 or more oil immersion fields at a magnification of ×1000). Some use a ×50 or ×60 oil immersion objective to screen stained blood films; however, the chance is greater that small parasites (e.g., *Plasmodium* spp., *Babesia* spp., *Leishmania donovani*) will be missed at the lower total magnification (×500 or ×600) compared with the ×1000 total magnification achieved using the ×100 oil immersion objective.

Before a smear is reported as negative for the presence of parasites, a minimum of 300 fields should be examined. The request for blood film examination should be considered a STAT procedure, and all results (negative and positive) should be reported by telephone to the physician as soon as possible. If a result is positive, the appropriate government agencies (local, state, and federal) should be notified within a reasonable time, in accordance with guidelines and laws. It is important to note that one negative set of blood films is not sufficient to rule out blood parasites.

**TABLE 47-11** Examination of Impression Smears

| Tissue | Possible Parasite | Stain* |
|---|---|---|
| Lung | Microsporidia | Modified trichrome, acid-fast stain, Giemsa, tissue Gram stain, optical brightening agent (calcofluor), methenamine silver, electron microscopy (EM) |
| | *Toxoplasma gondii* | Giemsa, immune-specific reagent |
| | *Cryptosporidium* spp. | Modified acid-fast stain, immune-specific reagent |
| | *Entamoeba histolytica* | Giemsa, trichrome |
| Liver | *Toxoplasma gondii* | Giemsa |
| | *Leishmania donovani* | Giemsa |
| | *Cryptosporidium* spp. | Modified acid-fast stain, immune-specific reagent |
| | *Entamoeba histolytica* | Giemsa, trichrome |
| Brain | *Naegleria fowleri* | Giemsa, trichrome |
| | *Acanthamoeba* spp. | Giemsa, trichrome |
| | *Balamuthia mandrillaris* | Giemsa, trichrome |
| | *Sappinia* spp. | Giemsa, trichrome |
| | *Entamoeba histolytica* | Giemsa, trichrome |
| | *Toxoplasma gondii* | Giemsa, immune-specific reagent |
| | Microsporidia | |
| | *Encephalitozoon* spp. | Modified trichrome, acid-fast stain, Giemsa, optical brightening agent (calcofluor), methenamine silver, EM |
| Skin | *Leishmania* spp. | Giemsa |
| | *Onchocerca volvulus* | Giemsa |
| | *Mansonella streptocerca* | Giemsa |
| | *Acanthamoeba* spp. | Giemsa, trichrome |
| Nasopharynx, sinus cavities | Microsporidia | Modified trichrome, acid-fast stain, Giemsa, optical brightening agent (calcofluor), methenamine silver, EM |
| | *Acanthamoeba* spp. | Giemsa, trichrome |
| | *Naegleria fowleri* | Giemsa, trichrome |
| **Intestine**<br>Small intestine | *Cryptosporidium parvum* (both small and large intestine) | Modified acid-fast, immune-specific reagent |
| Jejunum | *Cyclospora cayetanensis* | Modified acid-fast |
| | Microsporidia<br>*Enterocytozoon bieneusi*<br>*Encephalitozoon (Septata) intestinalis* | Modified trichrome, acid-fast stain, Giemsa, optical brightening agent (calcofluor), methenamine silver, EM |
| Duodenum | *Giardia lamblia* | Giemsa, trichrome |
| Colon | *Entamoeba histolytica* | Giemsa, trichrome |
| Cornea, conjunctiva | Various genera of microsporidia<br>*Acanthamoeba* spp. | Acid-fast stain, Giemsa, modified trichrome, methenamine silver, optical brightening agent (calcofluor), EM<br>Giemsa, trichrome, calcofluor (cysts) |
| Muscle | *Trichinella spiralis* | Wet examination, squash preparation |
| | Microsporidia<br>*Pleistophora* sp., *Brachiola* sp., *Trachipleistophora* sp. | Modified trichrome, acid-fast stain, Giemsa, optical brightening agent (calcofluor), methenamine silver, EM |

*Whenever Giemsa stain is mentioned in the table, any blood stain is acceptable: Giemsa, Wright's, Wright-Giemsa combination, rapid blood stains.

Both malaria and *Babesia* infections have been missed with automated differential instruments, delaying treatment. Although these instruments are not designed to detect intracellular blood parasites, the inability of the automated systems to distinguish between uninfected RBCs and those infected with parasites may pose diagnostic problems.

**Thick Blood Films.** In the preparation of a thick blood film, the greatest concentration of blood cells is in the center of the film. The examination should be performed at low magnification to detect microfilariae. Examination of a thick film usually requires 5 to 10 minutes (approximately 100 oil immersion fields). A search for malarial organisms and trypanosomes should be completed using oil immersion (total magnification of ×1000). Intact RBCs frequently are seen at the very periphery of the thick film; such cells, if infected, may prove useful in the diagnosis of malaria. These cells may demonstrate the characteristic organismic morphology required for speciation of the parasite (Box 47-7).

**Blood Film Stains.** To ensure accurate identification of blood parasites, a laboratory should demonstrate proficiency in the use of at least one good staining method. Selecting one method that provides reproducible results may improve identification. Blood films should be stained as soon as possible, because prolonged storage may result in stain retention. Failure to stain positive malarial smears within 1 month may result in failure to demonstrate typical staining characteristics for individual species.

The two most common types of stain are Wright's stain and Giemsa stain. In Wright's stain, the fixative is combined with the staining solution, which allows fixation and staining to occur at the same time; therefore, a thick film must be laked before staining. In Giemsa stain, the fixative and stain are separate, requiring fixation of a thin film with absolute methanol before staining.

**Buffy Coat Films.** *L. donovani*, trypanosomes, and *H. capsulatum* (a fungus with intracellular elements resembling those of *L. donovani*) occasionally may be detected in the peripheral blood. The parasite or fungus is detected in the large mononuclear cells found in the buffy coat (a layer of white blood cells resulting from centrifugation of whole citrated blood). Some microfilariae also may be found in a buffy coat preparation. With *L. donovani*, the nuclear material stains dark red-purple, and the cytoplasm is light blue. *H. capsulatum* appears as a large dot of nuclear material (dark red-purple) surrounded by a clear halo. Trypanosomes in the peripheral blood also concentrate with the buffy coat cells.

## DIRECT DETECTION METHODS

Progress has been made in the development and application of molecular methods for diagnosis of parasite

---

**BOX 47-7** Thick Blood Films: Review

**Principle**

To provide contrasting colors for background debris and parasites present. This technique is designed to allow examination and recognition of detailed organism morphology under oil immersion examination (×100 objective, for a total magnification of ×1000), primarily allowing recovery and identification of *Plasmodium* spp., *Babesia* spp., *Trypanosoma* spp., *Leishmania donovani,* and filarial blood parasites. The thick blood film is routinely used for detection of parasites, because the number of organisms per field is much greater than with the thin blood film. The primary purpose is to allow examination of a larger volume of blood than is seen with the thin blood film. Red blood cell (RBC) morphology is not preserved using this method. The blood films must be laked before or during staining (rupture of all RBCs); the only structures that are left on the blood film are white blood cells, platelets, and parasites.

**Specimen**

Finger-stick blood, whole blood, or anticoagulated blood (ethylenediaminetetraacetic acid [EDTA] recommended).

**Reagents**

Giemsa stain (water-based stain, laking of the RBCs occurs during staining process), Wright's stain (thick blood films must be laked before staining), or Wright-Giemsa stains and their associated solutions; mounting fluid (optional).

**Examination**

Oil immersion examination (×1000) of at least 300 fields; additional fields may be required if suspect organisms have been seen in the thin blood film. The slide may be screened using the newer ×50 or ×60 oil immersion objectives, but the results should not be reported until the examination has been completed using the ×100 oil immersion lens. A blood film must be examined totally at a lower power to rule out the presence of microfilariae. This is particularly true for proficiency testing specimens.

**Results**

The thick blood film is routinely used to detect the presence of parasites; final identification may require examination of the thin blood film. Both should be examined before the final result is reported.

**Notes and Limitations**

The thick blood film is prepared by spreading a few drops of blood (using a circular motion) over an area approximately 2 cm in diameter. If whole blood is used, the examiner should continue stirring about 30 seconds to prevent the formation of fibrin strands. The use of clean, grease-free slides is mandatory. The film is allowed to air-dry at room temperature (heat is never applied to these films). After the thick films are thoroughly dry, they can be laked to remove the hemoglobin. Although Giemsa stain is the stain of choice, blood parasites can be seen using other stains; however, the parasite morphology and color may not be consistent with that described for Giemsa-stained organisms. Giemsa stain does not stain the sheath of *Wuchereria bancrofti;* hematoxylin-based stains (e.g., Delafield's hematoxylin) are recommended for these organisms. The WBCs on the stained blood film serve as the quality control; if the WBC morphology and color are acceptable, then any parasites present will also appear normal and will be acceptable.

infections, including the use of purified or recombinant antigens and nucleic acid probes. Detection of parasite-specific antigen indicates current disease. Many of the assays originally were developed with polyclonal antibodies targeted to unpurified antigens, which markedly decreases the sensitivity and specificity of the tests. Nucleic acid–based parasitic diagnostic tests are primarily available in specialized research or reference centers. PCR and other nucleic acid probe tests have been reported for almost all species of parasites. An example is the commercially available, nucleic acid–based probe test for detecting *T. vaginalis*. The demand for implementation of direct detection using molecular methods will increase as the cost of these tests decreases and automation increases.

### Intestinal Parasites

Immunoassays generally are simple and allow simultaneous performance of many tests, thereby reducing overall costs. Antigen detection in stool specimens is limited to the detection of one or two pathogens simultaneously. A routine O&P examination should be performed to detect other parasitic pathogens. The current commercially available antigen tests (direct fluorescent antibody [DFA], enzyme immunoassay [EIA], indirect fluorescent antibody [IFA], and the cartridge formats) have excellent sensitivity and specificity compared with routine microscopy. The currently available antigen detection tests are listed in Table 47-12. Currently, the most common immunoassays are designed to confirm infection with *E. histolytica*, the *Entamoeba histolytica/Entamoeba dispar* group, *G. lamblia*, and *Cryptosporidium* spp. Test formats include fluorescence, enzyme immunoassays, immunochromatographic test strips, and rapid cartridges.

### Blood Parasites

Several new blood parasite antigen detection systems are available and have been effectively tested in field trials. Most of these procedures are designed as an antigen capture system and have been incorporated into a dipstick format (see Table 47-12).

## CULTIVATION

Nematode infections giving rise to larval stages that hatch in soil or in tissues can be diagnosed using fecal culture methods to increase the number of larvae. *S. stercoralis* larvae are generally the most common parasite identified in stool specimens. Depending on the fecal transit time through the intestine and the patient's condition, rhabditiform (and in rare cases filariform) larvae may be present. With hookworm, if stool examination is delayed, embryonated ova in addition to larvae may be present. Culture of feces for larvae is useful to (1) reveal their presence when the organisms are too scanty to be detected by concentration methods; (2) distinguish whether the infection is due to *S. stercoralis* or hookworm, based on rhabditiform larval morphology, by allowing hookworm eggs to hatch, releasing first-stage larvae; and (3) allow the development of larvae into the filariform stage for further differentiation.

Very few clinical laboratories offer specific culture techniques for protozoan parasites. The methods for in vitro culture are often complex, and quality control is difficult and not feasible in the routine diagnostic laboratory. Some techniques may be available in certain institutions, particularly those in which research and consulting services are available.

Cultures of parasites grown in association with an unknown flora are referred to as *xenic cultures*. An example of this type of culture is stool specimens cultured for *E. histolytica*. If the parasites are grown with a single known bacterium, the culture is referred to as *monoxenic*. An example of this type of culture is the clinical specimen (corneal biopsy) cultured with *Escherichia coli* as a means of recovering *Acanthamoeba* and *Naegleria* spp. If parasites are grown as pure culture without any bacterial associate, the culture is referred to as *axenic*. An example is the use of media for the isolation of *Leishmania* spp. or *T. cruzi*.

### Larval-Stage Nematodes

The use of certain fecal culture methods (sometimes referred to as *coproculture*) is especially helpful for detecting light infections of hookworm, *S. stercoralis*, and *Trichostrongylus* spp. The rearing of infective-stage nematode larvae improves the diagnosis of hookworm and trichostrongyle infections, because the eggs of these species are identical and differentiation is based on larval morphology. These techniques also are useful for obtaining infective-stage larvae for research purposes. Diagnostic methods available include the Harada-Mori filter paper strip culture, the Petri dish filter paper culture, the agar plate method, the charcoal culture, and the Baermann concentration.

### Protozoa

Few parasites can be routinely cultured, and the procedures more frequently available are specifically for *E. histolytica*, *N. fowleri*, *Acanthamoeba* spp., *T. vaginalis*, *Toxoplasma gondii*, *T. cruzi*, and the leishmaniae. Any laboratory providing these types of cultures must maintain stock quality control (QC) cultures of specific organisms, often obtained from the American Type Culture Collection (ATCC). The relevant QC organisms are cultured simultaneously with the patient specimen, thus providing some assurance that the culture system performed properly.

## SERODIAGNOSIS

Although parasites and their byproducts are immunogenic for the host, the host immune response usually is not protective. Host immunity usually is species specific and may be strain or stage specific. Human parasites generally are divided into two groups: (1) those that multiply in the host (e.g., protozoa) and (2) those that mature in the host without multiplying (e.g., schistosomes, *A. lumbricoides*). In protozoan infections in which the organism reproduces in the host, continuous antigenic stimulation of the host's immune system occurs as the infection progresses. In these cases, a positive correlation exists between clinical symptoms and serologic test

**TABLE 47-12** Antigen Detection Kits for Stool or Vaginal Discharge Specimens (may not be all-inclusive)*

| Organism/Kit Name | Company[†] | Test Format |
|---|---|---|
| **Protozoa** | | |
| *CRYPTOSPORIDIUM SPP.* | | |
| PARA-TECT Cryptosporidium | Medical Chemical | EIA |
| ProSpecT Cryptosporidium | Remel | EIA |
| Xpect Cryptosporidium RAPID | Remel | Rapid |
| Cryptosporidium II | TechLab–Inverness Medical Professional Diagnostics (formerly Wampole) | EIA |
| *CRYPTOSPORIDIUM SPP. AND GIARDIA LAMBLIA* | | |
| ColorPAC Giardia/Cryptosporidium RAPID | Becton Dickinson | Rapid |
| PARA-TECT Cryptosporidium/Giardia | Medical Chemical | DFA |
| Merifluor | Meridian Bioscience | DFA |
| ImmunoCardSTAT Cryptosporidium/Giardia | Meridian Bioscience | Rapid |
| ProSpecT Giardia/Cryptosporidium | Remel | EIA |
| Xpect Giardia/Cryptosporidium RAPID | Remel | Rapid |
| Giardia/Cryptosporidium CHEK | TechLab–Inverness Medical Professional Diagnostics (formerly Wampole) | EIA |
| *CRYPTOSPORIDIUM SPP., GIARDIA LAMBLIA, AND ENTAMOEBA HISTOLYTICA/E. DISPAR* GROUP | | |
| Triage (fresh, frozen) | BioSite/Alere | Rapid |
| Entamoeba histolytica | Remel | EIA |
| ProSpecT (fresh, frozen, Cary-Blair) | Remel | EIA |
| Entamoeba histolytica II (fresh, frozen) | Medical Professional Diagnostics (formerly Wampole) | EIA |
| *GIARDIA LAMBLIA* | | |
| PARA-TECT Giardia | Medical Chemical | EIA |
| ProSpecT Giardia | Remel | EIA |
| Xpect Giardia RAPID | Remel | Rapid |
| Giardia II | TechLab–Inverness Medical Professional Diagnostics (formerly Wampole) | EIA |
| *TRICHOMONAS VAGINALIS* | | |
| Affirm VPIII | Becton Dickinson | Probe |
| T. vaginalis | Chemicon | DFA |
| OSOM Trichomonas | Genzyme | Rapid |
| XenoStrip-Tv | Xenotope | Rapid |

*DFA,* Direct fluorescent antibody; *EIA,* enzyme immunoassay; *IFA,* indirect fluorescent antibody; *RAPID,* rapid immunochromatographic assay
*These kits are available commercially in the United States for immunodetection of parasitic organisms or antigens in stool or vaginal discharge. This is a representative list; not every available kit is listed. adapted from the Center for Disease Control and Prevention.
[†]Biosite, 11030 Roselle St., San Diego, CA 92121; Becton Dickinson Diagnostic Systems, 7 Loveton Circle, Sparks, MD 21152; Chemicon, 28835 Single Oak Dr., Temecula, CA 92590; Genzyme Diagnostics, One Kendall Square, Cambridge, MA 02139; Inverness Medical Professional Diagnostics (formerly Wampole), P.O. Box 1001, Cranbury, NJ 08512; Medical Chemical Corporation, 19430 Van Ness Ave., Torrance, CA 90501; Meridian Bioscience, 3471 River Hills Dr., Cincinnati, OH 45244; Remel, P.O. Box 14428, Lenexa, KS 66215; TechLab, VPI Research Park, 1861 Pratt Dr., Blacksburg, VA 24060; Xenotope Diagnostics, 3463 Magic Dr., Suite 350, San Antonio, TX 78229.

results. Infection caused by *T. gondii,* a tissue protozoon, is acquired by ingestion of infected meat, ingestion of oocysts from cat feces, transplacentally, and by blood transfusion or organ transplantation. Toxoplasmosis is diagnosed primarily serologically, rather than by identification of organisms in human clinical specimens.

In contrast to the protozoa, helminths often migrate through the body and pass through a number of developmental stages before becoming mature adults. These infections often are difficult to confirm serologically because of a limited antigenic response by the host or failure to use the appropriate antigen in the test system. Most parasitic antigens used in serologic procedures are undefined heterogeneous mixtures. Test results using such antigens may be invalid because of cross-reactions or poor sensitivity.

Serologic procedures have been available for many years; however, they are not routinely offered by most clinical laboratories because of the high cost, lack of trained personnel, difficulty in interpretation, low test volume, and decreased sensitivity and specificity. Standard techniques have been used in the laboratory for parasitic diagnostics, including complement fixation (CF), indirect hemagglutination (IHA), IFA, soluble antigen fluorescent antibody, bentonite flocculation, latex agglutination (LA), double diffusion, counterelectrophoresis, immunoelectrophoresis, radioimmunoassay, and intradermal tests.

The Centers for Disease Control and Prevention (CDC) offers a number of serologic procedures for diagnostic purposes, some of which are not available elsewhere. Regulations for submitting specimens to the CDC may vary from state to state. Each laboratory should check with the appropriate county or state department of public health for specific instructions. Additional information on procedures, the availability of skin test antigens, and interpretation of test results may be obtained directly from the CDC:

Serology Unit Parasitology Diseases Branch
Building 4 Room 1009
Mail Stop F13
Centers for Disease Control and Prevention
4770 Buford Highway
Atlanta, GA 30034
Serology (770) 488-7760
Chagas Disease and Leishmaniasis (770) 488-4474
Malaria (770) 488-7765

# PREVENTION

Prevention of human parasitic infections is directly linked to the various organism life cycles and modes of infection (see Table 47-4). Preventive measures include increased attention to personal hygiene, proper sanitation, and elimination of sexual activities that may involve fecal-oral contact. Adequate water treatment (including filtration) may be required, in addition to overall awareness of environmental sources of infection. In some cases, avoiding contaminated environmental water and soil sources may be important—it is mandatory when dealing with contact lens care systems and potential infection with free-living amebae.

Chemoprophylactic agents to prevent clinical symptoms are given to individuals traveling to areas in which malaria is endemic. The prophylactic medications are effective against the erythrocytic forms but do not prevent infection with malaria; that is, the drugs do not prevent sporozoites from entering the host, traveling to the liver, and beginning the preerythrocytic developmental cycle. In general, chloroquine is the drug of choice, although different regimens may be used in areas with chloroquine-resistant strains of malaria.

Vector control and awareness of transmission through blood transfusions, shared drug needles, congenital infections, and organ transplants are important considerations in preventing human parasitic disease. Careful monitoring of the blood supply is required to prevent transmission of parasites. This is particularly important in areas of the world in which blood-borne parasites play a large role in human disease.

Adequate cooking of meat that may be infected is also important; cultural habits may influence the handling and eating of raw or poorly cooked foods. Prevention depends on a thorough understanding of the life cycle and epidemiology of all parasites that cause human disease. This information is critical to the prevention of human disease caused either by parasites limited to the human host or by parasites that can cause disease in humans and other animal hosts.

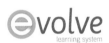 *Visit the Evolve site to complete the review questions.*

# BIBLIOGRAPHY

Alvar J, Aparicio P, Aseffa A, et al: The relationship between leishmaniasis and AIDS: the second 10 years, *Clin Microbiol Rev* 21:334, 2008.

Chen LH, Keystone JS: New strategies for the prevention of malaria in travelers, *Infect Dis Clin North Am* 19:185, 2005.

Clark DP: New insights into human cryptosporidiosis, *Clin Microbiol Rev* 12:554, 1999.

Clinical and Laboratory Standards Institute: *Procedures for the recovery and identification of parasites from the intestinal tract*, Approved guideline, second edition, M28-A2, Villanova, Pa, 2005, the Institute.

Clinical and Laboratory Standards Institute: *Laboratory diagnosis of blood-borne parasitic diseases*, Approved guideline, M15-A, Wayne, Pa, 2000, the Institute.

Fayer R: Cryptosporidium: a water-borne zoonotic parasite, *Vet Parasitol* 126:37, 2004.

Feng Y, Xiao L: Zoonotic potential and molecular epidemiology of *Giardia* species and giardiasis, *Clin Microbiol Rev* 24:110, 2011.

Fotedar R, Stark D, Beebe N, et al: Laboratory diagnostic techniques for *Entamoeba* species, *Clin Microbiol Rev* 20:511, 2007.

Garcia LS: Malaria, *Clin Lab Med* 30:93, 2010.

Garcia LS, editor: *Clinical microbiology procedures handbook*, ed 3, vol 1-3, Washington, DC, 2010, ASM Press.

Garcia LS: *Diagnostic medical parasitology*, ed 5, Washington, DC, 2007, ASM Press.

Garcia LS: *Practical guide to diagnostic parasitology*, ed 2, Washington, DC, 2009, ASM Press.

Garcia LS, Shimizu RY: Detection of *Giardia lamblia* and *Cryptosporidium parvum* antigens in human fecal specimens using the ColorPAC combination rapid solid-phase qualitative immunochromatographic assay, *J Clin Microbiol* 38:1267, 2000.

Garcia LS, Shimizu RY, Bernard CN: Detection of *Giardia lamblia, Entamoeba histolytica/E. dispar,* and *Cryptosporidium parvum* antigens in human fecal specimens using the EIA Triage Parasite Panel, *J Clin Microbiol* 38:3337, 2000.

Gottstein B, Pozio E, Nockler K: Epidemiology, diagnosis, treatment, and control of trichinellosis, *Clin Microbiol Rev* 22:127, 2009.

Herman JS, Chiodini PL: Gnathostomiasis, another emerging imported disease. *Clin Microbiol Rev* 22:484, 2009.

Isenberg HD, editor: *Clinical microbiology procedures handbook*, ed 2, vol 1-3, Washington, DC, 2005, ASM Press.

Isenberg HD, editor: *Essential procedures for clinical microbiology*, Washington, DC, 1995, ASM Press.

Keiser J, Utzinger J: Food-borne trematodiases, *Clin Microbiol Rev* 22:466, 2009.

Keiser PB, Nutman TB: *Strongyloides stercoralis* in the immunocompromised population, *Clin Microbiol Rev* 17:208, 2004.

Markell EK, Voge M, John DT: *Medical parasitology*, ed 7, Philadelphia, 1992, WB Saunders.

Melvin DM, Brooke MM: *Laboratory procedures for the diagnosis of intestinal parasites*, US Department of Health, Education, and Welfare Pub No

(CDC) 85-8282, Washington, DC, 1985, US Government Printing Office.

Modai S, Bhattacharya P, Ali N: Current diagnosis and treatment of visceral leishmaniasis, *Expert Rev Anti Infect Ther* 8:19, 2010.

Murray CK, Gasser RA Jr, Magill AJ, Miller RS: Update on rapid diagnostic testing for malaria, *Clin Microbiol Rev* 21:97, 2008.

Ortega YR, Sanchez R: Update on *Cyclospora cayetanensis*, a food-borne and waterborne parasite, *Clin Microbiol Rev* 23:218, 2010.

Pasvol G: Management of severe malaria: interventions and controversies, *Infect Dis Clin North Am* 19:211, 2005.

Paulinoa M, Iribarnea F, Dubinb M, et al: The chemotherapy of Chagas' disease: an overview, *Mini Rev Med Chem* 5:499, 2005.

Procop GW: North American paragonimiasis (caused by *Paragonimus kellicotti*) in the context of global paragonimiasis, *Clin Microbiol Rev* 22:415, 2009.

Scholz T, Garcia HH, Kuchta R, Wicht B: Update on the human broad tapeworm (genus *Diphyllobothrium*),including clinical relevance, *Clin Microbiol Rev* 22:322, 2009.

Schuster FL, Ramirez-Avila L: Current world status of *Balantidium coli*, *Clin Microbiol Rev* 21:626, 2008.

Schwebke JR, Burgess D: Trichomoniasis, *Clin Microbiol Rev* 17:794, 2004.

Tan KS: New insights on classification, identification, and clinical relevance of *Blastocystis* spp., *Clin Microbiol Rev* 21:639, 2008.

Wilson M, Schantz PM: Parasitic immunodiagnosis. In Strickland GT, editor: *Hunter's tropical medicine and emerging infectious diseases*, ed 8, Philadelphia, 2000, WB Saunders.

Xiao L, Ryan UM: Cryptosporidiosis: an update in molecular epidemiology, *Curr Opin Infect Dis* 17:483, 2004.

# Intestinal Protozoa

## OBJECTIVES

1. Describe the basic life cycle, distinguishing morphologic characteristics, clinical disease (if pathogenic), laboratory diagnosis, and prevention for the organisms listed in the following table.
2. Define and identify the following parasitic structures: trophozoite, cyst, oocyst, spore, pseudopodia, flagella, cilia, chromatoidal bars, karysome, central vacuole, cyst form, axoneme, cytostome, spiral groove, undulating membrane, ventral disc, shepherd's crook, axostyle, macronucleus, micronucleus, apical complex, sporocyst, sporozoite, spore, sarcocyst, and polar tubule.
3. Define life cycle processes, including merogony, gametogony, sporogony, schizogony, and the associated organism(s) and stages.
4. Correlate the parasitic life cycles with the specific diagnostic stages for the organisms listed.
5. Distinguish pathogenic from nonpathogenic protozoa.

---

### PARASITES TO BE CONSIDERED

**Protozoa**
Amebae (intestinal)
  *Entamoeba histolytica*
  *Entamoeba dispar**
  *Entamoeba coli*
  *Entamoeba hartmanni*
  *Endolimax nana*
  *Iodamoeba bütschlii*
  *Blastocystis hominis*
Flagellates (intestinal)
  *Giardia lamblia†*
  *Chilomastix mesnili*
  *Dientamoeba fragilis*
  *Pentatrichomonas hominis*
Ciliates (intestinal)
  *Balantidium coli*
Coccidia, Microsporidia (intestinal)
  *Cryptosporidium* spp.
  *Cyclospora cayetanensis*
  *Isospora (Cystoisospora) belli*
  *Sarcocystis hominis*
  *Sarcocystis suihominis*
Microsporidia (intestinal)
  *Enterocytozoon bieneusi*
  *Encephalitozoon* spp.

---

*Currently, the name *Entamoeba histolytica* is used to designate true pathogens, and *Entamoeba dispar* is used to designate nonpathogens. Unless trophozoites containing ingested red blood cells are seen *(E. histolytica)*, the two organisms cannot be differentiated based on the morphology revealed by permanent stained smears of fecal specimens. Immunoassay kits are available for identifying the *E. histolytica/E. dispar* group and for differentiating *E. histolytica* from *E. dispar*.

†Although some individuals have changed the species designation for the genus *Giardia* to *G. intestinalis* or *G. duodenalii*, no general agreement has been reached. Therefore, for this list we retain the name *Giardia lamblia*.

---

The protozoa are unicellular eukaryotic organisms, most of which are microscopic. They have a number of specialized organelles that are responsible for life functions and that allow further division of the group into classes. Most protozoa multiply by binary fission and are ubiquitous worldwide.

The important characteristics of the intestinal protozoa are presented in Tables 48-1 to 48-7. The clinically relevant intestinal protozoa are generally considered to be *Entamoeba histolytica, Blastocystis hominis, Giardia lamblia, Dientamoeba fragilis, Balantidium coli, Isospora (Cystoisospora) belli, Cryptosporidium* spp., *Cyclospora cayetanensis,* and the microsporidia. Nonpathogenic intestinal protozoa are listed in various figures and tables but are not discussed in detail.

## AMEBAE

The class Sarcodina, or Amebae, includes the organisms capable of movement by means of cytoplasmic protrusions called **pseudopodia**. This group includes free-living organisms, in addition to nonpathogenic and pathogenic organisms found in the intestinal tract and other areas of the body (see Tables 48-1 and 48-2). Occasionally, when fresh stool material is examined as a direct wet mount, motile trophozoites may be seen, as well as other, nonparasitic structures (Figure 48-1).

### ENTAMOEBA HISTOLYTICA

#### General Characteristics

Living trophozoites (motile feeding stage) of E. *histolytica* vary in size from about 12 to 60 μm in diameter. Organisms recovered from diarrheic or dysenteric stools generally are larger than those in formed stool from an asymptomatic individual. The motility has been described as rapid and unidirectional. Although this characteristic motility is often described, amebiasis rarely is diagnosed on the basis of motility seen in a direct mount. The cytoplasm is differentiated into a clear outer ectoplasm and a more granular inner endoplasm.

E. *histolytica* has directional and progressive motility, whereas the other amebae tend to move more slowly and at random. However, motility is rarely seen even in a fresh wet mount from a patient with diarrhea or dysentery. The cytoplasm is generally more finely granular, and the presence of red blood cells (RBCs) in the cytoplasm is considered diagnostic for E. *histolytica* (Figure 48-2).

Permanent stained smears demonstrate accurate morphology compared with other techniques. When the organism is examined on a permanent stained smear (trichrome or iron-hematoxylin stain), the morphologic

**TABLE 48-1**  Intestinal Protozoa: Trophozoites of Common Amebae

| Characteristic | Entamoeba histolytica | Entamoeba dispar | Entamoeba hartmanni | Entamoeba coli | Endolimax nana | Iodamoeba bütschlii |
|---|---|---|---|---|---|---|
| Size* (diameter or length) | 12-60 $\mu m$ (usual range, 15-20 $\mu m$); invasive forms may be > 20 $\mu m$ | Same size range as E. histolytica | 5-12 $\mu m$ (usual range, 8-10 $\mu m$) | 15-50 $\mu m$ (usual range, 20-25 $\mu m$) | 6-12 $\mu m$ (usual range, 8-10 $\mu m$) | 8-20 $\mu m$ (usual range, 12-15 $\mu m$) |
| Motility | Progressive, with hyaline, finger-like pseudopodia; motility may be rapid | Same motility as E. histolytica | Usually nonprogressive | Sluggish, nondirectional; blunt, granular pseudopodia | Sluggish, usually nonprogressive | Sluggish, usually nonprogressive |
| Nucleus (single) and visibility | Difficult to see in unstained preparations | Difficult to see in unstained preparations | Usually not seen in unstained preparations | Often visible in unstained preparation | Occasionally visible in unstained preparations | Usually not visible in unstained preparations |
| Peripheral chromatin (stained) | Fine granules, uniform in size and usually evenly distributed; may have beaded appearance | Fine granules, uniform in size and usually evenly distributed; may have beaded appearance | Nucleus may stain more darkly than in E. histolytica, although morphology is similar; chromatin may appear as solid ring rather than beaded (trichrome) | May be clumped and unevenly arranged on the membrane; may also appear as solid, dark ring with no beads or clumps | Usually no peripheral chromatin; nuclear chromatin may be quite variable | Usually no peripheral chromatin |
| Karyosome (stained) | Small, usually compact; centrally located but may also be eccentric | Small, usually compact; centrally located but may also be eccentric | Usually small and compact; may be centrally located or eccentric | Large, not compact; may or may not be eccentric; may be diffuse and darkly stained | Large, irregularly shaped; may appear blotlike; many nuclear variations are common; may mimic E. hartmanni or Dientamoeba fragilis | Large, may be surrounded by refractile granules that are difficult to see ("basket nucleus") |
| Cytoplasm appearance (stained) | Finely granular, "ground glass" appearance; clear differentiation of ectoplasm and endoplasm; if present, vacuoles are usually small | Finely granular, "ground glass" appearance; clear differentiation of ectoplasm and endoplasm; if present, vacuoles are usually small | Finely granular | Granular, with little differentiation into ectoplasm and endoplasm; usually vacuolated | Granular, vacuolated | Granular, may be heavily vacuolated |
| Inclusions (stained) | Noninvasive organism may contain bacteria; **presence of red blood cells (RBCs) is diagnostic;** presence of RBCs is the only characteristic that allows differentiation between pathogenic E. histolytica and nonpathogenic E. dispar | Organisms usually contain bacteria; RBCs **not** present in cytoplasm | May contain bacteria; no RBCs | Bacteria, yeast, other debris | Bacteria | Bacteria |

*These sizes refer to wet preparation measurements. Organisms on a permanent stained smear may be 1 to 1.5 $\mu m$ smaller as a result of artificial shrinkage.

TABLE 48-2  Intestinal Protozoa—Cysts of Common Amebae

| Characteristic | Entamoeba Histolytica/ Entamoeba dispar | Entamoeba hartmanni | Entamoeba coli | Endolimax nana | Iodamoeba bütschlii |
|---|---|---|---|---|---|
| Size* (diameter or length) | 10-20 μm (usual range, 12-15 μm) | 5-10 μm (usual range, 6-8 μm) | 10-35 μm (usual range, 15-25 μm) | 5-10 μm (usual range, 6-8 μm) | 5-20 μm (usual range, 10-12 μm) |
| Shape | Usually spherical | Usually spherical | Usually spherical; may be oval, triangular, or other shapes; may be distorted on permanent stained slide because of inadequate fixative penetration | Usually oval, may be round | May vary from oval to round; cyst may collapse because of large glycogen vacuole space |
| Nucleus (number and visibility) | Mature cyst: 4 nuclei Immature cyst: 1-2 nuclei; nuclear characteristics difficult to see on wet preparation | Mature cyst: 4 nuclei; Immature cyst: 1-2 nuclei (2-nucleated cysts very common) | Mature cyst: 8 (occasionally 16 or more nuclei may be seen) Immature cysts with 2 or more nuclei are occasionally seen | Mature cyst: 4 Immature cysts: 2 Very rarely seen and may resemble cysts of Enteromonas hominis | Mature cyst: 1 |
| Peripheral chromatin (stained) | Peripheral chromatin present; fine, uniform granules, evenly distributed; nuclear characteristics may not be as clearly visible as in trophozoite | Fine granules evenly distributed on the membrane; nuclear characteristics may be difficult to see | Coarsely granular; may be clumped and unevenly arranged on membrane; nuclear characteristics not as clearly defined as in trophozoite; may resemble E. histolytica | No peripheral chromatin | No peripheral chromatin |
| Karyosome (stained) | Small, compact, usually centrally located but occasionally may be eccentric | Small, compact, usually centrally located | Large, may or may not be compact and/or eccentric; occasionally may be centrally located | Smaller than karyosome seen in trophozoites but generally larger than those of genus Entamoeba | Larger, usually eccentric refractile granules may be on one side of karyosome ("basket nucleus") |
| Cytoplasm, chromatoidal bodies (stained) | May be present; bodies usually elongate, with blunt, rounded, smooth edges; may be round or oval | Usually present; bodies usually elongate with blunt, rounded, smooth edges; may be round or oval | May be present (less frequently than in E. histolytica); splinter shaped with rough, pointed ends | Rare chromatoidal bodies present; occasionally small granules or inclusions seen; fine linear chromatoidals may be faintly visible on well-stained smears | No chromatoidal bodies present; occasionally small granules may be present |
| Glycogen (stained with iodine) | May be diffuse or absent in mature cyst; clumped chromatin mass may be present in early cysts (stains reddish brown with iodine) | May or may not be present, as in E. histolytica | May be diffuse or absent in mature cyst; clumped mass occasionally seen in mature cysts (stains reddish brown with iodine) | Usually diffuse if present (stains reddish brown with iodine) | Large, compact, well-defined mass (stains reddish brown with iodine) |

*Wet preparation measurements; in permanent stains, organisms usually are 1 to 2 μm smaller.

**TABLE 48-3** Intestinal Protozoa—Trophozoites of Flagellates

| Protozoa | Shape and Size | Motility | Number of Nuclei and Visibility | Number of Flagella (Usually Difficult to See) | Other Features |
|---|---|---|---|---|---|
| *Dientamoeba fragilis* | Shaped like amebae; 5-15 $\mu$m (usual range, 9-12 $\mu$m) | Usually nonprogressive; pseudopodia are angular, serrated, or broad lobed and almost transparent | Percentage may vary, but 40% of organisms have 1 nucleus and 60% have 2 nuclei; not visible in unstained preparations; no peripheral chromatin; karyosome is composed of a cluster of 4-8 granules | Internal flagella; not visible | Cytoplasm finely granular and may be vacuolated with ingested bacteria, yeasts, and other debris; may be great variation in size and shape on a single smear |
| *Giardia lamblia* | Pear-shaped; length 10-20 $\mu$m; width, 5-15 $\mu$m | "Falling leaf" motility may be difficult to see if organism is in mucus; slight flutter of flagella may be visible using low light (duodenal aspirate or mucus from Entero-Test capsule) | 2; not visible in unstained mounts | 4 lateral; 2 ventral, 2 caudal | Sucking disk occupies one half to three fourths of ventral surface; pear-shaped front view, spoon-shaped side view |
| *Chilomastix mesnili* | Pear-shaped; length 6-24 $\mu$m (usual range, 10-15 $\mu$m); width, 4-8 $\mu$m | Stiff, rotary | 1; not visible in unstained mounts | 3 anterior, 1 in cytostome | Prominent cytostome extending one third to one half the length of the body; spiral groove across ventral surface |
| *Pentatrichomonas hominis* | Pear-shaped; length 5-15 $\mu$m (usual range, 7-9 $\mu$m); width 7-10 $\mu$m | Jerky, rapid | 1; not visible in unstained mounts | 3-5 anterior, 1 posterior | Undulating membrane extends the length of the body; posterior flagellum extends free beyond end of body |
| *Trichomonas tenax* | Pear shaped; length 5-12 $\mu$m; average of 6.5-7.5 $\mu$m; width, 7-9 $\mu$m | Jerky, rapid | 1; not visible in unstained mounts | 4 anterior, 1 posterior | Seen only in preparations from mouth; axostyle (slender rod) protrudes beyond the posterior end and may be visible; posterior flagellum extends only halfway down the body; no free end |
| *Enteromonas hominis* | Oval; 4-10 $\mu$m (usual range, 8-9 $\mu$m); width, 5-6 $\mu$m | Jerky | 1; not visible in unstained mounts | 3 anterior, 1 posterior | One side of the body is flattened; posterior flagellum extends free posteriorly or laterally |
| *Retortamonas intestinalis* | Pear-shaped or oval; 4-9 $\mu$m (usual range, 6-7 $\mu$m); width, 3-4 $\mu$m | Jerky | 1; not visible in unstained mount | 1 anterior, 1 posterior | Prominent cytostome extends approximately one half the length of the body |

**TABLE 48-4** Intestinal Protozoa—Cysts of Flagellates

| Protozoa | Size | Shape | Number of Nuclei | Other Features |
|---|---|---|---|---|
| *Dientamoeba fragilis, Pentatrichomonas hominis, Trichomonas tenax* | No cyst stage | | | |
| *Giardia lamblia* | 8-19 $\mu$m (usual range, 11-14 $\mu$m); width, 7-10 $\mu$m | Oval, ellipsoidal, or may appear round | 4; not distinct in unstained preparations; usually located at one end | Longitudinal fibers in cysts may be visible in unstained preparations; deep staining median bodies usually lie across the longitudinal fibers. Shrinkage is common, with the cytoplasm pulling away from the cyst wall; "halo" effect may be seen around the outside of the cyst wall because of shrinkage caused by dehydrating reagents |
| *Chilomastix mesnili* | 6-10 $\mu$m (usual range, 7-9 $\mu$m); width, 4-6 $\mu$m | Lemon or pear shaped with anterior hyaline knob | 1; not distinct in unstained preparations | Cytostome with supporting fibrils, usually visible in stained preparation; curved fibril along side of cytostome, usually referred to as a "shepherd's crook" |
| *Enteromonas hominis* | 4-10 $\mu$m (usual range, 6-8 $\mu$m); width, 4-6 $\mu$m | Elongate or oval | 1-4; usually 2 lying at opposite ends of cyst; not visible in unstained mounts | Resembles *Endolimax nana* cyst; fibrils or flagella usually not seen |
| *Retortamonas intestinalis* | 4-9 $\mu$m (usual range, 4-7 $\mu$m); width, 5 $\mu$m | Pear shaped or slightly lemon shaped | 1; not visible in unstained mounts | Resembles *Chilomastix* cyst; shadow outline of cytostome with supporting fibrils extends above nucleus; "bird beak" fibril arrangement |

**TABLE 48-5** Intestinal Protozoa—Ciliates

| Protozoa | Shape and Size | Motility | Number of Nuclei | Other Features |
|---|---|---|---|---|
| *Balantidium coli* trophozoite | Ovoid with tapering anterior end; 50-100 $\mu$m long, 40-70 $\mu$m wide (usual range, 40-50 $\mu$m) | Ciliates: rotary, boring; may be rapid | 1 large kidney-shaped macronucleus; 1 small round micronucleus, which is difficult to see even in stained smear; macronucleus may be visible in unstained preparation | Body covered with cilia, which tend to be longer near cytostome; cytoplasm may be vacuolated |
| Cyst | Spherical or oval; 50-70 $\mu$m (usual range, 50-55 $\mu$m) | | 1 large macronucleus visible in unstained preparation; micronucleus difficult to see | Macronucleus and contractile vacuole are visible in young cysts; in older cysts, internal structure appears granular; cilia difficult to see in cyst wall |

characteristics of *E. histolytica/E. dispar* are readily seen. The nucleus is characterized by evenly arranged chromatin on the nuclear membrane and a small, compact, centrally located karyosome (condensed chromatin). As mentioned, the cytoplasm usually is described as finely granular, with few ingested bacteria and scant debris in vacuoles. As stated previously, in organisms isolated from a patient with dysentery, RBCs may be visible in the cytoplasm, a feature diagnostic for *E. histolytica* (Figure 48-3).

Most often, infection with *E. histolytica* is diagnosed on the basis of the organism's morphology, without the presence of RBCs.

As part of the life cycle, the trophozoites may condense into a round mass (precyst), and a thin wall is secreted around the immature cyst. Two types of inclusions may be found in this immature cyst: a glycogen mass and highly refractile **chromatoidal bars** (refractile chromatin structure) with smooth, rounded edges. As

**TABLE 48-6** Morphologic Criteria Used to Identify Intestinal Protozoa (Coccidia, *Blastocystis hominis*)

| Protozoa | Shape and Size | Other Features |
|---|---|---|
| *Cryptosporidium* spp. *C. parvum* (humans and animals) *C. hominis* (humans) | Oocyst generally round, 4-6 $\mu$m; each mature oocyst contains four sporozoites | Oocyst, diagnostic stage in stool, sporozoites occasionally visible within oocyst wall; acid-fast positive using modified acid-fast stains; various other stages in life cycle can be seen in biopsy specimens taken from gastrointestinal tract (brush border of epithelial cells) and other tissues; disseminated infection well documented in compromised host; oocysts immediately infective (in both formed and/or watery specimens); nosocomial infections documented; use enteric precautions for inpatients. |
| *Cyclospora cayetanensis* | Oocyst generally round, 8-10 $\mu$m; oocysts are not mature, no visible internal structure; oocysts may appear wrinkled | Oocyst, diagnostic stage in stool; acid-fast variable using modified acid-fast stains; color range from clear to deep purple (tremendous variation); best results obtained with decolorizing solution consisting of 1% acid, 3% maximum; oocysts may appear wrinkled (like crumpled cellophane); mimic *Cryptosporidium* oocysts but are twice as large. |
| *Isospora (Cystoisospora) belli* | Ellipsoidal oocyst; range 20-30 $\mu$m long, 10-19 $\mu$m wide; sporocysts rarely seen broken out of oocysts but measure 9-11$\mu$m | Mature oocyst contains two sporocysts with four sporozoites each; usual diagnostic stage in feces is immature oocyst containing spherical mass of protoplasm (intestinal tract). Oocysts are modified acid-fast positive. Whole oocyst may stain pink, but just the internal sporocysts stain if the oocyst is mature. |
| *Sarcocystis hominis* *S. suihominis* *S. bovihominis* | Oocyst thin-walled and contains two mature sporocysts, each containing four sporozoites; frequently thin oocyst wall ruptures; ovoid sporocysts each measure 10-16 $\mu$m long and 7.5-12 $\mu$m wide | Thin-walled oocyst or ovoid sporocysts occur in stool (intestinal tract) |
| *S. "lindemanni"* | Shapes and sizes of skeletal and cardiac muscle sarcocysts vary considerably | Sarcocysts contain several hundred to several thousand trophozoites, each measuring 12-16$\mu$m long and 4-9$\mu$m wide. Sarcocysts may also be divided into compartments by septa, which are not seen in *Toxoplasma* cysts (tissue/muscle). |
| *Blastocystis hominis* | Organisms are generally round, measure approximately 6-40 $\mu$m, and are usually characterized by a large, central body (looks like a large vacuole); this stage has been called the *central body form* | The more amebic form can be seen in diarrheal fluid but is difficult to identify. The central body forms vary tremendously in size, even on a single fecal smear; this is the most common form seen. Routine fecal examinations may indicate a positive rate much higher than other protozoa; some laboratories report figures of 20% and higher. |

the cyst matures (metacyst) (see Figure 48-3; Figure 48-4), nuclear division occurs, with the production of four nuclei. Often chromatoidals may be absent in the mature cyst. Cyst morphology does not differentiate *E. histolytica* from *E. dispar*. Cyst formation occurs only in the intestinal tract; once the stool has left the body, cyst formation does not occur. The one-, two-, and four-nucleated cysts are infective and represent the mode of transmission from one host to another.

## Epidemiology

Amebiasis is caused by infection with the true pathogen, *Entamoeba histolytica*. Recent evidence from molecular studies confirms the differentiation of pathogenic *E. histolytica* and nonpathogenic *E. dispar* (Figure 48-5) as two distinct species. *E. histolytica* is considered the etiologic agent of amebic colitis and extraintestinal abscesses

(amebic liver abscess), whereas nonpathogenic *E. dispar* produces no intestinal symptoms and is not invasive in humans.

Infection is acquired through the fecal-oral route from infective cysts contained in the feces. These cysts can be ingested in contaminated food or drink or contracted from fomites or various sexual practices that could include accidental ingestion of fecal organisms. Flies and cockroaches have been implicated as mechanical vectors of contaminated fecal material.

The infection occurs worldwide, particularly in areas with poor sanitation. It is estimated that *E. histolytica* infection kills more than 100,000 people each year.

## Pathogenesis and Spectrum of Disease

The pathogenesis of *E. histolytica* is related to the organism's ability to directly lyse host cells and cause tissue

**TABLE 48-7** Microsporidia That Cause Human Infection

| Microsporidia | Immunocompromised Patient | Immunocompetent Patient | Comments |
|---|---|---|---|
| **Common**<br>**Enterocytozoon bieneusi** | Chronic diarrhea; wasting syndrome, cholangitis, acalculous cholecystitis, chronic sinusitis, chronic cough, pneumonitis; cause of diarrhea in organ transplant recipients | Self-limiting diarrhea in adults and children; traveler's diarrhea; asymptomatic carriers | Short-term culture only; three strains identified but not named; AIDS patients with chronic diarrhea (present in 5% to 30% of patients when CD4 lymphocyte counts are very low); pigs, nonhuman primates |
| **Encephalitozoon hellem** | Disseminated infection; keratoconjunctivitis; sinusitis, bronchitis, pneumonia, nephritis, ureteritis, cystitis, prostatitis, urethritis | Possibly diarrhea | Cultured in vitro; detected in people with traveler's diarrhea and co-infection with *E. bieneusi*; pathogenicity unclear; spores not reported yet from stool; psittacine birds |
| **Encephalitozoon intestinalis** | Chronic diarrhea, cholangiopathy; sinusitis, bronchitis, pneumonitis; nephritis, bone infection, nodular cutaneous lesions | Self-limiting diarrhea; asymptomatic carriers | Cultured in vitro; formerly *Septata intestinalis;* AIDS patients with chronic diarrhea; dogs, donkeys, pigs, cows, goats |
| **Encephalitozoon cuniculi** | Disseminated infection; keratoconjunctivitis, sinusitis, bronchitis, pneumonia; nephritis; hepatitis, peritonitis, symptomatic and asymptomatic intestinal infection; encephalitis | Not described. Two HIV-serologically negative children with seizure disorder (suspect *E. cuniculi* infection) presumably were immunocompromised | Cultured in vitro; wide mammalian host range |
| **Uncommon**<br>**Pleistophora sp.** | Myositis (skeletal muscle) | Not described | Tend to infect fish |
| **Pleistophora ronneafiei** | Myositis | Not described | |
| **Trachipleistophora hominis** | Myositis; myocarditis keratoconjunctivitis; sinusitis | Keratitis | Cultured in vitro; AIDS patients |
| **Trachipleistophora anthropophthera** | Disseminated infection; keratitis | Not described | AIDS patients |
| **Anncaliia connori** | Disseminated infection | Not described | (Formerly *Nosema connori*); often infects insects; disseminated in infant with SCID |
| **Anncaliia vesicularum** | Myositis | Not described | Formerly *Brachiola vesicularum* |
| **Anncaliia algerae** | Myositis; nodular cutaneous lesions | Keratitis | (Formerly *Nosema algerae* or *Brachiola algerae*); cultured in vitro; skin nodules in boy with acute lymphocytic leukemia; found in arthropods |
| **Nosema ocularum** | Not described | Keratitis | HIV–serologically negative individual |
| **Vittaforma corneae** | Disseminated infection; urinary tract infection | Keratitis | (Formerly *Nosema corneum*); cultured in vitro; non-HIV patient |
| **Microsporidium ceylonensis*** | Not described | Corneal ulcer, keratitis | HIV–serologically negative individual, autopsy |
| **Microsporidium africanum*** | Not described | Corneal ulcer, keratitis | HIV–serologically negative individual, autopsy |
| **Microsporidia (not classified)** | | Keratoconjunctivitis in a contact lens wearer | |

*AIDS,* Acquired immunodeficiency syndrome; *HIV,* human immunodeficiency virus; *SCID,* severe combined immunodeficiency
*\*Microsporidium* is a collective generic name for microsporidia that cannot be classified

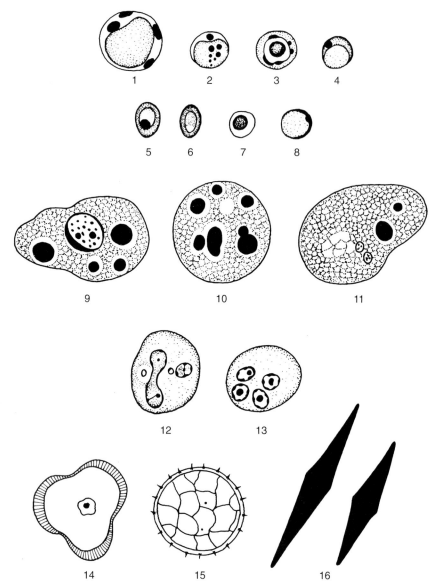

**Figure 48-1** Various structures that may be seen in stool preparations. **1, 2,** and **4,** *Blastocystis hominis.* **3** and **5** to **8,** Various yeast cells. **9,** Macrophage with nucleus. **10** and **11,** Deteriorated macrophage without nucleus. **12** and **13,** Polymorphonuclear leukocytes. **14** and **15,** Pollen grains. **16,** Charcot-Leyden crystals. (Modified from Markell EK, Voge M: *Medical parasitology,* ed 5, Philadelphia, 1981, WB Saunders.)

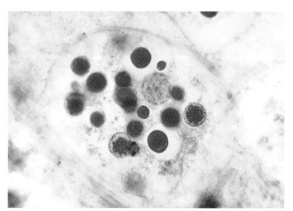

**Figure 48-2** *Entamoeba histolytica* trophozoite containing ingested red blood cells.

destruction. Amebic lesions show evidence of cell lysis, tissue necrosis, and damage to the extracellular matrix. Evidence indicates that *E. histolytica* trophozoites interact with the host through a series of steps: adhesion to the target cell, phagocytosis, and cytopathic effect. Numerous other parasite factors also play a role. From the perspective of the host, *E. histolytica* induces both humoral and cellular immune responses; cell-mediated immunity is the major human host defense against this complement-resistant cytolytic protozoan.

The presentations of disease are seen with invasion of the intestinal mucosa or dissemination to other organs (most often the liver) or both. However, it is estimated that a small proportion (2% to 8%) of infected individuals have invasive disease beyond the lumen of the bowel. Also, organisms may be spontaneously eliminated with no disease symptoms.

**Asymptomatic Infection.** Individuals harboring *E. histolytica* may have either a negative or a weak antibody titer and negative stools for occult blood. They also may be passing cysts detectable by a routine ova and parasite (O&P) examination. However, these cysts cannot be morphologically differentiated from those of the nonpathogen, *E. dispar*. Although trophozoites may be identified, they will not contain any phagocytized RBCs and cannot be differentiated from *E. dispar*. Molecular analyses of organisms isolated from asymptomatic individuals generally indicate that the isolates belong to the nonpathogenic *E. dispar*. Generally, asymptomatic patients never become symptomatic and may excrete cysts for a short period. This pattern is seen in patients infected with either nonpathogenic or pathogenic organisms.

**Intestinal Disease.** The incubation period varies from a few days to a much longer time; in an area where *E. histolytica* is endemic, it is impossible to determine exactly when exposure to the organism occurred. Normally, the incubation time ranges from 1 to 4 weeks. Although the exact mode of mucosal penetration is not known, microscopic studies suggest that amebae have enzymes that lyse. The enzymes are released from lysosomes on the surface of the amebae or from enzymes in the tissue released from ruptured organisms. Amebic ulcers often develop released the cecum, appendix, or adjacent portion of the ascending colon; however, they can also be found in the sigmoidorectal area. Other lesions may occur from these primary sites. Ulcers usually are raised, with a small opening on the mucosal surface and a larger area of destruction below the surface (i.e., flask shaped). The mucosal lining may appear normal between ulcers.

Invasive intestinal amebiasis has four clinical forms, all of which are generally acute: dysentery (bloody diarrhea), fulminating colitis, amebic appendicitis, and ameboma of the colon. Dysentery and diarrhea account for 90% of cases of invasive intestinal amebiasis. The severity of symptoms can range from asymptomatic to severe symptoms that mimic ulcerative colitis. Patients with colicky abdominal pain, frequent bowel movements, and tenesmus (a persistent feeling of needing to pass stool) may present with a gradual onset of disease. With the onset of dysentery, bowel movements are frequent (up to 10 per day). Although dysentery may last for months, it varies from severe to mild and may lead to weight loss and prostration. In severe cases, symptoms may begin very suddenly and include profuse diarrhea, fever, and dehydration with electrolyte imbalances.

**Hepatic Disease.** Blood flow from the mesenteric veins surrounding the intestine returns blood, via the portal vein, to the liver, most commonly the upper right lobe. Amebae in the submucosa can be carried by the bloodstream to the liver. The onset of symptoms may be gradual or sudden; upper right abdominal pain and fever (38° to 39°C) are the most consistent findings. Although the liver may be enlarged and tender, liver function tests may

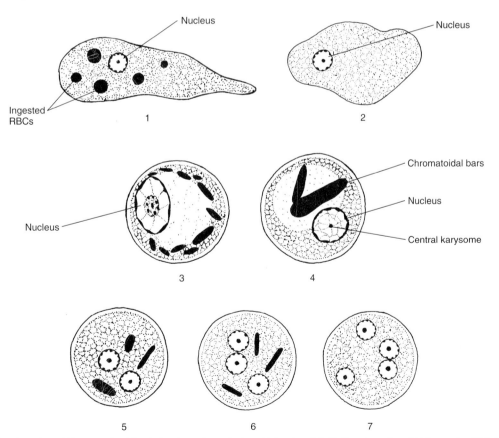

**Figure 48-3** **1,** Trophozoite of *Entamoeba histolytica* (note ingested red blood cells). **2,** Trophozoite of *Entamoeba histolytica/Entamoeba dispar* (morphology does not allow differentiation between the two species). **3** and **4,** Early cysts of *E. histolytica/E. dispar*. **5** to **7,** Cysts of *E. histolytica/E. dispar*.

*Continued*

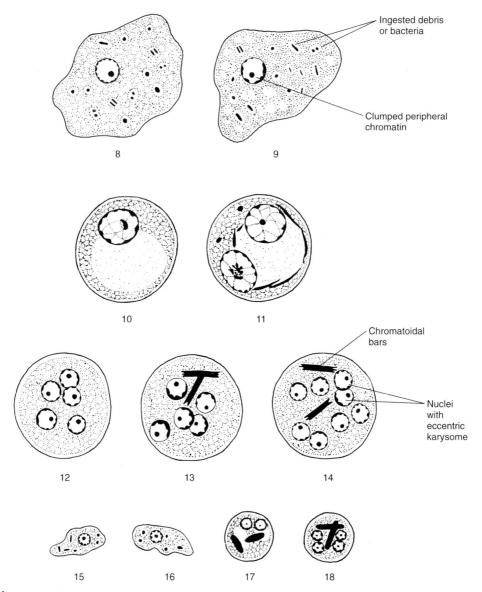

Ingested debris
or bacteria

Clumped peripheral
chromatin

Chromatoidal
bars

Nuclei
with
eccentric
karysome

**Figure 48-3, cont'd** **8** and **9,** Trophozoites of *Entamoeba coli.* **10** and **11,** Early cysts of *E. coli.* **12** to **14,** Cysts of *E. coli.* **15** and **16,** Trophozoites of *Entamoeba hartmanni.* **17** and **18,** Cysts of *E. hartmanni.* (From Garcia LS: *Diagnostic medical parasitology,* ed 4, Washington, DC, 2001, ASM Press. Illustrations **4** and **11** by Nobuko Kitamura.)

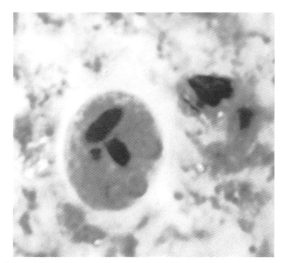

**Figure 48-4** *Entamoeba histolytica/Entamoeba dispar* cyst.

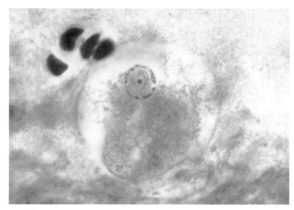

**Figure 48-5** *Entamoeba dispar* trophozoite; no ingested red blood cells are present.

be normal or slightly abnormal (jaundice is rare). The abscess can be visualized radiologically, sonically, or by radionuclear scan; most patients have a single abscess in the right lobe of the liver. The most common complication is rupture of the abscess into the pleural space. An abscess also can extend into the peritoneum and through the skin. Hematogenous spread to the brain, lung, pericardium, and other sites is possible.

Pyogenic and amebic liver abscesses are the two most common hepatic abscesses. The severity of a pyogenic abscess depends on the bacterial source and the patient's underlying condition. An amebic abscess tends to be more prevalent in those with suppressed cell-mediated immunity, men, and younger individuals. *E. histolytica* cysts and trophozoites are found in the stools of only a few patients with liver abscess. About 60% of these patients have no intestinal symptoms or any history of dysentery.

## Laboratory Diagnosis

**Routine Methods.** The standard O&P examination is the recommended procedure for recovery and identification of *E. histolytica* in stool specimens. Microscopic examination of a direct saline wet mount may reveal motile trophozoites, which may contain RBCs. However, trophozoites with RBCs are found only in a limited number of cases. In many patients who do not present with acute dysentery, trophozoites may be present but do not contain RBCs, and the organisms may be pathogenic *E. histolytica* or nonpathogenic *E. dispar*. An asymptomatic individual may have few trophozoites and possibly only cysts in the stool. Although the concentration technique is helpful for demonstrating cysts, the most important technique for the recovery and identification of protozoan organisms is the permanent stained smear (normally stained with trichrome or iron-hematoxylin). A minimum of three specimens collected over not more than 10 days may be required for identification.

Sigmoidoscopy specimens may be very helpful for identifying organisms. At least six areas of the mucosa should be sampled. Smears from these areas should be examined after permanent staining. However, these specimens are not considered a substitute for the recommended minimum of three stool specimens submitted for O&P examination (direct, concentration, and permanent stained smear).

Liver aspirate material is rarely examined, and often the specimen was not collected properly. Aspirated material must be aliquoted into several different containers as it is removed from the abscess; amebae may be found only in the last portion of the aspirated material, theoretically material from the abscess wall, not necrotic debris from the abscess center.

**Antigen Detection.** A number of enzyme immunoassay reagents are commercially available, and their specificity and sensitivity provide excellent options for the clinical laboratory. These tests can differentiate the *E. histolytica/ E. dispar* group from the rest of the *Entamoeba* species, such as nonpathogenic *Entamoeba coli* or *Entamoeba hartmanni*. Other test reagents can distinguish between *E. histolytica* and *E. dispar* (Entamoeba histolytica II test, TechLab, Blacksburg, VA or Entamoeba CELESA path, Cellabs, Brookvale, Australia). These kits require fresh or frozen stool; fecal preservatives have been found to interfere with the *Entamoeba* spp. reagents. Because of the specificity of the immunoassay reagents, the laboratory can inform the physician whether the *E. histolytica/ E. dispar* organisms seen in the stool specimen are pathogenic *E. histolytica* or nonpathogenic *E. dispar*. Without the use of these reagents, the only way to identify true pathogenic *E. histolytica* morphologically is to detect the rare presence of trophozoites containing ingested RBCs. If the laboratory does not use these reagents, the presence of *E. histolytica/E. dispar* should be reported to the physician, accompanied by commentary related to the newer information on pathogenicity. Depending on each state's requirements, pathogenic *E. histolytica* generally is reported to the public health facility (county).

**Antibody Detection.** Serologic testing for intestinal disease is rarely recommended unless the patient has true dysentery; even in these cases, the titer (e.g., indirect hemagglutination) may be low and thus difficult to interpret. A definitive diagnosis of intestinal amebiasis should not be made without demonstrating the presence of the organisms. In patients suspected of having extraintestinal disease, serologic tests are diagnostically more effective. Indirect hemagglutination and indirect fluorescent antibody tests have been reported positive with titers greater than or equal to 1:256 and greater than or equal to 1:200, respectively, in almost 100% of cases of amebic liver abscess. In the absence of STAT serologic tests for amebiasis (tests with very short turnaround times for results), the decision on diagnosis must be made on clinical grounds and on the basis of results of other diagnostic tests, such as scans.

**Histology.** A histologic diagnosis of amebiasis can be made when the trophozoites in the tissue are identified. Organisms must be differentiated from host cells, particularly histiocytes and ganglion cells. Periodic acid-Schiff (PAS) staining often is used to help locate the organisms, which appear bright pink with a green-blue background (depending on the counterstain used). Hematoxylin and eosin staining also allows visualization of the typical morphology, thus allowing accurate identification. As a result of sectioning, some organisms exhibit the evenly arranged nuclear chromatin with the central karyosome, and some no longer contain the nucleus.

## Nucleic Acid-Based Techniques

Nucleic acid-based amplification methods, including polymerase chain reaction (real-time and multiplex assays), have been developed for the identification of *E. histolytica*. Stool specimens, however, may contain inhibitors that would prevent accurate detection using amplification methods. These tests are not widely used, because they require more technical expertise and currently have not proven to be more sensitive than antigen-based immunoassays.

## Therapy

Two classes of drugs are used in the treatment of amebic infections: luminal amebicides, such as iodoquinol or diloxanide furoate, and tissue amebicides, such as metronidazole, chloroquine, or dehydroemetine. Because of the differences in drug efficacy, it is important that the laboratory report indicates whether cysts, trophozoites, or both are present in the stool specimen.

**Asymptomatic Infection.** Patients found to have true *E. histolytica* in the intestinal tract, even if asymptomatic, should be treated to eliminate the organisms. Both diloxanide furoate and iodoquinol or paromomycin are available for treatment of patients who have cysts in the lumen of the gut. In general, these treatments are ineffective against extraintestinal disease. If the patient is passing both trophozoites and cysts, the recommended treatment is metronidazole plus iodoquinol.

**Mild to Moderate Disease.** In patients with mild to moderate disease, metronidazole (Flagyl) should be used when tissue invasion occurs, regardless of the tissue involved. Drugs directed against the lumen organisms should also be used in these cases.

**Severe Intestinal Disease.** Metronidazole plus one of the luminal drugs should be used for therapy.

**Hepatic Disease.** Metronidazole plus one of the luminal drugs should be used to treat hepatic disease. Some other combinations also can be used; some contain emetine, in which case the patient must be monitored very carefully for possible cardiotoxicity. The importance of using both luminal and tissue amebicides is emphasized in patients with amebic liver abscesses. Asymptomatic colonization may be present with the true pathogen, *E. histolytica*. In patients treated with metronidazole (tissue amebicide), generally a 100% clinical response to the hepatic lesions is seen; however, failure to eliminate the organism from the bowel can lead to second bouts with invasive disease and intestinal colonization. Also, these carriers constitute a public health hazard because of continued shedding of infective cysts.

### Prevention

Humans are the reservoir host for *E. histolytica*, and infection can be transmitted to other humans, primates, dogs, cats, and possibly pigs. Accidental consumption of sewage-contaminated water provides another route of infection. Amebiasis is considered a zoonotic waterborne infection. The cyst stages are resistant to environmental conditions and can remain viable in the soil for 8 days at 28° to 34°C, for 40 days at 2° to 6°C, and for 60 days at 0°C. Cysts normally are removed by sand filtration or destroyed by 200 ppm of iodine, 5% to 10% acetic acid, or boiling. However, an asymptomatic carrier who is a food handler generally is thought to play the most important role in transmission. Proper disposal of contaminated feces is considered the most important preventive measure. Although vaccines have been discussed as a possibility for eliminating human disease, nothing currently is available.

## ENTAMOEBA COLI

### General Characteristics

The life cycle of *E. coli* is identical to that of *E. dispar*. After digestion of infective cysts, the organisms excyst in the intestinal tract and produce trophozoites. Cyst formation occurs as the gut contents move through the intestinal tract; the excreted cysts are the infective form that is transmitted to humans and some animals.

*E. coli* trophozoites are somewhat larger than those of *E. histolytica* and *E. dispar* and range from 15 to 50 μm in diameter (see Table 48-1; Figures 48-6 and 48-7; see Figure 48-3). Motility is sluggish with broad, short pseudopods. In wet preparations, differentiating nonpathogenic *E. coli* from pathogenic *E. histolytica* is almost impossible. On the permanent stained smear viewed at a higher magnification, the cytoplasm is granular with vacuoles containing bacteria, yeasts, and other food materials. The nucleus has a large blotlike karyosome that may be eccentric rather than centrally located. The chromatin on the nuclear membrane tends to be clumped and irregular. Although rare, if RBCs are present in the intestinal tract, *E. coli* may ingest them rather than bacteria.

Early cysts often contain chromatoidal bars, which tend to be splinter shaped and irregular. Eventually, the nuclei divide until the mature cyst, containing eight nuclei, is formed (see Table 48-2; see Figures 48-3 and 48-6). In rare cases, the number of nuclei reaches 16. The cysts measure 10 to 35 μm in diameter, and as they mature, the chromatoidal bars disappear. When the cyst of *E. coli* matures, it becomes more refractive to fixation; therefore, the cyst may be seen on the wet preparation but not on the permanent stained smear. Occasionally, on trichrome smears, the cysts appear distorted and somewhat pink (Figure 48-8).

### Epidemiology

Transmission occurs through the ingestion of mature cysts from contaminated food or water. The organism is readily acquired, and in some warmer climates or areas with primitive hygienic conditions, the colonization rate can be quite high.

### Pathogenesis and Spectrum of Disease

*E. coli* are considered nonpathogenic and do not cause disease.

### Laboratory Diagnosis

Unless the mature cyst with eight nuclei is seen, the morphologies of *E. histolytica*, *E. dispar*, *E. moshkovskii*, and *E. coli* are similar in the trophozoite and immature cyst stages. *E. moshkovskii* is typically a free-living amoeba isolated in river or stream sediment and rarely infects humans. Definitive identification relies on examination of permanent stained smears.

### Therapy

Specific treatment is not recommended for the nonpathogen *E. coli*. Correct differentiation among the species is critical to good patient care. Because the amebae are acquired through fecal-oral contamination, pathogens and nonpathogens can be found in the same patient. If few *E. histolytica*/*E. dispar* organisms are present among many *E. coli* organisms, extended microscopic examination and/or the use of species-specific immunoassay testing may be required to make the correct identification.

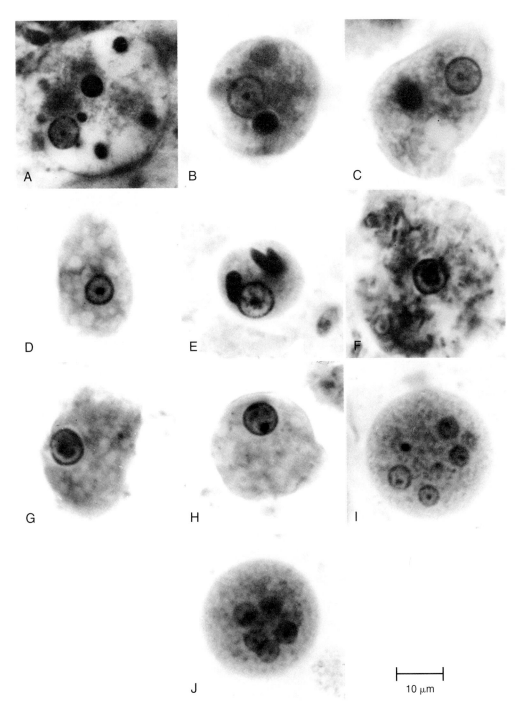

**Figure 48-6** **A** to **C,** Trophozoites of *Entamoeba histolytica* (note ingested red blood cells). **D,** Trophozoite of *E. histolytica/E. dispar.* **E,** Early cyst of *E. histolytica/E. dispar.* **F** to **H,** Trophozoites of *Entamoeba coli.* **I** and **J,** Cysts of *E. coli.*

### Prevention

Prevention depends on adequate disposal of human excreta and improved personal hygiene, preventive measures that apply to most of the intestinal protozoa.

## ENTAMOEBA HARTMANNI

### General Characteristics

The life cycle of *E. hartmanni* is similar to that of *E. dispar,* with differences in size (Figures 48-9 and 48-10). In wet

preparations, *E. hartmanni* trophozoites range in size from 4 to 12 μm in diameter, and cysts range in size from 5 to 10 μm in diameter. On the permanent stained smear, the cysts, primarily, tend to shrink as a result of dehydration; therefore, the sizes of all the organisms, including pathogenic *E. histolytica,* may be somewhat smaller (1 to 1.5 μm) than the wet preparation measurements.

Trophozoites do not ingest RBCs, and the motility is usually less rapid (see Table 48-1; see Figures 48-3, 48-9, and 48-10). The morphologic characteristics of *E. hartmanni* are very similar to those of *E. histolytica,* with two

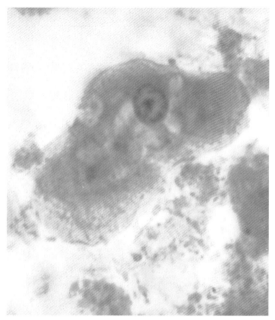

**Figure 48-7** *Entamoeba coli* trophozoite.

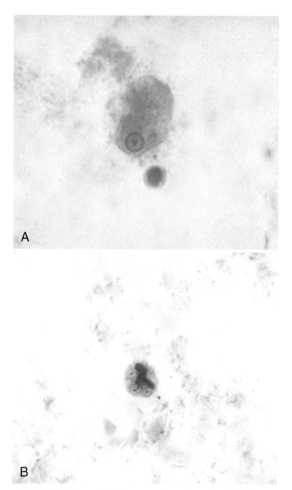

**Figure 48-9** **A,** *Entamoeba hartmanni* trophozoite. **B,** *E. hartmanni* cyst.

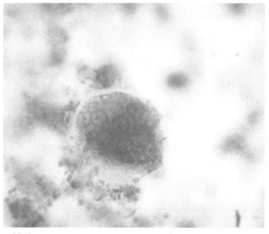

**Figure 48-8** *Entamoeba coli* cyst (trichrome stain) (poor preservation; typical appearance of some *E. coli* cysts).

identifications have been recorded, the colonization rate tends to match that of *E. histolytica*.

### Pathogenesis and Spectrum of Disease

*E. hartmanni* is considered nonpathogenic and does not cause disease.

### Laboratory Diagnosis

Unless the trophozoites and cysts match the size requirements, they are unlikely to be *E. hartmanni*. Definitive identification relies on examination of permanent stained smears and measurements made with the calibrated microscope.

## ENDOLIMAX NANA

### General Characteristics

*Endolimax nana*, one of the smaller nonpathogenic amebae, has a worldwide distribution and is seen as frequently as *E. coli*.

*E. nana* has the same life cycle stages as *E. dispar* and the other nonpathogenic amebae. The trophozoite usually measures 6 to 12 $\mu$m in diameter (normal range,

exceptions. Frequently, *E. hartmanni* cysts may contain only one or two nuclei, even though the mature cyst contains four nuclei. Mature cysts of *E. hartmanni* also retain their chromatoidal bars, a characteristic not usually seen in *E. histolytica/E. dispar*. *E. hartmanni*'s chromatoidal bars are similar to those of *E. histolytica* and *E. dispar* but smaller and more numerous (see Table 48-2; see Figures 48-9 and 48-10). At the species level, differentiation between *E. hartmanni* and *E. histolytica/E. dispar* depends on size; therefore, laboratories are required to use calibrated microscopes that are checked periodically for accuracy.

### Epidemiology

Transmission occurs through the ingestion of mature cysts from contaminated food or water. If accurate

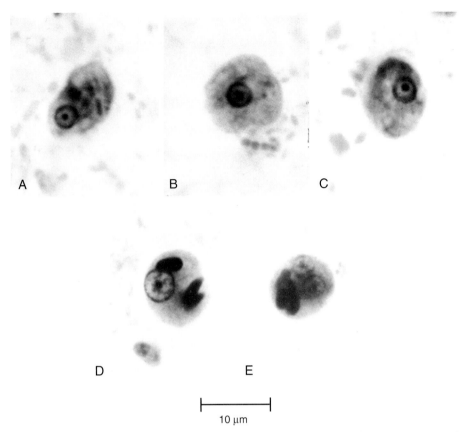

**Figure 48-10** **A** to **C,** Trophozoites of *Entamoeba hartmanni.* **D** and **E,** Cysts of *E. hartmanni.*

8 to 10 $\mu$m) (see Table 48-1; Figures 48-11 to 48-13). Although rarely seen, motility is sluggish and nonprogressive with blunt, hyaline pseudopods. In the permanent stained smear, normally no peripheral chromatin is seen on the nuclear membrane, and the karyosome is large, with either a central or an eccentric location in the nucleus (see Figures 48-12 and 48-13). *E. nana* shows more nuclear variation than any of the other amebae, and occasionally *E. nana* can mimic *D. fragilis* or *E. hartmanni.* The cytoplasm may have small vacuoles containing ingested debris or bacteria, but it also may appear relatively clean.

Cysts usually measure 5 to 10 $\mu$m in diameter (normal range, 6 to 8 $\mu$m) (see Table 48-2). Cysts as large as 14 $\mu$m have been seen. The cyst is usually oval to round, with the mature cyst containing four nuclei. The nuclei typically have no peripheral chromatin and are somewhat evenly distributed in the cyst. Occasionally, very small, slightly curved chromatoidal bars are present. The two-nucleated stage is not commonly seen, and frequently both trophozoites and cysts are present in clinical specimens.

### Epidemiology

Transmission occurs through the ingestion of mature cysts from contaminated food or water. The cysts of *E. nana* are less resistant to desiccation than those of *E. coli. E. nana* is also found in warm, moist climates and in other areas with a low standard of personal hygiene and poor sanitary conditions.

### Pathogenesis and Spectrum of Disease

*E. nana* is considered nonpathogenic and does not cause disease.

### Laboratory Diagnosis

Although cysts sometimes can be seen in a wet preparation, definitive identification of *E. nana* relies on examination of permanent stained smears.

## IODAMOEBA BÜTSCHLII

### General Characteristics

*Iodamoeba bütschlii,* one of the nonpathogenic amebae, has a worldwide distribution. Generally, the acquisition rate for this organism is not as high as that for *E. coli* and *E. nana.*

The life cycle stages of *I. bütschlii* are exactly the same as those of *E. nana.* The trophozoite varies from 8 to 20 $\mu$m in diameter and has fairly active motility in a fresh stool preparation (see Table 48-1). The cytoplasm is granular, containing numerous vacuoles with ingested debris and bacteria. The cytoplasm is more vacuolated than in *E. nana* trophozoites. The nucleus has a large karyosome, which can be either centrally located or eccentric (Figures 48-14 and 48-15). On the

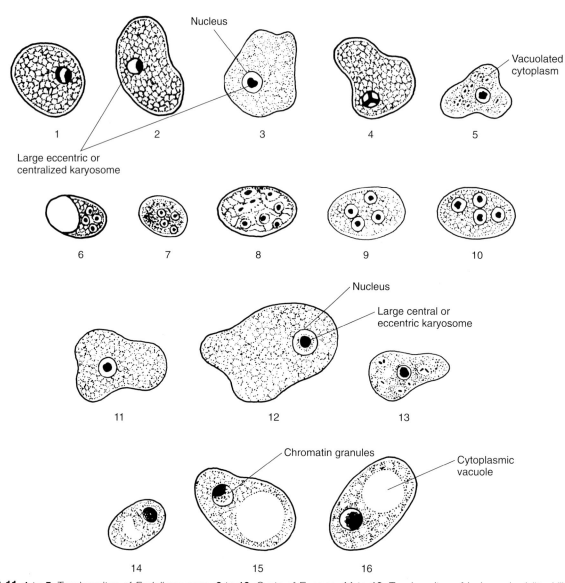

**Figure 48-11** **1** to **5,** Trophozoites of *Endolimax nana.* **6** to **10,** Cysts of *E. nana.* **11** to **13,** Trophozoites of *Iodamoeba bütschlii.* **14** to **16,** Cysts of *I. bütschlii.* (From Garcia LS: *Diagnostic medical parasitology,* ed 4, Washington, DC, 2001, ASM Press.)

permanent stained smear, the nucleus may appear to have a halo, and chromatin granules fan out around the karyosome. If the granules are on one side, the nucleus may appear to have a "basket nucleus" arrangement of chromatin, more commonly seen in the cyst stage. The trophozoites of *I. bütschlii* and *E. nana* may appear similar and are difficult to differentiate at the species level, even on the permanent stained smear. Both organisms are considered nonpathogenic. *E. nana* is recovered in clinical specimens much more frequently than is *I. bütschlii.*

*I. bütschlii* cysts are round to oval (see Table 48-2). The glycogen vacuole is so large that occasionally the cyst collapses on itself. Because nuclear multiplication does not occur in the cyst form, the mature cyst contains a single nucleus. The cysts measure approximately 5 to 20 μm in diameter and are rarely confused with those of other amebae (see Figures 48-14 and 48-15).

## Epidemiology

Transmission of *I. bütschlii* occurs through the ingestion of mature cysts from contaminated food or water. This organism is also found in warm, moist climates and in other areas with a low standard of personal hygiene and poor sanitary conditions.

## Pathogeneis and Spectrum of Disease

*I. bütschlii* is considered nonpathogenic and does not cause disease.

## Laboratory Diagnosis

Although *I. bütschlii* cysts sometimes can be seen in a wet preparation, definitive identification relies on the examination of permanent stained smears.

## Therapy

Specific treatment is not recommended for *I. bütschlii.* Because these nonpathogenic amebae are acquired

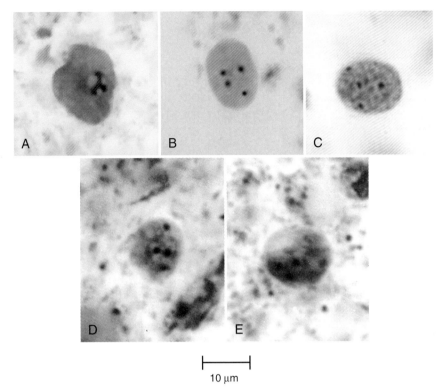

**Figure 48-12** **A** to **C,** Trophozoites of *Endolimax nana.* **D** and **E,** Cysts of *E. nana.* (**A-C** courtesy Lynne Garcia, Santa Monica, CA.)

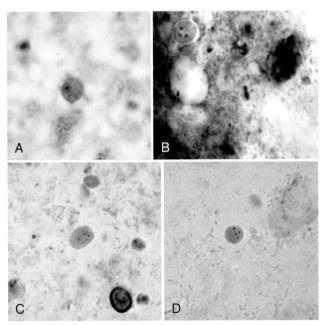

**Figure 48-13 A,** *Endolimax nana* trophozoite. **B,** *E. nana* cyst, iodine stain. **C,** *E. nana* cyst. **D,** *E. nana* cyst. (**B** courtesy Dr. Henry Travers, Sioux Falls, S.D.)

through fecal-oral contamination, both pathogens and nonpathogens can be found in the same patient. If few organisms are present, extended microscopic examination and multiple organism measurements are required for definitive identification. It is always important to report pathogens and nonpathogens, because they are acquired in similar ways.

### Prevention (*E. hartmanni, E. nana, I. bütschlii*)

Prevention depends on adequate disposal of human excreta and improved personal hygiene, preventive measures that apply to most of the intestinal protozoa.

## BLASTOCYSTIS HOMINIS

### General Characteristics

*Blastocystis hominis* (see Figure 48-1; see Table 48-6) comprises a number of different strains that are indistinguishable morphologically; some of which are pathogenic, and some are nonpathogenic. Although usually listed with the amebae, the organism's classification is still under review; different strains eventually may be classified as different species. Although the true role of this organism in terms of disease has been controversial, it is now generally considered a causative agent of intestinal disease. The current recommendation is to report the presence of *B. hominis* and quantitate from the permanent stained smear (i.e., rare, few, moderate, many, packed); this information may be valuable in helping to assess the pathogenicity of the organism in the individual patient.

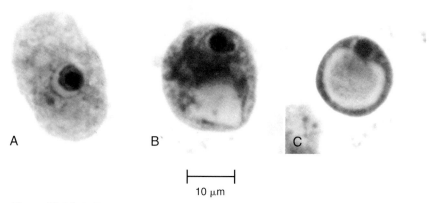

**Figure 48-14 A,** Trophozoites of *Iodamoeba bütschlii.* **B** and **C,** Cysts of *I. bütschlii.*

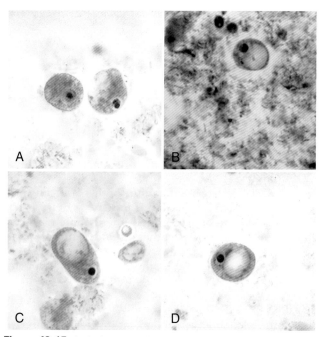

**Figure 48-15 A,** *Iodamoeba bütschlii* trophozoites. **B,** *I. bütschlii* cyst. **C,** *I. bütschlii* cyst. **D,** *I. bütschlii* cyst. (**B** courtesy Dr. Henry Travers, Sioux Falls, S.D.)

*B. hominis* consists of four major forms. The cyst form is the most recently described form of the life cycle stages. Thick-walled cysts are thought to be responsible for external transmission through the fecal-oral route; thin-walled cysts are thought to cause autoinfection. Cysts can vary in shape but are mostly ovoid or spherical. The central vacuole form (also referred to as the **central body form**) is the most common form found in clinical stool samples. The large central vacuole can occupy most of the cellular volume. The amoeboid form is rarely seen. The granular form can be seen in cultures of *B. hominis.*

### Epidemiology

Infection with *B. hominis* is acquired by the fecal-oral route from infective forms contained in the feces. The organisms can be ingested in contaminated food and drink or acquired from fomites or through various sexual practices that may include accidental ingestion of fecal organisms. As with *E. histolytica,* flies and cockroaches can be responsible for mechanical transmission. Human-to-human and animal-to-human transmission are probably more common than suspected.

*B. hominis* is a common intestinal parasite of humans and animals, with a worldwide distribution. Depending on the geographic location, it may be detected in 1% to 40% of fecal specimens. *B. hominis* may be the most common parasite found in the intestinal tract.

### Pathogenesis and Spectrum of Disease

*B. hominis* can cause diarrhea, cramps, nausea, fever, vomiting, abdominal pain, and urticaria and may require therapy. A possible relationship between *B. hominis* and intestinal obstruction and perhaps even infective arthritis has been suggested. In patients with other underlying conditions, the symptoms may be more pronounced. The incidence of this organism appears to be higher than suspected in stools submitted for parasite examination. In symptomatic patients in whom no other etiologic agent has been identified, *B. hominis* should certainly be considered the possible pathogen. It has been suggested that proteases of genetic subtype 3 could be considered a virulence factor responsible for protein degradation and subsequent pathogenesis.

### Laboratory Diagnosis

**Routine Methods.** Routine stool examinations are very effective in recovering and identifying *B. hominis;* the permanent stained smear is the procedure of choice, because examination of wet preparations may not easily reveal the organism. If the fresh stool is rinsed in water before fixation (for the concentration method), *B. hominis* organisms, other than the cysts, are destroyed, and a false-negative report may result. The organisms should be quantitated in the report (i.e., rare, few, moderate, or many). It is also important to remember that other possible pathogens should be adequately ruled out before a patient is treated for *B. hominis.*

**Antigen Detection.** Fecal immunoassays to detect *B. hominis* antigen have been developed but are not yet commercially available. The technique currently used is the enzyme-linked immunosorbent assay (ELISA).

**Antibody Detection.** ELISA and fluorescent antibody tests have been developed to detect serum antibody to *B. hominis* infections. A strong antibody response is consistent with the ability of this organism to cause symptoms. Also, demonstration of serum antibody production both during and after *B. hominis* symptomatic disease is immunologic evidence for the pathogenic role for this protozoan, although it may take 2 years or longer with chronic infections to develop a serologic response.

### Therapy

Although clinical evidence is limited, studies have been done on the in vitro susceptibility of *B. hominis* to numerous drugs. Currently, metronidazole (Flagyl) appears to be the most appropriate drug. Diiodohydroxyquin (Yodoxin) also has been effective, and dosage schedules for these two drugs are as recommended for other intestinal protozoa. The development of new drug sensitivity assays may improve researchers' ability to evaluate the activities of various drugs against this organism.

### Prevention

Prevention requires improved personal hygiene and sanitary conditions, in addition to proper disposal of fecal material.

## FLAGELLATES

The Mastigophora, or flagellates, have specialized locomotor organelles called **flagella;** these are long, thin, cytoplasmic extensions that may vary in number and position, depending on the species. Different genera of flagellates may live in the intestinal tract, the bloodstream, or various tissues.

Four common species of flagellates are found in the intestinal tract: *Giardia lamblia, Dientamoeba fragilis, Chilomastix mesnili,* and *Pentatrichomonas hominis* (Figures 48-16 to 48-23) (see Tables 48-3 and 48-4). Several other smaller, nonpathogenic flagellates, such as *Enteromonas hominis* and *Retortamonas intestinalis* (see Figure 48-16), are rarely seen, and none are identified in the intestinal tract. The **sucking disk** and **axonemes** of *G. lamblia,* the **cytostome** and **spiral groove** of *C. mesnili,* and the **undulating membrane** of *Trichomonas* spp. are all distinctive criteria for identification (see Figures 48-16 to 48-23).

*G. lamblia* and *D. fragilis* are the flagellates considered pathogenic. *D. fragilis* has been associated with diarrhea, nausea, vomiting, and other nonspecific intestinal complaints. *Trichomonas vaginalis* is pathogenic but occurs in the urogenital tract. *Trichomonas tenax* is occasionally found in the mouth and may be associated with poor oral hygiene.

## *GIARDIA LAMBLIA*

### General Characteristics

*G. lamblia* is the most common cause of intestinal infection worldwide. Other than *B. hominis, G. lamblia* (also called *G. duodenalis* and *G. intestinalis*) is probably the most common protozoan organism identified in individuals in the United States. It causes symptoms ranging from mild diarrhea, flatulence, and vague abdominal pains to acute, severe diarrhea to steatorrhea and a typical malabsorption syndrome. Various documented waterborne and food-borne outbreaks have occurred during the past several years. A number of animals may serve as reservoir hosts for *G. lamblia.* Differentiation of flagellates is based on overall shape, numbers, and arrangements of flagella.

Both the trophozoite and cyst stages are included in the life cycle of *G. lamblia.* Trophozoites divide by means of longitudinal binary fission, producing two daughter trophozoites. The organism is found most commonly in the crypts in the duodenum. Trophozoites are the intestinal dwelling stage and attach to the epithelium of the host villi by means of the **ventral disk.** The attachment is substantial and results in disk "impression prints" when the organism detaches from the surface of the epithelium. Trophozoites may remain attached to or may detach from the mucosal surface. Because the epithelial surface sloughs off the tip of the villus every 72 hours, the trophozoites apparently detach at that time. *G. lamblia* trophozoites are teardrop shaped and have been described as "someone looking at you" (see Figures 48-16 to 48-18).

Cyst formation takes place as the organisms move down through the jejunum after exposure to biliary secretions. The trophozoites retract the flagella into the axonemes, the cytoplasm becomes condensed, and the cyst wall is secreted (see Figures 48-16 to 48-18). As the cyst matures, the internal structures are doubled, so that when excystation occurs, the cytoplasm divides, producing two trophozoites. Excystation occurs in the duodenum or appropriate culture medium.

### Epidemiology

Transmission of *G. lamblia* occurs by ingestion of viable cysts. Although contaminated food or drink may be the source, intimate contact with an infected individual may also result in transmission of the organism. This organism is found more frequently in children or in groups living in close quarters. Outbreaks have been associated with poor sanitation facilities or sanitation breakdowns, as evidenced by infections of travelers and campers. Limited information is available on seasonal variations in giardiasis. Some data suggest an association with the cooler, wetter months of the year, which may implicate environmental conditions as advantageous to cyst survival. Certain occupations may place an individual at risk for infection, such as sewage and irrigation workers, who may be exposed to infective cysts. In situations in which young children are grouped together, such as in nursery schools, an increased incidence of exposure and subsequent infection of both children and staff members may be seen. A high incidence of giardiasis occurs in patients with immunodeficiency syndromes, particularly in those with common variable hypogammaglobulinemia. Giardiasis is the most common cause of diarrhea in these patients and may be associated with mild to severe villus atrophy.

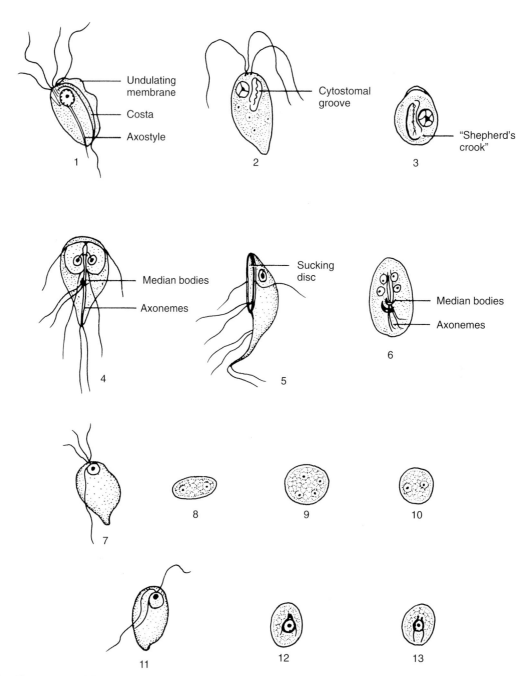

**Figure 48-16 1,** Trophozoite of *Pentatrichomonas hominis.* **2,** Trophozoite of *Chilomastix mesnili.* **3,** Cyst of *C. mesnili.* **4,** Trophozoite of *Giardia lamblia* (front view). **5,** Trophozoite of *G. lamblia* (side view). **6,** Cyst of *G. lamblia.* **7,** Trophozoite of *Enteromonas hominis.* **8** to **10,** Cysts of *E. hominis.* **11,** Trophozoite of *Retortamonas intestinalis.* **12** to **13,** Cysts of *R. intestinalis.* (From Garcia LS, Bruckner DA: *Diagnostic medical parasitology,* Washington, DC, 1993, ASM Press; illustration **5** by Nobuko Kitamura; illustrations **7** to **13** modified from Markell EK, Voge M: *Medical parasitology,* ed 5, Philadelphia, 1981, WB Saunders.)

An estimated 200 million people in Asia, Africa, and Latin America have symptomatic infections. In the United States, approximately 20,000 cases are reported yearly. However, an estimated 2 million cases may occur annually.

## Pathogenesis and Spectrum of Disease
The incubation period for giardiasis ranges from approximately 12 to 20 days. Giardiasis may not be recognized as the cause, because the infection mimics acute viral enteritis, bacillary dysentery, bacterial or other food poisonings, acute intestinal amebiasis, or "traveler's diarrhea" (toxigenic *Escherichia coli*). However, the type of diarrhea plus the lack of blood, mucus, and cellular exudate is consistent with giardiasis.

**Asymptomatic Infection.** Although the parasites in the crypts of the duodenal mucosa may reach very high numbers, they may not cause a pathologic condition. The organisms feed on the mucous secretions and do not penetrate the mucosa. Although organisms have been

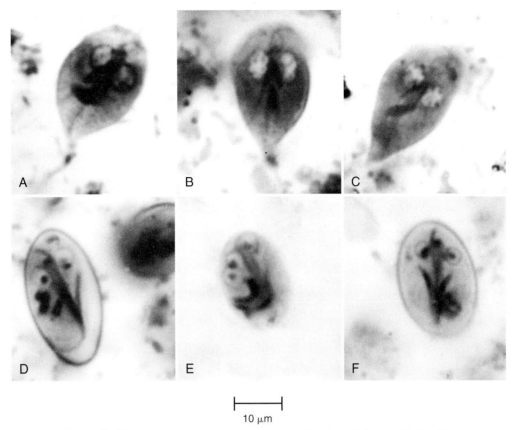

Figure 48-17 **A** to **C,** Trophozoites of *Giardia lamblia*. **D** to **F,** Cysts of *G. lamblia*.

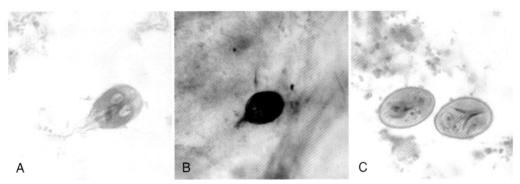

Figure 48-18 **A,** *Giardia lamblia* trophozoite. **B,** *G. lamblia* trophozoite, iodine stain. **C,** *G. lamblia* cysts. (**B** courtesy Dr. Henry Travers, Sioux Falls, S.D.)

seen in biopsy material obtained from inside the intestinal mucosa, others have been seen attached to the epithelium.

**Intestinal Disease.** For unknown reasons, symptomatic patients may have irritation of the mucosal lining, increased mucus secretion, and dehydration. The onset may be accompanied by nausea, anorexia, malaise, low-grade fever, and chills, in addition to a sudden onset of explosive, watery, foul-smelling diarrhea. Other symptoms include epigastric pain, flatulence, and diarrhea with increased amounts of fat and mucus in the stool but no blood. Weight loss often accompanies these

symptoms. Although some speculate that the organisms coating the mucosal lining may act to prevent fat absorption, this does not completely explain the prevention of the uptake of other substances normally absorbed at other intestinal levels. Severe malabsorption has also been linked with isolated levothyroxine malabsorption, leading to severe hypothyroidism and secondary impairment of pancreatic function. In both cases, treatment with metronidazole led to complete remission of symptoms. Occasionally the gallbladder is involved, resulting in gallbladder colic and jaundice. *G. lamblia* also has been identified in bronchoalveolar lavage fluid.

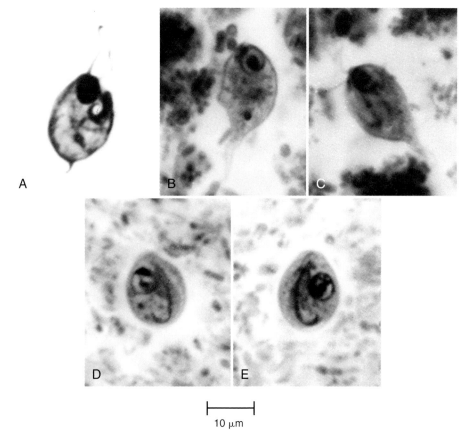

**Figure 48-19** **A** to **C,** Trophozoites of *Chilomastix mesnili* (**A,** silver stain). **D** and **E,** Cysts of *C. mesnili.*

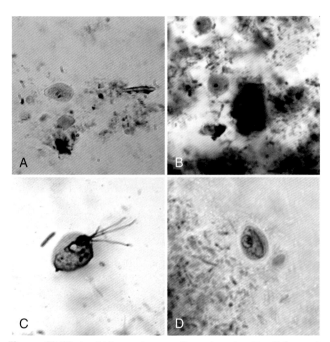

**Figure 48-20** **A,** *Chilomastix mesnili* trophozoite. **B,** *Chilomastix mesnili* cyst (both top figures are iodine stain). **C,** *Chilomastix mesnili* trophozoite (silver stain). **D,** *C. mesnili* cyst. (**A** and **B** courtesy Dr. Henry Travers, Sioux Falls, S.D.)

**Figure 48-21** Trophozoites of *Dientamoeba fragilis.*

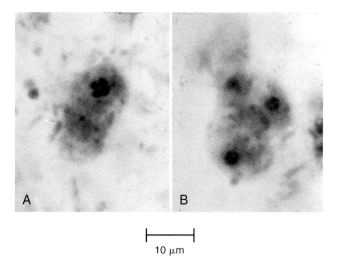

**Figure 48-22** **A** and **B,** Trophozoites of *Dientamoeba fragilis.*

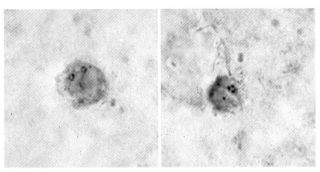

**Figure 48-23 A,** *Dientamoeba fragilis,* two nuclei. **B,** *D. fragilis,* one nucleus.

**Chronic Disease.** The acute phase often is followed by a subacute or chronic phase. Symptoms include recurrent, brief episodes of loose, foul-smelling stools and possibly increased distention and foul flatus. Between episodes of mushy stools, the patient may have normal stools or may be constipated. Abdominal discomfort includes marked distention and belching with a rotten-egg taste. Chronic disease must be differentiated from amebiasis; disease caused by other intestinal parasites (e.g., *D. fragilis, Cryptosporidium* spp., *Cyclospora cayetanensis, Isospora belli, Strongyloides stercoralis*); inflammatory bowel disease; and irritable colon. On the basis of symptoms such as upper intestinal discomfort, heartburn, and belching, giardiasis must also be differentiated from duodenal ulcer, hiatal hernia, and gallbladder and pancreatic disease.

**Antigenic Variation.** Variation of the surface antigen during human infections with *G. lamblia* has been documented. This capability suggests that variation may provide a mechanism for the organism to escape the host's immune response. The **variant-specific surface proteins** (VSPs) are a family of related, highly unusual proteins covering the surface of the organism. VSPs are resistant to the effects of intestinal proteases, which allows the parasites to survive in the protease-rich small intestine. Antigenic variation at the surface membrane of trophozoites occurs frequently; seemingly, the higher the rate of change, the more likely it is that a chronic infection would persist.

### Laboratory Diagnosis

**Routine Methods.** Routine stool examinations are normally recommended for the recovery and identification of intestinal protozoa. However, in the case of *G. lamblia*, because the organisms are attached securely to the mucosa by means of the sucking disk, a series of five or six stool samples may be examined without recovering the organism. The organisms also tend to be passed in the stool on a cyclic basis. The Entero-Test capsule can be helpful for recovering the organisms, as can the duodenal aspirate. Although cysts often can be identified on the wet stool preparation, many infections may be missed without examination of a permanent stained smear. If material from the string test (Entero-Test, HDC Corp., San Jose, CA) or mucus from a duodenal aspirate is submitted, it should be examined as a wet preparation for motility; however, motility may be represented by nothing more than a slight flutter of the flagella, because the organism is caught up in the mucus. After diagnosis, the positive specimen can be preserved as a permanent stain.

**Antigen Detection.** The development of fecal immunoassays to detect *Giardia* antigen in stool has dramatically improved the sensitivity seen with the routine O&P examination. The ELISA has been used to detect *Giardia* antigen in feces. Fluorescent methods with monoclonal antibodies have also proven extremely sensitive and specific in detecting *G. lamblia* in fecal specimens. Other products are available as a cartridge format that uses an immunochromatographic strip–based detection system for *G. lamblia* and/or *Cryptosporidium* spp. Any antigen detection system should always be reviewed for compatibility with stools submitted in preservatives rather than fresh specimens. Some limitations exist on the use of kits for organisms in the genus *Entamoeba.* However, commercial reagent kits for detecting *Giardia* and *Cryptosporidium* spp. can be used with formalin-based stool preservatives or with fresh or frozen specimens. Many of these cartridge format tests provide an answer within 10 minutes and are equal to or better than other immunoassays with regard to sensitivity and specificity. Many of these newer methods are being used to test patients suspected of having giardiasis or those who may be involved in an outbreak.

The detection of antigen in stool or visual identification of organisms by using monoclonal antibody reagents indicates current infection. The value of these detection assays as rapid, reliable immunodiagnostic procedures has been emphasized by the increase in *Giardia* infections and the greater awareness of particular incidences (e.g., nursery school settings). Because the organisms are shed so sporadically, use of a fecal immunoassay does not eliminate the need to analyze multiple stool specimens for sensitive detection of *G. lamblia;* a minimum of two stools should be tested. If the first specimen is negative, it may represent a false negative.

**Antibody Detection.** Unfortunately, serodiagnostic procedures for antibody detection do not fulfill the criteria necessary for wide clinical use, particularly because they may indicate either past or present infection.

**Histology.** Trophozoites are detectable in the duodenum and proximal jejunum; however, mucosal invasion generally has been found in areas where necrosis or mechanical trauma was present. Changes range from normal to almost complete villus atrophy, with a greater density of inflammatory infiltrate in the lamina propria when villus atrophy is present. The amount of villus damage seems to correlate with the degree of malabsorption. Apparently, patients with giardiasis also have reduced mucosal surface areas compared with control patients.

Histologic changes in the mucosal architecture in immunodeficient patients with giardiasis also range from mild to severe villus atrophy. It appears that giardiasis produces a more severe degree of villus damage in patients with hypogammaglobulinemia. In patients with acquired immunodeficiency syndrome (AIDS), giardiasis does not appear to be an important pathogen, although the infection has certainly been found in this group and in homosexual men.

### Nucleic Acid-Based Techniques

Currently, there are no molecular-based assays commercially available for the detection of *G. lamblia*.

### Prevention

The most effective practice for preventing the spread of infection in the child care setting is thorough hand washing by the children, staff members, and visitors. Rubbing the hands together under running water is the most important part of washing away infectious organisms. Premoistened towelettes or wipes and waterless hand cleaners should not be used as substitutes for washing the hands with soap and running water. These guidelines are not limited to giardiasis but include all potentially infectious organisms.

Because wild animals and possibly domestic animals serve as reservoir hosts, personal hygiene, improved sanitary measures, and safe drinking water are considerations. Iodine has been recommended as an effective disinfectant for drinking water. Filtration systems have also been recommended, although they have certain drawbacks, such as clogging.

## CHILOMASTIX MESNILI

### General Characteristics

*C. mesnili* has both trophozoite and cyst stages and is somewhat more easily identified than are some of the smaller flagellates, such as *E. hominis* and *R. intestinalis* (see Tables 48-3 and 48-4; see Figure 48-19). The *C. mesnili* trophozoite is pear shaped, measuring 6 to 24 μm long and 4 to 8 μm wide. It has a single nucleus and a distinct oral groove, or cytostome (mouth), close to the nucleus. Flagella are difficult to see without obvious motility in a wet preparation. The morphology can be seen on the permanent stained smear; the cytostome may be visible in some trophozoites. The cysts are pear or lemon shaped and range from 6 to 10 μm long and 4 to 6 μm wide (see Figure 48-20). They have a single nucleus and a typical curved cytostomal fibril, called the **shepherd's crook**. The cyst's definitive morphology can be seen on a permanent stain.

### Epidemiology

*C. mesnili* tends to have a cosmopolitan distribution, although it is found more frequently in warm climates. Transmission occurs through ingestion of infective cysts.

### Pathogeneis and Spectrum of Disease

*C. mesnili* is considered nonpathogenic and does not cause disease.

### Laboratory Diagnosis

Although cysts sometimes can be seen in a wet preparation, definitive identification of *C. mesnili* relies on examination of permanent stained smears.

### Therapy

Specific treatment is not recommended for *C. mesnili*. Because these nonpathogenic organisms are acquired through fecal-oral contamination, both pathogens and nonpathogens can be found in the same patient. If few organisms are present, extended microscopic examination and multiple organism measurements are required for definitive identification. It is always important to report pathogens and nonpathogens, because they are acquired the same way.

### Prevention

Prevention depends on adequate disposal of human excreta and improved personal hygiene, preventive measures that apply to most of the intestinal protozoa.

## DIENTAMOEBA FRAGILIS

### General Characteristics

*D. fragilis* was described in 1918. It has a worldwide distribution, and surveys report incidence rates of 1.4% to 19%. Much higher incidence figures have been reported for patients in mental institutions, missionaries, and Native Americans in Arizona. *D. fragilis* tends to be common in some pediatric populations, and the incidence is higher for patients under 20 years of age in some studies. Some speculate that *D. fragilis* may be infrequently recovered and identified; a low incidence or absence from survey studies may be due to poor laboratory techniques and a general lack of knowledge about the organism.

The *D. fragilis* trophozoite is characterized as having one nucleus (20% to 40%) or two nuclei (60% to 80%). The nuclear chromatin usually is fragmented into three to five granules, and normally no peripheral chromatin is seen on the nuclear membrane. In some organisms the nuclear chromatin tends to mimic that of *E. nana*, *E. hartmanni*, or even *C. mesnili*, particularly if the organisms are overstained with trichrome or iron-hematoxylin stain. The cytoplasm is usually vacuolated and may contain ingested debris and some large, uniform granules. The cytoplasm can also appear uniform and clean with few inclusions. Size and shape vary considerably among organisms, even on a single smear.

### Epidemiology

The life cycle and mode of transmission of *D. fragilis* are not known, although transmission in helminth eggs (e.g., *Ascaris* and *Enterobius* spp.) has been postulated (see Figures 48-21 to 48-23). The cyst stage has not been confirmed to date (see Tables 48-3 and 48-4).

### Pathogenesis and Spectrum of Disease

*D. fragilis* has been associated with a wide range of symptoms. Case reports of children infected with *D. fragilis* reveal a number of symptoms, including intermittent diarrhea, abdominal pain, nausea, anorexia, malaise, fatigue, poor weight gain, and unexplained eosinophilia. The most common symptoms in patients infected with this parasite appear to be intermittent diarrhea and fatigue. In some patients, both the organism and the symptoms persist or reappear until appropriate treatment is initiated.

## Laboratory Diagnosis

**Routine Methods.** Diagnosis of *D. fragilis* infections depends on proper collection and processing techniques (a minimum of three fecal specimens). Although the survival time for this parasite has been reported as 24 to 48 hours in the trophozoite form, the survival time in terms of morphology is limited, and stool specimens must be examined immediately or preserved in a suitable fixative soon after defecation. It is particularly important to examine permanent stained smears of stool with an oil immersion objective (×100).These trophozoites have been recovered in formed stool; therefore, a permanent stained smear must be prepared for every stool sample submitted for examination. Organisms seen in direct wet mounts may appear as refractile, round forms; the nuclear structure cannot be seen without examination of the permanent stained smear.

**Antigen Detection.** Although fecal immunoassays for antigen detection are not yet available commercially, they have been developed using several test formats. Detection of DNA from feces also is being used in some laboratories.

**Antibody Detection.** On indirect immunofluorescence assay, serum samples from patients with confirmed *D. fragilis* infections showed positive titers, and all matched controls had positive titers ranging from 20 to 160. However, these tests are not routinely used, nor are the reagents commercially available.

## Therapy

Clinical improvement has been seen in adults receiving tetracycline, and symptomatic relief has been observed in children receiving diiodohydroxyquin, metronidazole, or tetracycline. Current recommendations include iodoquinol, paromomycin, or tetracycline. Although limited studies have been undertaken on the efficacy of various therapies, information continues to support the finding that elimination of this organism from symptomatic patients leads to clinical improvement. Treatment of *D. fragilis* infection with iodoquinol, paromomycin, or combination therapy results in eradication of the parasite and complete resolution of symptoms.

## Prevention

Fecal-oral transmission has not been documented; therefore, it is difficult to speculate about preventive measures. However, if transmission does occur from ingestion of certain helminth eggs, the appropriate hygiene and sanitary measures to prevent contamination with fecal material are appropriate.

## *PENTATRICHOMONAS HOMINIS*

*P. hominis* is probably the most commonly identified flagellate, other than *G. lamblia* and *D. fragilis*. *P. hominis* has been recovered from all parts of the world, in both warm and temperate climates, and is considered nonpathogenic and noninvasive. It is not known to have a cyst stage (see Figure 48-16). *P. hominis* trophozoites live in the cecum and feed on bacteria. The trophozoite measures 5 to 15 μm long and 7 to 10 μm wide. It has a pyriform shape and has both an **axostyle** and an **undulating membrane,** which aid identification of the organism. The undulating membrane extends the entire length of the body, in contrast to that seen in the pathogen *T. vaginalis* (on which the membrane extends halfway down the body).

## Epidemiology

Because *P. hominis* is not known to have a cyst stage, transmission probably occurs in the trophic form. If ingested in a substance such as milk, these organisms apparently can survive passage through the stomach and small intestine in patients with achlorhydria. *P. hominis* cannot be transplanted into the vagina, the natural habitat of *T. vaginalis*. The incidence of this organism is relatively low, but it tends to be recovered more often than *E. hominis* or *R. intestinalis*, two small nonpathogenic flagellates that are rarely seen and extremely difficult to identify (see Figure 48-16).

## Pathogeneis and Spectrum of Disease

*P. hominis* is considered nonpathogenic and does not cause disease.

## Laboratory Diagnosis

*P. hominis* trophozoites can sometimes be seen on a permanent stained smear, but definitive identification can be difficult. However, it is important to report the presence of the organism if seen.

## Therapy

Specific treatment is not recommended for this nonpathogen.

## Prevention

Prevention depends on adequate disposal of human excreta and improved personal hygiene, preventive measures that apply to most of the intestinal protozoa.

# CILIATES

The class Ciliata, or ciliates, includes species that move by means of **cilia,** or short extensions of cytoplasm that cover the surface of the organism. The ciliates also have two different types of nuclei, one **macronucleus** and one or more **micronuclei**. This group includes only one organism that infects humans, *Balantidium coli*, which infects the intestinal tract and may produce severe symptoms.

## *BALANTIDIUM COLI*

### General Characteristics

The life cycle of *B. coli* includes both the trophozoite and cyst stages (Figures 48-24 and 48-25). The cyst form is the infective stage. After ingestion of the cysts and excystation, trophozoites secrete hyaluronidase, which aids the invasion of the colonic tissue.

The trophozoite is quite large, oval, and covered with short cilia. It measures approximately 50 to 150 μm long and 40 to 70 μm wide. The organism can be seen in a wet preparation on lower power. The anterior end is somewhat pointed and has a cytostome (primitive mouth opening); in contrast, the posterior end is broadly rounded. The cytoplasm contains many vacuoles with ingested bacteria and debris. The trophozoite has two nuclei: one very large, bean-shaped macronucleus and a smaller, round micronucleus. The organisms live in the large intestine. The trophozoites have a rapid, rotatory, boring motion because of the movement of the cilia. The cyst is formed as the trophozoite moves down the intestine. Nuclear division does not occur in the cyst; therefore, only two nuclei are present, the macronucleus and the micronucleus. The cysts measure 50 to 70 μm in diameter (see Table 48-5).

### Epidemiology

*B. coli* is widely distributed in hogs, particularly in warm and temperate climates, and in monkeys in the tropics. Human infection is found in warmer climates, sporadically in cooler areas, and in institutionalized groups with low levels of personal hygiene.

### Pathogenesis and Spectrum of Disease

Some individuals with *B. coli* infection are asymptomatic, whereas others have severe dysentery, similar to that seen in patients with amebiasis. Symptoms include diarrhea or dysentery, tenesmus, nausea, vomiting, anorexia, and headache. Insomnia, muscular weakness, and weight loss

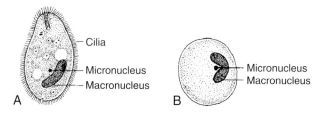

**Figure 48-24 A,** Trophozoite of *Balantidium coli*. **B,** Cyst of *B. coli*. (From Garcia LS: *Diagnostic medical parasitology,* ed 5, Washington, DC, 2007, ASM Press.)

also have been reported. Diarrhea may persist for weeks to months, with or without subsequent development of dysentery. Tremendous fluid loss may occur, with diarrhea similar to that seen in cholera or in some coccidial or microsporidial infections.

*B. coli* can invade tissue. It may penetrate the mucosa on contact, with cellular infiltration in the area of the developing ulcer. Some of the abscess formations may extend to the muscular layer. The ulcers may vary in shape, and the ulcer bed may be full of pus and necrotic debris. Although the number of cases is small, extraintestinal disease (peritonitis, urinary tract infection, inflammatory vaginitis) has been reported.

### Laboratory Diagnosis

Routine stool examinations, particularly wet preparation examinations of fresh and concentrated material, demonstrate the presence of organisms. Organism recognition and identification on a permanent stained smear is usually difficult. These protozoa are large and stain very darkly, which obscures any internal morphology. *B. coli* organisms may be confused with helminth eggs or debris because of their size, particularly when the cilia are not visible. Recovery of *B. coli* from specimens in the United States is rare. However, laboratories should be able to identify these organisms and are required to do so in proficiency testing specimens.

### Therapy

Tetracycline is the drug of choice for treating *B. coli* infection, although it is considered investigational for this infection. Iodoquinol or metronidazole may be used as an alternative. Nitazoxanide, a broad-spectrum antiparasitic drug, may be another alternative.

### Prevention

In areas where pigs are raised, the incidence of human infection can be quite high in pig farmers and slaughterhouse workers. Human infection is fairly rare in temperate areas, although infections can develop into an epidemic, particularly in areas of poor environmental

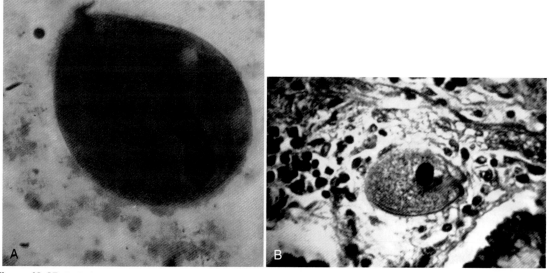

**Figure 48-25 A,** *Balantidium coli* trophozoite. **B,** *B. coli* trophozoite. (**B** courtesy Dr. Henry Travers, Sioux Falls, S.D.)

sanitation and personal hygiene. This situation has been seen in mental hospitals in the United States. Preventive measures involve increased attention to personal hygiene and sanitation measures, because the mode of transmission is ingestion of infective cysts through contaminated food or water.

# SPOROZOA (APICOMPLEXA)

All the Apicomplexa are unicellular and have an **apical complex.** These structures can be seen in electron microscopy studies and are used to help classify the various organisms. Genera that develop in the gastrointestinal tract of vertebrates throughout their entire life cycle include *Isospora, Cyclospora,* and *Cryptosporidium.* Genera capable of or requiring extraintestinal development are referred to as *cyst-forming coccidia;* they include *Sarcocystis* and *Toxoplasma* spp. The genera that cause disease in humans include *Cryptosporidium, Cyclospora, Isospora, Sarcocystis,* and *Toxoplasma* (see Chapter 50 for a discussion of *Toxoplasma*).

## *CRYPTOSPORIDIUM* SPP.

### General Characteristics

*Cryptosporidium* spp. are intracellular parasites that primarily infect epithelial cells of the stomach, intestine, and biliary ducts. The organism previously called *Cryptosporidium parvum,* thought to be the primary *Cryptosporidium* species infecting humans, now is classified as two species, *C. parvum* (mammals, including humans) and *C. hominis* (primarily humans) (see Table 48-6, Figures 48-26 to 48-28). Differentiation of these two species based on oocyst morphology is not possible. Currently, more than 20 established *Cryptosporidium* species

have been identified in vertebrates, and more than 10 *Cryptosporidium* spp. have been reported in humans.

*Cryptosporidium* infections begin with ingestion of viable oocysts. Upon contact with gastric and duodenal fluid, each oocyst releases four sporozoites, which invade

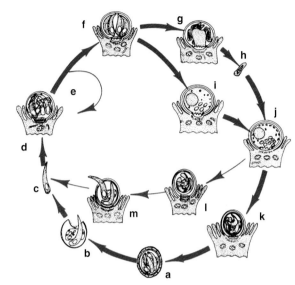

**Figure 48-26** Life cycle of *Cryptosporidium.* **(a)** Sporulated oocyst in feces. **(b)** Excystation in intestine. **(c)** Free sporozoite in intestine. **(d)** Type I meront (six or eight merozoites). **(e)** Recycling of type I merozoite. **(f)** Type II meront (four merozoites). **(g)** Microgametocyte with approximately 16 microgametes. **(h)** Microgamete fertilizes macrogamete **(i)** to form zygote **(j).** Approximately 80% of the zygotes form thick-walled oocysts **(k),** which sporulate within the host cell. About 20% of the zygotes do not form an oocyst wall; their sporozoites are surrounded only by a unit membrane **(l).** Sporozoites in "autoinfective," thin-walled oocysts **(l)** are released into the intestinal lumen **(m)** and reinitiate the endogenous cycle (at **c**). (Courtesy William L. Current, Lilly Research Laboratories, Greenfield, Ind.)

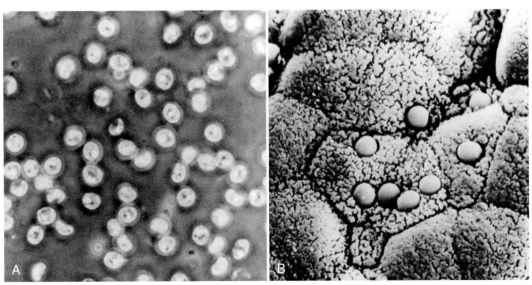

**Figure 48-27** *Cryptosporidium.* **A,** Oocysts recovered from a Sheather's sugar flotation; organisms measure 4 to 6 $\mu$m. **B,** Scanning electron microscopy view of organisms at brush border of epithelial cells. (From Garcia LS, Bruckner DA: *Diagnostic medical parasitology,* Washington, DC, 1993, ASM Press.)

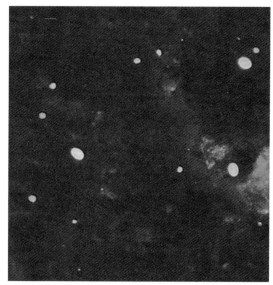

**Figure 48-28** *Cryptosporidium* oocysts and *Giardia* cysts stained with monoclonal antibody–conjugated fluorescent reagent. (Courtesy Merifluor, Meridian Diagnostics, Cincinnati, Ohio.)

the epithelial cells and develop into trophozoites surrounded by a parasitophorous vacuole (layers of endoplasmic reticulum around an intracellular parasite). In the epithelial cells, trophozoites undergo two or three generations of asexual amplification, called **merogony,** leading to the formation of different types of meronts containing four to eight merozoites. The merozoites differentiate into sexually distinct stages in a process called **gametogony.** New **oocysts** are then formed in the epithelial cells in a process called **sporogony.** About 20% of the oocysts are thin walled and may excyst in the digestive tract of the host, leading to the infection of new cells (autoinfection). The remaining 80% of the oocysts are excreted into the environment; are resistant to low temperature, high salinity, and most disinfectants; and can initiate infection in a new host. *Cryptosporidium* oocysts in humans measure 4 to 6 μm in diameter.

### Epidemiology

Humans can acquire cryptosporidiosis through several transmission routes, such as direct contact with infected people or animals or consumption of contaminated water (drinking or recreational) or food. The interval between ingestion of infective oocysts to completion of the life cycle and excretion of new oocysts usually is 4 to 10 days. The only extracellular stage in the *Cryptosporidium* life cycle is the oocysts; these are the environmental stage of the parasite and are immediately infectious when passed in the stool.

*Cryptosporidium* spp. have a worldwide distribution, and the oocysts are ubiquitous in the environment. In developing countries, human *Cryptosporidium* infection occurs mostly in children younger than 5 years, with peak occurrence of infections and diarrhea in children under 2 years of age. In developed countries, pediatric cryptosporidiosis occurs in older children, probably because, as a result of better hygiene, exposure to contaminated environments occurs later. Cryptosporidiosis

is also common in the elderly in nursing homes, where person-to-person transmission occurs. In the general population, sporadic infections occur in all age groups in the United States and the United Kingdom, and traveling to developing countries and consumption of contaminated food and water can lead to infection. Cryptosporidiosis is common in immunocompromised individuals, such as those with AIDS or primary immunodeficiency and cancer and transplant patients undergoing immunosuppressive therapy.

Calves and perhaps other animals serve as potential sources of human infection. Contact with these animals may be an unrecognized cause of gastroenteritis in humans in both rural and urban settings. Direct person-to-person transmission is also likely and may occur through direct or indirect contact with stool material. Direct transmission may occur during sexual practices involving oral-anal contact. Indirect transmission may occur through exposure to positive specimens in a laboratory setting or from contaminated surfaces or food or water.

### Pathogenesis and Spectrum of Disease

**Immunocompetent Individuals.** In immunocompetent people with sporadic cryptosporidiosis in industrialized nations, the most common symptom is diarrhea. Clinical symptoms include nausea, low-grade fever, abdominal cramps, anorexia, and five to 10 watery, frothy bowel movements per day, which may be followed by constipation. Some patients may have diarrhea, and others may have few symptoms, particularly later in the course of the infection. In patients with the typical watery diarrhea, the stool contains mainly water and mucus. Often the organisms are entrapped in the mucus, and diagnostic procedures are performed accordingly. Generally a patient with a normal immune system has a self-limited infection; however, patients who are immunocompromised may have a chronic infection with a wide range of symptoms. The illness usually lasts 9 to 21 days and may require hospitalization in up to 20% of those infected. Patients infected with *C. hominis* are more likely to have joint pain, eye pain, recurrent headache, dizziness, and fatigue than those infected with *C. parvum.*

**Immunocompromised Individuals.** Hemodialysis patients with chronic renal failure and renal transplant patients with cryptosporidiosis can have chronic, life-threatening diarrhea. In individuals infected with the human immunodeficiency virus (HIV), cryptosporidiosis increases as the CD4+ lymphocyte count falls, especially below 200 cells/μL. Sclerosing cholangitis and other biliary involvement are also seen in AIDS patients with cryptosporidiosis. The combination of AIDS and cryptosporidiosis often leads to increased mortality and diminished survival. In these patients, *Cryptosporidium* infections are not always confined to the gastrointestinal tract; additional symptoms (respiratory problems, cholecystitis, hepatitis, and pancreatitis) have been associated with extraintestinal infections. Although the clinical features of sclerosing cholangitis secondary to opportunistic infections of the biliary tree in patients with AIDS are well known, the mechanisms by which pathogens such as *Cryptosporidium* spp. actually cause disease are unclear.

## Laboratory Diagnosis

**Routine Methods.** Oocysts in clinical specimens are difficult to see without special staining techniques, such as the modified acid-fast, Kinyoun's, or Giemsa method, or the newer immunoassay methods. The four sporozoites may be seen in the oocyst wall in some of the organisms, although they are not always visible in freshly passed specimens.

**Antigen Detection.** Immunoassays are very helpful, because they are a more sensitive method of detecting organisms in stool specimens. A direct fluorescent antigen (FA) procedure with excellent specificity and sensitivity has been developed and results in a significantly increased detection rate over conventional staining and microscopy methods. Some of these reagents, particularly the combination direct FA product used to identify both *Giardia* spp. cysts and *Cryptosporidium* spp. oocysts, are being widely used in water testing and outbreak situations. Most antibodies in commercial direct fluorescent antibody (DFA) kits react with oocysts of almost all *Cryptosporidium* species, making identification to the species level impossible. Enzyme immunoassay (EIA) tests also provide excellent specificity and sensitivity for laboratories using this approach, as do the immunochromatographic cartridge rapid test formats. It is important to remember that if a patient is in the carrier state or undergoing self-cure, the number of oocysts may drop below the sensitivity levels of these kits, producing a false-negative result.

**Nucleic Acid-Based Methods.** Molecular techniques, especially polymerase chain reaction (PCR) and PCR-related methods, have been used to detect and differentiate *Cryptosporidium* spp., and a few of the PCR assays are commercially available. Several genus-specific PCR-restriction fragment length polymorphism–based genotyping tools have been developed for detecting and differentiating *Cryptosporidium* organisms at the species level. Other genotyping techniques are designed mostly for differentiation of *C. parvum* and *C. hominis* and cannot detect and differentiate other *Cryptosporidium* spp. or genotypes.

**Antibody Detection.** In the United States, drinking untreated surface water has been identified as a risk factor for cryptosporidiosis; residents living in cities with surface-derived drinking water generally have higher antibody levels against *Cryptosporidium* spp. in their blood than those living in cities with ground water as drinking water. However, antibody detection is not available on a routine basis and currently is not used in the diagnosis of cryptosporidiosis.

**Histology.** In the examination of histologic preparations, developmental stages (sporozoites, trophozoites, merozoites, and oocysts) in the life cycle of *Cryptosporidium* spp. can be found at all levels of the intestinal tract, with the jejunum being the most heavily infected site. Routine hematoxylin and eosin staining is sufficient to demonstrate these parasites. Under regular light microscopy, the organisms are visible as small, round structures (about 1 to 3 $\mu$m in diameter) aligned along the brush border. They are intracellular but extracytoplasmic and are found in parasitophorous vacuoles. Developmental stages are more difficult to identify without a transmission electron microscope. It also is important to remember that in severely compromised patients, *Cryptosporidium* spp. have been found in other body sites, primarily the lungs, as a disseminated infection.

### Therapy

Oral or intravenous rehydration and antimotility drugs are used whenever severe diarrhea is associated with cryptosporidiosis. Nitazoxanide is the only drug approved by the U.S. Food and Drug Administration (FDA) for the treatment of cryptosporidiosis in immunocompetent individuals. This drug can shorten the clinical disease and reduce the number of parasites present. However, nitazoxanide is not effective in treating cryptosporidiosis in immunodeficient patients; paromomycin and spiramycin have been used in these individuals.

In industrialized nations, the most effective prophylaxis and treatment for cryptosporidiosis in patients with AIDS is highly active antiretroviral therapy (HAART). Eradication and prevention of the infection are related to replenishment of CD4+ cells in treated individuals and the antiparasitic activities of the protease inhibitors used in HAART. Relapse of cryptosporidiosis is common in patients with AIDS who have stopped HAART.

### Prevention

Effective concentrations of most substances used for disinfection are not practical outside the laboratory, and high concentrations that significantly reduce oocyst infectivity are either very expensive or quite toxic. *Cryptosporidium* oocysts are highly resistant to most commercial disinfectants, including iodine water purification tablets. Although chlorine and related compounds can dramatically reduce the ability of oocysts to excyst or infect, high concentrations and long exposure times are required, making this approach impractical.

## *CYCLOSPORA CAYETANENSIS*

### General Characteristics

During the past few years, a number of outbreaks of diarrhea associated with *Cyclospora cayetanensis* have occurred; the distribution is worldwide (United States, Caribbean, Central and South America, Southeast Asia, Eastern Europe, Australia, Nepal). These organisms are acid-fast variable and have been found in the feces of immunocompetent travelers to developing countries, immunocompetent individuals with no travel history, and patients with AIDS. Cumulative evidence suggests that outbreaks in the United States and Canada during the spring months of 1996 and 1997 were related to the importation and ingestion of Guatemalan raspberries. An outbreak in Florida in 1995 quite likely was also attributable to contaminated food. The cases reported in all three outbreaks probably represented only a small fraction of incidences.

The life cycle of *C. cayetanensis* involves only humans as hosts. Oocysts are passed in the feces unsporulated (Figure 48-29). At room temperature (23° to 25°C), small numbers of oocysts may sporulate within 10 to 12 days.

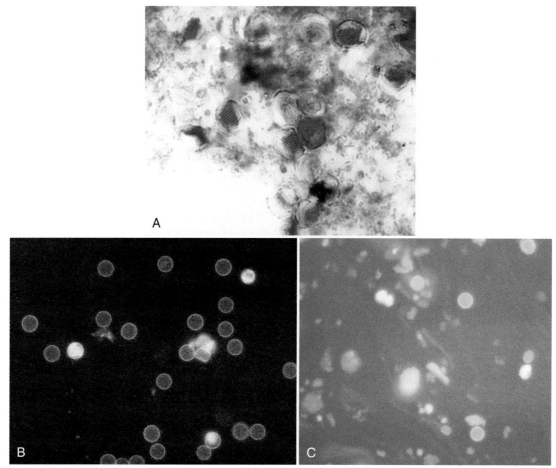

A

B

C

**Figure 48-29 A,** *Cyclospora cayetanensis* oocysts after modified acid-fast staining. Note the variability in the intensity of the stain. These oocysts measure 8 to 10 $\mu$m, twice the size of *Cryptosporidium* spp. (oil immersion, ×1000). **B** and **C,** *Cyclospora cayetanensis* oocysts exhibiting autofluorescence (high dry power, ×400). (**A** and **B** courtesy Charles R. Sterling, University of Arizona; **C** courtesy E. Long, Centers for Disease Control and Prevention, Atlanta, Ga.)

In clean wet mounts, *Cyclospora* organisms are seen as nonrefractile spheres, which are difficult to recognize as parasites. Unless a high number of oocysts are present, they may easily be mistaken for artifacts. They are acid-fast variable with the modified acid-fast stain; those that are unstained appear as glassy, wrinkled spheres (wrinkled cellophane). The oocysts are twice the size of those of *Cryptosporidium* spp. and measure 8 to 10 $\mu$m in diameter. Because it takes 10 days to 2 weeks for the oocysts to sporulate, no internal structures are visible (sporozoites), as can be seen in *Cryptosporidium* organisms.

### Epidemiology

Transmission of *C. cayetanensis* is thought to be by the fecal-oral route. However, direct person-to-person transmission has not been well documented and may not be a factor, because sporulation takes a number of days. Outbreaks linked to contaminated water and various types of fresh produce (raspberries, basil, baby lettuce leaves, and snow peas) have been reported. Information on reservoir hosts is not well defined; however, in some areas humans appear to be the only host.

*C. cayetanensis* is endemic in Central and South America, the Caribbean, Mexico, Indonesia, Asia, Nepal, Africa, India, Southern Europe, and the Middle East. In endemic areas, contact with soil and water increases the risk of *Cyclospora* infection. Infections in most temperate areas are correlated with the consumption of imported contaminated fruits and vegetables,

### Pathogenesis and Spectrum of Disease

Although some patients are asymptomatic, others report a flulike illness, marked by nausea, vomiting, anorexia, weight loss, and explosive diarrhea lasting 1 to 3 weeks. The incubation period is not yet known. However, the onset of symptoms after infection generally averages 7 to 8 days, and the symptoms last 2 to 3 weeks. Oocyst shedding in the feces is highly variable and may range from 7 days to several months. Indigenous infections are confined primarily to tropical, subtropical, or warm temperate regions of the world. Outbreaks occur in other areas of the world as a result of contaminated foodstuffs.

In immunocompromised and immunocompetent patients, *C. cayetanensis* infection can be associated with biliary disease. With light and transmission electron microscopy, developmental stages have been seen in the gallbladder epithelium of AIDS patients with acalculous cholecystitis. Also, oocysts have been seen in the bile of patients with active biliary disease.

### Laboratory Diagnosis

*C. cayetanensis* oocysts do not routinely stain with the trichrome fecal stain; special methods are required for identification. The oocysts can be concentrated using routine methods; special stains can then be used to enhance morphology. A single negative stool specimen is not conclusive in the examination of stools for coccidia; a total of three stool specimens collected on subsequent days must be examined before infection can be ruled out.

**Special Stains.** With modified acid-fast stains, the oocysts appear light pink to deep red, and some contain granules or have a bubbly appearance (described as wrinkled cellophane). It is very important to be aware of these organisms when the modified acid-fast stain is used, because *Cryptosporidium* spp. and other similar but larger structures (approximately twice the size of *Cryptosporidium* oocysts [8 to 10 $\mu m$]) are seen in the stained smear. Laboratories need to measure all acid-fast oocysts, particularly if they appear to be somewhat larger than those of *Cryptosporidium* spp. Variations on the safranin staining technique stain *C. cayetanensis* oocysts orange or pinkish orange, and heating and other treatments have been used to increase the staining frequency of oocysts. The oocysts autofluoresce green (450 to 490 DM excitation filter) or blue (365 DM excitation filter) under ultraviolet (UV) epifluorescence. It is strongly recommended that during concentration (formalin ethyl acetate) of stool specimens, centrifugation be carried out for 10 minutes at 500× *g*. The concentration sediment can then be stained, enhancing the sensitivity of the microscopy examinations.

**Flow Cytometry.** Flow cytometry is another diagnostic option. This approach appears to be a useful alternative to microscopy, particularly for screening large numbers of clinical specimens for *Cyclospora* oocysts in an outbreak situation. However, it is not commonly used.

**Other Diagnostic Methods.** Although culture, antigen detection, nucleic acid detection, and serologic tests for antibody have been developed, none of these methods is routinely available for most clinical laboratories.

### Therapy

Patients have been treated symptomatically with antidiarrheal preparations and have obtained some relief; however, the disease appears to be self-limiting within a few weeks. Trimethoprim (TMP-SMX), currently the drug of choice, is given orally twice daily for 7 days. Elimination of parasites, a decrease in diarrhea, and diminished abdominal pain occur within 2 to 3 days after treatment. Patients with AIDS may need higher doses and long-term maintenance treatment. However, more than 40% of patients have a recurrence of symptoms in 1 to 3 months after treatment.

### Prevention

Individuals in endemic areas should wear gloves when gardening to prevent exposure to oocysts of *C. cayetanensis*. Thorough washing of produce may help

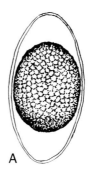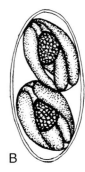

**Figure 48-30 A,** Immature concept of *Isospora belli*. **B,** Mature oocyst of *I. belli*. (Illustration by Nobuko Kitamura.)

remove oocysts. Most of the produce items implicated in the transmission of *C. cayetanensis* are consumed raw; thus cooking as a means of prevention is not relevant.

## ISOSPORA (CYSTOISOSPORA) BELLI

### General Characteristics

Although isosporiasis is found worldwide, certain tropical areas in the Western Hemisphere have specific locations where endemic infections occur. These organisms infect both adults and children, and intestinal involvement and symptoms are generally transient unless the patient is immunocompromised. *I. belli* has also been implicated in traveler's diarrhea. However, unlike with *Cryptosporidium* spp. and *C. cayetanensis*, large outbreaks of isosporiasis have not been reported (see Table 48-6, Figure 48-30).

*I. belli* oocysts are passed in the stool. They are long and oval, measuring 20 to 33 $\mu m$ long by 10 to 19 $\mu m$ wide. Usually the oocyst contains one immature **sporont,** but two may be present. Continued development occurs outside the body, with the development of two mature **sporocysts,** each containing four **sporozoites,** which can be recovered from the fecal specimen. The sporulated oocyst is the infective stage that excysts in the small intestine, releasing the sporozoites, which penetrate the mucosal cells and initiate the life cycle.

### Epidemiology

*I. belli* oocysts are passed in the feces unsporulated or partially sporulated. Oocysts complete sporulation within 72 hours, although it may take longer, depending on the temperature. The time required for unsporulated oocysts to appear in the feces after ingestion of sporulated oocysts is 9 to 17 days. Oocyst shedding is variable and depends on the immune status of the infected individual. Oocysts can be found for 30 to 50 days in immunocompetent patients, and immunosuppressed patients may continue to shed oocysts for 6 months or longer. Chronic infections can occur, and oocysts can be shed for months to years. In one particular case, an immunocompetent individual had symptoms for 26 years, and *I. belli* was recovered in stool a number of times over 10 years.

*I. belli* is thought to be the only species of *Isospora* that infects humans, and no other reservoir hosts are recognized for this infection. Transmission occurs through ingestion of water or food contaminated with mature, sporulated oocysts. Sexual transmission by direct oral contact with the anus or perineum also occurs, although this mode of transmission is probably much less common. The oocysts are very resistant to environmental conditions and may remain viable for months if kept cool and moist; oocysts usually mature within 48 hours after stool passage and are then infectious.

### Pathogenesis and Spectrum of Disease

Symptoms include diarrhea (most common), weight loss, abdominal colic, and fever. Stools (usually six to 10 per day) are watery to soft, foamy, and offensive smelling, suggesting a malabsorption process. Many patients have eosinophilia, recurrences are quite common, and the disease is more severe in infants and young children.

Patients who are immunosuppressed, particularly those with AIDS, often present with profuse diarrhea associated with weakness, anorexia, and weight loss. Biopsies reveal an abnormal mucosa with short villi, hypertrophied crypts, and infiltration of the lamina propria with eosinophils, neutrophils, and round cells. Physicians should consider *I. belli* in AIDS patients with diarrhea who have immigrated from or traveled to Latin America, are Hispanics born in the United States, are young adults, or who have not received prophylaxis with TMP-SMX for *Pneumocystis* infection. It has also been recommended that patients with AIDS traveling to Latin America and other developing countries be advised of the waterborne and food-borne transmission of *I. belli* and that chemoprophylaxis should be considered.

Extraintestinal infections in patients with AIDS have been reported. At autopsy, microscopic findings associated with *I. belli* infection were seen in the lymph nodes and walls of the small and large intestines, mesenteric and mediastinal lymph nodes, lymphatic channels, liver, and spleen. *I. belli* infections in the gallbladder epithelium and endometrial epithelium have also been reported, and oocysts have been recovered in bile specimens.

### Laboratory Diagnosis

Examination of fresh material, either as the direct smear or as concentrated material, is recommended rather than the permanent stained smear. The oocysts are very pale and transparent and can easily be overlooked. The light level should be reduced, and additional contrast should be obtained with the microscope for optimal examination conditions. On the permanent stained smear, the organisms may take up excess stain and resemble helminth eggs or artifacts.

It is possible to have a positive biopsy specimen but not recover the oocysts in the stool because of the small numbers of organisms present. The oocysts are acid-fast and can also be demonstrated by using auramine rhodamine stains. Organisms tentatively identified by using auramine rhodamine stains should be confirmed by wet smear examination or acid-fast stains, particularly if the stool contains other cells or excess artifact material (more normal stool consistency). Currently, there are no commercially available nucleic acid-based methods for the detection of *I. belli*. However, PCR assays have been developed for the detection of the organism in stool samples.

**Histology.** Developmental stages of *I. belli* have been reported for intestinal biopsy specimens of the duodenum, jejunum, and occasionally ileum. Intestinal development tends to occur in epithelial cells, although developing stages are occasionally reported from the lamina propria or submucosa. Extraintestinal infections in patients with AIDS have been reported; the organisms become dormant as cysts in a variety of tissues, including the intestine, mesenteric lymph nodes, liver, and spleen; these cysts are called *unizoite cysts*. In histologic sections, these cysts are thick walled and measure $12\text{-}22 \times 8\text{-}10$ μm, and each contains a single dormant sporozoite/merozoite of about $8\text{-}10 \times 5$ μm. As immunity declines, these cysts can reactivate patent infections.

### Therapy

The drug of choice to treat *I. belli* infection is trimethoprim-sulfamethoxazole, which is given two to four times a day for 10 to 14 days. With this approach, the parasites are eliminated, the diarrhea stops, and the abdominal pain decreases within a few days. Before the use of HAART, it was recommended that patients who were HIV positive and had a CD4+ cell count below 200 cells/mm$^3$ receive secondary prophylaxis with TMP-SMX once daily or three times a week to prevent relapse. Once the CD4 count exceeded 200 cells/mm$^3$, prophylaxis was no longer necessary.

### Prevention

Because transmission occurs through the infective oocysts, prevention includes improved personal hygiene measures and sanitary conditions to eliminate possible fecal-oral transmission from contaminated food, water, and possibly environmental surfaces.

## *SARCOCYSTIS* SPP.

### General Characteristics

Two well-described *Sarcocystis* species include *S. bovihominis* (cattle) and *S. suihominis* (pigs). (Some publications refer to *S. bovihominis* as *S. hominis.*) When uncooked meat from these infected animals is ingested by humans, gamogony (fission resulting in the production of sporozoan gametes) can occur in the intestinal cells, with eventual production of the sporocysts in stool.

*Sarcocystis* spp. have an obligatory two-host life cycle. Intermediate hosts (herbivores and omnivores) become infected through ingestion of sporocysts excreted in the feces of the definitive hosts (carnivores and omnivores). The definitive hosts become infected through ingestion of mature cysts found in the muscles of the intermediate hosts. In some intermediate hosts, such as cattle and sheep, all adult animals may be infected. Extraintestinal human sarcocystosis is rare, with a much lower incidence than is seen with the intestinal infection. Humans who have ingested meat containing the mature sarcocysts serve as the definitive hosts. Fever, severe diarrhea, abdominal pain, and weight loss have been reported in immunocompromised hosts, although the number of patients with these symptoms has been quite small.

The sporocysts found in the stool are broadly oval and slightly tapered at the ends. They measure 9 to 16 $\mu m$ long and contain four mature sporozoites and the residual body (see Table 48-6). Normally, the oocyst contains two sporocysts (similar to *I. belli*); however, in *Sarcocystis* infections, the sporocysts are released from the oocyst and normally are seen singly. These sporocysts tend to be larger than *Cryptosporidium* oocysts that contain four sporozoites, so they look totally different. The oocysts are fully sporulated when passed in the stool.

### Pathogenesis and Spectrum of Disease

When humans (intermediate host) ingest oocysts from other animal stool sources, the sarcocysts that develop in human muscle are 7 to 16 $\mu m$ long and cause few, if any, problems. Basically, no inflammatory response to these organisms occurs in the muscle, and no evidence of pathogenicity is seen. Patients demonstrate symptoms related to the disintegration of the sarcocysts and death of intracystic bradyzoites. Painful muscle swellings measuring 1 to 3 cm in diameter are associated with erythema of the overlying skin; these occur periodically and last 2 days to 2 weeks. Symptoms also include fever, diffuse myalgia, muscle tenderness, weakness, eosinophilia, and bronchospasm. Different types of skeletal and cardiac muscle sarcocysts have been found in humans. No specific therapy is required for this type of infection. Corticosteroids can reduce allergic inflammatory reactions.

Infections in humans can manifest primarily as intestinal disease if infected meat is ingested or as muscular disease if sporocysts are ingested. Intestinal disease occurs within a few hours after consumption of infected meat and is characterized by nausea, abdominal pain, and diarrhea. However, in both situations patients may be infected and asymptomatic.

### Laboratory Diagnosis

A presumptive diagnosis of intestinal disease may be based on the patient's symptoms, particularly with documented ingestion of raw or poorly cooked meat. Confirmation of the diagnosis may depend on finding human fecal specimens containing sporocysts, which are passed in the stool 11 to 18 days after ingestion of beef or pork. Sporocysts of the two *Sarcocystis* species are very difficult to differentiate.

A muscle biopsy is appropriate for suspected symptomatic intramuscular infection in a patient with a history of travel to or residence in a tropical location. Sarcocysts in biopsy specimens can be identified by microscopy on routine histologic sections stained with hematoxylin and eosin. Most sarcocysts in humans have been found in skeletal and cardiac muscle; however, muscles in the larynx, pharynx, and upper esophagus have also been involved. No molecular assays are currently available for the detection of sarcocystis in humans. However, several amplification methods have been used to detect sarcocystis in intermediate hosts.

### Therapy

No known treatment or prophylaxis is available for intestinal infection, myositis, vasculitis, or related lesions caused by human sarcocystosis. Supportive therapy for patients with severe diarrhea is indicated. It is also unclear whether immunosuppressives are effective at reducing the inflammatory reactions seen in vasculitis or myositis. Without more definitive data, no course of therapy currently can be recommended.

### Prevention

Cooking meat to an internal temperature higher than 67°C kills *Toxoplasma gondii* tissue cysts in meat; this temperature should also kill *Sarcocystis* tissue cysts in meat. Preventing cattle, buffalos, and swine from consuming human feces shedding infective oocysts also prevents animal infection. Most cases of human muscular *Sarcocystis* infection have been reported from the Far East. When humans are intermediate hosts, preventive measures involve careful disposal of animal feces that may contain the infective sporocysts. This may be impossible in wilderness areas, where wild animals may serve as reservoir hosts for many *Sarcocystis* spp.

# MICROSPORIDIA

Microsporidia are obligate intracellular, spore-forming parasites. More than 140 microsporidial genera and 1200 species have been identified. To date, seven genera (*Anncaliia*, *Encephalitozoon*, *Enterocytozoon*, *Nosema*, *Pleistophora*, *Vittaforma*, and *Trachipleistophora*) and unclassified microsporidia *(Microsporidium)* have been identified as causing human infections.

Although the microsporidia are true eukaryotes, they also have molecular and cytologic characteristics of prokaryotes. Microsporidia evolved from the fungi and are most closely related to the Zygomycetes. Features shared with fungi include the presence of chitin and trehalose, similarities in cell cycles, and certain gene organizations. Microsporidia are now considered highly derived fungi that underwent genetic and functional losses, resulting in one of the smallest eukaryotic genomes known. However, the life cycle of microsporidia is unique and unlike that of any fungal species. At this point, clinical and diagnostic issues and responsibilities may remain with the parasitologists, and we may be in a transition stage, similar to that seen with *Pneumocystis jirovecii* as it was moved from the parasites to fungi in terms of classification status.

## GENERAL CHARACTERISTICS

Human microsporidial infections have been documented worldwide. The spore, the only life cycle stage able to survive outside the host cell, is the infective stage (see Table 48-7 and Figures 48-31 to 48-35). Infection occurs with ingestion or inhalation of the infective spores, from which the infective sporoplasm (spore protoplasm) enters the host cell through the **polar tubule.** The microsporidia multiply extensively in the host cell cytoplasm; the life cycle includes repeated divisions by binary fission (merogony) or multiple fission (schizogony) and spore production (sporogony). Both merogony and sporogony

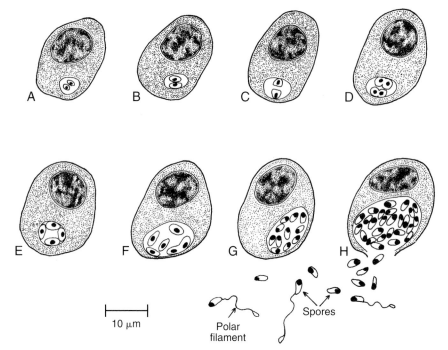

**Figure 48-31** Life cycle diagram of the microsporidia. **A** to **G,** Asexual development of sporoblasts. **H,** Release of spores. (Modified from Gardiner CH, Fayer R, Dubey JP: *An atlas of protozoan parasites in animal tissues,* Agriculture Handbook No 651, Washington, DC, 1988, US Department of Agriculture.)

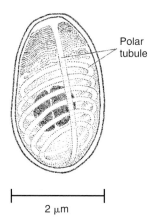

**Figure 48-32** Diagram illustrating the polar tubule in a microsporidian spore. (Modified from Bryan RT, Cali A, Owen RL, Spencer HC. In Sun T, editor: *Progress in clinical parasitology,* vol 2, New York, 1991, WW Norton.)

can occur in the same cell at the same time. During sporogony, a thick spore wall is formed, providing environmental protection for the spore.

Microsporidial spores measure 0.7 to about 4 μm in diameter. Mature spores contain a tubular extrusion apparatus (polar tube or tubule) for injecting infective spore contents (sporoplasm) into the host cell.

## EPIDEMIOLOGY

Transmission possibilities include human-to-human and animal-to-human routes. Many questions relating to reservoir hosts and possible congenital infections are still unanswered. Primary infection occurs through inhalation or ingestion of spores from environmental sources or by zoonotic transmission. The presence of *Encephalitozoon intestinalis* has been confirmed in tertiary sewage effluent, surface water, and groundwater; *Enterocytozoon bieneusi* has been confirmed in surface water; and *Vittaforma corneae* has been confirmed in tertiary effluent. This study represents the first confirmation, to the species level, of human-pathogenic microsporidia in water, indicating that these parasites are probably waterborne pathogens. Ingestion of the environmentally highly resistant spores is probably the normal mode of transmission.

*E. bieneusi*, an intestinal pathogen, serves as an example of infection potential. The spores are released into the intestinal lumen and are passed in the stool. These spores are environmentally resistant and can be ingested by other hosts. Zoonotic transmission of microsporidia infecting humans has not been verified but appears likely, because many microsporidial species can infect both humans and animals.

## PATHOGENESIS AND SPECTRUM OF DISEASE

Microsporidia were recognized as causing disease in animals as early as the 1920s but were not recognized as agents of human disease until the AIDS pandemic began in the mid-1980s. Before then, several earlier human cases had been reported but were thought to be very unusual.

### Enterocytozoon bieneusi

A number of cases of *E. bieneusi* infection have been reported in patients with AIDS. Chronic intractable

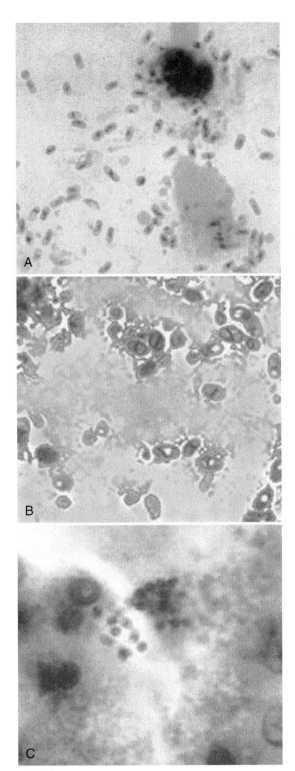

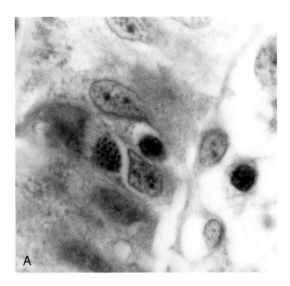

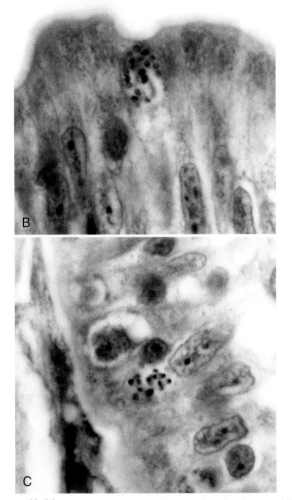

**Figure 48-33** Microsporidial spores stained with Ryan-blue modified trichrome stain. **A,** Nasopharyngeal aspirate. **B,** Stool (enlarged image). **C,** Urine.

**Figure 48-34** Routine histology micrograph of microsporidian spores in enterocytes (Giemsa stain). **A,** Note the small size. **B,** The spores are more easily seen; note the position between the nucleus and the brush border of the cell. **C,** In these spores, the granule is easily seen (stains positive with periodic acid-Schiff [PAS] stain).

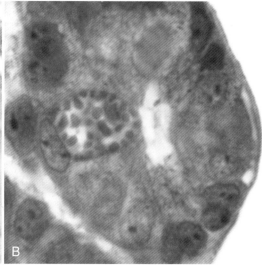

**Figure 48-35** Routine histology micrograph of microsporidian spores in enterocytes (Giemsa stain). **A,** Note the fully formed spores. **B,** These spores are not fully mature.

diarrhea, fever, malaise, and weight loss are symptoms of *E. bieneusi* infections, and these symptoms mimic those seen with cryptosporidiosis or isosporiasis. Often these patients have four to eight watery, nonbloody stools each day, accompanied by nausea and anorexia. Dehydration and D-xylose and fat malabsorption also may develop. These patients tend to be severely immunodeficient, with a CD4 count almost always below 200 cells/mm³ and often below 100 cells/mm³. Mixed infections with *E. bieneusi* and *E. intestinalis* have also been reported. *E. bieneusi* infection has been implicated in AIDS-related sclerosing cholangitis. However, demonstration of *E. bieneusi* spores in extraepithelial tissues does not always appear to be associated with subsequent development of systemic infection.

*E. bieneusi* spores have been identified in sputum and bronchoalveolar lavage fluid in addition to stool specimens. *E. bieneusi* can colonize the respiratory tract, and clinical specimens from these specimens may reveal the presence of spores. Multiorgan microsporidiosis caused by *E. bieneusi* has been diagnosed in patients infected with HIV; organisms have been recovered in stools, duodenal biopsy specimens, nasal discharge, and sputum.

Infection with *E. bieneusi* has also been reported in immunocompetent individuals; symptoms were self-limited, and diarrheal disease resolved within 2 weeks. *E. bieneusi* may be more commonly associated with sporadic diarrheal disease than was previously suspected, and the immune system may play a role in the control of this intestinal infection. It is also quite possible that *E. bieneusi* may persist as an asymptomatic infection in immunocompetent individuals.

### *Encephalitozoon* spp.

Both *Encephalitozoon cuniculi* and *Encephalitozoon hellem* have been isolated from human infections. The spectrum of disease in patients with AIDS, organ transplant recipients, and otherwise immunocompromised patients includes keratoconjunctivitis, intraocular infection,

sinusitis, bronchiolitis, pneumonitis, nephritis, ureteritis, cystitis, prostatitis, urethritis, hepatitis, sclerosing cholangitis, peritonitis, diarrhea, and encephalitis. Clinical manifestations may vary, ranging from an asymptomatic carrier state to organ failure.

### *Encephalitozoon (Septata) intestinalis*

*Encephalitozoon (Septata) intestinalis* infects primarily small intestinal enterocytes, but infection does not remain confined to epithelial cells. *E. intestinalis* is also found in lamina propria macrophages, fibroblasts, and endothelial cells. Dissemination to the kidneys, lower airways, and biliary tract appears to occur through infected macrophages. Fortunately, these infections tend to respond to therapy with albendazole, unlike infections caused by *E. bieneusi*.

### Other Microsporidia

Different microsporidial species have been isolated from immunocompetent individuals who presented with keratoconjunctivitis, severe keratitis, or corneal ulcers. Also, keratoconjunctivitis has been found in an immunocompetent contact lens wearer.

In immunocompromised patients, myositis has been seen in infections caused by *Pleistophora* sp., *Pleistophora ronneafiei*, *Trichomonas hominis*, *Anncaliia vesicularum*, and *Anncaliia algerae*. *Trachipleistophora anthropophthera* has been identified at autopsy in cerebral, cardiac, renal, pancreatic, thyroid, hepatic, splenic, lymphoid, and bone marrow tissue of patients with AIDS. Disseminated infection caused by *Anncaliia connori* was found at autopsy in a 4-month-old athymic male infant.

## LABORATORY DIAGNOSIS

The most commonly used stains are chromotrope-based stains (modified trichrome) and chemofluorescent optical brightening agents, including calcofluor white and other chemofluorescent stains. Regardless of the staining technique selected, the use of positive control material is highly recommended. Detection of the small microsporidial spores requires adequate illumination and magnification (i.e., magnification using the oil immersion objective [×100] for a total magnification of ×1000).

### Antigen Detection

Such tests have been developed, but the reagents are not widely available commercially.

### Antibody Detection

Although the detection of antibody using a number of methods has been documented, cross reactivity among the genera may occur. Currently, this approach is not commonly used.

### Molecular Methods

Molecular techniques have been quite successful in identifying a number of the microsporidia; however, this approach is not yet widely used.

### Histology

Microsporidia do not tend to stain predictably, if at all, in tissues. However, spores occasionally can be seen very well with use of the periodic acid-Schiff (PAS) stain, silver stains, or acid-fast stains. Modified Gram stains also have proved sensitive. The spore has a small, PAS-positive posterior body; the spore coat stains with silver, and the spores are acid-fast variable. Tissue examination by electron microscopy (EM) techniques is still considered the best approach for differentiation of genera; however, this option is not available to all laboratories, and the sensitivity of EM may not be equal to that of other methods when examining stool or urine.

## THERAPY

Albendazole therapy can result in clinical cure of HIV-associated infection with *Encephalitozoon* spp., along with elimination of spore shedding. Albendazole is not effective for *Enterocytozoon* infections, although clinical improvement occurs in some patients. Oral purified fumagillin appears to eradicate *Enterocytozoon bieneusi* in many patients, but serious adverse events and parasitic relapse have been seen. Antiretroviral combination therapy results in complete clinical response with elimination of intestinal microsporidia.

## PREVENTION

The presence of infective spores in human clinical specimens suggests that taking precautions when handling body fluids and following personal hygiene measures, such as hand washing, may be important in preventing primary infections in the health care setting. However, the establishment of comprehensive guidelines for disease prevention requires more definitive information about sources of infection and modes of transmission.

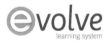 *Visit the Evolve site to complete the review questions.*

# CASE STUDY 48-1

A 34-year-old male presents to the emergency department with crampy abdominal pain and bloody diarrhea. The patient states that, over approximately 14 days, the symptoms have come and gone. During that time, he also has experienced a significant weight loss (approximately 6 pounds). Stool specimens are collected for routine ova and parasite (O&P) examination. Two cysts are identified in the samples (Figure 48-36). In addition, during the physical examination, the physician discovers a small rectal lesion. The biopsy specimen (Figure 48-37) indicates the presence of a significant parasite.

## QUESTIONS

1. What technique or techniques may be used to identify the infecting organism definitively?
2. The cysts identified in the stool specimens represent two species. What are the organisms and should the mixed infection cause any significant concern?
3. What treatment would be recommended for this individual?

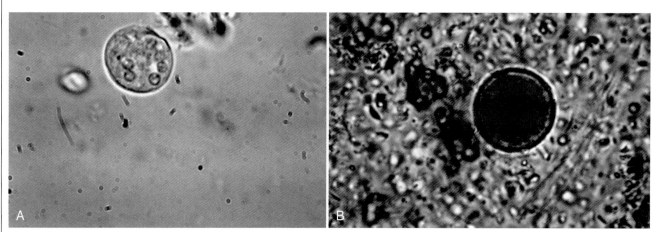

**Figure 48-36 A,** Cyst identified in stool specimen, **B,** Cyst identified in stool specimen (Courtesy Dr. Henry Travers, Sioux Falls, S.D.)

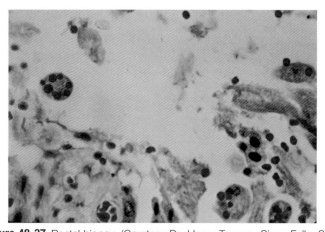

**Figure 48-37** Rectal biopsy. (Courtesy Dr. Henry Travers, Sioux Falls, S.D.)

# BIBLIOGRAPHY

Clark DP: New insights into human cryptosporidiosis, *Clin Microbiol Rev* 12:554, 1999.

Espinosa-Cantellano M, Martinez-Paloma A: Pathogenesis of intestinal amebiasis: from molecules to disease, *Clin Microbiol Rev* 13:318, 2000.

Fayer R: *Cryptosporidium*: a water-borne zoonotic parasite, *Vet Parasitol* 126:37, 2004.

Fayer R: *Sarcocystis* spp. in human infections, *Clin Microbiol Rev* 17:894, 2004.

Feng Y, Xiao L: Zoonotic potential and molecular epidemiology of *Giardia* species and giardiasis, *Clin Microbiol Rev* 24:110, 2011.

Fotedar R, Stark D, Beebe N, et al: Laboratory diagnostic techniques for *Entamoeba* species, *Clin Microbiol Rev* 20:511, 2007.

Garcia LS: *Diagnostic medical parasitology*, ed 5, Washington, DC, 2007, ASM Press.

Garcia LS: *Practical guide to diagnostic parasitology*, ed 2, Washington, DC, 2008, ASM Press.

Garcia LS, Shimizu RY: Detection of *Giardia lamblia* and *Cryptosporidium parvum* antigens in human fecal specimens using the ColorPAC combination rapid solid-phase qualitative immunochromatographic assay, *J Clin Microbiol* 38:1267, 2000.

Garcia LS, Shimizu RY, Bernard CN: Detection of *Giardia lamblia*, *Entamoeba histolytica/E. dispar*, and *Cryptosporidium parvum* antigens in human fecal specimens using the EIA Triage Parasite Panel, *J Clin Microbiol* 38:3337, 2000.

Johnson EH, Windsor JJ, Clark CG: Emerging from obscurity: biological, clinical, and diagnostic aspects of *Dientamoeba fragilis*, *Clin Microbiol Rev* 17:553, 2004.

Lindsay DS, Dubey JP, Blagburn BL: Biology of *Isospora* spp. from humans, nonhuman primates, and domestic animals, *Clin Microbiol Rev* 10:19, 1997.

Mathis A, Weber R, Deplazes P: Zoonotic potential of the microsporidia, *Clin Microbiol Rev* 18:423, 2005.

Ortega YR, Sanchez R: Update on *Cyclospora cayetanensis*, a food-borne and waterborne parasite, *Clin Microbiol Rev* 23:218, 2010.

Santi-Rocca J, Rigothier MC, Guillen N: Host-microbe interactions and defense mechanisms in the development of amoebic liver abscesses, *Clin Microbiol Rev* 22:65, 2009.

Schuster FL, Ramirez-Avila L: Current world status of *Balantidium coli*, *Clin Microbiol Rev* 21:626, 2008.

Shields JM, Olson BH: *Cyclospora cayetanensis*: a review of an emerging parasitic coccidian, *Int J Parasitol* 33:371, 2003.

Tan KS: New insights on classification, identification, and clinical relevance of *Blastocystis* spp, *Clin Microbiol Rev* 21:639, 2008.

Tanyuksel M, Petri WA Jr: Laboratory diagnosis of amebiasis, *Clin Microbiol Rev* 16:713, 2003.

ten Hove RJ, van Lieshout L, Brienen EA, et al: Real-time polymerase chain reaction for detection of *Isospora belli* in stool samples, *Diagn Microbiol Infect Dis* 61:280-283, 2008.

Thompson RC, Monis PT: Variation in *Giardia*: implications for taxonomy and epidemiology, *Adv Parasitol* 58:69, 2004.

Wilson M, Schantz PM: Parasitic immunodiagnosis. In Strickland GT, editor: *Hunter's tropical medicine and emerging infectious diseases*, ed 8, Philadelphia, 2000, WB Saunders.

Xiao L, Ryan UM: Cryptosporidiosis: an update in molecular epidemiology, *Curr Opin Infect Dis* 17:483, 2004.

## OBJECTIVES

1. Explain the general life cycle of *Plasmodium* spp. including both asexual and sexual stages, exoerythrocytic and erythrocytic cycle trophozoites, schizonts, hypnozoites, merozoites, gametocytes, and sporozoites.
2. Describe the distinguishing morphologic characteristics, clinical disease, vectors, stages of infectivity, and laboratory diagnosis for *Plasmodium* spp., *Babesia* spp., and *Trypanosoma* and *Leishmania* spp.
3. Define paroxysm in malarial periodicity.
4. Compare and contrast recrudescence and relapse including the physiologic basis for each during infection with malaria.
5. Compare and contrast the pathogenesis of infections with *P. falciparum*, *P. malariae*, *P. ovale*, *P. vivax*, and *P. knowlesi* including variation in signs and symptoms.
6. Differentiate intracellular forms of *Babesia* spp. from *Plasmodium* spp.
7. Define and describe the life cycle stages of *Trypanosoma* and *Leishmania* spp. including amastigotes, promastigotes, trypomastigotes, epimastigotes, and metacyclic trypanosome forms when appropriate.

---

### PARASITES TO BE CONSIDERED

**Protozoa**
Sporozoa, Flagellates (Blood, Tissue)
Sporozoa (Malaria and Babesiosis)
  *Plasmodium vivax*
  *Plasmodium ovale*
  *Plasmodium malariae*
  *Plasmodium falciparum*
  *Plasmodium knowlesi*
  *Babesia* spp.
Flagellates (Leishmaniae, Trypanosomes)
  *Leishmania tropica* complex
  *Leishmania mexicana* complex
  *Leishmania braziliensis* complex
  *Leishmania donovani* complex
  *Leishmania peruviana*
  *Trypanosoma brucei gambiense*
  *Trypanosoma brucei rhodesiense*
  *Trypanosoma cruzi*
  *Trypanosoma rangeli*

---

## PLASMODIUM SPP.

Malaria has been well documented as an ancient disease in Egyptian and Chinese writing beginning in 2700 BC. By 200 BC, malaria was identified in Rome, spread throughout Europe during the twelfth century, and arrived in England by the fourteenth century. By the early 1800s malaria was found worldwide.

Malaria has played a tremendous role in world history, influencing the outcome of wars, the movement of populations, and the development and decline of various nations. Before the American Civil War, malaria was found as far north as southern Canada; but it was no longer endemic within the United States by the 1950s.

It is estimated that more than 500 million individuals worldwide are infected with *Plasmodium* spp., and as many as 2.7 million people a year, most of whom are children, die from the infection. Malaria is endemic in more than 90 countries with a population of 2400 million people, representing 40% of the world's population. At least 90% of deaths caused by malaria occur in Africa. *Plasmodium falciparum* is the major species associated with deadly infections throughout the world. Unfortunately, prevention remains a complex problem, and no drug is universally effective for all *Plasmodium* species.

In addition, of the five species that infect humans, *P. vivax* and *P. falciparum* cause 95% of infections. *P. vivax* may be responsible for 80% of the infections, because this species has the widest distribution in the tropics, subtropics, and temperate zones. *P. falciparum* is generally confined to the tropics, *P. malariae* is sporadically distributed, and *P. ovale* is confined mainly to central West Africa and some South Pacific islands. The fifth human malaria, *Plasmodium knowlesi*, a malaria parasite of long-tailed macaque monkeys, has been confirmed in human cases from Malaysian Borneo, Thailand, Myanmar, and the Philippines.

The vector for malaria is the female anopheline mosquito. When the vector takes a blood meal, sporozoites contained in the salivary glands of the mosquito are discharged into the puncture wound (Figure 49-1). Within an hour, these infective sporozoites are carried via the blood to the liver, where they penetrate hepatocytes and begin to grow, initiating the **preerythrocytic** or **primary exoerythrocytic** cycle. The sporozoites become round or oval and begin dividing repeatedly. **Schizogony** results in large numbers of exoerythrocytic merozoites. Once these merozoites leave the liver, they invade the red blood cells (RBCs), initiating the **erythrocytic cycle**. A dormant schizogony may occur in *P. vivax* and *P. ovale* organisms, which remain quiescent in the liver. These resting stages have been termed **hypnozoites** and lead to a true relapse, often within 1 year or up to more than 5 years later. Delayed schizogony does not occur in *P. falciparum*, *P. malariae*, or *P. knowlesi*.

Once the RBCs and reticulocytes have been invaded, the parasites grow and feed on hemoglobin. Within the RBC, the merozoite (or young trophozoite) is vacuolated, ring shaped, more or less ameboid, and uninucleate. The excess protein and hematin present from the metabolism of hemoglobin combine to form malarial

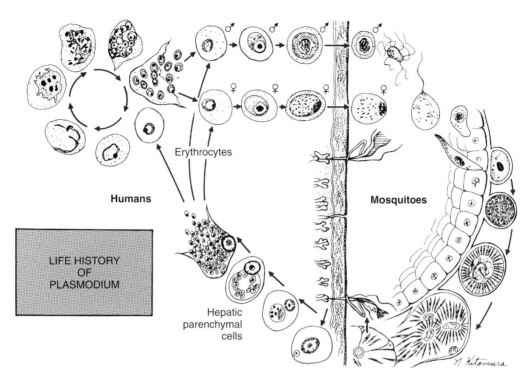

**Figure 49-1** Life cycle of *Plasmodium*. (Modified from Wilcox A: *Manual for the microscopical diagnosis of malaria in man,* Washington, DC, 1960, U.S. Public Health Service. Illustration by Nobuko Kitamura.)

pigment. Once the nucleus begins to divide, the trophozoite is called a developing schizont. The mature schizont contains merozoites (whose number depends on the species), which are released into the bloodstream. Many of the merozoites are destroyed by the immune system, but others invade RBCs and initiate a new cycle of erythrocytic schizogony. After several erythrocytic generations, some of the merozoites begin to undergo development into the male and female gametocytes.

Although malaria is often associated with travelers to endemic areas, other situations resulting in infection include blood transfusions, use of contaminated hypodermic needles, bone marrow transplantation, congenital infection, and transmission within the United States by indigenous mosquitoes that acquired the parasites from imported infections.

## *PLASMODIUM VIVAX* (BENIGN TERTIAN MALARIA)

### General Characteristics

*P. vivax* infects only the reticulocytes; thus, the parasitemia is limited to approximately 2% to 5% of the available RBCs (Tables 49-1 to 49-3, Figures 49-2 and 49-3). Splenomegaly occurs during the first few weeks of infection, and the spleen will progress from being soft and palpable to hard, with continued enlargement during a chronic infection. If the infection is treated during the early phases, the spleen will return to its normal size. A secondary or dormant schizogony occurs in *P. vivax* and *P. ovale,* which remain quiescent in the liver. These resting stages have been termed *hypnozoites.*

After a few days of irregular periodicity, a regular 48-hour cycle is established. An untreated primary attack may last from 3 weeks to 2 months or longer. Over time, the paroxysms (symptomatic period) become less severe and more irregular in frequency and then cease altogether. In approximately 50% of patients infected with *P. vivax,* relapses occur after weeks, months, or even after 5 years or more. The RBCs tend to be enlarged (young RBCs), there may be Schüffner's dots (exclusively found in *P. vivax* and *P. ovale*) after 8 to 10 hours, the developing rings are ameboid, and the mature schizont contains 12 to 24 merozoites (Figure 49-3 [3]).

### Pathogenesis and Spectrum of Disease

In patients who have never been exposed to malaria, symptoms such as headache, photophobia, muscle aches, anorexia, nausea, and sometimes vomiting may occur before organisms can be detected in the bloodstream. In other patients with prior exposure to the malaria, the parasites can be found in the bloodstream several days before symptoms appear.

Severe complications are uncommon in *P. vivax* infections, although coma and sudden death or other symptoms of cerebral involvement have been reported, particularly in patients with varying degrees of primaquine resistance. These patients can exhibit cerebral malaria, renal failure, circulatory collapse, severe anemia, hemoglobinuria, abnormal bleeding, acute respiratory distress syndrome, and jaundice. Acute cerebral malaria involves changes in mental status and if untreated may result in fatality within 3 days.

## *PLASMODIUM OVALE*

### General Characteristics

Although *P. ovale* and *P. vivax* infections are clinically similar, *P. ovale* malaria is usually less severe, tends to

**TABLE 49-1** *Plasmodium* spp.: Clinical Characteristics of the Five Human Infections

| Infection | P. vivax | P. ovale | P. malariae | P. falciparum | P. knowlesi | Comments |
|---|---|---|---|---|---|---|
| Incubation period | 8-17 days | 10-17 days | 18-40 days | 8-11 days | 9-12 days | All may be extended for months to years |
| Prodromal symptoms Severity / Initial fever pattern | Mild to moderate / Irregular (48 hr) | Mild / Irregular (48 hr) | Mild to moderate / Regular (72 hr) | Mild / Continuous remittent | Mild to moderate / Regular (24 hr) | All may mimic influenza symptoms / Early symptoms may reflect lack of regular periodicity |
| Symptom periodicity | 48 hr | 48 hr | 72 hr | 36-48 hr | 24-27 hr | |
| Initial paroxysm Severity / Mean duration | Moderate to severe / 10 h | Mild / 10 h | Moderate to severe / 11 h | Severe / 16-36 h | Moderate to severe / Not available | P. knowlesi might increase/lose virulence on passage in humans |
| Duration of untreated primary attack | 3-8+ wk | 2-3 wk | 3-24 wk | 2-3 wk | Not available | |
| Duration of untreated infection | 5-7 yr | 12 mo | 20+ yr | 6-17 mo | Not available | |
| Parasitemia limitations | Young RBCs | Young RBCs | Old RBCs | All RBCs | All RBCs | |
| Anemia | Mild to moderate | Mild | Mild to moderate | Severe | Moderate to severe | P. knowlesi can be as dangerous as P. falciparum |
| CNS involvement | Rare | Possible | Rare | Very common | Possible | |
| Nephrotic syndrome | Possible | Rare | Very common | Rare | Probably common | |

relapse less frequently, and usually ends with spontaneous recovery, often after no more than 6 to 10 paroxysms (see Tables 49-1 to 49-3, Figures 49-2 and 49-3). Like *P. vivax*, *P. ovale* infects only the reticulocytes, so that the parasitemia is limited to approximately 2% to 5% of the available RBCs. For many years the literature has stated that as with *P. vivax*, a secondary or dormant schizogony occurs in *P. ovale*, which remain quiescent in the liver. However, newer findings indicate that hypnozoites have never been demonstrated by biologic experiments.

After a few days of irregular periodicity, a regular 48-hour cycle is established. Over time, the paroxysms become less severe and more irregular in frequency and then stop altogether. In some patients infected with *P. ovale*, relapses occur after weeks, months, or up to 1 year or more. The RBCs tend to be enlarged (young RBCs), Schüffner's dots (also known as James stippling) are present from the beginning of the cycle, the developing rings are less ameboid than those of *P. vivax*, and the mature schizont contains an average of eight merozoites.

### Pathogenesis and Spectrum of Disease

The incubation period is similar to that for *P. vivax* malaria, but the frequency and severity of the symptoms are much less, with a lower fever and a lack of typical rigors. The geographic range is usually described as being limited to tropical Africa, the Middle East, Papua New Guinea, and Irian Jaya in Indonesia. However, *P. ovale* infections in Southeast Asia may cause benign and relapsing malaria in this area. In both Southeast Asia and Africa, two different types of *P. ovale* circulate in humans. Human infections with variant-type *P. ovale* are associated with a higher level of parasitemia.

## PLASMODIUM MALARIAE (QUARTAN MALARIA)

### General Characteristics

*P. malariae* invades primarily the older RBCs, limiting the number of infected cells (see Tables 49-1 to 49-3, Figures 49-2 and 49-3). The incubation period between infection and symptoms may be much longer than that for *P. vivax* or *P. ovale* malaria, ranging from about 27 to 40 days. A regular periodicity is seen from the beginning, with a more severe paroxysm, including a longer cold stage and more severe symptoms during the hot stage. Collapse during the sweating phase is not uncommon.

A regular periodicity of 72 hours is seen from the beginning of the erythrocytic cycle. The infection may end with spontaneous recovery, or there may be a recrudescence or series of recrudescence (recurrence of symptoms) over many years. These patients are left with a latent infection and persisting low-grade parasitemia for many, many years. The RBCs tend to be normal to small

TABLE 49-2   *Plasmodia* in Giemsa-Stained Thin Blood Smears

|  | *Plasmodium vivax* | *Plasmodium malariae* | *Plasmodium falciparum* | *Plasmodium ovale* | *Plasmodium knowlesi* |
|---|---|---|---|---|---|
| **Persistence of exoerythrocytic cycle** | Yes | No | No | Yes | No |
| **Relapses** | Yes | No, but long-term recrudescence is recognized | No long-term relapses | Possible, but usually spontaneous recovery | No |
| **Time of cycle** | 44-48 hr | 72 hr | 36-48 hr | 48 hr | 24 hr |
| **Appearance of parasitized RBCs; size and shape** | 1.5-2 times larger than normal; oval to normal; may be normal size until ring fills half of cell | Normal shape; size may be normal or slightly smaller | Both normal | 60% of cells larger than normal and oval; 20% have irregular, frayed edges | Normal shape, size |
| **Schüffner's dots (eosinophilic stippling)** | Usually present in all cells except early ring forms | None | None; occasionally comma-like red dots are present (Maurer's dots) | Present in all stages including early ring forms; dots may be larger and darker than in *P. vivax* | No true stippling; occasional faint dots |
| **Color of cytoplasm** | Decolorized, pale | Normal | Normal, bluish tinge at times | Decolorized, pale | Normal |
| **Multiple rings/ cell** | Occasional | Rare | Common | Occasional | Common |
| **All developmental stages present in peripheral blood** | All stages present | Ring forms few, since ring stage brief; mostly growing and mature trophozoites and schizonts | Young ring forms and no older stages; few gametocytes | All stages present | All stages present |
| **Appearance of parasite; young trophozoite (early ring form)** | Ring is ⅓ diameter of cell, cytoplasmic circle around vacuole; heavy chromatin dot | Ring often smaller than in *P. vivax*, occupying ⅙ of cell; heavy chromatin dot; vacuole at times "filled in"; pigment forms early | Delicate, small ring with small chromatin dot (frequently 2); scanty cytoplasm around small vacuoles; sometimes at edge of red cell (appliqué form) or filamentous slender form; may have multiple rings per cell | Ring is larger and more ameboid than in *P. vivax*; otherwise similar to *P. vivax* | Rings ⅓ to ½ diameter of RBC; double chromatin dots; appliqué forms rare; multiple rings per RBC |
| **Growing trophozoite** | Multishaped irregular ameboid parasite; streamers of cytoplasm close to large chromatin dot; vacuole retained until close to maturity; increasing amounts of brown pigment | Non-ameboid rounded or band-shaped solid forms; chromatin may be hidden by coarse dark brown pigment | Heavy ring forms; fine pigment grains | Ring shape maintained until late in development; non-ameboid compared to *P. vivax* | Slightly ameboid and irregular; band forms seen; very little pigment |

*Continued*

**TABLE 49-2** *Plasmodia* in Giemsa-Stained Thin Blood Smears—cont'd

| | *Plasmodium vivax* | *Plasmodium malariae* | *Plasmodium falciparum* | *Plasmodium ovale* | *Plasmodium knowlesi* |
|---|---|---|---|---|---|
| **Mature trophozoite** | Irregular ameboid mass; 1 or more small vacuoles retained until schizont stage; fills almost entire cell; fine brown pigment | Vacuoles disappear early; cytoplasm compact, oval, band shaped, or nearly round and almost filling cell; chromatin may be hidden by peripheral coarse dark brown pigment | Not seen in peripheral blood (except in severe infections); development of all phases following ring form occurs in capillaries of viscera | Compact; vacuoles disappear; pigment dark brown, less than in *P. malariae* | Denser cytoplasm (slightly ameboid) band forms seen; little to no malaria pigment (scattered, fine brown grains) |
| **Schizont (pre-segmenter)** | Progressive chromatin division; cytoplasmic bands containing clumps of brown pigment | Similar to *P. vivax* except smaller; darker, larger pigment granules peripheral or central | Not seen in peripheral blood (see above) | Smaller and more compact than *P. vivax* | Between 2 and 5 divided nuclear chromatin masses; abundant pigment granules occupy $\frac{2}{3}$ of RBC |
| **Mature schizont** | 16 (12-24) merozoites, each with chromatin and cytoplasm, filling entire red cell, which can hardly be seen | 8 (6-12) merozoites in rosettes or irregular clusters filling normal-sized cells, which can hardly be seen; central arrangement of brown-green pigment | Not seen in peripheral blood | $\frac{3}{4}$ of cells occupied by 8 (8-12) merozoites in rosettes or irregular clusters | RBCs normal size; distorted/fimbriated RBCs very rare; occupy whole RBC; maximum of 16 merozoites; no rosettes; grapelike clusters |
| **Macrogametocyte** | Rounded or oval homogeneous cytoplasm; diffuse delicate light brown pigment throughout parasite; eccentric compact chromatin | Similar to *P. vivax*, but fewer in number; pigment darker and more coarse | Gender differentiation difficult; "crescent" or "sausage" shapes characteristic; may appear in "showers" with black pigment near chromatin dot, which is often central | Smaller than *P. vivax* | Occupy most of RBC; bluish cytoplasm; dense pink chromatin at periphery of parasite |
| **Microgametocyte** | Large pink to purple chromatin mass surrounded by pale or colorless halo; evenly distributed pigment | Similar to *P. vivax*, but fewer in number; pigment darker and more coarse | Same as macrogametocyte (described above) | Smaller than *P. vivax* | Occupy most of RBC; cytoplasm pinkish purple; early forms similar to mature trophozoite |
| **Main criteria** | Large pale red cell; trophozoite irregular; pigment usually present; Schüffner's dots not always present; several phases of growth seen in one smear; gametocytes appear as early as third day | Red cell normal in size and color; trophozoites compact, stain usually intense, band forms not always seen; coarse pigment; no stippling of red cells; gametocytes appear after a few weeks | Development following ring stage takes place in blood vessels of internal organs; delicate ring forms and crescent-shaped gametocytes are only forms normally seen in peripheral blood; gametocytes appear after 7-10 days | Red cell enlarged, oval, with fimbriated edges; Schüffner's dots seen in all stages; gametocytes appear after 4 days or as late as 18 days | Ring forms compact; single/double chromatin dots, appliqué forms, multiple rings/RBC (mimic *P. falciparum*); overall RBCs not enlarged; developing stages mimic *P. malariae* (band forms, 16 merozoites in mature schizont, but no rosettes) |

**TABLE 49-3** Malaria Characteristics with Fresh Blood or Blood Collected Using EDTA with No Extended Lag Time*

| Type of Malaria | Characteristics |
|---|---|
| *Plasmodium vivax* (benign tertian malaria) | 1. 48-hour cycle<br>2. Tends to infect young cells<br>3. Enlarged RBCs<br>4. Schüffner's dots (true stippling) after 8-10 hours<br>5. Delicate ring<br>6. Very ameboid trophozoite<br>7. Mature schizont contains 12-24 merozoites |
| *Plasmodium malariae* (quartan malaria) | 1. 72-hour cycle (long incubation period)<br>2. Tends to infect old cells<br>3. Normal size RBCs<br>4. No stippling<br>5. Thick ring, large nucleus<br>6. Trophozoite tends to form "bands" across the cell<br>7. Mature schizont contains 6-12 merozoites |
| *Plasmodium ovale* | 1. 48-hour cycle<br>2. Tends to infect young cells<br>3. Enlarged RBCs with fimbriated edges (oval)<br>4. Schüffner's dots appear in the beginning (in RBCs with very young ring forms, in contrast to *P. vivax*)<br>5. Smaller ring than *P. vivax*<br>6. Trophozoite less ameboid than that of *P. vivax*<br>7. Mature schizont contains an average of 8 merozoites |
| *Plasmodium falciparum* (malignant tertian malaria) | 1. 36-48-hour cycle<br>2. Tends to infect any cell regardless of age, thus very heavy infection may result<br>3. All sizes of RBCs<br>4. No Schüffner's dots (Maurer's dots: may be larger, single dots, bluish)<br>5. Multiple rings/cell (only young rings, gametocytes, and occasional mature schizonts are seen in peripheral blood)<br>6. Delicate rings, may have two dots of chromatin/ring, appliqué or accolé forms<br>7. Crescent-shaped gametocytes |
| *Plasmodium knowlesi* (simian malaria)* | 1. 24-hour cycle<br>2. Tends to infect any cell regardless of age, thus very heavy infection may result<br>3. All sizes of RBCs, but most tend to be normal size<br>4. No Schüffner's dots (faint, clumpy dots later in cycle)<br>5. Multiple rings/cell (may have 2-3)<br>6. Delicate rings, may have two or three dots of chromatin/ring, appliqué forms<br>7. Band form trophozoites commonly seen<br>8. Mature schizont contains 16 merozoites, no rosettes<br>9. Gametocytes round, tend to fill the cell<br>Early stages mimic *P. falciparum*; later stages mimic *P. malariae* |

*Preparation of thick and thin blood films within <60 min of collection.

(old RBCs), there is no true stippling, the RBCs may have fimbriated edges, the developing rings tend to demonstrate "band" forms, and the mature schizont contains an average of 6 to 12 merozoites.

### Pathogenesis and Spectrum of Disease

Proteinuria is common in *P. malariae* infections and may be associated with clinical signs of nephrotic syndrome. With a chronic infection, kidney problems result from deposition within the glomeruli of circulating antigen-antibody complexes. A membrane proliferative type of glomerulonephritis is the most common lesion seen in quartan malaria. Because chronic glomerular disease associated with *P. malariae* infections is usually not reversible with therapy, genetic and environmental factors may play a role in the disease, as well. The patient may have a spontaneous recovery, or there may be a recrudescence or series of recrudescence over many years (>50 years). In these cases, patients are left with a latent infection and persisting low-grade parasitemia.

## PLASMODIUM FALCIPARUM (MALIGNANT TERTIAN MALARIA)

### General Characteristics

*Plasmodium falciparum* invades all ages of RBCs, and the number of infected cells may exceed 50% (see Tables 49-1 to 49-3, Figures 49-2 to 49-4). Schizogony occurs in the spleen, liver, and bone marrow rather than in the circulating blood. Ischemia caused by the obstruction of vessels within these organs by parasitized RBCs will produce various symptoms, depending on the organ involved. A decrease in the ability of the RBCs to change shape when passing through capillaries or the splenic filter may lead to plugging of the vessels Also, only *P. falciparum* causes cytoadherence, a feature that is associated with severe malaria.

The asexual and sexual forms circulate in the bloodstream during infections by four of the *Plasmodium* species. However, in *P. falciparum* infections, as the parasite grows, the RBC membrane becomes sticky and the cells adhere to the endothelial lining of the capillaries of the internal organs. Thus, only the ring forms and the gametocytes (occasionally mature schizonts) normally appear in the peripheral blood. Periodicity of the cycle will not be established during the early stages, and the presumptive diagnosis may be totally unrelated to a possible malaria infection. If the fever does develop a synchronous cycle, it is usually a cycle of 36 to 48 hours. Because *P. falciparum* infects young and old RBCs, very heavy parasitemia can occur. The RBCs are all sizes; there is no true stippling, but Maurer's dots (coarse granulation in the cytoplasm of RBCs) are sometimes present; often there are multiple rings per RBC and the rings are delicate and often have two dots of chromatin, appliqué or accolé forms (ring forms identified within the marginal regions of the erythrocytes); and the gametocytes are crescent-shaped.

### Pathogenesis and Spectrum of Disease

The onset of a *P. falciparum* malaria attack occurs 8 to 12 days after infection and is characterized by 3 to 4 days of

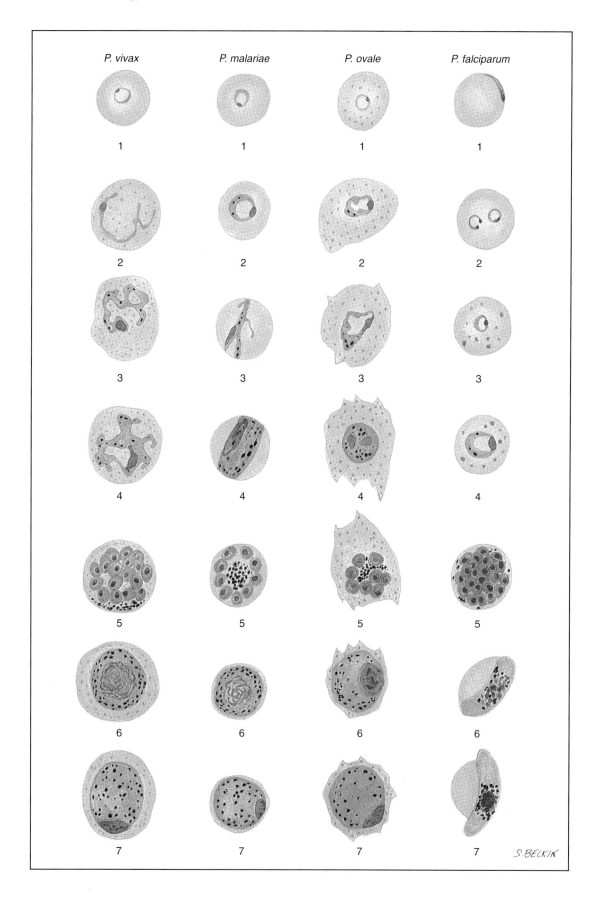

*P. vivax*  *P. malariae*  *P. ovale*  *P. falciparum*

S.BELKIN

**Figure 49-2** The morphology of malaria parasites. *Plasmodium vivax: 1,* Early trophozoite (ring form). *2,* Late trophozoite with Schüffner's dots (note enlarged red blood cell). *3,* Late trophozoite with ameboid cytoplasm (very typical of *P. vivax*). *4,* Late trophozoite with ameboid cytoplasm. *5,* Mature schizont with merozoites (18) and clumped pigment. *6,* Microgametocyte with dispersed chromatin. *7,* Macrogametocyte with compact chromatin. *Plasmodium malariae: 1,* Early trophozoite (ring form). *2,* Early trophozoite with thick cytoplasm. *3,* Early trophozoite (band form). *4,* Late trophozoite (band form) with heavy pigment. *5,* Mature schizont with merozoites (9) arranged in rosette. *6,* Microgametocyte with dispersed chromatin. *7,* Macrogametocyte with compact chromatin. *Plasmodium ovale: 1,* Early trophozoite (ring form) with Schüffner's dots. *2,* Early trophozoite (note enlarged red blood cell). *3,* Late trophozoite in red blood cell with fimbriated edges. *4,* Developing schizont with irregularly shaped red blood cell. *5,* Mature schizont with merozoites (8) arranged irregularly. *6,* Microgametocyte with dispersed chromatin. *7,* Macrogametocyte with compact chromatin. *Plasmodium falciparum: 1,* Early trophozoite (accolé or appliqué form). *2,* Early trophozoite (one ring is in headphone configuration/double chromatin dots). *3,* Early trophozoite with Maurer's dots. *4,* Late trophozoite with larger ring and Maurer's dots. *5,* Mature schizont with merozoites (24). *6,* Microgametocyte with dispersed chromatin. *7,* Macrogametocyte with compact chromatin. **Note:** Without the appliqué form, Schüffner's dots, multiple rings/cell, and other developing stages, differentiation among the species can be difficult. It is obvious that the early rings of all four species can mimic one another very easily. *Remember: One set of negative blood films cannot rule out a malarial infection.* (Reprinted by permission of the publisher from Garcia LS: *Diagnostic medical parasitology,* ed 5, Washington, DC, 2007, Copyright by American Society for Microbiology.)

---

vague symptoms such as aches, pains, headache, fatigue, anorexia, or nausea. This stage is followed by fever, a more severe headache, and nausea and vomiting, with occasional severe epigastric pain. At the onset of fever, there may be a feeling of chilliness. As with the other *Plasmodium* spp., periodicity of the cycle will not be established during the early stages.

Severe or fatal complications can occur at any time and are related to the obstruction of vessels in the internal organs (liver, intestinal tract, adrenal glands, intravascular hemolysis/black water fever, and kidneys). Blackwater fever is a complication of malaria that is a result of red blood cell lysis, releasing hemoglobin into the bloodstream and urine, causing discoloration. The severity of the complications may not correlate with the peripheral blood parasitemia, particularly in *P. falciparum* infections in a patient who has never been exposed to malaria before (immunologically naïve).

Disseminated intravascular coagulation is a rare complication and is seen with a high parasitemia, pulmonary edema, anemia, and cerebral and renal complications. Vascular endothelial damage from endotoxins and bound parasitized blood cells may lead to clot formation in small vessels. Cerebral malaria is more common in *P. falciparum* malaria, but can occur in the other species. If the onset is gradual, the patient becomes disoriented or violent or may develop severe headaches and pass into coma. However, some patients, including those with no prior symptoms, may suddenly become comatose. Physical signs of central nervous system involvement vary, and there is no correlation between the severity of the symptoms and the parasitemia.

Extreme fevers, 41.7° C (107° F) or higher, may occur in an uncomplicated malaria attack or in cases of cerebral malaria. Without vigorous therapy, the patient usually dies. Cerebral malaria is considered to be the most serious complication and the major cause of death with *P. falciparum*; it occurs in up to 10% of all *P. falciparum* patients admitted to the hospital and is responsible for 80% of fatal cases.

## *PLASMODIUM KNOWLESI* (SIMIAN MALARIA, THE FIFTH HUMAN MALARIA)

### General Characteristics

*P. knowlesi* invades all ages of RBCs, and the number of infected cells can be significantly more than seen in *P. vivax, P. ovale,* and *P. malariae. P. knowlesi* infection should be considered in patients with a travel history to forested areas of Southeast Asia, especially if *P. malariae* is diagnosed, unusual forms are seen with microscopy, or if a mixed infection with *P. falciparum/P. malariae* is diagnosed. Because the disease is potentially fatal, proper identification to the species level is critical.

The early blood stages of *P. knowlesi* resemble those of *P. falciparum*, whereas the mature blood stages and gametocytes resemble those of *P. malariae* (see Tables 49-1 to 49-3, Figures 49-2 to 49-4). Unfortunately, these infections are often misdiagnosed as the relatively benign *P. malariae*; however, infections with *P. knowlesi* can be fatal. The RBCs are all sizes, there is no true stippling (fine, granular, blue stippling in RBCs stained with Wright's stain or red when using eosin hematoxylin as seen in Figure 49-3 (*P. vivax* photo, third from the top), often there are multiple rings per RBC (there may be 2 to 3 rings), the rings are delicate and often have 2 to 3 dots of chromatin, band forms are typically seen with the developing trophozoites, and the mature schizont contains 16 merozoites. The early stages mimic *P. falciparum*, whereas the later stages mimic *P. malariae*.

Because of different levels of parasitemia, low organism densities, and confusion among various morphologic criteria for identification, detection of mixed infections can be quite difficult. Even if a mixed infection is suspected, identification to the species level may not be possible using routine microscopy methods. However, using polymerase chain reaction (PCR) methods, it is likely that higher detection and identification rates of chronic and mixed malarial infections will be possible.

### Pathogenesis and Spectrum of Disease

Patients exhibit chills, minor headaches, and daily low-grade fever. Patients who have been diagnosed with high numbers of *P. malariae* organisms by microscopy should receive intensive management as appropriate for severe *P. falciparum* malaria, assuming the infection is actually caused by *P. knowlesi*. Overall, these infections can be as severe as those caused by *P. falciparum*, with fatal outcomes.

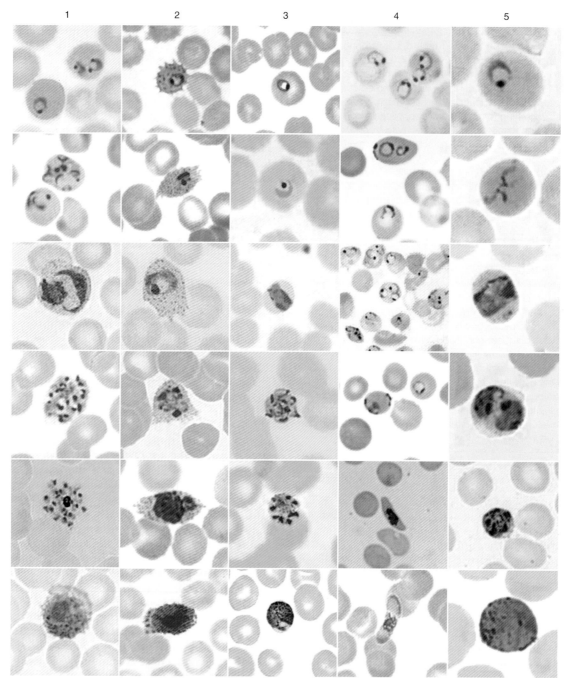

**Figure 49-3** Morphology of malaria parasites. **Column 1** (left to right): *Plasmodium vivax* (note enlarged infected RBCs). (1) Early trophozoite (ring form) (note one RBC contains 2 rings—not that uncommon); (2) older ring, note ameboid nature of rings; (3) late trophozoite with Schüffner's dots (note enlarged RBC); (4) developing schizont; (5) mature schizont with 18 merozoites and clumped pigment; (6) microgametocyte with dispersed chromatin. **Column 2:** *Plasmodium ovale* (note enlarged infected RBCs). (1) Early trophozoite (ring form) with Schüffner's dots (RBC has fimbriated edges); (2) early trophozoite (note enlarged RBC, Schüffner's dots, and RBC oval in shape); (3) late trophozoite in RBC with fimbriated edges; (4) developing schizont with irregular-shaped RBC; (5) mature schizont with 8 merozoites arranged irregularly; (6) microgametocyte with dispersed chromatin. **Column 3:** *Plasmodium malariae* (note normal or smaller than normal infected RBCs). (1) Early trophozoite (ring form); (2) early trophozoite with thick cytoplasm; (3) late trophozoite (band form); (4) developing schizont; (5) mature schizont with 9 merozoites arranged in a rosette; (6) microgametocyte with compact chromatin. **Column 4:** *Plasmodium falciparum*. (1) Early trophozoites (the rings are in the headphone configuration with double chromatin dots); (2) early trophozoite (accolé or appliqué form); (3) early trophozoites (note the multiple rings/cell); (4) late trophozoite with larger ring (accolé or appliqué form); (5) crescent-shaped gametocyte; (6) crescent-shaped gametocyte. **Column 5:** *Plasmodium knowlesi*—with the exception of image *5,* these were photographed at a higher magnification (note normal or smaller than normal infected RBCs). (1) Early trophozoite (ring form); (2) early trophozoite with slim band form; (3) late trophozoite (band form); (4) developing schizont; (5) mature schizont with merozoites arranged in a rosette; (6) microgametocyte with dispersed chromatin. **Note:** Without the appliqué form, Schüffner's dots, multiple rings per cell, and other developing stages, differentiation among the species can be very difficult. It is obvious that the early rings of all five species can mimic one another very easily. *Remember: One set of negative blood films cannot rule out a malaria infection.* (From Garcia LS: *Malaria Clin Lab Med* 30:93-129, 2010,with permission. Column 5 courtesy CDC.)

## LABORATORY DIAGNOSIS (ALL SPECIES)

### Routine Methods

Malaria is considered to be immediately life threatening, and a patient with the diagnosis of *P. falciparum* or *P. knowlesi* malaria should be considered a medical emergency because the disease can be rapidly fatal. This approach to the patient is also recommended in situations where *P. falciparum* or *P. knowlesi* cannot be ruled out as a possible diagnosis. Any laboratory providing the expertise to identify malarial parasites should do so on a 24-hour basis, 7 days a week.

Examination of a single blood specimen is not sufficient to exclude the diagnosis of malaria, especially when the patient has received partial prophylaxis or therapy and has a low number of organisms in the blood. Patients with a relapse case or an early primary case may also have few organisms in the blood smear. Regardless of the presence or absence of any fever periodicity, both thick (Figure 49-5) and thin blood films should be prepared immediately, and at least 200 to 300 oil immersion fields should be examined on both films before a negative report is issued. If the initial specimen is negative, additional blood specimens should be examined over a 36-hour time frame. Although Giemsa stain is recommended for all parasitic blood work, the organisms can also be seen with other blood stains, such as Wright's stain. Using any of the blood stains, the white blood cells (WBCs) serve as the built-in quality control; if the WBCs look good, any parasites present will also look good. Figure 49-6 compares the multinucleated stages (schizont) of *Plasmodium malariae* and *Plasmodium vivax*. Fluorescent nucleic acid stains, such as acridine orange, may also be used to identify organisms in infected RBCs. However, this may be more difficult to interpret because of the presence of white blood cell nuclei or RBC Howell-Jolly bodies.

Blood collected using ethylenediaminetetraacetic acid (EDTA) anticoagulant is preferred; however, if the blood remains in the tube for any length of time before blood film preparation, Schüffner's dots may not be visible after staining (*P. vivax*, as an example) and other morphologic changes in the parasites will be seen. Also, the proper ratio between blood and anticoagulant is required for good organism morphology, so each collection tube should be filled to the top. Finger-stick blood is recommended, particularly when the volume of blood required is minimal (i.e., when no other hematologic procedures have been ordered). The blood should be free flowing when taken for smear preparation, and should not be contaminated with alcohol used to clean the finger before the stick. However, the use of finger-stick blood is currently much less common, and venipuncture blood is the normal specimen collected for the laboratory. Identification to the species level is highly desirable, because this information determines which drug(s) is (are) recommended. In early infections, patients with *P. falciparum* infections may not have the crescent-shaped gametocytes in the blood. Also, low parasitemia with the delicate ring forms may be missed; consequently, oil immersion examination at 1000× is mandatory.

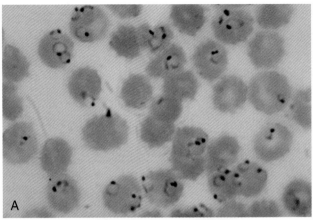

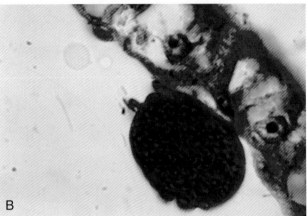

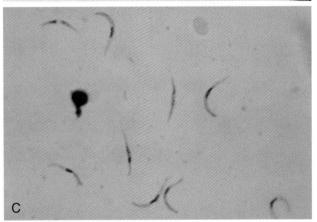

**Figure 49-4** *Plasmodium falciparum.* **A,** Ring forms; **B,** oocyte; and **C,** sporozoites. (Courtesy Dr. Henry Travers, Sioux Falls, S.D.)

### Serologic Methods

Several rapid malaria tests (RMTs) are now commercially available, some of which use monoclonal antibodies against the histidine-rich protein 2 (HRP2) whereas others detect species-specific parasite lactate dehydrogenase (pLDH). These procedures are based on an antigen capture approach in dipstick or cartridge formats. The BinaxNOW rapid malaria test (Alere, Waltham, MA) is FDA approved for use within the United States. The kit is designed to detect primarily *P. falciparum* and *P. vivax*; detection of the other species is less sensitive. However, because of sensitivity limitations in patients with a low parasitemia, the gold standard is still considered the examination of thick and thin blood films. If the rapid

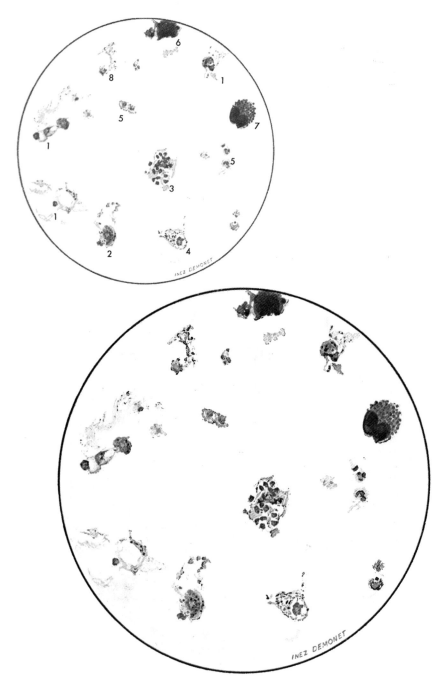

**Figure 49-5** *Plasmodium vivax* in thick smear. *1,* Ameboid trophozoites. *2,* Schizont, two divisions of chromatin. *3,* Mature schizont. *4,* Microgametocyte. *5,* Blood platelets. *6,* Nucleus of neutrophil. *7,* Eosinophil. *8,* Blood platelet associated with cellular remains of young erythrocytes. (From Wilcox A: *Manual for the microscopical diagnosis of malaria in man,* Washington, DC, 1960, U.S. Public Health Service.)

test is negative, the thick and thin blood films must be examined on a STAT basis.

### Molecular Diagnostics

Other methods include direct detection of the five species by using a specific DNA probe after PCR amplification of target DNA sequences. Some laboratories are now using PCR for detection of malaria; the high sensitivity, rapidity, and simplicity of some of the methods are becoming much more relevant for diagnosis. Detection is possible for as few as 5 or 10 parasites per microliter of blood; thus, PCR detects many more cases of low-level parasitemia than do thick blood films. This approach is

also valuable when the determination of species is questionable, or in situations where mixed infections are suspected.

### Automated Instruments

Using automated flow cytometry hematology instruments, there are potential limitations related to the diagnosis of blood parasite infections. *Plasmodium* spp. and *Babesia* infections have been completely missed using instruments. Failure to detect a light parasitemia is highly likely. Unfortunately, failure to make the diagnosis in many of these patients has resulted in delayed therapy. Although the majority of these instruments are not designed to detect intracellular blood parasites, the inability of the automated systems to discriminate between uninfected RBCs and those infected with parasites may pose serious diagnostic problems in situations where the parasitemia is 0.5% or less.

## THERAPY

Malaria has become a more serious health problem, both in residents of endemic areas and in travelers returning to nonendemic areas. Therapy has become more complex as a result of increased resistance of *P. falciparum* to a variety of drugs, resistance problems with *P. vivax,* and the need to treat severe disease complications. Antimalarial drugs are classified according to the stage of malaria against which they are targeted. These drugs are referred to as tissue schizonticides (which kill tissue schizonts), blood schizonticides (which kill blood schizonts), gametocytocides (which kill gametocytes), and sporonticides (which prevent formation of sporozoites within the mosquito). It is important for the clinician to know the species of *Plasmodium* involved in the infection, the estimated parasitemia, and the geographic and patient travel history to assess the possibility of drug resistance related to the organism and geographic area.

Chloroquine-resistant *P. falciparum* is present in almost all endemic areas other than Central America and the Caribbean. Increasing resistance to sulfadoxine-pyrimethamine and mefloquine has also been identified in *P. falciparum.* Therefore, treatment with ACT—including

artesunate-mefloquine, artemether-lumefantrine (Coartem), and artesunate-amodiaquine—has been instituted against *P. falciparum.* However, resistance to artesunate-mefloquine has already appeared in Southeast Asia. Current information on the distribution of drug-resistant *P. falciparum* is available from the Centers for Disease Control and Prevention (CDC) malaria hotline in Atlanta, Georgia [phone (770) 488-7788]. Therapy for chloroquine-resistant *P. falciparum* remains very complex with continual changes; thus consultation with an infectious disease specialist is highly recommended. Current treatment guidelines from the CDC are available at www.cdc.gov/malaria/pdf/clinicalguidance.pdf. Chloroquine resistance continues to evolve and spread. Primaquine tolerance has also been documented.

## BABESIA SPP.

The genus *Babesia* includes approximately 100 species transmitted by ticks of the genus *Ixodes.* In addition to humans, these blood parasites infect a variety of wild and domestic animals. Cases of babesiosis have been documented worldwide, and several outbreaks in humans have occurred in the northeastern United States, particularly in Long Island, Cape Cod, and the islands off the East Coast (Homer). Although there are many species of *Babesia, Babesia microti* is the cause of most human infections in the United States, whereas *B. divergens* tends to be more common in Europe, is often found in splenectomized patients, and causes a more serious form of the disease.

### GENERAL CHARACTERISTICS

#### Organism

Although the life cycle of *Babesia* spp. is similar to that of *Plasmodium* spp., no exoerythrocytic stage has been described; also, sporozoites injected by the bite of an infected tick invade erythrocytes directly. Once inside the erythrocytes, the trophozoites reproduce by binary fission rather than schizogony. Once the tick begins to take a blood meal; the sporozoites are injected into the host with the tick's saliva.

The trophozoites of *Babesia* can mimic *P. falciparum* rings; however, there are differences that can help differentiate the two organisms (Figure 49-7). *Babesia* trophozoites vary in size from 1 to 5 μm; the smallest are smaller than *P. falciparum* rings. Also, ring forms outside of the RBCs and two to three rings per RBC are much more common in *Babesia.* The ring forms of *Babesia* tend to be very pleomorphic and range in size, even within a single RBC. The diagnostic tetrads, the Maltese Cross, though not seen in every specimen or species, may be present (see Figure 49-7).

### PATHOGENESIS AND SPECTRUM OF DISEASE

Babesiosis is clinically similar to malaria, and symptoms include high fever, myalgias, malaise, fatigue, hepatosplenomegaly, and anemia. Usually, *B. microti* infections in the United States occur in nonsplenectomized individuals and are relatively mild. Infections with some of

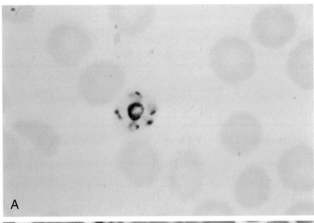

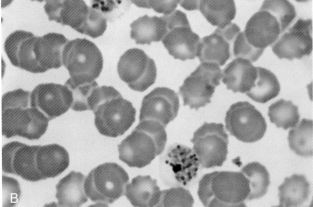

**Figure 49-6 A,** *Plasmodium malariae* schizont. **B,** *Plasmodium vivax* schizont. (Courtesy Dr. Henry Travers, Sioux Falls, SD.)

the other *Babesia* spp. from the United States and with *B. divergens* in Europe occur in splenectomized or immuno-compromised individuals and are clinically more serious. Mortality among symptomatic cases of *B. microti* infection in the United States is 5%, whereas that in *B. divergens* infection in Europe is around 40%. In both areas, risk factors for severe disease include increasing age, splenec-tomy, and a compromised immune system. Infections with *Babesia* species from California, Washington, and other western states tend to be more serious and can mimic the symptoms seen in *B. divergens*.

## LABORATORY DIAGNOSIS

### Routine Methods

The diagnosis of babesiosis should be considered for a patient with typical symptoms and a travel history includ-ing endemic areas, exposure to ticks, or recent blood transfusion. Examination of thick and thin stained blood films is the most direct approach to diagnosis. It is impor-tant to remember that the parasitemia may be low and these organisms tend to be routinely missed using auto-mated hematology instruments.

### Molecular Diagnostics

Although rare, molecular methods such as PCR are avail-able in some laboratories.

## THERAPY

Mild cases caused by *B. microti* usually resolve spontane-ously, and in more serious cases, treatment with clinda-mycin and quinine or atovaquone and azithromycin is used. In very severe cases of *B. microti* infection and in *B. divergens* splenectomized or immunosuppressed patients, exchange transfusion can also be used in addition to antimicrobials.

## PREVENTION

Personal protective measures, such as long pants, long-sleeved shirts, and insect repellant, may reduce the risk

of infection when outdoors in endemic areas for the tick vectors.

## *TRYPANOSOMA* SPP.

*Trypanosoma* spp. are hemoflagellate protozoa that live in the blood and tissue of the human host (Tables 49-4 and 49-5, Figures 49-8 to 49-10). African trypanosomiasis (sleeping sickness) is caused by *Trypanosoma brucei gam-biense* and *T. brucei rhodesiense* species belonging to the family Trypanozoon and is confined to the central belt of Africa. American trypanosomiasis (Chagas' disease) is produced by *Trypanosoma cruzi*, which belongs to the family Schizotrypanum and is confined to the American continent. *Trypanosoma rangeli* belongs to the family Tejaria, produces an asymptomatic infection, and is also

**TABLE 49-4** Characteristics of American Trypanosomiasis

| Characteristic | CAUSATIVE ORGANISM | |
| --- | --- | --- |
| | *Trypanosoma cruzi* | *Trypanosoma rangeli* |
| **Vector** | Reduviid bug | Reduviid bug |
| **Primary reservoirs** | Opossums, dogs, cats, wild rodents | Wild rodents |
| **Illness** | Symptomatic (acute, chronic) | Asymptomatic |
| **Diagnostic stage** | | |
| **Blood** | Trypomastigote | Trypomastigote |
| **Tissue** | Amastigote | None |
| **Recommended specimens** | Blood, lymph node aspirate, chagoma | Blood |

**TABLE 49-5** Characteristics of East and West African Trypanosomiasis

| Characteristic | East African | West African |
| --- | --- | --- |
| **Organism** | *Trypanosoma brucei rhodesiense* | *Trypanosoma brucei gambiense* |
| **Vector** | Tsetse fly, *Glossina morsitans* group | Tsetse fly, *Glossina palpalis* group |
| **Primary reservoirs** | Animals | Humans |
| **Illness** | Acute (early CNS invasion), <9 months | Chronic (late CNS invasion), months to years |
| **Lymphadenopathy** | Minimal | Prominent |
| **Parasitemia** | High | Low |
| **Epidemiology** | Anthropozoonosis, game parks | Anthroponosis, rural populations |
| **Diagnostic stage** | Trypomastigote | Trypomastigote |
| **Recommended specimens** | Chancre aspirate, lymph node aspirate, blood, CSF | Chancre aspirate, lymph node aspirate, blood, CSF |

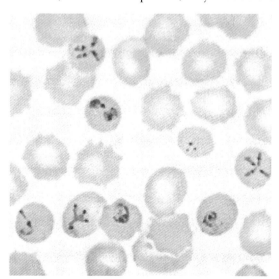

**Figure 49-7** *Babesia* in red blood cells.

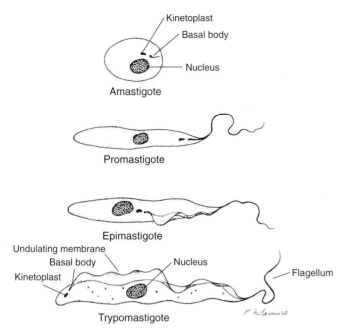

Figure 49-8 Characteristic stages of species of *Leishmania* and *Trypanosoma* in human and insect hosts. (Illustration by Nobuko Kitamura.)

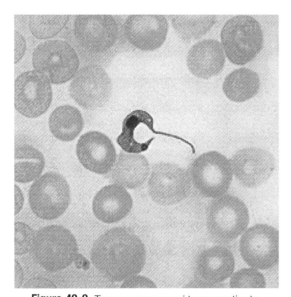

**Figure 49-9** *Trypanosoma cruzi* trypomastigote.

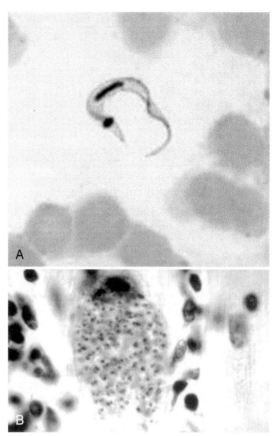

**Figure 49-10 A,** *Trypanosoma cruzi* in blood film (1600×). **B,** *Trypanosoma cruzi* parasites in cardiac muscle (2500×). (From Markell EK, Voge M: *Medical parasitology,* ed 5, Philadelphia, 1981, WB Saunders.)

present only on the American continent. African trypanosomes and *T. rangeli* are transmitted directly into the bite wound by salivary secretions from the insect vector, whereas *T. cruzi* is transmitted through contamination of the bite wound with the feces from the reduviid bug.

## AFRICAN TRYPANOSOMIASIS

The primary area of endemic infection with *T. brucei gambiense* (West African trypanosomiasis) coincides with the vector tsetse fly belt through the heart of Africa, where 300,000 to 500,000 people may be infected in Western and Central Africa. *T. brucei rhodesiense* (which causes Rhodesian trypanosomiasis or East African

sleeping sickness) is more limited in distribution than *T. brucei gambiense,* being found only in central East Africa, where the disease has been responsible for some of the most serious obstacles to economic and social development of Africa. Within this area, the tsetse flies prefer animal blood, which therefore limits the raising of livestock. The infection in humans has a greater morbidity and mortality than does *T. brucei gambiense* infection, and game animals, such as the bushbuck, and cattle are natural reservoir hosts.

A unique feature of African trypanosomes is their ability to change the antigenic surface coat of the outer membrane of the trypomastigote, helping to evade the host immune response. The trypomastigote surface is covered with a dense coat of variant surface glycoprotein (VSG). There are approximately 100 to 1000 genes in the genome, responsible for encoding as many as 1000 different VSGs. More than 100 serotypes have been detected in a single infection. It is postulated that the trypomastigote changes its antigenic coat about every 5 to 7 days (antigenic variation). This change is responsible for successive waves of parasitemia every 7 to 14 days and allows the parasite to evade the host humoral immune response. Each time the antigenic coat changes, the host does not recognize the organism and must mount a new immunologic response. The sustained high immunoglobulin M (IgM) levels are a result of the parasite producing variable antigen types, and in an immunocompetent host, the absence of elevated IgM levels in serum rules out trypanosomiasis.

### General Characteristics

Trypanosomal forms are ingested by the tsetse fly (*Glossina* spp.) when a blood meal is taken. The organisms multiply in the lumen of the midgut and hindgut of the fly. After approximately 2 weeks, the organisms migrate back to salivary glands where the organisms attach to the epithelial cells of the salivary ducts and then transform to their epimastigote forms. Multiplication continues within the salivary gland, and metacyclic (infective) forms develop from the epimastigotes in 2 to 5 days. While feeding, the fly introduces the metacyclic trypanosomal forms into the next victim in saliva injected into the puncture wound. The entire developmental cycle in the fly takes about 3 weeks, and once infected, the tsetse fly remains infected for life.

In fresh blood, the trypanosomes move rapidly among the red blood cells. An undulating membrane and flagellum may be seen with slower moving organisms. The trypomastigote forms are 14 to 33 μm long and 1.5 to 3.5 μm wide (see Table 49-4, Figure 49-8). With a blood stain, the granular cytoplasm stains pale blue. The centrally located nucleus stains reddish. At the posterior end of the organism is the kinetoplast, which also stains reddish, and the remaining intracytoplasmic flagellum (axoneme), which may not be noticeable. The flagellum arises from the kinetoplast, as does the undulating membrane. The flagellum runs along the edge of the undulating membrane until the undulating membrane merges with the trypanosome body at the anterior end of the organism. At this point, the flagellum becomes free to extend beyond the body.

### Pathogenesis and Spectrum of Disease

***Trypanosoma brucei gambiense.*** African trypanosomiasis caused by *T. brucei gambiense* (West African sleeping sickness) has a long, mild, chronic course that ends in death with central nervous system (CNS) involvement after several years' duration. This is unlike the disease caused by *T. brucei rhodesiense* (East African sleeping sickness), which has a short course and ends fatally within 1 year.

After the host has been bitten by an infected tsetse fly, a nodule or chancre at the site may develop after a few days. Usually, this primary lesion will resolve spontaneously within 1 to 2 weeks, and is rarely seen in patients living in an endemic area. Trypomastigotes may be detected in fluid aspirated from the ulcer. The trypomastigotes enter the bloodstream, causing a low-grade parasitemia that may continue for months with the patient remaining asymptomatic. This is considered stage I disease, where the patient can have systemic trypanosomiasis without CNS involvement. During this time, the parasites may be difficult to detect, even by thick blood film examinations. The infection may self-cure during this period without development of symptoms or lymph node invasion.

Symptoms may occur months to years after infection. When the lymph nodes are invaded, the first symptoms appear and include remittent, irregular fevers with night sweats. Headaches, malaise, and anorexia may also be present. The febrile periods of up to 1 week alternate with afebrile periods of variable duration. Many trypomastigotes may be found in the circulating blood during fevers, but few are seen during afebrile periods. Lymphadenopathy is a consistent feature of Gambian trypanosomiasis, and the enlarged lymph nodes are soft and painless. In addition to lymph node involvement, the spleen and liver become enlarged. With Gambian trypanosomiasis, the blood lymphatic stage may last for years before the sleeping sickness syndrome occurs.

When the organisms finally invade the CNS, the sleeping sickness stage of the infection is initiated (stage II disease). Behavioral and personality changes are seen during CNS invasion. This stage of the disease is characterized by steady progressive meningoencephalitis, apathy, confusion, fatigue, loss of coordination, and somnolence (state of drowsiness). In the terminal phase of the disease, the patient becomes emaciated and progresses to profound coma and death, usually from secondary infection. Thus, the typical signs of true sleeping sickness are seen in patients with Gambian disease.

***Trypanosoma brucei rhodesiense.*** *T. brucei rhodesiense* produces a more rapid, fulminating disease than does *T. brucei gambiense*. Fever, severe headaches, irritability, extreme fatigue, swollen lymph nodes, and aching muscles and joints are typical symptoms. Progressive confusion, personality changes, slurred speech, seizures, and difficulty in walking and talking occur as the organisms invade the CNS. The early stages of the infection are like those of *T. brucei gambiense* infections. However, CNS invasion occurs early, the disease progresses more rapidly, and death may occur before there is extensive CNS involvement. The incubation period is short, often within 1 to 4 weeks, with trypomastigotes being more numerous and appearing earlier in the blood. Lymph node involvement is less pronounced. Febrile episodes are more frequent, and the patients are more anemic and more likely to develop myocarditis or jaundice. Some patients may develop persistent tachycardia, and death may result from arrhythmia and congestive heart failure. Myocarditis may develop in patients with Gambian trypanosomiasis but is more common and severe with the Rhodesian form.

### Laboratory Diagnosis (All Species)

**Routine Methods.** Blood can be collected from either finger stick or venipuncture (use EDTA anticoagulant). Multiple thick and thin blood films should be made for examination, and multiple blood examinations should be done before trypanosomiasis is ruled out. Parasites will be found in large numbers in the blood during the febrile period and in small numbers when the patient is afebrile. In addition to thin and thick blood films, a buffy coat concentration method is recommended to detect the parasites. Parasites can be detected on thin blood films with a detection limit at approximately 1 parasite/200 microscopic fields (high dry power magnification, ×400) and thick blood smears when the numbers are greater than 2000/mL, and when they are greater than 100/mL with hematocrit capillary tube concentration.

**Antigen Detection.** A simple and rapid test, the card indirect agglutination trypanosomiasis test (TrypTect

CIATT), is available, primarily in areas of endemic infection, for the detection of circulating antigens in persons with African trypanosomiasis. The sensitivity of the test (95.8% for *T. brucei gambiense* and 97.7% for *T. brucei rhodesiense*) is significantly higher than those for lymph node puncture, micro hematocrit centrifugation, and cerebrospinal fluid examination (CSF) after single and double centrifugation. Its specificity is excellent, and it has a high positive predictive value.

**Antibody Detection.** Serologic techniques that have been widely used for epidemiologic screening include indirect fluorescent antibody assays (enzyme-linked immunosorbent assay [ELISA]), the indirect hemagglutination test, and the card agglutination trypanosomiasis test. A major problem in endemic areas is that individuals have elevated antibody levels attributable to exposure to animal trypanosomes that are noninfectious to humans. Serum and CSF IgM concentrations are of diagnostic value. However, CSF antibody titers should be interpreted with caution because of the lack of reference values and the possibility that the CSF will contain serum as the result of a traumatic tap.

**Molecular Diagnostics.** Referral laboratories have used molecular methods to detect infections and differentiate species, but these methods are not routinely used in the field. The PCR-based methods have not been standardized and validation studies have not been performed. There have been few studies where the various PCR methods used for diagnostic purposes have been compared. In general, these tests are not available in the routine laboratory.

## Therapy

All drugs used in the therapy of African trypanosomiasis are toxic and require prolonged administration. Treatment should be started as soon as possible, and the antiparasitic drug selected depends on whether the CNS is infected. Suramin or pentamidine isethionate can be used when the CNS is not infected. Melarsoprol, a toxic trivalent arsenic derivative, is effective for both blood and CNS stages but is recommended for treatment of late-stage sleeping sickness. Eflornithine (DL-α-difluoromethylornithine; DFMO) has been used for more than 10 years for melarsoprol-resistant *T. brucei gambiense* infection with or without CNS involvement. Any individual treated for African trypanosomiasis should be monitored for 2 years after completion of therapy.

## AMERICAN TRYPANOSOMIASIS

American trypanosomiasis (Chagas' disease) is a zoonosis occurring throughout the American continent and involves reduviid bugs/kissing bugs (vectors) living in close association with human reservoirs (dogs, cats, armadillos, opossums, raccoons, and rodents). Sylvatic cycles of *T. cruzi* transmission extend from southern Argentina and Chile to northern California. Transmission to humans depends on the defecation habits of the insect vector. In areas where the local species of reduviid bug does not ordinarily defecate while feeding, there are no human infections. This may explain why there are few human infections in the United States, even though sylvatic infections are known to occur in southern states. A number of autochthonous cases have been reported in the United States, in both Texas and California. The reduviid species involved in transmitting the infection to humans vary with the geographic area. A very serious problem is disease acquisition through blood transfusion and organ transplantation. A large number of patients with positive serologic results can remain asymptomatic. Patients can present with either acute or chronic disease.

### Trypanosoma cruzi

**General Characteristics.** Trypomastigotes (see Table 49-5 and Figures 49-9 and 49-10) are ingested by the reduviid bug (triatomids, kissing bugs, or conenose bugs) as it obtains a blood meal. The trypomastigotes transform into epimastigotes (see Figure 49-8) that multiply in the posterior portion of the bug's midgut. After 8 to 10 days, trypomastigotes develop from the epimastigotes. Humans contract Chagas' disease when the reduviid bug defecates while taking a blood meal and the parasites in the feces are rubbed or scratched into the bite wound or onto mucosal surfaces.

In humans, *T. cruzi* is found in two forms: amastigotes and trypomastigotes (see Figure 49-8). The trypomastigote form is present in the blood and infects the host cells. The amastigote form multiplies within the cell, eventually destroying the cell, and both amastigotes and trypomastigotes are released into the blood.

The trypomastigote (see Figures 49-9 and 49-10) is approximately 20 μm long, and it usually assumes a C or U shape in stained blood films. Trypomastigotes occur in the blood in two forms: a long slender form and a short stubby one. The nucleus is situated in the center of the body, with a large oval kinetoplast located at the posterior extremity. A flagellum arises from the kinetoplast and extends along the outer edge of an undulating membrane until it reaches the anterior end of the body, where it projects as a free flagellum. When the trypomastigotes are stained with any of the blood stains, the cytoplasm stains blue and the nucleus, kinetoplast, and flagellum stain red or violet.

When the trypomastigote penetrates a cell, it loses its flagellum and undulating membrane and divides by binary fission to form an amastigote (see Figure 49-10). The amastigote continues to divide and eventually fills and destroys the infected cell. Both amastigote and trypomastigote forms are released from the cell. The amastigote is indistinguishable from those found in leishmanial infections. It is 2 to 6 μm in diameter and contains a large nucleus and rod-shaped kinetoplast that stains red or violet with blood stains. The cytoplasm stains blue. Only the trypomastigotes are found free in the peripheral blood.

**Pathogenesis and Spectrum of Disease.** The clinical stages associated with Chagas' disease are categorized as acute, indeterminate, and chronic. The acute stage represents the initial encounter of the patient with the parasite, whereas the chronic phase is the result of late sequelae. In children under the age of 5, the disease is seen in its acute form, whereas in older children and adults, the disease is milder and is commonly diagnosed in the subacute or chronic form. The incubation period in humans is about 7 to 14 days but is somewhat longer in some patients.

Acute symptoms occur 2 to 3 weeks after infection and include high fevers, enlarged spleen and liver, myalgia, erythematous rash, acute myocarditis, lymphadenopathy, keratitis, and subcutaneous edema of the face, legs, and feet. There may be symptoms of CNS involvement, which carry a very poor prognosis. Myocarditis is confirmed by electrocardiographic changes, tachycardia, chest pain, and weakness. Amastigotes proliferate within the cardiac muscle cells and destroy the cells, leading to conduction defects and a loss of heart contractility (see Figure 49-10). Death may occur due to myocardial insufficiency or cardiac arrest. In infants and very young children, swelling of the brain can develop, causing death.

The chronic stage may be initially asymptomatic (indeterminate stage), and even though parasites are rarely seen in blood films, transmission by blood transfusion is a serious problem in endemic areas.

Chronic Chagas' disease may develop years after undetected infection or after the diagnosis of acute disease. Approximately 30% of patients may develop chronic Chagas' disease, including cardiac changes and enlargement of the colon and esophagus. Megacolon results in constipation, abdominal pain, and the inability to discharge feces. There may be acute obstruction leading to perforation, septicemia, and death. However, the most frequent clinical signs of chronic Chagas' disease involve the heart, where enlargement of the heart and conduction changes are commonly seen.

### Laboratory Diagnosis

***Routine Methods.*** Trypomastigotes may be detected in blood by using thick and thin blood films or the buffy coat concentration technique. Any of the blood stains can be used for both amastigote and trypomastigote stages.

***Molecular Diagnostics.*** Referral laboratories have used molecular methods to detect infections with as few as one trypomastigote in 20 mL of blood, but these methods are not routinely used in the field. The PCR-based methods have not been standardized and validation studies have not been performed. As with African trypanosomiasis, there have been few studies where the various PCR methods used for diagnostic purposes have been compared. In general, these tests are not available in the routine laboratory.

***Xenodiagnosis.*** In endemic areas where reduviid bugs are readily available, xenodiagnosis can be used to detect light infections; this technique is helpful in the diagnosis of chronic infections when there are few trypomastigotes in the blood. Trypanosome-free bugs are allowed to feed on individuals suspected of having Chagas' disease. If organisms are ingested in the blood meal, the parasites will multiply and be detected in the bug's intestinal contents, which should be examined monthly for flagellated forms over a period of 3 months.

***Antigen Detection.*** Immunoassays have been used to detect antigens in urine and sera in patients with congenital infections and those with chronic Chagas' disease. Antigen detection can also be valuable for early diagnosis

and for diagnosis of chronic cases in patients with conflicting serologic test results.

***Antibody Detection.*** Serologic tests for antibody detection include complement fixation, indirect fluorescent antibody, indirect hemagglutination tests, and ELISA. The use of synthetic peptides and recombinant antigens has improved the sensitivity and specificity of these tests. However, depending on the antigens used, cross reactions have been noted to occur in patients with *T. rangeli* infection, leishmaniasis, syphilis, toxoplasmosis, hepatitis, leprosy, schistosomiasis, infectious mononucleosis, systemic lupus erythematosus, and rheumatoid arthritis. The sensitivity and specificity of serologic tests for screening blood donors has improved; single-assay screening may be acceptable rather than the two-assay screening method previously recommended.

***Histology.*** In tissue, amastigotes can be differentiated from fungal organisms because they will not stain positive with periodic acid-Schiff, mucicarmine, or silver stains. Although the amastigotes of *T. cruzi* look like those in leishmaniasis, patient history, including geographic and/or travel history, and confirmation of organisms in striated muscle rather than reticuloendothelial tissues are very strong evidence for *T. cruzi* rather than *Leishmania donovani* as the causative agent.

***Therapy.*** Nifurtimox (Lampit) and benznidazole (Radamil) reduce the severity of acute Chagas' disease. Other drugs, allopurinol, fluconazole, itraconazole, and ketoconazole, have been used to treat a limited number of patients. However, drug therapy has little effect on reducing the progression of chronic Chagas' disease. In some cases, surgery has been successfully used to treat cases of chagasic heart disease, megaesophagus, and megacolon.

## *LEISHMANIA* SPP.

Leishmaniasis is caused by more than 20 species of the protozoan genus *Leishmania,* with a disease spectrum ranging from self-healing cutaneous lesions to debilitating mucocutaneous infections, subclinical viscerotropic dissemination, and fatal visceral involvement. Published disease burden estimates place leishmaniasis second in mortality and fourth in morbidity among all tropical diseases. Leishmaniasis is classified as one of the "most neglected diseases," based on its association with poverty and on the limited resources invested in diagnosis, treatment, and control. The World Health Organization (WHO) estimates that 1.5 million cases of cutaneous leishmaniasis (CL) and 500,000 cases of visceral leishmaniasis (VL) occur every year in 88 countries. Estimates indicate that approximately 350 million people are at risk for acquiring leishmaniasis, with 12 million currently infected.

Cases of leishmaniasis are seen each year in the United States and can be attributed to immigrants from countries with endemic infection, military personnel, and American travelers. Another concern is the potential for more infections occurring in areas of endemic infection in Texas and Arizona.

**TABLE 49-6** Features of Human Leishmanial Infections[a]

| Species | Disease Type | Humoral Antibodies | Delayed Hypersensitivity | Parasite Quantity | Self-Cure | Recommended Specimen |
|---|---|---|---|---|---|---|
| Leishmania donovani | VL | Abundant | Absent | Absent | Rare | Bone marrow, spleen |
| | CL | Variable | Present | Present | Yes | Skin macrophages |
| | DL | Variable | Variable | Variable | Variable | Skin macrophages |
| L. tropica | CL | Variable | Present | Present | Yes | Skin macrophages |
| L. major | CL | Present | Present | Present | Rapid | Skin macrophages |
| L. aethiopica | CL | Variable | Weak | Present | Slow | Skin macrophages |
| | DCL | Variable | Absent | Abundant | No | Skin macrophages |
| L. mexicana | CL | Variable | Present | Present | Yes | Skin macrophages |
| | DCL | Variable | Absent | Abundant | No | Skin macrophages |
| L. braziliensis | CL | Present | Present | Present | Yes | Skin macrophages |
| | MCL | Present | Present | Scant | No | Skin macrophages |

*CL,* Cutaneous leishmaniasis; *DCL,* diffuse cutaneous leishmaniasis; *DL,* dermal leishmanoid; *MCL,* mucocutaneous leishmaniasis; *VL,* visceral leishmaniasis.

[a]For culture, specimens must be collected aseptically; in older lesions, the number of parasites may be scant and difficult to recover. **Isolation:** Hamsters; culture media (Novy-MacNeal-Nicolle medium and Schneider's *Drosophila* medium with 30% fetal bovine serum). **Serology:** Most suitable for visceral leishmaniasis; little value for cutaneous leishmaniasis; limited value for mucocutaneous leishmaniasis. **Montenegro test:** Delayed hypersensitivity reaction to intradermal injection of cultured parasites.

## GENERAL CHARACTERISTICS

The parasite has two distinct phases in its life cycle: amastigote and promastigote (Table 49-6, Figure 49-11). The amastigote form is an intracellular parasite in the cells of the reticuloendothelial system and is oval, measuring 1.5 to 5 μm, and contains a nucleus and kinetoplast. *Leishmania* spp. exist as the amastigote in humans and as the promastigote in the insect host. As the vector takes a blood meal, promastigotes are introduced into the human host. Depending on the species, the parasites then move from the bite site to the organs within the reticuloendothelial system (bone marrow, spleen, liver) or to the macrophages of the skin or mucous membranes.

More than 90% of cutaneous leishmaniasis cases occur in Afghanistan, Algeria, Iran, Iraq, Saudi Arabia, Syria, Brazil, and Peru. There has been an increase in the number of cases among military personnel deployed in Afghanistan, Iraq, and Kuwait. Autochthonous (native to origin) human infections have been described in Texas. Most of the cases of mucocutaneous leishmaniasis occur in Bolivia, Brazil, and Peru. More than 90% of the cases of visceral leishmaniasis are found in Bangladesh, Brazil, India, Nepal, and Sudan.

Depending on the species involved, infection with *Leishmania* spp. can result in cutaneous, diffuse cutaneous, mucocutaneous, or visceral disease. In endemic areas with leishmaniasis, co-infection with human immunodeficiency virus (HIV)-positive patients is common. If co-infected patients are severely immunocompromised, up to 25% will die shortly after being diagnosed. The use of highly active antiretroviral therapy (HAART) has dramatically improved the prognosis of these co-infected patients.

## PATHOGENESIS AND SPECTRUM OF DISEASE

The first sign of cutaneous disease is a lesion (generally a firm, painless papule) at the bite site. Although a single lesion may appear insignificant, multiple lesions or disfiguring facial lesions may be devastating for the patient. Usually, the lesions will have a similar appearance and will progress at the same speed. The original lesion may remain as a flattened plaque or may progress to a shallow ulcer. As the ulcer enlarges, it produces exudate and often becomes secondarily infected with bacteria or other organisms.

In mucocutaneous leishmaniasis, the primary lesions are similar to those found in cutaneous leishmaniasis. Untreated primary lesions may develop into the mucocutaneous form in up to 80% of the cases. Dissemination to the nasal or oral mucosa may occur from the active primary lesion or may occur years later after the original lesion has healed. These mucosal lesions do not heal spontaneously, and secondary bacterial infections are common and may be fatal. Also, untreated visceral leishmaniasis will lead to death; secondary bacterial and viral infections are also common in these patients.

The incubation period ranges from 10 days to 2 years, usually being 2 to 4 months. Common symptoms include fever, anorexia, malaise, weight loss, and, frequently, diarrhea. Clinical signs include nontender enlarged liver and spleen, swollen lymph nodes, and occasional acute abdominal pain. Darkening of facial, hand, foot, and abdominal skin (kala-azar) is often seen in light-skinned persons in India. Death may occur after a few weeks or after 2 to 3 years in chronic cases. The majority of infected individuals will be asymptomatic or have very few or

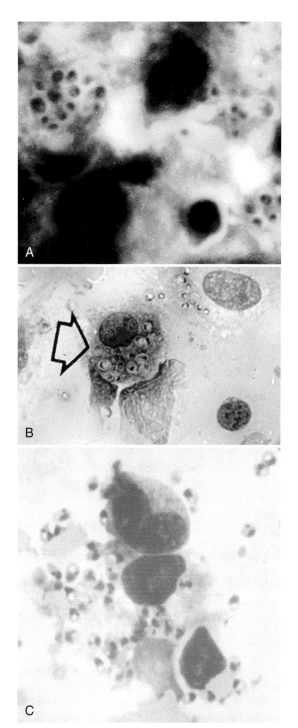

**Figure 49-11 A,** *Leishmania donovani* parasites in Küpffer cells of liver (2000×). **B,** *Leishmania* sp. **C,** *Leishmania donovani* amastigotes. (**B** courtesy Dr. Henry Travers, Sioux Falls, SD.)

minor symptoms that will resolve without therapy. Since 1990, an increase in leishmaniasis in organ transplant recipients has been documented. Most of these cases have been visceral leishmaniasis.

## LABORATORY DIAGNOSIS

After the cutaneous lesion exudate is removed, these lesions should be thoroughly cleaned with 70% alcohol.

Specimens can be collected from the margin of the lesion by aspiration, scraping, or punch biopsy or by making a slit with a scalpel blade. Smears can be prepared from the material obtained and stained with any of the blood stains; biopsy specimens should also be submitted for routine histologic examination. Specimens for visceral disease include lymph node aspirates, liver biopsy specimens, bone marrow specimens, and buffy coat preparations of venous blood. Amastigotes with reticuloendothelial cells have been detected in a number of different specimens from HIV-positive patients.

Stained smears can be examined for the presence of the amastigotes. Although the specimens can be cultured using special techniques, these procedures are not routinely available. PCR methods have excellent sensitivity and specificity for direct detection, for identification of causative species, and for assessment of treatment efficacy; although not routinely available, they can be performed at some reference centers. A rapid immunochromatographic dipstick test using the recombinant K39 antigen has become available for the qualitative detection of total anti–*Leishmania* immunoglobulins.

In patients with severe visceral leishmaniasis (kala-azar), there is a characteristic hypergammaglobulinemia, including both IgG and IgM. In highly suspect patients for the diagnosis of visceral leishmaniasis (assuming they are immunocompetent), if hypergammaglobulinemia is not present, this may be used to rule out the original diagnosis. Although serologic testing is available from some reference centers such as CDC, serologic assays are not very useful for the diagnosis of mucocutaneous and visceral leishmaniasis.

## THERAPY

In simple cutaneous leishmaniasis, lesions usually heal spontaneously, although treatment options include cryotherapy, heat, photodynamic therapy, surgical excision of lesions, and chemotherapy. Standard therapy consists of injections of antimonial compounds; however, relapse is quite common and the patient response varies depending on the *Leishmania* species and type of disease.

Patients clinically cured of mucocutaneous infection continue to be PCR positive for many years following therapy; this disease is characterized by chronicity, latency, and metastasis with mucosal membrane involvement.

For many years, pentavalent antimony compounds have been the drugs of choice for the treatment of visceral leishmaniasis. However, with the first reports of primary treatment failures in the mid-1990s, additional drugs have been used and include lipid-associated amphotericin B for Mediterranean and Indian disease.

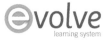

*Visit the Evolve site to complete the review questions.*

# ≡ BIBLIOGRAPHY

Alvar J, Aparicio P, Aseffa A, et al: The relationship between leishmaniasis and AIDS: the second 10 years, *Clin Microbiol Rev* 21:334-359, 2008.

Baird JK: Resistance to therapies for infection by *Plasmodium vivax, Clin Microbiol Rev* 22:508-534, 2009.

Chin-Hong PV, Schwartz BS, Bern C, et al: Screening and treatment of Chagas disease in organ transplant recipients in the United States: recommendations from the Chagas in transplant working group, *Am J Transplant* 2011 (Epub ahead of print).

Cogswell FB, Collins WE, Krotoski WA, et al: Hypnozoites of *Plasmodium simiovale, Am J Trop Med Hyg* 45:211-213, 1991.

Eliades MJ, Shah S, Nguyen-Dinh P, et al: Malaria surveillance—United States, 2003, *MMWR Surveill Summ* 54:25-40, 2005.

Garcia LS: *Diagnostic medical parasitology*, ed 5, Washington, DC, 2007, ASM Press.

Garcia LS: Malaria, *Clin Lab Med* 10:405-416, 2010.

Garcia LS: *Practical guide to diagnostic parasitology*, ed 2, Washington, DC, 2009, ASM Press.

Gemma S, Travagli V, Savini L, et al: Malaria chemotherapy: recent advances in drug development, *Recent Pat Antiinfect Discov* 5:195-225, 2010.

Hidron A, Vogenthaler N, Santos-Preciago JI, et al: Cardiac involvement with parasitic infections, *Clin Microbiol Rev* 23:324-349, 2010.

Jongwutiwes S, Putaporntip C, Iwasaki T, et al: Naturally acquired *Plasmodium knowlesi* malaria in human, Thailand, *Emerg Infect Dis* 10:2211-2213, 2004.

Koenderink JB, Kavishe RA, Rijpma SR, et al: The ABCs of multidrug resistance in malaria, *Trends Parasitol* 26:440-446, 2010.

Kribs-Zaleta C: Estimating contact process saturation in sylvatic transmission of *Trypanosoma cruzi* in the United States, *PLoS Negl Trop Dis* 4:e656, 2010.

Lescure FX, Le Loup G, Freilij H, et al: Chagas disease: changes in knowledge and management, *Lancet Infect Dis* 10:556-570, 2010.

Lou J, Lucas R, Grau GE: Pathogenesis of cerebral malaria: recent experimental data and possible applications for humans, *Clin Microbiol Rev* 14:810-820, 2001.

Murray CK, Gasser RA Jr, Magill AJ, et al: Update on rapid diagnostic testing for malaria, *Clin Microbiol Rev* 21:L466-472, 2008.

National Committee for Clinical Laboratory Standards: *Laboratory diagnosis of blood-borne parasitic diseases. Approved guideline M15-A*, Wayne, PA, 2000, National Committee for Clinical Laboratory Standards.

Richter J, Franken G, Mehlhorn H, et al: What is the evidence for the existence of *Plasmodium ovale* hypnozoites? *Parasitol Res* 107:1285-1290, 2010.

Rodgers J: Human African trypanosomiasis, chemotherapy and CNS disease, *J Neuroimmunol* 211:16-22, 2009.

Singh B, Kim Sung L, Matusop A, et al: A large focus of naturally acquired *Plasmodium knowlesi* infections in human beings, *Lancet* 363(9414):1017-1024, 2004.

## OBJECTIVES

1. Describe the distinguishing morphologic characteristics, clinical disease, basics of life cycle (source, stages of infectivity), and laboratory diagnosis for amebae, flagellates, and coccidia.
2. Compare and contrast the morphologic forms of the *Naegleria* trophozoites including specimens used for identification.
3. Compare and contrast *Naegleria fowleri*, *Balamuthia mandrillaris*, and *Ancanthamoeba* spp. including routes of transmission, specimens, risk factors, and disease presentation.
4. Compare and contrast the specimen requirements and morphologic characteristics of *Pentatrichomonas hominis* and *Trichomonas vaginalis*.
5. Identify the various morphologic forms of *Toxoplasma gondii* and correlate those with the clinical presentation of the infection (acute, chronic, and congenital).
6. Describe the various individual populations at risk for infection with *Toxoplasma* spp. and the disease symptoms and pathogenesis for each.
7. Define the following terms in relationship to the appropriate parasite discussed in this chapter: axostyle, bradyzoite, tachyzoite, ectocyst, mesocyst, endocyst, and oocyst.

---

### PARASITES TO BE CONSIDERED

**Amebae, Flagellates (Other Body Sites)**

Amebae
  *Naegleria fowleri*
  *Acanthamoeba* spp.
  *Balamuthia mandrillaris*
Flagellates
  *Trichomonas vaginalis*
  *Trichomonas tenax*

**Coccidia (Other Body Sites)**

Coccidia
  *Toxoplasma gondii*

---

## FREE-LIVING AMEBAE

Infections caused by small, free-living amebae belonging to the genera *Naegleria*, *Acanthamoeba*, and *Balamuthia* are generally not very well-known or recognized clinically. Also, methods for laboratory diagnosis are unfamiliar and not routinely offered by most laboratories. However, approximately 310 cases of primary amebic meningoencephalitis (PAM) caused by *Naegleria fowleri* and more than 150 cases of granulomatous amebic encephalitis (GAE) caused by *Acanthamoeba* spp. and *Balamuthia mandrillaris* (including several cases in patients with acquired

immunodeficiency syndrome [AIDS]) have been documented. Other infections caused by these organisms result in *Acanthamoeba* keratitis, now numbering more than 750 cases and related primarily to poor lens care in contact lens wearers. Additionally, both *Acanthamoeba* spp. and *B. mandrillaris* can cause cutaneous infections in humans. *Sappinia pedata*, a free-living ameba normally found in soil contaminated with the feces of elk and buffalo, was identified in an excised brain lesion from a 38-year-old immunocompetent man who developed a frontal headache, blurry vision, and loss of consciousness following a sinus infection. Additionally, *Paravahlkampfia francinae*, a new species of the free-living ameba genus *Paravahlkampfia*, was recently isolated from the cerebrospinal fluid (CSF) of a patient with a headache, sore throat, and vomiting, symptoms typical of primary amebic meningoencephalitis (PAM) caused by *Naegleria fowleri* from the environment.

---

## *NAEGLERIA FOWLERI*

### GENERAL CHARACTERISTICS

There are both trophozoite and cyst stages in the life cycle, with the stage present primarily dependent on environmental conditions. Trophozoites can be found in water or moist soil and can be maintained in tissue culture or other artificial media. The amebae may enter the nasal cavity by inhalation or aspiration of water, dust, or aerosols containing the trophozoites or cysts. *N. fowleri* is incapable of survival in clean, chlorinated water. Following inhalation or aspiration, the organisms then penetrate the nasal mucosa, probably through phagocytosis of the olfactory epithelium cells, and migrate via the olfactory nerves to the brain.

The trophozoites can occur in two forms: ameboid and flagellate (Table 50-1, Figure 50-1). The size ranges from 7 to 35 μm. The diameter of the rounded forms is usually 15 μm. There is a large, central karyosome and no peripheral nuclear chromatin. The cytoplasm is somewhat granular and contains vacuoles. The ameboid form organisms change to the transient, pear-shaped flagellate form when they are transferred from culture or teased from tissue into water and maintained at a temperature of 27° to 37° C. These flagellate forms do not divide, but when the flagella are lost, the ameboid forms resume reproduction. Cysts are generally round, measuring from 7 to 15 μm with a thick double wall.

### PATHOGENESIS AND SPECTRUM OF DISEASE

Primary amebic meningoencephalitis (PAM) caused by *N. fowleri* is an acute, suppurative infection of the brain

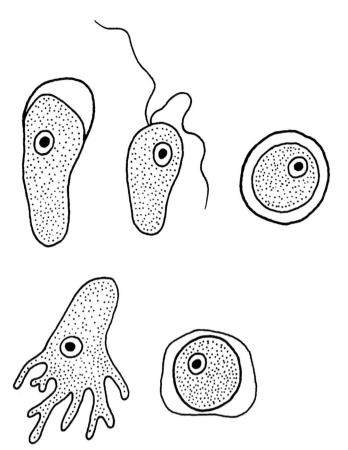

**Figure 50-1** *Naegleria fowleri, Acanthamoeba* spp. Diagram of trophozoites and cysts *(upper row)*. Flagellate and cyst forms of *Naegleria fowleri; (lower row)* trophozoite and cyst of *Acanthamoeba* spp. (Illustration by Sharon Belkin; from Garcia LS: *Diagnostic medical parasitology,* ed 5, Washington, DC, 2007, ASM Press.)

and meninges (Figure 50-2). With extremely rare exceptions, the disease is rapidly fatal in humans. The period between organism contact and onset of symptoms such as fever, headache, and rhinitis varies from a few days to 2 weeks. Early symptoms include vague upper respiratory tract distress, headache, lethargy, and occasionally olfactory problems. The acute phase includes sore throat; a stuffy, blocked, or discharging nose; and severe headache. Progressive symptoms include pyrexia, vomiting, and stiffness of the neck. Mental confusion and coma usually occur approximately 3 to 5 days before death, which is usually caused by cardiorespiratory arrest and pulmonary edema.

PAM resembles acute bacterial meningitis, and these conditions may be difficult to differentiate. Unfortunately, if the CSF Gram stain is interpreted incorrectly as a false positive, the resulting antibacterial therapy has no impact on the amebae and the patient will usually die within a few days.

## LABORATORY DIAGNOSIS

### Routine Methods

Clinical and laboratory data usually cannot be used to differentiate pyogenic meningitis from PAM. A high

index of suspicion is often critical for early diagnosis. Most cases are associated with exposure to contaminated water through swimming or bathing. There is normally an incubation period of 1 day to 2 weeks, and then a course of 3 to 6 days, most often ending in death.

Analysis of the CSF will show decreased glucose and increased protein concentrations. The leukocyte count will range from several hundred to >20,000 cells per mm³. Although Gram stains and bacterial cultures of CSF will be negative, serious patient complications can occur as the result of incorrect therapy if false-positive Gram stains are reported.

A confirmed diagnosis is made by the identification of amebae in the CSF or in biopsy specimens. CSF should be placed on a slide, under a cover slip, and observed for motile trophozoites; smears can be stained with any of the blood stains. It is important not to mistake leukocytes for actual organisms or vice versa. This type of misidentification often occurs when using a counting chamber and the amebae sink to the bottom and round up, hence the recommendation to use just a regular slide and cover slip. Depending on the temperature and lag time between specimen collection and examination, motility may vary. Slides may be warmed slightly to improve motility. The most important differential characteristic is the spherical nucleus with a large karyosome.

Specimens should never be refrigerated before examination, and CSF should be centrifuged at a slow speed (250× *g*). If *N. fowleri* is the causative agent, only trophozoites are normally seen, whereas cysts and trophozoites can be seen with *Acanthamoeba* spp.

### Other Methods

Most cases are diagnosed at autopsy; confirmation of tissue findings must include culture and/or special staining with monoclonal reagents in indirect fluorescent antibody procedures. Organisms can be cultured on nonnutrient agar plated with *Escherichia coli*. In tissue, the amebae can be identified using indirect immunofluorescence and immunoperoxidase techniques.

## THERAPY

Although many antimicrobial and antiparasitic drugs have been screened for activity against *N. fowleri*, only a few patients have recovered after receiving intrathecal and intravenous injections of amphotericin B or in combination with miconazole. Unfortunately, delay in diagnosis and the fulminant nature of PAM result in few survivors.

## *ACANTHAMOEBA* SPP.

### GENERAL CHARACTERISTICS

Unlike *N. fowleri, Acanthamoeba* spp. do not have a flagellate stage in the life cycle, only the trophozoite and cyst. Several species of *Acanthamoeba* cause granulomatous amebic encephalitis (GAE), primarily in immunosuppressed, chronically ill, or otherwise debilitated individuals. These patients usually have no relevant history

**TABLE 50-1**  Free-Living Amebae Causing Disease in Humans

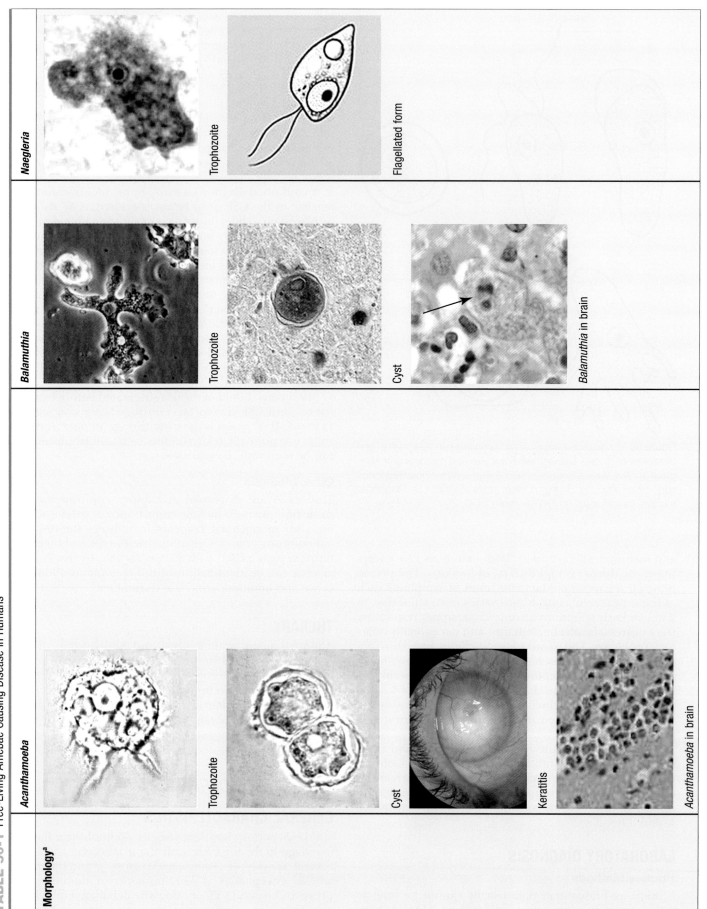

| Morphology[a] | *Acanthamoeba* | *Balamuthia* | *Naegleria* |
|---|---|---|---|
| | Trophozoite | Trophozoite | Trophozoite |
| | Trophozoite | Cyst | Flagellated form |
| | Cyst | *Balamuthia* in brain | |
| | Keratitis | | |
| | *Acanthamoeba* in brain | | |

| Disease parameter | Acanthamoeba | | | Balamuthia | Naegleria |
|---|---|---|---|---|---|
| **Disease parameter** | Granulomatous amebic encephalitis (GAE) | Acanthamoeba keratitis | Cutaneous lesions Sinusitis | GAE | Primary amebic meningoencephalitis (PAM) |
| **General disease description** | Chronic, protracted, slowly progressive CNS infection (may involve lungs); generally associated with individuals with underlying diseases | Painful, progressive, sight-threatening corneal disease; patients generally immunocompetent | Most common in patients with AIDS, with or without CNS involvement; those receiving immunosuppressive therapy for organ transplantation | Chronic, protracted, slowly progressive CNS infection (may involve lungs); generally associated with individuals with underlying diseases | Rare, but nearly always fatal infection; migration of amebae to brain through olfactory nerve; symptoms can mimic bacterial meningitis; death usually occurs 3-7 days after onset of symptoms; clinical suspicion based on history critical |
| **Entry into body** | Olfactory epithelium, respiratory tract, skin, sinuses | Corneal abrasion | Skin, sinuses, respiratory tract | Olfactory epithelium, skin, respiratory tract | Olfactory epithelium |
| **Incubation period** | Weeks to months | Days | Weeks to months | Weeks to months | Days |
| **Clinical symptoms** | Confusion, headache, stiff neck, irritability | Blurred vision, photophobia, inflammation, corneal ring, pain | Skin lesions, nodules, sinus lesions, sinusitis | Slurred speech, muscle weakness, headache, nausea, seizures | Headache, nausea, vomiting, confusion, fever, stiff neck, seizures, coma |
| **Disease pathology** | Focal necrosis, granulomas | Corneal ulceration | Granulomatous reaction in skin, inflammation | Multiple necrotic foci, inflammation, cerebral edema | Hemorrhagic necrosis |
| **Diagnostic methods** | Brain biopsy, CSF smear/wet prep, culture, indirect immunofluorescence on tissue,[b] PCR[b] | Corneal scrapings or biopsy, stain with calcofluor white, culture, confocal microscopy | Skin lesion biopsy, culture, indirect immunofluorescence of tissue[a] | Brain biopsy, culture on mammalian cells, indirect immunofluorescence of tissue[a] | Brain biopsy, CSF wet prep, culture, indirect immunofluorescence of tissue,[a] PCR[a] |

[a]Acanthamoeba in brain and Balamuthia in brain courtesy Dr. Govinda Visvesvara, Centers for Disease Control and Prevention.

[b]Indirect immunofluorescence on tissue and PCR methods available from Centers for Disease Control and Prevention.

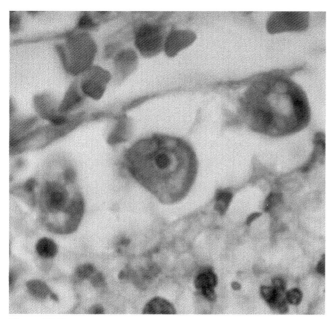

**Figure 50-2** *Naegleria fowleri* in brain tissue. Hematoxylin and eosin stain. Note the large karyosome.

involving freshwater exposure. *Acanthamoeba* spp. also cause amebic keratitis, and it is estimated that the incidence in the United States may be one to two cases per million contact lens users. Apparently, the incidence of *Acanthamoeba* keratitis in the United Kingdom is 15 times higher than that in the United States and 7 times higher than that in Holland.

Motile organisms have spine-like pseudopods; there is a wide organism size range (25 to 40 μm), with the average diameter of the trophozoites being 30 μm. The nucleus has the typical large karyosome, similar to that found in *N. fowleri*. This morphologic characteristic can be seen on a wet preparation.

The cysts are usually round with a single nucleus, also having the large karyosome as in the trophozoite nucleus. The double wall is usually visible, with the slightly wrinkled outer cyst wall and what has been described as a polyhedral inner cyst wall. This cyst morphology is identifiable in organisms cultured on agar plates.

## PATHOGENESIS AND SPECTRUM OF DISEASE

### GAE

Meningoencephalitis caused by *Acanthamoeba* spp. may present as an acute suppurative inflammation of the brain and meninges similar to *N. fowleri* infection. The incubation period of GAE is unknown; several weeks or months are probably necessary to establish disease. The clinical course tends to be subacute or chronic and is usually associated with trauma or underlying disease, not as a result of swimming. GAE may present with symptoms of confusion, dizziness, drowsiness, nausea, vomiting, headache, lethargy, stiff neck, seizures, and sometimes hemiparesis. Unlike PAM caused by *N. fowleri*, both trophozoites and cysts are found throughout the tissue. Also, dissemination to other tissues such as the liver, kidneys, trachea, and adrenals can occur in immunocompromised individuals; or additional unusual sites also include the ear and necrotic bone from a bone graft of the mandible. Some patients, especially those with AIDS, can develop erythematous nodules, chronic ulcerative skin lesions, or abscesses.

### Keratitis

*Acanthamoeba* spp. also cause keratitis and corneal ulceration. Clinicians need to consider acanthamoebic infection in the differential diagnosis of eye infections that are not responding to bacterial, fungal, or viral therapy. These infections are often due to direct exposure of the eyes to contaminated materials or solutions. Use of contact lenses is the leading risk factor for keratitis. Conditions that are linked with disease include the use of home-made saline solutions, poor contact lens hygiene, and corneal abrasions. A contact lens can act as a mechanical vector for transport of amebae present in the storage case onto the cornea. Subsequent multiplication and invasion of the tissue may occur. Decreased corneal sensation has contributed to the misdiagnosis of *Acanthamoeba* keratitis as herpes simplex keratitis. *Acanthamoeba* keratitis may be present as a secondary or opportunistic infection in patients with herpes simplex keratitis. Unfortunately, as a result, treatment can be delayed for 2 weeks to 3 months.

## LABORATORY DIAGNOSIS

### Routine Methods

The most effective culture approach uses non-nutrient agar plates with Page's saline and an overlay growth of *Escherichia coli* on which the amebae feed. Tissue stains are also effective, and cysts isolated from cultures can be stained with Gomori's silver methenamine, periodic acid-Schiff, and calcofluor white. Identification of *Acanthamoebae* in ocular samples and other tissues can be difficult, even for trained laboratory professionals; in histologic preparations, the organisms appear similar to keratoplasts, as well as neutrophils and monocytes. It has been estimated that up to 70% of clinical *Acanthamoeba* keratitis cases are misdiagnosed as viral keratitis. Also, the average time to diagnosis of keratitis attributable to *Acanthamoeba* infection can average 2.5 weeks longer for non–contact lens wearers than for contact lens users.

### Other Methods

CSF or bronchoalveolar lavage fluid cytospin preparations can be used to look for amebae in patients with GAE or respiratory symptoms. The characteristic morphology of the *Acanthamoeba* trophozoites, such as the prominent nucleolus, contractile vacuole, and cytoplasmic vacuoles, can be seen more easily using trichrome or hematoxylin and eosin stains on fixed preparations after cytocentrifugation.

In the differential diagnosis of GAE, other space-occupying lesions of the central nervous system (CNS) (e.g., tumor, abscess, fungal infection) must also be considered. Predisposing conditions include Hodgkin's disease, diabetes, alcoholism, pregnancy, and corticosteroid therapy. Organisms have also been found in the adrenal gland, brain, eyes, kidneys, liver, pancreas, skin, spleen, thyroid gland, and uterus.

In infections caused by *Acanthamoeba* spp., periodic acid-Schiff stains the cyst wall red and methenamine silver stains the cyst black. Normally, *Naegleria* and *Acanthamoeba* isolates are identified to the species level by a reference laboratory, such as the Centers for Disease Control and Prevention, using indirect fluorescent antibody procedures with a monoclonal or polyclonal antibody.

## THERAPY

### Disseminated Infections

Trophozoites and cysts of *Acanthamoeba* isolates vary in their sensitivity to antimicrobial agents. They are sensitive in vitro to ketoconazole, pentamidine, hydroxystilbamidine, paromomycin, 5-fluorocytosine, polymyxin, sulfadiazine, trimethoprim-sulfamethoxazole, azithromycin, and extracts of medicinal plants, especially, to combinations of these drugs. In vitro testing confirms strain and species differences in sensitivity.

## ACANTHAMOEBA KERATITIS

Prompt treatment is essential. Patients should be seen by an ophthalmologist immediately. Various prescription eye medications are available.

## BALAMUTHIA MANDRILLARIS

### GENERAL CHARACTERISTICS

*Balamuthia mandrillaris* is uncommon and was thought to be a harmless soil organism, with no relevance for infecting mammals. However, since the appearance of *B. mandrillaris* was first seen at the San Diego Wild Animal Park in a gibbon that died of meningoencephalitis, a number of primates, as well as dogs, sheep, and horses, have died of CNS infection caused by this organism. Approximately 100 cases of human amebic encephalitis worldwide have been identified with about half of the cases diagnosed within the United States. Death can occur from a week to several months after the onset of symptoms. Patients eventually die with a massive CNS infection. Genotyping studies indicate that lethal infections caused by *B. mandrillaris* are due to a single species with a global distribution.

The life cycle is similar to that of *Acanthamoeba* spp.; like *Acanthamoeba* spp., *Balamuthia* does not have a flagellated stage in the life cycle. Both trophozoites and cysts are found in CNS tissue, and their sizes are similar to those of *Acanthamoeba* trophozoites and cysts. It is difficult to differentiate *Balamuthia* from *Acanthamoeba* spp. in tissue sections under a light microscope. Using electron microscopy, the cysts are characterized by having three layers in the cyst wall: an outer wrinkled ectocyst, a middle structure–less mesocyst, and an inner thin endocyst. Under light microscopy, they appear to have two walls: an outer irregular wall and an inner round wall. In some cases, *Balamuthia* trophozoites in tissue sections appear to have more than one nucleolus in the nucleus. In such cases, it may be possible to distinguish *Balamuthia* amebae from *Acanthamoeba* organisms on the basis of nuclear morphology, because *Acanthamoeba* trophozoites have only one nucleolus.

## PATHOGENESIS AND SPECTRUM OF DISEASE

The disease is very similar to GAE caused by *Acanthamoeba* spp. The clinical presentation is subacute or chronic and is usually not associated with swimming in freshwater. No characteristic clinical symptoms, laboratory findings, or radiologic indicators have been found to be diagnostic for GAE. Whether single or multiple, the lesions in the brain involve mainly the cerebral cortex and subcortical white matter. Symptoms include headache, nausea, vomiting, fever, visual disturbances, dysphagia, seizures, and hemiparesis. The clinical course ranges from a few days to several months. In immunocompetent hosts, an inflammatory response occurs; however, with rare exceptions, these patients also tend to die with severe CNS disease.

## LABORATORY DIAGNOSIS

*B. mandrillaris* does not grow well on *E. coli*–seeded non-nutrient agar plates. However, these organisms can be cultured in mammalian cell cultures using monkey kidney cells and MRC, HEp-2, and diploid macrophage cell lines. Using human brain microvascular endothelial cells, *B. mandrillaris* has been cultured postmortem from brain and CSF from a case of granulomatous amebic meningoencephalitis. A cell-free growth medium is also commercially available. Although serum antibodies have been identified in infections, laboratory testing is not routinely available.

## THERAPY

In vitro studies indicate that *B. mandrillaris* is susceptible to pentamidine isethiocyanate and that patients may benefit from this treatment. Other studies indicate that ketoconazole, propamidine isethionate, clotrimazole, and certain biguanides have amebicidal activity.

## TRICHOMONAS VAGINALIS

### GENERAL CHARACTERISTICS

Infection is acquired primarily through sexual intercourse, hence the need to diagnose and treat asymptomatic males. The organism is capable of survival for extended periods in a moist environment such as damp towels and underclothes; however, this mode of transmission is thought to be very rare. Infection with *Trichomonas vaginalis* occurs worldwide. It is estimated that 5 million women and 1 million men in the United States have trichomoniasis, with an estimated 7.4 million new cases occurring annually. The prevalence of trichomoniasis

**TABLE 50-2** Characteristics of *Trichomonas vaginalis*

| | |
|---|---|
| Shape and size | Pear-shaped, 7-23 μm long (average, 13 μm); width, 5-15 μm |
| Motility | Jerky, rapid |
| Number of nuclei and visibility | 1; not visible in unstained mounts |
| Number of flagella (usually difficult to see) | 3-5 anterior, 1 posterior |
| Other features | Seen in urine, urethral discharge, and vaginal smears; undulating membrane extends ½ length of body; no free posterior flagellum; axostyle easily seen |
| Infective stage | Trophozoite |
| Usual location | Vagina (male, urethra) |
| Striking clinical findings | Leukorrhea, pruritus vulvae (thin white urethral discharge in male) |
| Other sites of infection | Urethra (prostate in male) |
| Stage usually recovered during clinical phase | Trophozoite only—no cyst |

*Trichomonas*, Wet Mount

*Trichomonas*, Giemsa stain

worldwide is estimated to be more than 170 million cases, which does not include the number of asymptomatic cases that remain untreated. In North America, more than 8 million new cases are reported yearly, with an estimated rate of asymptomatic cases being as high as 50%. Trichomoniasis is the primary non-viral sexually transmitted disease worldwide. Infection with *T. vaginalis* has major health consequences for women, including complications in pregnancy, association with cervical cancer, and predisposition to HIV infection.

The life cycle of *T. vaginalis* has a single trophozoite stage, and is very similar in morphology to other trichomonads (Table 50-2). The trophozoite is 7 to 23 μm long and 5 to 15 μm wide. The axostyle is usually obvious and protrudes through the bottom of the organism, whereas the undulating membrane ends halfway down the side of the trophozoite. There are a large number of granules evident along the axostyle.

## PATHOGENESIS AND SPECTRUM OF DISEASE

Growth of the organism results in inflammation and large numbers of trophozoites in the tissues and the secretions. As the acute infection becomes more chronic, the purulent discharge diminishes, with a decrease in the number of organisms. Symptoms such as vaginal or vulval pruritus and discharge are often sudden and occur during or after menstruation as a result of the increased vaginal acidity. Symptoms include vaginal discharge (42%), odor (50%), and edema or erythema (22% to 37%). Complaints also include dysuria and lower abdominal pain.

From 25% to 50% of infected women may be asymptomatic and have a normal vaginal pH of 3.8 to 4.2 and normal vaginal flora. Even in the carrier form, about 50% of women will become symptomatic during the following 6 months.

Although vaginitis is the most common finding in women with trichomoniasis, other complications include distention of a fallopian tube with pus, endometritis, infertility, low birth weight, and cervical erosion. There is also an increased association with HIV transmission and cervical dysplasia.

Dysuria, often the earliest symptom, occurs in about 20% of women with vaginal trichomoniasis. Infected males may be asymptomatic, or the infection may be self-limited, persistent, or result in recurring urethritis. In nonspecific urethritis, *T. vaginalis* has been detected in 10% to 20% of subjects and in 20% to 30% of those whose sexual partners had vaginitis. Once established, the infection persists for an extended period in females but only for about 10 days or less in males. *T. vaginalis* is the cause of 11% of all cases of non–gonococcal urethritis in males.

Respiratory distress has been reported in a full-term, normal male infant with *T. vaginalis* with severe respiratory problems following delivery. A wet preparation of thick, white sputum demonstrated few leukocytes and motile flagellates, which were identified as *T. vaginalis*. This study supports previous data confirming that the organism may cause neonatal pneumonia.

## LABORATORY DIAGNOSIS

Humans are the only natural host for *T. vaginalis*, and organisms reside in the vagina and prostate; they usually do not survive outside the urogenital tract. The parasites feed on the mucosal surface of the vagina, where bacteria and leukocytes are abundant. The preferred pH for good parasitic growth in females is slightly alkaline or acidic (6.0 to 6.3 optimal), not the normal pH (3.8 to 4.2) of the healthy vagina. The organisms can also be recovered in urine, in urethral discharge, or after prostatic massage. Often, the organisms are recovered in centrifuged urine sediment from both male and female patients.

### Wet Mounts

The identification of *T. vaginalis* is often based on the examination of wet preparations of vaginal and urethral discharges, urine, and prostatic secretions. This examination must be performed within 10 to 20 minutes after sample collection; if not, organisms lose motility and may not be identified. Several specimens may need to be examined for detection of the organisms. The sensitivity associated with wet mount examinations varies between 40% and more than 80%. Often, the percent detection from this procedure is quite low with limited sensitivity and specificity.

### Stained Smears

Giemsa or Papanicolaou stain can be used. However, atypical cellular changes can be misinterpreted, particularly on the Papanicolaou smear. The organisms are routinely missed on Gram stains. The number of false-positive and false-negative results reported on the basis of stained smears strongly suggests that confirmation should be accomplished by observation of motile organisms either from the direct wet mount or from appropriate culture media.

### Culture

A convenient plastic envelope method has been developed, which allows immediate examination and culture in one self-contained system. This system is commercially available as the InPouchTV (BIOMED Diagnostics, San Jose, Calif), which serves as the specimen transport container, the growth chamber during incubation, and the "slide" during microscopy. Once it is inoculated, it requires no opening for examination, and positive growth will occur within 5 days. The sensitivity of this system is reported to be superior to those of other available culture methods.

### Antigen Detection

Several diagnostic tests have been developed, including the XenoStrip-Tv (Xenotope Diagnostics, Inc., San Antonio, Tex) and the OSOM *Trichomonas* Rapid Test (Sekisui Diagnostics, Houston, TX), both of which are more sensitive than the wet mount.

### Molecular Diagnostics

The use of polymerase chain reaction (PCR) methods has led to improvements in *T. vaginalis* detection; nonviable organisms and cells and target sequences can also be detected. In addition to various culture and transport options, there are several other products available, including the Affirm VPIII probe from Becton Dickinson (Cockeysville, Md), the Quik-Tri/Can latex agglutination from Pan Bio InDX, Inc (Baltimore, Md), and the T.VAG DFA from Chemicon (Temecula, Calif). Depending on the patient population, client base, number of requests, and cost, one or more of these options may be appropriate for a particular diagnostic laboratory.

## THERAPY

Metronidazole is recommended for the treatment of urogenital trichomoniasis, although resistance to both metronidazole and other 5-nitromidazoles has been reported. It is also recommended that all sexual partners be treated simultaneously to avoid immediate reinfection. Metronidazole-resistant *T. vaginalis* has been implicated in an increased number of cases; unfortunately,

this drug is currently the only drug approved for the treatment of trichomoniasis in the United States. Tinidazole has also been used for therapy.

## PENTATRICHOMONAS HOMINIS

*Pentatrichomonas hominis* derives its name on the basis of the morphologic structure of the trophozoite. The organism has five anterior flagella and a parabasal body. The organism is recovered worldwide and is considered to be nonpathogenic although it has been isolated from patients with diarrhea.

### GENERAL CHARACTERISTICS

There is no known cyst stage. The trophozoite resides in the large intestine where it feeds on bacteria. The organism resembles *Trichomonas vaginalis,* measuring 5 to 15 μm in length and 7 to 10 μm in width with an undulating membrane and an axostyle. The organism's undulating membrane extends the entire length of the body, differentiating it from *Trichomonas vaginalis.*

### PATHOGENESIS AND SPECTRUM OF DISEASE

Although the organism is considered nonpathogenic, it is the most commonly identified flagellate other than *G. lamblia* and *Dientamoeba fragilis.* The organism may be associated with infections in warm climates.

### LABORATORY DIAGNOSIS

Similar to *Trichomonas vaginalis,* the wet preparation is commonly used to identify motile trophozoites. However, permanent stained smears provide the greatest sensitivity and specificity.

### THERAPY

Because the organism is nonpathogenic, it is important to differentiate it from *Trichmonas vaginalis.* However, if identified, no treatment is necessary.

## TOXOPLASMA GONDII

*Toxoplasma gondii* is a protozoan parasite that infects most species of warm-blooded animals, including humans. Members of the cat family, Felidae, are the only known definitive hosts for the sexual stages of *T. gondii* and serve as the main reservoirs of infection. Cats become infected with *T. gondii* through carnivorism or by ingestion of oocysts. Outdoor cats are much more likely to become infected than domestic cats that are confined indoors. After tissue cysts or oocysts are ingested by the cat, organisms are released and invade epithelial cells of the cat small intestine, where they undergo an asexual cycle followed by a sexual cycle with the formation of oocysts, which are excreted in the feces. The uninfective oocyst takes 1 to 5 days after excretion to become infective. Cats shed oocysts for 1 to 2 weeks and large numbers may be

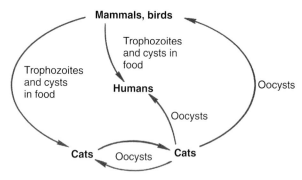

**Figure 50-3** Life cycle of *Toxoplasma gondii.*

shed, often more than 100,000 per gram of feces. Oocysts survive in the environment for several months to more than 1 year and are resistant to disinfectants, freezing, and drying. However, they are killed by heating to 70°C for 10 minutes. The life cycle in the cat takes approximately 19 to 48 days after infection with the oocysts but only 3 to 10 days after the ingestion of meat infected with cysts (e.g., a mouse) (Figure 50-3).

## GENERAL CHARACTERISTICS

There are three infectious stages of *T. gondii:* the tachyzoites (in groups or clones), the bradyzoites (in tissue cysts), and the sporozoites (in oocysts from cat feces). Tachyzoites rapidly multiply in any cell of the intermediate host and in epithelial cells of the definitive host (cats). Bradyzoites are found within the tissue cysts and usually multiply very slowly; the cyst may contain few to hundreds of organisms, and intramuscular cysts may reach 100 μm in size. The tissue cysts can be found in visceral organs such as the lungs, liver, and kidneys; however, they are more prevalent in the brain, eyes, and skeletal and cardiac muscle. Intact tissue cysts can persist for the life of the host and do not cause an inflammatory response.

Tachyzoites are crescent-shaped and are 2 to 3 μm wide by 4 to 8 μm long (Table 50-3). One end tends to be more rounded than the other. Giemsa is the stain of choice; the cytoplasm stains pale blue, and the nucleus stains red and is situated toward the broad end of the organism.

Cysts are formed in chronic infections, and the bradyzoites within the cyst wall are strongly periodic acid-Schiff positive. During the acute phase, there may be groups of tachyzoites that appear to be cysts; however, they are not strongly periodic acid-Schiff positive and have been termed pseudocysts.

## PATHOGENESIS AND SPECTRUM OF DISEASE

As the tachyzoites actively grow, increase in number, and eventually rupture from the cell, they invade adjacent cells. This process creates additional lesions. Once the cysts are formed, the process becomes quiescent, with little or no multiplication and spread. In the immunocompromised or immunodeficient patient, a cyst rupture or primary exposure to the organisms often leads to

**TABLE 50-3** Morphology of *Toxoplasma gondii* Stages Found in Humans

| Stage | Description |
|---|---|
| Tachyzoites<br />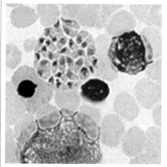 | Tachyzoites are crescent shaped and are 2-3 μm wide by 4-8 μm long. One end tends to be more rounded than the other. Giemsa is stain of choice; cytoplasm stains pale blue, and nucleus stains red and is situated toward broad end of organism. Tachyzoites are usually seen in early, more acute phases of infection. Tachyzoites rapidly multiply in any cell of the intermediate host (many animals and humans) and in nonintestinal epithelial cells of the definitive host (cats). |
| Bradyzoites<br />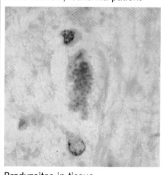<br />Bone marrow, leukemia patient<br />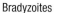<br />Bradyzoites in tissue | Bradyzoites are found within tissue cysts and multiply very slowly; cyst may contain few to hundreds of organisms, and intramuscular cysts may reach 100 μm in size. Although tissue cysts are seen in visceral organs such as lungs, liver, and kidneys, they are more common in brain, eyes, and skeletal and cardiac muscle. |

lesions. The organisms can be disseminated via the lymphatic system and the bloodstream to other tissues.

Toxoplasmosis can be categorized into four groups: (1) acquired in the immunocompetent patient; (2) acquired or reactivated in the immunodeficient patient; (3) congenital; and (4) ocular.

**TABLE 50-4** People at Risk for Severe Toxoplasmosis

| Category | Comments |
|---|---|
| Infants born to mothers who are first exposed to *Toxoplasma* infection several months before or during pregnancy | Mothers who are first exposed to *Toxoplasma* more than 6 months before becoming pregnant are not likely to pass infection to their children |
| Persons with severely weakened immune systems | Infection that occurred at any time during life can reactivate in an immunocompromised individual |

Diagnosis and their interpretations may differ for each clinical category.

### Immunocompetent Individuals

In almost all cases, no clinical symptoms are seen during the acute infection. However, 10% to 20% of these patients with acute infection may develop painless cervical lymphadenopathy and a flulike illness. This presentation is self-limited with symptoms resolving within weeks to months. Acute visceral manifestations are seen in rare cases. The majority of these patients remain asymptomatic or consider they have experienced nothing more than a common cold.

### Immunocompromised Individuals

Infections in the compromised patient can lead to severe complications (Table 50-4). Underlying conditions that may impact the disease outcome include Hodgkin's disease, non-Hodgkin's lymphomas, leukemia, solid tumors, collagen vascular disease, organ transplantation, and AIDS. In the immunocompromised patient, the CNS is primarily involved, but these patients may also have myocarditis or pneumonitis. More than 50% of these patients will show altered mental state, motor impairment, seizures, abnormal reflexes, and other neurologic sequelae. Toxoplasmosis in patients being treated with immunosuppressive drugs may be due to either newly acquired or reactivated latent infection.

In transplant recipients, the disease presentation depends on prior exposure to *T. gondii* by the donor and recipient, the type of organ involved, and the patient's level of immunosuppression. Reactivation of a latent infection or an acute primary infection acquired directly from the transplanted organ can lead to severe disease. Stem cell transplant (SCT) recipients are particularly susceptible to severe toxoplasmosis, primarily attributable to reactivation of a previously acquired latent infection.

Before the use of highly active antiretroviral therapies (HAARTs), *Toxoplasma* encephalitis (TE) was a life-threatening opportunistic infection among patients with AIDS and was usually fatal if not treated. In AIDS patients with reactivated latent infections, psychiatric manifestations of *T. gondii* are seen, including altered mental status (60%) with delusions, auditory hallucinations, and thought disorders. *T. gondii* enhances HIV-1 replication within reservoir host cells and, at the same time, HIV-1 undermines acquired immunity to the parasite, promoting reactivation of chronic toxoplasmosis.

### Congenital Infections

Congenital infection results when the mother acquires a primary infection during pregnancy. The majority of patients remain asymptomatic during the acute infection. However, congenital infections may be severe if the mother becomes infected during the first or second trimester. At birth or soon thereafter, symptoms in these infants may include retinochoroiditis, cerebral calcification, and occasionally hydrocephalus or microcephaly. Because treatment of the mother may reduce the severity of disease in the infant, prompt and accurate diagnosis is mandatory. Many infants who are asymptomatic at birth will subsequently develop symptoms of congenital toxoplasmosis; however, treatment may help prevent subsequent sequelae. Central nervous system involvement may not appear until several years later.

### Ocular Infections

Ocular toxoplasmosis, an important cause of chorioretinitis, may be the result of congenital or acquired infection, acquired infection being more common than congenital infection. Patients with congenital infection may be asymptomatic until the second or third decade; at that point, cysts may rupture with lesions and develop in the eye. Chorioretinitis is characteristically bilateral in patients with congenital infection but is often unilateral in individuals with acute acquired *T. gondii* infection.

## LABORATORY DIAGNOSIS

The most common method of diagnosis for toxoplasmosis is serologic testing for *T. gondii*–specific antibodies. Other procedures include PCR; examination of biopsy specimens, buffy coat cells, or cerebrospinal fluid; or isolation of the organism in tissue culture or in laboratory animals. It is important to remember that many individuals have been exposed to *T. gondii* and may have cysts within the tissues. Recovery of organisms from tissue culture or animal inoculation may be misleading, because the organisms may be isolated but may not be the etiologic agent of disease. However, two situations in which organism detection may be very significant are (1) tachyzoites in smears and/or tissue cultures inoculated from cerebrospinal fluid and (2) tachyzoites in patients with acute pulmonary disease and the demonstration of intracellular and extracellular tachyzoites in Giemsa-stained smears of bronchoalveolar lavage (BAL) fluid.

When laboratory personnel decide to initiate *Toxoplasma*-specific antibody testing or switch to a different antibody detection kit, the user must carefully review the manufacturer's package insert and published literature for information on the sensitivity and specificity rates.

An in-laboratory comparison of kits should be performed, using positive and negative samples confirmed by a toxoplasmosis reference laboratory.

The serologic diagnosis of toxoplasmosis is very complex and has been discussed extensively in the literature (Wilson & McAuley, 2003); a number of additional procedures include enzyme immunoassays, enzyme-linked immunosorbent assays (ELISAs), direct agglutination, an immunosorbent agglutination assay, an indirect immunofluorescence assay (IFA), immunocapture, and immunoblot tests.

## THERAPY

Treatment is recommended for the following conditions: clinically active disease, diagnosed congenital toxoplasmosis in newborns, pregnant women with infection during gestation, patients with chorioretinitis, and disease in symptomatic compromised patients. Therapy is also recommended for preventive or suppressive treatment in HIV-infected persons. The currently recommended drugs work primarily against the actively dividing tachyzoite form of *T. gondii* and do not eradicate encysted organisms (bradyzoites).

The most common drug combination used to treat congenital toxoplasmosis consists of pyrimethamine and a sulfonamide (sulfadiazine is recommended in the United States), plus folinic acid in the form of leucovorin calcium to protect the bone marrow from the toxic effects of pyrimethamine. Spiramycin is recommended for pregnant women with acute toxoplasmosis when fetal infection has not been confirmed in an attempt to prevent transmission of *T. gondii* from the mother to the fetus.

In immunosuppressed persons with toxoplasmosis, the combination of pyrimethamine and sulfadiazine plus leucovorin is the preferred treatment. Clindamycin is a second alternative for use in combination with pyrimethamine and leucovorin in those who cannot tolerate sulfonamides. Because relapse often occurs after toxoplasmosis in HIV-infected patients, maintenance therapy with pyrimethamine plus sulfadiazine or pyrimethamine plus clindamycin is recommended. For prophylaxis to prevent an initial episode of toxoplasmosis in *Toxoplasma*-seropositive persons with CD4+ T-lymphocyte counts of less than 100 cells/mL, trimethoprim-sulfamethoxazole is recommended as the first choice, with alternatives consisting of dapsone plus pyrimethamine or atovaquone with or without pyrimethamine. Leucovorin is given with all regimens, including pyrimethamine. HIV-infected persons who are serologically negative for *Toxoplasma* IgG should be advised to protect themselves from primary infection by eating well-cooked meats and washing their hands after possible soil contact. Cats kept as pets should be fed commercial or well-cooked food, should be kept indoors, and should have their litter box changed each day.

Pyrimethamine and sulfadiazine are often used for persons with ocular disease. Clindamycin, in combination with other antiparasitic medications, is frequently used for the treatment of ocular disease. In addition to antiparasitic drugs, physicians may add corticosteroids to reduce ocular inflammation.

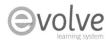 *Visit the Evolve site to complete the review questions.*

---

## CASE STUDY 50-1

A 16-year-old boy presented to the physician with a severe headache and nausea and vomiting. When he arrived at the emergency department he seemed somewhat confused and disoriented. He had chills but no fever. The physician noted that he was wearing swimming trunks under his clothes and upon physical exam had a few bruises on his arms. The young man said he had been staying at his friend's house for several days and while swimming in his friend's pool, he had slipped on the diving board.

### QUESTIONS

1. What are the potential causes for the young man's symptoms?
2. What laboratory tests would be the most useful for quick diagnosis?
3. The physician ruled out bacterial infection as the young man's complete blood count was normal, as was his CT scan result. A spinal tap was completed. Examine the cytospin photograph presented in Figure 50-4. What organism was identified and how should the young man be treated?

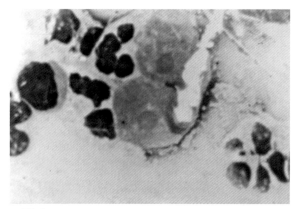

**Figure 50-4** Patient's specimen. (Photo courtesy Dr. Henry Travers, Sioux Falls, SD.)

# BIBLIOGRAPHY

Barratt JL, Harkness J, Marriott D, et al: Importance of nonenteric protozoan infections in immunocompromised people, *Clin Microbiol Rev* 23:795-836, 2010.

Booton C, Carmichael JR, Visvesvara GS et al: Genotyping of *Balamuthia mandrillaris* based on nuclear 18S and mitochondrial 16S rRNA genes, *Am J Trop Med Hyg* 68:65-69, 2003.

Boyer KM, Holfels E, Roizen N, et al: Risk factors for *Toxoplasma gondii* infection in mothers of infants with congenital toxoplasmosis: implications for prenatal management and screening, *Am J Obstet Gynecol* 192:564-571, 2005.

Centers for Disease Control and Prevention: Preventing congenital toxoplasmosis, *MMWR Recommend Rep* 49(RR-2):57-75, 2000.

Centers for Disease Control and Prevention: Guidelines for prevention and treatment of opportunistic infections among HIV-exposed and infected children, *MMWR Recommend Rep* 58(RR-11):1-176, 2009.

Clinical and Laboratory Standards Institute/NCCLS: *Clinical use and interpretation of serologic tests for Toxoplasma gondii; approved guideline*, Wayne, PA, 2004, Clinical and Laboratory Standards Institute.

Cudmore SL, Delgaty KL, Harward-McClelland SF et al: Treatment of infections caused by metronidazole-resistant *Trichomonas vaginalis*, *Clin Microbiol Rev* 17:783-793, 2004.

Dubey JP, Lindsay DS, Speer CAL: Structures of *Toxoplasma gondii* tachyzoites, bradyzoites, and sporozoites and biology and development of tissue cysts, *Clin Microbiol Rev* 11:267-299, 1988.

Garcia LS: *Diagnostic medical parasitology*, ed 5, Washington, DC, 2007, ASM Press.

Garcia LS: *Practical guide to diagnostic parasitology*, ed 2, Washington, DC, 2009, ASM Press.

Jayasekera S, Sissons J, Tucker J et al: Post-mortem culture of *Balamuthia mandrillaris* from the brain and cerebrospinal fluid of a case of granulomatous amoebic meningoencephalitis using human brain microvascular endothelial cells, *J Med Microbiol* 53:1007-1012, 2004.

Kilvington S, Gray T, Dart J et al: *Acanthamoeba* keratitis: the role of domestic tap water contamination in the United Kingdom, *Invest Ophthalmol Vis Sci* 45:165-169, 2004.

Marciano-Cabral F, Cabral G: *Acanthamoeba* spp. as agents of disease in humans, *Clin Microbiol Rev* 16:273-307, 2003.

Schuster FL, Dunnebacke TH, Booton GC et al: Environmental isolation of *Balamuthia mandrillaris* associated with a case of amebic encephalitis, *J Clin Microbiol* 41:3175-3180, 2003.

Schuster FL, Visvesvara GS: Free-living amoebae as opportunistic and non-opportunistic pathogens of humans and animals, *Int J Parasitol* 34:1001-1027, 2004a.

Schuster FL, Visvesvara GS: Opportunistic amoebae: challenges in prophylaxis and treatment, *Drug Resist Update* 7:41-51, 2004b.

Schwebke JR, Burgess D: Trichomoniasis, *Clin Microbiol Rev* 17:794-803, 2004.

Torrey EF, Yolken RH: *Toxoplasma gondii* and schizophrenia, *Emerg Inf Dis* 9:1375-1380, 2003.

Visvesvara GS: Amebic meningoencephalitides and keratitis: challenges in diagnosis and treatment, *Curr Opin Infect Dis* 23:590-594, 2010.

Wilson M, McAuley JB: Clinical use and interpretation of serologic tests for *Toxoplasma gondii*, M36-A, Wayne, PA, 2003, NCCLS.

## OBJECTIVES

1. Describe the distinguishing morphologic characteristics and basic life cycle (vectors, hosts, and stages of infectivity) for each of the parasites listed.
2. Define and identify the following parasitic structures when appropriate: mammillated ovum, gravid, rhabditiform larvae, buccal capsule, esophagus, genital primordia, polar hyaline plugs, copulatory bursa, embryonated egg, cutting plates, and filariform larvae.
3. Describe the diseases and mechanism of pathogenicity including route of transmission for each of the species listed.
4. Differentiate *Ascaris lumbricoides* adult male and female worms.
5. Define and differentiate direct versus indirect life cycle as related to nematodes and the routes of transmission including autoinfection and hyperinfections.
6. Identify and differentiate the characteristic morphologies and eggs for *A. lumbricoides*, *E. vermicularis*, and *T. trichiura*.
7. Compare clinical signs and symptoms, morphologic characteristics, and identification of hookworm's rhabditiform larvae for *Ancylostoma duodenale* and *Necator americanus*.
8. Compare and contrast the morphologic characteristics and identification of the larval forms of *Strongyloides stercoralis*.
9. List the various methods used to diagnosis intestinal nematode infections.
10. Identify the appropriate intestinal nematodes where the following techniques are useful and explain the principle for each including the Baermann concentration method, agar culture, and Harada-Mori filter paper method for the recovery of intestinal nematodes.

---

### PARASITES TO BE CONSIDERED

**Helminths**
*Nematodes*
Intestinal (roundworms)
   *Ascaris lumbricoides*
   *Enterobius vermicularis* (pinworm)
   *Strongyloides stercoralis* (threadworm)
   *Trichostrongylus* spp.
   *Trichuris trichiura* (whipworm)
   *Capillaria philippinensis* (hookworms)
   *Ancylostoma duodenale* (Old World)
   *Necator americanus* (New World)

---

There are more than 60 species of nematodes known to infect humans. *Ascaris lumbricoides,* hookworms (*Ancylostoma duodenale* and *Necator americanus*), and *Trichuris trichiura* are estimated to infect more than 1 billion people. Nematodes are nonsegmented, elongate, cylindrical worms with a well-developed digestive tract and reproductive system. The adult worms have separate sexes, with the male generally smaller than the female. Most nematodes are diagnosed by finding the characteristic eggs in the stool. The infective stage of the nematodes varies with species; for example, transmission may occur through the ingestion of eggs, whereas others burrow through the skin and migrate to the intestine. The nematodes have very diverse life cycles providing different routes of transmission as well as disease symptoms.

## ASCARIS LUMBRICOIDES

### GENERAL CHARACTERISTICS

*Ascaris lumbricoides* is the most common and the largest roundworm. The parasite has a worldwide distribution with higher prevalence in the tropical regions. Eggs are ingested and hatch in the duodenum, penetrate the intestinal wall, and migrate to the hepatic portal circulation. The adult worms live and reproduce in the lumen of the small intestine. The ovum is a thick, oval mammillated (outer protrusions) and embryonated egg. The eggs are passed in the feces and become infective 2 to 6 weeks following deposition, depending on the environment. The general life cycle is outlined in Figure 51-1. *A. lumbricoides* life cycle is classified as an indirect life cycle; transmission is not via a direct route from one host to the next.

### EPIDEMIOLOGY

Geographic distribution is associated with climate and poor sanitation. The eggs of *A. lumbricoides* require a warm humid environment in order for the embryonated ovum to mature and become infective. Infection rates are elevated in poverty-stricken areas that have poor sanitation. Transmission is through the fecal-oral route, usually through the ingestion of eggs on contaminated material. *Ascaris* eggs are capable of survival within harsh environmental conditions, including dry or freezing temperatures.

### PATHOGENESIS AND SPECTRUM OF DISEASE

Many *A. lumbricoides* infections are asymptomatic. The presentation of symptoms correlates with the length of infection, the number of worms present, and the overall health of the host. Intestinal symptoms range from mild to severe intestinal obstruction. Some patients will develop pulmonary symptoms and present with immune-mediated hypersensitivity pneumonia. The worms may cause an immune condition known as Löffler's syndrome characterized by peripheral eosinophilia. See Table 51-1 for a summarized detail of associated diseases.

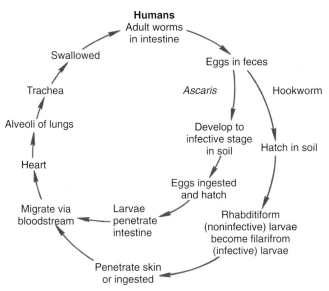

**Figure 51-1** Life cycle of *Ascaris lumbricoides* (indirect life cycle).

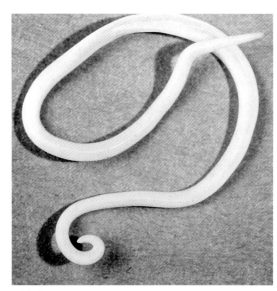

**Figure 51-3** *A. lumbricoides* adult male worm. Note the curved posterior end. (Courtesy Dr. Henry Travers, Sioux Falls, S.D.)

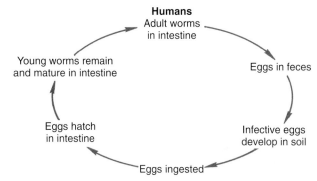

**Figure 51-4** Life cycles of *Enterobius vermicularis* and *Trichuris trichiura* (direct life cycle).

as a result of larval migration during development within the human host.

## THERAPY

Anthelmintic treatment is recommended for all infections. Preferred therapy includes oral albendazole, mebendazole, or pyrantel pamoate.

## PREVENTION

Prevention is managed through proper sanitation and good hygiene.

# ENTEROBIUS VERMICULARIS

## GENERAL CHARACTERISTICS

*Enterobius vermicularis* (pinworm) is distributed worldwide and commonly identified in group settings of children ages 5 to 10 years. The life cycle is considered direct; transmission occurs from an infected host to another individual (Figure 51-4). During the night, the mature

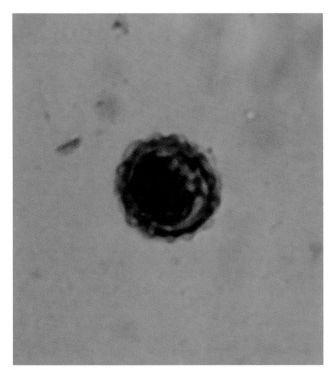

**Figure 51-2** Bile-stained mammillated *A. lumbricoides* ovum. (Courtesy Dr. Henry Travers, Sioux Falls, S.D.)

## LABORATORY DIAGNOSIS

Female worms have an extremely high daily output of eggs, making diagnosis relatively easy through the identification of eggs in feces. The large, broadly oval mammillated ova are typically stained brown from bile (Figure 51-2). Some eggs will be decorticated, or lacking the mammillated outer cover. Infertile eggs may be oval or irregular shaped with a thin shell and containing internal granules. Adult worms may also be identified in feces. The male is smaller (15 to 31 cm) with a curved posterior end (Figure 51-3) and contains three well-characterized lips. Larvae may be found in sputum or gastric aspirates

**TABLE 51-1** Pathogenesis and Spectrum of Associated Diseases

| Organism | Pathogenesis | Mode of Transmission and Spectrum of Disease |
|---|---|---|
| *Ascaris lumbricoides* | Attributed to four main factors:<br>1. Host immune response<br>2. Effects from larval migration<br>3. Mechanical disruption and blockage by worms<br>4. Nutritional deficiency associated with worm burden | Fecal-oral transmission<br>Reinfection possible<br>Children and young adolescents have higher infection rate<br>Pregnant women, unknown impact to unborn fetus<br>Potential tissue damage from migration to lungs, liver, and immune cell infiltration (pneumonitis)<br>Peripheral eosinophilia (Löffler's syndrome)<br>Nutritional impairment in young children<br>Hepatic ascariasis, including hepatic abscesses and obstructive cholangitis<br>Intestinal blockage, pancreatic or bile duct<br>Migration to other tissues may include kidneys, appendix, and pleural cavity |
| *Enterobius vermicularis* | Worm burden may be a single organism to thousands<br>Rarely migration occurs to nearby tissues | Fecal-oral or inhalation<br>Sexual transmission has been reported<br>Reinfection and autoinfection occur<br>Children and women more common than men<br>Mild nocturnal pruritus<br>Migration to vagina, uterus, and fallopian tubes where organisms become encapsulated granulomas<br>Hemorrhagic colitis and inflammation of ileum and colon in homosexual males<br>Uncommon sites include peritoneal cavity, lungs, liver, urinary tract, and natal cleft |
| *Strongyloides stercoralis* | Varies in severity dependent on worm burden and area of body infected<br>Immune response affects symptoms | Direct penetration<br>Chronic and hyperinfection may occur<br>May remain asymptomatic with peripheral eosinophilia<br>Cutaneous:<br>• Pruritus and erythema<br>• "Larva currens" tracks under skin from worm migration<br>Pulmonary:<br>• Asymptomatic to pneumonia<br>• Löffler's syndrome; shortness of breath and pulmonary infiltrates<br>Intestinal:<br>• Diarrhea, constipation, anorexia, and abdominal pain may occur<br>• Damage to mucosa may occur in heavy infections |
| *Trichostrongylus* spp. | Dependent on worm burden | Diarrhea, anorexia, and general malaise<br>Damage to intestinal mucosa may occur, resulting in hemorrhage and tissue desquamation<br>Heavy worm burden may result in anemia and cholecystitis |
| *Trichuris trichiura* | Dependent on worm burden<br>Mechanical damage to intestinal mucosa and allergic reaction<br>Migration of parasites | Fecal-oral transmission<br>Ingestion of embryonated eggs<br>Asymptomatic to mild symptoms associated with low worm burden<br>Heavy infections may result in hemorrhage, weight loss, abdominal pain, blood-tinged stools, and diarrhea<br>Rectal prolapse and hypochromic anemia in repeated heavy infections in children<br>Inflammation of mucosa |
| *Capillaria philippinensis* | Dependent on worm burden | Fecal-oral transmission<br>Ingestion of larvae-infected seafood such as fish, crab, shrimp, and snails<br>Malabsorption, fluid loss, and associated loss of electrolytes<br>Extended infections can result in organ failure and death |

**TABLE 51-1** Pathogenesis and Spectrum of Disease—cont'd

| Organism | Pathogenesis | Mode of Transmission and Spectrum of Disease |
|---|---|---|
| **Hookworms:** **A. duodenale** **N. americanus** | Vary according to life cycle phase and worm burden<br>Production of proteins that suppress host immune response<br>Hyaluronidase: facilitates digestion of connective tissue and penetration of epidermis and dermis<br>Migration of larvae to lungs<br>Mechanical: attachment, feeding, and anticoagulation production | Direct penetration<br>Mild to severe pruritus and potential secondary infections<br>Ground itch: Development of vesicles resulting from erythematous papular rash<br>Pneumonitis: decreased sensitization as compared to *A. lumbricoides* and *S. stercoralis.*<br>Gastrointestinal:<br>• Tissue damage at site of attachment<br>• Blood loss, anemia<br>• Acute gastrointestinal phase demonstrates increased eosinophilia<br>• Increased worm burden may result in death, particularly in young children |
| ***Ancylostoma duodenale*** | Period of arrested development | May be associated with vertical transmission and congenital infections<br>Eosinophilia peaks in approximately 1 month in gastrointestinal phase |
| ***Necator americanus*** | Proteolytic enzymes that degrade collagen, fibronectin, laminin, and elastin | Skin-associated symptoms as described for hookworms<br>Eosinophilia peaks in approximately 2 months in gastrointestinal phase |

female worm migrates out of the anus of the infected host and lays eggs in the perianal region. The embryonated eggs will mature and a third-stage larva stage develops, resulting in infectivity within hours. Transmission occurs by ingestion or inhalation of eggs. Reinfection may also occur when the eggs hatch and larvae return to the intestine where they mature.

## EPIDEMIOLOGY

Pinworm is more prevalent in school-age children up to about 14 years of age. Infections are associated with institutional crowding and are familial. Transmission is also associated with an increased rate of reinfection within a group or autoinfection from hatched larvae.

## PATHOGENESIS AND SPECTRUM OF DISEASE

Infections with *E. vermicularis* are typically asymptomatic. The most common complaint is perianal pruritus (itching) and resultant restless sleep. Occasionally, the parasite may migrate to other nearby tissues, causing pelvic, cervical, or peritoneal granulomas. See Table 51-1 for a summarized detail of associated diseases.

## LABORATORY DIAGNOSIS

Diagnosis is typically by microscopic identification of the characteristic flat-sided ovum (Figure 51-5). The eggs are collected using a sticky paddle or cellophane tape pressed against the perianal region. Eggs are not typically identified in feces, although they may occasionally be found in a stool specimen. Although adult pinworms may be visible, they can be easily confused with small pieces of thread. The female worm measures 8 to 13 mm long with a pointed "pin" shaped tail. In gravid females, almost the entire body will be filled with eggs (Figure 51-6). The males measure only 2 to 5 mm in length, die following fertilization, and may be passed in feces.

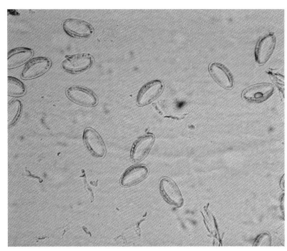

**Figure 51-5** *Enterobius vermicularis* eggs (cellophane [Scotch] tape preparation).

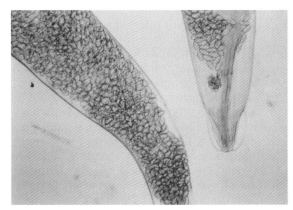

**Figure 51-6** *Enterobius vermicularis* gravid female. (Courtesy Dr. Henry Travers, Sioux Falls, S.D.)

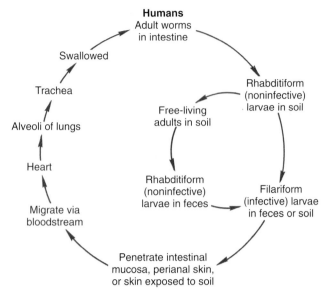

**Figure 51-7** *Strongyloides stercoralis* life cycle.

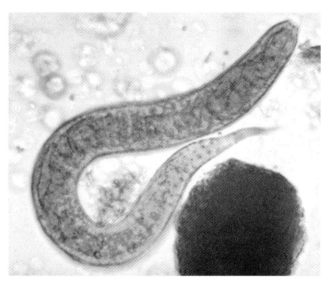

**Figure 51-8** *Strongyloides stercoralis* rhabditiform larva, iodine stain.

## THERAPY

Anthelmintic therapy is generally effective with one of the following agents: albendazole, mebendazole, pyrantel pamoate, or ivermectin.

## PREVENTION

Regular good personal hygiene is the major factor for prevention of continued reinfection and autoinfection.

# STRONGYLOIDES STERCORALIS

## GENERAL CHARACTERISTICS

Infection with *Strongyloides stercoralis* is less common than other intestinal nematodes. The organism is endemic in the tropics and subtropical regions of Asia, Latin America, and Africa. A limited geographic distribution exists in the United States and Europe.

*S. stercoralis*, commonly referred to as the threadworm, may inhabit the intestine or exist as a free-living organism in the soil. The life cycle can be classified as direct, indirect (free-living phase), or autoinfective (Figure 51-7). The filariform (infective larvae) penetrate the skin and migrate via the circulatory system to the heart and lungs. The organism enters the bronchial tree and then is swallowed, where it lives in the digestive tract and matures into an adult worm. In the intestine the filariform larvae may also penetrate the mucosa, resulting in autoinfection. The female worm produces eggs by parthenogenesis (a form of asexual reproduction where growth and development occur without fertilization), because parasitic adult male worms are nonexistent. Within the indirect life cycle, the rhabditiform (noninfective) larvae develop into mature males and egg-producing females (Figure 51-8). The free-living life cycle may revert to the production of infective larvae at any time.

## EPIDEMIOLOGY

*S. stercoralis* is transmitted via direct penetration in endemic areas. Person-to-person transmission occurs within institutionalized groups, in day care centers, and among homosexual men.

## PATHOGENESIS AND SPECTRUM OF DISEASE

Infections may be asymptomatic or consist of a variety of disseminated strongyloidiasis syndromes. Reinfection is more commonly associated with immunocompromised patients. Acute infections may develop a localized pruritic, erythematous papular rash. Some patients develop a macropapular or urticarial (red and raised) rash on the buttocks, perineum, and thighs. The migration of larvae may cause epigastric pain, nausea, diarrhea, and blood loss. Hyperinfection, an increased worm burden within the lungs and intestines, may occur. Disseminated infections may also result in larvae within the central nervous system, kidneys, and liver.

A second species, *Strongyloides fuelleborni*, a primate parasite, has been isolated from humans in Africa and causes a severe life-threatening condition called "swollen belly syndrome." See Table 51-1 for a summarized detail of associated diseases.

## LABORATORY DIAGNOSIS

The rhabditiform larva is the primary diagnostic stage for strongyloidiasis in humans through microscopic examination of stool. The larvae are 250 to 300 μm long with a short buccal capsule, a large bulb on the esophagus, and a prominent genital primordium (Figure 51-9). The filariform larvae are larger (up to 500 μm) and have a notched tail with an esophageal to intestinal ratio of 1 : 1. The eggs, which are rarely identified, are segmented with a thin shell.

*S. stercoralis* larvae are the most common found in human stool specimens. Depending on the fecal transit time though the intestine and the patient's condition,

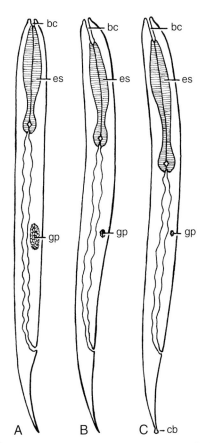

**Figure 51-9** Rhabditiform larvae. **A,** *Strongyloides.* **B,** Hookworm. **C,** *Trichostrongylus. bc,* Buccal cavity; *cb,* beadlike swelling of caudal tip; *es,* esophagus; *gp,* genital primordia. (Illustration by Nobuko Kitamura.)

both rhabditiform and rare filariform may be present. If stool examination is delayed, embryonated ova may be present. Parasite recovery from stool may be enhanced by the Baermann funnel technique. The basic method is to wrap the sample in a paper tissue or cloth and submerge it in a funnel filled with water. The nematodes will clump and sink to the bottom of the funnel where they can be recovered.

Culture of feces for larvae is useful to (1) reveal the presence of parasites when they are too scant to be detected by concentration methods; (2) distinguish whether the infection is due to *S. stercoralis* or hookworm based on rhabditiform larval morphology by allowing hookworm egg hatching to occur, releasing first-stage larvae; and (3) allow development of larvae into the filariform stage for further differentiation. In the agar culture method, a stool sample is placed on a nutrient agar dish and incubated for 48 hours. The larvae crawl over the top of the agar, leaving tracks in the bacterial growth. The modified Harada-Mori filter paper technique is the recommended culture method. This test uses filter paper smeared with fecal material inserted into a test tube containing distilled water. The capillary flow of water up through the filter paper provides soaking of the material. The capillary action provides a mechanism to move the soluble elements to the top of the paper,

capturing hatching ova and developing larvae. Because of low recovery of larvae, repeated examinations of stool may be required.

Serologic testing is indicated when infection is suspected and the organism cannot be isolated by repeated stool examinations, string test, or duodenal aspirates. The Centers for Disease Control and Prevention offers a highly sensitive (>95%) cross-reacting enzyme-linked immunosorbent assay (ELISA) with other parasites, including filaria, hookworm, Paragonimus, and Echinococcus.

Although not available in routine laboratories, real-time polymerase chain reaction (PCR) methods have been developed that amplify the small subunit of the rRNA gene. The assay is used to detect DNA in fecal samples and has a demonstrated sensitivity and specificity of 100%. A high throughput multiplex assay has also been developed that includes primer and probe pairs for *S. stercoralis* as well as other intestinal nematodes and protozoa.

Additional specimens such as sputum, body fluids, and tissues may be used for the diagnosis of hyperinfections.

## THERAPY

Ivermectin is the recommended treatment for uncomplicated infections. Albendazole is an alternative, but has not proven to be as effective. Hyperinfection and disseminated conditions require anthelmintic therapy in combination with broad-spectrum antibiotics to prevent secondary bacterial enteric infections. In addition, patients taking immunosuppressive medications should discontinue use during infection and treatment. Follow-up examinations are indicated and treatment should be reinstituted if larvae are identified within 2 weeks following cessation of therapy.

## PREVENTION

Immunocompromised individuals and patients taking immunosuppressive medications should avoid contaminated beaches and other areas.

# *TRICHOSTRONGYLUS* SPP.

## GENERAL CHARACTERISTICS

Although commonly found in mammals and birds worldwide, approximately 10 different species of *Trichostrongylus* have been found in human infections. The worms are small and live in the mucosa of the small intestine. The adult worm has no visible buccal capsule.

## EPIDEMIOLOGY

Human infections have been identified in areas within Asia and Africa. Additionally, approximately 70% of the human population is infected in southwest Iran and a village in Egypt. Infection in humans is acquired by ingestion of plant material contaminated with larvae.

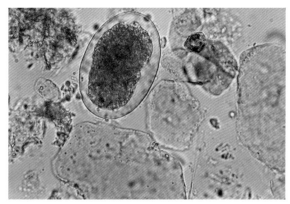

**Figure 51-10** *Trichostrongylus* sp. egg. (Courtesy Dr. Henry Travers, Sioux Falls, S.D.)

## PATHOGENESIS AND SPECTRUM OF DISEASE

Following ingestion of the larvae, the larvae mature and migrate through the lungs. Symptoms are related to the worm burden and the amount of damage within the intestine. See Table 51-1 for a summarized detail of associated diseases.

## LABORATORY DIAGNOSIS

Laboratory diagnosis includes identification of eggs or hatched larvae in the stool. The eggs are oval and resemble hookworm eggs except they are slightly longer and more pointed (Figure 51-10). Larvae should be differentiated from hookworm and *S. stercoralis* (see Figure 51-9).

## THERAPY

Anthelmintic agents are recommended including mebendazole and pyrantel pamoate. Albendazole is the treatment of choice.

## PREVENTION

Thorough washing of plant material, including cultivated vegetables, before handling or ingestion is recommended.

# TRICHURIS TRICHIURA

## GENERAL CHARACTERISTICS

*Trichuris trichiura*, whipworm, has a worldwide distribution. Unlike other intestinal nematodes discussed in this chapter, there is no tissue migration phase within the life cycle of *T. trichiura*.

## EPIDEMIOLOGY

*Trichuris trichiura* is typically found in moist, warm climates around the world. Infections are relatively common in Asia, Africa, and South America, with some cases identified in the southeastern United States. Often the nematode is identified in co-infections along with *A. lumbricoides*.

Poor hygiene is associated with increased transmission, especially in children. Humans are infected by ingestion of the eggs. Larvae are released in the intestine where they mature into adult worms. Eggs are then passed in the feces and deposited in the soil. The eggs require a warm, moist environment for embryonation in order to become infective to another host.

## PATHOGENESIS AND SPECTRUM OF DISEASE

Pathogenesis and severity of the disease are closely related to the worm burden. The lack of symptoms is related to the life cycle that does not include a tissue migration stage, as is seen in other nematode infections. Infections range from mild, very low worm burden, to severe infections with bleeding and weight loss in heavy worm infestations. The characteristic whiplike worm buries its threadlike anterior into the intestinal mucosa and feeds on tissue secretions, causing an inflammatory reaction and peripheral eosinophilia. See Table 51-1 for a summarized detail of associated diseases.

## LABORATORY DIAGNOSIS

Diagnosis is typically from the identification of eggs and rarely the adult worm within the feces. An adult female may produce up to 20,000 eggs per day. However, during the lengthy development of mature worms within the intestine, there may be no shedding of eggs for up to 3 months. Eggs appear as brown barrel-shaped structures. They are unembryonated and contain a thick wall with hyaline polar plugs at each end (Figure 51-11). The adult female worm ranges in size from 35 to 50 mm and demonstrates a gradually increasing width from anterior to posterior, with a straight end (Figure 51-12). The adult male ranges in size from 30 to 45 mm and demonstrates the same broadening morphology with a coiled posterior end.

## THERAPY

Therapy may or may not be indicated, dependent on the nutritional status of the host, the length of infection, and the level of worm burden. Anthelmintics such as albendazole are recommended when necessary.

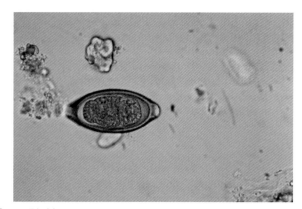

**Figure 51-11** *Trichuris trichiura* egg. Note the clearly evident polar hyaline plugs. (Courtesy Dr. Henry Travers, Sioux Falls, S.D.)

## PREVENTION

Prevention includes practicing proper hygiene and sanitation as well as the disposal of dirt or soil contaminated with feces.

# CAPILLARIA PHILIPPINENSIS

## GENERAL CHARACTERISTICS

*Capillaria philippinensis* was first recognized as a human parasite in the late 1960s and now has a well-known wide distribution. This parasite is prevalent in the northern Philippines, hence the name *C. philippinensis*, and has also been found in Thailand, Japan, Taiwan, Iran, and Egypt. The parasite reproduces in the gut, resulting in autoinfection and hyperinfection very similar to that observed in *S. stercoralis*.

## EPIDEMIOLOGY

Human infection is thought to occur from the ingestion of uncooked fish harboring infective larvae. In the Philippines, where the organism is prevalent, the people ingest a large spectrum of raw seafood, including fish, shrimp, crabs, and snails. In addition, defecation in the fields or water sources where snails, shrimp, and crabs are collected is common. The life cycle of the parasite is currently not fully understood.

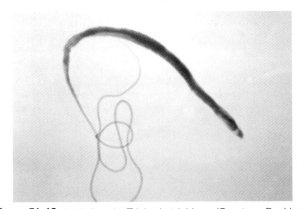

**Figure 51-12** Adult female *Trichuris trichiura*. (Courtesy Dr. Henry Travers, Sioux Falls, S.D.)

## PATHOGENESIS AND SPECTRUM OF DISEASE

Symptoms vary with the level of worm burden. The larvae are ingested and reside in the small intestine where they burrow into the mucosa. Because of the mechanical insertion into the intestinal wall, patients lose weight rapidly as a result of malabsorption and fluid loss. Long-term infections lasting weeks to months may result in death attributable to a severe loss of electrolytes, particularly potassium (hypokalemia), and associated organ failure. See Table 51-1 for a summarized detail of associated diseases.

## LABORATORY DIAGNOSIS

Diagnosis is typically from the identification of eggs, adult worms, or larvae in stool specimens. The eggs resemble those produced by *T. trichiura*. They are somewhat smaller with a thick, striated shell and less prominent polar plugs. Female worms produce the characteristic thick-shelled eggs as well as thin-shelled and free larvae.

## THERAPY

Anthelmintic agents including albendazole and mebendazole are recommended.

## PREVENTION

Adequate preparation and cooking of seafood, including fish, snails, crabs, and shrimp in endemic areas, are encouraged.

# HOOKWORMS

Hookworms are known to have a worldwide distribution with two species known to infect humans, *Ancylostoma duodenale* (Figure 51-13) and *Necator americanus* (Figure 51-14). They are the second most common helmintic infection reported in humans. The eggs and rhabditiform larvae of the two species are indistinguishable. Differentiation of the species is based on the morphology of the buccal capsule and the adult male copulatory bursa (see Figure 51-14, *B*).

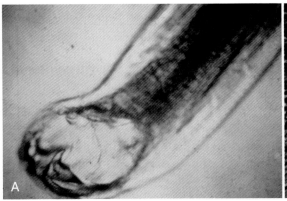
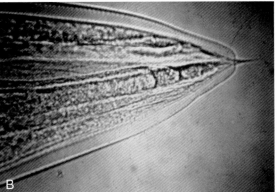

**Figure 51-13 A,** *Ancylostoma duodenale* head. **B,** Tail; note the appearance of the pointed tail. (Courtesy Dr. Henry Travers, Sioux Falls, S.D.)

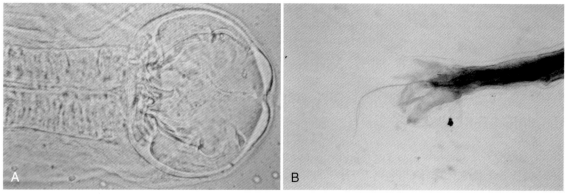

**Figure 51-14 A,** *Necator americanus* head; note the clearly evident rounded cutting plates protruding from the head. **B,** Copulatory bursa. (Courtesy Dr. Henry Travers, Sioux Falls, S.D.)

The parasites, infective filariform larvae, penetrate the skin and enter the circulation where the larvae are capable of breaking through the capillaries and entering the lungs of the host. The larvae migrate up the bronchial tree, over the epiglottis, and are swallowed. Upon entering the digestive system, the hookworms attach to the mucosa of the small intestine. Here they secrete anticoagulants and ingest blood as their source of nourishment. The worms mature and eggs are passed in the feces and deposited in soil where they mature into rhabditiform larvae. The noninfective rhabditiform larvae will then mature into filariform.

## EPIDEMIOLOGY

Hookworms are found in areas with moist, warm soil capable of supporting the life cycle of the parasite. Transmission is generally through direct skin penetration by filariform larvae.

## ANCYLOSTOMA DUODENALE

### GENERAL CHARACTERISTICS

*A. duodenale,* Old World hookworm, is prevalent in southern Europe, northern Africa, Southeast Asia, and South America. The adult male tends to be larger than the adult male of *N. americanus.* They attach to the intestinal mucosa by well-developed mouthparts, especially teeth (see Figure 51-13).

### PATHOGENESIS AND SPECTRUM OF DISEASE

*A. duodenale* is capable of maturation within the intestine without migrating through the lungs of the host. See Table 51-1 for a summarized detail of associated diseases.

## NECATOR AMERICANUS

### GENERAL CHARACTERISTICS

*N. americanus,* New World hookworm, is prevalent in Africa, Southeast Asia, and South and Central America as well as the southeastern United States. They attach to

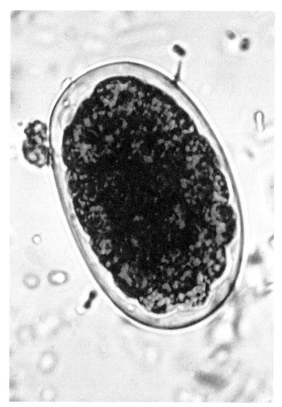

**Figure 51-15** Hookworm egg, iodine stain.

the intestinal mucosa by well-developed cutting plates (see Figure 51-14, *A*).

### PATHOGENESIS AND SPECTRUM OF DISEASE

See Table 51-1 for a summarized detail of associated diseases.

### LABORATORY DIAGNOSIS

Hookworms are typically diagnosed by the presence of eggs or rhabditiform larvae found in stool specimens. The eggs and larvae of the two species are indistinguishable. The eggs are oval and thin-shelled and contain a clearly visible four- to eight-cell stage embryo. There is a

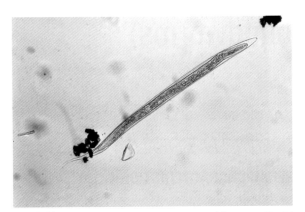

**Figure 51-16** Hookworm rhabditiform larvae. (Courtesy Dr. Henry Travers, Sioux Falls, S.D.)

characteristic clear space between the shell and the developing embryo (see Figure 51-14). Recovery and identification of eggs on direct smear or from concentration methods is recommended. Eggs may appear distorted on permanently stained smears. The rhabditiform larvae are typically 250 to 300 µm with a long buccal capsule and an inconspicuous genital primoridum (Figures 51-15 and 51-16). The larger filariform larvae are approximately 500 µm, with a pointed tail and a esophageal to intestinal ratio of 1:4. Both the rhabditiform and filariform larvae must be differentiated from *S. stercoralis.*

Fresh stool stored at room temperature may result in continued maturation and hatching of larvae. Larvae may be cultured according to the Harada-Mori method previously described within this chapter.

## THERAPY

Anthelmintic agents including albendazole, mebendazole, and pyrantel pamoate are indicated. However, as a result of variation in species and geographic distribution, some agents may not be effective in a specific population of parasites, and regional recommendations should be followed because of potential drug tolerance or resistance.

## PREVENTION

Avoid contaminated soil and beaches. Wear appropriate footwear such as enclosed shoes in potentially contaminated areas.

As a result of the immunosuppressive activity associated with the production of hookworm proteins, vaccination may only be partially effective. Currently no preventive vaccine exists. However, a protein, ASP-2, secreted by infective larvae of *N. americanus* is being investigated as a potential recombinant vaccine (see clinicaltrials.gov).

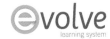 *Visit the Evolve site to complete the review questions.*

## CASE STUDY 51-1

A 56-year-old man presented to the emergency department with fever, chest discomfort, and a nonproductive cough. A complete blood count indicated a mild elevation in the level of eosinophils with no additional abnormalities. The patient's chest x-ray demonstrated patchy lobular infiltration. The patient was subsequently hospitalized for further evaluation. Three stool samples were collected over a period of 3 days with no evidence of parasitic infection. The patient died the following day.

### QUESTIONS

1. What, if any, additional laboratory tests may have been helpful to improve the diagnosis and evaluation of the patient's condition?
2. The autopsy revealed liver damage associated with deposition of the inclusions identified in Figure 51-17. Based on the morphologic appearance and the patient's initial symptoms, what is the likely parasite implicated in the patient's death?

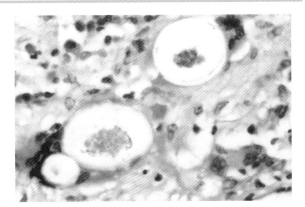

**Figure 51-17** Nematode eggs imbedded in liver tissue. (Courtesy Dr. Henry Travers, Sioux Falls, S.D.)

## BIBLIOGRAPHY

Garcia LS: *Diagnostic medical parasitology,* ed 5, Washington, DC, 2007, ASM Press.
Genta RM: Predictive value of an enzyme-linked immunosorbent assay (ELISA) for the serodiagnosis of strongyloides, *Am J Clin Pathol* 89:391-394, 1988.
Goncalves MLC, Araujo A, Ferreira LF: Human intestinal parasites in the past: new findings and a review, *Mem Inst Oswaldo Cruz* 98:21041-21210, 2003.
Mandell GL, Bennett JE, Dolin R, editors: *Principles and practice of infectious diseases,* ed 7, New York, 2010, Churchill Livingstone.
Taniuchi M, Verweij JJ, Noor Z, et al: High throughput multiplex PCR and probe-based detection with Luminex beads for seven intestinal parasites, *Am J Trop Med Hyg* 84:332-337, 2011.

## OBJECTIVES

1. Describe the distinguishing morphologic characteristics and basic life cycle (vectors, hosts, and stages of infectivity) for each of the parasites listed.
2. Describe the diseases and mechanism of pathogenicity, including route of transmission for each of the species listed.
3. Describe the life cycle of *Trichinella spiralis* in humans and swine, including the infectious form and location of adult worms.
4. Describe trichinosis and disease progression in humans, including body sites affected, peripheral blood presentation, severity of disease, and prognosis.
5. List the various methods used to diagnose tissue nematode infections.
6. Explain the diagnosis and recommended treatment for dracunculosis.
7. Define and differentiate visceral larva migrans, ocular larva migrans, and cutaneous larva migrans.
8. Correlate patient signs and symptoms and route of transmission with the correct organisms described in this chapter.

---

**PARASITES TO BE CONSIDERED**

**Helminths**
*Nematodes (Roundworms)*
Tissue
    *Trichinella spiralis*
    Visceral larva migrans (*Toxocara canis* or *Toxocara cati*)
    Ocular larva migrans (*Toxocara canis* or *Toxocara cati*)
    Cutaneous larva migrans (*Ancylostoma braziliense* or *Ancylostoma caninum*)
    *Dracunculus medinensis*
    *Parastrongylus (Angiostrongylus) cantonensis*
    *Parastrongylus (Angiostrongylus) costaricensis*
    *Gnathostoma spinigerum* (16)

---

Tissue nematodes have life cycles similar to those of intestinal nematodes, consisting of five distinct stages including adult male and female worms and four larval stages. These organisms are distributed worldwide, predominantly in the tropics and subtropics. The organisms are transmitted by three routes: biting and subsequent blood-feeding arthropods (filarial worms), as discussed in Chapter 53; ingestion of small freshwater crustaceans; and ingestion of contaminated meat. In most cases, adult worms do not multiply and develop within the human host. Clinical symptoms are dependent on the number of infecting parasites, the tissue invaded, and the host's general health and immune response. Diagnosis is typically by the microscopic visualization of the organisms in tissue when appropriate.

## TRICHINELLA SPIRALIS

### GENERAL CHARACTERISTICS

The family Trichinellidae contains 11 recognized species including *Trichinella spiralis, Trichinella nativa, Trichinella nelsoni, T. murrelli, T. papuae, T. zimbabwensis, T. pseudospiralis,* and *T. britovi,* all capable of causing trichinosis. However, *T. spiralis* is the most common human pathogen. The organism is unique in comparison to other helminths in that all stages of development, including the adult and larval stages, occur within a single host.

### EPIDEMIOLOGY

*Trichinella* occurs worldwide with the cycle maintained in several different mammalian species. The mammal serves as the definitive host for the adult worm and the intermediate host for the encysted larvae. Humans acquire the infection by eating undercooked meat that contains the infective encysted larvae. Although this is typically transmitted in pork, human cases have been associated with ingestion of bear, walrus, horsemeat, and other mammals.

The encysted larvae are ingested. When the undercooked meat is digested in the stomach, the larvae are resistant to the gastric pH and pass to the intestine, where they invade the mucosa. In about 1.5 days, the larvae mature and mate, and the female worm begins to release motile larvae. These larvae then migrate to the lymphatic system or mesenteric venules and become distributed throughout the body. The larvae then deposit in the striated muscle tissue, where they can continue development, coil, and encyst, becoming infective. The larvae encyst in the active striated muscle including the diaphragm, larynx, tongue, jaws, neck, ribs, biceps, and gastrocnemius. The generalized life cycle is depicted in Figure 52-1. The larvae may remain viable within the cyst for several years. The larvae eventually die and the encysted capsules become calcified.

### PATHOGENESIS AND SPECTRUM OF DISEASE

Trichinosis is a disease of the muscle caused by infection with the encysted larval form of *Trichinella* spp. (Figure 52-2). The adult stages reside in the human intestine. The disease ranges from mild to severe dependent on the number of parasites present. The intestinal stage lasts approximately 1 week and typically includes mild symptoms of nausea, abdominal discomfort, diarrhea, and/or constipation. Diarrhea may last as long as 14 weeks with no apparent muscle involvement. The migration of the larvae results in an intense inflammatory response causing periorbital edema, fever, muscle pain or

**Humans**
Ingestion of undercooked pork
containing encysted larvae

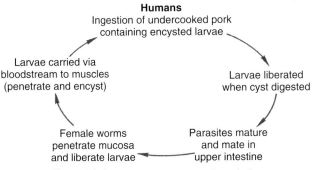

Larvae carried via
bloodstream to muscles
(penetrate and encyst)

Larvae liberated
when cyst digested

Female worms
penetrate mucosa
and liberate larvae

Parasites mature
and mate in
upper intestine

**Figure 52-1** Life cycle of *Trichinella spiralis*.

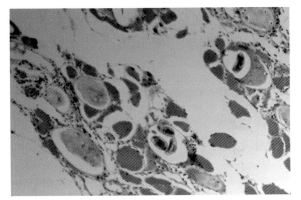

**Figure 52-2** Trichinosis. Encysted larvae within tissue. (Courtesy Dr. Henry Travers, Sioux Falls, S.D.)

tenderness, headache, and myalgia. A marked peripheral eosinophilia is often present. If the parasitic infection is low, eosinophilia may be the only diagnostic sign evident. Occasionally, splinter hemorrhages may be present below the nails.

In addition to the typical infection of the active striated muscle as previously indicated, occasionally larvae will migrate into the brain, meninges, and myocardium. However, the larvae will not encyst in these tissues. Brain and meningeal infections will result in neurologic symptoms, and infection of the myocardium may result in myocarditis and dysrhythmias leading to sudden death.

## LABORATORY DIAGNOSIS

Diagnosis may be difficult, because the symptoms may resemble a variety of flulike illnesses. A thorough patient history is required to assist the physician in diagnosing the condition in a timely fashion. Identification of encysted larvae through muscle biopsy provides definitive diagnosis. However, based on location, some tissues may be difficult to access and therefore the condition may not be diagnosed until the postmortem examination. Histologic examination of formalin-fixed or paraffin-imbedded tissue may be used to visualize encysted larvae. Occasionally, dependent on the length of infection, calcified larvae may be seen in x-rays.

Serologic diagnosis is sufficient in most cases. Patients will present with a specific antibody response in 3 to 5 weeks following acute illness. A negative serologic test

followed by a positive seroconversion is considered definitive diagnosis.

Molecular species–specific polymerase chain reaction (PCR) has been developed. Various techniques including RFLP (restriction fragment length polymorphism) and RAPD (rapid amplification of polymorphic DNA) have been investigated. Currently, these methods are predominantly used in animal epidemiologic studies and have not been implemented within the diagnostic laboratory.

## THERAPY

Thiabendazole is used during the intestinal phase to reduce the number of potentially infective larvae, and although the encysted larvae cannot be removed, albendazole is used to limit the continued pathologic development of the organism. Supportive measures including analgesics and steroids may be administered to lessen the effects of the generalized inflammatory response.

## PREVENTION

Most effective prevention relies on eating only thoroughly cooked meat as well as maintaining good animal husbandry for domestic swine.

## *TOXOCARA CANIS* (VISCERAL LARVA MIGRANS) AND *TOXOCARA CATI* (OCULAR LARVA MIGRANS)

### GENERAL CHARACTERISTICS

*Toxocara canis* (intestinal ascarid of dogs) and *Toxocara cati* (intestinal ascarid of cats) are the cause of a human syndrome resulting from larval migration within the host.

### EPIDEMIOLOGY

Toxocariasis is a zoonotic disease with worldwide distribution. Humans become infected with the accidental ingestion of eggs (Figure 52-3). The definitive hosts, dogs (*T. canis*) and cats (*T. cati*), pass the larvae transplacentally or lactogenically to their offspring and pass unembryonated eggs in the feces. The eggs mature in 10 to 20 days, and then become infective. Once the eggs are ingested, the larvae are released in the small intestine, penetrate the mucosa, and migrate to the liver, lungs, or other body sites. The larvae migrate up the respiratory tract and are swallowed, returning to the intestinal tract where they mature into adult worms. The adult worms are unable to mature in a human host and therefore wander throughout the body causing the migratory syndromes.

### PATHOGENESIS AND SPECTRUM OF DISEASE

Typically the infections are mild but may be severe. Severe life-threatening infections occur when there is involvement in the heart, brain, or other vital organs.

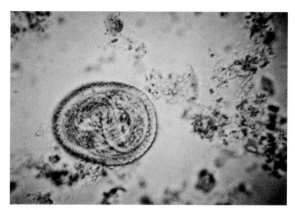

**Figure 52-3** *Toxocara canis* egg. Note the rough appearance on the outer surface of the egg. The egg also contains an infectious L2 larvae. (Courtesy Dr. Henry Travers, Sioux Falls, S.D.)

Disease is frequently found in young children and may persist for long periods with minimal pathologic manifestations. Larvae that remain in the liver or lungs may become encapsulated in fibrous tissue. Visceral (tissue) larva migrans (VLM) may result in a high degree of eosinophilia; however, this may be absent in ocular larva migrans (OLM). Symptoms may include fever, hepatomegaly, hyperglobulinemia, pulmonary infiltration, cough, neurologic symptoms, and endophthalmitis. OLM may result in the development of a granulomatous reaction in the retina of the eye.

## LABORATORY DIAGNOSIS

Toxocariasis must be differentiated from other migratory helmintic diseases including *A. lumbricoides*, *S. stercoralis*, and *Trichinella* spp. A history of exposure to dogs and cats is of importance when considering an infection with *Toxocara* spp. Because humans are an insufficient host for completion of the organism's life cycle, eggs are not passed in the stool. Diagnosis typically requires biopsy of tissue.

Serologic diagnosis has proven effective, particularly in OLM. Aqueous humor–elevated antibody titer specific for *Toxocara* spp., in comparison to serum levels, is considered diagnostic. Although serologic testing has been useful, it is important to note that antibody titers may vary depending on the location of the infection. A serum titer of 1:8 is considered significant for OLM; 1:32 is significant for VLM.

## THERAPY

Effective therapy depends on the location of infection but several anthelmintic medications have been used including thiabendazole, ivermectin, albendazole, and diethylcarbamazine. Antiinflammatory medications including corticosteroids may be used to reduce the pathology associated with inflammation. Photocoagulation has been used to treat OLM. The prognosis is good, even in cases of OLM, with prompt diagnosis and proper treatment.

## PREVENTION

Small children should be kept out of sandboxes and playgrounds frequented by dogs and cats. Sandboxes should be covered when not in use. Encouraging regular hand washing and teaching children to keep dirt out of their mouths will decrease the potential for infection. In addition, regular deworming of dogs and cats will reduce the spread of infective eggs.

# ANCYLOSTOMA BRAZILIENSE OR ANCYLOSTOMA CANINUM (CUTANEOUS LARVA MIGRANS)

## GENERAL CHARACTERISTICS

*Ancylostoma braziliense* and *Anycylostoma caninum* are common hookworms of dogs and cats. The parasites penetrate the skin and cause cutaneous larva migrans (CLM), also referred to as creeping eruption.

## EPIDEMIOLOGY

The organisms are found in warm climates within the Southeastern United States. Dogs and cats are the natural definitive host for *Ancylostoma* spp. The infective larvae penetrate the skin of the host and migrate in the circulation. The adult worms reside in the intestine. The eggs are shed in the feces of dogs and cats. The eggs undergo maturation in moist, sandy soil in areas protected from desiccation, such as under shady trees and houses. Children are often infected when playing in sandboxes that have been contaminated with dog and cat feces.

## PATHOGENESIS AND SPECTRUM OF DISEASE

The infective larvae penetrate the skin of the human host and migrate through the subcutaneous tissue. The host develops pruritic papules at the site of penetration, followed by serpiginous, vesicular, elevated linear tracks. The larvae will migrate several millimeters each day, forming these continued tracks. The area surrounding the tracks becomes inflamed with marked edema. The patient may present with a peripheral eosinophilia. Infection is typically self-limiting. As the larvae migrate, the host may scratch and scar the tissue, subjecting the host to potential secondary bacterial infections. The signs and symptoms resemble those of infection with similar insect larvae, *Strongyloides stercoralis*, and other animal hookworms.

Systemic involvement is rare; however, cases of pneumonitis resulting from larvae migration into the lungs have been identified. In addition, gastrointestinal discomfort including abdominal pain, diarrhea, and weight loss has been associated with *Ancylostoma* spp. infections. This condition is referred to as eosinophilic enteritis.

See Table 52-1 for a summarized detail of associated diseases.

**TABLE 52-1** Pathogenesis and Spectrum of Associated Diseases

| Organism | Pathogenesis | Mode of Transmission and Spectrum of Disease |
|---|---|---|
| **Tissue nematodes** | Attributed to three main factors:<br>1. **Host** immune response<br>2. Parasitic burden<br>3. General overall health of host | |
| *Trichinella* spp. | Worm burden may be small to several hundred<br>Migration and deposition of larvae in tissue depends on tissue involved in infection | Ingestion of poorly cooked meat, particularly domestic swine, but may be found in several mammalian species including bear, walrus, horse |
| *Toxocara canis* and *Toxocara cati* | Migration in host tissue and immune response | Accidental ingestion of eggs<br>Mild to severe disease dependent on tissue |
| *Ancylostoma braziliense* or *A. caninum* | Migration, inflammation, and edema<br>Secondary bacterial infections | Penetrate skin and migrate in circulation<br>Pneumonitis may occur<br>Systemic involvement is rare |
| *Dracunculus medinensis* | Larvae migration, inflammation, and secondary bacterial infections | Ingestion of infected copepods<br>Blisters develop where female exits the skin |
| *Parastrongylus cantonensis* | Migration to central nervous system | Ingestion of infected shrimp, fish, crabs, and frogs<br>Often self-limiting, but may cause meningoencephalitis or meningitis |
| *Parastrongylus costaricensis* | Migration resulting in inflammation and lesions in bowel | Ingestion of salad contaminated with infected slugs or snails |
| *Gnathostoma spinigerum* | Migration resulting in inflammation | Ingestion of contaminated fish<br>Tissue damage based on worm burden and migration pattern |

## LABORATORY DIAGNOSIS

Laboratory diagnosis is limited. Evidence of visible tracks and patient history of possible exposure are usually sufficient. The patient may present with a peripheral eosinophilia. In systemic cases, larvae may be recovered from sputum and Charcot-Leyden crystals may be evident.

## THERAPY

Anthelmintic therapy may include ivermectin or thiabendazole.

## *DRACUNCULUS MEDINENSIS*

### GENERAL CHARACTERISTICS

*Dracunculus medinensis*, commonly referred to as the guinea worm, is the cause of a subcutaneous infection known as dracunculiasis. The worm has a characteristic, thick cuticle and a large uterus that fills the body cavity and contains rhabditoid larvae.

### EPIDEMIOLOGY

The parasite was once known to have a worldwide distribution affecting millions of people. In 2008, the World Health Organization in collaboration with governmental groups and other organizations attempted to eradicate the organism. Efforts have reduced the incidence of infection, confining the remaining endemic area to Africa.

Humans are infected by the ingestion of freshwater from stagnant ponds containing larvae-infected copepods. The copepods are digested in the stomach, releasing the larvae. The larvae penetrate the small intestine and migrate through the thoracic musculature. Both adult male and female worms mature in approximately 2 to 3 months. The gravid female develops in approximately 10 to 14 months, migrating to the lower extremities. The gravid female produces a blister on the skin, and when the host submerges the affected area in water, the blister erupts and releases larvae into the water.

## PATHOGENESIS AND SPECTRUM OF DISEASE

The blisters formed by the gravid female worm cause burning and itching. Systemic symptoms may include fever, nausea, vomiting, diarrhea, headache, urticaria and eosinophilia. Secondary bacterial infections may occur. In addition, dead worms within the host may be absorbed or may calcify, causing secondary inflammatory symptoms.

## LABORATORY DIAGNOSIS

Diagnosis is by identification of larvae or adult worms.

## THERAPY

Treatment requires removal of the adult worms. The female worms are attached to a stick and slowly retracted from the host by gradual turning of the stick and removal of the worm. Although anthelmintic medications, such as metronidazole or thiabendazole, are not lethal, they are administered to assist with the retraction of the worms. Analgesics and antimicrobials are administered for discomfort and the prevention of secondary infections.

# PARASTRONGYLUS CANTONENSIS (CEREBRAL ANGIOSTRONGYLIASIS)

## GENERAL CHARACTERISTICS

*Parastrongylus cantonensis*, previously known as *Angiostrongylus* sp., is a filiarial worm commonly referred to as the rat lungworm.

## EPIDEMIOLOGY

The parasite has a worldwide distribution; however, it remains an endemic health threat in Southeast Asia and the Asian Pacific Islands. A variety of rodents serve as the definitive host. The adult worms reside in the pulmonary artery and right side of the heart. Eggs shed by the female lodge in the pulmonary capillaries, where the larvae hatch and migrate up the trachea. The larvae are swallowed and passed in the rodent feces. Once released the larvae infect the intermediate host, mollusks. The mollusks are consumed by a variety of paratenic hosts such as shrimp, fish, crabs, or frogs. The rodents then consume the paratenic hosts and the larvae penetrate the intestine, enter the circulation, and migrate to the central nervous system. Following two successive molts, the larvae then reenter the circulation and migrate to the pulmonary artery. Humans are infected by ingestion of either the intermediate or the paratenic host.

## PATHOGENESIS AND SPECTRUM OF DISEASE

The pathogenesis correlates with the worm burden and the site of infection. The larvae may migrate to the central nervous system, causing meningitis or meningoencephalitis. Symptoms include headache, fever, eosinophilia, increased cerebrospinal fluid (CSF) protein, and neurologic manifestations. Occasionally, the larvae may migrate to the eye, causing blindness. Most often the disease is self-limiting.

## LABORATORY DIAGNOSIS

Definitive diagnosis relies on histologic identification of the adult female worm. The adult female worm has a distinctive morphologic appearance with spiral, winding, "barber pole" appearing uterus. Highly specific serologic assays are available.

## THERAPY

Anthelmintic therapy may be helpful, such as mebendazole. It is important to closely monitor therapy, because the therapy may actually exacerbate the inflammatory response of the host and cause more systemic damage. If larvae are located within the eye, surgical removal is recommended.

# PARASTRONGYLUS COSTARICENSIS (ABDOMINAL ANGIOSTRONGYLIASIS)

## GENERAL CHARACTERISTICS

*Parastrongylus costaricensis* is found primarily in the cotton rat and the black rat.

## EPIDEMIOLOGY

The parasite is endemic in areas of Central and South America including Mexico and Costa Rica.

## PATHOGENESIS AND SPECTRUM OF DISEASE

The life cycle is very similar to that of *Parastrongylus cantonensis*. Human infection is typically by ingestion of salad contaminated with infected slugs or snails. The larvae create inflammatory lesions in the wall of the bowel, resulting in tissue inflammation, necrosis, vomiting, and diarrhea. The patient may experience lower right quadrant abdominal pain similar to that manifested in appendicitis.

## LABORATORY DIAGNOSIS

Histologic identification of larvae or eggs in tissue sections results in definitive diagnosis. Patients often present with leukocytosis and eosinophilia. Radiologic imaging may be useful.

## THERAPY

Traditional anthelmintic therapy is recommended.

# GNATHOSTOMA SPINIGERUM

## GENERAL CHARACTERISTICS

*Gnathostoma* spp., a gastric Spirurida, is found in a variety of mammals worldwide. Dogs and cats serve as the definitive host for *G. spinigerum*.

## EPIDEMIOLOGY

The adult worms reside in the stomach of the definitive host where they mate and produce eggs that are passed in the feces. When the feces are deposited in water, the larvae hatch and infect copepods. The larvae mature in the copepods and are then ingested by a variety of hosts including fish, snakes, and frogs. Inside the paratenic host the larvae then migrate to the musculature and encyst until the tissue is ingested by the definitive host. Once in the definitive host, the larvae excyst and penetrate the gastric wall, migrating and maturing in the stomach. Humans act as accidental hosts when they ingest larvae in contaminated fish.

## PATHOGENESIS AND SPECTRUM OF DISEASE

The worms are incapable of maturation within the human host and migrate aimlessly, causing tissue damage and inflammation. The infection is not typically fatal; however, it depends on the migration pattern and organs infected.

## LABORATORY DIAGNOSIS

The identification of the larvae in tissue is definitive for diagnosis. The head contains four rows of cephalic hooklets. The body is covered with transverse rows of spines that diminish anteriorly to posteriorly.

## THERAPY

Supportive corticosteroid treatment is recommended. Although anthelmintics are not lethal, they are often recommended. Surgical excision of the larvae is optimal treatment.

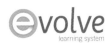 *Visit the Evolve site to complete the review questions.*

## BIBLIOGRAPHY

Garcia LS: *Diagnostic medical parasitology*, ed 5, Washington, DC, 2007, ASM Press.

Mandell GL, Bennett JE, Dolin R, editors: *Principles and practice of infectious diseases*, ed 7, New York, 2010, Churchill Livingstone.

Versalovic J: *Manual of clinical microbiology*, ed 10, Washington, DC, 2011, ASM Press.

Wu Z, Nagano I, Pozio E, et al: The detection of *Trichinella* with polymerase chain reaction (PCR) primers constructed using sequences of random amplified polymorphic DNA (RAPD) or sequences of complementary DNA coding excretory-secretory (E-S) glycoproteins, *Parasitology* 117:2, 1998.

Wu Z, Nagano I, Pozio E, et al: *Polymerase chain reaction-restriction fragment length polymorphism (PCR-RFLLP) for the identification of Trichinella isolates*, Vol 118, Issue 02, 1999, Cambridge University Press.

## OBJECTIVES

1. Describe the distinguishing morphologic characteristics and basic life cycle (vectors, hosts, and stages of infectivity) for each of the parasites listed.
2. Define microfilariae, hydrocele, chyluria, and sheath.
3. Describe the diseases and mechanism of pathogenicity, including route of transmission for each of the species listed.
4. Explain periodicity, including nocturnal and diurnal, as it relates to infection with microfilariae and correlate with the life cycle of the associated arthropod vector.
5. Differentiate the microfilariae based on the presence or absence of the sheath and the arrangement and number of tail nuclei.
6. Describe the two methods for concentration of blood specimens for the identification of organisms within the peripheral blood.
7. Determine the etiology of infection based on patient history, signs and symptoms, and laboratory results.

---

### PARASITES TO BE CONSIDERED

**Nematodes**

Blood and Tissues (Filarial Worms)

*Wuchereria bancrofti*
*Brugia malayi*
*Brugia timori*
*Loa loa*
*Onchocerca volvulus*
*Mansonella ozzardi*
*Mansonella streptocerca*
*Mansonella perstans*

---

**B**lood and tissue filarial nematodes are roundworms that infect humans. These organisms are transmitted via a blood-sucking arthropod vector such as a mosquito, midge, or fly. The filarial nematodes infect the subcutaneous tissues, deep connective tissues, body cavities, and lymphatic system. The life cycles of the filarial nematodes are complex (Figure 53-1). The infective larval stage resides in the insect vector with the adult worm stage, which is the pathogenic form in humans. When the arthropod vector feeds on a human blood meal, the infective larvae are injected into the bloodstream. The larvae are motile and migrate to the lymphatic vessels. The infective larvae grow and develop into the adult gravid worm in the human host over a period of months. The male and female adult worms mate in the definitive human host. The female worm produces large numbers of larvae called **microfilariae.** Depending on the species, the microfilariae may maintain the egg membrane as a sheath or may rupture the egg membrane, resulting in an unsheathed form. These parasites can reside in the host for many years and cause chronic, debilitating conditions and severe

inflammatory responses. Identification of the various species is based on the morphology of the microfilaria, the periodicity (defined circadian rhythm), and the location within the human host. Microfilariae morphologic characteristics are important in the identification and include the presence or absence of the sheath and the presence and arrangement of the nuclei in the tail of the worm (Figure 53-2). A comparison of the morphologic characteristics of the pathogenic filarial worms is depicted in Figure 53-3. Diagnosis of infection is based on the identification of the microfilariae in the blood or tissue of the host.

## WUCHERERIA BANCROFTI

### GENERAL CHARACTERISTICS

*Wuchereria bancrofti* is transmitted in a mosquito, the *Culex fatigans, Anopheles,* or *Aedes* spp. The adult worm has a sheath that stains faintly or not at all. It may grow to approximately 298 μm in length by 2.5 μm to 10 μm wide. The tail is pointed with no nuclei present (Figure 53-4).

### EPIDEMIOLOGY

*W. bancrofti* is the most common identified species of filarial worms that infect humans. It is widely distributed in the tropical and subtropics including Africa, South America, Asia, the Pacific Islands, and the Caribbean. The mosquito vectors have complex life cycles that include laying eggs and developing larvae on the surface of a water source. When the larvae mature into adult mosquitos, the male and females will swarm in the evening and mate. The female requires feeding on a blood meal in order to reproduce. The mosquito becomes the intermediate host for the microfilaria parasite. Humans are the definitive host and the reservoir for *W. bancrofti.* The parasite has two forms that demonstrate different periodicities. The nocturnal periodic form is found in the peripheral blood during the night between 10 PM and 4 AM. The second form is found only in the Pacific Islands and is present in the blood at all times, but more frequently during the day in the afternoon hours.

### PATHOGENESIS AND SPECTRUM OF DISEASE

Microfilaria clinical disease varies geographically based on the species of nematode causing the infection. The disease may present as acute or asymptomatic for many years. *W. bancrofti* causes bancroftian filariasis and elephantiasis. The adult worm resides in the lymphatic vessels distal to the lymph nodes. The presence of the organisms within the host results in an immunologic response including inflammation, hyperplasia, lymphedema, and hyperplasia. Lymphedema most often occurs in the lower extremities. Elephantiasis is a crippling condition that results from extended periods of filarial infection. The obstruction of the lymphatic vessels causes fibrosis and proliferation of dermal and connective tissue, resulting in the wrinkled, dry appearance of an "elephant" extremity. Lymphedema may also occur in the arms, female breasts, and scrotum of infected males.

Acute lymphatic filariasis results from worms residing within the lymph nodes. The lymph nodes swell and lymphangitis may appear peripherally from the infected node. Hydrocele formation, a fluid filled sac within the scrotum, may occur when adult worms block the retroperitoneal or subdiaphragmatic lymphatic vessels. Obstruction of the lymphatic vessels may result in a

condition referred to as chyluria. Chyluria is a result of the lymphatic rupture and fluid entering the urine. The urine will appear milky white. Resulting infection and changes in the skin may result in increased bacterial infections.

Patients residing in endemic tropical regions for filarial parasites may present with a syndrome referred to as tropical pulmonary eosinophilia (TPE). The microfilariae migrate through the pulmonary blood vessels, causing an allergic hypersensitivity in the host. The patients develop a strong immune response to the presence of the parasites with an elevated serum immunoglobulin E (IgE) level. Symptoms of TPE include weight loss, low-grade fever, cough and wheezing at night, and lymphadenopathy. Without treatment, patients may develop chronic and progressive respiratory complications resulting in death.

### Endosymbiont

*W. bancrofti*, *Brugia* spp., and *Onchocerca volvulus* harbor an endosymbiotic alpha-proteobacterium, *Wolbachia* sp. *Wolbachia* is an obligate intracellular organism.

The parasites require the endosymbiont for larval development, viability, and fertility. The bacteria have also been implicated in the pathogenesis of the infection with filarial parasites. The bacterial antigens enhance the host inflammatory response, leading to increased scarring and damage within the host lymphatic system. The bacterium is sensitive to tetracycline, azithromycin, and

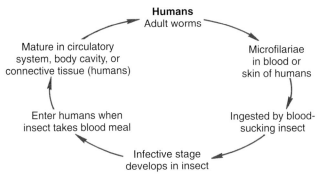

**Figure 53-1** Life cycle of human filarial worms.

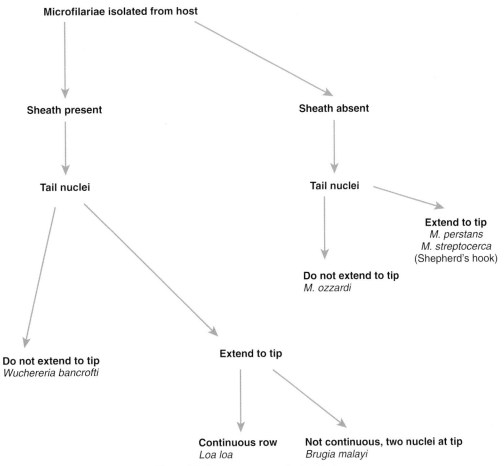

**Figure 53-2** Identification of microfilariae.

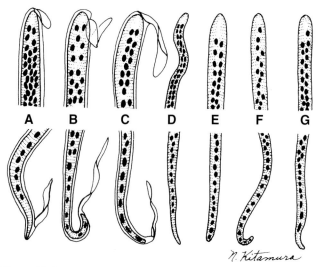

**Figure 53-3** Anterior and posterior ends of microfilariae found in humans. **A,** *Wuchereria bancrofti*. **B,** *Brugia malayi.* **C,** *Loa loa.* **D,** *Onchocerca volvulus.* **E,** *Mansonella perstans.* **F,** *Mansonella streptocerca.* **G,** *Mansonella ozzardi.*

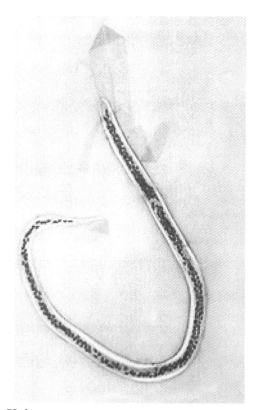

**Figure 53-4** Microfilaria of *Wuchereria bancrofti* in thick blood film.

rifampin. Combination antibiotic treatment in conjunction with treatment for the parasite infection improves clearance of the filarial parasite.

## LABORATORY DIAGNOSIS

### Direct Detection

Definitive laboratory diagnosis is based on the identification of the parasites in blood, fluids, or tissue. Blood samples should be drawn in accordance with the periodicity of the infection to optimize the likelihood of isolating the infecting organism. Direct examination of blood, urine, hydrocele fluid, or chyle (milky fluid produced in the small intestine for fat digestion and taken up by the lymphatic system) may be used for identification of the parasite. The fluid is placed on a slide and air-dried to prevent distortion of the parasite. The specimen should be stained with Giemsa, Wright's, or hematoxylin stain and examined microscopically. Ultrasound may be used to visualize the organisms within the tissues.

Nucleopore filtration or Knott's concentration may be used to increase the likelihood of isolating a filarial parasite from blood. The blood is passed through a polycarbonate filter that contains a 2-μm pore. Distilled water is passed through the filter, lysing the red blood cells and improving the visualization of the parasites. The filter is then air-dried, stained with Giemsa, and examined for the presence of microfilaria. Knott's concentration uses centrifugation to concentrate the organisms to a slide. One milliliter of anticoagulated blood is placed in 9 mL of 2% formalin, centrifuged at $500 \times g$ for 1 minute, and then applied to a microscope slide. The slide is then stained and examined microscopically. Sometimes adult worms may be visualized moving within the lymphatics, using high-frequency ultrasound.

### Serologic Detection

Serologic assays that measure antibody response have limited utility in the diagnosis of infections with microfilariae. The antibodies tend to demonstrate a high cross reactivity with other antibodies made in response to a wide variety of parasitic worm infections. The absence of an antibody reaction would, however, indicate the lack of infection by a microfilaria species. Laboratory detection of *W. bancrofti*-circulating antigens has demonstrated high specificity and sensitivity in detecting parasitic infections. However, the commercial testing formats available are not FDA-approved.

### Molecular Diagnostics

Polymerase chain reaction (PCR) amplification is available in reference laboratories for the rapid diagnosis of an infection with blood microfilariae including *W. bancrofti* and *Brugia* spp. Multiplex PCR has been developed to differentiate *W. bancrofti* and *Brugia malayi* in blood and mosquitos. The test results indicated that the reaction was highly sensitive and more efficient than traditional microscopic detection.

## *BRUGIA MALAYI* AND *BRUGIA TIMORI*

### GENERAL CHARACTERISTICS

The *Brugia* spp. are lymphatic filarial parasites resembling *W. bancrofti*. The adult parasites are somewhat smaller, (*B. timori*, 300 μm long and 5-6 μm wide; *B. malayi*, 270 μm long and 5-6 μm wide) have a different geographic distribution, and do not typically cause lymphadenitis in the genital regions.

### EPIDEMIOLOGY

The *Brugia* spp. are distributed throughout the Far East including China, Indonesia, Korea, Malaysia, Japan,

India, and the Philippines. The distribution of *B. timori* is limited to the two islands of Timor, an island of Indonesia. The organism is transmitted via mosquitos included in the genus *Anopheles* and *Mansonia*.

## PATHOGENESIS AND SPECTRUM OF DISEASE

As in infections with *W. bancrofti,* two periodic forms exist. The nocturnal form is the most common and located near areas of coastal rice fields, whereas the nonperiodic form is associated with infections in areas near swampy forests. The pathogenesis and spectrum of disease is essentially the same as for *W. bancrofti,* with the exception that involvement of the genital lymphatic vessels is predominantly associated with *W. bancrofti.* Clinical disease progresses faster following infection with *B. malayi* than with *W. bancrofti.* Microfilariae may appear in the blood in as little as 3 to 4 months.

Brugia spp. have been implicated in zoonotic infections of dogs, cats, rabbits, and raccoons worldwide. Cases of human infection have occurred in the United States in the northeastern region. Clinical disease is typically asymptomatic but may present with a tender region in the cervical, axillary, or inguinal region. The lymphatic mass may contain either a live or a dead worm. If the worm is no longer viable, the mass may be surrounded by a granulomatous reaction.

## LABORATORY DIAGNOSIS

Definitive diagnosis is generally by the identification of the adult worms in the blood of infected individuals. The adult worms can be distinguished from *W. bancrofti* morphologically. The *B. malayi* microfilariae are sheathed and contain 4 to 5 subterminal and 2 terminal nuclei in the tail. *B. timori* also contains 5 to 8 subterminal and terminal nuclei in the tail, but they are much larger than *B. malayi.* The *B. malayi* sheath will stain bright pink with Giemsa, whereas the *B. timori* sheath does not stain. The microfilariae of *B. timori* tend to be somewhat longer. High-frequency ultrasound has been useful in identifying adult worms in various locations within the patient, such as lymphatic vessels of the legs, inguinal area (groin or lower abdomen), lymph nodes, and female breasts. Nucleic acid-based methods have been developed but are not widely used in clinical laboratories.

## THERAPY

Diethylcarbamazine (DEC) is the treatment of choice for lymphatic filarial parasites including *W. bancrofti* and *Brugia* spp. Additionally, ivermectin and albendazole may be used. Death of the microfilarial worms may result in an increased hypersensitive reaction requiring the need for treatment with antihistamines to limit the inflammatory symptoms.

## PREVENTION

The use of insect repellent is recommended for travellers in areas where the parasites are endemic. DEC has also been used for prophylactic treatment before travel. Vector control studies in combination with mass

drug administration of DEC and ivermectin have successfully decreased the population of the arthropod vectors and decreased filarial infection in the human hosts.

# LOA LOA

## GENERAL CHARACTERISTICS

*Loa loa,* commonly referred to as the eye worm, is a microfilaria that circulates in the bloodstream and resides in the subcutaneous tissue in the human host. The worm may grow up to 300 μm.

## EPIDEMIOLOGY

The parasite is found within the rain forests of West and Central Africa. The organism is transmitted through a bite of the tabinid fly or deer fly of the genus *Chrysops.* The female lays her eggs on the leaves of small plants near the water. The larvae feed on small insects and develop in wet soil. The male fly feeds on pollen and the female feeds on a blood meal.

## PATHOGENESIS AND SPECTRUM OF DISEASE

The organism is often associated with asymptomatic infection. The larvae develop into adult worms in approximately 6 to 12 months, but can persist in the human host for up to 17 years. The infection is typically identified when the adult worm is seen migrating within the subconjunctiva of the host. Symptoms associated with infection include episodic "calabar swelling," which are localized areas of transient angioedema in response to the production of parasitic metabolic products. Predominant swelling on the extremities with inflammation of nearby joints and peripheral nerves may occur. Immune-mediated encephalopathy, nephropathy, and cardiomyopathy may occur.

## LABORATORY DIAGNOSIS

Infections with *Loa loa* may be asymptomatic for many years before the appearance of microfilariae in the peripheral blood. Therefore, patient diagnosis is often made on the basis of the patient's clinical symptoms including calabar swelling, eosinophilia, and travel or residency in an endemic area.

### Direct Detection

Definitive diagnosis is made by identification of the adult worm from the eye, in tissue or in the peripheral blood. The organism contains a sheath that does not stain with Giemsa. The adult females are larger than the adult males. The nuclei extend to the tail in an irregularly arranged fashion.

### Serologic Detection

As with other filarial infections, serologic assays have limited use for diagnosis. A *Loa*-specific recombinant protein has been used in the development of an enzyme-linked immunosorbent assay (ELISA) and has demonstrated improved specificity but limited sensitivity.

### Molecular Diagnostics

PCR assays are currently available but are limited to research laboratories.

## THERAPY

DEC is the treatment of choice. In heavy infections, inflammation and allergic reactions may occur, requiring the administration of antiinflammatory medications. Allergic responses can result in central nervous system damage, encephalitis, coma, and death.

## PREVENTION

Prophylactic treatment with DEC has been used to prevent infection.

# ONCHOCERCA VOLVULUS

## GENERAL CHARACTERISTICS

*Onchocerca volvulus* predominantly resides in tissue nodules within the host. Adult worms measure approximately 300 μm long by 5-9 μm wide.

## EPIDEMIOLOGY

*O. volvulus* is found throughout Africa, Central America, and South America. The parasite is transmitted by the black fly, *Simulium* spp. The black fly lays its eggs in running water where the larvae attach to the rocks. The larvae feed on algae and bacteria. The adults emerge as a flying insect. The females require a blood meal, whereas the males are nectar feeders. The flies feed predominantly during the day.

## PATHOGENESIS AND SPECTRUM OF DISEASE

Onchocerciasis, commonly referred to as river blindness, is a result of subcutaneous infection with the parasite. The infections are typically localized to the skin, lymph nodes, and eyes. Skin infections result in pruritus, edema, and erythema. Hypo- or hyperpigmentation can occur following a lengthy infection. Nodules, containing the adult worm, vary in size and are firm and tender. Lymphadenopathy may be found in the inguinal or femoral regions. Enlargement of the lymph node may result in a condition referred to as "hanging groin" that may result in a hernia. Onchocercal eye disease may be seen in moderate to heavy infections. Infections of the eye may lead to serious damage and blindness. Mortality increases in adults that experience blindness and systemic infection.

## LABORATORY DIAGNOSIS

### Direct Detection

Definitive diagnosis is made from the identification of the adult worm from tissue such as in a nodule or skin snip. Skin samples are placed in physiologic buffered saline for up to 24 hours. Following incubation, the

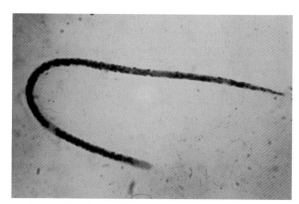

**Figure 53-5** Microfilaria of *Onchocerca volvulus*. (Courtesy Dr. Henry Travers, Sioux Falls, S.D.)

worms will emerge from the tissue and can be visualized microscopically. Occasionally the adult worms may be found in blood or urine following treatment. Microfilariae may also be visible in the cornea of the eye.

The microfilariae lack a sheath. The tail is tapered, appears bent or flexed, and does not include nuclei (Figure 53-5).

### Serologic Detection

Although serologic tests generally lack specificity, recombinant ELISAs using multiple antigens have demonstrated increased sensitivity and specificity for the diagnosis of onchocerciasis.

### Molecular Diagnostics

PCR amplification assays have been developed and are currently limited to research laboratories.

## THERAPY

Ivermectin is the recommended treatment. However, in Africa, where *O. volvulus* and *L. loa* are coendemic, ivermectin treatment is often associated with encephalopathy in patients with heavy microfilaria infections. Surgical excision of nodules containing adult worms is recommended when they are located on the head.

## PREVENTION

Mosquito control using insecticides in endemic areas has been used to assist in the control of transmission of *O. volvulus*. In addition, a mass-treatment program with ivermectin is effective in preventing infection.

# MANSONELLA SPP. (M. OZZARDI, M. STREPTOCERCA, M. PERSTANS)

## GENERAL CHARACTERISTICS

*Mansonella* spp. are generally not associated with serious infections. The adult worms of all species are very similar in size, ranging from approximately 200-225 μm long and 4-6 μm wide.

## EPIDEMIOLOGY

*Mansonella* spp. are distributed throughout varied geographic regions in Africa and South America. *M. ozzardi* is limited to Central and South America and the Caribbean islands. The parasites are transmitted by biting midges of the genus *Culicoides*. The female requires a blood meal for the maturation of eggs and typically bites in the early evening or morning hours. Transmission of *M. ozzardi* has also been associated with bites from the black fly *(Simulium amazonicum)*.

## PATHOGENESIS AND SPECTRUM OF DISEASE

*M. streptocerca* may be found in the skin; however, most infected individuals appear asymptomatic. Patients may present with a pruritic rash and pigmentation changes. In addition, lymphadenitis may occur. *M. perstans* resides in the pericardial, pleural, and peritoneal cavities. Symptomatic patients present with swelling of the arms or face similar to infection with *L. loa*. *M. ozzardi* and *M. perstans* are found in the blood.

*M. perstans* and *M. ozzardi* do not demonstrate periodicity when circulating within the bloodstream. *M. ozzardi* infections are not well characterized.

## LABORATORY DIAGNOSIS

*Mansonella* spp. microfilariae do not possess sheaths. *M. streptocerca* and *M. perstans* tails contain nuclei that extend to the end of the tail. The tail of *M. streptocerca* is often referred to as a "shepherd's crook." *M. ozzardi* have tails with nuclei that do not extend to the tip.

## THERAPY

Ivermectin is effective in the treatment of *M. streptocerca* and *M. ozzardi* infections. Treatment of *M. perstans* infections has not been effective in most cases.

## PREVENTION

Prevention relies on the use of insect repellents and adequate clothing.

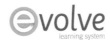 *Visit the Evolve site to complete the review questions.*

---

## CASE STUDY 53-1

A 45-year-old man returned to the United States following a 3-week safari in Central Africa. He presented to his physician complaining of a tender area near his groin and discomfort during urination. In addition, he was having difficulty sleeping at night because of intermittent periods of fever. A complete blood count was drawn and the patient exhibited a mild eosinophilia. All other results appeared normal. Urinalysis revealed no abnormal laboratory results. A CT scan of the man's lower abdomen and groin showed an unusual mass in his inguinal region. The physician admitted the patient for further observations and tests. Subsequent testing included additional peripheral blood collection during the periodic fevers. Thick and thin smears disclosed no unusual organisms. Following concentration of a blood sample and staining with Giemsa, the organism depicted in Figure 53-6 was identified.

### QUESTIONS

1. Identify the parasite depicted in Figure 53-6.
2. What is the recommended treatment for this patient?
3. What additional parasite could be associated with this patient's symptoms?

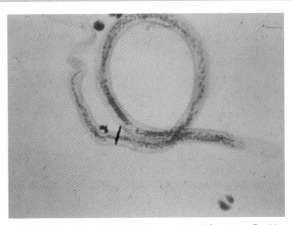

**Figure 53-6** Organism identified from patient. (Courtesy Dr. Henry Travers, Sioux Falls, S.D.)

---

## BIBLIOGRAPHY

Fischer P, Wibowo H, Pischke S, et al: PCR-based detection and identification of the filarial parasite *Brugia timori* from Alor Island, Indonesia, *Ann Trop Med Parasitol* 96(8):809-821, 2002.

Garcia LS: *Diagnostic medical parasitology*, ed 5, Washington, DC, 2007, ASM Press.

Mandell GL, Bennett JE, Dolin R, editors: *Principles and practice of infectious diseases*, ed 7, New York, 2010, Churchill Livingstone.

Mishra K, Raj DK, Hazra RK, et al: The development and evaluation of a single step multiplex PCR method for simultaneous detection of *Brugia malayi* and *Wuchereria bancrofti*, *Mol Cell Probes* 21:355, 2007.

Pani SP, Hoti SL, Elango A, et al: Evaluation of the ICT whole blood antigen card test to detect infection due to nocturnally periodic *Wuchereria bancrofti* in South India, *Trop Med Int Health* 5(5):359-363, 2000.

Sunish IP, Rajendran R, Mani TR, et al: Vector control complements mass drug administration against bancroftian filariasis in Tirukoilur, India, *Bull WHO* 85:138, 2007.

Versalovic J: *Manual of clinical microbiology*, ed 10, Washington, DC, 2011, ASM Press.

## OBJECTIVES

1. Describe the distinguishing morphologic characteristics, clinical disease, basic life cycle (vectors, hosts, and stages of infectivity), and laboratory diagnosis for the intestinal cestodes included in this chapter.
2. Define and identify (where appropriate) the following parasitic structures: scolex, proglottids, rostellum, hermaphroditic, oncosphere, hexacanth embryo, strobila, bothria, and coracidium.
3. Compare and contrast autoinfection and hyperinfection.
4. List several methods of control and prevention of tapeworm infection.
5. Correlate the life cycles with the specific diagnostic stage(s) for each organism.

---

### PARASITES TO BE CONSIDERED

**Intestinal Cestodes (Tapeworms)**
*Diphyllobothrium latum*
*Dipylidium caninum*
*Hymenolepis nana*
*Hymenolepis diminuta*
*Taenia solium*
*Taenia saginata*

---

The intestinal cestodes are commonly referred to as tapeworms. Tapeworms have a long, segmented, ribbonlike body with a specialized structure for attachment, or **scolex,** at the anterior end. The adult tapeworm consists of a chain of egg-producing units called **proglottids,** which develop posteriorly from the neck region of the scolex. The crown of the scolex, **rostellum,** may be smooth or armed with hooks. The body of the worm (proglottids) varies in the geometric characteristics or number of segments according to the genus and species of the cestode. The mature cestode is **hermaphroditic.** In other words, the organism contains both male and female reproductive organs. Food is absorbed from the host through the worm's **integument,** the outer covering or skin of the organism. Adult worms typically inhabit the small intestine; however, humans may be host to either the adult or the larval forms, depending on the infecting species. Humans infected with a cestode pass the eggs in the feces. The embryo may be visible within the tapeworm egg as an **oncosphere** (larva tapeworm within an embryonic envelope, infective stage) or **hexacanth** embryo. The intermediate host ingests feces containing the adult tapeworm eggs, which further develop into the larva of the cestode. Cestodes generally require one or more intermediate hosts for the completion of their life cycle. Intestinal tapeworm infections are generally asymptomatic. However, if the larval stage develops in human organs outside the intestine, they may cause additional life-threatening complications. Serologic tests are not available for the diagnosis of tapeworm infections, therefore requiring skilled laboratorians for proper morphologic identification of the organism. Fresh or preserved stools are the specimen of choice for ova and parasites (O&P) examination and cestode identification. Preserved stool containing adult worm segments **(strobila)** or the scolex may also be used for diagnosis. Chapter 47 describes the methods and specimen requirements in more detail as they relate to parasitology. This chapter describes the intestinal cestodes of public health importance.

## DIPHYLLOBOTHRIUM LATUM

### GENERAL CHARACTERISTICS

*Diphyllobothrium latum,* the freshwater broad fish tapeworm, is the largest human tapeworm. Adults have been known to reach up to 10 m in length, with more than 3000 to 4000 proglottids, and reside within a host for 30 years or more. The proglottids are characteristically wider than long with a central rosette-shaped uterine structure (Figure 54-1). The scolex is spatulate and contains two shallow sucking grooves referred to as **bothria** (Figure 54-1, *B*). *D. latum* has unembryonated eggs. The eggs are operculated with a terminal knob, similar to trematode eggs (Figure 54-1, *C*). The intermediate hosts include crustaceans and freshwater fish.

### EPIDEMIOLOGY

*Diphyllobothrium* is not found in the tropics; it is commonly found worldwide where cool lakes are contaminated by sewage. *D. latum* can be found wherever freshwater fish are eaten raw or marinated. This includes fish such as trout, pike, and salmon, which have been shipped to nonendemic areas. In the United States, *D. latum* is generally found in and around the Great Lakes.

### PATHOGENESIS AND SPECTRUM OF DISEASE

*Diphyllobothrium latum* is the only cestode to have an aquatic life cycle (Figure 54-2). Fish serve as the reservoir host, with humans serving as the definitive host. *D. latum* eggs are found in the feces of infected humans and other fish-eating mammals. Once passed into a water source, such as a lake, the life cycle requires two intermediate hosts. After incubation in freshwater for approximately 2 weeks, the mature eggs release the first larval stage (coracidium). The coracidia are ingested by

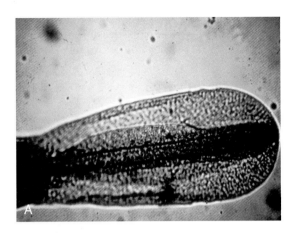

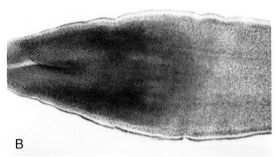

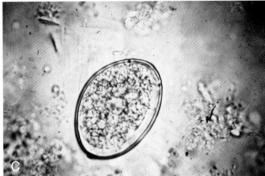

**Figure 54-1 A,** *Diphyllobothrium latum* scolex. **B,** *D. latum* scolex, bothria visible. **C,** *D. latum* ovum. (Courtesy Dr. Henry Travers, Sioux Falls, S.D.)

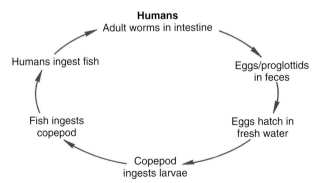

**Figure 54-2** Life cycle of *Diphyllobothrium latum.*

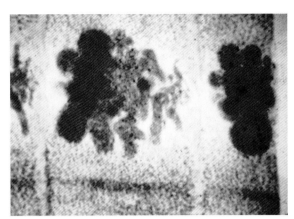

**Figure 54-3** Proglottid demonstrating rosette-shaped uterus in *D. latum.* (Courtesy Dr. Henry Travers, Sioux Falls, S.D.)

copepods. The fish feed upon the small crustaceans ingesting the procercoid larvae. Within the freshwater fish, the larvae develop into the infective larvae. *D. latum* infection occurs through the ingestion of poorly cooked freshwater fish containing the plerocercoid larval form. *D. latum* matures to an adult tapeworm within the human small intestine. Infection is usually asymptomatic, but mild gastrointestinal symptoms may occur such as diarrhea, abdominal pain, fatigue, vomiting, or dizziness. Symptoms vary depending on the worm burden and the host's immune response to the organism. The tapeworm nutritional requirements may decrease the host's vitamin $B_{12}$ level, resulting in megaloblastic anemia (Table 54-1).

## LABORATORY DIAGNOSIS

Both eggs and proglottids may be found in patient's feces. Visualization of the eggs is enhanced using a wet preparation of the patient's stool sample. Diagnosis is made by identification of the ovoid, operculated, yellow-brown eggs (58 to 75 μm by 40 to 50 μm) passed in abundance in the stool. They are sometimes confused with the eggs of *Paragonimus.* The mature gravid proglottids are wider than long (3 × 11 mm), often in chains, and contain a rosette-shaped central uterus (Figure 54-3). Species identification is through assessment of the morphologic characteristics of the proglottids as previously described (Tables 54-2 and 54-3).

## ANTIPARASITIC SUSCEPTIBILITY TESTING AND THERAPY

Humans infected with *D. latum* develop little or no protective immunity. Reinfection is common. Treatment with praziquantel or niclosamide is effective and nontoxic. Subsequent stool specimens should be reexamined 6 weeks following treatment. The patient may require a vitamin $B_{12}$ supplement if anemia develops.

## PREVENTION

Prevention simply includes avoiding the consumption of raw fish. The larva stage is destroyed when food is

**TABLE 54-1** Epidemiology of the Intestinal Cestodes That Cause Disease in Humans

| Parasite | Habitat (Reservoir) | Mode of Transmission |
|---|---|---|
| *Diphyllobothrium latum* | Adult tapeworms can be found in a number of wild animals, the most important being dogs, bears, seals, and walrus, that serve as reservoir hosts; the human serves as the definitive host. | Occurs via ingestion of poorly cooked freshwater fish containing the sparganum or plerocercoid larval form. |
| *Dipylidium caninum* | Humans serve as an accidental host for the dog tapeworm. Dogs, cats, and wild animals serve as a reservoir host. Arthropods such as the dog and cat flea serve as an intermediate host. | Transmitted to humans through the ingestion of dog/cat fleas. |
| *Hymenolepis nana* | The dwarf tapeworm can also occur in rodents; the human can serve as both intermediate and definitive host, with development from the egg to adult worm occurring in the human intestine. | Primarily acquired from accidental ingestion of eggs from an adult tapeworm, most commonly via fecal-oral exposure. |
| *Hymenolepis diminuta* | The rat tapeworm frequently infects rodents, and rarely infects humans. | Infects humans after infected mice and rats contaminate food with their feces. |
| *Taenia solium* | Humans serve as the definitive host for the pork tapeworm, whereas pigs and humans serve as intermediate hosts. | Humans become infected when cyst-infected pork is ingested. |
| *Taenia saginata* | Humans serve as the definitive host for the beef tapeworm, whereas cows/camels serve as intermediate hosts. | Humans become infected when cyst-infected beef is ingested. |

**TABLE 54-2** Common Human Parasites, Diagnostic Specimens, Tests, and Positive Findings

| Organism | Acquire Infection from: | Location in Host | Diagnostic Specimen | Diagnostic Test* | Positive Specimen | Comments |
|---|---|---|---|---|---|---|
| **Intestinal cestodes** *Taenia saginata* (beef) | Ingestion of raw beef | Intestine | Stool and/or proglottids | O&P, India ink proglottids | Eggs, proglottid branches | Both *Taenia* eggs look alike; need gravid proglottid or scolex for definitive identification. |
| *Taenia solium* (pork) | Ingestion of raw pork | | Stool and/or proglottids | O&P, India ink proglottids | Eggs, proglottid branches | |
| *Diphyllobothrium latum* | Ingestion of raw freshwater fish | | Stool and/or proglottids | O&P | Eggs, proglottid shape | |
| *Hymenolepis nana* | Tapeworm eggs | | Stool | O&P | Eggs | |
| *Hymenolepis diminuta* | Grain beetles | | Stool | O&P | Eggs | |
| *Dipylidium caninum* | Fleas from dogs/cats | | Stool and/or proglottids | O&P | Eggs, proglottid shape | |

*Although serologic tests are not always mentioned, they are available for a number of parasitic infections. Unfortunately, most are not routinely available. Contact your state public health laboratory or the Centers for Disease Control and Prevention in Atlanta, Georgia.

thoroughly cooked or frozen. Treatment of patients infected with adult tapeworms is indicated to prevent accidental autoinfection. Good hygiene and proper sanitation measures will also prevent reinfection. Treatment of sewage before it enters lakes may help reduce the prevalence of infection.

# DIPYLIDIUM CANINUM

## GENERAL CHARACTERISTICS

*D. caninum,* the cat or dog tapeworm (Figure 54-4), is a double-pored tapeworm consisting of many small proglottids. As the tapeworm matures, the proglottids separate and pass in the stool. They may be recognized on

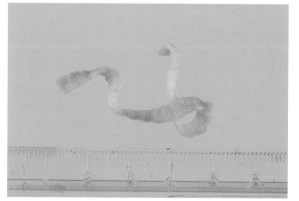

**Figure 54-4** *Dipylidium caninum* tapeworm. (Courtesy Dr. Henry Travers, Sioux Falls, S.D.)

**TABLE 54-3** Cestode Parasites of Humans (Intestinal)

| | *Diphyllobothrium latum* | *Taenia saginata* | *Taenia solium* | *Hymenolepis nana* | *Hymenolepis diminuta* | *Dipylidium caninum* |
|---|---|---|---|---|---|---|
| **Intermediate hosts (common)** | Two: copepods and fish | One: cattle | One: pig | One: various arthropods (beetles, fleas); or none | One: various arthropods (beetles, fleas) | One: various arthropods (fleas, dog lice) |
| **Mode of infection** | Ingestion of plerocercoid (sparganum) in flesh of infected fish | Ingestion of cysticercus in infected beef | Ingestion of cysticercus in infected pork | Ingestion of cysticercoid in infected arthropod or by direct ingestion of egg; autoinfection may also occur | Ingestion of cysticercoid in infected arthropod | Ingestion of cysticercoid in fleas, lice |
| **Prepatent period** | 3-5 weeks | 10-12 weeks | 5-12 weeks | 2-3 weeks | ≈3 weeks | 3-4 weeks |
| **Normal life span** | Up to 25 years | Up to 25 years | Up to 25 years | Perhaps many years as a result of autoinfection | Usually <1 year | Usually <1 year |
| **Length** | 4-10 m | 4-12 m | 1.5-8 m | 2.5-4.0 cm | 20-60 cm | 10-70 cm |
| **Scolex** | Spatulate, 3 × 1 mm; no rostellum or hooklets; has 2 shallow grooves (bothria) | Quadrate, 1-2 mm in diameter; no rostellum or hooklets; 4 suckers | Quadrate, 1-mm diameter; has rostellum and hooklets; 4 suckers | Knoblike but not usually seen; has rostellum and hooklets; 4 suckers | Knoblike but not usually seen; has rostellum but no hooklets; 4 suckers | 0.2-0.5 mm in diameter; has conical/retractile rostellum armed with 4-7 rows of small hooklets; 4 suckers |
| **Usual means of diagnosis** | Ovoid, operculate yellow-brown eggs (58-75 μm × 40-50 μm) in feces; egg usually has small knob at abopercular end; proglottids may be passed, usually in chain of segments (few cm to 0.5 m long); proglottids wider than long (3 × 11 mm) and have rosette-shaped central uterus | Gravid proglottids in feces; they are longer than wide (19 × 17 mm) and have 15-20 lateral branches on each side of central uterine stem; they usually appear singly; spheroidal yellow-brown, thick-shelled eggs (31-43 μm in diameter) containing an oncosphere may be found in feces | Gravid proglottids in feces; they are longer than wide (11 × 5 mm) and have 7-13 lateral branches on each side of central uterine stem; usually appear in chain of 5-6 segments; spheroidal, yellow-brown, thick-shelled eggs (31-43 μm) containing an oncosphere may be found in feces | Nearly spheroidal, pale, thin-shelled eggs (30-47 μm in diameter) in feces; oncosphere surrounded by rigid membrane, which has two polar thickenings from which 4-8 filaments extend into the space between the oncosphere and thin, outer shell | Large, ovoid, yellowish, moderately thick-shelled eggs (70-85 μm × 60-80 μm) in feces; egg contains oncosphere | Gravid proglottids (8-23 μm long) containing compartmented cluster of eggs in feces; proglottids have genital pores at both lateral margins; occasionally may see individual oncospheres (20-33 mm in diameter) in feces |
| **Diagnostic problems or notes** | Eggs are sometimes confused with eggs of *Paragonimus;* eggs are unembryonated when passed in feces | Eggs are identical to those of *Taenia solium;* ordinarily can distinguish between species only by examination of gravid proglottids; eggs can be confused with pollen grains (handle all proglottids with extreme care) | Eggs are identical to those of *T. saginata;* one is less likely to find eggs in feces than with *T. saginata* (handle all proglottids with extreme care since *T. solium* eggs are infective to humans) | Sometimes confused with eggs of *Hymenolepis diminuta;* rodents serve as reservoir hosts | Should not be confused with *H. nana* because eggs lack polar filaments; rodents serve as reservoir hosts | Gravid proglottids resemble rice grains (dry) or cucumber seeds (moist); dogs and cats serve as reservoir hosts |

the basis of their characteristic "cucumber seed" appearance when they are wet, as well as their resemblance to a dried grain of rice. Adult tapeworms measure 10 to 70 cm in length. The scolex contains four suckers and an armed rostellum. Egg packets may also be found in the feces of the host.

# EPIDEMIOLOGY

Infection is common worldwide. In the case of *Dipylidium caninum*, human infection is acquired through the accidental ingestion of fleas. Infection is most often seen in young children as a result of close contact with infected pets. The tapeworms are found in both wild and domestic dogs and cats.

## PATHOGENESIS AND SPECTRUM OF DISEASE

Ingestion of an infected flea may result in *D. caninum* infection. The flea is the intermediate host in which infective cysticercoids develop; humans, dogs, and cats are the reservoir hosts. The larval stage of the egg is ingested by a dog or cat and develops into cysticercoid larvae. The adult worm develops and matures within the reservoir host. An infected human host will usually pass proglottids in a bowel movement or they may stick to the skin around the anal area. Humans usually have very mild symptoms such as indigestion, appetite loss, weight loss, perianal itching, persistent diarrhea, and vague abdominal pain. The severity of the disease is dependent on the worm burden. Human infection is usually self-limited.

## LABORATORY DIAGNOSIS

Symptoms of *Dipylidium* infection are similar to those of pinworm infection; however, the treatments are very different. The laboratory should confirm suspected infections. Proglottids (8 to 23 µm) may be seen in the stool. *D. caninum* is also referred to as the "cucumber seed" tapeworm as previously described (see Figure 54-3). The first sign of infection may be the appearance of seedlike particles in the stool or undergarments of the patient. These particles are the egg-bearing segments of the tapeworm. Groups of egg packets may be found in the stool (Figures 54-5 and 54-6). The adult worms have a scolex with four suckers and a conical/retractile rostellum armed with four to seven rows of small hooklets (Figure 54-7). Patients may also develop a moderately elevated eosinophilia.

## ANTIPARASITIC SUSCEPTIBILITY TESTING AND THERAPY

*D. caninum* infection is usually asymptomatic and is self-limiting. When treated, praziquantel is typically effective. The medication causes the tapeworm to dissolve within the intestine. The drugs are generally well tolerated by the patient. Household pets should be treated simultaneously to prevent reinfection.

## PREVENTION

To reduce the risk of infection, flea control of pets in the household will reduce exposure to humans via the intermediate host. To limit the exposure to fleas by household cats, it is recommended to keep cats indoors to prevent infection.

# HYMENOLEPIS NANA

## GENERAL CHARACTERISTICS

*Hymenolepis nana*, also known as the dwarf tapeworm, is very small in comparison to other tapeworms. The organism may reach up to 4 cm in length. The proglottid contains a scolex with a short-armed rostellum. It is the most common tapeworm with worldwide distribution. An intermediate host is not required, thus making person-to-person spread possible. An adult dwarf tapeworm can live within the host for approximately 4 to 6 weeks.

## EPIDEMIOLOGY

*H. nana* is generally found in children. Although it is most prevalent in the southern United States, it has a wide distribution, particularly in crowded areas. It is more frequent in populations living in conditions of poverty or poor hygiene, in day care centers, and in persons living in institutional settings or prisons.

## PATHOGENESIS AND SPECTRUM OF DISEASE

*H. nana* has an unusual life cycle; ingestion of the egg can lead to the development of the adult worm in humans, thus bypassing the need for an intermediate host (Figure 54-8). Humans can serve as both intermediate and definitive hosts. Infection occurs by accidentally ingesting dwarf tapeworm eggs. This happens most commonly through direct fecal-oral transmission or accidental ingestion of an infected arthropod. The worm resides within the upper ileum of the intestinal tract. Once infected, the dwarf tapeworm may reproduce inside the body, thus causing **autoinfection.** Autoinfection is essentially a reinfection or constant reproduction of the parasite within the host. Massive infection with several thousand worms may follow autoinfection, resulting in **hyperinfection.** Hyperinfction refers to a large parasitic burden within the host. Autoinfection appears to initiate a cellular and humoral immune response. The immune response will provide the host with some protective immunity. Most patients are asymptomatic. Symptomatic patients may experience weight loss, nausea, weakness, loss of appetite, diarrhea, and abdominal discomfort. Young children, especially those with a heavy infection, may develop headache, itchy bottom, or difficulty sleeping. Dwarf tapeworm infection may be misdiagnosed as pinworm infection.

## LABORATORY DIAGNOSIS

Adult worms and proglottids are rarely seen in stool specimens. Diagnosis is typically through the identification

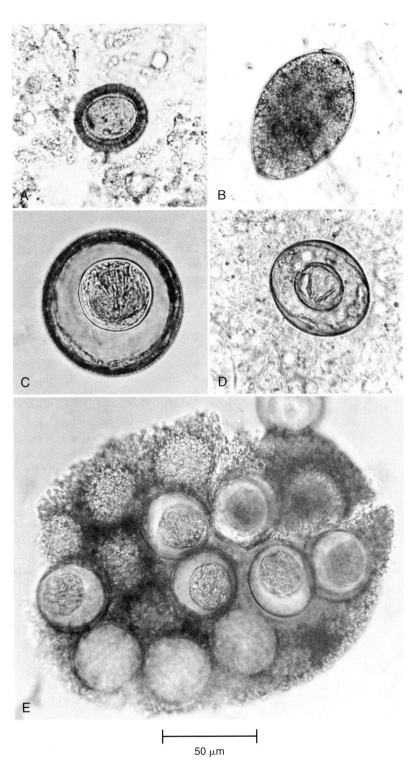

50 μm

**Figure 54-5 A,** *Taenia* spp. egg. **B,** *Diphyllobothrium latum* egg. **C,** *Hymenolepis diminuta* egg. **D,** *Hymenolepis nana* egg. **E,** *Dipylidium caninum* egg packet.

of eggs in stool specimens. Eggs are characterized by the presence of a thin shell enclosing an embryo (oncosphere) with six hooklets contained within two layers of membrane. The eggs are spheroidal, pale, and thin-shelled (30 to 47 μm in diameter). The eggs of *H. nana* and *Hymenolepis diminuta* are very similar. However, *H. nana* eggs are smaller and have polar filaments present in the space between the oncospheres and the eggshell (see Figure 54-5). The egg morphology is easily distinguishable in fresh or formalin-fixed fecal samples. It is important to note that eggs are infectious and therefore unpreserved specimens should be handled carefully. Concentration techniques and repeated examinations will increase the likelihood of detecting light infections. Some patients may demonstrate a low-grade eosinophilia.

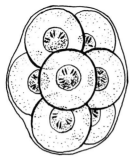

**Figure 54-6** *Dipylidium caninum* egg packet. (Illustration by Nobuko Kitamura.)

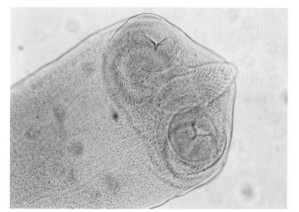

**Figure 54-7** *D. caninum* scolex demonstrating the armed rostellum. (Courtesy Dr. Henry Travers, Sioux Falls, SD.)

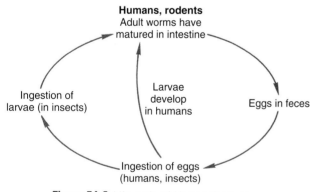

**Figure 54-8** Life cycle of *Hymenolepis nana.*

## ANTIPARASITIC SUSCEPTIBILITY TESTING AND THERAPY

Praziquantel remains the therapy of choice. Niclosamide is also effective and can be repeated with reinfection. Human adults living in endemic areas are provided some immunity as a result of their cellular and humoral immunologic responses.

## PREVENTION

Good hygiene is the best method for control and prevention. Preventing fecal contamination of food and water is the first line of defense. General sanitation measures, along with rodent control, are helpful in controlling the flea population.

# *HYMENOLEPIS DIMINUTA*

## GENERAL CHARACTERISTICS

*Hymenolepis diminuta,* the rat tapeworm, is larger than *H. nana* and can measure 20 to 60 cm in length. Outbreaks of human infection are rarely seen.

## EPIDEMIOLOGY

*H. diminuta* is a tapeworm infrequently seen in humans and frequently found in rodents including rats and mice. Rats are typically the natural reservoir. *H. diminuta* can infect humans following contamination of grains and flours with rodent feces.

## PATHOGENESIS AND SPECTRUM OF DISEASE

The life cycle of *H. diminuta* involves insects, similar to the life cycle of *H. nana. H. diminuta* rarely infects humans, but may do so if a human accidentally ingests an arthropod infected with cysticercoids. Multiple adult worms may mature in the human intestine. Infections are usually tolerated well by the host because of the small size of the organism. Symptoms may include diarrhea, anorexia, nausea, headache, and dizziness. The infection is more common in children, causing mild diarrhea, remittent fever, and abdominal pain.

## LABORATORY DIAGNOSIS

Proglottids are rarely seen in the stool; diagnosis is made by the identification of eggs. The eggs (70 to 85 μm by 60 to 80 μm) are large, ovoid, yellowish, and moderately thick-shelled. The eggs contain a six-hooked oncosphere with the absence of polar filaments in the space between the oncosphere and the eggshell (see Figure 54-5). The eggs are clearly differentiated from *H. nana* because of the absence of polar filaments.

## ANTIPARASITIC SUSCEPTIBILITY TESTING AND THERAPY

*H. diminuta* is readily treated with praziquantel, although the disease is self-limiting and treatment is often not necessary.

## PREVENTION

Prevention is attained primarily by controlling the mice and rat populations along with good hygiene and sanitation.

# TAENIA SOLIUM

## GENERAL CHARACTERISTICS

*T. solium*, the pork tapeworm, is the intestinal cestode capable of causing serious pathologic damage to the human host. Humans serve as the definitive host, whereas pigs serve as the intermediate host. Humans can also serve as the intermediate host. *T. solium* may result in an intestinal infection in which the larvae mature and reside in the small intestine for up to 25 years. The organisms can grow to be 1.5 to 8 m long and produce more than 1000 proglottids, each containing about 50,000 eggs. Cysticercosis is the extraintestinal form of the disease and can be much more severe. The disease is life threatening if the organism invades the central nervous system.

## EPIDEMIOLOGY

*T. solium* has a worldwide distribution. Higher rates of illness have been seen in Latin America. The parasite is found in the United States, typically among Latin American immigrants and Mexican agricultural workers. The tapeworm is more prevalent in underdeveloped communities with poor sanitation and when pork is ingested undercooked or raw.

## PATHOGENESIS AND SPECTRUM OF DISEASE

*T. solium* infection can result in the presence of both adult and larval stages in the human host (Figure 54-9). Infection begins when the intermediate host ingests embryonated eggs in feces. Once the egg is ingested, the hexacanth embryo is released into the intestine where the embryo penetrates the mucosa. The embryo then matures into a cyst (cysticercus) in the tissue. Humans may become infected when they eat raw or undercooked pork containing embedded cysts. Pork tapeworm infection is usually caused through the ingestion of multiple worms. During ingestion and subsequent digestion of the infected meat, the cysticercus is released and attaches to the mucosa within the small intestine of the human host. The cysticercus matures into an adult worm within approximately 5 to 12 weeks. The eggs are then released in the host's feces. Accidental ingestion of the eggs by the human host may also result in migration of the embryo through the intestine to other areas of the body, including the eyes, brain, muscle, or bone. In addition, the proglottids are motile and may migrate out of the anus. Infection of the adult tapeworm causes few clinical symptoms, although abdominal pain, diarrhea, indigestion, and loss of appetite may be present as a result of irritation to the mucosa of the intestinal wall. The major complication with *T. solium* is cysticercosis (larval forms throughout the body), in which the human host becomes the intermediate host and harbors the larvae in tissues as previously described. This infection is further discussed in Chapter 76.

## LABORATORY DIAGNOSIS

Serologic diagnosis is unreliable for infections with *T. solium*. Diagnosis of *Taenia* tapeworm infection is through the examination of stool samples. Individuals suspected of infection with *T. solium* should be asked if they have passed any notable tapeworm segments in their stool. Stool specimens should be collected on 3 different days and microscopically examined for the presence of *Taenia* eggs (see Figure 54-5). Tapeworm eggs can be detected in the stool 2 to 3 months after the tapeworm infection is established. Eggs are round or slightly oval (31 to 43 μm in diameter) and yellow-brown with a thick striated shell containing a six-hooked oncosphere. Diagnosis is based on the recovery of eggs or proglottids in stool or from the perianal area. *T. solium* and *T. saginata* cannot be differentiated on the basis of egg morphology. Speciation requires the examination of gravid proglottids or the scolices. *T. solium* gravid proglottids are longer than wide (19 × 17 mm) and may be distinguished from *T. saginata* according to the number of uterine branches. *T. solium* contains 7 to 13 lateral uterine branches along the proglottid (Figure 54-10), whereas *T. saginata* contains more than 13 branches. Uterine branches may be visualized by staining the proglottids with India ink. The scolex contains a neck region that is typically short and half the width of the scolex and differs from that of *T. saginata* by the presence of four suckers with hooks in a double row (Figure 54-11). The adult worm is usually 3 to 5 m long. Extreme care should be taken when handling infectious stool, since *T. solium* proglottids and eggs are extremely infectious. Additional laboratory findings may include a low-grade eosinophilia, increased serum IgE level, and the presence of atypical lymphocytes in the cerebrospinal fluid.

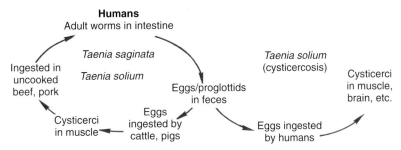

**Figure 54-9** Life cycle of *Taenia saginata* and *Taenia solium*.

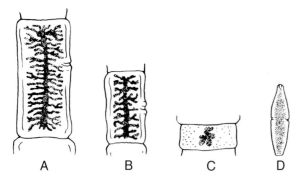

**Figure 54-10** Gravid proglottids. **A,** *Taenia saginata.* **B,** *Taenia solium.* **C,** *Diphyllobothrium latum.* **D,** *Dipylidium caninum.* (From Garcia LS: *Diagnostic medical parasitology,* ed 5, Washington, DC, 2007, ASM Press.)

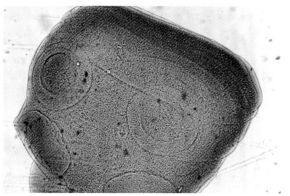

**Figure 54-11** *T. saginata* scolex with suckers. (Courtesy Dr. Henry Travers, Sioux Falls, S.D.)

## ANTIPARASITIC SUSCEPTIBILITY TESTING AND THERAPY

Adult worms can be eradicated with praziquantel or niclosamide. Expulsion of the scolex must be assured to assume satisfactory treatment.

## PREVENTION

Good hygiene and immediate treatment are essential for the prevention of autoinfection. Pork should be cooked or frozen thoroughly. Cysticerci do not survive temperatures below −10° C or above 50° C. Educational programs concerning the hazards associated with living near human sewage and contaminated drinking water are important in populations at risk. When traveling in countries where food is likely to be contaminated, wash, peel, or cook all raw vegetables and fruits with clean water before eating.

## *TAENIA SAGINATA*

### GENERAL CHARACTERISTICS

*T. saginata* or beef tapeworm has a worldwide distribution and is more common than *T. solium.* The worm can grow

4 to 12 m and contain 1000 to 2000 segments. *T. saginata* may produce 100,000 eggs and live up to 25 years in the human intestine.

## EPIDEMIOLOGY

*T. saginata* has a similar life cycle to that of *T. solium.* Cattle are the intermediate hosts and humans are infected through the ingestion of cysticerci (larval form) in raw or undercooked beef.

## PATHOGENESIS AND SPECTRUM OF DISEASE

The life cycle of *T. saginata* begins with human ingestion of undercooked or raw meet infected with larvae. The larvae are ingested in the meat and, following digestion, released into the small intestine where the worm attaches to the mucosa and matures. In about 3 months, the worm may grow up to 4 to 5 m in length and gravid segments begin to break off and pass in stool. Following deposition of gravid segments in the soil, an intermediate bovine host may ingest the segments. The segments are digested and the eggs hatch, releasing an oncosphere that penetrates the muscle tissue. Following penetration of the mucosa the organisms are carried via the lymphatic vessels and bloodstream throughout the intermediate host. Humans then ingest the infected meat of the intermediate host, as previously indicated. Humans typically are asymptomatic, or have very mild indigestion, loss of appetite, vomiting, and abdominal discomfort. A rare case of severe infection may result in intestinal obstruction and appendicitis. Patients are often unaware of their infection until gravid motile segments are passed in the feces and cause psychological distress.

## LABORATORY DIAGNOSIS

The stool should be examined for proglottids and eggs; eggs may also be present on anal swabs. The eggs of *T. saginata* are indistinguishable from those of *T. solium.* The uterus of *T. saginata* is longer than wide and typically contains 15 to 18 lateral branches on each side (see Figure 54-10). The scolex has four suckers and is unarmed or does not contain any hooklets (Figure 54-11). Stool specimens should be handled with care since the eggs cannot be distinguished from those of *T. solium.* Slight eosinophilia may develop.

## ANTIPARASITIC SUSCEPTIBILITY AND THERAPY

Recommended treatment includes praziquantel or niclosamide. Treatment of *T. saginata* can be considered successful when no proglottids are passed for 4 consecutive months.

## PREVENTION

Beef should be inspected for cysticerci and thoroughly cooked before ingesting.

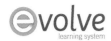 Visit the Evolve site to complete the review questions.

## CASE STUDY 54-1

A 50-year-old man presented to the physician complaining of headaches and difficulty maintaining his balance. On physical exam the physician noticed a lump in the man's left calf. Initial lab results including a complete blood count and differential were normal. The ESR (erythrocyte sedimentation rate) was slightly elevated, indicating generalized inflammation. The physician asked the man if he had traveled to any areas outside of the United States in the past 12 months. The man had recently returned from volunteering in Haiti. The physician prescribed niclosamide and had the patient collect three stool samples over the next 12 days. Following treatment the following parasite was recovered from the man's stool (see Figures 54-12 and 54-13).

**QUESTIONS**

1. Identify the parasite to the species level.
2. Explain the morphologic characteristics that would definitively provide a clear identification of the parasite.
3. What, if any, additional treatments are available for this patient?

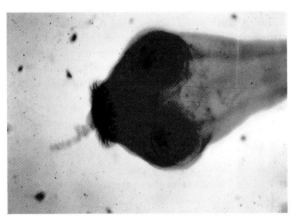

**Figure 54-12** Scolex. (Courtesy Dr. Henry Travers, Sioux Falls, S.D.)

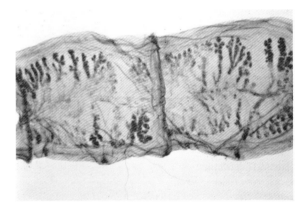

**Figure 54-13** Proglottid. (Courtesy Dr. Henry Travers, Sioux Falls, S.D.)

## BIBLIOGRAPHY

Garcia LS: *Practical guide to diagnostic parasitology,* Washington, DC, 1999, ASM Press.

Hyneman D: Chapter 89: Cestodes. In Baron S, editor: *Medical microbiology,* ed 4, Galveston, TX, 1996.

Mayta H, Talley A, Gilman RH: Differentiating *Taenia solium* and *Taenia saginata* infections by simple hematoxylin-eosin staining and PCR-restriction enzyme analysis, *J Clin Microbiol* 38:133, 2000.

Patamia I, Cappello E, Castellano-Chiodo D, et al: *Kor J Parasitol* 48:167, 2010.

Samkari A, Kiska DL, Riddell SW, et al: *Dipylidium caninum* mimicking recurrent *Enterobius vermicularis* (pinworm) infection, *Clin Pediatr* 47:397, 2008.

Schenone H: Praziquantel in the treatment of *Hymenolepis nana* infections in children, *Am J Trop Med Hyg* 29:320, 1980.

Scholz T, Garcia H, Kuchta R, et al: Update on the human broad tapeworm (genus *Diphyllobothrium*), including clinical relevance, *J Clin Microbiol* 22:146, 2009.

Sorvillo F, Wilkins P, Shafir S, et al: Public health implications of cysticercosis acquired in the United States, *Emerg Infect Dis* 17:1, 2011.

Tena D, Montserrat P, Carmen G, et al: Human infection with *Hymenolepis diminuta:* case report from Spain, *J Clin Microbiol* 136:2375, 1998.

Turner J: Human dipylidaisis (dog tapeworm infection) in the United States, *J Pediatr* 61:763, 1962.

Wicht B, Yanagida T, Ito A, et al: Multiplex PCR for differentiated identification of broadworm tapeworms (cestode: Diphyllobothrium) infecting humans, *J Clin Microbiol* 48:311, 2010.

Wiwanitkit V: Overview of *Hymenolepis diminuta* infection among Thai patients, *J Gen Med* 6:7, 2004.

# 55 Tissue Cestodes

## OBJECTIVES

1. Describe and compare the life cycles of the tissue cestodes, including reservoir and intermediate hosts.
2. Describe the clinical manifestations and complications of cysticercus in the human host.
3. List the various methods used to diagnose cystericercus infection.
4. Define and describe the morphologic characteristics of the following: oncosphere, brood capsule, hydatid cyst, and hydatid sand.
5. Describe hydatid disease, including laboratory diagnosis and the best course of treatment.
6. Compare and contrast the pathogenesis and spectrum of disease associated with direct tissue damage versus the immune response to *Echinococcus* spp.
7. Describe the tapeworm that causes coenurosis, including hosts and symptoms of disease.
8. Describe the preventive measures recommended to avoid infection with tissue cestodes.

---

### PARASITES TO BE CONSIDERED

**Cestodes (Tapeworms)**
Tissue (Larval Forms)
  *Taenia solium*
  *Echinococcus granulosus*
  *Echinococcus multilocularis*
  *Taenia multiceps*
  *Spirometra mansonoides*

---

Tissue cestodes do not reach the adult stage in the human host. The organisms infect the human in their intermediate or cyst stage. The infections are much more serious than those caused by the adult tapeworm. The parasites can cause serious disease, or even death. Larval cestodes cause infection by accidental ingestion of eggs excreted from the intermediate host (Table 55-1), and they lodge in various organs and tissues in the human body. Diagnosis of larval infections can be problematic.

## ▪ *TAENIA SOLIUM*

### GENERAL CHARACTERISTICS

*Taenia solium*, also known as the pork tapeworm, causes an intestinal infection from eating contaminated pork, as discussed in Chapter 54. The adult worm usually causes no clinical disease. Humans may accidentally become the intermediate host and ingest eggs from

human feces. This typically occurs when an individual is already infected with adult *T. solium*. Autoinfection occurs when the individual swallows eggs from improper hand washing. Humans may develop the larval infection, which could result in cysticercosis. Cysticercosis is usually asymptomatic unless larvae invade the central nervous system (CNS), the globe of the eye, or other muscle and tissues.

### EPIDEMIOLOGY

*T. solium* is found worldwide, with a higher incidence in Latin America. The larval form of the infection rarely occurs in the United States, but may be found among immigrants from Mexico. Following ingestion of *T. solium* eggs, the oncospheres hatch in the intestine and invade the intestinal wall. Once the larvae invade the tissue the organism is capable of spreading systemically by migration to the brain, liver, and other tissues, causing human cysticercosis. Cysticercosis is defined as larval forms distributed throughout the body. Human cysticercosis may also occur when reverse peristalsis returns gravid segments into the intestine, where the eggs hatch and release oncospheres. Cysticerci develop and may live many years. Cysticerci will eventually die and may calcify, which will aid in diagnosis.

### PATHOGENESIS AND SPECTRUM OF DISEASE

Clinical signs and symptoms depend on the location, viability, and number of the cysticerci present. Cysticerci can develop in any organ or tissue of the body. The severity of the symptoms depends on the body site involved and may not appear for years after the initial infection. The most severe cases are found in the central nervous system and the eye. Once cysticerci localize in the brain, the organism causes a condition referred to as **neurocysticercosis.** Infection can cause epileptic-type seizures, headaches, mental disturbances, meningitis, or sudden death. Cysticerci can also be found in the eye and must be removed to avoid permanent eye damage, including blindness. Much of the damage from cysticercosis is caused by the severe inflammatory host response that occurs after the cysticerci have died. Antibodies are produced and offer the patient secondary immunity.

### LABORATORY DIAGNOSIS

Cysticercosis can be difficult to diagnose. *T. solium* eggs are found in stools in fewer than half the patients with cysticercosis. Demonstration of eggs or proglottids in the feces is an indication of *Taenia* infection but does not provide a diagnosis for cysticercosis. Definitive diagnosis

**TABLE 55-1** Common Human Parasites, Diagnostic Specimens, Tests, and Positive Findings

| Organism | Acquired Infection | Location in Host | Diagnostic Specimen | Diagnostic Test* | Positive Specimen | Comments |
|---|---|---|---|---|---|---|
| **Tissue cestodes** | Ingestion of: | | | | | |
| *Echinococcus granulosus* | Eggs from dog tapeworm | Liver, lung, etc. | Serum, hydatid cyst aspirate; biopsy | Serology, centrifugation of fluid; histology | Positive serology; hydatid sand, tapeworm tissue | *E. granulosus* (enclosed cyst) |
| *E. multilocularis* | Eggs from fox tapeworm | CNS, subcutaneous tissues | Serum, scans, biopsy | Serology, films, histology | Positive serology, positive scans, tapeworm tissue | *E. multilocularis* (cyst develops throughout tissue) |
| *Taenia solium* (pork) | Eggs from human tapeworm | | | | | Small, enclosed cysticerci (cysticercosis) |

*Although serologic tests are not always mentioned, they are available for a number of parasitic infections. Unfortunately, most are not routinely available. Contact your state public health laboratory or the Centers for Disease Control and Prevention in Atlanta, Ga.

usually requires the identification of cysticercus in the tissue. The organism is surgically removed and microscopically examined for the presence of suckers and hooks on the scolex. The cysticercus is round to oval, translucent, and about 5 mm or more in diameter. The organism has a scolex with four suckers and a rostellum with a circle of hooks. Fine needle aspiration cytology may be helpful in the diagnosis and eliminates the need for surgical biopsy. Diagnosis may also be made using computed tomography (CT) scans and magnetic resonance imaging (MRI). Radiographs may also be useful in detecting calcifying cysticerci within tissue. Ocular cysticercosis may be diagnosed by visual identification of the larval worm. Serologic procedures (such as enzyme-linked immunosorbent assay [ELISA]) may also be used as a useful tool to aid in diagnosis, but may not be sensitive enough in light infections. The Centers for Disease Control and Prevention (CDC) offers an immunoblot assay that has demonstrated 100% specificity and 98% sensitivity. The assay uses purified antigen from *T. solium* containing seven different major glycoproteins. It is by far the test of choice over an ELISA. Nucleic acid-based methods and species-specific polymerase chain reaction (PCR) have been described to differentiate Taenia species.

## THERAPY

Cysticercosis should be treated with corticosteroids, anticonvulsants, and surgery if deemed appropriate. Treating nonviable cysticerci in the brain of asymptomatic patients has not been proven necessary. Not all patients respond to treatment and not all patients must be treated, because the inflammatory response as a result of the treatment may be more serious than the disease. Symptomatic neurocysticercosis should be managed using treatment that decreases the patient's symptoms. When treatment is suggested, albendazole is the drug of choice. If praziquantel is used, it should be combined with corticosteroids to reduce the inflammatory response and should not be used for ocular or spinal cord infections.

Surgery may be required for ocular, spinal, or brain involvement.

## PREVENTION

Education, meat inspection, and improvement of sanitation measures are the key preventive measures. Other prevention methods are discussed in Chapter 54.

# ECHINOCOCCUS GRANULOSUS

## GENERAL CHARACTERISTICS

*Echinococcus* is the smallest of all tapeworms (3 to 9 mm long) with three to five proglottids. It contains a scolex with four suckers and a rostellum with hooks to attach to the intestinal wall. *E. granulosus* is a tapeworm found in the small intestine of the definitive host, the canine. Eggs are ingested by the intermediate hosts and include a variety of mammals including sheep, cattle, moose, and humans. There are several strains of *Echinococcus granulosus* that have been identified, with the dog-sheep strain being the most common. Humans are typically accidental hosts and are considered a dead-end since the life cycle of the organism is unable to continue in a human host. Oncospheres hatch in the intestine of the intermediate host and invade the circulatory system, where they develop into hydatid cysts. Disease symptoms vary with the site and size of the cyst. Echinococcosis (**hydatid disease**) results from the presence of one or more cysts (**hydatids**), which can develop in any tissue.

## EPIDEMIOLOGY

*E. granulosus* is most common in cool, damp areas where sheep herds are prevalent, such as southern South America, Russia, East Africa, and the western United States. The eggs in the definitive host are passed through the feces and contaminate soil, water, or food. The eggs are able to survive freezing conditions and can remain viable within the environment for several years.

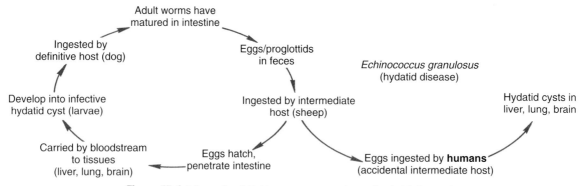

**Figure 55-1** Life cycle of *Echinococcus granulosus* (hydatid disease).

Adult worms are found only in the intermediate hosts (Figure 55-1).

## PATHOGENESIS AND SPECTRUM OF DISEASE

Hydatid disease in humans is potentially dangerous depending on the size and location of the cyst. Some cysts may remain undetected for many years until they grow large enough to affect other organs. Many humans live day-to-day without ever knowing they are infected. The cyst is very slow growing in humans. It is usually fluid-filled and has a germinal layer from which many thousands of scolices are budded. These are known as daughter cysts (**brood capsules**), which attach to the germinal layer or free-float in the cyst. The scolices in the hydatid fluid resemble grains of sand and are called **hydatid sand** (Figures 55-2, *A* and 55-3). The result is a unilocular cyst containing future adult worms. The cyst may resemble a slow-growing tumor. Infections in the liver or lungs may be asymptomatic for many years, but the pressure eventually causes noticeable symptoms. The majority of the hydatid cysts occur within the liver. Cysts within the liver cause chronic abdominal pain and allergic reactions and may result in cholangitis (infection of the common bile duct) and cholestasis (interference with flow of bile from the liver). Cysts that develop in the lungs may cause infections and abscesses and result in chronic cough, shortness of breath, and chest pain. During the life cycle of the cyst, there may be occasional seepage of fluid into the host tissue and circulation causing sensitization or activation of the immune response from the presence of the parasite. The rupture and release of the fluid of a hydatid cyst may cause anaphylactic shock as a result of the primary sensitization in a previously asymptomatic individual. If a cyst bursts within the human body, many new cysts may be released that are typically eliminated via the host's cellular immune response. Leaking fluid from a cyst may cause notable eosinophilia.

## LABORATORY DIAGNOSIS

Clinical symptoms of a slow-growing abdominal tumor with or without eosinophilia are suggestive of infection. Human infection ranges from asymptomatic to severe, including death. Diagnosis is made through the identification of cysts in the infected organ, accompanied with

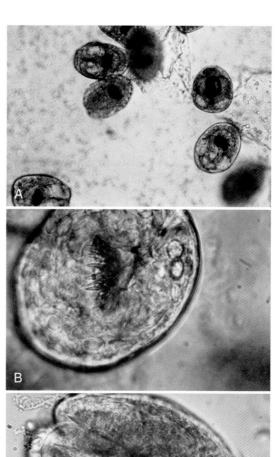

**Figure 55-2 A,** *Echinococcus* granules. **B,** Ovum. **C,** Scolex. (Courtesy Dr. Henry Travers, Sioux Falls, S.D.)

positive serologic tests. A variety of serologic tests are available including ELISA, indirect hemagglutination, and latex agglutination. Both false positives and false negatives may occur; therefore clinical history is extremely important for diagnosis. Ultrasound, magnetic resonance imaging (MRI), and computed tomography (CT) have

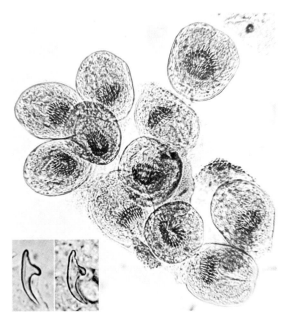

**Figure 55-3** *Echinococcus granulosus,* hydatid sand (300×). *(Inset)* Two individual hooklets (1000×).

improved the diagnosis and may provide visualization of the fluid-filled cysts. Calcified cysts can be visualized using conventional x-ray. Microscopic examination of the cyst fluid for the identification of the scolices can be useful in diagnosis. A 1% eosin stain may be added to the fluid to assist in the visualization and determination as to whether or not the cyst is viable. Nonviable scolices will stain with the eosin whereas viable scolices will not.

## THERAPY

Surgery is the most common form of treatment. The procedure involves surgical removal of cysts or inactivation of hydatid sand by injecting the cyst with 10% formalin and then removing it. Extreme care must be taken to avoid spillage. Albendazole is the drug of choice to kill the scolices within the cyst, reduce the size of the cyst, and prevent recurrence. Mebendazole and praziquantel have also been shown to be effective.

## PREVENTION

Preventive measures include avoiding contact with infected dogs and deworming animals regularly. Effective control includes educating the population concerning the danger and means of transmission of hydatid disease as well as maintaining good hygiene and practicing safe disposal of dog feces. Slaughtered animals must be disposed of properly, to prevent dogs from exposure to contaminated materials and interrupt the *Echinococcus* life cycle.

# ECHINOCOCCUS MULTILOCULARIS

## GENERAL CHARACTERISTICS

Although rarely found in the brain of humans, *E. multilocularis* causes alveolar hydatid disease, which is a fatal form of echinococcosis. It is the most lethal of all helmintic diseases. The cyst is extremely dangerous because it lacks a laminated membrane and develops a series of connected chambers. The chambers contain little or no fluid and rarely contain a scolex. The morphology of the cyst is very similar to that of *E. granulosus,* but the adult organisms are much smaller (1.2 to 3.7 mm). The cysts are very resistant to cold temperatures.

## EPIDEMIOLOGY

*E. multilocularis* is found in Asia, Europe, and northern North America, including areas such as Alaska, Montana, and Minnesota. Foxes, coyotes, and dogs are the definitive host for *E. multilocularis,* whereas rodents are the intermediate host. The parasite is occasionally transmitted to humans through the ingestion of contaminated food or water, and by handling infected animals. Fur trappers and veterinarians are at an increased risk of infection as a result of exposure to infected animals. The life cycle of *E. multilocularis* is essentially identical to that of *Echinococcus granulsosus.*

## PATHOGENESIS AND SPECTRUM OF DISEASE

Alveolar hydatid disease is a highly lethal, destructive disease. The cyst of *E. multilocularis* grows slowly and may take years to produce clinical symptoms. Many cysts are asymptomatic during the life of the infected individual and are sometimes found during autopsy, surgery, or imaging scans related to other clinical conditions. The severity of symptoms depends on the location of the cyst and the size, as seen with *E. granulosus.* Cysts form primarily in the liver and metastasize to the lung or brain. Cysts in the liver are not restricted with a laminated cyst wall and are capable of expansion into a multicystic structure. This **multilocular** (many chambers) hydatid cyst is often mistaken for a hepatic sarcoma, making diagnosis difficult. This disease is often fatal.

## LABORATORY DIAGNOSIS

Ultrasound, CT scans, and MRI are used to visualize the cyst and can be supported with serologic testing. Serologic tests, such as ELISA, are sensitive and highly specific.

## THERAPY

The most common treatment is to remove the parasite surgically; however, the disease is usually diagnosed late, when it is inoperable and results in a high rate of fatality. Treatment with mebendazole and albendazole has been used successfully and may be the preferred treatment in many cases. Surgery should follow and is the only means of removing the cyst.

## PREVENTION

Controlling rodents is an important means of prevention along with educating the public at risk to avoid exposure to infective feces. Practicing good hygiene and periodically deworming household pets are also helpful.

# TAENIA MULTICEPS

## GENERAL CHARACTERISTICS

*T. multiceps* is a tapeworm that causes coenurosis in humans. The **coenurus** (larval form) may cause destructive damage or death, but is an extremely rare disease in humans. The coenurus is a unilocular cyst similar to cysticercus, although the worm has multiple scolices. Daughter cysts may also be seen. The body of *T. multiceps* is 5 to 6 cm long and consists of 200 to 250 segments. The scolex has 4 suckers and a proboscis (tubular appendage) with 22 to 32 hooks arranged in 2 rows.

## EPIDEMIOLOGY

*T. multiceps* is most often found in Africa, although it may be seen in South America, the United States, and Canada. The adult worm is typically found in dogs and other canids. Many animals serve as the intermediate host, such as sheep, cattle, and deer. The animals become infected through the ingestion of eggs while grazing. Humans can also serve as an intermediate host. Human infection occurs from accidental ingestion of dog feces containing the eggs.

## PATHOGENESIS AND SPECTRUM OF DISEASE

The oncosphere hatches and penetrates the intestinal wall of the intermediate host. The embryo is carried via the bloodstream to various parts of the body including the brain, eyes, and central nervous system, where the organism lodges and the coenurus develops. The coenurus develops into multiple daughter cysts. Symptoms include headache, vomiting, paralysis, and blindness. The coenurus causes a serious disease called coenurosis in sheep and in dogs that have eaten the brains of infected sheep. This clinical condition is known as gid, sturdy, or staggers.

## LABORATORY DIAGNOSIS

Diagnosis is similar to that for *Echinococcus* infection. CT and MRI may be useful for detecting the cysts. Microscopic identification can be used if the cyst has been removed surgically. Currently, there are no serologic tests available.

## THERAPY

Treatment is similar to that for *Echinococcus*. The most common treatment is surgery if possible, although the drugs used for cysticercosis may also be effective against coenurus infection.

## PREVENTION

Dogs associated with sheep and other livestock should not be fed the brain or spinal cord from infected animals and should be dewormed regularly. Good hygiene should be practiced and care taken not to eat or drink anything contaminated with dog feces.

# SPIROMETRA MANSONOIDES

## GENERAL CHARACTERISTICS

Sparganosis is an infection caused by the plerocercoid larvae of *Spirometra*. The larvae (spargana) are white, wrinkled, and ribbon-shaped. They may be 3 mm wide and up to 30 cm long. The sparganum has **bothria** (longitudinal grooves) instead of suckers. No scolex is present, which can help differentiate *Spirometra* from *Taenia solium*.

## EPIDEMIOLOGY

*Spirometra* is found worldwide, with most human cases of sparganosis found in Asia. Sparganosis is endemic in animals throughout North America, but rare in humans. Adult spirometra live in the intestine of dogs and cats. Eggs are shed in feces, hatch in water, and release coracidia. The coracidia are then ingested by copepods, which become infected. Reptiles, fish, and amphibians ingest infected copepods containing the procercoid larvae. The procercoid larvae develop into plerocercoid larvae in the second intermediate host. Humans are accidental hosts; they acquire sparganosis following ingestion of contaminated water or by consuming undercooked fish. The life cycle is identical to that of the broad fish tapeworm, *Diphyllobothrium* spp. Humans are unable to serve as the definitive host for spirometra. However, spargana can live up to 20 years in the human host.

## PATHOGENESIS AND SPECTRUM OF DISEASE

Spargana migrate and lodge anywhere in the human body. Clinical symptoms depend on which organs or tissues are involved. Spargana can live for several years before symptoms develop. Sparganosis is usually asymptomatic until the larvae grow and cause an inflammatory reaction. Painful nodules can develop in the tissues. A variety of symptoms may occur, including seizure, weakness, headache, and eye pain that can lead to blindness if left untreated.

## LABORATORY DIAGNOSIS

Definitive diagnosis is usually made by removal and identification of the sparganum from infected tissue. Clinical history, ELISA, MRI, and CT can all be used together to presumptively diagnose sparganosis. Eosinophilia may also be present.

## THERAPY

Praziquantel has been used with limited success. Surgical removal of the complete sparganum is the treatment of choice.

## PREVENTION

Prevention strategies should include safe drinking water practices, and awareness of the dangers of consuming raw fish and amphibians. Water in contaminated areas should be boiled before consumption.

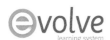

**Visit the Evolve site to complete the review questions.**

## CASE STUDY 55-1

A 65-year-old male from Montana was admitted to the emergency department in a local hospital. The patient is a sheepherder and owns dogs. He claims to have no travel history outside the local area. He enjoys hunting and trapping in the area and frequently enjoys eating his venison. He was admitted with upper right quadrant pain and vomiting. An abdominal mass was felt and an MRI ordered. MRI showed a 5-cm mass in the liver. Fluid-filled cysts and a scolex were surgically removed (Figure 55-4).

### QUESTIONS

1. What parasite should be considered?
2. What additional testing should be performed to aid in diagnosis?
3. Which preventive measures should be used to control the spread of this parasite?

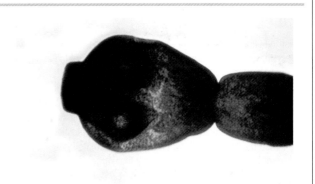

**Figure 55-4** Scolex collected from patient's liver biopsy. (Courtesy Dr. Henry Travers, Sioux Falls, SD.)

## BIBLIOGRAPHY

Beggs I: The radiology of hydatid disease, *Am J Roentgenol* 145:639, 1985.

Budke CM, White AC Jr, Garcia HH: Zoonotic larval cestode infections: neglected, neglected, tropical diseases, *Negl Trop Dis* 3:319, 2009.

Carroll CL, Connor DH: Sparganosis. In Connor DH, et al, editors: *Pathology of infectious disease*, Stamford, Conn, 1997, Appleton Lange.

Dahniya MH, Hanna RM, Askelou S et al: The imaging appearances of hydatid disease at some unusual sites, *Br J Radiol* 74:283, 2001.

Eckert J, Deplazes P: Biological, epidemiological, and clinical aspects of echinococcosis, a zoonosis of increasing concern, *Clin Microbiol Rev* 17:1077, 2004.

El-On J, Shelef I, Cagnano E, et al: *Taenia multiceps:* a rare human cestode infection in Israel, *Vet Ital* 44:621, 2008.

Garcia HH, Evans CA, Nast TE, et al: Current consensus guidelines for treatment of neurocysticercosis, *Clin Microbiol Rev* 15:747, 2002.

Garcia LS: *Diagnostic medical parasitology*, ed 5, Washington, DC, 2007, ASM Press.

Gonzalez LM, Montero E, Harrison LJ, et al: Differential diagnosis of *Taenia saginata* and *Taenia solium* infection by PCR, *J Clin Microbiol* 38:737-744, 2000.

Horton J: Albendazole for the treatment of echinococcosis, *Fundam Clin Pharmacol* 17:205, 2003.

Li M-W, Lin H-Y, Xie W-T, et al: Enzootic sparganosis in Guangdong People's Republic of China, *Emerg Infect Dis* 15:8, 2009.

Liance M, Janir V, Bresson-Hadni S, et al: Immunodiagnosis of *Echinococcus* infections: confirmatory testing and species differentiation by a new commercial western blot, *J Clin Microbiol* 38:3718, 2000.

McManus DP, Zhang W, Li J, et al: Echinococcosis, *Lancet* 362:1295, 2003.

Polat P, Kantarci M, Alper F, et al: Hydatid disease from head to toe, *Radiographics* 23:475, 2003.

Pedrosa I, Saiz A, Arrazola J, et al: Hydatid disease: radiologic and pathologic features and complications, *Radiographics* 20:795, 2000.

Rosas N, Sotelo J, Nieto D: ELISA in the diagnosis of neurocysticercosis, *Arch Neurol* 43:353, 1986.

Sorvillo F, Waterman S, Richards F, et al: Cysticercosis surveillance: locally acquired and travel-related infections and detection of intestinal tapeworm carriers in Los Angeles County, *Am J Trop Med Hyg* 47:365, 1992.

Versalovic J: *Manual of clinical microbiology*, ed 10, Washington, D.C., 2011, ASM Press.

Zhang W, Li J, McManus D: Concepts in immunology and diagnosis of hydatid disease, *Clin Microbiol Rev* 16:18, 2003.

## OBJECTIVES

1. List the clinically significant intestinal trematodes.
2. Describe the general life cycle of the intestinal trematodes and identify the life cycle stage infective for humans.
3. Describe the diagnostic methods used to identify intestinal trematodes.
4. Explain the pathogenesis of intestinal trematode infections.
5. List the drugs of choice for intestinal trematode infections.
6. Describe the environment where intestinal trematodes are found, the route of transmission, and preventive measures.

---

**PARASITES TO BE CONSIDERED**

**Helminths**
**Trematodes (Flukes)**
Intestinal
  *Fasciolopsis buski*
  *Heterophyes heterophyes*
  *Metagonimus yokogawai*

---

The intestinal trematodes (flukes) are members of the phylum Platehelminthes (flatworms), are dorsoventrically flattened, and require at least one intermediate host (a freshwater snail). Human infection occurs by ingestion of metacercariae encysted on freshwater vegetation or fish. Most trematodes are hermaphroditic (both ovaries and testes are contained within each adult worm). The parasites are typically identified from eggs shed in the feces.

The adult worms are located in the small intestine, where they lay eggs that may be embryonated or remain unembryonated until they are shed from the body via feces. The egg continues developing after reaching the water, and a ciliated, free-swimming miracidium larva is released. The miracidium enters a snail host and develops into a redia (cylindrical larvae), followed by development into tailed cercariae. The cercariae emerge from the snail and encyst as a metacercariae (encrusted larvae) on water plants or fish. A human host ingests raw or undercooked plants *(Fasciolopsis buski)* or fish *(Heterophyes heterophyes, Metagonimus yokogawai)* containing the metacercariae, which exycyst in the intestinal tract, attach, and mature into adults (Figure 56-1).

## FASCIOLOPSIS BUSKI

### GENERAL CHARACTERISTICS

The adults of *F. buski* have an elongated shape and range from 20 to 75 mm long to approximately 8 to 20 mm wide (Figure 56-2). They have an oral sucker at the anterior end and a ventral sucker located about midway to the posterior end. The eggs, which are indistinguishable from those of *Fasciola hepatica* (Figure 56-3), are oval and elongated, transparent, and yellow-brown with an operculum (lid) at one end, and they range in size from 130 to 140 μm long to 80 to 85 μm wide and may be unembryonated.

### EPIDEMIOLOGY

*Fasciolopsis buski* is found in Bangladesh, Cambodia, China, India, Indonesia, Laos, Malaysia, Pakistan, Taiwan, Thailand, and Vietnam, and is prevalent in school-aged children. Contaminated feces drains into the water from farm lands, where feces is used for fertilization, and defecation occurs in or near water sources. Reservoir hosts include pigs, dogs, and rabbits.

*F. buski* is the largest of the intestinal trematodes, and infection is acquired by ingestion of raw water chestnuts or caltrop. The definitive host is the pig, and fish-eating wild and domestic animals may serve as reservoir hosts. The water vegetation may become contaminated when feces is used for fertilization or where disposal of farm animal feces is inadequate.

### PATHOGENESIS AND SPECTRUM OF DISEASE

The intestinal attachment site of the adult worms often becomes locally inflamed and ulcerated, and may hemorrhage. Moderate to heavy infections may cause abdominal pain, diarrhea, intestinal obstruction, and edema of the abdomen and lower extremities, and may result in inadequate absorption of vitamin $B_{12}$. Eosinophilia is commonly observed.

### PREVENTION

Infection can be prevented by making sure that water plants and fish are properly cooked before eating. In addition, changes are needed in agricultural practices and health education in the endemic areas.

## HETEROPHYES HETEROPHYES AND METAGONIMUS YOKOGAWAI

### GENERAL CHARACTERISTICS

Adult *H. heterophyes* worms range in size from 1.0 to 1.7 mm in length by 0.3 to 0.4 mm in width, and have a broadly rounded posterior. *M. yokogawai* adults range in size from 1.0 to 2.5 mm long to approximately 0.4 to

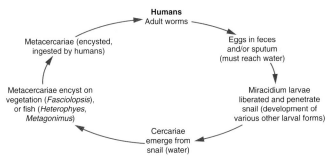

**Figure 56-1** Life cycle of trematodes acquired by humans through ingestion of raw fish, crabs, or crayfish and vegetation.

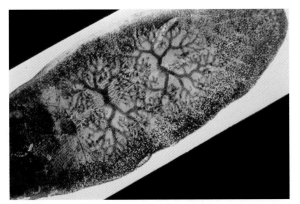

**Figure 56-2** Whole mount of *Fasciolopsis buski*. (Courtesy Dr. Henry Travers, Sioux Falls, S.D.)

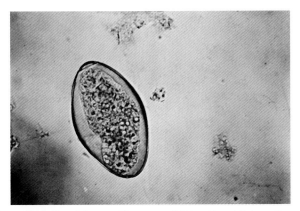

**Figure 56-3** *Fasciola* egg. The eggs of *F. buski* and *F. hepatica* are indistinguishable morphologically. (Courtesy Dr. Henry Travers, Sioux Falls, S.D.)

0.8 mm wide. The adult *H. heterophyes* also has an additional sucker, the genital sucker, which surrounds the genital pore. The eggs are small, yellow-brown, embryonated, and operculated and may have minimal opercular shoulders. Eggs range in size from 26 to 30 long μm to 15 to 17 μm wide, and may be indistinguishable between the two species.

## EPIDEMIOLOGY

*H. heterophyes* is found in China, Egypt, India, Iran, Israel, Japan, Korea, Sudan, Taiwan, the Philippines, Tunisia, and Turkey. *M. yokogawai* is found in the Balkans (a cultural region of southeastern Europe), China, Indonesia, Israel, Japan, Korea, Russia, Spain, and Taiwan, and is considered the most common intestinal fluke infection in the Far East. Reservoir hosts include cats, dogs, and birds, and a variety of freshwater fish may serve as the second intermediate host.

These are two very small trematodes acquired through ingestion of pickled or uncooked fish. A variety of fish-eating mammals may serve as reservoir hosts.

## PATHOGENICITY AND SPECTRUM OF DISEASE

Infections with a small number of worms may be asymptomatic. Symptoms in heavy infections may include abdominal pain, diarrhea with a large amount of mucus, and ulceration of the intestinal wall. Eggs may gain entry into intestinal capillaries and lymphatics, where they can be carried to the heart, brain, spinal cord, or other tissues, causing emboli or granuloma formation.

## PREVENTION

Avoid ingestion of raw, inadequately cooked, and pickled or salted fish. The risk of infection could be greatly reduced by improved sanitary conditions and health education programs.

## LABORATORY DIAGNOSIS

Identification of the intestinal trematodes is made by recovery of eggs, or in rare cases adults, from stool specimens using a sedimentation method such as formalin-ethyl acetate. The sediment may be examined in a wet mount with or without iodine. Because the eggs of *Fasciolopsis buski* are identical to those of *Fasciola hepatica*, and those of *Heterophyes heterophyes* and *Metagonimus yokogawai* are very similar, diagnosis may also require assessment of symptoms, obtaining a travel history, and/or recovery of adult worms. Table 56-1 shows the diagnostic characteristics of the intestinal trematodes.

## TREATMENT

The drug of choice for treatment of intestinal trematode infection is praziquantel (Biltricide), an isoquinoline derivative administered orally in three doses for 1 day. There may be some mild side effects, but these usually disappear within 48 hours, and may be more severe in those with heavy infections. An alternative drug is niclosamide (Niclocide), which is given for 1 to 2 days.

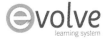 *Visit the Evolve site to complete the review questions.*

**TABLE 56-1** Diagnostic Characteristics of Intestinal Trematodes

| Intestinal Trematode | Food Source | Size of Egg | Description of Egg |
|---|---|---|---|
| *Fasciolopsis buski* | Freshwater vegetation | 80-85 μm × 130-140 μm | Operculated, yellow-brown, unembryonated |
| *Heterophyes heterophyes* | Pickled or uncooked fish | 15-17 μm × 26-30 μm | Operculated with slight opercular shoulders, yellow-brown, embryonated |
| *Metagonimus yokogawai* | Pickled or uncooked fish | 15-17 μm × 26-30 μm | Operculated with slight opercular shoulders, yellow-brown, embryonated |

## CASE STUDY 56-1

The husband of a 32-year-old woman is employed in the foreign service and the couple has recently been on assignment to Africa. The wife complained of a 2-month history of abdominal pain, vomiting, diarrhea, and weight loss. While in Africa she had often eaten the locally grown watercress. A stool specimen was collected for culture and ova and parasite examination. The bacterial culture was negative. A wet mount made during the parasite examination showed large, oval, operculated, and unembryonated helminth eggs.

QUESTIONS

1. What parasite is the probable cause of the patient's symptoms?
2. Another parasitic worm has indistinguishable eggs. How would the infections caused by these two worms differ?
3. How did the patient most likely acquire this infection?
4. What would be the preferred treatment for this infection?

## BIBLIOGRAPHY

Bogitsch BJ, Carter CE, Oeltmann TN, editors: *Human parasitology*, ed 3, San Diego, 2005, Academic Press.
Fried B, Graczyk TK, Tamang L: Food-borne intestinal trematodiases in humans, *Parasitol Res* 93:159-170, 2004.
Garcia LS: *Diagnostic medical parasitology*, ed 5, Washington, DC, 2006, ASM Press.
John DT, Petri WA: *Markell's and Voge's medical parasitology*, ed 9, St Louis, 2006, Saunders.
Keiser J, Utzinger J: Food-borne trematodiases, *Clin Microbiol Rev* 22(3):466-483, 2009.

# Liver and Lung Trematodes

## OBJECTIVES

1. List the clinically significant trematodes capable of infecting the liver and lungs.
2. Describe the general life cycle of the liver and lung flukes and identify the infective stage for humans.
3. Describe the diagnostic methods used to identify the liver and lung flukes including the microscopic differentiation of eggs and serologic methods.
4. Describe the pathogenesis of the liver and lung flukes including location and associated disease manifestations.
5. List the drug of choice for infections with liver and lung flukes.
6. Describe the transmission of the liver and lung flukes and discuss how infection may be prevented.

---

### PARASITES TO BE CONSIDERED

**Trematodes (Flukes)**
Liver/Lung
 *Clonorchis (Opisthorchis) sinensis*
 *Opisthorchis viverrini*
 *Fasciola hepatica*
 *Paragonimus westermani*
 *Paragonimus mexicanus*

---

The parasites within this chapter are typically foodborne and may result in serious economic impact. *Clonorchis* sp., *Opisthorchis* sp. and *Fasciola* sp. live in the biliary ducts of humans. *Paragonimus* spp. are found in the lungs and in other body sites.

## THE LIVER FLUKES

### GENERAL CHARACTERISTICS

The adults of these trematodes live in the biliary ducts and in heavy infections may be also found in the gallbladder. Two of these, *Clonorchis sinensis* (the Chinese liver fluke) and *Opisthorchis viverrini* (the Southeast Asian liver fluke), are elongated and narrow and much smaller than *Fasciola* (the sheep liver fluke). These flukes also all require a freshwater snail as an intermediate host.

### EPIDEMIOLOGY AND LIFE CYCLE

*Clonorchis sinensis* is found in China, Japan, Korea, Taiwan, and Vietnam. *Opisthorchis viverrini* is found in Cambodia, Laos, Thailand, and Vietnam. Reservoir hosts include dogs and cats. *Fasciola hepatica* has worldwide distribution and impacts the economics of the sheep and cattle

industries. Reservoir hosts include dogs, pigs, and rabbits. Infected feces enter the water system as a result of improper drainage and unsanitary practices.

The life cycle of the liver flukes is very similar to that of the intestinal flukes. The adult worms produce eggs in the biliary ducts that are then excreted from the body in the feces. The free-swimming miracidium is released from the egg in freshwater and enters the snail host where it develops into a redia and then a cercariae, which leaves the snail and enters the water (Figure 57-1). The cercariae of *Clonorchis* and *Opisthorchis* are ingested by a second intermediate host, a freshwater fish. The cercariae then encyst and develop into the metacercariae within the intermediate host. The metacercaria is the infective stage for humans. When infected freshwater fish are eaten raw or undercooked, the metacercariae will excyst in the duodenum and then travel to the bile duct where they mature. The cercariae of *Fasciola* encyst on freshwater vegetation, such as watercress and water chestnuts, and develop into metacercariae. When the infected vegetation is eaten raw, the metacercariae will excyst in the duodenum and then travel to the bile duct and mature. Figure 57-2 depicts the general life cycles of the liver and lung flukes.

### PATHOGENESIS AND SPECTRUM OF DISEASE

Light infections with *C. sinensis* or *O. viverrini* are most common, and may be asymptomatic. Heavier infections with these flukes may present with fever, abdominal pain, and jaundice. Eosinophilia and increased serum levels of immunoglobulin E (IgE) may be observed. Severe infections may cause obstruction of the biliary ducts, resulting in enlargement and tenderness of the liver, cirrhosis, cholecystitis (inflammation of the gallbladder), and cholangiocarcinoma (cancerous growth in bile duct epithelium).

Even light infections with *Fasciola* may cause fever, abdominal pain, nausea, diarrhea, enlargement and tenderness of the liver, jaundice, nonproductive cough, eosinophilia, and elevated serum IgE levels. More severe infections may result in obstruction of the biliary ducts, cirrhosis, cholecystitis, and cholangiocarcinoma. During migration in the human body, the larvae may penetrate the peritoneal cavity, and adult flukes may then be found in the intestinal walls, lungs, heart, or brain.

### LABORATORY DIAGNOSIS

Identification of the liver flukes is primarily made by recovery of the eggs in feces using a sedimentation method and a wet mount with or without iodine staining. Table 57-1 shows some diagnostic characteristics of the liver and lung flukes.

The adult worms of *Clonorchis* are elongated and narrow, and a transparent reddish-yellow color. Adult *Clonorchis* may vary in size from 10 to 25 mm × 3 to 5 mm. The eggs of *Clonorchis* are 28 to 30 µm × 14 to 18 µm. The eggs have shouldered opercula and a small knob at the end opposite the operculum, are yellow-brown in color, and are embryonated when they leave the body (Figure 57-3).

Like *Clonorchis*, the adult worms of *Opisthorchis* are elongated and narrow, and a transparent reddish-yellow color. Adult worms of *Opisthorchis*, however, are much smaller in size: 5 to 10 mm × 0.8 to 1.9 mm. The size of *Opisthorchis* eggs is slightly smaller than those of *Clonorchis*; *Opisthorchis* eggs are 19 to 29 µm × 12 to 17 µm. Also like *Clonorchis*, the eggs have shouldered opercula and a small knob at the end opposite the operculum, are yellow-brown in color, and are embryonated when they leave the body (see Figure 57-3).

The adult worm of *Fasciola* is much larger (2 to 5 cm × 0.8 to 1.3 cm), with a cephalic cone at the anterior end

**TABLE 57-1** Characteristics of Liver and Lung Trematodes

| Trematode | Adult Location | Food Source | Size of Egg | Description of Egg |
|-----------|---------------|-------------|-------------|--------------------|
| *Fasciola hepatica* | Bile ducts | Freshwater vegetation | 130-150 µm × 70-90 µm | Operculated, brownish-yellow, unembryonated |
| *Clonorchis sinensis* | Bile ducts | Freshwater fish | 28-34 µm × 14-18 µm | Operculated with shoulders, opposite end knob, yellow-brown, embryonated |
| *Opisthorchis viverrini* | Bile ducts | Freshwater fish | 19-29 µm × 12-17 µm | Operculated with shoulders, opposite end knob, yellow-brown, embryonated |
| *Paragonimus westermani* | Lungs | Freshwater crabs or crayfish | 80-120 µm × 45-60 µm | Operculated with shoulders, thick shelled, brownish-yellow, unembryonated |
| *Paragonimus mexicanus* | Lungs | Freshwater crabs | 40 µm × 80 µm | Operculated with shoulders, thick shelled, brownish-yellow, unembryonated |

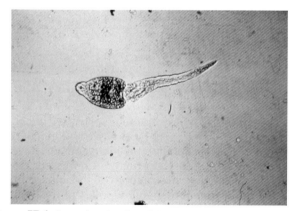

**Figure 57-1** Cercaria of a liver fluke. (Photo courtesy Dr. Henry Travers, Sioux Falls, S.D.)

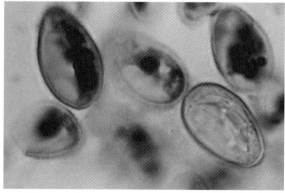

**Figure 57-3** *Clonorchis sinensis* egg. (Photo courtesy Dr. Henry Travers, Sioux Falls, S.D.)

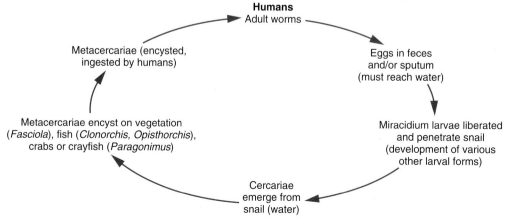

**Figure 57-2** Life cycle of the liver and lung flukes.

that contains the oral sucker. The eggs are 130 to 150 μm × 70 to 90 μm, operculated, brownish-yellow, and unembryonated when they leave the body. Because the eggs of *Fasciola* and *Fasciolopsis* are virtually indistinguishable, it may also be necessary to recover eggs from bile specimens, or to recover adult worms. Definitive identification of *Fasciola* is important because the treatment is different than that for *Fasciolopsis*. There is also serologic testing available in the United States for diagnosis of *Fasciola*. Enzyme immunoassay (EIA) and enzyme-linked immunosorbent assay (ELISA) serum IgG antibody testing is performed at private references laboratories; cross reactivity with other trematodes, such as the schistosomes, may be an issue. Figure 56-3 shows the eggs of *Fasciola hepatica*, and Figure 56-2 is a *Fasciolopsis buski* adult fluke.

## THERAPY AND PREVENTION

The drug of choice for treatment of infections with *Clonorchis* and *Opisthorchis* is praziquantel given orally three times for 1 day. An alternative drug is albendazole, a benzimidazole group drug, given once daily for 7 days. The drug of choice for *Fasciola* is bithionol (praziquantel is not effective) given orally every other day for 10 to 15 doses. A promising drug that has not yet been approved for human use in the United States or Canada, but is approved for veterinary use in the United States, and is recommended by the World Health Organization (WHO) for treatment of *Fasciola*, is triclabendazole, a benzimidazole compound.

Human infection can be prevented by ensuring that fish and aquatic vegetation are properly cooked before consumption, as well as by the improvement of sanitary conditions along with the education of good personal hygiene.

# ▌ THE LUNG FLUKES

## GENERAL CHARACTERISTICS

The genus *Paragonimus* contains several species known to infect humans. *Paragonimus westermani* is the most common and widely distributed lung fluke. The adult worms live in the lungs and produce eggs that may be present in sputum, or if expectorated and swallowed, may be present in feces. Like other trematodes, a freshwater snail is required as an intermediate host.

## EPIDEMIOLOGY AND LIFE CYCLE

*Paragonimus* is found primarily in the Far East (China, Japan, Korea, Manchuria, Papua New Guinea, and Southeast Asia), and certain species (such as *P. mexicanus*) are found in areas of Mexico and South America. Reservoir hosts for *P. westermani* include dogs and cats, and those for *P. mexicanus* include domestic and wild pigs, and dogs. Species of *Paragonimus* may also be found in other freshwater crab- or crayfish-eating mammals.

The adult worms, encapsulated in the lungs, produce eggs that leave the lung via the bronchioles, stimulating a cough response. The eggs are then swallowed and eventually excreted in the feces.* The free-swimming miracidium is released from the egg in freshwater and enters the snail host where it develops into a redia and then a cercariae, which leaves the snail and enters the water. The cercariae then enter a second intermediate host, a crab or crayfish, where they encyst and develop into metacercariae. The metacercaria is the infective stage for humans. When infected freshwater crabs and crayfish are eaten raw or undercooked, the metacercariae will excyst in the duodenum and then migrate through the intestinal wall, and eventually through the diaphragm and into the lungs where they encapsulate (usually in pairs) and mature (see Figure 57-2).

## PATHOGENESIS AND SPECTRUM OF DISEASE

Light infections may be asymptomatic. The migration of the metacercariae through muscle and tissue may cause local pain and immune response to tissue damage. In the lungs, the immune response causes infiltration of eosinophils and neutrophils. Serum IgE levels are usually elevated. Eventually the adult worms are encapsulated in a granuloma. Presence of the worms in the lungs usually results in a chronic cough, with possible production of blood-tinged sputum. The cough provides a mechanism to transport eggs up into the throat where they are swallowed and then may be excreted in the feces. The larvae of *P. mexicanus* may migrate to other areas of the body, frequently causing the formation of subcutaneous or lower abdominal nodules. The larvae of *Paragonimus* may even enter the brain (rarely), where they can cause severe damage.

## LABORATORY DIAGNOSIS

The adult worms of *Paragonimus* vary in size, 10 to 25 mm × 3 to 5 mm, and are a reddish-brown color. The eggs of *P. westermani* measure 80 to 120 μm × 45 to 60 μm, and those of *P. mexicanus* are approximately 80 μm × 40 μm. The eggs are unembryonated when they leave the body, operculated with opercular shoulders, thick shelled, and brownish-yellow. The eggs of *Paragonimus* are similar to those of *Diphyllobothrium* (freshwater fish tapeworm), but may be distinguished by the operculum, opercular shoulders, and thickened shell at the end opposite the operculum.

*Paragonimus* eggs (see Table 57-1) may be recovered from sputum, and occasionally in feces using a sedimentation concentration method. The eggs may be observed in a wet mount (with/without iodine stain) (Figure 57-4). Charcot-Leyden crystals may also be observed in sputum or lung tissue specimens. Charcot-Leyden crystals are slender and pointed at both ends. The crystals normally appear colorless and stain purplish to red with trichrome. Elevated levels of eosinophils in whole blood and elevated IgE levels in serum may be present. Lesions in the lungs may be observed in x-ray. There is also serologic testing available in the United States for diagnosis of

---

*Egg size varies with species from approximately 80 to 120 μm long and 45 to 70 μm wide.

*P. westermani.* The Division of Parasitic Disease at the Centers for Disease Control and Prevention (CDC) performs serum IgG EIA and immunoblot testing, and EIA serum and cerebrospinal fluid (CSF) IgG antibody testing is performed at private reference laboratories; cross reactivity with other species and trematodes may occur.

## TREATMENT AND PREVENTION

The drug of choice for treatment of *Paragonimus* infections is praziquantel given three times a day for 2 days. Alternative treatments are bithionol (which may have mild side effects such as skin rash) or a drug that has not yet been approved in the United States, triclabendazole.

Human infection can be prevented by not eating pickled, raw, or undercooked crabs and crayfish. Care should also be taken to properly clean utensils used in the preparation of these foods. Improvement of sanitary conditions and practices may also help to reduce the prevalence of these infections.

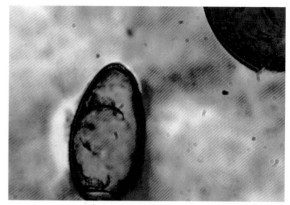

**Figure 57-4** *Paragonimus westermani* egg. (Photo courtesy Dr. Henry Travers, Sioux Falls, S.D.)

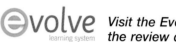

*Visit the Evolve site to complete the review questions.*

## CASE STUDY 57-1

A 50-year-old man visiting from Japan complained of fever, abdominal pain, and jaundice. A stool specimen was collected for ova and parasite examination. A blood specimen was also collected and sent to a clinical laboratory for testing. The blood work showed a slightly increased serum bilirubin level. The parasite examination showed small oval operculated eggs (approximately 80 μm × 45 μm), with opercular shoulders and a knob on the opposite end.

**QUESTIONS**

1. What parasite is the probable cause of this infection?
2. Another parasitic worm has eggs that are almost identical. What fact about the patient can aid in deciding which worm is responsible for his infection?
3. What other complications might be expected with this infection?
4. What would be the preferred treatment for this infection?

## BIBLIOGRAPHY

Bogitsch BJ, Carter CE, Oeltmann TN, editors: *Human parasitology*, ed 3, San Diego, 2005, Academic Press.

Fried B, Abruzzi A: Food-borne trematode infections of humans in the United States, *Parasitol Res* 106:1263-1280, 2010.

Garcia LS: *Diagnostic medical parasitology*, ed 5, Washington, DC, 2006, ASM Press.

John DT, Petri WA: *Markell's and Voge's medical parasitology*, ed 9, St Louis, 2006, Saunders.

Keiser J, Utzinger J: Food-borne trematodiases, *Clin Microbiol Rev* 22(3):466-483, 2009.

Zarrin-Khameh N, Citron DR, Stager CE, et al: Pulmonary paragonimiasis diagnosed by fine-needle aspiration biopsy, *J Clin Microbiol* 46(6):2137-2140, 2008.

# Blood Trematodes

## OBJECTIVES

1. List the clinically significant blood trematodes.
2. Describe the general life cycle of the blood trematodes and how human infection occurs.
3. Explain the diagnostic methods used to identify blood trematodes.
4. Differentiate the eggs of the five species of *schistosomes*.
5. Describe the pathogenesis of the blood trematodes.
6. List the drugs of choice for treatment of blood trematode infections.
7. Describe where blood trematodes are found and how infection may be prevented.

---

**PARASITES TO BE CONSIDERED**

**Trematodes**
Blood
  *Schistosoma mansoni*
  *Schistosoma haematobium*
  *Schistosoma japonicum*
  *Schistosoma intercalatum*
  *Schistosoma mekongi*

---

There are four species of blood flukes that are primarily associated with disease in humans (known as schistosomiasis, bilharziasis, or snail fever), all belonging to the genus *Schistosoma*. These four species are *Schistosoma haematobium*, *S. japonicum* (Oriental blood fluke), *S. mekongi*, and *S. mansoni*. A fifth species, *S. intercalatum*, is a pathogen primarily in animals but has been associated with human disease. The blood flukes differ in morphology and life cycle characteristics from the other trematodes, but because they all belong to the same genus, they are very similar, and may be difficult to distinguish from each other. They do, however, require a freshwater snail as the only intermediate host.

## GENERAL CHARACTERISTICS

Unlike the other trematodes, adult schistosomes are not flattened, but are rather long, thin, and rounded in shape. There is an oral sucker surrounding the mouth and a ventral sucker located just slightly below the oral sucker. The adult male averages 1.5 cm in length and is wider than the female, having a ventral fold that wraps around the female when they mate (Figure 58-1). The adult female averages 2 cm in length and is very thin. The eggs of each species are distinct, and can be distinguished by size, spine morphology, and sometimes specimen type (Figure 58-2). The size range for eggs of *S. haematobium* is 110 to 170 μm long by 40 to 70 μm wide,

and they have a sharply pointed terminal spine. They are fully embryonated without an operculum. The size range for the eggs of *S. japonicum* is 70 to 100 μm long by 50 to 65 μm wide, and they have a small lateral spine that is sometimes difficult to detect (Figure 58-3). *S. mekongi* eggs are smaller than those of *S. japonicum*, ranging in size from 50 to 65 μm long by 30 to 55 μm wide. They are fully embryonated without an operculum and have a small lateral spine. The size range for eggs of *S. mansoni* is 115 to 180 μm long by 40 to 75 μm wide, and they have a large lateral spine. *S. mansoni* eggs are unoperculate, immature when released, and take up to 8 to 10 days to develop a miracidium. *S. intercalatum* eggs are fully embryonated without an operculum, have a terminal spine, and range in size from 140 to 240 μm long by 50 to 85 μm wide. *S. intercalatum* eggs resemble those of *S. haematobium* and can be differentiated by Ziehl-Neelsen acid-fast positivity. In addition, *S. intercalatum* eggs are only found in feces, not in urine specimens. Table 58-1 provides a comparison of the schistosome eggs.

One of the main differences in the schistosomes from other trematodes is that instead of being hermaphroditic, there are separate male and female adult worms. In human infection, the adult worms live in either the veins that supply the intestine (*S. japonicum* and *S. mansoni*) or the veins that supply the urinary bladder (*S. haematobium*). The eggs are passed from the body in either the feces or the urine. To reach the inside of the intestine or bladder, the eggs must penetrate the tissue from the veins. This is accomplished via a spine that is distinctive among the major species. The embryonated egg will release the miracidium (Figure 58-4) once it reaches freshwater, and will enter the snail host, where it will develop into the infectious cercaria. The free-swimming cercariae are capable of penetrating through the human skin directly and do not encyst on aquatic vegetation or other aquatic wildlife (Figure 58-5). The cercariae penetrate the host tissue until they reach a vein; then they travel to capillaries near the lungs and then to the portal vein of the liver, where they mature. When they are mature, the adult males will pair with the females and then travel to the veins of either the intestine or the bladder, where the eggs are produced (Figure 58-6).

## EPIDEMIOLOGY

Schistosomes have a worldwide distribution from Egypt and China to Africa and the Americas. *S. haematobium* is found in Africa and the Arabian peninsula, and has no important reservoir hosts. *S. mansoni* is found in Africa, the Arabian peninsula, and Brazil. Reservoir hosts include wild rodents and marsupials. *S. japonicum* is found in China, Indonesia, and the Philippines. Many domestic animals (cats, dogs, cattle, horses, pigs) serve as reservoir hosts, as do some wild animals as well. *S. mekongi* primarily exists in the lower Mekong River basin in southern Laos and Cambodia. Reservoir hosts include dogs and domestic pigs. *S. intercalatum* is primarily found in central and western Africa. Reservoirs include rodents, marsupials, and nonhuman primates. Human schistosome infection is caused by fecal (and urine) contamination of small bodies of water that favor the growth of the snail hosts. Infection with *S. japonicum* is especially prevalent in areas where humans work in rice paddies.

# PATHOLOGY AND SPECTRUM OF DISEASE

Infection with only a small number of worms may be asymptomatic. Quite often, penetration of the skin by the cercariae causes localized swelling and itching. The migration of the larvae through the body may cause transient symptoms of fever, malaise, cough (when they migrate in the lungs), or hepatitis (when in the liver). The adults are able to acquire some host antigens on

**TABLE 58-1** Diagnostic Characteristics of the Blood Trematodes

| Blood Trematode | Adult Location | Size of Egg | Description of Egg |
|---|---|---|---|
| *Schistosoma haematobium* | Veins surrounding bladder | 110-170 µm × 40-70 µm | Pointed terminal spine, unoperculated, embryonated |
| *Schistosoma intercalatum* | Venules of colon | 140-240 µm × 50-85 µm | Resembles egg of *S. haematobium*, but acid-fast positive |
| *Schistosoma japonicum* | Venules of small intestine | 70-100 µm × 50-65 µm | Small lateral spine, unoperculated, embryonated |
| *Schistosoma mansoni* | Venules of large intestine | 115-180 µm × 40-75 µm | Large lateral spine, unoperculated, embryonated |
| *Schistosoma mekongi* | Venules of small intestine | 50-65 µm × 30-55 µm | Resembles egg of *S. mansoni*, but much smaller |

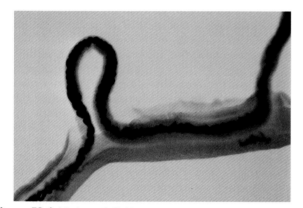

**Figure 58-1** Mating of *Schistosoma mansoni* male and female worms. (Photo courtesy Dr. Henry Travers, Sioux Falls, S.D.)

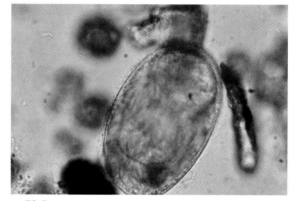

**Figure 58-3** *S. japonicum* egg. (Photo courtesy Dr. Henry Travers, Sioux Falls, S.D.)

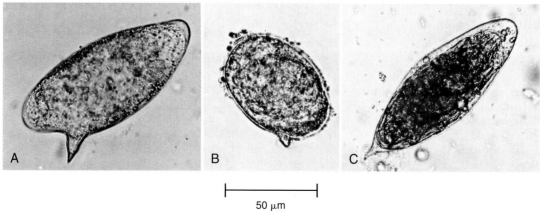

50 µm

**Figure 58-2** **A,** *Schistosoma mansoni* egg. **B,** *Schistosoma japonicum* egg. **C,** *Schistosoma haematobium* egg.

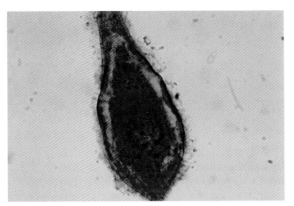

**Figure 58-4** *S. mansoni* miracidium. (Photo courtesy Dr. Henry Travers, Sioux Falls, SD.)

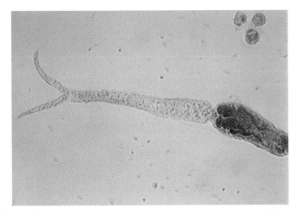

**Figure 58-5** *S. mansoni* cercaria. (Photo courtesy Dr. Henry Travers, Sioux Falls, SD.)

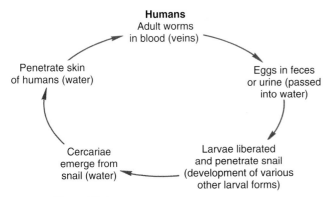

**Figure 58-6** Life cycle of human schistosomes.

their outer surface, and so may not elicit an immune response, although the eosinophil count may be high. Severe tissue damage, with associated pain, fever, and chills, may occur when the eggs travel through the tissue to reach the intestine or bladder. There may also be bloody diarrhea or blood in the urine (hematuria). Necrosis, lesions, and granulomas may develop, as well as obstruction of the bowel or ureters.

Penetration of human skin by the cercariae of blood flukes that commonly infect other mammals or aquatic birds may cause a schistosomal dermatitis known as "swimmer's itch." Erythema, edema, and intense itching may develop that usually disappear within 1 week. The cercariae of these species are not able to complete the life cycle by entering the human bloodstream, and are destroyed by the host immune system.

# LABORATORY DIAGNOSIS

The standard method of diagnosis is by the detection of characteristic eggs in feces or rectal biopsy, for *S. japonicum*, *S. mekongi*, *S. mansoni*, and *S. intercalatum* (and perhaps *S. haematobium* if these worms have migrated to a bladder vein that is close to the intestine); and in urine (usually concentrated before examination) or bladder tissue biopsy for *S. haematobium*. A wet mount with/without iodine from a sedimentation or concentration method can be examined for eggs. Figure 58-2 provides images of three different schistosome eggs. To optimize recovery of *S. haematobium* in urine, the specimen should be collected between noon and 2 PM.

There are some antibody-based assays that are available for diagnosis of schistosomal IgG antibody (enzyme immunoassay [EIA], enzyme-linked immunosorbent assay [ELISA], and immunoblot), but these methods cannot distinguish between current and previous infections. This type of assay may, however, be useful for travelers who have returned from endemic areas. These assays are performed at the Division of Parasitic Disease at the Centers for Disease Control and Prevention (CDC), and may be available at some private reference laboratories. Several nucleic acid-based testing methods have been developed that demonstrate high sensitivity and specificity using genomic or mitochondrial sequences. In addition, schistosome DNA has been identified in patients' plasma using real-time polymerase chain reaction (PCR).

# THERAPY

The drug of choice for treatment of schistosome infections is praziquantel, given in two or three doses in a single day. Infection with *S. mansoni* may require a larger dose than that for the other species. An alternative treatment for *S. haematobium* infections is metrifonate (Bilarcil), an organophosphorus compound, given once every other week in a total of three doses.

# PREVENTION

Because human infection is by direct penetration of the cercariae, prevention of schistosome infection is more difficult to achieve. Educational programs are required to help people in endemic areas understand how to help prevent infection. Sanitary conditions need to be improved with proper disposal not only of human wastes but also that of domestic animals (in areas with *S. japonicum* and *S. mekongi*). A safe water supply for bathing and washing clothes is also necessary. Various snail control methods have been tried, but these methods are very costly and would need to be repeated on a regular basis to have the desired effect.

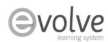 *Visit the Evolve site to complete the review questions.*

---

## CASE STUDY 58-1

An 18-year old man had recently been on 1 month long trip to Brazil with a group of volunteer workers, where he had enjoyed swimming in a nearby river with the local teenage volunteers. He complained of crampy abdominal pain, and twice noticed a small amount of blood in his feces. A stool specimen was collected for ova and parasite examination. A blood specimen was also collected and sent to a clinical laboratory for testing. The results of the blood tests showed increased eosinophil and IgE levels. The parasite examination showed large (115 μm × 75 μm), unoperculated, oval eggs with large lateral spines.

**QUESTIONS**

1. What parasite is the probable cause of this infection?
2. Where in the human host would the adults of this parasite be found?
3. What recent activity of this patient is probably responsible for his infection?
4. What is the drug of choice for treatment of infection with this parasite?

---

## BIBLIOGRAPHY

Bogitsch BJ, Carter CE, Oeltmann TN, editors: *Human parasitology*, ed 3, San Diego, 2005, Academic Press.

Garcia LS: *Diagnostic medical parasitology*, ed 5, Washington, DC, 2006, ASM Press.

Gobert GN, Chai M, Duke M, et al: Copro-PCR-based detection of Schistoma eggs using mitochondrial DNA markers, *Mol Cell Probes* 19:250-254, 2005.

Gryseels B, Polman K, Clerinx J, et al: Human schistosomiasis, *Lancet* 368(9541):1106-1118, 2006.

John DT, Petri WA: *Markell's and Voge's medical parasitology*, ed 9, St Louis, 2006, Saunders.

Pontes LA, Oliveira MC, Dias-Neto E, et al: Comparison of a polymerase chain reaction and the Kato-Katz technique for diagnosing infection with *Schistosoma mansoni, Am J Trop Med Hyg* 68:652-656, 2003.

Urbani C, Sinoun M, Socheat D, et al: Epidemiology and control of mekongi schistosomiasis, *Acta Trop* 82(2):157-168, 2002.

Van Dijk K, Starink MV, Bait A, et al: The potential of molecular diagnosis of cutaneous ectopic schistosomiases, *Am J Trop Med Hyg* 83(4):958-959, 2010.

Wichmann D, Panning M, Quack T, et al: Diagnosing schistosomiasis by detection of cell-free parasite DNA in human plasma, *PLoS Negl Trop Dis* 3:422, 2009.

Wilson M, Schantz PM, Nutman T, editors: *Molecular and immunological approaches for diagnosis of parasitic infection*, ed 7, Washington, DC, 2006, ASM Press.

# Overview of Fungal Identification Methods and Strategies

## OBJECTIVES

1. Define the terms *mycology, saprophytic, dermatophyte,* and *polymorphic, dimorphic,* and *thermally dimorphic fungi.*
2. Define and differentiate superficial, cutaneous, subcutaneous, and systemic mycoses, including the tissues involved.
3. Differentiate the colonial morphology of yeasts and filamentous fungi (molds).
4. Define and differentiate anamorph, teleomorph, and synanamorph.
5. Describe three ways in which fungi reproduce.
6. List the media that should be used for optimal recovery of fungi, including their incubation requirements.
7. List the common antibacterial agents used in fungal media.
8. Explain and differentiate the characteristic colonial morphology of fungi, including topography (rugose, umbonate, verrucose), texture (cottony, velvety, glabrous, granular, wooly) and surface described (front, reverse).
9. Describe and differentiate the sexual and asexual reproduction of the Ascomycota.
10. Define and differentiate rapid, intermediate, and slow growth rates with regard to fungal reproduction and cultivation.
11. Describe the proper method of specimen collection for fungal cultures, including collection site, acceptability, processing, transport, and storage.
12. Give the advantages and disadvantages of using screw-capped culture tubes, compared with agar plates, in the laboratory.
13. Describe the chemical principle and methodologies used to identify fungi, including calcofluor white–potassium hydroxide preparations, hair perforation, cellophane (Scotch) tape preparations, saline/wet mounts, lactophenol cotton blue, potassium hydroxide, Gram stain, India ink, modified acid-fast stain, periodic acid-Schiff stain (PAS), Wright's stain, Papanicolaou stain, Grocott's methenamine silver (GMS), hematoxylin and eosin (H&E) stain, Masson-Fontana stain, tease mount and microslide culture.

Mycology is a specialized discipline in the field of biology concerned with the study of fungi, including their taxonomy, environmental impact, and genetic and biochemical properties. Historically, the fungi were regarded as relatively insignificant causes of infection. However, in the early to mid-twentieth century, these microorganisms began to be recognized as important causes of disease, particularly because of changes in patient profiles, and this trend continues today. Because of the endemic systemic mycoses, which may cause disease in healthy hosts, a number of fungal species normally found in the environment have been recognized as important causes of human disease, particularly in the immunocompromised host. The modern clinical laboratory, therefore, must provide methods for isolating and identifying the common causes of mycologic disease. Susceptibility testing of these isolates is often necessary.

Some clinical microbiology laboratories have kept pace with changing times and have developed more extensive mycologic testing methods. However, the economic constraints of the current health care environment have prevented other laboratories from offering these services. In such cases, diagnostic clinical mycology is performed by reference laboratories, which have varying degrees of experience. The lack of experience in clinical mycology has been influenced by a shortage of trained individuals, lack of quality educational programs, and inability of clinical laboratories to support the cost of sending personnel to training courses. Commonly, individuals with experience who retire or leave their position are replaced by someone with considerably less experience. Training and continuing education programs are needed to assist in the development of such individuals, if quality laboratory services are to be offered. A real concern is that the changing health care environment and implementation of cost containment measures, without continuing education, will prevent future generations from being well trained in diagnostic clinical mycology.

This chapter is designed to assist technologists and microbiologists with the basics of diagnostic clinical mycology, in the hope that the information will allow some laboratories to offer clinical mycology services.

## EPIDEMIOLOGY

Fungal infections are an increasing threat to individuals. The number of nosocomial and community-acquired infections has increased dramatically. The major factors responsible for the increase in the number of fungal infections are alterations in the host, particularly the growing number of immunocompromised people. Whether caused by immunosuppressive agents or serious underlying diseases, these alterations may lead to infection by organisms normally nonpathogenic or part of the patient's normal microbiota (i.e., normal flora). These infections may occur in patients with debilitating diseases, such as progressive infection with the human immunodeficiency virus (HIV) or diabetes mellitus, or in patients with impaired immunologic function resulting from corticosteroid or antimetabolite chemotherapy. Other common predisposing factors include complex surgical procedures and antibacterial therapy. More than 200,000 valid species of fungi exist, but only 100 to 150 species are generally recognized as causes of human disease, and approximately 25 species cause most human disease. Most of these organisms normally live a **saprophytic** existence (living on dead or decayed organic matter) in nature.

Fungal infections generally are not communicable in the usual sense, through person-to-person transmission. Humans become accidental hosts for fungi by inhaling spores or through the introduction of fungal elements into tissue by trauma. Except for disease caused by the dimorphic fungi, humans are relatively resistant to infections caused by fungi. Classic infections are now appearing in new forms in patients, and the old "harmless" saprophytic molds are now being implicated in serious diseases. This ability of normally saprophytic fungi to cause disease in the immunocompromised patient means that laboratories now must be able to identify and report a wide array of fungi.

The primary pathogens appear to have well-defined geographic locations. An example of this is the dimorphic fungi *Coccidioides immitis*. *C. immitis* is usually found only in the United States in the desert Southwest, northern Mexico, and Central America. Opportunistic pathogens such as *Candida* and *Aspergillus* spp. are found all over the world.

# GENERAL FEATURES OF THE FUNGI

Fungi seen in the clinical laboratory generally can be categorized into two groups based on the appearance of the colonies formed. The **yeasts** produce moist, creamy, opaque or pasty colonies on media, whereas the **filamentous fungi** or **molds** (see Chapters 60 and 61) produce fluffy, cottony, woolly, or powdery colonies. Several systemic fungal pathogens exhibit either a yeast (or yeast-like) phase, and filamentous forms are referred to as **dimorphic.** When dimorphism is temperature dependent, the fungi are designated as **thermally dimorphic.** In general, these fungi produce a mold form at 25° to 30°C and a yeast form at 35° to 37°C under certain circumstances.

The medically important dimorphic fungi are *Histoplasma capsulatum*, *Blastomyces dermatitidis*, *C. immitis*, *Paracoccidioides brasiliensis*, *Sporothrix schenckii*, and *Penicillium marneffei* (see Chapter 60). *C. immitis* is not thermally dimorphic. Additionally, some of the medically important yeasts, particularly the *Candida* species, may produce yeasts forms, pseudohyphae, and/or true hyphae (see Chapter 62). Fungi that have more than one independent form or spore stage in their life cycle are called **polymorphic** fungi. The polymorphic features of this group of organisms are not temperature dependent.

# TAXONOMY OF THE FUNGI

Fungi are composed of a vast array of organisms that are unique compared with plants and animals. Included among these are the mushrooms, rusts and smuts, molds and mildews, and yeasts. Despite their great variation in morphologic features, most fungi share the following characteristics:

- Chitin in the cell wall
- Ergosterol in the cell membrane
- Reproduction by means of spores, produced asexually or sexually
- Lack of chlorophyll
- Lack of susceptibility to antibacterial antibiotics
- Saprophytic nature (derive nutrition from organic materials)

Traditionally, the fungi have been categorized into four well-established phyla: Zygomycota, Ascomycota, Basidiomycota, and Deuteromycota. The previous phylum, *Zygomycota*, has contained a very diverse group of organisms. Until further distinction is resolved, the organisms have been divided into the phylum, *Glomeromycota* and subphylum, *Mucoromycotina*, and *Entomophthoracortina*. This diverse group of fungi includes organisms that produce sparsely septate hyphae and exhibit asexual reproduction by sporangiospores and sexual reproduction by the production of zygospores. Some of the clinically important genera in this phylum are *Rhizopus*, *Mucor*, *Rhizomucor*, *Absidia*, and *Cunninghamella*.

The Ascomycota include many fungi that reproduce asexually by the formation of **conidia** (asexual spores) and sexually by the production of ascospores. The filamentous ascomycetes are ubiquitous in nature, and all produce true septate hyphae. All exhibit a sexual form **(teleomorph)** but also exist in an asexual form **(anamorph).** Fungi that have different asexual forms of the same fungus are called **synanomorphs.** In general, the anamorphic form correlates well with the teleomorphic classification. However, different anamorphic forms may have the same teleomorphic form. For example, *Pseudallescheria boydii* (Figure 59-1), in addition to having the *Scedosporium apiospermum* anamorph (Figure 59-2), may exhibit a *Graphium* anamorph (Figure 59-3). The latter anamorph may be seen with several other fungi.

An example of another clinically important fungi that belong to the phylum Ascomycota is *H. capsulatum*, which has a teleomorph designated as *Ajellomyces*. Some species of *Aspergillus* have a teleomorph, *Eurotium*.

Numerous yeast species also belong to the Ascomycota; these include *Saccharomyces* spp. and some species of *Candida*.

The phylum Basidiomycota includes fungi that reproduce sexually through the formation of basidiospores on a specialized structure called the **basidia.** The basidiomycetes are generally plant pathogens or environmental organisms that rarely cause disease in humans. This group includes smuts, rusts, mushrooms, and *Cryptococcus neoformans complex*. The teleomorphic form of *C. neoformans* is *Filobasidiella neoformans*.

The phylum Deuteromycota includes fungi that lack a sexual reproductive cycle and are characterized by their

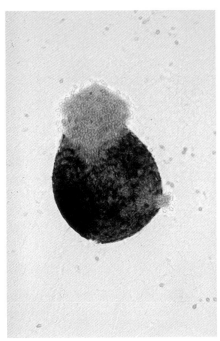

**Figure 59-1** A cleistothecium of *Pseudallescheria boydii* that has opened and is releasing numerous ascospores (×750).

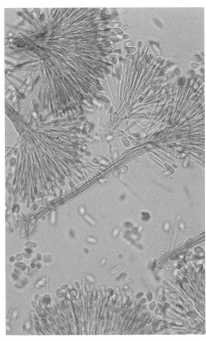

**Figure 59-3** *Graphium* anamorph of *P. boydii* (×500).

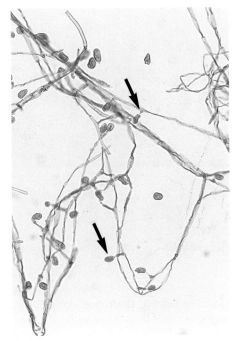

**Figure 59-2** *Scedosporium apiospermum* showing asexually produced conidia borne singly on conidiophores (anellophores *[arrows]*) (×430).

asexual reproductive structures, primarily conidia. The organisms in this group may have sexual forms that have not yet been described. The medically important fungus, *Blastomyces dermatitidis*, is a dimorphic fungus that has not been assigned to a phylum and is therefore placed in the order, *Incertae sedis* until the taxonomic placement is resolved.

# CLINICAL CLASSIFICATION OF THE FUNGI

The botanic taxonomic schema for grouping the fungi has little value in a clinical microbiology laboratory. Table 59-1 is a simplified taxonomic schema illustrating the major groups of fungi.

For clinicians, dividing the fungi into four categories of mycoses, according to the type of infection, is much more useful. The fungi are categorized as follows:

- Superficial (cutaneous) mycoses
- Subcutaneous mycoses
- Systemic mycoses
- Opportunistic mycoses

The superficial, or cutaneous, mycoses are fungal infections that involve the hair, skin, or nails without direct invasion of the deeper tissue. The fungi in this category include the dermatophytes (agents of ringworm, athlete's foot) and agents of infections such as tinea, tinea nigra, and piedra. All of these infect keratinized tissues.

Some fungi cause infections that are confined to the subcutaneous tissue without dissemination to distant sites. Examples of subcutaneous infections include chromoblastomycosis, mycetoma, and phaeohyphomycotic cysts (see Chapter 61).

As traditionally defined, agents of systemic fungal infections include the genera *Blastomyces*, *Coccidioides*, *Histoplasma*, and *Paracoccidioides*. Infections caused by these organisms primarily involve the lungs but also may become widely disseminated and involve any organ system. *P. marneffei*, a geographically limited cause of systemic mycosis in a select patient population, may also be considered a part of this group.

**TABLE 59-1** Phylogenetic Position of Medically Significant Fungi

| Phylum/Class | Order | Genus/Species |
|---|---|---|
| Phylum Glomeromycota<br>Subphylum Mucormycotina | Mucorales | *Absidia*<br>*Cunninghamella*<br>*Mucor*[†]<br>*Rhizopus*[†]<br>*Syncephalastrum* |
| Subphylum Entomophthoromycotina | Entomophthorales | *Basidiobolus*<br>*Conidiobolus* |
| Phylum Ascomycota<br>Dothideomycetes | Capnodiales<br><br>Dothideales<br>Pleosporales | *Cladosporium*<br>*Piedraia hortae*<br>*Aureobasidium*<br>*Alternaria*<br>*Bipolaris*<br>*Curvularia*<br>*Drechslera*<br>*Exserohilum*<br>*Helminthosporium*<br>*Stemphylium*<br>*Ulocladium*<br>*Epicoccum*<br>*Phoma* |
| Saccharomycetes | Saccharomycetales | *Endomyces (Geotrichum sp.)*\*<br>*Kluyveromyces (Candida pseudotropicalis)*\*<br>*Candida*[†]<br>*Geotrichum* |
| Sordariomycetes | Hypocreales<br><br><br><br><br><br>Microascales<br><br><br>Sordariales<br>Trichosphaeriales | *Acremonium*<br>*Gliocladium*<br>*Fusarium*[†]<br>*Scopulariopsis*<br>*Sepedonium*<br>*Trichoderma*<br>*Pseudallescheria boydii*[†]<br>*Scedosporium prolificans*<br>*Sporothrix*[†]<br>*Madurella*<br>*Nigrospora* |
| Eurotiomycetes | Chaetothyriales<br><br><br><br><br>Eurotiales<br><br><br><br>Onygenales | *Cladophialophora*<br>*Exophiala*<br>*Fonsecaea*<br>*Phialophora*<br>*Rhinocladiella*<br>*Emericella (Aspergillus nidulans)*\*<br>*Aspergillus*[†]<br>*Paecilomyces*<br>*Penicillium*<br>*Ajellomyces (Histoplasma capsulatum,*[†] *Blastomyces dermatitidis*[†]*)*\*<br>*Arthroderma (Trichophyton sp.*[†] *and Microsporum sp.*[†]*)*\*<br>*Chrysosporium*<br>*Coccidioides*[†]<br>*Epidermophyton*[†]<br>*Histoplasma*[†]<br>*Microsporum*[†]<br>*Paracoccidioides*[†]<br>*Trichophyton*[†] |
| Phylum Basidiomycota<br>Tremellomycetes | Filobasidiales | *Filobasidium (Cryptococcus neoformans*[†]*)*\* |
| Not assigned | Incertae sidis | *Blastomyces*[†] |

Modified from the Catalogue of Life. November 20, 2012. http://www.catalogueoflife.org/col/browse/classification and Hibbet DS, Binder M, Bischoff JF, et al. A higher-level of classification of the fungi, *Mycological Research*, 509-547, 2007.
\*When the sexual form is known.
[†]Most commonly encountered as causes of infection.

**TABLE 59-2** General Clinical Classification of Pathogenic Fungi

| Cutaneous | Subcutaneous | Opportunistic | Systemic |
|---|---|---|---|
| Superficial mycoses<br>Tinea<br>Piedra<br>Candidosis | Chromoblastomycosis<br>Sporotrichosis<br>Mycetoma (eumycotic)<br>Phaeohyphomycosis | Aspergillosis<br>Candidosis<br>Cryptococcosis<br>Geotrichosis | Aspergillosis<br>Blastomycosis<br>Candidosis<br>Coccidioidomycosis |
| Dermatophytosis | | Mucormycosis<br>Fusariosis<br>Trichosporonosis<br>Others* | Histoplasmosis<br>Cryptococcosis<br>Geotrichosis<br>Paracoccidioidomycosis<br>Mucormycosis<br>Fusariosis<br>Trichosporonosis |

*Virtually any fungus may cause disease in a profoundly immunocompromised host.

Any of the fungi could be considered an opportunistic pathogen in the appropriate clinical setting. The list of uncommon fungi found to cause disease in humans expands every year. Fungi previously thought to be nonpathogenic may be the cause of infections. The infections these organisms cause occur primarily in patients with some type of compromise of the immune system. This may occur secondary to an underlying disease process, such as diabetes mellitus, or it may be caused by an immunosuppressive agent. Although any fungus potentially can cause disease in these patients, the most commonly encountered genera in this group are *Aspergillus, Candida,* and *Cryptococcus,* among others. All of these organisms may cause disseminated (systemic) disease. Some of the dematiaceous fungi may cause deeply invasive phaeohyphomycoses (i.e., produce brown-pigmented structures) in this patient population.

Classification by type of infection allows the clinician to attempt to categorize organisms in a logical fashion into groups having clinical relevance. Table 59-2 presents an example of a clinical classification of infections and their etiologic agents that is useful to clinicians.

## PRACTICAL WORKING SCHEMA

To assist individuals working in clinical microbiology laboratories with the identification of clinically important fungi, Koneman and Roberts[1] have suggested a practical working scheme designed to do the following:

- Assist with the recognition of fungi most commonly encountered in clinical specimens
- Assist with the recognition of fungi recovered on culture media that are strictly pathogenic fungi
- Provide a pathway that allows an identification to be made based on a few colonial and microscopic features

Table 59-3 presents these features. However, the table includes only organisms commonly seen in the clinical laboratory. With practice, most laboratorians should be able to recognize these on a day-to-day basis. For other, less commonly encountered fungi, the microbiologist must use a variety of texts that have photomicrographs, which can aid identification.

Use of the identification scheme just described requires examination of the fungal culture for the presence, absence, and number of septa. If the hyphae appear to be broad and predominantly nonseptate (i.e., cells are not separated by a septum or wall), zygomycetes should be considered. If the hyphae are septate, they must be examined further for the presence or absence of pigmentation. If a dark pigment is present in the hyphae, the organism is considered to be dematiaceous, and the conidia are then examined for their morphologic features and their arrangement on the hyphae. If the hyphae are nonpigmented, they are considered to be hyaline. The fungi are then examined for the type and the arrangement of the conidia produced. The molds are identified by recognition of their characteristic microscopic features (see Table 59-3). Murray[2] has developed an expanded morphologic classification of medically important fungi based on general microscopic features and colonial morphology. The color pigmentation of colonies is presented as a useful diagnostic feature (Box 59-1).

## PATHOGENEIS AND SPECTRUM OF DISEASE

Fungal infection is caused by either primary pathogens or opportunistic pathogens. Infections caused by primary pathogens usually occur in immunocompetent hosts, are not always as virulent, and may lead to subclinical disease. Opportunistic pathogens infect immunocompromised hosts. Opportunistic pathogens include almost any fungus present in the environment. An increase in the number of opportunistic fungal infections in humans is due in large part to the immunocompromised nature of the host. However, certain factors, called virulence factors, make invading tissues and causing disease easier for these organisms. Some virulence factors have been known for years:

- The organism's size (with inhalation, the organism must be small enough to reach the alveoli)
- The organism's ability to grow at 37°C at a neutral pH

**TABLE 59-3**  Most Commonly Encountered Fungi of Clinical Laboratory Importance: a Practical Working Schema

| | MOLDS | | | Yeast | |
|---|---|---|---|---|---|
| **Aseptate Hyphae** | **SEPTATE HYPHAE** | | | | |
| | **Dematiaceous (Melanized)** | **Hyaline** | | | **Arthroconidia:** |
| **Glomeromycota (Mucorales)** | | | | | *Geotrichum* |
| | | | | | *Trichosporon* |
| Commonly encountered: *Rhizopus, Mucor* Rarely encountered: *Syncephalastrum Circinella Cunninghamella Absidia Rhizomucor* | Conidia multicelled: *Alternaria Stemphylium Epicoccum Curvularia Drechslera Bipolaris Exserohilum* Conidia single-celled: *Cladosporium Nigrospora,* and *Aureobasidium Scedosporium prolificans* Production of pycnidia: *Phoma* Production of perithecia: *Chaetomium* Production of cleistothecia: *Pseudallescheria boydii* Slow-growing species: *Cladosporium carrionii Phialophora verrucosa Exophiala jeanselmei Fonsecaea pedrosoi,* and *Cladophialophora bantiana* | Conidiophores terminating in a swollen vesicle: *Aspergillus* spp. *A. fumigatus A. flavus A. niger,* and *A. terreus* Conidiophores branching into a penicillus: *Penicillium Paecilomyces Scopulariopsis* Conidia in clusters: *Acremonium Trichoderma Gliocladium Fusarium* Conidia borne singly: *Chrysosporium Sepedonium* Scedosporium state of *Pseudallescheria boydii* | Dermatophytes: *Microsporum* spp.: *M. audouinii M. canis M. gypseum Trichophyton* spp.: *T. mentagrophytes T. rubrum T. tonsurans T. verrucosum T. schoenleinii T. violaceum* Epidermophyton species: *E. floccosum* Dimorphic molds: *Blastomyces dermatitidis Histoplasma capsulatum Coccidioides immitis Paracoccidioides brasiliensis Sporothrix schenckii* | Hyphae formed on cornmeal-Tween 80 agar: Pseudohyphae: *Candida* spp.: *C. albicans C. tropicalis C. parapsilosis C. kefyr (pseudotropicalis) C. krusei C. guilliermondii* | Hyphae not formed on cornmeal-Tween 80 agar: *Cryptococcus Rhodotorula Candida glabrata Saccharomyces** |

From Koneman EW, Roberts GD: *Practical laboratory mycology,* ed 3, Baltimore, 1985, Williams & Wilkins.
*Rudimentary hyphae may be present.

**BOX 59-1**   Phenotypic Classification of Medically Important Fungi

**Morphologic Classification of Medically Important Fungi, Monomorphic Yeasts, and Yeastlike Organisms**

1. Pseudohyphae with blastoconidia (genera)
   *Candida*
   *Hansenula*
   *Saccharomyces*
2. Yeastlike cells only (usually no hyphae or pseudohyphae) (genera)
   *Cryptococcus*
   *Hansenula*
   *Malassezia*
   *Prototheca*
   *Rhodotorula*
   *Saccharomyces*
   *Sporobolomyces*
   *Ustilago*
3. Hyphae and arthroconidia or annelloconidia (genera)
   *Blastoschizomyces*
   *Geotrichum*
   *Trichosporon*

**Thermally Dimorphic Fungi**

1. *Blastomyces dermatitidis*
2. *Histoplasma capsulatum*
3. *Paracoccidioides brasiliensis*
4. *Penicillium marneffei*
5. *Sporothrix schenckii*

**Thermally Monomorphic Molds**

1. White, cream, or light gray surface; nonpigmented reverse
   a. With microconidia or macroconidia (genera)
      *Acremonium*
      *Beauveria*
      *Chrysosporium*
      *Emmonsia*
      *Epidermophyton*
      *Fusarium*
      *Graphium*
      *Microsporum*
      *Pseudallescheria*
      *Sepedonium*
      *Stachybotrys*
      *Trichophyton*
      *Verticillium*
   b. Having sporangia or sporangiola (genera)
      *Absidia*
      *Apophysomyces*
      *Basidiobolus*
      *Conidiobolus*
      *Cunninghamella*
      *Mucor*
      *Rhizomucor*
      *Rhizopus*
      *Saksenaea*
   c. Having arthroconidia (genera)
      *Coccidioides*
      *Geotrichum*
   d. Having only hyphae with chlamydoconidia (genera)
      *Epidermophyton*
      *Microsporum*
      *Trichophyton*
2. White, cream, beige, or light gray surface; yellow, orange, or reddish reverse (genera)
   *Acremonium*
   *Chaetomium*
   *Microsporum*
   *Trichophyton*
3. White cream, beige, or light gray surface; red to purple reverse (genera)
   *Microsporum*
   *Penicillium*
   *Trichophyton*
4. White, cream, beige, or light gray surface; brown reverse (genera)
   *Chaetomium*
   *Chrysosporium*
   *Cokeromyces*
   *Emmonsia*
   *Madurella*
   *Microsporum*
   *Scopulariopsis*
   *Sporotrichum*
   *Trichophyton*
5. White, cream, beige, or light gray surface; black reverse (genera)
   *Chaetomium*
   *Graphium*
   *Nigrospora*
   *Phoma*
   *Pseudallescheria*
   *Scedosporium*
   *Trichophyton*
6. Tan to brown surface
   a. Having small conidia (genera)
      *Aspergillus*
      *Botrytis*
      *Chrysosporium*
      *Cladosporium*
      *Emmonsia*
      *Ochroconis*
      *Paecilomyces*
      *Phialophora*
      *Scedosporium*
      *Scopulariopsis*
      *Sporotrichum*
      *Trichophyton*
      *Verticillium*
   b. Having large conidia or sporangia (genera)
      *Alternaria*
      *Apophysomyces*
      *Basidiobolus*
      *Bipolaris*
      *Botrytis*
      *Cokeromyces*
      *Conidiobolus*
      *Curvularia*
      *Epicoccum*
      *Epidermophyton*
      *Fusarium*
      *Microsporum*
      *Rhizomucor*
      *Rhizopus*
      *Stemphylium*
      *Trichophyton*
      *Ulocladium*

*Continued*

---

**BOX 59-1** Phenotypic Classification of Medically Important Fungi—cont'd

c. Having miscellaneous microscopic morphology (genera)
*Chaetomium*
*Coccidioides*
*Madurella*
*Phoma*
*Ustilago*
7. Yellow to orange surface (genera)
*Aspergillus*
*Chrysosporium*
*Epicoccum*
*Epidermophyton*
*Microsporum*
*Monilia*
*Penicillium*
*Sepedonium*
*Sporotrichum*
*Trichophyton*
*Trichothecium*
*Verticillium*
8. Pink to violet surface (genera)
*Acremonium*
*Aspergillus*
*Beauveria*
*Chrysosporium*
*Fusarium*
*Gliocladium*
*Microsporum*
*Monilia*
*Paecilomyces*
*Sporotrichum*
*Trichophyton*
*Trichothecium*
*Verticillium*
9. Green surface; light reverse (genera)
*Aspergillus*
*Epidermophyton*
*Gliocladium*

*Penicillium*
*Trichoderma*
*Verticillium*
10. Dark gray or black surface; light reverse (genera)
*Aspergillus*
*Syncephalastrum*
11. Green, dark gray, or black surface; dark reverse
a. Having small conidia (genera)
*Aureobasidium*
*Botrytis*
*Cladosporium/Cladophialophora*
*Exophiala*
*Fonsecaea*
*Hortaea*
*Phialophora*
*Pseudallescheria*
*Scedosporium*
b. Having large conidia (genera)
*Alternaria*
*Bipolaris*
*Curvularia*
*Dactylaria*
*Epicoccum*
*Helminthosporium*
*Nigrospora*
*Pithomyces*
*Stachybotrys*
*Stemphylium*
*Ulocladium*
c. Having only hyphae (with or without chlamydoconidia) (genera)
*Hortaea*
*Madurella*
d. Having large fruiting bodies (genera)
*Chaetomium*
*Phoma*

From Murray PR: *ASM pocket guide to clinical microbiology,* vol 3, Washington, DC, 2004, ASM Press.

---

- Conversion of the dimorphic fungi from the mycelial form into the corresponding yeast or spherule form in the host
- Toxin production

Most of the fungi exist in environmental niches as saprophytic organisms (Table 59-4). Perhaps the fungi that cause disease in humans have developed various mechanisms that allow them to establish disease in the human host. Table 59-5 describes the known or speculative virulence factors of the fungi known to be pathogenic for humans.

# LABORATORY DIAGNOSIS

## COLLECTION, TRANSPORT, AND CULTURING OF CLINICAL SPECIMENS

The diagnosis of fungal infections depends entirely on the selection and collection of an appropriate clinical specimen for microscopic analysis and culture. Many fungal infections are similar clinically to mycobacterial infections, and often the same specimen is cultured for both fungi and mycobacteria. Many infections have a primary focus in the lungs; respiratory tract secretions are almost always included among the specimens selected for culture. It should be emphasized that dissemination to distant body sites may occur, and fungi may be recovered from nonrespiratory sites.

Proper collection of specimens and rapid transport to the clinical laboratory are crucial to the recovery of fungi. Specimens often contain not only the etiologic agent, but also contaminating bacteria or fungi that rapidly overgrow some of the slower-growing pathogenic fungi. The viability of fungi decreases over time. If processing will be delayed, specimens can be refrigerated for a short time, except for dermatologic specimens (skin, hair, nails), blood, and cerebrospinal fluid (CSF). Yeasts (e.g., *Candida* spp.) commonly are recovered on routine bacteriology media and fungal culture media. A few

**TABLE 59-4** Summary of Common Pathogens

| Organism | Natural Habitat | Infectious Form | Mode of Transmission | Common Sites of Infection | Clinical Form |
|---|---|---|---|---|---|
| *Aspergillus* spp. | Ubiquitous, plants | Conidia | Inhalation | Lungs, eyes, skin, nails | Hyphae |
| *Blastomyces dermatitidis* | Unknown(?), soil/wood | Probably conidia | Usually inhalation | Lungs, skin, long bones | Yeast |
| *Candida* spp. | Human flora | Yeast, pseudohyphae, and true hyphae | Direct invasion/dissemination | GI and GU tracts, nails, viscera, blood | Yeast, pseudohyphae, and true hyphae |
| *Coccidioides immitis* | Soil of many arid regions | Arthroconidia | Inhalation | Lungs, skin, meninges | Spherules, endospores |
| *Cryptococcus neoformans* complex | Bird feces, soil | Yeast* | Inhalation | Lungs, skin, meninges | Yeast |
| *Histoplasma capsulatum* | Bat and bird feces | Conidia | Inhalation | Lungs, bone marrow, blood | Yeast |
| *Paracoccidioides brasiliensis* | (?)Soil, plants | Conidia | Inhalation/trauma | Lungs, skin, mucous membranes | Yeast |
| *Sporothrix schenckii* | Soil, plants | Conidia/hyphae | Trauma/rarely inhalation | Skin and lymphatics, lungs, meninges | Yeast |
| Dermatophytes | Human disease, animals, soil | Conidia/hyphae | Contact | Skin, hair, or nails | Hyphae |

*GI,* Gastrointestinal; *GU,* genitourinary.
*Possibly the conidia of the teleomorphic stage *(Filobasidiella neoformans).*

**TABLE 59-5** Virulence Factors of Medically Important Fungi

| Fungal Pathogen | Putative Virulence Factor |
|---|---|
| *Aspergillus* spp. | Elastase-serine protease<br>Proteases<br>Toxins (Gliotoxin, —fumagillin, helvolic acid)<br>Elastase-metalloprotease<br>Aspartic acid proteinase<br>Aflatoxin<br>Catalase<br>Lysine biosynthesis<br>*p*-aminobenzoic acid synthesis |
| *Blastomyces dermatitidis* BAD-1 | Cell wall alpha-1,3-glucan<br>BAD-1, Adhesion and immune modulator |
| *Coccidioides immitis* | Extracellular proteinases |
| *Cryptococcus neoformans* complex | Capsule<br>Phenoloxidase melanin synthesis<br>Varietal differences |
| *Dematiaceous fungi* | Phenoloxidase melanin synthesis |
| *Histoplasma capsulatum* | Cell wall alpha-1,3-glucan<br>Intracellular growth<br>Thermotolerance<br>CBP, binds calcium |
| *Paracoccidioides brasiliensis* | Estrogen-binding proteins<br>Cell wall components<br>beta-glucan<br>alpha-1,3-glucan |
| *Sporothrix schenckii* | Thermotolerance<br>Extracellular enzymes |

Modified from Hogan LH, Klein BS, Levitz SM: Virulence factors of medically important fungi, Clin Microbiol Rev 9:469, 1966.

specific comments concerning specimen collection and culturing are included in this chapter.

### Respiratory Tract Secretions

Respiratory tract secretions (sputum, induced sputum, bronchial washings, bronchoalveolar lavage, and tracheal aspirations) are perhaps the most common specimens collected for fungal culture. To ensure optimal recovery of fungi and prevent overgrowth by contaminants, antibacterial antibiotics should be included in the battery of media used. The antifungal agent cycloheximide prevents overgrowth by rapidly growing molds and should be included in at least one of the culture media. As much specimen as possible (0.5 mL) should be used to inoculate each medium.

### Cerebrospinal Fluid

Cerebrospinal fluid collected for culture should be filtered through a 0.45-$\mu$m membrane filter attached to a sterile syringe. After filtration, the filter is removed and placed on the surface of an appropriate culture medium with the inoculum side down. Alternatively, the specimen may be centrifuged and the concentrated sediment used to inoculate the culture medium. Cultures should be examined daily. If plated using a filter, the filter should be moved to another location every other day. If less than 1 mL of specimen is submitted for culture, it should be centrifuged, and 1-drop aliquots of the sediment should be placed on several areas on the agar surface. Media used for the recovery of fungi from CSF should contain no antibacterial or antifungal agents. Once submitted to the laboratory, CSF specimens should be processed promptly. If prompt processing is not possible, samples should be kept at room temperature or placed in a 30°C incubator, because most organisms continue to replicate in this environment.

### Blood

Disseminated fungal infections are more prevalent than previously recognized, and blood cultures provide an accurate method for determining the etiology in many instances. Currently several automated blood culture systems, including the BACTEC (Becton Dickinson, Sparks, Maryland), BacT/ALERT (bioMérieux, Durham, North Carolina), and VersaTREK (Thermo Scientific, TREK Diagnostics, Cleveland, OH), are adequate systems for the recovery of yeasts.

Laboratories that frequently recover dimorphic fungi from blood are encouraged to use the lysis-centrifugation system, the Isolator (Alere Inc, Waltham, MA). The Isolator has been proven optimal for the recovery of *H. capsulatum* and other filamentous fungi. With this system, red blood cells and white blood cells, which may contain the microorganisms, are lysed, and centrifugation concentrates the organisms before culturing. The concentrate is inoculated onto the surface of appropriate culture media, and most fungi are detected within the first 4 days of incubation. However, occasional isolates of *H. capsulatum* may require approximately 10 to 14 days for recovery. The optimal temperature for fungal blood cultures is 30°C, and the suggested incubation time is 21 days.

### Hair, Skin, and Nail Scrapings

Specimens of hair, skin scrapings or biopsies, and nail clippings are usually submitted for dermatophyte culture and are contaminated with bacteria or rapidly growing fungi or both. Samples collected from lesions may be obtained by scraping the skin or nails with a scalpel blade or microscope slide; infected hairs are removed by plucking them with forceps. These specimens should be placed in a sterile container; they should not be refrigerated. Mycosel agar, which contains chloramphenicol and cycloheximide, is satisfactory for the recovery of dermatophytes. Cultures should be incubated for a minimum of 21 days at 30°C before being reported as negative.

### Vaginal

Vaginal samples should be transported to the laboratory within 24 hours of collection using culture transport swabs. Swabs should be kept moist in sterile tubes. This method of collection provides a specimen suitable for a wet preparation. Both selective and inhibitory agars should be plated. Vaginal cultures should be screened for yeasts and incubated at 30°C for 7 days.

### Urine

Urine samples collected for fungal culture should be processed as soon after collection as possible. The 24-hour urine sample is unacceptable for culture. The usefulness of quantitative cultures is undetermined. All urine samples should be centrifuged and the sediment cultured using a loop to provide adequate isolation of colonies. Because urine often is contaminated with gram-negative bacteria, media containing antibacterial agents must be used to ensure the recovery of fungi.

### Tissue, Bone Marrow, and Sterile Body Fluids

All tissues should be processed before culturing by mincing or placement in a high speed laboratory blender. Stomacher Lab Blenders, which are commercially available from various manufacturers, express the cytoplasmic contents of cells using pressure exerted from the action of rapidly moving metal paddles against the tissue in a broth suspension. (Large portions of tissue should be cut into smaller pieces if the Stomacher is to be used for processing.) After processing, at least 1 mL of specimen should be spread onto the surface of appropriate culture media, and the cultures should be incubated at 30°C for 21 days (incubation may be extended if clinical suspicion of a mycotic disease is high). Tissue samples should be inoculated onto an agar surface (i.e., not just the broth used to assist in the dissolution of the tissue in the Stomacher).

Bone marrow may be placed directly onto the surface of appropriate culture media and incubated in the manner previously mentioned. Sterile body fluids should be concentrated by centrifugation before culturing, and at least 1 mL of specimen should be placed on the surface of appropriate culture media. An alternative is to place bone marrow and other body fluids in an Isolator tube and process it as a blood culture. All specimens should be cultured as soon as possible to ensure the recovery of fungi.

## CULTURE MEDIA AND INCUBATION REQUIREMENTS

A number of fungal culture media are satisfactory for use in the clinical microbiology laboratory (Table 59-6). Most are adequate for the recovery of fungi, and the selection usually is left up to the laboratory director. For optimal recovery, a battery of media should be used; the following are recommended:

- Media with and without cycloheximide
- Media with and without an antibacterial agent (Media with an antibacterial agent are used for specimens likely to contain contaminating bacteria; they are not necessary for specimens from sterile sites.)

Agar plates or screw-capped agar tubes are satisfactory for the recovery of fungi; however, plates are preferred, because they provide better aeration of cultures, a large surface area for better isolation of colonies, and greater ease of handling by technologists when making microscopic preparations for examination. Agar tends to dehydrate during the extended incubation period required for fungal recovery, but this problem can be minimized by using culture dishes containing at least 40 mL of agar and placing them in a humidified incubator. Dishes should be opened and examined only in a certified biologic safety cabinet (BSC). Many laboratories discourage the use of culture dishes because of safety considerations; however, the advantages outweigh the disadvantages.

Compared with agar plates, screw-capped culture tubes are more easily stored, require less space for incubation, and are more easily handled. In addition, they

**TABLE 59-6** Fungal Culture Media: Indications for Use

| Media | Indications for Use | Media Composition | Mode of Action |
|---|---|---|---|
| **Primary Recovery Media** Brain-heart infusion agar | Primary recovery of saprobic and pathogenic fungi | Brain-heart infusion, enzymatic digest of animal tissue, enzymatic digest of casein; dextrose, sodium chloride | The agar provides a rich medium for bacteria, yeast, and pathogenic fungi. |
| Brain-heart infusion agar with antibiotics | Primary recovery of pathogenic fungi exclusive of dermatophytes | Brain-heart infusion, enzymatic digest of animal tissue, enzymatic digest of casein; dextrose, sodium chloride, antibiotics | The agar provides a rich medium for yeast and pathogenic fungi. |
| Brain-heart infusion biphasic blood culture bottles | Recovery of fungi from blood | Brain-heart infusion, peptone, glucose, disodium phosphate | Enhances the recovery of yeasts in blood |
| Chromogenic agar | Isolation and presumptive identification of yeast and filamentous fungi | Chromopeptone Glucose Chromogen mix Chloramphenicol | Chromogen mix contains substrates that react with enzymes produced by different organisms that result in the production of characteristic color changes. |
| Dermatophyte test medium | Primary recovery of dermatophytes; recommended as screening medium only | Dextrose, cycloheximide, gentamycin, chloramphenicol, phenol red | Dermatophytes produce alkaline metabolites, which raise the pH and change the medium from red to yellow. |
| Inhibitory mold agar | Primary recovery of pathogenic fungi exclusive of dermatophytes | Chloramphenicol, casein, dextrose, starch, sodium phosphate, magnesium sulphate, sodium chloride, manganese sulphate | Examine plates for growth. Chloramphenicol inhibits bacterial growth. |
| Potato flake agar | Primary recovery of saprobic and pathogenic fungi | Potato flakes, glucose, cycloheximide, chloramphenicol, bromthymol blue | Growth is enhanced by a pH alkaline reaction of fungus. Chloramphenicol and antibiotics inhibit the growth of bacteria and nonpathogenic fungi. |
| Mycosel | Primary recovery of dermatophytes | Cycloheximide, chloramphenicol, dextrose | Inhibits bacteria and saprophytic fungi |
| SABHI agar | Primary recovery of saprobic and pathogenic fungi | Sabourad dextrose, brain-heart infusion agar | Isolates and enhances growth of pathogenic fungi |
| Yeast-extract phosphate agar | Primary recovery of pathogenic fungi exclusive of dermatophytes | Yeast extract, dipotassium phosphate, chloramphenicol | Enhances the recovery of *Blastomyces dermatitidis* and *Histoplasma capsulatum* from contaminated specimens |
| **Differential Test Media** Ascospore agar | Detection of ascospores in ascosporogenous yeasts (e.g., *Saccharomyces* spp.) | Potassium acetate, yeast extract, dextrose | Potassium acetate is necessary, and yeast extract increases the sporulation of yeasts. |
| Christensen's urea agar | Identification of *Cryptococcus*, *Trichosporon*, and *Rhodotorula* spp. | 2% Urea, phenol red | Produces urease and a change in the pH |
| Cornmeal agar with Tween 80 and trypan blue | Identification of *Candida albicans* by chlamydospore production; identification of *C. albicans* by microscopic morphology | Cornmeal, Tween 80, trypan blue | Addition of Tween 80 enhances the production of chlamydospores, and the addition of trypan blue provides a contrasting background for observing the morphologic features of yeasts. |
| Cottonseed conversion agar | Conversion of the dimorphic fungus *B. dermatitidis* from mold to yeast form | Cottonseed meal, glucose | Allows conversion to yeast phase within 3 days |

*Continued*

**TABLE 59-6** Fungal Culture Media: Indications for Use—cont'd

| Media | Indications for Use | Media Composition | Mode of Action |
|---|---|---|---|
| Czapek's agar | Differential identification of *Aspergillus* spp. | Sodium nitrate, sucrose, yeast extract | Produces characteristic features of yeast and fungus |
| Niger seed agar (birdseed agar) | Identification of *Cryptococcus neoformans* complex | *Guizotia abysinica* seed, dextrose, chloramphenicol | *C. neoformans* produces a brown pigment through metabolism of caffeic acid. |
| Nitrate reduction medium | Detection of nitrate reduction to confirm *Cryptococcus* spp. | Potassium nitrate, peptone, meal extract, sulfanilic acid, N,N-dimethyl-1-naphthylamine | If the yeast produces nitrate reductase, a cherry red indicates a positive test result. |
| Potato dextrose agar | Demonstration of pigment production by *Trichophyton rubrum;* preparation of microslide cultures and sporulation of dermatophytes | Potato infusion, D(+) glucose **NOTE:** Some laboratories use potato flake agar, because it may be more stable. | Carbohydrate and potato infusion promotes the growth of yeasts and molds, and the low pH partially inhibits bacterial growth. |
| Rice medium | Identification of *Microsporum audouinii* | White rice extract, polysorbate 80 | Polysorbate 80 enhances chlamydospore formation by *C. albicans.* Differentiates *Microsporum canis,* which grows well with a yellow pigment, from *M. audouinii,* which shows no growth. |
| *Trichophyton* agars 1-7 | Identification of *Trichophyton* spp. | Casamino acids, dextrose, monopotassium phosphate, magnesium sulphate, amino acids (e.g., inositol, thiamine), ammonium nitrate | *Trichophyton* spp. may be differentiated by their growth in the presence of different amino acids. |
| Urea agar | Detection of *Cryptococcus* spp.; differentiate *Trichophyton mentagrophytes* from *T. rubrum;* detection of *Trichosporon* spp. | Peptone, dextrose, sodium chloride, monopotassium phosphate, urea, phenol red | Urea provides a nitrogen source for organisms producing urease. Urease releases ammonia, which increases the pH and is indicated by a color change from red to yellow. |
| Yeast fermentation broth | Identification of yeasts by determining fermentation | Yeast extract, peptone, bromcresol purple, and a specific carbohydrate (e.g., dextrose, maltose, sucrose) | Most yeasts produce acid, which is indicated by a change in the solution from purple to yellow as a positive fermenter. |
| Yeast nitrogen base agar | Identification of yeasts by determining carbohydrate assimilation | Ammonium sulphate, carbon source (e.g., glucose, sucrose, raffinose) | Assimilation of carbon by yeast cells produces a positive result. |

have a lower dehydration rate, and laboratory workers believe cultures are less hazardous to handle when in tubes. However, disadvantages, such as relatively poor isolation of colonies, a reduced surface area for culturing, and a tendency to promote anaerobiosis, discourage routine use in most clinical microbiology laboratories. If culture tubes are used, the tube should be as large as possible to provide an adequate surface area for isolation. After inoculation, tubes should be placed in a horizontal position for at least 1 to 2 hours to allow the specimen to absorb to the agar surface and avoid settling at the bottom of the tube. Cotton-plugged tubes are unsatisfactory for fungal cultures.

Cultures should be incubated at room temperature, or preferably at 30°C, for 21 to 30 days before they are reported as negative. A relative humidity in the range of 40% to 50% can be achieved by placing an open pan of water in the incubator. Cultures should be examined at least three times weekly during incubation.

As previously mentioned, some clinical specimens are contaminated with bacteria or rapidly growing fungi or both, requiring the use of antifungal and antibacterial agents. The addition of 0.5 $\mu$g/mL of cycloheximide and 16 $\mu$g/mL of chloramphenicol to media traditionally has been advocated to inhibit the growth of contaminating molds and bacteria, respectively. However, better results have been achieved using a combination of 5 $\mu$g/mL of gentamicin and 16 $\mu$g/mL of chloramphenicol as antibacterial agents. Ciprofloxacin at a concentration of 5 $\mu$g/mL may be used.

Cycloheximide may be added to any of the media that contain or lack antibacterial antibiotics. However, if cycloheximide is included in the battery of culture media, a medium lacking this ingredient should also be included.

Pathogenic fungi, such as *C. neoformans* complex, *Candida krusei* and other *Candida* spp., *Trichosporon* spp., *P. boydii*, and *Aspergillus* spp., are partially or completely inhibited by cycloheximide.

Although use of antibiotics in fungal culture media is necessary for optimal recovery of organisms, the use of decontamination and concentration methods advocated for the recovery of mycobacteria is not appropriate, because many fungi are killed by sodium hydroxide treatment.

## DIRECT MICROSCOPIC EXAMINATION

Direct microscopic examination of clinical specimens has been used for many years; however, its usefulness should be reemphasized. Because the mission of a clinical microbiology laboratory is to provide a rapid and accurate diagnosis, the mycology laboratory can provide this service in many instances by direct examination (particularly the Gram stain) of the clinical specimen submitted for culture. Microbiologists are encouraged to become familiar with the diagnostic features of fungi commonly encountered in clinical specimens and to recognize them when stained by various dyes. This important procedure often can provide the first microbiologic proof of the etiology of disease in patients with fungal infection. This is the most rapid method currently available.

Tables 59-7 and 59-8 present the methods available for direct microscopic detection of fungi in clinical specimens and a summary of the characteristic microscopic features of each. Figure 59-4 presents photomicrographs of some of the fungi commonly seen in clinical specimens.

Traditionally, the potassium hydroxide preparation has been the recommended method for direct microscopic examination of specimens. However, the calcofluor white stain now is believed to be superior (see Procedure 59-1 on the Evolve site). Slides prepared by this method may be observed using fluorescent or bright-field microscopy, as is used for the potassium hydroxide preparation; the former is optimal, because fungal cells fluoresce.

## SERODIAGNOSIS

Currently no commercially available procedures exist for serologic diagnosis of most fungi. However, serology testing may be a useful tool with a select few organisms, such as *Cryptococcus*, *Blastomyces*, *Histoplasma*, and *Aspergillus* spp.

Antibody testing has proven useful but not for immunocompromised patients, who are incapable of producing a measurable humoral response. Acute and convalescent titers need to be monitored during treatment of the fungal infection.

Complement fixation (CF) is a sensitive method that is difficult to perform and interpret. It requires a delay in testing that extends from exposure to the onset of symptoms; consequently, detection of antibody can take 2 to 3 months. Cross reactions with other fungal antibodies can also be a problem.

Immunodiffusion testing is a simple, cost-effective procedure. Although it is 100% specific, it is relatively insensitive and is not used as a screening tool. This test also requires 2 to 3 weeks to become positive.

Enzyme immunoassays for both antibody and antigen have been used. These tests are also frequently negative in immunocompromised patients, especially early in the infection.

### Molecular Detection

Molecular detection methods are becoming popular in all areas of clinical microbiology; however, none has been accepted as a routine diagnostic tool in clinical mycology. Ideally, a panel of primers specific for the detection of fungi in clinical specimens would include the most common organisms known to cause disease in immunocompromised patients (including the dimorphic fungi and *Pneumocystis jiroveci*). However, currently no commercial methods are available to the clinical laboratory, and reports in the literature deal predominantly with selected organisms such as the Advan Dx PNA fish for the identification of Cardida spp. from blood cultures (Advan Dx, Woburn, MA). The large number of fungi may limit the development of a cost-effective screening method. Studies by Hopfer,[4] Lu et al.,[5] Makimura et al.,[6] and Sandhu et al.[7] present examples of what has been done with molecular methods in mycology for the detection of fungi in clinical specimens.

### MALDI-TOF (Matrix-Assisted Laser Desorption Ionization)

MALDI-TOF is a biophysical method that significantly reduces the time required to specifically identify fungal organisms. An overview of the technique is discussed in more detail in Chapter 7.

# GENERAL CONSIDERATIONS FOR THE IDENTIFICATION OF YEASTS

Most often yeasts are identified through the use of a combination of tests (Figure 59-5). Identification factors and techniques include:

- Colonial morphologic features
- Microscopic morphologic features
- Physiologic studies
- Rapid commercial yeast identification tests

Several key characteristics can be seen macroscopically. Colonies have a wide variety of colors, shapes, and textures. Chromogenic agar can be used to differentiate yeast presumptively. Wet preps and lactophenol cotton blue stain can aid microscopic identification by improving the visualization of spore structure. Sexual and asexual characteristics are very important. Often a genus can be determined by the microscopic and macroscopic characteristics alone. India ink stain is useful when *Cryptococcus* organisms are suspected. Because carbon and nitrogen source differences are the key to differentiating yeasts, many automated and semiautomated commercial systems have been designed with assimilation and fermentation tests. Supplemental testing takes advantage of

**TABLE 59-7**  Summary of Methods Available for Direct Microscopic Detection of Fungi in Clinical Specimens

| Method | Use | Time Required | Advantages | Disadvantages |
|---|---|---|---|---|
| Acid-fast stain and partial acid-fast stain | Detection of mycobacteria and *Nocardia* spp., respectively | 12 min | Detects *Nocardia* spp.* and some isolates of *Blastomyces dermatitidis* | Tissue homogenates are difficult to observe because of background staining. |
| Auramine-rhodamine stain | Detection of mycobacteria and *Nocardia* spp., respectively | 10 min | Excellent screening tool; sensitive and affordable | Not as specific for acid-fast organisms as Ziehl-Neelsen stain |
| Calcofluor white stain | Detection of fungi | 1 min | Can be mixed with KOH: detects fungi rapidly because of bright fluorescence | Requires use of a fluorescence microscope; background fluorescence prominent, but fungi exhibit more intense fluorescence; vaginal secretions are difficult to interpret. |
| Gram stain | Detection of bacteria | 3 min | Commonly performed on most clinical specimens submitted for bacteriology; detects most fungi. | Some fungi stain well, but others (e.g., *Cryptococcus* spp.) show only stippling and stain weakly in some instances; some isolates of *Nocardia* spp. fail to stain or stain weakly. |
| India ink stain | Detection of *Cryptococcus neoformans* in CSF | 1 min | Diagnostic of meningitis when positive in CSF | Positive in fewer than 50% of cases of meningitis; not sensitive in non–HIV-infected patients |
| Lactophenol cotton blue wet mount | Most widely used method of staining and observing fungi | 1 min | Lactic acid preserves structures; slides can be made permanent. | Mechanical treatment dislodges fungal structures. |
| Potassium hydroxide | Clearing of specimen to make fungi more readily visible | 5 min; if clearing is not complete, an additional 5-10 min is necessary | Rapid detection of fungal elements | Requires experience, because background artifacts are often confusing; clearing of some specimens may require an extended time. |
| Masson-Fontana stain | Examination of melanin pigment in fungal cell walls | 1 hr, 10 min | Aids differentiation of melanin and hemosiderin pigments | Difficult to interpret when only rare granular staining is present |
| Methenamine silver stain | Detection of fungi in histologic section | 1 hr | Best stain for detecting fungal elements | Requires a specialized staining method that is not usually readily available to microbiology laboratories |
| Papanicolaou stain | Examination of secretions for malignant cells | 30 min | Cytotechnologist can detect fungal elements. | Fungal elements stain pink to blue. |
| Periodic acid-Schiff (PAS) stain | Detection of fungi | 20 min; 5 min additional if counterstain is used | Stains fungal elements well; hyphae of molds and yeasts can be readily distinguished. | *Nocardia* spp. do not stain well. |
| Saline wet mount | Examination of fungal elements | 1 min | Quickly performed and cost-effective | Specimen must be fresh; not all elements are visible with this preparation. |
| Wright's stain | Examination of bone marrow or peripheral blood smears | 7 min | Detects *Histoplasma capsulatum* and *C. neoformans* | Most often used to detect *H. capsulatum* and *C. neoformans* complex in disseminated disease. |

From Versalovic J: *Manual of clinical microbiology,* ed 10, Washington, DC, 2011, ASM Press.
*CSF,* Cerebrospinal fluid; *HIV,* human immunodeficiency virus; *KOH,* potassium hydroxide.
*Partially acid-fast bacterium.

**TABLE 59-8** Summary of Characteristic Features of Fungi Seen in Direct Examination of Clinical Specimens

| Morphologic Form Found in Specimens | Organism | Size Range (diameter, mm) | Characteristic Features |
|---|---|---|---|
| Yeastlike | Histoplasma capsulatum | 2-5 | Small; oval to round budding cells; often found clustered in histiocytes; difficult to detect when present in small numbers |
| | Sporothrix schenckii | 2-6 | Small; oval to round to cigar shaped; single or multiple buds present; uncommonly seen in clinical specimens |
| | Cryptococcus neoformans complex | 2-15 | Cells exhibit great variation in size; usually spherical but may be football shaped; buds single or multiple and "pinched off"; capsule may or may not be evident; occasionally, pseudohyphal forms with or without a capsule may be seen in exudates of cerebrospinal fluid |
| | Malassezia furfur (in fungemia) | 1.5-4.5 | Small; bottle-shaped cells, buds separated from parent cell by a septum; emerge from a small collar |
| | Blastomyces dermatitidis | 8-15 | Cells are usually large, double refractile when present; buds usually single; however, several may remain attached to parent cells; buds connected by a broad base |
| | Paracoccidioides brasiliensis | 5-60 | Cells are usually large and are surrounded by smaller buds around the periphery ("mariner's wheel appearance"); smaller cells may be present (2-5 $\mu$m) and resemble H. capsulatum; buds have "pinched-off" appearance |
| Spherules | Coccidioides immitis | 10-200 | Spherules vary in size; some may contain endospores, others may be empty; adjacent spherules may resemble B. dermatitidis; endospores may resemble H. capsulatum but show no evidence of budding; spherules may produce multiple germ tubes if a direct preparation is kept in a moist chamber ≥24 hr |
| | Rhinosporidium seeberi | 6-300 | Large, thick-walled sporangia containing sporangiospores are present; mature sporangia are larger than spherules of C. immitis; hyphae may be found in cavitary lesions |
| Yeast and pseudohyphae or hyphae | Candida spp. except C. glabrata | 5-10 (pseudohyphae) | Cells usually exhibit single budding; pseudohyphae, when present, are constricted at the ends and remain attached like links of sausage; hyphae, when present, are septate |
| | M. furfur (in tinea versicolor) | 3-8 (yeast) 2.5-4 (hyphae) | Short, curved hyphal elements are usually present, along with round yeast cells that retain their spherical shape in compacted clusters |
| Pauciseptate hyphae | Mucorales: Mucor, Rhizopus, and other genera | 10-30 | Hyphae are large, ribbonlike, often fractured or twisted; occasional septa may be present; smaller hyphae are confused with those of Aspergillus spp., particularly A. flavus |
| Hyaline septate hyphae | Dermatophytes, skin and nails | 3-15 | Hyaline, septate hyphae are commonly seen; chains of arthroconidia may be present |
| | Hair | 3-15 | Arthroconidia on periphery of hair shaft producing a sheath indicate ectothrix infection; arthroconidia formed by fragmentation of hyphae in the hair shaft indicate endothrix infection |
| | | 3-15 | Long hyphal filaments or channels in the hair shaft indicate favus hair infection |
| | Aspergillus spp. | 3-12 | Hyphae are septate and exhibit dichotomous, 45-degree branching; larger hyphae, often disturbed, may resemble those of zygomycetes |
| | Geotrichum spp. | 4-12 | Hyphae and rectangular arthroconidia are present and sometimes rounded; irregular forms may be present |
| | Trichosporon spp. | 2-4 by 8 | Hyphae and rectangular arthroconidia are present and sometimes rounded; occasionally, blastoconidia may be present |

*Continued*

**TABLE 59-8** Summary of Characteristic Features of Fungi Seen in Direct Examination of Clinical Specimens—cont'd

| Morphologic Form Found in Specimens | Organism | Size Range (diameter, mm) | Characteristic Features |
|---|---|---|---|
| Dematiaceous septate hyphae | *Bipolaris* spp., *Cladosporium* spp., *Curvularia* spp., *Drechslera* spp., *Exophiala* spp., *Exserohilum* spp., *Hortaea werneckii, Phialophora* spp. | 2-6 | Dematiaceous polymorphous hyphae are seen; budding cells with single septa and chains of swollen rounded cells are often present; occasionally, aggregates may be present in infection caused by *Phialophora* and *Exophiala* spp. |
| | *Wangiella dermatitidis* | 1.5-5 | Usually large numbers of frequently branched hyphae are present, along with budding cells |
| Sclerotic bodies | *Cladosporium carrionii* *Fonsecaea compacta* *Fonsecaea pedrosoi* *Phialophora verrucosa* *Rhinocladiella aquaspersa* | 5-20 | Brown, round to pleomorphic, thick-walled cells with transverse septations; commonly, cells contain two fission planes that form a tetrad of cells (sclerotic bodies) |
| Granules | *Acremonium* *A. falciforme* *A. kiliense* *A. recifei* | 200-300 | White, soft granules without a cementlike matrix |
| | *Aspergillus* *A. nidulans* | 500-1000 | Black, hard grains with a cementlike matrix at periphery |
| | *Curvularia* *C. geniculata* *C. lunata* | 65-160 | White, soft granule without a cementlike matrix |
| | *Exophiala* *E. jeanselmei* | 200-300 | Black, soft granules, vacuolated, without a cementlike matrix, made of dark hyphae and swollen cells |
| | *Fusarium* *F. moniliforme* | 200-500 | White, soft granules without a cementlike matrix |
| | *F. solani* | 300-600 | |
| | *Leptosphaeria* *L. senegalensis* | 400-600 | Black, hard granules with cementlike matrix present |
| | *L. tompkinsii* | 500-1000 | Periphery composed of polygonal swollen cells and center of a hyphal network |
| | *Madurella* *M. grisea* | 350-500 | Black, soft granules without a cementlike matrix, periphery composed of polygonal swollen cells and center of a hyphal network |
| | *M. mycetomatis* | 200-900 | Black to brown, hard granules, two types: (1) rust brown, compact, filled with cementlike matrix; (2) deep brown, filled with numerous vesicles, 6-14 $\mu$m in diameter, cementlike matrix in periphery, central area of light-colored hyphae |
| | *Neotestudina* *N. rosatii* | 300-600 | White, soft granules with cementlike matrix at periphery |
| | *Pseudallescheria* *P. boydii* | 200-300 | White, soft granules composed of hyphae and swollen cells at periphery in cementlike matrix |
| | *Pyrenochaeta* *P. romeroi* | 300-600 | Black, soft granules composed of polygonal swollen cells at periphery; center is network of hyphae; no cementlike matrix present |

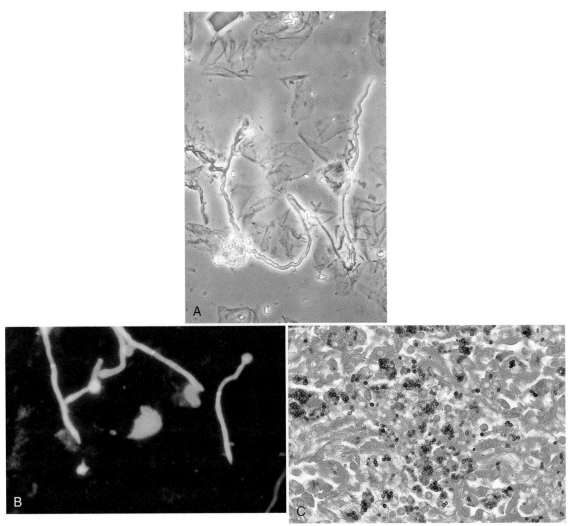

**Figure 59-4** Fungi commonly seen in clinical specimens. **A,** This potassium hydroxide preparation of a skin scraping from a patient with a dermatophyte infection shows septate hyphae intertwined among epithelial cells. (Phase-contrast microscopy; ×500.) **B,** This calcofluor white stain of urine demonstrates *Candida albicans*. **C,** The deeply staining, small, uniform yeast cells in this histologic section of lung tissue are typical of *Histoplasma capsulatum*. (Methenamine silver stain; ×430.)

restriction of a limited set of characteristics to further aid identification.

## GENERAL CONSIDERATIONS FOR THE IDENTIFICATION OF MOLDS

Filamentous fungi are also identified by a combination of tests (Figure 59-6). Molds are identified using a combination of the following:

- Growth rate
- Colonial morphologic features
- Microscopic morphologic features

In most cases the microscopic morphologic features provide the most definitive means of identification. Determination of the growth rate can be most helpful when a mold culture is examined. However, this may have limited value, because the growth rate of certain fungi varies, depending on the amount of inoculum present in a clinical specimen. Slow-growers form mature colonies in 11 to 21 days, and intermediate-growers form mature colonies in 6 to 10 days. Rapid-growers form mature colonies in 5 days or less.

The growth of *C. immitis* is often rapid and is hazardous to microbiologists. In general, the growth rate for the dimorphic fungi, *B. dermatitidis*, *H. capsulatum*, and *P. brasiliensis*, is slow; 1 to 4 weeks usually are required before colonies become visible. In some instances, cultures of *B. dermatitidis* and *H. capsulatum* may be detected within 3 to 5 days. This is a somewhat uncommon circumstance, encountered only when large numbers of the organism are present in the specimen. Colonies of Mucorales may appear within 24 hours, whereas the other hyaline and dematiaceous (melanized) fungi often exhibit growth in 1 to 5 days. The growth rate of an organism, therefore, is important, but it must be used in combination with other features before a definitive identification can be made.

The colonial morphologic features may have limited value for identifying molds because of natural variation

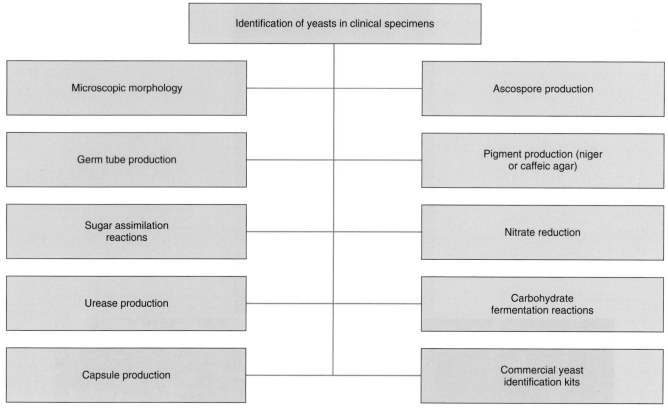

**Figure 59-5** Identification of yeasts in clinical specimens.

among isolates and colonies grown on different culture media. Although common organisms recovered repeatedly in the laboratory may be more easily recognized, colonial morphology is an unreliable criterion that should be used only to supplement the microscopic morphologic features of the organism.

The color of the colony can be important. The examiner must be sure to notice both the front and reverse sides of the culture. The colony topography describes the various elevations of the colony on the agar plate. Topography can be described as **verrucose** (furrowed or convoluted), **umbonate** (slightly raised in the center), and **rugose** (furrows radiate out from the center).

The colony's texture should also be noted. Various textures can be seen, such as **cottony** (loose, high aerial mycelium), **velvety** (low aerial mycelium resembling a velvet cloth), **glabrous** (smooth surface with no aerial mycelium), **granular** (dense, powdery, resembling sugar granules), and **wooly** (high aerial mycelium that appears slightly matted down).

Incubation conditions and culture media must also be considered. For example, *H. capsulatum*, which appears as a white-to-tan fluffy mold on brain-heart infusion agar, may have a yeastlike appearance when grown on the same medium containing blood enrichment.

In general, the microscopic morphologic features of the molds are stable and show minimal variation. Definitive identification is based on the characteristic shape, method of reproduction, and arrangement of spores; however, the size of the hyphae also provides helpful information. The large, ribbonlike, pauciseptate hyphae of the mucorales are easily recognized; small hyphae, approximately 2 $\mu$m in diameter, may suggest the presence of one of the dimorphic fungi or a dermatophyte.

The fungi may be prepared for microscopic observation using several techniques. The procedure traditionally used by most laboratories is the cellophane (Scotch) tape preparation (see Procedure 59-2 on the Evolve site; Figure 59-7). It can be done easily and quickly and often is sufficient to make the identification for most fungi. However, some laboratories prefer the wet mount (see Procedure 59-3 on the Evolve site; Figure 59-8) or tease mount (see Procedure 59-4 on the Evolve site). A microslide culture method (see Procedure 59-5 on the Evolve site; Figure 59-9) may be used when greater detail of the morphologic features is required.

## GENERAL MORPHOLOGIC FEATURES OF THE MOLDS

Specialized types of vegetative hyphae may be helpful for categorizing an organism into a certain group. For example, dermatophytes often produce several types of hyphae, including antler hyphae, so named because they are curved, freely branching, and have the appearance of antlers (Figure 59-10). Racquet hyphae are enlarged, club-shaped structures (Figure 59-11). In addition, certain dermatophytes produce spiral hyphae that are coiled or exhibit corkscrewlike turns in the hyphal strand

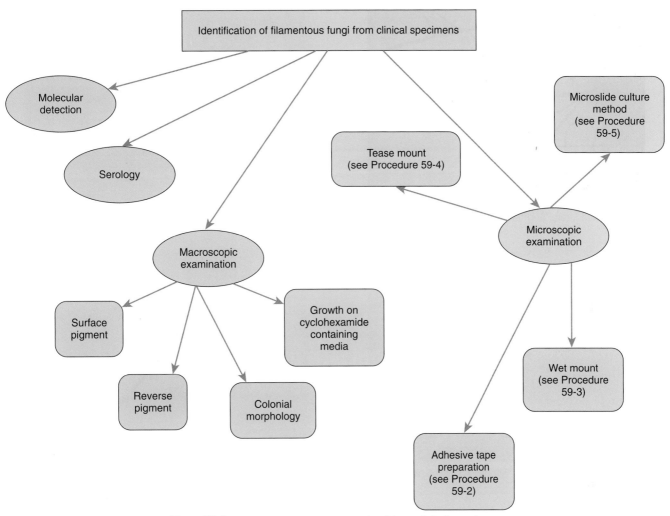

**Figure 59-6** Identification of filamentous fungi from clinical specimens.

(Figure 59-12). These structures are not characteristic for any certain group; however, they are found most commonly in dermatophytes.

Some species of fungi produce sexual spores in a large, saclike structure called an **ascocarp** (Figure 59-13). The ascocarp contains smaller sacs, called *asci,* each of which contains four to eight **ascospores.** This type of sexual reproduction is not commonly seen in the fungi recovered in the clinical microbiology laboratory; most exhibit only asexual reproduction. It is possible that all fungi have a sexual form, but for some species it has not yet been observed on artificial culture media. Conidia, which are produced by most fungi, represent the asexual reproductive cycle. The type of conidia and their morphology and arrangement are important criteria for definitively identifying an organism (Figure 59-14).

The simplest type of sporulation is the development of a spore directly from the vegetative hyphae. **Arthroconidia** are formed directly from the hyphae by fragmentation through the points of septation (Figure 59-15). When mature, they appear as square, rectangular, or barrel-shaped, thick-walled cells. These result from the simple fragmentation of the hyphae into spores, which are easily dislodged and disseminated into the environment. **Chlamydoconidia** (chlamydospores) are round, thick-walled spores formed directly from the differentiation of hyphae in which there is a concentration of protoplasm and nutrient material (Figure 59-16). These appear to be resistant resting spores produced by the rounding up and enlargement of the cells of the hyphae. Chlamydoconidia may be **intercalary** (within the hyphae) or **terminal** (on the end of the hyphae).

A variety of other types of spores occur with many species of fungi. Conidia are asexual spores produced singly or in groups by specialized hyphal strands, **conidiophores.** In some instances, the conidia are freed from their point of attachment by pinching off, or **abstriction.** Some conidiophores terminate in a swollen vesicle. From the surface of the vesicle are formed secondary small, flask-shaped phialides, which in turn give rise to long chains of conidia. This type of fruiting structure is characteristic of the aspergilli. A single, simple, slender, tubular conidiophore **(phialide)** that produces a cluster of conidia, held together as a gelatinous mass, is characteristic of certain fungi, including the genus *Acremonium* (Figure 59-17). In other instances, conidiophores

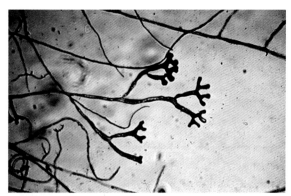

**Figure 59-10** Antler hyphae showing swollen hyphal tips, resembling antlers, with lateral and terminal branching (favic chandeliers) (×500).

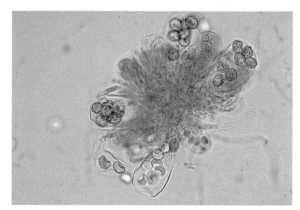

**Figure 59-13** Ascocarp showing dark-appearing ascospores (×430).

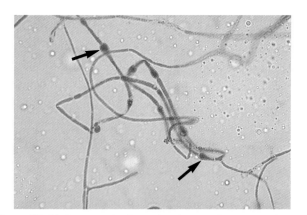

**Figure 59-11** Racquet hyphae showing swollen areas *(arrows)* resembling a tennis racquet.

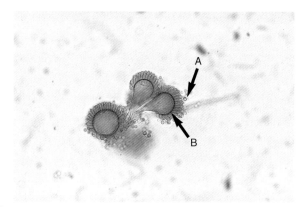

**Figure 59-14** Conidia (asexual spores [A]) produced on specialized structures (conidiophores [B]) of *Aspergillus* (×430).

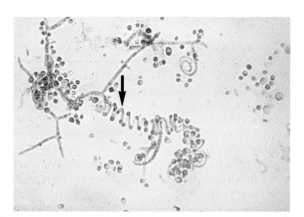

**Figure 59-12** Spiral hyphae *(arrow)* showing corkscrewlike turns (×430).

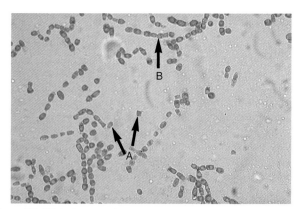

**Figure 59-15** Arthroconidia formation *(A)* produced by the breaking down of a hyphal strand *(B)* into individual rectangular units (×430).

form a branching structure called a **penicillus,** in which each branch terminates in secondary branches **(metulae)** and phialides, from which chains of conidia are borne (Figure 59-18). Species of *Penicillium* and *Paecilomyces* are representative of this type of sporulation. In other instances, fungi may produce conidia of two sizes: **microconidia,** which are small, unicellular, round, elliptical, or pyriform in shape, or **macroconidia,** which are large, usually multiseptate, and club or spindle shaped (Figure

59-19). Microconidia may be borne directly on the side of a hyphal strand or at the end of a conidiophore. Macroconidia are usually borne on a short to long conidiophore and may be smooth or rough walled. Microconidia and macroconidia are seen in some fungal species and are not specific, except as they are used to differentiate a limited number of genera.

The hyphae of the mucorales are sparsely septate. Sporulation takes place by progressive cleavage during

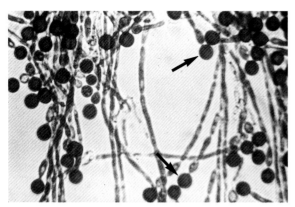

**Figure 59-16** Chlamydoconidia composed of thick-walled spherical cells *(arrows)* (×430).

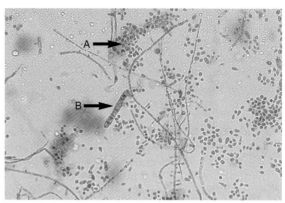

**Figure 59-19** In this preparation of a *Trichophyton* species, the numerous, small, spherical microconidia *(A)* are contrasted with a large, elongated macroconidium *(B)* (×430).

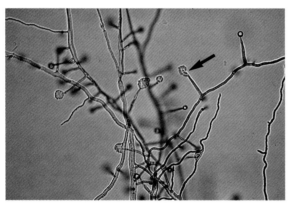

**Figure 59-17** Simple tubular phialide with a cluster of conidia at its tip *(arrow)* characteristic of *Acremonium* (×430).

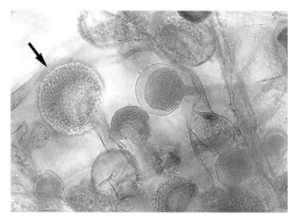

**Figure 59-20** Large, saclike sporangia that contain sporangio-spores *(arrow)* characteristic of the mucorales (×250).

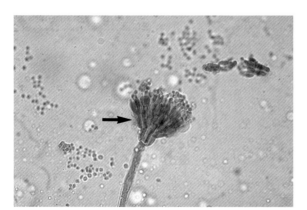

**Figure 59-18** Complex method of sporulation in which conidia are borne on phialides produced on secondary branches (metulae [*arrow*]) characteristic of *Penicillium* (×430).

the union of two matching types of a mucorales; this is an example of sexual reproduction.

## CLINICAL RELEVANCE FOR FUNGAL IDENTIFICATION

The question of when and how far to go with the identification of fungi recovered from clinical specimens presents an interesting challenge. The current emphasis on cost containment and the ever-increasing number of opportunistic fungi causing infection in compromised patients prompts consideration of whether all fungi recovered from clinical specimens should be thoroughly identified and reported. A study by Murray et al.[8] focused on the time and expense involved in identifying yeasts from respiratory tract specimens. Because these are the specimens most commonly submitted for fungal culture, the researchers questioned whether identifying every organism recovered was important. After evaluating the clinical usefulness of information provided through the identification of yeast recovered from respiratory tract specimens, they suggested the following:

maturation in the sporangium, a saclike structure produced at the tip of a long stalk **(sporangiophore).** Sporangiospores (spores produced in the sporangium) are produced and released by the rupture of the sporangial wall (Figure 59-20). In rare cases some isolates may produce **zygospores,** rough-walled spores produced by

- Routine identification of yeasts recovered in culture from respiratory secretions is not warranted, but all yeasts should be screened for *Cryptococcus neoformans* complex.
- All respiratory secretions submitted for fungal culture, regardless of the presence or absence of oropharyngeal contamination, should be cultured, because common pathogens, such as *H. capsulatum, B. dermatitidis, C. immitis,* and *S. schenckii,* may be recovered.
- Routine identification of yeast in respiratory secretions has little or no value for the clinician and probably represents "normal flora," except for *C. neoformans.*

The extent of identification of yeasts from other specimen sources is discussed in Chapter 63. The usefulness of identification and susceptibility testing of non-*Cryptococcus* yeast isolates was studied by Barenfenger.[9] She found that, compared with only superficial characterization (i.e., "Yeast present, not *C. neoformans*), identification and susceptibility testing of *Candida* isolates from respiratory secretions led to unnecessary treatment and increased costs. No statistical difference was seen in the mortality of these groups.

When and how far to proceed in the identification of a mold is a difficult question to answer. Except for obvious plate contaminants, all commonly encountered molds should be identified and reported if recovered from patients at risk for invasive fungal disease. Immunocompromised patients may have serious or even fatal disease caused by fungi that were once thought to be clinically insignificant. Organisms that fail to sporulate after a reasonable time should be reported as present, but identification is not required if the dimorphic fungi have been ruled out or if the clinician believes the organism is not clinically significant. Ideally, all laboratories should identify all fungi recovered from clinical specimens; however, the limits of practicality and economic considerations play a definite role in the decision-making process. The laboratory director, in consultation with the clinicians being served, must make this decision after considering the patient population, laboratory practice, and economic impact.

As shown in Table 59-9, an increasing number of fungi may be isolated in the clinical microbiology laboratory. They are considered environmental flora, but in reality must be regarded as potential pathogens because infections with a number of these organisms have been reported. Less commonly encountered fungal pathogens that have been shown to cause human infections include but are not limited to *P. boydii; Scedosporium prolificans; Bipolaris, Exserohilum, Trichosporon,* and *Aureobasidium* spp., and others. The laboratory must identify and report all organisms recovered from clinical specimens so that their clinical significance can be determined. In many instances, the presence of environmental fungi is unimportant; however, that is not always the case. Tables 59-10 and 59-11 present the molds and yeasts implicated in causing human infection, the time required for their identification, the most likely site for their recovery, and the clinical implications of each.

# ■ LABORATORY SAFETY

Although the handling of fungi recovered from clinical specimens poses risks, a common sense approach to the

**TABLE 59-9**  Fungi Most Commonly Recovered from Clinical Specimens

| Blood | Cerebrospinal Fluid | Genitourinary Tract | Respiratory Tract | Skin |
|---|---|---|---|---|
| Candida albicans | Cryptococcus neoformans | Candida albicans | Yeast, not Cryptococcus spp. | Trichophyton rubrum |
| Candida tropicalis | Candida albicans | Candida glabrata | Penicillium spp. | Trichophyton mentagrophytes |
| Candida parapsilosis | Candida parapsilosis | Candida tropicalis | Aspergillus spp. | Alternaria spp. |
| Cryptococcus spp. | Candida tropicalis | Candida parapsilosis | Aspergillus fumigatus | Candida albicans |
| Histoplasma capsulatum | Coccidioides immitis | Penicillium spp. | Cladosporium spp. | Penicillium spp. |
| Candida lusitaniae | Histoplasma capsulatum | Candida krusei | Alternaria spp. | Scopulariopsis spp. |
| Candida krusei | | Cryptococcus spp. | Aspergillus niger | Epidermophyton floccosum |
| Saccharomyces spp. | | Saccharomyces spp. | Geotrichum candidum | Candida parapsilosis |
| Candida kefyr | | Histoplasma capsulatum | Fusarium spp. | Aspergillus spp. |
| Candida zeylanoides | | Cladosporium spp. | Aspergillus versicolor | Acremonium spp. |
| Trichosporon spp. | | Aspergillus spp. | Aspergillus flavus | Aspergillus versicolor |
| Coccidioides immitis | | Trichosporon spp. | Acremonium spp. | Cladosporium spp. |
| Candida guilliermondii | | Alternaria spp. | Scopulariopsis spp. | Fusarium spp. |
| Malassezia furfur | | | Beauveria spp. | Trichosporon spp. |
| | | | Trichosporon spp. | Phialophora spp. |

**TABLE 59-10** Common Filamentous Fungi Implicated in Human Mycotic Infections

| Etiologic Agent | Time Required for Identification | Probable Recovery Sites | Clinical Implication |
|---|---|---|---|
| *Acremonium* spp. | 2-6 days | Skin, nails, respiratory secretions, cornea, vagina, gastric washings, blood | Skin and nail infections, mycotic keratitis, mycetoma |
| *Alternaria* spp. | 2-6 days | Skin, nails, conjunctiva, respiratory secretions, subcutaneous tissue | Skin and nail infections, sinusitis, conjunctivitis, hypersensitivity pneumonitis, skin abscess |
| *Aspergillus flavus* | 1-4 days | Skin, respiratory secretions, gastric washings, nasal sinuses, lung | Skin infections, allergic bronchopulmonary infection, sinusitis, myocarditis, disseminated infection, renal infection, subcutaneous mycetoma |
| *Aspergillus fumigatus* | 2-6 days | Respiratory secretions, skin, ear, cornea, gastric washings, nasal sinuses, lung | Allergic bronchopulmonary infection, fungus ball, invasive pulmonary infection, skin and nail infections, external otomycosis, mycotic keratitis, sinusitis, myocarditis, renal infection |
| *Aspergillus niger* | 1-4 days | Respiratory secretions, gastric washings, ear, skin | Fungus ball, pulmonary infection, external otomycosis, mycotic keratitis |
| *Aspergillus terreus* | 2-6 days | Respiratory secretions, skin, gastric washings, nails, lung | Pulmonary infection, disseminated infection, endocarditis, onychomycosis, allergic bronchopulmonary infection |
| *Bipolaris* spp. | 2-6 days | Respiratory secretions, skin, nose, bone, sinuses | Sinusitis, brain abscess, peritonitis, subcutaneous abscess, pulmonary infection, osteomyelitis, encephalitis |
| *Blastomyces dermatitidis* | 6-21 days (recovery time) (additional 1-2 days required for confirmatory identification) | Respiratory secretions, skin, oropharyngeal ulcer, bone, prostate, lung | Pulmonary infection, skin infection, oropharyngeal ulceration, osteomyelitis, prostatitis, arthritis, central nervous system (CNS) infection, disseminated infection |
| *Cladosporium* spp. | 6-10 days | Respiratory secretions, skin, nails, nose, cornea | Skin and nail infections, mycotic keratitis, chromoblastomycosis caused by *Cladophialophora carrionii* |
| *Coccidioides immitis* | 3-21 days | Respiratory secretions, skin, bone, cerebrospinal fluid (CSF), synovial fluid, urine, gastric washings, blood | Pulmonary infection, skin infection, osteomyelitis, meningitis, arthritis, disseminated infection |
| *Curvularia* spp. | 2-6 days | Respiratory secretions, cornea, brain, skin, nasal sinuses | Pulmonary infection, disseminated infection, mycotic keratitis, brain abscess, mycetoma, endocarditis |
| *Drechslera* spp. | 2-6 days | Respiratory secretions, skin, peritoneal fluid (after dialysis) | Pulmonary infection (rare) |
| *Epidermophyton floccosum* | 7-10 days | Skin, nails | Tinea cruris, tinea pedis, tinea corporis, onychomycosis |
| *Exophiala dermatitidis* | 5-21 days | Respiratory secretions, skin, eye | Phaeohyphomycosis, endophthalmitis, pneumonia |
| *Exserohilum* spp. | 2-6 days | Eye, skin, nose, bone | Keratitis, subcutaneous abscess, sinusitis, endocarditis, osteomyelitis |
| *Fusarium* spp. | 2-6 days | Skin, respiratory secretions, cornea, nails, blood | Mycotic keratitis, skin infection (in burn patients), disseminated infection, endophthalmitis |
| *Geotrichum* spp. | 2-6 days | Respiratory secretions, urine, skin, stool, vagina, conjunctiva, gastric washings, throat | Bronchitis, skin infection, colitis, conjunctivitis, thrush, wound infection |

*Continued*

**TABLE 59-10** Common Filamentous Fungi Implicated in Human Mycotic Infections—cont'd

| Etiologic Agent | Time Required for Identification | Probable Recovery Sites | Clinical Implication |
|---|---|---|---|
| *Histoplasma capsulatum* | ≤10-45 days (recovery time) (additional 1-2 days required for confirmatory identification) | Respiratory secretions, bone marrow, blood, urine, adrenals, skin, CSF, eye, pleural fluid, liver, spleen, oropharyngeal lesions, vagina, gastric washings, larynx | Pulmonary infection, oropharyngeal lesions, CNS infection, skin infection (rare), uveitis, peritonitis, endocarditis, brain abscess, disseminated infection |
| *Microsporum audouinii* | 10-14 days (recovery time) (additional 14-21 days required for confirmatory identification) | Hair (scalp) | Tinea capitis |
| *Microsporum canis* | 5-7 days | Hair, skin | Tinea corporis, tinea capitis, tinea barbae, tinea manuum |
| *Microsporum gypseum* | 3-6 days | Hair, skin | Tinea capitis, tinea corporis |
| *Mucor* spp. | 1-5 days | Respiratory secretions, skin, nose, brain, stool, orbit, cornea, vitreous humor, gastric washings, wounds, ear, lung | Rhinocerebral infection, pulmonary infection, gastrointestinal infection, mycotic keratitis, intraocular infection, external otomycosis, orbital cellulitis, disseminated infection |
| *Penicillium* spp. | 2-6 days | Respiratory secretions, gastric washings, skin, urine, ear, cornea | Allergy; human infections rare except with *P. marneffei* |
| *Phialophora* spp. | 6-21 days | Respiratory secretions, gastric washings, skin, cornea, conjunctiva | Some species produce chromoblastomycosis or mycetoma; mycotic keratitis, conjunctivitis, intraocular infection |
| *Pseudallescheria boydii* | 2-6 days | Respiratory secretions, gastric washings, skin, cornea | Pulmonary fungus ball, mycetoma, mycotic keratitis, endocarditis, disseminated infection, brain abscess |
| *Rhizopus* spp. | 1-5 days | Respiratory secretions, skin, nose, brain, stool, orbit, cornea, vitreous humor, gastric washings, wounds, ear, lung | Rhinocerebral infection, pulmonary infection, mycotic keratitis, intraocular infection, orbital cellulitis, external otomycosis, disseminated infection |
| *Scedosporium prolificans* | 2-6 days | Respiratory secretions, skin, nasal sinuses, bone | Arthritis, osteomyelitis, sinusitis, endocarditis |
| *Scopulariopsis* spp. | 2-6 days | Respiratory secretions, gastric washings, nails, skin, vitreous humor, ear | Pulmonary infection, nail infection, skin infection, intraocular infection, external otomycosis |
| *Sporothrix schenckii* | 3-12 days (recovery time) (additional 2-10 days required for confirmatory identification) | Respiratory secretions, skin, subcutaneous tissue, maxillary sinuses, synovial fluid, bone marrow, bone, CSF, ear, conjunctiva | Pulmonary infection, lymphocutaneous infection, sinusitis, arthritis, osteomyelitis, meningitis, external otomycosis, conjunctivitis, disseminated infection |
| *Trichophyton mentagrophytes* | 7-10 days | Hair, skin, nails | Tinea barbae, tinea capitis, tinea corporis, tinea cruris, tinea pedis, onychomycosis |
| *Trichophyton rubrum* | 10-14 days | Hair, skin, nails | Tinea pedis, onychomycosis, tinea corporis, tinea cruris |
| *Trichophyton tonsurans* | 10-14 days | Hair, skin, nails | Tinea capitis, tinea corporis, onychomycosis, tinea pedis |
| *Trichophyton verrucosum* | 10-18 days | Hair, skin, nails | Tinea capitis, tinea corporis, tinea barbae |
| *Trichophyton violaceum* | 14-18 days | Hair, skin, nails | Tinea capitis, tinea corporis, onychomycosis |

**TABLE 59-11** Common Yeastlike Organisms Implicated in Human Infection*

| Etiologic Agent | Probable Recovery Sites | Clinical Implication |
|---|---|---|
| *Candida albicans* | Respiratory secretions, vagina, urine, skin, oropharynx, gastric washings, blood, stool, transtracheal aspiration, cornea, nails, cerebrospinal fluid (CSF), bone, peritoneal fluid | Pulmonary infection, vaginitis, urinary tract infection, dermatitis, fungemia, mycotic keratitis, onychomycosis, meningitis, osteomyelitis, peritonitis, myocarditis, endocarditis, endophthalmitis, disseminated infection, thrush, arthritis |
| *Candida glabrata* | Respiratory secretions, urine, vagina, gastric washings, blood, skin, oropharynx, transtracheal aspiration, stool, bone marrow, skin (rare) | Pulmonary infection, urinary tract infection, vaginitis, fungemia, disseminated infection, endocarditis |
| *Candida tropicalis* | Respiratory secretions, urine, gastric washings, vagina, blood, skin, oropharynx, transtracheal aspiration, stool, pleural fluid, peritoneal fluid, cornea | Pulmonary infection, vaginitis, thrush, endophthalmitis, endocarditis, arthritis, peritonitis, mycotic keratitis, fungemia |
| *Candida parapsilosis* | Respiratory secretions, urine, gastric washings, blood, vagina, oropharynx, skin, transtracheal aspiration, stool, pleural fluid, ear, nails | Endophthalmitis, endocarditis, vaginitis, mycotic keratitis, external otomycosis, paronychia, fungemia |
| *Saccharomyces* spp. | Respiratory secretions, urine, gastric washings, vagina, skin, oropharynx, transtracheal aspiration, stool, blood | Pulmonary infection (rare), endocarditis |
| *Candida krusei* | Respiratory secretions, urine, gastric washings, vagina, skin, oropharynx, blood, transtracheal aspiration, stool, cornea | Endocarditis, vaginitis, urinary tract infection, mycotic keratitis |
| *Candida guilliermondii* | Respiratory secretions, gastric washings, vagina, skin, nails, oropharynx, blood, cornea, bone, urine | Endocarditis, fungemia, dermatitis, onychomycosis, mycotic keratitis, osteomyelitis, urinary tract infection |
| *Rhodotorula* spp. | Respiratory secretions, urine, gastric washings, blood, vagina, skin, oropharynx, stool, CSF, cornea | Fungemia, endocarditis, mycotic keratitis |
| *Trichosporon* spp. | Respiratory secretions, blood, skin, oropharynx, stool | Pulmonary infection, brain abscess, disseminated infection, piedra |
| *Cryptococcus* species complex (*C. neoformans*, var. neoformans; *C. neoformans*, var. grubii, *C. gatti*) | Respiratory secretions, CSF, bone, blood, bone marrow, urine, skin, pleural fluid, gastric washings, transtracheal aspiration, cornea, orbit, vitreous humor | Pulmonary infection, meningitis, osteomyelitis, fungemia, disseminated infection, endocarditis, skin infection, mycotic keratitis, orbital cellulitis, endophthalmic infection |
| *Cryptococcus albidus* subsp. *albidus* | Respiratory secretions, skin, gastric washings, urine, cornea | Meningitis, pulmonary infection |
| *Candida kefyr* (*pseudotropicalis*) | Respiratory secretions, vagina, urine, gastric washings, oropharynx | Vaginitis, urinary tract infection |
| *Cryptococcus luteolus* | Respiratory secretions, skin, nose | Not commonly implicated in human infection |
| *Cryptococcus laurentii* | Respiratory secretions, CSF, skin, oropharynx, stool | Not commonly implicated in human infection |
| *Cryptococcus albidus* subsp. *diffluens* | Respiratory secretions, urine, CSF, gastric washings, skin | Not commonly implicated in human infection |
| *Cryptococcus terreus* | Respiratory secretions, skin, nose | Not commonly implicated in human infection |

handling of these specimens protects the laboratory from contamination and workers from becoming infected.

Without exception, mold cultures and clinical specimens must be handled in a class II BSC. Some laboratory directors believe that mold cultures must be handled in an enclosed BSC equipped with gloves; however, this is not necessary if a laminar flow BSC is used. Yeast cultures may be handled on the bench top. An electric incinerator or a gas flame is suitable for decontaminating a loop used to transfer yeast cultures. Cultures of organisms suspected of being pathogens should be sealed with tape to prevent laboratory contamination and should be autoclaved as soon as the definitive identification is made. If common safety precautions are followed, few problems should occur with laboratory contamination or infection acquired by laboratory personnel.

# PREVENTION

Preventing and controlling fungal infections continue to be a challenge to individuals, researchers, laboratorians, and hospitals. Very few formal recommendations are available to prevent exposure to community-acquired fungal infections. Good personal hygiene may be the best course for prevention. However, many strategies can be followed to prevent nosocomial infections. Hospital staff members should be aware of the pathogenesis of fungal infections. Fungi are easily spread in ventilation systems, water, and skin-to-skin contact. Hospitals should follow

an infection control plan that includes periodic monitoring of air-handling systems and regular testing for environmental spores. Staff members, patients, and visitors should practice good personal hygiene to minimize exposure to potential fungal infections.

The laboratory also plays an important role in fungal prevention and control. Lack of rapid and specific testing continues to be a factor in a timely diagnosis. Early definitive diagnosis ensures that the appropriate therapy is given promptly and prevents mortality.

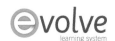 *Visit the Evolve site to complete the review questions.*

---

## CASE STUDY 59-1

A 5-year-old boy recently adopted from Haiti is seen by a primary care physician. The boy appears to have an infection of the hair and scalp. The physician suspects a dermatophyte and removes infected hairs by plucking them with forceps. The sterile container with the specimen is sent to the laboratory for culture.

### QUESTIONS

1. What agar and incubation temperature might the laboratorian choose for primary culture?

2. The laboratorian notices that the fungus is a slow grower, taking 12 days to grow. What other details should be noted?

3. The colony appears downy, flat, and spreading. It has a light tan front and red-brown reverse. What is the next step for identifying this fungus?

4. Rare club-shaped microconidia and sterile hyphae are noted with terminal chlamydospores. The laboratorian decides the dermatophyte is a *Microsporum* species. How might *M. canis* be differentiated from *M. audouinii*?

---

# BIBLIOGRAPHY

Adam RD, Paquin ML, Petersen EA, et al: Phaeohyphomycosis caused by the fungal genera Bipolaris and Exserohilum: a report of nine cases and review of the literature, *Medicine (Baltimore)* 65:203, 1986.

Alvarez M, Ponga BL, Rayon C, et al: Nosocomial outbreak caused by Scedosporium prolificans (inflatum): four fatal cases in leukemic patients, *J Clin Microbiol* 33:3290, 1995.

Barenfanger J, Arakere P, Dela Cruz R, et al: Improved outcomes associated with limiting identification of Candida spp. in respiratory secretions, *J Clin Microbiol* 41:5645, 2003.

Beck MR, Dekoster GT, Cistola DP, et al: NMR structure of a fungal virulence factor reveals structural homology with mammalian saposin B, *Mol Microbiol* 72(2):344-353, 2009.

Bernstein EF, Schuster MG, Stieritz, et al: Disseminated cutaneous Pseudallescheria boydii, *Br J Dermatol* 132:456, 1995.

Bille J, Stockman L, Roberts GD, et al: Evaluation of a lysis-centrifugation system for recovery of yeasts and filamentous fungi from blood, *J Clin Microbiol* 18:469, 1983.

Bille J, Edson RS, Roberts GD: Clinical evaluation of the lysis-centrifugation blood culture system for the detection of fungemia and comparison with a conventional biphasic broth blood culture system, *J Clin Microbiol* 19:126, 1984.

Bradsher R, McDonnell R: Blastomyces dermatitidis and Paracoccidioides brasiliensis. In Chmel H, Bendinelli M, Friedman I, editors: *Pulmonary infections and immunity*, New York, 1990, Plenum Press.

Brandhorst TT, Gauthier GM, Stein RA, et al: Calcium binding by essential virulence factor BAD-1 of *Blastomyces dermatitidis*, *J Biol Chem* 280(51):42156-42163, 2005.

Brasch J: Pathogens and pathogenesis of dermatophytoses, *Hautarzt* 41:9, 1990.

Brummer E, Castaneda E, Restrepo A: Paracoccidioidomycosis: an update, *Clin Microbiol Rev* 6:89, 1993.

Caporale NE, Calegari L, Perez D, et al: Peritoneal catheter colonization and peritonitis with Aureobasidium pullulans, *Perit Dial Int* 16:97, 1996.

Cherniak R, Sundstrom JB: Polysaccharide antigens of the capsule of Cryptococcus neoformans, *Infect Immun* 62:1507, 1994.

Cox R, Best G: Cell wall composition of two strains of Blastomyces dermatitidis exhibiting differences in virulence for mice, *Infect Immun* 5:449, 1972.

Cutler J: Putative virulence factors of Candida albicans, *Annu Rev Microbiol* 45:187, 1991.

Douer D, Goldschmied-Reouven A, Segev S, et al: Human Exserohilum and Bipolaris infections: report of Exserohilum nasal infection in a neutropenic patient with acute leukemia and review of the literature, *J Med Vet Mycol* 25:235, 1987.

Ener B, Douglas L: Correlation between cell-surface hydrophobicity of Candida albicans and adhesion to buccal epithelial cells, *FEMS Microbiol Lett* 78:37, 1992.

Frey C, Drutz D: Influence of fungal surface components on the interaction of Coccidioides immitis with polymorphonuclear neutrophils, *J Infect Dis* 153:933, 1986.

Girmenia C, Pagano L, Martino B, et al: Invasive infections caused by Trichosporon species and Geotrichum capitatum in patients with hematological malignancies: a retrospective multicenter study from Italy and review of the literature, *J Clin Microbiol* 43:1818, 2005.

Hageage G, Harrington B: Use of calcofluor white in clinical mycology, *Lab Med* 15:109, 1984.

Hibbett DS, Binder M, Bischoff JF, et al: A higher-level phylogenetic classification of the fungi, *Mycol Res* 111(5):509-547, 2007.

Hogan L, Klein B, Levitz S: Virulence factors of medically important fungi, *Clin Microbiol Rev* 9:469, 1996.

Hopfer R: Use of molecular biological techniques in the diagnostic laboratory for detecting and differentiating fungi, *Arch Med Res* 26:287, 1995.

Hopfer R, Walden P, Setterquist S: Detection and differentiation of fungi in clinical specimens using polymerase chain reaction (PCR) amplification and restriction enzyme analysis, *J Med Vet Mycol* 31:65, 1993.

Hostetter M: Adhesions and ligands involved in the interaction of Candida spp with epithelial and endothelial surfaces, *Clin Microbiol Rev* 7:29, 1994.

Huffnagle G, Chen G, Curtis J: Down-regulation of the afferent phase of T cell-mediated pulmonary inflammation and immunity by a high melanin–producing strain of Cryptococcus neoformans, *J Immunol* 155:3607, 1995.

Ibrahim AS, Mirbod F, Filler SG, et al: Evidence implicating phospholipase as a virulence factor of Candida albicans, *Infect Immun* 63:1993, 1995.

Kolattukudy PE, Lee JD, Rogers LM, et al: Evidence for possible involvement of an elastolytic serine protease in aspergillosis, *Infect Immun* 61:2357, 1993.

Koneman E, Roberts G: *Practical laboratory mycology*, ed 3, Baltimore, 1985, Williams & Wilkins.

Kozel TR, Gali ST, Pfrommer T, et al: Role of the capsule in phagocytosis of Cryptococcus neoformans, *Rev Infect Dis* 10:S436, 1988.

Kwon-Chung K, Bennet J: *Medical mycology*, Philadelphia, 1992, Lea & Febiger.

Lopez-Martinez R, Manzano Gayosso R, Mier T, et al: Exoenzymes of dermatophytes isolated from acute and chronic tinea, *Rev Latinoam Microbiol* 36:17, 1994.

Lu JJ, Chen CH, Bartlett MS, et al: Comparison of six different PCR methods for detection of Pneumocystis carinii, *J Clin Microbiol* 33:2785, 1995.

Lucas S, da luz Martins M, Flores O, et al: Differentiation of *Cryptococcus neoformans* varieties and *Cryptococcus gattii* using CAP59-based loop-mediated isothermal DNA amplification, *Clin Microbiol Infect* 16(6):711-714, 2010.

Madariaga MG, Tenorio A, Proia L: Trichosporon inkin peritonitis treated with caspofungin, *J Clin Microbiol* 41:5827, 2003.

Makimura K, Murayama SY, Yamaguchi H: Detection of a wide range of medically important fungi by the polymerase chain reaction, *J Med Microbiol* 40:358, 1994.

Mandell GL, Bennett JE, Dolin R: *Principles and practices of infectious diseases*, ed 7, Philadelphia, 2010, Churchill Livingstone/Elsevier.

Markaryan A, Morozova I, Yu H, et al: Purification and characterization of an elastinolytic metalloprotease from Aspergillus fumigatus and immunoelectron microscopic evidence of secretion of this enzyme by the fungus invading the murine lung, *Infect Immun* 62:2149, 1994.

McEwen JG, Bedoya V, Patino MM, et al: Experimental murine paracoccidioidomycosis induced by the inhalation of conidia, *J Med Vet Mycol* 25:165, 1987.

McGinnis MR, Rinaldi MG, Winn RE: Emerging agents of phaeohyphomycosis: pathogenic species of Bipolaris and Exserohilum, *J Clin Microbiol* 24:250, 1986.

Murray P: *ASM pocket guide to clinical microbiology*, Washington, DC, 1996, ASM Press.

Murray P, Van Scoy R, Roberts GD: Should yeasts in respiratory secretions be identified? *Mayo Clin Proc* 52:42, 1977.

Musial CE, Cockerill FR III, Roberts GD: Fungal infections of the immunocompromised host: clinical and laboratory aspects, *Clin Microbiol Rev* 1:349, 1988.

Neely AN, Orloff MM, Holder IA: Candida albicans growth studies: a hypothesis for the pathogenesis of Candida infections in burns, *J Burn Care Rehabil* 13:323, 1992.

Neilson JB, Fromtling RA, Bulmer GS: Cryptococcus neoformans: size range of infectious particles from aerosolized soil, *Infect Immun* 17:634, 1977.

Procop GW, Roberts GD: Emerging fungal diseases: the importance of the host, *Clin Lab Med* 24:691, 2004.

Roberts GD: Detection of fungi in clinical specimens by phase-contrast microscopy, *J Clin Microbiol* 2:261, 1975.

Roberts GD, Karlson AG, DeYoung DR: Recovery of pathogenic fungi from clinical specimens submitted for mycobacteriological culture, *J Clin Microbiol* 3:47, 1976.

Sandhu GS, Kline BC, Stockman L, et al: Molecular probes for diagnosis of fungal infections, *J Clin Microbiol* 33:2913, 1995.

Steinbach WJ, Schell WA, Miller JL, et al: Scedosporium prolificans osteomyelitis in an immunocompetent child treated with voriconazole and caspofungin, as well as locally applied polyhexamethylene biguanide, *J Clin Microbiol* 41:3981, 2003.

Stevens DA: The interface of mycology and endocrinology, *J Med Vet Mycol* 27:133, 1989.

Sugita T, Nishikawa A, Shinoda T, et al: Taxonomic position of deep-seated, mucosa-associated, and superficial isolates of Trichosporon cutaneum from trichosporonosis patients, *J Clin Microbiol* 33:1368, 1995.

Tomee J, Kauffman HF: Putative virulence factors of *Aspergillus fumigatus*, *Clin Exp Allergy* 30(4):476-484, 2000.

Vartivarian SE: Virulence properties and nonimmune pathogenetic mechanisms of fungi, *Clin Infect Dis* 14:S30, 1992.

Versalovic J: *Manual of clinical microbiology*, ed 10, Washington, DC, 2011, ASM Press.

Walsh TJ, Groll A, Hiemenz J, et al: Infections due to emerging and uncommon medically important fungal pathogens, *Clin Microbiol Infect* 10(Suppl 1):48, 2004.

Wang Y, Aisen P, Casadevall A: Cryptococcus neoformans melanin and virulence: mechanism of action, *Infect Immun* 63:3131, 1995.

Wu-Hsieh B, Howard D: Histoplasmosis. In Murphy J, Friedman H, Bendinelli M, editors: *Fungal infections and immune responses*, New York, 1993, Plenum Press.

Yuan L, Cole G, Sun S: Possible role of a proteinase endosporulation of Coccidioides immitis, *Infect Immun* 56:1551, 1988.

# Hyaline Molds, Mucorales (Zygomycetes), Dermatophytes, and Opportunistic and Systemic Mycoses

## OBJECTIVES

1. Describe where mucorales (zygomycetes) are found, how they are transmitted to humans, and the diseases they cause.
2. Describe the characteristic colony morphology of the mucorales (zygomycetes).
3. Outline the tests needed to diagnose a *Trichophyton* species.
4. List the key features that distinguish *Trichophyton rubrum* and *Trichophyton mentagrophytes*.
5. Compare and contrast the ways *Microsporum audouinii* and *Microsporum canis* are spread and the populations at risk.
6. Define ectothrix and endothrix.
7. Explain why diagnosing an opportunistic fungal infection in an immunocompromised patient is difficult.
8. Compare and contrast *Aspergillus* and *Penicillium* spp., both macroscopically and microscopically.
9. Discuss the dimorphic molds in relation to their endemic areas, disease states, and associated diagnostic methods for identification.

### HYALINE MOLDS TO BE CONSIDERED

| Current Name | Previous Name |
|---|---|
| **Mucorales** | Zygomycota |
| *Rhizopus* spp. | |
| *Mucor* spp. | |
| *Lichtheimia* spp. | |
| *Absidia* spp. | |
| **Dermatophytes** | |
| *Trichophyton* spp. | |
| *Microsporum* spp. | |
| *Epidermophyton* sp. | |
| **Opportunistic Mycoses** | |
| *Aspergillus* spp. | |
| *Fusarium* spp. | |
| *Geotrichum* spp. | |
| *Acremonium* spp. | |
| *Penicillium* spp. | |
| *Paecilomyces* spp. | |
| *Scopulariopsis* spp. | |
| **Systemic Mycoses** | |
| *Blastomyces dermatitidis* | |
| *Coccidioides immitis* | |
| *Histoplasma capsulatum* | |
| *Paracoccidioides brasiliensis* | |
| *Penicillium marneffei* | |
| *Sporothrix schenckii* | |

# THE MUCORALES

## GENERAL CHARACTERISTICS

The mucorales (zygomycetes) characteristically produce large, ribbonlike hyphae that are irregular in diameter and contain occasional septa. Because the septa may not be apparent in some preparations, this group sometimes has been characterized as aseptate. The specific identification of these organisms is confirmed by observing the characteristic saclike fruiting structures (**sporangia**), which produce internally spherical, yellow or brown spores (**sporangiospores**) (Figure 60-1). Each sporangium is formed at the tip of a supporting structure (**sporangiophore**). During maturation, the sporangium becomes fractured and sporangiospores are released into the environment. Sporangiophores are usually connected to one another by occasionally septate hyphae called **stolons,** which attach at contact points where root-like structures (**rhizoids**) may appear and anchor the organism to the agar surface. Identification of the mucorales (*Mucor, Rhizopus, Lichtheimia,* and *Absidia* spp.) is partly based on the presence or absence of rhizoids and the position of the rhizoids in relation to the sporangiophores.

## EPIDEMIOLOGY AND PATHOGENESIS

Although the mucorales (*Rhizopus, Mucor, Lichtheimia, Syncephalastrum, Cunninghamella* spp., and others) are a less common cause of infection than the aspergilli, they are an important cause of morbidity and mortality in immunocompromised patients, particularly patients with diabetes mellitus. The organisms involved have a worldwide distribution and are commonly found on decaying vegetable matter or old bread (they are a common bread mold) or in soil. The organism is generally acquired by inhalation or ingestion of spores or through percutaneous routes, followed by subsequent development of infection. Once established, the infection is rapidly progressive, particularly in patients with diabetes mellitus who have infections that involve the sinuses.

## SPECTRUM OF DISEASE

Immunocompromised patients are at greatest risk, particularly those who have uncontrolled diabetes mellitus and those who are undergoing prolonged corticosteroid, antibiotic, or cytotoxic therapy. The organisms that cause **mucormycosis** (an infection caused by mucorales) have a marked propensity for vascular invasion and rapidly produce thrombosis and necrosis of tissue. One of the most common presentations is the rhinocerebral form, in which the nasal mucosa, palate, sinuses, orbit, face, and brain are involved; each shows massive necrosis with vascular invasion and infarction. Perineural invasion also occurs in mucormycoses and is a potential means of retro-orbital spread (i.e., invasion into the brain). Other types of infection involve the lungs and gastrointestinal tract; some patients develop disseminated infection. The

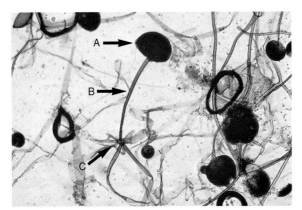

**Figure 60-1** *Rhizopus* spp. showing sporangium *(A)* on long sporangiophore *(B)* arising from pauciseptate hyphae. Note the characteristic rhizoids *(C)* at the base of the sporangiophore (×250).

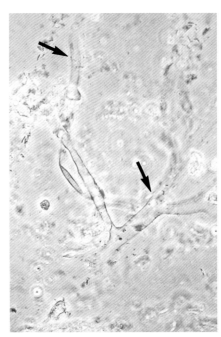

**Figure 60-2** Phase-contrast microscopy of a potassium hydroxide preparation of sputum. Note the fragmented portions *(arrows)* of broad, predominantly nonseptate hyphae of *Rhizopus* spp.

mucorales have also caused skin infections in patients with severe burns and infections of subcutaneous tissue in patients who have undergone surgery.

## LABORATORY DIAGNOSIS

### Specimen Collection and Transport

See General Considerations for the Laboratory Diagnosis of Fungal Infections in Chapter 59.

### Specimen Processing

See General Considerations for the Laboratory Diagnosis of Fungal Infections in Chapter 59.

### Direct Detection Methods

**Stains.** A mucormycosis may be diagnosed rapidly by examining tissue specimens or exudate from infected lesions in a calcofluor white or potassium hydroxide preparation. Branching, broad-diameter, predominantly nonseptate hyphae are observed (Figure 60-2). It is important that the laboratory notify the clinician of these findings, because mucorales grow rapidly, and vascular invasion occurs at a rapid rate.

**Antigen-Protein.** Antigen-protein–based assays are not used for the diagnosis of mucormycosis.

**Nucleic Acid Amplification.** Nucleic acid testing is not routinely used for the diagnosis of mucormycosis. These assays may be available in research settings.

**Cultivation.** The colonial morphologic features of the mucorales allow immediate suspicion that an organism belongs to this group. Colonies characteristically produce a fluffy, white to gray or brown hyphal growth that resembles cotton candy and that diffusely covers the surface of the agar within 24 to 96 hours (Figure 60-3). The hyphae can grow very fast and may lift the lid of the agar plate (also known as a "lid lifter"). The hyphae appear to be coarse. The entire culture dish or tube rapidly fills with loose, grayish hyphae dotted with brown or black sporangia. The different genera and species of mucorales cannot be differentiated by colonial morphologic features, because most are identical.

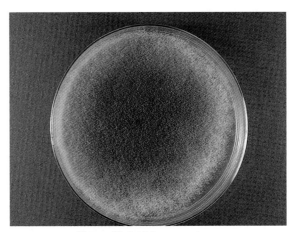

**Figure 60-3** *Rhizopus* colony.

### Approach to Identification

*Rhizopus* spp. have unbranched sporangiophores with rhizoids that appear opposite the point where the stolon arises, at the base of the sporangiophore (see Figure 60-1). In contrast, *Mucor* spp. are characterized by sporangiophores that are singularly produced or branched and have a round sporangium at the tip filled with sporangiospores. They do not have rhizoids or stolons, which distinguishes this genus from the other genera of the mucorales (Figure 60-4). *Lichtheimia* spp. and *Absidia* spp. are characterized by the presence of rhizoids that originate between sporangiophores (Figure 60-5). The sporangia of *Lichtheimia* spp. are pyriform and have a funnel-shaped area (**apophysis**) at the junction of the sporangium and the sporangiophore. Usually a septum is formed in the sporangiophore just below the

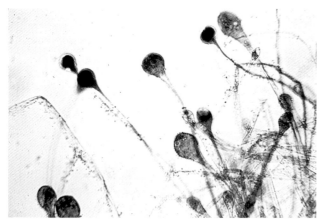

**Figure 60-4** *Mucor* spp. showing numerous sporangia without rhizoids (×430).

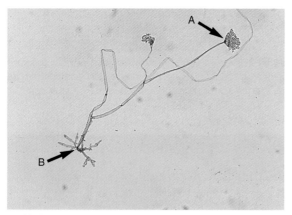

**Figure 60-5** *Lichtheimia* spp. *(A)* showing sporangia on long sporangiophores arising from pauciseptate hyphae *(B)*. Note that rhizoids are produced between sporangiophores and not at their bases (×250).

sporangium. Other genera of Glomeromycota that are encountered much less frequently in the clinical laboratory are *Rhizomucor, Saksenaea, Cunninghamella, Apophysomyces, Conidiobolus,* and *Basidiobolus* spp.

### Serodiagnosis

Serology is not useful for diagnosing zygomycosis.

## ▋ THE DERMATOPHYTES

### GENERAL CHARACTERISTICS

The dermatophytes produce infections involving the superficial areas of the body, including the hair, skin, and nails **(dermatomycoses).** The genera *Trichophyton, Microsporum,* and *Epidermophyton* are the principal etiologic agents of the dermatomycoses.

### EPIDEMIOLOGY AND PATHOGENESIS

The dermatophytes break down and utilize keratin as a source of nitrogen. They usually are incapable of penetrating the subcutaneous tissue, unless the host is immunocompromised, and even then penetration into the subcutis is rare. Species of the genus *Trichophyton* are capable of invading the hair, skin, and nails; *Microsporum* spp. involve only the hair and skin; and *Epidermophyton* sp. involves the skin and nails. Common species of dermatophytes recovered from clinical specimens, in order of frequency, are *Trichophyton rubrum, Trichophyton mentagrophytes, Epidermophyton floccosum, Trichophyton tonsurans, Microsporum canis,* and *Trichophyton verrucosum.* The frequency of recovery of these species may differ by geographic locale. Other geographically limited species are described elsewhere.

### SPECTRUM OF DISEASE

Cutaneous mycoses are perhaps the most common fungal infections of humans. They are usually referred to as **tinea** (Latin for "worm" or "ringworm"). The gross appearance of the lesion is an outer ring of the active, progressing infection, with central healing within the ring. These infections may be characterized by another Latin noun to designate the area of the body involved; for example, tinea corporis (ringworm of the body); tinea cruris (ringworm of the groin, or "jock itch"); tinea capitis (ringworm of the scalp and hair); tinea barbae (ringworm of the beard); tinea unguium (ringworm of the nail); and tinea pedis (ringworm of the feet, or "athlete's foot").

#### *Trichophyton* spp.

Members of the genus *Trichophyton* are widely distributed and are the most important and common causes of infections of the feet and nails; they may be responsible for tinea corporis, tinea capitis, tinea unguium, and tinea barbae. They are commonly seen in adult infections, which vary in their clinical manifestations. Most cosmopolitan species are **anthropophilic,** or "human loving"; few are **zoophilic,** primarily infecting animals.

Generally, hairs infected with *Trichophyton* organisms do not fluoresce under the ultraviolet (UV) light of a Wood's lamp. Fungal elements must be demonstrated inside, surrounding, and penetrating the hair shaft or within a skin scraping to diagnose a dermatophyte infection by direct examination. Confirmation requires recovery and identification of the causative organism.

### LABORATORY DIAGNOSIS

#### Specimen Collection and Transport

See General Considerations for the Laboratory Diagnosis of Fungal Infections in Chapter 59.

#### Specimen Processing

See General Considerations for the Laboratory Diagnosis of Fungal Infections in Chapter 59.

#### Direct Detection Methods

**Stains.** Calcofluor white or potassium hydroxide preparations reveal the presence of hyaline septate hyphae and/or arthroconidia (see Figures 59-4 and 60-6). Direct

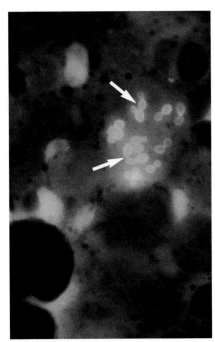

**Figure 60-6** Calcofluor white stain of sputum showing intracellular yeast cells of *H. capsulatum (arrows)*. The cells are 2 to 5 $\mu$m in diameter.

microscopic examination of infected hairs may reveal the hair shaft to be filled with masses of large arthroconidia (4 to 7 $\mu$m) in chains, characteristic of an **endothrix** type of invasion. In other instances, the hair shows external masses of spores that ensheath the hair shaft; this is characteristic of the **ectothrix** type of hair invasion. Hairs infected with *Trichophyton schoenleinii* reveal hyphae and air spaces within the shaft.

**Antigen-Protein.** Antigen-protein—based assays are not useful for the detection or identification of dermatophytes.

**Nucleic Acid Amplification.** Nucleic acid amplification assays for dermatophytes are not routine; these are available in research settings.

**Cultivation.** Because the dermatophytes generally present a similar microscopic appearance in infected hair, skin, or nails, final identification typically is made by culture. A summary of the colonial and microscopic morphologic features of these fungi is presented in Table 60-1. Figure 60-7 presents an identification schema useful to the clinical laboratory for identification of commonly encountered dermatophytes. The schema begins with the microscopic features of the dermatophytes that may be visible in the initial examination of the culture. In many instances, the primary recovery medium fails to function as well as a sporulation medium. Often the initial growth must be subcultured onto cornmeal agar or potato dextrose agar to induce sporulation.

### Approach to Identification

***Trichophyton* spp.** Microscopically, *Trichophyton* organisms are characterized by smooth, club-shaped, thin-walled macroconidia with three to eight septa ranging from 4 ×

8 $\mu$m to 8 × 15 $\mu$m. The macroconidia are borne singly at the terminal ends of hyphae or on short conidiophores; the microconidia (which may be described as "birds on a fence") predominate and are usually spherical, **pyriform** (teardrop shaped), or **clavate** (club shaped), and 2 to 4 $\mu$m (Figure 60-8). Only the common *Trichophyton* species are described here.

*T. rubrum* and *T. mentagrophytes* are the most common species recovered in the clinical laboratory. *T. rubrum* is a slow-growing organism that produces a flat or heaped-up colony, generally white to reddish, with a cottony or velvety surface. The characteristic cherry-red color is best observed on the reverse side of the colony; however, this is produced only after 3 to 4 weeks of incubation. Occasional strains may lack the deep red pigmentation on primary isolation. Two types of colonies may be produced: fluffy and granular. Microconidia are uncommon in most of the fluffy strains and more common in the granular strains; they occur as small, teardrop-shaped conidia often borne laterally along the sides of the hyphae (see Figure 60-8). Macroconidia are seen less commonly, although they are sometimes found in the granular strains, where they appear as thin-walled, smooth-walled, multicelled, cigar-shaped conidia with three to eight septa. *T. rubrum* has no specific nutritional requirements. It does not perforate hair in vitro or produce urease.

*T. mentagrophytes* produces two distinct colonial forms: the downy variety recovered from patients with tinea pedis and the granular variety recovered from lesions acquired by contact with animals. The rapidly growing colonies may appear as white to cream-colored or yellow, cottony or downy, and coarsely granular to powdery. They may produce a few spherical microconidia. The granular colonies may show evidence of red pigmentation. The reverse side of the colony is usually rose-brown, occasionally orange to deep red, and may be confused with *T. rubrum*. Granular colonies sporulate freely, with numerous small, spherical microconidia in grapelike clusters and thin-walled, smooth-walled, cigar-shaped macroconidia measuring 6 × 20 $\mu$m to 8 × 50 $\mu$m, with two to five septa (Figure 60-9). Macroconidia characteristically exhibit a definite narrow attachment to their base. Spiral hyphae may be found in one third of the isolates recovered.

*T. mentagrophytes* produces urease within 2 to 3 days after inoculation onto Christensen's urea agar. Unlike *T. rubrum*, *T. mentagrophytes* perforates hair (Figure 60-10), a feature that may be used to distinguish between the two species when differentiation is difficult.

*T. tonsurans* is responsible for an epidemic form of tinea capitis that commonly occurs in children and occasionally in adults. It has displaced *Microsporum audouinii* as a primary cause of tinea capitis in most of the United States. The fungus causes a low-grade superficial lesion of varying severity and produces circular, scaly patches of alopecia (loss of hair). The stubs of hair remain in the epidermis of the scalp after the brittle hairs have broken off, which may give the typical "black dot" ringworm appearance. Because the infected hairs do not fluoresce under a Wood's lamp, the physician should carefully search for the embedded stubs, using a bright light.

**TABLE 60-1** Characteristics of Dermatophytes Commonly Recovered in the Clinical Laboratory

| Dermatophyte | Colonial Morphology | Growth Rate | Microscopic Identification |
|---|---|---|---|
| *Microsporum audouinii** | Downy white to salmon-pink colony; reverse tan to salmon-pink | 2 weeks | Sterile hyphae; terminal chlamydoconidia, favic chandeliers, and pectinate bodies; macroconidia rarely seen (bizarre shaped if seen); microconidia rare or absent |
| *Microsporum canis* | Colony usually membranous with feathery periphery; center of colony white to buff over orange-yellow; lemon-yellow or yellow-orange apron and reverse | 1 week | Thick-walled, spindle-shaped, multiseptate, rough-walled macroconidia, some with a curved tip; microconidia rarely seen |
| *Microsporum gypseum* | Cinnamon-colored, powdery colony; reverse light tan | 1 week | Thick-walled, rough, elliptical, multiseptate macroconidia; microconidia few or absent |
| *Epidermophyton floccosum* | Center of colony tends to be folded and is khaki green; periphery is yellow; reverse yellowish brown with observable folds | 1 week | Macroconidia: large, smooth walled, multiseptate, clavate, and borne singly or in clusters of two or three; microconidia not formed by this species |
| *Trichophyton mentagrophytes* | Different colonial types; white, granular, and fluffy varieties; occasional light yellow periphery in younger cultures; reverse buff to reddish brown | 7-10 days | Many round to globose microconidia, most commonly borne in grapelike clusters or laterally along the hyphae; spiral hyphae in 30% of isolates; macroconidia are thin walled, smooth, club shaped, and multiseptate; numerous or rare, depending upon strain |
| *Trichophyton rubrum* | Colonial types vary from white downy to pink granular; rugal folds are common; reverse yellow when colony is young, but wine/red color commonly develops with age | 2 weeks | Microconidia usually teardrop-shaped, most commonly borne along sides of the hyphae; macroconidia usually absent but when present are smooth, thin walled, and pencil shaped |
| *Trichophyton tonsurans* | White, tan to yellow or rust, suedelike to powdery; wrinkled with heaped or sunken center; reverse yellow to tan to rust red | 7-14 days | Microconidia are teardrop or club shaped with flat bottoms; vary in size but usually larger than other dermatophytes; macroconidia rare (balloon forms found when present) |
| *Trichophyton schoenleinii** | Irregularly heaped, smooth, white to cream colony with radiating grooves; reverse white | 2-3 weeks | Hyphae usually sterile; many antler-type hyphae seen (favic chandeliers) |
| *Trichophyton violaceum** | Port wine to deep violet colony, may be heaped or flat with waxy-glabrous surface; pigment may be lost on subculture | 2-3 weeks | Branched, tortuous. sterile hyphae; chlamydoconidia commonly aligned in chains |
| *Trichophyton verrucosum* | Glabrous to velvety white colonies; rare strains produce yellow-brown color; rugal folds with tendency to skin into agar surface | 2-3 weeks | Microconidia rare, large and teardrop-shaped when seen; macroconidia extremely rare but form characteristic rat-tail types when seen; many chlamydoconidia seen in chains, particularly when colony is incubated at 37°C |

*These organisms are not commonly seen in the United States.

Cultures of *T. tonsurans* develop slowly and are typically buff to brown, wrinkled and suedelike in appearance. The colony surface shows radial folds and often develops a craterlike depression in the center with deep fissures. The reverse side of the colony is yellowish to reddish brown. Microscopically, numerous microconidia with flat bases are produced on the sides of hyphae. With age, the microconidia tend to become pleomorphic, are swollen to elongated, and are referred to as balloon forms (Figure 60-11). Chlamydoconidia are abundant in old cultures; swollen and fragmented hyphal cells resembling arthroconidia may be seen. *T. tonsurans* grows poorly on media lacking enrichments (casein agar); however, growth is greatly enhanced by the presence of thiamine or inositol in casein agar.

*T. verrucosum* causes a variety of lesions in cattle and in humans; it is most often seen in farmers, who acquire the infection from cattle. The lesions are found chiefly on the beard, neck, wrist, and back of the hands; they are deep, pustular, and inflammatory. With pressure,

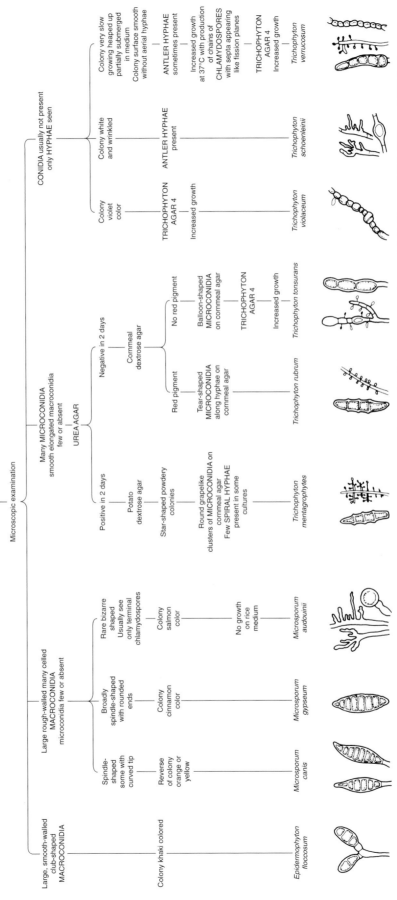

**Figure 60-7** Dermatophyte identification schema. (From Koneman EW, Roberts GD: *Practical laboratory mycology*, ed 3, Baltimore, 1985, Williams & Wilkins.)

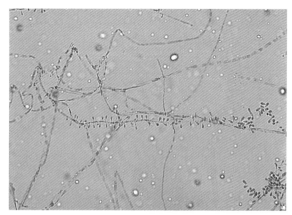

**Figure 60-8** *Trichophyton rubrum* showing numerous pyriform microconidia borne singly on hyphae (×750).

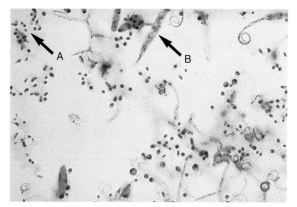

**Figure 60-9** *A, Trichophyton mentagrophytes* showing numerous microconidia in grapelike clusters. *B,* Several thin-walled macroconidia also are present (×500).

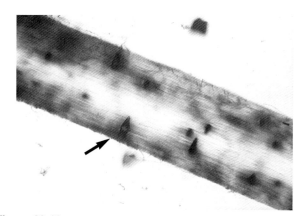

**Figure 60-10** Hair perforation by *Trichophyton mentagrophytes.* Wedge-shaped areas *(arrow)* illustrate hair perforation (×100).

short stubs of hair may be recovered from the purulent lesion. Direct examination of the hair shaft reveals sheaths of isolated chains of large spores (5 to 10 μm in diameter) surrounding the hair shaft (ectothrix), and hyphae within the hair (endothrix). Masses of these conidia may also be seen in exudate from the lesions.

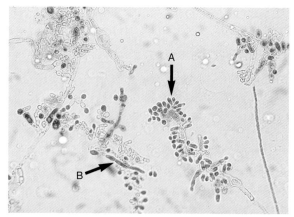

**Figure 60-11** *Trichophyton tonsurans* showing numerous microconidia *(A)* that are borne singly or in clusters. A single macroconidium *(B)* (rare) is also present (×600).

*T. verrucosum* grows slowly (14 to 30 days); growth is enhanced at 35° to 37°C and on media enriched with thiamine and inositol. *T. verrucosum* may be suspected when slowly growing colonies appear to embed themselves into the agar surface.

Kane and Smitka described a medium for the early detection and identification of *T. verrucosum*. The ingredients for this medium are 4% casein and 0.5% yeast extract. The organism is recognized by its early hydrolysis of casein and very slow growth rate. Chains of chlamydoconidia are formed regularly at 37°C. Early detection of hydrolysis, the formation of characteristic chains of chlamydoconidia, and the restrictive slow growth rate of *T. verrucosum* differentiate it from *T. schoenleinii*, another slowly growing organism. Colonies are small, heaped, and folded, occasionally flat and disk shaped. At first they are glabrous and waxy, with a short aerial mycelium. Colonies range from gray and waxlike to bright yellow. The reverse of the colony most often is nonpigmented but may be yellow.

Microscopically, chlamydoconidia in chains and antler hyphae may be the only structures observed microscopically in cultures of *T. verrucosum* (see Figures 59-10 and 59-16). Chlamydoconidia may be abundant at 35° to 37°C. Microconidia may be produced by some cultures if the medium is enriched with yeast extract or a vitamin (Figure 60-12). Conidia, when present, are borne laterally from the hyphae and are large and clavate. Macroconidia are rarely formed, vary considerably in size and shape, and are referred to as "rat tail" or "string bean" in appearance.

*T. schoenleinii* causes a severe type of infection called **favus.** It is characterized by the formation of yellowish cup-shaped crusts, or scutulae, on the scalp, considerable scarring of the scalp, and sometimes permanent alopecia. Infections are common among members of the same family. A distinctive invasion of the infected hair, the favic type, is demonstrated by the presence of large, inverted cones of hyphae and arthroconidia at the base of the hair follicle and branching hyphae throughout the length of the hair shaft. Longitudinal tunnels or empty spaces appear in the hair shaft where the

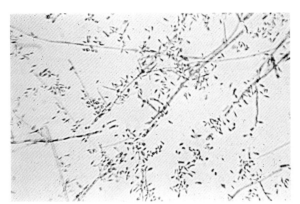

**Figure 60-12** *Trichophyton verrucosum* showing microconidia, which are rarely seen (×500).

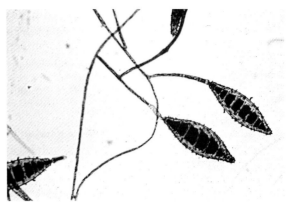

**Figure 60-14** Large, rough-walled macroconidia of *Microsporum canis* (×430).

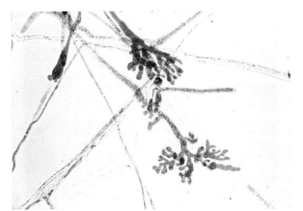

**Figure 60-13** *Trichophyton schoenleinii* showing swollen hyphal tips with lateral and terminal branching (favic chandeliers). Microconidia and macroconidia are absent (×500).

hyphae have disintegrated. In calcofluor white or potassium hydroxide preparations, these tunnels are readily filled with fluid; air bubbles may also be seen in these tunnels.

*T. schoenleinii* is a slowly growing organism (30 days or longer) that produces a white to light gray colony with a waxy surface. Colonies have an irregular border consisting mostly of submerged hyphae, which tend to crack the agar. The surface of the colony is usually nonpigmented or tan, furrowed, and irregularly folded. The reverse side of the colony is usually tan or nonpigmented. Microscopically, conidia commonly are not formed. The hyphae tend to become knobby and club shaped at the terminal ends, with the production of many short lateral and terminal branches (Figure 60-13). Chlamydoconidia are generally numerous. All strains of *T. schoenleinii* may be grown in a vitamin-free medium and grow equally well at room temperature or at 35° to 37°C.

*Trichophyton violaceum* causes an infection of the scalp and body and is seen primarily in people living in the Mediterranean region, the Middle and Far East, and Africa. Hair invasion is of the endothrix type; the typical "black dot" type of tinea capitis is observed clinically. Direct microscopic examination of a calcofluor white or potassium hydroxide preparation of the nonfluorescing hairs shows dark, thick hairs filled with masses of

arthroconidia arranged in chains, similar to those seen in *T. tonsurans* infections.

Colonies of *T. violaceum* are very slow growing, beginning as cone-shaped, cream-colored, glabrous colonies. Later these become heaped up, verrucous (warty), violet to purple, and waxy in consistency. Colonies may often be described as "port wine" in color. The reverse side of the colony is purple or nonpigmented. Older cultures may develop a velvety area of mycelium and sometimes lose their pigmentation. Microscopically, microconidia and macroconidia generally are not present; only sterile, distorted hyphae and chlamydoconidia are found. In some instances, however, swollen hyphae containing cytoplasmic granules may be seen. Growth of *T. violaceum* is enhanced on media containing thiamine.

***Microsporum* spp.** Species of the genus *Microsporum* are immediately recognized by the presence of large (8-15 × 35-150 μm), spindle-shaped, echinulate, rough-walled macroconidia with thick walls (up to 4 μm) containing four or more septa (Figure 60-14). The exception is *Microsporum nanum*, which characteristically produces macroconidia having two cells. Microconidia, when present, are small (3 to 7 μm) and club shaped and are borne on the hyphae, either laterally or on short conidiophores. Cultures of *Microsporum* spp. develop either rapidly or slowly (5 to 14 days) and produce aerial hyphae that may be velvety, powdery, glabrous, or cottony, varying in color from whitish, buff, to a cinnamon brown, with varying shades on the reverse side of the colony.

In past years, *M. audouinii* was the most important cause of epidemic tinea capitis among schoolchildren in the United States. This organism is anthropophilic and is spread directly by means of infected hairs on hats, caps, upholstery, combs, or barber clippers. Most infections are chronic; some heal spontaneously, whereas others may persist for several years. Infected hair shafts fluoresce yellow-green under a Wood's lamp. Colonies of *M. audouinii* generally grow more slowly than other members of the genus *Microsporum* (10 to 21 days), and they produce a velvety aerial mycelium that is colorless to light gray to tan. The reverse side often appears salmon-pink to reddish brown. Colonies of *M. audouinii* do not usually sporulate in culture. The addition of yeast extract may stimulate growth and the production of macroconidia in some instances. Most commonly, atypical vegetative forms, such as terminal chlamydoconidia and antler and racquet hyphae, are the only clues to the identification of this organism. *M. audouinii* often is identified as a cause of infection by exclusion of all the other dermatophytes.

*M. canis* is primarily a pathogen of animals (zoophilic); it is the most common cause of ringworm infection in dogs and cats in the United States. Children and adults acquire the disease through contact with infected animals, particularly puppies and kittens, although human-to-human transfer has been reported. Hairs infected with *M. canis* fluoresce a bright yellow-green under a Wood's lamp, which is a useful tool for screening pets as possible sources of human infection. Direct examination of a calcofluor white or potassium hydroxide preparation of infected hairs reveals small spores (2 to 3 μm) outside the hair. Culture must be performed to provide the specific identification.

Colonies of *M. canis* grow rapidly, are granular or fluffy with a feathery border, white to buff, and characteristically have a lemon-yellow or yellow-orange fringe at the periphery. On aging, the colony becomes dense and cottony and a deeper brownish-yellow or orange and frequently shows an area of heavy growth in the center. The reverse side of the colony is bright yellow, becoming orange or reddish-brown with age. In rare cases, strains are recovered that show no reverse side pigment. Microscopically, *M. canis* shows an abundance of large (15-20 × 60-125 μm), spindle-shaped, multisegmented (four to eight) macroconidia with curved ends (see Figure 60-14). These are thick walled with spiny (**echinulate**) projections on their surfaces. Microconidia are usually few in number, but large numbers occasionally may be seen.

*Microsporum gypseum*, a free-living organism of the soil (**geophilic**) that only rarely causes human or animal infection, occasionally may be seen in the clinical laboratory. Infected hairs generally do not fluoresce under a Wood's lamp. However, microscopic examination of the infected hairs shows them to be irregularly covered with clusters of spores (5 to 8 μm), some in chains. These arthroconidia of the ectothrix type are considerably larger than those of other *Microsporum* species.

*M. gypseum* grows rapidly as a flat, irregularly fringed colony with a coarse, powdery surface that appears to be buff or cinnamon color. The underside of the colony is conspicuously orange to brownish. Microscopically, macroconidia are seen in large numbers and are characteristically large, ellipsoidal, have rounded ends, and are multisegmented (three to nine) with echinulated surfaces (Figure 60-15). Although they are spindle shaped, these macroconidia are not as pointed at the distal ends as those of *M. canis*. The appearance of the colonial and microscopic morphologic features is sufficient to make the distinction between *M. gypseum* and *M. canis*.

**Epidermophyton sp.** *E. floccosum*, the only member of the genus *Epidermophyton*, is a common cause of tinea cruris and tinea pedis. Because this organism is susceptible to cold, specimens submitted for dermatophyte culture should not be refrigerated before culture, and cultures should not be stored at 4°C. In direct examination of skin scrapings using the calcofluor white or potassium hydroxide preparation, the fungus is seen as fine branching

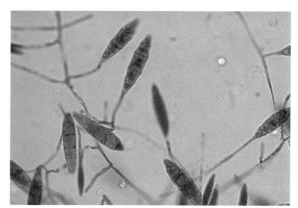

**Figure 60-15** *Microsporum gypseum* showing ellipsoidal, multi-celled macroconidia (×750).

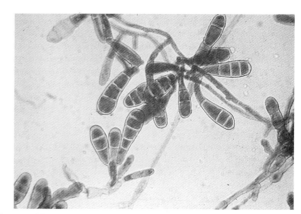

**Figure 60-16** *Epidermophyton floccosum* showing numerous smooth, multiseptate, thin-walled macroconidia that appear club shaped (×1000).

hyphae. *E. floccosum* grows slowly; the growth appears olive green to khaki, with the periphery surrounded by a dull orange-brown. After several weeks, colonies develop a cottony white aerial mycelium that completely overgrows the colony; the mycelium is sterile and remains so even after subculture. Microscopically, numerous smooth, thin-walled, club-shaped, multiseptate (2 to 4 μm) macroconidia are seen (Figure 60-16). They are rounded at the tip and are borne singly on a conidiophore or in groups of two or three. Microconidia are absent, spiral hyphae are rare, and chlamydoconidia are usually numerous. The absence of microconidia is useful for differentiating this organism from *Trichophyton* spp.; the morphology of the macroconidia (smooth, thin walled) is useful for differentiating it from *Microsporum* spp.

### Serodiagnosis

Serology is not useful for the diagnosis of disease caused by dermatophytes.

## THE OPPORTUNISTIC MYCOSES

### GENERAL CHARACTERISTICS

The tissue-invasive opportunistic mycoses are a group of fungal infections that occur almost exclusively in immunocompromised patients. Opportunistic fungal infections are typically identified in a host compromised by some underlying disease process, such as lymphoma, leukemia, diabetes mellitus, or another defect of the immune system. Many patients, particularly those who undergo some type of transplantation, are often placed on treatment with corticosteroids, cytotoxic drugs, or other immunosuppressive agents to control rejection of the transplanted organ. Many fungi previously thought to be nonpathogenic are now recognized as etiologic agents of opportunistic fungal infections. Because most of the organisms known to cause infection in this group of patients are commonly encountered in the clinical laboratory as **saprobes** (saprophytic fungi), it may be impossible for the laboratorian to determine the clinical significance of these isolates recovered from clinical specimens. Therefore, laboratories must identify and report completely the presence of all fungi recovered, because each is a potential pathogen. Many of the organisms associated with opportunistic infections are acquired during construction, demolition, or remodeling of buildings or are hospital acquired. Other information about the specific clinical aspects of the opportunistic fungal infections is discussed with the individual organism.

## EPIDEMIOLOGY AND PATHOGENESIS

### Aspergillus spp.

Several *Aspergillus* spp. are among the most frequently encountered fungi in the clinical laboratory (Table 60-2); any is potentially pathogenic in the immunocompromised host, but some species are more frequently associated with disease than others. The aspergilli are widespread in the environment, where they colonize grain, leaves, soil, and living plants. Conidia of the aspergilli are easily dispersed into the environment, and humans become infected by inhaling them. Assessing the significance of *Aspergillus* organisms in a clinical specimen may be difficult. They are found frequently in cultures of respiratory secretions, skin scrapings, and other specimens.

## PATHOGENESIS AND SPECTRUM OF DISEASE

### Aspergillus spp.

*Aspergillus* spp. are capable of causing disseminated infection, as is seen in immunocompromised patients, but also of causing a wide variety of other types of infections, including a pulmonary or sinus fungus ball, allergic bronchopulmonary aspergillosis, external **otomycosis** (a fungus ball of the external auditory canal), mycotic keratitis, **onychomycosis** (infection of the nail and surrounding tissue), sinusitis, endocarditis, and central nervous system (CNS) infection. Most often, immunocompromised patients acquire a primary pulmonary infection that becomes rapidly progressive and may disseminate to virtually any organ.

### Fusarium spp. and Other Hyaline Septate Opportunistic Molds

Infection caused by *Fusarium* spp. and other hyaline septate monomorphic molds is becoming more common, particularly in immunocompromised patients. These organisms are common environmental flora and have long been known to cause mycotic keratitis after traumatic implantation into the cornea. Disseminated fusariosis is commonly accompanied by fungemia, which is detected by routine blood culture systems. In contrast, the aspergilli are rarely recovered from blood culture, even in cases of endovascular infection. Necrotic skin lesions are common with disseminated fusariosis. Other types of infection caused by *Fusarium* spp. include sinusitis, wound (burn) infection, allergic fungal sinusitis, and endophthalmitis.

*Fusarium* spp. are commonly recovered from respiratory tract secretions, skin, and other specimens from patients who show no evidence of infection. Interpretation of culture results rests with the clinician and is often assisted by correlation with histopathology results. *Geotrichum candidum* is an uncommon cause of infection but has been shown to cause wound infections and oral thrush; it is an opportunistic pathogen in the immunocompromised host. *Acremonium* spp. are also recognized

**TABLE 60-2** Species of *Aspergillus* Recovered from Clinical Specimens During a 10-Year Period at the Mayo Clinic

| Organisms | CLINICAL SPECIMEN SOURCE | | | | |
|---|---|---|---|---|---|
| | Respiratory Secretions | Gastrointestinal | Genitourinary | Skin, Subcutaneous Tissue | Blood, Bone, CNS, Other |
| A. clavatus | *97/93* | 1/1 | – | 1/1 | – |
| A. flavus | 1298/740 | 10/10 | 11/11 | 177/131 | 2/2 |
| A. fumigatus | 3247/2656 | 11/9 | 14/14 | 175/137 | 8/8 |
| A. glaucus | 503/307 | 1/1 | – | 8/8 | 1/1 |
| A. nidulans | 52/48 | – | – | 5/3 | – |
| A. niger | 1484/1376 | 18/18 | 17/17 | 151/124 | 11/11 |
| A. terreus | 164/146 | – | – | 23/21 | 3/3 |
| A. versicolor | 1237/1202 | 6/6 | 24/22 | 226/224 | 16/16 |
| Other Aspergillus species | 3463/3418 | 18/14 | 32/32 | 319/314 | 16/16 |

*CNS,* Central nervous system.
*Numerator, Number of cultures; denominator, number of patients.

as important pathogens in immunocompromised hosts; these have been associated with disseminated infection, fungemia, subcutaneous lesions, and esophagitis. *Penicillium* spp. are among the most common organisms recovered by the clinical laboratory. In North America they are rarely associated with invasive fungal disease. However, they may be a cause of allergic bronchopulmonary penicilliosis or chronic allergic sinusitis. One species, *P. marneffei*, is an important and emerging pathogen in Southeast Asia and is discussed further in the section on dimorphic pathogens. Of the *Paecilomyces* species, *P. lilacinus* appears to be the most pathogenic species and has been associated with endophthalmitis, cutaneous infections, and arthritis. *P. variotii* has also been shown to be an important pathogen, causing endocarditis, fungemia, and invasive disease.

A variety of other saprobic fungi that are not discussed here may be encountered in the clinical laboratory but are seen less commonly. Other references are recommended for further information about identification of these organisms.

## LABORATORY DIAGNOSIS

### Specimen Collection and Transport

See General Considerations for the Laboratory Diagnosis of Fungal Infections in Chapter 59.

### Specimen Processing

See General Considerations for the Laboratory Diagnosis of Fungal Infections in Chapter 59.

### Direct Detection Methods

**Stains.** Specimens submitted for direct microscopic examination containing organisms in this group demonstrate septate hyphae that usually show evidence of dichotomous branching, often of 45 degrees (Figure 60-17). In addition, some hyphae may have rounded, thick-walled cells. Although often considered to represent an *Aspergillus* species, these cannot be reliably distinguished from hyphae of *Fusarium* spp., *Pseudallescheria boydii*, or other hyaline molds.

**Antigen-Protein.** Antigen-protein–based assays are beginning to be used to monitor patients at high risk for developing invasive fungal infections. One of these assays, the galactomannan assay, specifically targets antigens of *Aspergillus* spp., the most common source of invasive fungal infections caused by the hyaline septate molds (i.e., hyalohyphomycosis). The beta-glucan assay is designed to detect antigens common to all clinically important fungi. The ways these tests will be used in the future and how they will compare with nucleic acid amplification tests remain to be determined.

**Nucleic Acid Amplification.** Nucleic acid amplification assays are not commonly performed to detect or identify these fungi. However, a variety of both broad-range assays (those that detect all fungi) and species-specific assays have been developed and in specialized centers may be used for patient care.

**MALDI-TOF (Matrix-Assisted Laser Desorption Ionization).** MALDI-TOF is a biophysical method that significantly reduces the time required to specifically identify

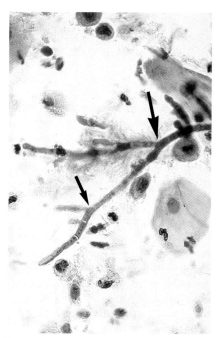

**Figure 60-17** Papanicolaou staining of sputum shows the dichotomously branching septate hyphae *(arrows)* of *Aspergillus fumigatus*.

fungal isolates and is being implemented in some large reference laboratories. An overview of the technique is discussed in more detail in Chapter 7.

**Cultivation.** Because aspergilli are recovered frequently, it is imperative that the organism be demonstrated in the direct microscopic examination of fresh clinical specimens and/or that it be recovered repeatedly from patients with a compatible clinical picture to ensure that the organism is clinically significant. Correlation with biopsy results is the best means of establishing the significance of an isolate. Most *Aspergillus* spp. are susceptible to cycloheximide. Therefore, specimens submitted for recovery or subculture of these species should be inoculated onto media that lack this ingredient.

*A. fumigatus* is the most commonly recovered species from immunocompromised patients; moreover, it is the species most often seen in the clinical laboratory. *Aspergillus flavus* sometimes is recovered from immunocompromised patients and represents a frequent isolate in the clinical microbiology laboratory. Recovery of *A. fumigatus* or *A. flavus* from surveillance (nasal) cultures has been correlated with subsequent invasive aspergillosis; however, the absence of a positive nasal culture does not preclude infection. *Aspergillus niger* is commonly seen in the clinical laboratory, but its association with clinical disease is somewhat limited; this organism is a cause of fungus ball and otitis externa. *Aspergillus terreus* is a significant cause of infection in immunocompromised patients, but its frequency of recovery is much lower than that of the previously mentioned species. However, correct identification of *A. terreus* is important, because it is innately resistant to ampicillin B.

### Approach to Identification

***Aspergillus* spp.** *A. fumigatus* is a rapidly growing mold (2 to 6 days) that produces a fluffy to granular, white to

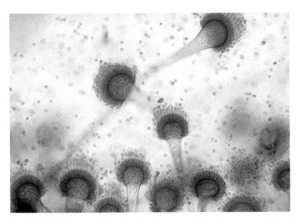

**Figure 60-18** *Aspergillus fumigatus* conidiophore and conidia (×400).

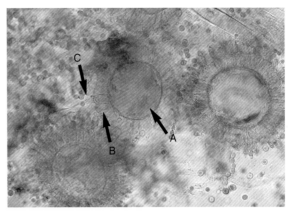

**Figure 60-19** *Aspergillus flavus* showing spherical vesicles *(A)* that give rise to metulae *(B)* and phialides *(C)* that produce chains of conidia (×750).

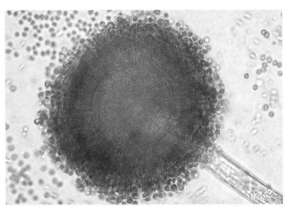

**Figure 60-20** *Aspergillus niger* showing larger spherical vesicle that gives rise to metulae, phialides, and conidia (×750).

blue-green colony. Mature sporulating colonies most often have a blue-green, powdery appearance. Microscopically, *A. fumigatus* is characterized by the presence of septate hyphae and short or long conidiophores with a characteristic "foot cell" at their base. The foot cell is T or L shaped at the base of the conidiophore, but it is not a separate cell. The tip of the conidiophore expands into a large, dome-shaped vesicle with bottle-shaped phialides covering the upper half or two thirds of its surface. Long chains of small (2 to 3 μm in diameter), spherical, rough-walled, green conidia form a columnar mass on the vesicle (Figure 60-18). Cultures of *A. fumigatus* are thermotolerant and able to withstand temperatures up to 45°C.

*A. flavus* is a somewhat more rapidly growing species (1 to 5 days) that produces a yellow-green colony. Microscopically, vesicles are globose, and phialides are produced directly from the vesicle surface (**uniserate**) or from a primary row of cells called metulae (**biserate**). The phialides give rise to short chains of yellow-orange elliptical or spherical conidia that become roughened on the surface with age (Figure 60-19). The conidiophore of *A. flavus* is also coarsely roughened near the vesicle.

*A. niger* produces darkly pigmented, roughened spores macroscopically, but microscopically its hyphae are hyaline and septate, as are those of other aspergilli (i.e., it is not melanized). *A. niger* produces mature colonies within 2 to 6 days. Growth begins initially as a yellow colony that soon develops a black, dotted surface as conidia are produced. With age, the colony becomes jet black and powdery but the reverse remains buff or cream colored; this occurs on any culture medium. Microscopically *A. niger* shows septate hyphae, long conidiophores supporting spherical vesicles giving rise to large metulae, and smaller phialides (biserate), from which long chains of brown to black, rough-walled conidia are produced (Figure 60-20). The entire surface of the vesicle is involved in sporulation.

*A. terreus* is less commonly seen in the clinical laboratory; it produces tan colonies that resemble cinnamon. Vesicles are hemispherical, as seen microscopically, and phialides cover the entire surface and are produced from a primary row of metulae (biserate). Phialides produce globose to elliptical conidia arranged in chains. This species produces larger cells, **aleurioconidia,** which are found on submerged hyphae (Figure 60-21).

***Fusarium* spp.** Colonies of *Fusarium* spp. grow rapidly, within 2 to 5 days, and are fluffy to cottony and may be pink, purple, yellow, green, or other colors, depending on the species. Microscopically the hyphae are small and septate and give rise to phialides producing either single-celled microconidia, usually borne in gelatinous heads similar to those seen in *Acremonium* spp. (see Figure 59-17) or large, multicelled macroconidia that are sickle or boat shaped and contain numerous septations (Figure 60-22). Some cultures of *Fusarium* spp. commonly produce numerous chlamydoconidia. The most common medium used to induce sporulation is cornmeal agar. The keys to identification of *Fusarium* spp. are based on growth on potato dextrose agar.

***Geotrichum candidum.*** *G. candidum* often initially appears as a white to cream-colored, yeastlike colony; some isolates may appear as white, powdery molds. Hyphae are septate and produce numerous rectangular to cylindrical to barrel-shaped arthroconidia (Figure 60-23). Arthroconidia do not alternate but are contiguous, in contrast to *Coccidioides immitis* (Figure 60-24). Blastoconidia are not produced.

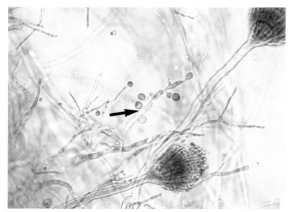

**Figure 60-21** *Aspergillus terreus* showing typical head of *Aspergillus* and aleurioconidia *(arrow)* found on submerged hyphae of this species (×500).

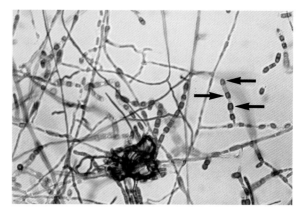

**Figure 60-24** Mycelial form of *Coccidioides immitis* showing numerous thick-walled, rectangular or barrel-shaped *(arrows)* alternate arthroconidia (×500).

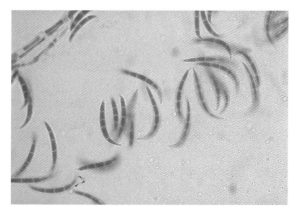

**Figure 60-22** *Fusarium* spp. showing characteristic multicelled, sickle-shaped macroconidia (×500).

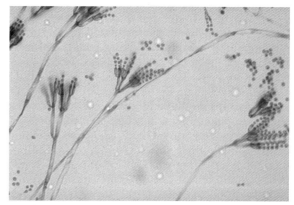

**Figure 60-25** *Penicillium* spp. showing typical brushlike conidiophores (penicilli) (×430).

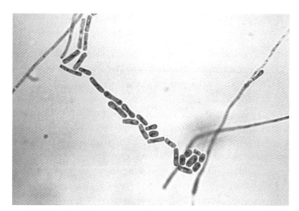

**Figure 60-23** *Geotrichum candidum* showing numerous arthroconidia. Note that arthroconidia do not alternate with a clear (dysjunctor) cell as in the case of *Coccidioides immitis* (×430).

gelatinous cluster at the tip of the phialide (see Figure 59-17).

***Penicillium* spp.** Colonies of *Penicillium* spp. are most commonly shades of green or blue-green, but pink, white, or other colors may be seen. The surface of the colonies may be velvety to powdery because of the presence of conidia. Microscopically hyphae are hyaline and septate and produce brushlike conidiophores (i.e., penicilli). Conidiophores produce metulae from which flask-shaped phialides producing chains of conidia arise (Figure 60-25). *P. marneffei,* a particularly virulent species in this genus, is discussed in the section on hyaline, septate, dimorphic molds.

***Paecilomyces* spp.** Colonies of *Paecilomyces* spp. are often velvety, tan to olive brown, and somewhat powdery. Colonies of *P. lilacinus* exhibit shades of lavender to pink. Microscopically *Paecilomyces* spp. resemble *Penicillium* spp. in that a penicillus is formed. However, the phialides of *Paecilomyces* spp. are long, delicate, and tapering (Figure 60-26), in contrast to the more blunted phialides of *Penicillium* spp.. The penicillus produces numerous chains of small, oval conidia that are easily dislodged. Single phialides producing chains of conidia may also be present.

***Scopulariopsis* spp.** *Scopulariopsis* spp. have been associated with onychomycosis, pulmonary infection, fungus ball and, more recently, invasive fungal disease in the

***Acremonium* spp.** Colonies of *Acremonium* spp. are rapid growing and also may appear yeastlike when initial growth is observed. Mature colonies become white to gray to rose or reddish-orange. Microscopically, small septate hyphae that produce single, unbranched, tubelike phialides are observed. Phialides give rise to clusters of elliptical, single-celled conidia contained in a

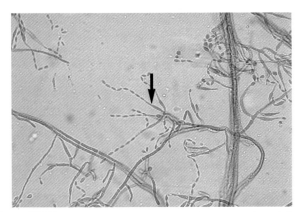

**Figure 60-26** *Paecilomyces* spp. showing long, tapering, delicate phialides *(arrow)*.

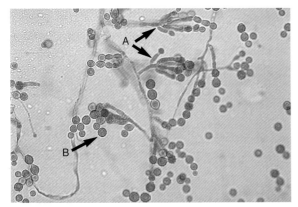

**Figure 60-27** *Scopulariopsis* spp. showing a large penicillus *(A)* with echinulate conidia *(B)* (×430).

immunocompromised host. Colonies of *Scopulariopsis* spp. initially appear white but later become light brown and powdery. Colonies often resemble those of *M. gypseum*. Microscopically a *Scopulariopsis* organism resembles a large *Penicillium* organism at first glance, because a rudimentary penicillus is produced. Annellophores produce the flask-shaped annellides, which support the lemon-shaped conidia in chains. Conidia are large, have a flat base, and are rough walled (Figure 60-27). The hyaline and septate species is *S. brevicaulis. S. brumptii* is a dematiaceous species and is occasionally recovered in the clinical laboratory; it has been reported to have caused a brain abscess in a liver transplant recipient.

### Serodiagnosis

The use of serology for *Aspergillus* spp. is limited to assistance in the diagnosis of bronchopulmonary aspergillosis and fungus ball. Serology currently has no value for the diagnosis of disseminated aspergillosis.

# SYSTEMIC MYCOSES

## GENERAL CHARACTERISTICS

Most of the dimorphic fungi produce systemic fungal infections that may involve any of the internal organs of the body, including lymph nodes, bone, subcutaneous tissue, meninges, and skin. The dimorphic fungal pathogens most commonly encountered in North America are *Histoplasma capsulatum, Blastomyces dermatitidis,* and *Coccidioides immitis.* Asymptomatic or subclinical infection is common with *H. capsulatum* and *C. immitis* and may go unrecognized clinically. These infections may be detectable only by serology or after histopathologic review of tissues removed because of lesions found during a roentgenographic examination.

Symptomatic infections may present signs of a mild or more severe but self-limited disease, with positive supportive evidence from cultural or immunologic findings. Patients with disseminated or progressive infection have severe symptoms, with spread of the initial disease, often from a pulmonary locus, to several distant organs. However, some cases of disseminated infection may show little in the way of signs or symptoms of disease for long periods, only to undergo exacerbation later. Immunocompromised patients most often present with disseminated infection, particularly those with advanced human immunodeficiency virus (HIV) infection (i.e., acquired immunodeficiency syndrome [AIDS]) or those receiving long-term corticosteroid therapy.

The classic term "systemic mycoses," used to refer to the dimorphic fungi, is somewhat misleading, because other fungi, including *Cryptococcus neoformans* complex and *Candida* spp. and *Aspergillus* spp., may also cause disseminated systemic infections.

## EPIDEMIOLOGY

### Blastomyces dermatitidis

*B. dermatitidis* commonly produces a chronic infection that contains a mixture of suppurative and granulomatous inflammation. The disease (**blastomycosis**) is most commonly found in North America and extends southward from Canada to the Mississippi, Ohio, and Missouri river valleys, Mexico, and Central America. Some isolated cases have also been reported from Africa. The largest numbers of cases occur in the Mississippi, Ohio, and Missouri river valley regions. The exact ecologic niche for this organism in nature has not been determined; however, patients with blastomycosis often have a history of exposure to soil or wood. Several outbreaks have been reported and have been related to a common exposure. Blastomycosis is more common in men than in women and seems to be associated with outdoor occupations or activities. The disease also occurs in dogs.

### Coccidioides immitis

*C. immitis* is found primarily in the desert portion of the southwestern United States and in the semiarid regions of Mexico and Central and South America. Although the geographic distribution of the organism is well defined, infection may be seen in any part of the world because of the ease of travel. The infection (**coccidioidomycosis**) is acquired by inhalation of the infective arthroconidia of *C. immitis.*

### Histoplasma capsulatum

Outbreaks of histoplasmosis have been associated with activities that disperse aerosolized conidia or small hyphal fragments. Infection is acquired through inhalation of these infective structures from the environment. The severity of the disease is generally related directly to the inoculum size and the immunologic status of the host. Numerous cases of histoplasmosis have been reported in people who clean out an old chicken coop or barn that has been undisturbed for long periods and in individuals who work in or clean areas that have served as roosting places for starlings and similar birds. Spelunkers (i.e., cave explorers) are commonly exposed to the organism when it is aerosolized from bat guano in caves. An estimated 500,000 people are infected with *H. capsulatum* annually. The history of exposure often is impossible to document, even though histoplasmosis is perhaps one of the most common systemic fungal infections seen in the Midwest and South in the United States, including areas along the Mississippi River, the Ohio River valley, and the Appalachian Mountains.

### Paracoccidioides brasiliensis

Infection caused by *P. brasiliensis* is most commonly found in South America, with the highest prevalences in Brazil, Venezuela, and Colombia. It also has been seen in many other areas, including Mexico, Central America, and Africa. Occasional imported cases are seen in the United States and Europe. The exact mechanism by which paracoccidioidomycosis is acquired is unclear; however, some speculate that it has a pulmonary origin and that it is acquired by inhalation of the organism from the environment. Because mucosal lesions are an integral part of the disease process, it also is speculated that the infection may be acquired through trauma to the oropharynx caused by vegetation commonly chewed by some residents of the endemic areas. The specific ecologic niche of the organism in nature is not known.

### Penicillium marneffei

*P. marneffei* is an emerging dimorphic pathogenic fungus endemic to Southeast Asia, particularly the Guangxi Zhuang Autonomous Region of the People's Republic of China. *P. marneffei* has been associated with the bamboo rat *(Rhizomys pruinosus)* and the Vietnamese bamboo rat *(Rhizomys sinensis)*.

### Sporothrix schenckii

*S. schenckii* has a worldwide distribution, and its natural habitat is living or dead vegetation. Humans acquire the infection (**sporotrichosis**) through trauma (thorns, splinters), usually to the hand, arm, or leg. The infection is an occupational hazard for farmers, nursery workers, gardeners, florists, and miners; it is commonly known as "rose gardener's disease." Pulmonary sporotrichosis rarely occurs as a result of inhalation of spores.

## PATHOGENESIS AND SPECTRUM OF DISEASE

Traditionally, the systemic mycoses have included only blastomycosis, coccidioidomycosis, histoplasmosis, and paracoccidioidomycosis. Of the species that cause these disorders, only *H. capsulatum* and *B. dermatitidis* are genetically related. Although these fungi are

morphologically dissimilar, they have one characteristic in common: dimorphism. Most of these organisms, except for *C. immitis*, are thermally dimorphic. The dimorphic fungi exist in nature as the mold form, which is distinct from the parasitic or invasive form, sometimes called the tissue form. Distinct morphologic differences may be observed with the dimorphic fungi both in vivo and in vitro, as discussed later in the chapter.

### Blastomyces dermatitidis

*B. dermatitidis* commonly produces an acute or chronic suppurative and granulomatous infection. Blastomycosis begins as a respiratory infection and is probably acquired by inhalation of the conidia or hyphal fragments of the organism. The infection may spread and involve secondary sites of infection in the lungs, long bones, soft tissue, and skin.

### Coccidioides immitis

Approximately 60% of patients with coccidioidomycosis are asymptomatic and have self-limited respiratory tract infections. However, the infection may become disseminated, with extension to visceral organs, meninges, bone, skin, lymph nodes, and subcutaneous tissue. Fewer than 1% of those who develop coccidioidomycosis ever become seriously ill; dissemination does occur, however, most frequently in individuals of dark-skinned races. Pregnancy also appears to predispose women to disseminated infection. This infection has been known to occur in epidemic proportions. In 1992, an epidemic occurred in northern California, with more than 4000 cases seen in Kern County near Bakersfield. People who visit endemic areas and return to a distant location may present to their local physician; therefore, the endemic mycoses should be considered in the differential diagnosis if the patient has the appropriate travel history. All laboratories should be prepared to deal with the laboratory diagnosis of coccidioidomycosis.

### Histoplasma capsulatum

*H. capsulatum* most commonly produces a chronic, granulomatous infection (histoplasmosis) that is primary and begins in the lung and eventually invades the reticuloendothelial system. Approximately 95% of cases are asymptomatic and self-limited, although chronic pulmonary infections occur. The disease can be disseminated throughout the reticuloendothelial system; the primary sites of dissemination are the lymph nodes, liver, spleen, and bone marrow. Infections of the kidneys and meninges are also possible. Resolution of disseminated infection is the rule in immunocompetent hosts, but progressive disease is more common in immunocompromised patients (e.g., patients with AIDS). Ulcerative lesions of the upper respiratory tract may occur in both immunocompetent and immunocompromised hosts.

### Paracoccidioides brasiliensis

*P. brasiliensis* produces a chronic granulomatous infection (paracoccidioidomycosis) that begins as a primary pulmonary infection. It often is asymptomatic and then disseminates to produce ulcerative lesions of the mucous membranes. Ulcerative lesions are commonly present in the nasal and oral mucosa, gingivae, and less commonly the conjunctivae. Lesions occur commonly on the face in association with oral mucous membrane infection. The lesions are characteristically ulcerative, with a serpiginous (snakelike) active border and a crusted surface. Lymph node involvement in the cervical area is common. Pulmonary infection is frequently seen, and progressive chronic pulmonary infection is found in approximately 50% of cases. In some patients dissemination occurs to other anatomic sites, including the lymphatic system, spleen, intestines, liver, brain, meninges, and adrenal glands.

### Penicillium marneffei

*P. marneffei* is an emerging pathogen that commonly infects immunosuppressed individuals. The organism causes either a focal cutaneous or mucocutaneous infection, or it may produce a progressive disseminated and frequently fatal infection. Granulomatous, suppurative, and necrotizing inflammatory responses have been demonstrated. The mode of transmission and the primary source in the environment are unknown, but the bamboo rat has been implicated.

### Sporothrix schenckii

*S. schenckii*, also a dimorphic fungus, is often associated with chronic subcutaneous infection. The primary lesion begins as a small, nonhealing ulcer, often of the index finger or the back of the hand. With time, the infection is characterized by the development of nodular lesions of the skin or subcutaneous tissues at the point of contact and later involves the lymphatic channels and lymph nodes that drain the region. The subcutaneous nodules ulcerate to form an infection that becomes chronic. Only rarely is the disease disseminated. Pulmonary infection may be seen in patients that inhale the spores of *S. schenckii*.

## LABORATORY DIAGNOSIS

### Specimen Collection and Transport

See General Considerations for the Laboratory Diagnosis of Fungal Infections in Chapter 59.

### Specimen Processing

See General Considerations for the Laboratory Diagnosis of Fungal Infections in Chapter 59.

### Direct Detection Methods

**Stains.** The microscopic morphologic features of the tissue forms, or what has been termed the parasitic forms, of the dimorphic fungi vary with the genus and are described for each.

**Blastomyces dermatitidis.** The diagnosis of blastomycosis may easily be made when a clinical specimen is observed by direct microscopy. *B. dermatitidis* appears as large, spherical, thick-walled yeast cells 8 to 15 μm in diameter, usually with a single bud that is connected to the parent cell by a broad base (Figures 60-28 to 60-30). A smaller form (2-8 μm) is seen in rare cases.

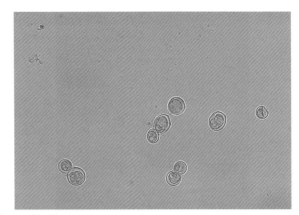

**Figure 60-28** *Blastomyces dermatitidis* yeast form showing thick-walled, oval to round, single-budding, yeastlike cells (×500).

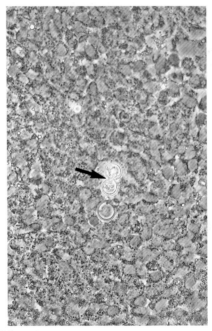

**Figure 60-29** Potassium hydroxide preparation of exudate shows a large budding yeast cell with a distinct broad base *(arrow)* between the cells, which is characteristic of *Blastomyces dermatitidis*. (Phase-contrast microscopy.)

**Coccidioides immitis.** In direct microscopic examinations of sputum or other body fluids, *C. immitis* appears as a nonbudding, thick-walled spherule, 20 to 200 μm in diameter, that contains either granular material or numerous small (2 to 5 μm in diameter), nonbudding endospores (Figures 60-31 to 60-33). The endospores are freed by rupture of the spherule wall; therefore, empty and collapsed "ghost" spherules may also be present. Small, immature spherules measuring 5 to 20 μm may be confused with *H. capsulatum* or *B. dermatitidis*. Two endospores or immature spherules lying adjacent to one another may give the appearance that budding yeast is present. When identification of *C. immitis* is questionable, a wet preparation of the clinical specimen may be made

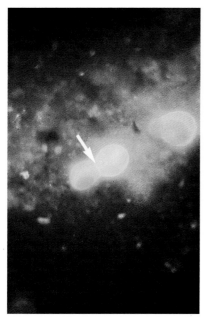

**Figure 60-30** Auramine-rhodamine preparation of specimen material from a bone lesion demonstrates the characteristic broad-based budding yeast *(arrow)* of *Blastomyces dermatitidis.*

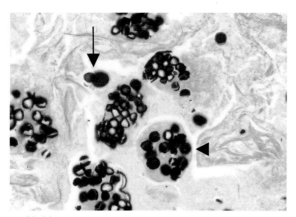

**Figure 60-31** Tissue form of *Coccidioides immitis* (i.e., the spherule). The external wall of the spherule does not stain with the silver stain, whereas the internal endospores do stain *(arrowhead).* Also note how the juxtaposed endospores, which have been released from a spherule that has burst, resemble budding yeast *(arrow).* (GMS stain; ×400).

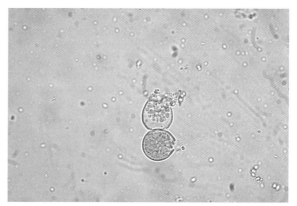

**Figure 60-32** Potassium hydroxide preparation of sputum demonstrates two spherules of *Coccidioides immitis* filled with endospores. When these lie adjacent to each other, they may be mistaken for *Blastomyces dermatitidis.* (Bright-field microscopy.)

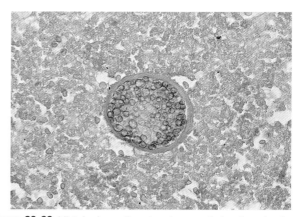

**Figure 60-33** Histologic section showing a well-developed spherule of *Coccidioides immitis* that is filled with endospores.

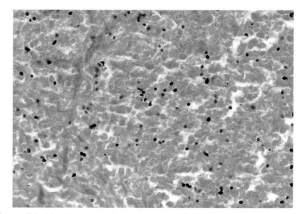

**Figure 60-34** These small, oval yeast cells that are relatively uniform in size are characteristic of *Histoplasma capsulatum* (×2000).

using sterile saline, and the edges of the coverglass may be sealed with petrolatum and incubated overnight. When spherules are present, the endospores produce multiple hyphal strands.

***Histoplasma capsulatum.*** Direct microscopic examination of respiratory tract specimens and other similar specimens often fails to reveal the presence of *H. capsulatum.* However, an astute laboratorian may detect the organism when examining Wright- or Giemsa-stained specimens of bone marrow and, in rare cases, peripheral blood. *H. capsulatum* is found intracellularly in mononuclear cells as small, round to oval yeast cells 2 to 5 μm in diameter (Figure 60-34; also see Figure 60-6).

***Paracoccidioides brasiliensis.*** Specimens submitted for direct microscopic examination are important for the diagnosis of paracoccidioidomycosis. Large, round or oval, multiple budding yeast cells (8 to 40 μm in diameter) are usually recognized in sputum, mucosal biopsy specimens, and other exudates. Characteristic multiply budding yeast forms resemble a "mariner's wheel"

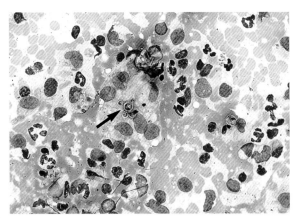

**Figure 60-35** *Paracoccidioides brasiliensis* in a bone marrow aspirate shows a yeast cell with multiple buds *(arrow)*.

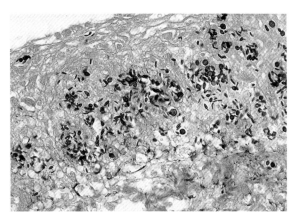

**Figure 60-37** The deeply staining bodies in this mouse testis are the yeast forms of *Sporothrix schenckii*.

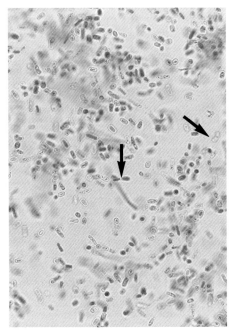

**Figure 60-36** *Penicillium marneffei* and binary fission *(arrows)* (×500).

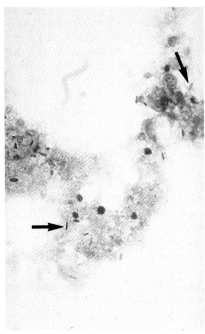

**Figure 60-38** Periodic acid-Schiff (PAS) staining of exudate shows the cigar-to-oval–shaped yeast cells *(arrows)* of *Sporothrix schenckii*.

(Figure 60-35). The yeast cells surrounding the periphery of the parent cell range from 8 to 15 $\mu$m in diameter. Some cells may be as small as 2 to 5 $\mu$m but still exhibit multiple buds.

**Penicillium marneffei.** Direct examination of infected tissues and exudates reveals that *P. marneffei* produces small, yeastlike cells (2 to 6 $\mu$m) that have internal crosswalls; no budding cells are produced (Figure 60-36). Like *H. capsulatum*, *P. marneffei* may be detected in peripheral blood smears with disseminated disease.

**Sporothrix schenckii.** Exudate aspirated from unopened subcutaneous nodules or from open draining lesions often is submitted for culture and direct microscopic examination. Direct examination of this material usually has little diagnostic value, because demonstrating the rare characteristic yeast forms is difficult. *S. schenckii* usually appears as small (2 to 5 $\mu$m in diameter), round

to oval, to cigar-shaped yeast cells (Figure 60-37). If stained using the periodic acid-Schiff (PAS) method in histologic section, an amorphous pink material may be seen surrounding the yeast cells (Figure 60-38).

**Antigen-Protein.** Immunodiffusion methods (the exoantigen test) may be used to identify isolates of these organisms based on precipitation bands of identity between specific antibodies and fungal antigen extracts. However, these assays have been largely replaced by the more rapid nucleic acid hybridization reactions.

**Nucleic Acid Amplification.** Nucleic acid amplification assays are not routinely performed but are available in some reference laboratories and in research settings. Real-time or homogeneous, rapid-cycle polymerase chain reaction (PCR) assays have been described for *H. capsulatum* and *C. immitis*. These assays have proved suitable for isolate identification. Perhaps the most significant advance in clinical mycology in the past few decades was the development of specific nucleic acid probes for identifying some of the dimorphic fungi (see Procedure 60-2 on the Evolve site). DNA probes (Gen-Probe, San Diego, California) are commercially available that are complementary to species-specific ribosomal RNA. Fungal cells are heat killed and disrupted by a lysing agent and sonication, and the nucleic acid is exposed to a species-specific DNA probe, which has been labeled with a chemiluminescent tag (acridinium ester). The labeled DNA probe combines with a ribosomal RNA of the organism to form a stable DNA:RNA hybrid. All unbound DNA probes are "quenched," and light generated from the DNA:RNA hybrids is measured in a luminometer. The total testing time is less than 1 hour.

Nucleic acid probe identification is sensitive, specific, and rapid. Colonies contaminated with bacteria or other fungi may be tested; however, results from colonies recovered on a blood-enriched media must be interpreted with caution, because hemin may cause false-positive chemiluminescence. Nonetheless, nucleic acid probes should be used whenever possible to confirm the identification of an organism suspected of being *H. capsulatum*, *B. dermatitidis*, or *C. immitis*.

**Cultivation.** The dimorphic fungi are regarded as slow-growing organisms, requiring 7 to 21 days for visible growth to appear at 25° to 30°C. However, exceptions to this rule occur with some frequency. Occasionally cultures of *B. dermatitidis* and *H. capsulatum* are recovered in as short a time as 2 to 5 days when many organisms are present in the clinical specimen. In contrast, when a small number of colonies of *B. dermatitidis* and *H. capsulatum* are present, sometimes 21 to 30 days of incubation are required before they are detected. *C. immitis* is consistently recovered within 3 to 5 days of incubation, but when many organisms are present, colonies may be detected within 48 hours. Cultures of *P. brasiliensis* are commonly recovered within 5 to 25 days, with a usual incubation period of 10 to 15 days. The growth rate, if slow, might lead the laboratorian to suspect the presence of a dimorphic fungus; however, considerable variation in the time for recovery exists. The exceptions to this slow growth are *C. immitis* and *P. marneffei*, which may be recovered within 3 to 5 days.

Textbooks present descriptions of the dimorphic fungi that the reader assumes are typical for each particular organism. As is true in other areas of microbiology, variation in the colonial morphologic features also occurs, depending on the strain and the type of medium used. The laboratorian must be aware of this variation and must not rely heavily on colonial morphologic features to identify members of this group of fungi.

The pigmentation of colonies is sometimes helpful but also varies widely; colonies of *B. dermatitidis* and *H. capsulatum* are described as being fluffy white, with a change in color to tan or buff with age. Some isolates initially appear darkly pigmented, with colors ranging from gray or dark brown to red. On media containing blood enrichment, these organisms may appear heaped, wrinkled, glabrous, neutral in color, and yeastlike; often tufts of aerial hyphae project from the top of the colony.

Some colonies may appear pink to red, possibly because of the adsorption of hemoglobin from the blood in the medium. *C. immitis* is described as fluffy white with scattered areas of hyphae adherent to the agar surface, giving an overall "cobweb" appearance to the colony. However, numerous morphologic forms have been reported, including textures ranging from wooly to powdery and pigmentation ranging from pink-lavender or yellow to brown or buff.

The definitive traditional identification method for dimorphic fungus includes observing both the mold and tissue or parasitic forms of the organism. In general 25° to 30°C is the optimal temperature for recovery and identification of the dimorphic fungi from clinical specimens. Temperature (35° to 37°C), certain nutritional factors, and stimulation of growth in tissue independent of temperature are among the factors necessary to initiate the transformation of the mold form to the tissue form. Previously, *B. dermatitidis* and *H. capsulatum* were identified definitively by the in vitro conversion of a mold form to the corresponding yeast form through in vitro conversion on a blood-enriched medium incubated at 35° to 37°C; definitive identification of *C. immitis* involved conversion to the spherule form by animal inoculation. Except for *C. immitis*, the conversion of dimorphic molds to the yeast form can be accomplished with some difficulty (see Procedure 60-3 on the Evolve site). Some laboratories use the exoantigen test (see Procedure 60-4 on the Evolve site) to identify the dimorphic pathogens. However, this test requires extended incubation before cultures may be identified.

***Blastomyces dermatitidis.*** *B. dermatitidis* commonly requires incubation for 5 days to 4 weeks or longer at 25°C before growth can be detected; however, it may be detected in as short a time as 2 to 3 days. On enriched culture media, the mold form develops initially as a glabrous or waxy-appearing colony and is off-white to white. With age, the aerial hyphae often turn gray to brown. The waxy, yeastlike appearance is typified on media enriched with blood. Tufts of hyphae often project upward from the colonies, and this has been referred to as the "prickly state" of the organism. However, some isolates appear fluffy on primary recovery and remain so throughout the incubation period. On blood agar at 37°C, colonies are waxy, wrinkled, and yeastlike. Mold-to-yeast conversion usually requires 4 to 5 days.

***Coccidioides immitis.*** Cultures of *C. immitis* are a biohazard to laboratory workers, and strict safety precautions must be followed when cultures are examined. Mature colonies may appear within 2 to 5 days of incubation and may be present on most media, including those used in bacteriology. Laboratory workers are cautioned not to open cultures of fluffy white molds unless they are placed inside a biologic safety cabinet (BSC). Colonies of *C. immitis* often appear as a delicate, cobweb-like growth after 3 to 21 days of incubation. Some portions of the colony exhibit aerial hyphae, whereas in others the hyphae adhere to the agar surface. Most isolates appear fluffy white; however, colonies of varying colors have been reported, ranging from pink to yellow to purple and black. Some colonies exhibit a greenish discoloration on blood agar, and others appear yeastlike, smooth, wrinkled, and tan.

**Histoplasma capsulatum.** *H. capsulatum* is easily cultured from clinical specimens; however, it may be overgrown by bacteria or rapidly growing molds. A procedure that is useful for recovering *H. capsulatum, B. dermatitidis,* and *C. immitis* from contaminated specimens (e.g., sputa) uses a yeast extract/phosphate medium and a drop of concentrated ammonium hydroxide ($NH_4OH$) placed on one side of the inoculated plate of medium. In the past it was recommended that specimens not be kept at room temperature before culture, because *H. capsulatum* would not survive. The organism survives transit in the mail for as long as 16 days. However, the current recommendation is that specimens be cultured as soon as possible to ensure optimal recovery of *H. capsulatum* and other dimorphic fungi.

*H. capsulatum* is usually considered a slow-growing mold at 25° to 30°C and commonly requires 2 to 4 weeks or more for colonies to appear. However, the organism may be recovered in 5 days or less if many yeast cells are present in the clinical specimen. Isolates of *H. capsulatum* have been reported to be recovered from blood cultures with the Isolator within a mean time of 8 days. *H. capsulatum* is a white, fluffy mold that turns brown to buff with age. Some isolates ranging from gray to red have also been reported. The organism also may produce wrinkle, moist, heaped, yeastlike colonies that are soft and cream colored, tan, or pink. Tufts of hyphae often project upward from the colonies, as described for *B. dermatitidis. H. capsulatum* and *B. dermatitidis* cannot be differentiated using colonial morphologic features.

**Paracoccidioides brasiliensis.** Colonies of *P. brasiliensis* grow very slowly (21 to 28 days) and are heaped, wrinkled, moist, and yeastlike. With age, colonies may become covered with a short aerial mycelium and turn tan to brown. The surface of colonies often is heaped with crater formations.

**Penicillium marneffei.** At 25°C, *P. marneffei* grows rapidly and produces blue-green to yellowish colonies on Sabouraud's agar. A soluble, red to maroon pigment that diffuses into the agar and is often best observed by viewing the reverse of the colony is suggestive of *P. marneffei.* Although the growth rate and colonial morphologic features may help the laboratorian recognize the possibility of a dimorphic fungus, they should be considered in combination with the microscopic morphologic features to make the identification. *P. marneffei* cannot be definitively identified by morphologic features alone; thermal conversion studies or nucleic acid–based testing is needed to confirm the identification of this pathogen.

**Sporothrix schenckii.** Colonies of *S. schenckii* grow rapidly (3 to 5 days) and initially are usually small, moist, and white to cream colored. On further incubation, these become membranous, wrinkled, and coarsely matted, with the color becoming irregularly dark brown or black and the colony becoming leathery in consistency. It is not uncommon for the clinical microbiology laboratory to mistake a young culture of *S. schenckii* for a yeast until the microscopic features are observed.

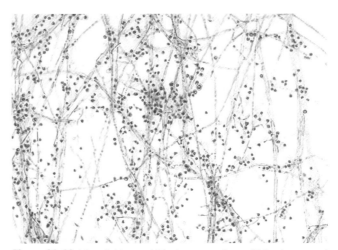

**Figure 60-39** Mycelial form of *Blastomyces dermatitidis* shows oval conidia borne laterally on branching hyphae (×1000).

## Approach to Identification

**Blastomyces dermatitidis.** Microscopically, hyphae of the mold form of *B. dermatitidis* are septate and delicate and measure approximately 2 *μm* in diameter. Commonly, ropelike strands of hyphae are seen; however, these are found with most of the dimorphic fungi. The characteristic microscopic morphologic features are single, circular to pyriform conidia produced on short conidiophores that resemble lollipops (Figure 60-39); less commonly, the conidiophores may be elongated. The production of conidia in some isolates is minimal or absent, particularly on a medium containing blood enrichment.

When incubated at 37°C, colonies of the yeast form develop within 7 days and appear waxy and wrinkled and cream to tan. Microscopically, large, thick-walled yeast cells (8 to 15 *μm* in diameter) with buds attached by a broad base are seen (see Figure 60-28). Some strains may produce yeast cells as small as 2 to 5 *μm*, called *microforms.* These small forms may resemble *C. neoformans* var. neoformans or *H. capsulatum.* Although these microforms may be present, a thorough search should reveal more typical yeast forms. During conversion, swollen hyphal forms and immature cells with rudimentary buds are also likely to be present. Because the conversion of *B. dermatitidis* is easily accomplished, this is feasible in the clinical laboratory; however, this is the most appropriate instance in which mold to yeast conversion should be attempted. *B. dermatitidis* may also be identified by the presence of a specific band (i.e., A band) in the exoantigen test or by nucleic acid probe testing. In some instances, *H. capsulatum, P. boydii,* or *T. rubrum* might be confused microscopically with *B. dermatitidis.* The site of infection and the relatively slow growth rate of *B. dermatitidis* and careful examination of the microscopic morphologic features usually differentiates it from these fungi.

**Coccidioides immitis.** Microscopically some *C. immitis* cultures show small, septate hyphae that often exhibit right-angle branches and racquet forms. With age, the hyphae form arthroconidia that are characteristically rectangular to barrel shaped. The arthroconidia are larger than the hyphae from which they were produced and stain darkly with lactophenol cotton or aniline blue. The arthroconidia are separated by clear or lighter staining, nonviable cells (disjunctor cells). These types of conidia are referred to as alternate arthroconidia (see Figure 60-24). Arthroconidia have been reported to range from 1.5 to 7.5 $\mu$m in width and 1.5 to 30 $\mu$m in length, whereas most are 3 to 4.5 $\mu$m in width and 3 $\mu$m in length. Variation has been reported in the shape of arthroconidia, ranging from rounded to square or rectangular to curved; however, most are barrel shaped. Even if alternate arthroconidia are observed microscopically, definitive identification should be made using nucleic acid probe testing. If a culture is suspected of being *C. immitis*, it should be sealed with tape to prevent chances of laboratory-acquired infection. Because *C. immitis* is the most infectious of all the fungi, extreme caution should be used in handling cultures of this organism. Safety precautions include the following:

1. If culture dishes are used, they should be handled only in a Level 3 BSC. Cultures should be sealed with tape if the specimen is suspected to contain *C. immitis*.
2. The use of cotton plug test tubes is discouraged, and screw-capped tubes should be used if culture tubes are preferred. All handling of cultures of *C. immitis* in screw-capped tubes should be performed inside a BSC.
3. All microscopic preparations for examination should be performed in a Level 3 BSC.
4. Cultures should be autoclaved as soon as final identification of *C. immitis* is made.

Other, usually nonvirulent fungi that resemble *C. immitis* microscopically may be found in the environment. Some molds, such as *Malbranchea* sp., also produce alternate arthroconidia, although these tend to be more rectangular; however, such species must be considered when making the identification. *G. candidum* and *Trichosporon* spp. produce hyphae that disassociate into contiguous arthroconidia; these should not be confused with *C. immitis* (Figure 60-40; see Figure 60-23). The colonial morphologic features of older cultures of these fungi may resemble *C. immitis*, but as noted, the arthroconidia are not alternate. It is also important to remember that if confusion in identification does arise, or when occasional strains of *C. immitis* that fail to sporulate are encountered, identification by exoantigen or nucleic acid probe testing may be performed.

***Histoplasma capsulatum.*** Microscopically the hyphae of *H. capsulatum* are small (approximately 2 $\mu$m in diameter) and are often intertwined to form ropelike strands. Commonly, large (8 to 14 $\mu$m in diameter) spherical or pyriform, smooth-walled macroconidia are seen in young cultures. With age, the macroconidia become roughened or tuberculate and provide enough evidence to make a tentative identification (Figure 60-41). The macroconidia are produced either on short or long conidiospores. Some isolates produce round to pyriform, smooth microconidia (2 to 4 $\mu$m in diameter), in addition to the characteristic tuberculate macroconidia. Some isolates of *H. capsulatum* fail to sporulate despite numerous attempts to induce sporulation.

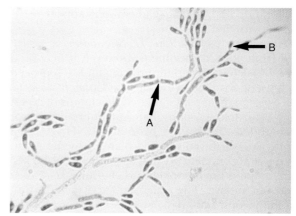

**Figure 60-40** *Trichosporon* spp. produce arthroconidia *(A)* and an occasional blastoconidium *(B)*.

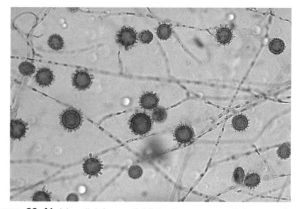

**Figure 60-41** Mycelial form of *Histoplasma capsulatum* produces characteristic tuberculate macroconidia (×1000).

Conversion of the mold to the yeast form is usually difficult and is not recommended. Microscopically a mixture of swollen hyphae and small budding yeast cells 2 to 5 $\mu$m in diameter should be observed. These are similar to the intracellular yeast cells seen in mononuclear cells in infected tissue. The yeast form of *H. capsulatum* cannot be recognized unless the corresponding mold form is present on another culture or unless the yeast is converted directly to the mold form by incubation at 25° to 30°C after yeast cells have been observed. The exoantigen test can be used for identification, but nucleic acid probe testing is now recommended as a definitive means of rapidly identifying this organism. *Sepedonium* sp., an environmental organism that grows on mushrooms, is always mentioned as being confused with *H. capsulatum*, because it produces similar tuberculate macroconidia. However, this organism is almost never recovered from clinical specimens, does not have a yeast form, fails to produce characteristic bands in the exoantigen test with *H. capsulatum* antiserum, and does not react in nucleic acid probe tests.

***Paracoccidioides brasiliensis.*** Microscopically the mold form is similar to that seen with *B. dermatitidis*. Small hyphae (approximately 2 $\mu$m in diameter) are seen, along

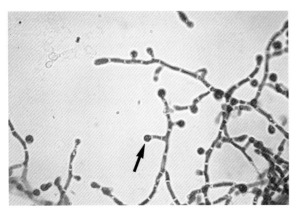

**Figure 60-42** Mycelial form of *Paracoccidioides brasiliensis* shows septate hyphae and pyriform conidia singly borne *(arrow)* (×430).

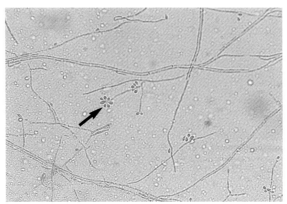

**Figure 60-43** Mycelial form of *Sporothrix schenckii* shows pyriform-to-ovoid microconidia in a flowerette morphology at the tip of the conidiophore *(arrow)* (×750).

with numerous chlamydoconidia. Small (3 to 4 μm), delicate, globose or pyriform conidia may be seen arising from the sides of the hyphae or on very short conidiophores (Figure 60-42). Most often cultures reveal only fine septate hyphae and numerous chlamydoconidia.

After temperature-based conversion on a blood-enriched medium, the colonial morphology of the yeast form is characterized by smooth, soft-wrinkled, yeastlike colonies that are cream to tan. Microscopically the colonies are composed of yeast cells 10 to 40 μm in diameter surrounded by narrow-necked yeast cells around the periphery, as previously described (see Figure 60-35). If in vitro conversion to the yeast form is unsuccessful, the exoantigen test (see Procedure 60-4 on the Evolve site) should be used to make the definitive identification of *P. brasiliensis*. Nucleic acid probe testing is not available for this organism. However, *P. brasiliensis* is known to cross react with *B. dermatitidis*. This cross reaction, in conjunction with microscopic and colonial morphology, epidemiologic data, and clinical features, may be used for definitive identification of this fungus.

**Penicillium marneffei.** At 25°C, *P. marneffei* grows rapidly and produces blue-green to yellowish colonies. A soluble red to maroon pigment, which diffuses into the agar, is highly suggestive of *P. marneffei*. At 37°C, conversion of mycelium to the infective, yeastlike form occurs in approximately 2 weeks. Oval, yeastlike cells (2 to 6 μm in diameter) with septa are seen; abortive, extensively branched, and highly septate hyphae may also be present (see Figure 60-36).

**Sporothrix schenckii.** Microscopically, hyphae are delicate (approximately 2 μm in diameter), septate, and branching. Single-celled conidia 2 to 5 μm in diameter are borne in clusters from the tips of single conidiophores (flowerette arrangement). Each conidium is attached to the conidiophore by an individual, delicate, threadlike structure (denticle) that may require examination under oil immersion to be visible. As the culture ages, single-celled, thick-walled, black-pigmented conidia may also be produced along the sides of the hyphae, simulating the arrangement of microconidia produced by *T. rubrum* (sleeve arrangement) (Figure 60-43).

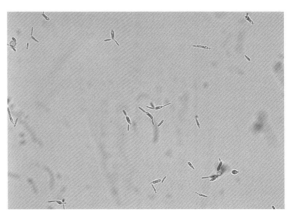

**Figure 60-44** Yeast form of *Sporothrix schenckii* consists of cigar-shaped and oval budding cells (×500).

Because of similar morphologic features, saprophytic species of the genus *Sporotrichum* may be confused with *S. schenckii*, and they must be differentiated. During incubation of a culture at 37°C, a colony of *S. schenckii* transforms to a soft, cream-colored to white, yeastlike appearance. Microscopically singly or multiply budding, spherical, oval, or elongate, cigar-shaped yeast cells are observed without difficulty (Figure 60-44). Conversion from the mold form to the yeast form is easily accomplished and usually occurs within 1 to 5 days after transfer of the culture to a medium containing blood enrichment; most isolates of *S. schenckii* are converted to the yeast form within 12 to 48 hours at 37°C. *Sporotrichum* spp. do not produce a yeast form.

Table 60-3 presents a summary of the colonial and microscopic morphologic features of the dimorphic fungi in addition to other organisms previously discussed.

## Serodiagnosis

Fungal serologies are rapid and useful tests that may aid the diagnosis of systemic fungal infections caused by *B. dermatitidis*, *H. capsulatum*, and *C. immitis*. These tests have also been useful to study the epidemiology of these fungal infections, because even individuals with

**TABLE 60-3**    Summary of the Characteristic Features of Fungi Known to Be Common Causes of Selected Fungal Infection in Humans

| Infection | Etiologic Agent | Growth Rate (Days) | CULTURAL CHARACTERISTICS AT 30°C | | | MICROSCOPIC MORPHOLOGIC FEATURES | | | Confirmatory Tests for Identification |
|---|---|---|---|---|---|---|---|---|---|
| | | | Blood-Enriched Medium | Medium Lacking Blood Enrichment | | Blood-Enriched Medium | Non-Blood-Enriched Medium | Recommended Morphologic Features of Tissue Form | |
| Blastomycosis | *Blastomyces dermatitidis* | 2-30 | Colonies are cream to tan, soft, moist, wrinkled, waxy, flat to heaped, and yeastlike; "tufts" of hyphae often project upward from colonies | Colonies are white to cream to tan, some with drops of exudate present, fluffy to glabrous, and adherent to the agar surface | | Hyphae 1-2 μm in diameter are present; some are aggregated in ropelike clusters; sporulation is rare | Hyphae 1-2 μm in diameter are present; single pyriform conidia are produced on short to long conidiophores; some cultures produce few conidia | 8-15 μm, broad-based budding cells with double-contoured walls are seen; cytoplasmic granulation is often obvious | 1. Specific nucleic acid probe 2. Broad-based budding cells may be seen after in vitro conversion on cottonseed agar 3. Exoantigen test |
| Histoplasmosis | *Histoplasma capsulatum* | 3-45 | Colonies are heaped, moist, wrinkled, yeastlike, soft, and cream, tan, or pink in color; "tufts" of hyphae often project upward from colonies | Colonies are white, cream, tan, or gray, fluffy to glabrous; some colonies appear yeastlike and adherent to the agar surface; many variations in colonial morphology occur | | Hyphae 1-2 μm in diameter are present; some are aggregated in ropelike clusters; sporulation is rare | Young cultures usually have a predominance of smooth-walled macroconidia that become tuberculate with age; macroconidia may be pyriform or spherical; some isolates produce small pyriform microconidia in the presence or absence of macroconidia | 2-5 μm, small, oval to spherical budding cells often seen inside of mononuclear cells | 1. Specific nucleic acid probe 2. Exoantigen test |

| Disease | Organism | Days | Colonial morphology | Microscopic morphology | Exoantigen test |
|---|---|---|---|---|---|
| Paracoccidioidomycosis | *Paracoccidioides brasiliensis* | 21-28 | Colonies are heaped, wrinkled, moist, and yeastlike; with age, colonies may become covered with short aerial mycelium and may turn brown | Hyphae 1-2 $\mu$m in diameter are present; some isolates produce conidia similar to those of *B. dermatitidis*; chlamydoconidia may be numerous, and multiple budding yeast cells 10-25 $\mu$m in diameter may be present | 10-25 $\mu$m, multiple budding cells (buds 1-2 $\mu$m), resembling a mariner's wheel, may be present; buds are attached to the parent cell by a narrow neck |
| Mucormycosis | *Rhizopus* spp., *Mucor* spp., and other mucorales | 1-3 | Colonies are extremely fast growing, wooly, and gray to brown to gray-black | *Rhizopus* spp.: Rhizoids are produced at the base of sporangiophore<br>*Mucor* spp.: No rhizoids are produced | Large, ribbonlike (10-30 $\mu$m), twisted, often distorted pieces of aseptate hyphae may be present; septa occasionally may be seen |
| Aspergillosis | *Aspergillus fumigatus, A. flavus, A. niger, A. terreus,* other *Aspergillus* spp. | 3-5 | Colonies of *A. fumigatus* are usually blue-green to gray-green, whereas those of *A. flavus* and *A. niger* are yellow-green and black, respectively; colonies of *A. terreus* resemble powdered cinnamon; other species of *Aspergillus* exhibit a wide range of colors; blood-enriched media usually have little effect on the colonial morphologic features | *A. fumigatus*: Uniserate heads with phialides covering the upper half to two thirds of the vesicle<br>*A. flavus*: Uniserate or biserate or both with phialides covering the entire surface of a spherical vesicle<br>*A. niger*: Biserate with phialides covering the entire surface of a spherical vesicle; conidia are black<br>*A. terreus*: Biserate with phialides covering the entire surface of a hemispherical vesicle; aleurioconidia are formed on submerged hyphae | Septate hyphae 5-10 $\mu$m in diameter that exhibit dichotomous branching |
| | | | | | Identification is based on characteristic morphologic features |
| | | | | | Identification is based on microscopic morphologic features and colonial morphology; *A. fumigatus* can tolerate elevated temperatures (≥45°C) |

*Continued*

**TABLE 60-3** Summary of the Characteristic Features of Fungi Known to Be Common Causes of Selected Fungal Infection in Humans—cont'd

| Infection | Etiologic Agent | Growth Rate (Days) | CULTURAL CHARACTERISTICS AT 30°C | | MICROSCOPIC MORPHOLOGIC FEATURES | | Recommended Morphologic Features of Tissue Form | Confirmatory Tests for Identification |
|---|---|---|---|---|---|---|---|---|
| | | | Blood-Enriched Medium | Medium Lacking Blood Enrichment | Blood-Enriched Medium | Non-Blood-Enriched Medium | | |
| Coccidioidomycosis | *Coccidioides immitis* | 2-21 | Colonies may be white and fluffy to greenish on blood-enriched media; some isolates are yeastlike, heaped, wrinkled, and membranous | Colonies usually are fluffy white but may be pigmented gray, orange, brown, or yellow; mycelium is adherent to the agar surface in some portions of the colony | | Chains of alternate, barrel-shaped arthroconidia are characteristic; some arthroconidia may be elongated; hyphae are small and often arranged in ropelike strands, and racquet forms are seen in young cultures | Round spherules 30-60 μm in diameter containing 2-5 μm endospores are characteristic; empty spherules are commonly seen | 1. Specific nucleic acid probe<br>2. Exoantigen test |

historically distant, asymptomatic, or subclinical infections often have developed an antibody response to the infecting pathogen. Unfortunately, these tests require detailed preparation and technical expertise. False-negative reactions may occur if serology specimens are drawn in immunocompromised individuals who are unable to produce an antibody response. False-positive reactions may occur because of cross reactivity with other fungi. For example, because the antigens of *H. capsulatum* are similar to those of *B. dermatitidis*, occasionally a specimen from a patient with histoplasmosis demonstrates a positive reaction for *B. dermatitidis* in serologic tests.

Two assays, complement fixation and immunodiffusion, should be used together to detect antibodies directed toward *B. dermatitidis*, *H. capsulatum*, and *C. immitis*. In the complement fixation assay, titers of 1:8 to 1:16 suggest active infection with *B. dermatitidis* and *H. capsulatum;* titers of 1:32 or greater indicate active disease. Titers as low as 1:2 to 1:4 have been identified in patients with coccidioidomycosis. Titers greater than 1:16 usually indicate active disease. Bands of identity form in the immunodiffusion test between known antisera, known fungal antigen, and the antibodies present in the patient's serum. Specific bands of identity are used for serologic detection of particular fungi, whereas nonspecific bands suggest the possibility of an infection by another fungal pathogen. One or two bands of identity, the H and M bands, may occur in patients with histoplasmosis. The presence of both bands indicates active infection. The presence of an M band may indicate early or chronic infection.

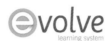 *Visit the Evolve site to complete the review questions.*

---

## CASE STUDY 60-1

An elderly woman with diabetes visits her clinician because she has a brown, dull, discolored toenail. The clinician takes nail clippings for culture. The laboratory places the clippings on media with no cycloheximide. SAB's agar reveals a rapid growing colony that is mature in 5 days. The colonies are initially white, become tan with age, and are velvety and powdery. The reverse is tan with a brown center. Microscopic examination reveals septate hyaline hyphae with annelides. Annelides are both solitary and in clusters that resemble a penicillus.

**QUESTIONS**

1. Why did the laboratory use agar without cycloheximide?
2. How would you distinguish between *Penicillium* and *Scopulariopsis* spp.?
3. One-celled conidia are rough walled, and spiny conidia in chains are seen. What organism is identified?

---

## BIBLIOGRAPHY

Bailek R, Kern J, Herrmann T, et al: PCR assays for identification of *Coccidioides posadasii* based on the nucleotide sequence of the antigen 2/proline-rich antigen, *J Clin Microbiol* 42:778, 2004.

Bille J, Stockman L, Roberts GD, et al: Evaluation of a lysis-centrifugation system for recovery of yeasts and filamentous fungi from blood, *J Clin Microbiol* 18:469, 1983.

Carey J, D'Amico R, Sutton DA, et al: *Paecilomyces lilacinus* vaginitis in an immunocompetent patient, *Emerg Infect Dis* 9:1155, 2003.

de Hoog G: *Atlas of clinical fungi,* t.N.a.R. Centraal bureau voor Schimell cultures/Universita Rovira i Virgili. Utrecht and Reus, Spain.

Deng Z, Ribas JL, Gibson DW, et al: Infections caused by *Penicillium marneffei* in China and Southeast Asia: review of eighteen published cases and report of four more Chinese cases, *Rev Infect Dis* 10:640, 1988.

Denz Z, Yun M, Ajello L: Human penicilliosis marneffei and its relation to the bamboo rat (*Rhizomys pruinosus*), *J Med Vet Mycol* 24:383, 1986.

Fleming RV, Walsh TJ, Anaissie EJ: Emerging and less common fungal pathogens, *Infect Dis Clin North Am* 16:915, 2002.

Friedank H: Hyalohyphomycoses due to *Fusarium* spp: two case reports and review of the literature, *Mycoses* 38:69, 1995.

Gray L, Roberts G: Laboratory diagnosis of systemic fungal disease, *Infect Dis Clin North Am* 2:779, 1988.

Guarro J, Gams W, Pujol I, et al: *Acremonium* species: new emerging fungal opportunists—in vitro antifungal susceptibilities and review, *Clin Infect Dis* 25:1222, 1997.

Gutierrez-Rodero F, Moragon M, Ortiz de la Tabla V, et al: Cutaneous hyalohyphomycosis caused by *Paecilomyces lilacinus* in an immunocompetent host successfully treated with itraconazole: case report and review, *Eur J Clin Microbiol Infect Dis* 18:814, 1999.

Harari AR, Hemple HO, Kimberlin CL, et al: Effects of time lapse between sputum collection and culturing on isolation of clinically significant fungi, *J Clin Microbiol* 15:425, 1982.

Heinic GS, Greenspan D, MacPhail LA, et al: Oral *Geotrichum candidum* infection associated with HIV infection: a case report, *Oral Surg Oral Med Oral Pathol* 73:726, 1992.

Huppert M, Sun S, Bailey J: Natural variability in *Coccidioides immitis.* In Ajello L, editor: *Coccidioidomycosis,* Tucson, 1967, University of Arizona Press.

Kane J, Smitka C: Early detection and identification of *Trichdophyton verrucosum,* *J Clin Microbiol* 8:740, 1978.

Kennedy M, Sigler L: *Aspergillus, Fusarium* and other moniliaceous fungi. In Murray P, Baron E, Pfaller M, editors: *Manual of clinical microbiology,* Washington, DC, 1995, American Society for Microbiology Press.

Kontoyiannis DP, Wessel VC, Bodey GP, et al: Zygomycosis in the 1990s in a tertiary-care cancer center, *Clin Infect Dis* 30:851, 2000.

Kwon-Chung K, Bennet J: *Medical mycology,* Philadelphia, 1992, Lea & Febiger.

Li JS, Pan LQ, Wu SX, et al: Disseminated penicilliosis marneffei in China: report of three cases, *Chin Med J (Engl)* 104:247, 1991.

Martagon-Villamil J, Shrestha N, Sholtis M, et al: Identification of *Histoplasma capsulatum* from culture extracts by real-time PCR, *J Clin Microbiol* 41:1295, 2003.

Meis JF, Kullberg BJ, Pruszczynski M, et al: Severe osteomyelitis due to the zygomycete *Apophysomyces elegans,* *J Clin Microbiol* 32:3078, 1994.

Nucci M: Emerging moulds: *Fusarium, Scedosporium,* and Zygomycetes in transplant recipients, *Curr Opin Infect Dis* 16:607, 2003.

Odabasi Z, Mattiuzzi G, Estey E, et al: Beta-D-glucan as a diagnostic adjunct for invasive fungal infections: validation, cutoff development, and performance in patients with acute myelogenous leukemia and myelodysplastic syndrome, *Clin Infect Dis* 39:199, 2004.

Ostrosky-Zeichner L, Alexander BD, Kett DH, et al: Multicenter clinical evaluation of the (1-3) beta-D-glucan assay as an aid to diagnosis of fungal infections in humans, *Clin Infect Dis* 41:654, 2005.

Patel R, Gustaferro CA, Krom RA, et al: Phaeohyphomycosis due to *Scopulariopsis brumptii* in a liver transplant recipient, *Clin Infect Dis* 19:198, 1994.

Pfeiffer CD, Fine JP, Safdar N: Diagnosis of invasive aspergillosis using a galactomannan assay: a meta-analysis, *Clin Infect Dis* 42:1417, 2006.

Procop GW, Cockerill III FR, Vetter EA, et al: Performance of five agar media for recovery of fungi from isolator blood cultures, *J Clin Microbiol* 38:3827, 2000.

Schell WA, Perfect JR: Fatal, disseminated *Acremonium strictum* infection in a neutropenic host, *J Clin Microbiol* 34:1333, 1996.

Skoulidis F, Morgan MS, MacLeod KM: *Penicillium marneffei:* a pathogen on our doorstep? *J R Soc Med* 97:394, 2004.

Smith C, Goodman N: Improved culture method for the isolation of *Histoplasma capsulatum* and *Blastomyces dermatitidis* from contaminated specimens, *Am J Clin Pathol* 68:276, 1975.

St. Germain G, Summerbell R: *Identifying filamentous fungi: a clinical handbook*, Belmont, Calif, 1996, Star Publishing.

Standard PG, Kaufman L: A rapid and specific method for the immunological identification of mycelial form cultures of *Paracoccidioides brasiliensis*, *Curr Microbiol* 4:297, 1980.

Stockman L, Clark KA, Hunt JM, et al: Evaluation of commercially available acridinium ester–labeled chemiluminescent DNA probes for culture identification of *Blastomyces dermatitidis, Coccidioides immitis, Cryptococcus neoformans,* and *Histoplasma capsulatum, J Clin Microbiol* 31:845, 1993.

Strimlan CV, Dines DE, Rodgers-Sullivan RF, et al: Respiratory tract *Aspergillus:* clinical significance, *Minn Med* 63:25, 1980.

Sun SH, Huppert M, Vukovich KR: Rapid in vitro conversion and identification of *Coccidioides immitis, J Clin Microbiol* 3:186, 1976.

Torres HA, Raad II, Kontoyiannis DP: Infections caused by *Fusarium* species, *J Chemother* 15(suppl 2):28, 2003.

Treger TR, Visscher DW, Bartlett MS, et al: Diagnosis of pulmonary infection caused by *Aspergillus:* usefulness of respiratory cultures, *J Infect Dis* 152:572, 1985.

Walsh TJ, Groll A, Heimenz J, et al: Infections due to emerging and uncommon medically important fungal pathogens, *Clin Microbiol Infect* 10(suppl 1):48, 2004.

Wang SM, Shieh CC, Liu CC: Successful treatment of *Paecilomyces variotii* splenic abscesses: a rare complication in a previously unrecognized chronic granulomatous disease child, *Diagn Microbiol Infect Dis* 53:149, 2005.

Willinger B: Laboratory diagnosis and therapy of invasive fungal infections, *Curr Drug Targets* 7:513, 2006.

Woo PC, Leung SY, Ngan A, et al: A significant number of reported *Absidia corymbifera* (*Lichtheimia corymbifera*) infections are caused by *Lichtheimia ramosa* (syn. *Lichtheimia hongkongensis*): an emerging cause of mucormycosis, *Emerg Microb Infect* 1.e15, 2012.

Zhiyong Z, Mei K, Yanbin L: Disseminated *Penicillium marneffei* infection with fungemia and endobronchial disease in an AIDS patient in China, *Med Princ Pract* 15:235, 2006.

# Dematiaceous (Melanized) Molds

---

### SEPTATE DEMATIACEOUS MOLDS TO BE CONSIDERED

**Superficial Infections**
*Hortaea werneckii*
*Piedraia hortae*

**Mycetoma**
*Pseudallescheria boydii*
*Acremonium* spp.
*Exophiala jeanselmei*
*Curvularia* spp.
*Madurella mycetomatis*

**Chromoblastomycosis**
*Cladosporium* spp.
*Cladophialophora* spp.
*Phialophora* spp.
*Fonsecaea* spp.

**Phaeohyphomycosis**
*Alternaria* spp.
*Bipolaris* spp.
*Drechslera* spp.
*Curvularia* spp.
*Exophiala jeanselmei*
*Exophiala dermatitidis*
*Exserohilum* spp.
*Ochroconis gallopava*

---

## GENERAL CHARACTERISTICS

The dematiaceous fungi indicate dark coloration as a result of their ability to produce melanin and are known agents of superficial and subcutaneous mycoses that involve the skin and subcutaneous tissues; less commonly, deeply invasive or disseminated disease may be caused by these fungi. These organisms are ubiquitous in nature and exist as saprophytes and plant pathogens. The etiologic agents are found in several unrelated fungal genera.

Humans and animals serve as accidental hosts after traumatic inoculation of the organism into cutaneous and subcutaneous tissues.

In the mycology laboratory, these fungal species often are initially separated by growth rate into the slow-growing dematiaceous molds, which may require 7 to 10 days to grow, and the rapid-growing dematiaceous molds, which usually grow in less than 7 days. When nonsterile body sites are cultured, determining the significance of these organisms is difficult or impossible. If colonies of common saprophytic molds occur near the edge of the plate and are clearly away from the inoculum, they should be considered contaminants unless additional evidence of infection is present.

## EPIDEMIOLOGY AND PATHOGENESIS

### SUPERFICIAL INFECTIONS (TINEA NIGRA AND BLACK PIEDRA)

Tinea nigra is a superficial skin infection caused by *Hortaea werneckii.* It is manifested by blackish brown, macular patches on the palm of the hand or the sole of the foot. Lesions have been compared with silver nitrate staining of the skin. Black piedra is a fungal infection of the hair, scalp, and occasionally the axillary and pubic hair caused by the dematiaceous fungus *Piedraia hortae.* These diseases occur primarily in tropical areas of the world, with cases reported from Africa, Asia, and Latin America.

### MYCETOMA

A mycetoma is a chronic granulomatous infection that usually involves the lower extremities but may occur in any part of the body. The infection is characterized by swelling, purplish discoloration, tumorlike deformities of the subcutaneous tissue, and multiple sinus tracts that drain pus containing yellow, white, red, or black granules. The color of the granules is partly due to the type of infecting organism. The infection gradually progresses to involve the bone, muscle, or other contiguous tissue and ultimately requires amputation in most progressive cases. Dissemination of the organism may occur but is uncommon. Mycetomas usually are seen among people living in tropical and subtropical regions of the world whose outdoor occupations and failure to wear protective clothing predispose them to trauma.

Two types of mycetomas have been described. Actinomycotic (bacterial) mycetomas are caused by the aerobic actinomycetes, including *Nocardia, Actinomadura,* and *Streptomyces* spp. (The aerobic *Actinomycetes* are described in detail in Chapter 19.) Eumycotic (fungal) mycetomas are caused by a heterogeneous group of fungi that have septate hyphae. Eumycotic mycetomas are subcategorized as white grain mycetomas or black grain mycetomas, a distinction determined by the pigmentation of the infecting agent's hyphae.

Some hyaline septate molds can cause mycetomas; however, the disease is covered in this section because many of the etiologic agents are dematiaceous fungi. Etiologic agents of eumycotic mycetoma to be discussed include *Pseudallescheria boydii* and *Acremonium* spp., causative agents of white grain mycetomas, and *Exophiala jeanselmei*, *Curvularia* spp., and *Madurella mycetomatis*, causative agents of black grain mycetomas.

Most patients with mycetomas live in tropical regions, but infections can occur in temperate zones. The most common etiologic agent of white grain mycetoma in the United States is *P. boydii*, a member of the Ascomycota. The organism is commonly found in soil, standing water, and sewage; humans acquire the infection through traumatic implantation of the organism into the skin and subcutaneous tissues.

## CHROMOBLASTOMYCOSIS

Chromoblastomycosis is a chronic fungal infection acquired through traumatic inoculation of an organism, primarily into the skin and subcutaneous tissue. The infection is characterized by the development of a papule at the site of the traumatic insult that slowly spreads to form warty or tumorlike lesions characterized as resembling cauliflower. Secondary infection and ulceration may occur. The lesions usually are confined to the feet and legs but may involve the head, face, neck, and other body surfaces.

Histologic examination of the lesion reveals characteristic **sclerotic bodies,** which are copper-colored, septate cells that appear to be dividing by binary fission and are thought by some to resemble copper pennies. These infections cause hyperplasia of the epidermis of the skin, which may be mistaken for squamous cell carcinoma. Fungal brain abscess, known in the past as cerebral chromoblastomycosis, may be caused by the dematiaceous fungi; however, it is more appropriately considered a type of phaeohyphomycosis and is discussed with that disease. Chromoblastomycosis is widely distributed, but most cases occur in tropical and subtropical areas of the world. Occasional cases are reported from temperate zones, including the United States. The infection is seen most often in areas in which agricultural workers do not wear protective clothing and suffer thorn or splinter puncture wounds.

## PHAEOHYPHOMYCOSIS

Phaeohyphomycosis is a general term used to describe any infection caused by a dematiaceous organism; it includes molds; brownish, yeastlike cells; pseudohyphae; and hyphae, except those described previously. These infections may be subcutaneous, localized, or systemic, and they may be caused by a number of dematiaceous fungi. They include phaeohyphomycotic cysts,

progressive soft tissue infection, brain abscess, sinusitis, endocarditis, mycotic keratitis, pulmonary infection, and systemic infection.

## PATHOGENESIS AND SPECTRUM OF DISEASE

The spectrum of disease caused by the dematiaceous fungi ranges from superficial infections (e.g., skin and hair) to emergent, rapidly progressive, and often fatal disease (e.g., brain abscess). The following list, which is not comprehensive, provides the common etiologic agents of diseases that may be caused by dematiaceous fungi (Table 61-1).

- Mycetoma
  - Bacterial: *Nocardia*, *Actinomadura*, and *Streptomyces* spp.
  - White grain mycetoma: *P. boydii* and *Acremonium* and *Fusarium* spp.
  - Black grain mycetoma: *Madurella mycetomatis*, *Exophiala jeanselmei*, and *Curvularia* spp.
- Chromoblastomycosis: *Cladosporium/Cladophialophora*, *Phialophora*, and *Fonsecaea* spp.
- Phaeohyphomycosis: *E. jeanselmei*; *Exophiala dermatitidis*; and *Curvularia*, *Bipolaris*, *Alternaria*, and *Exserohilum* spp.
- Sinusitis: *Alternaria*, *Bipolaris*, *Exserohilum*, and *Curvularia* spp.
- Mycotic keratitis and endophthalmitis: *E. dermatitidis* and *Bipolaris* and *Curvularia* spp.
- Brain abscess: *Cladophialophora bantiana*, *E. dermatitidis*, and *Bipolaris* spp.

## LABORATORY DIAGNOSIS

### SPECIMEN COLLECTION AND TRANSPORT

See General Considerations for the Laboratory Diagnosis of Fungal Infections in Chapter 59.

### SPECIMEN PROCESSING

See General Considerations for the Laboratory Diagnosis of Fungal Infections in Chapter 59.

### DIRECT DETECTION METHOD

#### Stains

In general, dematiaceous fungal hyphae are seen in clinical specimens by direct microscopic examination or by histopathologic examination of tissue obtained during surgery or autopsy. The dematiaceous character of the hyphae may not be appreciated if the examination is performed using calcofluor white/fluorescent microscopy alone, without observing the hyphae using traditional transmitted light microscopy.

**Superficial Infections.** Direct microscopic examination of a clinical specimen from a patient with tinea nigra may show dematiaceous hyphae and small budding yeast cells

**TABLE 61-1** Dematiaceous Fungi

| Organism | Disease | Site | Tissue Form |
|---|---|---|---|
| **Slow-Growing Species** | | | |
| Cladosporium spp. | Chromoblastomycosis | Subcutaneous | Sclerotic bodies |
| | Phaeohyphomycosis | Brain, subcutaneous | Septate hyphae |
| Ochroconis gallopava | Phaeohyphomycosis | Brain, subcutaneous, lungs | Septate hyphae |
| Exophiala dermatitidis | Phaeohyphomycosis | Brain, eye, subcutaneous, and dissemination | Hyphal fragments and budding yeast |
| | Pneumonial | Lungs | |
| Hortaea jeanselmei | Mycetoma phaeomycotic cyst | Subcutaneous | Hyphal fragments and budding yeasts |
| Hortaea werneckii | Tinea nigra | Skin | Hyphal fragments and budding yeast |
| Fonsecaea spp. | Chromoblastomycosis | Subcutaneous | Sclerotic bodies |
| | Phaeohyphomycosis | Brain | Septate hyphae |
| | Cavitary lung disease | Lungs | Septate hyphae |
| Phialophora spp. | Chromoblastomycosis | Subcutaneous | Sclerotic bodies |
| | Phaeohyphomycosis | Subcutaneous | Septate hyphae |
| | Septic arthritis | Joints | Septate hyphae |
| Piedraia hortae | Black piedra | Hair | Asci-containing nodules cemented to hair shafts |
| Madurella mycetomatis | Mycetoma | Subcutaneous | Hyphal fragments |
| **Rapid-Growing Species** | | | |
| Alternaria spp. | Phaeohyphomycosis | Subcutaneous | Septate hyphae |
| | Sinusitis | Sinuses | Septate hyphae, possibly fungus ball |
| | Nasal septal erosion | Nasal septum | Septate hyphae |
| | Ulcers and onychomycosis | Skin, nails | Septate hyphae |
| Bipolaris spp. | Phaeohyphomycosis | Subcutaneous, brain, eye, bones | Septate hyphae |
| | Sinusitis, fungus ball | Sinuses | Septate hyphae, possibly fungus ball |
| Curvularia spp. | Sinusitis | Sinuses | Septate hyphae; possibly fungus ball |
| | Phaeohyphomycosis | Subcutaneous, heart valves, eye, and lungs | Septate hyphae |
| Drechslera spp. | Phaeohyphomycosis | Subcutaneous and brain | Septate hyphae |
| | Sinusitis | Sinuses | Septate hyphae |
| Exserohilum spp. | Phaeohyphomycosis | Subcutaneous | Septate hyphae |
| Pseudallescheria boydii | Mycetoma | Subcutaneous | Granules of hyaline hyphae |
| | Phaeohyphomycosis | Subcutaneous, skin, joints, bones, brain, lungs | Septate, hyaline hyphae |
| Cladophialophora bantiana | Phaeohyphomycosis | Brain | Septate hyphae |

and/or hyphal fragments. Portions of hairs from a patient with black piedra are examined in wet mounts using potassium hydroxide that is gently heated for nodules composed of cemented mycelium. Crushing the mature nodules reveals oval asci, containing two to eight aseptate ascospores, 19 to 55 $\mu$m long by 4 to 8 $\mu$m in diameter. The asci are spindle shaped and have a filament at each pole.

**Chromoblastomycosis.** The laboratory diagnosis of chromoblastomycosis is made easily. Scrapings from crusted lesions added to 10% potassium hydroxide (KOH) show

sclerotic bodies, which are rounded, brown, 4 to 10 $\mu$m in diameter, and have fission planes. They resemble copper pennies (Figure 61-1).

**Mycetoma and Phaeohyphomycosis.** Direct examination of clinical specimens from patients with a eumycotic mycetoma or phaeohyphomycosis demonstrates yellowish brown, septate to moniliform hyphae, with or without budding yeast cells present. The presence of dematiaceous yeasts depends on the fungus. Dematiaceous yeasts are commonly seen in the direct examination of clinical

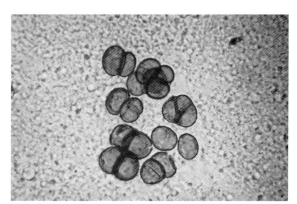

**Figure 61-1** Sclerotic bodies from the tissue of a patient with chromoblastomycosis (×400). (From Velasques LF, Restrepo A: Chromomycosis in the toad (*Bufo marinus*) and a comparison of the etiologic agent with fungi causing human chromomycosis, *Sabouraudia* 13:1,1975.)

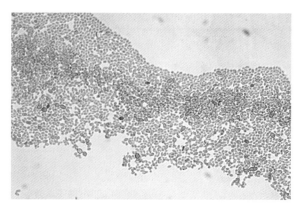

**Figure 61-2** Yeast forms of *Hortaea werneckii.*

specimens from patients with infections caused by *Exophiala* spp. Macroscopic examination of granules from mycetoma lesions caused by *P. boydii* reveal them to be white to yellow and 0.2 to 2 mm in diameter. Microscopically, the granules of *P. boydii* consist of loosely arranged, intertwined septate hyaline hyphae cemented together.

Observation of pigmented hyphae in hematoxylin-eosin or unstained histopathologic sections is presumptive for a diagnosis of dematiaceous fungal disease. The methenamine silver stain used to detect fungal elements in tissues stains fungi black, which makes determining whether they are hyaline septate or dematiaceous septate molds impossible. Fontana-Masson stain, which stains the melanin and melanin-like pigments in the cell walls of these organisms, may be used to confirm the presence of pigmented hyphae in histologic sections. Culture of the specific etiologic agent is necessary for final confirmation.

### Antigen-Protein

Antigen-protein–based assays are not used for the diagnosis of disease caused by these organisms.

### Nucleic Acid Amplification

Nucleic acid amplification assays are not routinely used for detection or identification of these organisms, although these tests may be available in research settings.

### Cultivation

Although dematiaceous molds recovered in the clinical mycology laboratory may represent true pathogens, more often they represent transient flora, inhaled spores, or contaminants. Cultures from sterile body sites, if aseptically obtained, should not contain these molds. Cultures should be interpreted in conjunction with the results of the direct examination for fungal elements, corresponding histopathology, and discussion with the clinician to most effectively establish the diagnosis of mycotic infection caused by these organisms.

**Superficial Infections.** *H. werneckii,* the causative agent of tinea nigra, may be recovered on common fungal media but grows very slowly. Initial colonies of *H. werneckii* may be olive to black, shiny, and yeastlike (Figure 61-2), and usually grow within 2 to 3 weeks. As the cultures age, colonies become filamentous, with velvety gray aerial hyphae. *P. hortae, the* causative agent of black piedra, is easily cultured on any fungal culture medium lacking cycloheximide. Colonies of this organism are also very slow growing, appear dark brown to black, and also produce aerial mycelium. Some isolates may produce a red to brown diffusible pigment.

### Mycetoma

**White Grain Mycetoma.** *P. boydii* grows rapidly (5 to 10 days) on common laboratory media. Initial growth begins as a white, fluffy colony that changes in several weeks to a brownish gray (the so-called mousy gray) colony; the reverse of the colony progresses from tan to dark brown. *Acremonium* spp. that cause mycetomas, such as *A. falciforme,* grow slowly and produce gray to brown colonies.

**Black Grain Mycetoma.** Colonies of *M. mycetomatis* and *E. jeanselmei* are slow growing, unlike colonies of *Curvularia* spp. Colonies of *M. mycetomatis* vary from white (during the early phases of growth) to olive-brown; a brown diffusible pigment is characteristic of this fungus. Colonies of *E. jeanselmei* appear yeastlike and darkly pigmented (olive to black), but in time develop a more velvety appearance with the production of aerial hyphae. *Curvularia* spp. produce a fluffy or downy, olive-gray to black colony, and growth is rapid.

**Chromoblastomycosis.** The fungi known to cause chromoblastomycosis, *Cladosporium, Cladophialophora, Phialophora* spp., and *Fonsecaea* spp., are all dematiaceous. These fungi are slow growing and produce heaped-up, slightly folded, darkly pigmented colonies with a gray to olive to black and velvety or suedelike appearance. The reverse side of the colonies is jet black. Microscopic examination is necessary to identify the pathogenic agent definitively.

**Phaeohyphomycosis.** The colonies of many of the rapidly growing dematiaceous molds are similar; therefore, identification relies on microscopic examination. The colonies of *Alternaria* spp. are rapidly growing, fluffy, and gray to gray-brown or gray-green. *Curvularia* spp. produce rapidly growing colonies that resemble those of *Alternaria* spp. *Bipolaris* spp. produce colonies that are gray-green to dark brown and slightly powdery, as do *Drechslera* spp. and *Exserohilum* spp.

The colonies of many of the slow-growing dematiaceous molds are also similar to one another and require identification based on microscopic morphology. *E. jeanselmei* and *E. dermatitidis* grow slowly (7 to 21 days) and initially produce shiny black, yeastlike colonies. *E. dermatitidis* often is mucoid and may be brown, compared with *E. jeanselmei*, but the two organisms are very similar in appearance. Colonies become filamentous and velvety with age as a result of the production of mycelium. The colonial morphology of other slowly growing dematiaceous fungi (e.g., *Fonsecaea* spp.) was described in the previous section.

## APPROACH TO IDENTIFICATION

### Superficial Infections

*H. werneckii* is a dematiaceous fungus that produces yeastlike cells that may be one or two celled. Conidia produced by this organism are produced by **annellophores** (conidia-forming cells that produce conidia containing transverse rings), which bear successive rings (**annellides**), which are difficult to see microscopically. The biophysical profile is used to differentiate this fungus from other *Exophiala* spp. In contrast, *P. hortae* usually does not sporulate on routine mycologic media but demonstrates highly septate, dematiaceous hyphae and swollen intercalary cells.

### Mycetoma

The specific etiologic agent of a eumycotic mycetoma cannot be determined without culturing the organism. Culture media containing antibiotics should not be used as the sole medium for culturing clinical specimens from a mycetoma, because species of the aerobic actinomycetes are susceptible to antibacterial antibiotics and may be inhibited by these agents. (See the bibliography for further information on other, less common fungi that cause mycetomas.)

**White Grain Mycetoma: *Pseudallescheria boydii* and *Acremonium* spp.** As previously mentioned, these fungi are hyaline molds that produce septate hyphae. The features described here are useful for identification regardless of the disease process (i.e., mycetoma or hyalohyphomycosis). *P. boydii* is also involved in causing a variety of infections elsewhere in the body. These include infections of the nasal sinuses and septum, meningitis, arthritis, endocarditis, mycotic keratitis, external otomycosis, brain abscess, and disseminated invasive infection. Most of these more serious infections occur primarily in immunocompromised patients.

*P. boydii* is an example of an organism that exhibits both asexual and sexual reproduction. The teleomorphic, or sexual, form of this fungus, which is evidenced by the production of cleistothecia, is *P. boydii*; if asexual reproductive structures alone are observed, the organism may be called *Scedosporium apiospermum*. The asexually produced conidia of *P. boydii/S. apiospermum* are

golden brown, elliptical to pyriform, and single celled and are borne singly from the tips of long or short conidiophores (annellophores) (see Figure 59-2). This **anamorph** (a fungus that disseminates reproductive structures without meiosis) predominates in cultures from clinical specimens. Another anamorphic form, the *Graphium* stage of *P. boydii*, may be seen less commonly. It consists of clusters of conidiophores with conidia produced at the ends; it has also been referred to as *coremia* (see Figure 59-3). The teleomorphic (sexual) form of the organism produces brown to black cleistothecia, which are pseudoparenchyatous, saclike structures containing asci and ascospores. When the latter are fully developed, the large (50 to 200 μm), thick-walled cleistothecia rupture, releasing the asci and ascospores (see Figure 59-1). Ascospores are oval and delicately pointed at each end. Isolates of *P. boydii* may be induced to form cleistothecia by culturing on plain water agar; however, they are seldom found on primary recovery of a culture from a clinical specimen. Recognition of *P. boydii* is important, because the organism is resistant to amphotericin B, an antifungal agent commonly used for systemic infections.

Another *Scedosporium* species, *S. prolificans*, has been associated with infections other than mycetomas, such as arthritis or invasive disease in immunocompromised patients. *S. prolificans* differs from *S. apiospermum* in that it produces inflated, flask-shaped annellophores. The obsolete or previous name for *S. prolificans* was *S. inflatum*, which more accurately reflects the morphology of the conidiophore. Recognition of this organism also is important, because it is resistant to most if not all the commonly used antifungal agents.

*Acremonium* spp. develops hyaline hyphae and produces simple, unbranched, erect conidiophores. Single-celled conidia are produced loosely or in gelatinous masses at the tip of the conidiophore (see Figure 59-17). Intercalary and terminal chlamydoconidia may also be produced.

**Black Grain Mycetoma: *Exophiala jeanselmei*, *Curvularia* spp., and *Madurella mycetomatis*.** Sterile hyphae are produced when *M. mycetomatis* is grown on rich fungal media. Nutritionally poor media may be used to induce sporulation. Long, tapering phialides with **collarettes** and **sclerotia** may be seen. Temperature tolerance, biochemical hydrolysis, and assimilation studies may be used to differentiate *M. mycetomatis* from *Madurella grisea*. (See Phaeohyphomycosis, later in the chapter, for the description of *E. jeanselmei* and *Curvularia* spp.)

**Chromoblastomycosis: *Cladosporium*, *Phialophora*, and *Fonsecaea* spp.** The taxonomy of the organisms that cause chromoblastomycosis is complex. Their identification is based on somewhat distinct microscopic morphologic features. These are polymorphic fungi that may produce more than one type of conidiation. The genus *Cladosporium* includes species that produce long chains of budding, often fusiform, conidia (blastoconidia) that have a dark septal scar. Some of these organisms have been reclassified into the genus *Cladophialophora*, because they also produce phialides; however, for the most part, the genus name *Cladosporium* is used in this chapter.

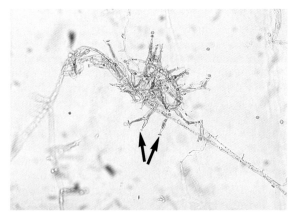

**Figure 61-3** *Phialophora richardsiae* showing phialides with prominent, saucerlike collarette *(arrows)* (×500).

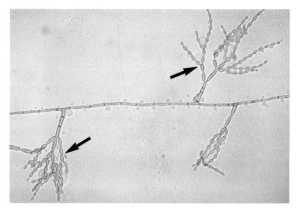

**Figure 61-4** *Cladosporium* spp. showing *Cladosporium* type of sporulation *(arrows)* with chains of elliptical conidia (×430).

The genus *Phialophora* includes species that produce short, flask-shaped to tubular phialides, each having a well-developed collarette. Clusters of conidia are produced by the phialides through an apical pore and often remain aggregated near the opening in a gelatinous mass. *Phialophora* spp. produce colonies that are wooly and olive-brown to brownish gray; some strains may appear to have concentric zones of color. Microscopically, hyphae are dematiaceous, and sporulation is common. *Phialophora richardsiae* produces phialides with distinct flattened or saucerlike collarettes (Figure 61-3). In contrast, *Phialophora verrucosa* produces deeper, more cup- or flask-shaped phialides. Pleomorphic phialides may also be seen with these species; however, all produce either or both hyaline elliptical conidia or brown elliptical conidia within the phialides.

The genus *Fonsecaea* includes organisms that exhibit a mixed type of sporulation. The genus produces a distinct *Fonsecaea*-type conidiophore, which somewhat resembles truncated *Cladosporium*-type sporulation. It may also produce a *Rhinocladiella*-type sporulation, in which single-celled conidia are produced on denticles that arise from all sides of conidiophores (sympodially). A mixture of the *Fonsecaea, Rhinocladiella,* and *Cladosporium* types may occur, and phialides with collarettes or *Phialophora*-type sporulation also may be present.

The diagnostic features of the *Cladosporium, Phialophora,* and *Fonsecaea* genera can be summarized as follows:

- *Cladosporium (Cladosporium carrionii):* Cladosporium type of sporulation with long chains of elliptical conidia (2-3 × 4-5 µm) borne from erect, tall, branching conidiophores (Figure 61-4).
- *Phialophora* spp.: *P. verrucosa* produces phialides, each with a distinct cup- or flask-shaped collarette (Figure 61-5); *P. richardsiae* produces phialides with a flattened collarette (see Figure 61-3). Conidia are produced endogenously and occur in clusters at the tip of the phialide.
- *Fonsecaea* spp.: Conidial heads with sympodial arrangement of conidia are seen, with primary conidia giving rise to secondary conidia (Figure 61-6). *Cladosporium*-type, *Phialophora*-type, and/or *Rhinocladiella*-type sporulation may also occur.

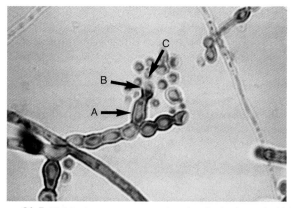

**Figure 61-5** *Phialophora verrucosa* showing flask-shaped phialide *(A)* with distinct collarette *(B)* and conidia *(C)* near its tip (×750).

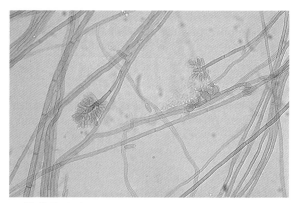

**Figure 61-6** Both the *Rhinocladiella* and *Phialophora* types of sporulation may be produced by *Fonsecaea pedrosoi* and are demonstrated here (×430).

**Phaeohyphomycosis:** *Alternaria, Bipolaris, Cladosporium, Curvularia, Drechslera, Exophiala, Exserohilum,* **and** *Phialophora* **spp.** A useful approach to identification of the dematiaceous molds is first to determine whether single-celled or multicelled conidia are produced. If conidia are produced singly, the laboratorian should determine whether they are produced individually or in chains

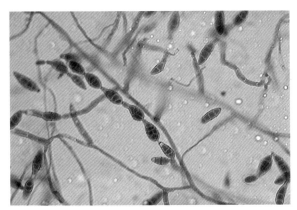

**Figure 61-7** *Alternaria* spp. showing chaining multiform dematiaceous conidia with horizontal and longitudinal septa.

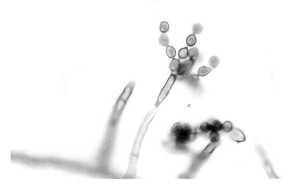

**Figure 61-9** *Cladosporium* spp. showing branching chains of dematiaceous blastoconidia that are easily dislodged during preparation of a microscopic mount (×430).

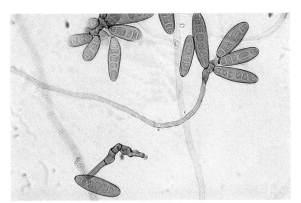

**Figure 61-8** *Bipolaris* spp. showing dematiaceous, multicelled conidia produced sympodially from geniculate conidiophores (×430).

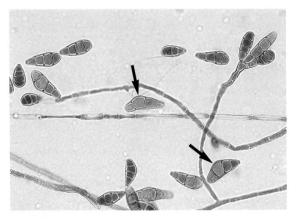

**Figure 61-10** *Curvularia* spp. showing twisted conidiophore and curved conidia with a swollen central cell *(arrows)* (×500).

(e.g., *Cladosporium* spp.). In cellophane tape preparations, the chains of conidia produced by *Cladosporium* spp. are easily disrupted. If multicellular conidia are produced, examining the septations within the conidium is useful. Multicellular conidia with septations in the horizontal axis of the conidium (i.e., the axis perpendicular to the longitudinal axis of the conidium) are characteristic of certain organisms, such as in *Bipolaris, Curvularia,* and *Drechslera* spp.; conidia with septations in both the longitudinal and horizontal axes of the conidium are characteristic of other fungi, such as *Alternaria* spp.

**Alternaria** **spp.** Microscopically hyphae are septate and golden brown pigmented; conidiophores are simple but sometimes branched. Conidiophores bear a chain of large, brown conidia resembling a drumstick and contain both horizontal and longitudinal septa (Figure 61-7). Observing chains of conidia sometimes is difficult, because they may be dislodged as the culture mount is prepared.

**Bipolaris** **spp.** Hyphae are dematiaceous and septate. Conidiophores, however, are characteristically bent **(geniculate)** at the locations where conidia are attached; conidia are arranged sympodially and are oblong to fusoid. The hilum protrudes slightly (Figure 61-8). Germ tubes are formed at one or both ends, parallel to the long axis of the conidium, when the fungus is incubated in water at 25°C for up to 24 hours (i.e., from both poles, thus the name *Bipolaris*).

**Cladosporium** **spp.** Microscopically hyphae are septate and brown. Conidiophores are long, branched, and give rise to branching chains of darkly pigmented, budding conidia. Conidia usually are single celled and exhibit prominent attachment scars **(dysjunctors).** The cells that produce the branch points are often referred to as **shield** cells (Figure 61-9). This organism frequently fails to reveal chains of conidia on wet mounts, because conidia are so easily dislodged.

**Curvularia** **spp.** Microscopically hyphae are dematiaceous and septate. Conidiophores are geniculate (i.e., bent where conidia are attached). Conidia are arranged sympodially and are golden brown, multicelled, and curved, with a central swollen cell (Figure 61-10). The end cells are lighter in color than the swollen cell.

**Drechslera** **spp.** Microscopically the hyphae are septate and darkly pigmented, and conidiophores are geniculate. Conidia are produced sympodially (Figure 61-11). However, sporulation is generally sparse with this organism and is not commonly seen. The conidia of *Drechslera* spp. are impossible to differentiate from those of *Bipolaris* spp. based on morphologic criteria alone.

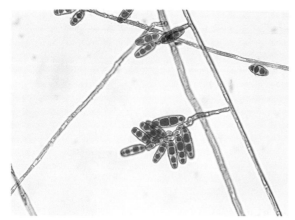

**Figure 61-11** *Drechslera* spp. showing dematiaceous, multicelled conidia. Most isolates produce only a few conidia.

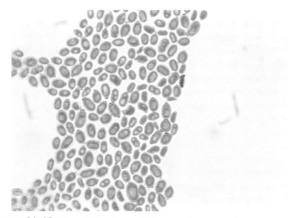

**Figure 61-12** *Exophiala dermatitidis* showing dematiaceous, yeast-like cells from a young culture. These forms asexually reproduce via annellides rather than through true buds (blastoconidiation) (×500).

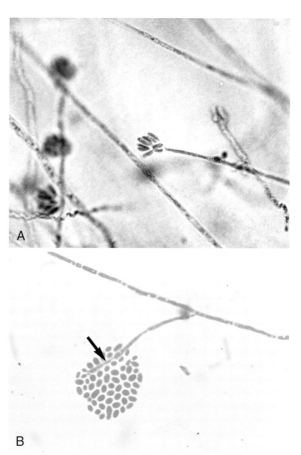

**Figure 61-13 A,** *Exophiala jeanselmei* showing elongated conidiophore (annellophore) with a narrow, tapered tip (×500). **B,** *Exophiala dermatitidis* showing elongated tubular annellophores *(arrow)*; morphologically very similar to *E. jeanselmei* (×500).

The germ tube test may be used to differentiate these organisms. Conidia are placed in a drop of water, a coverslip is applied, and the organism is observed after an incubation period of at least 24 hours. Any of the cells of the conidia belonging to *Drechslera* spp. may germinate, and these may grow perpendicular to the long axis of the conidium. In contrast, only the end cells of the conidia belonging to *Bipolaris* spp. germinate, and these grow predominantly parallel to the longitudinal axis of the conidium.

**Exophiala spp.** Only the *Exophiala* species *E. jeanselmei* and *E. dermatitidis* are considered here; although other species exist, they are recovered far less commonly in the clinical laboratory. The microscopic features of young colonies of *Exophilia sp.* exhibit dematiaceous, yeastlike cells (Figure 61-12). Although these may appear to be budding, close inspection may disclose that the daughter cells are produced by annellides rather than true buds. The microscopic features of young colonies of *Exophilia sp.* exhibit dematiaceous, yeastlike cells. Felt-like, filamentous colonies produce dematiaceous hyphae and conidiophores that are cylindrical and have a tapered tip.

Annellations may be visible at the tip, and clusters of oval to round conidia are apparent (Figure 61-13). Potassium nitrate is utilized by *E. jeanselmei* but not by *E. dermatitidis*. Temperature studies are also useful for differentiating the most common *Exophiala* species. Both *E. jeanselmei* and *E. dermatitidis* grow at 37°C, but only *E. dermatitidis* can grow at 40° to 42°C.

**Exserohilum spp.** Hyphae are septate and dematiaceous. Conidiophores are geniculate, and conidia are produced sympodially. Conidia are elongate, ellipsoid to fusoid, and exhibit a prominent hilum that is truncated and protruding (Figure 61-14). The conidia are multicellular, have perpendicular septa, and usually contain five to nine septa.

**Phialophora spp.** *P. richardsiae* is considered a cause of phaeohyphomycosis (see Chromoblastomycosis for a description of *P. richardsiae*).

## SERODIAGNOSIS

Some serologic and skin tests may be useful for the diagnosis of allergy to dematiaceous fungi. However, serology is not useful for the diagnosis of invasive dematiaceous fungal disease.

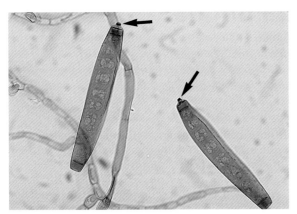

**Figure 61-14** *Exserohilum* spp. showing elongated, multicelled conidia with prominent hila *(arrows)*.

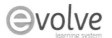
Visit the Evolve site to complete the review questions.

## CASE STUDY 61-1

A 54-year-old female presents to her physician with a mildly tender subcutaneous cyst on her right forefinger. She experienced trauma to her hand while gardening 6 weeks earlier. The cyst is punctured, and the exudate is examined microscopically and cultured. Direct microscopic examination reveals yeastlike cells and brown, pigmented, branching, septate hyphae. The culture is slow growing and initially develops a shiny black, yeastlike colony that ages to a filamentous, velvety texture with black reverse.

**QUESTIONS**

1. What genus of fungi should be considered?
2. If you saw cylindrical conidiophores that had annellations at the tips and clusters of conidia, what test or tests would you perform next to aid identification?
3. You find that this mold grows at 37°C but not at 42°C. What organism is this?

## ◼ BIBLIOGRAPHY

Abd El-Bagi ME, Abdul Wahab O, Al-Thaqafi MA, et al: Mycetoma of the hand, *Saudi Med J* 25:352, 2004.

Adam RD, Paquin ML, Petersen EA, et al: Phaeohyphomycosis caused by the fungal genera *Bipolaris* and *Exserohilum*: a report of 9 cases and review of the literature, *Medicine (Baltimore)* 65:203, 1986.

Ahmed AO, Van Leeuwen W, Fahal A, et al: Mycetoma caused by *Madurella mycetomatis*: a neglected infectious burden, *Lancet Infect Dis* 4:566, 2004.

Douer D, Goldschmied-Reouven A, Segev S, et al: Human *Exserohilum* and *Bipolaris* infections: report of *Exserohilum* nasal infection in a neutropenic patient with acute leukemia and review of the literature, *J Med Vet Mycol* 25:235, 1987.

McGinnis MR, Rinaldi MG, Winn RE: Emerging agents of phaeohyphomycosis: pathogenic species of *Bipolaris* and *Exserohilum*, *J Clin Microbiol* 24:250, 1986.

Palaoglu S, Sav AA, Basak TT, et al: Cerebral phaeohyphomycosis, *Neurosurgery* 33:894, 1993.

Pang KR, Wu JJ, Huang DB, et al: Subcutaneous fungal infections, *Dermatol Ther* 17:523, 2004.

Sakayama K, Kidani TT, Sugawara YY, et al: Mycetoma of the foot: a rare case report and review of the literature, *Foot Ankle Int* 25:763, 2004.

Spielberger RT, Tegtmeier BR, O'Donnell MR, et al: Fatal *Scedosporium prolificans (S. inflatum)* fungemia following allogeneic bone marrow transplantation: report of a case in the United States, *Clin Infect Dis* 21:1067, 1995.

Tintelnot K, von Hunnius P, de Hoog GS, et al: Systemic mycosis caused by a new *Cladophialophora* species, *J Med Vet Mycol* 33:349, 1995.

Whittle DI, Kominos S: Use of itraconazole for treating subcutaneous phaeohyphomycosis caused by *Exophiala jeanselmei*, *Clin Infect Dis* 21:1068, 1995.

Versalovic J: *Manual of clinical microbiology*, ed 10, Washington, DC, 2011, ASM Press.

# Opportunistic Atypical Fungus:
## *Pneumocystis jiroveci*

## OBJECTIVES

1. Describe the symptoms of *Pneumocystis jiroveci* infection and the cells affected by this organism.
2. List the appropriate specimen types collected for diagnosis of pneumocystis pneumonia.
3. Discuss the laboratory tests used in the diagnosis of *P. jiroveci* infection, including the methodology and biochemical principles.
4. List the four stains most commonly used in the diagnosis of *P. jiroveci* infection.

---

### GENUS AND SPECIES TO BE CONSIDERED

| Current Name | Previous Name |
| --- | --- |
| *Pneumocystis jiroveci* | *Pneumocystis carinii* |

---

## GENERAL CHARACTERISTICS

In 1999 the name of the organism that causes a pneumonia in immunocompromised humans, commonly called *pneumocystis pneumonia* (PCP), was changed from *Pneumocystis carinii* to *Pneumocystis jiroveci*. (The causative organism for the rodent form of pneumocystis is still called *P. carinii*.) *P. jiroveci* is an opportunistic, atypical fungus that infects immunocompromised hosts and mostly manifests as PCP.

*P. jiroveci* originally was thought to be a trypanosome, but its precise taxonomic categorization remains challenging. Several factors supported the notion that *P. jiroveci* was a protozoan parasite: its morphology is similar to that of microbes and protozoa, and clinically it responds to antiprotozoal drugs but not to antifungal drugs in patients with pneumocystosis. Inability to maintain and propagate the organism in routine culture has further limited its characterization, although cultivation is possible under special conditions. *P. jiroveci* exists as three forms in its life cycle: trophozoite, precyst (sporocyte), and cyst (the latter is the diagnostic form).

Although *P. jiroveci* has been shown to be a fungus, it differs from other fungi in various aspects. Its cell membrane contains cholesterol rather than ergosterol. The flexible-walled trophozoite is susceptible to osmotic disturbances. Also, *P. jiroveci* contains only one or two copies of the small ribosomal subunit gene, whereas most other fungi contain numerous copies of this gene. DNA sequence analysis of the small ribosomal subunit gene in *P. jiroveci* has disclosed a greater sequence homology with the fungi than with the protozoa. Two independent analyses that compared the DNA sequences of *P. jiroveci*

with those of other fungi confirmed the placement of *P. jiroveci* in the fungal kingdom, somewhere between the ascomycetes and the basidiomycetes (the closest yeast is the fission yeast, *Schizosaccharomyces pombe*). DNA analysis also confirmed the difference between the rodent and human forms of pneumocystis.

## EPIDEMIOLOGY

*P. jiroveci* has a worldwide distribution and most commonly presents as pneumonia in an immunocompromised host. As mentioned, infection appears to be species specific, with *P. carinii* causing disease in rodents and *P. jiroveci* causing human disease. The exact transmission of disease is still not known. Some speculate that pneumocystis is transmitted person to person. Immunocompetent mammals may be the reservoir for *P. jiroveci*, which is transmitted to immunodeficient individuals as a pathogen. Most children by age 2 to 4 have antibodies to pneumocystis. Vargas et al. showed that pneumocystis DNA was present in 24 of 72 infants, as determined from nasopharyngeal specimens, and that seroconversion occurred in 85% of infants by 20 months of age.

Since the onset of the human immunodeficiency virus/acquired immunodeficiency syndrome (HIV/AIDS) epidemic in the 1980s, pneumocystis has been defined as the most common opportunistic infection among those with HIV or AIDS in the United States. The introduction of highly active antiretroviral therapy (HAART) for patients with HIV has reduced the incidence of disease. However, PCP remains a significant medical problem, because numerous patients with HIV do not respond to therapy, do not comply with therapy, or do not know they are infected.

## PATHOGENESIS AND SPECTRUM OF DISEASE

After inhalation of *P. jiroveci*, the pathogen is thought to adhere to type I pneumocytes. The organisms replicate extracellularly while bathed in alveolar lining fluid. With successful replication of the organism, the alveolar spaces fill with foamy material, which can be detected with hematoxylin and eosin staining. These changes result in impaired oxygen-diffusing capacity and hypoxemia. A predominantly interstitial mononuclear inflammatory response is associated with this type of pneumonia. When first described, this pneumonia was known as interstitial plasma cell pneumonia.

Symptoms of PCP include a nonproductive cough, low-grade fever, dyspnea, chest tightness, and night sweats. In patients without HIV infection, the underlying conditions most commonly seen as risk factors for this opportunistic infection are asthma, chronic obstructive pulmonary disease (COPD), cystic fibrosis, systemic lupus erythematosus (SLE), pregnancy, rheumatoid arthritis, infection with Epstein-Barr virus, ulcerative colitis, and high-dose corticosteroid therapy.

# LABORATORY DIAGNOSIS

## SPECIMEN COLLECTION AND TRANSPORT

Respiratory specimens from the deep portions of the lung, such as bronchoalveolar lavage fluid (BALF), are best for detection of *P. jiroveci*. A sputum specimen submitted for direct examination should be an induced sputum obtained by a trained respiratory therapist; otherwise, the rate of false-negative results may be unacceptably high.

## SPECIMEN PROCESSING

See the following section for specific details for specimen processing required for different test methods.

## DIRECT DETECTION METHODS

### Stains

The diagnosis of *P. jiroveci* pneumonia currently is based on the clinical presentation, radiographic studies, and direct and/or pathologic examination of bronchoalveolar lavage fluid or biopsy material. The flexible-walled trophozoites are the predominant form of the organism, but these are difficult to visualize. They are somewhat discernible in Giemsa-stained material, but their pleomorphic appearance makes this form of the organism difficult to identify. A firm-walled cystic form also exists, although the cysts are outnumbered by the trophozoites 10 to 1. Cysts are more easily recognized than trophozoites and may be definitively identified using a variety of stains, such as calcofluor white, methenamine silver, and immunofluorescent staining (Figure 62-1). The cysts are spherical to concave, uniform in size (4 to 7 µm in diameter), do not bud, and contain distinctive intracystic bodies.

A comparison of the four most common staining methods used for *P. jiroveci* (i.e., Giemsa, immunofluorescent, calcofluor white, and methenamine silver) has demonstrated that immunofluorescent staining (Merifluor Pneumocystis; Meridian Bioscience, Cincinnati, Ohio), calcofluor white staining (Fungifluor; Polysciences, Warington, Pennsylvania), and methenamine silver staining (GMS and DiffQuick; Baxter Scientific, McGraw Park, Illinois) likely represent the best balance between sensitivity and specificity and have the best overall positive and negative predictive values. The

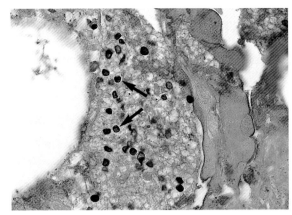

**Figure 62-1** Cystic forms of *Pneumocystis jiroveci (arrows)* stain well with methenamine silver and hematoxylin and eosin stain (×500).

immunofluorescent method showed greater sensitivity than the other three but a smaller negative predictive value. Therefore, if this method is used as a screening tool for pneumocystis, a confirmatory method should be performed because of the high number of false-positive results.

### Antigen-Protein

Commercial kits use monoclonal antibodies directed against *P. jiroveci* to stain both the cysts and the trophozoites. These tests are a highly sensitive microscopic method of detection, but they are expensive. Also, because they use nonspecific staining, which may be thought to represent the pleomorphic trophozoite forms, the specificity of this assay may be limited.

### Nucleic Acid Amplification

A variety of nucleic acid amplification assays for *P. jiroveci* have been developed, including, most recently, real-time polymerase chain reaction (PCR) methods. These methods are making their way from the research setting into the clinical molecular microbiology laboratory, but commercial kits are not yet available.

### Cultivation

*P. jiroveci* is very difficult to cultivate outside the lung; therefore, routine culture methods are not performed.

### Approach to Identification

See Direct Detection Methods.

### Serodiagnosis

Serology is not useful for the diagnosis of pneumocystosis.

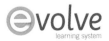 *Visit the Evolve site to complete the review questions.*

## CASE STUDY 62-1

A 69-year-old male is diagnosed with follicular lymphoma and placed on a 4-week regimen of combination chemotherapy. During the fourth week of treatment, the patient develops a fever that lasts 3 days. On the third day, he is admitted to the hospital. The findings from the initial physical exam are normal except for the fever. The following laboratory test results are obtained:

| | | |
|---|---|---|
| WBC count | 2500/$\mu$L | Normal: 4800-10,800/$\mu$L |
| Absolute neutrophil count | 1100/$\mu$L | Normal: 50% to 60% of WBCs |
| Serum beta-D glucan | 182 pg/mL | Normal: <20 pg/mL |
| CT scan of the lungs | Ground-glass opacities in the lung | |

These findings result in a diagnosis of interstitial pneumonia. The patient is treated with intravenous (IV) panipenem/betamipron, micafungin, and ganciclovir.

The patient does not seem to be recovering. After additional testing, he is switched to oral trimethoprim-sulfamethoxazole (TMP-SMX), and the lung infiltrates disappear within 2 weeks.

### QUESTIONS

1. What additional testing would have been performed to confirm the diagnosis of *Pneumocystis jiroveci*?
2. What patient characteristics would have contributed to the man's susceptibility to infection with *P. jiroveci*?

## ≡ BIBLIOGRAPHY

Bruns TD, Vilgalys R, Barns SM, et al: Evolutionary relationships within the fungi: analyses of nuclear small subunit rRNA sequences, *Mol Phylogenet Evol* 1:231, 1992.

Chagas C: Nova trypanosomiaze humana, *Mem Inst Oswaldo Cruz Rio J* 1:159, 1909.

Edman J, Kovacs JA, Masur H, et al: Ribosomal RNA sequence shows Pneumocystis to be a member of the fungi, *Nature* 334:519, 1988.

Edman J, Kovacs JA, Masur H, et al: Ribosomal RNA genes of Pneumocystis carinii, *J Protozool* 36:18S, 1989.

Giuintuli D, Stringer S, Stringer J: Extraordinary low number of ribosomal RNA genes in P. carinii, *J Eukaryot Microbiol* 41:88S, 1994.

Kaneshiro E, Ellis JE, Jayasimhulu K, et al: Evidence for the presence of "metabolic sterols" in Pneumocystis: identification and initial characterization of Pneumocystis carinii sterols, *J Eukaryot Microbiol* 41:78, 1994.

Kaplan JE, Hanson D, Dworkin MS, et al: Epidemiology of human immunodeficiency virus–associated opportunistic infections in the United States in the era of highly active antiretroviral therapy, *Clin Infect Dis* (30 Suppl 1):S5, 2000.

Procop GW, Haddad S, Quinn J, et al: Detection of Pneumocystis jiroveci in respiratory specimens by four staining methods, *J Clin Microbiol* 42:3333, 2004.

Stringer JR: Pneumocystis carinii: what is it, exactly? *Clin Microbiol Rev* 9:489, 1996.

Stringer SL, Stringer JR, Blase MA, et al: Pneumocystis carinii: sequence from ribosomal RNA implies a close relationship with fungi, *Exp Parasitol* 68:450, 1989.

Van der Peer Y, Hendriks L, Goris A, et al: Evolution of basidiomycetous yeasts as deduced from small ribosomal subunit RNA sequences, *Syst Appl Microbiol* 15:250, 1992.

Vargas SL, Hughes WT, Santolaya ME, et al: Search for primary infection by Pneumocystis carinii in a cohort of normal, healthy infants, *Clin Infect Dis* 32:855, 2001.

Walzer P: Pneumocystis carinii. In Mandell G, Bennett J, Dolin R, editors: *Principles and practice of infectious disease*, New York, 1995, Churchill Livingstone.

# The Yeasts

# GENERAL CHARACTERISTICS

Yeasts are eukaryotic, unicellular organisms that are round to oval and range in size from 2 to 60 $\mu$m. The microscopic morphologic features have limited usefulness in helping to differentiate or identify these organisms. The microscopic morphology on cornmeal agar is most useful when considered in conjunction with the biophysical profile (i.e., a combination of the biochemical and physical characteristics used in the identification of a microorganism) obtained using a commercial system. Differentiation of yeasts in direct microscopic and histopathologic examination of clinical specimens is often impossible, but sometimes particular characteristics are seen that suggest the identification or are pathognomonic (i.e., unique) for a particular organism. Important morphologic characteristics that are useful in differentiating yeasts include the size of the yeasts, the presence or absence of a capsule, and broad-based or narrow-necked budding. For example, variability in size with evidence of a capsule and narrow-necked budding are features that can be helpful for distinguishing *Cryptococcus* spp. from *Candida* spp. The medically important yeasts and yeastlike organisms belong to different taxonomic groups, including the Ascomycota, Basidiomycota, and Deuteromycota.

In general, the yeasts reproduce asexually by blastoconidia formation (budding) (Figure 63-1) and sexually by the production of ascospores or basidiospores. The process of budding begins with a weakening and subsequent outpouching of the yeast cell wall. This process continues until the bud, or daughter cell, is completely formed. The cytoplasm of the bud is contiguous with the cytoplasm for the original cell. Finally, a cell wall septum is created between mother and daughter yeast cells. The daughter cell often eventually detaches from the mother cell, and a residual defect occurs at the budding site (i.e., a bud scar).

With certain environmental stimuli, yeast can produce different morphologies. An outpouching of the cell wall that becomes tubular and does not have a constriction at its base is called a *germ tube;* it represents the initial stage of true hyphae formation (Figure 63-2). Alternatively, if buds elongate, fail to dissociate, and form subsequent buds, pseudohyphae are formed; to some, these resemble links of sausage (Figure 63-3). Pseudohyphae have cell wall constrictions rather than true intracellular septations delineating the fungal cell borders.

The number of fungal infections caused by yeasts and yeastlike fungi has increased significantly during recent years. Most of these infections have been caused by various *Candida* spp. However, other yeasts also cause significant disease, particularly in immunocompromised hosts, as yeasts are the cause of many opportunistic infections. In addition to causing disease in immunocompromised patients, infections also are common in postsurgical patients, trauma patients, and patients with long-term indwelling venous catheters. Some of these yeasts are resistant to commonly used antifungal agents, which emphasizes the need for prompt, appropriate identification and, in some cases, antifungal susceptibility testing.

The extent to which the laboratory should identify all yeast species is the subject of debate. Each laboratory director must decide how much time, effort, and expense is to be spent on the identification of yeasts in the laboratory.

The development of commercially available yeast identification systems has provided laboratories of all sizes with accurate, standardized methods. However, these methods should be used in conjunction with cornmeal agar morphology to prevent misidentifications. Some commercial systems have extensive computer databases that include biochemical profiles of a large number of yeasts. Variations in the reactions of carbohydrates and other substrates utilized are considered in the identification of yeasts provided by these systems.

Commercially available systems are recommended for all laboratories. They may be used in conjunction with some less expensive and rapid screening tests that provide presumptive identification of *C. neoformans* and definitive identification of *Candida albicans.*

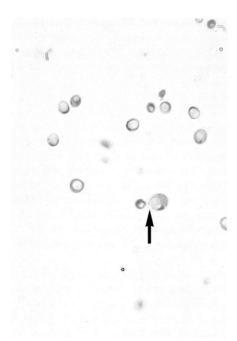

**Figure 63-1** Blastoconidia (budding cells *[arrow]*) characteristic of the yeasts.

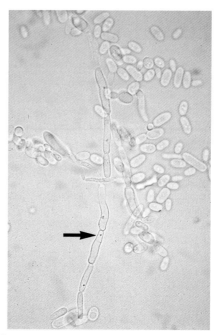

**Figure 63-3** Pseudohyphae consisting of elongated cells *(arrow)* with constrictions at attachment.

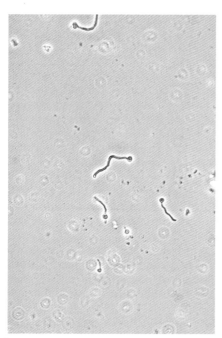

**Figure 63-2** Germ tube test for *C. albicans* showing yeast cells with germ tubes.

More recent diagnostic tools that have been introduced for quicker characterization of yeasts include CHROMagar Candida (BD Diagnostics, Sparks, Maryland) and *C. albicans* PNA FISH (AdvanDX, Woburn, Massachusetts). Because some laboratories might prefer to use conventional systems, the information presented in this section discusses rapid screening methods for presumptive identification of yeasts, commercially available systems, and a conventional schema for identifying commonly encountered yeast species.

# EPIDEMIOLOGY

## *CANDIDA* SPP.

*Candida* spp. are responsible for the most frequently encountered opportunistic fungal infections. Currently *Candida* spp. are the fourth most common cause of hospital-acquired bloodstream infections (BSIs) in the United States, and a mortality rate as high as 49% has been seen with these infections. *Candida* infections are caused by a variety of species. *C. albicans* is the most commonly isolated yeast, but other, emerging species include *Candida glabrata, Candida parapsilosis, Candida tropicalis, Candida dubliniensis,* and *Candida krusei.* The frequency with which these organisms are isolated varies by institution. Until recently *C. albicans* was the most common yeast isolated from infections, accounting for at least 60% to 70% of yeast infections. Epidemiologic data for the past decade reveal a paradigm shift in candidal infections. Studies from intensive care units (ICUs) confirm an increase in *C. glabrata* and *C. krusei* (isolated in approximately 25% of infections) and *C. albicans* (about 50% of infections). *C. albicans* and other *Candida* spp. are part of the human body's microbiota (i.e., normal flora), but they also have become endemic in most hospitals. Infections may be caused by endogenous yeasts or may be acquired in the hospital. Differentiating among the *Candida* spp. in the clinical laboratory is very important because of the differences in the virulence of the species and in their susceptibility to antifungal drugs.

## *CRYPTOCOCCUS* SPP.

*Cryptococcus neoformans-Cryptococcus gatti* complex has been divided into the two species and five serotypes. Serotype

A has been referred to as *C. neoformans* var. *grubii* with some groups recognizing the variant as a distinct species. Serotype D is now classified as *C. neoformans* var. *neoformans*. Both *C. neoformans* serotypes produce the teleomorphic state *Flobasidiella neoformans*. A *C. grubii/C. neoformans* hybrid exists that is a variant of serotypes A and D. Serotypes B and C are recognized as the independent species, *C. gattii*. Both serotypes B and C produce the teleomorph referred to as *Filobasidiella bacillispora*. Standard laboratory tests do not differentiate among the serotypes of *C. neoformans* and *C. gattii*.

*Cryptococcus* exists as a saprobe in nature. It is most associated with avian excreta, particularly pigeons. *C. neoformans* is thought to be widely distributed in nature, and aerosolization is a prerequisite to most infections.

### *TRICHOSPORON* AND *MALASSEZIA* SPP.

See the next section, Pathogenesis and Spectrum of Disease.

# PATHOGENESIS AND SPECTRUM OF DISEASE

## *CANDIDA ALBICANS*

Candidiasis is an infection caused by a *Candida* spp. It may include oroesophageal candidiasis, intertriginous candidiasis (in which skin folds are involved), paronychia, onychomycosis, perlèche respiratory infections, vulvovaginitis, thrush, pulmonary infection, eye infection, endocarditis, meningitis, fungemia or candidemia, or disseminated infection. Paronychia is an infection of the tissues surrounding the nails, and onychomycosis is an infection of the nail and nail bed. Thrush, an infection of the mucous membranes in the mouth, is considered a localized infection. Thrush can be seen in newborns, patients with human immunodeficiency virus (HIV) infection, individuals with diabetes, and patients undergoing chemotherapy. Creamy patches or colonies appear on the tongue and mucous membranes. *Candida* organisms may be recovered from the oropharynx, gastrointestinal (GI) tract, genitourinary tract, and skin.

The clinical significance of candidal organisms recovered from respiratory tract secretions is difficult to determine, because *Candida* spp. are considered part of the normal oropharyngeal flora of humans. A study at the Mayo Clinic evaluated the clinical significance of yeasts other than *C. neoformans* that are recovered from respiratory secretions. These researchers concluded that such yeasts are part of the normal flora and do not need to be routinely identified. Similarly, Barenfanger et al. demonstrated that routine identification of yeasts from respiratory specimens results in unnecessary antifungal therapy, an extended hospital stay, and increased health care costs without demonstrable benefit. Simultaneous recovery of the same species of yeast from several body sites, including urine, is a good indicator of disseminated infection and fungemia.

The pathogenesis of candidal infections is extremely complex and probably varies with each species. Adhesion of *Candida* organisms to the epithelium of the gastrointestinal or urinary tract is a crucial factor. *Candida* spp. commonly colonize mucosal surfaces. Their ability to invade and cause infection depends on adherence to the surface before infection. Three distinct aspartyl proteases have been described in *C. albicans*, and strains with high levels of proteases have been shown to have an increased ability to cause disease in experimental animal models. Hydrophobic molecules on the surface of *Candida* spp. also appear to be important in pathogenesis, and a strong correlation exists between adhesion and surface hydrophobicity. In addition, high levels of phospholipase, found in strains of *C. albicans*, have correlated with a higher mortality rate in experimental animals compared with experimental infections caused by strains that produce a lower level of phospholipase. Phenotypic switching (i.e., the ability to produce pseudohyphae and hyphae), seen in *C. albicans*, also may play a role in pathogenesis.

## NON-*ALBICANS* CANDIDA

The other *Candida* spp. (also called non-*albicans Candida*), once thought not to cause disease, are emerging as agents of infection in certain patient populations. The incidence of infection with *C. glabrata* is higher in older adults than in young adults and children. Recent studies have demonstrated the ability of *C. glabrata* to become resistant to common antifungal drugs. *C. tropicalis* has been shown to be prevalent in patients with hematologic malignancies, especially those who are neutropenic. Mouse models of infection and human studies have shown *C. tropicalis* in the tissues surrounded by necrotic tissues, which may indicate that the organism can invade the GI tract efficiently, particularly in oncology patients. This phenomenon most likely is due to the expression and secretion of aspartyl proteases and tropiase (acid proteinase), a virulence factor found in *Candida* organisms. Because *C. krusei* is inherently resistant to the azole class of antifungal drugs, identification of this species is essential to proper clinical management of the patient. *C. parapsilosis* is the primary cause of fungemia in the neonatal intensive care unit (NICU). *C. parapsilosis* is also the second most frequently isolated *Candida* spp. in positive blood cultures; this could be due partly to its known selective growth in hyperalimentation solutions and also to its ability to grow on intravascular catheters. Historically *C. parapsilosis* was categorized into three groups (I to III); however, it now has been typed by molecular methods into three different *Candida* species: *C. parapsilosis*, *C. orthopsilosis*, and *C. metapsilosis*.

## *CRYPTOCOCCUS NEOFORMANS*

### Genus Cryptococcus

Cryptococcoccosis is an acute, subacute, or chronic fungal infection that has several manifestations. *Crytococcus neoformans* var. *grubii*, *C. neoformans* var. *neofromans*, and *C. gatti* are considered the major human pathogens. Differences in the infections by *Cryptococcus neoformans* appear to be dependent on the host immune status and not the variant. *C. neoformans* infections can present initially as a chronic or subacute pulmonary infection. *C. neoformans* eventually makes its way to the central nervous system, where the yeast can cause cryptococcal meningitis. Disseminated disease with meningitis is commonly seen in immunocompromised patients. Patients with a moderately compromised immune system or who are early in the disease process of cryptococcal fungemia may present without concomitant meningitis. Disseminated cryptococcosis and cryptococcal meningitis became well recognized in patients with acquired immunodeficiency syndrome (AIDS), and they remain an important cause of morbidity and mortality in these patients in resource-poor countries that do not have access to highly active antiretroviral therapy.

Patients with disseminated infection may have painless papular skin lesions that may ulcerate. Other, less common manifestations of cryptococcosis include endocarditis, hepatitis, renal infection, and pleural effusion. Interestingly, a review of patient records at the Mayo Clinic revealed that more than 100 immunocompetent patients with *C. neoformans* colonization of the respiratory tract did not develop subsequent infection. Follow-up on these patients was as long as 6 years, and none in this group were considered to be immunocompromised. This makes the clinical significance of *C. neoformans* somewhat difficult to assess. However, given the severity of disease it can cause, its presence in clinical specimens should be considered significant. In many instances, the clinical symptoms are suppressed by corticosteroid therapy, which is a risk factor for disease, and culture or serologic evidence (detection of cryptococcal antigens) provides the earliest proof of infection. Cryptococcal infection is strongly associated with such debilitating diseases as leukemia and lymphoma and the immunosuppressive therapy that may be required for these and other underlying diseases. In some cases the presence of *C. neoformans* in clinical specimens precedes the symptoms of an underlying disease.

*C. neoformans* can exhibit a very characteristic polysaccharide capsule. The capsule collapses and protects the yeast from desiccation under drying conditions. The capsule of *C. neoformans* is thought to help the organism survive through the pigeon gut before it is excreted. The reduction in the yeast's cell size caused by capsular collapse places the organism in the ideal size range for alveolar deposition in the human host. In addition, a virulent property of the polysaccharide capsule is that it contains compounds that phagocytes do not recognize. The so-called acapsular strains of *C. neoformans*, which actually just have a very reduced capsule, are more easily phagocytosed. In some instances, *C. neoformans* elicits minimal tissue response in infected individuals, particularly severely immunocompromised patients.

Phenoloxidase, an enzyme found in *C. neoformans*, is responsible for melanin production. Some have speculated that melanin might act as a virulence factor by making the organism resistant to leukocyte attack. Evidence also has been presented that increased melanin production can decrease immune system functions, such as lymphocyte proliferation and tumor necrosis factor production. Whether phenoloxidase is truly a virulence factor has yet to be determined (Li SS, et al, 2010. (Cryptococcus. 2010 Proc Am Thorac Soc Vol 7 pp 186-196,

2010). An interesting question is whether the interactions of substances in the brain that are known to react with phenoloxidase may play a role in the affinity of *C. neoformans* and certain neurotropic dematiaceous fungi for invading the central nervous system (Li et al, 2010).

### CRYPTOCOCCUS GATTII

*C. gattii* was thought to be a variant of *C. neoformans* until genetic studies proved it to be a distinct species. Since the 1990s this organism has emerged in the Pacific Northwest as a pathogen in immunocompetent hosts—a major difference from *C. neoformans*, which causes disease in primarily immunodeficient hosts. Some speculate that *C. gattii* is able to modulate the host's immune system by reducing the inflammatory response or evading the immune system completely.

### TRICHOSPORON SPP.

Trichosporonosis is caused by a variety of *Trichosporon* spp., which have undergone changes in nomenclature based on DNA sequence comparisons. The yeastlike fungus causes disease almost exclusively in immunocompromised patients, particularly those with leukemia. Disseminated trichosporonosis is the most common clinical manifestation. Skin lesions accompanied by fungemia are frequently seen. Endocarditis, endophthalmitis, and brain abscess have been reported. *Trichosporon* organisms occasionally are recovered from respiratory tract secretions, skin, the oropharynx, and the stool of patients with no evidence of infection and may represent transient fungal colonization of those individuals.

White piedra, an uncommon fungal infection of immunocompetent patients, is found in both tropical and temperate regions of the world. It is characterized by the development of soft, yellow or pale brown aggregations around hair shafts in the axillary, facial, genital, and scalp regions of the body. The *Trichosporon* spp. that cause this disease frequently invade the cortex of the hair, causing damage.

### MALASSEZIA SPP.

*Malassezia furfur* causes tinea versicolor, a skin infection characterized by superficial, brownish, scaly areas on light-skinned individuals and lighter areas on dark-skinned people. The lesions occur on the smooth surfaces of the body, namely, the trunk, arms, shoulders, and face. The disorder has a worldwide distribution. *M. furfur* is also a cause of disseminated infection in infants and young children and even in adults given lipid replacement therapy. *Malassezia pachydermatis*, another species, may be recovered from skin lesions. In rare cases it may cause fungemia in immunocompromised patients.

## ▪ LABORATORY DIAGNOSIS

### SPECIMEN COLLECTION, TRANSPORT, AND PROCESSING

See Chapter 59.

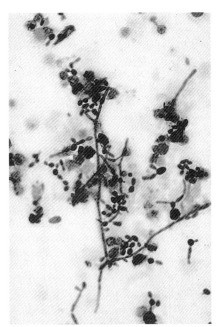

**Figure 63-4** Periodic acid-Schiff (PAS) staining of urine demonstrates blastoconidia and pseudohyphae of *Candida albicans*.

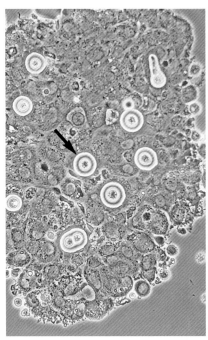

**Figure 63-5** Potassium hydroxide preparation of pleural fluid shows the encapsulated, variably sized, spherical yeast cells *(arrow)* of *Cryptococcus neoformans* (phase-contrast microscopy).

## Stains

***Candida* spp.** Direct microscopic examination of clinical specimens containing *Candida* organisms reveals budding yeast cells (blastoconidia) 2 to 4 μm in diameter and/or pseudohyphae (Figure 63-4) showing regular points of constriction, resembling links of sausage. True septate hyphae (filamentation) may also be produced by *C. albicans* and *C. dubliniensis*. The blastoconidia, hyphae, and pseudohyphae are strongly gram positive. The approximate number of such forms should be reported, because the presence of large numbers in a fresh clinical specimen may have diagnostic significance. Microscopically *C. glabrata* blastoconidia are notably smaller (at 1 to 4 μm) than those of other medically significant *Candida* spp.

***Cryptococcus* spp.** Traditionally, the India ink preparation has been the most widely used method for the rapid detection of *C. neoformans* in clinical specimens. This method is still used as a rapid and inexpensive assessment tool in many institutions and has considerable diagnostic value in resource-poor settings. This method delineates the large capsule of *C. neoformans*, because the ink particles cannot penetrate the capsular polysaccharide material. Although this test is useful, many laboratories have replaced it with the more sensitive cryptococcal latex agglutination test that detects cryptococcal antigen. (The cryptococcal antigen detection [CAD] test is described later in the chapter.) The India ink preparation is commonly positive in specimens from patients with AIDS and has been shown to have a sensitivity of 50% in patients who do not have HIV or AIDS. Laboratories that examine many specimens from these patients may want to continue using this procedure in combination with the CAD test and culturing.

Microscopic examination of other clinical specimens, including respiratory secretions, can be valuable for making a diagnosis of cryptococcosis. *C. neoformans* appears as a spherical, single or multiple budding, thick-walled yeast 2 to 15 μm in diameter. It usually is surrounded by a wide, refractile polysaccharide capsule (Figure 63-5). Perhaps the most important characteristic of *C. neoformans* is the extreme variation in the size of the yeast cells; this is unrelated to the amount of polysaccharide capsule present. It is important to remember that not all isolates of *C. neoformans* exhibit a discernible capsule.

***Trichosporon* spp.** Microscopic examination of clinical specimens that contain *Trichosporon* spp. reveals hyaline hyphae, numerous round to rectangular arthroconidia, and occasionally a few blastoconidia. Usually hyphae and arthroconidia predominate. In white piedra, white nodules are removed and observed using the potassium hydroxide (KOH) preparation after light pressure is applied to the coverslip to crush the nodule. Hyaline hyphae 2 to 4 μm wide and arthroconidia are found in the preparation of the cementlike material that binds the hyphae together. The organism may be identified in culture by the presence of true hyphae, blastoconidia, and arthroconidia in conjunction with a positive urease (see Figure 60-40). Although *Trichosporon asahii* may be distinguished from other *Trichosporon* species by its biophysical profile (carbohydrate and substrate utilization), these organisms are likely best distinguished at the species level with molecular tools, such as DNA sequencing.

***Malassezia* spp.** *M. furfur* most often is detected through direct microscopic examination of skin scrapings. The organism is easily recognized as oval- or bottle-shaped cells that exhibit monopolar budding in the presence of a cell wall with a septum at the site of the bud scar. Small hyphal fragments also are observed (Figure 63-6); the morphology is commonly described as "spaghetti and meatballs." In cases of fungemia, the morphologic form

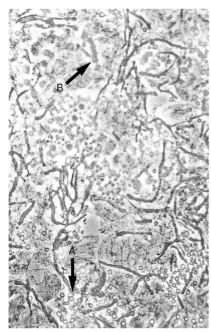

**Figure 63-6** Potassium hydroxide preparation of a skin scraping from a patient with tinea versicolor demonstrates spherical yeast cells *(A)* and short hyphal fragments *(B)* of *Malassezia furfur.* (Phase-contrast microscopy; ×500.)

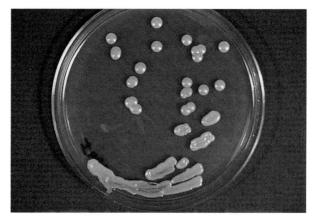

**Figure 63-7** Colonies of *Cryptococcus neoformans* appear shiny and mucoid because of the presence of a polysaccharide capsule.

seen in direct examination of blood cultures is small yeasts without the presence of pseudohyphae.

### Antigen Detection

The CAD test for *C. neoformans* may be performed on CSF or serum. In many laboratories this assay has replaced the use of India ink to screen for *C. neoformans*. It should be noted that *Trichosporon* spp. produce an antigen similar to that of *C. neoformans*. Sera from patients who have trichosporonosis often yield false-positive CAD tests when latex agglutination methods are used.

### Molecular Assays

Nucleic acid amplification tests (NAATs) have been developed for a variety of yeast species. However, these are usually performed in research settings. Most are labeled as "laboratory-developed tests" or "home-brewed tests," and few have been approved by the U.S. Food and Drug Administration (FDA). Real-time polymerase chain reaction (PCR) methods are now commercially available in the TaqMan system (Applied Biosystems, USA) and LightCycler (Roche Molecular Systems, Indianapolis, Indiana). These methods are very expensive but have proven to be much more specific than conventional yeast identification methods. Ligouri et al. recently demonstrated the Multiplex PCR method for identifying *Candida* spp. that has high concordance with commercially available phenotypic identification systems, such as the API 20C AUX (bioMérieux, Durham, North Carolina) and Vitek 2 YST card (bioMérieux, Durham, North Carolina). The Multiplex PCR method is much faster and more sensitive than the current phenotypic tests. A newer molecular test, the PNA FISH kit, uses in situ hybridization to detect *Candida* organisms in blood

culture bottles by targeting specific rRNA sequences. Subculturing should follow this method, because whether more than one species is present cannot be determined. Colonies may also display protrusions from the colony, resembling a star or foot-like projections on blood agar.

### Cultivation

***Candida* spp.** The colonial and microscopic morphologic features of *Candida* spp. have little value for making a definitive identification. Most *Candida* spp. produce smooth, creamy white colonies, but some produce dry, wrinkled, dull colonies. In 50% of autopsy-proven cases of invasive candidiasis, organisms could not be isolated from blood culture bottles. Newer blood culture systems, such as the automated BACTEC (Becton Dickinson, Franklin Lakes, NJ) and BacT/ALERT (Biomerieux, Durham, N.C.), have increased the recovery of *Candida* spp.

***Cryptococcus* spp.** *C. neoformans* is easily cultured on routine fungal culture media without cycloheximide. The organism is inhibited by the presence of cycloheximide at 25° to 30°C. For optimal recovery of *C. neoformans* from cerebrospinal fluid, a 0.45-mm membrane filter should be used with a sterile syringe. The filter is placed on the surface of the culture medium and is removed at daily intervals so that growth under the filter can be visualized. An alternative to the membrane filter technique is culture after centrifugation.

Colonies of *C. neoformans* usually appear on culture media within 1 to 5 days. The growth begins as a smooth, white to tan colony that may be mucoid to creamy (Figure 63-7). It is important to recognize the colonial morphology on different culture media, because variation does occur; for example, on inhibitory mold agar, *C. neoformans* appears as a golden yellow, nonmucoid colony. Textbooks typically characterize the colonial morphology as being *Klebsiella*-like because of the large amount of polysaccharide capsule material present. In reality, most isolates of *C. neoformans* do not have large capsules and may not have the typical mucoid appearance.

***Trichosporon* spp.** Colonies of *Trichosporon* spp. vary in their morphology; however, most are cream colored, heaped, dry to moist, and wrinkled. Some may appear white, dry, and powdery.

***Malassezia* spp.** *M. furfur* is infrequently cultured in the clinical laboratory. Recovery of the organism is not required to establish a diagnosis (in skin infections), and it is seldom attempted for this purpose. Cultivation, such as from a positive blood culture, requires an agar medium overlaid with a long-chain fatty acid (olive oil). The colonies are small compared with the colonies of *C. albicans* and are creamy and white to off-white.

## APPROACH TO IDENTIFICATION

The general approach to yeast identification consists of evaluating the carbohydrate and substrate utilization profile with a commercial system and observing the morphology in a cornmeal preparation. This latter aspect is particularly important for discovering any errors in identification that may have been made by the commercial system and prevents the release of an erroneous identification to the clinician. For example, if a commercial system designates an isolate as *C. glabrata* but pseudohyphae are seen in the cornmeal preparation, additional testing is needed to identify the isolate correctly, because *C. glabrata* does not produce pseudohyphae. This traditional approach could be modified to use newer methods of confirmation, such as CHROMagar Candida.

### *Candida* spp.

*C. albicans* may be identified by the production of germ tubes or chlamydoconidia (Figure 63-8; also see Figure 63-2). Other *Candida* spp. are most commonly identified by the utilization of specific substrates and the fermentation or assimilation of particular carbohydrates. For instance, *C. glabrata* ferments and assimilates only glucose and trehalose, whereas *C. tropicalis* ferments and assimilates sucrose and maltose. Another method of identifying *C. albicans* and differentiating it from other *Candida* spp. is based on the presence of chlamydoconidia (see Figure 63-8) on cornmeal agar containing 1% Tween 80 and trypan blue incubated at room temperature for 24 to 48 hours. (Many of the finer points of yeast identification are discussed in *The Yeasts: A Taxonomic Study*, by Kreger-Van Rij.) The morphologic features of yeasts on cornmeal agar containing Tween 80 often allow for tentative identification of selected species and, an important benefit, may detect misidentifications by commercial systems (Table 63-1).

Colonies that appear star-like or possess feet-like projections on agar, as previously described on blood agar, may be identified as *C. albicans*, according to the Clinical Laboratory Standards Institute document M35-A2. However, this method is not as sensitive as traditional methods when colonies are examined within 18 to 24 hours versus 24- to 48-hour incubation times. In addition, species such as *Trichosporon* spp. may give false-positive results for possessing the pseudohyphal fringe that appears as starting on blood agar. A Gram stain of the isolate would provide a means of differentiation of the isolate as *Trichosporon* spp. by the characteristic presence of arthroconidia. The susceptibility profiles of *C. albicans* and *Trichosporon* spp. would also be significantly different.

### Germ Tube Test

The germ tube test (see Procedure 63-1 on the Evolve site) is the most generally accepted and economical method used in the clinical laboratory to identify yeasts.

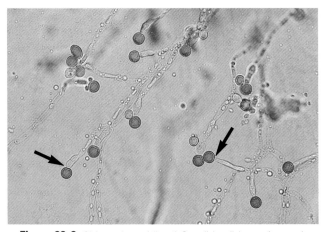

**Figure 63-8** Chlamydoconidia of *Candida albicans* (arrows).

**TABLE 63-1** Characteristic Microscopic Features of Commonly Encountered Yeasts on Cornmeal Tween 80 Agar

| Organism | Arthroconidia/ Blastoconidia | Pseudohyphae or Hyphae |
|---|---|---|
| Candida albicans | Spherical clusters at regular intervals on pseudohyphae | Chlamydoconidia present on hyphae |
| Candida glabrata | Small, spherical, and tightly compacted | None produced |
| Candida krusei | Elongated; clusters occur at septa of pseudohyphae | Branched pseudohyphae |
| Candida parapsilosis | Present but not characteristic | Sagebrush or "shaggy star" appearance; large (giant) hyphae present |
| Candida kefyr (pseudotropicalis) | Elongated, lie parallel to pseudohyphae | Pseudohyphae present but not characteristic |
| Candida tropicalis | Produced randomly along hyphae or pseudohyphae | Pseudohyphae present but not characteristic |
| Cryptococcus spp. | Round to oval, vary in size, separated by a capsule | Rare; usually not seen |
| Saccharomyces spp. | Large and spherical | Rudimentary hyphae sometimes present |
| Trichosporon spp. | Numerous, resemble Geotrichum spp.; septate hyphae present | May be present but difficult to find |

Approximately 75% of the yeasts recovered from clinical specimens are *C. albicans,* and the germ tube test usually provides sufficient identification of this organism within 3 hours.

Germ tubes appear as early hyphal-like extensions of yeast cells that are produced without a constriction at the point of origin from the yeast cell (see Figure 63-2). Another *Candida* species, *C. dubliniensis,* has been shown to also produce true germ tubes. Although *C. dubliniensis* is infrequently encountered, supplemental biochemical or morphologic testing may be needed to differentiate it from *C. albicans. C. tropicalis* produces what has been called "pseudo-germ tubes," which are constricted at the base or point of germ tube origin from the yeast cell. Unless this is recognized and the laboratorian has developed the skills to distinguish between true germ tubes and pseudo-germ tubes, *C. tropicalis* isolates will be misidentified as *C. albicans.*

The search for a more rapid, less subjective method of identifying *C. albicans* and other *Candida* spp. continues. *C. albicans* produces beta-galactose aminidase and L-proline aminopeptidase. Other *Candida* spp. may produce one enzyme but not both. Assays such as BactiCard Candida (Remel Laboratories, Lenexa, Kansas), were designed to detect these enzymes.

Heelan et al. compared the germ tube test to Bacti-Card, Murex C. albicans-50, Albicans-sure, and the API 20C AUX yeast identification systems. All rapid enzymatic screening methods were sensitive and specific for rapid identification of *C. albicans.* Compared with the germ tube test, all required less time (5 to 30 minutes), were more expensive, and required some additional equipment. Overall, all methods provided rapid and objective alternatives to the germ tube test.

CHROMagar Candida is another product that uses enzymatic reactions to differentiate *C. albicans* and several other yeast species. More recently C. albicans PNA FISH was released for detection and differentiation of *C. albicans* from non-*albicans* Candida spp. directly in positive blood cultures that contain yeast. The use of any new or additional testing for identification of yeasts should be submitted to a financial impact and outcomes analysis and should be compared with the traditional identification methods. Thereafter, the medical director, in conjunction with the medical staff, may determine the optimal approach for the laboratory.

### *Cryptococcus neoformans*

Microscopic examination of colonies of *C. neoformans* may be helpful for providing a tentative identification of *C. neoformans,* because the cells are spherical and vary considerably in size. A presumptive identification of *C. neoformans* may be based on rapid urease production and failure to utilize an inorganic nitrate substrate. Final identification of *C. neoformans* usually is based on typical substrate utilization patterns and, in some laboratories, pigment production on niger seed (thistle or birdseed) agar (Figure 63-9). Immunocompromised patients suffering from infection die each year, with an estimated 500,000 in Africa alone. Diagnosis is typically made by identifying the encapsulated yeast in the spinal fluid using India ink. The use of serological techniques for the

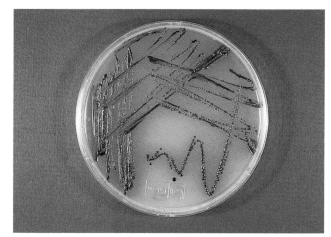

**Figure 63-9** *Cryptococcus neoformans* colonies are brown when grown on niger seed agar.

detection of the cryptococcal polysaccharide capsule glucuronoxylamannan (GXM) may be completed using latex agglutination or enzyme-linked immunosorbent assay (ELISA). A recent study demonstrated that plasma and urine can be used to identify cryptococcal antigen, thereby eliminating the need for the invasive spinal tap. The use of alternate specimens has the potential to improve screening of patients infected with HIV and reduced CD4 lymphocyte counts before the exacerbation of symptoms, which may not be apparent early enough for successful treatment of the infection. Additional tests useful for identifying *C. neoformans* and other species of cryptococci are discussed later in the chapter.

### Rapid Urease Test

The rapid urease test (see Procedure 63-2 on the Evolve site) is a most useful tool for screening for urease-producing yeasts recovered from respiratory secretions and other clinical specimens. Alternatives to this method include use of a heavy inoculum of the tip of a slant of Christensen's urea agar and subsequent incubation at 35° to 37°C. In many instances, a positive reaction occurs within several hours; however, 1 to 2 days of incubation may be required. Interestingly, strains of *Rhodotorula* spp., some *Candida* spp., and *Trichosporon* spp. hydrolyze urea with time, so a distinction should be made between a traditional urease test, which takes hours, and the rapid urease test.

The microscopic morphologic features of the yeast in question are helpful for interpreting the usefulness of the traditional urease test. An alternative to traditional urease testing is the rapid selective urease test (see Procedure 63-3 on the Evolve site). This method appears to be useful for rapidly detecting *C. neoformans.* These screening tests are helpful for making a presumptive identification of *C. neoformans.* When inoculum is limited, the laboratorian must use tests that can be performed and then prepare a subculture so that additional tests can be performed later. Often, inoculating the organism onto the surface of a plate of niger seed agar is just as fast, and results may be obtained during the same day of incubation at 25°C (this is discussed later in this section).

All the tests mentioned provide a tentative identification of *C. neoformans*; however, they must be supplemented with additional tests (usually the results of a commercial system in conjunction with cornmeal agar morphology) before a final identification can be reported. Additional tests useful in the identification of potential cryptococci are the nitrate reduction test and the detection of phenoloxidase production.

### *Trichosporon* spp.

The presence of contiguous arthroconidia that are rectangular, often with rounded ends, and predominate, along with septate hyaline hyphae, raises the possibility of *Trichosporon* spp. Blastoconidia are sometimes present but are not seen in all cultures. Urease production is helpful for differentiating *Trichosporon* spp., which are positive, from *Blastoschizomyces* and *Geotrichum* spp., which are negative. Final identification is based on the characteristic substrate utilization.

### *Malassezia* spp.

*M. furfur* may be recovered from the blood of patients who have fungemia. In most instances the residual lipid (from lipid replacement therapy) is adequate to support primary growth of the organism in the blood culture. However, subculture onto additional media requires overlaying of the inoculum by olive oil or another source of long-chain fatty acids. These findings, in conjunction with the "bowling pin" or "pop bottle" morphology, are sufficient for identification. Other *Malassezia* spp. do not require long-chain fatty acids and are traditionally identified using substrate utilization analysis in conjunction with cornmeal agar morphology.

# COMMERCIALLY AVAILABLE YEAST IDENTIFICATION SYSTEMS

Commercially available yeast identification systems have provided laboratories of all sizes with standardized identification methods. For the most part, the methods are rapid, providing results within 24 to 72 hours. The major advantage is that the systems provide an identification based on a database of thousands of yeast biotypes that considers a number of variations and substrate utilization patterns. Another advantage is that manufacturers of these products provide computer consultation services to help the laboratorian identify isolates that produce an atypical result. Although these systems are powerful tools, they should not be used as the sole method of identification; traditionally, they are most effectively used in conjunction with yeast morphology on blood, chocolate, or cornmeal agar.

## API-20C AUX YEAST SYSTEM

The API-20C AUX yeast identification system has perhaps the most extensive computer-based data set of all commercial systems available. The system consists of a strip that contains 20 microcupules, 19 of which contain dehydrated substrates for determining the utilization profiles of yeasts. Reactions are compared with growth (turbidity) in the first cupule, which lacks a carbohydrate substrate. Reactions are read and results are converted to a seven-digit biotype profile number. Most of the yeasts are identified within 48 hours; however, some *Cryptococcus* and *Trichosporon* spp. may require up to 72 hours. The API-20C AUX yeast identification system, as well as all other commercially available products, requires that the microscopic morphologic features of yeast grown on cornmeal agar containing 1% Tween 80 and trypan blue be used in conjunction with the substrate utilization patterns. This is particularly helpful when more than one possibility for an identification is provided; the microscopic morphologic features can be used to distinguish between the possibilities given by the profile register.

Several evaluations of the API-20C AUX yeast identification system have been performed, and the results have all been favorable. This system is limited in that it cannot identify unusual species; however, most of those seen in the clinical laboratory are accurately identified to the species level, especially the non-germ tube forming *Candida* spp. When this system is used to differentiate *C. albicans* from *C. dubliniensis*, assimilation results for xylose and alpha-methyl-D-glucoside may help distinguish between the two species. The results are negative for *C. dubliniensis* in 100% and 95% of the strains and positive for *C. albicans* in 100% and 95% of the strains.

## MICROSCAN YEAST IDENTIFICATION PANEL

The MicroScan Yeast Identification Panel (Siemens, Deerfield, Illinois) is a 96-well, microtiter plate containing 27 dehydrated substrates. It was introduced as an alternative to the API-20C AUX yeast identification system. It uses chromogenic substrates to assess specific enzyme activity, which can be detected within 4 hours. Specific enzyme profiles have been generated for many of the yeasts commonly encountered in the clinical microbiology laboratory. The most recent evaluation of the method showed that it was moderately accurate within 4 hours using no supplementary tests. When supplementary tests were used, the sensitivity was excellent compared with that of the API-20C AUX yeast identification system. Accuracy for identification of common yeasts was high, and uncommon yeasts were identified in most instances.

## VITEK BIOCHEMICAL CARDS

The Yeast Biochemical Card (bioMérieux, Durham, North Carolina) is a 30-well, disposable plastic card that contains conventional biochemical tests and negative controls. It is used with the automated Vitek II system (BioMérieux, Durham, North Carolina), which is used for bacterial identification and susceptibility testing in many laboratories. The most recent evaluation of this system showed an overall accuracy of identification near 100% compared with API-20C AUX. Fewer than one fourth of the yeasts required supplemental biochemical or morphologic features to confirm their identification. Of all correctly identified yeasts, more than half were reported after 24 hours of incubation. The accuracy of identification of common and uncommon species was satisfactory. Identifying germ tube–positive yeasts is not necessary with this system. For laboratories already using this system, accurate and reliable identification of most commonly encountered yeasts can be accomplished.

Interest in commercially available yeast identification systems has taken precedence over the more cumbersome, labor-intensive conventional yeast identification methods. Currently the rapid identification methods are financially feasible and provide laboratories of all sizes with the capability to identify yeasts. Commercially available systems, which provide accurate and rapid identification of yeasts and yeastlike organisms, are recommended for all laboratories. In general, they are easy to use, easy to interpret, and relatively inexpensive compared with conventional methods. In most cases they are faster than conventional systems, provide more standardized results, and require less technical skill to perform. As with any system, uncommon identifications should be scrutinized to prevent misidentifications.

## CHROMAGAR CANDIDA

CHROMagar is a differential medium useful for the recovery of *Candida* organisms in clinical specimens, differentiation of *Candida* spp., and isolation of colonies. Distinct enzymes of different *Candida* spp. react with chromogenic substrates to yield a characteristic colony color. When used with colonial morphologic features, this system can provide a presumptive identification. Sand-Millan et al. reported an evaluation of 1537 isolates of yeast, which after 48 hours of incubation at 37°C showed that CHROMagar had a sensitivity and specificity near 100% for *C. albicans*, *C. tropicalis*, and *C. krusei*. Another evaluation by Pfaller et al. showed that more than 95% of stock and clinical isolates of *C. albicans*, *C. tropicalis*, and *C. krusei* were correctly identified. A similar sensitivity was observed for *C. glabrata*. CHROMagar also was evaluated as a recovery medium and was found to detect mixed cultures of *Candida* spp. Considering that the previously mentioned species account for approximately 90% of the yeast recovered in the clinical laboratory, CHROMagar appears to be a suitable alternative to other yeast identification systems.

## MATRIX-ASSISTED LASER DESORPTION IONIZATION TIME-OF-FLIGHT (MALDI-TOF)

Matrix-assisted laser desorption ionization time-of-flight mass spectrometry (MALDI-TOF) is emerging as a potential rapid technique for the identification of yeast and fungal isolates within the microbiology laboratory. See Chapter 7 for more information. MALDI-TOF requires that isolates be cultured overnight and then processed using a standardized extraction procedure. Several studies report the correct identification of yeast to the species level up to approximately 98% in comparison to traditional culture methods. In addition, some laboratories have required the direct isolation of organisms from blood culture systems without subculturing to another medium to facilitate identification. Evidence suggests that MALDI-TOF is able to resolve species discrepancies more accurately than traditional culture methods and will reduce the time needed to identify an organism significantly.

## CONVENTIONAL YEAST IDENTIFICATION METHODS

A few laboratories still prefer to use conventional methods to identify yeasts. Regardless of the type of identification system used, the germ tube test often is the first step in screening a large number of isolates, unless another screening test for *C. albicans* has been used (e.g., PNA FISH). As previously mentioned, approximately 75% of yeasts recovered in the clinical laboratory can be identified using the germ tube test.

### CORNMEAL AGAR MORPHOLOGY

The second major step in this practical identification schema is to use cornmeal agar morphology as a means to determine whether the yeast produces blastoconidia, arthroconidia, pseudohyphae, true hyphae, and/or chlamydoconidia (see Procedure 63-4 on the Evolve site). Cornmeal agar morphology can be used to detect characteristic chlamydoconidia produced by *C. albicans*. This method currently is satisfactory for definitive identification of *C. albicans* when the germ tube test is negative. In other instances, microscopic morphologic features on cornmeal agar help differentiate the genera *Cryptococcus*, *Saccharomyces*, *Candida*, *Geotrichum*, and *Trichosporon*. Previously, it was believed that the morphologic features of the common *Candida* spp. were distinct enough to provide a presumptive identification. This can be accomplished for *C. albicans*, *C. glabrata*, *C. krusei*, *C. parapsilosis*, *C. tropicalis*, and *C. kefyr*, keeping in mind that numerous other species, uncommonly recovered in the clinical laboratory, might resemble microscopically any of the previously mentioned species. In general, this method performs well, because the previously mentioned genera and species are more commonly seen in clinical laboratories.

Cornmeal agar morphology has less value for uncommonly encountered isolates. It should be used as an adjunct test with most commercially available yeast identification systems (e.g., to differentiate *C. albicans* from *C. dubliniensis*). It aids the differentiation of yeasts that yield similar biochemical profiles and helps prevent misidentifications, particularly of less commonly encountered species that may not be well represented in the commercial database.

### CARBOHYDRATE UTILIZATION

Carbohydrate utilization patterns are the most commonly used conventional methods for definitive identification of yeasts recovered in a clinical laboratory. Various methods have been advocated for use in determining carbohydrate utilization patterns by clinically important yeasts, and all work equally well. Procedure 63-5, which can be found on the Evolve site, outlines the method previously found to be most useful by the Mayo Clinic

Mycology Laboratory; however, this method is not commonly used in clinical laboratories. Most use commercially available methods.

Once the carbohydrate utilization profile has been obtained, reactions may be compared with those listed in tables in most mycology laboratory manuals. In most instances, carbohydrate utilization tests provide definitive identification of an organism, and additional tests are unnecessary. Some laboratories prefer carbohydrate fermentation tests, which are simply performed using purple broth containing different carbohydrate substrates. In general, carbohydrate fermentation tests are unnecessary and are not recommended for routine use.

## PHENOLOXIDASE DETECTION USING NIGER SEED AGAR

Use of a simplified *Guizotia abyssinica* (niger seed) medium is a definitive method for detecting phenoloxidase production by yeasts (see Procedure 63-6 on the Evolve site). Most isolates of *C. neoformans* readily produce phenoloxidase; however, some do not. In addition, in some instances, cultures of *C. neoformans* have been shown to contain both phenoloxidase-producing and phenoloxidase-deficient colonies in the same culture.

If conventional methods are used, all criteria, including urease production, carbohydrate utilization, and the phenoloxidase test, must be met before a final identification of *C. neoformans* is made.

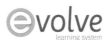 *Visit the Evolve site to complete the review questions.*

---

## CASE STUDY 63-1

A 48-year-old male recovering from liver transplantation in the intensive care unit (ICU) develops a persistent fever. In the initial physical examination, the only thing of note is inflammation surrounding a catheter. The catheter is removed and sent to the microbiology laboratory.

The diagnosis is systemic candidiasis originating from the catheter. The catheter is changed, and the patient is treated with fluconazole. Blood cultures are negative within 1 week.

### QUESTIONS

1. What tests were likely performed on the catheter to obtain a definitive diagnosis of candidiasis?
2. Given the limited information about the patient's history, what route of transmission of the organism probably resulted in the patient's infection?
3. Based on the patient history provided, what information would indicate that he is susceptible to yeast infection?

---

## BIBLIOGRAPHY

Alexander BD, Ashley ED, Reller LB, et al: Cost savings with implementation of PNA FISH testing for identification of Candida albicans in blood cultures, *Diagn Microbiol Infect Dis* 54:277, 2006.

Anaissie E, Gokaslan A, Hachem R, et al: Azole therapy for trichosporonosis: clinical evaluation of eight patients, experimental therapy for murine infection, and review, *Clin Infect Dis* 15:781, 1992.

Aubertine CL, Rivera M, Rohan SM, et al: Comparative study of the new colorimetric VITEK 2 yeast identification card versus the older fluorometric card and of CHROMagar Candida as a source medium with the new card, *J Clin Microbiol* 44:227, 2006.

Bader O, Weig M, Taverne-Ghadwal L, et al: Improved clinical laboratory identification of human pathogenic yeasts by matrix-assisted laser desorption ionization-time-of-flight spectrometry, *Clin Microbiol Infect* 17(9):1359-1365, 2012.

Barenfanger J, Arakere P, Dela Cruz R, et al: Improved outcomes associated with limiting identification of Candida spp. in respiratory secretions, *J Clin Microbiol* 41:5645, 2003.

Berenguer J, Buck M, Witebsky F, et al: Lysis-centrifugation blood cultures in the detection of tissue-proven invasive candidiasis: disseminated versus single-organ infection, *Diagn Microbiol Infect Dis* 17:103, 1993.

Bille E, Dauphin B, Leto J, et al: MALDI-TOF MS Andromas strategy for routine identification of bacteria, mycobacteria, yeasts, Aspergillus spp. and positive blood cultures, *Clin Microbial Infect* 18(11):1117-1125, 2012.

Calderone RA: Introduction and historical perspectives. In Calderone R, editor: *Candida and candidiasis*, Washington, DC, 2002, ASM Press.

Chan KS, Deepak RN, Tan MG, et al: Abbreviated identification of Candida albicans by the presence of a pseudohyphal fringe ("spiking" appearance)—some caveats, *J Med Microbiol* 60(5):687-688, 2011.

Cherniak R, Sundstrom JB: Polysaccharide antigens of the capsule of Cryptococcus neoformans, *Infect Immun* 62:1507, 1994.

Clinical Laboratory Standards Institute, *Abbreviated identification of bacteria and yeast, approved guidelines M35-A2 CLSI*, Wayne, Pennsylvania, 2008.

Currie B, Casadevall A: Estimation of the prevalence of cryptococcal infection among patients infected with the human immunodeficiency virus in New York City, *Clin Infect Dis* 19:1029, 1994.

Diamond R: Cryptococcus neoformans. In Mandell G, Bennett J, Dolin R, editors: *Mandell, Douglas, and Bennett's principles and practice of infectious diseases*, New York, 1995, Churchill Livingstone.

Dooley D, Beckius M, Jeffrey B: Misidentification of clinical yeast isolates by using updated Vitek Yeast Biochemical Card, *J Clin Microbiol* 32:2889, 1994.

El-Zaatari M, Pasarell L, McGinnis MR, et al: Evaluation of the updated Vitek Yeast Identification database, *J Clin Microbiol* 28:1938, 1990.

Ellepola ANB, Hurst SF, Ellie CM, et al: Rapid and unequivocal differentiation of Candida dubliniensis from other Candida species using species-specific DNA probes: comparison with phenotypic identification methods, *Oral Microbiol Immunol* 18:379, 2003.

Ellepola ANB, Morrison CJ. Laboratory diagnosis of invasive candidiasis, *J Microbiol* 43:65, 2005.

Ener B, Douglas L: Correlation between cell-surface hydrophobicity of Candida albicans and adhesion to buccal epithelial cells, *FEMS Microbiol Lett* 78:37, 1992.

Guinet R, Chanas J, Goullier A, et al: Fatal septicemia due to amphotericin B–resistant Candida lusitaniae, *J Clin Microbiol* 18:443, 1983.

Guiver M, Levi K, Oppenheim BA, et al: Rapid identification of Candida species by TaqMan PCR, *J Clin Pathol* 54:362, 2001.

Heelan J, Siliezar D, Coon K: Comparison of rapid testing methods for enzyme production with the germ tube method for presumptive identification of Candida albicans, *J Clin Microbiol* 34:2847, 1996.

Hostetter M: Adhesions and ligands involved in the interaction of Candida spp with epithelial and endothelial surfaces, *Clin Microbiol Rev* 7:29, 1994.

Hsu MC, Chen KW, Lo HJ, et al: Species identification of medically important fungi by use of real-time LightCycler PCR, *J Med Micriobiol* 52:1071, 2003.

Huffnagle G, Chen G, Curtis J: Down-regulation of the afferent phase of T cell–mediated pulmonary inflammation and immunity by a high melanin-producing strain of Cryptococcus neoformans, *J Immunol* 155:3607, 1995.

Jarvis JN, Percival A, Bauman S, et al: Evaluation of a novel point-of-care cryptococcal antigen test on serum, plasma, and urine from patients with HIV-associated cryptococcal meningitis, *Clin Infect Dis* 53(10):1019-1023, 2011.

Jin WY, Jang SJ, Lee MJ, et al: Evaluation of VITEK 2, Microscan, and Phoenix for identification of clinical isolates and reference strains, *Diagn Microb Infect Dis* 70(4):442-447, 2011.

Kathavade RJ, Kura MM, Valand AG, et al: Candida tropicalis: its prevalence, pathogenicity and increasing resistance to fluconazole, *J Med Microbiol* 59:873, 2010.

Kreger-Van Rij N: *The yeasts: a taxonomic study*, New York, 1984, Elsevier.

Kronstad JW, Attarian R, Cadieux B, et al: Expanding fungal pathogenesis: Cryptococcus breaks out of the opportunistic box, *Nature Rev Microbiol* 9:193, 2011.

Kwon-Chung K, Bennet J: *Medical mycology*, Philadelphia, 1992, Lea & Febiger.

Libertin CR, Wilson WR, Roberts GD: Candida lusitaniae: an opportunistic pathogen, *Diagn Microbiol Infect Dis* 3:69, 1985.

Liguori G, Di Onofrio V, Lucariello A, et al: Oral candidiasis: a comparison between conventional methods and multiplex polymerase chain reaction for species identification, *Oral Microbiol Immunol* 24:76, 2009.

Liguori G, Galle F, Lucariello A, et al: Comparison between multiplex PCR and phenotypic systems for Candida spp. identification, *New Microbiol* 33:63, 2010.

Loiex C, Wallet F, Sendid B, et al: Evaluation of VITEK 2 colorimetric cards versus fluorometric cards for identification of yeasts, *Diagnost Microbiol Infect Dis* 56(4):455-457, 2006.

Marcon MJ, Powell DA: Epidemiology, diagnosis, and management of Malassezia furfur systemic infection, *Diagn Microbiol Infect Dis* 7:161, 1987.

Murray CK, Beckius ML, Green JA, et al: Use of chromogenic medium in the isolation of yeasts from clinical specimens, *J Med Microbiol* 54:981, 2005.

Murray MP, Zinchuk R, Larone DH: CHROMagar Candida as the sole primary medium for isolation of yeasts and as a source medium for the rapid-assimilation-of-trehalose test, *J Clin Microbiol* 43:1210, 2005.

Murray P, Van Scoy R, Roberts GD: Should yeasts in respiratory secretions be identified? *Mayo Clin Proc* 52:42, 1977.

Neely AN, Orloff MM, Holder IA: Candida albicans growth studies: a hypothesis for the pathogenesis of Candida infections in burns, *J Burn Care Rehabil* 13:323, 1992.

Neilson JB, Fromtling RA, Bulmer GS: Cryptococcus neoformans: size range of infectious particles from aerosolized soil, *Infect Immun* 17:634, 1977.

Oliveira K, Haase G, Kurtzman C, et al: Differentiation of Candida albicans and Candida dubliniensis by fluorescent in situ hybridization with peptide nucleic acid probes, *J Clin Microbiol* 39:4138, 2001.

Paliwal DK, Randhawa HS: Evaluation of a simplified Guizotia abyssinica seed medium for differentiation of Cryptococcus neoformans, *J Clin Microbiol* 7:346, 1978.

Pfaller MA, Houston A, Coffmann S: Application of CHROMagar Candida for rapid screening of clinical specimens for Candida albicans, Candida tropicalis, Candida krusei, and Candida (Torulopsis) glabrata, *J Clin Microbiol* 34:58, 1996.

Pfaller MA, Diekema DJ, Gibbs DL, et al: Geographic variation in the frequency of isolation and fluconazole and voriconazole susceptibilities of Candida glabrata: an assessment from the ARTEMIS DISK Global Antifungal Surveillance Program, Global Antifungal Surveillance Group, *Diagn Microbiol Infect Dis* 67:162, 2010.

Pfaller MA, Diekema DJ, Gibbs DL, et al: Results from the ARTEMIS DISK Global Antifungal Surveillance Study, 1997 to 2007: a 10.5-year analysis of susceptibilities of Candida species to fluconazole and voriconazole as determined by CLSI standardized disk diffusion, Global Antifungal Surveillance Group, *J Clin Microbiol* 48:1366, 2010.

Pfaller MA, Moet GJ, Messer SA, et al: Candida bloodstream infections: comparison of species distribution and resistance to echinocandin and azole antifungal agents in intensive care unit (ICU) and non-ICU settings in the SENTRY Antimicrobial Surveillance Program (2008-2009), *Int J Antimicrob Agents* 38(1):65-69, 2011.

Rigby S, Procop GW, Haase G, et al: Fluorescence in situ hybridization with peptide nucleic acid probes for rapid identification of Candida albicans directly from blood culture bottles, *J Clin Microbiol* 40:2182, 2002.

Silva S, Negri M, Henriques M, et al: Candida glabrata, Candida parapsilosis and Candida tropicalis: biology, epidemiology, pathogenicity and antifungal resistance, *FEMS Microbiol Rev*, doi: 10.1111/j.1574-6976.2011.00278.x. [Epub ahead of print], 2011.

St Germain G, Beauchesne D: Evaluation of the MicroScan Rapid Yeast Identification panel, *J Clin Microbiol* 29:2296, 1991.

Tan GL, Peterson EM: CHROMagar Candida medium for direct susceptibility testing of yeast from blood cultures, *J Clin Microbiol* 43:1727, 2005.

Terreni AA, Strohecker JS, Dowda H Jr: Candida lusitaniae septicemia in a patient on extended home intravenous hyperalimentation, *J Med Vet Mycol* 25:63, 1987.

Trofa D, Gacser A, Nosanchuk JD, et al: Candida parapsilosis, an emerging fungal pathogen, *Clin Microbiol Rev* 21:606, 2008.

Van Herendael BH, Bruynseels P, Bensaid M, et al: Validation of a modified algorithm for the identification of yeast isolates using matrix-associated laser desorption ionization time-of-flight mass spectrometry (MALDI-TOF MS), *Eur J Clin Micorobiol* 31(5):841-848, 2012.

Vartivarian SE: Virulence properties and nonimmune pathogenetic mechanisms of fungi, *Clin Infect Dis* 14:S30, 1992.

Wang Y, Aisen P, Casadevall A: Cryptococcus neoformans melanin and virulence: mechanism of action, *Infect Immun* 63:3131, 1995.

Warren N, Hazen K: Candida, Cryptococcus and other yeasts of medical importance. In Murray P et al, editors: *Manual of clinical microbiology*, Washington, DC, 1995, ASM Press.

Wilson DA, Joyce MJ, Hall LS, et al: Multicenter evaluation of a C. albicans peptide nucleic acid fluorescent in situ hybridization probe for characterization of yeast isolates from blood cultures, *J Clin Microbiol* 43:2909, 2005.

Zilberberg MD, Shorr AF, Kollef MH, et al: Secular trends in candidemia-related hospitalization in the United States, 2000-2005, *Infect Control Hosp Epidemiol* 29:978, 2008.

Zilberberg MD, Kollef MH, Arnold H, et al: Inappropriate empiric antifungal therapy for candidemia in the ICU and hospital resource utilization: a retrospective cohort study, *BMC Infect Dis* 10:15, 2010.

# Antifungal Susceptibility Testing, Therapy, and Prevention

## OBJECTIVES

1. Name the documents available that contain the current guidelines for antifungal susceptibility testing.
2. Identify three circumstances in which antifungal susceptibility testing may be valuable.
3. List three areas of concern that complicate interpretive guidelines.
4. Explain how amphotericin B is produced, how it is administered, and its most significant adverse reaction.
5. Describe the mechanism of action of flucytosine and the drug's therapeutic use.
6. Identify three echinocandins and describe their mechanism of action.

## ANTIFUNGAL SUSCEPTIBILITY TESTING

Antifungal susceptibility tests are designed to provide information that helps the physician select the appropriate antifungal agent to treat a specific infection. Although antifungal susceptibility testing perhaps has not advanced as far as methods for determining the susceptibility of bacteria to antimicrobial agents, significant progress has been made. Substantial efforts have attempted to develop a standardized method that is reproducible among different laboratories. All of the technical variables in the testing process have been standardized, and efforts are underway to develop interpretative guidelines for different antifungal agents.

The Clinical Laboratory Standards Institute (CLSI) sets the standards for antifungal susceptibility testing. The current guidelines for these tests are provided in the following three documents, which are available on the CLSI website (www.clsi.org):

- Document M27-A3, *Reference Method for Broth Dilution Antifungal Susceptibility Testing of Yeasts*, Approved Standard, 3rd edition. This document covers requirements for use of the broth microdilution method. The standards for susceptibility testing are very specific about the inoculum size, test medium, incubation time and temperature, and end point of yeasts that cause invasive fungal infections.
- Document M38-A2, *Reference Method for Broth Dilution Antifungal Susceptibility Testing of Filamentous Fungi*, Approved Standard, 2nd edition. This standard is a microdilution method for molds that cause invasive and cutaneous infections.
- Document M44-A2, *Method for Antifungal Disk Diffusion Susceptibility Testing of Yeasts*, 2nd edition, Approved Guideline. This standard provides methodology for disk diffusion testing for *Candida* spp., including quality control and interpretation

guidelines. Also see the International Supplement M44S3.

It must be emphasized that the methodology and interpretation of antifungal susceptibility tests continue to evolve, and the laboratory should check for updated standards or a regular basis. Antifungal susceptibility tests are costly and time-consuming, but they may have value in the following circumstances:

- Determining antibiograms for isolates in an institution
- Aiding the management of patients with refractory oropharyngeal candidiasis
- Aiding the management of patients with invasive candidiasis caused by non-albicans *Candida* spp. when the use of the azoles is in question

The interpretative breakpoints for fluconazole, itraconazole, and flucytosine are based on experience in treating patients with mucosal infections, but they also appear to be consistent with information assembled for invasive infections. Problems that complicate the interpretative guidelines include:

- Patient's physical condition (i.e., immunologic status)
- Type of infection and the drug's ability to penetrate a closed space (in the case of an abscess)
- Dose of the drug and its pharmacokinetics
- Susceptibility testing method used and serum level of drug administered

Isolates of the same species may exhibit differences in minimum inhibitory concentrations (MICs) because of previous exposure to antifungal agents and/or acquisition of a genetic mechanism of resistance. For example, some isolates of *Candida glabrata* show susceptibility to fluconazole, but others do not. CLSI's interpretative guidelines should be followed whenever possible, but anecdotal experience also is useful.

Despite the problems associated with antifungal susceptibility testing, many physicians believe that these tests are important for selecting an appropriate antifungal agent and as a method to detect the development of resistance of certain organisms during chemotherapy. A laboratory that is not equipped to perform CLSI methods, or validated equivalent methods, for susceptibility of clinically important fungal isolates should be prepared to send the isolate to a reference laboratory for testing. Amphotericin B, 5-fluorocytosine, ketoconazole, itraconazole, voriconazole, and fluconazole are common antifungal agents that traditionally have been tested; the newer antifungal agents may now be added to this list. For those interested in further information on this topic, the susceptibilities of many of the newer antifungal agents to some of the more challenging fungal pathogens have been published in a minireview by Lass-Florl et al.

# ANTIFUNGAL THERAPY AND PREVENTION

Numerous antifungal agents have been developed, and newer agents are on the horizon. The increasing number of immunosuppressed patients and the expansion of drug resistance of microorganisms make the development and appropriate use of antimicrobial agents two of the most important areas in microbiology and infectious diseases. This section is meant only to introduce the reader to the more commonly used antifungal agents; it is by no means comprehensive. Also, this section is not to be used as a guide for therapy. Therapeutic guidelines may be found in the texts listed in the bibliography.

## POLYENE MACROLIDE ANTIFUNGALS

Polyene macrolide antifungal agents consist of a group of complex organic molecules, most of which contain multiple, conjugated, double-bond and one- to three-ring structures. This group includes many of the most commonly used antifungal agents, such as amphotericin B, the colloidal and liposomal preparations of amphotericin B, nystatin, and griseofulvin.

### Amphotericin B

Amphotericin B is produced by the actinomycete *Streptomyces nodosus*. It is commonly infused intravenously to treat deep-seated fungal infections (e.g., invasive aspergillosis), and those caused by *Candida* spp., *Cryptococcus* spp., and members of the Mucorales. Amphotericin B binds the ergosterol component of the fungal cell membrane and alters the selective permeability of this membrane. However, other sterols, including those present in mammalian cell membranes, are also bound. The most significant adverse reaction associated with amphotericin B therapy is renal insufficiency. The liposomal amphotericin B compounds reportedly diminish this adverse reaction. Although amphotericin B is active against a wide variety of fungi, resistant organisms exist, which the laboratory must be able to identify. Fungi resistant to amphotericin B include *Pseudallescheria boydii*, *Aspergillus terreus*, *Trichosporon* spp., and in most cases *Fusarium* spp.

### Nystatin

Nystatin, an antifungal antibiotic produced by *Streptomyces noursei*, is not absorbed in the gastrointestinal tract. It is principally used locally to treat oral or vulvovaginal candidiasis. The toxicity of this drug is prohibitive to parenteral use.

### Griseofulvin

Griseofulvin is an antifungal antibiotic produced by a species of *Penicillium*. Its mechanism of action consists of binding microtubular proteins, which are required for mitosis. Griseofulvin is an oral agent used to treat dermatophytoses, which are not responsive to azole antifungal therapy. Headache, gastrointestinal disturbances, and photosensitivity are a few of the adverse reactions that limit the usefulness of this drug.

### 5-Fluorocytosine (Flucytosine)

Flucytosine is a pyrimidine base, which is fluorinated in the fifth position. Flucytosine is metabolized to 5-fluorouracil, which is incorporated into fungal RNA. This subsequently inhibits protein synthesis. Flucytosine is also metabolized into fluorodeoxyuridine monophosphate, a potent inhibitor of DNA synthesis. Flucytosine and amphotericin B act synergistically and have been used in combination therapy for treating infections by *Candida* spp. and *Cryptococcus* spp. Side effects and the emergence of resistance have limited its usefulness.

## AZOLE ANTIFUNGAL DRUGS

The azole group of antifungal agents consists of the imidazoles and the triazoles. These compounds contain six carbon ring structures with conjugated double bonds, chloride residues, and five carbon ring structures that contain at least two nitrogen molecules. Traditionally used agents in this group include clotrimazole, miconazole, fluconazole, itraconazole, voriconazole and ketoconazole. The newer triazoles are voriconazole, posaconazole and, most recently, ravuconazole; of these only voriconazole is discussed here, because it was the first of the newer agents released and has been the most thoroughly reviewed. Azole antifungal agents disrupt the integrity of the fungal cell membrane by interfering with the synthesis of ergosterol.

### Clotrimazole and Miconazole

The synthetic imidazoles clotrimazole and miconazole are covered together because of their many similarities. These agents are available for topical or intravaginal application. They are useful in mild cases of dermatophytosis, including tinea versicolor. Adverse reactions are generally limited to burning, itching, and/or skin irritation.

### Fluconazole

Fluconazole, a triazole, is exceptionally soluble in water, which allows either oral or intravenous administration. Fluconazole has excellent activity against most *Candida* spp. and *Cryptococcus* spp. therapeutic levels are easily reached in the central nervous system. Side effects of fluconazole therapy are usually minimal. The susceptibility of *C. glabrata* to fluconazole is not predictable. Isolates of *C. glabrata* may be susceptible, dose-dependent susceptible, or resistant to fluconazole. Other notable yeasts or yeastlike fungi resistant to fluconazole are *Candida krusei* and *Rhodotorula* spp.

### Ketoconazole

Ketoconazole is an imidazole that is either taken orally or applied topically. It is useful in mild cases of paracoccidioidomycosis and is an alternative to amphotericin B for infections caused by *Blastomyces* or *Histoplasma* spp. Ketoconazole may be used if prolonged oral therapy for chronic mucocutaneous candidiasis is needed. One group has reported some success in the treatment of *P. boydii* infections with ketoconazole. In vivo, ketoconazole is fungistatic, because fungicidal levels are not achievable with therapeutic concentrations. Adverse reactions include transient elevations in liver enzymes, nausea, and dose-related gynecomastia, decreased libido, and oligospermia in males.

### Itraconazole

The triazole itraconazole has a spectrum of activity that encompasses that of ketoconazole. In addition, itraconazole has been shown to be effective in cases of aspergillosis, sporotrichosis, cryptococcosis, and onychomycosis. Adverse reactions principally include gastrointestinal disturbances; however, vestibular disturbances, edema, and skin irritations have been reported.

### Voriconazole

Voriconizole, one of the new triazoles, has an expanded spectrum of activity compared with itraconazole. In addition to the uses described previously for itraconazole, voriconazole demonstrates useful activity against some *Fusarium* strains and against fluconazole-resistant yeasts, such as *C. krusei* and *C. glabrata*. However, it is important to note that the Mucorales are resistant to voriconizole. Elevated liver enzymes may occur, as may transient visual disturbances, which can significantly alarm the patient if the individual is not forewarned.

### Posaconazole

Posaconazole is a triazole structurally similar to voriconazole. Posaconazole is an oral azole that is effective against dermatophytes, including *Candida* spp., *Aspergillus terreus*, *Fusarium* spp., and Mucorales.

### Anidulafungin

Anidulafungin is a broad-spectrum echinocandin. It is a selective inhibitor of the fungal enzyme beta-(1,3)-D-glucan synthase that is involved in fungal cell wall synthesis. The drug is effective against *Candida* spp., including strains that are resistant to fluconazole.

### Micafungin

Micafungin is an echonocandin. The drug is a selective inhibitor of the fungal enzyme beta-(1,3)-D-glucan synthase that is involved in fungal cell wall synthesis. It is used for the propylaxis and treatment of *Candida* spp. infections in adult and pediatric patients.

### OTHER

#### Terbinafine (Lamisil)

Terbinafine is a synthetic allylamine that is highy lipophilic, allowing it to accumulate in the skin, nails, and fatty tissue. The drug interferes with fungal cell wall synthesis and is an effective topical treatment for infections.

### ECHINOCANDINS

The echinocandins are glucan synthesis inhibitors. More specifically, they inhibit 1, 3 beta-glucan synthase, an enzyme important in fungal cell wall synthesis. These drugs lead to cellular osmotic instability. The three echinocandins are caspofungin, micafungin, and anidulafungin. Caspofungin was the first to be released and is the representative compound for this group.

#### Caspofungin

Caspofungin is fungicidal against *Candida* spp., including species that are or may be resistant to fluconazole (e.g. *C. krusei* and *C. glabrata*, respectively). It is fungistatic rather than fungicidal against *Aspergillus* spp. It is important to note that *C. neoformans* var. neoformans is intrinsically resistant to caspofungin. Caspofungin also is not likely to be useful against *Trichosporon* spp., *Rhodotorula* spp., or the Mucorales. Side effects are minimal.

#### Selenium Sulfide

Selenium sulfide shampoos, available commercially, disclose antifungal activity against *Malassezia furfur*, the causative agent of tinea versicolor. Additionally, selenium sulfide is sporicidal for *Trichophyton tonsurans* and therefore may be used as an adjuvant to griseofulvin therapy.

#### Potassium Iodide

Potassium iodide is the therapy of choice for cutaneous/lymphatic sporotrichosis. Localized heat therapy may be used adjunctively. Some individuals are allergic to potassium iodide. Adverse reactions include a bitter taste, allergic rash, and anorexia.

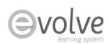 *Visit the Evolve site to complete the review questions.*

---

## BIBLIOGRAPHY

Beggs W, Andrews F, Sarosoi G: Actions of imidazole-containing antifungal drugs, *Life Sci* 28:111, 1981.

Espinel-Ingroff A: Antifungal susceptibility testing, *Clin Microbiol Newsl* 184:161, 1996.

Galgiani JN, Stevens DA, Graybill JR, et al: *Pseudallescheria boydii* infections treated with ketoconazole: clinical evaluations of seven patients and in vitro susceptibility results, *Chest* 86:219, 1984.

Korting HC, Kiencke P, Nelles S: Comparable efficacy and safety of various topical formulations of terbinafine in tinea pedis irrespective of the treatment regimen: results of a meta-analysis, *Am J Clin Derm* 8(6):357-364, 2007.

Lass-Florl C, Griff K, Mayr A, et al: Epidemiology and outcome of infections due to *Aspergillus terreus*: 10-year single centre experience, *Br J Haematol* 131:201, 2005.

Mayr A, Aigner M, Lass-Florl C: Anidulafungin for the treatment of invasive candidiasis, *Clin Microbiol Infect* 17(suppl 1):1-12, 2011.

O'Sullivan AK, Weinstein MC, Pandya A, et al: Cost-effectiveness of posaconazole versus fluconazole for prevention of invasive fungal infections in U.S. patients with graft-versus-host disease, *Am J Health Syst Pharm* 69(2):149-156, 2012.

Pfaller MA, Diekema DJ: Rare and emerging opportunistic fungal pathogens: concern for resistance beyond *Candida albicans* and *Aspergillus fumigatus*, *J Clin Microbiol* 4:4419, 2004.

Scott LJ: Micafungin: A review of its use in the prophylaxis and treatment of invasive Candida infections, *Drugs* 72(16):2141-2165, 2012.

Solovieva E, Olsufyeva EN, Preobrazhenskaya MN: Chemical modifications of antifungal polyene macrolide antibiotics, *Russ Chem Rev* 80(2):103-126, 2011.

Walsh M, White L, Atkinson K, et al: Fungal *Pseudoallescheria boydii* lung infiltrates unresponsive to amphotericin B in leukaemic patients, *Aust N Z J Med* 22:265, 1992.

Wolf DG, Falk R, Hacham M, et al: Multidrug-resistant *Trichosporon asahii* infection of nongranulocytopenic patients in three intensive care units, *J Clin Microbiol* 39:4420, 2001.

# Overview of the Methods and Strategies in Virology*

## OBJECTIVES

1. Describe the physical components that make up a virion and list a function for each component.
2. Define the viral infectious cycle, including naming the six steps in this process.
3. Explain viral tropism and provide a specific example.
4. Define the properties used to classify a virus and identify the person responsible for classification of a virus.
5. Explain the steps in viral pathogenesis.
6. List some of the reasons the clinical science industry has seen an increased demand for clinical viral services.
7. Name some of the equipment necessary to set up a clinical virology laboratory and give the function of each piece.
8. List some of the viruses associated with the following clinical specimens: throat or nasopharyngeal swab or aspirate, urine, stool, lesion, blood, bone marrow, and stool or rectal swab.
9. List some of the most efficient laboratory tests for detecting the following viruses: enterovirus, herpes simplex virus, influenza virus, norovirus, and respiratory syncytial virus (RSV).
10. Define the Tzanck test and list the viruses for which the test is used.
11. Define monolayer, primary cells, semicontinuous (low passage) cells, and continuous cells.
12. Explain the types of cell lines used in viral cell culture; describe their similarities and differences.
13. Define and differentiate cell culture growth medium and maintenance medium.
14. Explain the incubation conditions for routine cell cultures.
15. Define CPE and explain how it is rated when reading cell cultures.
16. Describe a shell vial cell culture and explain its advantages over conventional cell culture.
17. Define the hemadsorption procedure and name the viruses for which the test is used.
18. Name the virus family capable of establishing viral latency in the human dorsal nerve root ganglion and explain the possible consequence of the latency.
19. Name the preferred tissue type of cell culture for growth of the following viruses: influenza A virus, varicella-zoster virus, herpes virus, and cytomegalovirus (CMV).
20. Associate an appropriate viral pathogen with the following viral syndromes: infant croup, infant bronchiolitis, adult gastroenteritis, parotitis, infectious mononucleosis, and meningitis.

*Special thanks to the South Dakota Public Health Laboratory for contributing their expertise and photographs; information contributed by Danette M. Hoffman, B.S. MT(ASCP), Sr. Microbiologist, Technical Supervisor, Virology.

Evidence of viral disease exists in ancient records, dating back to as far as 23 BC, when the Eschunna Code of ancient Mesopotamia noted "the bite of mad dogs to affect disease on humans." Homer, author of the *Iliad*, characterizes Hector as "rabid." Aristotle's work, *The Natural History of Man*, written in the fourth century BC, describes a "madness" in dogs that "causes them to become very irritable and all mammals they bite become diseased." What remains apparent in all these early writings is that all writers realized the communicable nature of something unseen. These writings clearly refer to the rabies virus, transmitted through the saliva of an infected animal.

The survival of viral infectious agents depends on their ability to infect and reside in a living organism. These tiny organisms are thought to have evolved alongside humans and in conjunction with the domestication of animals. Throughout history, evidence shows that viruses are able to survive when established populations of humans are available to provide a means for continued propagation. Viruses that established a long-term relationship with their host (i.e., did not kill the host immediately upon infection) were the first to become adapted to co-evolution with the human race. Some of these earliest viruses were thought to be retroviruses, such as the herpes viruses, and papillomaviruses.

A virus is a submicroscopic, obligate intracellular parasite, among the smallest of all infectious agents, and capable of infecting any animal, plant, or bacterial cell. Viruses are found in every ecosystem. They are strict obligate intracellular parasites, incapable of replication without a living host cell. Virus types are very specific, and each has a limited number of hosts it can infect; this is referred to as viral **tropism.**

Much is still unknown about the origins of viral agents, although most speculation indicates that viruses affecting man established themselves in the human population through transmission of an animal virus to a human. Transmission of viruses from animals to humans still occurs, as demonstrated in the more recent viral outbreaks associated with the severe acute respiratory syndrome (SARS), West Nile, and influenza A H5 viruses, as well as the 2009 H1N1 virus, formerly known as the pandemic "swine flu." The influenza virus has proven to be one of the deadliest viruses to affect humans; its history dates back to the 1700s in Italy. The virus was named to indicate disease resulting from the "influence" of miasma (bad air).

The emergence of a new viral disease across a very large geographical region (worldwide) with prolonged human-to-human transmission is called a **pandemic.** To date, most of the pandemics recorded have been caused by an influenza virus. Pandemics result when an influenza virus undergoes a genetic shift and the reassortment of genes combines with those of another organism, usually an animal. The resulting virus emerges as a completely new or "novel" virus. The genetic changes in viral genomes may result from **antigenic shift** (major changes that result in novel viral antigens) and/or **antigenic drift** (minor changes that occur infrequently), which are discussed in Chapter 66. One of the most deadly influenza outbreaks was the Spanish Flu pandemic of 1918-1919. This pandemic was associated with infection with a novel influenza virus of avian origin. After a period of adaptation in humans, the virus emerged in pandemic form and was responsible for more than 50 million deaths worldwide, including 500,000 in the United States. What was so different about this pandemic was that it affected young and healthy individuals, not just the very young or very old. The more recent influenza pandemic of the twentieth century was associated with a human influenza virus in which genes reassorted in combination with an avian influenza virus.

Protection from viral infection has been successful for some viral pathogens. Vaccination (immunization) has proven to be a valuable tool in the control of viral diseases such as yellow fever and rabies and has been instrumental in the eradication of one of the most lethal viruses, smallpox. However, many viral diseases such as influenza, acquired immunodeficiency syndrome (AIDS), and hepatitis continue to pose challenges in treatment, prevention, and control.

The science of clinical virology has seen a rapid expansion in the past few years as new and emerging pathogenic viruses continue to evolve. Since 1988, 50 new viruses have been identified, making prevention and control more and more difficult. The science of virology will continue to evolve and clinicians will continue to rely on the laboratory scientist for the development and implementation of testing to diagnose, treat, and prevent viral disease.

# GENERAL CHARACTERISTICS

## VIRAL STRUCTURE

Virus particles, referred to as virions, consist of two or three parts:

- An inner nucleic acid core, consisting of either ribonucleic acid (RNA) or deoxyribonucleic acid (DNA)
- A protein coat that surrounds and protects the nucleic acid (the **capsid)**
- In some of the larger viruses, a lipid-containing envelope that surrounds the virus

Because enveloped viruses are very susceptible to drying out and destruction in the environment, they typically are transmitted by direct contact, such as respiratory, sexual, or parenteral contact. This prevents exposure to the environment and successful propagation of the viral agent to another susceptible host. Viruses that do not have an envelope are often referred to as "naked" viruses. Naked viruses are very resistant to environmental factors. Because of their stability, they typically are transmitted by the fecal-oral route. Many viruses have glycoprotein spikes extending from their surface. The term **nucleocapsid** is often used to describe the nucleic acid genome surrounded by a symmetric protein coat (Figure 65-1).

The function of the nucleic acid genome is to encode the proteins required for viral penetration, transmission, and replication. The viral genome structure determines the mechanism for viral replication. A variety of vial genome structures exist, including (+) sense strand RNA, (−) sense strand RNA, and DNA genomes. In addition, viral genomes may be single- or double-stranded molecules. The structural implications of variation in genome organization are discussed in more detail in the section on viral replication.

The viral capsid protects the viral genome and is responsible for the tropism to specific cell types in naked viruses. Viral capsids typically are composed of repeating structural subunits referred to as **capsomeres.** The capsomeres associate to form the capsid and a characteristic symmetric structure. The most common capsid structures geometrically form a helical or icosahedral structure (see Figure 65-1). Icosahedral capsids are cubical and have 20 flat sides; irregularly shaped capsids usually assume a helical form and are spiral shaped.

As mentioned, in some viruses the nucleocapsid is enclosed in a lipid envelope. The envelope is responsible for viral entry into the host cell (see Figure 65-1). During the infectious process, enveloped virions bud from a host cell's cytoplasmic, nuclear, or endoplasmic reticular membrane, and a portion of the membrane remains attached to the virion as the viral envelope. Inserted into this viral envelope are viral proteins, such as hemagglutinin (HA), neuraminidase, or glycoprotein spikes. The glycoprotein spikes assist in stabilization of attachment for the lipid envelope and for attachment to the host cell to facilitate viral entry. Some enveloped viruses also contain a matrix protein that lies between the envelope and the nucleocapsid. The matrix protein may have enzymatic activities and/or biologic functions related to infection, such as inhibition of host-cell transcription.

Viruses that cause disease in humans range from approximately 20 to 300 nm. Even the largest viruses, such as the poxviruses, cannot be detected with a light microscope, because they are less than one fourth the size of a staphylococcal cell (Figure 65-2). Not until the invention of the electron microscope in the 1930s were viruses visualized. The electron microscope's improved magnification (more than 100,000 times) allowed visualization of virus particles and paved the way for viral classification based on structural components.

## VIRUS TAXONOMY

Viral taxonomy is determined by the International Committee on Taxonomy of Viruses (ICTV) of the Virology

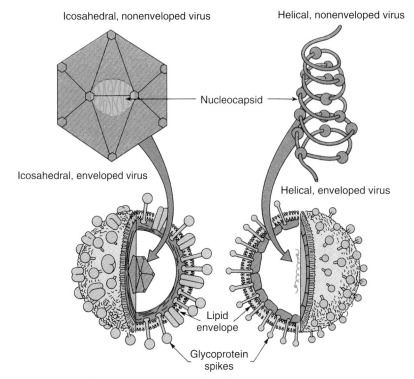

**Figure 65-1** Illustration of a viral particle. Enveloped and nonenveloped virions have an icosahedral or irregular (usually helical) shape. (Modified from Murray PR, Drew WL, Kobayashi GS, et al, editors: *Medical microbiology,* St Louis, 1990, Mosby.)

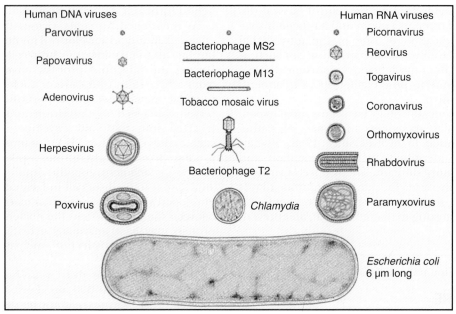

**Figure 65-2** Relative sizes of representative viruses, bacteriophages (bacterial viruses), and bacteria, including chlamydia. (From Murray PR, Drew WL, Kobayashi GS, et al, editors: *Medical microbiology,* St Louis, 1990, Mosby.)

Division of the International Union of Microbiological Societies. Viral taxonomy is divided into categories: six orders (-virales), 87 families (name ending in -viridae), 19 subfamilies (-virinae), 348 genera (-virus), and 2290 species. Classification of viral species can be problematic and therefore is often polythetic; that is, the members of a group share common characteristics but may not have

a single defining characteristic. In addition, some viral families currently are not assigned to an order, and some species are not assigned to a family.

Complex viral taxonomy incorporates a variety of categories, including information related to host range, transmission, disease pathology, antigenicity, and viral particle properties, such as size, envelope, capsid structure, physical properties, genome type, and configuration. For simplicity purposes, many texts limit viral classification to three basic properties: (1) viral morphology; (2) method of replication, including genome organization (whether the genome is RNA or DNA and single- or double-stranded); and (3) presence or absence of a lipid envelope. The term means of replication refers to the strategy the virus uses to duplicate the viral genome. For example, enteroviruses have single-stranded RNA genomes that synthesize additional strands of RNA, whereas retroviruses make RNA in a two-step process by first synthesizing DNA, which subsequently makes RNA.

Characterization of viral genomes has increasingly improved as a result of advances in molecular techniques. Molecular sequencing of viral genomes is becoming more and more common. However, because of the genetic instability of viral genomes, molecular sequencing is limited to providing evidence for species relationships and epidemiologic comparisons of isolates. As a result, clinical virologists generally categorize viruses as containing DNA or RNA and further organize by family and common names.

## VIRAL REPLICATION

Viruses are strict intracellular parasites, reproducing or replicating only inside a host cell. The six steps of virus replication, called the **infectious cycle,** proceed as follows (Figure 65-3).

1. **Attachment,** also referred to as adsorption, is the first step of the infectious cycle. It involves recognition of a suitable host cell and specific binding between viral capsid proteins (often the glycoprotein spikes) and the carbohydrate receptor of the host cell. Each type of virus specifically recognizes and attaches to a specific type of host cell, allowing infection of some

tissues but not others (viral tropism, as previously described).

2. **Penetration** is the process by which viruses enter the host cell. One mechanism of penetration involves fusion of the viral envelope with the host cell membrane. This method not only provides a mechanism for internalizing the virus, but also leads to fusion between the infected host cell and additional nearby host cells, forming multinucleated cells called **syncytia.** Detection of syncytia can be used to determine the presence of virus in cell cultures or stained smears of clinical specimens. Other mechanisms of viral penetration include phagocytosis by host cells (endocytosis) or injection of viral nucleic acid.

3. **Uncoating** occurs once the virus has been internalized. It is the process by which the capsid is removed; this may be by degradation of viral enzymes or host enzymes or by simple dissociation. Uncoating is necessary to release the viral genome before the viral DNA or RNA is delivered to its intracellular site of replication in the nucleus or cytoplasm.

4. **Macromolecular synthesis** involves the production of nucleic acid and protein polymers. Viral transcription leads to the synthesis of messenger RNA (mRNA), which encodes early and late viral proteins. Early proteins are nonstructural elements, such as enzymes, and late proteins are structural components. Rapid identification of virus in a cell culture can be accomplished by detecting early viral proteins in infected cells using immunofluorescent staining techniques. Replication of viral nucleic acid is necessary to provide genomes for progeny virus particles or virions. Macromolecular synthesis varies, depending on the organization of the viral genome.

5. **Viral assembly** is the process by which structural proteins, genomes, and in some cases viral enzymes are

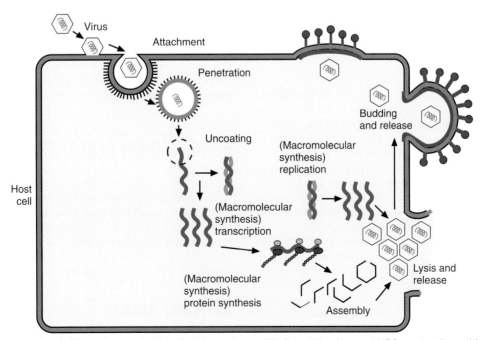

**Figure 65-3** Illustration of the viral infectious cycle. (Modified from Murray PR, Drew WL, Kobayashi GS, et al, editors: *Medical microbiology,* St Louis, 1990, Mosby.)

assembled into virus particles. Envelopes are acquired during viral "budding" from a host cell membrane. Nuclear endoplasmic reticulum and cytoplasmic membranes are common areas for budding. Acquisition of an envelope is the final step in viral assembly.

6. **Release** of intact virus particles occurs after cell lysis (lytic virus) or by budding from cytoplasmic membranes. Release by budding may not result in rapid host cell death, as does release by cell lysis. Detection of virus in cell cultures is facilitated by recognition of areas of cell lysis. Detection of virus released by budding is more difficult, because the cell monolayer remains intact. Influenza viruses, which are released by budding with minimal cell destruction, can be detected in cell culture by an alternative technique called **hemadsorption.** Influenza virus–infected cells contain virally encoded glycoprotein hemagglutinins inserted into the host cell's cytoplasmic membrane, preparing for inclusion in the viral envelope at the time of release by cytoplasmic budding. Red blood cells (RBCs) added to the culture medium adsorb to the outer membranes of infected cells but not to uninfected cells. Each infected host cell results in as many as 100,000 virions; however, as few as 1% of these may be infectious or "viable" in the practical sense. Noninfectious viral particles may result from errors or mutations that occur during the infectious cycle.

# EPIDEMIOLOGY

Viruses are transmitted from person to person by the respiratory, fecal-oral, and sexual contact routes; by trauma or injection with contaminated objects or needles; by tissue transplants (including blood transfusions); by arthropod or animal bites; and during gestation (transplacental transmission).

# PATHOGENESIS AND SPECTRUM OF DISEASE

Once introduced into a host, the virus infects susceptible cells, frequently in the upper respiratory tract. Viral infections may produce one of three characteristic clinical presentations: (1) acute viral infection, displaying evident signs and symptoms; (2) latent infection, which has no visible signs and symptoms, but the virus is still present in the host cell in a lysogenic state (inserted into the host genome in a resting state); and (3) chronic or persistent infection, in which low levels of virus are detectable and the degree of visible signs or symptoms varies.

After a local viral infection, a viremia occurs (viruses present in the patient's blood), which inoculates secondary target tissue distant from the primary site and releases mediators of human immune cell functions. Secondary viremia may occur in a variety of tissues, such as the skin, salivary glands, kidneys, and brain tissues. Symptomatic disease ensues. Disease resolves when specific antibody and cell-mediated immune mechanisms prevent continued replication of the virus. Tissue is damaged as a result of lysis of virus-infected cells or by immunopathologic mechanisms directed against the virus that are also destructive to neighboring tissue. Most DNA-containing viruses, such as those in the herpes group, remain latent in host tissue with no observable clinical impact. Retroviruses and most DNA viruses establish a latent state after primary infection. During the latent state, viral genome is integrated into the host cell's chromosome and no viral replication occurs. Latent viruses can reactivate silently, resulting in viral replication and shedding but no clinical symptoms, or they can reactivate and cause symptomatic, even fatal, disease. Reactivation may accompany immune suppression, resulting in the recurrence of clinically apparent disease.

Occasionally, pathogenic viruses stimulate an immune reaction that cross-reacts with related human tissue, resulting in damage to host function; this is called **autoimmune pathogenesis.** When present, it occurs well after the acute viral infection has resolved. Rare viral infection promotes transformation or immortalization of host cells, resulting in uncontrolled cell growth. Viruses with the ability to stimulate uncontrolled growth of host cells are referred to as **oncogenic** viruses. Some papillomaviruses (wart viruses) are oncogenic, giving rise to human cervical cancer.

Examples of the variety of pathogenic mechanisms of viral infection are illustrated in disease caused by infection with the measles virus. After replication in the upper respiratory tract and subsequent viremia, the virus infects many susceptible cells throughout the body, including endothelial cells in capillaries of the skin. This is accompanied by local inflammation and results in the characteristic rash of measles. Immunocompetent individuals eradicate the virus, resolving the infection, and have lifelong immunity. In some, antibody produced in response to the measles infection cross reacts with tissue in the central nervous system (CNS), causing a postinfectious encephalitis. In others, slow but continuing replication of damaged virus in the brain gives rise to subacute sclerosing panencephalitis. In severely immunocompromised individuals, ongoing primary infection is not aborted by the usual immune mechanisms, and the result is death (Figure 65-4). Because the measles virus is not an oncogenic virus, no cancers result from prolonged infection.

# PREVENTION AND THERAPY

Immunizations are available for some viruses capable of causing disease in humans. However, for viruses for which there are no available vaccines, the most effective means of preventing viral infection involves regular, thorough hand washing and avoiding contact with others during episodes of evident signs and symptoms, such as fever, cough, diarrhea, and respiratory infections.

## ANTIVIRAL AGENTS

An increased understanding of viral structure and replication has improved the availability of therapeutic agents for the treatment of viral infections. Approximately 40

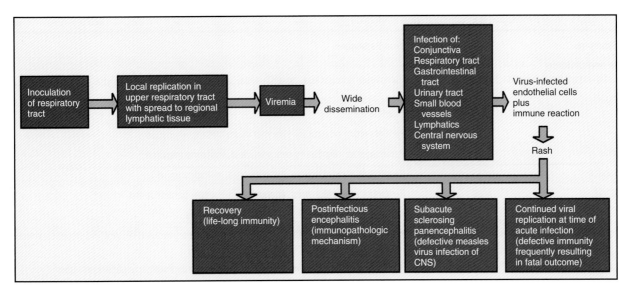

**Figure 65-4** Viral pathogenesis is illustrated by the mechanisms through which the measles virus spreads in the body. (From Murray PR, Drew WL, Kobayashi GS, et al, editors: *Medical microbiology,* St Louis, 1990, Mosby.)

antiviral drugs are formally licensed for clinical use, and about half of these are used in the treatment of human immunodeficiency virus (HIV) infections. Antivirals also are used in the treatment of herpes viruses (herpes simplex virus [HSV], varicella-zoster virus [VZV], and cytomegalovirus [CMV]), hepatitis B virus (HBV), hepatitis C virus (HCV), respiratory syncytial virus (RSV), and the influenza viruses. (Antiviral agents are reviewed in more detail in Chapter 67.)

# VIRUSES THAT CAUSE HUMAN DISEASES

Hundreds of viruses cause disease in humans. Viruses of human medical importance comprise four orders, 25 families, 13 subfamilies and 66 genera. Individual viruses may cause multiple different diseases, and conversely, many viruses may cause the same disease, all of which complicates the understanding of viral disease in humans. For example, viruses that can cause encephalitis include HSV, many arboviruses, rabies virus, HIV, and measles virus. However, HSV also can cause pharyngitis, genital infection, conjunctivitis, and encephalitis. Viruses that are important pathogens in humans and the viral syndromes they cause are summarized in Table 65-1. Specific viral agents and their role in human disease are discussed in Chapter 66.

# LABORATORY DIAGNOSIS

## SETTING UP A CLINICAL VIROLOGY LABORATORY

The demand for clinical virology laboratory services has skyrocketed during the past two decades. This growth has resulted from the introduction of virus-specific antiviral drugs; the commercial availability of reagents; the development of rapid diagnostic techniques using conventional methods such as fluorescence microscopy and enzyme immunoassays; the ready availability of cell lines for cell culture procedures; and the introduction of real-time polymerase chain reaction (PCR) assays for detecting viral genomes. Ironically, improved medical care, in the form of organ transplantation and immune suppression with cancer therapy, has resulted in an increased number of patients with viral disease. When these factors are considered along with the appearance of emerging viral pathogens that are threatening local and world populations (e.g., SARS, avian influenza, monkey pox), laboratory diagnosis of viral infection becomes far more important than in previous years.

When determining which virology tests to offer, each clinical laboratory should decide whether the test is required for the appropriate care of their patient population and whether techniques are available that provide an accurate, cost-effective test result. Viral diseases that require laboratory diagnosis include sexually transmitted diseases, diarrhea, respiratory disease in adults and children, aseptic meningitis, arbovirus encephalitides, congenital diseases, hepatitis, and infections in immunocompromised individuals. Table 65-2 presents a representative sample of viruses identified in a community clinical virology laboratory.

Laboratory scientists in a clinical virology laboratory must be familiar with cell culture, enzyme immunoassay, immunofluorescence methods, and molecular methods (e.g., PCR), in addition to other common laboratory techniques. Large equipment needed for a full-service virology laboratory includes a laminar flow biologic safety cabinet (BSC), fluorescence microscope, inverted bright field microscope, refrigerated centrifuge, incubator, refrigerator and freezer, roller drum

**TABLE 65-1** Viral Syndromes and Common Viral Pathogens

| Viral Syndrome | Viral Pathogens |
|---|---|
| **Infants and Children** Upper respiratory tract infection | Rhinovirus, coronavirus, parainfluenza, adenovirus, respiratory syncytial virus, influenza |
| Pharyngitis | Adenovirus, coxsackie A, herpes simplex virus, Epstein-Barr virus, rhinovirus, parainfluenza, influenza |
| Croup | Parainfluenza, respiratory syncytial virus, metapneumovirus |
| Bronchitis | Parainfluenza, respiratory syncytial virus, metapneumovirus |
| Bronchiolitis | Respiratory syncytial virus, parainfluenza, metapneumovirus |
| Pneumonia | Respiratory syncytial virus, adenovirus, influenza, parainfluenza |
| Gastroenteritis | Rotavirus, adenovirus 40-41, calicivirus, astrovirus |
| Congenital and neonatal disease | HSV-2, echovirus, and other enteroviruses, CMV, parvovirus B19, VZV, HIV, hepatitis viruses |
| **Adults** Upper respiratory tract infection | Rhinovirus, coronavirus, adenovirus, influenza, parainfluenza, Epstein-Barr virus |
| Pneumonia | Influenza, adenovirus, sin nombre virus (hantavirus), severe acute respiratory syndrome (SARS) coronavirus |
| Pleurodynia | Coxsackie B |
| Gastroenteritis | Noroviruses |
| Cervical cancer | Human papillomavirus |
| **All Patients** Parotitis | Mumps, parainfluenza |
| Myocarditis/pericarditis | Coxsackie B and echoviruses |
| Keratitis/conjunctivitis | Herpes simplex virus, VZV, adenovirus, enterovirus 70 |
| Pleurodynia | Coxsackie B |
| Herpangina | Coxsackie A |
| Febrile illness with rash | Echoviruses and coxsackie viruses |
| Infectious mononucleosis | Epstein-Barr virus and CMV |
| Meningitis | Echoviruses and coxsackie viruses, mumps, lymphocytic choriomeningitis, HSV-2 |
| Encephalitis | HSV-1, togaviruses, bunyaviruses, flaviviruses, rabies, enteroviruses, measles, HIV, JCV |
| Hepatitis | Hepatitis A, B, C, D (delta agent), E, and non-A, B, C, D, E |
| Hemorrhagic cystitis | Adenovirus, BK virus |
| Cutaneous infection with or without rash | HSV-1 and HSV-2; VZV; enteroviruses; measles; rubella; parvovirus B-19; human herpes virus 6 and 7; HPV; poxviruses, including smallpox, monkeypox, molluscum contagiosum; and orf |
| Hemorrhagic fever | Ebola, Marburg, Lassa, yellow fever, dengue, and other viruses |
| Generalized, no specific target organ | HIV-1, HIV-2, HTLV-1 |

*CMV,* cytomegalovirus; *HIV,* human immunodeficiency virus; *HPV,* human papillomavirus; *HSV-1,* herpes simplex virus type 1; *HSV-2,* herpes simplex virus type 2; *HTLV-1,* human T-lymphotropic virus type 1; *JCV,* JC virus; *SARS,* severe acute respiratory syndrome; *VZV,* varicella-zoster virus.

for holding cell culture tubes during incubation, and enzyme or molecular testing instrumentation (Figures 65-5 to 65-7).

Standard precautions and Biosafety Level 2 conditions are needed for community and most nonretroviral laboratories. Requirements include standard microbiologic practices, training in biosafety, protective clothing and gloves, limited access, decontamination of all infectious waste, and a class I or II BSC. Some viruses should not be propagated in Biosafety Level 2 laboratories, including influenza H5N1, SARS coronavirus, hemorrhagic fever viruses, and smallpox.

## SPECIMEN SELECTION AND COLLECTION

### General Principles

Specimen selection depends on the specific disease syndrome, viral etiologies suspected, and time of year. Selecting a specimen based on disease is confusing, because most viruses enter through the upper respiratory tract and infect tissues that may produce symptoms distant from the primary inoculation site. For example, aseptic meningitis, caused by infection with various types of enterovirus, may be identified by detecting virus in throat, rectal swab, or cerebrospinal fluid (CSF)

**TABLE 65-2** Viruses Detected by Culture, PCR, or Assay for Antigen in a Community Hospital Virology Laboratory*

| Infecting Virus | Number of Cases (Adults and Children) |
|---|---|
| Adenovirus | 25 |
| Cytomegalovirus | 30 |
| Enterovirus | 50 |
| Herpes simplex virus | 206 |
| Influenza virus | 426 |
| Parainfluenza virus | 41 |
| Respiratory syncytial virus | 151 |
| Rotavirus | 163 |
| Varicella-zoster virus | 38 |
| Total | 1130 |

*PCR,* Polymerase chain reaction.
*Data from 1 year of testing at Evanston Northwestern Healthcare, Evanston, Illinois.

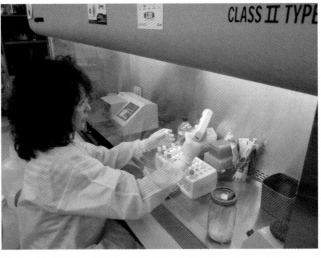

**Figure 65-7** Class II biological safety cabinet used in a clinical virology laboratory.

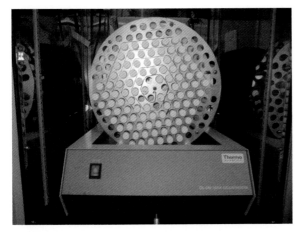

**Figure 65-5** Roller drum used to hold cell culture tubes during incubation. Slow rotation continually bathes the cells in the medium.

specimens. Pharyngitis and gastrointestinal symptoms may not be included in the patient's complaints.

Specimen selection based on the suspected viral etiology is complicated by the fact that similar clinical syndromes can be caused by many different viruses. When specimens required for identification of a specific virus are collected without thorough consideration of other possible viral agents, additional important etiologic agents may be missed. For example, testing smears of nasal secretions from an infant using fluorescence staining or enzyme immunoassay to detect RSV does not allow for diagnosis of similar disease resulting from infection with influenza virus, parainfluenza virus, or metapneumovirus.

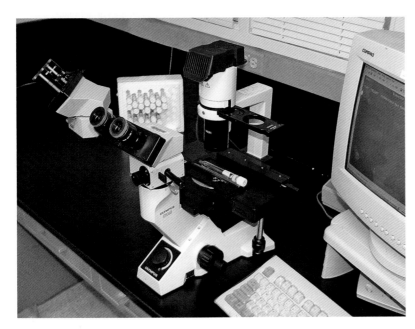

**Figure 65-6** Inverted microscope used to examine cell monolayers growing attached to the inside surface beneath the liquid medium. Note that the objective is under the glass test tube, facilitating observation of the cell monolayer.

Selection of the appropriate type of specimen is one of the keys to a correct test result. Selection should include the proper specimen source and the correct sample volume and timing of collection. This information should be reviewed institutionally on an annual basis and made available to clinicians.

Appropriate specimen selection dictates that the specimen type and suspected viruses should be included on the requisition. The laboratory should always be notified if rare agents representing a danger to laboratory workers are suspected (e.g., SARS coronavirus, H5N1 avian influenza virus, hemorrhagic fever viruses). Serum for serologic testing may be necessary, and some viral diseases should be considered during specific months. Table 65-3 presents specimens for the diagnosis of viral diseases, noting trends in seasonality.

Specimens for the detection of virus should be collected as early as possible after the onset of symptomatic disease. Virus may no longer be present as early

as 2 days after the appearance of symptoms. However, other factors, such as the patient's immune status or age, the type of virus, and the amount of systemic involvement, may play a role in the length of time viral shedding is evident, allowing effective laboratory detection. Certain viruses, such as West Nile virus, produce a brief, low viremia and undetectable levels at the onset of symptoms. Recommendations for collection of various specimens are summarized in this section.

In addition to the type of specimen and collection method, validated devices or containers can enhance the recovery and detection of the viral agent. Swab specimens should not contain chemicals or other compounds that may be toxic to cultured cells and therefore are unsuitable for viral specimen collection. Calcium alginate swabs interfere with PCR, the recovery of some enveloped viruses, and fluorescent-antibody tests and therefore should not be used.

**TABLE 65-3** Specimens for Diagnosis of Viral Diseases*

| Disease Categories and Probable Viral Agent | Season of Most Common Occurrence | Throat/ Nasopharynx | Stool | CSF | Urine | Other |
|---|---|---|---|---|---|---|
| **Respiratory** Adenoviruses | Y | ++++ | | | | |
| Influenza virus | W | ++++ | | | | |
| Parainfluenza virus | Y | ++++ | | | | |
| Respiratory syncytial virus (RSV) | W | ++++ | | | | |
| Metapneumovirus | W | ++++ | | | | |
| Rhinoviruses | Y | | | | | Nasal (+++) |
| SARS coronavirus | W | ++++ | | | | |
| Sin nombre virus | SP, S | | | | | Serum for antibody detection |
| **Dermatologic and Mucous Membrane** VESICULAR Enterovirus | S, F | ++ | +++ | | | Vesicle fluid or scraping |
| Herpes simplex virus[†] | Y | | | | | Vesicle fluid or scraping |
| Varicella-zoster virus[†] | Y | ++ | | | | Vesicle fluid or scraping |
| Monkeypox | Y | | | | | Vesicle fluid or scraping |
| EXANTHEMATOUS Enterovirus | S, F | +++ | ++ | | | |
| Measles | Y | ++ | | | ++ | Serum for antibody detection |
| Rubella | Y | | | | ++ | Serum for antibody detection |
| Parvovirus | Y | | | | | Serum for antibody detection, amniotic fluid (PCR) |
| PUSTULAR/NODULAR Molluscum contagiosum, orf | Y | | | | | Tissue |
| Warts Papillomavirus | Y | | | | | Tissue/cells, thin-prep cervical |
| **Meningoencephalitis/Encephalitis** Arboviruses | S, F | | | | | CSF/serum for antibody detection |

**TABLE 65-3** Specimens for Diagnosis of Viral Diseases—cont'd

| Disease Categories and Probable Viral Agent | Season of Most Common Occurrence | Throat/ Nasopharynx | Stool | CSF | Urine | Other |
|---|---|---|---|---|---|---|
| Enteroviruses | S, F | +++ | | ++ | ++++ | |
| Herpes simplex virus | Y | | | ++++ | | Brain biopsy (PCR) |
| Lymphocytic choriomeningitis | Y | | | | | Serum for antibody detection |
| Mumps virus | Y | | | | | Serum for antibody detection |
| HIV | Y | | | | | Brain biopsy (culture/PCR) |
| Polyomavirus (JC virus) | Y | | | | | Brain biopsy (EM/PCR) |
| Rabies virus | Y | | | | | Corneal cells, brain |
| **Gastrointestinal Disease** Adenoviruses (serotypes 40-41) | Y | | ++++ | | | Stool (EIA or EM) |
| Noroviruses | S | | ++++ | | | Stool (EM) |
| Rotavirus | W, SP | | ++++ | | | Stool (EIA, latex) |
| **Dermatologic and Mucous Membrane** CONGENITAL AND PERINATAL Cytomegalovirus | Y | | | | +++ | Serum for antibody (IgM) detection |
| Enteroviruses | S, F | +++ | | +++ | +++ | |
| Herpes simplex virus | Y | | | | | Vesicle fluid |
| Parvovirus | Y | | | | | Amniotic fluid, liver tissue |
| Rubella | Y | | | | ++ | Serum for antibody (IgM) detection |
| EYE (OCULAR DISEASE) Adenoviruses | Y | ++ | | | | Conjunctival swab or scraping |
| Herpes simplex virus | Y | | | | | Conjunctival swab or scraping |
| Varicella-zoster virus | Y | | | | | Conjunctival swab or scraping |
| POSTTRANSPLANTATION SYNDROME Cytomegalovirus | Y | | | | ++ | Blood (++++) shell vial and/or antigenemia; tissue (++++) |
| Epstein-Barr virus | Y | | | | | Serology, tissue (PCR) (EBV) |
| Human herpesvirus-6 (HH6) | Y | | | | | Serology, blood (PCR) |
| Herpes simplex | Y | | | | | Tissue (+++) virus |
| BK virus | Y | | | | ++++ | |
| **Myocarditis, Pericarditis, and Pleurodynia** Coxsackie B | S, F | +++ | | ++ | | Pericardial fluid (++++) |
| **Hemorrhagic Fevers** Ebola/Marburg viruses | Y | | | | | Tissue, respiratory secretions, serum for antibody detection |
| Lassa fever virus | | +++ | | | + | Serum/throat washes for viral detection Serum for antibody detection |
| **Hepatitis** Hepatitis | Y | | | | | Serology, blood (PCR) |

*CSF*, cerebrospinal fluid; *EBV,* Epstein-Barr virus*; EIA*, enzyme immunoassay; *EM*, electron microscopy; *F*, fall; *PCR*, polymerase chain reaction; *HIV,* human immunodeficiency virus; *S*, summer; *SARS,* severe acute respiratory syndrome; *SP*, spring; *W*, winter; *Y*, Year-round.
*Specimens indicated beside specific viruses should be obtained if that specific virus is suspected (++++, most appropriate; + least appropriate).
†Direct fluorescent antibody studies are available for herpes simplex virus and varicella-zoster virus.

## Throat, Nasopharyngeal Swab, or Aspirate

In general, nasopharyngeal aspirates are superior to throat or nasopharyngeal swabs for recovering viruses; however, swabs are considerably more convenient. Throat swabs are acceptable for the recovery of enteroviruses, adenoviruses, and HSV, whereas nasopharyngeal swab or aspirate specimens are preferred for the detection of RSV and influenza and parainfluenza viruses. Rhinovirus detection requires a nasal specimen. Throat specimens are collected with a dry, sterile swab by passing the swab over the inflamed, vesiculated, or purulent areas on the posterior pharynx. The swab should not be touched to the tongue, buccal mucosa, teeth, or gums. Nasopharyngeal secretion specimens are collected by inserting a swab with a flexible shaft through the nostril into the nasopharynx or by washing and collecting the secretions by rinsing with a bulb syringe and 3 to 7 mL of buffered saline. The saline is squirted into the nose by squeezing the bulb and aspirated with a small tubing inserted into the other nostril when the bulb or suction is released.

All respiratory specimens are acceptable for culture of most viruses. However, respiratory and oral samples often are contaminated with bacteria. Contaminants may be removed by concentrating the sample through centrifugation. However, this process may also result in removal of virus-infected cells and reduce the recovery of viral agents from the sample.

## Bronchial and Bronchoalveolar Washes

Washings and lavage fluid collected during bronchoscopy are excellent specimens for detecting viruses that infect the lower respiratory tract, especially influenza viruses and adenoviruses.

## Rectal Swabs and Stool Specimens

Stool and rectal swabs of fecal specimens are used to detect rotavirus, enteric adenoviruses (serotypes 40 and 41), and enteroviruses. Many agents of viral gastroenteritis do not grow in cell culture and require PCR or electron microscopy for detection (these are discussed later in the chapter). In general, stool specimens are preferable to rectal swabs and should be required for rotavirus and enteric adenovirus testing. Rectal swabs are acceptable for detecting enteroviruses in patients suspected of having an enteroviral disease, such as aseptic meningitis. The rectal swab is inserted 3 to 5 cm into the rectum and rotated against the mucosa to obtain feces. The swab should then be placed in appropriate transport media. A stool sample is preferred over a rectal swab because of the potential for decreased viral recovery from a small sample size. Five to 10 mL of freshly passed diarrheal stool or stool collected in a diaper from young infants is sufficient and preferred for rotavirus and enteric adenovirus detection.

## Urine

CMV; mumps, rubella, and measles viruses; polyomaviruses; and adenoviruses can be detected in urine. Virus often is shed intermittently or in low numbers. Viral recovery may be increased by processing multiple (two to three) specimens. Improved recovery results with a minimum specimen volume of 10 mL from a clean-catch first-morning urine. The urine pH and contaminating bacteria may interfere with viral replication. Virus recovery is improved by centrifugation or filtering to remove contaminants and neutralizing the pH with a 7.5% solution of sodium bicarbonate.

## Skin and Mucous Membrane Lesions

Enteroviruses, HSV, VZV, and in rare cases CMV or pox viruses can be detected in vesicular lesions of the skin and mucous membranes. Once the vesicle has ulcerated or crusted, detection of the virus is difficult.

Collection of specimens from cutaneous vesicles for detection of HSV or VZV may require a Tzanck smear if PCR testing is not available. Tzanck smears are prepared by carefully unroofing the vesicle. The procedure is as follows: If a tuberculin syringe is used, a small "drop" of vesicle fluid should be aspirated first and held for further use in the event a viral or bacterial culture is needed. The needle is flushed with a viral transport medium, and phosphate buffered saline or viral support media (EMEM) is added to the viral transport tube. With the roof of the vesicle folded back, excess fluid is carefully removed by dabbing with sterile gauze. A clean glass microscope slide is pressed against the base of the ulcer. The slide is lifted, moved slightly, and pressed again. Cells from the base of the ulcer stick to the slide, making an "impression smear" of infected and uninfected cells. Additional smears can be made from other vesicles. The slides are sent to the laboratory for fixation and staining. As an alternative, vesicle fluid and cells scraped from the base of an unroofed vesicle can be added to 2 to 3 mL of viral transport medium. Smears can be prepared in the laboratory with cytocentrifugation of fluid medium, or PCR can be performed from the specimen in the viral transport medium.

## Sterile Body Fluids Other Than Blood

Sterile body fluids, especially CSF and pericardial and pleural fluids, may contain enteroviruses, HSV, VZV, influenza viruses, or CMV. These specimens are collected aseptically by the physician and sent to the laboratory for processing.

## Blood

Viral culture of blood is used primarily to detect CMV; however, HSV, VZV, enteroviruses and adenovirus occasionally may be encountered. CMV viremia is associated with peripheral blood leucocytes. Five to 10 mL of anticoagulated blood collected in a whole blood tube is needed. Heparinized, citrated, or ethylenediaminetetraacetic acid (EDTA) anticoagulated blood is acceptable for CMV detection. Citrated blood should be used when other viruses are being considered. EDTA should be used for samples collected for nucleic acid testing, because other anticoagulants may interfere with the enzyme functions required for PCR amplification. Serum may be used for serologic tests and nucleic acid assays.

### Bone Marrow

Bone marrow for virus detection should be added to a sterile tube with anticoagulant. Heparin, citrate, or EDTA anticoagulants are acceptable. As previously described for blood, EDTA should be used if the specimen is intended for nucleic acid testing. Specimens are collected by aspiration. Except for parvovirus B19, most viruses are detected more readily from sites other than bone marrow.

### Tissue

Tissue specimens are especially useful for detecting viruses that commonly infect the lungs (CMV, influenza virus, adenovirus, sin nombre virus), brain (HSV), and gastrointestinal tract (CMV). Specimens are collected during surgical procedures. Fresh tissue is preferred for nucleic acid assays, but formalin-fixed and paraffin-embedded tissues may be used after removal of the paraffin (deparaffinization) and extraction.

### Genital Specimens

Genital specimens often are required for detection of HSV and human papillomavirus (HPV). Genital swabs should be used for ulcerations and placed in appropriate viral transport media. Cervical specimens may be collected using a swab or brush and placed in viral transport media. Some manufactured endocervical or liquid-based cytology devices are appropriate for nucleic acid testing. Following the manufacturer's recommended protocols is essential when processing such specimens.

### Serum for Antibody Testing

Acute and convalescent serum specimens may be needed to detect antibody to specific viruses. Acute specimens should be collected as soon as possible after the appearance of symptoms. The convalescent specimen is collected a minimum of 2 to 3 weeks after the acute specimen. In both cases, an appropriate specimen is 3 to 5 mL of serum collected by venipuncture.

## SPECIMEN TRANSPORT AND STORAGE

Ideally all specimens collected for detection of virus should be processed immediately. Although inoculation of specimens into cell culture at the bedside has been recommended in the past, potential biohazards, sophisticated processing steps, and necessary quality controls make this impractical. Specimens for viral isolation should not be allowed to sit at room or higher temperature. Specimens should be kept cool (4°C) and immediately transported to the laboratory. If a delay in transport is unavoidable, the specimen should be refrigerated, not frozen, until processed. Every attempt should be made to process the specimen within 12 to 24 hours of collection. Under unusual circumstances, specimens may need to be held for several days before processing. For storage up to 5 days, specimens are held at 4°C. Storage for 6 days or longer should be at −20° or preferably−70°C. Specimens for freezing should first be diluted or emulsified in viral transport medium. Significant loss of viral infectivity may occur during prolonged storage, regardless of conditions, especially for the more labile enveloped viruses.

If a commercial kit is used for viral identification (e.g., nucleic acid testing), the specimens should be transported and stored according to the manufacturer's instructions. Specimens for processing using commercial reagents that are not approved by the U.S. Food and Drug Administration (FDA), such as analyte-specific reagents, or assays that have been created and validated in the user's laboratory (laboratory-developed tests [LDTs]), are transported and stored at refrigeration temperatures. Freezing at −70°C is recommended if processing is delayed for longer than 2 to 3 days.

Many types of specimens for the detection of virus can be collected with a swab. Most types of synthetic swab material, such as rayon and Dacron, are acceptable. Swabs with cotton tips and wooden shafts are not recommended. Once collected, specimens on swabs should be emulsified in viral transport medium before transport to the laboratory, especially if transport will occur at room temperature and require longer than 1 hour. Calcium alginate is not acceptable for the detection of HSV, because it may inactivate the virus. Also, as previously mentioned, it is not recommended for PCR amplification of any respiratory viruses.

Commercially prepared transport media are useful for maintaining viral stability. They are used to transport small volumes of fluid specimens, small tissues and scrapings, and swab specimens, especially when contamination with microbial flora is expected. Transport media contain protein (e.g., serum, albumin, or gelatin) to stabilize the viral agents and antimicrobials to prevent overgrowth of bacteria and fungi. Penicillin (500 units/mL) and streptomycin (500 to 1000 mcg/mL) have been used traditionally; however, a more potent mixture is composed of vancomycin (20 mcg/mL), gentamicin (50 mcg/mL), and amphotericin (10 mcg/mL). If serum is added as the protein source, fetal calf serum is recommended, because it is less likely to contain inhibitors, such as antibodies. Examples of successful transport media include Stuart's medium, Amie's medium, Leibovitz-Emory medium, Hanks balanced salt solution (HBSS), Eagle's tissue culture medium, and the commercially available M4, M5, and universal transport media. Respiratory and rectal and stool specimens can be maintained in modified Stuart's medium, modified HBSS, or Leibovitz-Emory medium containing antimicrobials.

Blood for viral culture, transported in a sterile tube containing anticoagulant, must be kept at refrigeration temperature (4°C) until processed. Blood for viral serology testing should be transported to the laboratory in the sterile tube in which it was collected. Serum should be separated from the clot as soon as possible. Serum can be stored for hours or days at 4°C or for weeks or months at −20°C or below before testing. Testing for virus-specific IgM should be completed before freezing whenever possible, because IgM may form insoluble aggregates upon thawing, producing a false-negative result.

# SPECIMEN PROCESSING

## General Principles

Specimens for viral culture should be processed immediately upon receipt in the laboratory. This may be accomplished by combining bacteriology and virology processing responsibilities. Although the threat of cell culture contamination in the past dictated separation of virology procedures, the addition of broad-spectrum antimicrobials to cell cultures has significantly reduced the possibility of cross-contamination with bacteria and fungi. In most laboratories, processing with other microbiology specimens allows viral cultures to be processed 7 days a week. If delays must occur, specimens should be stored in a viral transport medium at 4°C as described previously. Delay in the processing of fluid specimens requires dilution in a transport medium (1:2 to 1:5) before storage.

In addition to patient identification and demographics, each specimen for virus isolation should be accompanied by a requisition that provides (1) the source of the specimen; (2) the clinical history or viruses suspected; and (3) the date and time of specimen collection. If this information is not available, a call for additional details should be made to the requesting physician or to the person caring for the patient.

Viral specimens should be processed in a BSC whenever possible (see Figure 65-7). This protects specimens from contamination by the processing technologist and protects those in the laboratory from infectious aerosols created when specimens are manipulated. Latex gloves and a laboratory coat should be worn during manipulation of all patient specimens. Vortexing, pipetting, and centrifugation can create dangerous aerosols. Vortexing should be done in a tightly capped tube behind a shield. After vortexing, the tube should be opened in a BSC. Pipetting should be performed behind a protective shield. Pipettes must be discarded into a disinfectant fluid so that the disinfectant reaches the inside of the pipette or into a leak-proof biosafety bag for autoclaving or incineration. When patient cell cultures are manipulated, such as during inoculation or feeding (exchange of cell culture medium), only one patient sample or series of cell culture tubes should be open at one time. Aerosols and microsplashes contribute to cross-contamination of cultures, especially during viral respiratory season when a high percentage of specimens are positive for influenza virus, RSV, and other viruses.

Processing virology specimens is not complicated (Table 65-4). In general, any primary specimen or swab specimen that may be contaminated with bacteria or fungi should be added to a viral transport medium. Normally sterile fluid specimens can be inoculated directly to cell culture. The viral transport medium or fluid specimens not in a transport medium should be vortexed immediately before inoculation to break up virus-containing cells and resuspend the inoculum. Adding sterile glass beads to the transport medium helps break up cell clumps and release virus from cell aggregates. This may not be necessary, because some commercially available mediums contain beads. Grossly contaminated or potentially toxic specimens, such as minced or ground tissue, can be centrifuged (1000× *g* for 15 minutes) and the virus-containing supernatant used as the inoculum. Each viral cell culture tube is inoculated with 200 to 400 μL of specimen. If insufficient specimen is available, the specimen obtained is diluted with a viral transport medium to increase the volume. Excess specimen can be stored at −70°C in the event the initial culture is contaminated. A set of uninoculated cultures should be maintained simultaneously for continual monitoring of sterility and contamination throughout the process.

Contaminated specimens can be reprocessed with an antibiotic-containing viral transport medium if they were not originally handled in this manner, or they can be filtered using a disposable, 0.22 to 0.45 μm filter and the filtrate recultured. In practice, virus is rarely detected in culture from most specimens requiring reprocessing because of the potential for contamination. When these specimens are processed, the specimen should be allowed to adsorb in an incubator at 35° to 37°C for 30 to 60 minutes; 1 to 1.5 mL of maintenance medium is then added, and the tubes are returned to the incubator, preferably in a roller rack in a rotating drum. Blood for viral culture requires special processing to isolate leukocytes, followed by inoculation into cell culture tubes (see Procedure 65-1 on the Evolve site). Rapid shell vial cell cultures are used to detect many viruses. (Handling and examination of cell cultures after inoculation with specimen are discussed later in this chapter.)

## Processing Based on Specimen Type

Virology laboratories should maintain a menu of individual virus detection and serology tests and an algorithm for their use, rather than using one test battery for all situations. Tables 65-5 and 65-6 present virus detection and serology assays that are useful in a community clinical virology laboratory. Molecular detection methods increasingly are being used for all infectious agents, particularly viruses. In some laboratories, more than half of all virus detection assays are molecular based (e.g., PCR or DNA probe detection). To optimize viral detection, an algorithm for the process should be based on the type of specimen or the specific virus suspected. However, this is often problematic, because most laboratories receive specimens with little or no clinical data. The algorithm in Figure 65-8 is designed for use with such specimens.

**Lip and Genital Specimens.** Lip and genital specimens should be tested for HSV using culture or molecular methods. Other etiologic agents associated with lip or genital infections, such as VZV or enterovirus, are unusual and are considered when specifically requested by the attending physician.

**Urine.** Urine specimens often are submitted for CMV detection. This sample typically is used in a shell vial cell culture or molecular assay.

**Stool.** Stool specimens from infants and young children (5 years of age and younger) in North America should be tested for rotavirus during the fall, winter, and spring. Enteric adenoviruses (serotypes 40 and 41) cause diarrhea in young children and infants throughout the year. Adenovirus gastroenteritis appears to be more common in some geographic areas. Routine testing is necessary in locations where disease is endemic. Stool or

**TABLE 65-4** Laboratory Processing of Viral Specimens

| Source | Specimen | Processing* | Cells for Detection of Common Viruses |
|---|---|---|---|
| Blood | Anticoagulated blood | Separate leukocytes (see Procedure 65-1) | PMK, HDF, HEp-2 |
| Cerebrospinal fluid (CSF) | 1 mL CSF | Inoculate directly | PMK, HDF, HEp-2 |
| Stool or rectal swab | Pea-sized aliquot of feces | Place in 2 mL of viral transport medium vortex. Centrifuge at 1000× *g* for 15 min and use supernatant fluid for inoculum | PMK, HDF, HEp-2 |
| Genital, skin | Vesicle fluid or scraping | Emulsify in viral transport medium | HDF |
| Miscellaneous | Swab, fluids | Emulsify in viral transport medium Fluid, inoculate directly | PMK, HDF, HEp-2 |
| Respiratory tract | Nasopharyngeal secretions, throat swab, respiratory tract washings, sputum | Dilute with viral transport medium | PMK, HDF, HEp-2 |
| Tissue | Tissue in sterile container | Mince with sterile scalpel and scissors and gently grind. Prepare 20% suspension in viral transport medium. Centrifuge at 1000× *g* for 15 min and use supernatant fluid for inoculum. | PMK, HDF, HEp-2 |
| Urine | Midstream specimen | Clear: Inoculate directly. Turbid: Centrifuge at 1000× *g* for 15 min and use supernatant fluid for inocula. | HDF, HEp-2 (if adenovirus suspected) |

*HDF*, Human diploid fibroblast; *HEp-2*, human epidermoid; *PMK*, primary monkey kidney.
*All inocula into tissue culture tubes are 0.25 mL volumes.

rectal swabs from adults, children, and infants should be examined for enterovirus in summer and fall as an aid to the diagnosis of aseptic meningitis. Stool for enterovirus should be collected in conjunction with throat and CSF specimens when possible.

**Respiratory Tract.** Respiratory specimens should be separated based on the patient's age and underlying medical condition. Immunocompromised patients require a comprehensive virus detection assay consisting of cell culture or corresponding molecular tests. Immunocompetent adults should be examined for influenza virus with culture or PCR during November to April in most areas. Children younger than 10 years of age are susceptible to serious infection caused by influenza virus, parainfluenza virus, RSV, and adenoviruses and require a full respiratory virus panel. Infants younger than 2 years of age are especially vulnerable to RSV bronchiolitis, which may require hospitalization and comprehensive supportive care. A rapid, nonculture RSV detection assay, such as PCR, fluorescent antibody (FA) staining or enzyme immunoassay, is appropriate in these situations.

**Specimens from Neonatal Patients.** When appropriate, specimens from newborns should be examined with a comprehensive virus culture, rapid shell vial cell culture for CMV, and appropriate molecular tests (e.g., enteroviruses) to determine whether congenital or perinatal disease is present. Consultation with the pediatrician or neonatologist is necessary to determine which diagnostics are required in light of the patient's specific clinical condition.

**Cerebrospinal Fluid.** CSF specimens can contain many different viral agents. HSV, enteroviruses, HIV, and arboviruses are the most prevalent viruses isolated from CSF. HSV, HIV, and enteroviruses can be quickly detected using molecular assays, whereas arboviruses require antibody testing. Testing for other, less frequently suspected viruses, such as CMV, VZV, JC virus (JCV), and many more, should be included after consultation with the patient's physician.

**Blood.** CMV, VZV, HCV, adenovirus, or enteroviruses may be isolated from blood; however, CMV is by far more frequently detected, and quantitation has proven clinically relevant for monitoring therapy. All specimens from immunocompromised patients and tissues or fluids from normally sterile sites should be processed for comprehensive virus detection. Processing of specimens (see Figure 65-8) should be modified to match the needs of local physicians and the endemic viral diseases.

### Processing Based on Requests for Specific Viruses

**Arboviruses.** Serologic tests for arboviruses are offered in public health laboratories and some commercial laboratories. Diagnosis of arbovirus encephalitis, such as Eastern, Western, Venezuelan, St. Louis, and California encephalitis, and also La Crosse and West Nile virus infection, requires detection of virus-specific IgM antibody in serum or a rise in IgG antibody titer in paired sera. Detection of virus-specific IgM in CSF is available for most agents. Culture of arboviruses for diagnostic purposes is not practical. PCR for some agents is available through state public health laboratories but may be less sensitive than serodiagnosis, because the virus and the viral nucleic acid are detectable only for brief periods during the course of infection.

**TABLE 65-5** Virus Detection or Quantitation Tests

| Test | Frequency of Request (%)* |
|---|---|
| **Culture/Antigen Detection** | |
| Blood culture (cytomegalovirus [CMV] shell vial/antigenemia) | 2 |
| Bronchial secretions culture | 5 |
| Enterovirus culture | 4 |
| Herpes simplex virus culture | 5 |
| Influenza culture/antigen detection | 12 |
| Pediatric respiratory viruses culture | 13 |
| Rotavirus antigen detection | 8 |
| Respiratory syncytial virus detection | 24 |
| Urine culture | 2 |
| Viral culture (tissue and fluids) | 12 |
| Varicella-zoster virus detection | 13 |
| **Total tests (N = 4776)** | 100 |
| **Molecular Detection/Quantitation** | |
| Cytomegalovirus detection | 5 |
| Enterovirus detection | <1 |
| Hepatitis C virus quantitation | 8 |
| Human immunodeficiency virus detection and quantitation | 7 |
| Human papillomavirus detection | 54 |
| Herpes simplex virus detection | 4 |
| Influenza virus detection | 22 |
| Parvovirus detection | <1 |
| **Total tests (N = 4842)** | 100 |

Data from 1 year of testing at Evanston Northwestern Healthcare, Evanston, Illinois.
*Frequency of request expressed as a percentage of all tests.

**TABLE 65-6** Viral Serology Tests

| Test | Frequency of Request (%)* |
|---|---|
| Cytomegalovirus IgM and/or IgG | 3 |
| Enterovirus antibody | <1 |
| Epstein-Barr virus panel or individual antibody | 1 |
| Hepatitis panel | 8 |
| Hepatitis A IgM and/or IgG | 1 |
| Hepatitis B panel or individual antigen/antibody test | 28 |
| Hepatitis C antibody | 7 |
| Human immunodeficiency virus antibody or antigen | 34 |
| Human T-lymphotropic virus type 1 antibody | <1 |
| Influenza A or B antibody | <1 |
| Measles antibody | 5 |
| Mumps antibody | 1 |
| Parvovirus antibody | <1 |
| Rubella antibody | 6 |
| Varicella-zoster antibody | 6 |
| **Total tests (N = 24,071)** | 100 |

Data from 1 year of testing at Evanston Northwestern Healthcare, Evanston, Illinois.
*Frequency of request expressed as percentage of all tests.

**Cytomegalovirus.** CMV can be detected in clinical specimens using conventional cell culture, shell vial assay, antigenemia immunoassay, or molecular methods. CMV produces cytopathic effects (CPE) in diploid fibroblast cells in 3 to 28 days, averaging 7 days. CMV shell vial assay sensitivity is equivalent to conventional cell culture, and results are available within 16 hours. The antigenemia immunoassay uses monoclonal antibody in an indirect immunoperoxidase or indirect immunofluorescent stain to detect CMV protein (pp65) in peripheral blood leukocytes. The antigenemia assay requires 3 to 5 hours and includes the sedimentation and separation of leukocytes, counting of leukocytes, and a standardized density smear preparation, followed by staining and counting of infected (fluorescing) cells (see Procedure 65-2 on the Evolve site). Results are reported as the number of positive leukocytes per total number of leukocytes in the smear. Quantitative CMV PCR and a commercially available CMV hybrid capture assay (Digene, Gaithersburg, Maryland) are also available for detection and quantitation of CMV viremia. Molecular assays have replaced the anteginemia assay in some laboratories.

**Enteroviruses.** Enteroviruses can be detected using conventional cell culture and PCR. Although most enteroviruses grow in primary monkey kidney (PMK) cells, some strains grow faster in diploid fibroblast, buffalo green monkey kidney, or rhabdomyosarcoma cell lines. To reduce waste and provide availability when needed, frozen "ready cells" (Diagnostic Hybrids, Athens, Ohio) may be used. Ready cells may be stored for up to 5 months and demonstrate comparable results as fresh cells. Presumptive diagnosis is based on CPE. Confirmation or definitive diagnosis is accomplished using commercially available FA stains. PCR is the preferred method for diagnosing enterovirus septic meningitis. Most enteroviruses are detected from June to December. The mean time from sample inoculation to detection in cell culture is 4 days.

**Epstein-Barr Virus.** Serology tests are useful in the diagnosis of Epstein-Barr virus (EBV)–associated diseases, including infectious mononucleosis. Isolation of EBV (in cultured B lymphocytes) is not routinely performed in clinical laboratories.

**Hepatitis Viruses.** Disease or asymptomatic carriage caused by hepatitis A, B, C, D, and E viruses is detected using serology, antigen detection, or PCR tests (Table 65-7). Even though hepatitis viruses are not routinely cultured, a variety of diagnostic tests are available for the detection of antibody and antigen. Hepatitis A, usually

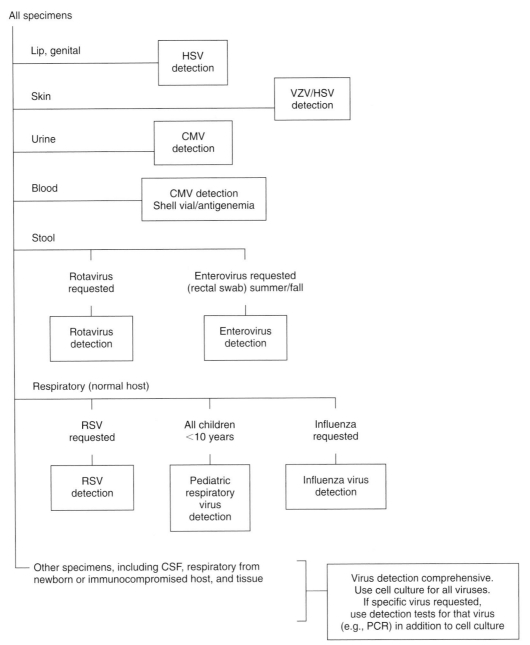

**Figure 65-8** Algorithm for the processing of viral specimens based on specimen type and suspected virus. Virus detection implies viral culture, antigen detection, or molecular testing (e.g., polymerase chain reaction [PCR] assay).

transmitted through contaminated food and water, is diagnosed by screening for the IgM antibody using serology. Hepatitis B produces acute and chronic infection and is associated with hepatocellular carcinoma; it is transmitted parenterally and by tattooing, acupuncture, sexual contact, and perinatal infection. Diagnosis of hepatitis B infection is made through the quantitation of antibody, and antibody to the surface, core, and e antigens. The first marker to appear in acute infection is the hepatitis B surface antigen (HBsAg); as the infection resolves, HBsAg disappears and HBsAb appears.

Hepatitis C is a RNA virus transmitted by blood transfusion, intravenous drug abuse, hemodialysis, and contaminated instruments, such as body piercing and tattooing devices. HCV infection becomes chronic in more than 80% of patients, and the diagnosis is made by antibody detection. HCV RNA can be measured by PCR to assess the patient's response to treatment.

**Herpes Simplex Virus.** HSV grows rapidly in most cell lines. MRC-5 or mink lung fibroblast cell lines are recommended, along with a continuous cell line such as A-549. Ready cells, as previously described, are also available for the cultivation of herpes viruses. Fifty percent of genital HSV isolates are detected within 24 hours and 100% within 3 to 5 days. Cultures should be examined daily and finalized if negative after 5 days of incubation. Real time-PCR detects HSV within hours, and the sensitivity is equal to or greater than cell culture.

**TABLE 65-7** Serology Tests for Hepatitis Viruses

| Disease | Virus | Diagnostic Tests |
|---|---|---|
| Hepatitis A | Enterovirus 72 | Antibody to Hepatitis A virus (IgG and IgM) |
| Hepatitis B | Hepadnavirus | Hepatitis B surface-antigen (HBsAg) Hepatitis B early-antigen (HBeAg) Anti-HBsAg Anti-HBeAg Anti-HB core antigen |
| Hepatitis C | Flavivirus | Antibody to hepatitis C virus |
| Hepatitis D | Delta agent (hepatitis D virus) | Antibody to delta agent |
| Hepatitis E | Calicivirus-like (herpes virus) | Antibody to hepatitis E virus |

Enzyme-linked viral-induced system (ELVIS; Diagnostic Hybrids, Athens, Ohio) is a special shell vial system available for detection of HSV in 24 hours. When the cells become infected with HSV, they accumulate β-galactosidase. Following incubation, the shell vial is fixed and stained with substrate for β-galactosidase, resulting in a visible blue color change that can be viewed using an inverted microscope. This technique is described in more detail later in this chapter. In addition, type-specific serology tests, such as HerpeSelect (Focus Diagnostics, Cypress, CA) are also available. More recently, a new isothermal nucleic acid-based test, BioHelix IsoAmp HSV assay, has been developed, It uses a proprietary amplification technology referred to as helicase-dependent amplification (HAD; BioHelix, Beverly, MA). The assay is capable of detecting HSVI and HSVII genital or oral lesions in approximately 1.5 hours.

**Human Immunodeficiency Virus and Other Retroviruses.** HIV type 1 (HIV-1) is detected by antibody, antigen, and reverse transcriptase PCR (RT-PCR). HIV-1 enzyme-linked immunosorbent assay (ELISA) antibody tests also detect antibody to HIV type 2 (HIV-2). The ELISA screening test is confirmed with an HIV-1–specific Western blot test or with an ELISA for HIV-2 followed by an HIV-2–specific Western blot test. Recently infected patients who have not seroconverted or newborn babies with maternal antibody can be identified as HIV infected using sensitive RT-PCR assays. HIV infection can also be monitored in those receiving antiviral therapy using quantitative molecular testing with serum specimens. Successful antiviral therapy should reduce the HIV serum viral load to undetectable levels.

Blood for transfusion is screened for antibody indicative of infection with HIV-1, HIV-2, and human T-lymphotropic virus type 1 (HTLV-1) and type 2 (HTLV-2). HTLV-1 ELISA screening tests also detect antibody to HTLV-2. In addition, an HIV antigen (p24) test is performed to determine whether donors have been recently infected. Units containing antigen or antibody are discarded to lower the risk of transferring latent virus from donor cells to the recipient. In 2012, the Food and Drug Administration approved the OraQuick in-home HIV test (OraSure Technologies, Bethlehem, PA). The test provides results within 20 minutes using an oral fluid sample. A positive result does not indicate a definitive infection with HIV. The Centers for Disease Control recommends early detection and testing by qualified personnel for management of infection and appropriate follow-up testing. Home testing does not replace professional diagnosis and patient care.

**Influenza A and B Viruses.** Influenza A and B viruses can be detected by using conventional cell culture, shell vial culture, membrane enzyme immunoassay (EIA), direct staining of respiratory tract secretions using FA methods (Figure 65-9), and RT-PCR. RT-PCR is the current recommended method of detection in most laboratories. PMK cells demonstrate improved detection compared with other cell lines. The median time to detection, using hemadsorption at day 2 or 3, is approximately 3 days. FA staining is used to confirm and type isolates as A or B. Nearly all positive influenza samples demonstrate detectable virus after 1 week of incubation.

**Pediatric Respiratory Viruses.** Influenza and parainfluenza viruses, RSV, and adenoviruses should be sought in specimens from hospitalized infants and children younger than 10 years of age with suspected viral lower respiratory tract disease. All viruses can be detected by fluorescent staining of respiratory secretions or rapid cell culture (shell vial). If direct fluorescent staining is used, cell culture confirmation of all negatives should be examined for children suspected of having viruses other than RSV. Many laboratories use R-Mix cells in a rapid shell vial format to detect respiratory viruses (Box 65-1). This approach mixes two cell lines (human lung carcinoma A549 and mink lung fibroblast Mv1Lu cells; Diagnostic Hybrids, Athens, Ohio) in a single shell vial. Two R-Mix shell vial tubes are inoculated for each specimen. After an 18- to 24-hour incubation, the cell mixture from one tube is stained with a pooled antibody reagent designed to detect all common respiratory viruses. Positive (fluorescent) specimens have the second tube scraped, spotted onto eight-well slides, and stained with individual antibody reagents to identify the specific virus.

If conventional cell culture is used, influenza and parainfluenza viruses are detected in PMK cells by CPE or hemadsorption. Fluorescent staining is used for confirmation and typing. Adenovirus and RSV are detected in HEp-2 cell culture and confirmed, if necessary, by fluorescent staining. Specimens from infants or young children sent for RSV detection should be tested by a rapid, nonculture RSV test. FA staining, conducted by experienced personnel, is equivalent to culture in sensitivity and should be used for single specimens or small batches. Conventional ELISA also is accurate and recommended for large batches of specimens. Membrane ELISA and related testing methods are less sensitive than culture, but results are available quickly (less than 1 hour). These methods are convenient for STAT testing. Figure 65-10 describes a comprehensive approach for the detection of pediatric respiratory viruses.

**Gastroenteritis Viruses.** Electron microscopy (EM) can be used to identify viral agents known to cause

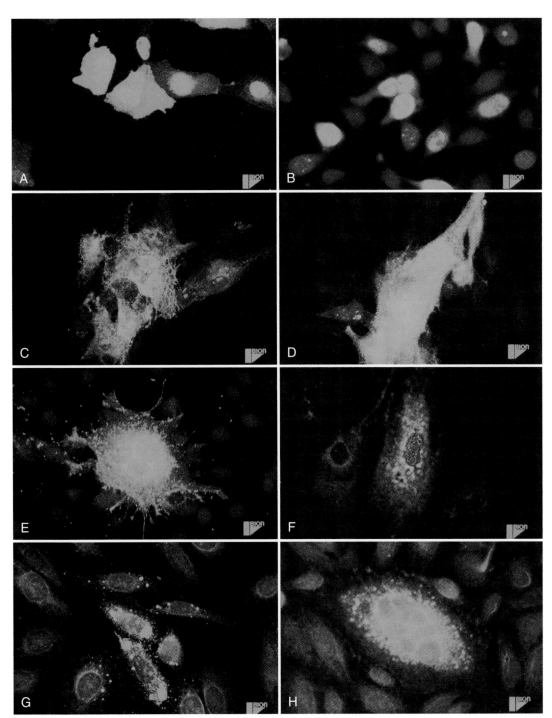

**Figure 65-9** Fluorescent antibody staining of virus-infected cells. **A,** Influenza virus. **B,** Adenovirus. **C,** Varicella-zoster virus. **D,** Herpes simplex virus. **E,** Respiratory syncytial virus. **F,** Parainfluenza virus. **G,** Mumps virus. **H,** Measles virus. (Courtesy Bion Enterprises, Park Ridge, Illinois.)

gastroenteritis (Table 65-8). However, EM is labor intensive and not widely available in clinical virology laboratories. Immunoassays for rotaviruses and enteric adenovirus types 40 and 41 are commercially available. Other viruses, such as noroviruses and astroviruses, do not cause life-threatening diarrheal disease; screening is not routinely done for astrovirus, but RT-PCR is used to detect norovirus, and the results are available the same day. RT-PCR has proven to be a valuable tool in epidemiologic

investigations of outbreaks in nursing homes and day care centers.

**TORCH.** TORCH is an acronym for *Toxoplasma*, rubella, cytomegalovirus, and herpes simplex virus. Testing for these agents and for other viral etiologies of infection in newborns is appropriate during pregnancy. Transplacental infection can result in congenital defects and postnatal complications. CMV frequently is associated with congenital infections.

## BOX 65-1  Overview of Respiratory Virus Detection by R-Mix Shell Vials

### Purpose

To rapidly detect respiratory viruses (influenza A and B viruses, respiratory syncytial viruses, parainfluenza virus types 1, 2, and 3, and adenovirus) using shell vial cell culture and fluorescent antibody staining.

### Principle

A shell vial incubated for 24 to 48 hours is stained with a pool of fluorescently conjugated antibodies capable of reacting with common respiratory viruses. If the result is positive, a second shell vial is scraped and applied as multiple spots to a microscope slide for staining with individual antibody conjugates, each specific for a different virus.

### Specimen

Lower respiratory tract secretions (sputum, endotracheal or bronchial washes, bronchoalveolar lavages), lung tissue, or nasopharyngeal secretions. Throat swabs and specimens are not recommended.

### Materials

- R-Mix shell vials containing a mixture of human lung carcinoma and mink lung cells (Diagnostic Hybrids, Athens, Ohio),
- Centrifuge
- Incubator
- Fluorescent microscope
- Monoclonal antibody screening reagent pool
- Specific virus monoclonal antibody staining reagents (all conjugated to fluorescein isothiocyanate [FITC])

### Methods

1. Thaw, wash, and add refeed medium to cells in shell vials.
2. Inoculate specimen to two duplicate vials.
3. Centrifuge shell vials at 700× *g* for 1 hour.
4. Incubate at 35° to 37°C for 24 to 48 hours.
5. Stain one vial with monoclonal antibody pool screening reagent; if the result is positive, scrape the other shell vial and spot onto an eight-well slide.
6. Stain with specific monoclonal staining reagent to detect the specific virus present.

### Interpretation

Report the specific virus detected with specific monoclonal staining reagent. If no fluorescence is detected with the monoclonal pool screening reagent, report as "No Respiratory Viruses Detected."

### Procedure Notes

R-Mix shell vials should be screened and stained at 24 hours for influenza A and B viruses. Respiratory syncytial viruses; parainfluenza virus types 1, 2, and 3; and adenovirus require 48 hours of incubation for maximum sensitivity.

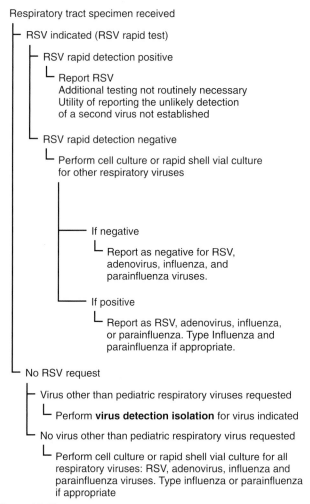

**Figure 65-10** Flowchart for the detection and identification of pediatric respiratory viruses.

A blanket request for TORCH assays should be avoided when possible, especially in specimens from newborns. Clinical presentation in the newborn may be characteristic for one or two of the viral agents, and tests for these etiologies should be pursued. Table 65-9 suggests laboratory tests for the diagnosis of the viral diseases in the newborn.

**Varicella-Zoster Virus.** VZV causes chickenpox (varicella) and shingles (zoster). Varicella (a vesicular eruption) is the clinical presentation associated with a primary VZV infection. VZV, a DNA-containing virus, establishes latency in a dorsal nerve root ganglion. Months to years later, during periods of relative immune suppression, VZV reactivates to cause zoster. Zoster is a modified or limited form of varicella, localized to a specific dermatome, the cutaneous area served by the infected nerve ganglion. Virus is present in the vesicular fluid and in the cells at the base of the vesicle. Material for virus detection should be collected from newly formed vesicles. Once the vesicle has opened and crusted over, detection is unlikely. Virus can be detected by staining cells from the base of the vesicles, by culturing cells and vesicular fluid, or by PCR testing of fluid and cells.

A stained smear of cells from the base of a skin vesicle used to detect VZV or HSV inclusions is referred to as a Tzanck test (described previously). Giemsa, Papanicolaou (Pap), or other suitable cytologic staining method is used for the Tzanck test, which detects typical multinucleated giant cells and inclusions (Figure 65-11, *A*). FA staining also can be used to detect VZV in Tzanck smears.

**TABLE 65-8** Tests for Human Gastroenteritis Viruses

| Virus | Relative Medical Importance | Epidemiology | Diagnostic Tests |
|---|---|---|---|
| Rotavirus | ++++ | Major cause of diarrhea in infants | EIA, LA |
| Enteric adenoviruses | ++ | Diarrhea in infants and young children | EIA, EM (especially types 40-41) |
| Noroviruses (caliciviruses) | +++ | Epidemics in children and adults | EM, RT-PCR |
| Astroviruses | + | Diarrhea in children | EM |

*EIA,* Enzyme immunoassay; *EM,* electron microscopy; *LA,* latex agglutination; *RT-PCR,* reverse transcription polymerase chain reaction (++++, most clinically significant; +, least clinically significant).

**TABLE 65-9** Laboratory Diagnosis of Viral Diseases in the Newborn

| Virus | Specimen | Diagnostic Tests |
|---|---|---|
| Rubella virus | Serum | Serology |
| CMV | Urine, Tissue | Cell culture (shell vial), PCR Cell culture (shell vial), histopathology |
| Enteroviruses | Cutaneous lesion, tissue, CSF | Cell culture, RT-PCR |
| HSV | Cutaneous lesion CSF | Cell culture, PCR PCR, cell culture |
| HIV | Blood, tissue Serum | RT-PCR, cell culture Serology |
| HBV | Blood | PCR, serology |
| VZV | Cutaneous lesion Tissue, fluid, or secretions | FA (Tzanck preparation), PCR Cell culture (shell vial), PCR |

*CMV,* Cytomegalovirus; *FA,* fluorescent antibody; *HBV,* hepatitis B virus; *HIV,* human immunodeficiency virus; *HSV,* herpes simplex virus; *PCR,* polymerase chain reaction; *RT-PCR,* reverse transcription PCR; *VZV,* varicella-zoster virus.

Traditionally, a diploid fibroblast cell culture (e.g., MRC-5) has been used to detect VZV, which requires up to 28 days before visible CPE are produced. The shell vial assay reduces the detection time to 48 hours and significantly increases sensitivity, identifying virus that fails to produce CPE in conventional cell culture. Comparison of FA staining of Tzanck smears, conventional cell culture, rapid shell vial culture, and PCR testing shows PCR to be the most sensitive detection method (Box 65-2). In laboratories in which PCR testing is not available, FA staining is the recommended method for diagnosis.

## VIRUS DETECTION METHODS

### Cytology and Histology

A readily available technique for detecting virus is cytologic or histologic examination for characteristic viral inclusions. This involves the morphologic study of cells or tissue, respectively. Viral inclusions are intracellular structures formed by aggregates of virus or viral

**BOX 65-2** Varicella-Zoster Virus Detection by Polymerase Chain Reaction Assay

**Purpose**

To detect varicella-zoster virus (VZV) in dermal lesions from patients with chickenpox (varicella) or shingles (zoster). Dermal swab specimens can be used. The real-time polymerase chain reaction (PCR) method detects VZV DNA in a 2-hour assay with greater sensitivity than do conventional cell culture, shell vial cell culture, VZV fluorescent antibody staining, and Papanicolaou smear.

**Specimen**

Dermal swab, vesicular scraping, or vesicular fluid.

**Materials**

- Nucleic acid extraction reagents or instrument (e.g., QIAamp DNA Mini Kit, Qiagen, Valencia, Calif.)
- Real-time PCR instrument (e.g., LightCycler System, Roche Diagnostics, Indianapolis, Ind.)
- Molecular laboratory for performance of PCR
- PCR reaction mixture containing polymerase, primers, and deoxynucleoside triphosphates

**Method**

1. Extract DNA.
2. Perform real-time PCR.
3. Computer analysis after each amplicon production cycle.

**Interpretation**

The presence of VZV-specific amplicons, detected by a fluorescent signal using crossover plot (see Figure 65-18), signifies a positive test result.

**Procedure Notes**

PCR provides a 1.9-fold increase in positive findings compared with shell vial culture. The assay is uniformly negative when other viruses, not VZV, are present in the specimen. The LightCycler is a closed system, which nearly eliminates carryover contamination. Amplicon identity is confirmed using melt curve analysis (see Figure 65-18).

components in an infected cell or abnormal accumulations of cellular materials resulting from virus-induced metabolic disruption. Inclusions occur in single or syncytial cells. Syncytial cells are aggregates of cells fused to form one large cell with multiple nuclei. Pap- or Giemsa-stained cytologic smears are examined for inclusions or syncytia. Inclusions resulting from infection with CMV, adenovirus, parvovirus, papillomavirus, and molluscum contagiosum virus are detected by histologic

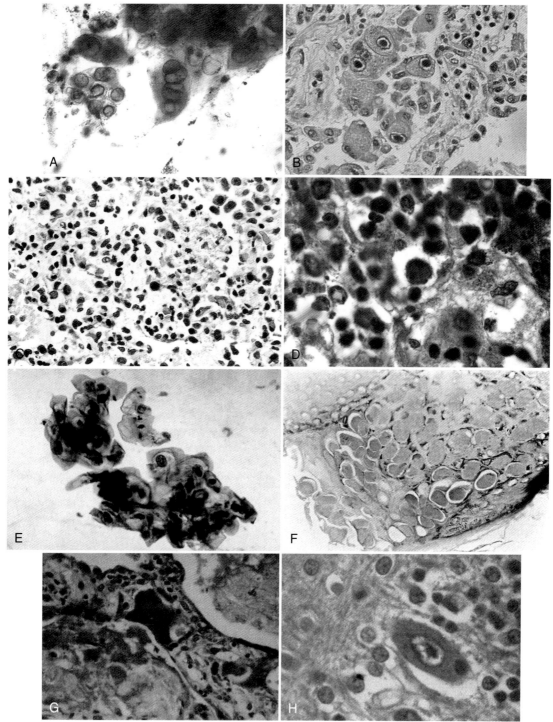

**Figure 65-11** Viral inclusions. **A,** Pap-stained smear showing multinucleated giant cells typical of herpes simplex or varicella-zoster viruses. **B,** Hematoxylin and eosin (HE)–stained lung tissue containing intranuclear inclusion within enlarged cytomegalovirus (CMV)–infected cells. **C,** HE-stained lung tissue containing epithelial cells with intranuclear inclusions characteristic of adenovirus. **D,** HE-stained liver from stillborn fetus showing intranuclear inclusions in erythroblasts (extramedullary hematopoiesis) resulting from parvovirus infection. **E,** Pap stain of exfoliated cervicovaginal epithelial cells showing perinuclear vacuolization and nuclear enlargement characteristic of human papillomavirus infection. **F,** HE-stained epidermis filled with molluscum bodies, which are large, eosinophilic, cytoplasmic inclusions resulting from infection with molluscum contagiosum virus. **G,** HE-stained cells infected with measles virus. **H,** HE-stained brain tissue showing oval, eosinophilic rabies cytoplasmic inclusion (Negri body). (**E** and **F** from Murray PR, Kobayashi GS, Pfaller MA, et al, editors: *Medical microbiology,* ed 2, St Louis, 1994, Mosby.)

examination of tissue stained with hematoxylin and eosin or Pap (see Figure 65-11, *B* through *F*). Less commonly, inclusions characteristic of measles and rabies viruses are detected by examining stained tissues (see Figure 65-11, *G* and *H*). Rabies virus inclusions in brain tissue are called Negri bodies. Cytology and histology are less sensitive than culture but are especially helpful for viruses that are difficult or dangerous to isolate in the laboratory, such as parvovirus and rabies virus, respectively.

## Electron Microscopy

Very few laboratories use electron microscopes (EM) to detect viruses, because it is labor intensive and relatively insensitive. EM is most helpful for detecting viruses that do not grow readily in cell culture and works best if the titer of virus is at least $10^6$ to $10^7$ particles per milliliter. Immune EM allows visualization of virus particles present in numbers too small for easy direct detection. The addition of specific antiserum to the test suspension causes the virus particles to form antibody-bound aggregates,

which are more easily detected than are single virus particles. In the clinical virology laboratory, EM is most useful for detecting gastroenteritis viruses that cannot be detected by other methods (e.g., astroviruses) and encephalitis-causing viruses that are undetectable with cell culture (HSV, measles virus, and JC polyomavirus) (Figure 65-12). In addition, the etiology of newly recognized viral syndromes can be recognized rapidly by identifying characteristic viral morphology by EM in infected tissue. This was exemplified by the early recognition of Ebola virus as the cause of an outbreak of viral hemorrhagic fever (Ebola hemorrhagic fever) in Africa in the 1970s and sin nombre virus (hanta pulmonary syndrome) as the cause of fatal pneumonia in the Four Corners area of the southwest United States in the 1990s.

## Immunodiagnosis (Antigen Detection)

High-quality, commercially available viral antibody reagents have led to the development of fluorescent antibody, enzyme immunoassay, latex agglutination, and

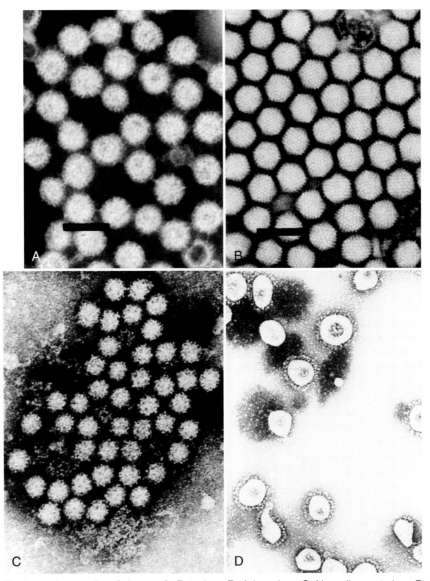

**Figure 65-12** Electron micrographs of viruses. **A,** Rotavirus. **B,** Adenovirus. **C,** Norwalk agent virus. **D,** Coronavirus.

*Continued*

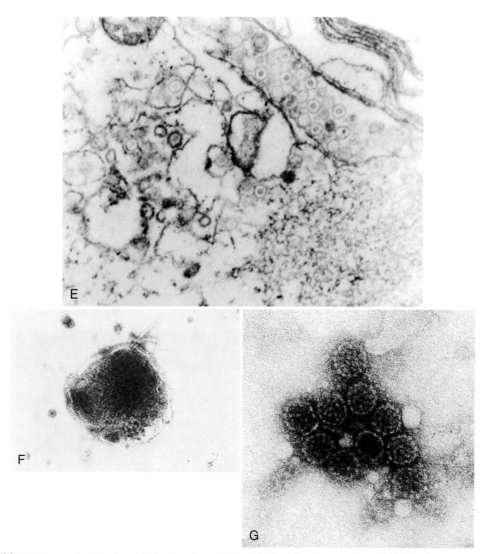

**Figure 65-12, cont'd E,** Herpes simplex virus. **F,** Measles virus. **G,** Negatively stained preparation of JC virus in brain tissue. (**C** from Howard BJ, Klaas J, Rubin SJ, et al: *Clinical and pathogenic microbiology,* St Louis, 1987, Mosby; **D** and **F** from US Department of Health, Education, and Welfare, Public Health Service, Centers for Disease Control, Atlanta, Ga; **G** courtesy Dr. Gabriele M. ZuRhein, UNW-Madison, Madison, Wisconsin.)

immunoperoxidase tests that detect viral antigen in patient specimens.

Direct and indirect immunofluorescent methods are used. Direct immunofluorescent testing involves the use of a labeled antiviral antibody; the label is usually fluorescein isothiocyanate (FITC), which is layered over a specimen suspected of containing a homologous virus. The indirect immunofluorescent procedure is a two-step test in which unlabeled antiviral antibody is added to the slide, followed by a labeled (FITC) antiglobulin that binds to the first-step antibody bound to virus in the specimen. Direct immunofluorescence is generally more rapid and specific than indirect immunofluorescence but less sensitive. The increased sensitivity of indirect immunofluorescence results from signal amplification that occurs with the addition of the second antibody. Signal amplification decreases specificity by increasing nonspecific background fluorescence.

Direct immunofluorescence is best suited to situations in which large quantities of virus are suspected or when high-quality, concentrated monoclonal antibodies are used, such as for the detection of RSV in a patient specimen or the identification of viruses growing in cell culture.

Indirect immunofluorescence should be used when lower quantities of virus are suspected, such as detection of respiratory viruses in specimens from adult patients. High-quality monoclonal antibodies improve the sensitivity and specificity of immunofluorescence testing.

Strict criteria for the interpretation of fluorescent patterns must be used. This includes standard interpretation of fluorescent intensity (Table 65-10) and recognition of viral inclusion morphology. Nuclear and cytoplasmic staining patterns are typical for influenza virus, adenovirus, and the herpes viruses; cytoplasmic staining is typical for RSV, parainfluenza, and mumps viruses; and staining

**TABLE 65-10** Interpretation of Fluorescence Intensity Using FITC

| Intensity | Interpretation |
|-----------|----------------|
| Negative | No apple-green fluorescence |
| 1+ | Faint yet unequivocal apple-green fluorescence |
| 2+ | Apple-green fluorescence |
| 3+ | Bright apple-green fluorescence |
| 4+ | Brilliant apple-green fluorescence |

within multinucleated giant cells is typical of measles virus or the herpes virus (see Figures 65-10 to 65-12; also Figure 65-13). False-positive staining can occur with specimens containing yeasts, certain bacteria, mucus, or leukocytes. Leukocytes, which contain Fc receptors for antibody, also can cause nonspecific binding of antibody conjugates. To verify employees' ability to interpret FA tests, every laboratory should perform viral culture or some alternative detection method along with immunofluorescence until in-house performance has been established.

The most useful immunofluorescent stains in the clinical virology laboratory are those for RSV, influenza and parainfluenza viruses, adenovirus, HSV, VZV, and CMV. A pool of antibodies can be used to screen a specimen for multiple viruses. A positive screen is tested with each individual reagent to identify the exact virus. Screening pools have been used successfully to detect respiratory viruses in specimens from children. Such pools are less sensitive when used with specimens from adults because of the lower numbers of viral particles in the specimens.

Enzyme immunoassay methods used in clinical virology include solid-phase enzyme-linked immunosorbent assay (solid-phase ELISA) and the membrane-bound enzyme-linked immunosorbent assay (membrane ELISA). Solid-phase ELISA is performed in a small test tube or microtiter tray. Breakaway strips of microtiter wells are available for low-volume test runs (Figure 65-14). The remaining, unused wells can be saved for future testing. Membrane ELISA tests have been developed for low-volume testing and for cases in which rapid results are needed. They can be performed by individuals with minimum training and usually require less than 30 minutes to complete. The membrane method uses a handheld reaction chamber with a cellulose-like membrane. Specimen and reagents are applied to the membrane. After a short incubation period, a chromogenic (color) reaction occurs on the surface of the membrane and is read visually. Built-in controls on the same membrane provide convenient monitoring of test procedures. Figure 65-15 illustrates a membrane ELISA used to detect rotavirus. The most used enzyme immunoassays for antigen detection are those for RSV (solid-phase and membrane), rotavirus (solid-phase and membrane), and influenza viruses (membrane).

Advantages of enzyme immunoassays are the use of relatively stable reagents and results that can be interpreted qualitatively (positive or negative) or quantitatively (titer or degree of positive reaction). It is important to note that enzyme immunoassays frequently have an indeterminate or borderline interpretative category. This result implies that low levels of viral antigen or background interference prevented a clear-cut positive or negative result. Such results usually require testing of a second specimen to avoid interference or to detect a rise in antigen level. ELISAs are sensitive and simple to perform and can be easily automated. However, specimen quality cannot be evaluated; that is, the number of cells cannot be assessed, as can be determined microscopically with fluorescent immunoassays.

Immunoperoxidase staining, and latex agglutination are additional techniques used to detect viral antigen. Immunoperoxidase staining is commonly used to stain histologic sections for virus but is less popular than immunofluorescence staining in clinical virology laboratories. Latex agglutination is an easy and inexpensive method but lacks sensitivity compared with ELISA and fluorescent immunoassays.

### Enzyme-Linked Virus-Inducible System

The enzyme-linked virus-inducible system (ELVIS) uses a baby hamster kidney (BHK) cell culture system with a cloned (added) beta-galactosidase gene that is expressed only when cells are infected with a virus. In the ELVIS-HSV test system (Diagnostic Hybrids, Athens, Ohio), the genetically engineered BHK cells are sold in multiwell microtiter plates. After inoculation of specimens and overnight incubation, growth of HSV results in production of the β-galactosidase enzyme by the BHK cells. β-galactosidase serves as the "reporter" molecule. When cells are fixed and stained for galactosidase activity, positive staining indicates the presence of HSV type 1 (HSV-1) or HSV type 2 (HSV-2). Wells that do not contain HSV show no staining.

### Molecular Detection Using Nucleic Acid Probes and Polymerase Chain Reaction Assays

During the past decade, the introduction of nucleic acid detection techniques into the clinical virology laboratory has resulted in a major shift in testing strategy. With the use of both nucleic acid detection and amplification-based systems, in conjunction with automated nucleic acid isolation techniques for sample preparation, nearly all virology laboratories have access to commercial or in-house molecular assays. These technologic improvements make it possible to generate results within 2 to 6 hours. Nucleic acid detection can be accomplished using nucleic acid probes, which are short segments of DNA that hybridize with complementary viral DNA or RNA segments. The probe is labeled with a fluorescent or chromogenic tag that allows detection if hybridization occurs. The probe reaction can occur in situ, such as in a tissue thin section; in liquid; or on a reaction vessel surface or membrane. A DNA probe test used to detect papillomavirus DNA in a smear of cervical cells is illustrated in Figure 65-16. Nucleic acid probes are most useful when the amount of virus is relatively abundant; viral culture is slow or not possible; and immunoassays lack sensitivity or specificity.

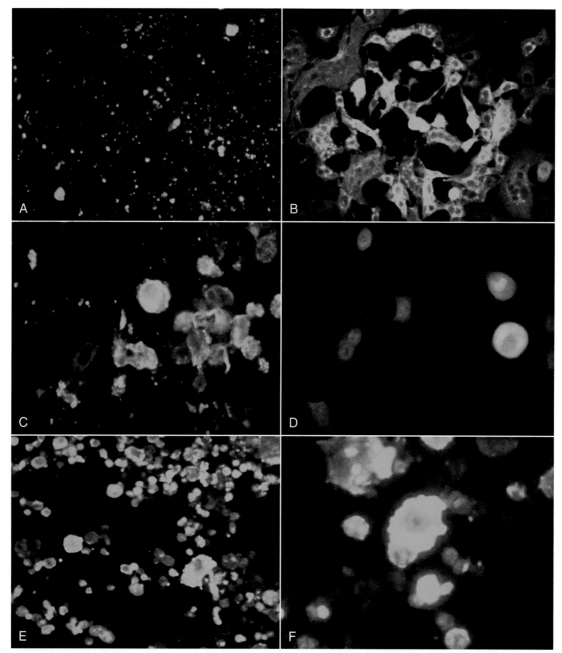

**Figure 65-13** **A,** RSV-infected RMK (rhesus monkey kidney) cells at 400×, stained with Light Diagnostics RSV MoAb. Fluorescence is seen in the cytoplasm and associated with syncytia. Cytoplasmic staining is often punctuate with small inclusions. **B,** HSV I: HSV I infected Vero cell control slide 200×. Stained with Pathfinder HSV 1 MoAb DFA assay. Fluorescent staining is cytoplasmic. **C,** Influenza B infected RMK cells at 400×. Stained with Light Diagnostics Influenza B MoAb. Fluorescence is nuclear, cytoplasmic, or both. Nuclear staining is uniformly bright and the cytoplasmic staining is often punctuate with l large inclusions. **D,** Herpes Simplex II infected A549 cells at 200×. Stained with Pathfinder HSV II MoAb DFA assay. Fluorescence may stain the cytoplasm, the nucleus, or both depending on the stage of the infection cycle. When infected cells are rounded, staining may appear nuclear due to cytoplasm covering the nucleus. **E,** HSV II Infected A549 cells at 200×. **F,** HSV II Infected A549 cells at 400×. Picture shows the multinucleated "giant" cells characteristic of HSV II CPE (cytopathogenic effect).

DNA target fragments that are too few in number in the original specimen to be detected by probes can be amplified using molecular techniques such as PCR, a method that duplicates short DNA targets thousands to a million-fold. The PCR procedure is described in more detail in Chapter 8. The PCR reaction with ensuing amplicon identification has been automated and made very rapid. Rapid PCR testing, referred to as real-time PCR, is illustrated in Figure 65-17. In real-time PCR, target amplification and detection occur simultaneously in the same tube; with conventional PCR, amplification and product detection take place separately. The PCR

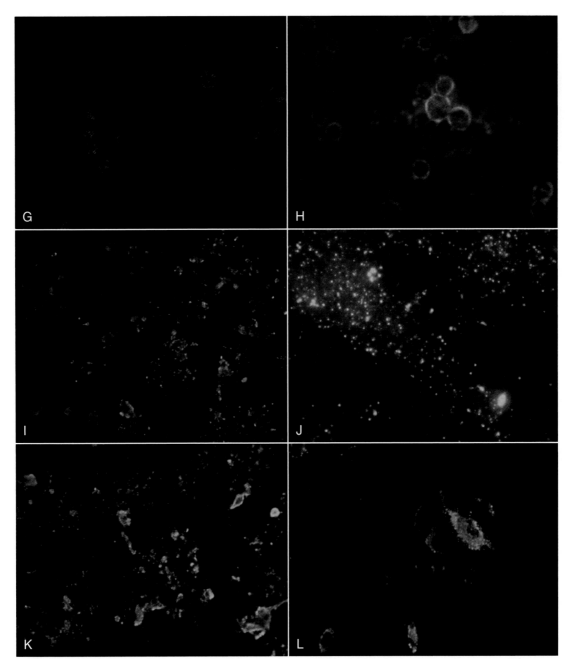

**Figure 65-13, cont'd G,** Uninfected cells, no fluorescence seen. **H,** Top Right: Adenovirus infected RMK cells at 400×. Stained with LD Adenovirus MoAb. Fluorescence is nuclear, cytoplasmic or both. Shows the characterictic rounding of infected cells. **I,** Parainfluenza 2 infected RMK cells 200×. Stained with LD Parainfluenza 2 MoAb. Fluorescence is confined to the cytoplasm and staining is punctuate with irregular inclusions. **J,** Rabies positive brain tissue using Fujeribio conjugated MoAb, 400×. Bright apple-green fluorescence of particles ranging in size and morphology from "dust particles" to prominent cytoplasmic inclusion "Negri bodies". **K,** Parainfluenza 3 infected RMK cells, 200×. Stained with LD Parainfluenza 3 MoAb. In a typical staining pattern, fluorescence is confined to the cytoplasm and staining is punctuate with irregular inclusions. **L,** Mumps IgM Bion IFA Control Slide, 200×. Stained with Bion Mumps IgM MoAb. Antigen/antibody complexes visualized by conjugation with fluorescent stain.

product can be detected as it is produced; novel fluorogenic probes or fluorescent dyes are used to monitor the product as it accumulates. This requires special thermal cyclers with precision optics that can monitor the fluorescence emission from the sample wells.

The PCR test can be used to amplify and detect RNA viruses by enzyme reverse transcriptase (RT). The first step in RT-PCR includes making a complementary DNA strand of the RNA segment in question. The usual PCR steps used to multiply the DNA target are then performed, leading to DNA amplicons that, when identified, signify the presence of the original RNA sequence. The rapid appearance and broad application of molecular diagnostics require the introduction and

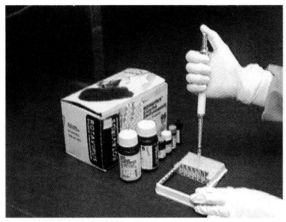

**Figure 65-14** Solid-phase enzyme immunoassay for detection of rotavirus with breakaway strips of microtiter wells for small-batch testing. (Courtesy Children's Hospital Medical Center of Akron, Akron, Ohio.)

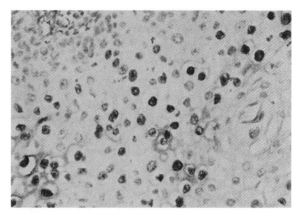

**Figure 65-16** Smear of cervical cells stained with probe for papillomavirus DNA. Dark-staining cells contain viral DNA. (Courtesy Children's Hospital Medical Center of Akron, Akron, Ohio.)

## Cell Culture

**Conventional Cell Culture.** Viruses are strict intracellular parasites, requiring a living cell for multiplication and reproduction. To detect virus using living cells, suitable host cells, cell culture media, and techniques in cell culture maintenance are necessary. Host cells, referred to as cell cultures (referred to by some as tissue cultures), originate as a few cells and grow into a monolayer (single confluent layer) on the sides of glass or plastic test tubes. The cells are kept moist and supplied with nutrients by keeping them continuously immersed in a cell culture medium (Figure 65-18). Cell cultures are routinely incubated in a roller drum that holds cell culture test tubes tilted 5 to 7 degrees while they slowly revolve (0.5 to 1 rpm) at 35° to 37°C (see Figure 65-5). Cell culture tubes can be incubated in a stationary rack rather than a roller drum. Rapidly growing viruses, such as HSV, appear to be detected equivalently by the two methods. Comparative studies are not available for most viruses.

Metabolism of growing cells in a closed tube results in the production of carbon dioxide and acidification of the growth liquid. To counteract the pH decrease, a bicarbonate buffering system is used in the culture medium to keep the cells at physiologic pH (7.2). Phenol red, a pH indicator that is red at physiologic pH, yellow at acidic pH, and purple at alkaline pH, is added to monitor adverse pH changes. Once inoculated with specimen, cell cultures are incubated for 1 to 4 weeks, depending on the viruses suspected. Periodically the cells are inspected microscopically with an inverted light microscope for the presence of virus, indicated by areas of dead or dying cells, called **cytopathic effect.** The degree of CPE is graded from 1+ to 4+; 1+ involves 25% of the cell monolayer; 2+ involves 50%; 3+ involves 75%; and 4+ involves 100% of the cell monolayer.

Virus-induced CPE also presents two other important considerations: the rate at which CPE progresses and whether the type of cell culture in which the virus grows may be used for presumptive identification. An example of rate can be seen with HSV, in which CPE progresses rapidly to involve the entire cell monolayer. In contrast, two other herpes viruses, VZV and CMV, grow slowly, mainly in human diploid fibroblast cells (HDFs), and

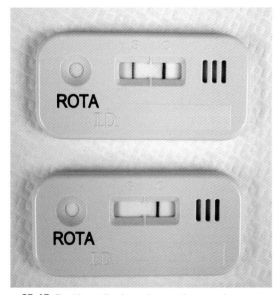

**Figure 65-15** Positive- *(top)* and negative-membrane enzyme-linked immunoassays (ELISAs) for detection of rotavirus. The red line in the reaction area on the left represents a positive test result. A red line in the reaction area on the right represents an internal test control ensuring that the test has been carried out correctly. If the test control line is not present, the test is invalid and must be repeated.

use of standardized materials and external quality control programs. In addition, the use of universal internal controls throughout the procedure ensures accuracy. In addition, several new multiplex assays and microassays capable of detecting multiple viruses in a single reaction have been developed. These assays are particularly useful for the diagnosis of respiratory pathogens and are described in more detail in Chapter 66. Finally, isothermal amplification reactions, as previously described for HSV and included in Chapter 8, are becoming more popular.

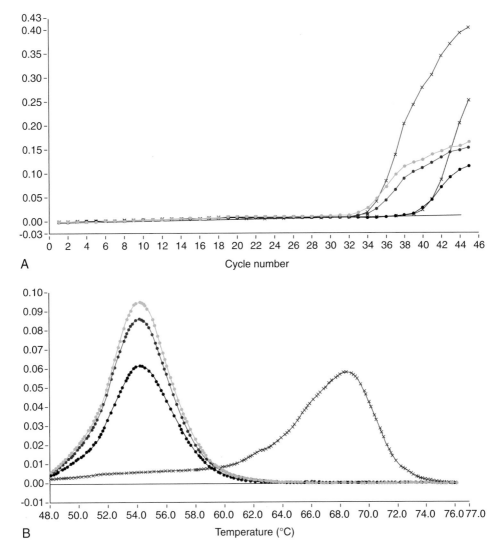

**Figure 65-17** Real-time polymerase chain reaction (PCR) detection of herpes simplex virus (HSV). Black, red, and light green lines represent three different HSV type 1 (HSV-1) viruses. Pink and dark green lines represent two different HSV type 2 (HSV-2) viruses. **A,** Cycle crossover detection of HSV-1 and HSV-2 amplicons, with all viruses detected between cycles 34 and 40. **B,** Melt curve confirmation of the presence of HSV-1 and HSV-2 viruses. HSV-1 amplicons melt at approximately 54°C (three HSV-1 viruses confirmed), and HSV-2 amplicons melt at approximately 68°C (one HSV-2 virus confirmed).

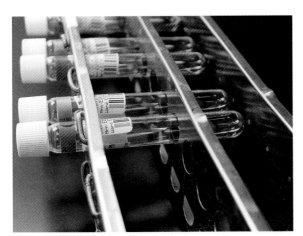

**Figure 65-18** Cell culture tubes incubating on their sides in a stationary rack. Tubes are oriented with the same glass surface facing downward, because an emblem printed on one side of the glass near the neck is used for correct positioning in the rack.

CPE progresses over a number of days or weeks. The fact that the cell culture type may serve as an indicator of the presumptive identification can be seen with poliovirus and echovirus. Poliovirus and echovirus produce similar CPE in primary rhesus monkey kidney (RMK) cells, but echovirus does not induce CPE in continuous cell lines, whereas poliovirus does. A trained virologist can determine whether CPE is due to viral growth or is nonspecific because of toxicity of specimens, contamination with bacteria or fungi, or simply old cells. Inoculation into fresh cells should amplify viral effects and dilute toxic effects.

Two kinds of media, growth medium and maintenance medium, are used for cell culture. Both are prepared with Eagle's minimum essential medium (EMEM) in Hanks' or Earle's balanced salt solution (HBSS or EBSS, respectively) and include antimicrobials to prevent bacterial contamination. HBSS has a better buffering capacity with carbon dioxide ($CO_2$), whereas EBSS has a better buffering capacity in ambient air. Typical added antimicrobials include vancomycin (10 $\mu g/mL$), gentamicin (20 $\mu g/mL$), and amphotericin (2.5 $\mu g/mL$). Growth medium is a serum-rich nutrient medium (10% fetal, newborn, or agammaglobulinemic calf serum) designed to support rapid cell growth. This medium is used to initiate the growth of cells in a tube when cell cultures are prepared in-house or to feed tubes of purchased cell cultures that have incomplete cell monolayers. "Feeding" refers to the removal of old medium, followed by the addition of fresh culture medium.

Maintenance medium is similar to growth medium but contains less serum (0% to 2%) and is used to keep cells in a steady state of metabolism. Fetal, newborn, or agammaglobulinemic calf serum is used to avoid inhibitors, such as specific antibody, and because it is free of mycoplasmas present in the serum of older animals.

Several kinds of cell cultures are routinely used for isolation of viruses. A cell culture becomes a cell line once it has been passed, or subcultured, in vitro. Cell lines are classified as primary, diploid (semicontinuous), or continuous. Primary cell lines have been passed only once or twice since harvesting (e.g., PMK cells). Further passage of primary cells results in a decreased receptivity to viral infection. Diploid cell lines remain virus sensitive through 20 to 50 passages. HDF cells, such as lung fibroblasts, are a commonly used diploid cell line. Continuous cell lines, such as human epidermoid carcinoma (HEp-2) cells, can be passed and remain sensitive to virus infections indefinitely. Unfortunately, most viruses do not grow well in continuous cell lines. Most clinically significant viruses can be recovered using one cell culture type from each group. A combination frequently used by clinical laboratories is RMK cells, MRC-5 lung fibroblast cells, and HEp-2 cells or A-549 cells (Table 65-11).

Inoculated cell cultures should be incubated immediately at 35°C. After allowing virus to adsorb to the cell monolayer for 12 to 24 hours, the remaining inoculum and culture medium commonly are removed and replaced with fresh maintenance medium. This avoids most inoculum-induced cell culture toxicity and improves virus recovery. Incubation should be continued for 5 to 28 days, depending on the suspected agent (see Table 65-11). Maintenance medium should be changed periodically (usually once or twice weekly) to provide fresh nutrients to the cells.

Blind passage refers to passing cells and fluid to a second cell culture tube. Blind passage is used to detect viruses that may not produce CPE in the initial culture tube but produce CPE when the "beefed-up" inoculum is passed to a second tube. Cell cultures that show nonspecific or ambiguous CPE are also passed to additional cell culture tubes. Toxicity, which causes ambiguous CPE, is diluted during passage and should not appear in the second cell culture tube. In both instances, passage is performed by scraping the monolayer off the sides of the tube with a pipette or disrupting the monolayer by vortexing with sterile glass beads added to the culture tube, followed by inoculation of 0.25 mL of the resulting suspension into new cell cultures. Blind passage is less frequently used today, because the added time and expense

do not justify detection of a few additional isolates after extended incubation in two cell culture tubes.

**Shell Vial Cell Culture.** The shell vial cell culture is a rapid modification of conventional cell culture. Virus is detected more quickly using the shell vial technique, because the infected cell monolayer is stained for viral antigens produced soon after infection, before the development of CPE. Viruses that normally take days to weeks to produce CPE can be detected within 1 to 2 days by detecting early produced viral antigens. A shell vial culture tube, a $15 \times 45$ mm 1-dram vial, is prepared by adding a round coverslip to the bottom of the tube, covering this with growth medium, and adding appropriate cells (Figure 65-19). During incubation, a cell monolayer forms on top of the coverslip. Shell vials should be used 5 to 9 days after cells have been inoculated. Shell vials can be purchased with the monolayer already formed. Specimens are inoculated onto the shell vial cell monolayer by low-speed centrifugation. This enhances viral infectivity for reasons that are not well understood. Coverslips are stained using virus-specific immunofluorescent conjugates. The presence and visualization of characteristic fluorescing inclusions are used to confirm the presence of an infecting virus (Figure 65-20). The shell vial procedure for detecting CMV is presented in detail in Procedure 65-3, which can be found on the Evolve site.

The shell vial culture technique can be used to detect most viruses that grow in conventional cell culture. It is best used for viruses requiring relatively long incubation before producing CPE, such as CMV and VZV. The advantage of the shell vial procedure is its speed; most viruses are detected within 24 hours. The disadvantage is that only a single type of virus can be detected per shell vial. For example, a specimen that might contain influenza A or B or adenovirus would need to be inoculated to three separate shell vials so that each vial could be stained with a separate virus-specific conjugate. Other strategies pool antibody for detection of many viruses with a single vial. Additional vials from positive specimens are then stained with individual conjugates to identify the specific virus present. The shell vial procedure with mixed cell types used to detect seven different respiratory viruses is outlined in Box 65-1.

**Identification of Viruses Detected in Cell Culture.** Viruses are most often detected in cell culture by the recognition of CPE. Virus-infected cells change their usual morphology and eventually lyse or detach from the glass surface while dying. Viruses have distinct CPEs, just as colonies of bacteria on agar plates have unique morphologies (Figure 65-21). CPE may be quantitated as indicated in Table 65-12. Preliminary identification of a virus frequently can be made based on the cell line that supports viral replication, how quickly the virus produced CPE, and a description of the CPE (see Table 65-11). Experienced virologists can presumptively identify most viruses isolated in clinical laboratories based on these criteria. When confirmation or definitive identification is required, additional testing can be performed. Fluorescent-labeled antisera, available for most viruses, are used for confirmation. In addition, acid lability is used to differentiate enteroviruses from rhinoviruses, and neutralization is

**TABLE 65-11** Isolation and Identification of Common Clinically Encountered Viruses

| Virus | PMK | HEp-2 | HDF | CPE Description | Rate of Growth (days) | Identification and Comments |
|---|---|---|---|---|---|---|
| Adenovirus | ++* | +++ | ++ | Rounding and aggregation of infected cells in grapelike clusters | 2-10 | Confirm by FA test; serotype by cell culture neutralization |
| Cytomegalovirus (CMV) | − | − | ++++ | Discrete, small foci of rounded cells | 5-28 | Distinct CPE sufficient to identify; confirm by FA test |
| Enterovirus | ++++ | + | ++ | Characteristic refractile angular or tear-shaped CPE; progresses to involve entire monolayer | 2-8 | Confirm by FA test; stable at pH 3 |
| Herpes simplex (HSV) | + | ++++ | ++++ | Rounded, swollen refractile cells; occasional syncytia, especially with HSV-2; rapidly involves entire monolayer | 1-3 (may take up to 7) | Distinct CPE sufficient to identify; confirm by FA test |
| Influenza | ++++ | − | ± | Destructive degeneration with swollen, vacuolated cells | 2-10 | Detect by hemadsorption or hemagglutination with guinea pig RBCs; identify by FA test |
| Mumps | +++ | ± | ± | CPE usually absent; syncytia occasionally seen | 5-10 | Detect by hemadsorption with guinea pig RBCs; confirm by FA test |
| Parainfluenza | +++ | − | − | CPE usually minimal or absent | 4-10 | Detect by hemadsorption with guinea pig RBCs; identify by FA test |
| Respiratory syncytial virus (RSV) | + | +++ | + | Syncytia in HEp-2 cells | 3-10 | Distinct CPE in HEp-2 cells sufficient for presumptive identification; confirm by FA test |
| Rhinovirus | ++ | − | +++ | Characteristic refractile rounding of cells; in PMK, CPE is identical to that produced by enteroviruses | 4-10 | Labile at pH 3; growth optimal at 32° to 33°C |
| Varicella-zoster virus | − | − | ++ | Discrete foci of rounded, swollen, refractile cells; slowly involves entire monolayer | 5-28 | Confirm by FA test |

*CPE,* Cytopathic effects; *FA,* fluorescent antibody; *HDF,* human diploid fibroblast; *HEp-2,* human epidermoid; *PMK,* primary monkey kidney; *RBCs,* red blood cells.
*Relative sensitivity of cell cultures for recovering the virus: −, None recovered; ±, rare strains recovered; +, few strains recovered; ++++, ≥80% of strains recovered.

**TABLE 65-12** Quantitation of Cell Culture Cytopathic Effects

| Quantitation | Interpretation |
|---|---|
| Negative | Uninfected monolayer |
| Equivocal (±) | Atypical alteration of monolayer involving few cells |
| 1+ | 1% to 25% of monolayer exhibits cytopathic effects (CPE) |
| 2+ | 25% to 50% of monolayer exhibits CPE |
| 3+ | 50% to 75% of monolayer exhibits CPE |
| 4+ | 76% to 100% of monolayer exhibits CPE |

used to identify viruses with many serotypes for which fluorescent-labeled antisera are not available. Some viruses that produce little or no CPE (e.g., influenza, parainfluenza, and mumps viruses) can be detected by hemadsorption, because infected cells contain viral hemadsorbing glycoproteins in their outer membranes. The addition of guinea pig red blood cells (RBCs) to the cell culture tube, followed by a wash to remove nonadsorbed RBCs, results in a ring of RBCs around infected cells (see Figure 65-21, *G*). Cell cultures demonstrating hemadsorption can be stained with fluorescent-labeled antisera to identify the specific hemadsorbing virus present. Detailed procedures for culture confirmation by FA staining and hemadsorption for the detection of

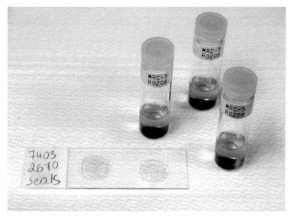

**Figure 65-19** Shell vial cell culture tubes and stained coverslips. At the bottom of each shell vial tube under the culture medium is a round coverslip with a cell monolayer on the top surface. After incubation, the coverslip is removed, stained, and placed on a microscope slide for fluorescence viewing. Note that two stained coverslips are on the glass slide.

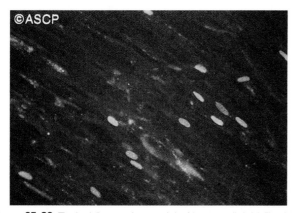

**Figure 65-20** Typical fluorescing nuclei of human diploid fibroblast cells infected with cytomegalovirus as seen in the shell vial assay. (Courtesy Bostick CC: Laboratory detection of CMV, 1992, Microbiology Tech Sample No MB-3.)

influenza and parainfluenza viruses are presented in Procedures 65-4 and 65-5, which can be found on the Evolve site.

## VIRAL SEROLOGY

### General Principles

Serology was the primary means of laboratory diagnosis of viral infections until the mid-1970s. At that time, culture and detection of viral antigen became more widely available because of commercially available reagents, such as cell cultures, and a broad range of immunodiagnostic test kits and the production of virus-specific monoclonal antibodies to detect viral antigen in patient specimens. Viral serology is now used primarily to determine immune status and to confirm the diagnosis of infection when the virus cannot be cultivated in cell culture or detected readily by immunoassay or molecular assays.

In most viral infections, IgM is undetectable 1 to 4 months after the acute infection resolves, but detectable levels of IgG remain for the life of the patient. If a patient is infected with an antigenically similar virus or the original strain has remained latent and reactivates at a later time, these virus-specific IgG and IgM antibody levels may again rise. The secondary IgM response may be difficult to detect; however, a significant (fourfold) IgG titer rise is readily apparent in immunocompetent patients.

An immune status check measures whether a particular virus has previously infected a patient. A positive result with a sensitive, virus-specific IgG test indicates past infection. Some immune status tests include methods that can detect both IgG and IgM; these are used to identify recent or active infections.

To diagnose active disease, two approaches are helpful. Detection of virus-specific IgM in an acute-phase specimen collected at least 7 to 14 days after the onset of infection indicates current or very recent disease. Detection of a fourfold (or equivalent increase if twofold dilutions are not tested) antibody titer rise between acute and convalescent sera also indicates current or recent disease. Acute-phase serum should be collected as soon as possible after the onset of symptoms. The convalescent specimen should be collected 2 to 3 weeks after the acute-phase specimen. If a single postacute serum, collected between acute and convalescent times, or a convalescent specimen is all that is available for testing, an extremely high, virus-specific IgG titer may suggest infection. The exact titer specific for active disease, if known at all, varies with each testing method and virus. In general, titers high enough to be diagnostic are unusual, and single specimens should not be tested. A reasonable policy would involve using IgM tests, where available, and performing IgG tests only on paired acute and convalescent specimens. IgG tests are not needed on the first, acute specimen until receipt of the convalescent specimen. This eliminates useless testing of single specimens when a second sample is never submitted for analysis.

Many serologic methods are or have been routinely used to detect antiviral antibody. Prominent among these are complement fixation (CF), ELISA, indirect immunofluorescence, anticomplement immunofluorescence (ACIF), and Western immunoblotting. CF is a labor-intensive, technically demanding method best fitted to batch testing. As less demanding, easily automated techniques for batch testing are developed (e.g., ELISA), the need for CF testing will disappear. Additional advantages of ELISA are that it can be used to detect IgM-specific antibodies free of common interfering factors, particularly through use of an antibody-capture technique. Indirect immunofluorescence is best used for individual specimens or small-batch testing.

Immunofluorescence also can be used to detect virus-specific IgM; however, it requires prior separation and elimination of the IgG fraction, which if present can result in both false-positive and false-negative results. IgM and IgG can be separated by ion exchange chromatography (Figure 65-22), by immune precipitation, or with an IgG inactivation reagent, such as Gullsorb, (Meridian

Bioscience) a reagent containing an anti-human IgG reagent (caprine) capable of neutralizing up to 15 mg/mL of IgG antibody in human serum.

IgG indirect FA testing is subject to false-positive results because of antibody-Fc receptors that occur in cells infected with virus. Indirect immunofluorescence antibody (IFA) testing is performed using virus-infected substrate cells fixed to a microscope slide. When the substrate cells are overlaid with patient serum, the Fc portion of the antibody molecule binds to these receptors. Fluorescent-labeled antiglobulin attaches to both homologous antibody (bound to viral antigen) and to Fc-bound antibody. Subsequent fluorescence of Fc-bound antibody results in a false-positive or falsely elevated reading. To avoid this complication, the ACIF test can be used. Because fluorescent-labeled complement binds

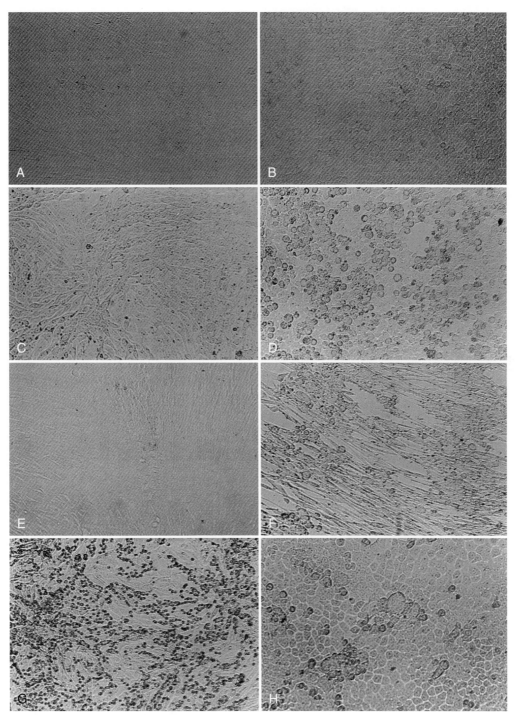

**Figure 65-21** Cell culture morphology and viral cytopathic effects (CPE). **A,** Normal human diploid lung fibroblast cells (HDF). **B,** Normal HEp-2 cells. **C,** Normal primary monkey kidney cells (PMK). **D,** HEp-2 cells infected with adenovirus. **E,** HDF cells infected with cytomegalovirus. **F,** HDF cells infected with herpes simplex virus. **G,** PMK cells infected with hemadsorbing virus, such as influenza, parainfluenza, or mumps, plus guinea pig erythrocytes. **H,** HEp-2 cells infected with respiratory syncytial virus.

*Continued*

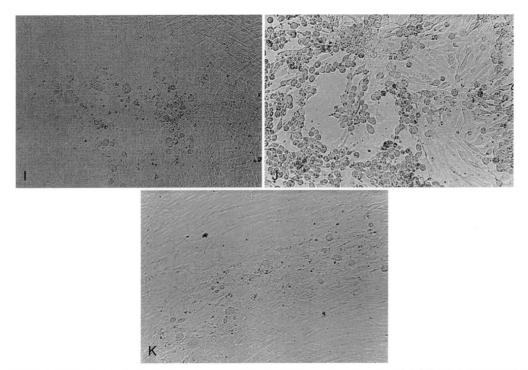

**Figure 65-21, cont'd** **I,** HDF cells infected with rhinovirus. **J,** PMK cells infected with echovirus. **K,** HDF cells infected with varicella-zoster virus. (From US Department of Health, Education, and Welfare, Public Health Service, Centers for Disease Control, Atlanta, Ga.)

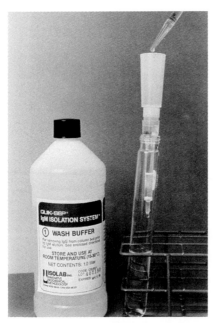

**Figure 65-22** IgM is separated from human serum by passing the serum through an ion exchange column.

only to antigen-antibody complexes, the nonspecific antibody attached by Fc receptors, which is complement free, does not fluoresce. Western immunoblotting is also used for viral antibody detection. Because complex antigens are separated into individual components during the Western blot procedure, and positive or negative reactions are observed with each of these components, the Western blot provides a more specific result than other serologic tests, such as EIA.

False-positive and false-negative results can occur when testing for virus-specific IgM antibodies. False-positive results occur when rheumatoid factor, an anti-IgG/IgM-type globulin, combines with homologous or virus-specific IgG present in the patient specimen. Labeled anti-IgM combines with either bound virus-specific IgM or rheumatoid factor, causing falsely positive fluorescence. False-negative IgM test results occur when high levels of strongly binding homologous IgG antibodies prevent binding of IgM molecules, decreasing or eliminating IgM-specific fluorescence. Both problems can be eliminated by testing the IgG-free serum fraction.

### Immune Status Testing

Immune status tests (Table 65-13) are used to detect patients who have been infected with (or vaccinated for) a virus in the past, conferring lifelong immunity to reinfection. Rubella antibody immune status testing is used with women of childbearing age. A positive result (presence of IgG antibody) indicates past infection or immunization and implies that congenital infection will not occur during subsequent pregnancies. Absence of IgG antibody implies susceptibility to infection and should prompt rubella vaccination if the woman is not pregnant. Varicella and measles immune status assays are used most commonly to test health care workers. Those with no IgG antibody must avoid diseased patients and receive a booster or secondary vaccination. CMV immune status is useful for organ transplant donors and recipients, and premature babies hospitalized in newborn intensive care nurseries, who are likely to receive blood transfusions. Transplant recipients are susceptible to life-threatening CMV infection. Knowing the CMV status of the donor and recipient enables the physician to better diagnose

**TABLE 65-13** Serology Panels and Immune Status Testing for Common Viral Syndromes

| Condition | Viruses Under Consideration |
|---|---|
| Acquired immunodeficiency syndrome (AIDS) | Human immunodeficiency virus (HIV) |
| Central nervous system (CNS) infections | Arboviruses, especially Eastern and Western equine encephalitis viruses, St. Louis encephalitis virus, La Crosse virus, West Nile virus<br>Lymphocytic choriomeningitis virus<br>Enteroviruses<br>Measles<br>Mumps<br>Herpes simplex virus (HSV) and other herpes viruses<br>Rabies |
| Exanthems | Measles<br>Rubella<br>Parvovirus |
| Vesicular conditions | HSV<br>Varicella-zoster virus (VZV) |
| Hepatitis A | Hepatitis A virus |
| Hepatitis B | Hepatitis B virus |
| Heterophile-negative infectious mononucleosis syndromes | Cytomegalovirus (CMV)<br>Epstein-Barr virus |
| Myocarditis-pericarditis | Group B coxsackievirus, types 1-5<br>Influenza A and B<br>CMV |
| Respiratory conditions | Influenza A and B<br>Respiratory syncytial virus (RSV)<br>Parainfluenza types 1-3<br>Adenovirus |
| Serology needed to determine immune status | Rubella<br>Hepatitis B<br>VZV<br>CMV<br>Measles |

and treat this disease. Newborns whose mothers were never infected with CMV are susceptible to serious, primary CMV infection that can be transmitted in white blood cells during blood transfusion. CMV-negative babies should receive only CMV-negative blood.

### Serology Panels

In some cases, testing for antibody to an individual virus is less helpful than using a battery of antigens to test for antibody to many viruses. The use of a combination of serologic tests to diagnose a clinical syndrome (see Table 65-13) may be useful when the viruses under consideration cannot be cultured; specimens of infected tissue are not available (e.g., brain tissue); antiviral agents have been administered; or the patient is convalescing and isolation of virus is unlikely. In most cases, some but not all viruses in the battery require testing. Consultation with the patient's physician can narrow the list of potential etiologies.

## PRESERVATION AND STORAGE OF VIRUSES

Clinical virology laboratories must have a method for storing and retrieving viruses, along with an accurate inventory system from which to identify and locate stored viruses. Isolates should be kept as control strains and, in rare instances, for epidemiologic investigations. Public health laboratories may use current enterovirus or influenza virus strains for typing. Viruses can be stored by freezing at −70°C or in liquid nitrogen. Freezing at −70°C is more practical for clinical laboratories. A method for preserving and storing viruses by freezing is described in Procedure 65-6, which can be found on the Evolve site.

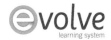 *Visit the Evolve site to complete the review questions.*

---

## CASE STUDY 65-1

A previously healthy, 19-year-old college student presents to the emergency department (ED) with symptoms of a respiratory tract infection. While in the ED, the patient experiences severe shortness of breath. He is transferred to the intensive care unit and is intubated and placed on a ventilator. A chest radiograph reveals left lung infiltrates.

QUESTIONS

1. What viruses cause serious respiratory tract disease in young adults?

2. What specimens are recommended to aid the diagnosis of viral respiratory tract infection?

3. What viral diagnostic tests are appropriate for detecting respiratory tract viruses?

# BIBLIOGRAPHY

Balfour H: Drug therapy, *N Engl J Med* 340:1255, 1999.

Carr J, Gyorfi T: Human papillomavirus, *Clin Lab Med* 20:235, 2000.

Cockerill FR: Application of rapid-cycle real-time polymerase chain reaction for diagnostic testing in the clinical microbiology laboratory, *Arch Pathol Lab Med* 127:1112, 2003.

Constantine N, Zhao R: Molecular-based laboratory testing and monitoring for human immunodeficiency virus infections, *Clin Lab Sci* 18:263, 2005.

Debiasi RL, Tyler KL: Molecular methods for diagnosis of viral encephalitis, *Clin Microbiol Rev* 17:903, 2004.

De Clercq E: Antiviral drugs in current clinical use, *J Clin Virol* 30:115, 2004.

Espy MJ, Uhl JR, Sloan M, et al: Real-time PCR in clinical microbiology: applications for routine laboratory testing, *Clin Microbiol Rev* 19:165, 2006.

Flint SJ, Enquist LW, Krug RM, et al: *Principles of virology: molecular biology, pathogenesis and control*, Washington, DC, 2000, ASM Press.

Forbes BA: Introducing a molecular test into the clinical microbiology laboratory: development, evaluation, and validation, *Arch Pathol Lab Med* 127:1106, 2003.

Gavin PJ, Thomson RB: Review of rapid diagnostic tests for influenza, *Clin Appl Immunol Rev* 4:151, 2003.

Harris KR, Dighe AS: Laboratory testing for viral hepatitis, *Am J Clin Pathol* 118(Suppl 1):S18, 2002.

Johnson FB: Transport of viral specimens, *Clin Microbiol Rev* 3:120, 1990.

Kowalski RP, Karenchak LM, Shah C, et al: ELVIS: A new 24-hour culture test for detecting herpes simplex virus from ocular samples, *Arch Ophthalmol* 120(7):960-963, 2002.

Lauer GM, Walker BD: Hepatitis C virus infection, *N Engl J Med* 345:41, 2001.

Lee W: Hepatitis B virus infection, *N Engl J Med* 337:1733, 1997.

Lesprit P, Scieux C, Lemann M, et al: Use of the cytomegalovirus (CMV) antigenemia assay for the rapid diagnosis of primary CMV infection in hospitalized adults, *Clin Infect Dis* 26:646, 1998.

Liang TJ, Rehermann B, Seeff L, et al: Pathogenesis, natural history, treatment, and prevention of hepatitis C, *Ann Intern Med* 132:296, 2000.

McIntosh K, McAdam AJ: Human metapneumovirus: an important new respiratory virus, *N Engl J Med* 350:431, 2004.

Miller NS, Yen-Lieberman B, Poulter MD, et al: Comparative clinical evaluation of the IsoAmp HSV Assay with ELVIS HSV culture/ID/typing test system for the detection of herpes simplex virus in genital and oral lesions, *J Clin Virol* 54(4):355-358, 2012.

Niesters HG: Molecular and diagnostic clinical virology in real-time, *Clin Microbiol Infect* 10:5, 2004.

Paltiel DA, Walensky RP: Home HIV testing: good news but not a game changer, *Ann Intern Med* 157(10):744-746, 2012.

Petersen LR, Marfin AA: West Nile virus: a primer for the clinician, *Ann Intern Med* 137:173, 2002.

Pigott DC: Hemorrhagic fever viruses, *Crit Care Clin* 21:765, 2005.

Poon LL, Guan Y, Nicholls JM, et al: The aetiology, origins, and diagnosis of severe acute respiratory syndrome, *Lancet Infect Dis* 4:663, 2004.

Schiffman M, Castle PE: Human papillomavirus epidemiology and public health, *Arch Pathol Lab Med* 127:930, 2003.

Schmaljohn C, Hjelle B: Hantaviruses: a global disease problem, *Emerg Infect Dis* 3:95, 1997.

Sejvar JJ, Chowdary Y, Schomogyi M, et al: Human monkeypox infections: a family cluster in the Midwestern United States, *J Infect Dis* 190:1833, 2004.

Storch GA: Diagnostic virology, *Clin Infect Dis* 31:739, 2000.

Thomson RB, Bertram H: Laboratory diagnosis of central nervous system infections, *Infect Dis Clin North Am* 15:1047, 2001.

Van Helvoort T: When did virology start? *ASM News* 62:142, 1996.

Versalovic J: *Manual of clinical microbiology*, ed 10, Washington, DC, 2011, ASM Press.

Warrell MJ, Warrell DA: Rabies and other lyssavirus diseases, *Lancet* 363:959, 2004.

Wilder-Smith A, Schwartz E: Dengue in travelers, *N Engl J Med* 353:924, 2005.

Writing Committee of the World Health Organization Consultation on Human Influenza A/H5: Avian influenza A (H5N1) infection in humans, *N Engl J Med* 353:1374, 2005.

# Viruses in Human Disease

## OBJECTIVES

1. List the common human respiratory viruses and modes of transmission.
2. Differentiate between viral *antigenic shift* and *antigenic drift*. Explain how each occurs, its effect on the production of vaccine, and why is it an important consideration in the study of the influenza virus.
3. Define the term "pandemic" and identify historical pandemics within the past century, including the latest influenza pandemic.
4. List the serotypes of rhinovirus and explain how testing for rhinovirus is accomplished and how it differs from testing for the other respiratory viruses.
5. List some of the most common human arboviruses.
6. Define arbovirus and describe the mode of transmission.
7. List the viruses responsible for viral encephalitis.
8. Name the most common sexually transmitted viral diseases.
9. Define tissue tropism associated with human papillomavirus (HPV) and explain the relationship between HPV and cervical cancer.
10. Define skin exanthema and identify the most common types affecting children.
11. Compare human gastrointestinal viruses, stating the types that affect adults more frequently and those that affect children.
12. Define hanta pulmonary syndrome; identify the disease-causing virus and the mode of transmission.
13. Name the family of viruses responsible for the skin eruptions orf and molluscum contagiosum.
14. List the family of viruses responsible for outbreaks of severe disease among military recruits and describe the recommended preventive measures.
15. Define the viral proteins hemagglutinin and neuraminidase; explain how these proteins function to ensure the transmissibility and reproducibility of the influenza virus.
16. Correlate the agents of specific infections shown in the following box with diseases and pathologic manifestations, including routes of transmission and appropriate diagnostic tests.

---

### VIRUSES TO BE CONSIDERED

**DNA Viruses**
*Family*
Adenoviridae
Hepadnaviridae
Herpesviridae
Papillomaviridae
Parvoviridae
Polyomaviridae
Poxviridae

**RNA Viruses**
*Family*
Arenaviridae
Astroviridae

---

### VIRUSES TO BE CONSIDERED—cont'd

Bunyaviridae
Caliciviridae
Coronaviridae
Filoviridae
Flaviviridae
Orthomyxoviridae
Paramyxoviridae
Picornaviridae
Reoviridae
Retroviridae
Rhabdoviridae
Togaviridae

---

## VIRUSES IN HUMAN DISEASE

Viruses of medical importance to humans comprise seven families of deoxyribonucleic acid (DNA) viruses and fourteen families of ribonucleic acid (RNA) viruses. This chapter examines the specific families of viruses, including the diseases and the symptoms associated with the viral infection. Tables 66-1 and 66-2 present a quick reference to the viral families and syndromes caused by these viruses. Table 66-1 divides the virus families according to the makeup of the viral genome, either RNA or DNA. Table 66-2 lists some of the common human viral infections.

## ADENOVIRUSES

Adenoviruses (Table 66-3) are medium-sized (70 to 90 nm), icosahedral, nonenveloped, double-stranded, linear DNA viruses. This virus was first isolated from cultures of human adenoids and tonsils in the early 1950s, hence the name adenovirus. The adenoviruses belong to the family Adenoviridae and are widely distributed in nature. However, only members of the genus *Mastadenovirus* cause human infection. Currently, 52 serotypes of human adenoviruses have been described. Most human disease is associated with one third of the viral types. These types are then divided into seven species, A through G, with species B subdivided into two subspecies; virus serotypes are then numbered within the species classification. The viruses can cause a broad range of disease in humans. Respiratory and gastrointestinal diseases are the most common clinical manifestation associated with adenovirus infection.

Adenoviruses cause less than 5% of all acute respiratory disease in the general population, however, they account for up to 18% of respiratory infections in

**TABLE 66-1** DNA and RNA Viruses That Cause Serious Disease in Humans

| Family | Viral Members |
|---|---|
| **DNA Viruses** | |
| Adenoviridae | Human adenoviruses |
| Hepadnaviridae | Hepatitis B virus |
| Herpesviridae | HSV types I and II, VZV, CMV, EBV, human herpes viruses 6, 7, and 8 |
| Papillomaviridae | Human papilloma viruses |
| Parvoviridae | Parvovirus B-19 |
| Polyomaviridae | BK and JC polyomaviruses |
| Poxviridae | Variola, vaccinia, orf, molluscum contagiosum, monkeypox viruses |
| **RNA Viruses** | |
| Arenaviridae | Lymphocytic choriomeningitis virus, Lassa fever virus |
| Astroviridae | Gastroenteritis-causing astroviruses |
| Bunyaviridae | Arboviruses, including California encephalitis and Lacrosse viruses; nonarboviruses, including sin nombre and related hantaviruses |
| Caliciviridae | Noroviruses and hepatitis E virus |
| Coronaviridae | Coronaviruses, including SARS coronavirus |
| Filoviridae | Ebola and Marburg hemorrhagic fever viruses |
| Flaviviridae | Arboviruses, including yellow fever, dengue, West Nile, Japanese encephalitis, and St. Louis encephalitis viruses; nonarboviruses, including hepatitis C virus |
| Orthomyxoviridae | Influenza A, B, and C viruses |
| Paramyxoviridae | Parainfluenza viruses, mumps virus, measles virus, RSV, metapneumovirus, Nipah virus |
| Picornaviridae | Polio viruses, coxsackie A viruses, coxsackie B viruses, echoviruses, enteroviruses 68-71, enterovirus 72 (hepatitis A virus), rhinoviruses |
| Reoviridae | *Rotavirus* spp., Colorado tick fever virus |
| Retroviridae | HIV types 1 and 2, HTLV types 1 and 2 |
| Rhabdoviridae | Rabies virus |
| Togaviridae | Eastern, Western, and Venezuela equine encephalitis viruses, rubella virus |

*CMV,* Cytomegalovirus; *EBV,* Epstein-Barr virus; *HIV,* human immunodeficiency virus; *HSV,* herpes simplex virus; *HTLV,* human T-lymphotropic viruses; *RSV,* respiratory syncytial virus; *SARS,* severe acute respiratory syndrome; *VZV,* varicella-zoster virus.

children. By the age of 10, most children have been exposed to and infected with at least one of the adenovirus species. In addition, adenovirus serotypes 40 and 41 cause gastroenteritis in infants and young children, and other serotypes are associated with conjunctivitis and keratitis. Although respiratory and gastrointestinal diseases are most common, disseminated disease in multiple organ systems may develop in compromised hosts.

Transmission of the virus may occur as an aerosolized droplet or maybe airborne. Respiratory disease caused by adenovirus is usually acquired through contact with contaminated respiratory secretions, stool, and fomites. The virus is very stable and can remain viable for weeks at variable temperatures on surfaces and in solution. The incubation period for respiratory disease is 2 to 14 days. Common upper respiratory tract infections caused by adenovirus include colds, tonsillitis, pharyngitis, pharyngoconjunctival fever, and sometimes croup (viral infection of the larynx). Infections of the eye and conjunctivitis often accompany respiratory infection, and in children, otitis media (ear infection) is often a complication of the respiratory disease. Lower respiratory tract infections can be quite severe in children, and adenovirus pneumonia is often fatal in infants and young children.

A unique feature of the adenoviruses is the ability to cause severe, acute respiratory disease epidemics in military recruits, often resulting in considerable morbidity and mortality. A highly effective vaccine to control the outbreaks was developed for serotypes 4 and 7 and administered to recruits from 1971 to 1996. Once the vaccination program was discontinued, the outbreaks resumed. The current adenovirus contains live serotypes 4 and 7 and is approved for military personnel between the ages of 17 and 50. In addition to the reemergence of epidemics, the emergence of a new, unusually severe lower respiratory tract infection caused by adenovirus type 14 has been identified in healthy individuals of all ages in several areas of the United States.

Adenoviruses can be detected from respiratory secretions or stool in cell culture using various epithelial cell lines, such as A-549, HEp-2, and He-La cells. Growth is usually apparent in 2 to 5 days. Adenovirus produces a characteristic grapelike cluster cytopathic effect (CPE). Viral confirmation follow-up is performed using an indirect fluorescent antibody (IFA) technique or enzyme immunoassay (EIA). Nucleic acid testing for adenovirus is becoming more popular because of the s' detection time and the increased sensitivity over traditional cell culture. Rapid cell culture (i.e., shell vials) using centrifugation reduces detection time but is less sensitive than tube culture.

# ARENAVIRUSES

Arenaviruses, of the family Arenaviridae, include 29 spherical, enveloped RNA viruses that have T-shaped glycoprotein spikes 7 to 10 nm long surrounding the surface membrane of the virion (Table 66-4). The viruses can readily infect a variety of mammalian species, especially rodents and bats, often resulting in a deleterious effect on the reservoir rodent host. Human transmission usually occurs through inhalation of aerosols of infected rodent excrement (urine, saliva, feces, nasal secretions) or by direct contact with infected rodents. Disease in humans clinically displays a broad range of symptoms, from asymptomatic (no symptoms) to fever, prostration, headache and vomiting, to the more severe cases of meningitis and hemorrhagic fever.

**TABLE 66-2** Viral Syndromes and Common Viral Pathogens

| Viral Syndrome | Viral Pathogens |
|---|---|
| **Infants and Children**<br>Upper respiratory tract infection | Rhinovirus, coronavirus, parainfluenza, adenovirus, RSV, influenza |
| Pharyngitis | Adenovirus, coxsackie A, HSV, EBV, rhinovirus, parainfluenza, influenza |
| Croup | Parainfluenza, RSV, metapneumovirus |
| Bronchitis | Parainfluenza, RSV, metapneumovirus |
| Bronchiolitis | RSV, parainfluenza, metapneumovirus |
| Pneumonia | RSV, adenovirus, influenza, parainfluenza |
| Gastroenteritis | Rotavirus, adenovirus 40-41, calicivirus, astrovirus |
| Congenital and neonatal disease | HSV-2, echovirus, and other enteroviruses, CMV, parvovirus B-19, VZV, HIV, hepatitis viruses |
| **Adults**<br>Upper respiratory tract infection | Rhinovirus, coronavirus, adenovirus, influenza, parainfluenza, EBV |
| Pneumonia | Influenza, adenovirus, sin nombre virus (hantavirus), SARS coronavirus |
| Pleurodynia | Coxsackie B |
| Gastroenteritis | Noroviruses |
| **All Patients**<br>Parotitis | Mumps, parainfluenza |
| Myocarditis/pericarditis | Coxsackie B and echoviruses |
| Keratitis/conjunctivitis | HSV, VZV, adenovirus, enterovirus 70 |
| Pleurodynia | Coxsackie B |
| Herpangina | Coxsackie A |
| Febrile illness with rash | Echoviruses and coxsackie viruses |
| Infectious mononucleosis | EBV, CMV |
| Meningitis | Echoviruses and coxsackie viruses; mumps, lymphocytic choriomeningitis viruses; HSV-2 |
| Encephalitis | HSV-1, togaviruses, bunyaviruses, flaviviruses, rabies virus, enteroviruses, measles virus, HIV, JC virus |
| Hepatitis | Hepatitis A, B, C, D (delta agent), E, and non-A, B, C, D, E viruses |
| Hemorrhagic cystitis | Adenovirus, BK virus |
| Cutaneous infection with or without rash | HSV types 1 and 2; VZV; enteroviruses; measles, rubella viruses; parvovirus B-19; human herpes virus 6 and 7; HPV; poxviruses, including smallpox, monkeypox, molluscum contagiosum, and orf |
| Hemorrhagic fever | Ebola, Marburg, Lassa, yellow fever, dengue, and other viruses |
| Generalized, no specific target organ | HIV-1, HIV-2, HTLV-1 |

*CMV,* Cytomegalovirus; *EBV,* Epstein-Barr virus; *HIV,* human immunodeficiency virus; *HPV,* human papillomavirus; *HSV,* herpes simplex virus; *HTLV,* human T-lymphotropic viruses; *RSV,* respiratory syncytial virus; *SARS,* severe acute respiratory syndrome; *VZV,* varicella-zoster virus.

The arenaviruses capable of causing disease in humans include lymphocytic choriomeningitis (LCM) virus and Lassa fever virus (first detected in Lassa, Nigeria). LCM has been identified in cases of aseptic meningitis in Europe and the Americas. Lassa has been associated with hemorrhagic fever, shock, and death in 5% to 15% of symptomatic patients (80% of cases are asymptomatic). Lassa fever virus is a significant cause of morbidity and mortality in West Africa, where economic resources are limited. Capillary leak and widespread organ involvement, accompanied by shock, respiratory distress, and/or hemorrhage, are responsible for most deaths from Lassa fever. Other, less commonly reported arenaviruses may also cause hemorrhagic fever.

Arenavirus infection is diagnosed using serologic tests or reverse transcriptase polymerase chain reaction (RT-PCR) to detect viral nucleic acid. Viral isolation using cell culture is not routinely recommended. Cell culture for viral isolation has proven to be unreliable because of inconsistent sensitivity. In addition, handling cultures and specimens puts laboratory personnel at high risk. Samples and cultures containing LCM virus require Biosafety Level (BSL) 3 facilities, and Lassa fever virus requires a BSL 4 laboratory. Serologic diagnosis is also difficult because the immunologic antibody response is delayed for several days and often weeks following symptomatic illness. An RT-PCR assay has been developed to detect arenaviruses, but it is not widely available in the acute care setting.

**TABLE 66-3** Adenoviruses

| | |
|---|---|
| **Family** | Adenoviridae |
| **Common name** | Adenovirus |
| **Virus** | Adenovirus |
| **Characteristics** | Double-stranded DNA genome; icosahedral capsid, no envelope; approximately 50 human serotypes |
| **Transmission** | Respiratory, fecal-oral, and direct contact (eye) |
| **Site of latency** | Replication in oropharynx |
| **Disease** | Pharyngitis, pharyngoconjunctival fever, keratoconjunctivitis, pneumonia, hemorrhagic cystitis, disseminated disease, and gastroenteritis in children |
| **Diagnosis** | Cell culture (HEp-2 and other continuous human epithelial lines), enzyme immunoassay (EIA) for gastroenteritis serotypes 40-41 |
| **Treatment** | Supportive |
| **Prevention** | Vaccine (adenovirus serotypes 4 and 7) for military recruits |

**TABLE 66-4** Arenaviruses

| | |
|---|---|
| **Family** | Arenaviridae |
| **Common name** | Arenavirus |
| **Virus** | Lymphocytic choriomeningitis (LCM) and Lassa fever (Lassa, Nigeria) viruses |
| **Characteristics** | Enveloped, irregular-shaped capsid containing a two-segmented (each segment is circular), single-stranded RNA genome |
| **Transmission** | From rodent to human through contamination of human environment with rodent urine; virus enters through skin abrasions or inhalation |
| **Disease** | LCM causes asymptomatic to influenza-like to aseptic meningitis–type disease; Lassa fever virus causes influenza-like disease to severe hemorrhagic fever |
| **Diagnosis** | Serology, polymerase chain reaction |
| **Treatment** | Supportive for LCM; ribavirin and immune plasma for Lassa fever |
| **Prevention** | Avoid contact with virus, institute rodent control; isolation and barrier nursing prevent nosocomial spread |

# BUNYAVIRUSES

Bunyaviruses, first detected in Bunyamwera, Uganda, belong to the family Bunyaviridae (Table 66-5). The virus is an RNA virus consisting of three, single-stranded RNA segments enclosed in a helical nucleocapsid that is surrounded by a lipid envelope. A unique feature of this family of viruses is their tripartite genome. The genomic structure provides a mechanism for genetic reassortment

**TABLE 66-5** Bunyaviruses

| | |
|---|---|
| **Family** | Bunyaviridae |
| **Common name** | Bunyavirus |
| **Virus** | Arboviruses,* including the California encephalitis group containing Lacrosse virus, and non–arthropod-borne viruses, including hantaviruses (containing sin nombre virus) |
| **Characteristics** | Segmented, single-stranded, RNA genome; spherical or pleomorphic capsid with envelope |
| **Transmission** | Mosquito, tick, and sandfly vectors, except for hantaviruses, which are zoonoses transmitted by contact with rodent host and/or their excretions |
| **Disease** | Encephalitis for arboviruses; pneumonia or hemorrhagic fever for hantaviruses |
| **Diagnosis** | Serology and antibody detection in cerebrospinal fluid, reverse transcriptase polymerase chain reaction (RT-PCR) for hantaviruses (serology [IgM and IgG]) also available for hantavirus (sin nombre virus) |
| **Treatment** | Supportive |
| **Prevention** | Avoid contact with arthropod vector. Vector control programs; hantaviruses, avoid rodent urine and feces |

*Arthropod-borne viruses (arboviruses) are taxonomically heterogeneous but were once grouped together because of their common mode of transmission. Viruses adapted to arthropod vectors occur in several taxonomic families, including the Togaviridae, Flaviviridae, and Bunyaviridae. The virus group in Togaviridae that includes arboviruses is the alphavirus group. Common arboviruses are referred to as bunyaviruses, flaviviruses, and alphaviruses.

in nature, much like the orthomyxovirus family of viruses. Bunyaviruses comprise a large, diverse group of viruses (approximately 300 total members with 12 human pathogens), most of which are transmitted by mosquitoes (arboviruses).

The most important human pathogens in the United States consist of the California serogroup (CAL), which includes the California encephalitis and Lacrosse viruses (LAC). Although the name California encephalitis implies that these cases are related to the state of California, they are identified primarily in Minnesota, Wisconsin, Iowa, Illinois, Indiana, and Ohio. Disease is typically mild and self-limiting; however, severe, even fatal, encephalitis ensues in approximately 2% of patients infected. Other human disease–causing members of the family Bunyaviridae include the Cache Valley (CV), Jamestown Canyon (JC), Snowshoe hare (SSH), Tahyna, Rift Valley fever, and Inkoo viruses.

Bunyaviruses that belong to the *Hantavirus* genus are not arboviruses. The viruses are rodent borne and transmitted through exposure (inhalation) to aerosolized rodent excreta. Rodents develop a chronic infection that results in shedding of the virus in saliva, feces, and urine. Disruption of these animal excreta by vacuuming, sweeping, or shaking rugs aerosolizes infected particles, which are then inhaled. Evidence indicates that the chance of inhaling these particles is greater in indoor, poorly ventilated spaces than through outdoor exposure.

The disease that ensues is called hantavirus pulmonary syndrome (HPS). It was originally discovered in 1993 in the four corners area of the southwestern United States (Arizona, New Mexico, Colorado, and Utah). The discovery of this virus resulted from the outbreak of an unexplained pulmonary illness among several young, healthy people who died from acute respiratory failure. Diagnostic testing failed to identify a known cause of death. Through exhaustive analysis by the virologists at the Centers for Disease Control and Prevention (CDC) using molecular testing, the scientists were able to link the pulmonary syndrome with a previously unknown type of hantavirus. The new virus originally was called Muerto Canyon virus, but later the name was changed to sin nombre (no name) virus (SNV).

HPS begins with generalized symptoms that include headache, fever, and body aches, typically after an incubation period of 11 to 32 days. Subsequently, the symptoms become much more severe, leading to hemorrhagic fever, kidney disease, and acute respiratory failure. The deer mouse (Peromyscus maniculatus) is the primary host for the sin nombre virus. Transmission of the virus from rodent to human has been the only documented mode of human infection. No person-to-person transmission of HPS has ever been documented in the United States.

Since the discovery of SNV, several hantaviruses that cause HPS have been discovered throughout the United States. The Bayou virus, carried by the rice rat (Oryzomys palustris), was first discovered in a male from the state of Louisiana. The cotton rat (Sigmodon hispidus) is the carrier of the Black Creek Canal virus, discovered in a resident from Florida. The white-footed mouse (Peromyscus leucopus) has been implicated in a case of a hantavirus infection called the New York-1 virus. Cases of HPS stemming from related hantaviruses have been documented in Argentina, Brazil, Canada, Chile, Paraguay, and Uruguay, making HPS a panhemispheric disease.

Laboratory diagnosis relies on the identification of hantavirus-specific IgM and or IgG antibody. By the time symptoms have appeared, all patients have formed hantavirus-specific IgM antibody, and most have also developed hantavirus-specific IgG antibody. Enzyme-linked immunosorbent assay (ELISA) is usually the method of choice for diagnosis. Other available diagnostic methods include identification of viral antigen in tissue using immunohistochemistry or the presence of amplifiable viral RNA sequences in blood or tissues. Although RT-PCR assays have been developed for some hantaviruses, the variation in the viral genome reduces sensitivity, making routine identification by RT-PCR complicated for the diagnosis of hantavirus infections. Virus isolation from human sources is difficult, and to date no isolates of SNV-like viruses have been recovered from humans.

# CALICIVIRUSES

Caliciviruses are small (30 to 38 nm), rounded, nonenveloped, single-stranded, positive RNA viruses that cause acute gastroenteritis in humans. Caliciviruses (Table

**TABLE 66-6** Caliciviruses

| | |
|---|---|
| **Family** | Caliciviridae |
| **Common name** | Calicivirus |
| **Virus** | Noroviruses |
| **Characteristics** | Nonenveloped, icosahedral capsid surrounding single-stranded RNA genome |
| **Transmission** | Fecal-oral |
| **Disease** | Nausea, vomiting, and diarrhea |
| **Diagnosis** | EM, RT-PCR, EIA for noroviruses |
| **Treatment** | Supportive |
| **Prevention** | Avoid contact with virus |

EIA, Enzyme immunoassay; EM, electron microscopy; RT-PCR, reverse transcriptase polymerase chain reaction.

66-6) have been previously recognized as major animal pathogens and have a broad host range and disease manifestation. The virus causes respiratory disease in cats, a vesicular disease in swine, and a hemorrhagic disease in rabbits. Not until the 1990s did the taxonomic status of noroviruses (formerly known as Norwalk-like viruses, named after Norwalk, Ohio) and hepatitis E virus result in classification in the family Caliciviridae. Hepatitis E virus has since been removed from the calicivirus family and included in a new family, the Hepeviridae. (Hepatitis E virus is discussed later in this chapter.)

Members of the Norovirus and Sapovirus genera are the primary cause of viral gastroenteritis in humans and are referred to as the human caliciviruses (HuCV). Previously called "Norwalk-like viruses" and "Sapporo-like viruses," the viruses were named after their prototype strains, the Norwalk virus and the Sapporo virus, respectively. These viruses are now referred to as the "norovirus" and "sapovirus." The HuCVs are further classified into genogroups, and within the genogroups, into genetic clusters. Human isolates in the norovirus genogroup include genogroups I, II, and IV and in the sapovirus genogroup, I, II, IV, and V.

The clinical symptoms associated with norovirus infection include nausea, abdominal cramps, vomiting, and watery diarrhea. Symptoms usually occur after a 1- to 2-day incubation period and continue for approximately 1 to 3 days. Vomiting occurs more often in children than in adults. Infection with sapovirus is similar to that with norovirus; however, sapoviruses more frequently cause disease in infants and toddlers than in school-age children, whereas norovirus infections are common to all age groups. Maximum viral shedding in the feces occurs early, at the onset of clinical symptoms, but viral shedding can occur for up to 2 to 3 weeks after cessation of the clinical symptoms. As a result, control of viral transmission is problematic, and infection does not confer long-lasting immunity.

Norovirus is the source of more than 80% of nonbacterial acute gastroenteritis cases and more than 50% of food-borne outbreaks for all ages in developed and underdeveloped countries. A major public health concern is its ability to cause large outbreaks in semiclosed environments. In recent years, noroviruses have been implicated in large outbreaks of disease on cruise ships, in nursing homes, in schools, summer camps, hospitals, and restaurants. Several factors contribute to the rapid spread of infection: fecal-oral transmission, the low infectious dose (fewer than 100 virus particles), and the virus's high environmental stability. Noroviruses are easily transmitted in water, person to person, or in airborne droplets of vomitus. The virus persists in water despite treatment processes.

Norovirus cannot be cultivated using cell culture. The most widely used identification method is RT-PCR. Commercially available ELISA kits that use monoclonal antibodies (MoAbs) or hyperimmune sera are also available to detect norovirus but are inferior in sensitivity and specificity to RT-PCR. RT-PCR may also be used to detect the HuCVs in environmental specimens, such as drinking water or contaminated food or both.

# CORONAVIRUSES

The family Coronaviridae includes the genera *Torovirus* and *Coronavirus* (CoV) and contains many species of both human and animal origin (Table 66-7). Once considered a harmless virus capable of causing the human "cold," the CoVs cause a wide variety of disease in animals and birds. Interest in this virus and its relationship with animals and humans was renewed after the global outbreak of the novel coronavirus severe acute respiratory syndrome (SARS) in 2002 that resulted in severe respiratory distress in the human population. (The SARS outbreak is discussed in detail later in this chapter.) Coronaviruses are pleomorphic, roughly spherical, medium-sized, enveloped RNA viruses. The prefix corona- results from the viral structure and the crownlike surface projections on the external surface of the virus that can be seen with electron microscopy. Human respiratory coronaviruses cause colds and occasionally pneumonia in adults. Together the rhinoviruses and coronaviruses cause more than 55% of the "common colds" in the human populations. Viral transmission is person to person via

contaminated respiratory secretions or aerosols. The virus is present in the highest concentration in the nasal passages, where it infects the nasal epithelial cells. Coronaviruses are thought to cause diarrhea in infants based on the presence (as seen with electron microscopy) of coronavirus-like particles in the stool of symptomatic patients. Although antigen detection is available, the technique lacks sensitivity compared with nucleic acid–based testing. No practical diagnostic methods other than electron microscopy and RT-PCR are available. Many CoVs do not grow in routine cell culture. Modified cell cultures have been useful when confirmatory testing with antigen- or nucleic acid–based methods are used.

In November, 2002, SARS was identified as the cause of a worldwide outbreak. It first emerged in the Guangdong province in China. The virus is believed to have mutated and crossed into the human population from palm civets, an exotic mammal present in the live animal markets of China. More than 80% of these animals showed evidence of coronavirus infection. The proximity of humans to animals during exposure in the live animal markets probably facilitated the initial human infection. The outbreak started as a single case in a hotel in China and then snowballed, with a subsequent outbreak in a Hong Kong hospital as the virus evolved and was able to propagate through person-to-person transmission. Within months, more than 8000 patients worldwide were affected, and approximately 700 people died. The disease was characterized by a rapid onset of high fever, followed by a dry cough and dyspnea. The severe respiratory syndrome followed an incubation period of approximately 2 to 7 days after the appearance of the initial symptoms (fever, headache, myalgia, and malaise). Frequently the illness would progress to severe respiratory distress, requiring the patient to be hospitalized for supportive care and mechanical ventilation. During the hospitalizations of several patients, a secondary attack rate of more than 50% was noted among health care workers caring for the SARS patients. This secondary attack rate is a result of SARS being an unusual respiratory virus. The period of maximum infectivity and highest viral loads in the upper airways begins in the second week of illness, during the time the patients often were severely ill. The CDC soon established a case definition, and a worldwide effort in infection control began in order to stop the spread of the virus. The worldwide SARS outbreak was finally considered "contained" in July, 2003. Since the initial outbreak, the virus has not been detected in humans, but the animal reservoir and live animal markets in China are still present. This indicates that future viral strains may emerge if animal-to-human transmission occurs.

Low levels of virus in the respiratory tract during early disease provide a diagnostic challenge. Because of its sensitivity and specificity, molecular testing by RT-PCR remains the recommended method for laboratory diagnosis. The nonspecific symptoms associated with a SARS infection make laboratory testing crucial in the diagnosis and control of the virus. Although nucleic acid testing by RT-PCR is the most useful diagnostic test available, the virus is capable of growth in cell culture using the Vero-E6 cell line. The characteristic viral CPE appears as a rapid cell rounding, refractivity and detachment. BSL 3 or

## TABLE 66-7  Coronaviruses

| Family | Coronaviridae |
|---|---|
| Common name | Coronaviruses |
| Virus | Coronavirus |
| Characteristics | Single-stranded, RNA genome; helical capsid with envelope |
| Transmission | Unknown, probably direct contact or aerosol |
| Disease | Common cold; possibly gastroenteritis, especially in children; SARS |
| Diagnosis | EM, RT-PCR |
| Treatment | Supportive |
| Prevention | Avoid contact with virus |

*EM,* Electron microscopy; *RT-PCR,* reverse transcriptase polymerase chain reaction; SARS, severe acute respiratory syndrome.

higher is required for propagation and manipulation of cell cultures containing this virus.

# FILOVIRUSES

The Filoviridae family of viruses (Table 66-8) is considered the most pathogenic of the hemorrhagic fever viruses. The term *filo* means threadlike, referring to the virus's long, filamentous structural morphology seen with electron microscopy. The viruses are pleomorphic, enveloped, nonsegmented, single-stranded, negative sense RNA viruses. The filamentous morphology appears in many forms or configurations under the electron microscope, such as the number "6," "U," or circular. Marburg hemorrhagic fever virus displays the characteristic "shepherd's hook" morphology. The term "viral hemorrhagic fever" is used to describe a severe multisystem syndrome in which multiple organ systems are affected throughout the body. The patient's vascular system becomes damaged, and the body's ability to regulate itself is impaired. Infection with the Marburg or Ebola virus, endemic in Africa, results in severe hemorrhages, vomiting, abdominal pain, myalgia, pharyngitis, conjunctivitis, and proteinuria. Human case fatality rates for Ebola virus infection exceed 80%; the toll for Marburg virus infection is somewhat lower, with a case fatality rate of 23% to 25%. These diseases have no cure or established drug treatment.

The first filovirus was detected in Marburg, Germany, when a group of German laboratory workers became ill and developed hemorrhagic fever after handling imported African green monkeys or monkey tissue while preparing polio vaccine. Simultaneous hemorrhagic fever outbreaks occurred in laboratories in Frankfurt, Germany, and Belgrade, Yugoslavia (now Serbia). Thirty-one individuals became symptomatic, and seven individual fatalities were recorded. Symptomatic individuals included the laboratory workers, their family members, and medical personnel. The Marburg virus was isolated from the African green monkeys and determined to be the etiologic agent of infection.

Ebola virus is the only other member of the Filovirus family. It is named after a river in Zaire (now the Democratic Republic of the Congo), where it was first identified. The genus *Ebolavirus* has five subspecies, based on the first location where the virus was identified: *Zaire ebolavirus, Sudan ebolavirus, Cote d'Ivoire ebolavirus* (formerly referred to as Ebola–Ivory Coast), *Bundibugyo ebolavirus,* and *Reston ebolavirus.* All of the Ebola subspecies cause disease in humans and nonhuman primates (i.e., chimpanzees, gorillas, and monkeys) except for *Reston ebolavirus,* which causes disease only in nonhuman primates. The Ebola virus was first recognized in 1976, when a total of 602 people became ill in Zaire and Sudan. Infections are acute, with no carrier state, and humans become ill after contact with an infected animal, usually a primate. Transmission of the virus is rapid. Individuals caring for the sick who come in contact with the patient's secretions quickly develop symptoms. In fact, many of the early Ebola outbreaks were attributed to "nosocomial" infections. Personal protective equipment (e.g., gowns, masks, and gloves) often were not used by those caring for sick patients. Also, objects such as needles and syringes often were not sterilized before reuse, and many people were exposed to the virus through contaminated syringes and needles. In the initial Ebola outbreak, 431 people died, a fatality rate greater than 70%.

The natural animal reservoir for the Ebola and Marburg viruses has never been determined, although the animal source is believed to be native to Africa. Disease outbreaks in monkeys have occurred in the United States in research facilities. Several monkeys housed in separate cages became ill simultaneously. Laboratory workers working in these facilities were also infected and developed antibodies but never developed symptoms of the disease. Reston ebolavirus is known to have caused infections through aerosolization of secretions.

RT-PCR is used to identify the Ebola and Marburg viruses. Electron microscopy is also available in some research facilities. Cell culture is available in laboratories with BSL 4 facilities. Antibody production occurs after an Ebola virus infection, and an antigen-capture ELISA is available to detect IgM and IgG antibodies to Ebola virus.

# FLAVIVIRUSES

The flaviviruses (family Flaviviridae; Table 66-9) include viruses that cause arbovirus diseases, such as yellow fever, dengue, West Nile viral encephalitis, and Japanese and St. Louis encephalitis. Hepatitis C virus (HCV) is a flavivirus but not an arbovirus. Flaviviruses are small, single-stranded, positive sense RNA, enveloped, icosahedral viruses. The name is derived from the Latin word *flavus,* which means yellow. The first disease identified in this group was yellow fever, which causes yellow jaundice in humans. Diseases in this viral group are transmitted to humans through the bite of an infected arthropod, usually the mosquito.

Yellow fever has been one of the great plagues throughout history. In 1900, thousands of individuals died during

**TABLE 66-8** Filoviruses

| Family | Filoviridae |
|---|---|
| Common name | Filovirus |
| Virus | Ebola (or Ebola-Reston) and Marburg viruses |
| Characteristics | Enveloped, long, filamentous and irregular capsid forms with single-stranded RNA |
| Transmission | Transmissible to humans from monkeys and, presumably, other wild animals; human-to-human transmission via body fluids and respiratory droplets |
| Disease | Severe hemorrhage and liver necrosis; mortality as high as 90% |
| Diagnosis | Electron microscopy, cell culture in monkey kidney cells; Biosafety Level 4 required |
| Treatment | Supportive |
| Prevention | Avoid contact with virus; export prohibitions on wild monkeys |

**TABLE 66-9** Flaviviruses

| Family | Flaviviridae |
|---|---|
| Common name | Flavivirus |
| Characteristics | Single-stranded RNA genome surrounded by spherical and icosahedral capsid with envelope |
| Virus | Arboviruses,* including yellow fever, dengue, West Nile, Japanese encephalitis, and St. Louis encephalitis viruses |
| Transmission | Arthropod vector, usually mosquito |
| Disease | St. Louis and West Nile encephalitis, dengue and yellow fever |
| Diagnosis | Serology and antibody detection in cerebrospinal fluid; reverse transcriptase polymerase chain reaction (RT-PCR) for dengue and yellow fever |
| Treatment | Supportive |
| Prevention | Avoid contact with vector; vector control programs |
| Virus | Hepatitis C virus |
| Transmission | Parenteral or sexual |
| Disease | Acute and chronic hepatitis; strong correlation between chronic HCV infection and hepatocellular carcinoma |
| Diagnosis | Serology, RT-PCR and viral genotyping |
| Treatment | Supportive, interferon |
| Prevention | Avoid contact with virus; blood supply screened for antibody to hepatitis C virus |

*Arthropod-borne viruses (arboviruses) are taxonomically heterogeneous but were once grouped together because of their common mode of transmission. Viruses adapted to arthropod vectors occur in several taxonomic families, including the Togaviridae, Flaviviridae, and Bunyaviridae. The virus group within Togaviridae that includes arboviruses is the alphavirus group. Common arboviruses are referred to as bunyaviruses, flaviviruses, and alphaviruses.

the construction of the Panama Canal. An army physician, Dr. Walter Reed, uncovered the source of the infection. In the jungle habitat, monkeys serve as the reservoir and the vector is a mosquito. This was the first virus clearly associated with transmission by a mosquito. The yellow fever virus also is the first flavivirus for which an effective vaccine has been developed. In urban outbreaks, humans can serve as the reservoir, as long as the mosquito vector is present.

The yellow fever virus primarily infects liver cells, resulting in fever, jaundice, and hemorrhage. Transmission through the mosquito bite is followed by a 3- to 6-day incubation period. The onset of symptoms is sudden and includes fever, rigors, headache, and backache. The patient's clinical condition progresses rapidly, and the patient becomes intensely ill with nausea, vomiting, facial edema, dusky pallor, swollen, bleeding gums, and hemorrhagic tendencies with black vomit, melena (black, tarry feces), and ecchymoses (bruising). Mortality rates range from 5% to 50%; when death occurs, it is usually

within 6 to 7 days following the onset of symptoms but rarely after 10 days. The characteristic yellow jaundice typically is seen in convalescing patients. Prevention in urban areas depends on elimination of the yellow fever vector, the mosquito, *Aedes aegypti*. The current vaccine is very effective at preventing infection.

Diagnosis of yellow fever infection is often a result of correlation of the patient's clinical symptoms with the patient's location and travel history. Laboratory testing on serum or cerebrospinal fluid (CSF) is available for detection of virus-specific antibodies or neutralizing antibodies. Serologic testing is also available using IgM-capture ELISA, microsphere-based immunoassays (MIAs), and IgG ELISA. In fatal cases of yellow fever, patient tissues may be sent to reference laboratories for nucleic acid amplification, histopathology, and cell culture.

The dengue virus is the most prevalent arbovirus in the world; more than 100 million people are infected annually. It is the leading cause of illness and death in the tropics and subtropics. The virus is endemic in Latin America, Puerto Rico, and Mexico. Most cases reported in the United States (more than 90%) are travel related. Humans are the main reservoir for this virus, and person-to-person transmission occurs through a mosquito vector. Dengue virus has four serotypes that cause a variety of clinical manifestations, including nonlethal fever, arthritis, and rash. Infection with one serotype confers immunity only to the infecting serotype. Subsequent infection with one of the three remaining serotypes results in immune-enhanced disease in the form of severe hemorrhagic fever or dengue shock syndrome. Of the more than 100 million cases of dengue fever, 250,000 cases result in dengue hemorrhagic fever, resulting in approximately 25,000 deaths annually. Dengue normally affects adults and older children. The infection begins with a sudden onset of fever, severe headache, chills, and general myalgia. Often a macropapular rash may be visible on the trunk of the body, which then spreads to the face and extremities. No vaccine is available for dengue. Laboratory diagnosis is based on the presence of virus-specific IgM antibody, a fourfold rise in specific IgG antibody, or a positive RT-PCR amplification for dengue genomic sequences.

Scores of other arthropod-borne flaviviruses, most transmitted by mosquitoes or ticks, cause encephalitis, hemorrhagic fever, or milder disease characterized by fever, arthralgia, and rash. West Nile virus (first isolated in the West Nile district of Uganda), a flavivirus closely related to the Japanese and St. Louis encephalitis viruses, is endemic in Africa, Israel, and Europe. West Nile virus has been endemic in the United States since 1999. Since the virus was identified in New York City in 1999, it has spread westward across the entire United States and into Canada, Mexico, Central America, South America, and some Caribbean islands. The virus accounts for the largest number of cases of viral encephalitis in the United States.

West Nile virus is maintained in a bird-mosquito cycle. Birds are the natural reservoir for the virus. Currently, 59 species of mosquitos and more than 300 species of birds are infected with the West Nile virus. Amplification of virus during warm months results in the death of bird hosts, most commonly crows, ravens, and jays. Bridge

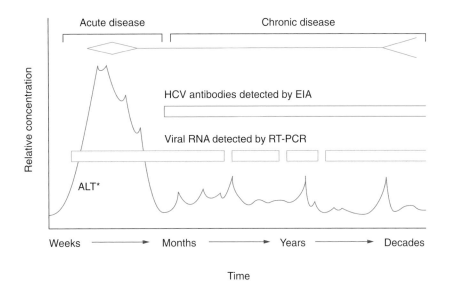

*Alanine aminotransferase marker for liver necrosis.

**Figure 66-1** Time course of immune response and disease caused by hepatitis C virus.

mosquitos (those that bite both humans and birds) are responsible for transmission to humans; as the viral populations in birds increases, more humans become infected. Interestingly, West Nile virus also has been transmitted person to person through blood transfusions, tissue transplantation, and in human breast milk. Infection is often accompanied by fever, leukopenia, and malaise and may progress to encephalitis.

Laboratory diagnosis typically involves detection of IgM antibody to West Nile virus in the patient's serum or CSF. Several commercial kits are available for detection of West Nile IgM and IgG specific antibodies using ELISA or IFA methods. Nucleic acid amplification testing has been very successful in detecting the arbovirus from the tissues of fatal cases and has also been used to detect the virus from the tissues of birds. Additionally, molecular testing has used to detect West Nile virus in mosquito pools. West Nile mosquito surveillance has become increasingly important in the attempt to control this disease.

The hepatitis C virus causes hepatitis. Worldwide, an estimated 170 million people are HCV carriers, and about 4 million of those live in the United States. Acute infection with HCV progresses to a chronic infection in 50% to 90% of infected individuals (Figure 66-1). The acute infection with HCV often goes undiagnosed, because it is often asymptomatic. When clinical illness is present, it is generally mild. Chronic infection with HCV is an important cause of liver disease and is associated with the development of end-stage liver disease and hepatocellular carcinoma. The virus is transmitted predominantly by exposure to infected blood, such as during intravenous drug use and administration of contaminated blood products. The screening of blood products for HCV has eliminated the risk of transmission through contaminated blood products. Less efficient modes of transmission include sexual contact with infected partners, acupuncture, tattooing, and sharing of razors.

HCV disease is identified with screening antibody tests, anti-HCV EIA, confirmatory antibody testing, anti-HCV immunoblot, and RT-PCR. In addition, RT-PCR and quantitative bDNA (branched chain DNA) is used to quantitate virus in the blood to monitor viral therapy. Finally, viral genotyping using molecular techniques is available for identifying genotypes that do not respond appropriately to therapy. The full benefits of modern laboratory testing, including the application of molecular methods, has significantly improved the recognition, monitoring, and treatment of HCV disease.

# HEPEVIRUS

Hepatitis E virus (HEV) is the type species of the new genus *Hepevirus*, in the family Hepeviridae (Table 66-10). Previously classified in the family of caliciviruses, HEV is a small, nonenveloped virus with a single-stranded RNA genome. The only other member of this virus family is an avian HEV known to cause enlarged liver and spleen disease in chickens. Several genetic and antigenic variants or strains of HEV exist and are referred to as genotypes. The different viral strains are common to different geographic locations. Genotype 3 is the strain found in the United States. HEV has also been isolated from swine worldwide and from wild deer in Japan. This indicates that the potential for transmission from animal to humans, resulting in a zoonotic human infection.

HEV was discovered in Asia by a Russian virologist who volunteered to drink stool filtrates from a patient with an unidentified form of hepatitis. The virus is waterborne. The primary mode of transmission is the consumption of water contaminated with feces. HEV is not endemic in the United States and other developed areas of the world. HEV infection results in an acute and generally self-limiting viral hepatitis (inflammation of the liver). Most infected patients do not progress to a long-term carrier

**TABLE 66-10** Hepevirus

| Family | Hepeviridae |
|---|---|
| Common name | Hepatitis E |
| Virus | Hepevirus |
| Characteristics | Nonenveloped, icosahedral capsid surrounding single-stranded RNA genome |
| Transmission | Fecal-oral |
| Disease | Hepatitis similar to that caused by hepatitis A virus except for extraordinarily high case fatality rate (10% to 20%) among pregnant women |
| Diagnosis | Serology |
| Treatment | Supportive |
| Prevention | Avoid contact with virus |

**TABLE 66-11** Hepadnaviruses

| Family | Hepadnaviridae |
|---|---|
| Common name | Hepadnavirus |
| Virus | Hepatitis B virus (HBV) |
| Characteristics | Partly double-stranded DNA genome; icosahedral capsid with envelope; virion (also called Dane particle); surface antigen originally termed "Australia antigen" |
| Transmission | Humans are reservoir and vector; spread by direct contact, including exchange of body secretions, recipient of contaminated blood products, percutaneous injection of virus, and perinatal exposure |
| Site of latency | Liver |
| Disease | Acute infection with resolution (90%); fulminant hepatitis, most co-infected with delta virus (1%); chronic hepatitis, persistence of hepatitis B surface antigen (HBsAg) (9%) followed by resolution (disappearance of HBsAg), asymptomatic carrier state, chronic persistent (systemic disease without progressive liver disease), or chronic active disease (progressive liver damage) |
| Diagnosis | Serology, viral antigen detection, and polymerase chain reaction (PCR) |
| Oncogenic | Liver cancer |
| Treatment | Antivirals and liver transplant for fulminant disease |
| Prevention | HBV vaccine; hepatitis B immune globulin |

status. This virus is well established in developing countries as a cause of hepatitis clinically similar to infection with the hepatitis A virus (HAV). It differs from HAV in that the virus can cause an exceptionally high fatality rate among pregnant women. Fulminant hepatitis develops rapidly and is fatal in approximately 30% of women when infected during the third trimester of pregnancy. The reason for this high rate of mortality among pregnant women is not known. Women should take all possible precautions to avoid exposure to HEV while pregnant, including refraining from traveling to areas of the country where HEV is endemic, such as India and Pakistan.

HEV infection typically begins with nonspecific symptoms common to many viral illnesses, such as fever, headache, nausea, and stomach pain. One of the first signs of a potential hepatitis infection is dark urine, pale feces, yellow discoloration of the skin and sclera. However, not all patients develop jaundice. The liver of infected individuals typically is enlarged and tender.

Clinical diagnosis of HEV infection is important not only to control outbreaks, but also to clinical management of the disease. During patient diagnosis, it is imperative to rule out the other types of hepatitis that can cause a more serious form of disease. With HEV infection, liver function tests typically demonstrate increased levels of serum bilirubin, aspartate aminotransferase (AST) and alanine aminotransferase (ALT) at the time of disease onset. The diagnosis is confirmed using serologic testing. High levels of both IgM and IgG antibodies are produced at disease onset. Although the high levels of IgG confer lifetime immunity to those infected with hepatitis A, whether the antibodies produced in HEV infection do the same is not known. A variety of commercial immunoassays are available that vary in sensitivity and specificity, primarily because of the antigenic variability of the virus. Nucleic acid testing is recommended to confirm positive serology results in areas where HEV is not endemic. Studies are underway to develop a vaccine against HEV, prompted by the highly successful immunization program against HAV.

# HEPADNAVIRUSES

Hepatitis B virus (HBV) (Table 66-11) is the prototype virus of the Hepadnaviridae family (hepa- from hepatitis and dna from the genome type). The virus has long been recognized as a significant cause of liver damage associated with morbidity and mortality. Other mammalian and avian hepadnaviruses are known to exist. Hepadnavirus is a pleomorphic, enveloped virus containing circular, partially double-stranded DNA that replicates through an RNA intermediate. Replication occurs by means of reverse transcription and then DNA replication.

Although a successful vaccine against HBV exists, the number of humans infected with HBV worldwide is nearly 400 million, and approximately 50 million new cases occur annually. Humans are the only source of the virus. Percutaneous exposure to blood or blood products is the primary route of transmission. However, the virus may also be contracted through perinatal or sexual contact. HBV is a relatively heat-stable virus and can retain its infectivity in drying blood and other bodily fluids for several days. HBV infection previously was associated with blood transfusion, but this is now rare because of the screening of blood products and vaccination program.

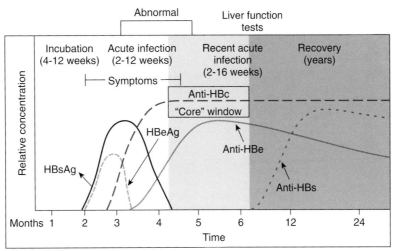

**Figure 66-2** Time course of antigenemia and immune response in a patient demonstrating recovery from acute hepatitis B infection.

The incubation period for an acute HBV infection usually is 1 to 3 months but may be considerably longer. The initial symptoms of acute infection often are nonspecific, much like mild, flulike symptoms (Figure 66-2). Many cases are asymptomatic, especially in children. The infection presents as an acute or chronic hepatitis with a pathologic effect on the liver, resulting in self-limited or fatal outcomes. Fatal disease is most likely to occur in people co-infected with the hepatitis D virus (delta agent), a deficient RNA virus capable of replication in cells infected with HBV. Chronic HBV infection remains a significant worldwide cause of liver cirrhosis and hepatocellular carcinoma despite the availability of an effective vaccine.

Because of the generality of HBV symptoms and the similarities it shares with other causative agents of hepatitis, clinicians rely extensively on the laboratory for confirmation of the clinical diagnosis of acute or chronic infection and identification of the virus. Laboratory diagnosis typically uses immunoassays. Immunoassays are available for specific identification of viral antigens or antibodies (viral markers) in a patient's blood. Several commercial types of assays exist. The most common type uses the EIA format. Most of the commercially available serologic assays demonstrate excellent specificity and sensitivity. HBV is not cultivatable in vitro.

Hepatitis B surface antigen (HBsAg) is the most reliable marker for identifying HBV infection. The antigen becomes evident in the patient's serum weeks before any biochemical evidence associated with liver damage (biochemical liver assays may show only minimal elevation). HBsAg remains in the serum during the acute and chronic stages of hepatitis B. The presence of HBsAg 6 months after acute infection indicates that the patient is a chronic carrier. IgM (anti-HBcAg) to hepatitis B core antigen (HBcAg) appears early in the course of disease, during the acute infection. Anti-HBsAg (antibody to surface antigen) indicates the patient is in convalescence and has developed immunity. The presence of HBeAg (hepatitis B "e" antigen) indicates high infectivity and a chronic carrier state. The best indication of active viral replication and a high state of infectivity is the presence of HBV DNA in the serum. Viral DNA may be detected by a number of molecular tests, including PCR. A number of user-friendly molecular assays are now widely available. The molecular assays provide a quick turnaround time. Also, detection of HBV DNA in serum is used to resolve questionable serologic results, and quantitation is helpful for predicting the patient's response to treatment.

# HERPES VIRUSES

The word "herpes" is derived from the Greek word meaning "to creep" and was historically used to describe the spreading, ulcerative skin lesions typically seen in a herpes simplex virus (HSV) infection. Herpes viruses are large (150 to 200 nm), double-stranded DNA, enveloped viruses. The virion consists of four components, the nucleic acid core, the capsid, the tegument, and the envelope. The tegument, an asymmetric structure made of a fibrous-like material, surrounds the capsid and contains 20 different proteins. These proteins enter the host cell upon fusion of the envelope and cell membrane and initiate the viral replication cycle.

Eight human herpes group viruses have been described (Table 66-12). Herpes viruses are widely disseminated among animal species. However, the zoonotic forms of herpes do not infect humans, except for herpes B virus from nonhuman primates (not counted among the eight human herpes viruses). Herpes B virus causes a severe, usually fatal encephalitis in humans. Human herpes viruses include HSV types 1 and 2 (HSV-1 and HSV-2), varicella-zoster virus (VZV), Epstein-Barr virus (EBV), and cytomegalovirus (CMV). More recently detected herpes viruses include human herpes virus (HHV) types 6 (HHV-6), 7 (HHV-7), and 8 (HHV-8). HHV-6 and HHV-7 are lymphotropic viruses acquired early in life. HHV-8, Kaposi's sarcoma–associated herpes virus (KSHV), causes a tumor of the connective tissue. HHV-6 and HHV-7 are associated with the childhood disease roseola (exanthem subitum). The disease is characterized by a short period of fever and a skin rash.

HSV-1 and HSV-2 share several viral characteristics, including a variable host range, a short replication cycle, rapid spread in cell culture, efficient destruction of

**TABLE 66-12** Herpesviruses

| | |
|---|---|
| **Family** | Herpesviridae |
| **Common name** | Herpesvirus |
| **Characteristics** | Double-stranded DNA genome; icosahedral capsid with envelope; at least eight human herpes viruses known: HSV-1, HSV-2, VZV, Epstein-Barr virus (EBV), CMV, HHV-6, HHV-7, and HHV-8 |
| **Virus** | **Herpes simplex virus types I and II (HSV-1 and HSV-2)** |
| Transmission | Direct contact with infected secretions |
| Site of latency | Sensory nerve ganglia |
| Disease | Predominant virus in parentheses. Gingivostomatitis (HSV-1), pharyngitis (HSV-1), herpes labialis (HSV-1), genital infection (HSV-2), conjunctivitis (HSV-1), keratitis (HSV-1), herpetic whitlow (HSV-1 and HSV-2), encephalitis (HSV-1 in adults), disseminated disease (HSV-1 or HSV-2 in neonates) |
| Detection | Cell culture (HDF, others), EIA, FA stain, IH stain, PCR |
| Treatment | Acyclovir, valacyclovir, famciclovir |
| Prevention | Avoid contact |
| **Virus** | **Varicella-zoster virus (VZV)** |
| Transmission | Close personal contact, especially respiratory |
| Site of latency | Dorsal root ganglia |
| Disease | Chicken pox (varicella), shingles (zoster) |
| Detection | FA stain, cell culture (HDF), shell vial culture, PCR |
| Treatment | Acyclovir and famciclovir |
| Prevention | Vaccine |
| **Virus** | **Epstein-Barr virus (EBV)** |
| Transmission | Close contact with infected saliva |
| Site of latency | B lymphocytes |
| Disease | Infectious mononucleosis, progressive lymphoreticular disease, oral hairy leukoplakia in patients with HIV |
| Detection | Serology, PCR |
| Oncogenic | Burkitt's lymphoma, nasopharyngeal carcinoma |
| Treatment | Supportive |
| Prevention | Avoid contact |
| **Virus** | **Cytomegalovirus (CMV)** |
| Transmission | Close contact with infected secretions, blood transfusions (WBCs), organ transplants, transplacental |
| Site of latency | WBCs, endothelial cells, cells in a variety of organs |
| Disease | Asymptomatic infection, congenital disease of newborn, symptomatic disease of immunocompromised host, heterophile-negative infectious mononucleosis |
| Diagnosis | Cell culture (HDF), shell vial culture, CMV antigenemia, FA stain, PCR |
| Treatment | Supportive; decrease immune suppression; ganciclovir and foscarnet |
| Prevention | Use CMV antibody-negative blood and tissue for transfusion and transplantation, respectively |
| **Virus** | **Human herpesviruses 6 and 7 (HHV-6 and HHV-7)** |
| Transmission | Most likely close contact via respiratory route; almost all children infected by age 2 to 3 years |
| Site of latency | T lymphocytes (CD4 cells) |
| Disease | Roseola (exanthem subitum), fever, malaise, rash, leukopenia, and interstitial pneumonitis in organ transplant recipients |
| Detection | Detection of virus in peripheral blood specimens by PCR, cell culture using lymphocyte lines |
| Treatment | Susceptible to ganciclovir and foscarnet |
| Prevention | None practical |

**TABLE 66-12** Herpesviruses—cont'd

| Virus | Human herpesvirus 8 (HHV-8) |
|---|---|
| Transmission | Not known; much less widely disseminated than other herpes viruses |
| Site of latency | Viral genome found in Kaposi's tumor cells, endothelial cells, and tumor-infiltrating leukocytes |
| Disease | Kaposi's sarcoma |
| Detection | PCR or in situ by hybridization |
| Treatment | None known |
| Prevention | Avoid contact with virus |

*EIA,* Enzyme immunoassay; *FA,* fluorescent antibody; *HDF,* human diploid fibroblast; *HIV,* human immunodeficiency virus; *IH,* iron hematoxylin; *PCR,* polymerase chain reaction; *WBCs,* white blood cells.

infected cells, and the ability to establish latency in the sensory ganglia. These viruses affect individuals of all ages and are the cause of a wide variety of disease, including mucous membrane and skin lesions and ocular, visceral, and central nervous system (CNS) disease. HSV-1 and HSV-2 are transmitted during close personal contact; HSV-1 infection occurs at the oropharyngeal mucosa, and HSV-2 infection occurs at genital sites. Primary HSV-1 infection usually occurs by the time a child reaches the age of 5, and more than 50 million people in the United States are thought to have oral herpes. A subset of primary infections, 10% to 15%, actually produces clinical disease.

Although HSV-2 has been primarily linked to genital herpes, the incidence of genital herpes associated with HSV-1 infection has increased in the U.S. college population from 31% in 1993 to 78% in 2001. HSV-2 is the primary cause of genital herpes and is often associated with sexual promiscuity. Women are 45% more likely to become infected with HSV-2 than are men. The risk of contracting herpes from an infected male after a single sexual contact is 80%.

The defining characteristic associated with herpes infection is the reoccurrence of skin lesions following the primary infection. More than 50% of infected individuals have a recurrent episode of a lesion outbreak within 1 year following initial infection. HSV-1 is associated with mucosal lesions that resemble small vesicles that last 4 to 7 days. The lesions are referred to as herpes labialis, facialis, or febrilis; cold sores, or fever blisters. In women, HSV-2 produces vesicles on the mucosal membranes, labia, and vagina. In men, vesicles form on the shaft of the penis, the prepuce (foreskin), and the glans penis. Systemic symptoms often accompany the primary infection in women, including fever, headache, malaise, and generalized myalgias.

HSV-1 is the most commonly reported viral CNS infection and usually occurs as a result of viral neurotropic spread through the olfactory bulb. This type of infection often occurs in infants and immunocompromised patients. Without treatment, mortality rates associated with HSV infection may be as high as 80%. After appropriate treatment, the mortality rate typically is reduced to 15% in newborns and 20% in other patients. Even when treated, individuals who survive often suffer neurologic, lasting effects, experiencing difficulties in memory, cognition, and personality disorders.

Laboratory diagnosis of herpes infection is available using a variety of diagnostic methodologies. Cell culture traditionally has served as the "gold standard" for herpes virus identification. However, it is important to note that the success of the cell culture depends on the sample collection procedure and the quality of the specimen. The herpes lesion or vesicle should be punctured and the vesicular fluid absorbed with a swab, making sure to swab the base of the vesicle. Samples should be inoculated into cell culture within 1 hour after collection. If this is not possible, the swab should be placed in viral transport media and either refrigerated or frozen at −70°C to preserve the specimen until it can be properly processed and inoculated into cell culture. Herpes is readily grown in cell culture using A-549 or MRC-5 cell lines. The virus is fast growing and typically produces a characteristic rounding, refractile CPE within 1 to 2 days after inoculation of the cell culture. The virus also can be detected using direct antigen testing or nucleic acid amplification systems (PCR), and paired serologic assays of acute and convalescent serum specimens. Direct antigen detection is a rapid, sensitive, and inexpensive method for diagnosis. The antigen present in the lesion is mixed with HSV-specific antibody. If the viral antigen is present, it forms a complex with the antibody that can be identified using immunofluorescent (IF) or immunoperoxidase (IP) staining. This same reaction can be applied in an immunoassay, usually ELISA. Immunoassay offers the additional benefit of adaptability to automation. Nucleic acid testing for the herpes virus has become more widely used and is more sensitive than cell culture and antigen detection. Molecular amplification can be especially beneficial for rapid diagnosis and treatment of herpes viral encephalitis. Both qualitative and quantitative molecular assays exist for identification and diagnosis of herpes viral infection.

The varicella-zoster virus causes what is known as a "classic" childhood disease, chicken pox, and is characterized by the appearance of a maculopapular rash. Before the introduction of the vaccine for VZV, more than 90% of the adults in the United States demonstrated immunity to VZV as a result of childhood infection. Virus transmission is increased during the inclement months, because individuals remain indoors in proximity. The virus is transmitted person to person via respiratory secretions.

VZV infects the conjunctiva or mucosa of the upper respiratory tract and then travels to the lymph nodes. Four to 6 days after the initial infection, infected T cells enter the bloodstream and cause a primary viremia. The infected T cells invade the liver, spleen, and other organs, causing a second round of infection. A secondary viremia ensues, 14 days after the initial infection. This secondary wave infects cells in the skin, causing the characteristic vesicular rash of chicken pox. Symptoms at the onset of infection are usually general and include fever and malaise that appear before the onset of the maculopapular rash on the patient's trunk and scalp. The lesions usually crust over in 1 to 2 days but do not resolve for approximately 3 weeks. After the acute viral replication in the skin, VZV affects the sensory ganglia in the CNS, where it establishes latency; that is, the virus "hides" in the CNS, which is not subject to vigorous immune surveillance. After a period of latency, the virus may initiate another acute infectious cycle. This reactivation produces the characteristic recurrent disease known as "shingles," which occurs predominately in immunocompetent people over age 45. Shingles follows an anatomic route around the torso along the dorsal ganglia, as the virus spreads cell to cell along the neurons to epithelial cells in the skin. This condition results in vesicular lesions similar to those produced during the primary infection. Shingles may be accompanied by a painful condition known as postherpetic neuralgia. This condition causes a chronic, debilitating pain that can persist long after other symptoms of shingles have resolved. This pain is believed to be caused by VZV destruction of neurons.

Laboratory diagnosis is not recommended for uncomplicated cases of VZV infection in healthy children or adults. However, in certain situations, such as infection in an immunosuppressed patient or neonate, laboratory diagnosis of VZV may be beneficial.

The virus produces inclusions and giant cells. The traditional method for identifying VZV was to scrape the base of a fresh vesicular lesion and stain the scrapings with Tzanck, Giemsa, or hematoxylin-eosin stain to identify the inclusions or giant cells. This method was complicated by the fact that HSV also produces inclusion bodies. An additional rapid method for identification of VZV is direct identification of viral antigens. Samples of vesicle epithelial cells are collected and smears are prepared and stained with fluorescent, dye-conjugated, monoclonal antibodies to VZV and then observed with a fluorescent microscope. This is a fairly rapid method, because it can be performed within hours of receiving the specimen. However, interpretation and sensitivity can be questionable if not enough epithelial cells are collected.

VZV can grow in cell culture. It produces a characteristic CPE of small clusters of ovoid cells in fibroid cells such as MRC-5, HF, and A549. However, the virus grows slowly, and positivity of the culture may take 7 to 10 days. Shell vial cultures are a simplified method of detecting VZV compared with regular cell culture. Shell vials use cover slips with MRC-5 cells attached in a monolayer across the surface. After inoculation, the cover slip is fixed with acetone after 3 and 6 days of viral growth. The cover slip then is stained with fluorescein isothiocyanate–conjugated (FITC) monoclonal IgG antibody specific for VZV. Positive specimens exhibit a cytoplasmic, apple-green fluorescence when viewed under a fluorescent microscope. Serologic assays for VZV IgG and IgM antibodies are also available to determine the patient's immune status. Several commercial ELISAs are available for detection and quantitation of VZV antibodies.

Molecular diagnostic testing for VZV is becoming increasingly popular and replacing conventional methods of identifying the virus. This is a result of improvements in diagnostic testing, such as rapid detection time and increased sensitivity and specificity associated with real-time PCR compared with conventional methods of antigen detection or cell culture. In addition, molecular methods can detect multiple human herpes viruses in a single clinical specimen, a technique referred to as multiplex PCR. An automated DNA microarray PCR method has been developed for high-throughput detection of multiple herpes viruses, including VZV, in clinical samples. Molecular diagnostics also can quantitate viral VZV DNA in the blood. Molecular testing is useful for monitoring patients considered high risk for severe VZV infection.

Epstein-Barr virus was discovered four decades ago during a search for the cause of Burkitt's lymphoma, a disease that predominately affects children in Africa. EBV is responsible for the disease infectious mononucleosis (IM). The virus, which is transmitted in the saliva of infected patients, typically affects adolescents and young adults. The major symptoms include fever, sore throat, headache, malaise, and fatigue. Lymphadenopathy (swollen lymph nodes) and splenomegaly also may result during the disease. Mononucleosis typically is diagnosed through serologic methods that detect antibodies to EBV (Figure 66-3). Nonspecific heterophile antibodies (also referred to as Paul-Bunnell antibodies) appear early on during the disease, making the diagnosis difficult. Antibody production to the virus typically follows the classic immune response, resulting in specific IgM production followed by IgG production. Antibody to the viral capsid (IgM) appears within 4 weeks after infection. This is followed by IgG and IgA antibody to the early antigen (EA), indicating acute or recent infection. Both the EA-IgG and IgA may be undetectable after approximately 6 months. Some Anti-EA IgG antibodies may persist in the patient's serum for life. These persistent antibodies typically are elevated in patients with Burkitt's lymphoma. The final diagnostic serologic marker is the antibody to the nuclear antigen (EBNA) that appears within 1 month of infection and peaks approximately 6 to 12 months after infection. In addition to Burkitt's lymphoma, other cancers have been associated with EBV infection (e.g., nasopharyngeal carcinoma), and the virus is recognized as an important agent in the development of lymphoma or other lymphoproliferative disorders in transplant recipients.

Molecular assays have become instrumental in the diagnosis of herpes viruses. Box 66-1 provides an outline for the basic procedure for EBV PCR amplification.

CMV infection is a common cause of congenital birth defects. The virus is included in the TORCH panel for disease screening in infants. (TORCH is an acronym for toxoplasma, rubella, CMV and HSV-1). Besides being the

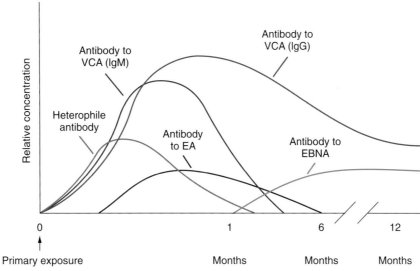

**Figure 66-3** Time course of immune response to Epstein-Barr (EBV) infection.

---

**BOX 66-1** Basic Outline for Epstein-Barr Virus PCR Amplification

**Principle**

Nucleic acid extracted from patient specimens is amplified and detected by polymerase chain reaction (PCR) and fluorescent resonance energy transfer (FRET) probe detection. The procedure is both qualitative and quantitative.

**Specimen**

5 mL ethylenediaminetetraacetic acid (EDTA) whole blood
Cerebrospinal fluid (CSF)

**Method**

1. Specimens should be processed in a laboratory area away from where the extracts are placed in the thermocycler. Gloves should be worn for all procedural steps involving patient specimens, including DNA extraction.
2. PCR master mix should be prepared in a PCR clean area. Master mix should be prepared in a batch from reagent components and stored in aliquots to prevent repeat freezing and thawing. A single specimen reaction typically includes 15 μL of mix plus 5 μL of sample. Master mix contains primer-probes, internal control, DNA polymerase, and magnesium chloride ($MgCl_2$). Quantities should be determined based on the initial concentration of reagents included in the kit or separate analytic components.

3. The PCR master mix should have limited exposure to light to prevent degradation of fluorescent tags on primer-probe pairs.
4. Each assay should include a positive and negative control, qualitative assay.
5. The quantitative assay should include standards that are sufficient to detect low-level viremia consistent with the sensitivity of the assay, in addition to the linearity limits as predetermined by validation testing and verification studies.
6. Samples should be placed in a thermal cycler. A sample thermocycling program should include an initial denaturation cycle at 94°C, followed by 30 to 45 cycles for amplification, and then a cooling cycle.

**Limitations of Procedure**

The test should be used as an aid in diagnosis and should not be considered diagnostic alone. The single assay should not be used as the only evidence to form a clinical conclusion. The test should be correlated with serologic tests, the patient's symptoms, and the clinical presentation. A negative result does not negate the presence of the organism or disease.

---

cause of congenital infection in infants, CMV has been found to cause an infectious mononucleosis–like illness in immunocompromised patients. The disease may be extremely serious in immunosuppressed organ transplant recipients. CMV may be identified using viral cell culture, serologic tests for IgM and IgG antibodies, direct antigen detection, and nucleic acid testing. Although the virus grows in cell culture using human fibroblasts, it is a slow-growing virus that requires 1 to 2 weeks of incubation before CPE is evident, and in some cases CPE may not be visible for a month. Centrifugation-amplified shell vials, a modification of conventional cell culture, can provide a diagnosis within 24 to 48 hours. CMV antigenemia (see Chapter 65 and Procedure 65-2) is routinely used to

monitor therapy for CMV infection. A positive CMV antigenemia result is shown in Figure 66-4. Molecular qualitative and quantitative PCR amplification using analyte-specific reagents is available in some clinical laboratories. In addition, a fully automated quantitative CMV assay is available (COBAS AmpliPrep/COBAS TaqMan CMV Test, Roche Molecular Systems, Inc; Pleasanton, CA). Research studies indicate that nucleic acid-based methods are more sensitive for the detection of CMV in symptomatic and asymptomatic patients.

A unique feature of the herpes virus family is their "hallmark" characteristic of latency, or the virus's ability to reside in the infected host while staying in a repressed state. Reactivation of the virus can be caused by various

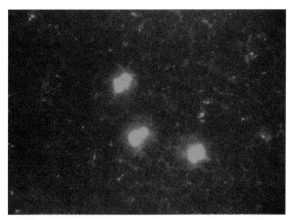

**Figure 66-4** Typical fluorescing white blood cells containing cytomegalovirus (CMV) antigen, as seen in the CMV antigenemia stain.

stimuli, including fever, emotional stress, exposure to UV light, or axonal injury. Recurrence of viral replication at subsequent times results in disease that may be present differentially as a result of the host's immune response. Viruses in this family are capable of viral recurrence or reactivation. HSV-1 may reactivate, causing mucous membrane disease or life-threatening encephalitis. Encephalitis caused by HSV is the most common viral encephalitis, with 2.3 per million cases reported annually. HSV-2 reactivates, causing mucous membrane vesicles or aseptic meningitis. VZV reactivates as localized lesions (shingles). EBV reactivates, causing asymptomatic shedding of virus in the oropharynx or as disseminated disease in immunocompromised patients. As does EBV, CMV recurs symptomatically in compromised hosts as a pathogen in many tissues (e.g., heart, gastrointestinal tract, lung, brain). HHV-6 and HHV-7 also cause reactivation disease in compromised hosts.

# ORTHOMYXOVIRUSES

The influenza virus is a member of the family Orthomyxoviridae (Table 66-13). The members of this family are pleomorphic, spherical, enveloped, single-stranded, segmented, negative sense RNA viruses. Of all the respiratory viruses known to infect humans, influenza is the cause of the greatest number of serious acute illnesses; more than 200,000 hospitalizations and more than 30,000 deaths occur in the United States every year. Although three types of influenza viruses are known to infect humans (A, B, and C), type C usually causes subclinical infections and is not known to pose a threat to human health. The three genera Influenza virus A, Influenza virus B, and Influenza virus C can be distinguished based on the antigenic differences in the matrix protein (M) and the nucleoprotein (NP). Influenza virus A is further subdivided based on the major surface glycoproteins, hemagglutinin (HA) and neuraminidase (NA). Influenza A naturally infects many bird species, swine, seals, felines, and horses. Influenza B and C are only known to infect humans.

Projecting from the envelope of the virion are the two major surface glycoproteins, HA and NA. The HA proteins are rod-shaped spikes that enable viral attachment to sialic acid containing cellular receptors. Once attached to the receptors, the virus can initiate infection. The NA proteins are mushroom-shaped spikes. They facilitate the release of mature virions from infected cells and assist in viral movement through mucus to adjacent cells. Sixteen different HA molecules and nine different NA molecules have been identified. All of the different viral protein antigenic types can be found in the avian species. However, only H1, H2, H3, and N1 or N2 currently circulate in the human population. Strains of influenza A currently found in the human population are H1N1, H3N2, and H1N2. With the rise of the novel influenza A strain of 2009, it is important to separate the types of H1N1 that circulate through various groups of individuals. (This is discussed later in this chapter.) Influenza A H3N2 is a highly pathogenic virus. Infection with H3N2 results in greater mortality than infection with influenza A H1N1 or influenza B.

A unique property of influenza A and influenza B is the organization of the viral genome. It is composed of an eight-part, segmented RNA genome, each segment essentially serving as a single gene. This property, combined with the influenza viruses' unique ability to alter their HA and NA antigens, results in the production of an antigenically different virus from year to year. This is termed antigenic drift. Antigenic drift is a continuous, gradual form of change in the viral genome during replication. Antigenic drift occurs in all viral influenza types.

Influenza A undergoes a seasonal antigenic drift every year, making the formulation of an effective vaccine challenging. Antigenic shift is a much more dramatic change in the viral genome and only occurs with influenza A viruses. Antigenic shift occurs when a circulating influenza A strain acquires a completely new or "novel" subtype. This phenomenon occurs when two different strains of influenza virus simultaneously infect a single host. During viral replication the segmented genome of the influenza virus may reassort, mixing segments from the different strains during the infection, resulting in a unique antigenic combination. Avian influenza and human influenza reassortment of genes have been the cause of several pandemics throughout history. Often swine act as the intermediate, or "mixing vessel," for these reassortment events. Viruses from avian and human origin can infect and replicate in the swine respiratory epithelium. When these reassortments occur, a virus emerges against which the population does not have immune protection because of the new antigenic structure. When this happens, a pandemic can occur if the virus is able to sustain human-to-human transmission. A **pandemic** is a virulent human influenza virus that causes a global outbreak of serious illness, against which there is little natural immunity, and has sustained person-to-person transmission. Often pandemics result in high rates of human mortality with significant social, infrastructure, and economic consequences.

Six pandemics occurred during the past century. Of these the most devastating was the Spanish flu pandemic of 1918, which caused 25 million to 50 million deaths worldwide, more than 500,000 of them in the United

**TABLE 66-13** Orthomyxoviruses

| | |
|---|---|
| **Family** | Orthomyxoviridae |
| **Common name** | Orthomyxovirus |
| **Characteristics** | Segmented (eight separate molecules), single-stranded, RNA genome; helical capsid with envelope; three major antigenic types, influenza A, B, and C; types A and B cause nearly all human disease |
| **Virus** | **Influenza A** |
| Transmission | Contact with respiratory secretions |
| Disease | Influenza (fever, malaise, headache, myalgia, cough); primary influenza pneumonia; in children, bronchiolitis, croup, otitis media |
| Detection | Cell culture (PMK), EIA, FA stain, RT-PCR |
| Epidemiology | Viral subtypes based on hemagglutinin and neuraminidase glycoproteins abbreviated "H" and "N," respectively (e.g., H1N1 or H3N2); infects humans and other animals; antigenic drift, resulting in minor antigenic change, causes local outbreaks of influenza every 1-3 years; antigenic shift, resulting in major antigenic change, causes periodic worldwide outbreaks |
| Treatment | Supportive; antivirals amantadine and rimantadine (influenza A only), and zanamivir and oseltamivir influenza A and B |
| Prevention | Influenza vaccine or antiviral prophylaxis |
| **Virus** | **Influenza B** |
| Transmission | Contact with respiratory secretions |
| Disease | Similar to "mild" influenza |
| Detection | Cell culture (PMK), EIA, FA stain, RT-PCR |
| Epidemiology | Antigenic drift only, resulting in local outbreaks every 1-3 years |
| Treatment | Supportive; antivirals zanamivir and oseltamivir |
| Prevention | Influenza vaccine or antiviral prophylaxis |
| **Virus** | **Influenza C** |
| Transmission | Contact with respiratory secretions |
| Disease | Mild form of influenza causing URTIs |
| Detection | Testing not routinely requested, so virus is infrequently detected; only valid test is NAAT |
| Epidemiology | Most cases occur in children; occurs sporadically or as localized outbreaks |
| Treatment | Supportive |
| Prevention | Avoid contact with virus |

*EIA,* Enzyme immunoassay; *FA,* fluorescent antibody; *NAAT,* nucleic acid amplified testing; *RT-PCR,* reverse transcriptase polymerase chain reaction; *PMK,* primary monkey kidney; *URTIs,* upper respiratory tract infections.

States. The cause of this pandemic was the novel H1N1 virus, which emerged from a reassortment of human and avian influenza components. The survivors of an influenza pandemic develop immunity to the infecting strain. The virus then typically evolves into a "seasonal" circulating strain. Such is the case with the pandemic outbreak of influenza H1N1 in Mexico in 2009. This virus was a triple reassortment of human, avian, and swine viruses capable of human-to-human transmission. The triple reassortment was the result of an interaction between the recent North American H3N2 and H1N2 swine (avian, human, swine triple reassortment viruses) with a Eurasian avian-like swine virus. Although the mortality rate of this pandemic was not as significant as predicted, more than 214 countries and overseas territories reported laboratory-confirmed cases of pandemic influenza A H1N1 2009, resulting in approximately 18,449 deaths. These statistics may be an underestimate of the number of deaths resulting from this outbreak. Many individuals

with influenza do not seek medical care, and a relatively small number of those who do are actually tested for influenza infection. Children and young adults, people with underlying health conditions, pregnant women and indigenous populations were more affected than the general population. The World Health Organization (WHO) officially declared the pandemic over in May, 2010. The virus continues to circulate as a "seasonal" strain throughout the world.

Enhanced surveillance for the next pandemic strain of influenza was preceded by the appearance of the avian influenza "bird flu" circulating in Asia. This influenza strain stems from the avian population. The virus is a highly pathogenic avian influenza that has reassorted multiple times with other avian influenza strains capable of causing disease in poultry and other birds. The first cases of human infection with "bird flu" were reported in Hong Kong, where 18 people became ill and six died. H5N1 influenza was identified as the cause. Infection control practices and prompt slaughter of infected domestic fowl halted the outbreak. Although the major outbreak seems to have been prevented, migratory birds have spread the virus along natural flyways to more than 30 countries. Despite the high prevalence of H5N1 among avian populations, human infection remains low, and the low transmissibility suggests a natural barrier to cross-species infection. Most human infections are acquired as a result of contact with infected poultry raised inside or outside the home. As of February, 2011, WHO reported 522 cases of H5N1 viral infection, with 309 associated deaths in 15 countries. The case fatality rate for this disease is close to 60%. This virus has significantly affected the worldwide economy. It has caused the death and destruction of more than 500 million wild and domestic birds worldwide and losses to the poultry industry of more than $10 billion.

Influenza normally is transmitted person to person through inhalation of aerosolized droplets of infected secretions. The incubation period is 1 to 4 days, with rapid onset of symptoms, including fever, nonproductive cough, sore throat, rhinitis, headache, malaise, and myalgia. The illness usually resolves within a week, although some symptoms may persist longer.

Bacterial co-infections are common with influenza, possibly because of viral NA-induced changes in the respiratory epithelium that allow increased bacterial adherence or decreased mucociliary clearance. Recently, clusters of fatal methicillin-resistant *Staphylococcus aureus* (MRSA) infections secondary to seasonal influenza A have been reported in otherwise healthy children and adults.

Testing for influenza can be completed by viral culture, detection of viral nucleic acid or antigen, and serology. Optimal testing requires proper collection and timing of specimens. Virus is shed 3 to 5 days after the onset of symptoms. Optimal specimens are collected from the posterior nasopharynx. The epithelium of the nasopharynx usually contains high titers of virus and large amounts of infected cells. A variety of other respiratory samples, including nasal aspirates, nasal wash, throat swabs, and throat washes, may be used for viral identification. The samples should be placed in viral transport media and may be stored at 4°C for up to 5 days. If the sample must be stored longer, it should be stored in a freezer at −70°C until processed.

Cell culture is available for influenza virus using a variety of cell lines. Primary monkey kidney (PMK) cell lines have demonstrated a consistent season-to-season isolation frequency of influenza virus. Sometimes the influenza viruses fail to produce a CPE in cell culture, requiring additional testing by hemadsorption with guinea pig red blood cells for viral detection. Follow-up confirmatory methods include assays (e.g., IFA). RT-PCR is rapidly replacing cell culture and is becoming the new gold standard for identification of respiratory viruses. The technique is effective when specimens are compromised, such as when they are collected late in the course of the disease or when appropriate collection and transportation requirements have not been met. Sensitivity has proven to be equal to or better than that of cell culture. Because the time from collection to detection is reduced compared to viral culture, nucleic acid testing

likely will become more widely available for the detection of the respiratory virus causing infection.

In addition to immunization, antiviral treatment of influenza has proven to be effective in limiting the duration and severity of the disease. Treatment options are discussed in Chapter 67.

# PAPILLOMAVIRUSES

Papilloma viruses are small, nonenveloped, circular, double-stranded DNA viruses. These viruses are abundant in nature and cause infections in humans, dogs, cattle, monkeys, and many other species. The Papillomaviridae family (Table 66-14) includes the human papillomaviruses (HPVs). HPVs cause human warts. They exhibit a tissue tropism for either cutaneous or mucosal tissue. The viruses have not been cultivated in cell culture, which prevents the production of type-specific antigens and corresponding typing antisera. HPVs are divided into more than 200 genotypes based on the viral DNA sequences; approximately 80 of those have been well characterized. Much attention has been focused on the more than 30 sexually transmitted genotypes and their role in the pathogenesis of cancer. The various HPV genotypes have differing cellular tropisms, resulting in defined variation in the clinical presentation of the warts. For example, HPV-1 is associated with plantar warts; HPV-2 and HPV-4 are associated with common warts of the hands; and HPV-6, HPV-11, and others are associated with genital warts. Fifteen to 20 types of HPV cause virtually all cases of cervical cancer, with types 16 and 18 causing more than 60% of cases. Type 16 is also responsible for a subset of cancers of the oropharynx and penile cancer in men (Table 66-14).

HPV infection is the most prevalent sexually transmitted viral disease in the United States; it is estimated that

**TABLE 66-14** Papillomaviruses

| Family | Papovaviridae |
|---|---|
| **Common name** | Papillomavirus |
| **Characteristics** | Double-stranded DNA genome; icosahedral capsid, no envelope; includes papilloma viruses |
| **Virus** | Human papilloma virus (HPV) |
| **Characteristics** | Contains more than 200 DNA types |
| **Transmission** | Direct contact, sexual contact for genital warts |
| **Site of latency** | Epithelial tissue |
| **Disease** | Skin and genital warts, benign head and neck tumors, anogenital warts |
| **Diagnosis** | Cytology, DNA probes |
| **Oncogenic** | Cervical and penile cancer (especially HPV types 16 and 18) |
| **Treatment** | Spontaneous disappearance the rule; surgical or chemical removal may be necessary |
| **Prevention** | Avoid contact with infected tissue, vaccination |

more than 65 million Americans are living with an incurable STD, such as HPV or HSV infection. Infection is detected using histopathologic or cytologic examination of cutaneous biopsy or cells, respectively, and DNA probe assays for identification of specific genotypes in infected epithelial cells. A single, liquid-based cytology sample can be used for cytology and genotyping. Several commercial HPV assays currently are available in the United States, including HC2 (Qiagen), Cervista HPR HR (Hologic), Roche Amplicor HPV Test (Roche Molecular Diagnostics), GenProbe Aptima HPV Test (GenProbe), Abbott RealTime High Risk HPV Test (Abbott Molecular), PreTect HPV-Proofer (Norchip) and NucliSENS Easy Q HPV v1 Test (bioMeriéux). Two vaccines for HPV are currently licensed by the FDA: Cervarix (Glaxo Smith Kline, United Kingdom and Gardasil (Merck & Co., Inc, Whitehouse Station, N.J.). The vaccines are a derivative of the protein viral coat and provide some protective immunity to HPV16.

# PARAMYXOVIRUSES

The Paramyxoviridae family (Table 66-15) includes many pathogenic viruses. Many of these viruses are identified more often in young children, including measles, mumps, parainfluenza viruses, and respiratory syncytial virus (RSV). Recently, human metapneumovirus and Nipah virus (Nipah is the area in Malaysia where the virus first was isolated) have been recognized as disease-causing paramyxoviruses. Paramyxoviruses do not have a segmented genome, as do the orthomyxoviruses, and therefore do not undergo antigenic shift. Paramyxoviruses are spherical, enveloped RNA viruses, and all members of this group can cause respiratory disease.

Human parainfluenza viruses are important pathogens in children. Viral infection may present as either croup or other upper respiratory diseases in children and adults. The paramyxoviruses are second only to RSV in causing bronchiolitis and pneumonia in infants and young children. The parainfluenza virus has four subtypes; parainfluenza 1 is the most common cause of croup, and parainfluenza 3 is second in prevalence to RSV as a disease of infants and very young children. Most children have had an infection with parainfluenza 3 by 2 years of age. Parainfluenza 3 is most often associated with severe disease and fatalities. Not much is known about parainfluenza 4, which is difficult to grow in cell culture. Serologic studies have shown the virus to be as prevalent as parainfluenza 2.

Parainfluenza viral infection is acquired through inoculation of mucous membranes of the respiratory tract with infectious secretions transmitted on fomites or as large, droplet aerosols. Parainfluenza virus can live up to 10 hours on varying surfaces. Laboratory identification is accomplished through the use of cell culture, using primary or continuous cell lines, followed by confirmatory testing using IFA or other methods of antigen detection. Recently, a multiplex molecular diagnostic test that can differentiate the three major types of parainfluenza was approved for clinical use in the United States.

RSV causes bronchiolitis in young children and is the most significant cause of acute lower respiratory tract infection in children under 5 years of age worldwide. Each year in the United States, RSV is responsible for more than 100 deaths and approximately 60,000 to 100,000 hospitalizations. The virus contains a surface protein called F (fusion) protein. F protein mediates host cell fusion into syncytial cells, which are a hallmark of RSV infection and so named because of the CPE syncytia formation in monolayer cell culture. RSV immune serum prevents severe RSV bronchiolitis during the early months of life in susceptible newborns at risk for RSV disease and those with underlying medical conditions, especially in premature children with underdeveloped lungs. Diagnostic testing for RSV also is performed using cell culture and direct antigen detection. Amplified nucleic acid detection is becoming more readily available and desirable because of its increased sensitivity and specificity and faster turnaround time.

Mumps is an acute, self-limiting disease characterized by parotitis (inflamed salivary gland) accompanied by a high temperature (fever) and fatigue. The mumps virus is transmitted through droplets and contact with infected saliva. The measles virus causes an acute, generalized infection often accompanied by a characteristic rash. The hallmark rash of measles infection is referred to as Koplik's spots, which are bluish white spots with a red halo located on the buccal or labial mucosa. These spots are found on the inner lip or opposite the lower molars in the mouth. The virus is transmitted from person to person through aerosols and infects the mucosal cells of the respiratory tract.

Measles is one of six classic childhood diseases capable of causing a rash or skin eruption (exanthem). The other diseases that cause an exanthem are scarlet fever (which is caused by a bacterium, Group A *Streptococcus*); rubella (German measles), referred to as atypical scarlet fever; erythema infectiosum (or fifth disease, caused by parvovirus B-19); and roseola (caused by HHV-6).

Since the introduction of the live attenuated childhood trivalent vaccine against measles, mumps, and rubella (MMR), cases of mumps have dropped by more than 99% and measles infections are rare in the United States and Europe. However, these viruses continue to circulate and remain a common illness in developing countries. Mortality rates from measles infections can be as high as 20% as a result of contributing factors such as poor hygiene and malnutrition. These viruses are often brought into the United States by travelers or people from other countries. The potential for an outbreak arises when infected individuals come in contact with unvaccinated individuals, and prompt laboratory investigation of suspect cases is required. Diagnostic testing for these viruses involves serologic analysis of patient serum for IgM and IgG antibodies and cell culture for virus detection and, recently, nucleic acid detection. For measles cell culture, the specimens of choice are respiratory or throat specimens; for mumps cell culture, buccal swabs collected from the inside of the cheek are recommended. These viruses are also shed in the urine; therefore, urine specimens can be examined for their presence.

**TABLE 66-15** Paramyxoviruses

| Family | Paramyxoviridae |
|---|---|
| **Common name** | Paramyxoviruses |
| **Characteristics** | Single-stranded, RNA genome; helical capsid with envelope; no segmented genome (e.g., orthomyxoviruses) |
| **Virus** | **Measles virus** |
| Transmission | Contact with respiratory secretions; extremely contagious |
| Disease | Measles, atypical measles (occurs in those with waning "vaccine" immunity), and subacute sclerosing panencephalitis |
| Detection | Cell culture (PMK) and serology |
| Treatment | Supportive; immunocompromised patients can be treated with immune serum globulin |
| Prevention | Measles vaccine |
| **Virus** | **Mumps virus** |
| Transmission | Person-to-person contact, presumably respiratory droplets |
| Disease | Mumps |
| Detection | Cell culture (PMK) and serology |
| Treatment | Supportive |
| Prevention | Mumps vaccine |
| **Virus** | **Parainfluenza virus** |
| Transmission | Contact with respiratory secretions |
| Disease | Adults: Upper respiratory disease, rarely pneumonia<br>Children: Respiratory including croup, bronchiolitis, and pneumonia |
| Detection | Cell culture (PMK), shell vial culture, and FA stain |
| Epidemiology | Four serotypes, disease occurs year-round |
| Treatment | Supportive |
| Prevention | Avoid contact with virus |
| **Virus** | **Respiratory syncytial virus (RSV)** |
| Transmission | Person-to-person by hand and respiratory contact |
| Disease | Primarily in infants and children.<br>Infants: Bronchiolitis, pneumonia, and croup<br>Children: Upper respiratory disease |
| Detection | Cell culture (HEp-2), EIA, and FA stain |
| Epidemiology | Disease occurs annually late fall through early spring; nosocomial transmission can occur readily |
| Treatment | Supportive; treat severe disease in compromised infants with ribavirin |
| Prevention | Avoid contact with virus; immune globulin for infants with underlying lung disease; prevent nosocomial transmission with isolation and cohorting |
| **Virus** | **Metapneumovirus** |
| Transmission | Person to person |
| Disease | Primarily in infants and children; bronchiolitis and pneumonia |
| Detection | RT-PCR |
| Epidemiology | Winter epidemics, severity varies from year to year |
| Treatment | Supportive |
| Prevention | Avoid contact with virus |

*EIA,* Enzyme immunoassay; *FA,* fluorescent antibody; *HEp-2,* human epidermoid carcinoma; *PMK,* primary monkey kidney; *RT-PCR,* reverse transcriptase polymerase chain reaction.

Metapneumovirus is a newly discovered virus closely related to RSV. It has caused disease presumably throughout human history but has avoided detection in clinical specimens because it is difficult to grow in cell culture. In infections in children, this virus appears to be less common than RSV but more common than parainfluenza virus, making it an important, medically relevant infectious agent. The virus causes bronchiolitis and pneumonia in infants and most likely lower respiratory tract disease in older adults. In infants 6 to 12 months of age, infection with metapneumovirus is likely to show more lower airway involvement. The virus is considered the second or third most common cause of hospitalization for lower airway disease in pediatric patients. Like RSV, metapneumovirus is associated with winter epidemics that vary in severity from year to year. As stated previously, isolation of metapneumovirus from cell culture is difficult, because the virus is very slow to grow and often takes longer than 2 weeks to develop detectable CPE. Nucleic acid testing for viral RNA is becoming more widely available because of the reduced detection time and improved sensitivity of the assays.

Nipah virus is a recently discovered paramyxovirus capable of causing respiratory disease in pigs and acute, febrile encephalitis in humans. The first human outbreak was identified in 1999. The outbreak was a result of direct contact and viral transmission from diseased pigs and accounted for 265 human cases of viral infection and 108 deaths. Multiple outbreaks have been described in subsequent years. The reservoir for Nipah virus is presumed to be fruit bats, and pigs and other animals are intermediate hosts.

# PARVOVIRUSES

Parvoviruses (the Latin term parvus means small) have a wide distribution among warm-blooded animals (Table 66-16). Parvovirus B-19 is the single human pathogen among the Parvoviridae. The virus is a nonenveloped, icosahedral, single-stranded DNA virus that may appear spherical on electron microscopy. Because its replication in human cells is largely restricted to erythroid progenitor cells, adult bone marrow and fetal liver cells (the site of erythropoiesis during fetal development) are the major sites of viral replication. Important diseases associated with parvovirus B-19 infection are fifth disease (the fifth of the childhood exanthems), aplastic crisis in patients with underlying hemoglobinopathies, and fetal infection (hydrops fetalis) resulting from transplacental inoculation. Parvovirus causes a biphasic illness in humans. The first phase, marked fever, malaise, myalgia, and chills, corresponds to peak levels of virus and destruction of erythroblasts. This phase, when mild, may be overlooked or considered a nonspecific viral disease. The second phase involves rash and arthralgia, which occur after the virus has disappeared but at a time when parvovirus-specific antibody can be detected. This is consistent with the appearance of the rash caused by immune complex deposition in the capillaries of the skin. IgM antibodies appear within 7 days after infection, followed by IgG at approximately 14 days. Laboratory diagnosis is

**TABLE 66-16** Parvoviruses

| Family | Parvoviridae |
|---|---|
| Common name | Parvovirus |
| Virus | Parvovirus B-19 |
| Characteristics | Single-stranded DNA virus; icosahedral capsid, no envelope; parvovirus B-19 is the only known human parvovirus |
| Transmission | Close contact, probably respiratory |
| Disease | Erythema infectiosum (fifth disease), aplastic crises in patients with chronic hemolytic anemias, and fetal infection and stillbirth |
| Detection | Serology, polymerase chain reaction (PCR), histology |
| Treatment | Supportive |
| Prevention | Avoid contact |

accomplished using parvovirus-specific IgM or virus-specific IgG antibody testing with paired acute and convalescent sera or by detection of viral DNA using PCR. Parvovirus cannot be cultivated in the typical cells available in clinical virology laboratories.

# PICORNAVIRUSES

Picornaviruses (Table 66-17) are small (from the Italian word piccolo, meaning small), nonenveloped, single-stranded RNA viruses. They are among the simplest of the RNA viruses, with a highly structured capsid that has limited surface elaboration. This family of viruses includes the enteroviruses, rhinoviruses, and HAV. Enterovirus infections are among the most common human viral infections (Table 66-18), and although these infections often are mild, the viruses also can cause serious disease. Enteroviruses are responsible for a variety of diseases and conditions, including aseptic meningitis, paralytic poliomyelitis, and encephalitis, in addition to respiratory illness, myocarditis, and pericarditis. Enteroviruses are the most common cause of aseptic meningitis, an inflammation of the brain parenchyma, and have been isolated from more than 40% of patients with this disease.

Before the development of the polio vaccine, the polio enterovirus was responsible for paralytic poliomyelitis around the world. Polio virus infections were identified as early as the 1800s, when cases involving paralysis with fever were noted. During the polio outbreaks of the first half of the twentieth century, thousands of people, especially children, developed an acute, flaccid (relaxed, "rag doll") paralysis that affected their ability to breathe. To assist these patients with breathing during viral infection, the "iron lung," or tank respirator, was invented. The iron lung was an airtight chamber that encased the patient and created negative air pressure around the thoracic cavity, causing air to rush into the lungs. Control of polio through a vaccine began in 1955 with the Salk inactivated polio vaccine, which was administered by intramuscular injection. In 1961 the Sabin oral live

**TABLE 66-17** Picornaviruses

| Family | Picornaviridae |
|---|---|
| Common name | Picornaviruses |
| Characteristics | Single-stranded RNA genome; icosahedral capsid with no envelope |
| Virus | **Enteroviruses**<br>**Poliovirus (3 types)**<br>**Coxsackie virus, group A (23 types)**<br>**Coxsackie virus, group B (6 types)**<br>**Echovirus (31 types)**<br>**Enteroviruses (5 types)** |
| Transmission | Fecal-oral |
| Disease | Predominant virus in parentheses: polio (poliovirus), herpangina (coxsackie A), pleurodynia (coxsackie B), aseptic meningitis (many enterovirus types), hand-foot-mouth disease (coxsackie A), pericarditis and myocarditis (coxsackie B), acute hemorrhagic conjunctivitis (enterovirus 70), and fever, myalgia, summer "flu" (many enterovirus types), neonatal disease (echoviruses and coxsackie viruses) |
| Detection | Cell culture (PMK and HDF), PCR, and serology |
| Treatment | Supportive, pleconaril in development |
| Prevention | Avoid contact with virus; vaccination for polio |
| **Virus** | **Hepatitis A virus (enterovirus type 72)** |
| Transmission | Fecal-oral |
| Disease | Hepatitis with short incubation, abrupt onset, and low mortality; no carrier state |
| Detection | Serology |
| Treatment | Supportive |
| Prevention | Vaccine; prevent clinical illness with serum immunoglobulin |
| **Virus** | **Rhinovirus (common cold virus)** |
| Characteristics | Approximately 100 serotypes |
| Transmission | Contact with respiratory secretions |
| Disease | Common cold |
| Detection | Cell culture (usually not clinically necessary), RT-PCR |
| Treatment | Supportive |
| Prevention | Avoid contact with virus |

*EIA,* Enzyme immunoassay; *FA,* fluorescent antibody; *HDF,* human diploid fibroblasts; *HEp-2,* human epidermoid carcinoma; *PCR,* polymerase chain reaction; *PMK,* primary monkey kidney; *RT-PCR,* reverse transcriptase polymerase chain reaction.

**TABLE 66-18** Enterovirus Infections

| Central nervous system | Aseptic meningitis, encephalitis, flaccid paralysis |
|---|---|
| Respiratory | Mild upper respiratory tract (URT) illness (common cold), lymphonodular pharyngitis, bronchiolitis, bronchitis, pneumonia |
| Exanthems | Hand-foot-mouth disease, herpangina |
| Cardiac | Myocarditis, pericarditis |
| Other | Pleurodynia, acute hyperemia conjunctivitis (AHC), neonatal disseminated disease, chronic infection of agammaglobulinemic patients |

Afghanistan, India, Nigeria, and Pakistan. A global effort to eradicate this disease through continued surveillance and vaccination programs continues.

The early studies of poliovirus are landmarks in the discipline of the virology and the understanding of the pathogenesis, treatment. and control of enteroviruses. Investigation of this virus started in the early twentieth century. From the evidence they collected, scientists were able to prove the communicable nature of the disease and the importance of asymptomatic infection in the transmission of the disease. These studies also provided breakthrough observations related to the propagation of viruses and cell culture.

The enteroviruses originally were divided into poliovirus, coxsackie virus, and echovirus groups based on similarity of characteristics in cell culture and disease in humans. Classification based on these criteria resulted in the definition of 67 serogroups of enterovirus. Genetic diversity among these viruses, recognized through the application of modern molecular techniques, dictates that newly characterized strains be given enterovirus-type designations rather than serotype status in one of the three original groups. The molecular and serotype designations provide an improved classification system because of the previously poor disease- and phenotype-based classification system. Human enteroviruses have now been reclassified into five species, human enteroviruses A to D, and poliovirus.

The virus is transmitted by the respiratory and fecal-oral routes. Therefore, the primary site for enterovirus infection is the respiratory epithelium or the gastrointestinal tract. Specimens of choice for detecting enterovirus are (in order of preference) stool specimens or rectal swabs, throat swabs or washings, and CSF. For cases of acute hyperemia conjunctivitis caused by enterovirus 70, conjunctival swabs or tears can be used. Several enterovirus species can be readily grown in cell culture and produce a characteristic CPE of visible cell rounding and shrinking, as well as refractility and cell degeneration. However, no one cell line supports the growth of all types of enteroviruses. A variety of primate and human cell lines may be used for virus isolation. CPE can be observed within 24 hours if the inoculum contains substantial

attenuated vaccine was licensed in the United States. This drug frequently was administered as a sugar cube coated with the vaccine. In the later 1980s, WHO began a massive campaign to eradicate polio from the world population. By 2006 the number of countries where polio was still endemic had been reduced to four:

infectious particles. CPE appears rapidly and often destroys the entire monolayer of cells within hours.

An enterovirus diagnosis is confirmed using a panenterovirus IFA, and specific confirmation of enterovirus identification is completed using cell culture neutralization and type-specific antisera. These confirmatory tests often are available only in specialty laboratories. Molecular testing is fast replacing traditional cell culture for confirmation of an enterovirus diagnosis, especially in CSF from patients showing symptoms of meningitis. Some molecular procedures are also capable of further characterizing the enterovirus into the specific type using genomic sequencing. The major advantages of using nucleic acid testing for enterovirus are faster detection of the virus, increased sensitivity, and the ability to detect enterovirus types incapable of growth in cell culture. Serologic testing for the presence of IgM antibody with ELISA can be used for suspect cases of enterovirus infection, and has been used as an epidemiologic tool in enterovirus outbreaks.

Rhinovirus is the cause of the "common cold." Its name reflects the fact that the primary infection and replication site is the epithelium cells in the nose. Rhinoviruses are responsible for more than 50% of viral colds and cause more upper respiratory viral infections than any other virus. Although frequently mild, rhinovirus infections can cause complications such as otitis media and sinusitis and can exacerbate previously existing conditions such as asthma, chronic obstructive pulmonary disease (COPD), and cystic fibrosis, in which the risk of severe lower respiratory disease is significantly increased and morbidity can result. Considerably more cases of lower respiratory tract disease in adults are caused by rhinovirus than was previously known. Infection occurs by person-to-person transmission of infected respiratory secretions. Infection usually occurs through self-inoculation through the eyes or nose and also occurs through contact with infectious aerosols. Symptoms usually begin 2 to 3 days after exposure. The clinical presentation includes a profuse, watery nasal discharge frequently accompanied by symptoms of headache, malaise, sneezing, nasal congestion, sore throat, and cough. Illness generally lasts 10 days to 2 weeks.

Neutralization studies have defined more than 100 serotypes of rhinovirus, making development of antigen detection tests difficult. As a result of the numerous serotypes, infections continue to occur year after year. It is also important to note that a previous infection with one serotype of rhinovirus does not confer immunity to a subsequent infection with a different serotype. Confirmation of rhinovirus infection is infrequently required for clinical reasons, because the infection typically is self-limiting. However, the specimen of choice for diagnosis is nasal secretions. Culture can be performed for rhinovirus using human cell lines such as MRC-5. CPE usually occurs 1 to 4 days after inoculation. CPE appears as large and small round refractile cells in the fibroblast cell line. The rhinoviruses grow best or exclusively at lower temperatures (30°C); therefore, detection in clinical virology laboratories often is unlikely because typical incubation temperatures for viral cell culture are 35° to 37°C. If required, cell culture conditions should resemble the physiologic environment in the nasal passages, including a pH of 7 and a temperature of 33° to 35°C. An acid treatment of the clinical sample before culture inoculation may be used to distinguish rhinovirus growth from acid-stable enteroviruses. However, this test is not readily available in clinical laboratories because of its complexity and long turnaround time. IFA cannot be used to confirm rhinovirus in cell culture, because no monoclonal antibodies or antigen detection assays are available. The use of PCR to detect rhinoviruses has expanded understanding of the range of diseases caused by this group. PCR frequently is used for detection of rhinovirus because of its faster detection time and increased sensitivity.

Hepatitis A virus, another member of the picornaviruses, causes an infectious nonchronic hepatitis. HAV is usually transmitted through contaminated food or water or household contact with an infected person. Other transmission routes include sharing of contaminated needles (illicit drug use), travel to endemic countries, and homosexual male intercourse. The virus is significantly different from the other picornavirus based on the liver tissue tropism, high thermal stability, and viral assembly. This is the only hepatitis group of viruses capable of growth in cell culture. However, currently diagnosis is still completed using a serologic assay to identify the IgM antibody (Figure 66-5). A vaccine against this virus for adults and for children older than 2 years of age became available during the 1990s.

# POLYOMAVIRUSES

The polyomaviruses (Table 66-19) are small, nonenveloped, circular, double-stranded DNA viruses that have been isolated from many species, including humans. The first human viruses included the JC and BK viruses, named with the initials of the patients from whom the viruses were first isolated. Infection with these viruses usually occurs during childhood and has little clinical significance. These viral infections include latent states in the kidney and B lymphocytes and can result in symptomatic reactivation during periods of immune suppression.

Immunocompromised individuals almost always present with the pathologic effects of infections caused by the JC and BK viruses. JC virus reactivates, resulting in disease in the CNS; BK virus causes a hemorrhagic cystitis. Recently other viruses in this family have been discovered, including the KI virus, MC virus, and WU virus. Both the KI and WU viruses were detected independently through the use of molecular methods and in clinical specimens of respiratory secretions and stool specimens. The pathogenicity and prevalence of these viruses is not yet known. The MC virus, which causes Merkel cell carcinoma, is associated with a high percentage of tumors and has also been detected in respiratory specimens. In the late 1950s and early 1960s, millions of people were inadvertently exposed to a simian polyomavirus (SV40) as a result of administration of SV40-contaminated Salk polio vaccine. This virus has been shown to induce tumors in animals in the research laboratory and has since been periodically associated with several human tumors.

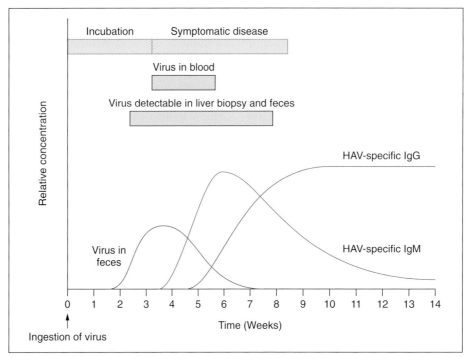

**Figure 66-5** Time course of disease and immune response to hepatitis A virus. (Modified from Murray PR, Kobayashi GS, Pfaller MA et al, editors: *Medical microbiology,* ed 2, St Louis, 1994, Mosby.)

**TABLE 66-19** Polyomaviruses

| Family | Polyomaviridae |
|---|---|
| Common name | Polyomavirus |
| Virus | Polyomavirus (BK virus [BKV] and JC virus [JCV] infect humans) |
| Characteristics | Double-stranded DNA genome; icosahedral capsid, no envelope; includes BK and JC polyomaviruses |
| Transmission | Probably direct contact with infected respiratory secretions; both viruses are ubiquitous in humans |
| Site of latency | Kidney |
| Disease | Mild or asymptomatic primary infection, virus remains dormant in kidneys; reactivation in immunocompromised patients causes hemorrhagic cystitis (BKV) or progressive multifocal leukoencephalopathy (JCV) |
| Detection | JCV by polymerase chain reaction (PCR) (cerebrospinal fluid) or electron microscopy (EM) (brain tissue); BKV by PCR or cytology (urine) |
| Treatment | Supportive; decrease immune suppression |
| Prevention | Avoid contact with virus; prevention of acquisition of virus unlikely |

Laboratory detection of the JC virus is completed using PCR on CSF samples or electron microscopy of brain tissue. BK virus is detected using PCR or cytologic examination of urine. Because these are infrequent infections, testing is most likely to be referred to a reference laboratory.

# POXVIRUSES

The poxviruses (Table 66-20) are the largest and most complex of all viruses. The virions consist of a double-stranded DNA genome. The virions appear as oval or brick-shaped structures 200 to 400 nm in length. Because of their large size, poxvirus virions may be visualized through a light microscope.

One of the most feared viruses of history, smallpox, is a member of this family. Smallpox played a crucial role in demonstrating the importance of vaccination to protect against disease. In 1798 Edward Jenner recognized that milkmaids previously infected with cowpox were immune to the disease of smallpox. This discovery led to the practice of inoculating humans against smallpox by using the actual organism (virus) responsible for the disease. Smallpox is known to infect only humans and exists as two distinct subtypes. Variola major, which caused the most severe disease (case fatality rate of 30%), occurred mainly in Asia; variola minor was associated with less severe disease and case fatality rates of 0.1% to 2%. As a result of an intensive vaccination campaign, WHO declared naturally occurring variola virus eradicated in 1980. The variola virus no longer circulates in nature. The virus is feared as a possible biologic weapon,

**TABLE 66-20** Poxviruses

| Family | Poxviridae |
|---|---|
| Common name | Poxvirus |
| Virus | Smallpox, molluscum contagiosum, orf, and monkeypox viruses |
| Characteristics | Largest and most complex of all viruses; brick-shaped virion with nonconforming symmetry, referred to as complex; double-stranded DNA genome |
| Transmission | Respiratory droplets (smallpox); direct contact (molluscum contagiosum, orf, monkeypox) |
| Disease | All are diseases of the skin; smallpox is a generalized infection with pustular rash (10% to 25% fatal); molluscum contagiosum manifests as benign nodules; orf manifests as localized papules/vesicles; monkeypox manifests as a generalized infection that includes the skin |
| Detection | Electron microscopy (EM) of material from a skin lesion; polymerase chain reaction (PCR) |
| Epidemiology | Smallpox was eradicated in 1977; smallpox and molluscum contagiosum are limited to humans; orf and monkeypox are zoonoses |
| Treatment | Supportive |
| Prevention | Vaccine for smallpox; avoid contact for all viruses |

and testing capability for this organism is maintained by hundreds of Laboratory Response Network (LRN) laboratories throughout the nation. All known stocks of the virus are held at two WHO collaborating laboratories: the Centers for Disease Control and Prevention (CDC) in Atlanta, Georgia, and the State Center of Virology and Biotechnology (VECTOR) in Kotsovo, Russia. WHO has requested destruction of the remaining stocks of this virus, but that has been postponed to evaluate the need for developing vaccines, rapid diagnostics, and antiviral therapy. Since the eradication of smallpox in 1980, most vaccination campaigns against this virus have stopped, and most of the world's population lacks any protective immunity against this disease or any related poxviruses.

Besides the smallpox virus, 10 other poxviruses are capable of infecting humans. Except for the smallpox virus and the molluscum contagiosum virus, most of these are zoonoses, or infections that result from contact with animals. Fortunately, other than monkeypox and the eradicated smallpox virus, none of these viruses can sustain human-to-human transmission. The viruses normally are acquired through abrasions of the skin and contact with an infected animal, or in the case of human monkeypox, through the oropharynx or nasopharynx in addition to through abrasions on the skin. Poxvirus replicates in the epidermal cells and causes change in the cellular structure, characterized by the "pocks" on the skin. Poxvirus infection can take one of two courses: it can cause a localized infection at the site of inoculation, with little spread from the original site of inoculation, or

it can cause a fulminant, systemic infection with spread of the virus throughout the body. The second type of infection is associated with variola virus (smallpox) and also monkeypox, and an increased mortality rate. Monkeypox is almost indistinguishable from smallpox infection except that it lacks the same level of mortality and transmissibility. The monkeypox virus is found in the tropical rain forests of Africa, and its host reservoir is one or more rodent species.

After the individual is exposed to the virus, symptoms of fever and headache occur first, followed by the development of a rash and lymphadenopathy. The rash typically first appears on the face, beginning as macules (small, round changes in skin color), progressing to papules (slightly elevated with no fluid) to vesicles (containing a bubble of fluid) and then pustules (containing purulent material consisting of necrotic inflammatory cells). Depending on the severity of the disease, the illness can last 2 to 4 weeks. Two clades of monkeypox exist, and the Congo Basin clade has the highest fatality rate (up to 12%). In 2003 the importation of rats as pets led to an outbreak of monkeypox in the United States, proving that international travel can be a significant portal of disease from anywhere and to anywhere in the world. RT-PCR (real-time) offers a rapid diagnostic identification tool for cases of monkeypox.

Another member of the poxvirus family is the molluscum contagiosum virus, which causes single or small clusters of lesions. Its only host is humans, and infection occurs either nonsexually, through direct contact or fomites, or sexually, through intimate contact. Usually a self-limiting disease in healthy individuals, molluscum contagiosum can cause a more severe form of disease in immunocompromised patients, resulting in large lesions, especially on the face, neck, scalp, and upper body. Laboratory diagnosis of molluscum contagiosum usually is through biopsy of the lesions and histologic examination. Molecular assays, such as traditional PCR, restriction fragment length polymorphism (RFLP), and real-time-PCR, are still under development.

Orf is another member of the poxvirus family and is transmitted from sheep to humans through human direct contact with infected sheep. This virus causes single or multiple nodules, usually on the hands. These nodules may be painful and may be accompanied by symptoms such as low-grade fever and lymph node swelling. The infection usually resolves in 4 to 6 weeks without further complication, although autoinoculation of the eye can have more serious consequences. An orf diagnosis is made through direct examination of the nodule, along with epidemiologic evidence of a recent history of contact with sheep or lambs. Continued development of PCR assays for identification of parapoxviruses will aid the diagnosis and identification of these viruses.

# REOVIRUSES

The reoviruses (Table 66-21) were first isolated from respiratory and enteric specimens and therefore are referred to as respiratory-enteric-orphan viruses (reoviruses). The term "orphan" originally was included in the description of the virus as a result of the absence of an associated disease when the viruses were first described. Reoviruses infect most mammalian species and are readily detected in water contaminated with animal feces. Common human pathogens of this family include the rotavirus and the agent of Colorado tick fever. Rotaviruses are nonenveloped, double-stranded RNA viruses composed of three concentric protein shells, the outer shell, the inner shell, and the core. Based on the proteins present in these shells, rotavirus is further classified into seven distinct groups, A through G; groups A, B and C cause human disease. Rotavirus is now recognized as the major causative agent of infantile severe gastroenteritis throughout the world. Worldwide, rotavirus is responsible for more than 111 million cases per year, resulting in more than 2 million hospitalizations and 352,000 to 592,000 deaths. Gastroenteritis caused by rotavirus can occur in children of all ages but is most common in infants from 6 months to 3 years old. The disease is characterized by sudden onset of vomiting, followed by explosive, watery diarrhea and moderate to high fever, often accompanied by dehydration. The severity of the disease often is worse for children in developing countries because of malnutrition and limited or delayed health care. Rotaviruses are transmitted by the fecal-oral route, although airborne transmission has been suspected as the cause of nosocomial infections and outbreaks in nursing homes, hospitals, and day care centers. Rotavirus occurs more frequently in the winter months in temperate climates.

Many methods of laboratory testing are available for the diagnosis of rotavirus. Rotavirus can be detected directly in the stool using ELISA, latex agglutination, RT-PCR, cell culture, and electrophoretic separation of the viral genome or electron microscopy. The latex agglutination test offers rapid results with limited laboratory equipment, an advantage in developing countries where resources are limited. Rotavirus is difficult to cultivate from human specimens. Viral isolation is not normally attempted.

**TABLE 66-21** Reoviruses

| Family | Reoviridae |
|---|---|
| Common name | Reovirus |
| Virus | Rotavirus |
| Characteristics | Segmented, double-stranded, RNA genome; icosahedral capsid with no envelope |
| Transmission | Fecal-oral; survives well on inanimate objects |
| Disease | Gastroenteritis in infants and children 6 months to 2 years |
| Detection | Enzyme immunoassay (EIA), latex agglutination (LA) |
| Epidemiology | Winter-spring seasonality in temperate climates; nosocomial transmission can occur easily |
| Treatment | Supportive, especially fluid replacement |
| Prevention | Avoid contact with virus; vaccination |

# RETROVIRUSES

The retrovirus family Retroviridae (Table 66-22) constitutes a large group of viruses that primarily infect vertebrates. They are enveloped RNA viruses, and each virion contains two identical copies of single-stranded RNA. The viral nucleic acid strands are surrounded by the structural proteins that form the nucleocapsid and the matrix shell. On the outer surface of the nucleocapsid and matrix protein is the lipid envelope derived from the host cell membrane. Proteins that mediate adsorption and penetration into the host cell membrane are inserted into the viral envelop. Retroviruses are unique, because they have the enzyme reverse transcriptase. Reverse transcriptase allows the viral RNA genome to be replicated into DNA and then RNA rather than directly into RNA.

Amino acid sequencing of the reverse transcriptase protein divides the retrovirus family into groups. The human immunodeficiency viruses types 1 and 2 (HIV-1 and HIV-2) are members of this family as are the human T cell lymphoma viruses types 1 and 2 (HTLV-1 and HTLV-2). HIV-1 (Figure 66-6) is the more aggressive virus and is responsible for the acquired immunodeficiency syndrome (AIDS) pandemic. The virus was first isolated in 1983, and a year later was proven to be associated with early and late stages of AIDS. HIV-2 was discovered in 1986 and is less pathogenic. AIDS is the end stage of a process in which the immune system and its ability to control infections and malignant proliferation is destroyed. The virus has an affinity for the CD4+ surface marker of T lymphocytes. As the number of CD4+ T lymphocytes decreases, the risk and severity of opportunistic infections increases. Some of the most common opportunistic infections associated with HIV infection include disseminated coccidioidomycosis, cryptococcosis, cryptosporidiosis, histoplasmosis, recurrent pneumonia, and pneumocystis pneumonia. Detection of the HIV antibody is the mainstay of clinical diagnosis. Repeatedly reactive antibody tests done with EIA should be confirmed using Western blot testing (Figure 66-7). Clinical management of infected individuals involves the use of highly active antiretroviral therapy (HAART) and depends on the measurement of CD4+ lymphocytes and the viral load. Molecular methods often are used to quantify the viral load. Diagnosis of HIV infection in babies born to HIV-positive mothers is problematic because of maternal IgG in the baby's blood; therefore, PCR for identification of viral DNA or RNA is recommended. Genome sequencing is used to establish susceptibility to antiviral agents.

The risk of laboratory-acquired infections with these viruses is a critical consideration; the greatest caution must be exercised in handling any specimens capable of harboring a blood-borne agent. Infection occurs through contamination of the hand and mucous membranes of the eyes, nose, or mouth with infected blood or other body fluids. No evidence exists of airborne transmission. Proper personal protective equipment must always be worn, including a laboratory gown, good-quality gloves, and eye protection. Disposable, unbreakable plastic ware

**TABLE 66-22** Retroviruses

| Family | Retroviridae |
|---|---|
| **Common name** | Retroviruses |
| **Characteristics** | Single-stranded, RNA genome; icosahedral capsid with envelope; reverse transcriptase converts genomic RNA into DNA |
| **Virus** | **Human immunodeficiency virus types 1 and 2 (HIV-1, HIV-2)** |
| Transmission | Sexual contact, blood and blood product exposure, and perinatal exposure |
| Site of latency | CD4 T lymphocytes |
| Disease | Most disease in humans caused by HIV-1; infected cells include CD4$^+$ (helper) T lymphocytes, monocytes, and some cells of the central nervous system; asymptomatic infection, acute flulike disease, acquired immunodeficiency syndrome (AIDS)–related complex, and AIDS-associated infections and malignancies |
| Detection | Serology, antigen detection, reverse transcriptase polymerase chain reaction (RT-PCR) |
| Epidemiology | Those at risk of infection are homosexual or bisexual males, intravenous drug abusers, sexual contacts of individuals infected with HIV, and infants of infected mothers |
| Treatment | Many, including nucleoside reverse transcriptase inhibitors, nonnucleoside reverse transcriptase inhibitors, protease inhibitors, and inhibitors of viral entry into host cells; treat infections resulting from immunosuppression |
| Prevention | Avoid contact with infected blood/blood products and secretions; blood for transfusion is screened for antibody to HIV-1 and -2 |
| **Virus** | **Human T-lymphotropic viruses types 1 and 2 (HTLV-1, HTLV-2)** |
| Transmission | Known means of transmission are similar to those for HIV |
| Disease | T-cell leukemia and lymphoma, and tropical spastic paraparesis for HTLV-1; no known disease associations for HTLV-2 |
| Detection | Serology |
| Epidemiology | HTLV-1 is present in 0.025% of volunteer blood donors in the United States. Blood is screened for antibody to HTLV-1 and HTLV-2; rates of HTLV-1 infection in areas of Japan and the Caribbean are considerably higher than those in the United States. |
| Oncogenic | T-cell lymphoma (HTLV-1) |
| Treatment | Supportive |
| Prevention | Avoid contact with virus |

should always be used in the handling of blood or bodily fluids.

HTLV-1 is endemic in the Caribbean, Africa, South and Central America, Melanesia, and Japan. However, only a small percentage of people infected (fewer than 4%) develop symptoms and disease. Cell-to-cell contact and TAX-induced clonal expansion of infected cells are the major avenues for viral replication, making detection of the virus difficult. As a result, serologic detection has remained the gold standard for diagnosis. Molecular detection and the development of PCR assays are being investigated in research laboratories. The average time from infection to the development of adult T-cell leukemia is approximately 40 years.

# RHABDOVIRUSES

Rhabdoviruses (Table 66-23) infect plants, arthropods, fish, and mammals. The virion consists of single-stranded RNA with a helical nucleocapsid surrounded by a lipid bilayer envelope. Spikelike projections approximately 10 nm long extend from the surface of the lipid bilayer. Electron microscopy has shown that the virion has a bullet-shaped or conical appearance. The rabies virus is a neurotropic virus that infects all mammals; with very

**TABLE 66-23** Rhabdoviruses

| Family | Rhabdoviridae |
|---|---|
| **Common name** | Rhabdovirus |
| **Virus** | Rabies virus |
| **Characteristics** | Single-stranded, RNA genome; helical capsid with envelope, bullet-shaped |
| **Transmission** | Bite of rabid animal most common; 20% of human rabies cases have no known exposure to rabid animal |
| **Disease** | Rabies |
| **Detection** | Fluorescent antibody (FA) staining, polymerase chain reaction (PCR) |
| **Treatment** | Supportive |
| **Prevention** | Avoid contact with rabid animals; vaccinate domestic animals; postexposure prophylaxis with hyperimmune antirabies globulin and immunization with rabies vaccine |

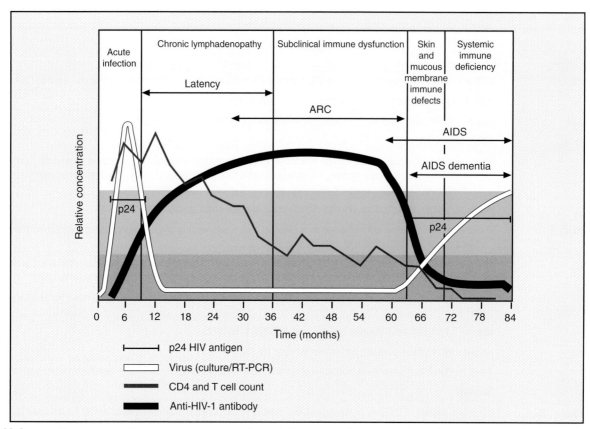

**Figure 66-6** Usual time course of immune response, viremia, and disease resulting from untreated human immunodeficiency virus type 1 (HIV-1) infection. (Redrawn from Murray PR, Kobayashi GS, Pfaller MA et al, editors: *Medical microbiology,* ed 2, St Louis, 1992, Mosby.)

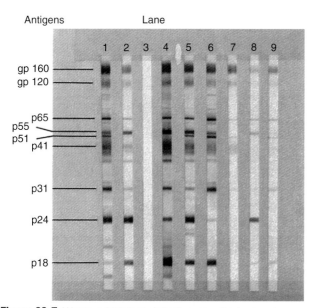

**Figure 66-7** Western blot test detecting specific human immunodeficiency virus (HIV) antibody. Lane 1 is the high-positive control; lane 2 is the low-positive control; lane 3 is the negative control; lanes 4 through 8 are positive sera; lane 9 is an indeterminate serum. Numbers at left refer to approximate molecular weights of HIV antigens. (Courtesy R.L. Hodinka, Children's Hospital of Philadelphia.)

few exceptions, infection terminates in the death of the infected mammal. The rabies virus is transmitted through the saliva of infected animals, usually by a bite. After inoculation, the virus may invade the peripheral nerves or nerve endings directly. Following infection of the nerve cells, the viral genome progresses centripetally transneuronally, through retrograde axoplasmal flow to the central nervous system. In the CNS it proceeds from first-order neurons to second-order neurons. the neurons are the site of viral replication, mainly in the brain and spinal cord; from there the virus spreads to peripheral nerves and to some nonnervous tissue, including the salivary glands. After a variable incubation period, human disease usually begins with generalized symptoms of malaise, fever, fatigue, anorexia, and headache. Frequently (and characteristically for this disease), symptoms include pain and sometimes "tingling" at the site of exposure, which can be the first "rabies-specific" symptom. After this prodromal phase, behavioral changes may start to manifest, followed by rapidly progressing neurologic symptoms that lead to coma and death.

Only six cases of survival of a rabies infection have been documented worldwide. These cases include patients who survived without any complications; other patients have experienced significant neurologic impairment. In 2004, Randy Willoughby developed a treatment protocol for rabies referred to as "The Milwaukee Protocol." This protocol requires that the patient remain in a prolonged state of generalized anesthesia, anti-viral drugs, and supportive, life-sustaining care until the individual's natural active immunity is capable of clearing and/or fighting the infection. Updated protocol and statistics related to patient treatment and survival are maintained by the Medical College of Wisconsin and can be accessed at mcw.edu/Pediatrics/Infectious Diseases/PatientCare/Rabies.htm

Animal rabies presents much as do human rabies cases. After the prodromal phase of the disease, a period of increased excitation occurs, with or without aggression. Clinical presentations of rabies often are described as "furious" or "dumb"; the furious type is associated with heightened aggression and agitation, and the dumb type with lethargy and paralysis.

Rabies is diagnosed by postmortem examination of brain tissue using a direct immunofluorescent assay. Specific sections of the brain are examined for the rabies antigen using fluorescent-tagged monoclonal antibodies and a fluorescent microscope. Prompt, accurate diagnosis of rabies infections in animals is important to ensure the success of postexposure prophylaxis for human victims of animal bites and injuries.

# TOGAVIRUSES

The Togaviridae family (Table 66-24) includes rubella virus and the alpha viruses, a large group of mosquito-borne arboviruses. Rubella is found only in the human population and is transmitted through direct contact with nasopharyngeal secretions or by congenital transmission. Rubella, sometimes called the "German measles," is usually a benign disease characterized by fever and rash. Before the trivalent vaccine, MMR (measles, mumps, and rubella), was developed, rubella was an epidemic disease. A risk associated with this disease is exposure and infection of pregnant women. The virus can infect the developing fetus, causing multiple congenital anomalies. Intrauterine infection during the first trimester may result in low birth weight, mental retardation, deafness, congenital heart disease, and neurologic defects. Infection that occurs later in pregnancy may result in splenomegaly or osteomyelitis, among other birth deficiencies. Fetal infection can be prevented through vaccination of all women before pregnancy.

In arbovirus infections, mosquitoes infect a vertebrate host (e.g., birds and rodents), the virus multiplies (amplifies) in this host and is picked up and passed along in subsequent mosquito bites. Humans are infected incidentally and are not amplifiers of the virus; rather, they are dead-end hosts, unable to pass on the virus to other humans or animals. Human disease varies from asymptomatic infection to fatal encephalitis and includes Eastern, Western, and Venezuelan equine encephalitides. Togavirus disease is diagnosed through detection of specific serum IgG and IgM antibodies. Virus isolation is not practical in clinical laboratories.

# MISCELLANEOUS VIRUSES

Additional viruses detected in humans include the astroviruses and potential agents of hepatitis,

**TABLE 66-24** Togaviruses

| Family | Togaviridae |
|---|---|
| **Common name** | Togaviruses |
| **Characteristics** | Single-stranded RNA genome and icosahedral capsid with envelope; family contains arboviruses and non–arthropod-borne rubella virus |
| **Virus** | **Rubella virus** |
| Transmission | Respiratory, transplacental |
| Disease | Rubella (mild exanthematous disease), congenital rubella |
| Detection | Serology |
| Treatment | Supportive |
| Prevention | Rubella vaccine |
| **Virus** | **Arboviruses referred to as alphaviruses*** |
| Transmission | Arthropod vector, usually mosquito |
| Disease | Eastern, Western, and Venezuelan equine encephalitis |
| Detection | Serology and antibody detection in cerebrospinal fluid (CSF) |
| Treatment | Supportive |
| Prevention | Avoid contact with vector; vector control programs |

*Arthropod-borne viruses (arboviruses) are taxonomically heterogeneous but were once grouped together because of their common mode of transmission. Viruses adapted to arthropod vectors occur in several taxonomic families, including the Togaviridae, Flaviviridae, and Bunyaviridae. The virus group in Togaviridae that includes arboviruses is the alphavirus group. Common arboviruses are referred to as bunyaviruses, flaviviruses, and alphaviruses.

transfusion-transmitted virus (TTV), and hepatitis G virus (HGV). The astrovirus is a single-stranded RNA virus found in the gastrointestinal tract of many animals, including humans. Human astroviruses are ubiquitous in children, causing a minority of childhood diarrheas. Astroviruses are detected using electron microscopy.

TTV and HGV are DNA and RNA viruses, respectively. They are detected commonly in human blood specimens but have not yet been associated with any disease. HGV is a flavivirus, similar to HCV. TTV resembles a new group of animal viruses called circoviruses.

# INTERPRETATION OF LABORATORY TEST RESULTS

Interpretation of laboratory test results must be based on knowledge of the normal viral flora in the clinical specimen, the clinical findings, and the epidemiology of viruses. Serologic testing, in addition to virus detection assays, may be needed to support or refute the association of a virus isolate with a disease state.

## VIRUSES IN TISSUE AND BODY FLUIDS

In general, detection of any virus in host tissues, CSF, blood, or vesicular fluid is significant. Recovery of adenovirus or mumps virus in urine is usually diagnostic of disease; in contrast, detection of CMV may merely reflect asymptomatic reactivation. Occasionally, enteroviruses are detected in urine as a result of fecal contamination, or HSV from symptomatic or asymptomatic infection of the external urogenital tract. Interpretation of these culture results requires correlation with clinical data. CMV viruria (virus in the urine) during the first 2 weeks of life establishes a diagnosis of congenital CMV infection, whereas detection at 4 weeks or later suggests intrapartum or postpartum acquisition.

## VIRUSES IN THE RESPIRATORY TRACT

Detection of the measles, mumps, influenza, parainfluenza, and respiratory syncytial viruses is significant, because asymptomatic carriage and prolonged shedding is unusual. Conversely, HSV, CMV, and adenoviruses can be shed in the absence of symptoms for periods ranging from a few days to many months. Adenoviruses are detected commonly from asymptomatic infants and young children. Simultaneous detection of this virus from both throat and feces in febrile patients with respiratory syndromes increases the probability of association with illness. Isolation from throat but not feces has a lesser probability of association, and isolation from feces alone has the least diagnostic significance.

## VIRUSES IN THE EYE

Detection of adenoviruses, HSV, VZV, and some enteroviruses from diseased cornea and conjunctiva usually establishes the etiology of the infection. Enterovirus type 70 is known to cause a particularly contagious form of viral conjunctivitis referred to as acute hyperemia conjunctivitis (AHC).

## DETECTION OF EPSTEIN-BARR VIRUS

Disease caused by EBV is established by detecting antibody to multiple antigens (see Figure 66-3). Detection of antibody to viral capsid antigen, early antigen, and Epstein-Barr nuclear antigen is interpreted as shown in Table 66-25.

## DETECTION OF ENTEROVIRUSES

Enteroviruses are most commonly found in asymptomatic infants and children, particularly during the late summer and early fall. Knowledge of the relative frequency of virus shedding is extremely helpful in assessing the significance of results of throat or stool cultures. The prevalence of enteroviruses in the stools of infants and toddlers may approach 30% during peak periods. Shedding of enteroviruses in the throat is relatively transient, usually 1 to 2 weeks, whereas fecal shedding may last 4 to 16 weeks. Thus, isolation of an enterovirus from the throat supports an etiology of a clinically compatible illness more than isolation from the feces alone. If live attenuated oral poliovirus vaccine is used, vaccine strains can be detected in stools of recently vaccinated children and their contacts (e.g., siblings). Typing identifies the enteroviruses as a poliovirus serotype and, in absence of clinical findings that suggest polio along with a setting of recent vaccination, the isolate can be considered "normal."

## DETECTION OF HEPATITIS VIRUSES

Disease caused by HAV is detected using serology tests specific for viral-induced IgM and IgG (see Figure 66-5; Table 66-26). In addition to clinical findings consistent with disease, the presence of HAV-specific IgM is diagnostic of current, active disease. HBV requires detection of antigen and antibody to multiple antigens to classify the disease type. HDV co-infection with HBV relies on detection of anti-HDV antibodies. Diagnostic tests for HCV include RT-PCR and antibody detection. PCR is used to detect early acute hepatitis C disease, because antibody detection tests may be negative. ELISA testing for antibody is used to detect chronic hepatitis C disease (see Figure 66-1). HCV RNA levels in serum, detected by a number of highly sensitive molecular biopsy methods, are used to differentiate patients who are likely to respond to therapy from those with lower response rates. All patients with sustained response to therapy became negative for HCV RNA within 6 months. HCV genotyping is used to identify genotypes more or less likely to respond to therapy. For example, patients with HCV genotype 1 have significantly lower response rates to therapy. Antibody tests are used to detect patients infected with hepatitis E; however, disease is rare in the United States.

**TABLE 66-25** Interpretation of Serology Results for Epstein-Barr Virus Infection

| Clinical Situation | Heterophile Antibody | IgG-VCA | IgM-VCA | EA | EBNA |
|---|---|---|---|---|---|
| No past infection | Usually negative | − | − | − | − |
| Acute infection | Usually positive | + | + | + | − |
| Convalescence phase | +/− | + | + or − | + or − | + |
| Past infection | Usually negative | + | − | − or W+ | + |
| Chronic or reactivation | Not useful | + | − | + | + |

*EA*, Early antigen; *EBNA*, Epstein-Barr nuclear antigen; *VCA*, viral capsid antigen; *W+*, weakly positive.

**TABLE 66-26** Serologic Profiles After Typical Hepatitis B Virus (HBV) Infection

| HBsAg | Anti-HBsAg | HBeAg | Anti-HBeAg | Anti-HBcAg | Most Likely Interpretation |
|:---:|:---:|:---:|:---:|:---:|:---|
| − | − | − | − | − | No (or very early) exposure to HBV |
| + | − | +/− | − | − | Early acute hepatitis B (HB) |
| + | − | + | − | + | Acute or chronic HB |
| + | − | − | + | + | Chronic HBV carrier state |
| − | − | − | + | + | Early recovery phase from acute HB |
| − | + | − | + | + | Recovery from HB with immunity |
| − | + | − | − | − | Distant HBV infection or HB vaccine |

## DETECTION OF VARICELLA-ZOSTER VIRUS AND HERPES SIMPLEX VIRUS

Detection of VZV is always significant. Asymptomatic shedding does not appear to occur with this virus, as it does with other herpes viruses. Detection of HSV from cutaneous or mucocutaneous vesicles also is significant, implying primary or reactivation disease. HSV may be detected in respiratory secretions during asymptomatic "stress" reactivation unless typical vesicles or ulcers are present. HSV in stool usually represents either severe disseminated infection or infection of the anus or perianal areas. Isolation from any specimen from a newborn infant suggests potentially severe infection.

## DETECTION OF CYTOMEGALOVIRUS

Interpretation of results of specimens containing CMV is most difficult. Primary CMV infection is usually asymptomatic and is commonly followed by silent reactivation of the latent virus throughout the patient's life. CMV disease in immunocompromised patients can be life-threatening, and antiviral therapy may be warranted. Detection of CMV in urine or respiratory secretions, however, is not diagnostic of significant disease. Detection of CMV in tissue (e.g., lung) by culture or histopathology or in blood collected by venipuncture suggests an active role in disease. Detection of CMV antigenemia or DNA in the blood by a molecular method is highly suggestive of active disease, and quantitative results can be used to evaluate therapeutic intervention and the patient's prognosis. Interpretation of the CMV antigenemia assay depends on the patient population and laboratory expertise. In general, detectable virus in peripheral leukocytes is seen with CMV disease. Disease severity is roughly proportional to the quantity of virus (i.e., the number of fluorescing cells. As the disease is treated and resolves, the number of positive cells decreases. Antigenemia levels should decrease to zero as the patient's immune function is restored and antiviral therapy is introduced. The presence of virus-specific IgM or a fourfold increase in IgG antibodies may indicate disease. However, positive serology results must be interpreted with caution. False-positive IgM results have been attributed to infections caused by other viruses, such as EBV, and rises in both IgM and IgG may result from transfusions or immune globulin therapy.

## DETECTION OF HUMAN IMMUNODEFICIENCY VIRUS

The HIV-1 Western blot test provides a method of antibody-specific identification of several HIV antigens (see Figure 66-7). The presence of antibody to HIV p24 and to either gp41 or gp160 is sufficient to confirm HIV-1 infection. HIV-1 p24 antigen testing is used to detect acutely infected patients before the appearance of antibody. PCR testing for HIV is useful for newborns, whose maternal HIV antibody may confound interpretation of serology tests, and for all patients because detectable antibody may not be produced for months after primary infection. The quantitative plasma RNA test (viral load) is used to measure the amount of HIV in the blood. As many as 10 billion new HIV virions may be produced daily in the blood of untreated patients. Viral load testing has become an essential parameter in guiding decisions to begin or change antiviral therapy. Plasma HIV RNA can be quantified with various assays approved by the U.S. Food and Drug Administration, including the Roche Monitor RT-PCR (Roche Molecular Diagnostics), Bayer Versant HIV-1 (bDNA) Assay (Bayer Diagnostics), and NucliSense EasyQ HIV-1 (NASBA) Assay (bioMérieux). Viral load testing is performed at the time of diagnosis of HIV infection and periodically thereafter. Successful antiretroviral therapy should reduce plasma RNA to undetectable levels (less than 50 copies/mL).

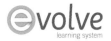 *Visit the Evolve site to complete the review questions.*

## CASE STUDY 66-1

A 74-year-old male presents to the emergency department with his family. The patient reports having confusion and fever for approximately 2 days. The onset of symptoms was gradual, over several hours, and included frontal headache, fever of greater than 100°F, and myalgias. His wife notes that he has been sleeping a great deal, and she has had trouble waking him to take Tylenol for his headache. Originally the patient believed that this was simply a case of the "flu" and would resolve without a doctor's care.

Upon examination by the physician and during an extensive interview, the patient reveals that he has dysnomia, or difficulty finding the right words to describe his condition. He complains primarily of headache and denies GI or respiratory symptoms.

His physical exam results are positive for nuchal rigidity, but no other significant findings are noted.

A lumbar puncture is performed for probable meningitis. The laboratory results are as follows:

Cerebrospinal fluid (CSF): Appears as clear fluid
Red blood cells (RBCs): 112/$\mu$L
White blood cells (WBCs): 96/$\mu$L, 78% lymphs
Glucose: 78 mg/dL (reference range, 50-80 mg/dL)
Serum glucose: 110 mg/dL (reference range, 70-140 mg/dL)
Protein: 94 (reference range, 15-60 mg/dL)
CSF presentation indicates a potential viral infection because of the WBC count and high percentage of lymphocytes, along with the increased protein content.

Other laboratory results include:
WBC: 13k with normal differential
Hemoglobin (Hgb): 15.8 g/dL
Liver function tests (LFTs): Normal

Creatinine (Cr): 1.4 mg/dL (adult male reference range, 0.8-1.4 mg/dL)
Blood urea nitrogen (BUN): 34 mg/dL (reference range, 7-10 mg/dL)
Electrolytes: Normal
C-reactive protein (CRP): 7.5 mg (reference range, 1-3 mg)
Erythrocyte sedimentation rate (ESR): 25 mm/hr (age-normalized reference range, 0-20 mm/hr)
CRP and ESR consistent with generalized inflammation.
Chest x-ray: Normal
Head computed tomography (CT) scan with and without contrast: Normal

Clinical Summary: The patient has a clinical presentation of meningitis, given the examination finding of nuchal rigidity. This is complicated by confusion and abnormal findings on CSF consistent with a viral infection. Moreover, his confusion is concerning and is an indication for viral encephalitis. An MRI of the brain was ordered, and additional studies on the CSF were performed.

Additional laboratory tests included:
Viral culture, serology and molecular testing
Magnetic resonance imaging (MRI): Brain scan reveals right temporal lobe enhancement.

### QUESTIONS

1. List some viral agents that may be associated with the patient's symptoms and with probable viral encephalitis.
2. What distinguishing symptoms led the physician to consider a diagnosis of viral encephalitis?
3. Are any notable risk factors associated with this case that typically would alert the physician to a viral infection?

## ⊟ BIBLIOGRAPHY

Alexander LN, Seward JF, Santibanez TA, et al: Vaccine policy changes and epidemiology of poliomyelitis in the United Sates, *JAMA* 292:1696, 2004.

Binda S, Mammoliti A, Primache V, et al: Pp65 antigenemia plasma real-time PCR and DBS test in symptomatic and asymptomatic cytomegalovirus congenitally infected newborns, *BMC Infect Dis* 10(1):24-28, 2010.

Cabral F, Arruda LB, de Araujo ML, et al: Detection of T-cell lymphotropic virus type 1 in plasma samples, *Virus Res* 163(1):87-90, 2012.

Centers for Disease Control and Prevention: Outbreak of severe acute respiratory syndrome: worldwide, 2003, *Morb Mortal Wkly Rep* 52:226, 2003.

Centers for Disease Control and Prevention: Resurgence of wild poliovirus type 1 transmission and consequences of importation: 21 countries, 2002-2005, *Morb Mortal Wkly Rep* 55:145, 2006.

Centers for Disease Control and Prevention: Revised US surveillance case definition for severe acute respiratory syndrome (SARS) and update on SARS cases: United States and worldwide, December, 2003, *Morb Mortal Wkly Rep* 52:1202, 2003.

Cockerill FR: Application of rapid-cycle real-time polymerase chain reaction for diagnostic testing in the clinical microbiology laboratory, *Arch Pathol Lab Med* 127:1112, 2003.

Constantine N, Zhao R: Molecular-based laboratory testing and monitoring for human immunodeficiency virus infections, *Clin Lab Sci* 18:263, 2005.

Debiasi RL, Tyler KL: Molecular methods for diagnosis of viral encephalitis, *Clin Microbiol Rev* 17:903, 2004.

De Clercq E: Antiviral drugs in current clinical use, *J Clin Virol* 30:115, 2004.

Dufresne AT, Gromeier M: Understanding polio: new insights from a cold virus, *Microbe* 1:13, 2006.

Espy MJ, Uhl JR, Sloan M, et al: Real-time PCR in clinical microbiology: applications for routine laboratory testing, *Clin Microbiol Rev* 19:165, 2006.

Henrickson KJ: Parainfluenza viruses, *Clin Microbiol Rev* 16:242, 2003.

Kahn JS: Epidemiology of human metapneumovirus, *Clin Microbiol Rev* 19:546, 2006.

Lauer GM, Walker BD: Hepatitis C virus infection, *N Engl J Med* 345:41, 2001.

McIntosh K, McAdam AJ: Human metapneumovirus: an important new respiratory virus, *N Engl J Med* 350:431, 2004.

Nainan OV, Xia F, Vaughan G, et al: Diagnosis of hepatitis A virus infection: a molecular approach, *Clin Microbiol Rev* 19:64, 2006

Niesters HG: Molecular and diagnostic clinical virology in real-time, *Clin Microbiol Infect* 10:5, 2004.

Pigott DC: Hemorrhagic fever viruses, *Crit Care Clin* 21:765, 2005.

Poon LL, Guan Y, Nicholls JM, et al: The aetiology, origins, and diagnosis of severe acute respiratory syndrome, *Lancet Infect Dis* 4:663, 2004.

Rubin J, David D, Willoughby RE, Jr., et al: Applying the Milwaukee Protocol to treat canine rabies in Equatorial Guinea, *Scand J Infect Dis* 41:372-380, 2009.

Schiffman M, Castle PE: Human papillomavirus epidemiology and public health, *Arch Pathol Lab Med* 127:930, 2003.

Storch GA: Diagnostic virology, *Clin Infect Dis* 31:739, 2000.

Thomson RB, Bertram H: Laboratory diagnosis of central nervous system infections, *Infect Dis Clin North Am* 15:1047, 2001.

Wilder-Smith A, Schwartz E: Dengue in travelers, *N Engl J Med* 353:924, 2005.

Writing Committee of the World Health Organization Consultation on Human Influenza A/H5: avian influenza A (H5N1) infection in humans, *N Engl J Med* 353:1374, 2005.

# Antiviral Therapy, Susceptibility Testing, and Prevention

## OBJECTIVES

1. Define antiviral resistance and explain what may lead a health care provider to believe that resistance to antiviral therapy is occurring?
2. Define antiviral susceptibility testing and list some of the factors that may vary the end results of testing.
3. Explain the lack of standardization of protocols for antiviral susceptibility testing.
4. Define the criteria that determine whether antiviral susceptibility testing should be performed.
5. Explain the difference between phenotypic and genotypic antiviral susceptibility testing.
6. Name some of the types of phenotypic susceptibility testing and list some of the advantages and disadvantages of this method of susceptibility testing.
7. Describe the methodology of genotypic susceptibility testing and list some of the illnesses for which it is used.
8. List the reasons for drug susceptibility testing for individuals infected with the human immunodeficiency virus (HIV).
9. List the vaccinations used to prevent influenza infection. Also, explain why this vaccine must be reformulated every year and why ongoing surveillance of influenza isolates is crucial to the global vaccination program.
10. Name the two classes of antiviral medications used to treat and prevent influenza. Also, list the four antiviral medications that have been approved by the U.S. Food and Drug Administration (FDA) and briefly explain their mode of action.

## ANTIVIRAL THERAPY

Antiviral therapy has expanded over the past several years as a treatment for a number of viral infections. Although most of the population is susceptible to such treatments, overuse of these agents has led to the emergence of drug-resistant strains, especially in immunocompromised patients. Resistance is known to develop to all agents and may be detected in vitro by using antiviral susceptibility testing. Virology laboratories are increasingly being asked to perform in vitro testing of antiviral agents when a patient's infection fails to respond clinically to antiviral therapy, but testing for antiviral resistance is not currently available in many clinical settings. This chapter provides an overview of the viral diseases in which antiviral resistance has emerged, the need for in vitro susceptibility testing, and the phenotypic and genotypic susceptibility testing methods currently available.

## ANTIVIRAL RESISTANCE

Antiviral resistance means that a virus has changed in such a way that the antiviral drug is less effective in preventing illness. Antiviral resistance is indicated if a patient is taking an antiviral drug that has been proven in vitro to be effective against a virus, but the patient shows no improvement and continues to deteriorate clinically. Drug resistance must be distinguished from clinical resistance. With clinical resistance, the viral infection fails to respond to the antiviral therapy because of factors other than a change in the virus; such factors may include the patient's immunologic status, the pharmacokinetics of the antiviral drug in the individual patient, and, if a combination of drugs is administered, potential antagonism and interference with the absorption of one or more drugs. Other patient factors that also affect the success of drug therapy include nonadherence to or intolerance of a specific drug and prescriptive errors, such as inappropriate doses or route of administration. In addition, infections in immunocompromised patients may fail to respond to therapy that has proven effective in immunocompetent individuals.

Very few standards have been established for antiviral susceptibility testing. The development of such protocols began in 2004 with the establishment of an approved standard for susceptibility testing for herpes simplex virus (HSV) by the Clinical and Laboratory Standards Institute (CLSI).

The final result of antiviral susceptibility testing is determined by many variables, and these variables also hinder the standardization of antiviral susceptibility testing. Some of these variables include the following:

- Cell line used to grow the virus
- Viral inoculum titer
- Incubation time of the culture
- Concentration range of the antiviral drug tested
- Reference strains
- Assay method
- End-point criteria
- Calculation of the end point
- Interpretation of the end point

Each of these categories in turn has variables that affect the final results. For example, if the inoculum quantity is too large, a susceptible isolate may appear resistant; if the inoculum quantity is too small, the isolate may appear susceptible. The complexity of all these variables makes it imperative that established control strains also be tested when antiviral susceptibility testing is performed. Controls should include both drug-resistant and drug-susceptible isolates that have been well characterized. Several research laboratories across the nation can provide reference and drug-resistant strains of a virus for susceptibility testing; they include the National Institute of Allergy and Infectious Diseases AIDS Research and Reference Reagent Program (niaid.nih.gov) and the American Type Culture Collection (atcc.org). Pharmaceutical companies also are a source.

# METHODS OF ANTIVIRAL SUSCEPTIBILITY TESTING

The purpose of antiviral susceptibility testing is to evaluate new antiviral chemoprophylaxis, to test for cross resistance or cross reactivity to alternate agents, and to determine how frequently drug-resistance viral mutations occur.

The two general types of antiviral susceptibility testing are phenotypic testing and genotypic testing. Phenotypic susceptibility assays measure viral replication in the presence of antiviral agents; they measure the inhibitory effect of an antiviral agent on the entire virus population in a clinical isolate. Genotypic susceptibility assays use polymerase chain reaction (PCR) to detect genes known to be responsible for resistance, coupled with molecular sequencing to determine whether genome alterations associated with resistance have occurred. These assays use the virus's nucleic acid to determine whether the virus has mutations capable of causing viral drug resistance. Alternately, a combination of the two general types of antiviral susceptibility, known as a virtual phenotype resistance assay, may be performed. This assay is a characterization of the patient's virus genotype compared to a data base that includes paired genotypic and phenotypic information. This information is then used to estimate the most likely phenotype of the patient's virus. The success of this approach varies with the virus type and antiviral drugs examined.

Each of these types of susceptibility testing has unique properties that can be used to complement each other. Phenotypic assays are better used to assess the combined effect of multiple-resistance mutations on drug susceptibility, but they are labor intensive, expensive, and have lengthy end result times. Genotypic assays have a shorter turnaround time and are less expensive than phenotypic assays, but they can detect only defined viral mutations.

## PHENOTYPIC ASSAYS

Phenotypic assays use a variety of end-point measurements to determine whether a virus is inhibited by an antiviral drug or demonstrates drug resistance. Some of these end-point measurements include a reduction in the number of plaques, inhibition of viral DNA synthesis, a reduction in the yield of a viral structural protein, or a reduction of the enzymatic activity of a functional protein. As mentioned, an advantage of phenotypic assays is that they are much better for assessing the combined effect of multiple-resistance mutations on drug susceptibility. This is useful for assaying viruses such as hepatitis B virus (HBV), human immunodeficiency virus type 1 (HIV-1), and human cytomegalovirus (HCMV), which acquire resistance mutations in multiple genes. The disadvantages of phenotypic assays are that they are labor intensive, expensive, and require weeks to perform.

### Plaque Reduction Assay

The plaque reduction assay (PRA) is the standard method of antiviral susceptibility testing to which new methods are compared. CLSI has developed standardized PRA protocols for antiviral susceptibility testing of HSV. This test is based on the principle of inhibition of viral plaque formation in the presence of an antiviral agent. The concentration of antiviral drug that inhibits plaque formation by 50% is the IC50; that is, the 50% inhibitory concentration and 50% effective concentration.

### DU Assay

The dye uptake (DU) assay has been used for years in the susceptibility testing of HSV. When the virus is in the presence of an antiviral drug, only cells that are alive and viable take up a vital dye called neutral red. Following infection with HSV, the relative amount of dye bound to viable cells compared with that bound to uninfected cells determines the extent of the viral lytic activity. The drug concentration that inhibits viral lytic activity by 50% is the IC50.

### DNA Hybridization

The DNA hybridization assay measures the effect of antiviral reagents on the synthesis of viral DNA. The assay semiquantitatively measures how much viral DNA is produced in the presence of antiviral agents compared with how much is produced in the absence of antiviral agents; the IC50 is calculated from these comparisons. These assays have been successfully used for susceptibility testing of HSV, varicella zoster virus (VZV), and HCMV.

### Enzyme Immunoassay

The enzyme immunoassay (EIA) uses spectrophotometry analysis to quantitatively measure the amount of viral activity. The concentration of antiviral agent that reduces the amount of absorbance by 50% compared with the absorbance values of a viral control is the IC50. This method of susceptibility testing has been used for influenza A, HSV, and VZV.

### Flow Cytometry

Flow cytometry readily distinguishes drug-resistant isolates from drug-susceptible isolates; in addition, it is time-saving, and it has been used to detect viral susceptibility in HCMV infections and in treatment with the drug ganciclovir. It uses a fluorochrome-labeled monoclonal antibody to an HCMV early antigen. Flow cytometry is used to quantitate the number of virus-infected cells; the instrument quantitates the number of antigen-positive cells in the absence and the presence of antiviral compounds. The advantages of this assay are that it can be automated; it is time-saving; and it is easier to use and less objective than other phenotypic susceptibility assays.

### Neuraminidase Inhibition Assay

The neuraminidase inhibition assay is used to detect neuraminidase (NA) inhibition resistance when the drugs oseltamivir and zanamivir are used to treat influenza A and influenza B infections. Oseltamivir and zanamivir act by inhibiting the influenza viral protein neuraminidase. Resistance to these drugs is measured by incubating cultured influenza isolates containing neuraminidase with varying concentrations of the drugs. A fluorogenic substrate is then added, allowing the fluorescence to be quantitated by a fluorimeter. The IC50 is calculated by comparing the activity of viral NA to a control reaction that does not use any neuraminidase inhibitors.

## GENOTYPIC SUSCEPTIBILITY ASSAYS

Genotypic susceptibility assays use PCR to detect genes known to be responsible for resistance, coupled with genetic sequencing to determine whether genome alterations associated with resistance have occurred. Genotypic assays use DNA sequencing by automated sequencers, PCR amplification and restriction enzyme digestion of the products, and hybridization to microarrays containing multiple oligonucleotide probes. These assays are rapid, because isolation of the virus in culture is not necessary for testing.

The response to an antiviral agent is also measured by quantitative monitoring of the viral load (by means of the nucleic acid concentration) in the patient's blood. Such testing is common in patients infected with HBV, hepatitis C virus (HCV), and cytomegalovirus (CMV). The viral load should diminish significantly after addition of an antiviral agent to which the virus is susceptible. Using molecular testing (e.g., quantitative PCR) to measure the amount of virus in serum is a surrogate test for resistance to antiviral agents. The viral load rises quickly when resistance appears.

### Pyrosequencing

DNA sequencing is among the most important testing methods for the study of biologic entities. Pyrosequencing, which is relatively new, is a sequence-based detection method that allows rapid, accurate quantification of sequence variation. It allows rapid acquisition of short reads (100 to 200 bp) of genomic sequence to identify known mutations. It is based on the technology of detection of released pyrophosphate (PPi) during DNA synthesis. In a sequence of enzymatic reactions, a enzyme (polymerase) catalyzes the addition of nucleotides into a nucleic acid chain. As a result of this addition, a PPi molecule is released and converted to adenosine triphosphate (ATP) by the ATP enzyme sulfurylase. Visible light is produced when a luciferin molecule is oxidized during the luciferase reaction. The visible light or signal strength generated is proportional to the number of nucleotides incorporated into the final product.

The two types of pyrosequencing methods currently available are solid-phase pyrosequencing and liquid-phase pyrosequencing. Solid-phase pyrosequencing involves a three-enzyme system that uses immobilized DNA, and a washing step is performed to remove excess substrate after each nucleotide addition. In liquid-phase pyrosequencing, a fourth nucleotide-degrading enzyme (made from potato) is added. The advantage of the liquid-phase system is that it eliminates the need for solid support and the intermediate washing step, allowing the reaction to be performed in a single tube.

Because of its rapid, accurate quantification of sequence variation, pyrosequencing is an adaptable tool that can be used for a wide range of applications.

Automation with pyrosequencing is made possible by the liquid-phase methodology. Pyrosequencing signals are quantitative, which allows a large number of people to be screened through examination of the allelic frequency in a population. This technique also is used taxonomically to group different organisms into strains or subtypes, and it can be applied to bacteria, yeasts, and viruses. It is currently the fastest method for sequencing a PCR product and can be applied to the resequencing of PCR-amplified disease genes for mutation screening. It also is used to screen clinical isolates for the genes that confer resistance to antiviral therapy, such as for analysis of influenza specimens for the adamantine resistance mutation.

## HUMAN IMMUNODEFICIENCY VIRUS

Patients infected with HIV frequently develop resistance to the antiretroviral drugs, which often results in treatment failure. Testing for antiretroviral resistance is crucial to the assessment of a regimen of drugs intended to suppress HIV replication and to testing for cross resistance to alternative antiretroviral drugs. The U.S. Department of Health and Human Services and a European panel of experts have developed guidelines and established protocols to monitor patients with acute and chronic HIV infection. Susceptibility testing should proceed as follows:

1. Before the initiation of therapy
2. When antiretroviral regimens are changed in cases of virologic failure
3. When suboptimal viral load reduction is seen after beginning or changing therapy

The recombinant virus assay (RVA) is a phenotypic type of susceptibility test for HIV. It is used to test the reaction of HIV-1 isolates to nucleoside analog reverse transcription (RT) inhibitors. RVA uses reverse transcription PCR (RT-PCR) amplification of the RT and pathogenesis-related (PR) gene coding sequences directly from the patient's plasma. An advantage of this assay is that in a single test, a virus's ability to replicate in the presence of various levels of an antiretroviral drug is measured by the detection of luciferase activity in the target cells. Two types of commercial kits are available for this method of testing.

Genotypic susceptibility testing has become a routine component of the management of patients infected with HIV. Genotypic assays for mutations that confer resistance are useful because of their rapid turnaround time. Several genotypic methods and commercial assays are available to test for these mutations in HIV; they include sequencing, selective PCR, oligonucleotide-specific hybridization, microarray hybridization, and reverse hybridization.

## INFLUENZA

Currently, two main approaches are used in health care to control the spread of influenza: vaccination and the use of antiviral drugs. The influenza virus has the unique capability of being able to change its antigenic makeup; this mechanism, known as antigenic drift, occurs with all three types of influenza virus (A, B, and C). Influenza A shows the greatest rate of antigenic change. Antigenic drift is caused by sequential point mutations in the hemagglutination (HA) or NA genes that arise during viral ribonucleoprotein (RNP) replication and immune selection, giving rise to new strains; this gives the virus the ability to reinfect "nonimmune" susceptible hosts each season. Another phenomenon, antigenic shift, is manifested only by the influenza A virus. It involves complete reassortment of the segmented viral genome during a co-infection with a nonhuman animal, which results in major antigenic change and periodic worldwide outbreaks (pandemics) of a never before circulated type of influenza A virus. Influenza B undergoes antigenic change very slowly.

Antigenic drift requires the reformulation of the influenza vaccine each year to ensure maximum efficacy against the currently circulating strains of influenza A and influenza B, because the vaccine is only as efficient as the influenza strains selected for it. This is accomplished by global surveillance of the yearly influenza epidemics to evaluate the strains that are circulating and provide early detection of viruses that may have pandemic potential. The World Health Organization (WHO) coordinates a influenza surveillance program in more than 80 countries. In the United States, the surveillance program established by the Centers for Disease Control and Prevention (CDC) includes monitoring of pneumonia and influenza deaths above a calculated "epidemic threshold." It also includes tallying pediatric deaths, assessment of weekly virology data, and typing of influenza virus isolates submitted by reference laboratories. This extensive surveillance system provides the data for determining and predicting the influenza strains likely to be circulating in the upcoming winter, and vaccine components are chosen annually by WHO based on the analysis of these strains. The summer months are used to manufacture the vaccine so that it is ready for early autumn distribution to health care providers. In the United States, the vaccine is prepared from viruses grown in embryonated chicken eggs; this is a trivalent vaccine containing two influenza A strains with the newest HA and NA surface antigens and a current type B strain.

Currently two types of vaccine are used to prevent influenza infection: the trivalent inactivated influenza vaccine (TIV) and the live attenuated influenza virus vaccine (LAIV). The TIV is a noninfectious vaccine administered intramuscularly. It currently is approved in the United States for individuals 6 months or older, including those with chronic medical conditions. It is 70% to 100% effective in preventing infection among healthy adults and 30% to 60% effective in the elderly and pediatric populations. The LAIV contains live whole infectious virus. It is administered intranasally and currently is approved in the United States for healthy individuals 2 to 49 years of age. Because it contains live virus, it is not recommended for immunocompromised individuals, the elderly, or people with reactive airway disease. The LAIV causes shedding of the virus that is detectable in rapid antigen assays for about a week.

Two classes of antiviral drugs, the adamantanes and the neuraminidase inhibitors, currently are used to treat influenza infections. The adamantanes, which include the drugs amantidine and rimantadine, were the first antiinfluenza class of antiviral treatment developed. Their mechanism of viral defense is blockage of the virion M2 ion channel, which prevents the virus from uncoating. This class of drugs is effective only at treating influenza A infections; it has never had any effect on influenza B infections. The neuraminidase inhibitors include the drugs zanamivir (Relenza) and oseltamivir (Tamiflu). Both of these drugs inhibit the viral protein neuraminidase, which prevents release of the virus from infected cells. The neuraminidase inhibitors are used to treat both influenza A and influenza B infections, although oseltamivir has been reported to have lower efficacy against influenza B. Both classes of drugs have proven to be most effective when administrated within 48 hours of symptoms. The drugs shorten the duration of the infection and reduce complications.

The need for effective influenza antiviral susceptibility surveillance has increased around the world, and its importance is validated by the emergence of universal resistance to the adamantine antiviral therapy for influenza A (H3N2). Samples of viruses collected from around the United States and worldwide are studied to determine whether they are resistant to any of the four influenza antiviral drugs approved by the U.S. Food and Drug Administration (FDA). The CDC, in collaboration with state public health departments and WHO, conducts ongoing surveillance and performs testing of influenza viruses to monitor for antiviral resistance. The number of surveillance sites, both domestically and globally, are being increased, and the data from this surveillance are used to make public health policy recommendations on the use of these antiviral medications. The CDC is constantly improving its methods of rapidly detecting and monitoring antiviral resistance. Laboratory methods for testing also are being improved, and the number of laboratories capable of testing for antiviral resistance is rising.

Antiviral resistance to the adamantanes among circulating influenza A (H3N2) viruses rapidly increased worldwide beginning in the 2003-2004 influenza season. Data from the CDC's World Health Organization (WHO) Collaborating Center for Surveillance, Epidemiology and Control of Influenza reports that the percentage of influenza A (H3N2) virus isolates submitted from around the world that were adamantine resistant increased from 0.4% in the 1994-1995 season to 12.3% in the 2003-2004 season. This resistance continued to increase; during the 2005-2006 influenza season, the CDC reported that of 209 isolates, 193 (92%) of the influenza A (H3N2) isolates carried a change at amino acid 31 in the M2 gene that confers resistance to the adamantanes. At the end of the 2008-2009 influenza season, 100% of influenza A H3N2, along with novel 2009 influenza A H1N1, were resistant to the adamantanes.

Resistance to oseltamivir appeared in the seasonal influenza A/H1N1 virus subtype during the 2007-2008 season. Oseltamivir resistance can result from a number

**TABLE 67-1** Antiviral Agents

| Virus | Mode of Action | Target | Examples of Common Drugs |
|---|---|---|---|
| CMV | Nucleoside analog | Viral DNA | Ganciclovir |
| HIV* | Nucleoside analog<br>Nucleotide analog<br>Nonnucleoside analog<br>Protease inhibitor<br>Fusion inhibitor | Viral DNA<br>Viral DNA<br>Reverse transcriptase<br>Viral protease<br>Virus, host cell membrane | Efavirenz<br>Tenofovir disoproxil fumarate<br>Emtricitabine |
| HSV/VZV | Nucleoside analog<br>Pyrophosphate analog | Viral DNA<br>DNA polymerase | Acyclovir<br>Foscarnet |
| Hepatitis B | Nucleoside analog<br>Nucleotide analog | Reverse transcriptase<br>DNA polymerase | Lamivudine<br>Adefovir dipivoxil |
| Influenza A | Inhibit penetration and uncoating of virus | Host cell membrane | Amantadine, imantadine |
| Influenza A and B | Prevent release of virus | Neuraminidase inhibitors | Zanamivir, oseltamivir |
| RSV | Inhibit expression of viral mRNA and protein synthesis | Viral mRNA | Ribavirin |
| HCV | Inhibit expression of viral mRNA; increase resistance to virus | Viral mRNA or neighboring host cells | Ribavirin plus interferon-alpha |
| Picornaviruses (enteroviruses and rhinoviruses) | Inhibit attachment and uncoating of virus | Binds to virus | Pleconaril |

*CMV*, Cytomegalovirus; *HIV*, human immunodeficiency virus; *HSV*, herpes simplex virus; *VZV*, varicella-zoster virus; *RSV*, respiratory syncytial virus; *HCV*, hepatitis C virus.
*More than 20 antiretroviral drugs in six different mechanistic classes are available to design treatment regimens. See the most recent guidelines at http://aidsinfo.nih.gov/guidelines

of mutations in the neuraminidase gene, and for the 2007-2008 season, the CDC reported a nationwide resistance of 10.9% of the isolates submitted. This resistance also continued to increase; at the end of the 2008-2009 influenza season, the CDC reported that of 825 isolates of seasonal influenza A H1N1, 820 (99.4%) were resistant to oseltamivir. None of the other strains of influenza (i.e., influenza H3N2, novel 2009 influenza A H1N1, and influenza B) showed any resistance to the neuraminidase inhibitors (neither oseltamivir nor zanamivir).

For the 2010 influenza season, resistance to the adamantanes remained high; both circulating influenza A viruses (H3N2 and 2009 H1N1) showed high levels of resistance to the these drugs. These viruses are still susceptible to the neuraminidase inhibitors, and this class of antiviral medication is the current therapy of choice for antiviral treatment and for chemoprophylaxis of current circulating influenza A virus strains (Table 67-1).

At the end of the 2009-2010 season, almost all (98.9%) of the 2009 H1N1 isolates characterized at the CDC were susceptible to oseltamivir (Tamiflu), and all (100%) were susceptible to oseltamivir (Relenza). The rare 2009 H1N1 oseltamivir-resistant influenza A viruses shared a single genetic mutation, causing them to be resistant to this antiviral medication. Many of the influenza A H5N1 strains (avian influenza) are resistant to the adamantanes, so oseltamivir is the current antiviral of choice. Early treatment with oseltamivir improves the chance of survival in individuals infected with this type of influenza virus, but the mortality rate for the disease remains high.

**TABLE 67-2** Examples of Vaccines for Preventing Viral Diseases

| Disease | Type of Vaccine |
|---|---|
| Yellow fever | Attenuated-live |
| Poliomyelitis | Attenuated-live and inactivated |
| Measles | Attenuated-live |
| Mumps | Attenuated-live |
| Rubella | Attenuated-live |
| Hepatitis B | Inactivated |
| Influenza | Inactivated |
| Smallpox | Attenuated-live |
| Chickenpox | Attenuated-live |
| Hepatitis A | Inactivated |
| Rabies | Inactivated |
| Rotavirus | Attenuated-live |

# PREVENTION OF OTHER VIRAL INFECTIONS

## VACCINATION

Control of many viral diseases has been accomplished by vaccination. Since Jenner developed the first vaccine against smallpox 200 years ago, attenuated-live or inactivated-dead viral vaccines have been used successively to prevent yellow fever, poliomyelitis, measles, mumps, rubella, hepatitis B, and influenza (Table 67-2).

**TABLE 67-3** Immune Prophylaxis or Therapy for Viral Diseases

| Disease | Circumstances of Use |
|---|---|
| **Prophylaxis** Hepatitis A | Traveler to developing country |
| Hepatitis B | Newborns of infected mothers or unimmunized laboratory worker following needlestick |
| Rabies | After bite from potentially rabid animal |
| Measles | Unimmunized close contact with infected individual |
| Varicella | Newborns of infected mothers at time of delivery |
| Respiratory | Infants younger than 2 years of age with underlying lung syncytial disease virus |
| **Therapy** Lassa fever | During disease to reduce severity |

Smallpox was eliminated in 1977 by an effective vaccination program. Additional vaccines continue to appear. New smallpox vaccines with fewer side effects are being developed to prevent outbreaks in the event of bioterrorism. A live-attenuated varicella (chickenpox) vaccine is now recommended for all children, and an inactivated hepatitis A vaccine is available for travelers and others entering areas of higher endemicity. Rotavirus vaccines are approved by the FDA and are now available. Recombinant vaccines are also available for the prevention of HPV infection.

## IMMUNE PROPHYLAXIS AND THERAPY

Immune prophylaxis is used to prevent serious viral infection in patients who are immunocompromised or functionally compromised. Instead of actively immunizing an individual with an antiviral vaccine, limited protection can be conferred by intramuscular inoculation of human immunoglobulin. Pooled human immunoglobulin contains antibody against all common viruses. Specific high-titered immunoglobulin can be collected from patients recovering from a specific infection to ensure maximum antibody levels. Immune prophylaxis should be considered an emergency procedure. Table 67-3 lists immune prophylaxis available for viral infections.

Passive immunoprophylaxis of respiratory syncytial virus (RSV) infection in infants younger than 2 years who have underlying lung disease resulting from premature birth or congenital heart disease is particularly effective at preventing life-threatening bronchiolitis and pneumonia in this patient group. The drug, palivizumab (Synagis), is a manufactured antibody to RSV. It is used in certain infants and young children to prevent RSV infections of the breathing tubes and lungs; it cannot be used to treat a child already sick with RSV.

Passive immunization occasionally is effective as therapy for viral infection (see Table 67-3). Therapy with immune serum for some hemorrhagic fevers, such as Lassa fever, has also been successful in reducing mortality associated with the disease.

## ERADICATION

Global eradication of a viral disease has occurred only with smallpox. Factors that result in eradication of any viral disease include no animal reservoir, a lack of recurrent infectivity, one or few stable serotypes, and an effective vaccine. Viral diseases currently considered candidates for eradication include measles and poliomyelitis. Poliomyelitis has been known and feared by humans for thousands of years. Infection with the poliovirus causes an acute flaccid paralysis that can affect the ability to breathe. Years ago, it was often seen in children. In the mid-1950s, Jonas Salk developed the first polio vaccine from dead virus, and in 1960, Sabin developed an oral polio vaccine using a live-attenuated virus. These developments allowed the United States to launch a massive vaccination program against polio, and the last case of indigenous polio was reported in the United States in 1979 (other reports of polio cases were due to vaccination or occurred in individuals who had emigrated from other countries).

In 1988 WHO resolved to eradicate acute paralytic poliomyelitis from the rest of the world and staged a massive vaccination campaign to accomplish this. At the time, poliomyelitis was endemic in 125 countries on five continents and was responsible for an estimated 350,000 cases annually. The success of this program reduced the number of polio-endemic countries to six by 2003, and by 2006 the disease remained endemic in only four countries: Afghanistan, India, Nigeria, and Pakistan. The strategies used to eradicate the disease included surveillance of acute flaccid paralysis, routine vaccination with the oral polio vaccine, and supplementary immunization activities.

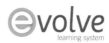 *Visit the Evolve site to complete the review questions.*

## BIBLIOGRAPHY

Balfour H: Drug therapy, *N Engl J Med* 340:1255, 1999.
Bryant B, Payne D: Possible resistance comparison of possible HIV resistance results derived from a genotyping report versus the IC50 virtual phenotype, *Lab Med* 38(1):26-28, 2002.
Centers for Disease Control and Prevention: Influenza antiviral drug resistance Available at www.cdc.gov/flu/about/qa/antiviralresistance.htm. Accessed 6/23/2011.
De Clercq E: Antiviral drugs in current clinical use, *J Clin Virol* 30:115, 2004.

Constantine N, Zhao R: Molecular-based laboratory testing and monitoring for human immunodeficiency virus infections, *Clin Lab Sci* 18:263, 2005.
De Clercq E: Antiviral drugs in current clinical use, *J Clin Virol* 30:115, 2004.
Fields BN, Howley PN, Griffin DN et al, editors: *Virology*, ed 3, Philadelphia, 2001, Lippincott Williams & Wilkins.
Flint SJ, Enquist LW, Krug RM et al: *Principles of virology: molecular biology, pathogenesis and control*, Washington, DC, 2000, ASM Press.
Hodinka RL: What clinicians need to know about antiviral drugs and viral resistance, *Infect Dis Clin North Am* 11:945, 1997.
Lee W: Hepatitis B virus infection, *N Engl J Med* 337:1733, 1997.
Levine AJ: *Viruses*, New York, 1991, Scientific American Library.

Liang TJ, Rehermann B, Seeff L et al: Pathogenesis, natural history, treatment, and prevention of hepatitis C, *Ann Intern Med* 132:296, 2000.

McSharry J, Lurain N, Drusanao G et al: Rapid ganciclovir susceptibility assay using flow cytometry for HCMV isolates, *Antimicrob Agents Chemother* 42:2326, 1998.

Niesters HG: Molecular and diagnostic clinical virology in real-time, *Clin Microbiol Infect* 10:5, 2004.

Ronaghi M: Pyrosequencing sheds light on DNA sequencing. Available at http://genome.schlp.org/content/11/1/3.full. Accessed 6/23/2011.

Specter S, Hodinka RL, Young SA, et al: *Clinical virology manual*, ed 4, Washington, DC, 2009, ASM Press.

Storch GA: Diagnostic virology, *Clin Infect Dis* 31:739, 2000.

Versalovic J: *Manual of clinical microbiology*, ed 10, Washington, DC, 2011, ASM Press.

## OBJECTIVES

1. Identify and describe some of the medical consequences that occur when the bloodstream is infected by microorganisms.
2. Name the most common causes of bacterial bloodstream infection, and explain the route of transmission and source of infection.
3. Define the following bloodstream infections: bacteremia, fungemia, and septicemia.
4. List the most common fungi associated with bloodstream infections and the population of patients most often affected by this type of infection.
5. Explain what causes mortality in most cases of parasitic blood-borne infections.
6. Differentiate between intravascular and extravascular bloodstream infections.
7. Define continuous bacteremia, and provide an example.
8. Describe the development of infective endocarditis, including the contributing factors and the microorganisms that are the primary cause for the condition.
9. Define mycotic aneurysms and suppurative thrombophlebitis, and describe the causes for these conditions.
10. Explain the pathogenic features of *S. epidermidis* that make it uniquely suited for causing catheter-related infections.
11. Explain the importance of collection parameters associated with blood cultures for suspected cases of bloodstream infections, including collection time, the number of cultures, and the volume of blood required.
12. List and briefly describe some of the blood culture systems available to the microbiologist, including the self-contained systems, the lysis centrifugation systems, and instrument-based systems.
13. List some of the most common causes of bloodstream infection associated with the blood cultures from HIV-infected patients.
14. Define the acronym AACEK, and describe the type of blood-borne infections these organisms are most often associated with.
15. Outline the guidelines used to determine if agents isolated from blood cultures are true pathogens or probable contaminants.

Invasion of the bloodstream by microorganisms constitutes one of the most serious situations in infectious disease. Microorganisms present in the circulating blood—whether continuously, intermittently, or transiently—are a threat to every organ in the body. The suffix *emia* is derived from the Greek word meaning "blood" and refers to the presence of a substance in the blood; *bacteremia* refers to the presence of bacteria in the blood, *fungemia* refers to the presence of fungi in

the bloodstream, and *septicemia* indicates bacteria are present in the blood, producing an infection and reproducing within the bloodstream. Microbial invasion of the bloodstream resulting from any organism can have serious immediate consequences, including shock, multiple organ failure, disseminated intravascular coagulation (DIC), and death. Approximately 200,000 cases of bacteremia and fungemia occur annually, with mortality rates ranging from 20% to 50%. Timely detection and identification of blood-borne pathogens are two of the most important functions of the microbiology laboratory. Pathogens of all four major groups of microbes—bacteria, fungi, viruses, and parasites—may be found circulating in blood during the course of many diseases. Positive blood cultures may help provide a clinical diagnosis, as well as a specific etiologic diagnosis.

## GENERAL CONSIDERATIONS

The successful recovery of microorganisms from blood by the laboratory depends on many, often complex, factors: the type of bacteremia, the specimen collection method, the blood volume, the number and timing of blood cultures, the interpretation of results, and the type of patient population being served by the laboratory. All of these parameters must be considered in the development of the blood culture protocol within the laboratory in order to maximize the detection and recovery of microorganisms and ensure quality patient care.

### ETIOLOGY

As previously mentioned, all major groups of microbes can be present in the bloodstream during the course of many diseases.

#### Bacteria

The organisms most commonly isolated from blood are gram-positive cocci, including coagulase-negative staphylococci, *Staphylococcus aureus*, and *Enterococcus* spp., and other organisms likely to be inhabitants of the hospital environment that colonize the skin, oropharynx, and gastrointestinal tract of patients. Some of the most common, clinically significant bacteria isolated from blood cultures are listed in Box 68-1. In general, the number of fungi and coagulase-negative staphylococci has increased, whereas the number of clinically significant anaerobic isolates has decreased since the early 2000s.

Of importance, the laboratory isolation of certain bacterial species from blood can indicate the presence of an underlying, occult, or undiagnosed neoplasm. Alterations in local conditions at the site of the neoplasm allowing bacteria to proliferate and seed the bloodstream have been suggested as a potential mechanism for the association between bacteremia and cancer. Another possible mechanism is reduced killing of bacterial cells by the host phagocytes. Organisms associated with neoplastic disease include *Clostridium septicum* and other uncommonly isolated clostridial species, *Streptococcus galldyticus*, *Aeromonas hydrophila*, *Plesiomonas shigelloides*, and *Campylobacter* spp. Finally, if *Streptococcus anginosis* group bacteria are isolated from blood, the possibility of an abscess should be considered.

## Fungi

Fungemia (the presence of fungi in blood) is usually a serious condition, occurring primarily in immunosuppressed patients and in those with serious or terminal illness. *Candida albicans* is by far the most common species, but *Malassezia furfur* can often be isolated in patients, particularly neonates, receiving lipid-supplemented parenteral nutrition. *Candida* spp. account for approximately 8% to 10% of all nosocomial bloodstream infections.

Except for *Histoplasma*, which multiply in leukocytes (white blood cells), fungi do not invade blood cells, but their presence in the blood usually indicates a focus of infection elsewhere in the body. Fungi in the bloodstream can disseminate (be carried) to all organs of the host, where they may grow, invade normal tissue, and produce toxic products. Fungi gain entrance to the circulatory system via loss of integrity of the gastrointestinal or other mucosa; through damaged skin; from primary sites of infection, such as the lung or other organs; or by means of intravascular catheters.

Systemic fungal infections begin as pneumonia and may disseminate from the lungs, which serve as the portal of entry. Arthroconidia of *Coccidioides immitis* and microconidia of *Histoplasma capsulatum* and *Blastomyces dermatitidis* are ingested by alveolar macrophages in the lung. These macrophages carry the fungi to nearby lymph nodes, usually the hilar nodes. The fungi multiply within the node tissue and ultimately are released into the circulating blood, from which they are capable of seeding other organs or are destroyed by the body's defenses. Molds are particularly insensitive to host defenses such as antibody and phagocytic cells because of their large size and their sterol containing cell wall structure.

## Parasites

Eukaryotic parasites may be found transiently in the bloodstream as they migrate to other tissues or organs. Their presence, however, cannot be considered consistent with a state of good health. For example, tachyzoites of the parasite *Toxoplasma gondii* may be found in circulating blood. They invade cells within lymph nodes and other organs, including the lungs, liver, heart, brain, and eyes. The resulting cellular destruction accounts for the manifestations of toxoplasmosis. Also, microfilariae are seen in peripheral blood during infection with *Dipetalonema*, *Mansonella*, *Loa loa*, *Wuchereria*, or *Brugia*.

Malarial parasites invade host erythrocytes and hepatic parenchymal cells. The significant anemia and subsequent tissue hypoxia (reduction in oxygen levels) may result from destruction of red blood cells by the parasite. Vascular trapping of normal erythrocytes by the infected red blood cells, which are less flexible and tend to clog small capillaries, is a major cause of morbidity. The host's immunologic response is to remove the parasites and damaged red blood cells; the immune response may also have deleterious effects.

Parasites in the bloodstream are usually detected by direct visualization. Those parasites for which traditional diagnosis is dependent on observation of the organism in peripheral blood smears include *Plasmodium*, *Trypanosoma*, and *Babesia*. Patients with malaria or filariasis may display a periodicity in their episodes of fever that allows the physician to time the collection of blood for microscopic examination intended for optimal detection. Rapid serological methods and molecular methods are currently used to detect malaria, babesiosis, and trypanosomiasis. These tests are described in Chapter 49.

## Viruses

Although many viruses do circulate in the peripheral blood at some stage of disease, the primary pathology relates to infection of the target organ or cells. Those viruses that preferentially infect blood cells are Epstein-Barr virus (invades lymphocytes), cytomegalovirus (invades monocytes, polymorphonuclear cells, and lymphocytes), and human immunodeficiency virus (HIV) (involves only certain T lymphocytes and perhaps macrophages) and other human retroviruses that attack lymphocytes. The pathogenesis of viral diseases of the blood is the same as that for viral diseases of any organ; by diverting the cellular machinery to create new viral components or by other means, the virus may prevent the host cell from performing its normal function. The cell may be destroyed or damaged by viral replication, and immunologic responses of the host may also contribute to the pathogenesis.

Although many viral diseases have a viremic stage, recovery of virus particles or detection of circulating viruses is used in the diagnosis of only a few diseases. Chapter 66 discusses the recovery of viruses from blood in greater detail.

## TYPES OF BACTEREMIA

Bacteremia may be transient, continuous, or intermittent. Most people have experienced transient bacteremia; teething infants and people having dental procedures have had oral flora gain entry to the bloodstream through breaks in the gums. Other conditions in which bacteria are only transiently present in the bloodstream include manipulation of infected tissues, devices or instrumentation inserted through contaminated mucosal surfaces, and surgery involving nonsterile sites. These circumstances may also lead to significant septicemia, although normally the bacteria are cleared from the blood by scavenging leukocytes, resulting in no infection. Septicemia can occur when the bacteria multiply more rapidly than the immune system is capable of killing and removing the organism.

In septic shock, bacterial endocarditis, and other endovascular infections, organisms are released into the bloodstream at a fairly constant rate (continuous bacteremia). Also, during the early stages of specific infections, including typhoid fever, brucellosis, and leptospirosis, bacteria are continuously present in the bloodstream.

In most other infections, such as in patients with undrained abscesses, bacteria can be found intermittently in the bloodstream. Of note, the causative agents of meningitis, pneumonia, pyogenic arthritis, and osteomyelitis are often recovered from blood during the early course of these diseases. In the case of transient seeding of the blood from a sequestered focus of infection, such as an abscess, bacteria are released into the blood approximately 45 minutes before a febrile episode.

The symptoms of septicemia are fever, chills, and malaise; these are caused by the presence of the invading microorganism and the toxins produced by these microorganisms. The older the patient is, the greater the risk and the rate of mortality as a result of septicemia.

## TYPES OF BLOODSTREAM INFECTIONS

The two major categories of bloodstream infections are intravascular (those that originate within the cardiovascular system) and extravascular (those that result from bacteria entering the blood circulation through the lymphatic system from another site of infection). Of note, other organisms, such as fungi, may also cause intravascular or extravascular infections. However, because bacteria account for the majority of significant vascular infections, these types of bloodstream infections are discussed in more detail. Factors contributing to the initiation of bloodstream infections are immunosuppressive agents, widespread use of broad-spectrum antibiotics that suppress the normal flora and allow the emergence of resistant strains of bacteria, invasive procedures allowing bacteria access to the interior of the host, more extensive surgical procedures, and prolonged survival of debilitated and seriously ill patients.

---

**BOX 68-2** Agents of Infective Endocarditis

*Aggregatibacter aprophilus*
Viridans streptococci*
Nutritionally deficient streptococci (*Abiotrophia* spp. and *Granulicatella* spp.)
Enterococci*
*Streptococcus bovis*
*Staphylococcus aureus**
Staphylococci (coagulase-negative)
Enterobacteriaceae
*Pseudomonas* spp. (usually in drug users)
*Haemophilus* spp.
Unusual gram-negative bacilli (e.g., *Actinobacillus, Cardiobacterium, Eikenella, Coxiella burnetii*)
Yeast
Other (including polymicrobial infectious endocarditis)

*Most common organisms associated with native valve endocarditis in non-drug-using adults.

---

### Intravascular Infections

Intravascular infections include infective endocarditis, mycotic aneurysm, suppurative thrombophlebitis, and intravenous (IV), catheter-associated bacteremia. Because these infections are within the vascular system, organisms are present in the bloodstream at a fairly constant rate (i.e., a continuous bacteremia). These infections in the cardiovascular system are extremely serious and considered life threatening.

**Infective Endocarditis.** The development of infective endocarditis (infection of the endocardium most commonly caused by bacteria) is believed to involve several independent events. Cardiac abnormalities, such as congenital valvular diseases that lead to turbulence in blood flow or direct trauma from IV catheters, can damage cardiac endothelium. This damage to the endothelial surface results in the deposition of platelets and fibrin. If bacteria transiently gain access to the bloodstream (this can occur after an innocuous procedure such as brushing the teeth) after alteration of the capillary endothelial cells, the organisms may stick to and then colonize the damaged cardiac endothelial cell surface. After colonization, the surface will rapidly be covered with a protective layer of fibrin and platelets. This protective environment is favorable to further bacterial multiplication. This web of platelets, fibrin, inflammatory cells, and entrapped organisms is called a vegetation (Figure 68-1). The resulting vegetations ultimately seed bacteria into the blood at a slow but constant rate.

The primary causes of infective endocarditis are the viridans streptococci, comprising several species (Box 68-2). These organisms are normal inhabitants of the oral cavity, often gaining entrance to the bloodstream as a result of gingivitis, periodontitis, or dental manipulation. Heart valves, especially those previously damaged, present convenient surfaces for attachment of these bacteria. *Streptococcus sanguis* and *Streptococcus mutans* are frequently isolated in streptococcal endocarditis. Gram-negative bacilli, known as the AACEK group, *Aggregatibacter aphrophilus, Actinobacillus actinomycetemcomitans,*

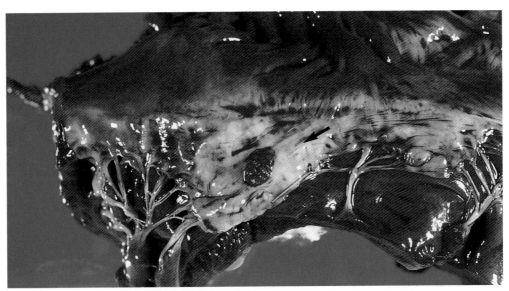

**Figure 68-1** Vegetations of bacterial endocarditis. Arrow indicates the vegetations. (Courtesy Celeste N. Powers, MD, PhD, Virginia Commonwealth University Medical Center, Medical College of Virginia Campus, Richmond, Va.)

*Cardiobacterium hominis, Eikenella corrodens,* and *Kingella kingae,* can also be associated with endocarditis.

With the ever-increasing use of IV catheters, arterial lines, and vascular prostheses, organisms considered normal or hospital-acquired inhabitants of the human skin are able to gain access to the bloodstream and attach to various surfaces, including heart valves and vascular endothelium. It has been estimated that more than 200,000 nosocomial infections (bloodstream) occur annually in the United States in adults and children. The majority of these infections are caused by the use of intravascular catheters. *Staphylococcus epidermidis* and other coagulase-negative staphylococci have been increasingly implicated as the cause of infection associated with intravascular catheters. *S. epidermidis* is the most common etiologic agent identified in prosthetic valve endocarditis, with *S. aureus* being the second most common. *S. aureus* is an important cause of septicemia without endocarditis and is found in association with other foci, such as abscesses, wound infections, and pneumonia, as well as sepsis related to indwelling intravascular catheters.

**Mycotic Aneurysm and Suppurative Thrombophlebitis.** Two other intravascular infections, mycotic aneurysms and suppurative thrombophlebitis, result from damage to the endothelial cells lining blood vessels. With respect to mycotic aneurysm, an infection causes inflammatory damage and weakening of an arterial wall; this weakening causes a bulging of the arterial wall (i.e., aneurysm) that can eventually rupture. The etiologic agents are similar to those that cause endocarditis.

Suppurative thrombophlebitis is an inflammation of a vein wall. The pathogenesis of this intravascular infection involves an alteration in the vein's endothelial lining followed by clot formation. The site is then seeded with organisms, thereby establishing a primary site of infection. Suppurative thrombophlebitis represents a frequent complication of hospitalized patients caused by the increasing use of IV catheters.

***Intravenous Catheter–Associated Bacteremia.*** IV catheters are an integral part of the care for many hospitalized patients. More than 3 million central venous catheters are used annually in the United States. For example, central venous catheters are used to administer fluids, blood products, medications, antibiotics, and nutrition, and for hemodynamic monitoring. A short-term, triple-lumen (channel opening within a tube) central venous catheter is shown in Figure 68-2. Unfortunately, a major consequence of these medical devices is colonization of the catheter by either bacteria or fungi, which can lead to catheter infection and serious bloodstream infection. This consequence is a major nosocomial source of illness and even death.

IV catheter–associated bacteremia (or fungemia) is believed to occur primarily by two routes (Figure 68-3). The first route involves the movement of organisms from the catheter entry site through the patient's skin and down the external surface of the catheter to the catheter tip within the bloodstream. After arriving at the tip, the organisms multiply and may cause a bacteremia. The second way that IV catheter–associated bacteremia may occur is by migration of organisms along the inside of the catheter (the lumen) to the catheter tip. The catheter's hub, where tubing connects into the IV catheter, is considered the site at which organisms gain access to the patient's bloodstream through the catheter lumen. The most common etiologic agents for IV catheter–associated bloodstream infections, regardless of the route of infection, are organisms found on the skin (Box 68-3). Certain strains of *S. epidermidis* appear to be uniquely suited for causing catheter-related infections because of their ability to produce a biofilm or "slime" that consists of complex sugars (polysaccharides) believed to help the organism adhere to the catheter's surface. The initial attachment of *S. epidermidis* to the catheter's polystyrene surface is related to a cell surface protein. Once attached, the organism

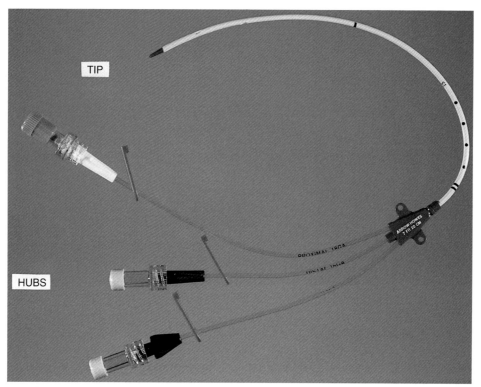

**Figure 68-2** Short-term, triple-lumen central venous catheter. The ends from which the catheter is accessed are usually referred to as the hubs. After the catheter is inserted, the tip resides within the bloodstream.

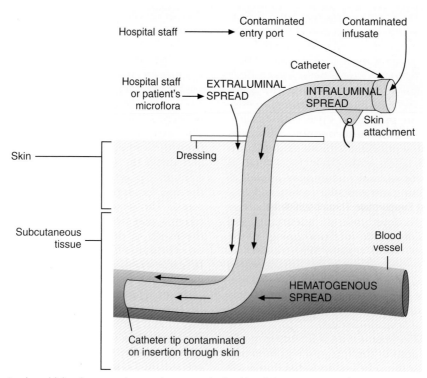

**Figure 68-3** Possible routes by which microorganisms gain access to the bloodstream to cause intravenous catheter–associated bacteremias. (Modified from Elliott TS: PHLS Communicable disease report: line-associated bacteremias, *CDR Review* 3:R91, 1993.)

**TABLE 68-1** Organisms Commonly Associated with Bloodstream Invasion from Extravascular Sites of Infection

| Organism | Extravascular Site of Infection |
| --- | --- |
| **Anaerobic organisms** | Wound, soft tissue |
| ***Brucella* spp.** | Reticuloendothelial system |
| ***Candida albicans*** | Genitourinary tract |
| ***Chlamydia pneumoniae*** | Respiratory |
| ***Clostridium* spp.** | Wound, soft tissue |
| **Coagulase negative staphylococci** | Wound, soft tissue |
| **Enterobacteriaceae (*E.coli*, *Klebsiella* spp., *Enterobacter* spp., *Proteus* spp., *Enterococcus* spp.)** | Genitourinary tract infections, central nervous system |
| ***Haemophilus influenzae*** | Meninges (CNS), epiglotitis, periorbital region, respiratory |
| ***Legionella* spp.** | Respiratory |
| ***Listeria monocytogenes*** | Meninges (CNS) |
| ***Neisseria meningitidis*** | Meninges (CNS) |
| ***Pseudomonas aeruginosa*** | Wound, soft tissue, central nervous system |
| ***Salmonella enterica typhi*** | Small intestine, regional lymph nodes of the intestine, reticuloendothelial system |
| ***Streptococcus penumoniae*** | Meninges (CNS), respiratory |
| ***Streptococcus pyogenes*** | Wound, soft tissue |
| ***Staphylococcus aureus*** | Wound, soft tissue, meninges (CNS) |

proliferates, subsequently forming a biofilm. Uncommon routes of IV catheter–tip infection include contaminated fluids or blood-borne seeding from another infection site.

## Extravascular Infections

Except for intravascular infections, bacteria usually enter the circulation through the lymphatic system. Most cases of clinically significant bacteremia are a result of extravascular infection. When organisms multiply at a local site of infection such as the lung, they are drained by the lymphatics and reach the bloodstream. In most individuals, organisms in the bloodstream are effectively and rapidly removed by the reticuloendothelial system in the liver, spleen, and bone marrow and by circulating phagocytic cells. Depending on the extent of immunologic control of the infection, the organism may be circulated more widely, thereby causing a bacteremia or fungemia.

The most common portals of entry for bacteremia are the genitourinary tract (25%), respiratory tract (20%), abscesses (10%), surgical wound infections (5%), biliary tract (5%), miscellaneous sites (10%), and uncertain sites (25%). For the most part, the probability of bacteremia occurring from an extravascular site depends on the site of infection, its severity, and the organism. For example, any organism producing meningitis is likely to produce bacteremia at the same time. Of importance, certain organisms causing extravascular infections commonly invade the bloodstream; some of these organisms are listed in Table 68-1. In addition to these organisms, a large number of other bacteria and fungi that cause extravascular infections are also capable of invading the bloodstream. Whether these organisms invade the bloodstream depends on the host's ability to control the infection and the organism's pathogenic potential. Some of the organisms associated with potential bloodstream infections from a localized site include members of the family Enterobacteriaceae, *Streptococcus pneumoniae*, *Staphylococcus aureus*, *Neisseria gonorrhoeae*, anaerobic cocci, *Bacteroides*, *Clostridium*, beta-hemolytic streptococci, and *Pseudomonas*. These are only some of the organisms frequently isolated from blood. Almost every known bacterial species and many fungal species have been implicated in extravascular bloodstream infections.

## CLINICAL MANIFESTATIONS

As previously discussed, bacteremia may indicate the presence of a focus of disease, such as intravascular infection, pneumonia, or liver abscess, or it may represent transient release of bacteria into the bloodstream. Septicemia or sepsis indicates a condition in which bacteria or their products (toxins) are causing harm to the host. Unfortunately, clinicians often use the terms *bacteremia* and *septicemia* interchangeably. Signs and symptoms of septicemia may include fever or hypothermia (low body temperature), chills, hyperventilation (abnormally increased breathing leading to excess loss of carbon dioxide from the body) and subsequent respiratory alkalosis (a condition caused by the loss of acid leading to an increase in pH), skin lesions, change in mental status, and diarrhea. More serious manifestations include hypotension or shock, DIC, and major organ system failure. The syndrome known as septic shock, characterized by fever, acute respiratory distress, shock, renal failure, intravascular coagulation, and tissue destruction, can be initiated by either exotoxins or endotoxins. Septic shock is mediated by the production of cytokines from activated mononuclear cells, such as tumor necrosis factor and interleukins.

Shock is the gravest complication of septicemia. In septic shock, the presence of bacterial products and the host's response act to shut down major host physiologic systems. Clinical manifestations include a drop in blood pressure, increase in heart rate, functional impairment in vital organs (brain, kidney, liver, and lungs), acid-base alterations, and bleeding problems. Gram-negative bacteria contain a substance in their cell walls, called endotoxin, which has a strong effect on several physiologic functions. This substance, a lipopolysaccharide (LPS) comprising part of the cell wall structure (see Chapter 2), may be released during the normal growth cycles of bacteria or after the destruction of bacteria by host defenses. Endotoxin (or the core of the LPS, lipid A) has been shown to mediate numerous systemic reactions, including a febrile response, and the activation of complement and certain blood-clotting factors. Although gram-positive bacteria do not contain the lipid A endotoxin, many produce exotoxins, and the effects of their presence in the bloodstream may be equally devastating to the patient.

Disseminated intravascular coagulation (DIC) is a disastrous complication of sepsis. DIC is characterized by numerous small blood vessels becoming clogged with blood clots and bleeding as a result of the depletion of coagulation factors. DIC can occur with septicemia involving any circulating pathogen, including parasites, viruses, and fungi, although it is most often a consequence of gram-negative bacterial sepsis.

## IMMUNOCOMPROMISED PATIENTS

One of the greatest challenges facing microbiologists is the handling of blood cultures from immunocompromised patients. The number of immunocompromised patients has steadily increased in recent years in large part as the result of advances in medicine. People undergoing organ transplantation, elderly persons, individuals with malignant disease (e.g., malignancies and cancer), and those receiving therapy for the malignancy are examples of immunosuppressed patients. Acquired immunodeficiency syndrome (AIDS) has also contributed to the increase in the number of immunocompromised individuals. The marked immunosuppression brought about by infection with the human immunodeficiency virus (HIV) in patients with AIDS is a result of this virus' profound impairment of cellular immunity. Patients with AIDS have the greatest diversity of pathogens recovered from blood, including mycobacterial species, *Bartonella henselae*, *Corynebacterium jeikeium*, *Shigella flexneri*, unusual *Salmonella* species, *Histoplasma capsulatum*, *Cryptococcus neoformans*, and cytomegalovirus.

As is typically observed in other hospitalized patients, organisms such as gram-positive aerobic bacteria (e.g., *Staphylococcus aureus*, *Enterococcus*) and gram-negative aerobic bacteria (e.g., Enterobacteriaceae, *Pseudomonas aeruginosa*) are common causes of bloodstream infections in immunocompromised patients. In addition, bloodstream infections in immunocompromised patients are frequently caused by either unusual pathogens whose recovery from blood requires special techniques or by organisms normally considered contaminants when

isolated from blood cultures. Therefore, microbiologists must be aware of the potential pathogenicity of organisms in immunosuppressed patients that are typically considered as probable blood culture contaminants. Without this knowledge, aerobic gram-positive rods isolated from blood cultures may be dismissed as contaminating diphtheroids, when, in fact, the organism is *C. jeikeium*, known to cause bacteremia in immunosuppressed patients. Microbiologists must be familiar with the unusual pathogens isolated from blood cultures obtained from immunocompromised patients and organisms that require special techniques for isolation (some of the special considerations are covered later in this chapter).

## DETECTION OF BACTEREMIA

Mortality rates associated with bloodstream infection range from 20% to 50%. Because bacteremia frequently provides evidence of a life-threatening infection, the prompt detection and recovery of microorganisms from blood is of paramount importance.

To detect bloodstream infections, a patient's blood must be obtained by aseptic venipuncture and then incubated in culture media. Bacterial growth can be detected using techniques ranging from manual to totally automated methods. Once growth is detected, the organism is isolated, identified, and if considered pathogenic or treatment is necessary for the patient, the organism is then tested for susceptibility to various antimicrobial agents.

### SPECIMEN COLLECTION
#### Preparation of the Site
Because blood culture media have been developed as enrichment broths to encourage the multiplication of as few as a single organism, these media will enhance growth of contaminating organisms, including a normal inhabitant of human skin. Therefore, careful skin preparation before collecting the blood sample is of paramount importance to reduce the risk of introducing contaminants into blood culture media.

The vein from which the blood is to be drawn must be chosen before the skin is disinfected. If a patient has an existing IV line, the blood should be drawn below the existing line; blood drawn above the line will be diluted with fluid being infused. It is less desirable to draw blood through a vascular shunt or catheter, because these prosthetic devices are difficult to decontaminate completely.

**Antisepsis.** Once a vein is selected, the skin site is defatted (fat removal) with 70% isopropyl alcohol and an antiseptic is applied to kill surface and subsurface bacteria. Regardless of the antiseptic used, it is critical to follow the manufacturer's recommendation for the length of time the antiseptic is allowed to remain on the skin. Available data indicate that iodine tincture (iodine in alcohol) and chlorhexidine are equivalent for skin preparation before drawing blood cultures. The steps necessary for drawing blood for culture are given in Procedure 68-1, which can be found on the Evolve site.

As part of ongoing quality assurance, laboratories should determine the rate of blood culture contamination by clinically evaluating patients' conditions in conjunction with the organism isolated from culture. Laboratories that recover contaminants at rates greater than 3% should suspect improper phlebotomy techniques and should institute measures to educate the phlebotomists in proper skin preparation methods.

**Precautions.** Standard precautions require that phlebotomists wear gloves for blood drawing. Because blood for culture must be obtained aseptically, it is important that contaminated surfaces that might come in contact with the disinfected venipuncture site be disinfected. For example, if the site must be touched after preparation, the phlebotomist must disinfect the gloved fingers used for palpation. Also, if the rubber stopper or septum of the container into which blood is to be inoculated (e.g., test tubes or commercial culture bottles) is potentially contaminated, the phlebotomist must disinfect the septum.

## Specimen Volume

**Adults.** For many years, it has been recognized that most bacteremias in adults have a low number of colony-forming units (CFU) per milliliter (mL) of blood. For example, in several studies, fewer than 30 CFU per mL of blood were commonly found in patients with clinically significant bacteremia. Therefore, a sufficient sample volume is critical for the successful detection of bacteremia.

There is a direct relationship between the volume of blood and an increased probability that the laboratory will isolate the infecting the organism. Therefore, collection of two sets of cultures using 10 to 20 mL of blood per culture is strongly recommended for adults. To illustrate, Cockerill and colleagues reported that in patients without infective endocarditis, volumes of 20 mL increased the yield, identification of the organism, by 30% compared with 10-mL volumes. Unfortunately, a study confirmed that it is common practice to under inoculate blood culture bottles; findings from this study suggested that the yield increases by 3.2% for each milliliter of blood cultured.

**Children.** It is not safe to take large samples of blood from children, particularly infants. The optimal volume of blood required for successful identification of organisms from infants and children has not been clearly delineated. Similar to adults, this patient population has low level (small numbers of organisms) bacteremia. In light of low-level bacteremia in infants and children and based on the premise that it is safe to obtain as much as 4% to 4.5% of a patient's known total blood volume for culture and the relationship between blood volume and patient weight, Baron and colleagues have determined recommendations for blood volumes for cultures from infants and children (Table 68-2). For infants and small children, only 1 to 5 mL of blood should be drawn for bacterial culture. Blood culture bottles are available designed specifically for the pediatric patient. Because blood specimens from septic children may yield fewer than 5 CFU/mL of the organism, quantities less than 1 mL may not be adequate to detect pathogens. Nevertheless, smaller volumes should still be cultured because high levels of bacteremia (more than 1000 CFU/mL of blood) are detected in some infants.

## Number of Blood Cultures

Because periodicity of microorganisms in the bloodstream may be characteristic for some diseases, continuous for some and random in others, patterns of bacteremia must be considered in establishing standards for the timing and number of blood cultures. If the volume of blood is adequate, usually two or three blood cultures are sufficient to achieve the optimum blood culture sensitivity. In patients with endocarditis who have not received antibiotics, a single blood culture is positive in 90% to 95% of the cases, whereas a second blood culture establishes the diagnosis in at least 98% of patients, depending on the study. For patients who have received prior antibiotic therapy, three separate blood collections of 16 to 20 mL each, and an additional blood culture or two taken on the second day, if necessary, detects most etiologic agents of endocarditis. This presumes use of a culture system adequate for growth of the

**TABLE 68-2** Suggested Blood Volumes for Cultures from Infants and Children

| WEIGHT OF PATIENT | | Total Blood Volume (mL) | RECOMMENDED VOLUME OF BLOOD FOR CULTURE (mL) | | | % of Total Blood Volume |
|---|---|---|---|---|---|---|
| kg | lb | | Culture No. 1 | Culture No. 2 | Total Volume for Culture (mL) | |
| ≤1 | ≤2.2 | 50-99 | 2 | | 2 | 4 |
| 1.1-2 | 2.2-4.4 | 100-200 | 2 | 2 | 4 | 4 |
| 2.1-12.7 | 4.5-27 | >200 | 4 | 2 | 6 | 3 |
| 12.8-36.3 | 28-80 | >800 | 10 | 10 | 20 | 2.5 |
| >36.3 | >80 | >2200 | 20-30 | 20-30 | 40-60 | 1.8-2.7 |

From Baron EJ, Weinstein MP, Dunne WM, et al: Blood cultures IV. In Baron EJ, coordinating editor, *Cumitech 1C,* Washington, DC, 2005, American Society for Microbiology, reprinted with permission.
Note: Volumes and recommendations may vary based on automated system and manufacturer's guidelines.

organism involved, which often entails extending the incubation period. Similarly, for patients without infective endocarditis, 65.1% are detected in the first culture, 80% by the first two cultures, and 95.7% were detected in the first three blood cultures.

### Timing of Collection

The timing of cultures is not as important as other factors in patients with intravascular infections because organisms are released into the bloodstream at a fairly constant rate. Because the timing of intermittent bacteremia is unpredictable, it is generally accepted that two or three blood cultures be spaced an hour apart. However, a study found no significant difference in the yield between multiple blood cultures obtained simultaneously or those obtained at intervals. The authors concluded that the overall volume of blood cultured was more critical to increasing organism yield than timing.

When a patient's condition requires therapy to be initiated as rapidly as possible, little time is available to collect multiple blood culture samples over a timed interval. An acceptable compromise is to collect 40 mL of blood at one time, 20 mL from each of two separate venipuncture sites, using two separate needles and syringes before the patient is given antimicrobial therapy. Regardless, blood should be transported immediately to the laboratory and placed into the incubator or instrument as soon as possible. With blood culture instrumentation, a delay beyond 2 hours can delay the detection of positive cultures.

### Miscellaneous Matters

**Anticoagulation.** Blood drawn for culture must not be allowed to clot. If bacteria become entrapped within a clot, their presence may go undetected. Thus, blood drawn for culture may be either inoculated directly into the blood culture broth media or into a sterile blood collection tube containing an anticoagulant for transport to the laboratory for subsequent inoculation. Heparin, ethylenediaminetetraacetic acid (EDTA), and citrate inhibit numerous organisms and are not recommended for use. Sodium polyanethol sulfonate (SPS, Liquoid) in concentrations of 0.025% to 0.03% is the best anticoagulant available for blood cultures. As a result, the most commonly used preparation in blood culture media today is 0.025% to 0.05% SPS. In addition to its anticoagulant properties, SPS is also anticomplementary and antiphagocytic, and interferes with the activity of some antimicrobial agents, notably aminoglycosides. SPS, however, may inhibit the growth of a few microorganisms, such as some strains of *Neisseria* spp., *Gardnerella vaginalis*, *Streptobacillus moniliformis*, and all strains of *Peptostreptococcus anaerobius*. Because of the inhibitory effect of SPS on some organisms in conjunction with the necessity for an additional step to transfer the blood to the ultimate culture bottles that increases the risk of exposure to blood-borne pathogens as well as contamination, using collection tubes instead of direct inoculation into culture bottles may compromise organism recovery. For these reasons, the use of intermediate collection tubes is discouraged. Although the addition of 1.2% gelatin has been shown to counteract the

inhibitory action of SPS, the recovery of other organisms decreases.

**Dilution.**   In addition to the volume of blood collected and type of medium chosen, the dilution factor for the blood in the medium must be considered. To conserve space and materials, it is desirable to combine the largest feasible amount of blood from the patient (usually 10 mL) with the smallest amount of medium that will still encourage the growth of bacteria and dilute out or inactivate the antibacterial components of the blood. Traditionally, a 1:10 ratio of blood to medium was required for successful bacterial growth; however, several new commercial media containing resins or other additives have demonstrated enhanced recover with as low as a 1:5 ratio. For this purpose, a 1:5 ratio of blood to unmodified medium has been found to be adequate in conventional blood cultures. All commercial blood culture systems (discussed later in this chapter) specify the appropriate dilution.

**Blood Culture Media.**   The diversity of bacteria recovered from blood requires an equally diverse and large number of media to enhance the growth of these bacteria. Basic blood culture media contain a nutrient broth and an anticoagulant. Several different broth formulations are commercially available. Most blood culture bottles available commercially contain trypticase soy broth, brain-heart infusion broth, supplemented peptone, or thioglycolate broth. More specialized broth bases include Columbia or Brucella broth.

## TYPES OF BLOOD CULTURE BOTTLE

The addition of penicillinase to blood culture media for inactivation of penicillin has been largely superseded in recent years by the availability of a resin-containing medium that inactivates most antibiotics nonselectively by adsorbing them to the surface of the resin particles. Resin-containing media may enhance isolation of staphylococci, particularly when patients are receiving bacteriostatic drugs. The BACTEC system (Becton Dickinson Microbiology Systems, Sparks, Maryland) offers several resin-containing media. In addition to resin-containing media, BacT/ALERT has a blood culture bottle with supplemented brain heart infusion (BHI) broth containing activated charcoal particles that significantly increase the yield of microorganisms over standard blood culture media. In addition, resins or charcoal may be added to commercial media to absorb and inactivate antimicrobial agents within the patient's blood. Care should be exercised when interpreting gram stains from resin- and charcoal-containing bottles. The additives may be confused with gram-positive organisms.

In general, each blood culture set includes a blood culture bottle designated for aerobic recovery and one for anaerobic recovery of bacteria. Because of the decline in the late 1990s in the proportion of positive blood cultures yielding anaerobic bacteria coupled with the increasing pressure for laboratories to be cost effective, some investigators have recommended laboratories discard this routine practice of processing all blood samples aerobically and anaerobically. It has been proposed that anaerobic cultures should be selectively performed and, in place of the anaerobic blood culture, a second aerobic bottle be included. Because this is a controversial proposal, laboratories must deal with conflicting recommendations as they attempt to provide clinically useful blood culture results. Also, depending on the patient population served by the laboratory, numbers of blood cultures submitted, and personnel and financial resources, the laboratory may have one or more methods available to ensure detection of the broadest range of organisms in the least possible time.

## CULTURE TECHNIQUES

Special blood culture broth systems are available for the isolation of mycobacteria. The systems are useful in detecting disseminated infections caused by Mycobacterium tuberculosis and non-tuberculosis mycobacteria.

### Conventional Blood Cultures

**Incubation Conditions.**  The atmosphere in commercially prepared blood culture bottles is usually at a low oxidation-reduction potential, permitting the growth of most facultative and some anaerobic organisms. To encourage the growth of obligate (strict) aerobes, such as yeast and *Pseudomonas aeruginosa*, transient venting of the bottles with a sterile, cotton-plugged needle may be necessary. Constant agitation of the bottles during the first 24 hours of incubation also enhances the growth of most aerobic bacteria.

### Self-Contained Subculture System

A modification of the biphasic blood culture medium is the BD Septi-Chek system (Becton Dickinson Microbiology Systems, Sparks, Maryland) (Figure 68-4) consisting of a conventional blood culture broth bottle with an attached chamber containing a slide coated with agar or several types of agars. Special media for isolation of fungi and mycobacteria are also available. To subculture, the entire broth contents are allowed to contact the agar surface by inverting the bottle, a simple procedure that does not require opening the bottle or using needles. The large volume of broth subcultured and the enclosed method provide faster detection for many organisms than is possible with conventional systems. The Septi-Chek system appears to enhance the recovery of *Streptococcus pneumoniae*, but such biphasic systems do not efficiently recover anaerobic isolates.

### Lysis Centrifugation

The Isolator (Alere, Waltham, MA) is a lysis centrifugation system commercially available. The Isolator consists of a stoppered tube containing saponin to lyse blood cells and SPS as an anticoagulant (Figure 68-5). After centrifugation, the supernatant is discarded, the sediment containing the pathogen is vigorously vortexed, and the entire sediment is plated to solid agar. Benefits of this system include rapid and improved recovery of filamentous fungi, the presence of actual colonies for direct identification and susceptibility testing after initial incubation, the ability to quantify the colony-forming units present in the blood, rapid detection of polymicrobial bacteremia, dispensing with the need for a separate antibiotic-removal step, the ability to choose special

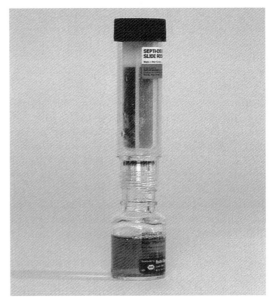

**Figure 68-4** Becton Dickinson Septi-Chek pediatric-size biphasic blood culture bottle. The medium-containing base bottle is inoculated with blood, and the top piece containing agar paddles is added in the laboratory. The agar is inoculated by tipping the bottle to allow the blood-containing medium to flow over the agar.

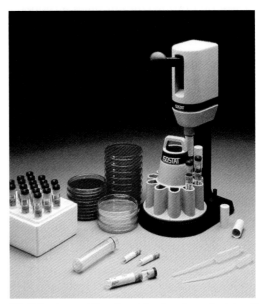

**Figure 68-5** Lysis centrifugation blood culture (Isolator System, Alere, Waltham, MA) uses vacuum-draw collection tubes with a lysing agent and special apparatus (Isostat Press) to facilitate removal of the supernatant without use of needles. (Courtesy Wampole Laboratories, Cranbury, NJ.)

media for initial culture setup based on clinical impression (e.g., direct plating onto media supportive of *Legionella* spp. or *Mycobacterium* spp.), and potential enhanced recovery of intracellular microorganisms caused by lysis of host cells. Possible limitations of the system seem to be a relatively high rate of plate contamination and a decreased ability to detect certain bacteria, such as *Streptococcus pneumoniae, Listeria monocytogenes, Haemophilus influenzae,* and anaerobic bacteria, compared with conventional systems. If a mixed infection is suspected, an additional blood culture collection tube should be inoculated simultaneously.

### Instrument-Based Systems

Conventional blood culture techniques are labor intensive and time consuming. During these times of cost constraints in health care and a corresponding requirement for clinically relevant care, the development of improved instrumentation for blood cultures was needed. Instruments are capable of rapid and accurate detection of organisms in blood specimens. By using newer instrumentation, laboratories processing a large volume of blood cultures can also provide results cost effectively.

**BACTEC Systems.** Many laboratories use the BACTEC system (Becton Dickinson Microbiology Systems, Sparks, Maryland), which measures the production of carbon dioxide ($CO_2$) by metabolizing organisms. Blood or sterile body fluid for routine culture is inoculated into bottles containing appropriate substrates.

The first BACTEC systems were semiautomated. Vials, containing 14C-labeled substrates (glucose, amino acids, and alcohols) were incubated and often agitated on a rotary shaker. At predetermined time intervals thereafter, the bottles were placed into the monitoring module, where they were automatically moved to a detector. The detector inserted two needles through a rubber septum seal at the top of each bottle and withdrew the accumulated gas above the liquid medium and replaced it with fresh gas of the same mixture (aerobic or anaerobic). Any amount of radiolabeled $CO_2$, the final end product of metabolism of the 14C-labeled substrates (above a preset baseline level), was considered to be suspicious for microbial growth. Microbiologists retrieved suspicious bottles and worked them up (performed subcultured and identification procedures) for possible microbial growth.

Subsequent modifications further automated the incubation and measuring device, and detection was accomplished by nonradioactive means. The BACTEC blood culture systems are fully automated with the incubator, shaker, and detector all in one instrument. These fully automated blood culture systems use fluorescence to measure $CO_2$ released by organisms; a gas-permeable fluorescent sensor is on the bottom of each vial (Figure 68-6). As $CO_2$ diffuses into the sensor and dissolves in water present in the sensor matrix, hydrogen (H+) ions are generated. These H+ ions cause a decrease in pH, which, in turn, increases the fluorescent output of the sensor. There is continuous monitoring of each bottle and detection is external to the bottle. Of importance, the noninvasion of the blood culture bottle eliminates the potential for cross-contamination of cultures.

**BacT/ALERT Microbial Detection System.** Other laboratories use the BacT/Alert System (bioMérieux, Durham, North Carolina), which measures $CO_2$-derived pH changes with a colorimetric sensor in the bottom of each bottle (see Figure 68-6). The sensor is separated from the broth medium by a membrane permeable to $CO_2$. As organisms grow, they release $CO_2$, which diffuses across the membrane and is dissolved in water present in the matrix of the sensor. As $CO_2$ is dissolved, free hydrogen ions are generated. These free hydrogen ions cause a color change in the sensor (blue to light green to yellow as the pH decreases); a sensor in the instrument reads this color change.

**Versa TREK System.** The Versa TREK system (Thermo Scientific, TREK Diagnostics, Cleveland, Ohio) utilizes a unique agitation system during blood culture inoculation. The aerobic media bottles each contain a small magnetic stir bar enhancing oxygenation during incubation. Like the other systems, this is also a continuously monitoring instrument. Table 68-3 summarizes characteristics of some blood culture instruments that are available at the time of printing of the text.

### Techniques to Detect IV Catheter–Associated Infections

The insertion of an IV catheter during hospitalization is common practice. Infection, either locally at the catheter insertion site or sepsis, caused by bacteremia, is one of the most common complications of catheter placement. Because the skin of all patients is colonized with microorganisms that are also common pathogens in catheters, techniques used to diagnose catheter-related infections attempt to quantitate bacterial growth. Diagnosis of an IV catheter–related bacteremia (or fungemia) is difficult, because there are often no signs of infection at the catheter insertion site and the typical signs and symptoms of sepsis can overlap with other clinical manifestations; even the finding of a positive blood culture does not identify the catheter as the source. To date, various methods, such as semiquantitative cultures, Gram stains of the skin entry site, and culture of IV catheter tips following catheter removal. The terminal end of the IV catheter is removed and rolled several times across a blood agar plate. The tip is then removed from the agar plate and placed in enrichment broth. Both the plate and enrichment broth are incubated at 37° C for 18 to 24 hours. Following inoculation, the blood agar plates are examined, and any isolates are identified according to the laboratory protocol. The enrichment broth may be subcultured to blood agar and anaerobic media for further analysis and potential detection of intraluminal colonization. Many methods involve some type of quantitation in an attempt to differentiate colonization of the catheter from probable infection. Two major approaches to the diagnosis of catheter-related infection (CRI) in which the catheter remains in place are based on the premise that a greater number of organisms will be present in the intravascular catheter compared to the number found in blood specimens obtained from distant peripheral veins. The first approach, differential quantitative cultures, involves drawing two blood cultures—one from a peripheral site and the other from the suspected infected line. Quantitative cultures are processed for each specimen by inoculating the same volume of blood to standard microbiology media and colonies counted the following day. A colony count ratio greater than 4 to 10:1 between the central venous blood and a peripheral blood specimen indicates a probable CRI with a sensitivity of 78% to 94% and a specificity of 99% to 100%. The second approach involves the comparison of the differential time to positivity of blood specimens obtained from a peripheral and

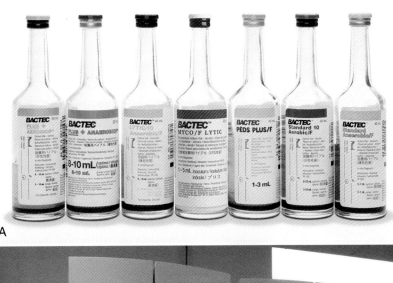

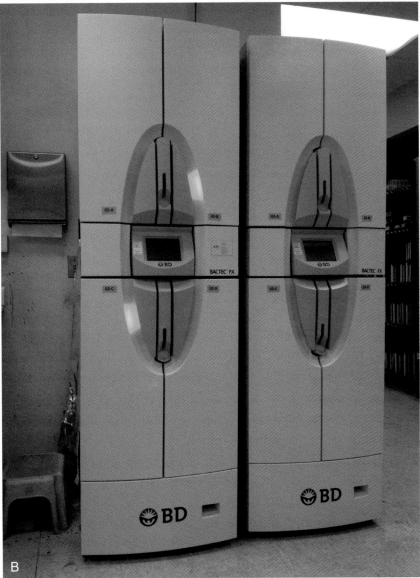

**Figure 68-6 A,** Blood culture bottles for the BACTEC 9240, 9120, and 9050 continuous monitoring instruments. **B,** The BD BACTEC FX continuous monitoring blood culture system.

*Continued*

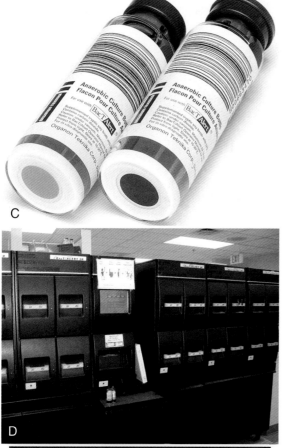

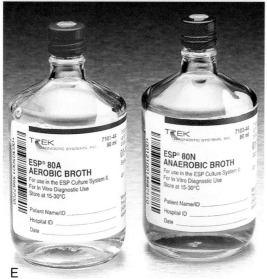

**Figure 68-6, cont'd**   **C,** Blood culture bottles for the BacT/Alert continuous monitoring blood culture instruments. **D,** The BacT/Alert continuous monitoring blood culture system. **E,** Blood culture bottles for Trek Diagnostic Systems, Inc., ESP Culture System II continuous monitoring instrument. (**A** courtesy Becton Dickinson Microbiology Systems, Sparks, Md; BACTEC is a trademark of Becton Dickinson Microbiology Systems. **B** courtesy steven D. Dallas, PhD, UT Health Science Center San Antonio, San Antonio, Texas. **C** courtesy bioMérieux, Durham, NC. **D** courtesy of Stacie Lansink, Sioux Falls, SD. **E** courtesy Trek Diagnostic Systems, Inc., Cleveland, Ohio.)

intravascular site; a differential time to positivity greater than 2 hours between bottles inoculated with blood from the catheter and those from a peripheral vein indicates a probable CRI. Unfortunately, no single method has demonstrated a clear clinical benefit in diagnosing CRI, and the debate remains unsettled.

### Handling Positive Blood Cultures

Most laboratories use a broth-based automated blood culture method. When a positive culture is indicated according to the automated detection system, a Gram-stained smear of an air-dried drop of medium should be performed. Methanol fixation of the smear preserves bacterial and cellular morphology, which may be especially valuable for detecting gram-negative bacteria among red cell debris. Designed to maximize sensitivity, detection algorithms of automated blood culture instruments lead to a certain percentage of false-positive results. Thus, in addition to performance of a Gram stain using methanol fixation, acridine orange (AO) staining is also useful for those blood culture bottles flagged by the instrument as positive but Gram stain-negative for organisms. Adler and colleagues found that AO staining proved particularly helpful in the early detection of candidemia—one third of all microorganisms missed by Gram stain of instrument-positive bottles were yeasts detected by AO staining. As soon as a morphologic description can be tentatively assigned to an organism detected in blood, the physician should be contacted and given all available information. Determining the clinical significance of an isolate is the physician's responsibility. If no organisms are seen on microscopic examination of a bottle that appears positive, subcultures should be performed anyway.

Subcultures from blood cultures suspected of being positive, whether proved by microscopic visualization or not, should be made to various media that would support the growth of most bacteria, including anaerobes. Initial subculture may include chocolate agar, 5% sheep blood agar, MacConkey agar (if gram-negative bacteria are seen), and supplemented anaerobic blood agar. In addition, some laboratories are subculturing to specialized chromogenic agar for the isolation of specific pathogenic organisms such as MNSA, yeast (*Candida* spp.). The incidence of polymicrobial bacteremia or fungemia ranges from 3% to 20% of all positive blood cultures. For this reason, samples must be resubcultured for isolated colonies.

Numerous rapid tests for identification and presumptive antimicrobial susceptibilities can be performed from the broth blood culture if a monomicrobic infection is suspected (based on microscopic evaluation). A suspension of the organism that approximates the turbidity of a 0.5 McFarland standard, obtained directly from the broth or by centrifuging the broth and resuspending the pelleted bacteria, can be used to perform either disk diffusion (qualitative) or broth dilution (quantitative) antimicrobial susceptibility tests. These suspensions may also be used to perform preliminary tests such as coagulase, thermostable nuclease, esculin hydrolysis, bile solubility, antigen detection by fluorescent-antibody stain or agglutination procedures for gram-positive bacteria, oxidase,

**TABLE 68-3** Summary Characteristics of the More Commonly Used Continuous-Monitoring Blood Culture Systems

| System | Bottles Available* | Inoculum Volume (mL)** | Blood: Broth | Detection |
|--------|-------------------|------------------------|--------------|-----------|
| BacT/ALERT | SA Aerobic | 5-10 | 1:4 | Colorimetric detection of $CO_2$ |
| | SN Anaerobic | 5-10 | 1:4 | |
| | FA, FN (aerobic and anaerobic bottles) | 5-10 | 1:4 | |
| | PF Pediatric | 1-4 | 1:5 | |
| | MB (mycobacteria whole blood) | 0.50 | ~1:5 | |
| | MP (mycobacteria processed specimen or body fluid other than blood) | 0.50 | — | |
| BACTEC | Standard aerobic/F | 8-10 | 1:4 | Fluorescent detection of $CO_2$ |
| | Standard anaerobic/F | 5-7 | 1:4 | |
| | Plus aerobic/F | 8-10 | 1:2.5 | |
| | Plus anaerobic/F | 5-7 | 1:2.5 | |
| | Peds Plus/F | 0.5-5 | 1:8 | |
| | Lytic/10 anaerobic/F | 8-10 | 1:4 | |
| | Myco/F Lytic medium (for fungi and mycobacteria) | 1-5 | 1:8 | |
| VersaTREK | REDOX (aerobic) | 10 | 1:9 | Detection of $O_2$ consumption and/or $CO_2$, $H_2$, and/or $N_2$ production |
| | REDOX (anaerobic) | 10 | 1:9 | |
| | EZ Draw REDOX 1 aerobic | 5 | 1:9 | |
| | EZ Draw REDOX 2 anaerobic | 5 | 1:9 | |

*No venting required on any bottles listed.
**Minimum sample volumes. Increased volume will enhance the recovery of the organisms.
NOTE: Due to the modular design of automated blood culture systems, various models and arrangements of modular units provide a customized specimen capacity to suit the laboratories needs.

and commercially available rapid identification kits for gram-negative bacteria. Presumptive results must be verified with conventional procedures using pure cultures. In addition to these approaches, the introduction of a number of molecular methods, including conventional and peptide nucleic acid hybridization assays using specific probes, conventional and real-time polymerase chain reaction assays and microarrays have been used to directly identify microorganisms in blood culture bottles.

In the event of possible future studies (e.g., additional susceptibility testing), all isolates from blood cultures should be stored for a minimum of 6 months by freezing at −70°C in 10% skim milk. A commercial preservation system, Microbank beads, is available for the preservation and storage or bacterial and fungal isolates (Pro-Lab Diagnostics, Austin, Texas). The vials contain pretreated beads and a cryopreservative solution that improves storage of microorganisms. Storing an agar slant of the isolate under sterile mineral oil at room temperature is a good alternative to freezing. It is often necessary to compare separate isolates from the same patient or isolates of the same species from different patients months after the bacteria were isolated.

### Interpretation of Blood Culture Results

Because of the increasing incidence of blood/vascular infection caused by bacteria normally considered avirulent, indigenous microflora of a healthy human host, interpretation of the significance of growth of such bacteria in blood cultures has become increasingly difficult. On one hand, contaminants may lead to unnecessary antibiotic therapy, additional testing and consultation, and increased length of hospital stay. Costs related to false-positive blood culture results (i.e., contaminants) are associated with 40% higher charges for IV antibiotics and microbiology testing. On the other hand, failure to recognize and appropriately treat indigenous microflora can have dire consequences. Guidelines that can assist in distinguishing probable pathogens from contaminants are as follows:

- Probable contaminant
  - Growth of *Bacillus* spp., *Corynebacterium* spp., *Propionibacterium acnes*, or coagulase-negative staphylococci in one of several cultures

Note: *Bacillus anthracis* must be ruled out before dismissing *Bacillus* species as a probable contaminant.

  - Growth of multiple organisms from one of several cultures (polymicrobial bacteremia is uncommon)
  - The clinical presentation or course is not consistent with sepsis (physician-based, not laboratory-based criteria)
  - The organism causing the infection at a primary site of infection is not the same as that isolated from the blood culture

- Probable pathogen
  - Growth of the same organism in repeated cultures obtained either at different times or from different anatomic sites
  - Growth of certain organisms in cultures obtained from patients suspected of endocarditis, such as enterococci, or gram-negative rods in patients with clinical gram-negative sepsis
  - Growth of certain organisms such as members of Enterobacteriaceae, *Streptococcus pneumoniae*, gram-negative anaerobes, and *Streptococcus pyogenes*
  - Isolation of commensal microbial flora from blood cultures obtained from patients suspected to be bacteremic (e.g., immunosuppressed patients or those having prosthetic devices)

# SPECIAL CONSIDERATIONS FOR OTHER RELEVANT ORGANISMS ISOLATED FROM BLOOD

The organisms discussed in this section require somewhat different conditions for their successful recovery from blood culture samples. Most of these organisms are infrequently isolated from blood. Therefore, it is important for the physician to notify the laboratory of remarkable patient history, such as travel abroad. In light of recent events and concerns about bioterrorism, it is also important the laboratory be aware of organisms isolated from blood cultures that are considered potential agents for bioterrorist attacks. These bacteria include *Bacillus anthracis*, *Francisella tularensis*, *Brucella* spp., and *Yersinia pestis*. Finally, in addition to the organisms discussed later that require special different conditions for isolation from blood, a number of organisms are unable to grow on artificial media and are best diagnosed by alternative methods such as serology or molecular amplification assays; these organisms are listed in Box 68-4.

## HACEK (AACEK) BACTERIA

As mentioned earlier in the chapter, the term HACEK refers to a group of fastidious, gram-negative bacilli including *Aggregatibacter aphrophilus*, *Actinobacillus actinomycetemcomitans*, *Cardiobacterium hominis*, *Eikenella corrodens*, and *Kingella kingae*. Recovery of these organisms from blood cultures is usually associated with infective

---

**BOX 68-4** Microorganisms That Cause Bloodstream Infections but Do Not Grow on Artificial Media

*Coxiella burnetii*
*Chlamydophila* spp. (*C. pneumoniae* and *C. psittaci*)
*Rickettsia* spp.
*Tropheryma whippelii*

---

endocarditis. Other fastidious organisms, such as *Capnocytophaga* spp., *Rothia dentocariosa*, *Flavobacterium* spp., and *Chromobacterium* spp., may also be isolated from blood cultures. In the past, if the clinician suspected any of these organisms, the laboratory held the blood cultures for an extended period beyond the first week and made blind subcultures to several enriched media, including more supportive media such as buffered charcoal-yeast extract. However, recent studies using continuous monitoring blood culture systems have indicated that almost all bloodstream infections, including endocarditis, were detected within 5 days of incubation.

## CAMPYLOBACTER AND HELICOBACTER

Several species of *Campylobacter* and *Helicobacter* are occasionally isolated from blood cultures, usually growing within the 5-day incubation protocol. However, these organisms are small, thin, curved, gram-negative rods, which may only be visualized using an AO stain following detection by continuous monitoring instruments. Because of the fastidious nature of these organisms, appropriate media and atmospheric conditions for subculture from blood culture bottles must be employed (see Chapter 34).

## FUNGI

Even though all disseminated fungal disease is preceded by fungemia, only recently have the microorganisms been recovered from blood cultures. One reason for this may be that cultures were not often collected during the fungemia stage, because clinical symptoms had not yet developed. However, introduction of better methods for isolating fungi from blood, including the lysis centrifugation system, has resulted in greater recovery of fungi from peripheral blood and greater physician awareness to order fungal blood cultures.

Many fungi, particularly yeast, can be recovered in standard blood culture media, if the bottle is incubated at the appropriate temperature and has been vented and agitated to allow sufficient oxygenation for fungal growth. However, some fungi may grow slowly and poorly in these media, which best support bacterial growth. Optimal isolation of fungi in blood cultures is achieved with either agitated incubation of a commercial biphasic system, such as the Septi-Chek, or by using the lysis centrifugation system. Manufacturers of media for automated blood culture systems have developed specific media for fungal isolation. These new formulas have dramatically increased the numbers of fungi isolated from patients with fungemia and have shortened the incubation time required for detection of the fungi. Blood specimens for detecting fungemia are collected in the same manner as for bacterial culture.

## MYCOBACTERIA

Patients with HIV infection can have disseminated infection with species of nontuberculous mycobacteria, predominantly *Mycobacterium avium* complex. Isolation of *M. tuberculosis* from the blood of these patients also occurs; as many as 42% of HIV-positive patients with tuberculosis have positive blood cultures.

In the past, the use of special media was recommended, such as Middlebrook 7H9 broth with 0.05% SPS or brain-heart infusion broth with 0.5% polysorbate 80, with or without a Middlebrook 7H11 agar slant. However, newer methods of detection have increased sensitivity in the ability to detect mycobacteria present in blood specimens and have significantly shortened the time required for mycobacterial blood cultures to become positive.

## BRUCELLA

Brucellosis is a common disease in many developing countries but is uncommon in developed countries. Because brucellosis may be included in the differential diagnosis of many infections, microbiologists should be prepared to process blood cultures suspected of having Brucella; blood cultures are positive in 70% to 90% of patients with brucellosis. Septicemia occurs primarily during the first 3 weeks of illness. Special handling may be required for recovering *Brucella* spp. from blood because these organisms are fastidious, often slow-growing, intracellular parasites. Best recovery is obtained with Brucella or trypticase soy broth. The use of biphasic media may enhance growth, or the Isolator system may allow release of intracellular bacteria.

The use of continuous monitoring systems has enhanced recovery of *Brucella* spp. For example, the use of the BACTEC instruments makes possible the diagnosis of more than 95% of positive cultures within a 5-day period without routine subcultures of negative vials.

## SPIROCHETES

### Borrelia

Visualization in direct preparations is diagnostic for 70% in cases of relapsing fever, a febrile disease caused by *Borrelia recurrentis*. Organisms may be seen in direct wet preparations of a drop of anticoagulated blood diluted in saline as long, thin, unevenly coiled spirochetes that seem to push the red blood cells around as they move. Thick and thin smears of blood, prepared as for malaria testing and stained with Wright's or Giemsa stain, are also sensitive for the detection of *Borrelia*.

### Leptospira

Leptospirosis can be diagnosed by isolating the causative spirochete from blood during the first 4 to 7 days of illness. Leptospires will grow 1 to 3 cm below the surface, usually within 2 weeks. The organisms remain viable in blood with SPS for 11 days, allowing for transport of specimens from distant locations. Direct dark-field examination of peripheral blood is not recommended because many artifacts are present that resemble spirochetes. If blood must be shipped to a reference laboratory for culture, blood may be collected into heparin, oxalate, or citrate tubes

and maintained at ambient temperature. One to two drops of blood are inoculated into semi-solid oleic acid-albumin medium at the patient's bedside. Various commercial mediums are available, such as Fletcher's medium (BD Diagnostics, Sparks, MD). Multiple cultures are recommended to improve recovery of the organisms. Due to the organism's failure to grow in conventional blood culture systems, molecular assays may improve detection of the organism, as well as the use of serological markers for rapid diagnosis. (Further information about *Borrelia* and *Leptospira* is provided in Chapter 46.)

## VITAMIN B6-DEPENDENT STREPTOCOCCI

*Granulicatella* spp. and *Abiotrophia* spp. are unable to multiply without the addition of 0.001% pyridoxal hydrochloride (also called thiol or vitamin B6). These streptococci are known as "nutritionally variant" or "satelliting" streptococci and have been associated with bacteremia and endocarditis. Although human blood introduced into the blood culture medium provides enough of the pyridoxal to allow the organisms to multiply in the bottle, standard sheep blood agar plates may not support their growth. Subculturing the broth to a 5% sheep blood agar plate and either overlaying a streak of *Staphylococcus aureus* or dropping a pyridoxal disk to produce the supplement generally demonstrates colonies of the streptococci growing as tiny satellites next to the streak. Some commercial media may be supplemented with enough pyridoxal (0.001%) to support growth of nutritionally variant streptococci.

## MYCOPLASMA HOMINIS

*Mycoplasma hominis* can be recovered during postabortal or postpartum fever, following gynecologic or urologic procedures, or in patients who were immunocompromised. Isolates can be recovered from manual and automated blood culture systems. However, because so few clinical isolates have been recovered to date, it has not been determined which blood culture system is optimal for recovering *M. hominis*. Although some studies report that *M. hominis* can produce sufficient $CO_2$ to be detected by instrumentation, the majority of isolates have been recovered only by subculture; in some cases, 7 days of incubation were required before growth was detected. It should be noted that *M. hominis* should be suspected if there are colonies on subculture yet no organisms seen on Gram stain. Thus, if *M. hominis* bacteremia is suspected, routine blind and terminal subcultures to special media to support the growth of *M. hominis* (e.g., arginine broth) and at least 7 days of incubation are recommended.

## BARTONELLA

Based on phenotypic and genotypic characteristics, bacteria of the genus *Rochalimaea* were reclassified into the genus *Bartonella*. *Bartonella* previously contained only a single species, *B. bacilliformis*, the agent of verruga peruana and a septicemic, hemolytic disease known as Oroya fever (see Chapter 33). New species such as *Bartonella henselae* and *B. elizabethae*, as well as *Bartonella quintana*, have been reported to cause bacteremia and endocarditis in both immunocompetent and immunocompromised patients. *B. henselae* has also been linked to cat-scratch disease, a common infectious disease in the United States. Cat-scratch disease is characterized by a persistent necrotizing inflammation of the lymph nodes. For the most part, the most reliable method for diagnosis of *Bartonella bacteremia* is serology.

Because experience in successful primary isolation of *Bartonella* from blood using either broth-based or biphasic blood culture systems is limited to date, use of the Isolator system was historically recommended. Of importance, use of the Isolator overrides the inhibition of *B. henselae* growth by SPS concentrations present in broth-based systems. Acridine orange, DNA staining, and blind subculture from negative bottles may improve the identification. Newer approaches using specialized pre-enrichment media (e.g., alphaproteobacteria growth media) has improved isolation and the molecular detection of Bartonella spp. Once processed, blood is plated onto enriched (chocolate or blood-containing) media, incubated at 35° to 37° C under elevated $CO_2$ and humidity. For optimal growth, media should be freshly prepared. Plates can be sealed with either Parafilm or Shrink seals after the first 24 hours of incubation and incubated up to 30 days.

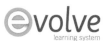

*Visit the Evolve site to complete the review questions.*

---

## CASE STUDY 68-1

A college student was admitted to the hospital with fever and chills. He also appeared disoriented and complained of chest pain. Blood cultures were collected on admission, and he was started on cefazolin therapy. His condition worsened, and within 12 hours the blood cultures were reported positive for a gram-positive cocci, suggestive of *Staphylococcus* spp. Two hours later the laboratory confirmed the identification of *Staphylococcus aureus*. An echocardiogram was performed that showed multiple vegetations on his tricuspid and aortic valves (see Figure 68-1). Surgery was planned to repair the valves, but the patient died within 48 hours of admission. It was discovered that the student had been injecting cocaine with his friends.

### QUESTIONS

1. How did the laboratory identify the organism so quickly?
2. How many blood cultures should be submitted to diagnose bacteremia?
3. If the isolate had been coagulase negative, what would indicate that this was a true infection with the organism?

---

## ▤ BIBLIOGRAPHY

Adler H, Baumlin N, Frie R: Evaluation of acridine orange staining as a replacement of subcultures for BacT/ALERT-positive, Gram stain-negative blood cultures, *J Clin Microbiol* 41:5238, 2003.

Agan BK, Dolan MJ: Laboratory diagnosis of Bartonella infections, *Clin Lab Med* 22:937-962, 2002.

Barenfanger J, Drake C, Lawhorn J, et al: Comparison of chlorhexidine and tincture of iodine for skin antisepsis in preparation for blood sample collection, *J Clin Microbiol* 42:2216, 2004.

Baron EJ, Weinstein MP, Dunne WM, et al: Blood cultures IV. In Baron EJ, coordinating editor: *Cumitech 1C*, Washington, DC, 2005, American Society for Microbiology.

Beebe JL, Koneman EL: Recovery of uncommon bacteria from blood: association with neoplastic disease, *Clin Microbiol Rev* 8:336, 1995.

Calfee DP, Farr BM: Comparison of four antiseptic preparations for skin in the prevention of contamination of percutaneously drawn blood cultures: a randomized trial, *J Clin Microbiol* 40:1660, 2002.

Centers for Disease Control and Prevention: Guidelines for the prevention of intravascular catheter-related infections, *Morb Mortal Wkly Rep* 51:RR-10, 2002.

Cockerill FR, Wilson JW, Vetter EA, et al: Optimal testing parameters for blood cultures, *Clin Infect Dis* 38:1724, 2004.

Fernandez-Guerrero ML, Ramos J, and Soriano F: Mycoplasma hominis bacteraemia not associated with genital infections, *J Infect* 39:91, 1999.

Isaacman DJ, Karasic RB: Lack of effect of changing needles on contamination of blood cultures, *Pediatr Infect Dis J* 9:274, 1990.

Krumholz HM, Cummings S, York M: Blood culture phlebotomy: switching needles does not prevent contamination, *Ann Intern Med* 113:290, 1990.

Lamey JR, Eschenbach DA, Mitchell SH, et al: Isolation of mycoplasmas and bacteria from the blood of postpartum women, *Am J Obstet Gynecol* 143:104, 1982.

Levett PN: Usefulness of serologic analysis as a predictor of the infecting serovar in patients with severe leptospirosis, *Clin Infect Dis* 36:447-452, 2003.

Levett PN, Morey RE, Galloway RL, et al: Detection of pathogenic leptospires by real-time quantitative PCR, *J Med Microbiol* 54:45-49, 2005.

Li J, Plourde JL, Carlson LG: Effects of volume and periodicity on blood cultures, *J Clin Microbiol* 32:2829, 1994.

Maggi RG, Duncan AW, Breitschwerdt EB: Novel chemically modified liquid medium that will support the growth of seven bartonella species, *J Clin Microbiol* 43:2651-2655, 2005.

Mermel LA, Farr BM, Sheretz RJ, et al: Guidelines for the management of intravascular catheter-related infections, *Clin Infect Dis* 32:1249, 2001.

Mermel LA, Maki DG: Detection of bacteremia in adults: consequences of culturing an inadequate volume of blood, *Ann Intern Med* 119:270, 1993.

Meyer RD, Clough W: Extragenital Mycoplasma hominis infections in adults: emphasis on immunosuppression, *Clin Infect Dis* 17(Suppl 1):243, 1993.

Morris AJ, Wilson ML, Mirrett S, et al: Rationale for selective use of anaerobic blood cultures, *J Clin Microbiol* 31:2110, 1993.

National Committee for Clinical Laboratory Standards: *Procedures for the collection of diagnostic blood specimens by venipuncture: approved standard H3-A5*, ed 5, Wayne, Pa, 2003, National Committee for Clinical Laboratory Standards.

Needlestick Safety and Prevention Act, *http://thomas.loc.gov.*

Pfaller MA, Diekema DJ: Twelve years of fluconazole in clinical practice: global trends in species distribution and fluconazole susceptibility of bloodstream isolates of Candida, *Eur Soc Clin Microbiol Infect Dis* 10(Suppl 1):11, 2004.

Salzman MB, Rubin LG: Intravenous catheter-related infections, *Adv Pediatr Infect Dis* 10:337, 1995.

Wenzel RP, Edmond MB: The impact of hospital-acquired bloodstream infections, *Emerg Infect Dis* 7:174, 2001.

Wisplinghoff H, Bischoff T, Tallent SM, et al: Nosocomial bloodstream infections in U.S. hospitals: analysis of 24,179 cases from a prospective nationwide surveillance study, *Clin Infect Dis* 39:309, 2004.

Wisplinghoff H, Seifert H, Tallent SM, et al: Nosocomial bloodstream infections in pediatric patients in United States Hospitals; epidemiology, clinical features and susceptibilities, *Pediatr Infect Dis J* 22:686, 2003.

Yagupsky P: Detection of Brucellae in blood cultures, *J Clin Microbiol* 37:3437, 1999.

## OBJECTIVES

1. Define the trachea, bronchi, bronchioles, and alveoli, and explain the anatomic structure of the lower respiratory system.
2. List the most common etiologic agents responsible for lower respiratory disease and pneumonia in patients of various ages and categories: children <5 years of age, school-age children, young adults, older adults, and immunocompromised patients.
3. Describe the virulence factors found in bacteria and viruses associated with infection of the lower respiratory tract.
4. List the four possible routes of transmission or dissemination within the body that allow organisms to cause an infection in the lungs.
5. Name the most important decision for physicians regarding the treatment of pneumonia in older individuals, and list the three-step process used to guide them in this decision.
6. List the most prevalent cause of community-acquired pneumonia in adults.
7. Differentiate between community-acquired and hospital-acquired pneumonia.
8. State the factors anaerobic bacteria possess that enhance their ability to produce disease; explain how these anaerobes gain entrance to the lungs.
9. Define Lukens trap, and explain the type of patient or specimen associated with the method.
10. Describe the difference between early-onset or late-onset hospital- or ventilator-associated pneumonia.
11. List the etiologic agent of lung infections identified in cystic fibrosis patients.
12. Name the organisms most often associated with pneumo-opportunistic infection in HIV-positive individuals.
13. Explain the mechanisms that, because of the bacterial production of toxins, enable microorganisms to produce respiratory-associated disease.
14. Explain how the host immune system can contribute to microorganism growth in the respiratory disease process.
15. Explain why *Mycobacterium tuberculosis* is a classic representative of an intracellular pathogen.
16. Describe specimens collected for respiratory infections including determination of specimen quality and rejection criteria for the following: sputum, induced sputum, endotracheal suction, pleural fluid, bronchoalveolar lavage, bronchial washing, and bronchial brush sample.
17. Explain how the microbiologist would test for the less common causes of respiratory infection, including *Pneumocystis jiroveci*, *Legionella* spp., *Chlamydophila pneumonia*, *Bordetella pertussis*, *Mycoplasma pneumonia*, and *Norcardia*.

## GENERAL CONSIDERATIONS

### ANATOMY

The respiratory tract can be divided into two major areas: the upper respiratory tract consists of all structures above the larynx, whereas the lower respiratory tract follows airflow below the larynx through the trachea to the bronchi and bronchioles and then into the alveolar spaces where gas exchange occurs (Figure 69-1). The respiratory and gastrointestinal tracts are the two major connections between the interior of the body and the outside environment. The respiratory tract is the pathway through which the body acquires fresh oxygen and removes unneeded carbon dioxide. It begins with the nasal and oral passages, which humidify inspired air, and extends past the nasopharynx and oropharynx to the trachea and then into the lungs. The trachea divides into bronchi, which subdivide into bronchioles, the smallest branches that terminate in the alveoli. Some 300 million alveoli are estimated to be present in the lungs; these are the primary microscopic gas exchange structures of the respiratory tract.

Familiarization with the anatomic structure of the thoracic cavity ensures proper specimen collection from various sites in the lower respiratory tract for processing by the laboratory. The thoracic cavity, which contains the heart and lungs, has three partitions separated from one another by pleura (see Figure 69-1). The lungs occupy the right and left pleural cavities, whereas the mediastinum (space between the lungs) is occupied mainly by the esophagus, trachea, large blood vessels, and heart.

## PATHOGENESIS OF THE RESPIRATORY TRACT: BASIC CONCEPTS

Microorganisms primarily cause disease by a limited number of pathogenic mechanisms (see Chapter 3). Because these mechanisms relate to respiratory tract infections, they are discussed briefly. Encounters between the human body and microorganisms occur many times each day. However, establishment of infection after such contact tends to be the exception rather than the rule. Whether an organism is successful in establishing an infection depends not only on the organism's ability to cause disease (pathogenicity) but also on the human host's ability to prevent the infection.

### Host Factors

The human host has several mechanisms that nonspecifically protect the respiratory tract from infection: the nasal hairs, convoluted passages, and the mucous lining of the nasal turbinates; secretory IgA and nonspecific antibacterial substances (lysozyme) in respiratory secretions; the cilia and mucous lining of the trachea; and reflexes such as coughing, sneezing, and swallowing. These mechanisms prevent foreign objects or organisms from entering the bronchi and gaining access to the lungs, which remain sterile in the healthy host.

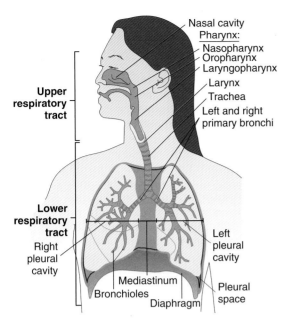

**Figure 69-1** Anatomy of the respiratory tract, including upper and lower respiratory tract regions.

**BOX 69-1** Organisms Present in the Nasopharynx and Oropharynx of Healthy Humans

**Possible Pathogens**
*Acinetobacter* spp.
Viridans streptococci, including *Streptococcus anginosus* group
Beta-hemolytic streptococci
*Streptococcus pneumoniae*
*Staphylococcus aureus*
*Neisseria meningitidis*
*Mycoplasma* spp.
*Haemophilus influenzae*
*Haemophilus parainfluenzae*
*Moraxella catarrhalis*
*Candida albicans*
Herpes simplex virus
Enterobacteriaceae
*Mycobacterium* spp.
*Pseudomonas* spp.
*Burkholderia cepacia*
Filamentous fungi
*Klebsiella ozaenae*
*Eikenella corrodens*
*Bacteroides* spp.
*Peptostreptococcus* spp.
*Actinomyces* spp.
*Capnocytophaga* spp.
*Actinobacillus* spp., *A. actinomycetemcomitans*
*Haemophilus aphrophilus*
*Entamoeba gingivalis*
*Trichomonas tenax*

**Rarely Pathogens**
Nonhemolytic streptococci
Staphylococci
Micrococci
*Corynebacterium* spp.
Coagulase-negative staphylococci
*Neisseria* spp., other than *N. gonorrhoeae* and *N. meningitidis*
*Lactobacillus* spp.
*Veillonella* spp.
Spirochetes
*Rothia dentocariosa*
*Leptotrichia buccalis*
*Selenomonas*
*Wolinella*
*Stomatococcus mucilaginosus*
*Campylobacter* spp.

Aspiration of minor amounts of oropharyngeal material, as occurs often during sleep, plays an important role in the pathogenesis of many types of pneumonia. Once particles escape the mucociliary sweeping activity and enter the alveoli, alveolar macrophages ingest them and carry them to the lymphatics.

In addition to these nonspecific host defenses, normal flora of the nasopharynx and oropharynx help prevent colonization by pathogenic organisms of the upper respiratory tract. Normal bacterial flora prevent the colonization by pathogens by competing for the same space and nutrients as well as production of bacteriocins and metabolic products that are toxic to invading organisms. Some of the bacteria that can be isolated as part of the indigenous flora of healthy hosts, as well as many species that may cause disease under certain circumstances and are often isolated from the respiratory tracts of healthy persons, are listed in Box 69-1. Under certain circumstances and for unknown reasons, these colonizing organisms can cause disease—perhaps because of previous damage by a viral infection, loss of some host immunity, or physical damage to the respiratory epithelium (e.g., from smoking). Differentiation of normal flora of the respiratory tract is important for determining the importance of an isolate in the clinical laboratory. Colonization does not always represent an infection. It is important to differentiate colonization from infection based on the specimen source, number of organisms present, and presence or quantity of white blood cells. (Organisms isolated from normally sterile sites in the respiratory tract by sterile methods that avoid contamination with normal flora should be definitively identified and reported to the clinician.)

## Microorganism Factors

Organisms possess traits or produce products that promote colonization and subsequent infection in the host. The virulence, or disease-producing capability of an organism, depends on several factors including adherence, production of toxins, amount of growth or proliferation, tissue damage, avoiding the host immune response, and ability to disseminate.

**Adherence.** For any organism to cause disease, it must first gain a foothold within the respiratory tract to grow to sufficient numbers to produce symptoms. Therefore, most etiologic agents of respiratory tract disease must first adhere to the mucosa of the respiratory tract. The presence of normal flora and the overall state of the host affect the ability of microorganisms to adhere. Surviving or growing on host tissue without causing overt harmful effects is termed *colonization*. Except for those microorganisms inhaled directly into the lungs, all etiologic agents of disease must first colonize the respiratory tract before they can cause harm.

*Streptococcus pyogenes* possess specific adherence factors such as fimbriae comprised of molecules such as lipoteichoic acids and M proteins. These molecules appear as a thin layer of fuzz surrounding the bacteria. *Staphylococcus aureus* and certain viridans streptococci are other bacteria that posses these lipoteichoic acid adherence complexes. Many gram-negative bacteria (which do not have lipoteichoic acids), including Enterobacteriaceae, *Legionella* spp., *Pseudomonas* spp., *Bordetella pertussis*, and *Haemophilus* spp., also adhere by means of proteinaceous finger-like surface fimbriae. Viruses possess either a hemagglutinin (influenza and parainfluenza viruses) or other proteins that mediate their epithelial attachment.

**Toxins.** Certain microorganisms are almost always considered to be etiologic agents of disease if they are present in any numbers in the respiratory tract because they possess virulence factors that are expressed in every host. These organisms are listed in Box 69-2. The production of extracellular toxin was one of the first pathogenic mechanisms discovered among bacteria. *Corynebacterium*

*diphtheriae* is a classic example of a bacterium that produces disease through the action of an extracellular toxin. Once the organism colonizes the upper respiratory epithelium, it produces a toxin that is disseminated systemically, adhering preferentially to central nervous system cells and muscle cells of the heart. Systemic disease is characterized by myocarditis, peripheral neuritis, and local disease that can lead to respiratory distress. Growth of *C. diphtheriae* causes necrosis and sloughing of the epithelial mucosa, producing a "diphtheritic (pseudo) membrane," which may extend from the anterior nasal mucosa to the bronchi or may be limited to any area between—most often the tonsillar and peritonsillar areas. The membrane may cause sore throat and interfere with respiration and swallowing. Although nontoxic strains of *C. diphtheriae* can cause local disease, it is much milder than disease associated with toxigenic strains.

Some strains of *Pseudomonas aeruginosa* produce a toxin similar to diphtheria toxin. Whether this toxin actually contributes to the pathogenesis of respiratory tract infection with *P. aeruginosa* has not been established. *Bordetella pertussis*, the agent of whooping cough, also produces toxins. The role of these toxins in production of disease is not clear. They may act to inhibit the activity of phagocytic cells or to damage cells of the respiratory tract. *Staphylococcus aureus* and beta-hemolytic streptococci produce extracellular enzymes capable of damaging host cells or tissues. Extracellular products of staphylococci aid in the production of tissue necrosis and the destruction of phagocytic cells and contribute to the abscess formation associated with infection caused by this organism. Although *S. aureus* can be recovered from throat specimens, it has not been proved to cause pharyngitis. Enzymes of streptococci, including hyaluronidase, allow rapid dissemination of the bacteria. Many other etiologic agents of respiratory tract infection also produce extracellular enzymes and toxins.

**Microorganism Growth.** In addition to adherence and toxin production, pathogens cause disease by merely growing in host tissue, interfering with normal tissue function, and attracting host immune effectors, such as neutrophils and macrophages. Once these cells begin to attack the invading pathogens and repair the damaged host tissue, an expanding reaction ensues with more nonspecific and immunologic factors being attracted to the area, increasing the amount of host tissue damage. Respiratory viral infections usually progress in this manner, as do many types of pneumonias, such as those caused by *Streptococcus pneumoniae, S. pyogenes, Staphylococcus aureus, Haemophilus influenzae, Neisseria meningitidis, Moraxella catarrhalis, Mycoplasma pneumoniae, Mycobacterium tuberculosis,* and most gram-negative bacilli.

**Avoiding the Host Response.** Another virulence mechanism present in various respiratory tract pathogens is the ability to evade host defense mechanisms. *S. pneumoniae, N. meningitidis, H. influenzae, Klebsiella pneumoniae,* mucoid *P. aeruginosa, Cryptococcus neoformans,* and others possess polysaccharide capsules that serve both to prevent engulfment by phagocytic host cells and to protect somatic antigens from being exposed to host immunoglobulins. The capsular material is produced in such abundance by certain bacteria, such as pneumococci, that soluble polysaccharide antigen particles can bind host antibodies, blocking them from serving as opsonins. Vaccine consisting of capsular antigens provides host protection to infection, indicating that the capsular polysaccharide is a major virulence mechanism of *H. influenzae, S. pneumoniae,* and *N. meningitidis.*

Some respiratory pathogens evade the host immune system by multiplying within host cells. *Chlamydia trachomatis, Chlamydia psittaci, Chlamydia pneumoniae,* and all viruses replicate within host cells. They have evolved methods for being taken in by the "nonprofessional" phagocytic cells of the host to where they thrive within the intracellular environment. Once within these cells, the organism is protected from host humoral immune factors and other phagocytic cells. This protection lasts until the host cell becomes sufficiently damaged that the organism is then recognized as foreign by the host and is attacked. A second group of organisms that cause respiratory tract disease comprises organisms capable of survival within phagocytic host cells (usually macrophages). Once inside the phagocytic cell, these respiratory tract pathogens are able to multiply. *Legionella, Pneumocystis jiroveci (Pneumocystis carinii),* and *Histoplasma capsulatum* are some of the more common intracellular pathogens.

*Mycobacterium tuberculosis* is the classic representative of an intracellular pathogen. In primary tuberculosis, the organism is carried to an alveolus in a droplet nucleus, a tiny aerosol particle containing tubercle bacilli. Once phagocytized by alveolar macrophages, organisms are carried to the nearest lymph node, usually in the hilar or other mediastinal chains. In the lymph node, the organisms slowly multiply within macrophages. Ultimately, *M. tuberculosis* destroys the macrophage and is subsequently taken up by other phagocytic cells. Tubercle bacilli multiply to a critical mass within the protected environment of the macrophages, which are prevented from accomplishing phagosome-lysosome fusion capable of destroying the bacteria. Having reached a critical mass, the organisms spill out of the destroyed macrophages, through the lymphatics, and into the bloodstream, producing mycobacteremia and carrying tubercle bacilli to many parts of the body. In most cases, the host immune system reacts sufficiently at this point to kill the bacilli; however, a small reservoir of live bacteria may be left in areas of normally high oxygen concentration, such as the apical (top) portion of the lung. These bacilli are walled off, and years later, an insult to the host, either immunologic or physical, may cause breakdown of the focus of latent tubercle bacilli, allowing active multiplication and disease (secondary tuberculosis). In certain patients with primary immune defects, the initial bacteremia seeds bacteria throughout a compromised host, leading to disseminated or miliary tuberculosis. Growth of the bacteria within host macrophages and histiocytes in the lung causes an influx of more effector cells, including lymphocytes, neutrophils, and histiocytes, eventually resulting in granuloma formation, then tissue destruction and cavity formation. The lesion consists of a semisolid, amorphous tissue mass resembling semisoft cheese, from which it received the name caseating necrosis (death of cells or tissues). The infection can extend into bronchioles and bronchi from which bacteria are disseminated via respiratory secretions and coughing. Aerosolized droplets are produced by coughing and contain organisms that are inhaled by the next susceptible host. Other portions of the patient's lungs may become infected as well through aspiration (inhalation of a fluid or solid).

# DISEASES OF THE LOWER RESPIRATORY TRACT

## BRONCHITIS

### Acute

Acute bronchitis is characterized by acute inflammation of the tracheobronchial tree. This condition may be part of, or preceded by, an upper respiratory tract infection such as influenza (the "flu") or the common cold. Most infections occur during the winter when acute respiratory tract infections are common.

The pathogenesis of acute bronchitis has no specific documented etiology but appears to be a mixture of viral cytopathic events and a response by the host immune system. Regardless of the cause, the protective functions of the bronchial epithelium are disturbed and excessive fluid accumulates in the bronchi. Depending on the etiology, destruction of the bronchial epithelium may be either extensive (e.g., influenza virus) or minimal (e.g., rhinovirus colds).

Clinically, bronchitis is characterized by cough, variable fever, and sputum production. Sputum (pus from the lungs) is often clear at the onset but may become purulent as the illness persists. Bronchitis may manifest as croup (a clinical condition marked by a barking cough or hoarseness).

The value of microbiologic studies to determine the cause of acute bronchitis in otherwise healthy individuals has not been established. Acute bronchitis is caused by viral agents, such as influenza and respiratory syncytial virus (RSV). The bacterium *Bordetella pertussis* is often associated with bronchitis in infants and preschool children (Table 69-1). The best specimen for diagnosis of pertussis is a deep nasopharyngeal specimen collected with a calcium alginate swab (see Chapter 37).

### Chronic versus Acute

Chronic bronchitis is a common condition affecting about 10% to 25% of adults. This disease is defined by clinical symptoms in which excessive mucus production leads to coughing up sputum on most days during at least 3 consecutive months for more than 2 successive years.

**TABLE 69-1** Major Causes of Acute Bronchitis

| Bacteria | Viruses |
|---|---|
| *Bordetella pertussis, B. parapertussis, Mycoplasma pneumoniae, Chlamydia pneumoniae* | Influenza virus, adenovirus, rhinovirus, coronavirus (other less common viruses: respiratory syncytial virus, human metapneumovirus, coxsackie A21 virus) |

Cigarette smoking, infection, and inhalation of dust or fumes are important contributing factors. Acute bronchitis is not related to long-term etiologies causing damage to the lungs, but is typically a result of an infectious process.

Patients with chronic bronchitis can suffer from acute flare-ups of infection, but determination of the cause of the infection is difficult. Potentially pathogenic bacteria, such as nonencapsulated strains of *Haemophilus influenzae, Streptococcus pneumoniae,* and *Moraxella catarrhalis,* are frequently cultured from the bronchi of these patients. Because of chronic colonization, it is difficult to incriminate one of these organisms as the specific cause of an acute infection in patients with chronic bronchitis. Although the role of bacteria in acute infections in these patients is questionable, viruses are frequent causes.

# BRONCHIOLITIS

Bronchiolitis, the inflammation of the smaller diameter bronchiolar epithelial surfaces, is an acute viral lower respiratory tract infection that primarily occurs during the first 2 years of life. Characteristic clinical manifestations include an acute onset of wheezing and hyperinflation as well as cough, rhinorrhea (runny nose), tachypnea (rapid breathing), and respiratory distress. The disease is primarily caused by viruses including a recently discovered virus, human metapneumovirus. RSV accounts for 40% to 80% of cases of bronchiolitis and demonstrates a marked seasonality; the etiologic agents of bronchiolitis are listed in Box 69-3. Like other viral infections, bronchiolitis shows a marked seasonality in temperate climates with a yearly increase in cases during winter to early spring.

Initially, the virus replicates in the epithelium of the upper respiratory tract, but in the infant it rapidly spreads to the lower tract airways. Early inflammation of the bronchial epithelium progresses to necrosis. Symptoms such as wheezing may be related to the type of inflammatory response to the virus as well as other host factors. For the most part, patients are managed based on clinical parameters, with the laboratory having a role in cases that require hospitalization; a specific viral etiology can be identified in a large number of infants by viral isolation from respiratory secretions, preferably from a nasal wash (see Chapter 65).

# PNEUMONIA

Pneumonia (inflammation of the lower respiratory tract involving the lung's airways and supporting structures) is a major cause of illness and death. There are two major categories of pneumonias: those considered community-acquired pneumonia (patients are believed to have acquired their infection outside the hospital setting) and those including hospital- or ventilator-associated (patients are believed to have acquired their infection within the hospital setting, usually at least 2 days following admission) or health care–associated pneumonia (affects only patients hospitalized in an acute care hospital for 2 or more days within 90 days of infection from a long-term care facility, or patients who have received recent intravenous antibiotic therapy, chemotherapy, or wound care within 30 days of the current infection, or who have attended a hospital or hemolysis clinic). Nevertheless, once a microorganism has successfully invaded the lung, disease can follow affecting the alveolar spaces and their supporting structure, the interstitium, and the terminal bronchioles.

## Pathogenesis

Organisms can cause infection of the lung by four possible routes: by upper airway colonization or infection that subsequently extends into the lung, by aspiration of organisms (thereby avoiding the upper airway defenses), by inhalation of airborne droplets containing the organism, or by seeding of the lung via the blood from a distant site of infection. Viruses cause primary infections of the respiratory tract, as well as inhibit host defenses that, in turn, can lead to a secondary bacterial infection. For example, viruses may destroy respiratory epithelium and disrupt normal ciliary activity. Presumably, the growth of viruses in host cells disrupts the function of the latter and encourages the influx of nonspecific immune effector cells exacerbating the damage. Damage to host epithelial tissue by virus infection is known to predispose patients to secondary bacterial infection.

Aspiration of oropharyngeal contents is important in the pathogenesis of many types of pneumonia. Aspiration may occur during a loss of consciousness such as during anesthesia or a seizure, or after alcohol or drug abuse, but other individuals, particularly geriatric patients, may also develop aspiration pneumonia. Neurologic disease or esophageal pathology and periodontal disease or gingivitis are other important risk factors. Aided by gravity and often by loss of some host nonspecific protective mechanisms, organisms reach lung tissue, where they multiply and attract host inflammatory cells. Other mechanisms include inhalation of aerosolized material and hematogenous seeding. The buildup of cell debris and fluid contributes to the loss of lung function and thus to the pathology.

Furthermore, regarding the pathogenesis of hospital-associated, health care–associated, and ventilator-associated pneumonias, health care devices, the environment, and the transfer between the patient and staff or other patients can serve as sources of pathogens causing pneumonia. The primary routes for bacterial entry into the lower respiratory tract are by aspiration of oropharyngeal organisms or leakage of secretions containing bacteria around an endotracheal tube. For these reasons, intubation and mechanical ventilation significantly increase the risk of pneumonia (6- to 21-fold). In addition, bacterial and viral biofilm in the endotracheal tube with subsequent spread to distal airways may be important in the pathogenesis of ventilator-associated pneumonia.

## Clinical Manifestations

The symptoms suggestive of pneumonia include fever, chills, chest pain, and cough. In the past, pneumonias were classified into two major groups: (1) typical or acute pneumonias (e.g., *Streptococcus pneumoniae*) and (2) atypical pneumonias, based on whether the cough was productive or nonproductive of mucoid sputum. However, analysis of symptoms of pneumonia caused by the atypical pneumonia pathogens (*Mycoplasma pneumoniae*, *Legionella pneumophila*, and *Chlamydophila pneumoniae*) has revealed no significant differences from those symptoms of patients with typical bacterial pneumonias. Because of this overlap in symptoms, it is important to consider all possible etiologies associated with the patient's clinical presentation.

Some patients with pneumonia exhibit no signs or symptoms related to their respiratory tract (i.e., some only have fever). Therefore, physical examination of the patient, chest radiograph findings, patient history, and clinical laboratory findings are important. In addition to respiratory symptoms, 10% to 30% of patients with pneumonia complain of headache, nausea, vomiting, abdominal pain, diarrhea, and myalgias.

## Epidemiology/Etiologic Agents

As previously mentioned, there are two major categories of pneumonias: those considered community-acquired pneumonias and hospital-, ventilator-, or health care–associated pneumonias. Because the epidemiology and etiologies can differ, these two categories are discussed separately. Pneumonia in the immunocompromised patient is addressed separately in this chapter. Emerging viral infections associated with severe acute respiratory syndrome (SARS) and influenza outbreaks (H1N1) are typically associated with upper respiratory infections but may lead to serious lower respiratory infections in the young, elderly, or immunocompromised patient. See Chapter 66 for detailed information related to these emerging viral infectious diseases and diagnostic recommendations.

**Community-Acquired Pneumonia.** In the United States, pneumonia is the sixth leading cause of death and the number one cause of death from infectious diseases. It is estimated that as many as 2 million to 3 million cases of community-acquired pneumonia occur annually, and roughly one fifth of these require hospitalization; 45,000 pneumonia-related deaths occur in the United States each year. The etiology of acute pneumonias is strongly dependent on age. More than 80% of pneumonias in infants and children are caused by viruses, compared to less than 10% to 20% of pneumonias in adults.

**Children.** Community-acquired pneumonia in children is a common and potentially serious infection. The annual incidence of pneumonia in children younger than 5 years of age is 34 to 40 cases per 1000 in Europe and North America. Determining the cause of pneumonia is challenging because the lungs are rarely sampled

directly and sputum is difficult to obtain from children. Among previously healthy patients 2 months to 5 years old, RSV, human metapneumovirus, parainfluenza, influenza, and adenoviruses are the most common etiologic agents of lower respiratory tract disease. Children suffer less commonly from bacterial pneumonia, usually caused by *H. influenzae*, *S. pneumoniae*, or *S. aureus*. Neonates may acquire lower respiratory tract infections with *C. trachomatis* or *P. jiroveci* (which likely indicates an immature immune system or an underlying immune defect).

*M. pneumoniae* and *C. pneumoniae* are the most common causes of bacterial pneumonia in school-age children (5-14 years of age). The four most common causes of community-acquired viral pneumonia in children include influenza, RSV, parainfluenza, and adenovirus. The agents associated with nosocomial outbreaks in children include the influenza virus, RSV, and adenovirus. Mixed viral and bacterial infections have been documented in 35% of patients, with the majority of these (81%) being mixed viral-bacterial infections. In addition, the time of onset of hospital- or ventilator-associated pneumonia is an important epidemiologic variable and risk factor: early-onset pneumonia (defined as occurring within the first 4 days of hospitalization), usually carries a better prognosis, being more likely to be caused by antibiotic-sensitive bacteria, whereas late-onset pneumonia (5 days or more) is more likely to be caused by multidrug-resistant organisms and is associated with increased patient morbidity and mortality.

**Young Adults.** The most common etiologic agent of lower respiratory tract infection among adults younger than 30 years of age is *Mycoplasma pneumoniae*, which is transmitted via close contact. Contact with secretions seems to be more important than inhalation of aerosols for transmission and infection. After contact with respiratory mucosa, *Mycoplasma* are able to adhere to and colonize respiratory mucosal cells. Both a protein adherence factor and gliding motility determine virulence. *Mycoplasma* attach to the cilia of respiratory mucosal cells; once there, they multiply and destroy ciliary function. Attachment and cytotoxins produced by the organisms induce cell damage. *Chlamydia pneumoniae* is the third most common agent of lower respiratory tract infection in young adults, following mycoplasmas and influenza viruses; it also affects older individuals. *Chlamydia* spp., intracellular pathogens capable of disrupting cellular function and causing respiratory disease, are similar to viral pathogens.

The epidemiology and treatment of community-acquired and hospital-acquired pneumonia have changed dramatically as a result of improvements in diagnostics, antimicrobial therapy, and supportive care modalities. The changes in the organization of health care has made the distinction between community-acquired and hospital-acquired pneumonia less clear. However, pneumonia still remains an important cause of morbidity and mortality in elderly patients. The American Thoracic Society and the Infectious Disease Society of America guidelines have suggested that patients who have been hospitalized in the last 90 days, reside in a nursing home or long-term care facility, or have had a recent intravenous antibiotic therapy or hemodialysis, be classified as a patient with health care-associated pneumonia (HCAP). Patients with health care-associated pneumonia have a higher incidence of cardiopulmonary and neurodegenerative diseases, cancer, chronic kidney disease, chronic obstructive pulmonary disease, and immunosuppression than elderly patients with community-acquired pneumonia. Both populations become infested with various organisms. The organisms most frequently responsible for community-acquired pneumonia include *S. pneumoniae, H. influenzae, M. pneumoniae, C. pneumoniae, M. catarrhalis,* and *Legionella spp.* Factors that contribute to the onset include decreased mucociliary function, decreased cough reflex, decreased level of consciousness, periodontal disease, and decreased general mobility. Health care-associated patients have been found to be more frequently colonized with gram-negative bacilli and other multidrug resistant pathogens, perhaps because of poor oral hygiene, decreased saliva, or decreased epithelial cell turnover. The microorganisms associated with these infections, in addition to those previously mentioned, may include methicillin-resistant *S. aureus* (MRSA), *Pseudomonas aeruginosa,* a variety of Enterobacteriaceae, *Acinetobacter* spp., anaerobic bacteria, carbapenamase-resistant *Klebsiella pneumonia,* and extended spectrum beta-lactamase resistant Enterobacteriaceae (ESBLS). According to the Infectious Diseases Society of America (IDSA), the decision to hospitalize a patient or to treat him or her as an outpatient is possibly the single most important clinical decision made by physicians during the course of illness. This decision in turn impacts the subsequent site of treatment (home, hospital, or intensive care unit), intensity of laboratory evaluation, antibiotic therapy, and cost. Thus, the IDSA has developed management guidelines for community-acquired pneumonia in adults based on a three-step process: (1) assessment of preexisting conditions that might compromise safety of home care, (2) quantification of short-term mortality (referred to as the pneumonia port severity index [PSI] and based on a prediction rule derived from more than 14,000 patients) with subsequent assignment of patients to five risk classes (classes I through V), and (3) clinical judgment usually require hospitalization. The PSI, however, is not useful for patients in nursing homes or other health care facilities. It is therefore essential to properly assess the severity of the disease in both cases of community-acquired and health care associated pneumonia in elderly patients that clearly includes the three major management guidelines as outlined by the IDSA.

Pneumonia secondary to aspiration of gastric or oral sections is common and occurs in the community setting.

Pneumonia secondary to aspiration of gastric or oral secretions is common and occurs in the community setting. The most common agents include the oral anaerobes such as black-pigmented *Prevotella* and *Porphyromonas* spp., *Prevotella oris, P. buccae, P. disiens, Bacteroides gracilis,* fusobacteria, and anaerobic or microaerophilic streptococci. The anaerobic agents possess many factors, such as extracellular enzymes and capsules enhancing their ability to produce disease. It is their presence, however, in an abnormal site within the host producing lowered oxidation-reduction potential secondary to

tissue damage that contributes to their pathogenicity. *Staphylococcus aureus,* various Enterobacteriaceae, and *Pseudomonas* may also be acquired by aspiration; *Haemophilus influenzae, Legionella* spp., *Acinetobacter, Moraxella catarrhalis, Chlamydia pneumoniae,* meningococci, and other agents may also be implicated. Pnuemonia is the leading cause of death among patients with nosocomial infections (hospital- ventilator- and health care-associated) (as high as 50%) mortality among patients in intensive care units. Some of these pneumonias are secondary to sepsis, and some are related to contaminated inhalation therapy equipment, particularly for intubated patients. Hospitalized patients or long-term care patients may experience asymptomatic colonization of the upper airway and result in aspiration of microorganisms into the lower respiratory tract. In addition to those organisms previously listed, these patients are more prone to infections with the multi-drug resistant strains of bacteria (ESBLS and MRSA) including *Providencia stuartii, Morganella morganii, E. coli, Proteus mirabilis, K. pneumoniae, Enterobacter* spp., and *Staphylococcus aureus.*

**Adults (Viral pneumonia).** Adults may suffer from an estimated 100 million cases annually of community-acquired viral pneumonia cased by influenza, adenovirus, enteroviruses (coxsackieviruses and rhinoviruses), coronaviruses, human metapneumovirus, parainfluenza, varicella, rubeola or RSV, particularly during epidemics. Influenza associated viral pneumonia poses an increased risk for pregnant women of approximately 4-9 times greater than the general public, with the greatest risk associated with the third trimester. RSV is considered the third most common cause of community-acquired pneumoniae with 78% of the deaths occurring in patients over the age of 65. Similarly to RSV, human metapneumovirus has been associated with outbreaks in long-term care facilities. Following viral pneumonia, secondary bacterial disease caused by beta-hemolytic streptococci, *S. aureus, M. catarrhalis, H. influenzae,* and *Chlamydia pneumoniae.* Other agents may be considered depending on the geographic location and clinical presentation are viruses in the *Hantavirus* group, the most common of which is sin nombre virus as well as severe acute respiratory syndrome (SARS). (See Chapter 65.)

Of these agents, influenza virus, RSV and adenovirus have been implicated in nosocomial outbreaks. The time of onset of hospital- or ventilator-associated pneumonia is an important epidemiologic variable and risk factor; early onset pneumonia (defined as occurring within the first 4 days of hospitalization.

**Adults (Fungal pneumonia).** Unusual causes of acute lower respiratory tract infection in adults include Actinomyces and *Nocardia* spp. Other agents may rarely be recovered from sputum and include the agents of plague, tularemia, melioidosis (*Burkholderia pseudomallei*), Brucella, Salmonella, *Coxiella burnetii* (Q fever), *Bacillus anthracis, Pasteurella multocida,* and certain parasitic agents such as *Paragonimus westermani, Entamoeba histolytica, Ascaris lumbricoides,* and *Strongyloides* spp. (the latter may cause fatal disease in immunosuppressed patients). A high index of suspicion by the clinician is usually a prerequisite to a diagnosis of parasitic pneumonia in the United States. Psittacosis should be ruled out as a cause of acute lower respiratory tract infection in patients who have had recent contact with birds. Among the fungal etiologies, *Histoplasma capsulatum*, *Blastomyces dermatitidis*, *Paracoccidioides brasiliensis*, *Coccidioides immitis*, *Cryptococcus neoformans*, and, occasionally, *Aspergillus fumigatus* may cause acute pneumonia. Therefore, occupational history and history of exposure to animals are important in suggesting specific potential infectious agents.

**Chronic Lower Respiratory Tract Infections.** *Mycobacterium tuberculosis* is the most likely etiologic agent of chronic lower respiratory tract infection, but fungal infection and anaerobic pleuropulmonary infection may also run a subacute or chronic course. Mycobacteria other than *M. tuberculosis* may also cause such disease, particularly *M. avium* complex and *M. kansasii*. Although possible causes of acute, community-acquired lower respiratory tract infections, fungi and parasites are more commonly isolated from patients with chronic disease. *Actinomyces* and *Nocardia* may also be associated with gradual onset of symptoms. *Actinomyces* is usually associated with an infection of the pleura or chest wall, and *Nocardia* may be isolated along with an infection caused by *M. tuberculosis*. The pathogenesis of many of the infections caused by agents of chronic lower respiratory tract disease is characterized by the requirement for breakdown of cell-mediated immunity in the host or the ability of these agents to avoid being destroyed by host cell-mediated immune mechanisms. This may be caused by an effect on macrophages, the ability to mask foreign antigens, sheer size, or some other factor, allowing microbes to grow within host tissues without eliciting an overwhelming local immune reaction.

Cystic fibrosis (CF) is a genetic disorder that leads to persistent bacterial infection in the lung, causing airway wall damage and chronic obstructive lung disease. Eventually, a combination of airway secretions and damage leads to poor gas exchange in the lungs, cardiac malfunction, and subsequent death. Patients with CF may present as young adults with chronic respiratory tract disease or, more commonly, as children with gastrointestinal problems and stunted growth. *Staphylococcus aureus* is the most prevalent opportunistic bacterial pathogen infecting 55% of children 0–9 years of age with CF, with *Pseudomonas aeruginosa* the most prevalent (81%) in older children. A very mucoid *Pseudomonas*, characterized by production of copious amounts of extracellular capsular polysaccharide, can be isolated from the sputum of almost all patients with CF who are older than 18 years of age, becoming more prevalent with increasing age after 5 years. Even if CF has not been diagnosed, isolation of a mucoid *Pseudomonas aeruginosa* from sputum should alert the clinician to the possibility of underlying disease. Microbiologists should always report this unusual morphologic feature. In addition to mucoid *Pseudomonas* and *Staphylococcus aureus*, important pathogens in patients with CF are likely to harbor *Haemophilus influenzae*, *Streptococcus pneumoniae*, *Stenotrophomonas maltophilia*, *Achromobacter xylosoxidans*, *Ralsotnia* spp. *Cupriavidus* spp., *Pandoraea* spp., *Escherichia coli*, strains of *Burkholderia cepacia* complex, fast growing mycobacteria, RSV, influenza and fungi including *Aspergillu*, *Scedosporium* spp., and *Exophiala dermatidis*. In addition, due to the viscous mucous plugs associated with CF, several anaerobic organisms have been detected in the lungs of CF patients

including *Prevotella*, *Bifidobacterium*, *Veillonella*, *Peptostreptococcus* and *Fusobacterium*. Using advanced diagnostic molecular methods, additional organisms have also been identified in chronic polymicrobial CF infections including viridans streptococci, *Streptococcus constellatus*, *Streptococcus intermedius* and *Streptococcus anginosus*.

Lung abscess is usually a complication of acute or chronic pneumonia. In these circumstances, organisms infecting the lung cause localized destruction of the lung parenchyma (functional elements of the lung). Symptoms associated with lung abscess are similar to those of acute and chronic pneumonia, except symptoms fail to resolve with treatment.

**Immunocompromised Patients. *Patients with Neoplasms.*** Patients with cancer are at high risk to become infected because of either granulocytopenia or other defects in phagocytic defenses, cellular or humoral immune dysfunction, damage to mucosal surfaces and the skin, and various medical procedures such as blood product transfusion. In these patients, the nature of the malignancy often determines the etiology (Table 69-2) and pneumonia is a frequent clinical manifestation.

***Transplant Recipients.*** For successful organ transplantation, the recipient's immune system must be suppressed. As a result, these patients are predisposed to infection. Regardless of the type of organ transplant (heart, renal, bone marrow, heart/lung, liver, pancreas), most infections occur within 4 months following transplantation. Major infections can occur within the first month but are usually associated with infections carried over from the pretransplant period. Pulmonary infections are of great importance in this patient population. Some of the most common causes of pneumonia include *S. aureus* *Streptococcus pneumoniae*, *Haemophilus influenzae*, *Pneumocystis jiroveci*, and cytomegalovirus. In addition, other organisms such as *Cryptococcus neoformans*, *Aspergillus* spp., *Candida* spp., *Nocardia* sp. and over, can cause life-threatening pulmonary infection.

***HIV-Infected Patients.*** Patients who are infected with human immunodeficiency virus (HIV) are at high risk for developing pneumonia. As discussed in the previous chapter, opportunistic infections as a result of severe immunodeficiency are a major cause of illness and death among these patients. In the United States, the most common opportunistic infection among patients with acquired immunodeficiency syndrome is *Pneumocystis jiroveci* pneumonia. Although *P. jiroveci* remains a major pulmonary pathogen, other organisms must be considered in this patient population, including *Mycobacterium tuberculosis* and *Mycobacterium avium* complex, as well as common bacterial pathogens such as *Streptococcus pneumoniae* and *Haemophilus influenzae*. In addition to these common pathogens, many other organisms can cause lower respiratory tract infections, including *Nocardia* spp., *Rhodococcus equi* (a gram-positive, aerobic, pleomorphic organism), and *Legionella* spp.

## PLEURAL INFECTIONS

As a result of an organism infecting the lung and subsequently gaining access to the pleural space via an abnormal passage (fistula), the patient may develop an empyema (pus in a body cavity such as the pleural cavity).

**TABLE 69-4** Examples of Infectious Agents Frequently Associated with Certain Malignancies

| Malignancy (site and type of infections) | Pathogens |
|---|---|
| Acute nonlymphocytic leukemia (pneumonia, oral lesions, cutaneous lesions, urinary tract infections, hepatitis, most often sepsis without obvious focus) | Enterobacteriaceae<br>*Pseudomonas*<br>Staphylococci<br>*Corynebacterium jeikeium*<br>*Candida*<br>*Aspergillus*<br>Mucor<br>Hepatitis C and other non-A, non-B |
| Acute lymphocytic leukemia (pneumonia, cutaneous lesions, pharyngitis, disseminated disease) | Streptococci (all types)<br>*Pneumocystis jiroveci* (*P. carinii*)<br>Herpes simplex virus<br>Cytomegalovirus<br>Varicella zoster virus |
| Lymphoma (disseminated disease, pneumonia, urinary tract infections, sepsis, cutaneous lesions) | *Brucella*<br>*Candida* (mucocutaneous)<br>*Cryptococcus neoformans*<br>Herpes simplex virus (cutaneous)<br>Varicella zoster virus<br>Cytomegalovirus<br>*Pneumocystis jiroveci* (*P. carinii*)<br>*Toxoplasma gondii*<br>*Listeria monocytogenes*<br>Mycobacteria<br>*Nocardia*<br>*Salmonella*<br>Staphylococci<br>Enterobacteriaceae<br>*Pseudomonas*<br>*Strongyloides stercoralis* |
| Multiple myeloma (pneumonia, cutaneous lesions, sepsis) | *Haemophilus influenza*<br>*Streptococcus pneumoniae*<br>*Neisseria meningitides*<br>Enterobacteriaceae<br>*Pseudomonas*<br>Varicella zoster virus<br>*Candida*<br>*Aspergillus* |

Symptoms in these patients are insidious because early in the course of disease they are related to the primary infection in the lung. Once enough purulent exudate is formed, typical physical and radiographic findings indicative of an empyema are produced.

# LABORATORY DIAGNOSIS OF LOWER RESPIRATORY TRACT INFECTIONS

## SPECIMEN COLLECTION AND TRANSPORT

Although rapid determination of the etiologic agent is of paramount importance in managing pneumonia, the responsible pathogen is not identified in as many as 50% of patients, despite extensive diagnostic testing.

Unfortunately, no single test is capable of identifying all potential lower respiratory tract pathogens. Refer to Table 5-1 for an overview of the method used to collect, transport, and process specimens from the lower respiratory tract.

### Sputum

**Expectorated.** The examination of expectorated sputum has been the primary means of determining the causes of bacterial pneumonia. However, lower respiratory tract secretions will be contaminated with upper respiratory tract secretions, especially saliva, unless they are collected using an invasive technique. For this reason, sputum is among the least clinically relevant specimens received for culture in microbiology laboratories, even though it is one of the most numerous and time-consuming specimens.

Good sputum samples depend on thorough health care worker education and patient understanding throughout all phases of the collection process. Food should not have been ingested for 1 to 2 hours before expectoration and the mouth should be rinsed with saline or water just before expectoration. Patients should be instructed to provide a deep-coughed specimen. The material should be expelled into a sterile container, with an attempt to minimize contamination by saliva. Specimens should be transported to the laboratory immediately. Even a moderate amount of time at room temperature can result in the loss of viable infectious agents and the recovery of pathogens.

**Induced.** Patients unable to produce sputum may be assisted by respiratory therapists, who use postural drainage and thoracic percussion to stimulate production of acceptable sputum. Before specimen collection, patients should brush the buccal mucosa, tongue, and gums with a wet toothbrush. As an alternative, an aerosol-induced specimen may be collected for the isolation of mycobacterial or fungal agents. Induced sputum is also recognized for its high diagnostic yield in cases of *Pneumocystis jiroveci* pneumonia. Aerosol-induced specimens are collected by allowing the patient to breathe aerosolized droplets, using an ultrasonic nebulizer containing 10% 0.85% NaCl or until a strong cough reflex is initiated. Lower respiratory secretions obtained in this way appear watery, resembling saliva, although they often contain material directly from alveolar spaces. These specimens are usually adequate for culture and should be accepted in the laboratory without prescreening. Obtaining such a specimen may obviate the need for a more invasive procedure, such as bronchoscopy or needle aspiration.

The gastric aspirate is used exclusively for isolation of acid-fast bacilli and may be collected from patients who are unable to produce sputum, particularly young children. Before the patient wakes up in the morning, a nasogastric tube is inserted into the stomach and contents are withdrawn (on the assumption that acid-fast bacilli from the respiratory tract were swallowed during the night and will be present in the stomach). The relative resistance of mycobacteria to acidity allows them to remain viable for a short period. Gastric aspirate specimens must be delivered to the laboratory immediately so that the acidity can be neutralized. Specimens can be

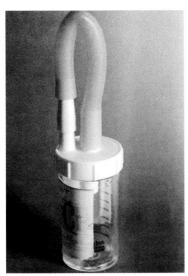

**Figure 69-2** Tracheal secretions received in the laboratory in a Lukens trap.

neutralized and then transported if immediate delivery is not possible.

### Endotracheal or Tracheostomy Suction Specimens

Patients with tracheostomies are unable to produce sputum in the normal fashion, but lower respiratory tract secretions can easily be collected in a Lukens trap (Figure 69-2). Tracheostomy aspirates or tracheostomy suction specimens should be treated as sputum by the laboratory. Patients with tracheostomies rapidly become colonized with gram-negative bacilli and other nosocomial pathogens. Such colonization per se is not clinically relevant, but these organisms may be aspirated into the lungs and cause pneumonia. Culture results should be correlated with clinical signs and symptoms.

**Bronchoscopy.** Bronchoscopy specimens include bronchoalveolar lavage (BAL), bronchial washing, bronchial brushing, and transbronchial biopsies. The diagnosis of pneumonia, particularly in HIV-infected and other immunocompromised patients, often necessitates the use of more invasive procedures. Fiberoptic bronchoscopy has dramatically affected the evaluation and management of these infections. With this method, the bronchial mucosa can be directly visualized and collected for biopsy, and the lung tissue can be sent for transbronchial biopsy for the evaluation of lung cancer and other lung diseases. Although transbronchial biopsy is important, the procedure is often associated with significant complications such as bleeding. The sample should be transported in sterile 0.85% saline.

During bronchoscopy, physicians obtain bronchial washings or aspirates, bronchoalveolar lavage (BAL) samples, protected bronchial brush samples, or specimens for transbronchial biopsy. Bronchial washings or aspirates are collected using a small amount of sterile physiologic saline inserted into the bronchial tree and withdrawing the fluid. These specimens will be contaminated with upper respiratory tract flora such as viridans streptococci and *Neisseria* spp. Recovery of potentially pathogenic organisms from bronchial washings should be attempted.

A deep sampling of desquamated host cells and secretions can be collected through bronchoscopy and BAL. Lavages are especially suitable for detecting Pneumocystis cysts and fungal elements. During this procedure, a high volume of saline (100 to 300 mL) is infused into a lung segment through the bronchoscope to obtain cells and protein of the pulmonary interstitium and alveolar spaces. It is estimated that more than 1 million alveoli are sampled during this process. The value of this technique in conjunction with quantitative culture for the diagnosis of most major respiratory tract pathogens, including bacterial pneumonia, has been documented. Scientists have found significant correlation between acute bacterial pneumonia and greater than $10^3$ to $10^4$ bacterial colonies per milliliter of BAL fluid. BAL has been shown to be a safe and practical method for diagnosing opportunistic pulmonary infections in immunosuppressed patients. At bedside, nonbronchoscopic "mini BAL" using a Metras catheter has been introduced; typically 20 mL or less of saline is instilled.

Another type of respiratory specimen is obtained via a protected catheter bronchial brush as part of a bronchoscopy examination. Specimens obtained by this moderately invasive collection procedure are suited for microbiologic studies, particularly in aspiration pneumonia. Protected specimen brush bristles collect from 0.001 to 0.01 mL of material. An overview of the collection process is shown in Figure 69-3. Upon receipt, contents of the bronchial brush may be suspended in 1 mL of broth solution with vigorous vortexing and inoculated onto culture media using a 0.01-mL calibrated inoculating loop. Some researchers have indicated that specimens obtained via double-lumen–protected catheters are suitable for both anaerobic and aerobic cultures. Colony counts of greater than or equal to 1000 organisms per milliliter in the broth diluent (or $10^6/$ mL in the original specimen) have been considered to correlate with infection. All facets of the bronchoscopic procedure—such as order of sampling, use of anesthetic, and rapidity of plating—should be rigorously standardized.

**Transtracheal Aspirates.** Percutaneous transtracheal aspirates (TTAs) are obtained by inserting a small plastic catheter into the trachea via a needle previously inserted through the skin and cricothyroid membrane. This invasive procedure, although somewhat uncomfortable for the patient and not suitable for all patients (it cannot be used in uncooperative patients, in patients with bleeding tendency, or in patients with poor oxygenation), reduces the likelihood that a specimen will be contaminated by upper respiratory tract flora and diluted by added fluids, provided care is taken to keep the catheter from being coughed back up into the pharynx. Although this technique is rarely used, anaerobes, such as *Actinomyces* and those associated with aspiration pneumonia, can be isolated from TTA specimens.

**Other Invasive Procedures.** When pleural empyema is present, thoracentesis may be used to obtain infected fluid for direct examination and culture. This constitutes an excellent specimen that accurately reflects the bacteriology of an associated pneumonia. Laboratory examination of such material is discussed in Chapter 77. Blood

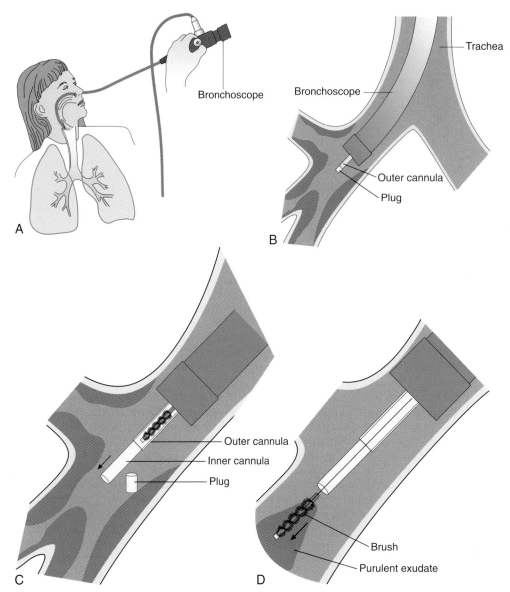

**Figure 69-3** Overview for obtaining a protected catheter bronchial brush during a bronchoscopy examination. **A,** The bronchoscope is introduced into the nose and advanced through the nasopharyngeal passage into the trachea. The bronchoscope is then inserted into the lung area of interest. **B,** A small brush that holds 0.001 to 0.01 mL of secretions is placed within a double cannula. The end of the outermost tube or cannula is closed with a displaceable plug made of absorbable gel. The cannula is inserted to the proper area. **C,** Once in the correct area, the inner cannula is pushed out, dislodging the protective plug as it is extruded. **D,** The brush is then extended beyond the inner cannula, and the specimen is collected by "brushing" the involved area. The brush is withdrawn into the inner cannula, which is withdrawn into the outer cannula to prevent contamination by upper airway organisms as it is removed.

cultures, of course, should always be obtained from patients with pneumonia.

For patients with pneumonia, a thin needle aspiration of material from the involved area of the lung may be performed percutaneously. If no material is withdrawn into the syringe after the first try, approximately 3 mL of sterile saline can be injected and then withdrawn into the syringe. Patients with emphysema, uremia, thrombocytopenia, or pulmonary hypertension may be at increased risk of complication (primarily pneumothorax [air in the pleural space] or bleeding) from this procedure. The specimens obtained are very small in volume, and protection from aeration is usually impossible. This

technique is more frequently used in children than in adults.

The most invasive procedure for obtaining respiratory tract specimens is the open lung biopsy. Performed by surgeons, this method is used to procure a wedge of lung tissue. Biopsy specimens are extremely helpful for diagnosing severe viral infections, such as herpes simplex pneumonia, for rapid diagnosis of *Pneumocystis* pneumonia, and for other hard-to-diagnose or life-threatening pneumonias. Ramifications of this and all other specimen collection techniques are discussed in *Cumitech 7B,* "Laboratory Diagnosis of Lower Respiratory Tract Infections."

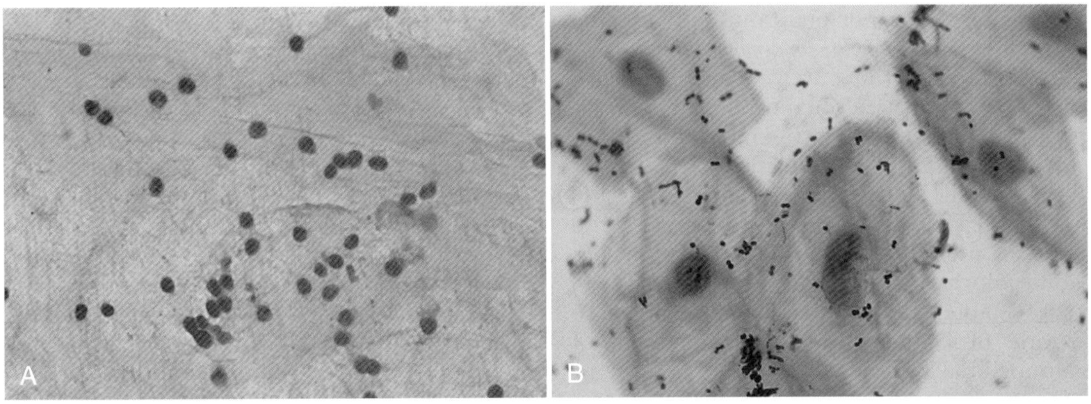

**Figure 69-4** Gram stain of sputum specimens. **A,** This specimen contains numerous polymorphonuclear leukocytes and no visible squamous epithelial cells, indicating that the specimen is acceptable for routine bacteriologic culture. **B,** This specimen contains numerous squamous epithelial cells and rare polymorphonuclear leukocytes, indicating an inadequate specimen for routine sputum culture.

## SPECIMEN PROCESSING

### Direct Visual Examination

Lower respiratory tract specimens can be examined by direct wet preparation for parasites and special procedures for *Pneumocystis*. Fungal elements can be visualized under phase microscopy with 10% potassium hydroxide, under ultraviolet light with calcofluor white, or using periodic acid-Schiff–stained smears.

For most other evaluations, the specimen must be fixed and stained. Bacteria and yeasts can be recognized on Gram stain. One of the most important uses of the Gram stain, however, is to evaluate the quality of expectorated sputum received for routine bacteriologic culture. A portion of the specimen consisting of purulent material is chosen for the stain. The smear can be evaluated adequately even before it is stained, thus negating the need for Gram stain of specimens later judged unacceptable. An acceptable specimen yields fewer than 10 squamous epithelial cells per low-power field (100×). The number of white blood cells may not be relevant, because many patients are severely neutropenic and specimens from these patients will not show white blood cells on Gram stain examination. On the other hand, the presence of 25 or more polymorphonuclear leukocytes per 100× field, together with few squamous epithelial cells, implies an excellent specimen (Figure 69-4). Samples that contain predominantly upper respiratory tract material should be rejected. Previously, only expectorated sputa were suitable for rejection based on microscopic screening. However, endotracheal aspirates (ETAs) from mechanically ventilated adult patients can be screened by Gram stain. Criteria used to reject ETAs from adult patients include greater than 10 squamous epithelial cells per low-power field or no organisms seen under oil immersion (1000×). In *Legionella* pneumonia, sputum may be scant and watery, with few or no host cells. Such specimens may be positive by direct fluorescent antibody stain and culture, and they should not be subjected to screening procedures. Conversely, sputum from patients with CF should be screened. A throat swab is an acceptable specimen from patients with CF in selected clinical settings and should be processed in a similar manner as CF sputum. Staining of respiratory samples is useful and

should be compared to culture results to reveal errors in procedures, specimen collection, and transport or specimen identification.

Respiratory secretions may need to be concentrated before staining. The cytocentrifuge instrument has been used successfully for this purpose, concentrating the cellular material in an easily examined monolayer on a glass slide. As an alternative, specimens are centrifuged, and the sediment is used for visual examinations and cultures. For screening purposes, the presence of ciliated columnar bronchial epithelial cells, goblet cells, or pulmonary macrophages in specimens obtained by bronchoscopy or BAL indicates a specimen from the lower respiratory tract.

In addition to the Gram stain, respiratory specimens may be stained for acid-fast bacilli with either the classic Ziehl-Neelsen or the Kinyoun carbolfuchsin stain. Auramine or auramine-rhodamine is also used to detect acid-fast organisms. Because they are fluorescent, these stains fluorescent superior already here comment only are more sensitive than the carbolfuchsin formulas and are preferable for rapid screening. Slides may be restained with the classic stains directly over the fluorochrome stains as long as all of the immersion oil has been removed carefully with xylene. All of the acid-fast stains will reveal *Cryptosporidium* spp. if they are present in the respiratory tract, as may occur in immunosuppressed patients. These patients are often at risk of infection with *P. jiroveci*. Although the modified Gomori methenamine silver stain has been used traditionally to recognize *Nocardia*, *Actinomyces*, fungi, and parasites, it takes approximately 1 hour of the technologist's time to perform, is technically demanding, and is not suitable as an emergency procedure. A fairly rapid stain, toluidine blue O, has been used in many laboratories with some success. Toluidine blue O stains *Pneumocystis*, *Nocardia asteroides*, and some fungi. A monoclonal antibody stain is the optimum stain for *Pneumocystis* (see Chapter 59) for less invasive specimens such as BAL and induced sputa.

Direct fluorescent antibody (DFA) staining has been used to detect *Legionella* spp. in lower respiratory tract specimens. Sputum, pleural fluid, aspirated material, and tissues are all suitable specimens. Because there are so many different serotypes of legionellae, polyclonal antibody reagents and a monoclonal antibody directed against all serotypes of *Legionella pneumophila* are used. Because of low sensitivity (50% to 75%), DFA results should not be relied on in lieu of culture. Rather, *Legionella* culture, DFA or urinary antigen, and serology should be performed for optimum sensitivity. See Chapter 35 for details regarding detection of *Legionella* spp.

Commercially available DFA reagents are also used to detect antigens of numerous viruses, including herpes simplex, cytomegalovirus, adenovirus, influenza viruses, and RSV (see Chapter 65). Commercial suppliers of reagents provide procedure information for each of these tests. Monoclonal and polyclonal fluorescent stains for *Chlamydia trachomatis* are available and may be useful for staining respiratory secretions of infants with pneumonia. A number of molecular amplification techniques (see Chapter 8) for the direct detection of respiratory pathogens have been described; however, the sensitivity and specificity of these assays vary greatly from one study to another. Amplification assays are also available for the direct detection of *Mycobacterium tuberculosis* on smear-positive specimens (see Chapter 43).

Rapid direct detection from respiratory samples is now available using nucleic acid-based methods. The xTAG Respiratory Viral Panel (RVP) (Luminex Corporation, Austin, TX), can be used for the simultaneous detection of influenza (four types), RSV, human metapneumovirus, and adenovirus from nasopharyngeal swabs. In addition, the FilmArray Respiratory Panel (BIOFIRE Diagnostics, Salt Lake City, UT ) is capable of detecting upper respiratory tract infections associated with coronavirus (four types) , adenovirus, influenza (five types), rhinovirus, parainfluenza virus (four types), enterovirus, human metapneumovirus, RSV, *Bordetella pertussis*, *Mycoplasma pneumoniae*, and *Chlamydophila pneumoniae* in approximately 1 hour directly from patient samples. Smaller molecular panels are also available such as the real-time multiplex amplification kit for influenza A, B, and RSV (Hologic-Gen-Probe, San Diego, CA). All of the previously mentioned methods are FDA-approved. In addition to these, there are a variety of research-use-only and other molecular respiratory panels in clinical validation studies. It is important when considering the use of a molecular assay that the laboratory consider their patient population including severity of illness, immune status, and transplant histories.

### Routine Culture

Most of the commonly sought etiologic agents of lower respiratory tract infection are isolated on routine media: 5% sheep blood agar, MacConkey agar for the isolation and differentiation of gram-negative bacilli, and chocolate agar for *Haemophilus* and *Neisseria* spp. Because of contaminating oral flora, sputum specimens, specimens obtained by bronchial washing and lavage, tracheal aspirates, and tracheostomy or endotracheal tube aspirates are not inoculated to enrichment broth or incubated

anaerobically. Only specimens obtained by percutaneous aspiration (including transtracheal aspiration) and protected bronchial brush are suitable for anaerobic culture; the latter must be done quantitatively for proper interpretation (refer to prior discussion). Transtracheal and percutaneous lung aspiration material may be inoculated to enriched thioglycollate as well as to solid media. For suspected cases of Legionnaires' disease, buffered charcoal-yeast extract (BCYE) agar and selective BCYE should be inoculated. Plates should be streaked in four quadrants to provide a basis for objective semiquantitation to define the amount of growth. After 24 to 48 hours of incubation, the numbers and types of colonies are recorded. For *Legionella* cultures, colonies form on the selective agar after 3 to 5 days at 35° C.

Sputum specimens from patients known to have CF should be inoculated to selective agar, such as specific chromagenic agar, for recovery of *S. aureus* and selective horse blood–bacitracin, incubated anaerobically and aerobically, for recovery of *H. influenzae* that may be obscured by the mucoid *Pseudomonas* on routine media. The use of a selective medium for *B. cepacia*, such as PC or OFPBL agars, is also necessary.

For interpretation of culture results on those specimens contaminated by normal oropharyngeal flora (e.g., expectorated and induced sputum, bronchial washings), growth of the predominant aerobic and facultative anaerobic bacteria is reported. To ensure optimum culture reporting, conditions must be well defined in terms of an objective grading system for streaked plates. Finally, the clinical significance of culture findings depends not only on standardized and appropriate laboratory methods but also on how specimens are collected and transported, other laboratory data, and the patient's clinical presentation.

Numerous bacterial agents that cause lower respiratory tract infections are not detected by routine bacteriologic culture. Mycobacteria, *Chlamydia*, *Nocardia*, *Bordetella pertussis*, *Legionella*, and *Mycoplasma pneumoniae* require special procedures for detection; this also applies to viruses and fungi. Optimal recovery for *Mycobacterium tuberculosis* requires multiple specimens for acid-fast staining culture, and at least one sample for molecular testing as recommended by the Centers for Disease Control. Refer to the appropriate chapter section for more information regarding these organisms. Finally, one must keep in mind those potential agents for bioterrorist attack, such as *Bacillus anthracis*, *Francisella tularensis*, and *Yersinia pestis*, that might be recovered from respiratory specimens (see Chapter 80).

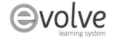 *Visit the Evolve site to complete the review questions.*

# CASE STUDY 69-1

A 16-month-old boy was admitted with fever, lethargy, and trouble breathing. A diagnosis of pneumonia was made by physical examination. The child had recently been to Panama and was treated with ceftriaxone for cough and fever. His fever continued, despite treatment. On admission, he was given erythromycin therapy. Tracheal aspirate and blood cultures were obtained, but the respiratory specimen contained numerous epithelial cells and yielded normal respiratory flora on culture. A pleural aspirate and blood cultures were positive for *Streptococcus pneumoniae,* which was resistant to erythromycin and penicillin and intermediate in susceptibility to ceftriaxone. The patient was given high doses of ceftriaxone and vancomycin and responded to this therapy.

**QUESTIONS**

1. What criteria are used in laboratories to reject sputum and tracheal aspirates for culture?
2. If greater than 10 squamous epithelial cells per low-power field are seen in a Gram stain but the smear also has numerous white blood cells (greater than 25 per low-power field), should the specimen be rejected for culture?
3. In cases of pneumococcal pneumonia, what percentage of blood and sputum cultures is positive for *S. pneumoniae?*
4. The organism was reported as resistant to penicillin (MIC of 4 μg/mL) and intermediate in susceptibility to third-generation cephalosporins (minimum inhibitory concentration to ceftriaxone of 2 μg/mL). How does the laboratory test for this organism?

# BIBLIOGRAPHY

American Thoracic Society and the Infectious Diseases Society of America: Guidelines for the management of adults with hospital-acquired, ventilator-associated, and healthcare-associated pneumonia, *Am J Respir Crit Care Med* 171:388, 2005.

Bartlett JG, Dowell SF, Mandell LA, et al: Practice guidelines for the management of community-acquired pneumonia in adults, *Clin Infect Dis* 31:347, 2000.

Boivin G, Abed Y, Pelletier G, et al: Virological features and clinical manifestations associated with human metapneumovirus: a new paramyxovirus responsible for acute respiratory tract infections in all age groups, *J Infect Dis* 186:1330, 2002.

Broughton WA, Middleton RM III, Kirkpatrick MB, et al: Bronchoscopic protected specimen brush and bronchoalveolar lavage in the diagnosis of bacterial pneumonia, *Infect Dis Clin North Am* 5:437, 1991.

Caliendo AM: Enhanced diagnosis of *Pneumocystis carinii:* promises and problems, *Clin Microbiol Newsletter* 18:113, 1996.

Campbell S, Forbes BA: The clinical microbiology laboratory in the diagnosis of lower respiratory tract infections, *J Clin Microbiol* 49(9):S30-S33, 2011.

Cantral DE, Tape TG, Reed EC, et al: Quantitative culture of bronchoalveolar lavage fluid for the diagnosis of bacterial pneumonia, *Am J Med* 95:601, 1993.

Carroll KA: Laboratory diagnosis of lower respiratory tract infections: controversy and conundrums, *J Clin Microbiol* 40:3115, 2002.

Centers for Disease Control and Prevention: National Nosocomial Infections Surveillance (NNIS) System Report, data summary from January 1992 through June 2004, issued October 2004, *Am J Infect Control* 32:470, 2004

Cesario TC: Viruses associated with pneumonia in adults, *Clin Pract* 55:107-113, 2012.

Current topics: atypical pneumonia agents are joining the mainstream, *ASM News* 61:621, 1995.

Denny F, Clyde WJ: Acute lower respiratory tract infections in non-hospitalized children, *J Pediatr* 108:635, 1989.

Doring G, Parameswaran IG, Murphy TF: Differential adaptation of microbial pathogens to airways of patients with cystic fibrosis and chronic obstructive pulmonary disease, *FEMS Microbiol Reviews* 35(1):124-146, 2010.

Falcone M, Blasi F, Menichetti F, et al: Pneumonia in frail older patients: an up to date, *Intern Emerg Med* 7(5):415-424, 2012.

Gilligan P: Report on the consensus document for microbiology and infectious diseases in cystic fibrosis, *Clin Microbiol Newsletter* 18:11, 1996.

Kahn FW, Jones JM: Analysis of bronchoalveolar lavage specimens from immunocompromised patients with a protocol applicable in the microbiology laboratory, *J Clin Microbiol* 26:1150, 1988.

Kauppinen M, Saikku P: Pneumonia due to *Chlamydia pneumoniae:* prevalence, clinical features, diagnosis, and treatment, *Clin Infect Dis* 21:244, 1995.

Kuo CC, Jackson LA, Campbell LA, et al: *Chlamydia pneumoniae* (TWAR), *Clin Microbiol Rev* 8:451, 1995.

Lentino JR: The nonvalue of unscreened sputum specimens in the diagnosis of pneumonia, *Clin Microbiol Newsletter* 9:70, 1987.

Mandell LA, Bartlett JG, Dowell SF, et al: Update of practice guidelines for the management of community-acquired pneumonia in immunocompetent adults, *Clin Infect Dis* 37:1405, 2003.

Marrie TJ: Community-acquired pneumonia, *Clin Infect Dis* 18:501, 1994.

Marrie TJ, Durant H, Bates L: Community-acquired pneumonia requiring hospitalization: a 5-year prospective study, *Rev Infect Dis* 11:586, 1989.

McIntosh K: Community-acquired pneumonia in children, *N Engl J Med* 346:429, 2002.

Morris AJ, Tanner DC, Reller RB: Rejection criteria for endotracheal aspirates from adults, *J Clin Microbiol* 31:1027, 1993.

Mosenifau Z, Jeng A, Kamangar N, et al: Viral pneumonia, Medscape; emedicine.medscape.com/article/300455-overview. 2012.

Navarro D, Garcia-Maset L, Gimenao C, et al: Performance of the Binax NOW *Streptococcus pneumoniae* urinary antigen assay for diagnosis of pneumonia in children with underlying pulmonary diseases in the absence of acute pneumococcal infection, *J Clin Microbiol* 42:4853, 2004.

Niederman MS, Bass JB Jr, Campbell GD, et al: Guidelines for the initial management of adults with community-acquired pneumonia: diagnosis, assessment of severity, and initial antimicrobial therapy, *Am Rev Respir Dis* 148:1418, 1993.

Pinner RW, Teutsch SM, Simonsen I, et al: Trends in infectious diseases mortality in the United States, *JAMA* 275:189, 1996.

Pisani RJ, Wright AJ: Clinical utility of bronchoalveolar lavage in immunocompromised hosts, *Mayo Clin Proc* 67:221, 1992.

Poe R: Management of lower respiratory tract infections, *Guthrie J* 65:40, 1996.

Pollock HM, Hawkins EL, Bonner JR, et al: Diagnosis of bacterial pulmonary infections with quantitative protected catheter cultures obtained during bronchoscopy, *J Clin Microbiol* 17:255, 1983.

Roson B, Fernandez-Sabe N, Carratala J, et al: Contribution of a urinary antigen assay (Binax NOW) to the early diagnosis of pneumococcal pneumonia, *Clin Infect Dis* 38:222, 2004.

Sadeghi E, Matlow A, MacLusky I, et al: Utility of Gram stain in evaluation of sputa from patients with cystic fibrosis, *J Clin Microbiol* 32:54, 1994.

Salemi C, Morgan J, Padilla S, et al: Association between severity of illness and mortality from nosocomial infection, *Am J Infect Control* 23:188, 1995.

Sharp SE, Robinson A, Saubolle M, et al: Lower respiratory tract infections. In Sharp SE, coordinating editor: *Cumitech 7B*, Washington, DC, 2004, ASM Press.

Stuckey-Schrock K, Hayes BL, George CM: Community-acquired pneumonia in children, *Am Fam Physician* 86(7):661-667, 2012.

Thoulouze MI, Alcover A: Can viruses form biofilms? *Trends Microbiol* 19(6):257-262, 2011.

Tollemar J: Prophylaxis against fungal infections in transplant recipients: possible approaches, *Biodrugs* 11(5):309-318, 1999.

Tsolia MN, Psarras S, Bossios A, et al: Etiology of community-acquired pneumonia in hospitalized school-age children: evidence for high prevalence of viral infections, *Clin Infect Dis* 39:681, 2004.

Versalovic J: Manual of clinical microbiology, ed 10, Washington, DC, 2011, ASM Press.

## OBJECTIVES

1. Explain the anatomy and structures of the upper respiratory tract, including the three parts of the pharynx.
2. Identify the principal causative organism of pharyngitis; name other organisms capable of causing pharyngitis.
3. Define the following conditions: laryngitis, epiglottis, and parotitis. List the etiologic organisms associated with these conditions.
4. Explain the pathogenic mechanisms (virulence factors) associated with *Streptococcus pyogenes* pharyngitis.
5. Define Vincent's angina and peritonsillar abscesses. What organism do they share as the causative agent of disease?
6. Describe the disease process caused by pharyngeal infection with *Corynebacterium diphtheriae*; name the hallmark symptom of this infection and list the complications associated with infection.
7. Differentiate between stomatitis and thrush, and explain the testing process for each disease.
8. Outline the steps used in the culture of specimens for the isolation of *Streptococcus pyogenes*.
9. Explain the signs and symptoms and pathogenic mechanisms associated with disease caused by *Bordetella pertussis*. What special requirements are needed to detect this organism in culture?
10. List three types of periodontal infections that require culture to identify the causative agent of infection; name the bacteria associated with these infections.
11. Explain the unique characteristics of C and G *streptococcus*, and explain how they contribute to their pathogenesis.

## GENERAL CONSIDERATIONS

### ANATOMY

The respiratory tract is generally divided into two regions, the upper and the lower.

The upper respiratory tract includes all the structures down to the larynx: the sinuses, throat, nasal cavity, epiglottis, and larynx; the throat is also called the pharynx. These anatomic structures are shown in Figure 70-1.

The pharynx is a tubelike structure that extends from the base of the skull to the esophagus (see Figure 70-1). Made of muscle, this structure is divided into three parts:
- Nasopharynx (portion of the pharynx above the soft palate)
- Oropharynx (portion of the pharynx between the soft palate and epiglottis)
- Laryngopharynx (portion of the pharynx below the epiglottis that opens into the larynx)

The oropharynx and nasopharynx are lined with stratified squamous epithelial cells that are teeming with microbial flora. The tonsils are contained within the oropharynx; the larynx is located between the root of the tongue and the upper end of the trachea.

## PATHOGENESIS

An overview of the pathogenesis of respiratory tract infections is presented in Chapter 69. It is important to keep in mind that upper respiratory tract infections may spread and become more serious because the mucosa (mucous membrane) of the upper tract is continuous with the mucosal lining of the sinuses, eustachian tube, middle ear, and lower respiratory tract.

## DISEASES OF THE UPPER RESPIRATORY TRACT, ORAL CAVITY, AND NECK

### UPPER RESPIRATORY TRACT

Diseases of the upper respiratory tract are named according to the anatomic sites involved. Most of these infections are self-limiting, and the majority of infections are of viral origin.

#### Laryngitis

Acute laryngitis is usually associated with the common cold or influenza syndromes. Characteristically, patients complain of hoarseness and lowering or deepening of the voice. Acute laryngitis is generally a benign illness.

Acute laryngitis is almost exclusively associated with viral infection. Although numerous viruses can cause laryngitis, influenza and parainfluenza viruses, rhinoviruses, adenoviruses, coronavirus, and human metapneumovirus are the most common etiologic agents. If examination of the larynx reveals an exudate or membrane on the pharyngeal or laryngeal mucosa, streptococcal infection, mononucleosis, or diphtheria should be suspected (see the discussion about miscellaneous infections caused by other agents, presented later in this chapter). Chronic laryngitis, although less frequently associated with infectious agents, may be caused by bacteria or fungal isolates. Infections have been identified that are associated with methicillin-resistant *Staphylococcus aureus* (MRSA) and *Candida* spp.

#### Laryngotracheobronchitis

Another clinical syndrome closely related to laryngitis is acute laryngotracheobronchitis, or croup. Croup is a relatively common illness in young children, primarily those younger than 3 years of age. Of significance, croup can represent a potentially more serious disease if the infection extends downward from the larynx to involve the trachea or even the bronchi. Illness is characterized by variable fever, inspiratory stridor (difficulty in moving enough air through the larynx), hoarseness, and a harsh, barking, nonproductive cough. These symptoms last for 3 to 4 days, although the cough may persist for a longer period. In young infants, severe respiratory distress and fever are common symptoms.

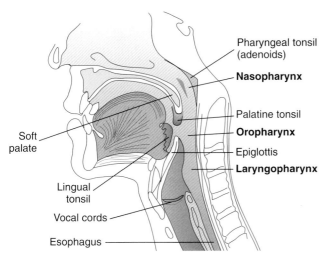

**Figure 70-1** The pharynx, including its three divisions and nearby structures.

Similar to the etiologic agents of laryngitis, viruses are a primary cause of croup; parainfluenza viruses are the major etiologic agents. In addition to parainfluenza viruses, influenza viruses, respiratory syncytial virus, and adenoviruses can also cause croup.

Also capable of causing croup, though not as frequently, are *Mycoplasma pneumoniae*, rhinoviruses, and enteroviruses.

### Epiglottitis

Epiglottitis is an infection of the epiglottis and other soft tissues above the vocal cords. Infection of the epiglottis can lead to significant edema (swelling) and inflammation. Most commonly, children between the ages of 2 and 6 years of age are infected. These children typically present with fever, difficulty in swallowing because of pain, drooling, and respiratory obstruction with inspiratory stridor. Epiglottitis is a potentially life-threatening disease because the patient's airway can become completely obstructed (blocked) if not treated.

In contrast to laryngitis, epiglottitis is usually associated with bacterial infections. In the past, 2- to 4-year-old children were typically infected with *Haemophilus influenzae* type b as the primary cause of epiglottitis. However, due to the common use of *Haemophilus influenzae* type b conjugated vaccine, the typical patient is an adult with a sore throat. Other organisms occasionally implicated are streptococci and staphylococci. Diagnosis is established on clinical grounds, including the visualization of the epiglottis, which appears swollen and bright red in color. Bacteriologic culture of the epiglottis is contraindicated because swabbing of the epiglottis may lead to respiratory obstruction. Of importance, *H. influenzae* bacteremia usually occurs in children with epiglottitis caused by this organism.

### Pharyngitis, Tonsillitis, and Peritonsillar Abscesses

**Pharyngitis and Tonsillitis.** Pharyngitis (sore throat) and tonsillitis are common upper respiratory tract infections affecting both children and adults. Acute pharyngitis is an illness that frequently causes people to seek medical care.

**Clinical Manifestations.** Infection of the pharynx is associated with pharyngeal pain. Visualization of the pharynx reveals erythematous (red) and swollen tissue. Depending on the causative microorganism, either inflammatory exudate (fluid with protein, inflammatory cells, and cellular debris), vesicles (small blister-like sacs containing liquid) and mucosal ulceration, or nasopharyngeal lymphoid hyperplasia (swollen lymph nodes) may be observed.

**Pathogenesis.** Pathogenic mechanisms differ and depend on the organism causing the pharyngitis. For example, some organisms directly invade the pharyngeal mucosa (e.g., *Arcanobacterium haemolyticum*), others elaborate toxins and other virulence factors at the site (e.g., *Corynebacterium diphtheriae*), and still others invade the pharyngeal mucosa and elaborate toxins and other virulence factors (e.g., group A streptococci [*Streptococcus pyogenes*]). Pathogenic mechanisms are reviewed in Part III according to various organism groups.

**Epidemiology/Etiologic Agents.** Most cases of pharyngitis occur during the colder months and often accompany other infections, primarily those caused by viruses. Patients with respiratory tract infections caused by influenza types A and B, parainfluenza, coxsackie A, rhinoviruses, or coronaviruses frequently complain of a sore throat. Pharyngitis, often with ulceration, is also commonly found in patients with infectious mononucleosis caused by either Epstein-Barr virus or cytomegalovirus. Although less common, pharyngitis caused by adenovirus or herpes simplex virus is clinically severe. Finally, acute retroviral syndrome caused by human immunodeficiency virus 1 (HIV-1) is associated with acute pharyngitis.

Although different bacteria can cause pharyngitis or tonsillitis, the primary cause of bacterial pharyngitis is *Streptococcus pyogenes* (or group A beta-hemolytic streptococci). Viral pharyngitis or other causes of pharyngitis/tonsillitis must be differentiated from that caused by *S. pyogenes*, because pharyngitis resulting from *S. pyogenes* is treatable with penicillin and a variety of other antimicrobials, whereas viral infections are not. In addition, treatment is of particular importance because infection with *S. pyogenes* can lead to complications such as acute rheumatic fever and glomerulonephritis. These complications are referred to as poststreptococcal sequelae (diseases that follow a streptococcal infection) and are primarily immunologically mediated; these sequelae are discussed in greater detail in Chapter 15. *S. pyogenes* may also cause pyogenic infections (suppurations) of the tonsils, sinuses, and middle ear, or cellulitis as secondary pyogenic sequelae after an episode of pharyngitis. Accordingly, streptococcal pharyngitis is usually treated to prevent both the suppurative and nonsuppurative sequelae, as well as to decrease morbidity.

Although bacteria other than group A streptococci may cause pharyngitis, this occurs less often. Large colony isolates of groups C and G streptococci (classified as *Streptococcus dysgalactiae* subsp. *equisimilis*) are pyogenic streptococci with similar virulence traits as *S. pyogenes*; symptoms of pharyngitis caused by these agents are also similar to *S. pyogenes*. In contrast to *S. pyogenes*, these agents are rarely associated with poststreptococcal sequelae, namely glomerulonephritis and possibly

**TABLE 70-1** Examples of Bacteria That Can Cause Acute Pharyngitis and/or Tonsillitis

| Organism | Disease | Relative Frequency |
|---|---|---|
| *Streptococcus pyogenes* | Pharyngitis/tonsillitis/ rheumatic fever/ scarlet fever | 15% to 35% |
| Group C and G beta-hemolytic streptococci | Pharyngitis/tonsillitis | <3% to 11% |
| *Arcanobacterium (Corynebacterium) haemolyticum* | Pharyngitis/tonsillitis/ rash | <1% to 10% |
| *Neisseria gonorrhoeae* | Pharyngitis/ disseminated disease | Rare* |
| *Corynebacterium ulcerans* | Pharyngitis | Rare |
| *Mycoplasma pneumoniae* | Pneumonia/ bronchitis/ pharyngitis | Rare |
| *Yersinia enterocolitica* | Pharyngitis/ enterocolitis | Rare |
| Human immunodeficiency virus-1 | Pharyngitis/acute retroviral disease | Rare |

*Less than 1%.

rheumatic fever. Recent studies have demonstrated that these streptococci can exchange genetic information with *S. pyogenes* and thus potentially obtain virulence factors usually associated with *S. pyogenes* such as M proteins, streptolysin O, and superantigen genes. *Arcanobacterium haemolyticum* is also a cause of pharyngitis among adolescents. Examples of agents that can cause pharyngitis or tonsillitis are listed in Table 70-1.

Although *H. influenzae*, *S. aureus*, and *S. pneumoniae* are frequently isolated from nasopharyngeal and throat cultures, they have not been shown to cause pharyngitis. Carriage of any of these organisms, as well as *Neisseria meningitidis*, may have clinical importance for some patients. Cultures of specimens obtained from the anterior nares often yield *S. aureus*. The carriage rate for this organism is especially high among health care workers, and 10%-30% of the general population can be colonized with this microbe, depending on the population characteristics.

Vincent's angina, also called acute necrotizing ulcerative gingivitis, or trench mouth, is a mixed bacterial-spirochetal infection of the gingival edge. The infection is relatively rare today, but it is considered a serious disease because it is often complicated by septic jugular thrombophlebitis, bacteremia, and widespread metastatic infection. Adults are more often affected than children; poor oral hygiene is a predisposing factor. Multiple anaerobes, especially *Fusobacterium necrophorum*, are implicated in this syndrome. Although Gram stain of a throat specimen is usually not predictive, in those patients with symptoms suggestive of Vincent's angina, Gram stain reveals numerous fusiform, gram-negative bacilli, and spirochetes.

**BOX 70-1** Viral Agents That Can Cause Rhinitis

Rhinoviruses
Coronaviruses
Adenoviruses
Parainfluenza and influenza viruses
Respiratory syncytial virus
Enterovirus

**Peritonsillar Abscesses.** Peritonsillar abscesses are generally considered a complication of tonsillitis. This infection is most common in children older than 5 years of age and in young adults. It is important to treat these infections because they can spread to adjacent tissues, as well as erode into the carotid artery to cause an acute hemorrhage. The predominant organisms isolated in peritonsillar abscesses include non–spore-forming anaerobes, such as *Fusobacterium* (especially *F. necrophorum*), *Bacteroides* (including the *B. fragilis* group), and anaerobic cocci. *Streptococcus pyogenes* and viridans streptococci may also be involved.

### Rhinitis

Rhinitis (common cold) is an inflammation of the nasal mucous membrane or lining. Depending on the host response and the etiologic agent, rhinitis is characterized by variable fever, increased mucous secretions, inflammatory edema of the nasal mucosa, sneezing, and watery eyes. With rare exceptions, rhinitis is typically associated with viral infections (20%-25%); some of these agents are listed in Box 70-1. Rhinitis is common because of the large number of different causative viruses, and reinfections may occur. Bacterial agents associated with rhinitis (10%-15%) include *Chlamydia pneumoniae*, *Mycoplasma pneumoniae*, and Group A streptococci.

**Miscellaneous Infections Caused by Other Agents.**

***Corynebacterium diphtheriae.*** Pharyngitis caused by *Corynebacterium diphtheriae* is less common than streptococcal pharyngitis. After an incubation period of 2 to 4 days, diphtheria usually presents as pharyngitis or tonsillitis. Patients are often febrile and complain of sore throat and malaise (body discomfort). The hallmark for diphtheria is the presence of an exudate or membrane that is usually on the tonsils or pharyngeal wall. The gray-white membrane is a result of the action of diphtheria toxin on the epithelium at the site of infection. Complications occur frequently with diphtheria and are usually seen during the last stage of the disease (paroxysmal stage). The most feared complications are those involving the central nervous system such as seizures, coma, or blindness. Information as to how this organism causes disease is discussed in Chapter 69. Additional specifics regarding this organism are provided in Chapter 17.

***Bordetella pertussis.*** Although mass immunization programs have greatly reduced the incidence of pertussis, enough cases (because of outbreaks and regional epidemics) still occur. In 2010, the CDC reported 27,500 cases of pertussis. This increased number of identifiable cases may be due to improved awareness and improved diagnostic methods, such as nucleic acid-based testing. It is important that laboratories are capable of detecting, isolating, and identifying the organism, or the specimen should be referred to a reference laboratory.

Characteristically, pertussis, or whooping cough, is a prolonged disease (lasting as long as 6 to 8 weeks) marked by paroxysmal (sudden or intense) coughing.

Following an incubation period of 7 to 13 days, the patient with symptomatic infection develops upper respiratory symptoms, including a dry cough, fever, runny nose, and sneezing. After about 2 weeks, this may progress to spells of paroxysmal coughing. As these episodes worsen, the characteristic whoop, caused by attempted inspiration through an epiglottis undergoing spasm, begins. Vomiting may occur, and usually a lymphocytosis is present. This phase of the illness may last as long as 6 weeks. Bacterial culture for *B. pertussis* is effective using nasopharyngeal specimens during the first 2 weeks when symptoms are evident. Amplification and polymerase chain reaction may demonstrate positive results within 0-4 weeks of the onset of symptoms. However, positive results should be interpreted with caution and in correlation with patient signs and symptoms. More information regarding B. *pertussis* is provided in Chapter 37.

**Klebsiella spp.** Rhinoscleroma is a rare form of chronic, granulomatous infection of the nasal passages, including the sinuses and occasionally the pharynx and larynx. Associated with *Klebsiella rhinoscleromatis* and *Klebsiella ozaenae*, the disease is characterized by nasal obstruction appearing over a long period, caused by tumor-like growth with local extension. *K. ozaenae* may contribute to another infrequent condition called ozena, characterized by a chronic, mucopurulent nasal discharge that is often foul smelling. It is caused by secondary, low-grade anaerobic infection.

## ORAL CAVITY

### Stomatitis

Stomatitis is an inflammation of the mucous membranes of the oral cavity. Herpes simplex virus is the primary agent of this disease, in which multiple ulcerative lesions are seen on the oral mucosa. These lesions are painful and can be found in the mouth and in the oropharynx. Herpetic infections of the oral cavity are prevalent among immunosuppressed patients.

### Thrush

*Candida* spp. can also invade the oral mucosa. Immunosuppressed patients, including very young infants, may develop oral candidiasis, called thrush. Oral thrush can extend to produce pharyngitis or esophagitis, a common finding in patients with acquired immunodeficiency syndrome and in other immunosuppressed patients. Thrush is suspected if whitish patches of exudate on an area of inflammation are observed on the buccal (cheek) mucosa, tongue, or oropharynx. Oral mucositis or pharyngitis in the granulocytopenic patient may be caused by Enterobacteriaceae, *S. aureus*, or *Candida* spp. and is manifested by erythema, sore throat, and possibly exudate or ulceration.

### Periodontal Infections

**Types.** The three dental problems that may require culture and identification in a clinical laboratory include (1) root canal infections, with or without periapical abscess; (2) orofacial odontogenic infections, with or without osteomyelitis (inflammation of a bone) in the jaw; and (3) perimandibular space infections. Oral bacteria are clearly important in other dental processes, such as caries (destruction of the mineralized tissues of the tooth; a cavity), periodontal (tissues in, around, and supporting the tooth) disease, and localized juvenile periodontitis, but clinical laboratories are not involved in culturing in such cases.

**Etiologic Agents.** The bacteriology is similar in all of these infections and involves primarily anaerobic bacteria and streptococci except for perimandibular space infections, which may also involve staphylococci and *Eikenella corrodens* in about 15% of patients. The streptococci are microaerobic or facultative and are usually alpha-hemolytic (particularly the *Streptococcus anginosus* group—see Chapter 15); they are usually found in 20% to 30% of dental infections.

Members of the *Bacteroides fragilis* group are found in root canal infections, orofacial odontogenic infections, and bacteremia secondary to dental extraction in 5% to 10% of patients. Anaerobic cocci (both *Peptostreptococcus* and *Veillonella*), pigmented *Prevotella* and *Porphyromonas*, the *Prevotella oralis* group, and *Fusobacterium* are found in about 20% to 50% of the three conditions mentioned, as well as in postextraction bacteremia. Infection with *Actinomyces israelii* may complicate oral surgery.

### Salivary Gland Infections

Acute suppurative parotitis (inflammation of the salivary glands located under the cheek in front of and below the external ear) is seen in very ill patients, especially those who are dehydrated, malnourished, elderly, or recovering from surgery. It is associated with painful, tender swelling of the parotid gland; purulent drainage may be evident at the opening of the duct of the gland in the mouth. *Staphylococcus aureus* is the major pathogen but on occasion Enterobacteriaceae, other gram-negative bacilli, and oral anaerobes may play a role in infection. A chronic bacterial parotitis has been described involving *Staphylococcus aureus*. Less often, other salivary glands may be involved with a bacterial infection, usually because of ductal obstruction.

The mumps virus is traditionally the major viral agent involved in parotitis; however, since the advent of childhood vaccination, infection with mumps virus is rarely diagnosed. Influenza virus and enteroviruses may also cause this syndrome. Viral parotitis is typically diagnosed using serology. Infrequently, *Mycobacterium tuberculosis* may involve the parotid gland in conjunction with pulmonary tuberculosis.

## NECK

Infections of the deep spaces of the neck are potentially serious because they may spread to critical structures such as major vessels of the neck or to the mediastinum, leading to mediastinitis, purulent pericarditis, and pleural empyema. Oral flora is responsible for these infections. Accordingly, the predominant organisms are anaerobes, primarily *Peptostreptococcus*, various *Bacteroides*, *Prevotella*, *Porphyromonas*, *Fusobacterium* spp., and *Actinomyces*.

Streptococci, chiefly of the viridans variety, are also important. *Staphylococcus aureus* and various aerobic, gram-negative bacilli may be recovered, particularly from patients developing these problems in the hospital.

Scrofula is a tuberculous infection in the lymph nodes of the neck that may be associated with *Mycobacterium tuberculosis, Mycobacterium scrofulaceum,* or *Mycobacterium avium.* The characteristic signs and symptoms include painless swelling of the lymph nodes with the rare appearance of fever or ulcerations. Diagnosis may require bacterial culture of the lymph nodes, computed tomography (CT) of the neck, biopsy, and chest x-ray or PPD (purified protein derivative) testing associated with *M. tuberculosis.*

# DIAGNOSIS OF UPPER RESPIRATORY TRACT INFECTIONS

## COLLECTION AND TRANSPORT OF SPECIMENS

Sterile, Dacron, or Rayon swabs with plastic shafts are suitable for collecting most upper respiratory tract microorganisms. Flocked swabs may also be used when available. If the swab remains moist, no further precautions need to be taken for specimens cultured within 4 hours of collection. After that period, transport medium is required to maintain viability and prevent overgrowth of contaminating organisms. Swabs for detection of group A streptococci (*Streptococcus pyogenes*) are the only exception. This organism is highly resistant to desiccation and remains viable on a dry swab for as long as 48 to 72 hours. These throat swabs can be placed in glassine paper envelopes for mailing or transport to a distant laboratory. Throat swabs are also adequate for recovery of adenoviruses and herpes viruses, *Corynebacterium diphtheriae, Mycoplasma, Chlamydia,* and *Candida* spp. Recovery of *C. diphtheriae* is enhanced by culturing both the throat and nasopharynx.

Nasopharyngeal swabs are better suited for recovery of *Bordetella pertussis, Neisseria* spp., along with several viruses including respiratory syncytial virus, parainfluenza virus, and the other viruses causing rhinitis. Optimum conditions for the collection and transport of specimens for viral detection or culture are described in Chapter 65. Although swabs made of calcium alginate are commonly used to collect nasopharyngeal specimens (excluding those specimens for chlamydia or viral culture), nasopharyngeal secretions collected by either aspiration or washing will improve recovery for *Bordetella pertussis* because a larger amount of material is obtained.

The type of swab used for collection is very important. For example, cotton swabs should never be used for culture because fibers contain fatty acids on the surface, which are capable of killing *Bordetella.* Calcium alginate or Dacron swabs are acceptable for obtaining nasopharyngeal swab specimens, with calcium alginate being optimal for culture. However, if polymerase chain reaction (PCR) is to be performed, Dacron or rayon swabs on plastic shafts are preferred. Specimens for *B. pertussis* ideally should be inoculated directly to fresh culture media at the patient's bedside. If this is not possible, transport for less than 2 hours in 1% Casamino acid medium at room temperature

is acceptable. If specimens are plated on the day of collection, Amies transport medium with charcoal is acceptable. If specimens are plated more than 24 hours after collection, Regan-Lowe or Jones-Kendrick transport medium is optimal; both contain charcoal, starch, and nutrients as well as cephalexin. If lengthy delays in transport are expected, transport of specimens in Regan-Lowe medium at 4°C is recommended.

## DIRECT VISUAL EXAMINATION OR DETECTION

A Gram stain of material obtained from upper respiratory secretions or lesions may not improve diagnosis. Yeast-like cells can be identified, which are helpful in identifying thrush, and the characteristic pattern of fusiform and spirochetes of Vincent's angina may be visualized. Gram's crystal violet (allowed to remain on the slide for 1 minute before rinsing with tap water) and the Gram stain can be used to identify the spirilla and fusiform bacilli of Vincent's angina. However, if crystal violet is used, the smear should be very thin because everything will be intensely Gram positive, making a thick smear difficult to read. Additionally, spirilla and bacilli may be stained using a dilute solution of carbol fuchsin.

For causes of pharyngitis, Gram stains are unreliable. Direct smears of exudate from membrane-like lesions used to differentiate diphtheria from other causes are also not reliable or recommended.

Fungal elements, including yeast cells and pseudohyphae, may be visualized with a 10% potassium hydroxide (KOH) preparation, calcofluor white fluorescent stain, or periodic acid-Schiff (PAS) stain. Direct examination of material obtained from the nasopharynx of suspected cases of whooping cough using a fluorescent antibody stain (see Chapter 37) has been shown to yield some early positive results for detection of *B. pertussis.* However, direct fluorescent antibody (DFA) staining of nasopharyngeal secretions often lack sensitivity and specificity depending on the antibody used. Numerous studies have demonstrated that PCR-based assays for *B. pertussis* in nasopharyngeal secretions are superior to both DFA and culture. Various methods, including fluorescent antibody stain reagents, enzyme immunoassays, and nucleic acid amplification methods are also commercially available to detect numerous viral agents (see Chapter 65).

Improvement in the development of rapid methods for detection of group A streptococcal antigen or nucleic acid has obviated the need for culture of pharyngeal specimens. At least 40 commercial products are available to identify group A streptococcal antigens using membrane enzyme immunoassays or liposomal and optical immunoassay techniques. Although the specific procedures vary with the products, several generalizations can be made. Throat swabs are incubated in an acid reagent or enzyme to extract the group A specific carbohydrate antigen. Dacron swabs seem to be most efficient at releasing antigen, although other types of swabs may yield acceptable results. In laboratory comparisons between a rapid antigen method and conventional culture methods for detecting the presence of group A streptococci in throat swabs, the commercial kits have shown relatively acceptable (62% to more than 90%) sensitivity and specificity.

Specimens with a negative direct antigen test for group A streptococci should be cultured (requires collection of specimen with two swabs) or confirmed using a nucleic acid method. Group A streptococci can be directly detected from pharyngeal specimens by nucleic acid testing using different molecular assay formats. The commercially available assay (Probe Group A Strep Direct Test (GAS Direct), Hologic-GenProbe, Inc., San Diego, California) that employs a nonisotopic, chemiluminescent, single-stranded DNA probe complementary to the rRNA target of the group A *Streptococcus*. The assay detects organisms directly from swab specimens by lysing the bacterial cells before amplification. Dacron swabs are acceptable for use with this assay. Sensitivities of the Gen-Probe Group A Strep Direct Test range from 91.7% to 99.3% when compared with culture. A rapid-cycle real-time PCR method, the Light Cycler Strep-A (Roche Applied Science, Indianapolis, Indiana), also detects *S. pyogenes* directly from throat swabs. Using this technology, 32 samples (including controls) can be tested per run in about 1.5 hours. Isothermol DNA amplification is also available for the detection of Group A Streptococcus from throat swabs (Illumigene Group A Streptococcus, Meridian Bioscience, Inc., Cincinnati, Ohio) and demonstrates sensitivity equal to the Group A Strep Direct test. See Chapter 8 for more information on isothermal DNA amplification.

## CULTURE

### *Streptococcus pyogenes* (Beta-Hemolytic Group A Streptococci)

Because the primary cause of bacterial pharyngitis in North America is *Streptococcus pyogenes*, most laboratories routinely screen throat cultures for this organism. Group A streptococci are usually beta-hemolytic, with less than 1% being nonhemolytic. Three variables must be taken into consideration regarding successful culture of group A streptococci from pharyngeal specimens: medium, atmosphere, and duration of incubation. Kellogg recommended four combinations of media and atmosphere of incubation for throat specimens; these are listed in Table 70-2. Regardless of the medium and atmosphere of incubation employed, culture plates should be incubated for at least 48 hours before reporting as negative for group A streptococci. In addition, the incubation of sheep blood agar in 5% to 10% $CO_2$ was strongly discouraged.

Drawbacks to culture include an extended incubation time of 24 to 48 hours for visible colony formation with

**TABLE 70-2** Medium and Atmosphere for Incubation of Cultures to Recover Group A Streptococci from Pharyngeal Specimens

| Media | Atmosphere of Incubation |
| --- | --- |
| Sheep blood agar | Anaerobic |
| Sheep blood agar with coverslip over the primary area of inoculation | Aerobic |
| Sheep blood agar with trimethoprim-sulfamethoxazole | 5%-10% $CO_2$ or anaerobic |

additional manipulations of the beta-hemolytic organisms for definitive identification (see Chapter 15). If sufficient numbers of pure colonies are not available for identification, a subculture requiring additional incubation is necessary. By placing a 0.04-unit differential bacitracin filter paper disk, available commercially directly on the area of initial inoculation, presumptive identification of *S. pyogenes* can be made after overnight incubation (all of group A and a very small percentage of group B streptococci are susceptible). However, use of the bacitracin disk in the primary area of inoculation reduces the sensitivity and specificity of culture and identification of *S. pyogenes*. Sometimes growth of too few beta-hemolytic colonies or overgrowth of other organisms makes interpretation difficult. Therefore, using the bacitracin disk as the only method of identification of *S. pyogenes* is not recommended. New selective agars, such as streptococcal selective agar, have been developed that suppress the growth of almost all normal flora and beta-hemolytic streptococci except for groups A and B and *Arcanobacterium haemolyticum*. Direct antigen or nucleic detection tests or the PYR test (see Chapter 15) can also be carried out on isolated beta-hemolytic colonies.

### *Corynebacterium diphtheriae*

If diphtheria is suspected, the physician must communicate this information to the clinical laboratory. Because streptococcal pharyngitis is included in the differential diagnosis of diphtheria and because dual infections do occur, cultures for *Corynebacterium diphtheriae* should be plated onto sheep blood agar or streptococcal selective agar, as well as onto special media for recovery of this agent. These special media include a Loeffler's agar slant and a cystine-tellurite agar plate. Chapter 17 discusses the identification of the organism. Recovery of this organism is improved when culturing specimens from the throat and nasopharynx of potentially infected patients. In addition to culture, rapid toxigenicity assays, including immunoassays and polymerase chain reaction, may be used to assist in the diagnosis. Caution should be used when interpreting molecular assays, because positive results have been associated with related species of Corynebacteria.

### *Bordetella pertussis*

Freshly prepared Bordet-Gengou agar was the first medium developed for isolation of *Bordetella pertussis*. However, because it was inconvenient to use, other media were subsequently developed (see Chapter 37). Today, Regan-Lowe or charcoal horse blood agar is recommended for use in diagnostic laboratories. Because the organisms are extremely delicate, specimens should be plated directly onto media, if possible. The yield of positive isolations from clinical cases of pertussis seems to vary from 20% to 98% depending on the stage of disease, previous treatment of the patient, age of the patient, and laboratory techniques. Due to the fastidious growth requirements, additional methods, including 16SrRNA sequencing and matrix-assisted laser desorption ionization time-of-flight mass spectrometry (MALDI-TOF) have proven effective. See Chapter 7 for a description of MALDI-TOF methodology.

### Neisseria

Specimens received in the laboratory for isolation of *Neisseria meningitidis* (for detection of carriers) or *N. gonorrhoeae* should be plated to a selective medium, either modified Thayer-Martin or Martin-Lewis agar. After 24 to 48 hours of incubation in 5% to 10% carbon dioxide, typical colonies of *Neisseria* spp. may be visible (see Chapter 40).

### Epiglottitis

Clinical specimens from cases of epiglottitis (swabs obtained by a physician) should be plated to sheep blood agar, chocolate agar (for recovery of *Haemophilus* spp.), and a streptococcal selective medium. *Staphylococcus aureus*, *Streptococcus pneumoniae*, and beta-hemolytic streptococci are all potential etiologic agents of this disease. Refer to Table 5-1 for an overview of the methods used to collect, transport, and process different specimens from the upper respiratory tract.

# DIAGNOSIS OF INFECTIONS IN THE ORAL CAVITY AND NECK

## COLLECTION AND TRANSPORT

It is important to avoid or minimize contamination with oral flora when collecting oral and dental material for diagnosis of infection. For collection of material from root canal infection, the tooth is isolated by means of a rubber dam. A sterile field is established, the tooth is swabbed with 70% alcohol, and after the root canal is exposed, a sterile paper point is inserted, removed, and placed into semisolid, nonnutritive, anaerobic transport medium. Alternatively, needle aspiration can be used if sufficient purulent material is present. Completely defining the flora of such infections is beyond the scope of routine clinical microbiology laboratories.

Specimens from neck space infections can usually be obtained with a syringe and needle or by biopsy during a procedure by the surgeon. Transport must be under anaerobic conditions.

## DIRECT VISUAL EXAMINATION

All material submitted for culture should be smeared and examined by Gram stain and other appropriate techniques for fungi (i.e., calcofluor white, KOH, or PAS stains), if requested.

## CULTURE

Infections such as peritonsillar abscesses, oral and dental infections, and neck space infections usually involve anaerobic bacteria. The anaerobes involved typically originate in the oral cavity and are often more delicate than anaerobes isolated from other clinical material. Very careful methods are required in order to provide optimal specimens for anaerobic cultivation, as well as collection and transport for the recovery and identification of the etiologic agents. See Chapter 41 for more information related to anaerobic organisms.

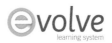 *Visit the Evolve site to complete the review questions.*

---

## CASE STUDY 70-1

A 2-year-old girl presented to her physician with a sore throat and fever. On examination, her tonsils were enlarged and inflamed. A rapid test was performed for group A streptococci; the test result was negative. The physician decided to treat with amoxicillin regardless of the test results and asked that a culture be performed. The next day the laboratory reported that moderate growth of beta-hemolytic group A streptococcus was present.

### QUESTIONS

1. List the tests that rapidly identify group A *Streptococcus* (*Streptococcus pyogenes*).

2. Not all group A streptococci are *S. pyogenes*. How can the nonpathogenic group A streptococci be differentiated from the pathogenic strains?
3. Not all *S. pyogenes* are beta-hemolytic. What is the reason for this phenomenon, and how can the laboratory ensure detection of the nonhemolytic strains?
4. What is the sensitivity of rapid diagnostic tests to detect group A streptococcal antigen?

---

# BIBLIOGRAPHY

Bourbeau PP: Role of the microbiology laboratory in diagnosis and management of pharyngitis, *J Clin Microbiol* 41:3467, 2003.
Bourbeau PP, Heiter BJ: Use of swabs without transport media for the Gen-Probe Group A Strep Direct Test, *J Clin Microbiol* 42:3207, 2004.
Cambier M, Janssens M, Wauters G: Isolation of *Arcanobacterium haemolyticum* from patients with pharyngitis in Belgium, *Acta Clin Belg* 47:303, 1992.
Cassiday PK, Sanden GN, Kane CT, et al: Viability in *Bordetella pertussis* in four suspending solutions at three temperatures, *J Clin Microbiol* 32:1550, 1994.
Cloud JL, Hymas W, Carroll KC: Impact of nasopharyngeal swab types on detection of *Bordetella pertussis* by PCR and culture, *J Clin Microbiol* 40:3838, 2002.
Hallander HO, Reizenstein E, Renemar B, et al: Comparison of nasopharyngeal aspirates with swabs for culture of *Bordetella pertussis*, *J Clin Microbiol* 31:50, 1993.

Kellogg JA: Suitability of throat culture procedures for detection of group A streptococci and as reference standards for evaluation of streptococcal antigen kits, *J Clin Microb* 28:165, 1990.
Kobayashi RH, Rosenblatt HM, Carney JM, et al: Candida esophagitis and laryngitis in chronic mucocutaneous candidiasis, *Pediatrics* 66(3):380-384, 1980.
Liakos T, Kaye K, Rubin AD: Methicillin-resistant Staphylococcus aureus laryngitis, *Ann Otol Rhinol Laryngol* 119(9):590-593, 2010.
Mandell GL, Bennett JE, Dolin R, editors: *Principles and practice of infectious diseases*, ed 7, Philadelphia, 2010, Elsevier Churchill Livingstone.
McGowan KL: Diagnostic tests for pertussis: culture vs. DFA vs. PCR, *Clin Microbiol Newsl* 24:143, 2002.
Moulis G, Martin-Blondel G: Scrofula, the king's evil, *CMAJ* 184(9):2012.
Sachse S, Seidel P, Gerlach D, et al: Superantigen-like gene(s) in human pathogenic *Streptococcus dysgalactiae*, subsp. *equisimilis*: genomic localization of the gene encoding streptococcal pyrogenic exotoxin G (spe Gdys), *FEMS Immunol Med Microbiol* 34:159, 2002.
Versalovic J: *Manual of clinical microbiology*, ed 10, Washington, DC, 2011, ASM Press.

# Meningitis, Encephalitis, and Other Infections of the Central Nervous System

# GENERAL CONSIDERATIONS

## ANATOMY

Diagnosis of an infection involving the central nervous system (CNS) is of critical importance. Most clinicians consider infection in the CNS to be a medical emergency. An understanding of the basic anatomy and physiology of the CNS is helpful for the microbiologist to ensure appropriate specimen processing and interpretation of laboratory results.

### Coverings and Spaces of the CNS

The central nervous system consists of the brain and the spinal cord. Because of the vital and essential role of the CNS in the body's regulatory processes, the brain and spinal cord have two protective coverings: an outer covering consisting of bone and an inner covering of membranes called the *meninges*. The outer bone covering encases the brain (i.e., cranial bones or skull) and spinal cord (i.e., the vertebrae). The meninges is a collective term for the three distinct membrane layers surrounding the brain and spinal column:

- Dura mater (outermost membrane layer)
- Arachnoid
- Pia mater (innermost membrane layer)

The pia mater and the arachnoid membrane are collectively called the *leptomeninges*. The portion of the arachnoid that covers the top of the brain contains arachnoid villi, which are special structures that absorb the spinal fluid and allow it to pass into the blood.

Between and around the meninges are spaces that include the epidural, subdural, and subarachnoid spaces. The relative location of the meninges and spaces to one another in the brain are depicted in Figure 71-1. The location and nature of the meninges and spaces are summarized in Table 71-1.

### Cerebrospinal Fluid

Cerebrospinal fluid (CSF) surrounds the brain and spinal cord and has several functions. The CSF provides cushioning and buoyancy for the bulk of the brain, reducing the effective weight of the brain by a factor of 30. CSF carries essential metabolites into the neural tissue and cleanses the tissues of wastes as it circulates around the brain, ventricles, and spinal cord. Every 3 to 4 hours, the entire volume of CSF is exchanged. In addition to these functions, CSF provides a means by which the brain monitors changes in the internal environment.

CSF is found in the subarachnoid space (see Table 71-1) and within cavities and canals of the brain and spinal cord. There are four large, fluid-filled spaces within the brain referred to as ventricles. Specialized secretory cells, called the choroid plexus, produce CSF. The choroid plexus is located centrally within the brain in the third and fourth ventricles. Approximately 23 mL of CSF are contained within these ventricles in an adult. The fluid travels around the outside areas of the brain within the subarachnoid space, driven primarily by the pressure produced initially at the choroid plexus (Figure 71-2). By virtue of its circulation, chemical and cellular changes in the CSF may provide valuable information about infections within the subarachnoid space.

### ROUTES OF INFECTION

One of the most important defense mechanisms of the CNS is the blood-brain barrier. The blood-brain barrier functions to maintain homeostasis in the brain through restricting the flow of chemical constituents from the blood to the CNS. In order for the CNS to become infected with bacteria, parasite, or virus, the blood-brain barrier must be penetrated.

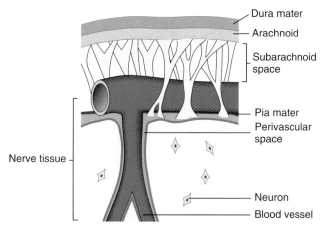

**Figure 71-1** Cross section of the brain shows the important membrane coverings and spacing and other key structures.

**TABLE 71-1** Inner Coverings (Meninges) of the Brain, Spinal Cord, and Surrounding Spaces

| Anatomic Structure | Relative Location | Key Features |
|---|---|---|
| Epidural space | Outside the dura mater yet inside the skull | Cushion of fat and connective tissues |
| Dura mater | Outermost membrane | Membrane that adheres to the skull; white fibrous tissue |
| Subdural space | Between the dura mater and the arachnoid membrane | Cushion of lubricating serous fluid |
| Arachnoid membrane | Between the dura mater and pia mater | Delicate, cobweb-like membrane covering the brain and spinal cord |
| Subarachnoid space | Beneath the arachnoid membrane | Contains a significant amount of CSF in an adult (~125-150 mL) |
| Pia mater | Beneath the subarachnoid space | Adheres to the outer surface of the brain and spinal cord; contains blood vessels |

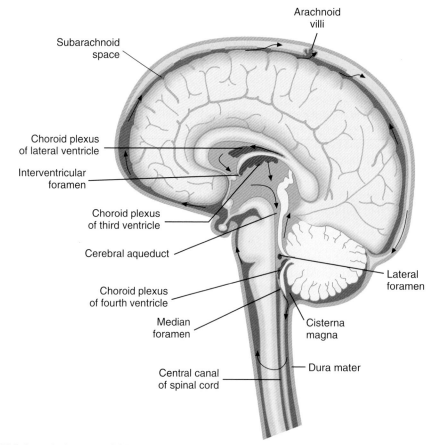

**Figure 71-2** Flow of CSF through the brain. CSF originates in the choroid plexus and then flows through the ventricles and subarachnoid space and into the bloodstream.

Organisms may gain access to the CNS through several primary routes:

- Hematogenous spread: followed by entry into the subarachnoid space through the choroid plexus or through other blood vessels of the brain. This is the most common route of infection for the CNS.
- Direct spread from an infected site: the extension of an infection close to or contiguous with the CNS can occasionally occur; examples of such infections include otitis media (infection of middle ear), sinusitis, and mastoiditis.
- Anatomic defects in CNS structures: anatomic defects as a result of surgery, trauma, or congenital abnormalities can allow microorganisms easy and ready access to the CNS.
- Travel along nerves leading to the brain (direct intraneural): the least common route of CNS infection caused by organisms such as rabies virus, which travels along peripheral sensory nerves, and herpes simplex virus.

## DISEASES OF THE CENTRAL NERVOUS SYSTEM

### Meningitis

Infection within the subarachnoid space or throughout the leptomeninges is called meningitis. Based on the host's response to the invading microorganism, meningitis is divided into two major categories: purulent and aseptic meningitis.

**Purulent Meningitis.** A patient with purulent meningitis typically has a marked, acute inflammatory exudative cerebral spinal fluid containing large numbers of polymorphonuclear cells (PMNs). Frequently, the underlying CNS tissue, in particular the ventricles, may be involved. If the ventricles become involved, this process is referred to as ventriculitis. Bacterial organisms are usually the cause of these infections.

***Pathogenesis.*** The outcome of a host-microbe interaction depends on the characteristics of both the host and the microorganism. As previously indicated, an important host defense mechanism within the CNS is the blood-brain barrier; this barrier involves the choroid plexus, arachnoid membrane, and the cerebral microvascular endothelium. The unique structural properties of the vascular endothelium, such as the continuous intercellular tight junctions, provide a barrier minimizing the passage of infectious agents into the CSF. The normal function of the vascular endothelium includes regulating the transport of nutrients in and out of the CSF, including low-molecular-weight plasma proteins, glucose, and electrolytes.

The host's age and other underlying factors contribute to whether an individual is predisposed to the development of infectious meningitis. Neonates have the highest infection rate for meningitis, because of the immature neonatal immune system, the increased permeability of the blood-brain barrier in newborns, and the presence of colonizing bacteria in the female vaginal tract that can pass to the infant during childbirth. The most common bacterial pathogens responsible for meningitis in newborns are group B streptococci, *Escherichia coli*, and *Listeria monocytogenes*. Prior to the advent of the Hib vaccine in the United States in 1985, *Haemophilus influenza* type b (Hib) was a common cause of meningitis in children 4 months to 5 years of age. Because of the incorporation of Hib into childhood immunization programs, childhood Hib disease has dramatically declined.

Among young adults, *Neisseria meningitidis* is typically the agent that is associated with meningitis. *N. meningitidis* has been identified in epidemics among young adults in crowded conditions (e.g., military recruits and college dormitory mates). There are two meningococcal vaccines (vaccines for *N. meningitidis*) available in the United States. The meningococcal polysaccharide vaccine (MPSV4) is used for individuals older than 55 years of age, and the meningococcal conjugate vaccine (MCV4) is used for adolescents. *Streptococcus pneumoniae* is frequently the cause of meningitis in young children and the elderly; often this meningitis develops from bacteremia or from infection of the sinuses or middle ear. There are two pneumococcal vaccines (vaccines for *S. pneumoniae*) that are recommended currently in the United States. The pneumococcal conjugate vaccine (PCV13) protects against infection from 13 different serotypes of *S. pneumoniae* and is used for vaccination of children and adults. The second vaccine, pneumococcal polysaccharide vaccine (PPSV), provides protection from 23 serotypes of *S. pneumoniae*, including those associated with serious life-threatening infections. This vaccine is recommended for adults 65 years of age and older or anyone over the age of 2 who has long-term health problems or is immunocompromised.

Because the respiratory tract is the primary portal of entry for many etiologic agents of meningitis, factors that predispose adults to meningitis are often the same factors that increase the likelihood for the development of pneumonia or other respiratory tract colonization or infection. Alcoholism, splenectomy, diabetes mellitus, prosthetic devices, and immunosuppression contribute to increased risk. Finally, patients with prosthetic devices, particularly CNS and ventriculoperitoneal shunts, are at increased risk for developing meningitis.

For organisms to reach the CNS (primarily by the blood-borne route), host defense mechanisms must be overcome. Most cases of meningitis are a result of bacteria that share a similar pathogenesis. The successful meningeal pathogen must first sequentially colonize and cross host mucosal epithelium, then enter and thrive within the bloodstream. The most common causes of meningitis possess the ability to evade host defenses at each of these levels. For example, clinical isolates of *Streptococcus pneumoniae* and *N. meningitidis* secrete IgA proteases capable of destroying the host's secretory IgA, thereby facilitating bacterial attachment to the epithelium. In addition, all of the most common etiologic agents of bacterial meningitis possess an antiphagocytic capsule that allows the organisms to evade destruction by the host immune system.

Organisms appear to enter the CNS by interacting and subsequently breaking down the blood-brain barrier at the level of microvascular endothelium. One of the least understood processes in the pathogenesis of meningitis is how organisms cross this barrier into the subarachnoid space. Nevertheless, there appear to be specific bacterial

**TABLE 71-2** Guidelines for Interpretation of Results Following Hematologic and Chemical Analysis of Cerebrospinal Fluid (CSF) from Children and Adults (Excluding Neonates)

| Clinical Setting | Leukocytes/mm$^3$ | Predominant Cell Type | Protein | Glucose* |
|---|---|---|---|---|
| Normal | 0-5 | None | 15-50 mg/dL | 45-100 mg/dL |
| Viral infection | 2-2000 (mean of 80) | Mononuclear$^†$ | Slightly elevated (50-100 mg/dL) or normal | Normal |
| Purulent infection | 5-20,000 (mean of 800) | PMN | Elevated (>100 mg/dL) | Low (<45 mg/dL), but may be normal early in the course of disease |
| Tuberculosis and fungi | 5-2000 (mean of 100) | Mononuclear | Elevated (>50 mg/dL) | Normal or often low (>45 mg/dL) |

*Must consider CSF glucose level in relation to blood glucose level. Normally, the CSF glucose serum ratio is 0.6, or 50% to 70% of the blood glucose normal value.
$^†$About 20% to 75% of cases may have PMN leukocytosis early in the course of infection.

surface components, such as pili, polysaccharide capsules, and lipoteichoic acids, that facilitate adhesion of the organisms to the microvascular endothelial cells and subsequent penetration into the CSF. Organisms can enter (1) through loss of capillary integrity by disrupting tight junctions of the blood-brain barrier, (2) through transport within circulating phagocytic cells, or (3) by crossing the endothelial cell lining within endothelial cell vacuoles. After gaining access, the organism multiplies within the CSF, a site initially free of antimicrobial antibodies or phagocytic cells.

**Clinical Manifestations.** Meningitis can be classified as either an acute or a chronic disease in the onset and overall progression within the host.

**Acute.** Symptoms of acute meningitis include fever, stiff neck, headache, nausea and vomiting, neurologic abnormalities, and change in mental status.

In acute bacterial meningitis, the CSF usually contains large numbers of inflammatory cells (>1000/mm$^3$), primarily polymorphonuclear cells (PMNs). The CSF shows a decreased glucose level relative to the serum glucose level and an increase in protein concentration. In a healthy individual, the normal CSF glucose level is 0.6 of the serum glucose level and ranges from 45 to 100 mg/dL; the CSF protein range in an adult is 15 to 50 mg/dL; newborn CSF protein ranges run as high as 170 mg/dL with an average of 90 mg/dL.

The sequelae of acute bacterial meningitis in children are frequent and serious. Seizures can occur in 20% to 30% of patients, and other neurologic changes are common. Acute sequelae include cerebral edema, hydrocephalus, cerebral herniation, and focal neurologic changes. Permanent deafness can occur in 10% of children who recover from bacterial meningitis. Other subtle physiologic and psychological sequelae may also follow an episode of acute bacterial meningitis.

**Chronic.** Chronic meningitis can often occur in patients who are immunocompromised, although this is not always the case. Patients experience an insidious onset of disease, with some or all of the following symptoms: fever, headache, stiff neck, nausea and vomiting, lethargy, confusion, and mental deterioration. Symptoms may persist for a month or longer before treatment is sought. The CSF usually manifests an abnormal number of white blood cells (usually lymphocytic), elevated protein, and decrease in glucose content (Table 71-2). The pathogenesis of chronic meningitis is similar to that of acute disease.

**Epidemiology/Etiologic Agents-Acute Meningitis.** The etiology of acute meningitis depends on the age of the patient. Most cases in the United States occur in children younger than 5 years of age. Before 1985, *H. influenzae* type b *H. influenzae* type b was the most common infectious agent in children between 1 month and 6 years of age within the United States. Ninety-five percent of all cases were due to *H. influenzae* type b, *Neisseria meningitidis*, and *Streptococcus pneumoniae*. In 1985, the first Hib vaccine, a polysaccharide vaccine, was licensed for use in children 18 months of age or older but was not efficacious in children younger than 18 months. However, the widespread use of conjugate vaccine, Hib polysaccharide-protein conjugate, in children as young as 2 months of age has significantly affected the incidence of invasive *H. influenzae* type b disease; the total number of annual cases of *H. influenzae* disease in the United States have been reduced by 55% and the number of cases of *H. influenzae* meningitis by 94%. However, the risks for meningococcal and pneumococcal diseases resulting from agents other than *H. influenzae* have remained level. Children older than 6 years of age are less likely to develop meningitis, but the risk for meningitis infection increases when the child reaches early adulthood. As previously mentioned, neonates have the highest incidence of acute meningitis, with a concomitant increased mortality rate (as high as 20%). Organisms causing disease in the newborn are different from those that affect other age groups; many of them are acquired by the newborn during passage through the mother's vaginal vault. Neonates are likely to be infected with, in order of incidence, group B streptococci, *Escherichia coli*, other gram-negative bacilli, and *Listeria monocytogenes*; occasionally other organisms may be involved. For example, *Elizabethkingia meningoseptica* has been associated with nursery outbreaks of meningitis. This organism is a normal inhabitant of water in the environment and is presumably acquired as a nosocomial infection.

Important causes of meningitis in the adult, in addition to the meningococcus in young adults, include

**Viral**
HIV cytomegalovirus
Enterovirus
HSV
*Mycobacterium tuberculosis*
*Cryptococcus neoformans*
*Coccidioides immitis*
*Histoplasma capsulatum*
*Blastomyces dermatitidis*
*Candida* spp.
Aspergillosis
Mucormycosis
Miscellaneous other fungi
*Nocardia*
*Actinomyces*
*Treponema pallidum*
*Brucella*
*Borrelia burgdorferi*
*Sporothrix schenckii*
Rare parasites—*Toxoplasma gondii,* cysticercus,
   *Paragonimus westermani, Trichinella spiralis, Schistosoma*
   spp., *Acanthamoeba*

---

pneumococci, *Listeria monocytogenes,* and, less commonly, *Staphylococcus aureus* and various gram-negative bacilli. Meningitis caused by the latter organisms results from hematogenous seeding from various sources, including urinary tract infections. The percentage of adults with nosocomial bacterial meningitis at large urban hospitals has been increasing. The various etiologic agents of chronic meningitis are listed in Box 71-1.

**Aseptic Meningitis.** Aseptic meningitis is usually viral and characterized by an increase of lymphocytes and other mononuclear cells (pleocytosis) in the CSF; bacterial and fungal cultures are negative. (This is in contrast to bacterial meningitis, which is characterized by purulence and the polymorphonuclear [PMN] cell response in the CSF.) Aseptic meningitis is usually self-limiting with symptoms that may include fever, headache, stiff neck, nausea, and vomiting.

In addition to the increase of lymphocytes and other mononuclear cells in the CSF, the glucose level remains normal, whereas the protein CSF level may remain normal or be slightly elevated. Aseptic meningitis can also be a symptom for syphilis and some other spirochete diseases (e.g., leptospirosis and Lyme borreliosis). Stiff neck and CSF pleocytosis may also be associated with other disease processes, such as malignancy.

## ENCEPHALITIS/MENINGOENCEPHALITIS

Encephalitis is an acute inflammation of the brain parenchyma and is usually caused by direct viral invasion. Concomitant meningitis occurring with encephalitis is known as meningoencephalitis, and the cellular infiltrate present in the CSF is typically lymphocytic rather than polymorphonuclear cells.

The host response to these CNS infections can differ somewhat from those associated with purulent or aseptic meningitis. Early in the course of viral encephalitis, or when considerable tissue damage occurs as a part of encephalitis, the nature of the inflammatory cells found in the CSF may be no different from that associated with bacterial meningitis; cell counts, however, are typically much lower.

### Viral.

Viral encephalitis, which cannot always be distinguished clinically from meningitis, is common in the warmer months. The primary agents are enteroviruses (coxsackie viruses A and B, echoviruses), mumps virus, herpes simplex virus, and arboviruses (West Nile virus, togavirus, bunyavirus, equine encephalitis, St. Louis encephalitis, and other encephalitis viruses). Other viruses—such as measles, cytomegalovirus, lymphocytic choriomeningitis, Epstein-Barr virus, hepatitis, varicella-zoster virus, rabies virus, myxoviruses, and paramyxoviruses—are less commonly encountered. Any preceding viral illness and exposure history are important considerations in establishing a cause by clinical means. Since 1999, with the first debut of West Nile in the United States, the West Nile virus has been an important consideration in the diagnosis of viral encephalitis. The Centers for Disease Control and Prevention (CDC) reports that the incidence of West Nile infection peaked in 2003 with 9862 cases of West Nile infection; 2860 were reported cases of meningitis and encephalitis, resulting in 264 deaths. Since then the rates of infection have dropped: human cases reported to the CDC in 2010 were significantly lower with 1021 total reported cases of West Nile; 629 were neuroinvasive cases resulting in 57 deaths; a state-by-state breakdown of the disease incidence is outlined in Table 71-3. In 2012, a deadly resurgence of West Nile virus occurred, including neuroinvasive and non-neuroinvasive, for a total of 4531 cases through mid-October, according to the CDC.

Neuroinvasive infection with West Nile presents with symptoms of headache, fever, and a change in consciousness along with altered mental status. The examination of the CSF shows an increase in leukocytes with a marked increase in lymphocytes. Chemistries demonstrate an elevated protein count and normal glucose levels. Definitive diagnosis requires testing for the presence of the IgM antibody to West Nile in the serum or CSF, and because IgM does not cross the blood-brain barrier, presence of IgM antibody to West Nile in the CSF is a strong indicator for CNS infection. Polymerase chain reaction (PCR) can also be used to test for West Nile infection, but because West Nile infections have a transient and low viremia, results must be interpreted with caution. A negative result does not necessarily rule out West Nile infection.

Involvement of the nervous system in patients who are infected with the human immunodeficiency virus (HIV) is common. HIV is a neurotropic (attracted to nerve cells) virus capable of entering the CNS by macrophage transport and the cause of various neurologic syndromes. As HIV-infected individuals become progressively more immunosuppressed, the CNS becomes a target for opportunistic pathogens, such as cytomegalovirus, BK virus, and JC (John Cunningham) virus, which

**TABLE 71-3** Final 2010 West Nile Virus Human Infections in the United States*

| State | Neuroinvasive Disease Cases | Non-neuroinvasive Disease Cases | Total Cases | Deaths | Presumptive Viremic Donors* |
|---|---|---|---|---|---|
| Alabama | 1 | 2 | 3 | 0 | 0 |
| Arizona | 107 | 60 | 167 | 15 | 31 |
| Arkansas | 6 | 1 | 7 | 1 | 0 |
| California | 72 | 39 | 111 | 6 | 24 |
| Colorado | 26 | 55 | 81 | 4 | 1 |
| Connecticut | 7 | 4 | 11 | 0 | 5 |
| District of Columbia | 3 | 3 | 6 | 0 | 0 |
| Florida | 9 | 3 | 12 | 2 | 1 |
| Georgia | 4 | 9 | 13 | 0 | 1 |
| Idaho | 0 | 1 | 1 | 0 | 0 |
| Illinois | 45 | 16 | 61 | 4 | 5 |
| Indiana | 6 | 7 | 13 | 1 | 0 |
| Iowa | 5 | 4 | 9 | 2 | 1 |
| Kansas | 4 | 15 | 19 | 0 | 1 |
| Kentucky | 2 | 1 | 3 | 1 | 7 |
| Louisiana | 20 | 7 | 27 | 0 | 7 |
| Maryland | 17 | 6 | 23 | 2 | 0 |
| Massachusetts | 6 | 1 | 7 | 0 | 1 |
| Michigan | 25 | 4 | 29 | 3 | 2 |
| Minnesota | 4 | 4 | 8 | 0 | 1 |
| Mississippi | 3 | 5 | 8 | 0 | 2 |
| Missouri | 3 | 0 | 3 | 0 | 0 |
| Nebraska | 10 | 29 | 39 | 2 | 10 |
| Nevada | 0 | 2 | 2 | 0 | 0 |
| New Hampshire | 1 | 0 | 1 | 0 | 0 |
| New Jersey | 15 | 15 | 30 | 2 | 0 |
| New Mexico | 21 | 4 | 25 | 1 | 6 |
| New York | 89 | 39 | 128 | 4 | 16 |
| North Dakota | 2 | 7 | 9 | 0 | 0 |
| Ohio | 4 | 1 | 5 | 0 | 0 |
| Oklahoma | 1 | 0 | 1 | 0 | 1 |
| Pennsylvania | 19 | 9 | 28 | 0 | 0 |
| South Carolina | 1 | 0 | 1 | 0 | 0 |
| South Dakota | 4 | 16 | 20 | 0 | 0 |
| Tennessee | 2 | 2 | 4 | 0 | 1 |
| Texas | 77 | 12 | 89 | 6 | 14 |
| Utah | 1 | 1 | 2 | 0 | 3 |
| Virginia | 4 | 1 | 5 | 1 | 2 |
| Washington | 1 | 1 | 2 | 0 | 0 |
| Wisconsin | 0 | 2 | 2 | 0 | 1 |
| Wyoming | 2 | 4 | 6 | 0 | 0 |
| **Totals** | **629** | **392** | **1021** | **57** | **144** |

*Neuroinvasive disease* refers to severe cases of disease that affect a person's nervous system. These include encephalitis, meningitis, and acute flaccid paralysis that is an inflammation of the spinal cord that can cause a sudden onset of weakness in the limbs or breathing muscles.
*Human Cases Reported to CDC.

can produce meningitis or encephalitis. BK virus is named after the initials of the first renal transplant patient where the virus was identified in association with clinical disease.

### Parasitic

Parasites can cause meningoencephalitis, brain abscess (see the following discussion), or other CNS infection via two routes. A rare but devastating meningoencephalitis is caused by the free-living amebae, *Naegleria fowleri* and *Acanthamoeba* spp., which invade the brain via direct extension from the nasal mucosa. These organisms are acquired during swimming or diving in natural, stagnating freshwater ponds and lakes.

Other parasites reach the brain via hematogenous spread. Toxoplasmosis, caused by an intracellular parasite that destroys brain parenchyma, is a common CNS affliction in HIV-infected patients with acquired immunodeficiency syndrome (AIDS). *Entamoeba histolytica* and *Strongyloides stercoralis* have been identified in brain tissue, and the larval form of *Taenia solium* (the pork tapeworm), called a cysticercus, can travel to the brain via the bloodstream and encyst within the brain tissue. Amebic brain infection and cysticercosis cause changes in the CSF similar to meningitis.

## BRAIN ABSCESS

Brain abscesses (localized collections of pus in a cavity formed by the breakdown of tissue) may occasionally cause changes in the CSF and clinical symptoms similar to meningitis. Brain abscesses result from contiguous infection of the sinuses, middle ear, or mastoids (25%-50%), hematogeneously (15%-30%), or through direct inoculation as a result of trauma or surgery (8%-19%). Brain abscesses may rupture into the subarachnoid space, producing severe meningitis with a high mortality rate. If anaerobic organisms or viridans streptococci are recovered from CSF cultures, the diagnosis of brain abscess should be considered; however, CSF culture is typically negative in brain abscess. Patients who are immunosuppressed or who have diabetes with ketoacidosis may present with a rapid progressive fungal infection (phycomycosis) of the nasal sinuses or palatal region capable of traveling directly to the brain. The complex polymicrobial infections isolated from brain abscesses are far too extensive to list.

## SHUNT INFECTIONS

Information and studies related to infections involving CSF shunts is limited. The organisms reported most frequently associated with infections include coagulase-negative staphylococcus, *Staphylococcus aureus*, *Propionibacterium acnes,* and viridians group streptococci, A few Gram-negative rods have been identified, including *Pseudomonas aeruginosa*, *Klebsiella* spp., *Escherichia coli*, and *Serratia marcescens*. Positive cultures were most often associated with shunt tip cultures, shunt valves, and cerebral ventricle fluid.

## LABORATORY DIAGNOSIS OF CENTRAL NERVOUS SYSTEM INFECTIONS

### MENINGITIS

Except in unusual circumstances, a lumbar puncture (spinal tap) is one of the first steps in the diagnosis of a patient with suspected CNS infection, in particular, meningitis. Refer to Table 5-1 to review the procedure for collecting, transporting, and processing specimens obtained from the central nervous system.

#### Specimen Collection and Transport

CSF is collected by aseptically inserting a needle into the subarachnoid space (lumbar puncture), at the lumbar spine region between L3, L4, or L5. Three or four tubes of CSF should be collected into sterile collection tubes that contain no additives. The tubes are numbered sequentially in the order in which they were collected along with the patient's name. When processing the CSF collection tubes in the laboratory, tube 1 is used for chemistry studies, glucose and protein count, as well as immunology studies, as these tests are least affected by the presence of blood cells or bacteria introduced as a result of the spinal tap procedure; tube 2 is used for culture, allowing a larger proportion of the total fluid to be concentrated, which can facilitate the detection of infectious agents present in low numbers; tubes 3 and 4 are used for cell count and differential, as these tubes are least likely to contain cells introduced by the collection procedure. If a small capillary blood vessel is inadvertently broken during the spinal tap, blood cells picked up from this source will usually be absent from the last tube collected; comparison of counts between tubes 1 and 3 (4) is occasionally needed if a traumatic tap is suspected as well as to differentiate a traumatic bloody tap from a true subarachnoid hemorrhage. In a traumatic tap, the red blood cells will be unevenly distributed among the three tubes, with the heaviest concentration of red blood cells being in tube 1 and diminishing amounts in tubes 2 and 3. In an intracranial hemorrhage, the red blood cells will be evenly distributed among the three tubes. The volume of CSF that can be collected is based on the volume available in the patient (adult versus neonate) and the opening pressure of the CSF when the needle first punctures the subarachnoid space. An elevated pressure requires the CSF fluid to be withdrawn more slowly, which may prevent the collection of a larger volume. The volume of CSF is critical for detecting certain microorganisms, such as mycobacteria and fungi. A minimum of 5 to 10 mL is recommended for detecting these agents by centrifugation and subsequent culture. When the laboratory receives an inadequate volume of CSF , the physician should be consulted regarding the order of priority for laboratory tests. Processing too little specimen lowers the sensitivity of laboratory tests, which may lead to false-negative results. This is potentially more harmful to patient care than performing an additional lumbar puncture to obtain the necessary or required amount of sample.

CSF should be hand-delivered immediately to the laboratory. Certain agents, such as *Streptococcus pneumoniae,* may not be detectable after an hour or longer. Specimens for microbiology studies should never be refrigerated; if not rapidly processed, CSF should be incubated (35°C) or left at room temperature. One exception to this rule involves CSF for viral studies. These specimens may be refrigerated for as long as 23 hours after collection or frozen at −70°C if a longer delay is anticipated until they are processed and inoculated into culture media. CSF for viral studies should never be frozen at temperatures above −70°C. If not processed immediately, CSF specimen for hematology studies can be refrigerated, whereas the CSF for chemistry and serology can be frozen (−20°C).

Information gathered from specimen analysis should be promptly relayed to the clinician who can directly affect therapeutic outcome. Such specimens should be processed immediately upon receipt in the laboratory (STAT) and results reported to the physician as soon as possible.

### Initial Processing

Initial processing of CSF for bacterial, fungal, or parasitic studies includes centrifugation of all specimens with a volume greater than 1 mL for at least 15 minutes at 1500× *g*. Specimens in which cryptococci or mycobacteria are suspected require special handling. (Discussions of techniques for culturing CSF for mycobacteria and fungi are found in Chapters 43 and 59, respectively.) If fewer than 1 mL of CSF is available, the specimens should be gram stained and plated directly to blood and chocolate agar plates. The supernatant is removed to a sterile tube, leaving approximately 0.5 mL of fluid. The remaining fluid is used to suspend the sediment for visual examination or culture. Mixing of the sediment after the supernatant has been removed is critical. Forcefully aspirating the sediment up and down into a sterile pipette several times will adequately disperse the organisms that remained adherent to the bottom of the tube after centrifugation. Laboratories that use a sterile pipette to remove portions of the sediment from underneath the supernatant will miss a significant number of positive specimens. The supernatant can be used to test for the presence of antigens, rapid diagnostic test (vertical flow immunochromatography), for *N. meningitidis,* or for chemistry evaluations (e.g., protein, glucose, lactate, C-reactive protein). As a safeguard, keep the supernatant even if it has no immediate use.

### CSF Laboratory Results

As previously mentioned, CSF is also removed for analysis of cells, protein, and glucose. Ideally, the glucose content of the peripheral blood is determined simultaneously for comparison to CSF levels. General guidelines for the interpretation of results are shown in Table 71-2.

Because the results of hematologic and chemical tests directly relate to the probability of infection, communication between the physician and the microbiology laboratory is essential. Among 555 cerebrospinal fluid samples from patients older than 4 months of age tested at the University of California–Los Angeles, only 2 showed normal cell count and protein in the presence of bacterial meningitis. Thus, the diagnosis of acute bacterial

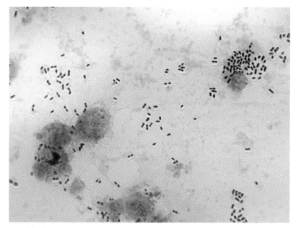

**Figure 71-3** Gram stain of cerebrospinal fluid showing white blood cells and many gram-positive diplococci. This specimen subsequently grew *Streptococcus pneumoniae.*

meningitis can be excluded in patients with normal fluid parameters in almost all cases, precluding further expensive and labor-intensive microbiologic processing beyond a standard smear and culture (which must be included in all cases). Similar criteria have been used to exclude performance of smear and culture for tuberculosis, as well as syphilis serology, on CSF specimens.

### Visual Detection of Etiologic Agents

Following centrifugation, the resulting CSF sediment may be visually examined for the presence of cells and organisms.

**Stained Smear of Sediment.** Gram stain must be performed on all CSF sediments. False-positive smears have resulted from inadvertent use of contaminated slides. Therefore, use of alcohol-dipped and flamed or autoclaved slides is recommended. After thoroughly mixing the sediment, a heaped drop is placed on the surface of a sterile or alcohol-cleaned slide. The sediment should never be spread out on the slide surface, because this increases the difficulty of finding small numbers of microorganisms. The drop of sediment is allowed to air dry, is heat or methanol fixed, and is stained by either Gram (Figure 71-3) or acridine orange. The acridine orange fluorochrome stain may allow faster examination of the slide under high-power magnification (400×) and thus a more thorough examination. The brightly fluorescing bacteria will be easily visible. All suspicious smears can be stained using the Gram stain (directly over the acridine orange) to confirm the presence and morphology of organisms.

Using a cytospin centrifuge to prepare slides for staining has also been found to be an excellent alternative procedure. This method for preparing smears for staining concentrates cellular material and bacterial cells up to a 1000-fold. By centrifugation, a small amount of CSF (or other body fluid) is concentrated onto a circular area of a microscopic slide (Figure 71-4), fixed, stained, and then examined.

The presence or absence of bacteria, inflammatory cells, and erythrocytes should be reported following examination. Based on demographic and clinical patient

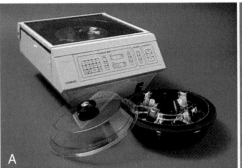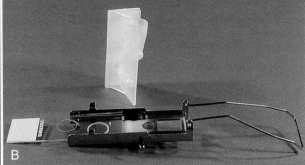

**Figure 71-4 A,** Cytocentrifuge. **B,** Device used to prepare the concentrated smears of material from body fluid specimens such as CSF by cytocentrifugation. (**A** courtesy Cytospin 2, Shandon, Inc., Pittsburgh, Pa.)

data and Gram stain morphology, the etiology of the majority of bacterial meningitis cases can be presumptively determined within the first 30 minutes following receipt of the specimen.

**Wet Preparation.** Amoebas are best observed by examining thoroughly mixed sediment as a wet preparation under phase-contrast microscopy. If a phase-contrast microscope is not available, observing under light microscopy with the condenser closed slightly can be used as an alternative. Amoebas are identifiable by their typical slow, methodical movement in one direction via pseudopodia. (The organisms may require a little time under the warm light of the microscope before they begin to move.) Organisms must be distinguished from motile macrophages, which occasionally occur in CSF. Following a suspicious wet preparation, a trichrome stain can assist in the differentiation of amoebas from somatic cells. The pathogenic amoebas can be cultured on a lawn of *Klebsiella pneumoniae* or *Escherichia coli* (see Chapter 47).

**India Ink Stain.** The large polysaccharide capsule of *Cryptococcus neoformans* allows these organisms to be visualized by the India ink stain. However, latex agglutination testing for capsular antigen is more sensitive and extremely specific. Antigen testing is recommended over the use of an India ink stain. Furthermore, strains of *C. neoformans* that infect patients with AIDS may not possess detectable capsules making culture essential. To perform the India ink preparation, a drop of CSF sediment is mixed with one-third volume of India ink (Pelikan Drawing Ink, Block, Gunther, and Wagner; available at art supply stores). The India ink can be protected against contamination by adding 0.05 mL thimerosal (Merthiolate, Sigma Chemical Co., St. Louis, Missouri) to the stain. After mixing the CSF and ink to make a smooth suspension, a coverslip is applied to the drop and the preparation is examined under high-power magnification (400×) for characteristic encapsulated yeast cells, which can be confirmed by examination under oil immersion. The inexperienced microbiologist must be careful not to confuse white blood cells with yeast. The presence of encapsulated buds, smaller than the mother cell, is diagnostic.

## Direct Detection of Etiologic Agents

**Antigen.** Commercial reagents and kits are available for the rapid detection of antigen in the CSF; a review of the

methodologies used will be discussed in the following sections; for more detailed specifics, please refer back to Chapter 9.

***Bacteria.*** Rapid antigen detection from CSF has been largely accomplished by the techniques of latex agglutination (see Chapter 9). All commercial agglutination systems use the principle of an antibody-coated particle capable of binding to specific antigen, resulting in macroscopically visible agglutination. The soluble capsular polysaccharide found in the common etiologic agents of meningitis, including the group B streptococcal polysaccharide, are well suited to serve as bridging antigens. The agglutination assays may contain either a polyclonal or monoclonal antibody or an antigen from an infectious agent.

In general, the commercial systems have been developed for use with CSF, urine, or serum, although results with serum have not been as diagnostically useful as those with CSF. Soluble antigens from *Streptococcus agalactiae* and *Haemophilus influenzae* may concentrate in the urine. Urine, however, seems to produce a higher incidence of nonspecific reactions than either serum or CSF. The manufacturers' directions must be followed for performance of antigen detection test systems for different specimen types. Although some of the systems require pretreatment of samples (usually heating for 5 minutes), not all manufacturers recommend such a step. The reagents, however, may yield false positive or cross-reactions unless the specimen is pretreated. Interference by rheumatoid factor and other substances, more often present in body fluids other than CSF, has also been reported. The method of Smith and colleagues has been shown to effectively reduce a substantial portion of nonspecific and false-positive reactions, at least for tests performed with latex particle reagents. This pretreatment, called rapid extraction of antigen procedure (REAP; see Procedure 71-1 on the Evolve site), is recommended for laboratories that use commercial body fluid antigen detection kits. Certain commercial systems have an extraction procedure included in the protocol.

Based on the findings of several studies, only a limited number of clinically useful situations warrant bacterial antigen testing (BAT). Examples include CSF specimens from previously treated patients and Gram stain–negative CSF specimens with abnormal parameters (elevated protein, decreased glucose, or an abnormal white blood cell count). The assays are not substitutes for properly performed smears and cultures. Some of the assays demonstrate a decreased sensitivity and specificity. In light of these limitations, practice guidelines for the diagnosis and management of bacterial meningitis do not recommend routine use of BAT.

**Cryptococcus neoformans.** Reagents for the detection of the polysaccharide capsular antigen of *Cryptococcus neoformans* are available commercially. CSF specimens that yield positive results for cryptococcal antigen should be tested with a second latex agglutination test for rheumatoid factor. The commercial test systems incorporate rheumatoid factor testing in the protocol. A positive rheumatoid factor test renders the cryptococcal latex test unable to interpret, and the results should be reported as such, unless the rheumatoid factor antibodies have been inactivated. Both latex agglutination assays (numerous commercial manufacturers) and enzyme immunoassays are available for the detection of cryptococcus antigen. Undiluted specimens containing large amounts of capsular antigen may yield a false-negative reaction caused by a prozone phenomenon. Patients with AIDS may have an antigen titer in excess of 100,000 requiring many dilutions to reach an end point. Serial dilution protocols are useful for monitoring a patient's response to treatment, as well as for initial diagnosis.

**Molecular Methods.** With the introduction of amplification technologies, such as polymerase chain reaction (PCR), many reports in the literature recommend the application of molecular technologies for the diagnosis of CNS infections caused by various microorganisms. Published data indicate that molecular assays demonstrate increased sensitivity and specificity compared with presently available techniques, particularly of CNS infections caused by herpes simplex virus and enteroviruses. PCR testing for HSV, EBV, CMV, and enterovirus in CNS infections has a sensitivity nearing 100%. Reagents for some of these amplification assays are commercially available for both conventional and real-time PCR assays.

## Miscellaneous Tests

Other tests—such as the limulus lysate test, CSF lactate determinations, C-reactive protein, mass spectrometry, and gas-liquid chromatography—have been evaluated for use in the diagnosis of CNS infections. However, the utility and value of these tests are either controversial or remain to be defined, or these tests are impractical for routine use in the clinical laboratory.

## Culture

The majority of cases of bacterial meningitis is usually caused by a single organism and requires a limited number of culture media.

**Bacteria and Fungi.** Routine bacteriologic media should include a chocolate agar plate, 5% sheep blood agar plate, and an enrichment broth, usually thioglycolate without indicator. The chocolate agar plate is needed to recover fastidious organisms, most notably *H. influenzae* and isolates of *N. meningitidis*, which are unable to grow on blood agar plates; the use of the blood agar plate aids

in the recognition of *S. pneumoniae*. After vortexing the sediment and preparing smears, several drops of the sediment should be inoculated to each medium. Plates should be incubated at 37°C in 5% to 10% carbon dioxide ($CO_2$) for at least 72 hours. If a $CO_2$ incubator is not available, a candle jar can be used. The broth should be incubated in air at 37°C for at least 5-10 days. The broth cap must be loose to allow free exchange of air. If organisms morphologically resembling anaerobic bacteria are seen on the Gram stain or if a brain abscess is suspected, an anaerobic blood agar plate may also be inoculated. These media will support the growth of almost all bacterial pathogens and several fungi.

The symptoms of chronic meningitis that prompt a physician to request fungal cultures are the same as those for tuberculous meningitis. Cultures for mycobacteria are addressed in Chapter 43. For CSF fungal cultures, two drops of the well-mixed sediment should be inoculated onto Sabouraud dextrose agar or other non-blood-containing medium and brain-heart infusion with 5% sheep blood. Fungal media should be incubated in air at 30°C for 4 weeks. If possible, two sets of media should be inoculated, with one set incubated at 30°C and the other at 35°C.

**Parasites and Viruses.** Conditions for the culture of free-living amoebae and viral agents are discussed in Chapters 47 and 65, respectively. The physician must notify the laboratory to culture these agents.

### Brain Abscess/Biopsies

***Specimen Collection, Transport and Processing.*** Whenever possible, biopsy specimens or aspirates from brain abscesses should be submitted to the laboratory under anaerobic conditions. Several devices are commercially available to transport biopsy specimens under anaerobic conditions. Swabs are not considered an optimum specimen, but if used to collect abscess material they should be sent in a transport device that maintains an anaerobic environment.

Biopsy specimens should be homogenized in sterile saline before plating and smear preparation. This processing should be kept to a minimum to reduce oxygenation.

Abscess and biopsy specimens submitted for culture should be inoculated onto 5% sheep blood and chocolate agar plates. Plates should be incubated in 5% to 10% $CO_2$ for 72 hours at 35°C. In addition, an anaerobic agar plate and broth with an anaerobic indicator, vitamin K, and hemin should be inoculated and incubated in an anaerobic environment at 35°C. Anaerobic culture plates are incubated for a minimum of 72 hours but are examined after 48 hours of incubation. Anaerobic broths should be incubated for a minimum of 5 days. If a fungal etiology is suspected, fungal media, such as brain-heart infusion with blood and antibiotics or inhibitory mold agar, should be inoculated.

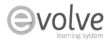 *Visit the Evolve site to complete the review questions.*

## CASE STUDY 71-1

A 2-year-old girl presented at midnight to the hospital emergency department with a temperature of 104° F. She was diagnosed with bilateral otitis. She was treated with amoxicillin/clavulanic acid and retained for observation in the hospital. During the night, the child became lethargic. She developed purpura and nuchal rigidity. A CSF sample was collected, and the child was started on ceftriaxone. No organisms were noted on gram stain. The following day, the laboratory reported growth of a gram-negative diplococcus.

### QUESTIONS

1. What is the suspected organism in this infection, and how can the laboratory rapidly identify it?
2. Is it recommended that laboratories do susceptibility testing for *N. meningitidis*?
3. How can the laboratory improve the speed with which it detects this organism in CSF?
4. What measures are taken to prevent the spread of infection among health care workers who are exposed to patients with *N. meningitidis*?

## BIBLIOGRAPHY

Albright RE, Christenson RH, Emlet JL, et al: Issues in cerebrospinal fluid management: acid-fast bacillus smear and culture, *Am J Clin Pathol* 95:418, 1991.

Albright RE, Graham CB, Christenson RH, et al: Issues in cerebrospinal fluid management: CSF venereal disease research laboratory testing, *Am J Clin Pathol* 95:387, 1991.

Al Masalma MA, Lonjon M, Richet H, et al: Metagenomic analysis of brain abscesses identifies specific bacterial associations, *Clin Infect Dis* 54(2):202-210, 2011.

Centers for Disease Control and Prevention: *Epidemic/epizootic West Nile virus in the United States: guidelines for surveillance, prevention and control*–3rd revision, 2003, available at www.cdc.gov/ncidod/dvbid/westnile/resources/wnvguidelines2003.pdf.

Conen A, Walti LN, Merlo A, et al: Characteristics and treatment outcome of cerebrospinal fluid shunt-associated infections in adults: a retrospective analysis over an 11-year period, *Clin Infect Dis* 47(1):73-82, 2008.

Gradon JD, Timpone JG, Schnittman SM: Emergence of unusual opportunistic pathogens in AIDS: a review, *Clin Infect Dis* 15:134, 1992.

Hariharan S: BK virus nephritis after renal transplantation: a review, *Kidney International* 69:655, 2006.

Hayward RA, Shapiro MF, Oye RK: Laboratory testing on cerebrospinal fluid: a reappraisal, *Lancet* 1:1, 1987.

Huang C, Morse D, Slater B, et al: Multiple-year experience in the diagnosis of viral central nervous system infections with a panel of polymerase chain reaction assays for detection of 11 viruses, *Clin Infect Dis* 39:630, 2004.

Korimbocus J, Scaramozzino N, Lacroix B, et al: DNA probe array for the simultaneous identification of herpesviruses, enteroviruses, and flaviviruses, *J Clin Micrbiol* 43: 3779, 2005.

Parkkinen J, Korhonen TK, Pere A, et al: Binding sites in the rat brain for *Escherichia coli* S fimbriae associated with neonatal meningitis, *J Clin Invest* 81:860, 1988.

Plaut AG: The IgA1 proteases of pathogenic bacteria, *Ann Rev Microbiol* 37:603, 1983.

Poppert S, Essig A, Stoehr B, et al: Rapid diagnosis of bacterial meningitis by real-time PCR and fluorescence in situ hybridization, *J Clin Microbiol* 43:3390, 2005.

Schwartz MN: Bacterial meningitis—a view of the past 90 years, *N Engl J Med* 351:1826, 2004.

Smith LP, Hunter KW Jr, Hemming VG, et al: Improved detection of bacterial antigens by latex agglutination after rapid extraction from body fluids, *J Clin Microbiol* 20:981, 1984.

Strasinger S, DiLorenzo M: *Urinalysis and body fluids*, ed 5, Philadelphia, 2008, FA Davis.

Tunkel AR, Hartman BJ, Kaplan SL, et al: Practice guidelines for the management of bacterial meningitis, *Clin Infect Dis* 39:1267, 2004.

van de Beek D, de Gan J, Spanjaard L, et al: Clinical features and prognostic factors in adults with bacterial meningitis, *N Engl J Med* 351:1849, 2004.

Virji M, Alexandrescu C, Ferguson DJ, et al: Variations in the expression of pili: the effect on adherence of *Neisseria meningitidis* to human epithelial and endothelial cells, *Mol Microbiol* 6:1271, 1992.

Virji M, Kayhty H, Ferguson DJ, et al: The role of pili in the interactions of pathogenic Neisseria with cultured human endothelial cells, *Mol Microbiol* 5:1831, 1991.

Wilhelm C, Ellner JJ: Chronic meningitis, *Neurol Clin* 4:115, 1986.

# Infections of the Eyes, Ears, and Sinuses

## OBJECTIVES

1. Describe the anatomy of the eye, including naming the external and internal structures.
2. Name the three tissues, outer to inner, of the eyeball.
3. Differentiate normal flora of the eye and potential pathogens.
4. Describe the defense mechanisms of the eye for the protection from infective agents.
5. Define the following diseases of the eye: blepharitis, conjunctivitis, keratitis, and endophthalmitis.
6. List the common types of eye infections, the associated etiologic agents, and the at-risk patient population for each.
7. Define keratitis, and identify the organisms associated with the infection, the virulence factors, and the antimicrobial-resistant properties for each.
8. Define endophthalmitis, explain how it is contracted, and identify the etiologic agents.
9. Explain mycotic endophthalmitis, and list the risk factors that may predispose an individual to this type of infection.
10. Define a periocular infection, and list some of the associated infectious agents and the different types of clinical presentations of the infection.
11. Identify the anatomic parts of the ear, and list the structures associated with each region within the ear.
12. Define the following external ear infections: acute externa otitis and chronic externa otitis; list the potential pathogens.
13. Define otitis media; differentiate acute and chronic otitis media, and name the most frequently encountered pathogens and the age group most often affected by this disease.
14. Explain the laboratory method used to culture the eye and the ear, including appropriate media; describe collection and transportation requirements.
15. Differentiate acute and chronic sinusitis.
16. Explain why the organisms causing otitis media are often the same ones responsible for sinusitis.
17. List the collection methods and culture media used for cases of sinusitis.
18. Correlate signs and symptoms of infection with the results of laboratory diagnostic procedures for the identification of the etiologic agent associated with infections of the eye, ear, and sinuses.

## EYES

### ANATOMY

Eye (ocular) infections can be divided based on the area of the eye infected and the exposed or external structures or the internal sites of the eye.

The external structures of the eye—eyelids, conjunctiva, sclera, and cornea—are depicted in Figure 72-1. The eyeball comprises three layers. From the outside in, these tissues are the sclera, choroid, and retina. The sclera is a tough, white, fibrous tissue (i.e., "white" of the eye). The anterior (toward the front) portion of the **sclera** is the **cornea**, which is transparent and has no blood vessels. A mucous membrane, called the **conjunctiva**, lines each eyelid and extends onto the surface of the eye itself.

Only a small portion of the eye is exposed to the environment; about five sixths of the eyeball is enclosed within bony orbits shaped like four-sided pyramids. The large interior space of the eyeball is divided into two sections: the anterior and posterior cavities (see Figure 72-1). The anterior cavity is filled with a clear and watery substance called **aqueous humor;** the posterior cavity is filled with a soft, gelatin-like substance called **vitreous humor.**

Infections can occur in the eye's **lacrimal** (pertaining to tears) system. The major components of the lacrimal apparatus include the lacrimal gland, lacrimal canaliculi (short channel), and lacrimal sac.

### RESIDENT MICROBIAL FLORA

Rather sparse indigenous flora is present in the conjunctiva sac. *Staphylococcus epidermidis* and *Lactobacillus* spp. are the most frequently encountered organisms; *Propionibacterium acnes* may also be present. *Staphylococcus aureus* is found in less than 30% of individuals, and *Haemophilus influenzae* colonizes 0.4% to 25%. *Moraxella catarrhalis,* various *Enterobacteriaceae,* and various streptococci (*Streptococcus pyogenes, Streptococcus pneumoniae,* other alpha-hemolytic and gamma-hemolytic forms) are found in a very small percentage of individuals.

### DISEASES

The eye and its associated structures are uniquely predisposed to infection by various microorganisms. The major infections of the eye are listed in Table 72-1 along with a brief description of the disease.

### PATHOGENESIS

The eye has a number of defense mechanisms. The eyelashes prevent entry of foreign material into the eye. The lids blink 15 to 20 times per minute, during which time secretions of the lacrimal glands and goblet cells wash away bacteria and foreign matter. Lysozyme and immunoglobulin A (IgA) are secreted locally and serve as part of the eye's natural defense mechanisms. Also, the eyes themselves are enclosed within the bony orbits. The delicate intraocular structures are enveloped in a tough collagenous coat (sclera and cornea). If these barriers are broken by a penetrating injury or ulceration, infection may occur. Infection can also reach the eye via the bloodstream from another site of infection. Finally, because

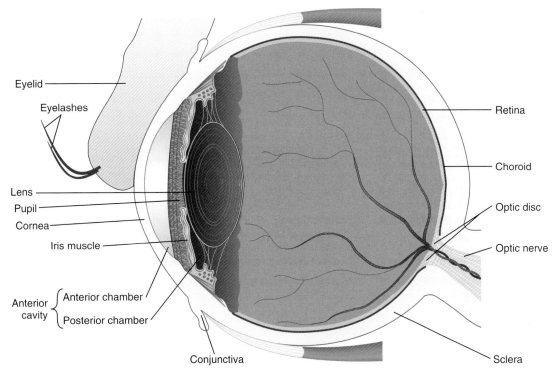

**Figure 72-1** Key anatomic structures of the eye. (Modified from Thibodeau GA, Patton KT: *Anatomy and physiology*, ed 2, St Louis, 1993, Mosby.)

three of the four walls of the orbit are contiguous with the paranasal (facial) sinuses, sinus infections may extend directly to the periocular orbital structures.

## EPIDEMIOLOGY AND ETIOLOGY OF DISEASE

### Blepharitis

Blepharitis is a bump that appears on the eyelid that is red, swollen, and resembles a pimple. Most bumps on the eyelid are caused by an inflamed oil gland on the edge of the eyelid commonly referred to as a stye. Bacteria, viruses, and, occasionally, lice can cause blepharitis, an infection of the eyelid surrounding the eye. Although occasionally isolated from surfaces surrounding the healthy eye, *Staphylococcus aureus* and *S. epidermidis* are the most common infectious agents associated with blepharitis in developed countries. Symptoms include burning, itching, the sensation of the presence of a foreign body, and crusting of the eyelids.

Viruses can also cause a vesicular (blister-like) eruption of the eyelids. Herpes simplex virus (HSV) produces vesicles on the eyelids that typically crust and heal with scarring within 2 weeks. Unfortunately, once this vesicular stage has resolved, the lesions can be confused with bacterial blepharitis.

Finally, the pubic louse *Phthirus pubis* has a predilection for eyelash hair. The presence of this organism produces irritation, itch, and swelling of the lid margins (edges).

### Conjunctivitis

Bacterial conjunctivitis, commonly referred to as "pink eye," is the most common type of ocular infection and may be caused by allergies or bacterial or viral infection. The principal causes of acute conjunctivitis in the normal host are listed in Table 72-1. Age-related factors are key in the identification of the etiologic agent. In neonates, neisserial and chlamydial infections are frequent and are acquired during passage through an infected vaginal canal. With the common practice of instilling antibiotic drops into the eyes of newborns in the United States, the incidence of gonococcal and chlamydial conjunctivitis has dropped dramatically. However, *Chlamydia trachomatis* remains responsible for one of the most important types of conjunctivitis, trachoma, one of the leading causes of blindness in the world, primarily in underdeveloped countries.

In children the most common causes of bacterial conjunctivitis includes *Haemophilus influenzae*, *S. pneumoniae*, and perhaps *S. aureus*. *S. pneumoniae* and *H. aegyptius* have been isolated from conjunctivitis epidemics. Inflammation of the conjunctiva is characterized by redness, itching, and discharge, and the condition is highly contagious; it can be transferred from one eye to the other by rubbing the infected eye and can easily be transferred to other individuals.

Numerous other bacteria may also cause conjunctivitis. For example, diphtheritic conjunctivitis may occur in conjunction with diphtheria elsewhere in the body. *Moraxella lacunata* produces a localized conjunctivitis with little discharge from the eye. Distinctive clinical pictures may also occur with conjunctivitis caused by *Mycobacterium tuberculosis*, *Francisella tularensis*, *Treponema pallidum*, and *Yersinia enterocolitica*.

Fungi may be responsible for this type of infection as well, often in association with a foreign body that has

**TABLE 72-1** Infections of the Eye

| Infection | Description | Bacteria | Viruses | Fungi | Parasites |
|---|---|---|---|---|---|
| Blepharitis | Inflammation of the margins (edges) of the eyelids; (eyelids, eye lashes or associated pilosebaceous glands or meibomiam glawds) symptoms include irritation, redness, burning sensation, and occasional itching. Condition is typically bilateral | *Staphylococcus aureus* | Herpes simplex virus | Staphylococcues epidermidrs *Malassezia furfar* | *Phthirus pulis* |
| Conjunctivitis | Inflammation of the conjunctiva; symptoms vary according to the etiologic agent, but most patients have swelling of the conjunctiva, inflammatory exudates, and burning and itching | *Streptococcus pneumoniae, Haemophilus influenzae, S. aureus, Haemophilus* spp., *Chlamydia trachomatis, Neisseria gonorrhoeae, Streptococcus pyogenes, Moraxella* spp., *Corynebacterium* spp. | Adenoviruses, herpes simplex (HSV), varicella zoster. Epstein-Barr virus (EBV) influeza vius, pararryxovirus, rubella, HIV enterovirus, coxscukie A | | |
| Keratitis | Inflammation of the cornea; although there are no specific clinical signs to confirm infection, most patients complain of pain and usually some decrease in vision, with or without discharge from the eye | *S. aureus S. pneumoniae, Pseudomonas, aeruginosa Moraxella lacunata, Bacillus* spp. | HSV, adenoviruses, varicella zoster | *Fusarium solani, Aspergillus* spp., *Candida* spp., *Acremonium, Curvularia* | *Acanthamoeba* spp. |
| Keratoconjunctivitis | Infection involving both the conjunctiva and cornea; ophthalmia neonatorum is an acute conjunctivitis or keratoconjunctivitis of the newborn caused by either *N. gonorrhoeae* or *C. trachomatis* | Refer to agents for keratitis/ conjunctivitis | Refer to agents for keratitis/ conjunctivitis | Refer to agents for keratitis | *Toxoplasma gondii, Toxocara* |
| Chorioretinitis and uveitis | Inflammation of the retina and underlying choroid or the uvea; infection can result in loss of vision | *Mycobacterium tuberculosis Treponema pallidum, Borrelia burgdorferi* | Cytomegalovirus, HSV | *Candida* spp. | *Toxoplasma gondii, Toxocara* Treponema pallidum Brucella spp. |
| Endophthalmitis | Infection of the aqueous or vitreous humor. This infection is usually caused by bacteria or fungi, is rare, develops suddenly and progresses rapidly, often leading to blindness. Pain, especially while moving the eye, and decreased vision, are prominent features. | *S. aureus, S. epidermidis, S. pneumoniae,* other streptococcal spp., *P. aeruginosa,* other gram-negative organisms, Nocardia spp. | HSV Varicella zoster | *Candida* spp., *Aspergillus* spp., *Volutella* spp., *Acremonium* spp. | *Toxocara, Onchocerca volvulus* |
| Lacrimal infections, canaliculitis | A rare, chronic inflammation of the lacrimal canals in which the eyelid swells and there is a thick, mucopurulent discharge | *Actinomyces, Propionibacterium propionicum* | | | |
| Dacryocystis | Inflammation of the lacrimal sac that is accompanied by pain, swelling, and tenderness of the soft tissue in the medial canthal region | *S. pneumoniae, S. aureus, S. pyogenes, Haemophilus influenzae* | | *C. albicans, Aspergillus* spp. | |
| Dacryoadenitis | Acute infection of the lacrimal gland; these infections are rare and can be accompanied by pain, redness, and swelling of the upper eyelid, conjunctiva discharge | *S. pneumoniae, S. aureus, S. pyogenes* | | | |

been introduced into the eye or an underlying host immunologic problem. However, these infections are infrequently encountered.

In adults, the etiology of conjunctivitis is usually viral, with adenovirus being the most common viral cause; 20% of such infections in children resulted from adenoviruses in one large U.S. study and 14% of infections in adult patients in another study. Adenoviruses types 4, 3, and 7A are common. Most viral conjunctivitis is self-limited but is highly contagious, with the potential to cause major outbreaks. Worldwide, enterovirus 70 and Coxsackie virus A24 are responsible for outbreaks and epidemics of acute hemorrhagic conjunctivitis.

## Keratitis

Keratitis (corneal infection) may be caused by a variety of infectious agents, usually following some type of trauma to the ocular surface. Keratitis should be regarded as an emergency, because corneal perforation and loss of the eye can occur within 24 hours when organisms such as *Pseudomonas aeruginosa*, *Staphylococcus aureus*, or HSV are involved. Bacteria account for 65% to 90% of corneal infections.

In the United States, *S. aureus*, *S. pneumoniae*, and *P. aeruginosa* account for more than 80% of all bacterial corneal ulcers. Many culture-positive cases are now being recognized as polymicrobial. A toxic factor known as exopeptidase has been implicated in the pathogenesis of corneal ulcer produced by *S. pneumoniae*. With *P. aeruginosa*, proteolytic enzymes (*Neisseria gonorrhoeae*) are responsible for the corneal destruction. Gonococcus may cause keratitis in the course of inadequately treated conjunctivitis. *Acinetobacter*, which may look identical microscopically to gonococcus and is resistant to penicillin and many other antimicrobial agents, can cause corneal perforation. Many other bacteria, several viruses other than HSV, and many fungi may cause keratitis. Fungal keratitis is usually a complication of trauma.

Although still unusual, a previously rare etiologic agent of corneal infections has become more common in users of soft and extended-wear contact lenses. *Acanthamoeba* spp., free living amebae, can survive in improperly sterilized cleaning fluids and be introduced into the eye with the contact lens. The fungus, *Fusarium*, is emerging as an infectious disease associated with contact lens use or contact lens solutions. This genus of fungus is ubiquitous and can be found in soil and tap water and on many plants; fungal keratitis is rare but usually associated with trauma to the eye from an object contaminated with plant matter. This infection can be serious and can lead to the loss of vision. Other bacterial and fungal causes of infections have also been traced to inadequate cleaning of lenses.

## Endophthalmitis

Surgical trauma, nonsurgical trauma (infrequently), and hematogenous spread from distant sites of infection are the typical routes of transmission for endophthalmitis. The infection may be limited to specific tissues within the eye or may involve all of the intraocular contents. Bacteria are the most common infectious agents responsible for endophthalmitis.

After surgery or trauma, evidence of the disease is usually identified within 24 to 48 hours. Postoperative infection involves primarily normal flora bacteria from the ocular surface. Although *Staphylococcus epidermidis* and *S. aureus* are responsible for the majority of cases of endophthalmitis following cataract removal, any bacterium, including those considered to be saprophytic, may cause endophthalmitis. In hematogenous endophthalmitis, a septic focus elsewhere is usually evident before onset of the intraocular infection. *Bacillus cereus* has caused endophthalmitis in people addicted to narcotics and following transfusion with contaminated blood. Endophthalmitis associated with meningitis may involve various organisms, including *Haemophilus influenzae*, streptococci, and *Neisseria meningitidis*. *Nocardia* endophthalmitis may follow pulmonary infection with this organism.

Mycotic infection of the eye has increased significantly since the 1980s because of the increased use of antibiotics, corticosteroids, antineoplastic chemotherapy, addictive drugs, and hyperalimentation (overeating). Fungi generally considered to be saprophytic are important causes of postoperative endophthalmitis (see Table 72-1). Endogenous mycotic endophthalmitis is most often caused by *Candida albicans*. High-risk patients include those with diabetes or some other chronic underlying disease. Other causes of hematogenous ocular infection include *Aspergillus*, *Cryptococcus*, *Coccidioides*, *Sporothrix*, and *Blastomyces*.

Endophthalmitis may be a result of viral or parasitic infections. Viral causes of endophthalmitis include HSV, varicella (herpes) zoster virus (VZV), cytomegalovirus, and measles viruses. The most common parasitic agent associated with endophthalmitis is *Toxocara*. *Toxoplasma gondii* is a well-known cause of chorioretinitis. Thirteen percent of patients with cysticercosis (*Taenia solium*) have ocular involvement. *Onchocerca* usually produces keratitis, but intraocular infection also occurs.

## Periocular

Canaliculitis, one of three infections of the lacrimal apparatus (see Table 72-1), is an inflammation of the lacrimal canal and is usually caused by *Actinomyces* or *Propionibacterium propionicum* (formerly *Arachnia*). Infection of the lacrimal sac (dacryocystitis) may involve numerous bacterial and fungal agents; the major causes are listed in Table 72-1. Dacryoadenitis is an uncommon infection of the lacrimal gland characterized by pain of the upper eyelid with erythema and often involves pyogenic bacteria such as *S. aureus* and streptococci. Chronic infections of the lacrimal gland occur in tuberculosis, syphilis, leprosy, and schistosomiasis. Acute inflammation of the gland may occur during the course of the mumps and infectious mononucleosis.

Orbital cellulitis is an acute infection of the orbital contents and is most often caused by bacteria. This is a potentially serious infection because it may spread posteriorly to produce central nervous system complications. Most cases involve spread from contiguous sources such as the paranasal sinuses. In children, blood-borne bacteria, notably *Haemophilus influenzae*, may lead to orbital cellulitis. *S. aureus* is the most common etiologic agent; *Streptococcus pyogenes* and *S. pneumoniae* are also common.

Anaerobes may cause a cellulitis secondary to chronic sinusitis, primarily in adults. Mucormycosis of the orbit is a serious, invasive fungal infection seen particularly in patients with diabetes who have poor control of their disease, patients with acidosis from other causes, and patients with malignant disease receiving cytotoxic and immunosuppressive therapy. *Aspergillus* may produce a similar infection in the same settings but also can cause mild, chronic infections of the orbit.

Newer surgical techniques involving the ocular implantation of prosthetic or donor lenses have resulted in increasing numbers of iatrogenic (resulting from the activities of a physician) infections. Isolation of *Propionibacterium acnes* may have clinical significance in such situations, in contrast to many other sites in which it is usually considered to be a contaminant. Nontuberculous mycobacterial periocular infections have become increasingly important in patients with systemic disease. These infections are more prevalent in immunocompromised patients.

### Other Infections

Opportunistic infections in human immunodeficiency virus (HIV)-infected individuals can involve the eye. Ocular manifestations were previously reported in up to 70% of HIV-infected patients. Systemic infections that involve the eye included cytomegalovirus, *Pneumocystis jiroveci*, *Cryptococcus neoformans*, *Mycobacterium avium* complex, and *Candida* spp. Most often the retina, choroid, and optic nerve may be infected with these agents, resulting in significant visual morbidity (unhealthy condition) if left untreated. However, because of widespread use of highly active antiretroviral therapy capable of assisting in immune system recovery and lowering the viral load in patients with HIV infection, the incidence of acquired immunodeficiency syndrome (AIDS) and related ophthalmic infections has declined sharply.

## LABORATORY DIAGNOSIS

### Specimen Collection and Transport

Purulent material from the surface of the lower conjunctiva sac and inner canthus (angle) of the eye is collected on a sterile swab for cultures. Both eyes should be cultured separately. Chlamydial cultures are taken with a dry calcium alginate swab and placed in 2-SP (2-sucrose phosphate) transport medium. An additional swab may be rolled across the surface of a slide, fixed with methanol, and sent if direct fluorescent antibody (DFA) chlamydia stains are used for detection.

In the patient with keratitis, an ophthalmologist collects scrapings of the cornea with a heat-sterilized platinum spatula. Multiple inoculations with the spatula are made to blood agar, chocolate agar, an agar for the isolation of fungi, thioglycollate broth, and an anaerobic blood agar plate. Other special media may be used if indicated. Corneal specimens for culture of HSV and adenovirus are placed in viral transport media. Recently, the collection of two corneal scrapes (one used for Gram stain and the other transported in brain heart infusion medium and used for culture) was determined to provide a simple method for diagnosis of bacterial keratitis.

Cultures of endophthalmitis specimens are inoculated with material obtained by the ophthalmologist from the anterior and posterior chambers of the eye, wound abscesses, and wound dehiscence (splitting open). Lid infection material is collected on a swab in the conventional manner. For microbiologic studies of canaliculitis, material from the lacrimal canal should be transported under anaerobic conditions. Aspiration of fluid from the orbit is contraindicated in patients with orbital cellulitis. A patient history of sinusitis in association with orbital cellulitis is an indication for obtaining an otolaryngologist's assistance in the collection of material from the maxillary sinus by antral puncture. Blood cultures should also be obtained. Tissue biopsy is essential for the microbiologic diagnosis of mucormycosis. Because cultures are usually negative, the diagnosis is made by histologic examination.

### Direct Visual Examination

All material submitted for culture should be smeared and examined directly by Gram stain or other appropriate microscopic techniques. In bacterial conjunctivitis, polymorphonuclear leukocytes predominate; in viral infection, the host cells are primarily lymphocytes and monocytes. Specimens in which *Chlamydia* is suspected can be stained immediately with monoclonal antibody conjugated to fluorescein for the detection of elementary bodies or inclusions. Using histologic stains, basophilic intracytoplasmic inclusion bodies are seen in epithelial cells. Cytologists and anatomic pathologists usually perform these tests. Direct examination of conjunctivitis specimens using histologic methods (Tzanck smear; a scraping from the lesion for collection of cells) may reveal multinucleated epithelial cells typical of herpes group viral infections. However, DFA stains available for both HSV and VZV are recommended for rapid diagnosis of viral infections. In patients with keratitis, scrapings may be examined using Gram, Giemsa, periodic acid-Schiff (PAS), and methenamine silver stains. If *Acanthamoeba* or other amebae are suspected, a direct wet preparation should be examined for motile trophozoites, and a trichrome stain should be added to the regimen. For this diagnosis, however, culture is by far the most sensitive detection method for the identification of the organism. In patients with endophthalmitis, the specimen is examined using Gram, Giemsa, periodic acid-schiff (PAS), and methenamine silver stains. When submitted in large volumes of fluid, ophthalmic specimens must be concentrated by centrifugation before additional studies are performed.

### Culture

Because of the constant washing action of the tears, the number of organisms recovered from cultures of eye infections may be relatively low. Unless the clinical specimen is obviously purulent, using a relatively large inoculum and a variety of media is recommended to ensure recovery of the etiologic agent. Conjunctival scrapings placed directly onto media yield the best results. At a minimum, blood and chocolate agar plates should be inoculated and incubated under increased carbon dioxide tension (5% to 10% $CO_2$). Because potential pathogens may be present in an eye without causing infection, it may be very helpful to culture both eyes. If a potential pathogen grows in cultures of the infected and the uninfected eye, the organism may not be causing the infection; however, if the organism only grows in culture from the infected eye, it is most likely the causative agent. When *Moraxella lacunata* is suspected, Loeffler's medium may prove useful; the growth of the organism often leads to proteolysis and pitting of the medium, although nonproteolytic strains may be isolated. If diphtheritic conjunctivitis is suspected, Loeffler's or cystine-tellurite medium should be used. For more serious eye infections, such as keratitis, endophthalmitis, and orbital cellulitis, one should always include a reduced anaerobic blood agar plate, a medium for the isolation of fungi, and a liquid medium such as thioglycolate broth. Blood cultures are also important in serious eye infections.

Specimen cultures for *chlamydia* and viruses should be inoculated to appropriate media from transport broth.

For *Chlamydia* isolation use cycloheximide-treated McCoy cells; for viral isolation the use of human embryonic kidney, primary mondey kidney and Hep-2 cell lines is recommended.

### Nonculture Methods

Although acute and convalescent serologic tests for viral agents might be used in the event of epidemic conjunctivitis, they typically are not performed because the infections are self-limited. Enzyme-linked immunosorbent assay (ELISA) tests and DFA staining are available for the detection of *Chlamydia trachomatis*. An ELISA test of aqueous humor is available for the diagnosis of *Toxocara* infection. Finally, single and multiplex polymerase chain reaction (PCR) assays including both conventional and real-time formats have been used to diagnose viral and chlamydial keratoconjunctivitis and other ophthalmic infections including uveitis (inflammation in the middle layer of the eye).

# EARS

## ANATOMY

The ear is divided into three anatomic parts: the external, middle, and inner ear. Important anatomic structures are depicted in Figure 72-2.

The middle ear is part of a continuous system including the nares, nasopharynx, auditory tube, and the mastoid air spaces. These structures are lined with respiratory epithelium (e.g., ciliated cells, mucus-secreting goblet cells).

## RESIDENT MICROBIAL FLORA

The normal flora within the external ear canal is rather sparse, similar to flora of the conjunctiva sac. Pneumococci, *Streptococcus pneumoniae*, *Propionibacterium acnes*, *Staphylococcus aureus*, and *Enterobacteriaceae* are encountered somewhat more frequently. *Pseudomonas aeruginosa* is found on occasion. *Candida* spp. (non-*C. albicans*) is also common.

## DISEASES, EPIDEMIOLOGY, AND ETIOLOGY OF DISEASE

### Otitis Externa (External Ear Infections)

Otitis externa is similar to skin and soft tissue infection. Two major types of external otitis exist: acute or chronic.

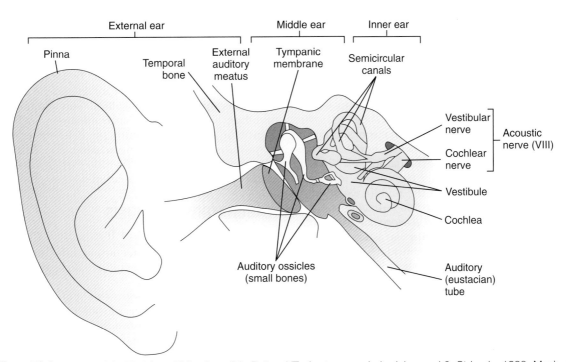

**Figure 72-2** The ear. (Modified from Thibodeau GA, Patton KT: *Anatomy and physiology*, ed 2, St Louis, 1993, Mosby.)

Acute external otitis may be localized or diffuse. Acute localized disease occurs in the form of a pustule or furuncle and typically is caused by *Staphylococcus aureus*. Erysipelas caused by group A streptococci may involve the external ear canal and the soft tissue of the ear. Acute diffuse otitis externa (swimmer's ear) is related to maceration (softening of tissue) of the ear from swimming or hot, humid weather. Gram-negative bacilli, particularly *Pseudomonas aeruginosa*, play an important role. A severe, hemorrhagic external otitis caused by *P. aeruginosa* is difficult to treat and has occasionally been related to hot tub use.

Chronic otitis externa results from the irritation of drainage from the middle ear in patients with chronic, suppurative otitis media and a perforated eardrum. Malignant otitis externa is a necrotizing infection that spreads to adjacent areas of soft tissue, cartilage, and bone. If allowed to progress and spread into the central nervous system or vascular channel, a life-threatening condition may develop. *P. aeruginosa*, in particular, and anaerobes are frequently associated with this process. Malignant otitis media is seen in patients with diabetes who have blood vessel disease of the tissues overlying the temporal bone in which poor local perfusion of tissues results in an environment conducive for invasion by bacteria. On occasion, external otitis can extend into the cartilage of the ear, usually requiring surgical intervention. Certain viruses may infect the external auditory canal, the soft tissue of the ear, or the tympanic membrane; influenza A virus is a suspected, but not an established, cause. VZV may cause painful vesicles within the soft tissue of the ear and the ear canal. Viral agents such as influenza are the bacterial agents typically associated with acute otitis media (*S. pneumoniae*, *H. influenzae*, and *M. catarrhalis*). *Mycoplasma pneumoniae* is rarely associated with this condition.

### Otitis Media (Middle Ear Infections)

In children (in whom otitis media is most common), pneumococci (33% of cases) and *Haemophilus influenzae* (20%) are the usual etiologic agents in acute disease. Group A streptococci (*Streptococcus pyogenes*) are the third most frequently encountered agents, found in 8% of cases. Other organisms, encountered in 1% to 6% of cases, include *Moraxella catarrhalis*, *Staphylococcus aureus*, gram-negative enteric bacilli, and anaerobes; in one recent study, *M. catarrhalis*, *S. pneumoniae*, and *H. influenzae* were the most common bacterial pathogens. Viruses, chiefly respiratory syncytial virus (RSV) and influenza virus, have been recovered from the middle ear fluid of 4% of children with acute or chronic otitis media. *Chlamydia trachomatis* and *Mycoplasma pneumoniae* have occasionally been isolated from middle ear aspirates. Otitis media with effusion (fluid) is considered a chronic sequela of acute otitis media. A slowly growing organism, *Alloiococcus otitis* is a pathogen that has been isolated from patients with otitis media with effusion.

Chronic otitis media yields a predominantly anaerobic flora, with *Peptostreptococcus* spp., *Bacteroides fragilis* group, *Prevotella melaninogenica* (pigmented, anaerobic, gram-negative rods), *Porphyromonas*, other *Prevotella* spp., and *Fusobacterium nucleatum* as the principal pathogens; less

**TABLE 72-2** Major Infectious Causes of Ear Disease

| Disease | Common Causes |
|---|---|
| *Otitis externa* | Acute: *Staphylococcus aureus, Streptococcus pyogenes, Pseudomonas aeruginosa;* other gram-negative bacilli |
| | Chronic: *P. aeruginosa;* anaerobes |
| *Otitis media* | Acute *Streptococcus pneumoniae; Haemophilus influenzae; Moraxella catarrhalis; S. pyogenes;* respiratory syncytial virus; influenza virus |
| | Chronic: Anaerobes |

frequently present are *S. aureus*, *Pseudomonas aeruginosa*, *Proteus* spp., and other gram-negative facultative bacilli. Table 72-2 summarizes the major causes of ear infections.

The mastoid is a portion of the temporal bone (lower sides of the skull) containing the mastoid sinuses (cavities). Mastoiditis is a complication of chronic otitis media in which organisms find their way into the mastoid sinuses. To prevent the further spread of this infection to the central nervous system, a mastoidectomy is performed.

## PATHOGENESIS

Local trauma, the presence of foreign bodies, or excessive moisture can lead to otitis externa (external ear infections). Infrequently, an infection from the middle ear can extend by purulent drainage to the external ear.

Anatomic or physiologic abnormalities of the auditory tube can predispose individuals to develop otitis media. The auditory tube is responsible for protecting the middle ear from nasopharyngeal secretion, draining secretions produced in the middle ear into the nasopharynx, and ventilating the middle ear and equilibrate air pressure with the external ear canal. If any of these functions becomes compromised and fluid develops in the middle ear, infection may occur. To illustrate, if a person has a viral upper respiratory infection, the auditory tube becomes inflamed and swollen. This inflammation and swelling may, in turn, compromise the auditory tube's ventilating function, resulting in a negative, rather than a positive, pressure in the middle ear. This change in pressure can then allow for potentially pathogenic bacteria present in the nasopharynx to enter the middle ear.

## LABORATORY DIAGNOSIS

### Specimen Collection and Transport

Although middle ear infection or otitis media is usually not diagnosed by culture, culture can be used for the laboratory diagnosis of external otitis; the external ear should be cleansed with a mild germicide such as 1 : 1000 aqueous solution of benzalkonium chloride to reduce the numbers of contaminating skin flora before obtaining the specimen. Material from the ear, especially that obtained after spontaneous perforation of the eardrum or by needle aspiration of middle ear fluid (tympanocentesis), should be collected by an otolaryngologist, using sterile equipment. Specimens from the mastoid are generally taken on swabs during surgery, although actual bone is preferred. Specimens should be transported anaerobically.

### Direct Visual Examination

Material aspirated from the middle ear or mastoid is also examined directly for bacteria and fungi. The calcofluor white or PAS stains can reveal fungal elements. Methenamine silver stains have the added efficiency of staining most bacterial, fungal, and several parasitic species.

### Culture and Nonculture Methods

Ear specimens submitted for culture should be inoculated to blood, MacConkey, and chocolate agars. Anaerobic cultures should also be set up on those specimens obtained by tympanocentesis or those obtained from patients with chronic otitis media or mastoiditis. Because cultures of middle ear effusions are culture positive for only 20% to 30% of patients, conventional and real-time PCR assays have been used to detect the common middle ear pathogens.

## SINUSES

### ANATOMY

The sinuses, like the mastoids, are unique, air-filled cavities within the head (Figure 72-3). The sinuses are normally sterile. These structures, as well as the eustachian tube, the middle ear, and the respiratory portion of the pharynx, are lined by respiratory epithelium. The clearance of secretions and contaminants depends on normal ciliary activity and mucous flow.

### DISEASES

The pathogens associated with otitis media are the same ones associated with sinusitis; bacteria from the nose and throat make their way to the inner ear and sinuses. Acute sinusitis usually develops during the course of a cold or influenza illness and tends to be self-limited, lasting 1 to 3 weeks, and is usually more prevalent in winter and spring. Acute sinusitis is often difficult to distinguish from the primary illness. Symptoms include purulent nasal and postnasal discharge, a feeling of pressure over the sinus areas of the face, cough, and a nasal quality to the voice. Fever is sometimes present.

Occasionally, acute sinusitis persists and reaches a chronic state in which bacterial colonization occurs and the condition no longer responds to antibiotic treatment. Ordinarily, surgery or drainage is required for successful management. Patients with chronic sinusitis may have acute exacerbations (flare-ups). Other complications include local extension into the orbit, skull, meninges, or brain, and development of chronic sinusitis.

### PATHOGENESIS

Most cases of acute sinusitis are believed to be bacterial complications following a viral respiratory infection. The exact mechanisms involved are unknown. About 5% to 10% of acute maxillary sinus infections result from infection originating from a dental source. The maxillary sinuses are close to the roots of the upper teeth, providing a mechanism for dental infections to extend into the sinuses. The primary problems associated with the development of chronic sinusitis include inadequate drainage, impaired mucociliary clearance, and mucosal damage.

### EPIDEMIOLOGY AND ETIOLOGY OF DISEASE

Although difficult to access, the actual incidence of acute sinusitis parallels that of acute upper respiratory tract infections (i.e., being most prevalent in the fall through spring).

Most studies of the microbiology of acute sinusitis are associated with maxillary sinusitis because it is the most common type and specimen collection available through puncture and aspiration. Acute viral sinusitis is one of the most common causes of respiratory tract infection and in most cases resolves without treatment. However, published estimates indicate that 0.5% to 2% of cases of acute viral sinusitis in adults are complicated by bacterial sinusitis. This scenario is even more common in children. Bacterial cultures are positive in about three fourths of patients. Studies have indicated that *Streptococcus pneumoniae* and *Haemophilus influenzae* are the major bacterial pathogens in adults with acute sinusitis; other species such as beta-hemolytic and alpha-hemolytic streptococci, *Staphylococcus aureus*, and anaerobes have also been cultured but less frequently. The predominant bacterial organisms associated with chronic sinusitis include *S. pneumoniae, H. influenzae, and M. catarrhalis;* less frequently isolated organisms include anaerobic streptococci, Prevotella spp., and Fusobacterium spp. Fungal pathogens such as Aspergillus, Fusarum, and *Candida albicans* have also been identified in cases of chronic sinusitis using culture and polymerase chain reaction (PCR).

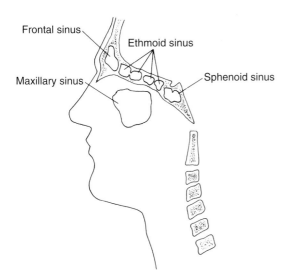

Frontal sinus
Ethmoid sinus
Maxillary sinus
Sphenoid sinus

**Figure 72-3** Location of the paranasal sinuses. (From Milliken ME, Campbell G: *Essential competencies for patient care,* St Louis, 1985, Mosby.)

**TABLE 72-3** Major Infectious Causes of Acute Sinusitis

| Age Group | Common Causes |
|---|---|
| Young adults | *Haemophilus influenzae, Streptococcus pneumoniae, Streptococcus pyogenes, Moraxella catarrhalis* |
| Children | *S. pneumoniae, H. influenzae, M. catarrhalis,* rhinovirus |

Among children, *S. pneumoniae*, *H. influenzae*, and *M. catarrhalis* are most common. Rhinovirus is found in 15% of patients, influenza virus in 5%, parainfluenza virus in 3%, and adenovirus in less than 1%. The major causes of acute sinusitis are summarized in Table 72-3. *M. catarrhalis* has been isolated in chronic sinusitis in children.

## LABORATORY DIAGNOSIS

In most cases, a diagnosis can be made on the basis of physical findings, history, radiograph studies, and other imaging techniques such as magnetic resonance imaging. However, if a laboratory diagnosis is needed, an otolaryngologist collects a specimen from the maxillary sinus by puncture and aspiration or during surgery. Sinus drainage is unacceptable for smear or culture because this material will be contaminated with aerobic and anaerobic normal respiratory flora; sinus washings or aspirates surgically collected are the specimens of choice. Gram-stained smears and aerobic and anaerobic cultures should be performed on each specimen. Aerobic culture media should include blood, chocolate, and MacConkey agar.

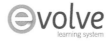

*Visit the Evolve site to complete the review questions.*

---

## CASE STUDY 72-1

A 12-year-old boy complained of severe ear pain of 4 days duration. He was afebrile, but his tympanic membrane was erythematous and bleeding. The boy had been swimming a few days earlier in a local lake. His physician collected samples, which grew a gram-negative rod with a pleasant odor. The patient was given antibiotic eardrops and did well, with resolution of his symptoms.

**QUESTIONS**

1. What organism caused this infection?
2. How can this isolate be identified rapidly?
3. If the characteristic odor is lacking, what characteristics of the organism make it easy to identify?
4. Name the other fluorescent *Pseudomonas* spp.

---

## BIBLIOGRAPHY

Bernardes TF, Bonfioli AA: Blepharitis, *Semin Ophthalmol* 25(3):79-83, 2010.

Cramer L, Emara DM, Gadre AK: Mycoplasma an unlikely cause of bullous myringitis, *Ear Nose Throat J* 91(6):E30-31, 2012.

Finegold SM, Flynn MJ, Rose FV, et al: Bacteriologic findings associated with chronic bacterial maxillary sinusitis in adults, *Clin Infect Dis* 35(4):428-433, 2002.

Hendolin PH, Paulin L, Ylikoski J: Clinically applicable multiplex PCR for four middle ear pathogens, *J Clin Microbiol* 38:125, 2000.

Henry CR, Flynn HW, Miller D, et al: Infectious keratitis progressing to endophthalmitis: A 15-year study of microbiology, associated factors, and clinical outcomes, *Ophthalmology* 119(12):2443-2449, 2012.

Kaye SB, Rao PG, Smith G, et al: Simplifying collection of corneal specimens in cases of suspected bacterial keratitis, *J Clin Microbiol* 41:3192, 2003.

Kim ST, Choi JH, Jeon HG, et al: Comparison between polymerase chain reaction and fungal culture for the detection of fungi in patients with chronic sinusitis and normal controls, *Acta Otolaryngol* 125(1):72-75, 2005.

Lynn WA, Lightman S: The eye in systemic infection, *Lancet* 364(9443):1439-1450, 2004.

Mandell GL, Bennett JE, Dolin R, editors: *Principles and practice of infectious diseases*, ed 7, Philadelphia, 2010, Elsevier Churchill Livingstone.

Marciano-Cabral F, Cabral G: *Acanthamoeba* spp as agents of disease in humans, *Clin Microbiol Rev* 16:273, 2003

Moorthy RS, Valluri S, Rao NA: Nontuberculous mycobacterial ocular and adnexal infections, *Surv Ophthalmol* 57(3):202-235, 2012.

Palmu AA, Herva E, Savolainen H, et al: Association of clinical signs and symptoms with bacterial findings in acute otitis media, *Clin Infect Dis* 38:234, 2004.

Piccirillo JF: Acute bacterial sinusitis, *N Engl J Med* 351:902, 2004.

Roels P: Ocular infections of AIDS: new considerations for patients using highly active anti-retroviral therapy (HAART), *Optometry* 75:624, 2004.

Sande M, Gwaltney JM: Acute community-acquired bacterial sinusitis: continuing challenges and current management, *Clin Infect Dis* 39:S151, 2004.

Skevaki CL, Galani IE, Pararas MV, et al: Treatment of viral conjunctivitis with antiviral drugs, *Drugs* 71(3):331-347, 2011.

Solomon AW, Peeling RW, Foster A, et al: Diagnosis and assessment of trachoma, *Clin Microbiol Rev* 17:982, 2004.

Versalovic J: *Manual of clinical microbiology*, ed 10, Washington, DC, 2011, ASM Press.

# Infections of the Urinary Tract

1. Describe the anatomy and identify the structures of the urinary tract, for both males and females.
2. Name the organisms that colonize the urethra and are considered normal flora.
3. Explain how the female urinary tract anatomy may predispose women to urinary tract infections.
4. Differentiate between community-acquired urinary tract infections and hospital-acquired urinary tract infections.
5. List the routes of transmission that allow bacteria to invade and cause a urinary tract infection.
6. Name the physical and chemical properties of urine that contribute to its role in the body's defense mechanism against the bacteria capable of causing urinary tract infections.
7. Explain host and microbial factors that determine whether bacteria will be able to colonize and cause a urinary tract infection.
8. Name the properties bacteria possess that predispose them to having greater pathogenicity in causing urinary tract infections.
9. Define the five major types of urinary tract infections: pyelonephritis, cystitis, urethritis, acute urethral syndrome, and asymptomatic bacteriuria.
10. Compare and contrast complicated and uncomplicated urinary tract infections.
11. Explain the collection methods for urine specimens, including clean catch midstream urine, straight catheterized urine, a suprapubic bladder aspiration, and an indwelling catheter collection.
12. Describe the urine-screening methods available to determine bacteriuria and pyuria.
13. Explain the nitrate reductase test, the leukocyte esterase test, and the catalase test in regard to their urine-screening capability.
14. Name the media required for urine cultures.
15. Explain the proper methodology for plating and interpreting a quantitative urine culture.
16. Correlate signs and symptoms with the results of laboratory diagnositc procedures for the identification of the etilogic agent associated with infections of the urinary tract.

# GENERAL CONSIDERATIONS

## ANATOMY

The urinary tract consists of the kidneys, ureters, bladder, and urethra (Figure 73-1). The function of the urinary tract is to make and process urine. Urine is an ultrafiltrate of blood that consists mostly of water but also contains nitrogenous wastes, sodium, potassium, chloride, and other analytes. Urine is normally a sterile fluid, Often, urinary tract infections (UTIs) are characterized as being either upper (U-UTI) or lower (L-UTI) based primarily on the anatomic location of the infection: the lower urinary tract encompasses the bladder and urethra, and the upper urinary tract encompasses the ureters and kidneys. Upper urinary tract infections affect the ureters (ureteritis) or the renal parenchyma (pyelonephritis). Lower urinary tract infections may affect the urethra (urethritis), the bladder (cystitis), or the prostate in males (prostatitis).

The anatomy of the female urethra is of particular importance to the pathogenesis of UTIs. The female urethra is relatively short compared with the male urethra and also lies in close proximity to the warm, moist, perirectal region, which is teeming with microorganisms. Because of the shorter urethra, bacteria can reach the bladder more easily in the female host, thus urinary tract infections are primarily a disorder of women. For men, the incidence of urinary tract infections increases after the age of 60, when the enlargement of the prostate interferes with the removal of urine from the bladder.

## RESIDENT MICROORGANISMS OF THE URINARY TRACT

The urethra has resident microflora that colonize its epithelium in the distal portion; these organisms are lactobacilli, corynebacteria, and coagulase-negative staphylococci (Box 73-1). Potential pathogens, including gram-negative aerobic bacilli (primarily Enterobacteriaceae) and occasional yeasts, are also present as transient colonizers. All areas of the urinary tract above the urethra in a healthy human are sterile. Urine is typically sterile, but noninvasive methods for collecting urine must rely on a specimen that has passed through a contaminated milieu. Therefore, quantitative cultures for the diagnosis of UTIs have been used to discriminate among contamination, colonization, and infection.

# INFECTIONS OF THE URINARY TRACT

## EPIDEMIOLOGY

UTIs are among the most common bacterial infections that lead patients to seek medical care. It has been estimated that more than 7 million outpatient visits, 1 million visits to the emergency department, and 100,000 hospital stays every year in the United States are due to UTIs. Approximately 10% of humans will have a UTI at some time during their lives. Of note, UTIs are also the most common hospital-acquired infection, accounting for as many as 35% of nosocomial infections.

The exact prevalence of UTIs is age and sex dependent. During the first year of life, UTIs are less than 2% in males and females. The incidence of UTIs among males remains relatively low after 1 year of age and until

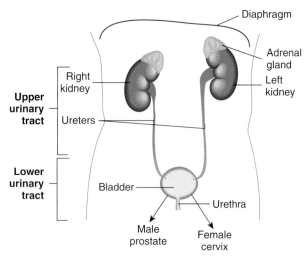

**Figure 73-1** Overview of the anatomy of the urinary tract. (From Potter PH, Perry AG: *Fundamentals of nursing,* St. Louis, 1985, Mosby.)

---

**BOX 73-1** Resident Microflora of the Urethra

Coagulase-negative staphylococci (excluding
  *S. saprophyticus*)
Viridans and nonhemolytic streptococci
Lactobacilli
Diphtheroids (*Corynebacterium* spp.)
Nonpathogenic (saprobic) *Neisseria* spp.
Anaerobic cocci
*Propionibacterium* spp.
Anaerobic gram-negative bacilli
Commensal *Mycobacterium* spp.
Commensal *Mycoplasma* spp.

---

approximately 60 years of age when enlargement of the prostate interferes with emptying of the bladder. Extensive studies have shown that the incidence of bacteriuria (presence of bacteria in urine) among girls 5 through 17 years of age is 1% to 3%. The prevalence of bacteriuria in females increases gradually with time to as high as 10% to 20% in older women. In women between 20 and 40 years of age who have had UTIs, as many as 50% may become reinfected within 1 year. The association of UTIs with sexual intercourse may also contribute to this increased incidence because sexual activity increases the chances of bacterial contamination of the female urethra. Finally, as a result of anatomic and hormonal changes that favor development of UTIs, the incidence of bacteriuria increases during pregnancy. These infections can lead to serious infections in both mother and fetus.

UTIs are important complications of diabetes, renal disease, renal transplantation, and structural and neurologic abnormalities that interfere with urine flow. In 40% to 60% of renal transplant recipients, the urinary tract is the source of bacteremia, and in these patients, the recurrence rate is about 40%. In addition, UTIs are a leading cause of gram-negative sepsis in hospitalized patients and are the origin for about half of all nosocomial infections caused by urinary catheters.

## ETIOLOGIC AGENTS

### Community-Acquired

*Escherichia coli* is by far the most frequent cause of uncomplicated community-acquired UTIs. At the molecular level, the *E. coli*, designated uropathogenic *E. coli* (UPEC), that causes UTIs is sufficiently different from other types of *E. coli*. Other bacteria frequently isolated from patients with UTIs are *Klebsiella* spp., other *Enterobacteriaceae, Staphylococcus saprophyticus,* and enterococci. In more complicated UTIs, particularly in recurrent infections, the relative frequency of infection caused by *Proteus, Pseudomonas, Klebsiella,* and *Enterobacter* spp. increases. In addition, community-acquired urinary tract infections are increasingly associated with multidrug-resistant organisms such as extended β-lactamase-resistant *E. coli.*

### Hospital-Acquired

The hospital environment plays an important role in determining the organisms involved in UTIs. Hospitalized patients are most likely to be infected by *E. coli, Klebsiella* spp., *Proteus* spp., staphylococci, other Enterobacteriaceae, *Pseudomonas aeruginosa,* enterococci, and *Candida* spp. The introduction of a foreign body into the urinary tract, especially one that remains in place for an extended period (e.g., Foley catheter), carries a substantial risk of infection, particularly if obstruction is present. Thirty five percent of all hospital-acquired infections are urinary tract infections. Eighty percent of those infections are associated with the use of an indwelling catheter. Consequently, UTI is the most common nosocomial infection in the United States, and the infected urinary tract is the most frequent source of bacteremia.

### Miscellaneous

Other less frequently isolated agents are other gram-negative bacilli, such as *Acinetobacter* and *Alcaligenes* spp., other *Pseudomonas* spp., *Citrobacter* spp., *Gardnerella vaginalis, Aerococcus urinae,* and beta-hemolytic streptococci. Bacteria such as mycobacteria, *Chlamydia trachomatis, Ureaplasma urealyticum, Campylobacter* spp., *Haemophilus influenzae, Leptospira,* and certain *Corynebacterium* spp. (e.g., *C. renale*) are rarely recovered from urine. Because renal transplant recipients are immunosuppressed, these patients not only suffer from common uropathogens but are also susceptible to opportunistic infections with unusual pathogens. A study involving renal transplant recipients showed that for culture-negative urine, amplification of regions in bacterial 16S rRNA and subsequent analysis by high-performance liquid chromatography detected the presence of a number of known uropathogens as well as unusual agents. *Salmonella* spp. may be recovered during the early stages of typhoid fever; their presence should be immediately reported to the physician. If anaerobes are suspected, the physician should perform a percutaneous bladder tap unless urine can be obtained from the upper urinary tract by another means (e.g., from a nephrostomy tube). Communication by the clinician to the laboratory that such an agent is suspected is important for detecting such agents. In patients with "sterile pyuria," Gram stain may reveal unusual organisms with distinctive morphology (e.g., *H. influenzae,* anaerobes). The presence of any organisms on smear that do not grow in culture is an important clue to the cause of the infection. The laboratory can then take the action necessary to optimize chances for recovery.

In general, viruses and parasites are not usually considered urinary tract pathogens. *Trichomonas vaginalis* may occasionally be observed in urinary sediment, and *Schistosoma haematobium* can lodge in the urinary tract and release eggs into the urine. Adenoviruses types 11 and 21 have been implicated as causative agents in hemorrhagic cystitis in children.

## PATHOGENESIS

### Routes of Infection

Bacteria can invade and cause a UTI via three major routes: ascending, hematogenous, and lymphatic pathways. Although the ascending route is the most common course of infection in females, ascent in association with instrumentation (e.g., urinary catheterization, cystoscopy) is the most common cause of hospital-acquired UTIs in both sexes. For UTIs to occur by the ascending pathway, enteric gram-negative bacteria and other microorganisms that originate in the gastrointestinal tract must be able to colonize the vaginal cavity or the periurethral area. Once these organisms gain access to the bladder, they may multiply and then pass up the ureters to the kidneys. UTIs occur more often in women than men, at least partially because of the short female urethra and its proximity to the anus. As previously mentioned, sexual activity can increase chances of bacterial contamination of the female urethra.

In most hospitalized patients, UTI is preceded by urinary catheterization or other manipulation of the urinary tract. The pathogenesis of catheter-associated UTI is not fully understood. It is certain that soon after hospitalization, patients become colonized with bacteria endemic to the institution, often gram-negative aerobic and facultative bacilli carrying resistance markers. These bacteria colonize the patient's skin, gastrointestinal tract, and mucous membranes, including the anterior urethra. With insertion of a catheter, the bacteria may be pushed along the urethra into the bladder or, with an indwelling catheter, may migrate along the track between the catheter and the urethral mucosa, gaining access to the bladder. It is estimated that approximately 10% to 30% of catheterized patients will develop bacteriuria (presence of bacteria in urine).

UTIs may also occur by the hematogenous, or bloodborne, route. Hematogenous spread usually occurs as a result of bacteremia. Any systemic infection can lead to seeding of the kidney, but certain organisms, such as *Staphylococcus aureus* or *Salmonella* spp., are particularly invasive. Although most infections involving the kidneys are acquired through the ascending route, yeast (usually *Candida albicans*), *Mycobacterium tuberculosis*, *Salmonella* spp., *Leptospira* spp., or *Staphylococcus aureus* in the urine often indicates pyelonephritis acquired via hematogenous spread, or the descending route. Hematogenous spread accounts for less than 5% of UTIs.

Finally, increased pressure on the bladder can cause lymphatic flow into the kidneys, resulting in UTI.

However, evidence for the significance of this potential route is insufficient, indicating that the ascending route remains the major mechanism for the development of UTI.

### The Host-Parasite Relationship

Many individuals, women in particular, are colonized in the vaginal or periurethral area with organisms originating from the gastrointestinal tract, yet they do not develop urinary infections. Whether an organism is able to colonize and then cause a UTI is determined in large part by a complex interplay of host and microbial factors.

In most cases, the host defense mechanisms are able to eliminate the organisms. Urine itself is inhibitory to some of the urethral flora such as anaerobes. In addition, if urine has a low pH, high or low osmolality, high urea concentration, or high organic acid content, even organisms capable of growth in the urinary tract may be inhibited. If bacteria do gain access to the bladder, the constant flushing of contaminated urine from the body either eliminates bacteria or maintains their numbers at low levels. Clearly, any interference with the act of normal voiding, such as mechanical obstruction resulting from kidney stones or strictures, will promote the development of UTI. Also, the bladder mucosal surface has antibacterial properties. If the infection is not eradicated, the site of infection remains in the superficial mucosa; deep layers of the bladder are rarely involved.

In addition to the previously described host defenses, a valvelike mechanism at the junction of the ureter and bladder prevents the reflux (backward flow) of urine from the bladder to the upper urinary tract. Therefore, if the function of these valves is inhibited or compromised in any way, such as by obstruction or congenital abnormalities, urine reflux provides a direct route for organisms to reach the kidney. Hormonal changes associated with pregnancy and their effects on the urinary tract increase the chance for urine reflux to the upper urinary tract.

Activation of the host immune response by uropathogens also plays a key role in fending off infection. For example, bacterial contact with urothelial cells initiates an immune response via a variety of signaling pathways. Bacterial lipopolysaccharide (LPS; see Chapter 2) activates host cells to ultimately release cytokines such as tumor necrosis factor and interferon-gamma. In addition, bacteria can activate the complement cascade, leading to the production of biologically active components such as opsonins, as well as augment the host's adaptive immune response. Host factors that lead to host susceptibility or resistance to uropathogens have been identified. For example, a glycoprotein synthesized exclusively by epithelial cells in a specific anatomic location in the kidney, referred to as Tamm-Horsfall protein or uromodulin, serves as an anti-adherence factor by binding to *E. coli*–expressing type 1 fimbriae (discussed later). Defensins, a group of small antimicrobial peptides, are produced by a variety of host cells such as macrophages, neutrophils, and cells in the urinary tract and attach to the bacterial cell, eventually causing its death.

Although many microorganisms can cause UTIs, most cases are a result of infection by a few organisms. To illustrate, only a limited number of serogroups of *E. coli* cause a significant proportion of UTIs. Numerous investigations indicate that UPEC possesses virulence factors that enhance their ability to colonize and invade the urinary tract. Some of these virulence factors include increased adherence to vaginal and uroepithelial cells by bacterial surface structures (adhesins, in particular, pili), alpha-hemolysin production, and resistance to serum-killing activity (Box 73-2). Also, genome sequences of some UPEC strains have been determined, indicating that several potential virulence factor genes associated with the acquisition and development of UTIs are encoded on pathogenicity islands (e.g., hemolysins and *E. coli P. fimbriae*). Uropathogenic E. coli (UPEC) possess pathogenicity islands containing a variety of virulence factors. By definition, pathogenicity islands (see Chapter 3) contain genes that are associated with virulence and are absent from avirulent or less virulent strains of the same species.

The importance of adherence in the pathogenesis of UTIs has also been demonstrated with other species of bacteria. Once introduced into the urinary tract, *Proteus* strains appear to be uniquely suited to cause significant disease in the urinary tract. Data indicate that these strains are able to facilitate their adherence to the mucosa of kidneys. Also, *Proteus* is able to hydrolyze urea via urease production. Hydrolysis of urea results in an increase in urine pH that is directly toxic to kidney cells and also stimulates the formation of kidney stones. Similar findings have been made with *Klebsiella* spp. *Staphylococcus saprophyticus* also adheres better to uroepithelial cells than does *S. aureus* or *S. epidermidis*.

Other bacterial characteristics may be important in the pathogenesis of UTIs. Motility may be important for organisms to ascend to the upper urinary tract against the flow of urine and cause pyelonephritis. Some organisms demonstrate greater production of K antigen (capsule or outer cell wall); this antigen protects bacteria from being phagocytosed.

Finally, despite numerous host defenses and even antibiotic treatments that can effectively sterilize the urine, a significant proportion of patients have recurrent UTIs. Studies show that uropathogens can invade superficial epithelial cells in the bladder and replicate, forming large foci of intracellular *E. coli*. This invasion of bladder epithelial cells triggers the host immune response, which in turn causes the superficial cells to exfoliate within hours following infection. Although this exfoliation is considered a host defense mechanism by eliminating infected cells, intracellular organisms are able to

reemerge from the bladder epithelial cells and invade the underlying, new superficial layer of epithelial cells, consequently persisting within the urinary tract. Anderson and colleagues reported that intracellular bacteria mature into numerous, large protrusions on the bladder surface they referred to as "pods." This bacterial organization—in which the intracellular bacteria are embedded in a fibrous, polysaccharide-rich matrix resembling that of a biofilm—may help further explain the persistence of bladder infections despite strong host defenses.

## TYPES OF INFECTION AND THEIR CLINICAL MANIFESTATIONS

UTI encompasses a broad range of clinical entities that differ in terms of clinical presentation, degree of tissue invasion, epidemiologic setting, and requirements for antibiotic therapy. There are several types of UTIs: urethritis, ureteritis, asymptomatic bacteriuria, cystitis, the urethral syndrome, and pyelonephritis. Sometimes UTIs are classified as uncomplicated or complicated. Uncomplicated infections occur primarily in otherwise healthy females and occasionally in male infants and adolescent and adult males. Most uncomplicated infections respond readily to antibiotic agents to which the etiologic agent is susceptible. Complicated infections occur in both sexes. In general, individuals who develop complicated infections often have certain risk factors. Some of these risk factors are listed in Box 73-3. In general, complicated infections are more difficult to treat and have greater morbidity (e.g., kidney damage, bacteremia) and mortality compared with uncomplicated infections.

The clinical presentation of UTIs may vary, ranging from asymptomatic infection to full-blown pyelonephritis (infection of the kidney and its pelvis). Some UTI symptoms may be nonspecific, and frequently symptoms overlap considerably in patients with lower UTIs and in those with upper UTIs.

### Urethritis

Symptoms associated with urethritis (infection of the urethra), dysuria (painful or difficult urination), and frequency are similar to those associated with lower UTIs. Urethritis is a common infection. Because *Chlamydia trachomatis*, *Neisseria gonorrhoeae*, and *Trichomonas vaginalis* are common causes of urethritis and considered to be sexually transmitted, urethritis is discussed as a sexually transmitted disease in Chapter 74.

## Ureteritis

Inflammation or infection within the ureters is considered in combination with kidney infections. UTI within the ureters indicates that organisms have begun or are in the process of ascending into the kidneys and should be treated similarly to prevent further infection.

## Asymptomatic Bacteriuria

Asymptomatic bacteriuria or asymptomatic UTI is the isolation of a specified quantitative count of bacteria in an appropriately collected urine specimen obtained from a person without symptoms or signs of urinary infection. Asymptomatic bacteriuria is common, but its prevalence varies widely with age, gender, and the presence of genitourinary abnormalities or underlying diseases. For example, the prevalence of bacteriuria increases with age in healthy women from as low as about 1% among school-age females to greater than or equal to 20% among women 80 years of age or older living in the community, whereas bacteriuria is rare in healthy young men. Because its clinical significance was controversial (asymptomatic bacteriuria precedes UTI but does not always lead to asymptomatic infection), guidelines have been published for the diagnosis and treatment of asymptomatic bacteriuria in adults older than 18 years of age. The foundation of these guidelines rests on the premise that screening of asymptomatic subjects for bacteriuria is appropriate if bacteriuria has adverse outcomes that can be prevented by antimicrobial therapy. Thus, screening and treatment for asymptomatic bacteriuria is recommended for pregnant women (because the risk of progression to severe symptomatic UTI and possible harm to the fetus), males undergoing transurethral resection of the prostate, and individuals undergoing urologic procedures for which mucosal bleeding is anticipated. In contrast, screening for or treatment of asymptomatic bacteriuria is not recommended for premenopausal, nonpregnant women, diabetic women, older persons living in the community, older institutionalized subjects, persons with spinal cord injury, or catheterized patients while the catheter is in place.

## Cystitis

Typically, patients with cystitis (infection of the bladder) complain of dysuria, frequency, and urgency (compelling need to urinate). These symptoms are due not only to inflammation of the bladder but also to multiplication of bacteria in the urine and urethra. Often, there is tenderness and pain over the area of the bladder. In some individuals, the urine is grossly bloody. The patient may note urine cloudiness and a bad odor. Because cystitis is a localized infection, fever and other signs of a systemic (affecting the body as a whole) illness are usually not present.

## Acute Urethral Syndrome

Another UTI is acute urethral syndrome. Patients with this syndrome are primarily young, sexually active women, who experience dysuria, frequency, and urgency but yield fewer organisms than $10^5$ colony-forming units of bacteria per milliliter (CFU/mL) urine on culture. (The criterion of greater than $10^5$ CFU/mL of urine is highly indicative of infection in most patients with UTIs.) Almost 50% of all women who seek medical attention for complaints of symptoms of acute cystitis fall into this group. Although *Chlamydia trachomatis* and *N. gonorrhoeae* urethritis, anaerobic infection, genital herpes, and vaginitis account for some cases of acute urethral syndrome, most of these women are infected with organisms identical to those that cause cystitis but in numbers less than $10^5$ CFU/mL of urine. One must use a cutoff of $10^2$ CFU/mL, rather than $10^5$ CFU/mL, for this group of patients but must insist on concomitant pyuria (presence of eight or more leukocytes per cubic millimeter on microscopic examination of uncentrifuged urine). Approximately 90% of these women have pyuria, an important discriminatory feature of infection.

## Pyelonephritis

Pyelonephritis refers to inflammation of the kidney parenchyma, calices (cup-shaped division of the renal pelvis), and pelvis (upper end of the ureter that is located inside the kidney) and is usually caused by bacterial infection. The typical clinical presentation of an upper urinary tract infection includes fever and flank (lower back) pain and, frequently, lower tract symptoms (frequency, urgency, and dysuria). Patients can also exhibit systemic signs of infection such as vomiting, diarrhea, chills, increased heart rate, and lower abdominal pain. Of significance, 40% of patients with acute pyelonephritis are bacteremic.

## Urosepsis

Approximately 25% of sepsis cases (severe blood infection) are a result of urosepsis, a systemic infection that may develop from community- or hospital-acquired urinary tract infections. Early diagnosis and treatment of urinary tract infections are essential in preventing urosepsis.

# LABORATORY DIAGNOSIS OF URINARY TRACT INFECTIONS

As previously mentioned, because noninvasive methods for collecting urine must rely on a specimen that has passed through a contaminated milieu, quantitative cultures for the diagnosis of UTI are used to discriminate between contamination, colonization, and infection. Refer to Table 5-1 for a quick reference for collecting, transporting, and processing urinary tract specimens.

## SPECIMEN COLLECTION

Prevention of contamination by normal vaginal, perineal, and anterior urethral flora is the most important consideration for collection of a clinically relevant urine specimen.

### Clean-Catch Midstream Urine

The least invasive procedure, the clean-catch midstream urine specimen collection, must be performed carefully

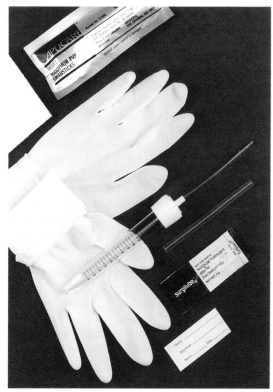

**Figure 73-2** Collection device to obtain urine by "in and out" or "straight" catheterization. (Courtesy Tristate Hospital Supply Corp., Howell, Mich.)

for optimal results, especially in females. Good patient education is essential. Guidelines for proper specimen collection should be prepared on a printed card (bilingual, if necessary), with the procedure clearly described and preferably illustrated to help ensure patient compliance. The patient should be instructed to clean the periurethral area well with a mild detergent to avoid contamination. Of importance, the patient should also be instructed to rinse well because the detergent may be bacteriostatic. Once cleansing is completed, the patient should retract the labial folds or glans penis, begin to void, and then collect a midstream urine sample. Studies showed that uncleansed, first-void specimens from males were as sensitive as (but less specific than) midstream urine specimens.

### Straight Catheterized Urine

Although slightly more invasive, urinary catheterization provides a method for the collection of uncontaminated urine from the bladder. Either a physician or another trained health professional performs this procedure. Risk exists, however, that urethral organisms will be introduced into the bladder with the catheter. An example of a collection device to obtain "straight," or "in and out," catheterized urine is shown in Figure 73-2.

### Suprapubic Bladder Aspiration

With suprapubic bladder aspiration, urine is withdrawn directly into a syringe through a percutaneously inserted needle, thereby ensuring a contamination-free specimen. The bladder must be full before performing the procedure. This collection technique may be indicated in certain clinical situations, such as pediatric practice, when urine is difficult to obtain. In brief, the full bladder is punctured using a needle and syringe and sampled following proper skin preparation (antisepsis). If good aseptic techniques are used, this procedure can be performed with little risk in premature infants, infants, small children, and pregnant women and other adults with full bladders.

### Indwelling Catheter

The number of patients in hospitals and nursing homes with long-term, indwelling urinary catheters continues to increase. These patients ultimately develop bacteriuria, which predisposes them to more severe infections.[5] Specimen collection from patients with indwelling catheters requires scrupulous aseptic technique. Health care workers who manipulate a urinary catheter in any way should wear gloves. The catheter tubing should be clamped off above the port to allow the collection of freshly voided urine. The catheter port or wall of the tubing should then be cleaned vigorously with 70% ethanol, and urine aspirated via a needle and syringe; the integrity of the closed drainage system must be maintained to prevent the introduction of organisms into the bladder. Specimens obtained from the collection bag are inappropriate, because organisms can multiply there, obscuring the true relative numbers. Cultures should be obtained when patients are ill; routine monitoring does not yield clinically relevant data.

### Specimen Transport

Because it is an excellent supportive medium for growth of most bacteria, urine must be immediately refrigerated or preserved. Bacterial counts in refrigerated (4°C) urine remain constant for as long as 24 hours. Urine transport tubes (BD Urine Culture Kit [Becton Dickinson Vacutainer Kits, Rutherford, New Jersey]) containing boric acid, glycerol, and sodium formate have been shown to preserve bacteria without refrigeration for as long as 24 hours when greater than $10^5$ CFU/mL (100,000 organisms per milliliter) were present in the initial urine specimen. The system may inhibit the growth of certain organisms, and it must be used with a minimum of 3 mL of urine. Another preservative system (Starplex Scientific, Inc., Etobicoke, Cleveland, TN) is also available. Both boric acid products preserve bacterial viability in urine for 24 hours in the absence of antibiotics. For patients from whom colony counts of organisms of less than 100,000/mL might be clinically significant, plating within 2 hours of collection is recommended. The kits provide a convenient method for preserving and transporting urine from remote areas where refrigeration is not practical.

## SCREENING PROCEDURES

As many as 60% to 80% of all urine specimens received for culture by the acute care medical center laboratory may contain no etiologic agents of infection or contain only contaminants. Procedures developed to identify quickly those urine specimens that will be negative on culture and circumvent excessive use of media, technologist time, and the overnight incubation period are discussed in this section. A reliable screening test for the presence or absence of bacteriuria provides physicians important same-day information that a conventional urine culture may take a day or longer to provide. Many screening methods have been advocated for use in detecting bacteriuria and/or pyuria. These include microscopic methods, colorimetric filtration, bioluminescence, electrical impedance, enzymatic methods, photometric detection of growth, and enzyme immunoassay. Because a discussion of all available urine-screening methods is beyond the scope of this chapter, only the more commonly used methods are highlighted.

## Gram Stain

A Gram stain of urine is an easy, inexpensive means to provide immediate information as to the nature of the infecting organism (bacteria or yeast) to guide empiric therapy. After a drop of well-mixed urine is allowed to air-dry, the smear is fixed, stained, and examined under oil immersion (1000×) for the presence of 1 or 5 bacteria per oil immersion field (OIF). The performance characteristics of the urine Gram stain are not well defined in that different criteria have been used to define a positive result (1 or 5 bacteria per OIF). Using either 1 or 5 bacteria/OIF has a sensitivity of 96% and 95%, respectively, and a specificity of 91% when correlated with significant bacteriuria ($>10^5$ CFU/mL). The Gram stain should not be relied on for detecting polymorphonuclear leukocytes in urine because leukocytes deteriorate quickly in urine that is not fresh or not adequately preserved. Many microbiologists have not adopted Gram stain examination of urine specimens because of its unreliability in detecting lower yet clinically significant numbers of organisms and because of its labor intensity. If employed, urine Gram stain should be limited to patients with acute pyelonephritis, patients with invasive UTIs, or other patients for whom immediate information is necessary for appropriate clinical management.

## Pyuria

Pyuria is the hallmark of inflammation, and the presence of polymorphonuclear neutrophils (PMNs) can be detected and enumerated in uncentrifuged specimens. This method of screening urine correlates fairly well with the number of PMNs (neutrophils) excreted per hour, the best indicator of the host's state. Patients with more than 400,000 PMNs excreted into the urine per hour are likely to be infected, and the presence of more than 8 PMNs/mm$^3$ correlates well with this excretion rate and with infection. This test can be performed using a hemocytometer, but it is not easily incorporated into the workflow of most microbiology laboratories. The standard urinalysis (usually done in hematology or chemistry sections) includes an examination of the centrifuged sediment of urine for enumeration of PMNs, results of which do not correlate well with either the PMN excretion rate or the presence of infection. Pyuria also can be associated with other clinical diseases, such as vaginitis, and therefore is not specific for UTIs.

## Indirect Indices

Frequently, screening tests detect bacteriuria or pyuria by examining for the presence of bacterial enzymes or PMN enzymes rather than the organisms or PMNs themselves.

**Nitrate Reductase (Greiss) Test.** This screening procedure looks for the presence of urinary nitrite, an indicator of UTI. Nitrate-reducing enzymes that are produced by the most common urinary tract pathogens reduce nitrate to nitrite. This test has been incorporated onto a paper strip that also tests for leukocyte esterase, an enzyme produced by PMNs (discussed next).

**Leukocyte Esterase Test.** As previously mentioned, evidence of a host response to infection is the presence of PMNs in the urine. Because inflammatory cells produce leukocyte esterase, a simple, inexpensive, and rapid method that measures this enzyme has been developed. Studies have shown that leukocyte esterase activity correlates with hemocytometer chamber counts. The nitrate reductase and leukocyte esterase tests have been incorporated into a paper strip. Numerous manufacturers sell these strips commercially, and the strips are one of the most widely used enzymatic tests. Although the sensitivity of the combination strip is higher than either test alone, the sensitivity of this combination screening is not great enough to recommend its use as a stand-alone test in most circumstances. Of note, the leukocyte esterase test is not sensitive enough for determining pyuria in patients with acute urethral syndrome.

**Catalase.** The Accutest *Uriscreen* (JANT Pharmacal Crop., Encino, Calif.) is another rapid urine-screening system based on the detection of catalase present in somatic (pertaining to the body) cells and in most bacterial species commonly causing UTIs except for streptococci and enterococci. Approximately 1.5 to 2 mL of urine is added to a tube containing dehydrated substrate. Hydrogen peroxide is added to the urine, and the solution is mixed gently. The formation of bubbles above the liquid surface is interpreted as a positive test. Some studies have reported that this system does not offer significant advantages over the leukocyte esterase-nitrite strip.

## Automated and Semiautomated Systems

Automated screening systems offer the promise of a large throughput with minimal labor and a rapid turnaround time compared with conventional cultures. However, these advantages may be offset by a substantial cost for the instrumentation. Often these costs can be justified only in laboratories that receive many specimens.

Various automated or semi-automated urine-screening systems are commercially available, such as the iRIcell Systems (IRIS International, Inc., Chatsworth, Calif.) and are capable of analyzing a urine or body fluid sample in one instrument. The instrument analyzes both the microscopic components and the urine chemistries by combining technology of both types of analyzers into one automated system. The Sysmex *UF-100* (TOA Medical

Electronics; Kobe, Japan) are able to recognize many cellular structures, including leukocytes and bacteria.

### General Comments Regarding Screening Procedures

In general, screening methods are insensitive at levels below $10^5$ CFU/mL. Therefore, they are not acceptable for urine specimens collected by suprapubic aspiration, catheterization, or cystoscopy. Screening methods may also fail to detect a significant number of infections in symptomatic patients with low colony counts ($10^2$ to $10^3$ CFU/mL) such as young, sexually active females with acute urethral syndrome. Further complicating the laboratory's decision as to whether to adopt a screening method is whether screening results will be used to rule out infection in asymptomatic patients. Under these circumstances, testing for pyuria is essential.

Therefore, given the importance of the $10^2$ CFU/mL count and the PMN count, no screening test should be used indiscriminantly. Selecting a screening method largely depends on the laboratory and the patient population being served by the laboratory. For example, there will be a cost advantage in screening urine in laboratories that receive many culture-negative specimens. On the other hand, urine from patients with symptoms of UTI plus a selected group expected to have asymptomatic bacteriuria should be cultured. For example, patients in their first trimester of pregnancy should be cultured because these women might appear asymptomatic but have a covert infection and become symptomatic later; UTIs in pregnant women may lead to pyelonephritis and the likelihood of a premature birth. Other situations in which patients with no symptoms of UTI might be cultured include the following:

- Bacteremia of unknown source
- Urinary tract obstruction
- Follow-up after removal of an indwelling catheter
- Follow-up of previous therapy

Other factors that must be considered when selecting a rapid urine screen include accuracy, ease of test performance, reproducibility, turnaround time, and whether bacteriuria or pyuria is detected.

## URINE CULTURE

### Inoculation and Incubation of Urine Cultures

Once it has been determined that a urine specimen should be cultured for isolation of the common agents of UTI, a measured amount of urine is inoculated to each of the appropriate media. The urine should be mixed thoroughly before plating. The plates can be inoculated using disposable sterile plastic tips with a displacement pipetting device calibrated to deliver a constant amount, but this method is somewhat cumbersome. Most often, microbiologists use a calibrated loop designed to deliver a known volume, either 0.01 or 0.001 mL of urine. These loops, made of platinum, plastic, or other material, can be obtained from laboratory supply companies.

The calibrated loop that delivers the larger volume of urine (0.01 mL) is recommended to detect lower numbers of organisms in certain specimens. For example, urine collected from catheterization, nephrostomies,

ileal conduits, and suprapubic aspirates should be plated with the larger calibrated loop. The communication of pertinent clinical history to the laboratory is essential so that appropriate processing can be performed.

The choice of media to inoculate depends on the patient population served and the microbiologist's preference. The use of a 5% sheep blood agar plate and a MacConkey agar plate allows detection of most gram-negative bacilli, staphylococci, streptococci, and enterococci. To save cost and somewhat streamline culture processing, many laboratories use an agar plate split in half (biplate); one side contains 5% sheep blood agar and the other half contains MacConkey agar.

In some circumstances, enterococci and other streptococci may be obscured by heavy growth of *Enterobacteriaceae*. Because of this possibility, some laboratories add a selective plate for gram-positive organisms, such as Columbia colistin-nalidixic acid agar (CNA) or phenylethyl alcohol agar. Although some discriminatory capability may be added, cost is also added to the procedure. In addition to increased cost, inclusion of plated media selective for gram-positive organisms generally provides no or limited additional information. Many European laboratories use cystine-lactose electrolyte-deficient (CLED) agar. In recent years, chromogenic media have been introduced and become commercially available from a number of manufacturers, allowing for more specific direct detection and differentiation of urinary tract pathogens on primary plates, such as BD CHROMagar (Becton Dickison, Heidelberg, Germany). This medium uses enzymatic reactions to identify *E. coli* and *Enterococcus* without additional confirmatory testing from urine specimens as well as providing presumptive identification of *S. saprophyticus*, *Streptococcus agalactiae*, *Klebsiella-Enterobacter-Serratia* and the *Proteus-Morganella-Providencia* groups.

Before inoculation, urine is mixed thoroughly and the top of the container is then removed. The calibrated loop is inserted vertically into the urine in a cup. Otherwise, more than the desired volume of urine will be taken up, potentially affecting the quantitative culture result (Figure 73-3). A widely used method is described in

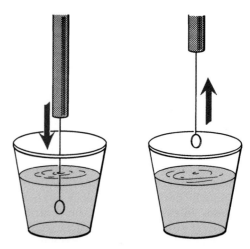

**Figure 73-3** Method for inserting a calibrated loop into urine to ensure that the proper amount of specimen adheres to the loop.

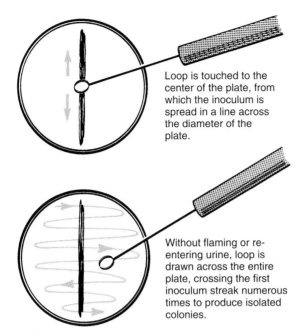

Loop is touched to the center of the plate, from which the inoculum is spread in a line across the diameter of the plate.

Without flaming or re-entering urine, loop is drawn across the entire plate, crossing the first inoculum streak numerous times to produce isolated colonies.

**Figure 73-4** Method for streaking with calibrated urine loop to produce isolated colonies and countable colony-forming units.

**TABLE 73-1** Criteria for Classification of Urinary Tract Infections by Clinical Syndrome

| Category | Clinical | Laboratory |
|---|---|---|
| Acute, uncomplicated UTI in women | Dysuria, urgency, frequency, suprapubic pain<br>No urinary symptoms in last 4 weeks before current episode<br>No fever or flank pain | ≥10 WBC/mm³<br>≥10³ CFU/mL uropathogens* in CCMS urine |
| Acute, uncomplicated pyelonephritis | Fever, chills<br>Flank pain on examination<br>Other diagnoses excluded<br>No history or clinical evidence of urologic abnormalities | ≥10 WBC/mm³<br>≥10⁴ CFU/mL uropathogens in CCMS urine |
| Complicated UTI and UTI in men | Any combination of symptoms listed above<br>One or more factors associated with complicated UTI† | ≥10 WBC/mm³<br>≥10⁵ CFU/mL uropathogens in CCMS urine |
| Asymptomatic bacteriuria | No urinary symptoms | ± >10 WBC/mm³<br>≥10⁵ CFU/mL in two CCMS cultures >24 hours apart |

*Uropathogens: Organisms that commonly cause UTIs.
†Factors associated with complicated UTI include any UTI in a male, indwelling or intermittent urinary catheter, >100 mL of postvoid residual urine, obstructive uropathy, urologic abnormalities, azotemia (excess urea in the blood, even without structural abnormalities), and renal transplantation.
*UTI,* Urinary tract infection; *WBC,* white blood cells; *CFU,* colony-forming unit; *CCMS,* clean-catch midstream urine.
From Stamm WE: Criteria for the diagnosis of urinary tract infection and for the assessment of therapeutic effectiveness, *Infection* 20 (suppl 3): S151, 1992.

Procedure 73-1, which can be found on the Evolve site. If the urine is in a small-diameter tube, the surface tension will alter the amount of specimen picked up by the loop. A quantitative pipette should be considered if the urine cannot be transferred to a larger container. Once inoculated, the plates are streaked to obtain isolated colonies (Figure 73-4).

Once plated, urine cultures are incubated overnight at 35° C. For the most part, incubation for a minimum of 24 hours is necessary to detect uropathogens. Thus, some specimens inoculated late in the day cannot be read accurately the next morning. These cultures should either be reincubated until the next day or interpreted later in the day when a full 24-hour incubation has been completed.

### Interpretation of Urine Cultures

As previously mentioned, UTIs may be completely asymptomatic, produce mild symptoms, or cause life-threatening infections. Of importance, the criteria most useful for microbiologic assessment of urine specimens is dependent not only on the type of urine submitted (e.g., voided, straight catheterization) but the clinical history of the patient (e.g., age, sex, symptoms, antibiotic therapy).

One major problem in interpreting urine cultures arises because urine cultures collected by the voided technique may be contaminated with normal flora, including *Enterobacteriaceae.* Determining what colony count represents true infection from contamination is of utmost importance and is related to the patient's clinical presentation. A number of studies have proposed the use of different cutoffs in colony counts based on clinical presentation; an example of one such set of guidelines is given in Table 73-1.

Ideally, the clinician caring for the patient should provide the laboratory with enough clinical information to allow specimens from different patient populations to be identified. These specimens could then be selectively processed using the guidelines in Table 73-1. However, because microbiology laboratories frequently receive little or no clinical information about patients, questions have been raised as to whether these cutoffs are practical and realistic for routine laboratory use. Further complicating urine culture interpretation is the increasing difficulty in distinguishing between infection and contamination as the criterion for a positive culture is lowered from 10⁵ CFU/mL to 10² CFU/mL. Because of these issues, many laboratories establish their own interpretative criteria for urine cultures based on the type of urine submitted (e.g., clean-catch midstream, catheterized, and surgically obtained specimens such as suprapubic aspirates). Variations in interpretative guidelines

**TABLE 73-2** General Interpretative Guidelines for Urine Cultures

| Result | Specific Specimen Type/Associated Clinical Condition, if Known | Workup |
|---|---|---|
| $\geq 10^4$ CFU/mL of a single potential pathogen or for each of two potential pathogens | CCMS urine/pyelonephritis, acute cystitis, asymptomatic bacteriuria, or catheterized urines | Complete* |
| $\geq 10^3$ CFU/mL of a single potential pathogen | CCMS urine/symptomatic males or catheterized urines or acute urethral syndrome | Complete |
| $\geq$Three organism types with no predominating organism | CCMS urine or catheterized urines | None; because of possible contamination, ask for another specimen |
| Either two or three organism types with predominant growth of one organism type and $<10^4$ CFU/mL of the other organism type(s) | CCMS urine | Complete workup for the predominating$^\dagger$ organism(s); description of the organism(s) |
| $\geq 10^2$ CFU/mL of any number of organism types (set up with a 0.001- and 0.01-mL calibrated loop) | Suprapubic aspirates, any other surgically obtained urines (including ileal conduits, cystoscopy specimens) | Complete |

*A complete workup includes identification of the organism and appropriate susceptibility testing.
$^\dagger$Predominant growth = $10^4$ to $\geq 10^5$ CFU/mL.
*CFU*, colony-forming unit; *CCMS*, clean-catch midstream urine.

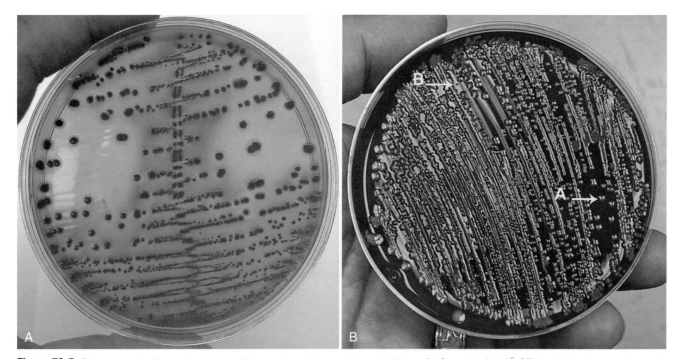

**Figure 73-5** Culture results illustrating some of the various interpretative guidelines. **A,** Growth of $\geq 10^5$ CFU/mL of a lactose-fermenting gram-negative rod in a clean-catch midstream (CCMS) urine from a patient with pyelonephritis; complete workup would be done. **B,** Growth of $\geq 10^5$ CFU/mL of a lactose-fermenting gram-negative rod (*arrow A*) and $<10^4$ CFU/mL of another organism type (*arrow B*) from a CCMS urine; only the organism with a colony count of $>10^4$ to $10^5$ CFU/mL would be worked up completely.

occur from one laboratory to another but some generalities can be made; these are listed in Table 73-2. Some examples of urine culture results are shown in Figure 73-5 to illustrate some of these interpretations. See the Evolve site for a semi-quantitative procedure for inoculation of urine cultures.

In addition to the previously described guidelines, a pure culture of *S. aureus* is considered to be significant regardless of the number of CFUs, and antimicrobial susceptibility tests are performed. The presence of yeast in any number is reported to physicians, and pure cultures of yeast may be identified to the species level. In all urine, regardless of the extent of final workup, all isolates should be enumerated (e.g., three different organisms present at $10^3$ CFU/mL), and those present in numbers greater than $10^4$ CFU/mL should be described morphologically (e.g., non-lactose-fermenting gram-negative rods).

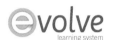 *Visit the Evolve site to complete the review questions.*

---

## CASE STUDY 73-1

A 25-year-old woman presented to her physician with severe suprapubic pain that increased during urination. Her physician diagnosed this as her fourth episode of bladder infection in the past year. He decided to order a urinalysis and a culture. The urinalysis was positive for leukocyte esterase, and the patient was treated with nitrofurantoin. The culture subsequently grew $10^3$ staphylococci/mL.

QUESTIONS

1. Is this organism significant?
2. What would you do to identify it to species?
3. Is susceptibility testing indicated for this organism?
4. Would a rapid urine screen be helpful in diagnosing the infection in this young woman?

---

## BIBLIOGRAPHY

Anderson AC, Martin SM, Hultgren SJ: Host subversion by formation of intracellular bacterial communities in the urinary tract, *Microbes Infect* 6:1094, 2004.

Bernard MS, Hunter KF, Moore KN: A review of strategies to decrease the duration of indwelling urethral catheters and potentially reduce the incidence of catheter-associated urinary tract infections, *Urol Nurs* 32(1):29-37, 2012.

Carroll KC, Hale DC, Von Boerum DH, et al: Laboratory evaluation of urinary tract infections in an ambulatory clinic, *Am J Clin Pathol* 101:100, 1994.

Churchill D, Gregson D: Screening urine samples for significant bacteriuria in the clinical microbiology laboratory, *Clin Microbiol Newsl* 26:179, 2004.

Domann E, Hong G, Imirzalioglu C, et al: Culture-independent identification of pathogenic bacteria and polymicrobial infections in the genitourinary tract of renal transplant recipients, *J Clin Microbiol* 41:5500, 2003.

Falkiner FR: The insertion and management of indwelling urethral catheters: minimizing the risk of infection, *J Hosp Infect* 25:79, 1993.

Foxman B, Brown P: Epidemiology of urinary tract infections: transmission and risk factors, incidence, and costs, *Infect Dis Clin North Am* 17:227, 2003.

Hamilton-Miller JM: The urethral syndrome and its management, *J Antimicrob Chemother* 33(suppl A):63, 1994.

Kucheria R, Dagsupta P, Sacks SH, et al: Urinary tract infections: new insights into a common problem, *Postgrad Med J* 81:83, 2004.

Kunin CM: Urinary tract infections in females, *Clin Infect Dis* 18:1, 1994.

Kunin CM, White LV, Hua TH: A reassessment of the importance of "low-count" bacteriuria in young women with acute urinary symptoms, *Ann Intern Med* 119:454, 1993.

Morgan MG, McHenzie H: Controversies in the laboratory diagnosis of community-acquired urinary tract infection, *Eur J Clin Microbiol Infect Dis* 12:491, 1993.

Murray PR, Traynor P, Hopson D: Evaluation of microbiological processing of urine specimens: comparison of overnight versus two-day incubation, *J Clin Microbiol* 30:1600, 1992.

Nicolle LE, Bradley S, Colgan R, et al: Infectious Diseases Society of America guidelines for the diagnosis and treatment of asymptomatic bacteriuria in adults, *Clin Infect Dis* 40:643, 2005.

Nosseir SB, Lind LR, Winkler HA: Recurrent uncomplicated urinary tract infections in women: a review, *J Womens Health* 21(3):347-354, 2012.

Parham NJ, Pollard SJ, Chaudhuri RR, et al: Prevalence of pathogenicity isolate II$_{CFT073}$ genes among extraintestinal clinical isolates of *Escherichia coli, J Clin Microbiol* 43:2425, 2005.

Pezzlo M: Detection of urinary tract infections by rapid methods, *Clin Microbiol Rev* 1:268, 1988.

Pezzlo M, York MK: Urine cultures. Section 3.12. In Isenberg HD, editor: *Clinical microbiology procedures handbook*, vol 1, Washington, DC, 2004, American Society for Microbiology.

Sobel JD: Pathogenesis of urinary tract infections: host defenses, *Infect Dis Clin North Am* 1:751, 1987.

Stamm WE: Criteria for the diagnosis of urinary tract infection and for the assessment of therapeutic effectiveness, *Infection* 20(suppl 3):S151, 1992.

Stamm WE: Protocol for the diagnosis of urinary tract infection: reconsidering the criterion for significant bacteriuria, *Urology* 32(suppl):6, 1988.

Stevens M: Evaluation of Questor urine screening for bacteriuria and pyuria, *J Clin Pathol* 46:817, 1993.

Wagenlehner FM, Pilatz A, Weidner W: Urosepsis—from the view of the urologist, *Int J Antimicrob Agents* S38:51-57, 2011.

Wilson ML, Gaido L: Laboratory diagnosis of urinary tract infections in adult patients, *Clin Infect Dis* 38:1150, 2004.

Wong ES: Guideline to prevention of catheter-associated urinary tract infections, *Am J Infect Control* 11:28, 1983.

# Genital Tract Infections

## OBJECTIVES

1. Describe the basic anatomy of the male and female reproductive systems.
2. Define the following conditions: vaginitis, cervicitis, proctitis, bartholinitis, pelvic inflammatory disease (PID), epididymitis, prostatitis, orchitis, neoplasia, urethritis, and dysuria.
3. List microorganisms that commonly are associated with vaginitis, cervicitis, and PID.
4. Describe the normal flora of the male and female genital tracts, and differentiate normal flora from pathogenic organisms.
5. List the media used to selectively isolate and differentiate genital tract pathogens including Modified Thayer-Martin (MTM), New York City (NYC), Colistin Nalidixic Agar (CNA), and JEMBEC System and the organisms capable of growth on each.
6. Compare and contrast the recommended use of various collection swabs for genital tract specimens including the organisms inhibited by each (cotton-tipped, with or without charcoal; calcium alginate; Dacron; rayon).
7. Determine specimen acceptability based on collection, transport, and diagnostic test orders for a genital tract specimen.
8. Explain the significance of gram-negative intracellular diplococci in genital specimens from both men and women.
9. Correlate signs and systems of infections with the results of laboratory diagnostic procedures for identification of the etiologic agent associated with infections of the genital tract.

## GENERAL CONSIDERATIONS

### ANATOMY

Familiarity with the anatomic structures is important for appropriate processing of specimens from genital tract sites and interpretation of microbiologic laboratory results. The key anatomic structures for the female and male genital tract in relation to other important structures are shown in Figure 74-1.

The female reproductive system consists of two main parts: the uterus and the ovaries. The uterus produces vaginal and uterine secretions and is the location where the human fetus grows and matures during reproduction. The ovaries connect to the uterus and the fallopian tubes. The ovary produces the female eggs that pass through the fallopian tubes and will imbed in the uterus when fertilized by the male sperm. The uterus connects to the vaginal opening through the cervix.

The male reproductive system, unlike the female, consists of a number of organs that are located external to the abdominal cavity. The main organs consist of the penis and the testis that produce the semen and sperm for fertilization of the female egg. The sperm is stored in a small gland coiled around the testis, the epididymis. The prostate gland surrounds the ejaculatory duct and produces semen, prostatic fluid, and seminal fluid.

## RESIDENT MICROBIAL FLORA

The lining of the human genital tract consists of a mucosal layer of transitional, columnar, and squamous epithelial cells. Various species of commensal bacteria colonize these surfaces, causing no harm to the host except under abnormal circumstances. The colonization of the surface by resident flora produces a biologic barrier preventing the adherence of pathogenic organisms. Normal urethral flora includes coagulase-negative staphylococci and corynebacteria, as well as various anaerobes. The vulva and penis, especially the area underneath the prepuce (foreskin) of the uncircumcised male, may harbor *Mycobacterium smegmatis* along with other gram-positive bacteria.

The flora of the female genital tract varies with the pH and estrogen concentration of the mucosa, which depends on the host's age. Prepubescent and postmenopausal women harbor primarily staphylococci and corynebacteria (the same flora present on surface epithelium), whereas women of reproductive age may harbor large numbers of facultative bacteria such as Enterobacteriaceae, streptococci, and staphylococci, as well as anaerobes such as lactobacilli, anaerobic non-spore-forming bacilli and cocci, and clostridia. Lactobacilli are the predominant organisms in secretions from normal, healthy vaginas. Recent studies have shown that hydrogen peroxide–producing lactobacilli are associated with a healthy state. The numbers of anaerobic organisms remain constant throughout the monthly cycle. Many women carry group B beta-hemolytic streptococci (*Streptococcus agalactiae*), which may be transmitted to the neonate. Although yeasts (acquired from the gastrointestinal tract) may be transiently recovered from the female vaginal tract, they are not considered normal flora.

## SEXUALLY TRANSMITTED DISEASES AND OTHER GENITAL TRACT INFECTIONS

Genital tract infections may be classified as endogenous or exogenous. Exogenous infections may be acquired as people engage in sexual activity, and these infections are referred to as sexually transmitted diseases (STDs). In contrast, endogenous infections result from normal genital flora.

In the female, genital tract infections can be divided between lower genital tract (vulva, vagina, and cervix) and upper genital tract (uterus, fallopian tubes, ovaries, and abdominal cavity) infections. Lower genital tract infections are commonly acquired by sexual or direct contact. Although the organisms that cause lower genital tract infections are not usually part of the normal genital tract flora, some organisms normally present in very low numbers can increase sufficiently to cause disease. Upper genital tract infections are frequently an extension of a

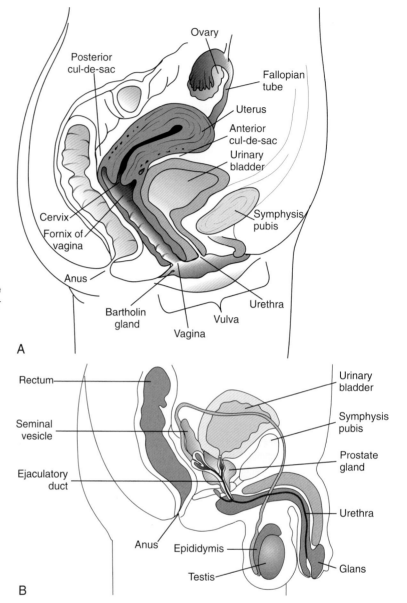

**Figure 74-1** Location of key anatomic structures of the female (**A**) and male (**B**) genital tracts in relation to other major anatomic structures.

lower tract infection in which organisms from the vagina or cervix travel into the uterine cavity and on through the endometrium to the fallopian tubes and ovaries. Similarly, an organism can spread along contiguous mucosal surfaces in the male from a lower genital tract site of infection (i.e., urethra) and cause infection in a reproductive organ such as the epididymis.

# GENITAL TRACT INFECTIONS

## SEXUALLY TRANSMITTED DISEASES AND OTHER LOWER GENITAL TRACT INFECTIONS

Lower genital tract infections may be acquired either through sexual contact with an infected partner or through nonsexual means. These infections are some of the most common infectious diseases.

### Epidemiology/Etiologic Agents

STDs are major public health problems in all populations and socioeconomic groups worldwide. An estimated 448 million new cases of curable STDs occur each year worldwide. The incidence and spread of STDs are greatly influenced by numerous factors such as the availability of multiple sexual partners, the presence of asymptomatic infection, the frequent movement of people within populations, and increasing affluence.

The number of microorganisms that can cause genital tract infections is large. These organisms are diverse, representing all four major groups of microorganisms (bacteria, viruses, fungi, and parasites). The major causes of genital tract infections are listed in Table 74-1.

### Routes of Transmission

Although genital tract infections can be caused by members of the patient's genital flora (endogenous

**TABLE 74-1** Major Causes of Genital Tract Infections and Sexually Transmitted Diseases

| Frequency | Disease | Agent | Organism Group |
|---|---|---|---|
| **More Common** | Genital and anal warts (condyloma); cervical dysplasia; cancer | Human papillomavirus | Viruses |
| | Vaginitis | *Gardnerella/Mobiluncus, Trichomonas vaginalis, Candida albicans* | Bacteria, parasites, fungi |
| | Urethritis/cervicitis (also acute salpingitis, acute perihepatitis, urethritis, pharyngitis) | *Neisseria gonorrhoeae, Chlamydia trachomatis, Ureaplasma urealyticum* | Bacteria |
| | Herpes genitalis (genital/skin ulcers) | Herpes simplex virus type 2 (less commonly type 1) | Viruses |
| | AIDS | Human immunodeficiency virus (HIV) | Viruses |
| | Hepatitis (acute and chronic infection) | Hepatitis B virus | Viruses |
| **Less Common** | Lymphogranuloma venereum | *C. trachomatis* (L-1, L-2, L-3 serovars) | Bacteria |
| | Granuloma inguinale | *Klebsiella granulomatis* (Donovania) | Bacteria |
| | Syphilis | *Treponema pallidum* | Bacteria |
| | Chancroid | *Haemophilus ducreyi* | Bacteria |
| | Scabies, mites | *Sarcoptes scabiei* | Ectoparasites |
| | Pediculosis pubis, "crabs" infestation | *Phthirus pubis* | Ectoparasites |
| | Enteritis (homosexuals/proctitis) | *Giardia lamblia, Entamoeba histolytica, Shigella* spp., *Salmonella* spp. *Enterobius vermicularis, Campylobacter* spp., *Helicobacter* spp. | Bacteria, parasites |
| | Molluscum contagiosum | Poxlike virus | Viruses |
| | Heterophile-negative mononucleosis, congenital infections | Cytomegalovirus | Viruses |

infections), the overwhelming majority of lower genital tract infections are sexually transmitted.

**Sexually Transmitted.** *Chlamydia trachomatis, Neisseria gonorrhoeae, Trichomonas vaginalis,* human immunodeficiency virus (HIV), *Treponema pallidum, Ureaplasma urealyticum, Mycoplasma hominis,* other mycoplasmas, herpes simplex virus (HSV), and others may be acquired during sexual activity. In addition, other agents that cause genital tract disease and may be sexually transmitted include adenovirus, coxsackievirus, molluscum contagiosum virus (a member of the poxvirus group), the human papillomaviruses (HPVs) of genital warts (condylomata acuminata; types 6, 11, and others), and those associated with cervical carcinoma (predominantly types 16 and 18, but numerous others are also implicated), *Klebsiella granulomatis,* and ectoparasites such as scabies and lice. Some of these agents are not routinely isolated from clinical specimens. Infections with more than one agent may occur; therefore, dual or concurrent infections should always be considered.

An individual's sexual habits and practices dictate potential sites of infection. Homosexual practices and increasingly common heterosexual practices of anal-genital or oral-genital intercourse allow for transmission of a genital tract infection to other body sites such as the pharynx or anorectic region. In addition, these practices have required that other gastrointestinal and systemic pathogens also be considered etiologic agents of STDs. The intestinal protozoa *Giardia lamblia,*

*Entamoeba histolytica,* and *Cryptosporidium* spp. are significant causes of STDs, especially among homosexual populations. In the same group of patients, fecal pathogens, such as *Salmonella, Shigella, Campylobacter,* and *Microsporidium,* are often transmitted sexually. Oral-genital practices may provide an opportunity for *N. meningitidis* to colonize and infect the genital tract. Viruses shed in secretions or present in blood (cytomegalovirus [CMV]; hepatitis B, possibly C and E; other non-A, non-B hepatitis viruses; human T-cell lymphotropic virus type I [HTLV-I]; and HIV) are spread by sexual practices.

Certain infections that are sexually transmitted occur on the surface epithelium of or near the lower genital tract. The major pathogens of these types of infections include HSV, *Haemophilus ducreyi,* and *T. pallidum.*

**Other Routes.** Organisms may also be introduced into the genital tract by instrumentation, presence of a foreign body, or irritation and can subsequently cause infection. These infections are often a result of infection with the same organisms capable of causing skin or wound infections. Infection can also be transmitted from mother to infant either in vivo (within the living body) or during delivery. For example, transplacental infection may occur with syphilis, HIV, CMV, or HSV. Infection in the newborn can also be acquired during delivery by direct contact with an infectious lesion or discharge in the mother and a susceptible mucous membrane such as the eye in the infant. STDs, such as HSV, *C. trachomatis,* and *N. gonorrhoeae,* may be transmitted from mother to newborn in this manner. Other organisms, such as group B streptococci, *Escherichia coli*, and *Listeria monocytogenes* originating from the mother may also be transmitted to the infant before, during, or after birth. (Infections in the fetus and newborn are discussed later in this chapter.)

### Clinical Manifestations

Clinical manifestations of lower genital tract infections are as varied and diverse as the etiologies.

**Asymptomatic.** Although symptoms of genital tract infections generally cause the patient to seek medical attention, a patient with an STD, especially a female, may be free of symptoms (i.e., asymptomatic). For example, gonorrhea (*Neisseria gonorrhoeae*) or chlamydia (*Chlamydia trachomatis*) infection in the male is usually obvious because of a urethral discharge, yet females with either or both of these infections may have either minimal symptoms or no symptoms at all. Also, the primary lesion of syphilis (chancre) can be unremarkable and go unnoticed by the patient. Therefore, the lack of symptoms does not guarantee the absence of disease. Unfortunately, these asymptomatic individuals can serve as reservoirs for infection and unknowingly spread the pathogen to other individuals. Asymptomatic infections in the female caused by *N. gonorrhoeae* or *C. trachomatis* that go untreated can lead to serious sequelae such as pelvic inflammatory disease or infertility.

**Dysuria.** Although a frequent presenting symptom associated with urinary tract infection, dysuria (painful urination) can commonly result from an STD caused by organisms such as *N. gonorrhoeae*, *C. trachomatis*, and HSV.

**Urethral Discharge.** The presence of an inflammatory exudate at the tip of the urethral meatus is generally observed in males; the symptoms of urethral infection in females are infrequently localized. Most males complain of discomfort at the penile tip as well as dysuria. Urethritis (swelling and irritation of the urethra) may be gonococcal, caused by *N. gonorrhoeae*, or nongonococcal. Nongonococcal urethritis can be caused by *C. trachomatis*, *Trichomonas vaginalis* (less frequently), and genital mycoplasmas such as *Mycoplasma hominis*, *Mycoplasma genitalium*, and *Ureaplasma urealyticum*.

**Lesions of the Skin and Mucous Membranes.** Numerous organisms can cause genital lesions that are diverse in both their appearance and their associated symptoms (Figure 74-2). The agents and their features of infection are summarized in Table 74-2. Some of these infections, such as genital herpes (caused by HSV) or genital warts (caused by HPVs and discussed in Chapter 66), are common, whereas others, such as lymphogranuloma venereum and granuloma inguinale, are uncommon in

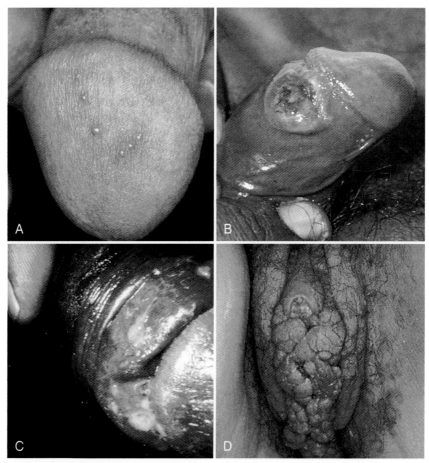

**Figure 74-2** Genital lesions of the skin and mucous membranes that are sexually transmitted. **A,** Genital herpes showing vesicular lesions. **B,** Typical chancre of primary syphilis. **C,** Early chancroid lesion of the penis. **D,** Condyloma acuminatum. (From Farrar WE, Wood MJ, Innes JA, Hubbs H: *Infectious diseases text and color atlas,* ed 2, London, 1992, Gower Medical Publishing.)

**TABLE 74-2** Summary of Common Causes of Genital Lesions of the Skin and Mucous Membranes

| Agent | Disease | Lesion | Major Associated Symptoms |
|---|---|---|---|
| Herpes simplex virus | Genital herpes | Papules, vesicles (blisters), pustules, or ulcers | Multiple lesions that are usually painful and tender, can recur (see Figure 74-2, A) |
| *Treponema pallidum* | Primary syphilis | Genital ulcer (chancre) | Usually a single lesion, painless; lesion has even edges, represents the first of three stages of syphilis (see Figure 74-2, B) |
| *Haemophilus ducreyi* | Chancroid | Papule that becomes pustular and ulcerates (chancroid); multiple ulcers may develop | Ulcer is deeply invasive, tender, painful, and purulent in appearance; edges of lesion are ragged (see Figure 74-2, C) |
| *Chlamydia trachomatis* serotype L1, L2, and L3 | Lymphogranuloma venereum | Small ulcer or vesicle that heals spontaneously without leaving a scar | After lesion heals, painful, swollen lymph nodes (lymphadenopathy) develop 2-6 weeks later; fever and chills; severe lymphatic obstruction and lymphedema can develop |
| *Klebsiella* | Granuloma inguinale | Single or multiple subcutaneous nodules | Indolent and chronic course; nodules enlarge granulomatis and erode through the skin, producing a deep red, sharply defined ulcer that is painless |
| Human papillomavirus | *Condylomata acuminate* (primary genotypes 6 and 11) | Genital warts | Warts have a cauliflower-like appearance; usually multiple lesions that can be flat or elevated; usually asymptomatic apart from physical presence (see Figure 74-2, D) |
| | *Condylomata planum* (primary genotypes 16, 18, 31, 33) | Flat, genital warts | Cervical warts that must be visualized by using a magnifying lens after the application of acetic acid (called colposcopy); infections can cause neoplasias that in some cases can progress to cervical cancer |

the United States. Specific HPV genotypes infect mucosal cells in the cervix and can cause a progressive spectrum of abnormalities classified as low-grade and high-grade squamous intraepithelial neoplasia (process of rapid cell growth that is faster than normal and continues to grow, i.e., a tumor) and in some cases, progress to invasive cervical cancer.

**Vaginitis.** Inflammation of the vaginal mucosa, called vaginitis, is a common clinical syndrome accounting for approximately 10 million office visits each year. Women who present with vaginal symptoms often complain of an abnormal discharge and additional symptoms such as an offensive odor or itching. Vulvitis, local irritation of external genitalia, may be associated with vaginitis. The three most common causes of vaginitis in premenopausal women are vaginal candidiasis, bacterial vaginosis (group B streptococci, *E. coli*, and enterococci), and trichomoniasis.

*Candida albicans* causes about 80% to 90% of cases of vaginal candidiasis; other species of *Candida* account for the remaining cases. Yeast can be carried vaginally in small numbers and produce no symptoms. Most patients experiencing candidiasis complain of perivaginal itching, often with little or no discharge. Irritating symptoms such as erythema are also associated with candidiasis. Frequently, discharge is classically thick and "cheesy" in appearance.

Vaginal infection with *T. vaginalis*, a protozoan parasite, produces a profuse, slightly offensive, yellow-green discharge; patients frequently complain of itching. About 25% of women carrying trichomonads are asymptomatic.

The World Health Organization has ranked trichomoniasis as the most prevalent, nonviral, sexually transmitted disease in the world with an estimated 172 million new cases a year.

In addition to vaginitis caused by these two organisms, there is a third type referred to as bacterial vaginosis (BV). Initially, BV was thought to be associated with *Gardnerella vaginalis* infection, but *G. vaginalis* was isolated from 40% of women without vaginitis. Bacterial vaginosis is polymicrobial in etiology, involving *G. vaginalis* and other facultative and anaerobic organisms. A study using three different molecular methods, including broad-range polymerase chain reaction (PCR) amplification of the 16S rDNA gene, confirms the bacterial diversity of organisms involved in this infection; 35 unique bacterial species were detected including many newly recognized species in women with BV. This study also confirmed the loss of vaginal lactobacilli and concomitant overgrowth of anaerobic and facultative bacteria. The exact mechanism for the onset of BV is unknown, although it appears to be associated with a reduction in lactobacilli and hydrogen peroxide production, a rise in the vaginal pH, and the overgrowth of BV-associated organisms. Synergistic activity of various anaerobic organisms, including *Prevotella* spp., *Porphyromonas* spp., *Bacteroides* spp., *Peptostreptococcus* spp., *Mobiluncus* spp. (curved, motile rods), and *Mycoplasma* spp., as well as *G. vaginalis*, seems to contribute to the pathology of BV. BV is characterized by perivaginal irritation that is considerably milder than trichomoniasis or candidiasis and is usually associated with a foul-smelling discharge often described as having

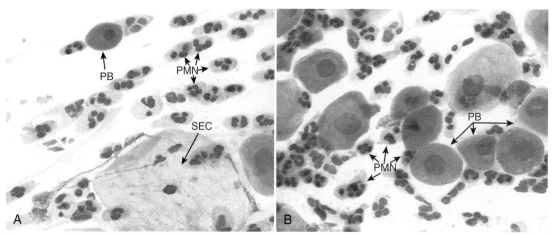

**Figure 74-3** Gram stain of vaginal secretions from a patient with desquamate inflammatory vaginitis. **A,** Numerous polymorphonuclear cells *(PMNs),* a squamous epithelial cell *(SEC),* a parabasal cell *(PB),* and the absence of lactobacilli are observed. **B,** Numerous PMNs, several PBs, and the absence of lactobacilli are observed.

a "fishy" odor. This odor is a result of products of bacterial metabolism (polyamines) being volatilized by vaginal fluids. Some patients also complain of abdominal discomfort. It appears that BV and trichomoniasis frequently coexist. Because BV can recur in the absence of sexual reexposure and other settings (e.g., nonsexually active women, virgins), BV is not exclusively sexually transmitted. BV also increases a woman's risk of acquiring HIV, is associated with increased complications in pregnancy, and may be involved in the pathogenesis of pelvic inflammatory disease.

Although uncommon, there are other infectious causes of vaginitis. Three are briefly mentioned here because Gram stain of vaginal secretions may be helpful. First, Sobel described a number of premenopausal patients with a diffuse, exudative vaginitis with massive vaginal cell exfoliation, purulent vaginal discharge, and an occasional vaginal and cervical spotted rash. Laboratory findings included elevated pH of vaginal secretions. Also, numerous polymorphonuclear cells, an increased number of parabasal cells, the absence of gram-positive bacilli, and their replacement by occasional gram-positive cocci are observed on direct Gram stain (Figure 74-3). Basal cells appear as a result of the extensive exfoliation of epithelial cells. This clinical syndrome is referred to as desquamate inflammatory vaginitis. Symptoms associated with another disorder, lactobacillosis, resemble those of candidiasis and often follows antifungal therapy. Gram stain or wet mount typically reveals a large number of very long lactobacilli. These predominately anaerobic lactobacilli are 40 to 75 µ in length and are significantly longer than the average normal flora lactobacillus (5 to 15 µ). Finally, preexisting lesions due to other diseases may become secondarily infected with a mixed anaerobic flora of fusobacteria and spirochetes. This is referred to as fusiform-spirochete disease; this infection can progress rapidly. Gram stain examination reveals inflammatory cells in conjunction with gram-negative, fusiform bacterial morphotypes and spirochetes.

**Cervicitis.** Polymorphonuclear neutrophils (PMNs) are normally present in the endocervix; however, an abnormally increased number of PMNs may be associated with cervicitis (inflammation of the cervix). Therefore, a purulent discharge from the endocervix can be observed in some cases of cervicitis. The endocervix is the site from which *N. gonorrhoeae* is most frequently isolated in women with gonococcal infections. In patients presenting with cervicitis, *C. trachomatis* can also be isolated; chlamydia have not been associated with vaginitis. Frequently, patients are infected with both pathogens. Because most women with cervicitis caused by gonococci or chlamydia are asymptomatic and cervical abnormalities are either subtle or absent in these women, an appropriate laboratory diagnosis to detect these organisms must be performed.

HSV and human papillomavirus (HPV) can also infect the cervix. In women with herpes cervicitis, the cervix is friable (bleeds easily) and may have ulcers. Affected patients may also have lower abdominal pain.

**Anorectal Lesions.** As previously mentioned, because of the homosexual practice and increasingly common heterosexual practice of anal-genital intercourse, sites of infection in addition to those in the genital tract must be considered. The anorectum and pharynx are commonly infected with the classic STDs, including anal warts caused by HPV, as well as other viruses and parasites. Patients with symptoms of proctitis (inflammation of the rectum) caused by *N. gonorrhoeae* or *C. trachomatis* complain of itching, mucopurulent anal discharge, anal pain, bleeding, and tenesmus (painful straining during a bowel movement). Anorectal infection caused by HSV is associated with severe anal pain, rectal discharge, tenesmus, and systemic signs and symptoms such as fever, chills, and headaches.

In HIV-infected individuals and other immunocompromised patients, these infections tend to last longer, be more severe, and are more difficult to treat compared with infection in immunocompetent individuals. Anorectal lesions are common in HIV-infected patients and include anal condylomata, anal abscesses, and ulcers. Anal abscesses and ulcers can be due to various organisms, including CMV, *Mycobacterium avium* complex, HSV, *Campylobacter* spp., and Shigella, as well as traditional etiologic agents of STDs.

**Bartholinitis.** In adult women, the Bartholin's gland is a 1-cm mucus-producing gland on each side of the vaginal orifice. Each gland has a 2-cm duct that opens on the inner surface of the labia minora. If infected, this duct can become blocked and result in a Bartholin's gland abscess. Although *N. gonorrhoeae* and *C. trachomatis* can cause infection, anaerobic and polymicrobic infections originating from normal genital flora are more common.

## Infections of the Reproductive Organs and Other Upper Tract Infections

Besides the lower genital tract, infections can occur in the reproductive organs of both males and females.

**Females.** Infection of the female reproductive organs (i.e., uterus, fallopian tubes, ovaries, and even the abdominal cavity) can occur. The organisms spread as they ascend from lower-tract sites of infection. Organisms may also be introduced to the reproductive organs by surgery, instrumentation, or during childbirth.

***Pelvic Inflammatory Disease.*** Pelvic inflammatory disease (PID) is an infection that results when cervical microorganisms travel upward to the endometrium (inner membrane of the uterus), fallopian tubes, and other pelvic structures. This infection can produce one or more of the following inflammatory conditions: endometritis, salpingitis (inflammation of the fallopian tubes), localized or generalized peritonitis, or abscesses involving the fallopian tubes or ovaries. Patients with PID often have intermittent abdominal pain and tenderness, vaginal discharge, dysuria, and possibly systemic symptoms such as fever, weight loss, and headache. Serious complications, such as permanent scarring of the fallopian tubes and infertility, can arise if PID is untreated.

Infection with *N. gonorrhoeae* or *C. trachomatis* in the lower genital tract can lead to PID if a woman is not adequately treated. Other organisms, such as anaerobes, gram-negative rods, streptococci, and mycoplasmas, may ascend through the cervix, particularly after parturition (childbirth), dilation of the cervix, or abortion. The presence of an intrauterine device (IUD) is associated with a slightly higher rate of PID. Such infections caused by *Actinomyces* have been associated with the use of IUDs.

***Infections after Gynecologic Surgery.*** Following gynecologic surgery, such as a vaginal hysterectomy, women frequently develop postoperative infections including pelvic cellulitis or abscesses. The major pathogens include the normal flora organisms: aerobic gram-positive cocci, gram-negative bacilli, anaerobes such as *Peptostreptococcus* spp., and genital mycoplasmas.

***Infections Associated with Pregnancy.*** Infections can also occur in women during pregnancy (prenatal) or following the birth (postpartum) of a child. These infections may, in turn, be transmitted to the infant and are not only capable of compromising the mother's health but also the health of the developing fetus or neonate.

While developing within the uterus, the fetus is protected from most environmental factors, including infectious agents. The human immune system does not become fully competent until several months following birth. Immunoglobulins that cross the placental barrier, primarily immunoglobulin G (IgG), protect the newborn

**TABLE 74-3** Common Etiologic Agents of Prenatal and Neonatal Infections

| Time of Infection* | Route of Infection | Common Agents |
|---|---|---|
| **Prenatal** | Transplacental | Bacteria: *Listeria monocytogenes, Treponema pallidum, Borrelia burgdorferi* Viruses: Cytomegalovirus (CMV), rubella, HIV, parvovirus B19, enteroviruses Parasites: *Toxoplasma gondii, Plasmodium* spp. |
| | Ascending | Bacteria: Group B streptococci, *Escherichia coli, L. monocytogenes, Chlamydia trachomatis*, genital mycoplasmas Viruses: CMV, herpes simplex virus (HSV) |
| **Natal** | Passing through the birth canal | Bacteria: Group B streptococci, *E. coli, L. monocytogenes, N. gonorrhoeae, C. trachomatis* Viruses: CMV, HSV, enteroviruses, hepatitis B virus, HIV |
| **Postnatal** | All of the above routes, from the nursery environment, or from maternal contact (e.g., breastfeeding) | All agents listed above and various organisms from the nursery environment, including gram-negative bacteria and viruses such as respiratory syncytial virus |

*Some newborns develop infections during the first 4 weeks of postnatal life. Infections may be delayed manifestations of earlier prenatal (before birth), natal, or postnatal (after birth) acquisition of pathogens.

from many infections until the infant begins to produce immunoglobulins of his or her own in response to antigenic stimuli. This unique environmental niche, however, does expose the vulnerable fetus to pathogens present in the mother.

Prenatal infections (those that occur any time before birth) may be acquired hematogenously (circulation) or ascending genital tract routes from mother to infant. If the mother has a bloodstream infection, organisms can reach and cross the placenta, with possible spread of infection to the developing fetus. Organisms that can cross the placenta are listed in Table 74-3. Alternatively, organisms can also infect the fetus by the ascending route from the vagina through torn or ruptured fetal membranes. Chorioamnionitis is an infection of the uterus and its contents during pregnancy. This infection is commonly acquired when organisms spread from the vagina or cervix after premature or prolonged rupture of the membranes or during labor. Organisms that are commonly isolated from amniotic fluid are listed in Box 74-1. Other maternal infections associated with adverse pregnancy outcomes that are not generally sexually transmitted include parvovirus B19, rubella, and *Listeria monocytogenes*.

---

---

**Males.** Infections in male reproductive organs can also occur and include epididymitis, prostatitis, and orchitis (testicular swelling). Epididymitis, an inflammation of the epididymis, is commonly seen in sexually active men. Patients complain of fever and pain and swelling of the testicle. *N. gonorrhoeae* and *C. trachomatis* are common causes of epididymitis. However, enterics and coagulase-negative staphylococci can also cause infection in men older than 35 years of age and in homosexual men; these infections are often associated with obstruction by the prostate gland.

Prostatitis is a term to clinically describe adult male patients who have perineal, lower back, or lower abdominal pain, urinary discomfort, or ejaculatory complaints. Prostatitis is caused by both infectious and noninfectious means. Bacteria can cause an acute or chronic prostatitis. Patients with acute bacterial prostatitis have dysuria and urinary frequency, symptoms typically associated with lower urinary tract infection. Frequently, these patients have systemic signs of illness such as fever. Chronic bacterial prostatitis is an important cause of persistent bacteriuria in the male that leads to recurrent bacterial urinary tract infections. The common causes of these infections are similar to the bacterial causes of lower urinary tract infections such as *Escherichia coli* and other enterics.

Finally, inflammation of the testicles, orchitis, is uncommon and generally acquired by the blood-borne dissemination of viruses. Mumps is associated with most cases. Patients exhibit testicular pain and swelling following infection. Infections range from mild to severe.

**Gonorrhea.** Gonorrhea is a common sexually transmitted infection caused by the bacterium *Neisseria gonorrhoeae*. The infection may be spread by direct contact with secretions within the mouth, vagina, penis, or perianal region. The organism reproduces in warm moist areas of the body including the urethra of men and women, fallopian tubes, uterus, and cervix.

Symptoms occur 2 to 5 days following infection in women. Men may not display symptoms for up to one month following infection. Symptoms in women include a vaginal discharge, pain and frequency on urination, sore throat, abdominal pain, fever, and painful sexual intercourse. Males experience pain and frequency during urination, a penile discharge, red or swollen urethra, and tenderness in the testes.

Gonorrhea can be directly diagnosed by gram-staining a sample of urethral discharge, cervical specimens, or joint fluids. *Neisseria gonorrhoeae* is a gram-negative diplococcus with a characteristic kidney bean shape on Gram stain. The detection of intracellular diplococci in male secretions is diagnostic for *N. gonorrhoeae*. Extracellular diplococci in women is an indication of normal genital flora; however, intracellular diplococci indicates the presence of pathogenic organisms. Definitive

diagnosis in females must include confirmation by culture. Infection with *N. gonorrhoeae* can lead to increased complications including pelvic inflammatory disease and gonorrheal ophthalmia neonatorum (eye infections) in newborns.

**Syphilis.** Syphilis is a sexually transmitted disease that is caused by the bacterium *Treponema pallidum*. The organism is transmitted from person to person through direct contact with infected lesions on the external genital area, vagina, anus or rectum. Syphilis may also be transmitted from mother to baby during pregnancy.

Many individuals can be infected and remain asymptomatic for years, making the control of this disease difficult. The disease is characterized by three stages: primary, secondary, and tertiary (also referred to as late or latent syphilis). Direct diagnosis may be accomplished by dark-field microscopy of material from an infectious lesion. However, serology provides a more accurate and reliable method for diagnosis. See Chapter 46 for a more detailed description of the disease and laboratory diagnosis.

---

# LABORATORY DIAGNOSIS OF GENITAL TRACT INFECTIONS

## LOWER GENITAL TRACT INFECTIONS

### Urethritis, Cervicitis, and Vaginitis

**Specimen Collection.** This discussion focuses on those specimens submitted for culture or direct examination. Procedures for the collection and transport of specimens for detection of agents by other noncultural methods (e.g., detection of *Chlamydia trachomatis* by amplification) should be followed according to the respective manufacturer's instructions. Refer to Table 5-1 for a review of collection, transport, and processing of genital tract specimens.

**Urethral.** Urethral discharge may occur in both males and females infected with pathogens such as *Neisseria gonorrhoeae* and *Trichomonas vaginalis*. The presence of infection is more likely to be asymptomatic in females because the discharge is usually less profuse and may be masked by normal vaginal secretions. *Ureaplasma urealyticum* can also be isolated from male urethral discharge.

A urogenital swab designed expressly for collection of such specimens should be used. These swabs are made of cotton or rayon treated with charcoal to adsorb material toxic to gonococci and wrapped tightly over one end of a thin wire shaft. Cotton- or rayon-tipped swabs on a thin wire may also be used to collect specimens for isolation of mycoplasmas and chlamydiae. Calcium alginate swabs are generally more toxic for HSV, gonococci, chlamydiae, and mycoplasmas than are treated cotton swabs. Because Dacron swabs are least toxic, they are recommended for viral specimens. Dacron-tipped swabs on plastic shafts are also acceptable for chlamydiae and genital mycoplasmas.

To obtain a urethral specimen, a swab is inserted approximately 2 cm into the urethra and rotated gently before withdrawing. Because chlamydiae are intracellular pathogens, it is important to remove epithelial cells (with the swab) from the urethral mucosa. Separate swabs for cultivation of gonococci, chlamydiae, and ureaplasma are required. When profuse urethral discharge is present, particularly in males, the discharge may be collected externally without inserting a sampling device into the urethra. However, a urethral swab for chlamydiae must be collected on males. A few drops of first-voided urine have also been used successfully to detect gonococci in males.

Because *T. vaginalis* may be present in urethral discharge, material for culture should be collected by swab as described and another specimen collected on a swab and placed into a tube containing 0.5 mL of sterile physiologic saline. This specimen should be delivered to the laboratory immediately. Direct wet mounts and cultures for *T. vaginalis* can be performed from this second specimen. Commercial media for culture of *Trichomonas* are available. The first few drops of voided urine is a suitable specimen for recovery of *Trichomonas* from infected males, if it is inoculated into culture media immediately. Alternatively, material may be smeared onto a slide for a fluorescent antibody stain. Plastic envelopes for direct examination and subsequent culture are also available (InPouch TV, BIOMED, White City, Oregon); sensitivity of this system is superior to other available methods, and organism viability is maintained up to 48 hours (Figure 74-4). In addition, several other techniques are available, including enzyme immunoassay, latex agglutination tests, and the Affirm VPIII probe (Becton Dickinson, Cockeysville, Maryland); polymerase chain reaction (PCR) has also been used to detect *T. vaginalis* directly in clinical specimens.

*N. gonorrhoeae* may be detected from clinical specimens using nucleic acid-based methods, including PACE 2 and APTIMA GC (Hologic/GenProbe, San Diego, CA) using a DNA probe that hybridizes to organismal rRNA. Additional nucleic acid-based tests include Roche AMPLICOR (Roche Diagnostics, Indianapolis, IN) and the BD ProbeTecET (BD Diagnostics, Sparks, MD). Fully automated systems for complete sample processing are now available that reduce technical time, such as the BD Viper System (BD Diagnostics, Sparks, MD) and the PANTHER System (Hologic/GenProbe, San Diego, CA). These tests are widely used for quick detection of *N. gonorrhoeae* from vaginal, urethral, thin-prep, and urine specimens.

***Cervical/Vaginal.*** Organisms that cause purulent vaginal discharge (vaginitis) include *T. vaginalis*, gonococci, and, rarely, beta-hemolytic streptococci. The same organisms that cause purulent infections in the urethra may also infect the epithelial cells in the cervical opening (os), as can HSV. Mucus is removed by gently rubbing the area with a cotton ball. The urethral swab is inserted into the cervical canal and rotated and moved from side to side for 30 seconds before removal.

Swabs are handled as previously described for urethral swabs for isolation of *Trichomonas* and gonococci. Chlamydiae cause a mucopurulent cervicitis with discharge. Endocervical specimens are obtained after the cervix has been exposed with a speculum, which allows visualization of vaginal and cervical architecture, and after ectocervical mucus has been adequately removed. The speculum

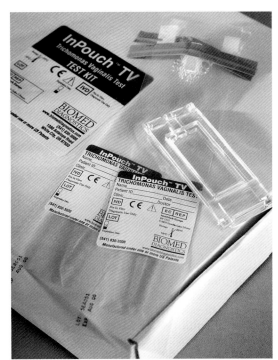

**Figure 74-4** InPouch TV diagnostic system for wet mount examination and culture of *Trichomonas vaginalis*. The swab collected from the patient is inserted into liquid medium in the upper chamber of the plastic pouch and swirled. The top of the pouch is folded over and then sealed with the tabs. Once received in the laboratory, the upper chamber is examined for motile organisms; if no motile organisms are observed by microscopy, the upper chamber material is inoculated into the lower chamber and then incubated for up to 5 days. The lower chamber is similarly examined daily by microscopy for the presence of motile *T. vaginalis*. (Courtesy BioMed Diagnostics, White City, Ore.)

is moistened with warm water, because many lubricants contain antibacterial agents. Because normal vaginal secretions contain great quantities of bacteria, care must be taken to avoid or minimize contaminating swabs for culture by contact with these secretions. A small, nylon-bristled cytology brush, or Cytobrush, may be used to ensure that cellular material is collected. Collection may result in patient discomfort and bleeding.

In addition to cervical specimens, which are particularly useful for isolating herpes, gonococci, mycoplasmas, and chlamydiae, vaginal discharge specimens may be collected. Organisms likely to cause vaginal discharge include *Trichomonas*, yeast, and the agents of BV. Swabs for diagnosis of BV are dipped into the fluid that collects in the posterior fornix of the vagina.

Genital tract infections caused by sexually transmitted agents in children (preadolescents) are most often the result of sexual abuse. Because of medico-legal implications, the laboratory should treat specimens from such patients with extreme care, carefully identifying and documenting all isolates. Although nucleic acid-based testing methods are available for the identification of organisms associated with sexual abuse cases, culture remains the preferred method of detection for *C. trachomatis and N. gonorrhoeae*. In addition, cultivation of the isolate may be

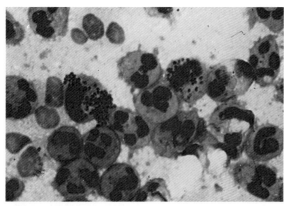

**Figure 74-5** Gram-negative intracellular diplococci, which are diagnostic for gonorrhea in urethral discharge and presumptive for gonorrhea in vaginal discharge.

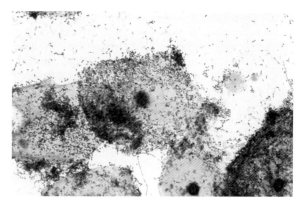

**Figure 74-6** Clue cells in vaginal discharge suggestive of bacterial vaginosis.

required to link the specific isolate to the perpetrator using epidemiologic studies.

Because it is impossible to exclude contamination with vaginal flora, obtaining swabs of Bartholin gland exudate is not recommended. Infected Bartholin glands should be aspirated with needle and syringe after careful skin preparation, and cultures should be evaluated for anaerobes and aerobes.

***Transport.*** Swabs collected for isolation of gonococci may be transported to the laboratory in modified Stuart's or Amies' charcoal transport media and held at room temperature until inoculated to culture media. Good recovery of gonococci is possible if swabs are cultured within 12 hours of collection. Material that must be held longer than 12 hours should be inoculated directly to one of the commercial systems designed for recovery of gonococci, described later in this chapter.

Swabs for isolation of chlamydiae and mycoplasmas are transported in specific transport media containing antibiotics and other essential components. Specimens for chlamydia culture should be transported on ice. (Specimens transported at room temperature should be inoculated within 15 minutes of collection.) Specimens can be stored at 4° C for up to 24 hours. If culture inoculation will be delayed more than 24 hours, specimens should be quick-frozen in a dry ice and 95% ethanol bath and stored at −70° C until cultured. If collected and transported in specific transport media, specimens for genital mycoplasma culture may be transported on ice or at room temperature. If not in genital mycoplasma transport media, specimens should be transported on ice to suppress the growth of contaminating flora.

**Direct Microscopic Examination.** In addition to culture, urethral discharge may be examined by Gram stain for the presence of gram-negative intracellular diplococci (Figure 74-5), usually indicative of gonorrhea in males. After inoculation to culture media, the swab is rolled over the surface of a glass slide, covering an area of at least 1 cm². If the Gram stain is characteristic, cultures of urethral discharge need not be performed. Urethral smears from females may also be examined. If extracellular organisms resembling *N. gonorrhoeae* are seen, the microbiologist should continue to examine the smear for intracellular diplococci. Presumptive diagnosis can be

useful when decisions are to be made regarding immediate therapy, but confirmatory cultures or an alternative nonculture method should always be performed on specimens from females. Some strains of *N. gonorrhoeae* are sensitive to the amount of vancomycin present in selective media. If suspicious organisms seen on smear fail to grow in culture, re-culture on chocolate agar without antibiotics may be warranted.

Fluorescein-conjugated monoclonal antibody reagents are sensitive and specific for visualization of the inclusions of *Chlamydia trachomatis* in cell cultures or elementary bodies in urethral and cervical specimens containing cells. Reagents for direct staining of specimens are available commercially in complete collection and test systems, but the increased technologist time required limits the usefulness of this method for laboratories that receive many specimens, except as a confirmatory test for other antigen detection systems with borderline results. In some studies, the sensitivity of visual detection of chlamydia with these reagents has been similar to that of culture. False-positive results should not occur if at least 10 morphologically compatible fluorescing elementary bodies are seen on the smear. No direct visual methods exist for detection of mycoplasmas, but molecular assays have been evaluated.

Direct microscopic examination of a wet preparation of vaginal discharge provides the simplest rapid diagnostic test for *Trichomonas vaginalis* and can be examined immediately. The plastic envelope method combines direct visualization with culture. Motile trophozoites of *Trichomonas* can be visualized in a routine wet preparation in two thirds of cases or a direct fluorescent antibody (DFA) stain, Merifluor (chlamydia) (Meridian Diagnostics, Cincinnati, Ohio) may be used.

Budding cells and pseudohyphae of yeast can also be easily identified in wet preparations by adding 10% potassium hydroxide (KOH) to a separate preparation, thereby dissolving host cell protein and enhancing the visibility of fungal elements.

BV, characterized by a foul-smelling discharge, can be diagnosed microscopically or clinically. The discharge is primarily sloughed epithelial cells, many of which are completely covered by tiny, gram-variable rods, and coccobacilli. These cells are called clue cells (Figure 74-6). The absence of inflammatory cells in the vaginal discharge is another sign of BV. Although *Gardnerella*

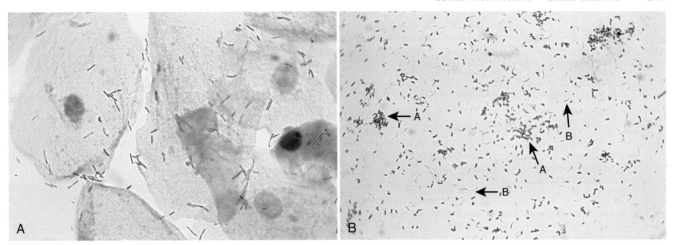

**Figure 74-7 A,** Predominance of lactobacilli in Gram stain from healthy vagina. **B,** Absence of lactobacilli and presence of *Gardnerella vaginalis* (*A arrows*) and *Mobiluncus* spp. (*B arrows*) morphologies.

*vaginalis* has been historically associated with the syndrome and can be cultured on a human blood bilayer plate, culture is not recommended for diagnosis of BV. A clinical diagnosis of BV is dependent on the presence of three or more of the following criteria: homogeneous, gray discharge; clue cells seen on wet mount or Gram stain; a pH greater than 4.5; and an amine or fishy odor elicited by the addition of a drop of 10% KOH to the discharge on a slide or on the speculum.

Bacterial vaginosis may be differentiated from other vaginal infection by Gram stain (Figure 74-7). Nugent and colleagues have developed a grading system for Gram stains of vaginal discharge (see Procedure 74-1 on the Evolve site). This system is based on the presence or absence of certain bacterial morphologies. Typically, in patients with BV, lactobacilli are either absent or few in number, whereas curved, gram-variable rods (*Mobiluncus* spp.) or *G. vaginalis* and *Bacteroides* morphotypes predominate. The Gram stain is more sensitive and specific than either the wet mount for detection of clue cells or culture for *G. vaginalis,* and the smear can be saved and reexamined later.

**Culture.** Samples for isolation of gonococci may be inoculated directly to culture media, obviating the need for transport medium. Commercially produced systems have been developed for this purpose, and many clinicians inoculate standard plates directly if convenient access to an incubator is available. Modified Thayer-Martin medium is most often used, although New York City (NYC) medium has the added advantage of supporting the growth of mycoplasmas and gonococci. Excellent recovery of gonococci results from direct inoculation to any of these media in self-contained incubation systems such as JEMBEC plates (Figure 74-8). The specimen swab is rolled across the agar with constant turning to expose all surfaces to the medium. The JEMBEC plate, which generates its own increased carbon dioxide atmosphere by means of a sodium bicarbonate tablet, is inoculated in a W pattern. The plate may be cross-streaked with a sterile loop in the laboratory (Figure 74-9).

Specimens must be inoculated to additional media for isolation of yeast, streptococci, and mycoplasmas. Yeast grows well on Columbia agar base with 5% sheep blood and colistin and nalidixic acid (CNA), although more

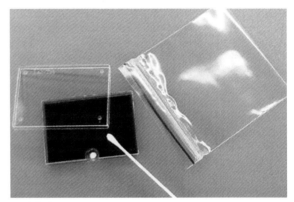

**Figure 74-8** JEMBEC plate containing modified Thayer-Martin medium in a plastic, snap-top box with a self-contained $CO_2$-generating tablet, all sealed inside a Zip-Lok plastic envelope after inoculation.

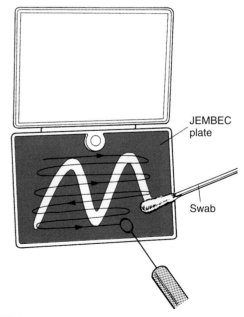

**Figure 74-9** Method of cross-streaking JEMBEC plate after original specimen has been inoculated by rolling the swab over the surface of the agar in a W pattern.

selective media are available. Most yeast and streptococci also grow on standard blood agar; thus, adding special fungal media such as Sabouraud brain-heart infusion agar (SABHI) is unwarranted.

A specimen from the lower vagina followed by the rectum using the same swab at 35 to 37 weeks' gestation reliably predicts the presence of group B streptococci at delivery. The swab should be transported to the laboratory in a nonnutritive transport medium such as Amies' or Stuart's without charcoal and then inoculated into a recommended selective broth medium such as Todd-Hewitt broth supplemented either with gentamicin and nalidixic acid or with colistin and nalidixic acid. Selective enrichment broths are subcultured to agar the next day to isolate and identify group B streptococci. In addition, the presence of group B streptococci in urine in any concentration from a pregnant woman is a marker for heavy genital tract colonization. Any quantity of group B streptococci in urine from pregnant women should be worked up in the laboratory (see Chapter 73).

*T. vaginalis* may be cultured in Diamond's medium (available commercially) or plastic envelopes inoculated with discharge material. Culture techniques are most sensitive. A commercially available biphasic genital mycoplasma culture system (Mycotrim-GU, Irvine Scientific, Santa Ana, California) can be used to culture *Mycoplasma hominis* and *Ureaplasma urealyticum,* although commercially prepared media are not as sensitive as fresh media. *Mycoplasma genitalium* may not grow on commercial media because of the presence of thallium acetate.

**Nonculture Methods.** Various nonculture methods may be used to diagnose genital tract diseases, including serology, latex agglutination, nucleic acid hybridization and amplification assays, and enzyme immunoassays. Most assays detect a single or possibly two genital tract pathogens, and most are commercially available. These methods are described in more detail in chapters relating to individual pathogens.

As previously discussed, BV involves several organisms. Besides the Gram stain, BV can be diagnosed by using the Amsel criteria, which include pH measurement, performance of an amine test, and wet mount microscopy

of vaginal secretions. However, this approach has been considered unreliable because of the lack of microscopy-related skills and availability of pH paper in most doctors' offices. Although the Gram stain offers high sensitivity and specificity, it is not immediately available. Currently, commercial laboratory tests are available to aid in the diagnosis of BV, but not all are available in the United States; a test for sialidase (OSOM BVBLUE, Sekisui Diagnostics, Farmingham, Massachusetts) in conjunction with measuring pH has been reported to be a rapid, highly sensitive, and specific means to diagnose BV. (Sialidases are secreted from anaerobic gram-negative rods such as *Bacteroides* and *Prevotella* as well as *Gardnerella* and play a role in bacterial nutrition, cellular interactions, and immune response evasion, which in turn improves the ability of bacteria to adhere, invade, and destroy mucosal tissue.) A hybridization assay (Affirm VP III Microbial Identification Test; Becton Dickinson Microbiology Systems, Sparks, Maryland) is commercially available to diagnose BV, as well as genital tract infections caused by *Candida* spp. and *Trichomonas vaginalis.* Once the appropriate reagents and specimen are added to special trays, the entire hybridization assays are then performed by instrumentation (Figure 74-10). Evaluations indicate this system is sensitive and specific.

### Genital Skin and Mucous Membrane Lesions

External genital lesions are usually either vesicular or ulcerative. Causes of lesions can be determined by physical examination, histologic/cytologic examination, or microscopic examination or culture of exudate.

Vesicles in the genital area are almost always attributable to viruses, and herpes simplex is the most common cause. Epithelial cells from the base of a vesicle may be spread onto the surface of a slide and examined for the typical multinucleated giant cells of HSV or stained by immunofluorescent antibody stains for viral antigens. Additionally or alternatively, the material may be transported for culture of the virus, as outlined in Procedure 74-2, which can be found on the Evolve site.

Several commercial fluorescein-conjugated monoclonal and polyclonal antibodies directed against herpetic

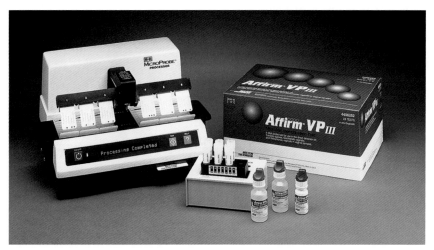

**Figure 74-10** Affirm VP III Microbial Identification Test used to differentiate the three major causes of vaginitis/bacterial vaginosis from a single sample within 1 hour. (Courtesy Becton Dickinson Microbiology Systems. Affirm is a trademark of Becton Dickinson and Company.)

antigens of either type 1 or 2 are available. When fluorescent antibody–stained lesion material containing enough cells is viewed under ultraviolet light, the diagnosis can be made in 70% to 90% of patients. Laboratories that routinely process genital material for herpes should be using immunofluorescent staining reagents when a rapid answer is desired; otherwise, culture, which is generally positive in 2 days, is the method of choice. Nonfluorescent markers, such as biotin-avidin-horseradish peroxidase or alkaline phosphatase, have also been conjugated to these specific antibodies, often allowing earlier detection of herpes-infected cells in tissue culture monolayers. Such reagents have been developed for use directly on clinical material, although their sensitivity is not great enough to forego culture if a definitive diagnosis is necessary.

Material from lesions suggestive of syphilis should be examined by dark-field or fluorescent microscopy. These procedures are described in Chapter 46.

All lesions suspected of infectious etiology may be Gram stained in addition to the procedures described. The smear of lesion material from a patient with chancroid may show many small, pleomorphic, gram-negative rods and coccobacilli arranged in chains and groups, characteristic of *H. ducreyi*. However, culture has been shown to be more sensitive for diagnosis of this agent. Material collected on cotton or Dacron swabs may be transported in modified Stuart's medium. Specimens should be inoculated to culture media within 1 hour of collection. A special agar, consisting of chocolate agar enriched with 1% IsoVitaleX (BBL Microbiology Systems) and vancomycin (3 mg/mL), has yielded good isolation if cultures are incubated in 5% to 7% carbon dioxide in a moist atmosphere, such as a candle jar. *H. ducreyi* grows best at 33° C.

Granuloma inguinale (*Klebsiella granulomatis*) is diagnosed by staining a crushed preparation of a small piece of biopsy tissue obtained from the edge of the base of the ulcer with Wright's or Giemsa stain and finding characteristic Donovan bodies (bipolar staining rods within macrophages). No acceptable media for isolation of *K. granulomatis* are available.

### Bubo

Buboes, swollen lymph glands in the inguinal (pelvic) region, are often evidence of a genital tract infection. Buboes are common in patients with primary syphilis, genital herpes, lymphogranuloma venereum, and chancroid. Patients with AIDS may show generalized lymphadenopathy. Other diseases that are not sexually transmitted, such as plague, tularemia, and lymphoma, can also produce buboes. Material from buboes may be aspirated for microscopic examination and culture.

## INFECTIONS OF THE REPRODUCTIVE ORGANS

### Pelvic Inflammatory Disease

Pelvic inflammatory disease is often caused by the same organisms that cause cervicitis or by organisms that make up the normal flora of the vaginal mucosa. Because of the profuse normal flora of the vaginal tract, specimens must be collected in such a way as to prevent vaginal flora contamination. Aspirated material collected by needle and syringe represents the best specimen. If this cannot be obtained at the time of surgery or laparoscopy, collection of intrauterine contents using a protected suction curetting device or double-lumen sampling device inserted through the cervix is also acceptable. Culdocentesis (aspiration of fluid in the cul-de-sac), after decontamination of the vagina by povidone-iodine, is satisfactory but rarely practiced today.

Aspirated material should be placed into an anaerobic transport container. The presence of mixed anaerobic flora, gonococci, or both can be rapidly detected from a Gram stain. Direct examination with fluorescent monoclonal antibody stain may also detect chlamydiae. All specimens should be inoculated to media that allow the recovery of anaerobic, facultative, and aerobic bacteria, gonococci, fungi, mycoplasmas, and chlamydiae. All material collected from normally sterile body sites in the genital tract should be inoculated to chocolate agar and placed into a suitable broth, such as chopped meat medium or thioglycollate, in addition to the other types of media noted. If only specimens obtained on routine swabs inserted through the cervix are available, cultures should be performed for detection of gonococci and chlamydiae.

### Miscellaneous Infections

Infections of the male prostate, epididymis, and testes are usually bacterial. In younger men, chlamydia predominates as the cause of epididymitis and possibly of prostatitis. Urine or discharge collected via the urethra is the specimen of choice unless an abscess is drained surgically or by needle and syringe. The first few milliliters of voided urine may be collected before and after prostatic massage to try to pinpoint the anatomic site of the infection. Cultures are inoculated to support the growth of anaerobic, facultative, and aerobic bacteria, as well as gonococci.

### Infections of Neonates and Human Products of Conception

Suspected infections acquired by the fetus as a result of a maternal infection that crosses the placenta (congenital infection) can be diagnosed culturally or serologically in the newborn. Because maternal IgG crosses the placenta, serologic tests are often difficult to interpret (see Chapter 10). For culturable agents, the most definitive diagnoses involve recovery of the pathogen in culture. HSV, varicella-zoster virus (VZV), enteroviruses, and cytomegalovirus (CMV) can be cultured easily, as can most bacterial agents. Rubella and parvovirus B19 are more difficult to culture. Nasal and urine specimens offer the greatest yield for viral isolation, although blood, cerebrospinal fluid, and material from a lesion can also be productive. Systemic neonatal herpes without lesions may be difficult to diagnose unless tissue biopsy material is examined, because the viruses may not be present in cerebrospinal fluid or blood. Bacteria and fungi can be isolated from lesions, blood, and other normally sterile sites.

Determining the presence of fetal immunoglobulin M (IgM) directed against the agent in question establishes the serologic diagnosis of congenital infection. Until recently, ultracentrifugation was required for separation of IgM from IgG, the only definitive means of preventing false-positive results caused by maternal IgG or fetal rheumatoid factor. Ion-exchange chromatography columns, antihuman IgG, and bacterial proteins that bind to IgG are commercially available for removing cross-reactive IgG and rheumatoid factor to obtain more homogeneous IgM for differentiation of fetal antibody. Indirect fluorescent antibody and enzyme-linked immunosorbent assay (ELISA) test systems are commercially available to detect IgM against *T. gondii*, rubella, CMV, HSV, and VZV. Interference by rheumatoid factor is still a consideration in most commercial IgM test systems (see Chapter 9). Our ability to detect viral inclusions in tissue, conjunctiva scrapings, and vesicular lesions, traditionally performed with Giemsa stain, has been improved as a result of monoclonal and polyclonal fluorescent antibody reagents, which are described in the chapters that discuss individual agents.

Infections that infants can acquire as they pass through an infected birth canal or are related to difficult labor, premature birth, premature rupture of the membranes, or other events include the following:

- HSV and CMV infections
- Gonorrhea
- Group B streptococcal sepsis
- Chlamydial conjunctivitis and pneumonia
- *Escherichia coli* or other neonatal meningitis

In the laboratory, these infections are diagnosed by direct detection or culturing for the agents when possible, or by performing serologic tests. The appropriate specimens (e.g., cerebrospinal fluid, serum, pus, tracheal aspirate) should be examined and inoculated immediately. Routine body surface cultures of infants in intensive care have not been shown to be helpful for predicting subsequent disease.

Finally, certain infectious agents are known to cause fetal infection and even abortion. For example, *Listeria monocytogenes*, although usually the causative agent of mild flulike symptoms in the mother, can cause extensive disease and abortion of the fetus if infection occurs late in the pregnancy. Therefore, isolation of the organism from the placenta and from tissues of the fetus is important.

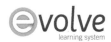 **Visit the Evolve site to complete the review questions.**

---

## CASE STUDY 74-1

A 19-year-old woman presented to the clinic with low-grade fever and abdominal pain of 2 days' duration. She had a vaginal discharge for the previous 4 days and was sexually active with multiple partners in the past 2 months. She used no contraceptives. Urine was collected for an amplified probe assay for *Chlamydia trachomatis* and for *Neisseria gonorrhoeae*. Routine genital culture of the cervix was also collected. She was given an injection of ceftriaxone and placed on doxycycline for 2 weeks.

**QUESTIONS**

1. DNA probe assays are routinely performed from urine specimens from teenagers, because they are easily obtained. Why did the physician also do a culture in this woman?
2. This woman likely has pelvic inflammatory disease (PID). If left untreated, many cases result in infertility. What are the causes of this infection?
3. In this case, the culture was positive for an oxidase-positive, gram-negative diplococci. What is the likely agent?

---

## ▓ BIBLIOGRAPHY

Anderson MR, Klink K, Cohrssen A: Evaluation of vaginal complaints, *JAMA* 291:1368, 2004.

Clarridge JE, Shawar R, Simon B: *Haemophilus ducreyi* and chancroid: practical aspects for the clinical microbiology laboratory, *Clin Microbiol Newsl* 12:137, 1990.

Creatsas G, Deligeoroglou E: Microbial ecology of the lower genital tract in women with sexually transmitted diseases, *J Med Microbiol* 61:1347-1351, 2012.

Fredricks DN, Fiedler TL, Marrazzo JM: Molecular identification of bacteria associated with bacterial vaginosis, *N Engl J Med* 353:1899, 2005.

Hammerschlag MR, Guillen CD: Medical and legal implications of testing for sexually transmitted infections in children, *Clin Microbiol Rev* 23(3):493-506, 2010.

Hillier SL, Krohn MA, Rabe LK, et al: Normal vaginal flora, H₂O₂-producing lactobacilli and bacterial vaginosis in pregnant women, *Clin Infect Dis* 16(suppl 4):S273, 1993.

Horowitz BJ, Mårdh P-A, Nagy E, et al: Vaginal lactobacillosis, *Am J Obstet Gynecol* 170:857, 1994.

Johnson RE, Newhall WJ, Rapp JR, et al: Screening tests to detect *Chlamydia trachomatis* and *Neisseria gonorrhoeae* infections—2002, *MMWR* 51(RR-15):1, 2002.

Kellogg JA, Seiple JW, Klinedinst JL, et al: Comparison of cytobrushes with swabs for recovery of endocervical cells and for Chlamydiazyme detection of *Chlamydia trachomatis*, *J Clin Microbiol* 30:2988, 1992.

Nugent RP, Krohn MA, Hillier SL: Reliability of diagnosing bacterial vaginosis is improved by a standardized method of Gram stain interpretation, *J Clin Microbiol* 29:297, 1991.

Romanowski B, Harris JR: Sexually transmitted diseases, *Clin Symp* 36:1, 1984.

Schmid GP, Faur YC, Valu JA, et al: Enhanced recovery of *Haemophilus ducreyi* from clinical specimens by incubation at 33° versus 35° C, *J Clin Microbiol* 33:3257, 1995.

Schrag S, Gorwitz R, Fultz-Butts K, et al: Prevention of perinatal group B streptococcal disease, revised guidelines from CDC, *MMWR* 51(RR-11):1, 2002.

Sobel JD: What's new in bacterial vaginosis and trichomoniasis? *Infect Dis Clin North Am* 19:387, 2005.

Spiegel CA: Bacterial vaginosis: changes in laboratory practice, *Clin Microbiol Newsl* 21:33, 1999.

Taylor-Robinson D, Bebear C: Antibiotic susceptibilities of mycoplasmas and treatment of mycoplasmal infections, *J Antimicrob Chemo* 40:622, 1997.

Warford A, Chernesky M, Peterson EM: Laboratory diagnosis of *Chlamydia trachomatis* infections. In Gleaves CA, coordinating editor, *Cumitech 19A*, Washington, DC, 1999, American Society for Microbiology.

Weiss EG, Wexner SD: Surgery for anal lesions in HIV-infected patients, *Ann Med* 27:467, 1995.

Wilson J: Managing recurrent bacterial vaginosis, *Sex Transm Infect* 80:8, 2004.

Wood JC, Lu RM, Peterson EM, et al: Evaluation of Mycotrim-GU for isolation of *Mycoplasma* species and *Ureaplasma urealyticum*, *J Clin Microbiol* 22:789, 1985.

# Gastrointestinal Tract Infections

## OBJECTIVES

1. Describe the general anatomy of the gastrointestinal tract and the relationship to transmission of infectious disease.
2. Differentiate normal flora from pathogenic organisms, and describe the relative numbers of organisms distributed throughout the gastrointestinal tract.
3. Identify nonbacterial agents of infection of the gastrointestinal tract, and name their associated diseases.
4. Describe the innate immunity as it relates to the gastrointestinal tract, including physical, chemical, and bacterial components.
5. Differentiate infections of the upper and lower gastrointestinal tract based on clinical manifestations including watery diarrhea and bloody diarrhea (dysentery).
6. Identify the major cause for antimicrobial therapy–associated diarrhea and the proper laboratory diagnostic procedure for identification, including the toxin assay.
7. Identify the most common causes for watery diarrhea, dysentery, pseudomembranous colitis, and infant botulism.
8. Describe the bacterial pathogenic mechanisms associated with gastrointestinal disease, including the presence and function of enterotoxins, attachment, and invasion mechanisms.
9. Determine the adequacy of a specimen based on collection, transport, and specimen type for the diagnosis of gastrointestinal infections.
10. Define the following media, including the organisms identified and the chemical properties associated with the selection and differentiation within the media (MAC, SMAC, EMB, HEK, XLD, SS, and Campy).
11. List the organisms and microbial products that can be detected by non-culture methods.
12. Correlate patient signs and symptoms with laboratory results for the identification of the gastrointestinal pathogen.

## ANATOMY

We are all connected to the external environment through our gastrointestinal (GI) tract (Figure 75-1). What we swallow enters the GI tract and passes through the esophagus into the stomach, through the small and large intestines, and finally to the anus. During passage, fluids and other components are added to this material as secretory products of individual cells and as enzymatic secretions of glands and organs, and they are removed from this material by absorption through the gut epithelium.

The major components of the tract are listed in Box 75-1. The nature of the epithelial cells lining the GI tract varies with each portion. The lining of the GI tract is called the mucosa. Because of the differing nature of the mucosal surfaces of various segments of the bowel, specific infectious disease processes tend to occur in each segment.

The wall of the small intestine has folds that have millions of tiny, hairlike projections called villi. Each villus contains an arteriole, venule, and lymph vessel (Figure 75-2). The function of villi is to absorb fluids and nutrients from the intestinal contents. Epithelial cells lining the surface of villi have a surface resembling a fine brush, referred to as a brush border. The brush border is formed by nearly 2000 microvilli per epithelial cell. Intestinal digestive enzymes are produced in brush border cells toward the top of the villi. Villi and microvilli help make the small intestine the primary site of digestion and absorption by significantly increasing the surface area; more than 90% of physiologic net fluid absorption occurs here. Mucus-secreting goblet cells are found in large numbers of villi and intestinal crypts.

Similar to the small intestine, the large intestine is composed of several segments (see Box 75-1). The wall of the large intestine consists of columnar epithelial cells, many of which are mucus-producing goblet cells. In contrast to the small intestine, there are no villous projections into the lumen. The remaining excess fluid within the GI tract is resorbed through the cells lining the large intestine before waste is finally discharged through the rectum.

In addition to the previously discussed components of the GI tract, numerous other organs and structures are either located in the main digestive organs or open into them. These accessory organs and structures include the salivary glands, tongue, teeth, liver, gallbladder, and pancreas. Except for the teeth and salivary glands, these organs are illustrated in Figure 75-1.

## RESIDENT MICROBIAL FLORA

The GI tract contains vast, diverse normal flora. Although the acidity of the stomach prevents any significant colonization in a normal host under most circumstances, many species can survive passage through the stomach to become resident within the lower intestinal tract. Normally, the upper small intestine contains only sparse flora (bacteria, primarily streptococci; lactobacilli; and yeasts; $10^1$ to $10^3$/mL), but in the distal ileum, counts are about $10^6$ to $10^7$/mL, with Enterobacteriaceae and *Bacteroides* spp. predominantly present.

Infants usually are colonized by normal human epithelial flora, such as staphylococci, *Corynebacterium* spp., and other gram-positive organisms (bifidobacteria, clostridia, lactobacilli, streptococci), within a few hours of birth. Over time, the content of the intestinal flora changes. The normal flora of the adult large bowel (colon) is established relatively early in life and consists predominantly of anaerobic species, including *Bacteroides, Clostridium, Peptostreptococcus, Bifidobacterium,* and *Eubacterium.*

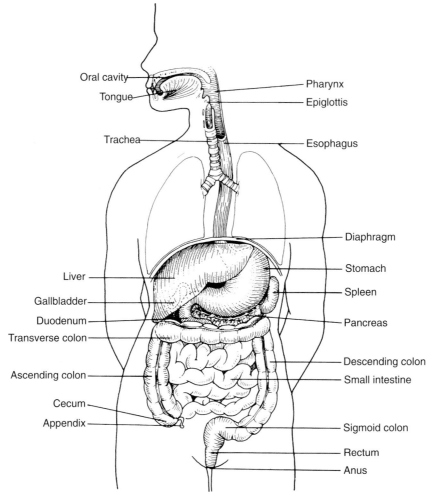

**Figure 75-1** General anatomy of the gastrointestinal tract. (From Broadwell DC, Jackson BS: *Principles of ostomy care,* 1982, St Louis, Mosby.)

---

**BOX 75-1** Components of the Gastrointestinal Tract

Mouth
Oropharynx
Esophagus
Stomach
- *Fundus:* enlarged portion of the stomach to the left and above the opening of the esophagus into the stomach
- *Body:* central part of the stomach
- *Pylorus:* lower portion of the stomach

Small intestine
- *Duodenum:* uppermost division; attached to pyloric end of the stomach
- *Jejunum:* midsection of the small intestine
- *Ileum:* lower portion of the small intestine

Large intestine
- Cecum
- Colon

*Ascending colon:* lies on the right side of the abdomen and extends up to the lower portion of the liver; the ileum joins the large intestine at the junction of the cecum and the ascending colon
*Transverse colon:* passes horizontally across the abdomen
*Descending colon:* lies on the left side of the abdomen in a vertical position
*Sigmoid colon:* extends downward, subsequently joining the rectum
- Rectum
- Anal canal

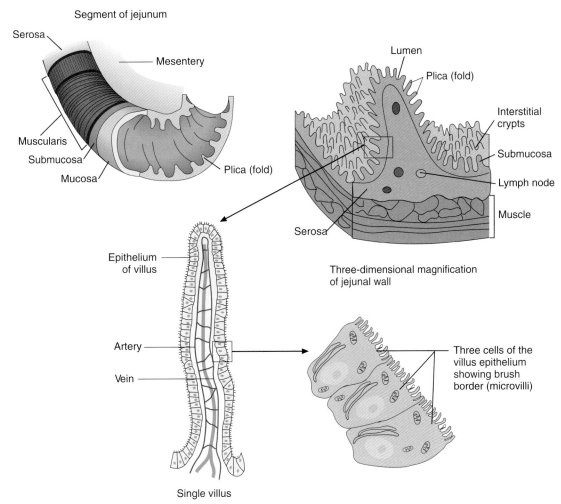

**Figure 75-2** Wall of the small intestine. Villi cover the folds of the mucosal layer; in turn, each villus is covered with epithelial cells.

Aerobes, including *Escherichia coli,* other Enterobacteriaceae, enterococci, and streptococci, are outnumbered by anaerobes 1000:1. The number of bacteria per gram of stool within the bowel lumen increases steadily as material approaches the sigmoid colon (the last segment). Eighty percent of the dry weight of feces from a healthy human consists of bacteria, which can be present in numbers as high as $10^{11}$ to $10^{12}$ colony-forming units (CFU)/g of stool.

# GASTROENTERITIS

Worldwide, diarrheal diseases are the second leading cause of death; about 48 million enteric infections occur each year. These infections cause significant morbidity and death, particularly in elderly people and children younger than 5 years of age. It has been estimated that 4 million to 6 million children die each year of diarrheal diseases, particularly in developing countries in Asia and Africa. Even in developed countries, significant morbidity occurs as a result of diarrheal illness. Although acute diarrheal syndromes are usually self-limited, some patients with infectious diarrhea require diagnostic studies and treatment.

# PATHOGENESIS

Similar to the pathogenesis of urinary tract infections, the host and the invading microorganism possess key features that determine whether an enteric pathogen is able to cause microbial diarrhea.

## Host Factors

The human host has numerous defenses that normally prevent or control disease produced by enteric pathogens. For example, the acidity of the stomach effectively restricts the number and types of organisms that enter the lower GI tract. Normal peristalsis helps move organisms toward the rectum, interfering with their ability to adhere to the mucosa. The mucous layer coating the epithelium entraps microorganisms and helps propel them through the gut. The normal flora prevents colonization by potential pathogens.

Mucous membranes line the GI tract, as well as the respiratory and urogenital tracts. These membranes are exposed to the external environment in the form of food, water, and air. These membranes contain multiple cell types; some are secreting or absorbing cells that perform physiologic functions of the membrane, while others serve as protective barriers. For example, sets of specialized cells called follicles are part of the mucous membrane lining the GI tract and serve a protective function. Collections of follicles are called Peyer's patches. Follicles contain M cells, macrophages, and B and T cells. As a result of the collective action of the follicle components following uptake and processing of the bacteria or antigens, secretory immunoglobulin A (sIgA) is released. Phagocytic cells and sIgA within the gut help destroy etiologic agents of disease, as do eosinophils, which are particularly active against parasites. Follicles and Peyer's patches are found in the small and large intestines.

Other factors that determine the progression and potential invasion by pathogenic organisms include the host's personal hygiene and age. An initial step in the pathogenesis of enteric infections is ingestion of the pathogen. The majority of enteric pathogens, including bacteria, viruses, and parasites, are transmitted by the fecal-oral route. Enteric infections can be spread by contamination of food products or drinking water and then subsequent ingestion. The age of the host also plays a role in whether disease is established. For example, diarrheal infections caused by rotavirus or enteropathogenic *Escherichia coli* tend to affect young children.

Finally, the normal intestinal flora is an important factor in the host protection from the introduction of a potentially harmful microorganism. Whenever a reduction in normal flora occurs as a result of antibiotic treatment or some host factor, resistance to GI infection is significantly reduced. The most common example of the protective effect of normal flora is the development of the syndrome pseudomembranous colitis (PMC). This inflammatory disease of the large bowel is caused by the toxins of the anaerobic organism *Clostridium difficile* and occasionally other clostridia and perhaps even *Staphylococcus aureus*. The inflammatory disease seldom occurs except following antimicrobial or antimetabolite treatment that has altered the normal flora. Almost every antimicrobial agent and several cancer agents have been associated with the development of PMC. *C. difficile*, usually acquired from the hospital environment, is suppressed by normal flora. When normal flora is reduced, *C. difficile* is able to multiply and produce its toxins. This syndrome is also known as antibiotic-associated colitis. Other microorganisms that may gain a foothold when released from selective pressure of normal flora include *Candida* spp., staphylococci, *Pseudomonas* spp., and various Enterobacteriaceae.

## Microbial Factors

The ability of an organism to cause GI infection depends not only on the susceptibility of the human host to the invading organism but also on the organism's virulence traits. To cause GI infection, a microorganism must possess one or more factors that allow it to overcome host defenses or it must enter the host at a time when one or more of the innate defense systems are inactive. For example, certain stool pathogens are able to survive gastric acidity only if the acidity has been reduced by bicarbonate, other buffers, or by medications for ulcers (e.g., cimetidine, ranitidine, H₂ blockers). Pathogens ingested with milk have a better chance of survival, because milk neutralizes stomach acidity. Organisms such as *Mycobacterium tuberculosis*, *Shigella*, *E. coli* O157:H7,

and *C. difficile* (a spore-forming *Clostridium* spp.) are able to withstand exposure to gastric acids and thus require much smaller infectious doses than do acid-sensitive organisms such as *Salmonella*.

**Primary Pathogenic Mechanisms.** Because the normal adult GI tract receives up to 8 L of ingested fluid daily, plus the secretions of the various glands that contribute to digestion (salivary glands, pancreas, gallbladder, stomach), of which all but a small amount must be resorbed, any disruption of the normal flow or reabsorption of fluid will profoundly affect the host. Depending on how they interact with the human host, enteric pathogens may cause disease in one or more of the following three ways:

- By changing the delicate balance of water and electrolytes in the small bowel, resulting in massive fluid secretion. In many cases, this process is mediated by enterotoxin production. This is a noninflammatory process.
- By causing cell destruction or a marked inflammatory response following invasion of host cells and possible cytotoxin production, usually in the colon.
- By penetrating the intestinal mucosa, with subsequent spread and multiplication in lymphatic or reticuloendothelial cells outside of the bowel; these infections are considered systemic infections.

Examples of microorganisms for each of these pathogenic mechanisms are listed in Table 75-1.

### Toxins

*Enterotoxins.* Enterotoxins alter the metabolic activity of intestinal epithelial cells, resulting in an outpouring of electrolytes and fluid into the lumen. They act primarily in the jejunum and upper ileum, where most fluid transport takes place. The stool of patients with enterotoxic diarrheal disease involving the small bowel is profuse and watery, and blood or polymorphonuclear neutrophils are not prominent features.

The classic example of an enterotoxin is that of *Vibrio cholerae* (Figure 75-3). This toxin consists of two subunits, A and B. The A subunit is composed of one molecule of A₁, the toxic moiety, and one molecule of A₂, which binds an A₁ subunit to five B subunits. The B subunits bind the toxin to a receptor (a ganglioside, an acidic glycolipid) on the intestinal cell membrane. Once bound, the toxin acts on adenylate cyclase enzyme, which catalyzes the transformation of adenosine triphosphate (ATP) to cyclic adenosine monophosphate (cAMP). Increased levels of cAMP stimulate the cell to actively secrete ions into the intestinal lumen. To maintain osmotic stabilization, the cells then secrete fluid into the lumen. The fluid is drawn from the intravascular fluid store of the body. Patients therefore can become dehydrated and hypotensive rapidly. *V. cholerae* inhabits sea and stagnant water and is spread in contaminated water. The organisms have been isolated from coastal waters of several states, and sporadic cases of cholera occur in the United States. Additional information about *V. cholerae* is provided in Chapter 26.

Other organisms also produce a cholera-like enterotoxin. A group of vibrios similar to *V. cholerae* but serologically different, known as the noncholera vibrios, produce

**TABLE 75-1** Examples of Microorganisms That Cause GI Infection for Each Primary Pathogenic Mechanism

| Mechanism | Examples of Microorganisms |
|---|---|
| **Toxin Production** Enterotoxin | *Vibrio cholera* Noncholera vibrios *Shigella dysenteriae* type 1 Enterotoxigenic *Escherichia coli* *Salmonella* spp. *Clostridium difficile* (toxin A) *Aeromonas* *Campylobacter jejuni* |
| Cytotoxin | *Shigella* spp. *Clostridium difficile* (toxin B) Enterohemorrhagic *Escherichia coli* |
| Neurotoxin | *Clostridium botulinum* *Staphylococcus aureus* *Bacillus cereus* |
| **Attachment Within or Close to Mucosal Cells/Adherence** | Enteropathogenic *Escherichia coli* Enterohemorrhagic *Escherichia coli* *Cryptosporidium parvum* *Isospora belli* Rotavirus Hepatitis A, B, C Norwalk virus |
| Invasion | *Shigella* spp. Enteroinvasive *Escherichia coli* *Entamoeba histolytica* *Balantidium coli* *Campylobacter jejuni* *Plesiomonas shigelloides* *Yersinia enterocolitica* *Edwardsiella tarda* |

disease clinically identical to cholera, effected by a very similar toxin. The heat-labile toxin (LT) elaborated by certain strains of *E. coli*, called enterotoxigenic *E. coli* (ETEC), is similar to cholera toxin, sharing cross-reactive antigenic determinants. The enterotoxins of some *Salmonella* spp. (including *S. enterica* subsp. *arizonae*), *Vibrio parahaemolyticus*, the *Campylobacter jejuni* group, *Clostridium perfringens*, *Clostridium difficile*, *Bacillus cereus*, *Aeromonas*, *Shigella dysenteriae*, and many other Enterobacteriaceae also cause positive reactions in at least one of the tests for enterotoxin (discussed later). The exact contribution of these enterotoxins to the pathogenicity of most stool pathogens remains to be elucidated.

Certain strains of *E. coli*, in addition to producing a heat-labile toxin (LT) similar to cholera toxin, also produce a heat-stable toxin (ST) with other properties. Although ST also promotes fluid secretion into the intestinal lumen, its effect is mediated by activation of guanylate cyclase, resulting in increased levels of cyclic guanylate monophosphate (GMP), which yields the same net effect as increased cAMP. Tests for ST include enzyme-linked immunosorbent assay (ELISA), immunodiffusion and cell culture. Molecular techniques, including the use of DNA probes as well as several amplification assays, have

been used to identify ETEC directly in clinical samples or isolated bacterial colonies.

Several tests are available for the detection of enterotoxin. Immunodiffusion, ELISA, and latex agglutination tests are all available to identify specific toxins. Molecular probes and amplification assays for toxin detection are also available, primarily for research use.

***Cytotoxins.*** Cytotoxins, which constitute the second category of toxins, disrupt the structure of individual intestinal epithelial cells. When destroyed, these cells slough from the surface of the mucosa, leaving it raw and unprotected. The secretory or absorptive functions of the cells are no longer performed. The damaged tissue evokes a strong inflammatory response from the host, further inflicting tissue damage. Numerous polymorphonuclear neutrophils and blood are often seen in the stool, and pain, cramps, and tenesmus (painful straining during a bowel movement) are common symptoms. The term *dysentery* refers to this destructive disease of the mucosa, almost exclusively occurring in the colon. Cytotoxin has not yet been shown to be the sole virulence factor for any etiologic agent of GI disease, because most agents produce a cytotoxin in conjunction with other factors.

*E. coli* strains seem to possess virulence mechanisms of many types. Some strains produce a cytotoxin capable of destroying epithelial cells and blood cells. Certain strains produce a cytotoxin that affects Vero cells (African green monkey kidney cells) and resemble the cytotoxin produced by *Shigella dysenteriae* (Shiga toxin); such strains of *E. coli* are associated with hemorrhagic colitis and the sequelae following infection of hemolytic-uremic syndrome (HUS) and thrombotic thrombocytopenia purpura (TTP). These strains of *E. coli* are referred to as enterohemorrhagic *E. coli* (EHEC), also referred to as serotoxigenic or STET/VTEC. See Chapter 20 for more information related to toxigenic *E. coli*. Table 75-2 summarizes the key pathogenic features of the primary groups of diarrheogenic *E. coli*.

*C. difficile* produces a cytotoxin, the presence of which is a most useful marker for diagnosis of PMC. *S. dysenteriae*, *Staphylococcus aureus*, *C. perfringens*, and *V. parahaemolyticus* produce cytotoxins that contribute to the pathogenesis of diarrhea, although they may not be essential for initiation of disease. Other vibrios, *Aeromonas hydrophila* (a relatively newly described agent of GI disease), and *Campylobacter jejuni*, the most common cause of GI disease in many areas of the United States, have been shown to produce cytotoxins. The role that these toxins play in the pathogenesis of the disease syndromes is not yet completely delineated.

***Neurotoxins.*** Food poisoning, or intoxication, may occur as a result of ingesting toxins produced by microorganisms. The microorganisms usually produce their toxins in foodstuffs before they are ingested; thus, the patient ingests preformed toxin. Strictly speaking, these syndromes are not GI infections but rather intoxications; because they are acquired by ingestion of microorganisms or their products, they are considered in this chapter. Particularly in staphylococcal food poisoning and botulism, the causative organisms may not be present in the patient's bowel.

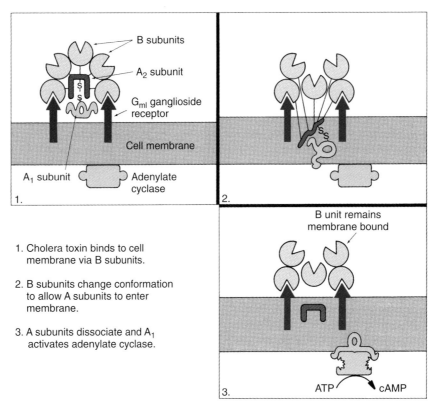

**Figure 75-3** Diagrammatic representation of the structure and action of cholera toxin.

**TABLE 75-2** Overview of the Primary Groups of *E. coli* That Cause Diarrhea in Humans

| Type | Primary Mode of Pathogenesis | Other Comments |
|------|------------------------------|----------------|
| Enterotoxigenic (ETEC) | Produces heat-labile (LT) or heat stable (ST) enterotoxins; genes of both toxins reside on a plasmid; LTs are closely related in structure and function to cholera toxin; STs result in net intestinal fluid secretion by stimulating guanylate cyclase | Common cause of traveler's diarrhea; infects all ages |
| Enteroaggregative (EAEC) | Binds to small intestine cells via fimbriae encoded by a large molecular weight plasmid, forming small clumps of bacteria on the cell surface; other plasmid-borne virulence factors include structured pilin, a heat-stable enterotoxin, novel anti-aggregative protein, and a heat-labile enterotoxin, all believed to be the cause of the associated diarrhea | Infects primarily young children |
| Enteroinvasive (EIEC) | Pathogenesis has yet to be totally elucidated; studies suggest that mechanisms by which diarrhea results are virtually identical to those of *Shigella* spp. | Very difficult to distinguish from *Shigella* spp. and other *E. coli* strains |
| Enteropathogenic (EPEC) | Initially attaches in the colon and small intestine and then becomes intimately adhered to intestinal epithelial cells, subsequently causing the loss of enterocyte microvilli (effacement); genes for attachment/effacement reside in a cluster on the bacterial chromosome (i.e., pathogenicity island) | Diarrhea in infants, particularly in large urban hospitals |
| Enterohemorrhagic (EHEC) OR | Attaches to and effaces gut epithelial cells in a similar manner as EPEC; in addition, EHEC elaborates shiga toxins | Although many outbreaks are caused by *E. coli* 0157:H7, other serotypes have been implicated in outbreaks and sporadic cases Gene recombination among strains makes classification difficult |
| Enterohemorrhagic (EHEC); or serotoxigenic (STEC); verotoxigenic (VTEC) (newest, terminology) | Produce one or more shiga toxins referred to as verocytotoxins. Attaches to and effaces gut epithelial cells in a similar manner as EPEC | 0157 STEC serotypes; contains most common serotypes 0157:H7 and nonmotile 0157:NM. There are more than 150 non-0157 serotypes that have been isolated from patients with diarrhea or hemolytic uremic syndrome |

Bacterial agents of food poisoning that produce neurotoxins include *Staphylococcus aureus* and *Bacillus cereus.* Toxins produced by these organisms cause vomiting, independent of other actions on the gut mucosa. Staphylococcal food poisoning is one of the most frequently reported categories of food-borne disease. The organisms grow in warm food, primarily meat or dairy products, and produce the toxin. Onset of disease is usually within 2 to 6 hours of ingestion. *B. cereus* produces two toxins, one of which is preformed, called the emetic toxin, because it produces vomiting. The second type, probably involving several enterotoxins, causes diarrhea. Often acquired from eating rice, *B. cereus* has also been associated with cooked meat, poultry, vegetables, and desserts.

Perhaps the most common cause of food poisoning is from type A *Clostridium perfringens,* which produces toxin in the host after ingestion. As a result, a relatively mild, self-limited (usually 24-hour) gastroenteritis occurs, often in outbreaks in hospitals. Meats and gravies are typical foods associated with this type of food poisoning.

One of the most potent neurotoxins is produced by the anaerobic organism *Clostridium botulinum.* This toxin prevents the release of the neurotransmitter acetylcholine at the cholinergic nerve junctions, causing flaccid paralysis. The toxin acts primarily on the peripheral nerves but also on the autonomic nervous system. Patients exhibit descending symmetric paralysis and ultimately die of respiratory paralysis unless they are mechanically ventilated. In most cases, adult patients who develop botulism have ingested the preformed toxin in food (home-canned tomato products and canned, cream-based foods are often implicated), and the disease is considered intoxication, although *C. botulinum* has been recovered from the stools of many adult patients. A relatively recently recognized syndrome, infant botulism, is a true GI infection. In adults, the normal flora probably prevents colonization by *C. botulinum,* whereas the organism is able to multiply and produce toxin in the infant bowel. Infant botulism is not an infrequent condition; babies acquire the organism by ingestion, although the source of the bacterium is not always clear. Because an association has been found with honey and corn syrup, infants younger than 9 months of age should not be fed honey. The effect of the toxin is the same, whether ingested in food or produced by growing organisms within the bowel.

**Attachment.** An organism's ability to cause disease can also depend on its ability to colonize and adhere to the bowel. To illustrate, ETEC must be able to adhere to and colonize the small intestine, as well as produce an enterotoxin. These organisms produce an adherence antigen, called colonization factor antigen (CFA). Certain strains of *E. coli* referred to as the enteropathogenic *E. coli* (EPEC) attach and then adhere to the intestinal brush border. This localized adherence is mediated by the production of pili. Subsequent to attaching, EPEC disrupts normal cell function by effacing the brush epithelium, thereby causing diarrheal disease. This complete process is referred to as attachment and effacement. Genes responsible for the initial adherence of ETEC, EHEC, and EPEC to intestinal epithelial cells

## Origins of EHEC/VTEC

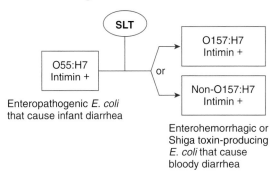

**Figure 75-4** It appears that the presence of EHEC/VTEC strain O157:H7 has actually increased in recent years and was not simply overlooked before 1982. *E. coli* O157:H7 strains are closely related to a Shiga toxin–negative EPEC strain O55:H7. It is proposed that this EPEC strain O55:H7 became infected by a bacteriophage that encoded Shiga toxin (SLT); it is now recognized that more than 100 different *E. coli* serotypes can express Shiga toxin.

reside on a transmissible plasmid. EHEC has the same ability to attach to intestinal epithelial cells and cause effacement. In addition, EHEC produces a Shiga toxin that spreads to the bloodstream, causing systemic damage to vascular endothelial cells of various organs, including kidney, colon, small intestine, and lung. EHEC is believed to have arisen as a result of an EPEC strain having become infected with a bacteriophage carrying the Shiga toxin gene (Figure 75-4).

*Giardia lamblia,* a parasite, has increasingly become more common as an etiologic agent of GI disease in the United States. Excreted into fresh water by natural animal hosts such as the beaver, the organism can be acquired by drinking stream water or even city water in some localities, particularly in the Rocky Mountain states. The organism, a flagellated protozoan, adheres to the intestinal mucosa of the small bowel, by means of a ventral sucker, destroying the mucosal cells' ability to participate in normal secretion and absorption. No evidence indicates invasion or toxin production.

*Cryptosporidia* and *Isospora* spp., parasitic etiologic agents of diarrhea in animals and poultry and more recently recognized as causing human disease, probably also act by adhering to intestinal mucosa and disrupting function. Cryptosporidia are often seen in the diarrhea of patients with acquired immunodeficiency syndrome (AIDS), as well as in travelers' diarrhea, day care epidemics, and diarrhea in people with animal exposure. Cryptosporidia and *Isospora* spp. may cause severe, protracted diarrhea in AIDS patients. Other coccidian parasites, such as microsporidia, produce diarrhea by destroying intestinal cell function.

**Invasion.** Following initial and essential adherence to GI mucosal cells, some enteric pathogens are able to gain access to the intracellular environment. Invasion allows the organism to reach deeper tissues, access nutrients for growth, and possibly avoid the host immune system.

In the case of diarrhea caused by *Shigella,* the primary mechanism of disease production consists of (1) the triggering and directing by *Shigella* entry into colonic

**TABLE 75-3** Types of Enteric Infections

| Pathogenic Mechanism | Major Symptoms | Examples of Etiologic Agents |
|---|---|---|
| Upsetting of fluid and electrolyte balance/ noninflammatory | Watery diarrhea No fecal leukocytes No fever | *Vibrio cholerae* Rotavirus Norwalk virus Enterotoxigenic *Escherichia coli* *Giardia lamblia* *Bacillus cereus* |
| Invasion and possible cytotoxin production/ inflammatory (dysentery) | Dysenteric-like diarrhea (mucus, blood, white cells) Fever Fecal leukocytes | *Shigella* spp. Enteroinvasive *E. coli* *Salmonella enteritidis* *Entamoeba histolytica* |
| Penetration with subsequent access to the bloodstream (enteric fever) | Signs of systemic infection (headache, malaise, sore throat) Fever | *Salmonella typhi* *Yersinia enterocolitica* |

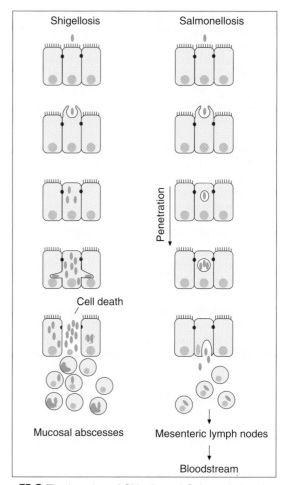

**Figure 75-5** The invasion of *Shigella* and *Salmonella* into intestinal epithelial cells. (Modified from Sansonetti PJ: Genetic and molecular basis of epithelial invasion by *Shigella* species, *Rev Infect Dis* 13[suppl 4]:S282, 1991, University of Chicago Press.)

epithelial cells by genes located on a plasmid, and once internalized, (2) the rapid multiplication of *Shigella* in the submucosa and lamina propria and its intracellular and extracellular spread to other adjacent colonic epithelial cells. Once in the host cell cytoplasm, *Shigella* spp. cause apoptosis and release of the cytokines interleukin (IL)-1 and IL-8. The inflammatory response to these cytokines damages the colonic mucosa and exacerbates (aggravates) the infection. The genes for invasiveness are located on a large invasion plasmid. These activities lead to extensive superficial tissue destruction. If these two steps do not occur, one does not get the clinical presentation of classic dysentery (Table 75-3). The entry process is illustrated in Figure 75-5.

Salmonellae interact with the apical (top) microvilli of colonic epithelial cells, disrupting the brush border. Similar to *Shigella*, *Salmonella* spp. also stimulate the host cell to internalize through rearrangements of host actin filaments and other cytoskeleton proteins. Once the whole bacteria are internalized within endocytic vesicles of the host epithelial cell, organisms begin to multiply within the vacuoles. In contrast to *Shigella* spp. that use the colonic mucosal epithelium as a site of multiplication, certain serotypes of *Salmonella*, such as Salmonella enterica serotype Typhi and S. *choleraesuis,* use the colonic epithelium as a route to gain access to the submucosal layers, mesenteric lymph nodes, and subsequently the bloodstream. The entry of *Salmonella* is a complex process involving several essential genes, as well as particular environmental conditions of the host cell; this process is still being delineated. Many virulence factors for invasion of salmonellae into nonphagocytic cells as well as their ability to cause systemic infections by surviving in phagocytic cells and replicating within the *Salmonella*-containing vesicle in a variety of eukaryotic cells are determined by chromosomal genes, many of which are located within pathogenicity islands. Invasiveness is also thought to

contribute to the pathogenesis of disease associated with species of vibrios, campylobacters, *Yersinia enterocolitica*, *Plesiomonas shigelloides*, and *Edwardsiella tarda*.

Certain parasites, particularly *Entamoeba histolytica* and *Balantidium coli*, invade the intestinal epithelium of the colon. The ensuing amebic dysentery is characterized by blood and numerous white blood cells, and the patient experiences cramping and tenesmus. Other parasites acquired by ingestion, such as *Trichinella*, may cause transient bloody diarrhea and pain during migration through the intestinal mucosa to their preferred sites within the host.

Other organisms selectively destroy absorptive cells (e.g., villus tip cells) in the mucosa, disrupting their normal cell function and thereby causing diarrhea. Rotaviruses and Norwalk-like viruses are both visualized by electron microscopy within the absorptive cells at the ends of the intestinal villi, where they multiply and destroy cellular function. As a result, the villi become shortened, and inflammatory cells infiltrate the mucosa, further contributing to the pathologic condition. In addition to these viral agents, hepatitis A, B, and C and occasionally enteric adenoviruses have been associated with diarrheal symptoms in patients.

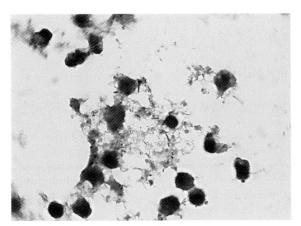

**Figure 75-6** Wright's stain of stool from a patient with shigellosis showing moderate numbers of polymorphonuclear cells.

**Miscellaneous Virulence Factors.** Other virulence traits appear to be involved in the development of GI infections and include characteristics such as motility, chemotaxis, and mucinase production. Also, the possession of certain antigens, such as the Vi antigen of *Salmonella typhi* and certain cell wall components, are also associated with virulence.

## CLINICAL MANIFESTATIONS

The clinical symptoms experienced by a patient are largely dependent on how the enteric pathogen causes disease. To illustrate, patients infected with an enteric pathogen that upsets fluid and electrolyte balance have no fecal leukocytes present in the stool and complain of watery diarrhea; fever is usually absent or mild. Although nausea, vomiting, and abdominal pain may also be present, the dominant feature is intestinal fluid loss. In contrast, patients infected with an enteric pathogen that causes significant cell destruction and inflammation have fecal leukocytes present in the stool (Figure 75-6). Their diarrhea is often characterized by the presence of mucus and blood; in many of these patients, fever is a prominent component of their disease, as well as abdominal pain, cramps, and tenesmus. Finally, patients who become infected with a pathogen capable of penetrating the intestinal mucosa of the small intestine without producing enterocolitis and then subsequently spreading and multiplying at other sites will present with signs and symptoms of a systemic illness such as headache, sore throat, malaise, and fever; diarrhea in these patients is not a prominent feature and is absent or mild in many cases. Features of these three types of enteric infections are summarized in Table 75-3.

## EPIDEMIOLOGY

Gastrointestinal infections occur in numerous epidemiologic settings. Awareness of these different settings is important because knowledge of a particular epidemiologic setting can help provide a basis for the diagnosis and clues to possible etiologies. When this knowledge is combined with clinical findings, the etiology of the infection can often be narrowed to three or four organisms.

### Institutional Settings

Diarrheal illness can be a major problem in institutional settings such as day care centers, hospitals, and nursing homes. Because individual hygiene is often difficult to maintain in these settings, coupled with the presence of several organisms with relatively low infecting doses such as *Shigella* and *Giardia lamblia*, numerous outbreaks of diarrheal illness caused by various organisms have been reported. Organisms such as Shigella, *Campylobacter jejuni*, *Giardia lamblia*, *Cryptosporidium*, and rotaviruses have been reported to cause outbreaks in day care centers. Of significance, these infections can be spread to family members. Similarly, outbreaks caused by these organisms, as well as hemorrhagic *E. coli* O157:H7, have been reported in nursing homes and other extended-care facilities.

Nosocomial diarrheal illness is also a problem for hospital patients and personnel. Rotaviruses, adenoviruses, and Coxsackie viruses have also been identified in nosocomial settings. In addition to these organisms, *Clostridium difficile* is a major nosocomial enteric pathogen in hospitals and other settings, including nursing homes and extended-care facilities. This organism is a hardy pathogen that readily survives on fomites (inanimate objects) such as floors, bed rails, call buttons, and door-knobs, and on the hands of hospital personnel caring for the patient. Of clinical concern is the emergence of a strain of *C. difficile* with increased virulence and fluoroquinolone resistance. By virtue of partial deletions in a toxin regulatory gene, tcdC, these isolates are able to produce 16- to 23-fold more toxin A and B. In addition, a separate binary toxin has been described that is encoded by cdtA and cdtB genes; cdtB mediates cell surface binding and cellular translocation, whereas cdtA disrupts the assembly of the actin filament, causing cell death. These strains have emerged as a cause of geographically dispersed outbreaks of *C. difficile*–associated disease. Many of the reported cases caused by these strains were in otherwise healthy patients with minimal or no exposure to a health care setting. *C. difficile* is the most common pathogen isolated in patients with antibiotic-associated diarrhea. However, antibiotic-associated hemorrhagic colitis (AAHC) is not linked to *C. difficile infection*. AAHC symptoms include a sudden onset of bloody diarrhea and abdominal cramps during antibiotic therapy. Toxin-producing *Klebsiella oxytoca* has been identified as a causative agent of AAHC.

### Traveler's Diarrhea

Individuals who travel into developing geographic areas with poor sanitation are at particularly high risk for developing diarrhea. In areas with poor sanitation, enteric pathogens heavily contaminate the water and food. Although many types of enteric pathogens can cause diarrhea in travelers, enterotoxigenic *E. coli* is a leading cause in Asia, Africa, and Latin America, accounting for about 50% of cases. Salmonellae, shigellae, *Campylobacter* spp., vibrios, rotavirus, and Norwalk virus can also cause diarrhea in travelers, depending on the area or country they visit.

### Food- and Water-Borne Outbreaks

The Centers for Disease Control and Prevention indicate that more than 48 million cases of food-borne illness are reported in the United States each year. Eating raw or undercooked fish, shellfish, or meats and drinking unpasteurized milk increases the risks of certain bacterial, parasitic, and viral infections. Many food-borne outbreaks can be traced to poor hygienic practices of food handlers such as not washing hands after using the toilet; hepatitis A, Norwalk virus, and *Salmonella* are a few examples of organisms that have contaminated food during preparation by a food handler and causing diarrheal disease. The number of cases of salmonellosis has gradually increased, with many of these infections associated with eating raw or undercooked eggs. Also, the potential for widespread dissemination of food-borne pathogens has increased because of factors such as the tendency to eat outside the home, the export and import of food sources worldwide, and travel.

In addition to food-borne outbreaks of GI tract infections, water-borne outbreaks of diarrheal disease caused by *Giardia lamblia* and *Cryptosporidium* have been traced to inadequately filtered surface water. Recreational waters, including swimming pools, can also become contaminated with enteric pathogens such as *Shigella* and *G. lamblia* because of poor toilet facilities or practices.

### Immunocompromised Hosts

GI tract infections in individuals infected with human immunodeficiency virus (HIV) and other patients who are immunosuppressed, such as organ transplant recipients or individuals receiving chemotherapy, are a diagnostic challenge for the clinician and microbiologist. For example, cytotoxic chemotherapy or antibiotic therapy may predispose patients to develop *C. difficile* colitis.

Diarrhea is a common clinical manifestation of infection with HIV. Numerous pathogens and opportunistic pathogens have been identified and are believed to cause recurrent or chronic diarrhea. Commonly reported etiologic agents include the following:

- Species of *Salmonella*, *Shigella*, and *Campylobacter*
- Cytomegalovirus
- Cryptosporidia, *Isospora belli*
- Microsporidia
- *Entamoeba histolytica*
- *Mycobacterium* spp.
- *Giardia lamblia*

## ETIOLOGIC AGENTS

Many microorganisms are able to cause enteric infections. A discussion of each organism is beyond the scope of this chapter. Rather, these organisms are addressed in Parts III through VI of the textbook. Table 75-4 summarizes the general characteristics of the more common agents of enteric infections.

## ▐ OTHER INFECTIONS OF THE GASTROINTESTINAL TRACT

Besides causing disease in the small and large intestine, microorganisms can also infect other sites of the GI tract, as well as the GI tract's accessory organs.

## ESOPHAGITIS

Infections of the mucosa of the esophagus (esophagitis) can cause painful or difficult swallowing or the sensation that something is lodged in the throat while swallowing. Individuals who have esophagitis usually have local or systemic underlying illnesses such as hematologic malignancies or HIV infection, or they are receiving immunosuppressive therapy. The most common etiologic agents are *Candida* spp. (primarily *C. albicans*), herpes simplex virus, and cytomegalovirus.

## GASTRITIS

Gastritis refers to inflammation of the gastric mucosa. This illness is associated with nausea and upper abdominal pain; vomiting, burping, and fever may also be present. A curved organism called *Helicobacter pylori* is seen on the surface of gastric epithelial cells of patients with gastritis. The organism is recovered from gastric biopsy material obtained endoscopically but not from stool. Following acute infection, *H. pylori* can persist for years in most individuals, with many remaining asymptomatic. *H. pylori* is also the causative agent of peptic ulcer disease and a significant risk factor for the development of stomach cancer.

## PROCTITIS

Proctitis is the inflammation of the rectum (distal portion of the large intestine). Common symptoms associated with proctitis are itching and a mucous discharge from the rectum; if the infection progresses, ulcers and abscesses may form in the rectum. The majority of infections are sexually transmitted through anal intercourse. *Chlamydia trachomatis*, herpes simplex, *T. pallidum*, and *N. gonorrhoeae* are the most common etiologic agents.

## MISCELLANEOUS

Unusual agents and those that have not been cultured, such as mycobacteria that may be associated with Crohn's disease and the bacterium associated with Whipple's disease, identified by molecular methods as a new agent, *Tropheryma whipplei*, are also candidates as etiologic agents of GI disease. Occasionally, stool cultures from patients with diarrheal disease yield heavy growth of organisms such as enterococci, *Pseudomonas* spp., or *Klebsiella pneumoniae*, not usually found in such numbers as normal flora. Only anecdotal evidence suggests that these organisms actually contribute to the pathogenesis of the diarrhea. Agents of sexually transmitted disease may cause GI symptoms when they are introduced into the colon via sexual intercourse. *Mycobacterium avium* intracellulare complex may be sexually transmitted, resulting in systemic disease in patients with AIDS. The pathogenesis of infections resulting from *Blastocystis hominis* (a possible coccidian etiologic agent of human diarrheal disease) is not well documented, although these organisms are associated with GI symptoms.

**TABLE 75-4** General Characteristics of the Common Agents of Enteric Infections

| Organism | Common Sources or Predisposing Condition | Distribution | Clinical Presentation | Predominant Pathogenic Mechanism | Fecal Leukocytes |
|---|---|---|---|---|---|
| Bacillus cereus | Meats, vegetables, rice | Worldwide | Intoxication: vomiting or watery diarrhea | Ingestion of preformed toxin (food poisoning) | − |
| Clostridium botulinum | Improperly preserved vegetables, meat, fish | Worldwide | Neuromuscular paralysis | Ingestion of preformed toxin (food poisoning) | − |
| Staphylococcus aureus | Meats, salads, dairy products | Worldwide | Intoxication: vomiting | Ingestion of preformed toxin (food poisoning) | − |
| Clostridium perfringens | Meats, poultry | Worldwide | Watery diarrhea | Ingestion of organism followed by toxin production | − |
| Aeromonas | Water | Worldwide | Watery diarrhea or dysentery | ? Enterotoxin ? Cytotoxin | − |
| Campylobacter spp. | Water, poultry, milk | Worldwide | Dysentery | ? Invasion ? Cytotoxins | + |
| Clostridium difficile | Antimicrobial therapy | Worldwide | Dysentery | Enterotoxin and cytotoxin | +/− |
| **Diarrheogenic Escherichia coli** Enteropathogenic (EPEC) | ? | Worldwide | Watery diarrhea | Adherence/? invasion without multiplication | − |
| Enterotoxigenic (ETEC) | Food, water | Worldwide—more prevalent in developing countries | Watery diarrhea | Enterotoxin | − |
| Enteroinvasive (EIEC) | Food | Worldwide | Dysentery | Invasion, enterotoxin | + |
| Enterohemorrhagic (VTEC/STEC/ EHEC) | Meats | Worldwide | Watery, often bloody diarrhea | Cytotoxin | −/+ |
| Plesiomonas shigelloides | Fresh water, shellfish | Worldwide | ? Dysentery | Unknown ? Enterotoxin | +/− |
| Salmonella spp. (nontyphoidal) | Food, water | Worldwide | Dysentery | Invasion | + |
| Salmonella enterica Typhi | Food, water | Tropical, developing countries | Enteric fever | Penetration | + (monocytes, not PMNs) |
| Shigella spp. | Food, water | Worldwide | Dysentery | Invasion | + |
| Shigella dysenteriae | Water | Tropical, developing countries | Dysentery | Invasion, cytotoxin | + |
| Vibrio cholerae | Water, shellfish | Asia, Africa, Middle East, South and North American (along coastal areas) | Watery diarrhea | ? Enterotoxin Cytotoxin | −/+ |
| Yersinia enterocolitica | Milk, pork, water | Worldwide | Watery diarrhea and/ or enteric fever | ? Invasion ? Penetration | − |
| Giardia lamblia | Food, water | Worldwide | Watery diarrhea | Unknown-impaired absorption | − |
| Cryptosporidium parvum | Animals, water | Worldwide | Watery diarrhea | ? Adherence | − |

*Continued*

**TABLE 75-4** General Characteristics of the Common Agents of Enteric Infections—cont'd

| Organism | Common Sources or Predisposing Condition | Distribution | Clinical Presentation | Predominant Pathogenic Mechanism | Fecal Leukocytes |
|---|---|---|---|---|---|
| *Entamoeba histolytica* | Food, water | Worldwide (more common in developing countries) | Dysentery | Invasion, cytotoxin | −/+ (amebae destroy the white cells) |
| Rotavirus | ? | Worldwide | Watery diarrhea | Mucosal damage leading to impaired absorption in small intestine | − |
| Norwalk viruses | Shellfish, salads | Worldwide | Watery diarrhea | Mucosal damage leading to impaired absorption in small intestine | − |

# LABORATORY DIAGNOSIS OF GASTROINTESTINAL TRACT INFECTIONS

## SPECIMEN COLLECTION AND TRANSPORT

If enteric pathogens are to be detected by the laboratory, adherence to appropriate guidelines for specimen collection and transport is imperative (see Table 5-1 for a quick guide to specimen collection, transport, and processing). If an etiologic agent is not isolated with the first culture or visual examination, two additional specimens should be submitted to the laboratory over the next few days. Because organisms may be shed intermittently, collection of specimens at different times over several days enhances recovery. Certain infectious agents, such as *Giardia*, may be difficult to detect, requiring the processing of multiple specimens over weeks, duodenal aspirates (in the case of *Giardia*), or additional alternative methods.

### General Comments

Specimens delivered to the laboratory within 30 minutes may be collected in a clean plastic container. Stool for direct wet-mount examination, *Clostridium difficile* toxin assay, immunoelectron microscopy for detection of viruses, and ELISA or the latex agglutination test for rotavirus must be sent to the laboratory without any added preservatives or liquids. Volume of a liquid stool at least equal to 1 teaspoon (5 mL) or a pea-sized piece of formed stool is necessary for most procedures.

### Stool Specimens for Bacterial Culture

If a delay longer than 2 hours is anticipated for stools for bacterial culture, the specimen should be placed in transport medium. The Cary-Blair transport medium preserves the viability of intestinal bacterial pathogens, including *Campylobacter* and *Vibrio* spp. However, the media produced by different manufacturers can vary. Most workers recommend reducing the agar content of Cary-Blair medium from 0.5% to 0.16% (modified) for maintenance of *Campylobacter* spp. Buffered glycerol transport medium does not maintain these bacteria. Several manufacturers produce a small vial of Cary-Blair

with a self-contained plastic scoop suitable for collecting samples.

Because *Shigella* spp. are sensitive to environmental factors, a transport medium of equal parts of glycerol and 0.033 M phosphate buffer (pH 7.0) increases the viability of *Shigella* in comparison to Cary-Blair. For this purpose, maintaining the glycerol transport medium at refrigerator or freezer temperatures also improves recovery.

If stool is unavailable, a rectal swab may be substituted for bacterial or viral culture, but it is not as good, particularly for diagnosis in adults. For suspected intestinal infection with *Campylobacter*, the swab must be placed in Cary-Blair transport medium immediately to avoid drying. Swabs are not acceptable for the detection of parasites, toxins, or viral antigens.

### Stool Specimens for Ova and Parasites

For detection of ova and parasites, specimen preservation with a fixative is recommended for visual examination (see Chapter 47).

### Stool Specimens for Viruses

Stools for virus culture must be refrigerated if they are not inoculated into cell cultures within 2 hours. A rectal swab, transported in modified Stuart's transport medium or another viral transport medium, is adequate for recovery of most viruses from feces. See Chapter 65 for more information regarding the collection and transport of specimens for viral culture.

### Miscellaneous Specimen Types

Other specimens that may be obtained for diagnosis of GI tract infection include duodenal aspirates. These samples should be examined immediately using direct microscopy for the presence of motile protozoan trophozoites, cultured for bacteria, and placed into polyvinyl alcohol (PVA) fixative for subsequent parasitic examination. The laboratory should be informed in advance so that the specimen can be processed and examined efficiently.

The string test has proved useful for diagnosing duodenal parasites, such as *Giardia*, and for isolating *Salmonella enterica* Typhi from carriers and patients with acute typhoid fever. The patient swallows a weighted gelatin capsule containing a tightly wound length of string, which is left protruding from the mouth and taped to the cheek. After a predetermined period, during which the capsule reaches the duodenum and dissolves, the string, now covered with duodenal contents, is retracted and delivered immediately to the laboratory. There the technologist, using sterile-gloved fingers, strips the mucus and secretions attached to the string and deposits some material on slides for direct examination and some material into fixative for preparation of permanent stained mounts. The technologist also inoculates some material to appropriate media for isolation of bacteria.

## DIRECT DETECTION OF AGENTS OF GASTROENTERITIS IN FECES

### Wet Mounts

A direct wet mount of fecal material, particularly with liquid or unformed stool, is the fastest method for detecting motile trophozoites of *Dientamoeba fragilis, Entamoeba, Giardia,* and other intestinal parasites. Occasionally the larvae or adult worms of other parasites may be visualized. Experienced observers can also see the refractile forms of Cryptosporidia and many types of cysts on the direct wet mount, including *Cyclospora cayetanensis,* a parasite that is associated with the consumption of contaminated food such as raspberries. If present in sufficient numbers, the ova of intestinal parasites can be seen.

Examination of a direct wet mount of fecal material containing blood or mucus, with the addition of an equal portion of Loeffler's methylene blue, is helpful for detection of leukocytes, which occasionally aids in differentiating among the various types of diarrheal syndromes. Another commercially available test detects lactoferrin, which is a glycoprotein released from neutrophil granules into the stool sample. This assay demonstrates improved sensitivity and specificity as compared to detection of intact WBCs. Under phase-contrast and dark-field microscopy, the darting motility and curved forms of *Campylobacter* may be observed in a warm sample. Water or saline, which will immobilize *Campylobacter,* should not be used. However, for practical reasons most laboratories do not use a wet mount.

### Stains

Feces may be Gram stained for detection of certain etiologic agents. For example, many thin, comma-shaped, gram-negative bacilli may indicate *Campylobacter* infection (if vibrios have been ruled out). In addition, polymorphonuclear cells may also be detected. An acid-fast stain can be used to detect *Cryptosporidium* spp., mycobacteria, and *Isospora* spp. Examination of fixed fecal material for parasites by trichrome or other stains is covered in Chapter 47. A permanent stained preparation should be made from all stool specimens received for detection of parasites.

### Antigen Detection

An accurate, sensitive, indirect fluorescent antibody stain for giardiasis and cryptosporidiosis is commercially available. These organisms can be visualized easily and unequivocally with a monoclonal antibody fluorescent stain (Meridian Diagnostics, Cincinnati, Ohio). Park and colleagues described a simple and rapid screening procedure using a direct fluorescent antibody stain for *E. coli* O157:H7.

Enzyme immunoassays (EIAs) can detect numerous microorganisms capable of causing GI tract infections. For example, EIAs are commercially available to detect *E. coli* O157:H7 and *Campylobacter* spp., the presence of the Shiga toxins produced by EHEC, or the presence of *C. difficile* toxins A or A and B. In addition, rotavirus is detected using a solid-phase EIA procedure. EIA methods are also available for detection of antigens of *Cryptosporidium* and *Giardia lamblia* as well as *E. histolytica.* EIA methods have also been evaluated for detection of certain bacterial pathogens. The laboratory diagnosis of *Clostridium difficile* has been inadequate when using traditional EIAs. Newer kits are coupling glutamate dehydrogenase (GDH) and A/B toxin in a combination assay. However, the combination kits do not seem to be more specific than a GDH assay alone. Laboratories have demonstrated excellent sensitivity and specificity using the GDH assay followed with PCR for definitive confirmation.

### Molecular Biologic Techniques

The development of amplification techniques has led to numerous publications for the direct detection of many enteric pathogens, including all major organism groups—bacteria, viruses, and parasites. A disadvantage with probe technology is that the organism itself is not available for susceptibility testing, which is important for certain bacterial pathogens (e.g., *Shigella*) for which susceptibility patterns vary.

## CULTURE OF FECAL MATERIAL FOR ISOLATION OF ETIOLOGIC AGENTS

### Bacteria

Fecal specimens for culture should be inoculated to several media for maximal yield, including solid agar and broth. The choice of media is arbitrary and based on the particular requirements of the clinician and the laboratory. Recommendations for selection of media are included in this section.

**Organisms for Routine Culture.** Stools received for routine culture in most clinical laboratories in the United States should be examined for the presence of *Campylobacter, Salmonella,* and *Shigella* spp. under all circumstances. Detection of *Aeromonas* and *Plesiomonas* spp. should be incorporated into routine stool culture procedures. The cost of doing a stool examination on every patient for all potential enteric pathogens is prohibitive. The decision as to what other bacteria are routinely cultured should take into account the incidence of GI tract infections caused by particular etiologic agents in the area served by the laboratory. For example, if the incidence of *Yersinia enterocolitica* gastroenteritis is high enough in the area served by the laboratory, then this agent should also be sought routinely. Similarly, because of the increasing prevalence of disease caused by *Vibrio* spp. in individuals living in high-risk areas of the United States (sea coast), laboratories in these localities may routinely look for these organisms. Conversely, unless a patient has a significant travel history, a laboratory located in the Midwestern United States should not routinely look for these organisms except by special request. Protocols for culture of enterohemorrhagic *E. coli* (e.g., *E. coli* O157:H7) vary greatly; based on incidence of disease, laboratories routinely culture for this organism when cases of severe diarrhea are implicated. Selective or screening media to detect *E. coli* O157:H7 also vary greatly, including using a 1% sorbitol-containing medium (most O157:H7 *E. coli* are sorbitol-negative), a specific trypticase blood agar (Unipath GmbH, Wesel, Germany), RambaCHROM (Gibson Laboratories, LLC, Lexington, Ky), CHROMagar (BD Diagnostics, Franklin Lakes, N.J.) or Rainbow Agar O157 (Bio-log, Inc., Hayward, California).

**Routine Culture Methods.** An in-depth discussion regarding culture of all enteric pathogens is beyond the scope of this chapter. Because U.S. laboratories should routinely examine stools for the presence of *salmonella*, *Shigella*, and *Campylobacter* spp., culture of these organisms is addressed. Culture conditions for all other pathogens, including viruses, are covered in Parts III, IV, and VI. Specimens received for detection of the most frequently isolated Enterobacteriaceae and *Salmonella* and *Shigella* spp. should be plated to a supportive medium, a slightly selective and differential medium, and a moderately selective medium.

Blood agar (tryptic soy agar with 5% sheep blood) is an excellent general supportive medium. Blood agar medium allows growth of yeast species, staphylococci, and enterococci, in addition to gram-negative bacilli. The absence of normal gram-negative fecal flora or the presence of significant quantities of organisms such as *Staphylococcus aureus*, yeasts, and *Pseudomonas aeruginosa* can be evaluated. The use of blood agar also provides colonies for oxidase testing. Several colonies that do not resemble Pseudomonas from the third or fourth quadrant should be routinely screened for production of cytochrome oxidase. If numerous colonies are present, *Aeromonas*, *Vibrio*, or *Plesiomonas* spp. should be suspected.

The slightly selective agar should support growth of most Enterobacteriaceae, vibrios, and other possible pathogens; MacConkey agar works well. Some laboratories use eosin-methylene blue (EMB), which is slightly more inhibitory. All lactose-negative colonies should be tested further, ensuring adequate detection of most vibrios and most pathogenic Enterobacteriaceae. Lactose-positive vibrios *(V. vulnificus)*, pathogenic *E. coli*, some *Aeromonas* spp., and *Plesiomonas* spp. may not be distinctive on MacConkey agar.

**Salmonella/Shigella.** The specimen should also be inoculated to a moderately selective agar such as Hektoen enteric (HE) or xylose-lysine desoxycholate (XLD) media. These media inhibit growth of most Enterobacteriaceae, allowing *Salmonella* and *Shigella* spp. to be detected. Colony morphologies of lactose-negative, lactose-positive, and H$_2$S-producing organisms are illustrated in Figure 75-7. Other highly selective enteric media, such as salmonella-shigella, bismuth sulfite, deoxycholate, or brilliant green, may inhibit some strains of *Salmonella* or *Shigella*. All these media are incubated at 35° to 37°C in ambient air and examined at 24 and 48 hours for suspicious colonies.

**Campylobacter.** Cultures for isolation of *Campylobacter jejuni* and *Campylobacter coli* should be inoculated to a selective agar containing antimicrobial agents that suppress the growth of normal flora. The introduction of a blood-free, charcoal-containing medium containing selective antibiotic components has improved recovery of most enteropathogenic *Campylobacter* spp. Brucella broth base has yielded less satisfactory recovery of *Campylobacter* spp. Commercially produced agar plates for isolation of campylobacters are available from several manufacturers. These plates are incubated in a microaerophilic atmosphere at 42°C and examined at 24 and 48 hours for suspicious colonies. Culture methods for other campylobacters associated with GI disease, such as *C. hyointestinalis* and *C. fetus* subsp. fetus, are provided in Chapter 34.

**Enrichment Broths.** Enrichment broths are sometimes used for enhanced recovery of *Salmonella*, *Shigella*, *Campylobacter*, and *Y. enterocolitica*, although *Shigella* usually does not survive enrichment. Gram-negative broth (Hajna GN) or selenite F broth yields good recovery. Enrichment broths for Enterobacteriaceae should be incubated in air at 35°C for 6 to 8 hours and then several drops should be subcultured to at least two selective media. A commercial system that allows broth to be tested for antigen of *Salmonella* or *Shigella* directly has been described; however, the reported sensitivity is lower than desired. Stool would be inoculated to broth initially; those broths that test negative could be discarded without subculturing. Campy-thioglycollate enrichment broth increases the yields of positive cultures for *Campylobacter* spp., although it is not necessary for routine use. Enrichment broth for *Campylobacter* is refrigerated overnight or for a minimum of 8 hours before a few drops are plated to Campylobacter agar and incubated at 42°C in a microaerophilic atmosphere.

## LABORATORY DIAGNOSIS OF CLOSTRIDIUM DIFFICILE–ASSOCIATED DIARRHEA

The definitive diagnosis of *C. difficile*–associated diarrhea is based on clinical criteria combined with laboratory testing. Visualization of a characteristic pseudomembrane or plaque on endoscopy is diagnostic for pseudomembranous colitis and, with the appropriate history of prior antibiotic use, meets the criteria for diagnosis of antibiotic-associated pseudomembranous colitis. No single laboratory test will establish the diagnosis unequivocally. Two tests are available for routine use: culture, detection of cytotoxin by tissue culture, and antigen detection assays (e.g., enzyme immunoassay, latex agglutination) for *C. difficile* toxin. In addition, many laboratories are now using polymerase chain reaction and the technically less demanding loop-mediated isothermal amplification. Commercially available PCR assays include BD Gene Ohm (BD Diagnostics, La Jolla, CA), Cepheid Xpert (Cepheid, Sunnyvale, CA), Roche Lightcycler (Roche Applied Science), and Progastro (Hologic-Gen-Probe (San Diego, CA). According to a recent study, PCR demonstrates high sensitivity and specificity for the diagnosis of *C. difficile*-associated diarrhea. Insufficient data are not currently available to determine the diagnostic usefulness of LAMP; additional studies are needed.

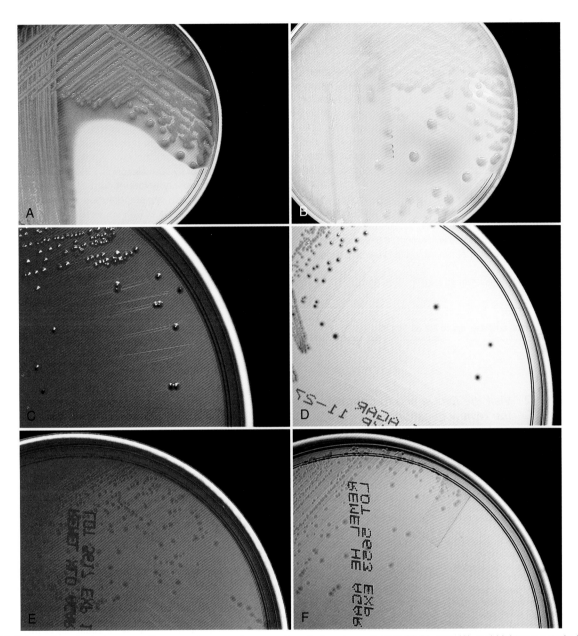

**Figure 75-7** Colonies of a lactose-positive organism growing on xylose-lysine deoxycholate (XLD) agar (**A**) and Hektoen enteric (HE) agar (**B**). Colonies of *Salmonella enteritidis* (lactose-negative) growing on XLD (**C**) and HE agar (**D**). (Note how both agars detect $H_2S$ production.) Colonies of *Shigella* (lactose-negative) growing on XLD (**E**) and HE agar (**F**).

## CASE STUDY 75-1

A 30-year-old man developed diarrhea with severe abdominal cramping 3 days after eating in a local restaurant. He became febrile and weak and went to his physician. A stool specimen was collected and immediately hand-carried to the laboratory. Numerous white blood cells and bacteria were seen in a wet mount, but the bacteria were noteworthy in that they were nonmotile. The patient was treated with ciprofloxacin. A culture was performed that grew a non-lactose-fermenting gram-negative rod that was identified as *Shigella sonnei*.

**QUESTIONS**

1. What agent of diarrhea becomes nonviable in a stool that has not been cultured within 30 minutes of collection?
2. If the culture is going to be delayed in transit, what preservative and storage temperature is best for preservation of the specimen?
3. What method is used to identify *Shigella* to the species level, and what is the importance of such identifications?

## CASE STUDY 75-2

A 52-year-old female on immune-suppressive therapy for rheumatoid arthritis presents with a 2-day history of severe, watery diarrhea. This is accompanied by chills and reported fever of 101° F. She has no complaints of nausea or myalgias, but she does have severe abdominal cramps and loss of appetite. She had recently visited her niece who had just purchased a pet turtle. She reports no other significant travel history or ill contacts and is treated with antidiarrheal medications as an outpatient.

On the third day of illness she returns in a worsening condition with the following physical exam and laboratory results:

- Vitals: Temp 102°F, respiration 20, BP 90/56, pulse 98
- Exam is essentially unremarkable with exception of diffusely tender abdomen; there is no rash or adenopathy, and the patient appears dehydrated
- WBC 16K (reference range 5 to $10 \times 10^9$/L ) with 82% granulocytes
- Hbg = 14.5
- Liver function tests: amylase, lipase are all normal

- Sodium is 144 (reference range 135 to 145 mEq/L)
- K = 3.0 (reference range 3.6 to 5.0 mEq/L)

She is admitted to the hospital for rehydration, potassium replacement, and additional investigation. The initial diagnosis is sepsis syndrome. Because diarrhea is the major feature of her illness, a stool sample is submitted for culture and fecal WBC count.

The patient rapidly convalesced by the second day of admission on empiric triple antibiotic therapy. While hospitalized, her niece became ill with severe diarrhea and was successfully treated as an outpatient.

### QUESTIONS

1. What is the likely agent of infection in this case?
2. Did the administration of antibiotics improve or worsen the patient's condition? Explain your answer.
3. Why did the niece recover so quickly, whereas the initial patient suffered a much more severe disease including dehydration and sepsis?

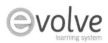 *Visit the Evolve site to complete the review questions.*

## BIBLIOGRAPHY

Abbott SL: Laboratory aspects of non-O157 toxigenic *E. coli, Clin Microbiol Newsl* 19:105, 1997.

Buvens G, Pierard D: Low prevalence of STEC autotransporter contributing to biofilm formation (Sab) in verocytotoxin-producing E. coli. isolates of humans and raw meats, *Eur J Clin Micro Infect Dis* 31(7):1463-1465, 2012.

Endtz HP, Ruijs GJ, Zwinderman AH, et al: Comparison of six media, including a semisolid agar, for the isolation of various *Campylobacter* species from stool specimens, *J Clin Microbiol* 29:1007, 1991.

Finlay BB, Falkow S: Salmonella interactions with polarized human intestinal Caco-2 epithelial cells, *J Infect Dis* 162:1096, 1990.

Galán JE, Ginocchio C, Costeas P: Molecular and functional characterization of the *Salmonella typhimurium* invasion gene invA: homology of invA to members of a new protein family, *J Bacteriol* 17:4338, 1992.

Gavin PJ, Thomson RB: Diagnosis of enterohemorrhagic *Esche-richia coli* infection by detection of Shiga toxins, *Clin Microbiol Newsl* 26:49, 2004.

Ginocchio C, Pace J, Galan JE: Identification and molecular characterization of a Salmonella typhimurium gene involved in triggering the internalization of Salmonellae into cultured epithelial cells, *Proc Natl Acad Sci U S A* 89:5976, 1992.

Goldenberg SD, Cliff PR, French GL: Glutamate dehydrogenase for laboratory diagnosis of *Clostridium difficile* infection, *J Clin Microbiol* 48:3050, 2010.

Guerrant RL: Bacterial and protozoal gastroenteritis, *N Engl J Med* 325:327, 1991.

Herwaldt BL, Beach MJ: The return of Cyclospora in 1997: another outbreak of cyclosporiasis in North America associated with imported raspberries, *Ann Intern Med* 130:210, 1999.

Kaplan BS: Commentary on the relationships between HUS and TTP. In Kaplan BS, et al, editors: *Hemolytic-uremic syndrome and thrombotic thrombocytopenic purpura*, New York, 1992, Marcel Dekker.

Kaye SA, Obrig TG: Pathogenesis of *E. coli* hemolytic-uremic syndrome, *Clin Microbiol Newsl* 18:49, 1996.

Kehl SC: Role of the laboratory in the diagnosis of entero-hemorrhagic *Escherichia coli* infections, *J Clin Microbiol* 40:2711, 2002.

Loo VG, Poirier L, Miller MA, et al: A predominantly clonal multi-institutional outbreak of *Clostridium difficile*-associated diarrhea with high morbidity and mortality, *N Engl J Med* 353:2442, 2005.

MacKenzie AM, Orrbine E, Hyde L, et al: Performance of the ImmunoCard STAT! *E. coli* O157:H7 test for detection of *Esche-richia coli* O157:H7 in stools, *J Clin Microbiol* 38:1866, 2000.

McDonald LC, Killgore GE, Thompson A, et al: An epidemic, toxin gene-variant of *Clostridium difficile, N Engl J Med* 353:2433, 2005.

Mundy LS, Shanholtzer CJ, Willard KE, et al: An evaluation of three commercial fecal transport systems for the recovery of enteric pathogens, *Am J Clin Pathol* 96:364, 1991.

Nataro JP, Kasper JB: Diarrheagenic *Escherichia coli, Clin Microbiol Rev* 11:142, 1998.

Novicki TJ, Daly JA, Mottice SL, et al: Comparison of sorbitol MacConkey agar and a two-step method which utilizes enzyme-linked immunosorbent assay toxin testing and a chromogenic agar to detect and isolate enterohemorrhagic *Escherichia coli, J Clin Microbiol* 38:547, 2000.

O'Horo JC, Jones A, Sternke M, et al: Molecular techniques for diagnosis of Clostridium difficile infection: systematic review and meta-analysis, *Mayo Clin Proc* 87(7):643-651, 2012.

Pal T, Pacsa AS, Emody L, et al: Modified enzyme-linked immunosorbent assay for detecting enteroinvasive *Escherichia coli* and virulent *Shigella* strains, *J Clin Microbiol* 26:948, 1985.

Park CH, Hixon DL, Morrison WL, Cook CB: Rapid diagnosis of entero-hemorrhagic *Escherichia coli* O157:H7 directly from fecal specimens using immunofluorescence stain, *Am J Clin Pathol* 101:91, 1994.

Sansonetti PJ: Genetic and molecular basis of epithelial cell invasion by *Shigella* species, *Rev Infect Dis* 13(suppl 4):S282, 1991.

Schmidt H, Hensel M: Pathogenicity islands in bacterial patho-genesis, *Clin Microbiol Rev* 17:14, 2004.

Sears CL, Kaper JB: Enteric bacterial toxins: mechanisms of action and linkage to intestinal secretion, *Microbiol Rev* 60:167, 1996.

Versalovic J. *Manual of clinical microbiology*, ed 10, Washington, DC, 2011, ASM Press.

Voth DE, Ballard JD: *Clostridium difficile* toxins: mechanisms of action and role in disease, *Clin Microbiol Rev* 18: 247, 2005.

Wilkins TD, Bartlett JG: *Clostridium difficile* testing: after 20 years, still challenging, *J Clin Microbiol* 41:531, 2003.

Zollner-Schwetz I, Hogenauer C, Joainig M, et al: Role of Klebsiella oxytoca in antibiotic-associated diarrhea, *Clin Infect Dis* 47(9):e74-e78, 2008.

# Skin, Soft Tissue, and Wound Infections

## OBJECTIVES

1. Identify the three layers of the skin and describe the function of the skin in host defense including the physical and chemical properties.
2. List the organisms that colonize the skin and are considered normal flora.
3. Describe the mechanisms for the transmission that allow bacteria to invade and cause skin and soft tissue infections.
4. Define each of the following manifestations of skin infection:
   - Macule
   - Papule
   - Nodule
   - Pustule
   - Vesicle
   - Bulla
   - Scales
   - Ulcer
5. Characterize each of the following types of infection, and describe the associated laboratory diagnosis:
   - Folliculitis
   - Furuncle
   - Carbuncle
   - Erysipelas
   - Erythrasma
   - Erysipeloid
   - Impetigo
   - Cellulitis
   - Dermatophytoses
   - Necrotizing fasciitis
   - Myositis
6. List an organism that commonly causes the following types of infection, and describe the associated laboratory diagnosis:
   - Postoperative
   - Bite
   - Burn
7. Define sinus tract, including organisms associated with this condition.
8. Identify the pathogens most frequently associated with infections in patients with diabetes mellitus.
9. Describe and evaluate a specimen submitted for culture from the following types of infection: ulcers, nodules or abscess, pyoderma or cellulitis, vesicles or bullae, sinus tracts, fistula, burns, postsurgical wounds, and bite infections.
10. Correlate patient signs and symptoms with laboratory results to identify the etiologic agent associated with the skin, soft tissue, or wound infection.

## GENERAL CONSIDERATIONS

The skin serves as a barrier between the internal organs and the external environment. Skin is often subjected to frequent trauma and therefore at frequent risk of infections. In addition, manifestations visible on the surface of the skin can also provide clues for the identification of an internal systemic disease.

## ANATOMY OF THE SKIN

The skin is divided into three distinct layers: the epidermis (the outermost layer), the dermis, and the subcutaneous tissue (Figure 76-1). The epidermis is made up of layered squamous epithelium. Hair follicles, sebaceous glands (oil-producing), and sweat glands open to the skin surface through the epidermis. The dermis is composed of dense connective tissue rich in blood and nerve endings, and this is where some hair follicles and sebaceous glands originate. The subcutaneous tissue contains loose connective tissue and is rich in fat. Deeper hair follicles and sweat gland originate in this layer. Below the subcutaneous layer are thin fascial membranes (sheets or bands of fibrous tissue) covering muscles, ligaments, and other connective tissues.

## FUNCTION OF THE SKIN

The skin is the body's largest and thinnest organ. It forms a self-repairing and protective boundary between the body's internal environment and the external environment. Skin plays a crucial role in the control of body temperature, excretion of water and salts, synthesis of important chemicals and hormones, and as a sensory organ. The skin has an important protective function because of the composition of the outermost layer of the epidermis, which is composed of cells containing keratin, a water-repellent protein. The skin's normal microbial flora, pH, and chemical defenses (high salt and acidic environment) also help prevent colonization by many pathogens. The resident microbial flora is listed in Box 76-1.

## PREVALENCE, ETIOLOGY, AND PATHOGENESIS

Approximately 15% of all patients who seek medical attention have either some skin disease or skin lesion, many of which are infectious. Various bacteria, fungi, and viruses may be involved. These infections can include one or several causative agents. Because of the diversity of etiologic agents and the potential complexity of these infections, only the most common infections involving the skin and subcutaneous tissues will be addressed.

Skin infections can arise from the invasion of certain organisms from the external environment through breaks in the skin or from organisms that reach the skin through the blood as part of a systemic disease. In some infections, such as staphylococcal scalded-skin syndrome, toxins produced by the bacteria cause skin lesions. In

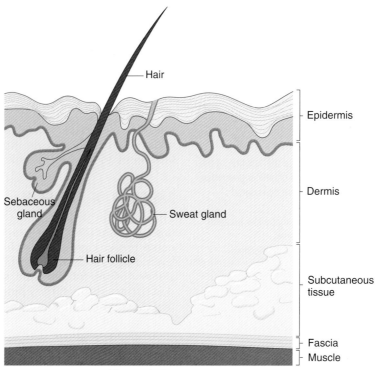

**Figure 76-1** Diagram of the skin.

---

BOX 76-1   Resident Microbial Flora of the Skin

Diphtheroids
*Staphylococcus epidermidis*
Other coagulase-negative staphylococci
*Propionibacterium acnes*

---

others, lesions are a result of the host's immune response to microbial antigens.

Because of the diversity of etiologic agents, clinicians will often rely on the appearance of skin lesions for diagnostic clues in order to determine the required laboratory testing. The physical characteristics of the lesions can indicate the need for smear, culture, biopsy, or surgical procedures. Some of the terms most frequently used to describe manifestations of skin infections are provided in Table 76-1. Figure 76-2 shows examples of some skin lesions.

# SKIN AND SOFT TISSUE INFECTIONS

## INFECTIONS OF THE EPIDERMIS AND DERMIS

Numerous infections of the skin may occur. Several of the most common are discussed here.

### Infections in or around Hair Follicles

Folliculitis, furuncles, and carbuncles are localized abscesses either in or around hair follicles. These infections are distinguished from one another based on size and the extent of involvement in subcutaneous tissues. Table 76-2 summarizes each infection's respective clinical

features. For the most part, these infections are precipitated by blockage of the hair follicle with skin oils (sebum) or because of minor trauma resulting from friction such as that caused by clothes rubbing the skin. *Staphylococcus aureus* is the most common etiologic agent for all three infections. Members of the Enterobacteriaceae family may also cause folliculitis. Outbreaks of folliculitis caused by *Pseudomonas aeruginosa* have been reported to be associated with the use of whirlpools, swimming pools, and hot tubs.

### Infections in the Keratinized Layer of the Epidermis

Because of their ability to utilize the keratin in the epidermal cells, the dermatophyte fungi are significant and well-suited pathogens for infection. Unlike the previously discussed infections, dermatophytes do not invade the deeper layers of skin. Because keratin is also present in hair and nails, these fungi may also cause superficial infections at these sites (see Chapter 61 for more information).

### Infections in the Deeper Layers of the Epidermis and Dermis

Most infections in the deeper layers of the epidermis and dermis result from the inoculation of microorganisms by traumatic breaks in the skin. These superficial skin infections usually do not require surgical intervention. Table 76-3 summarizes these infections. In most instances, these infections resolve with local care and only occasionally require antimicrobial therapy.

Cutaneous ulcers usually involve a loss of epidermal and part of the dermal tissues. In contrast, nodules are inflammatory foci in which the epidermal and dermal layers remain largely intact. Various bacteria and fungi can cause ulcerative or nodular skin lesions following

**TABLE 76-1** Manifestations of Skin Infections

| Term | Description | Possible Etiologic Agents (Infections) |
|---|---|---|
| Macule | A circumscribed (limited), flat discoloration of the skin | Dermatophytes<br>*Treponema pallidum* (secondary syphilis)<br>Viruses such as enteroviruses (exanthems rashes) |
| Papule | An elevated, solid lesion ≤5 mm in diameter | Human papillomavirus types 3 and 10 (flat warts)<br>Pox virus (Molluscum contagiosum)<br>*Sarcoptes scabiei* (scabies)<br>*S. aureus, P. aeruginosa*, etc. (folliculitis) |
| Nodule | A raised, solid lesion >5 mm in diameter | *Corynebacterium diphtheriae*<br>*Sporothrix schenckii*<br>Miscellaneous fungi (subcutaneous mycoses)<br>*Mycobacterium marinum*<br>*Nocardia* spp.<br>*S. aureus* (furuncle) |
| Pustule | A circumscribed, raised, pus-filled (leukocytes and fluid) lesion | *Candida* spp.<br>Dermatophytes<br>Herpes simplex virus<br>*Neisseria gonorrhoeae* (gonorrhea)<br>*S. aureus* (folliculitis)<br>*S. aureus* or group A streptococci (impetigo)<br>Varicella-zoster virus (chickenpox) |
| Vesicle | A circumscribed, raised, fluid-filled (blister-like) lesion ≤5 mm in diameter | Herpes simplex virus<br>Varicella-zoster virus (chickenpox and shingles) |
| Bulla | A circumscribed, raised, fluid-filled lesion >5 mm in diameter | Clostridial species (necrotizing gas gangrene)<br>Herpes simplex virus<br>Other gram-negative rods<br>*S. aureus* (bullous impetigo and scalded skin syndrome)<br>*Vibrio vulnificus* and other vibrios |
| Scales | Dry, horny, platelike lesions | Dermatophytes (tinea) |
| Ulcer | A lesion with loss of epidermis and dermis | *Bacillus anthracis* (cutaneous anthrax)<br>Bowel flora (decubiti)<br>*Haemophilus ducreyi* (chancroid)<br>*T. pallidum* (chancre of primary syphilis) |

Adapted from Lazar AJF: *Robbins Basic Pathology*, ed 8, St. Louis, 2007, Saunders.

**TABLE 76-2** Infections Involving Hair Follicles

| Infection | Skin Manifestations |
|---|---|
| Folliculitis—(minor infection of hair follicles) | Papules or pustules that are pierced by a hair and surrounded with redness |
| Furuncle (boil) | Abscess that begins as a red nodule in a hair follicle that ultimately becomes painful and full of pus |
| Carbuncle | Furuncles that coalesce and spread more deeply to the dermis and subcutaneous tissues; they usually have multiple sites, which drain to the skin surface (sinuses) |

direct traumatic inoculation. Examples of these causative agents include *Bacillus anthracis, Corynebacterium diphtheriae, Mycobacterium marinum, Nocardia* spp., and *Sporothrix schenckii.*

## INFECTIONS OF THE SUBCUTANEOUS TISSUES

Infections of the subcutaneous tissues may manifest as abscesses, ulcers, or boils. The most common etiologic agent of subcutaneous abscesses in healthy individuals is *S. aureus.* Many subcutaneous abscesses contain mixed bacteria. To a large degree, the organisms isolated from these abscesses depend on the site of infection. For example, anaerobes are commonly isolated from abscesses of the perineal, inguinal, and buttock area, whereas nonperineal infection is commonly caused by a mixed infection containing facultative organisms.

Progressive synergistic gangrene, or Meleney's ulcer, is a slowly progressive infection of the subcutaneous tissue that usually begins as an ulcer following trauma or surgery. The infection leads to subcutaneous necrosis and enlargement of a visible ulcer. This is a true

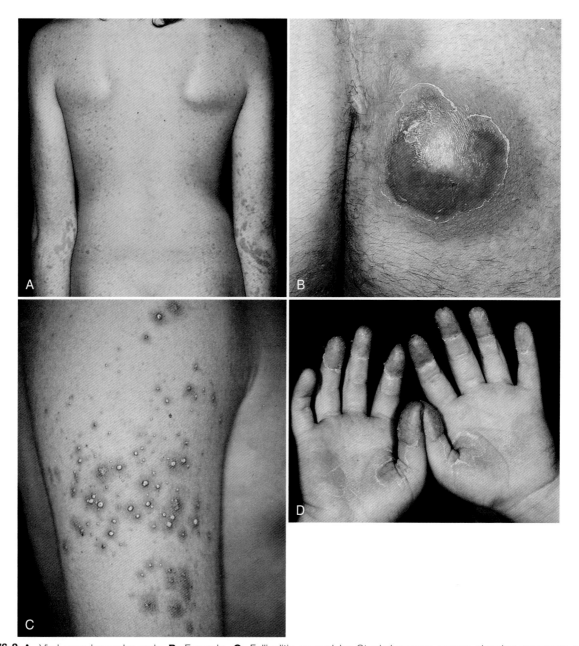

**Figure 76-2 A,** Viral maculopapular rash. **B,** Furuncle. **C,** Folliculitis caused by *Staphylococcus aureus* showing numerous pustules. **D,** Desquamation (shedding or scaling) of the skin resulting from scarlet fever caused by group A streptococci. (**A** and **D** from Habif TB: *Clinical dermatology: a color guide to diagnosis and therapy,* ed 3, St. Louis, 1996, Mosby.)

polymicrobial infection in which microaerophilic streptococci grow synergistically with *S. aureus*. The infection may also include other facultative or anaerobic organisms.

In many instances, infections of the epidermis and dermis extend deeper and become subcutaneous infections and may even reach the fascia or muscle. For example, erysipelas (Figure 76-3) can develop into subcutaneous cellulitis and eventually necrotizing fasciitis. Similarly, folliculitis can readily develop into a subcutaneous abscess or carbuncle that can extend to the fascia. Cellulitis can also extend to the subcutaneous tissues (Figure 76-4). Anaerobic cellulitis is associated with the production of large amounts of gas by organisms that may be present in the subcutaneous tissue. This type of

infection is most often located in the extremities and is particularly common among patients with diabetes. The infection may involve the neck, abdominal wall, perineum, connective tissue, or be present in other areas. Anaerobic cellulitis may also occur as a postoperative condition. The onset and spread of the lesion is usually slow and patients may not immediately show obvious systemic effects. The causative agents in deep tissue infections are almost always a mixture of aerobic/facultative and anaerobic organisms. Common aerobic/facultative organisms include *Escherichia coli*, alpha-hemolytic and nonhemolytic streptococci, and *S. aureus*, but group A streptococci and other members of the Enterobacteriaceae may be encountered as well. The anaerobes are typically found in greater numbers and in more variety, and include

**TABLE 76-3** Infections of the Epidermal and Dermal Layers of the Skin

| Infection | Key Features of Infection | Etiologies | Other Comments |
|---|---|---|---|
| Erysipelas | Primarily involves the dermis and most superficial parts of the subcutaneous tissue; lesions are painful, red, swollen, and indurated; patients are febrile, and regional lymphadenopathy (swollen glands) is often present; lesion has a marked, well-demarcated, raised border (see Figure 76-3) | Group A streptococci (*Streptococcus pyogenes* [sometimes groups B, C, or G streptococci]) | Infants, children, and elderly individuals are most affected; primarily a clinical diagnosis |
| Erythrasma | Chronic infection of the keratinized layer of the epidermis; lesions are dry, scaly, itchy, and reddish brown | *Corynebacterium minutissimum*— possible cause | Common in diabetics; resembles dermatophyte infection |
| Erysipeloid | Purplish-red, nonvesiculated skin lesion with an irregular, raised border; the lesions itch and burn; fever and other systemic symptoms are uncommon | *Erysipelothrix rhusiopathiae* | Uncommon; considered an occupational disease |
| Impetigo | Erythematous (red) lesions that may be bullous (less common) or nonbullous | Nonbullous—group A streptococci (*Streptococcus pyogenes*) Bullous—*Staphylococcus aureus* | |
| Cellulitis | Diffuse, spreading infection involving the deeper layers of the dermis; lesions are ill-defined, flat, painful, red, and swollen; patients have fever, chills, and regional lymphadenopathy (see Figure 76-4) | Commonly: Group A streptococci, *Staphylococcus aureus* Less common: *Aeromonas, Vibrio* spp., and *Hemophilus influenzae* (typically affects young children) | Primarily a clinical diagnosis |
| Dermatophytoses | Superficial fungal infections of the skin and its appendages (i.e., ringworm, athlete's foot, jock itch, as well as infections of nails and hair) | *Epidermophyton, Microsporum,* and *Trichophyton*, spp. | |
| Hidradenitis | Chronic infection of obstructed apocrine (sweat) glands in the axillas, genital, or perianal areas with intermittent discharge of often foul-smelling pus | *S. aureus, Streptococcus anginosus* group, anaerobic streptococci, and *Bacteroides* spp. | |
| Infected pilonidal tuft cyst or hairs | Pain and swelling, redness | Anaerobes, including *Bacteroides fragilis* group, *Prevotella, Fusobacterium*, anaerobic gram-positive cocci, and *Clostridium* spp. | |

*Peptostreptococcus* spp., *Bacillus fragilis* group strains, *Prevotella, Porphyromonas,* other anaerobic gram-negative bacilli, and clostridia. Bacteremia is not usually present.

# INFECTIONS OF THE MUSCLE FASCIA AND MUSCLES

There are several uncommon, yet serious or potentially serious, forms of deep and often extensive soft tissue and skin infections.

## Necrotizing Fasciitis

Necrotizing fasciitis is a serious infection that occurs relatively infrequently. The basic pathology involves infection of the fascia overlying the muscles, often with involvement of the overlying soft tissue. At the fascial level, no barrier exists to prevent the spread of infection, so fasciitis may extend widely and rapidly to involve large areas of the body in a short amount of time. This process typically involves group A streptococci or *S. aureus*. Necrotizing fasciitis frequently involves anaerobic bacteria, especially *Bacteroides* and *Clostridium* species.

## Progressive Bacterial Synergistic Gangrene

Progressive bacterial synergistic gangrene is usually a chronic necrotic condition of the skin most often encountered as a postoperative complication, particularly after abdominal or thoracic surgery. The lesions may be extensive and, with involvement of the abdominal wall, may lead to evisceration (extrusion of the internal organs). As the name implies, this is a synergistic mixed infection with microaerophilic streptococci and *S. aureus*. Other organisms may also be present, including anaerobic streptococci, *Proteus*, and other facultative and anaerobic bacteria. This infection occurs infrequently. Cultures should be taken from the advancing outer edge of the lesion (not the central portion of the wound). This prevents missing cultivation of microaerophilic streptococci that may be involved in the infection.

## Myositis

Myositis (inflammation of muscle) can be caused by a variety of organisms. The nature of the pathologic process is variable, sometimes involving extensive necrosis of muscle or focal collections of suppuration in muscle

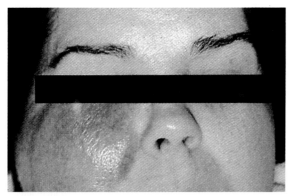

**Figure 76-3** Erysipelas caused by group A streptococci.

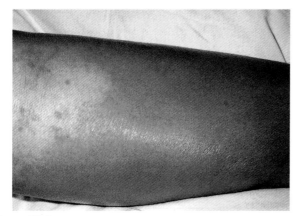

**Figure 76-4** Cellulitis. (From Farrar WE, et al: *Infectious diseases: text and color atlas*, ed 2, London, 1992, Mosby-Wolfe.)

**BOX 76-2** Organisms Producing Myositis or Other Muscle Pathology

*Clostridium perfringens*
*C. novyi*
*C. septicum*
*C. bifermentans*
*C. histolyticum*
*C. sordellii*
*C. sporogenes*
*Bacillus* spp.
*Aeromonas* spp.
*Peptostreptococcus* spp.
Microaerobic streptococci
*Bacteroides* spp.
Enterobacteriaceae
*Staphylococcus aureus*
Group A streptococci (*Streptococcus pyogenes*)
*Pseudomonas mallei*
*P. pseudomallei*
*Vibrio vulnificus*
*Mycobacterium tuberculosis*
*Salmonella typhi*
*Legionella* spp.
*Rickettsia* spp.
Viruses
*Trichinella*
*Taenia solium*
*Toxoplasma*

(pyomyositis). The most common cause of acute bacterial myositis from hematogenous spread is *S. aureus*. Categories of bacterial myositis include pyomyositis, psoas abscess, *S. aureus* myositis, group A streptococcal necrotizing myositis, group B streptococcal myositis, clostridial gas gangrene, and nonclostridial myositis. Serious vascular problems resulting from loss of blood supply may lead to death of muscle tissue, leading to a secondary infection (vascular gangrene). Organisms that cause myositis or other muscle pathology are listed in Box 76-2.

## WOUND INFECTIONS

Besides skin and soft tissue infections, wound infections occur primarily from breaks in the skin as a result of complications associated with surgery, trauma, and bites, or from diseases that interrupt the mucosal or skin surface.

### Postoperative Infections

Surgical site infections are among the most common nosocomial infections and occur after nearly 3% of all surgical procedures. Sources of surgical wound infections can include the patient's normal flora or organisms present in the hospital environment. These organisms are introduced to the patient by medical procedures or underlying disease or trauma (e.g., burns). The nature of the infecting flora depends on the patient's underlying condition and the location of the medical treatment

or procedure. The most common organism involved in postoperative infections is *S. aureus*. Surgical procedures in the colorectal or other lower gastrointestinal areas have the highest incidence of postoperative infections because of the presence of intestinal flora. These infections are most likely to be caused by enteric gram-negative bacteria, anaerobes, and enterococci. Principal pathogens are listed in Box 76-3.

### Bites

Human bite (Figure 76-5) infections can be attributed to occlusion bites or closed-fist injuries. Not surprisingly, the most commonly isolated organisms are normal oral flora. Most commonly isolated are viridans streptococci (particularly *S. anginosus*), *S. aureus*, and *Eikenella corrodens*. Common anaerobes isolated include *Prevotella*, *Fusobacterium*, *Veillonella*, and *Peptostreptococcus* species. These infections are usually polymicrobial and contain both aerobic and anaerobic organisms.

The most common animal bites are from domestic cats and dogs. Bites from these animals (Figure 76-6) usually are infected with organisms commonly found in the animal's oral and nasal fluids. The most frequently isolated aerobes are *Pasteurella*, *Streptococcus*, and *Staphylococcus* species. The most frequently isolated anaerobes are *Fusobacterium*, *Bacteroides*, and *Porphyromonas* species. Similar to human bites, animal bite wound infections are usually polymicrobial and include aerobes and anaerobes. Other far less common animal bites may also become infected. Rat bite infections are usually caused by *Streptobacillus moniliformis*. Snakebites may become infected with *Aeromonas hydrophilia*.

## Burns

Infected burn wounds may be associated with many organisms, causing significant mortality, and may interfere with the success of skin grafts. Burn wound infections are caused by bacteria (70%), fungi (20%-25%), and anaerobic organisms and viruses (5%-10%). Burn wound infections can commonly be identified as four types: impetigo, surgical infections, cellulitis, and invasive, systemic infections. Factors that contribute to the development of infection include loss of the skin barrier, coagulated proteins and other microbial nutrients, loss of vascularity of the wound, dehydration of surrounding tissue, and the inflammatory response of the patient's immune system. The organisms isolated most frequently from burns include *S. aureus*, *P. aeruginosa*, enterococci, *Enterobacter* spp., and *E. coli*. Other organisms such as fungi (e.g. *Candida* spp., *Aspergillus niger*, Fusarium spp., and Mucor spp.) and viruses may also be involved in invasive burn infections.

### Special Circumstances Regarding Skin and Soft Tissue Infections

In addition to the infections previously discussed, other circumstances can cause skin and underlying soft tissue to become infected. Some of these infections are associated with an immunocompromised host; others are manifestations of systemic infection.

### Infections Related to Vascular and Neurologic Problems

Frequently, a patient with infections associated with vascular or neurologic problems has diabetes mellitus. These patients have a high risk of developing infections, especially in their lower extremities. The excess glucose present in their blood can result in impaired microvascular circulation and peripheral motor neuropathy, leading to an increased risk of infection. Any skin-damaging injury or surgery greatly increases that risk. In addition, because of the complications associated with impaired circulation and neuropathy, the infected tissue of a diabetic patient does not heal as rapidly as that of a healthy individual. An estimated 25% of adults with diabetes will develop a foot infection, and the risk increases with age. Foot infections can lead to amputations and greatly increased mortality. Periodically, an acute cellulitis and lymphangitis may be associated with chronic, low-grade infection, thereby making control of the patient's diabetes difficult. Peripheral vascular disease unrelated to diabetes may also predispose a patient to skin and soft tissue infections, but usually these infections are easier to manage because there is no associated neuropathy.

Foot infections in diabetic patients can accelerate dramatically with devastating consequences without proper treatment. Therefore, appropriate techniques used to obtain a microbiologic sample are critical. Culture of aspirated fluid or pus, not surface swabbing, is more likely to yield a causative agent, particularly if taken from a deep pocket within the wound. In addition, culture of debrided infected tissue improves the diagnosis of these infections. The most common bacteria isolated from mild to moderate diabetic foot infections include *S. aureus*, group B streptococci, members of the Enterobacteriaceae, and

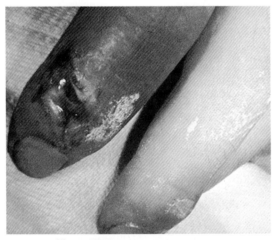

**Figure 76-5** Human bite infection.

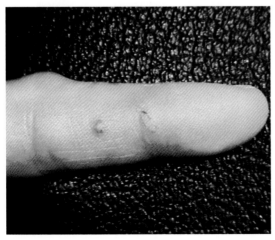

**Figure 76-6** Animal bite infection caused by *Pasteurella* spp.

anaerobes. More severe infections are usually polymicrobial. Extension of the infection into the underlying bone produces a difficult-to-manage osteomyelitis. Definitive diagnosis of this infection requires a specimen of bone obtained during open or percutaneous biopsy.

Venous insufficiency may also predispose an individual to infection, again primarily in the lower extremities (often in the calf or lower leg rather than the foot). Infections related to poor blood supply often involve *S. aureus* and group A streptococci. Those with open ulcers may become colonized with Enterobacteriaceae and *P. aeruginosa*. Anaerobes are also frequently involved in these infections, as a result of the blood supply creating anaerobic conditions. Anaerobes that may be involved include *Bacteroides fragilis* group, *Prevotella*, *Porphyromonas*, *Peptostreptococcus*, and, less frequently, *Clostridium* species.

Another common type of infection in this general category, especially in the elderly or chronically ill, bedridden patient, is infected decubitus ulcer (pressure sore; Figure 76-7). Anaerobic conditions are present in the lesions as a result of tissue necrosis. Most of these lesions are located near the anus or on the lower extremities. Because these patients are relatively helpless and have limited mobility, the ulcers may become contaminated with gastrointestinal flora, leading to chronic infection. These conditions contribute to further death of tissue and extension of the decubitus ulcer. Bacteremia is a possible complication, with *B. fragilis* group often involved, along with clostridia and other enteric bacteria. Nosocomial pathogens such as *S. aureus* and *P. aeruginosa* may also be recovered.

### Sinus Tracts and Fistulas

Sometimes, a deep-seated infection will develop a channel, called a sinus tract, to the skin surface. The sinus tract will drain fluid and pus onto the skin. The infections involved are often chronic and may include osteomyelitis. The organisms frequently involved in sinus tract formation with an underlying osteomyelitis include *S. aureus*, various members of the Enterobacteriaceae, *P. aeruginosa*, anaerobic gram-negative bacilli and anaerobic gram-positive cocci. In the case of actinomycosis (Figure 76-8), with or without bone involvement, the organisms involved include *Actinomyces* spp., *Aggregatibacter actinomycetemcomitans*, *Propionibacterium propionicum*, *Prevotella* or *Porphyromonas* species, and other non-spore-forming anaerobes. Chronic draining sinuses may also be found in patients with tuberculosis and atypical mycobacterial infection, *Nocardia* infection, and infections associated with implanted foreign bodies. Curetting or biopsy specimens from the debrided, cleansed sinus should be used for culture.

Abnormal channels connecting epithelial surfaces, either between two internal organs or between an organ and the skin epithelium, are known as fistulas. Infections associated with fistulas often pose insurmountable problems in terms of collection of a meaningful specimen because the organ involved may contain indigenous flora. Examples include perirectal fistulas from the small bowel to the skin associated with Crohn's disease or chronic intra-abdominal infection. When the bowel is involved, cultures for specific organisms, such as mycobacteria or *Actinomyces*, are useful. An attempt should always be made

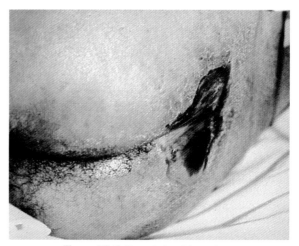

**Figure 76-7** Sacral decubitus ulcer.

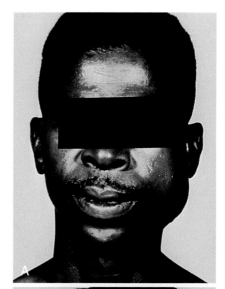
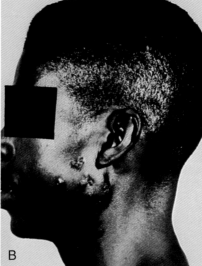

**Figure 76-8** Actinomycosis. **A,** Note "lumpy jaw." **B,** Side view. Note sinuses in skin of face and neck.

to rule out specific associated underlying causes such as tuberculosis, actinomycosis, and malignancy. A biopsy should be performed in these situations.

### Systemic Infections and Skin Manifestations

Cutaneous manifestations of systemic infections, such as bacteremia or endocarditis, may be important clues for the clinician. These represent an opportunity for direct detection or culture for the presence of a particular organism. For example, a scraping of petechiae (tiny red hemorrhagic spots in the skin) from patients with meningococcemia may demonstrate the presence of gram-negative diplococci. In other patients, the skin lesion may represent a metastatic infection. In *Vibrio vulnificus* sepsis, dramatic-appearing cutaneous ulcers with necrotizing vasculitis or bullae may be seen (Figure 76-9). In some patients, skin lesions may actually represent a noninfectious complication of a local or systemic infection such as scarlet fever or toxic shock syndrome. Various organisms involved in systemic infections capable of producing cutaneous lesions are listed in Box 76-4.

## LABORATORY DIAGNOSTIC PROCEDURES

### INFECTIONS OF THE EPIDERMIS AND DERMIS

For many of the infections of the epidermis and dermis, such as impetigo, folliculitis, cellulitis, and erysipelas, diagnosis is generally based on clinical observations. Table 76-3 provides the key features and etiologic agents of these infections.

#### Erysipeloid

Usually, a Gram stain or culture of superficial wound drainage is negative. However, culture of a full-thickness skin biopsy taken at the margin of the lesion can confirm the clinical diagnosis.

#### Superficial Mycoses and Erythrasma

If a dermatophyte infection is suspected, the lesion is cleaned and scrapings are obtained from the active border of the lesion. These scrapings should be treated with 10% potassium hydroxide and examined for the presence of hyphae. The specimen may also be cultured if necessary (see Chapter 60). A Wood's lamp examination of the skin lesions for tinea versicolor may show golden-yellow fluorescence.

Erythrasma, which is caused by infection with *Corynebacterium minutissimum*, can be diagnosed by making smears from the lesion revealing gram-positive pleomorphic bacilli. If necessary, skin scrapings may be cultured in media containing serum. Wood's lamp examination of these skin lesions may reveal a coral red fluorescence resulting from the production of porphyrin by *C. minutissimum*.

#### Erysipelas and Cellulitis

As previously mentioned, diagnosis of erysipelas and cellulitis can generally be made on the basis of clinical observation. Swab specimens from bullae, pustules, or ulcers

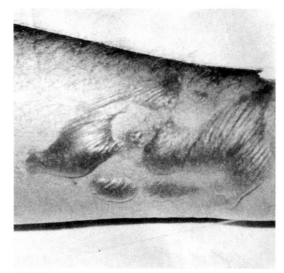

**Figure 76-9** Bullae on the arm of a patient with *Vibrio vulnificus* sepsis. (From Pollak SJ, Parrish EF III, Barrett TJ, et al: *Vibrio vulnificus* septicemia: isolation of organism from stool and demonstration of antibodies by direct immunofluorescence, *Arch Intern Med* 143:837, 1983. Copyright 1983, American Medical Association.)

---

**BOX 76-4** Organisms Involved in Systemic Infection with Cutaneous Lesions

Viridans streptococci
*Staphylococcus aureus*
Enterococci
Group A and other beta-hemolytic streptococci
*Neisseria gonorrhoeae*
*N. meningitidis*
*Haemophilus influenzae*
*Pseudomonas aeruginosa*
*P. mallei*
*P. pseudomallei*
*Listeria monocytogenes*
*Vibrio vulnificus*
*Salmonella typhi*
*Mycobacterium tuberculosis*
*M. leprae*
*Treponema pallidum*
*Leptospira*
*Streptobacillus moniliformis*
*Bartonella bacilliformis*
*Bartonella* (Rochalimaea) *henselae*
*Rickettsia*
*Candida* spp.
*Cryptococcus neoformans*
*Blastomyces dermatitidis*
*Coccidioides immitis*
*Histoplasma capsulatum*

---

may be cultured. Culturing of needle aspiration or punch biopsy specimens is not recommended and rarely informative. Blood cultures are also most often negative.

#### Vesicles and Bullae

These fluid-filled lesions characteristically involve specific organisms (see Table 76-1). Material in a blister-like lesion may vary from serous (resembling serum) fluid to serosanguineous (composed of serum and blood) fluid or hemorrhagic (bloody) fluid. Large bullae may permit withdrawal of fluid by needle and syringe aspiration. Specimens from tiny vesicles may need to be collected with a swab. The clinician can usually anticipate whether the lesion is viral or bacterial and may even suspect a particular organism. Specimens should be submitted for viral or bacterial culture based on the clinical presentation.

Bullous lesions are often associated with sepsis, requiring the collection of blood cultures. Gas gangrene caused by *Clostridium perfringens* and other clostridia is characterized by bronzed skin with bullous lesions. Gram stain of the fluid from the lesions typically reveals gram-positive bacilli.

## INFECTIONS OF THE SUBCUTANEOUS TISSUES

Proper collection and transport of specimens are important factors in the laboratory diagnosis of all infections. Specimen collection for the diagnosis of subcutaneous tissue infection is particularly difficult because many of these lesions are open and readily colonized by nosocomial pathogens that may not be involved in the systemic, underlying infection. The most reliable specimens for determining the etiology of ulcers and nodules are those obtained from the base of the ulcer or nodule following removal of overlying debris, or by surgical biopsy of deep tissues avoiding contact with the superficial layers of the lesion. A Gram stain of the specimen should be performed and material aerobically cultured on blood and MacConkey agar. If fungi, *Nocardia* spp., or mycobacterial infection is suspected, appropriate fungal media or mycobacterial media should be used. These culture methods are addressed in greater detail in Chapters 60 and 41, respectively.

Similar issues are faced when trying to collect material for culture from sinus tracts. The material should be obtained from the deepest portion of the sinus tract. If systemic symptoms such as fever are present, blood cultures should also be collected. A Gram stain should be routinely performed. Cultures should be inoculated to recover both facultative and anaerobic bacteria in the same manner as for surgical wounds. Molecular assays may be used to directly identify organisms such as *S. aureus* in wound infections. In addition, when deep tissue or bone infections are suspected and yield negative culture results, molecular assays may provide assistance in the identification of the infectious agent.

## INFECTIONS OF THE MUSCLE FASCIA AND MUSCLES

Blood cultures should always be collected from patients with significant myonecrosis. Transport of material (tissue is recommended, followed by purulent material, and then a swab) should be under anaerobic conditions.

Gram stains should be routinely performed. Cultures should be inoculated to recover both facultative and anaerobic bacteria in the same manner as for surgical wounds.

## WOUND INFECTIONS

### Postoperative

Because anaerobic bacteria are involved in many of these infections, specimen collection should be careful to avoid indigenous flora. Specimen transport in anaerobic conditions is essential. Unusual organisms associated with postsurgical wound infections, such as *Mycoplasma hominis*, *Mycobacterium chelonae*, *Mycobacterium fortuitum*, fungi, and even *Legionella* spp., should not be overlooked. A Gram-stained smear of material submitted for culture should be examined. Exudates from superficial wounds should routinely be inoculated to blood, MacConkey, and Colistin-nalidixic acid (CNA) agars, as well as an enrichment broth. Material from deep wounds should be inoculated onto media for both anaerobic and aerobic cultures. More detailed information regarding the processing of specimens for anaerobic cultures is presented in Chapters 41 and 42.

### Bites

Bite wound infections usually involve relatively small lesions and minimal exudate. A swab specimen in anaerobic transport media is usually appropriate. Surrounding skin should be thoroughly disinfected before the specimen is obtained. The best material for culture is purulent exudate aspirated from the depth of the wound or samples obtained during surgery involving incision and drainage or debridement (removal of all dead and necrotic tissue). Gram-stained smears should be prepared and examined. For aerobic cultures, a minimum of blood, MacConkey and chocolate agar should be inoculated.

### Burns

For many burn patients, diagnosis of infection is based on clinical symptoms, signs, and examination of the burn wound. When possible, cultures should be performed on any purulent wound exudates, and blood cultures should also be collected. Surface specimens should be collected with a moistened sterile swab using a minimal amount of pressure. Sometimes a quantitative or semiquantitative culture (see Procedure 76-1 on the Evolve site) of a tissue biopsy specimen is used for infection surveillance or to identify the most prevalent organism in a polymicrobial infection. This type of culture is reported in colony-forming units (CFUs) per gram of tissue, with a result of $\geq 10^5$ CFUs/g indicative of a potentially serious infection.

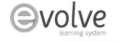 *Visit the Evolve site to complete the review questions.*

## CASE STUDY 76-1

A 59-year-old female teacher presented with swelling and pain in an injured left hand and enlarged lymph nodes in the axial region of her left arm. Her hand was injured when she stopped on her way home from school to rescue a small kitten that had wandered into the road. When she attempted to pick up the frightened kitten, it scratched her left hand. A specimen for culture was obtained by aspiration from the wound. A Gram stain showed small, gram-negative bacilli. The culture showed no growth on blood and MacConkey agar and sparse growth on chocolate agar.

**QUESTIONS**

1. The isolate was oxidase negative and catalase negative. Given this information, what is the suspected causative bacterium?
2. What would be the expected results if urease and nitrate reductase tests were performed?
3. What serology tests could be performed to identify this bacterium?

## CASE STUDY 76-2

A 45-year-old female presented to the clinic with complaint of a painful skin lesion on her back. This developed spontaneously 24 hours earlier. One month prior, she had a similar lesion on her thigh that was treated successfully with a sulfa drug but was not cultured.

Evaluation revealed no fever and she appeared to be in mild distress. Laboratory results revealed the following: CBC: WBC 12K, HGB 13K, HCT 39, PLTS 325K.

The abscess was drained. A Gram stain of the thick, cream-colored purulent drainage revealed gram-positive cocci in clusters. The lesion was thoroughly irrigated and the patient was started on oral sulfa antimicrobial therapy. The lesion resolved, and the woman returned 2 months later with another lesion.

**QUESTIONS**

1. Given the patient's clinical presentation and previous complaint of a lesion on her thigh, what would be the suspected infecting organism?
2. Because of the recurring nature of her infection, how would the physician determine if the patient was colonized with the organism?

## CASE STUDY 76-3

A 50-year-old man presented with extreme pain in his left thigh. He had an elevated measurement of creatine phosphokinase (CPK), an enzyme found predominantly in the heart, brain, and skeletal muscle. When the CPK is elevated, it usually indicates injury or stress to one or more of these areas. His heart muscle CPK fraction was normal. A biopsy specimen was collected by fine-needle aspiration. Gram stain showed gram-positive rods with subterminal spores. The aerobic culture was sterile, but the anaerobic culture grew a pure culture of bacteria with the same Gram stain morphology as seen in the direct smear. The colony had irregular edges like a medusa head; a film of growth swarmed over the entire plate by 24 hours (Figure 76-10).

**QUESTIONS**

1. The isolate was indole negative. Given this information, what are the genus and species of these bacteria?
2. What does the positive test for CPK indicate in this patient?
3. Infections with *C. septicum* are an indication of what underlying diseases?

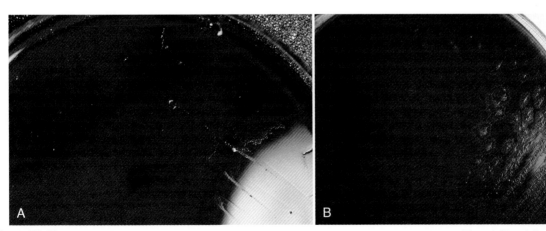

**Figure 76-10** Demonstration of the swarming film of growth of *Clostridium septicum* at 24 hours (**A**) and *Clostridium sporogenes* (**B**).

# ▤ BIBLIOGRAPHY

Bailey E, Kroshinsky D: Cellulitis: diagnosis and management, *Dermatol Ther* 24(2):229-239, 2011.

Buchanan K, Heimbach DM, Minshew BH, et al: Comparison of quantitative and semi quantitative culture techniques for burn biopsy, *J Clin Microbiol* 23:258, 1986.

Capoor MR, Sarabahi S, Tiwari VK, et al: Fungal infections in burns: diagnosis and management, *Indian J Plast Surg* 43(suppl):S37-S42, 2010.

Crum-Cianflone NF: Bacterial, fungal, parasitic, and viral myositis, *Clin Microbiol Rev* 21(3):473-494, 2008.

Humphreys H: Preventing and controlling the risk of post-operative surgical-site infections, *Eur Infect Dis* 2(2):110-112, 2008.

Lazar, AJF: The skin. *In Robbins basic pathology*, ed 8, St. Louis, 2007, Saunders.

Levy PY, Fenollar F: The role of molecular diagnostics in implant-associated bone and joint infection, *Clin Microbiol Infect* 18(12):1168-1175, 2012.

Lipsky BA: Medical treatment of diabetic foot infections, *Clin Infect Dis* 39(S2):S104-114, 2004.

Mayhall CG: The epidemiology of burn wound infections: then and now, *Clin Infect Dis* 37(4):543-550, 2003.

Mena KD, Gerba CP: Risk assessment of Pseudomonas aeruginosa in water, *Rev Environ Contam Toxicol* 201:71-115, 2006.

Murphy E: Microbiology of animal bites, *Clin Microbiol Newsl* 30(7):47-50, 2008.

ODell P, Corsten M: Postoperative Meleney's ulcer, *J Otolaryngol* 27(2):97-99, 1998.

Oehler RL, Velez AP, Mizrachi M, et al: Bite-related and septic syndromes caused by cats and dogs, *Lancet Infect Dis* 9(7):439-447, 2009.

Polavarapu N, Ogilvie MP, Panthaki ZJ: Microbiology of burn wound infections, *J Craniofac Surg* 19(4):899-902, 2008.

Salkind AR, Rao KC: Antibiotic prophylaxis to prevent surgical site infections, *Am Fam Physician* 83(5):585-590, 2011.

Talan AD, Abrahamian FM, Moran GJ, et al: Clinical presentation and bacteriologic analysis of infected human bites in patients presenting to emergency departments, *Clin Infect Dis* 37(11):1481-1489, 2003.

Williams DT, Hilton JR, Harding KG: Diagnosing foot infection in diabetes, *Clin Infect Dis* 39(S2):S83-86, 2004.

# Normally Sterile Body Fluids, Bone and Bone Marrow, and Solid Tissues

## OBJECTIVES

1. Describe the fine main cavities of the human body; also name the membranes associated with these cavities and state the function of these membranes.
2. Define each of the following body cavity fluids, and explain the diagnostic culture methods for each: pleural fluid, pericardial fluid, peritoneal fluid, joint fluid, and dialysis fluid.
3. Define parietal and visceral pleura.
4. Define cellulitis; name the etiologic agents of this illness, and explain the associated risk factors for the development of disease.
5. Define pleural effusion; explain the difference between exudative pleural effusion and transudative pleural effusion.
6. Explain when a pleural effusion becomes an empyema and what medical condition contributes to the development of an empyema?
7. Define pericarditis and myocarditis; explain the physical conditions that may contribute to the accumulation of pericardial fluid.
8. Define peritonitis and differentiate between primary and secondary peritonitis.
9. Name the etiologic agents most commonly isolated from primary peritonitis cases in children, adults, sexually active females, and immunocompromised patients.
10. Define osteomyelitis; explain how this infection is transmitted, the diagnostic method, and the organisms most frequently responsible for this type of infection.
11. Explain the process for culturing organisms from the following specimens: bone, tissue, and bone marrow.
12. Correlate patient signs and symptoms with laboratory results to identify the etiologic agent associated with the body fluid, bone and bone marrow, and other solid tissue infection.

The human body is divided into five main body cavities: cranial, spinal, thoracic, abdominal, and pelvic. Each cavity is lined with membranes, and within the body wall and these membranes, or between the membranes and organs, are small spaces filled with minute amounts of fluid. The purpose of this fluid is to bathe the organs and membranes, reducing the friction between organs.

Bacteria, fungi, virus, or parasite can invade any body tissue or sterile body fluid site. Although from different areas of the body, all specimens discussed in this chapter are considered normally sterile. Therefore, even one colony of a potentially pathogenic microorganism may be significant. (Refer to Table 5-1 for a quick guide regarding collection, transport, and processing of specimens from sterile body sites.)

## SPECIMENS FROM STERILE BODY SITES

### FLUIDS

In response to infection, fluid may accumulate in any body cavity. Infected solid tissue often presents as cellulitis or with abscess formation. Areas of the body from which fluids are typically sent for microbiologic studies (in addition to blood and cerebrospinal fluid [see Chapters 68 and 71]) include those in Table 77-1.

### Pleural Fluid

Lining the entire thoracic cavity (see Chapter 69) of the body is a serous membrane called the parietal pleura. Covering the outer surface of the lung is another membrane called the visceral pleura (Figure 77-1). Within the pleural space between the lung and chest wall is a small amount of fluid called pleural fluid that lubricates the surfaces of the pleura (the membranes surrounding the lungs and lining the chest cavity). Normally, equilibrium exists among the pleural membranes, but in certain disease states, such as cardiac, hepatic, or renal disease, excess amounts of this fluid can be produced and accumulates in the pleural space; this is known as a pleural effusion. Pleural effusions can either be exudative or transudative. Exudative pleural effusions are caused by inflammation, infection, and cancer, whereas transudative effusions are due to systemic changes, such as congestive heart failure.

Normal pleural fluid contains few or no cells and has a consistency similar to serum, but with a lower protein count. Pleural fluid containing numerous white blood cells is indicative of infections. Pleural fluid specimens are collected by thoracentesis, a procedure in which a needle is inserted through the chest wall into the pleural space and the excess fluid aspirated. This fluid is then submitted to the laboratory as thoracentesis fluid, pleural fluid, or empyema fluid. The fluid, or effusion, can then be analyzed for cell count, total protein, glucose, lactate dehydrogenase, amylase, cytology, and culture. The total protein and glucose results determine if the effusion is transudate or exudate. The patient's serum or plasma glucose level is needed to compare with the results indicated in the body fluid. Several characteristics can be used to determine whether a fluid is a transudate or exudate (Table 77-2). When effusions are extremely purulent or full of pus, the effusion is referred to as an empyema. Empyema often arises as a complication of pneumonia, but other infections near the lung (e.g., subdiaphragmatic infection) may seed microorganisms into the pleural cavity. It has been estimated that 50% to 60% of patients develop empyema as a complication of pneumonia.

### Peritoneal Fluid

The peritoneum is a large, moist, continuous sheet of serous membrane lining the walls of the abdominal-pelvic cavity and the outer coat of the organs contained within the cavity (Figure 77-2). In the abdomen, these two membrane linings are separated by a space called the peritoneal cavity, which contains or abuts the liver, pancreas, spleen, stomach and intestinal tract, bladder, and fallopian tubes and ovaries. The kidneys occupy a retroperitoneal (behind the peritoneum) position. Within the healthy human peritoneal cavity is a small amount of fluid that maintains the surface moisture of the peritoneum. Normal peritoneal fluid may contain as many as 300 white blood cells per milliliter, but the protein content and specific gravity of the fluid are low. During an infectious or inflammatory process, increased amounts of fluid accumulate in the peritoneal cavity, a condition called ascites. Most cases of ascites are due to liver disease, and in severe cases, the abdomen is often distended. The fluid can be collected for testing by paracentesis (the insertion of a needle into the abdomen and removal of fluid). The peritoneal or ascites fluid can then be analyzed for amylase, protein, albumin, cell count, culture, and cytology. Often ascitic fluid contains an increased number of inflammatory cells and an elevated protein level.

Agents of infection gain access to the peritoneum through a perforation of the bowel, through infection within abdominal viscera, by way of the bloodstream, or by external inoculation (as in surgery or trauma). On occasion, as in pelvic inflammatory disease (PID),

organisms travel through the natural channels of the fallopian tubes into the peritoneal cavity.

**Primary Peritonitis.** Peritonitis results when the peritoneal membrane becomes inflamed and can be either primary or secondary. Primary peritonitis is rare and results when infection spreads from the blood and lymph nodes with no apparent evidence of infection. The organisms likely to be recovered from patient specimens

**TABLE 77-1** Microbiology Laboratory Body Fluid Collection Sites

| Body Area | Fluid Name(s) |
|---|---|
| Thorax | Thoracentesis or pleural or empyema fluid |
| Abdominal cavity | Paracentesis or ascitic or peritoneal fluid |
| Joint | Synovial fluid |
| Pericardium | Pericardial fluid |

**TABLE 77-2** Pleural Fluid Effusion Characteristics

| | Transudate | Exudate |
|---|---|---|
| **Appearance** | Clear | Cloudy |
| **Specific Gravity** | <1.015 | >1.015 |
| **Total Protein** | <3.0 mg/dL | >3.0 mg/dL |
| **LD Fluid: Serum Ratio** | <0.6 | >0.6 |
| **Cholesterol** | <60 mg/dL | >60 mg/dL |
| **Cholesterol Fluid: Serum Ratio** | <0.3 | >0.3 |
| **Bilirubin Fluid:Serum Ratio** | <0.6 | >0.6 |
| **Total Protein Fluid: Serum Ratio** | <0.5 | >0.6 |
| **White Blood Cells** | <1000/μL (all white blood cell types, all <50%) | >1000/μL |
| **Red Blood Cells** | <10,000/μL = because of traumatic tap | >100,000/μL |
| **Clotting** | Will not clot | May clot |

Modified from Strasinger SK, Di Lorenzo MS: *Urinalysis and body fluids,* ed 5, Philadelphia, 2008, F.A. Davis.

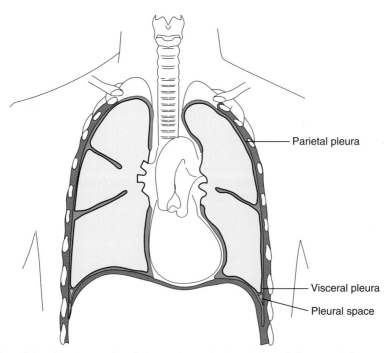

**Figure 77-1** The location of the pleural space in relation to the parietal and visceral pleura and the rest of the respiratory tract.

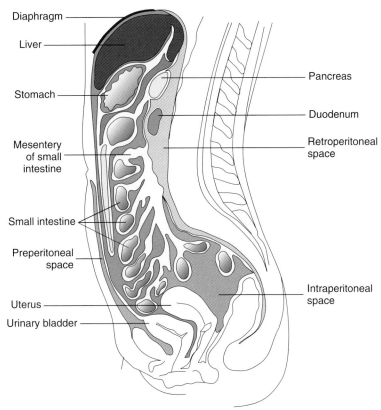

**Figure 77-2** The abdominal cavity. The retroperitoneal and preperitoneal spaces are considered as extraperitoneal (outside) spaces. (Modified from Thibodeau GA: *Anatomy and physiology,* St. Louis, 1993, Mosby.)

with primary peritonitis vary with the patient's age. The most common etiologic agents in children are *Streptococcus pneumoniae* and group A streptococci, Enterobacteriaceae, other gram-negative bacilli, and staphylococci. In adults, *Escherichia coli* is the most common bacterium, followed by *S. pneumoniae* and group A streptococci. Polymicrobic peritonitis is unusual in the absence of bowel perforation or rupture. Among sexually active young women, *Neisseria gonorrhoeae* and *Chlamydia trachomatis* are common etiologic agents of peritoneal infection, often in the form of a perihepatitis (inflammation of the surface of the liver, called Fitz-Hugh–Curtis syndrome). Tuberculous peritonitis occurs infrequently in the United States and is more likely to be found among individuals that have recently traveled in South America, Southeast Asia, or Africa. Fungal causes of peritonitis are not common, but *Candida* spp. may be recovered from immunosuppressed patients and patients receiving prolonged antibacterial therapy.

**Secondary Peritonitis.** Secondary peritonitis is a complication of a perforated viscus (organ), surgery, traumatic injury, loss of bowel wall integrity following a destructive disease (e.g., ulcerative colitis, ruptured appendix, carcinoma), obstruction, or a preceding infection (liver abscess, salpingitis, septicemia). The nature, location, and etiology of the underlying process govern the agents recovered from peritoneal fluid. With PID as the background, gonococci, anaerobes, or chlamydiae are isolated. With peritonitis or intra-abdominal abscess, anaerobes generally are found in peritoneal fluid, usually together with Enterobacteriaceae and enterococci or

other streptococci. In patients whose bowel flora has been altered by antimicrobial agents, more resistant gram-negative bacilli and *Staphylococcus aureus* may be encountered. Because anaerobes outnumber aerobes in the bowel by 1000-fold, it is not surprising that anaerobic organisms play a prominent role in intra-abdominal infection, perhaps acting synergistically with facultative bacteria. The organisms likely to be recovered include *E. coli*, the *Bacteroides fragilis* group, enterococci and other streptococci, *Bilophila* spp., other anaerobic gram-negative bacilli, anaerobic gram-positive cocci, and clostridia.

### Peritoneal Dialysis Fluid

More than 900,000 patients with end-stage renal disease are maintained on continuous ambulatory peritoneal dialysis (CAPD). One in every 10 American adults, totaling more than 20 million, suffer from some type of chronic kidney disease. In this treatment, fluid is injected into the peritoneal cavity and subsequently removed, which allows exchange of salts and water and removal of various wastes in the absence of kidney function. Because the dialysate fluid is injected into the peritoneal cavity via a catheter, the break in the skin barrier places the dialysis patient at significant risk for infection. The average incidence of peritonitis in these patients is up to two episodes per year per patient. Peritonitis is diagnosed by the presence of two of the following: cloudy dialysate, abdominal pain, or a positive culture from dialysate. Although white blood cells are usually plentiful (a value of leukocytes >100/mL is usually indicative of infection), the number of organisms is usually too low for detection on Gram stain of the peritoneal fluid sediment unless a concentrating technique is used; fungi are more readily detected. Many recent studies show that improved sensitivity can be achieved by using automated blood culture systems in which 10 mL of fluid is inoculated into culture bottles.

Most infections originate from the patient's own skin flora; *Staphylococcus epidermidis* and *S. aureus* are the most common etiologic agents, followed by streptococci, aerobic or facultative gram-negative bacilli, *Candida* spp., *Corynebacterium* spp., and others. The oxygen content of peritoneal dialysate is usually too high for the development of anaerobic infection. Among the gram-negative bacilli isolated, *Pseudomonas* spp., *Acinetobacter* spp., and the Enterobacteriaceae are frequently observed.

### Pericardial Fluid

The heart and contiguous major blood vessels are surrounded by the pericardium, a protective tissue. The area between the epicardium, which is the membrane surrounding the heart muscle, and the pericardium is called the pericardial space and normally contains 15 to 20 mL of clear fluid. If an infectious agent is present within the fluid, the pericardium may become distended and tight, and eventually tamponade (interference with cardiac function and circulation) can ensue. Up to 500 mL of fluid can accumulate during infection, which may seriously complicate cardiac function.

Agents of pericarditis (inflammation of the pericardium) are usually viruses, especially Coxsackie virus. Parasites, bacteria, certain fungi, and noninfectious causes are also associated with this disease.

Myocarditis (inflammation of the heart muscle itself) may accompany or follow pericarditis. The pathogenesis of disease involves the host inflammatory response contributing to fluid buildup as well as cell and tissue damage. Common causes of myocarditis include viral infections with Coxsackie virus, echoviruses, or adenovirus. The most common etiologic agents of pericarditis and myocarditis are listed in Box 77-1. Other bacteria, fungi, and parasitic agents have been recovered from pericardial effusions.

Patients who develop pericarditis resulting from agents other than viruses are often immunocompromised or suffering from a chronic disease. An example is infective endocarditis, in which a myocardial abscess develops and then ruptures into the pericardial space.

### Joint Fluid

Arthritis is an inflammation in a joint space. Infectious arthritis may involve any joint in the body. Infection of the joint usually occurs secondary to hematogenous spread of bacteria or, less often, fungi, as a direct extension of infection of the bone. It may also occur after injection of material, especially corticosteroids, into joints or after insertion of prosthetic material (e.g., total hip replacement). Although infectious arthritis usually occurs at a single site (monoarticular), a preexisting bacteremia or fungemia may seed more than one joint to establish polyarticular infection, particularly when multiple joints are diseased, such as in rheumatoid arthritis.

---

**BOX 77-1** Common Etiologic Agents of Pericarditis and Myocarditis

**Viruses**
Enteroviruses (primary Coxsackie A and B and, less frequently, echoviruses)
Adenoviruses
Influenza viruses

**Bacteria (relatively uncommon)**
*Mycoplasma pneumoniae*
*Chlamydia trachomatis*
*Mycobacterium tuberculosis*
*Staphylococcus aureus*
*Streptococcus pneumoniae*
Enterobacteriaceae and other gram-negative bacilli

**Fungi (relatively uncommon)**
*Coccidioides immitis*
*Aspergillus* spp.
*Candida* spp.
*Cryptococcus neoformans*
*Histoplasma capsulatum*

**Parasites (relatively uncommon)**
*Entamoeba histolytica*
*Toxoplasma gondii*

---

In bacterial arthritis, the knees and hips are the most commonly affected joints in all age groups.

In addition to active infections associated with viable microorganisms within the joint, sterile, self-limited arthritis caused by antigen-antibody interactions may follow an episode of infection, such as meningococcal meningitis. When an etiologic agent cannot be isolated from an inflamed joint fluid specimen, either the absence of viable agents or inadequate transport or culturing procedures may be the cause. For example, even under the best circumstances, *Borrelia burgdorferi* is isolated from the joints of fewer than 20% of patients with Lyme disease. Nonspecific test results, such as increased white blood cell count, decreased glucose, or elevated protein, may indicate that an infectious agent is present but inconclusive.

Overall, *Staphylococcus aureus* is the most common etiologic agent of septic arthritis, accounting for approximately 70% of infections. In adults younger than 30 years of age, however, *Neisseria gonorrhoeae* is isolated most frequently. *Haemophilus influenzae* has been the most common agent of bacteremia in children younger than 2 years of age, and consequently it has been the most frequent cause of infectious arthritis in these patients, followed by *S. aureus*. The widespread use of *H. influenzae* type B vaccine should contribute to a change in this pattern. Streptococci, including groups A (*Streptococcus pyogenes*) and B (*Streptococcus agalactiae*), pneumococci, and viridans streptococci, are prominent among bacterial agents associated with infectious arthritis in patients of all ages. Among anaerobic bacteria, *Bacteroides*, including *B. fragilis*, may be recovered and *Fusobacterium necrophorum*, which usually involves more than one joint in the course of sepsis. Among people living in certain endemic areas of the United States and Europe,

BOX 77-2 Most Frequently Encountered Etiologic Agents of Infectious Arthritis

**Bacterial**
*Staphylococcus aureus*
Beta-hemolytic streptococci
Streptococci (other)
*Haemophilus influenzae*
*Haemophilus* spp. (other)
*Bacteroides* spp.
*Fusobacterium* spp.
*Neisseria gonorrhoeae*
*Pseudomonas* spp.
*Salmonella* spp.
*Pasteurella multocida*
*Moraxella osloensis*
*Kingella kingae*
*Moraxella catarrhalis*
*Capnocytophaga* spp.
*Corynebacterium* spp.
*Clostridium* spp.
*Peptostreptococcus* spp.
*Eikenella corrodens*
*Actinomyces* spp.
*Mycobacterium* spp.
*Mycoplasma* spp.
*Ureaplasma urealyticum*
*Borrelia burgdorferi*

**Fungal**
*Candida* spp.
*Cryptococcus neoformans*
*Coccidioides immitis*
*Sporothrix schenckii*

**Viral**
Hepatitis B
Mumps
Rubella
Other viruses (rarely)

infectious arthritis is a prominent feature associated with Lyme disease. Chronic monoarticular arthritis is frequently due to mycobacteria, *Nocardia asteroides*, and fungi. Some of the more frequently encountered etiologic agents of infectious arthritis are listed in Box 77-2.

These agents act to stimulate a host inflammatory response, which is initially responsible for the pathology of the infection. Arthritis is also a symptom associated with infectious diseases caused by certain agents, such as *Neisseria meningitidis*, group A streptococci (rheumatic fever), and *Streptobacillus moniliformis*, in which the agent cannot be recovered from joint fluid. Presumably, antigen-antibody complexes formed during active infection accumulate in a joint, initiating an inflammatory response that is responsible for the ensuing damage.

Infections in prosthetic joints are usually associated with somewhat different etiologic agents than those in natural joints. After insertion of the prosthesis, organisms that gained access during the surgical procedure slowly multiply until they reach a critical mass and produce a host response. This may occur long after the initial surgery; approximately half of all prosthetic joint infections occur more than 1 year after surgery. Skin flora is the most common etiologic agent, with *Staphylococcus epidermidis*, other coagulase-negative staphylococci, *Corynebacterium* spp., *and Propionibacterium* spp. as the most common. However, *Staphylococcus aureus* is also a major pathogen in this infectious disease. Alternatively, organisms may reach joints during hematogenous spread from distant, infected sites.

Diagnosis of joint infections requires an aspiration of joint fluid for culture and microscopic examination. Inoculating the fluid directly into blood culture bottles may prevent the fluid from clotting. Some of the fluid may be Gram stained and inoculated onto blood as well as chocolate and anaerobic media. The use of AFB (acid fast bacteria) and fungal media must also be considered.

## BONE

### Bone Marrow Aspiration or Biopsy

Diagnosis of diseases, including brucellosis, histoplasmosis, blastomycosis, tuberculosis, and leishmaniasis, can sometimes be made by detection of the organisms in the bone marrow. *Brucella* spp. can be isolated on culture, as can fungi, but parasitic agents must be visualized in smears or sections made from bone marrow material. Many of the etiologic agents associated with disseminated infections in patients with human immunodeficiency virus (HIV) may be visualized or isolated from the bone marrow. Some of these organisms include cytomegalovirus, *Cryptococcus neoformans*, and *Mycobacterium avium* complex.

### Bone Biopsy

A small piece of infected bone is occasionally sent to the microbiology laboratory to identify the etiologic agent of osteomyelitis (infection of bone). Patients develop osteomyelitis from hematogenous spread of an infectious agent, invasion of bone tissue from an adjacent site (e.g., joint infection, dental infection), breakdown of tissue caused by trauma or surgery, or lack of adequate circulation followed by colonization of a skin ulceration with microorganisms. Once established, infections in bone may progress toward chronicity, particularly if blood supply is insufficient in the affected area.

*Staphylococcus aureus*, seeded during bacteremia, is the most common etiologic agent of osteomyelitis among patients of all age groups. The toxins and enzymes produced by this bacterium, as well as its ability to adhere to smooth surfaces and produce a protective glycocalyx coating, seem to contribute to the organism's pathogenicity. Osteomyelitis in younger patients is often associated with a single agent. Such infections are usually of hematogenous origin. Other organisms recovered from hematogenously acquired osteomyelitis include *Salmonella* spp., *Haemophilus* spp., Enterobacteriaceae, *Pseudomonas* spp., *Fusobacterium necrophorum*, and yeasts. *S. aureus* or *P. aeruginosa* is often recovered from cases in patients with drug addictions. Parasites or viruses are rarely, if ever, etiologic agents of osteomyelitis.

Bone biopsies from infections that have spread to a bone from a contiguous source or that are associated with poor circulation, especially in patients with diabetes, are likely to yield multiple isolates. Gram-negative bacilli are increasingly common among hospitalized patients; a break in the skin (surgery or intravenous line) may precede establishment of gram-negative osteomyelitis. Breaks in skin from other causes, such as a bite wound or trauma, also may be the initial event leading to underlying bone infection. For example, a human bite may lead to infection with *Eikenella corrodens*, whereas an animal bite may result in *Pasteurella multocida* osteomyelitis. Poor oral hygiene may lead to osteomyelitis of the jaw with *Actinomyces* spp., *Capnocytophaga* spp., and other oral flora, particularly anaerobes. Pigmented *Prevotella* and *Porphyromonas*, *Fusobacterium*, and *Peptostreptococcus* spp. are often involved. Pelvic infection in the female may result in a mixed aerobic and anaerobic osteomyelitis of the pubic bone.

Patients with neuropathy (pathologic changes in the peripheral nervous system) in the extremities, notably patients with diabetes, who may have poor circulation, may experience an unrecognized or notable trauma. They develop ulcers on the feet that do not heal, become infected, and may eventually progress to involve underlying bone. These infections are usually polymicrobial, involving anaerobic and aerobic bacteria. *Prevotella* or *Porphyromonas*, other gram-negative anaerobes, including the *Bacteroides fragilis* group, *Peptostreptococcus* spp., *Staphylococcus aureus*, and group A and other streptococci are frequently encountered.

Molecular testing, such as polymerase chain reaction, may be useful in determining the infectious organism associated with the patient's condition when the laboratory is unable to recover the organism by traditional culture.

## SOLID TISSUES

Pieces of tissue are removed from patients during surgical or needle biopsy procedures or may be collected at autopsy. Any agent of infection may cause disease in tissue, and laboratory practices should be adequate to recover bacteria, fungi, and viruses and detect the presence of parasites. Fastidious organisms (e.g., *Brucella* spp.) and agents of chronic disease (e.g., systemic fungi and mycobacteria) may require special media and long incubation periods for isolation. Some agents requiring special supportive or selective media are listed in Box 77-3.

---

**BOX 77-3** Infectious Agents in Tissue Requiring Special Media

*Actinomyces* spp.
*Brucella* spp.
*Legionella* spp.
*Bartonella* (Rochalimaea) *henselae* (cat-scratch disease bacilli)
Systemic fungi
*Mycoplasma* spp.
*Mycobacterium* spp.
Viruses

---

# LABORATORY DIAGNOSTIC PROCEDURES

## SPECIMEN COLLECTION AND TRANSPORT

Requirements for the collection and transport of specimens from sterile body sites vary because of the numerous types of specimens that can be collected and submitted to the laboratory for testing.

### Fluids and Aspirates

Most specimens (pleural, peritoneal, pericardial, and synovial fluids) are collected by aspiration with a needle and syringe. Collecting pericardial fluid is not without risk to the patient because the sample is collected from the cavity immediately adjacent to the heart. Collection is performed by needle aspiration with electrocardiographic monitoring or as a surgical procedure. Laboratory personnel should be alerted in advance of the procedure, ensuring that the appropriate media, tissue culture media, and stain procedures are available immediately.

Body fluids from sterile sites should be transported to the laboratory in a sterile tube or airtight vial. From 1 to 5 mL of specimen is adequate for isolation of most bacteria, but the larger the specimen, the better, particularly for isolation of *M. tuberculosis* and fungi; at least 5 mL should be submitted for recovery of these organisms. Ten milliliters of fluid is recommended for the diagnosis of peritonitis. Anaerobic transport vials are available from several sources. These vials are prepared in an oxygen-free atmosphere and are sealed with a rubber septum or short stopper through which the fluid is injected. Transportation of fluid in a syringe capped with a sterile rubber stopper is not recommended. Most clinically significant anaerobic bacteria survive adequately in aerobic transport containers (e.g., sterile, screw-capped tubes) for short periods if the specimen is purulent and of adequate volume. However, collection in anaerobic transport media is recommended, and procedures vary in different laboratories. Specimens received in anaerobic transport vials should be inoculated to routine aerobic (an enriched broth, blood, chocolate, and sometimes MacConkey agar plates) and anaerobic media as quickly as possible. Specimens for recovery of fungi or mycobacteria may be transported in sterile, screw-capped tubes. At least 5 to 10 mL of fluid are required for adequate recovery of small numbers of organisms. If gonococci or chlamydia are suspected, additional aliquots should be sent to the laboratory for smears and appropriate cultures.

Percutaneous catheters are placed during many surgical procedures to prevent the accumulation of exudate and blood at the operative site. Often, the laboratory receives drainage fluids from these catheters for culture when signs and symptoms suggest infection. However, culture of such fluid is potentially misleading when the fluid becomes contaminated within the catheter or collection device, or when the fluid does not originate from a site of the infection. Everts and colleagues confirmed that direct aspiration of potentially infected fluid collections rather than catheter drainage fluid should be submitted for culture for the assessment of deep tissue infections in patients.

With respect to pericardial, pleural, synovial, and peritoneal fluids, the inoculation of blood culture broth bottles at the bedside or in the laboratory may be beneficial. An additional specimen should be submitted to the laboratory for a Gram stain. The specimen in the blood culture bottle is processed as a blood culture, facilitating the recovery of small numbers of organisms and diluting out the effects of antibiotics. Citrate or sodium polyanetholsulfonate (SPS) may be used as an anticoagulant. Specimens collected by percutaneous needle aspiration (paracentesis) or at the time of surgery should be inoculated into aerobic and anaerobic blood culture bottles immediately at the bedside.

Fluid from CAPD patients can be submitted to the laboratory in a sterile tube, urine cup, or the original bag. The bag is entered with a sterile needle and syringe to withdraw fluid for culture. Fluid should be directly inoculated into blood culture bottles (at least 20 mL [10 mL in each of two culture bottles]). Numerous studies indicate that in addition to blood culture bottles, an adult Isolator tube is a sensitive and specific method for culture.

## Bone

Bone marrow is typically aspirated from the interstitium of the iliac crest. Usually, this material is not processed for routine bacteria, because blood cultures are equally useful, and false-positive cultures for skin bacteria (*Staphylococcus epidermidis*) are frequent. Some laboratories report good recovery from bone marrow material injected into a pediatric Isolator tube (ISOLATOR 1.5 mL, Alere, Waltham, MA) as a collection and transport device. The lytic agents within the Isolator tube are thought to lyse cellular components, presumably freeing intracellular bacteria for enhanced recovery. Bone removed at surgery or by percutaneous biopsy is sent to the laboratory in a sterile container.

## Tissue

Tissue specimens are obtained following careful preparation of the skin. It is critical that biopsy specimens be collected aseptically and submitted to the microbiology laboratory in a sterile container. A wide-mouthed, screwcapped bottle or plastic container is recommended. Anaerobic organisms survive within infected tissue long enough to be recovered from culture. A small amount of sterile, nonbacteriostatic saline may be added to keep the specimen moist. Because homogenizing with a tissue grinder can destroy some organisms by the shearing forces generated during grinding, it is often best to use a sterile scissors and forceps to mince larger tissue specimens into small pieces suitable for culturing (Figure 77-3). Note that *Legionella* spp. may be inhibited by saline; a section of lung should be submitted without saline for *Legionella* isolation.

If anaerobic organisms are of concern, a small amount of tissue can be placed into a loosely capped, wide-mouthed plastic tube and sealed into an anaerobic pouch system, which also seals in moisture enough for survival of organisms in tissue until the specimen is plated. The

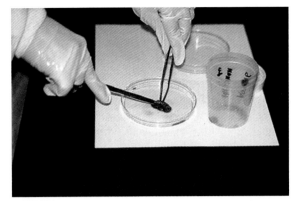

**Figure 77-3** Mincing a piece of tissue for culture using a sterile forceps and scissors. Note: Perform this procedure in a biosafety cabinet.

surgeon should take responsibility for seeing that a second specimen is submitted to anatomic pathology for histologic studies. Formaldehyde-fixed tissue is not useful for recovery of viable microorganisms, although some organisms can be recovered after very short periods. Material from draining sinus tracts should include a portion of the tract's wall obtained by deep curettage. Tissue from infective endocarditis should contain a portion of the valve and vegetation if the patient is undergoing valve replacement.

In some instances, contaminated material may be submitted for microbiologic examination. Specimens, such as tonsils or autopsy tissue, may be surface cauterized with a heated spatula or blanched by immersing in boiling water for 5 to 10 seconds to reduce surface contamination. The specimen may then be dissected with sterile instruments to permit culturing of the specimen's center, which will not be affected by the heating. Alternatively, larger tissues may be cut in half with sterile scissors or a blade and the interior portion cultured for microbes.

Because surgical specimens are obtained at great risk and expense to the patient, and because supplementary specimens cannot be obtained easily, it is important that the laboratory save a portion of the original tissue (if enough material is available) in a small amount of sterile broth in the refrigerator and at −70° C (or, if necessary, at −20° C) for at least 4 weeks in case additional studies are indicated. If the entire tissue must be ground up for culture, a small amount of the suspension should be placed into a sterile tube and refrigerated.

## SPECIMEN PROCESSING, DIRECT EXAMINATION, AND CULTURE

### Fluids and Aspirates

Techniques for laboratory processing of sterile body fluids are similar except for those previously discussed that are directly inoculated into blood culture bottles. Clear fluids may be concentrated by centrifugation or filtration, whereas purulent material can be inoculated directly to media. Any body fluid received in the laboratory that is already clotted must be homogenized to release trapped bacteria and minced or cut to release fungal cells. Either processing such specimens in a motorized tissue homogenizer or grinding them manually in a mortar and pestle or glass tissue grinder allows better recovery of bacteria. Hand grinding is often preferred, because motorized grinding can generate considerable heat and thereby kill microorganisms in the specimen. Grinding may lyse fungal elements; therefore, it is not recommended with specimens processed for fungi. Small amounts of whole material from a clot should be aseptically cut with a scalpel and placed directly onto media for isolation of fungi.

All fluids should be processed for direct microscopic examination. In general, if one organism is seen per oil immersion field, at least $10^5$ organisms per milliliter of specimen are present. In such cases, often only a few organisms are present in normally sterile body fluids. Therefore, organisms must be concentrated in body fluids. For microscopic examination, cytocentrifugation (see Figure 71-4) should be used to prepare Gram-stained smears because organisms can be further concentrated up to 1000-fold. Body fluids should be concentrated by either filtration or high-speed centrifugation. Once the sample is concentrated, the supernatant is aseptically decanted or aspirated with a sterile pipette, leaving approximately 1 mL liquid in which to thoroughly mix the sediment. Vigorous vortexing or drawing the sediment up and down into a pipette several times is required to adequately suspend the sediment. This procedure should be done in a biologic safety cabinet. The suspension is used to inoculate media. Direct potassium hydroxide (KOH) or calcofluor white preparations for fungi and acid-fast stain for mycobacteria can also be performed. See Chapter 6 for detailed descriptions related to the preparation of smears for staining procedures.

Specimens for fungi should be examined by direct wet preparation or by preparing a separate smear for periodic acid-Schiff (PAS) staining in addition to Gram stain. Either 10% KOH or calcofluor white is recommended for visualization of fungal elements from a wet preparation. In addition to hyphal forms, material from the thoracic cavity may contain spherules of *Coccidioides* or budding yeast cells.

Lysis of leukocytes before concentration of CAPD effluents can significantly enhance recovery of organisms. Filtration of CAPD fluid through a 0.45-mm pore membrane filter allows a greater volume of fluid to be processed and usually yields better results. Because the numbers of infecting organisms may be low (fewer than 1 organism per 10 mL of fluid), a large quantity of fluid must be processed. Sediment obtained from at least 50 mL of fluid has been recommended. If the specimen is filtered, the filter should be cut aseptically into three pieces, one of which is placed on chocolate agar for incubation in 5% carbon dioxide, one on MacConkey agar, and the other on a blood agar plate for anaerobic incubation.

If fluids have been concentrated by centrifugation, the resulting sediment should be inoculated to an enrichment broth, blood, and chocolate agars. Because these specimens are from normally sterile sites, selective media are inadvisable because they may inhibit the growth of some organisms. Appropriate procedures for the isolation of anaerobes, mycobacteria, fungi, *Chlamydia* spp., and viruses should be used when such cultures are clinically indicated.

## Bone

Clotted bone marrow aspirates or biopsies must be homogenized or ground to release trapped microorganisms. Specimens are inoculated to the same media as for other sterile body fluids. A special medium for enhancement of growth of *Brucella* spp. and incubation in 10% carbon dioxide may be needed. A portion of the specimen may be inoculated directly to fungal media. Sections are also made from biopsy material (bone) for fixation, staining, and examination (usually by anatomic pathologists) for the presence of mycobacterial, fungal, or parasitic agents. With respect to obtaining specimens from patients suspected of having osteomyelitis, cultures taken from open wound sites above infected bone or material taken from a draining sinus leading to an area of osteomyelitis may not reflect the actual etiologic agent of the underlying osteomyelitis. Cultures of samples of bone obtained during wound debridement surgery appear to be more useful for directing antibiotic therapy for better clinical outcome.

Diagnosis of prosthetic (artificial) joint infections is often difficult. Unfortunately, there is no universally accepted definition for the diagnosis of infection in the absence of microbiologic evidence because clinical symptoms such as pain do not differentiate infection from mechanical joint failure. There is no standardized approach to the laboratory diagnosis of these infections, and published data are conflicting. Further complicating the diagnosis is that the most common bacteria causing prosthesis infections are common skin contaminants such as coagulase-negative staphylococci. Some studies have reported that culture is relatively insensitive, possibly because of the organisms residing in biofilms, whereas polymerase chain reaction (PCR) assays were able to detect a majority of prosthetic joint infections. Atkins and colleagues recommended that five or six operative bone specimens be submitted for culture and that the cutoff for a definite diagnosis of infection be three or more of these specimens yielding the same organism. However, a recent study using PCR and culture using multiple media types and prolonged incubation found that appropriate culture was adequate to exclude bacterial infection in hip prostheses and PCR did not enhance diagnostic sensitivity for infection.

Normal bone is difficult to break up; however, most infected bone is soft and necrotic. Therefore, grinding the specimen in a mortar and pestle may break off some pieces. Small shavings from the most necrotic-looking areas of the bone specimen may sometimes be scraped off aseptically and inoculated to media. Pieces should be placed directly into media for recovery of fungi. Small bits of bone can be ground with sterile broth to form a suspension for bacteriologic and mycobacterial cultures. If anaerobes are to be recovered, all manipulations are best performed in an anaerobic chamber. If such an environment is unavailable, microbiologists should work quickly within a biosafety cabinet to inoculate prereduced anaerobic plates and broth with material from the bone.

## Solid Tissue

Tissue should be manipulated in a laminar flow biologic safety cabinet. Processing tissue within an anaerobic chamber is even better. The microbiologist should cut through the infected area (which is often discolored) with a sterile scalpel blade. Half of the specimen can be used for fungal cultures and the other half for bacterial cultures. Both types of microbial agents should be considered in all tissue specimens. Some samples should also be sent to surgical pathology for histologic examination. Specimens should be cultured for viruses or acid-fast bacilli when requested. Material that is to be cultured for parasites should be finely minced or teased before inoculation into broth. Direct examination of stained tissue for parasites is often performed in the anatomic pathology lab. Imprint cultures of tissues may yield bacteriologic results identical to homogenates and may help differentiate microbial infection within the tissue's center from surface colonization (growth only at the edge). Additional media can be inoculated for incubation at lower temperatures, which may facilitate recovery of certain systemic fungi and mycobacteria.

Tissue may also be inoculated to tissue culture cells for isolation of viruses. Brain, lung, spinal fluid, and blood are generally good specimens for viral isolation. Tissue may be examined by immunofluorescence for the presence of herpes simplex virus, varicella-zoster virus, cytomegalovirus, or rabies viral particles. Lung tissue should be examined by direct fluorescent antibody test for *Legionella* spp.

The tissues of all fetuses, premature infants, and babies who have died of an infectious process should be cultured for *Listeria*. Specimens of the brain, spinal fluid, blood, liver, and spleen are most likely to contain the organism. The isolation procedure may be reviewed in the reference by Seeliger and Cherry.

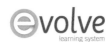 *Visit the Evolve site to complete the review questions.*

---

## CASE STUDY 77-1

A 79-year-old woman had left-knee arthroplasty to replace an arthritic joint with a prosthetic joint. The surgery was complicated and lasted more than 1 hour. She received antibiotics at the time of the surgery but not postoperatively, in accordance with usual protocols for this type of surgery. She did well post-operatively and went home in 7 days. After several weeks, she complained of low-grade fevers and pain in the joint. Her physician aspirated 50 mL of fluid from the knee and inoculated 10 mL into each of both aerobic and anaerobic blood culture bottles. Some fluid was also sent to the laboratory, where numerous white blood cells were found but no organisms were seen on Gram stain. The anaerobic blood culture bottle turned positive at 48 hours. A gram-positive cocci was identified. The aerobic bottle remained negative.

### QUESTIONS

1. What is the likely genus of the organism in the blood culture bottle?
2. What is the likely source of the infection in this patient?
3. The physician wanted the laboratory to be sure that the organism was not isolated because of poor technique in collection of the joint fluid specimen. Because the diagnosis of a septic joint means that the patient must have more surgery and long-term therapy, the physician wanted to be certain of the diagnosis. How can the laboratory ascertain that the organism caused the infection?

---

## BIBLIOGRAPHY

Alfa MJ, Degagne P, Olson N, et al: Improved detection of bacterial growth in continuous ambulatory peritoneal dialysis effluent by use of BacT/Alert FAN bottles, *J Clin Microbiol* 354:862, 1997.

Atkins BL, Athanasou N, Deeks JL, et al: Prospective evaluation of criteria for microbiological diagnosis of prosthetic-joint infection at revision arthroplasty, *J Clin Microbiol* 36:2932, 1998.

Bobadilla M, Sifuentes J, Garcia-Tsao G: Improved method for the bacteriological diagnosis of spontaneous bacterial peritonitis, *J Clin Microbiol* 27:2145, 1989.

Bourbeau P, Riley J, Heiter BJ, et al: Use of the BacT/Alert Blood Culture System for culture of sterile body fluids other than blood, *J Clin Microbiol* 36:3273,1998.

Centers for Disease Control Department of Health and Human Services: *The prevention and treatment of complication of diabetes: a guide for primary care practitioners*, Atlanta, 1996, Public Health Service.

Chapin-Robertson K, Dahlberg SE, Edberg SC: Clinical and laboratory analyses of cytospin-prepared Gram stains for recovery and diagnosis of bacteria from sterile body fluids, *J Clin Microbiol* 30:377, 1992.

Everts RJ, Heneghan JP, Adholla PO, et al: Validity of cultures of fluid collected through drainage catheters versus those obtained by direct aspiration, *J Clin Microbiol* 39:66, 2001.

Ince A, Rupp J, Frommelt L, et al: Is "aseptic" loosening of the prosthetic cup after total hip replacement due to nonculturable bacterial pathogens in patients with low-grade infection? *Clin Infect Dis* 39:1599, 2004.

Khatri G, Wagner DK, Sohnle PG: Effect of bone biopsy in guiding antimicrobial therapy for osteomyelitis complicating open wounds, *Am J Med Sci* 321:367, 2001.

Levy PY, Fenollar F: The role of molecular diagnostics in implant-associated bone and joint infection, *Clin Microbiol Infect* 18(12):1168-1175, 2012.

Ludlam HA, Price TN, Berry AJ, et al: Laboratory diagnosis of peritonitis in patients on continuous ambulatory peritoneal dialysis, *J Clin Microbiol* 26:1757, 1988.

Maderazo EG, Judson S, Pasternak H: Late infections of total joint prostheses, *Clin Orthop* 229:131, 1988.

Marinella MA: Electrocardiographic manifestations and differential diagnosis of acute pericarditis, *Am Fam Physician* 15:699, 1998

National Kidney and Urologic Diseases: Kidney disease statistics for the United States, 2009.

Reinhold CE, Nickolai DJ, Piccinini TE, et al: Evaluation of broth media for routine culture of cerebrospinal fluid and joint fluid specimens, *Am J Clin Pathol* 89:671, 1988.

Runyon B, Antillon MR, Akriviadis EA, et al: Bedside inoculation of blood culture bottles with ascitic fluid is superior to delayed inoculation in the detection of spontaneous bacterial peritonitis, *J Clin Microbiol* 28:2811, 1990.

Seeliger HPR, Cherry WB: *Human listeriosis: its nature and diagnosis*, Washington, DC, 1957, US Government Printing Office.

Teitelbaum I, Burkart J: Peritoneal dialysis, *Am J Kid Dis* 42:1082, 2003.

Von Essen R, Holtta A: Improved method of isolating bacteria from joint fluids by the use of blood culture bottle, *Ann Rheum Dis* 45:454, 1986.

CHAPTER

# 78 Quality in the Clinical Microbiology Laboratory

## OBJECTIVES

1. Distinguish between the terms *total quality management (TQM)*, *continuous quality improvement (CQI)*, *performance improvement (PI)*, *quality assurance (QA)*, *LEAN*, and Six Sigma.
2. Describe the quality program associated with the microbiology laboratory.
3. Identify acceptable guidelines for specimen collection and transport, and give examples of unacceptable specimens.
4. State the purpose of the Standard Operating Procedure Manual.
5. Explain the requirements for laboratory personnel, use of reference laboratories, and elements of patient reports.
6. Define *proficiency testing (PT)*, and outline the necessary steps to achieve successful results.
7. Design a log to check performance for instruments and media used in the microbiology laboratory.
8. Explain the requirements for Antimicrobial Susceptibility Tests (AST).
9. Compare the maintenance of reference quality control stocks in bacteriology, mycology, mycobacteriology, virology, and parasitology.
10. Outline a QA program for the microbiology laboratory to include all phases of infectious disease diagnosis, and differentiate between external and in-house QA audit programs.
11. Describe daily monitoring activities by microbiologists and supervisors that result in providing quality care to the patient population.

Since the publication of the report "To Err is Human" by the Institute of Medicine, the endeavor for a safer and a more efficient health care delivery system has been in full force. The issue of quality in the medical laboratory has evolved over more than four decades following the publication of the recommendations for quality control (QC) in 1965. Just as microbial taxonomy has changed over the years, the approach to quality has evolved as well. QC is now seen as only one part of the total laboratory quality program. Quality also includes total quality management (TQM), continuous quality improvement (CQI) or performance improvement (PI), and quality assurance (QA). TQM, CQI, and PI are umbrella terms, encompassing the entire institution's quality program. TQM evolved as an activity to improve patient care by having the laboratory monitor its work to detect deficiencies and subsequently correct them. CQI and PI went a step further by seeking to improve patient care by placing the emphasis on preventing mistakes; CQI and PI advocate continuous training to guard against having to correct deficiencies.

The LEAN methodology concentrates on eliminating redundant motion, recognizing waste, and identifying what creates value from the client's perspective. The main objective for the medical laboratory is to deliver quality patient results at the lowest cost, within the shortest time frame, while maintaining client satisfaction. It involves five principles: value, value stream, flow, pull, and continuous improvement. The first principle is to define the value in the process from the client's perspective, which is what the patient knowingly pays for the attributes of service. Next, identify the value stream for each process providing that value, challenge the wasted steps, and eliminate all of the waste. Then make sure the service flows continuously through the remaining value-added step. Now it is time to pull it all together by introducing a continuous flow of events between all steps of the process where continuous flow is possible. The last principle is continuous improvement by management working toward perfection on an ongoing basis so the number of steps and time is constantly under scrutiny. The scope of resources and the information needed to provide the service to the client needs to be monitored also. These principles can increase quality, throughput, capacity, and efficiency while decreasing cost, inventory, space, and lead time. Ultimately it would provide better patient care within the clinical laboratory.

Six Sigma is a relatively new concept as compared to TQM. Six Sigma originated in 1986 from Motorola's drive to reduce defects by minimizing variation in processes through metrics measurement. The process focuses on continuous quality improvements for achieving near perfection by restricting the number of possible defects to fewer than 3.4 defects per million. Six Sigma is based on DMAIC (define, measure, analyze, improve, control), which helps in making precise measurements, identifying exact problems, and providing measurable solutions. When implemented correctly, Six Sigma can help organizations reduce operational costs by focusing on reducing defects, minimizing turnaround time, and trimming costs. The main difference between TQM and Six Sigma is the approach. TQM tries to improve quality by ensuring conformance to internal requirements, whereas Six Sigma focuses on improving quality by reducing the number of defects and impurities. Six Sigma is also fact-based, data-driven, and results-oriented, providing quantifiable and measurable bottom-line results, linked to strategy and related to customer requirements.

QC is associated with the internal activities that ensure diagnostic test accuracy. QA is associated with the external activities that ensure positive patient outcomes. Positive patient outcomes in the microbiology laboratory are as follows:

- Reduced length of stay
- Reduced cost of stay
- Reduced turnaround time for diagnosis of infection
- Change to appropriate antimicrobial therapy
- Customer (physician or patient) satisfaction

CQI and PI, through well-thought-out programs of QC and QA, are part of the requirements for laboratory accreditation under Clinical Laboratory Improvement Amendments (CLIA, 1988).

## QUALITY PROGRAM

Each laboratory must establish and maintain written policies and procedures that implement and monitor quality systems for all phases of the total testing process (preanalytic, analytic, and postanalytic) as well as general laboratory systems. The laboratory director is primarily responsible for the QC and QA programs. However, all laboratory personnel must actively participate in both programs. Federal guidelines (CLIA, 1988) are considered minimum standards and are superseded by higher standards imposed by states or private certifying agencies such as the College of American Pathologists (CAP) or The Joint Commission (TJC).

The basic elements of a QC program are described in the following sections.

## SPECIMEN COLLECTION AND TRANSPORT

The laboratory is responsible for providing written policies and procedures that ensure positive identification and optimum integrity of a patient's specimen from the time of collection or receipt of the specimen through completion of testing and reporting of results.

These guidelines and instructions should be available to health care providers for use when specimens are collected. The written collection instructions should be in detail and include the following:

- Test purpose and limitations
- Patient selection criteria
- Timing of specimen collection (e.g., before antimicrobials are administered)
- Optimal specimen collection sites
- Approved specimen collection methods
- Specimen transport medium criteria
- Specimen transport time and temperature
- Specimen holding instructions if it cannot be transported immediately (e.g., hold at 4° C for 24 hours)
- Minimum acceptable volume requirements where applicable
- Availability of test (onsite or sent to reference laboratory)
- Turnaround time
- Result reporting procedures

The collection instructions should include information on how a requisition should be filled out electronically or by hand, and the laboratory must include a statement indicating that the requisition must be filled out entirely. In addition to standard information, such as patient name, hospital or laboratory number, and ordering physician, other critical information includes (1) whether the patient is receiving antimicrobial therapy, (2) the suspect agent or syndrome, (3) immunization history (if applicable), and (4) travel history when certain microorganisms or parasites are suspected. The laboratory should also establish criteria for unacceptable specimens. Examples of unacceptable specimens include the following:

- Unlabeled, mislabeled, or incompletely labeled specimens
- Quantity not sufficient for testing (QNS)
- Use of an improper transport medium such as stool for ova and parasites not submitted in preservative(s)
- Use of improper swab such as use of wooden shaft or calcium alginate tip for viruses
- Specimen inappropriately handled with respect to temperature, timing, or storage requirements.
- Improper collection site for test requested such as stool for respiratory syncytial virus
- Specimen leakage from transport container
- Sera excessively hemolyzed, lipemic, or contaminated with bacteria

Sometimes, even though the specimen is not acceptable, the physician may ask that it be processed anyway. If this happens, a disclaimer should be put on the final report, indicating that the specimen was not collected properly and the results should be interpreted with caution.

## STANDARD OPERATING PROCEDURE MANUAL

The requirement for a Standard Operating Procedure Manual (SOPM) is considered part of the QC program. The SOPM should define test performance, tolerance limits, reagent preparation, required quality control, result reporting, and references. The SOPM should be written in the format of Clinical and Laboratory Standards Institute (CLSI), and must be reviewed and signed annually or bi-annually by the laboratory director who appears on the CLIA certificate; in addition, all changes must be approved and dated by the laboratory director. The SOPM should be available in the work areas. It is the definitive laboratory reference and is used often for questions relating to individual tests. Any obsolete procedure should be dated when removed from the SOPM and retained for at least 2 years.

## PERSONNEL

It is the laboratory director's responsibility to employ sufficient qualified personnel for the volume and complexity of the work performed. For example, published studies regarding staffing of virology laboratories suggest one technologist per 500 to 1000 specimens per year.

Technical on-the-job training must be documented, and the employee's competency must be assessed twice in the first year and annually thereafter. Continuing education programs should be provided, and verification of attendance should be maintained in the employee's personnel file. CLIA has improved the regulations associated with personnel competency (CLIA subpart K:493.1235). Laboratory employee competency assessment must include the following: (1) Direct observation of test performance, to include patient preparation (if applicable), specimen handling, processing, and testing; (2) monitoring the recording and reporting of test results; (3) review of intermediate test results or work sheets, QC results, patient results, and preventative maintenance records; (4) direct observation of performance or instrument maintenance and function checks; (5) assessment of test performance through testing previously analyzed specimens, internal blind testing of samples or external patients samples, and; (6) assessment of problem-solving skills. These competency assessments must be documented and completed by qualified personnel.

## REFERENCE LABORATORIES

Not all testing can be completed in one facility. A laboratory test that cannot be performed in-house and needs to be sent somewhere else is considered a reference laboratory test. The reference laboratory is a separate entity from the facility that collects and sends the specimen. It must be accredited or licensed. The referral laboratory's name, address, and licensure numbers should be included on the patient's final report.

## PATIENT REPORTS

There should be an established system for supervisory review of all laboratory reports. This review involves checking the specimen workup to verify that the correct conclusions were drawn and no clerical errors were made in reporting results. Reports should be released only to individuals authorized by law to receive them (physicians and various midlevel practitioners). Clinicians should be notified about "panic values" immediately. Panic values are potential life-threatening results, for example, positive Gram stain for cerebrospinal fluid (CSF) or a positive blood culture. Reference ranges must be included on the report where appropriate. All patient records should be maintained for at least 2 years. In reality, records should be maintained for at least 10 years because they may be needed to support medical necessity in the event of a postpayment billing audit by the Centers for Medicare and Medicaid Services.

## PROFICIENCY TESTING (PT)

Proficiency testing (PT) is a quality assurance measure used to monitor the laboratory's analytic performance in comparison to its peers and reference standards. It provides an external validation tool and objective evidence of the laboratory competence for patients and accrediting and oversight agencies. Laboratories are required to participate in a PT program for each analyte (test) for which a program is available; the laboratory must maintain an average score of 80% to maintain licensure in any subspecialty area. The federal government no longer maintains a PT program, but some states, such as New York, as well as several private accrediting agencies, such as the College of American Pathologists (CAP), send out "blind unknowns." These unknowns are to be treated exactly as patient specimens, from accessioning into the laboratory computer or manual logbook through workup and reporting of results. The testing personnel and laboratory director are required to sign a statement when the PT is completed attesting to the fact that the specimen was handled exactly like a patient specimen. In this way, PT specimens establish the accuracy and reproducibility of a laboratory's day-to-day performance. The laboratory's procedures, reagents, equipment, and personnel are all checked in the process. Furthermore, errors on PT help point out deficiencies, and the subsequent education of the staff can lead to overall improvements in laboratory quality. When grades (evaluations) come back, critiques (summaries) accompanying them should be discussed with the entire technical staff. Evidence of corrective action in the event of problems should be documented, including changes in procedures, retraining of personnel, or the purchase of alternative media and reagents.

Some laboratories have a system of internal PT in addition to those received from external agencies. When external audit is not available for a particular test method, laboratories are required by law to set up an internal program to revalidate the test at least semiannually. Internal PT samples can be set up by (1) seeding a simulated specimen and labeling it as an autopsy specimen so that no one panics if a pathogen is recovered, (2) splitting a routine specimen for workup by two different technologists, or (3) sending part of a specimen to a reference laboratory to compare and confirm the laboratory's result.

## PERFORMANCE CHECKS

### INSTRUMENTS

Equipment logs should contain the following information:

- Instrument name, serial number, and date of implementation in the laboratory
- Procedure and periodicity of function checks with at least the frequency specified by the manufacturer; function checks must be within the manufacturer's established limits before patient testing is conducted
- Acceptable performance ranges
- Instrument function failures, including specific details of steps taken to correct the problems (corrective action)
- Date and time of service requests and response
- Maintenance records as defined and with at least the minimum frequency specified by the manufacturer

Maintenance records should be retained in the laboratory for the life of the instrument. Specific guidelines regarding the periodicity of testing for autoclaves, biologic safety cabinets, centrifuges, incubators, microscopes, refrigerators, freezers, water baths, heat blocks, and other microbiology laboratory equipment can be found in a number of the references listed at the end of this chapter.

## COMMERCIALLY PREPARED MEDIA EXEMPT FROM QC

The CLSI Subcommittee on Media Quality Control collected data over several years regarding the incidence of QC failures of commonly used microbiology media. Based on its findings, the subcommittee published a list of media that did not require retesting in the user's laboratory if purchased from a manufacturer who follows CLSI guidelines. The laboratory must inspect each shipment for cracked media or Petri dishes, hemolysis, freezing, unequal filling, excessive bubbles, clarity, and visible contamination. The manufacturer must supply written assurance that CLSI standards were followed; this verification must be maintained along with the laboratory's QC protocol.

## USER-PREPARED AND NONEXEMPT, COMMERCIALLY PREPARED MEDIA

QC forms for user-prepared media should contain the amount prepared, the source of each ingredient, the lot number, the sterilization method, the preparation date, the expiration date (usually 1 month for agar plates and 6 months for tubed media), and the name of the preparer. Both user-prepared and nonexempt, commercially prepared media should be checked for proper color, consistency, depth, smoothness, hemolysis, excessive bubbles, and contamination. A representative sample of the lot should be tested for sterility; 5% of any lot is tested when a batch of 100 or fewer units is received, and a maximum of 10 units are tested in larger batches. A batch is any one shipment of a product with the same lot number; if a separate shipment of the same lot number of product is received, then it is considered a different batch and needs to be tested separately.

Sterility is examined by incubating the medium for 48 hours under the environmental conditions and temperature routine used within the laboratory. Both user-prepared and nonexempt, commercially prepared media should also be tested with QC organisms of known physiologic and biochemical properties. Tables listing specific organisms to test for various media can be found in a number of the references listed at the end of this chapter.

## ANTIMICROBIAL SUSCEPTIBILITY TESTS

The goal of quality control testing of antimicrobial susceptibility tests (ASTs) is to ensure the precision and accuracy of the supplies and microbiologists performing the test. The laboratory must check each lot number and shipment of antimicrobial agent(s) before, or concurrent with, initial use, using approved control organisms. Criteria regarding frequency of testing are the same regardless of the methodology, such as minimum inhibitory concentration (MIC) broth dilution or Kirby-Bauer (see Chapter 12). Each new shipment of microdilution trays or Mueller-Hinton plates should be tested with

CLSI-approved American Type Culture Collection (ATCC [Rockville, Maryland]) reference strains.

Reference strains for MIC testing are selected for genetic stability and give MICs within the midrange of each antimicrobial agent tested. Reference strains for Kirby-Bauer testing have clearly defined mean diameters for the respective zone of inhibition for each antimicrobial tested. ATCC numbers of reference strains are different for various AST methods. Quality control MICs and zone diameters are annually updated and published by the CLSI Subcommittee on Antimicrobial Susceptibility Testing. New tables should be obtained from the CLSI regularly.

Each susceptibility test system must also be tested with use (usually daily) for 20 consecutive days. If three or fewer MICs or zone of inhibition diameters per drug-reference strain combination are outside the reference range during the 20-day testing period, laboratories may switch to weekly QC testing. Thereafter, aberrant results obtained during the weekly testing must be vigorously investigated. If a source of error, such as contamination, incorrect reference strain used, or incorrect atmosphere of incubation, is found, quality control testing may simply be repeated. However, if no source of error is uncovered, 5 consecutive days of retesting must be performed. If accuracy and precision are again acceptable, weekly QC testing may resume; if the problem drug/organism combinations are still outside the reference ranges, 20 days of consecutive testing must be reinitiated before weekly testing can be reinstated. Under no circumstances should any drug/organism combination be reported for a patient isolate if QC testing has failed.

## STAINS AND REAGENTS

Containers of stains and reagents should be labeled as to contents, concentration, storage requirements, date prepared (or received), date placed in service (commonly called the date opened), expiration date, source (commercial manufacturer or user prepared), and lot number. All stains and reagents should be stored according to manufacturer's recommendations and tested with positive and negative controls before use. Tables listing specific organisms to test for various stains or reagents can be found in a number of the references at the end of this chapter. Outdated materials or reagents that fail QC even after retesting with fresh organisms should be discarded immediately. Patient specimens should not be tested using the lot number in question until the problem is resolved; in the case of a repeat failure, an alternative method should be used or the patient's specimen should be sent to a reference laboratory.

## ANTISERA

The lot number, date received, condition received, and expiration date must be recorded for all shipments of antisera. In addition, the antisera should be dated when opened. New lots must be tested concurrently with previous lots, and testing must include positive and negative controls. Periodicity of testing thereafter should follow the requirements of agencies that inspect an individual laboratory (including the Centers for Medicare and

Medicaid Services) and may include, with use, monthly or semiannual checks.

## KITS

Kits that have been approved by the U.S. Food and Drug Administration need to be tested as specified in the manufacturer's package insert. Each shipment of kits must be tested even if it is the same lot number as a previously tested lot, because temperature changes during shipment may affect the performance. Components of reagent kits of different lot numbers must not be interchanged unless otherwise specified by the manufacturer.

## MAINTENANCE OF QC RECORDS

All QC results should be recorded and, when applicable, must include a review of the effectiveness of corrective actions taken to resolve problems, revision of policies and procedures necessary to prevent recurrence of problems, and discussion with appropriate staff. If temperature is adjusted or a biochemical test is repeated, the new readings within the tolerance limits should be listed. In many laboratories, the supervisor reviews and initials all forms weekly and the director then reviews each one monthly. QC records should be maintained for at least 2 years except those on equipment, which must be saved for the life of each instrument.

## MAINTENANCE OF REFERENCE QC STOCKS

Stock organisms may be obtained from the ATCC, commercial vendors, or PT programs; well-defined clinical isolates may also be used. The laboratory should have enough organisms on hand to cover the full range of testing of all necessary materials such as media, kits, and reagents.

### BACTERIOLOGY

Nonfastidious (rapidly growing), aerobic bacterial organisms can be saved up to 1 year on trypticase soy agar (TSA) slants. Long-term storage (less than 1 year) of aerobes or anaerobes can be accomplished either by lyophilization (freeze drying) or freezing at –70° C. Frozen, nonfastidious organisms should be thawed, reisolated, and refrozen every 5 years; fastidious organisms should be thawed, reisolated, and refrozen every 3 years. Stock isolates may be maintained by freezing them in 10% skim milk, trypticase soy broth (TSB) with 15% glycerol, 10% horse blood in sterile, screw-cap vials or Microbank commercially available system (Pro-Lab Diagnostics, Round Rock, Texas).

### MYCOLOGY

Yeasts may be treated as nonfastidious bacterial organisms for maintaining stock cultures. Molds can be stored on potato dextrose agar (PDA) slants at 4° C for 6 months to 1 year. For longer-term storage, PDA slants may be overlaid with sterile mineral oil and stored at room temperature. Alternatively, sterile water can be added to an actively sporulating culture on PDA, the conidia (spores) can be teased apart to dislodge them from the agar surface, and the water can then be dispensed to sterile, screw-top vials. These vials should be capped tightly and stored at room temperature.

## MYCOBACTERIOLOGY

Acid-fast bacilli (AFB) may be kept on Lowenstein-Jenson (LJ) agar slants at 4° C for up to 1 year. They may also be frozen at –70° C in 7H9 broth with glycerol.

## VIROLOGY

Viruses may be stored indefinitely at –70° C in a solution containing a cryoprotectant, such as 10% dimethyl sulfoxide (DMSO) or fetal bovine serum.

## PARASITOLOGY

Slides and photographs must be available for QC purposes. Trichrome and other permanent slides may be purchased from commercial vendors. Clinical slides may be preserved indefinitely by adding a drop of Permount and a coverslip. Clinical slides prepared in-house should be inspected periodically as the preservation solution may deteriorate and crack over time.

## QA PROGRAM

Because QA is the method by which the overall process of infectious disease diagnosis is reviewed, any of the steps involved in the diagnosis of an infectious disease may be studied. These steps include the following:
- Preanalytic
  - Ordering of test by the clinician
  - Processing of test request by the clerical staff
  - Collection of specimen by health care providers or patients
  - Transport of specimen to the laboratory
  - Initial processing of specimen in the laboratory, including specimen accessioning
- Analytic
  - Examination and workup of culture by the microbiologist
  - Interpretation of specimen results by the microbiologist
- Postanalytic
  - Formulation of a written or printed report by the microbiologist
  - Communication of the microbiologist's conclusions to the clinician in written or printed format
  - Interpretation of report by the clinician
  - Institution of appropriate therapy by the clinician

Analytic testing (the work actually done in the microbiology laboratory) is now seen as only one part of a continuing spectrum of steps that begins when the physician orders the test and ends when he or she receives the results and treats the patient.

QA audits are planned and conducted by examining the three stages of testing. The goal is to look at the proficiency with which the patient is served by the whole facility, including the laboratory. The outcome is to look at the consequences to the patient of the work that has been performed. QA audits involve the analysis of how the system works and how it can be improved.

# Q-PROBES

One way to conduct a QA audit is to subscribe to the Q-Probes program, which is a national interlaboratory QA program developed and administered by CAP. CAP selects topics to be audited and provides instructions and worksheets for the collection of data as well as data entry forms. Data are collected for a specified period and then returned to CAP for analysis. CAP returns a summary of the institution's performance as well as a comparison with other facilities of similar size and scope of service. That way, an individual facility can compare its results with those of its peers, a process called benchmarking. Q-Probes are designed for all areas of laboratory medicine. Since inception of the program, microbiology Q-Probe audits have included areas such as (1) blood culture utilization, (2) health care–associated (formerly nosocomial or hospital-acquired) infections, (3) cumulative susceptibility results, (4) antibiotic usage, (5) turnaround time of CSF Gram stains, (6) viral hepatitis test utilization, (7) laboratory diagnosis of tuberculosis, (8) blood culture contamination rates, (9) appropriateness of the ordering of stools for microbiology testing, and (10) sputum quality. Other laboratory-wide audits are also applicable to the microbiology laboratory, including error reporting, quality of reference laboratories, and effects of laboratory computer downtime.

# IN-HOUSE QA AUDITS

A facility that does not subscribe to the Q-Probe program may select topics for audits through suggestions from the medical, nursing, or pharmacy staff; complaints from the medical or nursing staff; or deficiency or observations noted in the laboratory.

Physicians may suggest an audit to measure the transcription accuracy of their orders by nursing unit clerical personnel. Nursing administrators may suggest an audit of contaminated urine cultures to access the compliance of the nursing staff in instructing patients about proper urine culture collection techniques. Pharmacists may notice improper antibiotic utilization by the clinical staff—for example, a patient was not placed on the appropriate therapy after the pathogen was reported or the patient remains on antibiotic therapy to which his or her organism is resistant after the susceptibility report has been charted. Complaints from the medical or nursing staff can involve failure of the laboratory to conduct all the tests requested on the requisition, performance of the wrong test, or an unexpected delay in turnaround time of test results. All complaints to the laboratory must be documented. Corrective action and follow-up with the laboratory, medical, and nursing staff must also be documented.

Deficiencies or problems in the laboratory performance should also be documented. If, for example, the laboratory notices a dramatic rise in the number of positive respiratory syncytial virus (RSV) direct antigen tests in the summer (not RSV season) and the problem is traced back to a quality control problem that a new employee did not recognize, a QA audit might be indicated to study the outcome of the patients, including inappropriate treatment for RSV and failure to institute treatment for the true causative agent. Alternatively, microbiologists may notice they are receiving many ova and parasite (O&P) examinations and stool cultures on patients hospitalized for more than 3 days. Because current cost containment guidelines suggest that this is inappropriate, the microbiology laboratory personnel could undertake a study to determine the percentage of positive results and the number of patients who tested positive for *Clostridium difficile* cytotoxin, which is the more likely cause of diarrhea in patients hospitalized for more than 3 days. If the audit showed that none of the stool cultures or O&P examinations tested positive and no stools were analyzed for *C. difficile* cytotoxin, then these findings would be presented to the medical staff. Some months following the medical staff in-service, the number of stool culture and O&P requests on patients hospitalized longer than 3 days would be reevaluated. It is hoped this would result in a dramatic decrease in numbers of inappropriate tests.

# CONDUCTING A QA AUDIT

Box 78-1 is an example of how an in-house QA audit may be conducted.

# CONTINUOUS DAILY MONITORING

Daily activities of microbiologists and supervisory personnel ensure that patients get the best quality care. These activities include (1) comparing results of morphotypes seen on direct examinations with what grows on the culture to ensure that all organisms have been recovered, (2) checking antimicrobial susceptibility reports to verify that profiles match those expected from a particular species, and (3) studying culture and susceptibility reports for clusters of patients with unusual infections or multiple-drug–resistant organisms. These and many other processes result in continual improvement to all test systems, ultimately resulting in quality patient care.

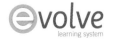 *Visit the Evolve site to complete the review questions.*

---

**BOX 78-1**   QA (Quality Assurance) Audit on STAT (Immediately; derived from Latin statim) Turnaround Times

**Background**

Following a complaint regarding turnaround time for STAT RSV direct antigen tests one winter, the microbiology laboratory at General Hospital has decided to audit its turnaround time. The medical staff indicated that it would like to turn the test around in 2.5 hours (150 minutes) from the time of collection to the time the physician is notified; the medical staff feels that this will ensure the maximum patient benefits.

**Study Design**

All RSV requests for direct antigen testing were evaluated for a 3-month period to determine if laboratory personnel were meeting this turnaround time.

**Results**

| Month | Reports Given in <150 Minutes | | Report Time Exceeding 150 Minutes | | Combined Averages | |
|---|---|---|---|---|---|---|
| | Number of Specimens | Average Time | Number of Specimens | Average Time | Number of Specimens | Average Time |
| December | 57 | 114 min | 15 | 195 min | 72 | 130 min |
| January | 114 | 108 min | 14 | 179 min | 128 | 116 min |
| February | 70 | 114 min | 3 | 165 min | 73 | 116 min |

**Analysis**

In all, 273 reports were reviewed. The average reporting time for the 3-month period was under the acceptable 150 minutes. In December and January, 15 and 14 specimens, respectively, had turnaround times that exceeded 150 minutes, with an average of 195 minutes in December and 179 minutes in January; in February, 3 reports exceeded 150 minutes.

**Conclusions**

The overall (combined) average reporting time, while remaining within 150 minutes, could be improved. There was a dramatic drop in February after the medical staff complaint. This was undoubtedly a result of in-services given to courier and clerical staff regarding the need to transport and accession the stat specimens quickly.

**Recommendations**

Because hospital-wide systems have been improved, appropriate follow-up would be to audit the STAT turnaround time for another test—for example, Gram stain of CSF—in 3 to 6 months to verify that it also meets the 150-minute turnaround time requirement.

---

# BIBLIOGRAPHY

Anderson NL, Noble MA, Weissfeld AS, et al: Quality systems in the clinical microbiology laboratory. In Sewell DL, coordinating editor: *Cumitech 3B*, Washington, DC, 2005, ASM Press.

Clinical and Laboratory Standards Institute: *Methods for dilution antimicrobial susceptibility tests for bacteria that grow aerobically*; approved standard M7-A7, Wayne, Pa, 2006, Clinical and Laboratory Standards Institute.

Clinical and Laboratory Standards Institute: *Performance standards for antimicrobial disk susceptibility tests*; approved standard M2-A9, Wayne, Pa, 2006, Committee for Clinical and Laboratory Standards Institute.

Clinical Laboratory Improvement Amendments (CLIA) regulations, *Subpart K* 493:1235, 2011.

International Organization for Standardization: *Medical laboratories—particular requirements for quality and competence*; ISO 15189:2003(E), Geneva, Switzerland, 2003, International Organization for Standardization.

Jenkins SG: Quality assurance, quality control, laboratory records, and water quality. In Isenberg HD, editor: *Clinical microbiology procedure handbook*, ed 2, Washington, DC, 2004, ASM Press.

LaRocco ML: Quality and productivity in the microbiology laboratory: continuous quality improvement, *Clin Microbiol Newsletter* 17:129, 1995.

National Committee for Clinical Laboratory Standards: *Application of a quality management system model for laboratory services*; approved guideline GP26-A3, Wayne, Pa, 2004, National Committee for Clinical Laboratory Standards.

National Committee for Clinical Laboratory Standards: *Assessment of laboratory tests when proficiency testing is not available*; approved guideline GP29-A, Wayne, Pa, 2002, National Committee for Clinical Laboratory Standards.

National Committee for Clinical Laboratory Standards: *Clinical laboratory technical procedure manuals*; approved guideline GP2-A3, Wayne, Pa, 1996, National Committee for Clinical Laboratory Standards.

National Committee for Clinical Laboratory Standards: *Continuous quality improvement: integrating five key quality system components*; approved guideline, GP22-A2, Wayne Pa, 2004, National Committee for Clinical Laboratory Standards.

National Committee for Clinical Laboratory Standards: *Development of in vitro susceptibility testing criteria and quality control parameters*; approved guideline M23-A2, Wayne, Pa, 2001, National Committee for Clinical Laboratory Standards.

National Committee for Clinical Laboratory Standards: *Methods for antimicrobial susceptibility testing of anaerobic bacteria*; approved standard M11-A6, Wayne, Pa, 2004, National Committee for Clinical Laboratory Standards.

National Committee for Clinical Laboratory *Standards: quality assurance for commercially prepared microbiological culture media*; approved standard M22-A3, Wayne, Pa, 2004, National Committee for Clinical Laboratory Standards.

National Committee for Clinical Laboratory Standards: *Quality control of microbiological transport systems*; approved standard M40-A, Wayne, Pa, 2003, National Committee for Clinical Laboratory Standards.

National Committee for Clinical Laboratory Standards: *Selecting and evaluating a referral laboratory*; approved guideline GP9-A, Wayne, Pa, 1998, National Committee for Clinical Laboratory Standards.

National Committee for Clinical Laboratory Standards: *Training and competence assessment*; approved guideline GP21-A2, Wayne, Pa, 2004, National Committee for Clinical Laboratory Standards.

National Committee for Clinical Laboratory Standards: *Using proficiency testing (PT) to improve the clinical laboratory*; approved guideline GP27-A, Wayne, Pa, 1999, National Committee for Clinical Laboratory Standards.

U.S. Department of Health and Human Services: Medicare, Medicaid and CLIA programs: Regulations implementing the Clinical Laboratory Improvement Amendments of 1988 (CLIA). Final rule. *Federal Register* 57:7002-7186, 1992.

Warford A: Quality assurance in clinical virology. In Specter S, Hodinka RL, Young SA, editors: *Clinical virology manual*, ed 3, Washington, DC, 2000, ASM Press.

Westgard, S: Quality management cocktail ISO, lean, and six sigma. Retrieved from www.westgard.com/guest30.htm.

# Infection Control

## OBJECTIVES

1. Define and compare health care–associated infections and community-acquired infections.
2. List three factors determining the likelihood that a given patient would acquire a health care–associated infection.
3. State the most common types of health care–associated infections, and identify the risk factors that predispose patients to acquire each infection.
4. Explain the emergence of antibiotic-resistant microorganisms and their impact on health care.
5. Describe hospital infection control programs, and outline the structure and responsibilities of the infection control committee in a medical facility.
6. Identify means of transmission for microorganisms within a health care facility.
7. Interpret the role of the microbiology laboratory in an infectious outbreak.
8. Compare the two major ways to characterize strains involved in an outbreak.
9. Discuss techniques for isolation precautions used to prevent the spread of health care–associated infections.
10. Identify potential useful applications for surveillance cultures.

It is estimated that between 1.75 and 3 million (5% to 10%) of the 35 million patients admitted annually to acute-care hospitals in the United States acquire an infection that was neither present nor in the prodromal (incubation) stage when they entered the hospital. These infections are called health care–associated infections (HAIs). HAI has replaced old confusing terms such as nosocomial, hospital-acquired or hospital-onset infections. Treatment of HAI is estimated to add between $4.5 and $15 billion annually to the cost of health care and represents an enormous economic problem in today's environment of cost containment. In addition, many of these infections lead to the death of hospitalized patients (patient mortality) or, at minimum, additional complications (patient morbidity) and further antimicrobial chemotherapy.

Some of the earliest efforts to control infection followed the recognition in the nineteenth century that women were dying in childbirth from bloodstream infections caused by group A *Streptococcus* (*Streptococcus pyogenes*) because physicians were spreading the organism by failing to wash their hands between examinations of different patients. Hand washing is still the cornerstone of modern infection control programs. Moreover, the first recommendations for isolation precautions in U.S. hospitals were published in the late 1800s, when guidelines appeared advocating placement of patients with infectious diseases in separate hospital facilities. By the late 1950s, the advent of HAI caused by *Staphylococcus aureus* finally ushered in the modern age of infection

control. In the past four decades, we have learned that, in addition to hospitalized patients acquiring infections, health care workers are also at risk of acquiring infections from patients. Thus, present-day infection control programs have evolved to prevent the acquisition of infection by patients and caregivers.

In contrast, *community-acquired infection* is an infection contracted outside a health care setting or an infection present on admission. Community-acquired infections are often distinguished from HAIs by the types of organisms that affect patients who are recovering from a disease or infection. Community-acquired respiratory infections commonly involve strains of *Haemophilus influenzae* or *Streptococcus pneumoniae* and are usually more antibiotic sensitive.

The American Recovery and Reinvestment Act of 2009 was signed into law on February 17, 2009. The Recovery Act was designed to stimulate economic recovery in various ways including strengthening the nation's health care infrastructure and reducing health care costs. Within the Recovery Act, $50 million was authorized to support states in the prevention and reduction of HAI. The HAI Recovery Act funds would be invested in efforts that support surveillance and prevention of HAIs, encourage collaboration, train the workforce in HAI prevention, and measure outcomes.

## INCIDENCE OF HAI

The Centers for Disease Control and Prevention (CDC) has established the National Healthcare Safety Network (NHSN) program to monitor the incidence of HAI in the United States. Data collected in NHSN are used to improve patient safety at the local and national levels. In aggregate, the CDC analyzes and publishes surveillance data to estimate and characterize the national burden of health care–associated infections. Regardless of a hospital's size or medical school affiliation, the rates of infections at each body site are consistent across institutions. The majority of HAIs are urinary tract infections (33%), followed by pneumonia (15%), surgical site infections (15%), and bloodstream infections (13%). The remaining 24% are other miscellaneous infections. Each HIA adds 5 to 10 days to the affected patient's hospital stay. Of individuals with hospital-acquired bloodstream or lung infections, 40% to 60% die each year. Likewise, patients with indwelling urinary catheters have a threefold increased chance of dying from urosepsis—a bloodstream infection that is a complication of a urinary tract infection—than those who do not have one.

Attack rates vary according to the type of hospital. Large, tertiary-care hospitals that treat the most seriously ill patients often have higher rates of HIA than do small, acute-care community hospitals; large medical school–affiliated (teaching) hospitals have higher infection rates than do small teaching hospitals. This difference in the risk of infection is probably related to several factors, including but not limited to the severity of illness, the frequency of invasive diagnostic and therapeutic procedures, and variation in the effectiveness of infection control programs. Within hospitals, the surgical and medical services have the highest rates of infection; the pediatric and nursery services have the lowest. Moreover, within services, the predominant type of infections varies—that is, surgical site infections are the most common on the surgical service, whereas urinary tract or bloodstream infections are the most common on medical services or in the nursery.

## TYPES OF HAI

The majority of HAIs are endogenous in origin—that is, they involve the patient's own microbial flora. Three principal factors determine the likelihood that a given patient will acquire an infection:

- Susceptibility of the patient to the infection
- The virulence of the infecting organism
- The nature of the patient's exposure to the infecting organism

In general, hospitalized individuals have increased susceptibility to infection. Corticosteroids, cancer chemotherapeutic agents, and antimicrobial agents all contribute to the likelihood of HAI by suppressing the immune system or altering the host's normal flora to that of resistant microbes. Likewise, foreign objects, such as urinary or intravenous catheters, break the body's natural barriers to infection. Nonetheless, these medications or devices are necessary to cure the patient's primary medical condition. Finally, exerting influence over the virulence of the pathogens is not possible because it is not possible to immunize patients against HAI. Patients with serious community-acquired infections are frequently admitted to the hospital, and the disease may spread by either direct contact; by contact with contaminated food, water, medications, or medical devices (fomites); or by airborne transmission. Thus, the HAI may never be completely eliminated, only controlled.

## URINARY TRACT INFECTIONS

Gram-negative rods produce the majority of health care–associated urinary tract infections, and *Escherichia coli* is the number one organism involved. Gram-positive organisms, *Candida* spp., and other fungi cause the remainder of the infections. The risk factors that predispose patients to acquire a health care–associated urinary tract infection include advanced age, female gender, severe underlying disease, and the placement of indwelling urinary catheters.

## LUNG INFECTIONS

The most common HAI pathogens causing pneumonia include gram-negative rods, *S. aureus*, and *Moraxella catarrhalis*. *Streptococcus pneumoniae* and *Haemophilus influenzae*, which cause the majority of community-acquired pneumonias, are not important etiologic agents in hospital-acquired infections except very early during the hospital course (first 2 to 5 days); these infections probably represent infections that were already incubating at the time of the hospital admission. The risk factors that predispose patients to acquire a health care–associated lung infection include advanced age, chronic lung disease, large-volume aspiration (the microorganisms in the upper respiratory tract are coughed up and lodge in the lungs instead of being spit out or swallowed), chest surgery, hospitalization in intensive care units, and intubation (placement of a breathing tube down a patient's throat) or attachment to a mechanical ventilator (which controls breathing).

## SURGICAL SITE INFECTIONS

Approximately 4% of surgical patients develop surgical site infections; 50% of these infections develop after the patient has left the hospital, so this number may be an underestimate. Gram-positive organisms (*S. aureus*, coagulase-negative staphylococci, and enterococci) cause the majority of these infections, followed by gram-negative rods and *Candida* spp. The risk factors that predispose patients to acquire a health care–associated wound infection include advanced age, obesity, infection at a remote site (that spreads through the bloodstream), malnutrition, diabetes, extended preoperative hospital stay, greater than 12 hours between preoperative shaving of site and surgery, extended time of surgery, and inappropriate timing of prophylactic antibiotics (given to prevent common infections before they seed the surgical site). Surgical wounds are classified as clean, clean-contaminated, contaminated, or dirty, depending on the number of contaminating organisms at the site. Bowel surgery is considered dirty, for example, whereas surgery for a total hip replacement is considered clean.

## CENTRAL LINE-ASSOCIATED BLOODSTREAM INFECTION

A central line-associated bloodstream infection (CLABSI) is a serious infection that occurs when microbes enter the bloodstream through a central line. A central line is a tube that health care providers place in a large vein in the neck, chest, or arm to give fluids, blood, or medications or to do certain medical tests quickly. CLABSIs result in thousands of deaths each year and billions of dollars in added costs to the U.S. health care system, yet these infections are preventable. The risk factors that predispose patients to acquire a CLABSI include age 1 year of age or younger or 60 years of age and older, malnutrition, immunosuppressive chemotherapy, loss of skin integrity (e.g., burn or decubiti [bedsore]), severe underlying illness, indwelling device (e.g., catheter), intensive care unit stay, and prolonged hospital stay.

# EMERGENCE OF ANTIBIOTIC-RESISTANT MICROORGANISMS

The organisms that cause HAIs have changed over the years because of selective pressures from the use (and overuse) of antibiotics (see Chapter 11). Risk factors for the acquisition of highly resistant organisms include prolonged hospitalization and prior treatment with antibiotics. In the pre-antibiotic era, most HAIs were caused by *S. pneumoniae* and group A *Streptococcus* (*Streptococcus pyogenes*). In the 1940s and 1950s, with the advent of treatment of patients with penicillin and sulfonamides, resistant strains of *S. aureus* appeared. Then, in the 1970s, treatment of patients with narrow-spectrum cephalosporins and aminoglycosides led to the emergence of resistant aerobic gram-negative rods, such as *Klebsiella*, *Enterobacter*, *Serratia*, and *Pseudomonas*. During the late 1970s and early 1980s, the use of more potent cephalosporins played a role in the emergence of antibiotic-resistant, coagulase-negative staphylococci, enterococci, methicillin-resistant *S. aureus* (MRSA), and *Candida* spp. The 1990s witnessed the emergence of beta-lactamase–producing, high-level gentamicin-resistant, and vancomycin-resistant enterococci (VRE). The twenty-first century has seen the emergence of vancomycin-resistant *Staphylococcus aureus* (VRSA).

Patients' normal flora will change quickly after hospitalization from viridans streptococci, saprophytic *Neisseria* spp., and diphtheroids to potentially resistant microorganisms found in the hospital environment. The colonized nares, skin, gastrointestinal tract, or genitourinary tract can later serve as reservoirs for endogenously acquired infections. Moreover, if patients colonized with resistant microorganisms return to nursing homes in the community harboring these organisms, they can also transfer them to other patients. This further increases the pool of patients who harbor multidrug-resistant organisms when they, in turn, are hospitalized. These new patients recontaminate the hospital environment and serve as potential reservoirs for spread to additional patients.

# HOSPITAL INFECTION CONTROL PROGRAMS

Hospital infection control programs are designed to detect and monitor HAIs and to prevent or control their spread. The infection control committee is multidisciplinary and should include a microbiologist, an infection control practitioner (often a nurse with special training), a hospital epidemiologist (usually an infectious disease physician), and a pharmacist. The infection control practitioner collects and analyzes surveillance data, monitors patient care practices, and participates in epidemiologic investigations. Daily review of charts of patients with fever or positive microbiology cultures allows the infection control practitioner to recognize problems with HAIs and to detect outbreaks as early as possible. The infection control practitioner is also responsible for the education of health care providers in techniques, such as hand washing and isolation precautions, that minimize the acquisition and spread of infections.

It is the infection control practitioner's job to identify all cases of an outbreak. The investigation of the cluster of cases during a particular outbreak involves its characterization in terms of commonalities, such as location in the hospital (nursery, intensive care unit), same caregiver, or prior respiratory or physical therapy. Risk factors—including underlying diseases, current or prior antimicrobial therapy, and placement of a urinary catheter—are also assessed. This information helps the infection control committee determine the reservoir of the organism in the hospital—that is, the place where it exists and the means by which the organism is transmitted from its reservoir to the patient.

Microorganisms are spread in hospitals through several modes:

- Direct contact—for example, in contaminated food or intravenous solutions
- Indirect contact, for example, from patient to patient on the hands of health care workers (MRSA, rotavirus)
- Droplet contact—for example, inhalation of droplets (>5 μm in diameter) that cannot travel more than 3 feet (pertussis)
- Airborne contact—for example, inhalation of droplets (>5 μm) that can travel large distances on air currents (tuberculosis)
- Vector-borne contact—for example, disease spread by vectors, such as mosquitoes (malaria) or rats (rat-bite fever); this mode of transmission is rare in hospitals in developed countries

Once the reservoir is known, the infection control practitioner can implement control measures, such as reeducation regarding hand washing (in the case of spread by health care workers) or hyperchlorination of cooling towers in the case of legionellosis.

# ROLE OF THE MICROBIOLOGY LABORATORY

The microbiology laboratory supplies the data on organism identification and antimicrobial susceptibility profile that the infection control practitioner reviews daily for evidence of HAI. Thus, the laboratory personnel must be able to detect potential microbial pathogens and then accurately identify them to species level and perform appropriate susceptibility testing. The microbiology laboratory staff should also monitor multidrug-resistant organisms by tabulating data on antimicrobial susceptibilities of common isolates and studying trends indicating emerging resistance. Significant findings should be immediately reported to the infection control practitioner. If an outbreak is suspected, the laboratory works in tandem with the infection control committee by (1) saving all isolates, (2) culturing possible reservoirs (patients, personnel, or the environment), and (3) performing typing of strains to establish relatedness between isolates of the same species. Microbiology laboratories are also obligated by law to report certain isolates or syndromes to public health authorities. For example, Table 79-1 lists organisms to be reported to state health authorities in Texas. Other states have similar criteria.

## CHARACTERIZING STRAINS INVOLVED IN AN OUTBREAK

The ideal system for typing microbial strains involved in outbreaks should be standardized, reproducible, sensitive, stable, readily available, inexpensive, applicable to a wide range of microorganisms, and field tested in other epidemiologic investigations. Although no such perfect system is currently available, a number of methods are used to aid in typing epidemic strains. There are two major ways to type strains using either phenotypic traits or molecular typing methods.

Classic phenotypic techniques include biotyping (analyzing unique biologic or biochemical characteristics), the use of antibiograms (analyzing antimicrobial susceptibility patterns), and serotyping (serologic typing of bacterial or viral antigens, such as bacterial cell wall [O] antigens). Bacteriocin typing, which examines an organism's susceptibility to bacterial peptides (proteins), and bacteriophage typing, which examines the ability of bacteriophages (viruses capable of infecting and lysing bacterial cells) to attack certain strains, have been useful for typing *Pseudomonas aeruginosa* and *S. aureus*, respectively; these techniques, however, are not widely available.

Genotypic, or molecular, methods have largely replaced phenotypic methods as a means of confirming the relatedness of strains involved in an outbreak. Plasmid analysis and restriction endonuclease analysis of chromosomal DNA are widely used. Plasmids are extrachromosomal pieces of genetic material (nucleic acids) that self-replicate (reproduce). Plasmids may be transferred from one bacterial cell to another by conjugation or transduction (see Chapter 2). Plasmid analysis has often been used to explain the occurrence of unusual or multiple-antibiotic resistance patterns. It has been shown that plasmids or R factors (resistance genes carried on plasmids) can cause outbreaks when a specific plasmid is transmitted from one genus of bacteria to another. Plasmid profiles, patterns created when plasmids are separated based on molecular weight by agarose gel electrophoresis, can also be used to characterize the similarity of bacterial strains. Relatedness of strains is based on the number and size of plasmids, with strains from identical sources showing identical plasmid profiles. Plasmids themselves or chromosomal DNA may also be typed by means of restriction endonuclease digestion patterns. Restriction enzymes recognize specific nucleotide sequences in DNA and produce double-stranded cleavages that break the DNA into smaller fragments. The fragments of various sizes are separated using gel electrophoresis based on molecular weight. The specific recognition sequence and cleavage site have been defined for a great many of these enzymes.

Modifications of the basic restriction endonuclease technique have been developed to reduce the number of bands generated to fewer than 20 in an attempt to make the gels easier to interpret. These include pulsed-field gel electrophoresis (PFGE) and hybridization of ribosomal RNA with short fragments of DNA. Plasmid restriction digests have been used to type *S. aureus* and coagulase-negative staphylococci, and PFGE is the preferred method for typing enterococci, enteric gram-negative rods, and other gram-negative rods.

Other molecular methods, such as PCR (polymerase chain reaction), are used in conjunction with these methods for strain typing. Molecular methods are discussed in more detail in Chapter 8.

## PREVENTING HAI

The CDC published guidelines in the 1970s specifying isolation precautions in hospitals. Techniques for isolation precautions included (1) health care workers washing their hands between caring for different patients; (2) segregation of infected patients in private rooms or cohorting of patients (placing patients with the same clinical syndrome in semiprivate rooms) if private rooms are not available; (3) wearing of masks, gowns, and gloves when caring for infected patients; (4) bagging of contaminated articles, such as bed linens, when removed from the room; (5) cleaning of all isolation rooms after the patient is discharged; and (6) placement of cards on the patient's door specifying the type of isolation and instructions for visitors and health care workers. Categories of isolation were also established and included (1) strict isolation for highly contagious diseases such as chickenpox, pneumonic plague, and Lassa fever; (2) respiratory isolation for diseases such as measles or *Haemophilus influenzae* or *Neisseria meningitidis*; (3) enteric precautions for diseases such as amebic dysentery, *Salmonella*, and *Shigella*; (4) contact isolation for patients infected with multidrug-resistant bacteria; (5) acid-fast bacilli (AFB) (tuberculosis) isolation for persons with *M. tuberculosis*; (6) drainage and secretion precautions for persons with conjunctivitis and burns; and (7) blood and body fluid precautions for individuals with acquired immunodeficiency syndrome (AIDS). Over time, a system of disease-specific precautions was added to the category-specific ones, and hospitals were given the option of using one of the two systems. Disease-specific precautions were more cost-effective, in that only those precautions specifically necessary were used to interrupt the transmission of a single disease.

In 1996, the CDC developed a new system of standard precautions synthesizing the features of universal precautions (described in Chapter 4) and body substance isolation. Standard precautions are used in the care of all patients and apply to blood; all body fluids, secretions, and excretions except sweat, regardless of whether they contain visible blood; nonintact skin; and mucous membranes.

**TABLE 79-1** Examples of Notifiable Infectious Conditions in Texas*

| Diseases to Be Reported Immediately by Telephone/Fax† | Diseases to Be Reported within 1 Working Day | Diseases to Be Reported within 1 Week | Diseases to Be Reported Quarterly |
|---|---|---|---|
| Anthrax | Brucellosis | Acquired immunodeficiency syndrome (AIDS) | Vancomycin-resistant *Enterococcus* (VRE) |
| Botulism, food-borne | Hepatitis A (acute) | Amebiasis | Penicillin-resistant *Streptococcus pneumoniae* |
| Diphtheria | Q fever | Botulism, infant | |
| *H. influenzae*, type b invasive infections | Rubella (including congenital) | Campylobacteriosis | |
| Measles (rubeola) | Tuberculosis | Chancroid | |
| Meningococcal infections, invasive | Tularemia | *Chlamydia trachomatis* infections | |
| Pertussis | *Vibrio* infection, including cholera | Creutzfeldt-Jakob disease | |
| Plague | | *Cryptosporidium* infections | |
| Poliomyelitis, acute paralytic | | Cyclospora | |
| Rabies in humans | | Dengue | |
| Severe acute respiratory syndrome (SARS) | | Encephalitis (specify etiology) | |
| Smallpox | | Ehrlichiosis | |
| Viral hemorrhagic fevers | | *Escherichia coli* O157:H7 | |
| Yellow fever | | Gonorrhea | |
| Vancomycin-resistant *Staphylococcus aureus* (VRSA) | | Hansen's disease (leprosy) | |
| Vancomycin-resistant coagulase-negative *Staphylococcus* spp. | | Hantavirus infection<br>Hemolytic-uremic syndrome (HUS)<br>Hepatitis B, D, E, and unspecified (acute)<br>Hepatitis B (chronic) identified prenatally or at delivery<br>Hepatitis C (newly diagnosed infection)<br>Human immunodeficiency virus (HIV) infection<br>Legionellosis<br>Listeriosis<br>Lyme disease<br>Malaria<br>Meningitis (specify type)<br>Mumps<br>Relapsing fever<br>Salmonellosis, including typhoid fever<br>Shigellosis<br>Spotted fever group rickettsioses<br>Streptococcal disease, invasive (group A or B or *S. pneumoniae*)<br>Syphilis<br>Tetanus<br>Trichinosis<br>Typhus<br>Varicella (chickenpox)<br>Yersiniosis | |

*In addition to individual case reports, any outbreak, exotic disease, or unusual group expression of disease that may be of public health concern should be reported by the most expeditious means. This list is not all-inclusive and is updated annually.
†Report even if only suspected; waiting for confirmation may hamper public health intervention activities.

---

**BOX 79-1** Infection Control Measures for Standard Precautions

- Health care workers (HCWs) should wash hands frequently using a plain soap except in special circumstances—for example, preoperatively or after handling dressings from patients on contact isolation.
- HCWs should wear gloves when touching blood, body fluids, secretions, excretions, and contaminated items.
- HCWs should wear a mask, gown, eye protection, or face shield as appropriate.
- Each hospital should ensure that it has adequate procedures for routine care, cleaning, and disinfection of environmental surfaces, beds, bed rails, and bedside equipment.
- Hospitals should handle, transport, and launder used linen soiled with blood, body fluids, secretions, and excretions in a manner that prevents skin and mucous membrane exposure and contamination of clothing, and that avoids the transfer of microorganisms to other patients or the environment.
- HCWs should take care to prevent injuries when using needles, scalpels, and other sharp instruments or devices.
- HCWs should use equipment, such as mouthpieces and resuscitation bags, instead of mouth-to-mouth resuscitation.
- HCWs should refrain from handling patient care equipment if they have exudative lesions or weeping dermatitis.
- Hospitals should place incontinent or nonhygienic patients in a private room.
- Hospitals should ensure that reusable equipment is properly sterilized.
- Hospitals should ensure that single-use items are discarded properly.

Modified from Healthcare Infection Control Practices Advisory Committee (HICPAC), 2007.

---

In addition, transmission-based precautions are used for patients known (or suspected) to be infected with pathogens spread by airborne or droplet transmission or by contact with dry skin or fomites. Box 79-1 lists infection control measures for standard precautions. Table 79-2 lists the infectious agents or syndromes along with the respective infection control measures for each transmission-based precaution. Many infection control practitioners find these guidelines a lot less cumbersome to implement than the old category- and disease-specific measures. Hospitals, however, may modify these guidelines to fit their individual situations as long as their number of HAIs remains low.

Some of the potential agents of bioterrorism can be transmitted person to person (smallpox, pneumonic plague, and viral hemorrhagic fevers) and some cannot (anthrax). The ones that can be easily transmitted have specific transmission-based precautions—that is, airborne precautions for smallpox, droplet precautions for patients for pneumonic plague, and contact precautions for individuals with one of the viral hemorrhagic fevers (Ebola, Marburg).

# SURVEILLANCE METHODS

Most routine environmental cultures in the hospital are now considered to be of little use and should not be performed unless there are specific epidemiologic reasons. The decision to perform these cultures should be determined by the microbiologist, infection control practitioner, and hospital epidemiologist. However, certain surveillance cultures are still performed as a method of limiting outbreaks. These include culturing cooling towers or hot water sources for *Legionella* spp., culturing water and dialysis fluids for hemodialysis as well as endotoxin testing, culturing blood bank products, especially platelets, and surveillance cultures for vancomycin-resistant enterococci (VRE), methicillin (or oxacillin)-resistant *S. aureus* (MRSA), and vancomycin-resistant *S. aureus* (VRSA) using rectal and oropharyngeal swabs. Physical rehabilitation centers often culture hydrotherapy equipment (whirlpools) quarterly to verify that cleaning methods are adequate; some centers culture more frequently.

Routine surveillance of air handlers, food utensils, food equipment surfaces, and respiratory therapy equipment is no longer recommended; neither is monitoring infant formulas prepared in-house nor items purchased as sterile. A better approach is for the infection control team to monitor patients for the development of an HAI that might be related to the use of contaminated commercial products. In the event of an outbreak or an incident related to suspected contamination, a microbiologic study would be indicated. However, most often, such infections are actually caused by in-use contamination, rather than contamination during the manufacturing process. Suspect lots of fluid and catheter trays should be saved, and the U.S. Food and Drug Administration should be notified if contamination of an unopened product is suspected.

Although some institutions still require preemployment stool cultures and ova and parasite examinations on food handlers, most now recognize that this is of limited value. It is much more important for food handlers to submit specimens for these tests if they develop diarrhea. Similarly, most hospitals no longer screen personnel routinely for nasal carriage of *S. aureus*. Although a significant percentage of the general population, including hospital personnel, are known to carry this organism, most individuals rarely shed enough organism to pose a hazard and there is no simple way to predict which nasal carriers will disseminate staphylococci.

All steam and dry-heat sterilizers and ethylene oxide gas sterilizers should be checked at least once each week with a liquid spore suspension.

Hospitals that perform bone marrow transplantation or treat hematologic malignancies may also conduct surveillance cultures of severely immunocompromised patients who occupy laminar flow rooms. In these instances, the isolation of specific organisms may have predictive value for subsequent systemic infection. Air sampling for fungi during construction is also indicated, especially if patients are immunocompromised and are being treated near the construction site.

**TABLE 79-2** Transmission-Based Precautions

| Type of Precaution | Specific Etiologic Agents or Syndromes | Infection Control Measure to Be Undertaken by Hospital |
|---|---|---|
| Airborne | Measles<br>Varicella<br>Tuberculosis<br>Smallpox | Place patient in private room that has monitored negative air pressure, 6-12 air changes per hour, and appropriate discharge of air outdoors or monitored HEPA filtration of room air before air is circulated to other areas of the hospital or cohorting of patients—that is, placing patients with the same infection in the same room, if private rooms are not available<br>Health care workers (HCWs) to wear respiratory protection when entering room of patient with known or suspected tuberculosis and, if not immune, for patients with measles or varicella as well<br>Transport patients out of their room only after placement of a surgical mask |
| Droplet | Invasive *Haemophilus influenzae* type b infection, including meningitis, pneumonia, epiglottitis, and sepsis<br>Invasive *Neisseria meningitidis* infection, including meningitis, pneumonia, and sepsis<br>Diphtheria (pharyngeal)<br>*Mycoplasma pneumoniae*<br>Pertussis<br>Pneumonic plague<br>Streptococcal pharyngitis, pneumonia, or scarlet fever in infants and young children<br>Adenovirus, influenza virus<br>Mumps<br>Parvovirus B19<br>Rubella | Place patient in private room without special air handling or ventilation or cohort patients<br>HCWs should wear mask when working within 3 feet of patient<br>Transfer patients out of their room only after placement of a surgical mask |
| Contact | Gastrointestinal, respiratory, skin, or wound infections, or colonization with multidrug-resistant bacteria<br>*Clostridium difficile*<br>For diapered or incontinent patients: *Escherichia coli* O157:H7, *Shigella*, hepatitis A virus, or rotavirus<br>Respiratory syncytial virus, parainfluenza virus, and enterovirus infections in infants and young children<br>Skin infections such as diphtheria (cutaneous), herpes simplex virus (neonatal or mucocutaneous), impetigo, major abscesses, cellulitis, or decubiti, pediculosis (lice infestation), scabies (mite infestation), staphylococci furunculosis (boils) in infants and young children, zoster (disseminated or in the immunocompromised host)<br>Viral hemorrhagic infections (Ebola, Lassa, or Marburg) | Place patient in private room without special air handling or ventilation or cohort patients<br>HCWs should wear gloves when entering patient's room<br>HCWs should wash hands with a special antimicrobial agent or a waterless antiseptic agent<br>HCWs should wear a mask and eye protection during activities that are likely to generate splashes of blood, body fluids, secretions, or excretions<br>HCWs should wear a gown during procedures likely to generate splashes<br>HCWs should ensure reusable equipment is properly sterilized<br>HCWs should ensure that single-use items are properly discarded |

Modified from Healthcare Infection Control Practices Advisory Committee (HICPAC), 2007.

The U.S. Pharmacopeia published requirements for monitoring of sterile compounding in hospital pharmacies. The laminar flow hoods, biologic safety cabinets, clean rooms, and donning areas must be monitored weekly or monthly so that intravenous or intrathecal products and drugs used in the operating room are made (compounded) under sterile conditions.

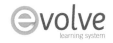

*Visit the Evolve site to complete the review questions.*

# BIBLIOGRAPHY

Banerjee SN, Emori TG, Culver DH, et al, and the National Nosocomial Infection Surveillance System: Secular trends in nosocomial primary bloodstream infections in the United States, 1980-1989, *Am J Med* 91(suppl 3B):86S, 1991.

Centers for Disease Control and Prevention: Public health focus: surveillance, prevention and control of nosocomial infections, *MMWR* 41:783, 1992.

Coffin SE, Zaoutis TE: Healthcare-associated infections. In Long SS, Pickering LK, Prober CG: *Principles and practice of pediatric infectious diseases*, ed 3, 2008, Churchill Livingstone, New York, Chapter 101.

Craven DE, Chroneou A, Zias N, Hjalmarson KI: Ventilator-associated tracheobronchitis: the impact of targeted antibiotic therapy on patient outcomes, *Chest* 135(2):521-528, 2009.

Craven DE, Steger KA, Barber TW: Preventing nosocomial pneumonia: state of the art and perspectives for the 1990s, *Am J Med* 91(suppl 3B):44S, 1991.

Edwards JR, Peterson KD, Andrus ML, et al, and the National Health-care Safety Network (NHSN) Report, data summary for 2006 through 2007, issued November 2008, *Am J Infect Control* 36(9):609-626, 2008.

Emori TG, Gaynes RP: An overview of nosocomial infections, including the role of the microbiology laboratory, *Clin Microbiol Rev* 6:428, 1993.

Garibaldi RA, Cushing D, Lerer T: Risk factors for postoperative infection, *Am J Med* 91(suppl 3B):158S, 1991.

Garner JS, Favero MS: *Guideline for hand washing and hospital environmental control, 1985*, PB85-923404, Atlanta, 1985, Centers for Disease Control.

Garner JS, Simmons BP: *CDC guideline for isolation precautions in hospitals*, PB85-923401, Atlanta, 1983, Centers for Disease Control.

Gastmeier P, Geffers C, Brandt C, et al: Effectiveness of a nationwide nosocomial infection surveillance system for reducing nosocomial infections, *J Hosp Infect.* 64(1):16-22, 2006.

Guidelines for the management of adults with hospital-acquired: ventilator-associated, and healthcare-associated pneumonia, *Am J Respir Crit Care Med* 171(4):388-416, 2005.

Guidelines for the prevention of intravascular catheter-related infections: Centers for Disease Control and Prevention. Available at www.cdc.gov/mmwr/PDF/rr/rr5110.pdf. Accessed December 31, 2010.

Horan TC, Andrus M, Dudeck MA: CDC/NHSN surveillance definition of health care-associated infection and criteria for specific types of infections in the acute care setting, *Am J Infect Control* 36(5):309-332, 2008.

Hospital Infection Control Practices Advisory Committee: Guideline for infection control in health care personnel, *Am J Infect Control* 26:289, 1998.

Hospital Infection Control Practices Advisory Committee: Guideline for isolation precaution in hospitals, *Infect Control Hosp Epidemiol* 17:53, 1996.

Hospital Infection Control Practices Advisory Committee: Guideline for prevention of intravascular device-related infections, *Am J Infect Control* 24:262, 1996.

Hospital Infection Control Practices Advisory Committee: *Guideline for prevention of nosocomial pneumonia, PB95-176970*, Atlanta, 1994, Centers for Disease Control and Prevention.

Hospital Infection Control Practices Advisory Committee: Guideline for prevention of surgical site infection, *Infect Control Hosp Epidemiol* 20:247, 1999.

Hospital Infection Control Practices Advisory Committee: Recommendations for preventing the spread of vancomycin resistance, *Infect Control Hosp Epidemiol* 16:105, 1995.

Hospital Infections Program, National Center for Infectious Diseases, Centers for Disease Control and Prevention: Public Health Focus: surveillance, prevention, and control of nosocomial infections, *MMWR* 41(42):783-787, 1992.

Javis WR: Infection control and changing health-care delivery systems, *Emerg Infect Dis* 7:170, 2001.

Jewett JF, Reid DE, Safon LE, et al: Childbed fever: a continuing entity, *JAMA* 206:344, 1968.

Klevens RM, Edwards JR, Richards CL, et al: Estimating healthcare-associated infections in US hospitals, 2002, *Public Health Rep* 122(2):160-166, 2007.

McGowan JE Jr, Weinstein RA: The role of the laboratory in control of nosocomial infection. In Bennett JV, Brachman PS, editors: *Hospital infections*, ed 3, Boston, 1992, Little, Brown.

Miller JM, Bell M, editors: Epidemiologic and infection control microbiology. In Isenberg HD, editor: *Clinical microbiology procedures handbook*, ed 2, Washington, DC, 2004, ASM Press.

Nichols RL: Surgical wound infection, *Am J Med* 91(suppl 3B): 54S, 1991.

Scott RD: The direct medical costs of healthcare-associated infections in US hospitals and the benefits of prevention, 2008, Centers for Disease Control and Prevention. Available at www.cdc.gov/ncidod/dhqp/pdf/Scott_CostPaper.pdf. Accessed December 31, 2010.

Siegel JD, Rhinehart E, Jackson M, Chiarello L, and the Healthcare Infection Control Practices Advisory Committee: *2007 Guideline for Isolation Precautions: Preventing Transmission of Infectious Agents in Healthcare Settings*, Centers for Disease Control and Prevention. Available at www.cdc.gov/ncidod/dhqp/pdf/guidelines/Isolation2007.pdf. Accessed December 31, 2010.

Stamm WE: Catheter-associated urinary tract infections: epidemiology, pathogenesis, and prevention, *Am J Med* 91 (suppl 3B):65S, 1991.

US Pharmacopeial Convention, Inc: Pharmaceutical compounding—sterile preparations. In *United States pharmacopeia 27*, pp 2350, Rockville, Md, 2004, US Pharmacopeial Convention, Inc.

US Pharmacopeial Convention, Inc: Pharmaceutical compounding—sterile preparations. In *United States pharmacopeia 27*, Supplement 1, pp 3121, Rockville, Md, 2004, US Pharmacopeial Convention, Inc.

Wenzel RP, editor: *Prevention and control of nosocomial infections*, ed 3, Baltimore, 1997, Williams & Wilkins.

Wenzel RP, Edmond MB: The impact of hospital-acquired bloodstream infections, *Emerg Infect Dis* 7(2):174-177, 2001.

Wong ES, Hooton TM: *Guideline for prevention of catheter-associated urinary tract infections*, Centers for Disease Control and Prevention. Available at www.cdc.gov/ncidod/dhqp/gl_catheter_assoc.html. Accessed December 31, 2010.

# Sentinel Laboratory Response to Bioterrorism

## OBJECTIVES

1. Define and give examples of a biocrime.
2. Define and give examples of select agents.
3. Site two laws that govern the possession of select agents.
4. List the government agencies that must be notified, by registration, before a laboratory may possess a select agent.
5. State the components of a biosecurity plan.
6. Summarize the standard operating procedures required for laboratories that maintain select agents.
7. Diagram and give a brief description of the Laboratory Response Network.
8. Outline the steps microbiology laboratories must follow if a select agent is isolated from a clinical specimen.
9. Explain the requirements for operation as a sentinel laboratory.
10. Name the government agencies responsible for the investigation and management of a bioterrorism event.

## GENERAL CONSIDERATIONS

The practice of clinical microbiology changed significantly after *Bacillus anthracis* was intentionally released into the United States postal system in October 2001. Prior to this release there were two events in which microorganisms were used to intentionally harm the civilian population in the United States.

The first incident, in 1984, was a large community outbreak of salmonellosis caused by the intentional contamination of restaurant salad bars in The Dalles, Oregon. In this incident, a cult leader, Baghwan Sri Rajneesh, set out to influence the outcome of a local election by incapacitating voters. Cultures of Salmonella *enterica* Thyphimurium were grown at a laboratory within the cult's compound. Ultimately, 751 individuals fell ill; luckily there were no deaths.

In 1996 an outbreak among laboratory workers was caused when a microbiology technologist in Dallas, Texas, purposely contaminated muffins and donuts with *Shigella dysenteriae* type 2. Forty-five laboratory workers developed gastroenteritis; four individuals were hospitalized.

The event in October 2001 stunned the country. Although there had previously been sporadic instances of suspicious letters, those events proved to be hoaxes. This outbreak resulted from the delivery of weaponized anthrax spores in mailed letters or packages; ultimately there were 11 cases of inhalational anthrax and 11 of cutaneous disease. Five individuals died. The attacks prompted institutions to implement or modify bioterrorism readiness plans. The United States government also reviewed the public health response and identified areas for improvement.

## BIOCRIME

A bioterrorism event, also known as a biocrime, is an intentional assault on a person, or group of people, using a pathogen or toxin. The assault may be overt or covert. An overt attack is announced. The letters sent to Senators Daschle and Leahy in 2001 are examples of an overt event; a note inside each envelope announced that the individual opening it had been exposed to *Bacillus anthracis* spores. A covert attack is unannounced; the recipient receives no indication that a threat is present. The package sent to the journalist at American Media Inc. is an example of a covert event; an environmental investigation of his office uncovered the anthrax spores following his death and the illness of a coworker.

## GOVERNMENT LAWS AND REGULATIONS

The bombings at the World Trade Center in 1993 and the federal building in Oklahoma City in 1995 led Congress to pass the Antiterrorism and Effective Death Penalty Act of 1996. Section 511 (d) restricts the possession and use of materials capable of producing catastrophic damage in the hands of terrorists by requiring their registration. A companion law, the Uniting and Strengthening America by Providing Appropriate Tools Required to Intercept and Obstruct Terrorism (USA PATRIOT) Act of 2001 prohibits any person to knowingly possess any biologic agent, toxin, or delivery system of a type or in a quantity that, under the circumstances, is not reasonably justified by prophylactic, protective, bona fide research, or other peaceful purpose. Later, the Public Health Security and Bioterrorism Preparedness and Response Act of 2002 required institutions to notify the Department of Health and Human Services (DHHS) or the United States Department of Agriculture (USDA) of the possession of specific pathogens or toxins called *select agents*. Therefore, clinical laboratories possessing any select agents must register with the Centers for Disease Control and Prevention (CDC), a branch of the DHHS. Violation of any of these statutes carries criminal penalties. The pathogens and toxins classified as select agents are listed in Box 80-1. List is updated as needed.

Bioterrorism agents are divided into three categories: A, B, or C. Category A agents are considered those presenting the highest risk to public health and national security because they are easily disseminated or transmitted from person to person and have high mortality rates. Category A includes pathogens such as *Bacillus anthracis* and *Yersinia pestis*. Category B agents are moderately easy to disseminate and have moderate to low mortality rates. This category includes *Brucella* species and *Clostridium*

---

**BOX 80-1** List of Select Agents*

**Viruses**
Crimean-Congo hemorrhagic fever virus
Eastern equine encephalitis virus
Ebola viruses
Hendra virus
Herpesvirus 1 (Herpes B virus)
Lassa fever virus
Marburg virus
Monkeypox virus
Nipah virus
Rift Valley fever virus
South American hemorrhagic fever viruses (Junin, Machupo,
   Sabia, Flexal, Guanarito)
Tick-borne encephalitis complex viruses
Variola major virus (smallpox virus)
Variola minor virus (Alastrim)
Venezuelan equine encephalitis virus

**Bacteria**
*Bacillus anthracis*
*Brucella abortus, B. melitensis, B. suis*
*Burkholderia (Pseudomonas) mallei*
*Burkholderia (Pseudomonas) pseudomallei*
*Clostridium botulinum*

*Francisella tularensis*
Reconstructed 1918 influenza virus
*Yersinia pestis*

**Rickettsiae**
*Coxiella burnetii*
*Rickettsia prowazekii*
*Rickettsia rickettsii*

**Toxins**
Abrin
Botulinum toxins
*Clostridium perfringens* epsilon toxin
Conotoxins
Diacetoxyscirpenol
Ricin
Saxitoxin
Shiga-like ribosome inactivating proteins
Shigatoxin
*Staphylococcal enterotoxins*
T-2 toxin
Tetrodotoxin

---
*HHS and USDA Select Agents and Toxins, 7 CFR Part 331, 9 CFR Part 121, and 42 CFR Part 73.

---

*perfringens* toxin. Category C contains emerging pathogens that could be engineered for mass spread in the future. Additional information may be found in Appendix F of the fifth edition of the CDC and the National Institutes of Health (NIH) manual *Biosafety in Microbiological and Biomedical Laboratories* (BMBL).

## BIOSECURITY

Biosecurity is the latest issue of concern for microbiology laboratory directors and managers. Laboratories must conduct a risk assessment and threat analysis in order to write a security plan. This plan must include physical security (e.g., electronic card key access and locked freezers and refrigerators), and data system (laboratory information system) security and security policies for personnel.

Most hospital clinical laboratories have made a decision not to store any select agents. Some commercial laboratories, on the other hand, store select agents for use as positive controls for comparison with suspect samples. These laboratories must write standard operating procedures for (1) the access of select agents; (2) specimen accountability; (3) the receipt of select agents into the laboratory; (4) the transfer or shipping of select agents from the laboratory; (5) the reporting of incidents, injuries, and breaches of security; and (6) an emergency response plan if security is breached or the isolate is unintentionally released during an accident. They must also register the agents with the CDC.

Each clinical laboratory should have a bioterrorism response plan. The plan should include policies and procedures to be enacted when a suspicious isolate cannot be ruled out as a biothreat agent. If a laboratory has any questions about isolating, identifying, or submitting an organism that may be an agent of bioterrorism, laboratory personnel should call the state public health laboratory. The select agent must be either sent to a public health laboratory or destroyed within 7 days of identification. If the agent is autoclaved, its destruction must be documented using Animal and Plant Health Inspection Service (APHIS)/CDC Form 4, which can be downloaded at www.selectagents.gov/CDForm.html.

## LABORATORY RESPONSE NETWORK

Laboratory testing and communication between clinical and public health laboratories is critical when responding to a bioterrorism event. To address this issue, the CDC, in partnership with the Association of Public Health Laboratories and the Federal Bureau of Investigation, established the Laboratory Response Network (LRN). The LRN is a three-tier system. Sentinel (formerly level A) laboratories receive patient samples, rule out pathogens, and transfer suspicious specimens to reference laboratories. References laboratories possess the required reagents and technology to perform confirmatory testing on pathogens. These labs may be local public health, military, international, veterinary, agriculture, food, or water testing laboratories. Confirmed bioterrorism agents are sent to a national laboratory. National laboratories, such as those at the CDC, U.S. Army Medical Research Institute for Infectious Diseases, or the Naval

Medical Research Center, are responsible for the definitive characterization of agents (Figure 80-1).

## ROLE OF THE SENTINEL LABORATORY

The main role of sentinel microbiology laboratories is to determine if a targeted agent is suspected in a human specimen. Detection and recognition of a possible bioterrorism event will depend on the following:

- A laboratory having an active microbial surveillance and monitoring program
- Vigilant technologists looking for a disease that (1) does not occur naturally in a particular geographic region (e.g., plague in New York City); (2) is transmitted by an aerosol route of infection; and (3) is a single case of disease caused by an unusual agent (e.g., *Burkholderia mallei*)
- Good communication with infection control practitioners, infectious disease physicians, and local or regional public health laboratories

Sentinel laboratories must have a class II biologic safety cabinet, copies of level A protocols containing the algorithms for ruling out suspicious microorganisms (Table 80-1), and participate in an applicable proficiency testing program such as the College of American Pathologist's Laboratory Preparedness Survey. Because sentinel laboratories rule out and refer microorganisms, proper knowledge of appropriate packaging and shipping is critical (see Chapter 4); all specimens must be classified as infectious. Sentinel laboratories should never accept nonhuman specimens such as those from animals or the

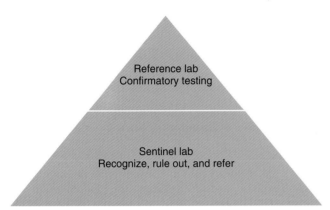

**Figure 80-1** Laboratory Network for Biological Terrorism.

**TABLE 80-1** Algorithm for Sentinel Laboratories for Likely Bioterrorism Agents*

| Agent | Sentinel Lab Procedures | Comments |
|---|---|---|
| *Bacillus anthracis* | Colony: large, nonhemolytic, stands up like beaten egg (Figure 80-2)<br>Gram stain: large, gram-positive rods (Figure 80-3)<br>Catalase: positive<br>Motility: nonmotile<br>Optional: use of the Red Line Alert Test (Tetracore, Inc.), cleared by the Food and Drug Administration, to rule out *B. anthracis* (see Chapter 16 for a fuller discussion of this test) | May be mistaken for *Bacillus megaterium* |
| *Brucella* spp. | Colony: small, nonhemolytic<br>Gram stain: lightly staining tiny gram-negative coccobacilli<br>Oxidase: positive<br>Urease: positive<br>Motility: nonmotile | May be mistaken for *Haemophilus* or *Francisella* |
| *Francisella tularensis* | Colony: pinpoint growth after 48 hours<br>Gram stain: pleomorphic, minute, faintly staining gram-negative coccobacilli<br>Oxidase: negative<br>Urease: negative<br>β-lactamase: positive | May be mistaken for *Haemophilus* or *Actinobacillus* |
| *Yersinia pestis* | Colony: pinpoint growth on blood agar after 24 hours<br>Gram stain: gram-negative rods exhibiting bipolar staining<br>Catalase: positive<br>Oxidase: negative<br>Urease: negative<br>Indole: negative | Rapid systems may misidentify as *Shigella* spp., H2S-negative *Salmonella* spp., *Acinetobacter* spp., and *Yersinia pseudotuberculosis* |
| *Clostridium botulinum* | None | Send all specimens to reference laboratory; patient must get antitoxin immediately |
| Smallpox and hemorrhagic fever viruses | None | Smallpox can be mistaken for herpes virus if inoculated into routine tissue culture cells |

*See individual chapters for a more detailed discussion of each organism.

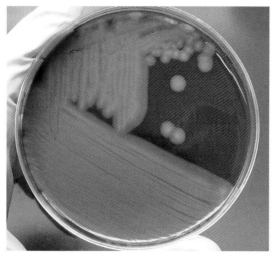

**Figure 80-2** Colony of *Bacillus anthracis*.

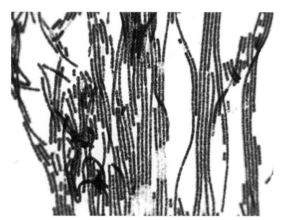

**Figure 80-3** Gram stain of *Bacillus anthracis*.

environment. Such specimens should be submitted directly to the nearest reference laboratory.

Rapid communication between LRN sentinel members and their reference public health laboratories is essential. Each sentinel laboratory must know how to contact public health officials 24 hours/day. Sentinel laboratories, however, do not make the determination that a bioterrorist event has occurred and do not notify law enforcement. The Federal Bureau of Investigation (FBI) has primary responsibility when a bioterrorism event occurs as outlined in Presidential Decision Directive 39. A bioterrorist event is first and foremost a criminal investigation. The Federal Emergency Management Agency (FEMA) has the lead role in consequence management. FEMA receives assistance from the Department of Defense (DOD), Department of Energy (DOE), USDA, Department of Transportation (DOT), DHHS, and Environmental Protection Agency (EPA). FEMA, for example, calls for the deployment of the National Pharmaceutical Stockpile by the CDC so victims may be appropriately treated. Early recognition is the key to saving lives, and sentinel laboratorians are on the front lines in the fight against bioterrorism.

Because sentinel laboratories are charged with ruling out possible bioterrorism agents and referring suspicious isolates to reference laboratories for confirmatory testing, each sentinel laboratory's bioterrorism response plan must include a telephone and pager number for the reference laboratory.

A sentinel laboratory's key responsibility is to be familiar with likely agents involved in a biocrime; it must have standard operating procedures (SOPs) to accomplish this task. To standardize the process nationwide, the American Society for Microbiology (ASM) has compiled a series of guidelines. These guidelines are listed in Box 80-2 and may be accessed on the ASM website at www.asm.org/index.php/what-s-new-in-public-policy/sentinel-level-clinical-microbiology-laboratory-guidelines.html. Algorithms for the identification of likely bioterrorism agents are provided in Table 80-1.

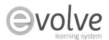 *Visit the Evolve site to complete the review questions.*

# BIBLIOGRAPHY

Centers for Disease Control and Prevention: Biological and chemical terrorism: strategic plan for preparedness and response, *MMWR* 49(RR-4):1, 2000.

Centers for Disease Control and Prevention: Laboratory security and emergency response guidance for laboratories working with select agents, *MMWR* 51(RR19):1, 2002.

Christopher GW, Cieslak TJ, Pavlin JA, et al: Biological warfare: a historical perspective, *JAMA* 278:412, 1997.

English JF: Overview of bioterrorism readiness plan: a template for healthcare facilities, *Am J Infect Cont* 27:468, 1999.

Franz DR, Jahrling PB, Friedlancder AM, et al: Clinical recognition and management of patients exposed to biological warfare agents, *JAMA* 278:399, 1997.

Gilchrist MJR, McKinney WP, Miller JM, et al: Laboratory safety, management and diagnosis of biological agents associated with bioterrorism. In Snyder JW, coordinating editor: *Cumitech* 33, Washington DC, 2000, ASM Press.

Hawley RJ, Eitzen EM Jr: Biological weapons—a primer for microbiologists, *Ann Rev Microbiol* 55:235, 2001.

Jernigan JA, Stephens DS, Ashford DA, et al: Bioterrorism-related inhalational anthrax: the first 10 cases reported in the United States, *Emerg Infect Dis* 7:933, 2001.

Klietmann WF, Ruoff KL: Bioterrorism: implications for the clinical microbiologist, *Clin Microbiol Rev* 14:364, 2001.

Kolavic SA, Kimura A, Simons SL, et al: An outbreak of Shigella dysenteriae type 2 among laboratory workers due to intentional food contamination, *JAMA* 278:396, 1997.

Morse SA: Bioterrorism: laboratory security, *Lab Med* 32:303, 2001.

Sewell DL: Laboratory safety practices associated with potential agents of biocrime or bioterrorism, *J Clin Microbiol* 41: 2801, 2003.

Snyder JW: Role of the hospital-based microbiology laboratory in preparation for and response to a bioterrorism event, *J Clin Microbiol* 41:1, 2003.

Torok TJ, Tauxe RV, Wise RP, et al: A large community outbreak of salmonellosis caused by intentional contamination of restaurant salad bars, *JAMA* 278:389, 1997.

US Department of Health and Human Services/CDC and National Institutes of Health, Chosewood LC, Wilson DE, editors: *Biosafety in microbiological and biomedical laboratories (BMBL)*, ed 5, Washington, DC, 2009, US Department of Health and Human Services.

Versalovic J: *Manual of clinical microbiology*, ed 10, Washington, DC, 2011, ASM Press.

# Glossary

**Abscess:** Localized collection of pus.

**Accessioning:** Receipt and recording of specimens delivered to the laboratory.

**Accuracy:** Ability of a test under evaluation to match the results of an accepted standard test (i.e., "gold standard").

**Acid-fast:** Characteristic of certain bacteria, such as mycobacteria, that involves resistance to decolorization by acids when stained by an aniline dye, such as carbolfuchsin.

**Acquired immunity:** The specific response of the host to the infecting organism.

**Acquired immunodeficiency syndrome (AIDS):** Severe immune deficiency disease caused by human immunodeficiency virus (HIV-1) infection of T cells, characterized by opportunistic infections and other complications.

**Acute serum:** Serum collected for antibody determination early in the course of an illness when little or no antibody would have been produced.

**Acute urethral syndrome:** Lower urinary tract infection that may be difficult to differentiate from cystitis; seen most commonly in younger, sexually active females and caused by *Escherichia coli* (counts as low as 100 per milliliter may be significant in this situation), Chlamydia, and other organisms.

**Aerobe, obligate:** Microorganism that lives and grows freely in air and cannot grow anaerobically.

**Aerosol:** Atomized particles suspended in air; in context of this textbook, microorganisms suspended in air.

**Aerotolerant:** Ability of an anaerobic microorganism to grow in air, usually poorly, especially after initial anaerobic isolation.

**Agarose gel electrophoresis:** Separation of proteins based on molecular weight by electrical current-stimulated movement through a semisolid gel matrix.

**Agglutination:** Aggregation or clumping of particles, such as bacteria when exposed to a specific antibody.

**AIDS:** Acquired immunodeficiency syndrome.

**Aminoglycosides:** Group of related antibiotics including streptomycin, kanamycin, neomycin, tobramycin, gentamicin, and amikacin.

**Amniotic:** Pertaining to the innermost fetal membrane forming a fluid-filled sac.

**Amplicon:** Amplified nucleic acid product.

**Anaerobe, obligate:** Microorganism that grows only in complete or nearly complete absence of air or molecular oxygen.

**Anamnestic response:** More rapid production of antibodies in response to exposure to an antigen previously encountered.

**Anamorph:** Asexual fungal form.

**Anergy:** Absence of reaction to antigens or allergens.

**Angiogenesis:** Forming new capillaries from preexisting ones.

**Antibiogram:** A cumulative susceptibility report that tracks resistance or susceptibility of commonly isolated organisms to commonly administered antimicrobials.

**Antibiotic:** Substance produced by a microorganism that inhibits or kills other microorganisms; a broad-spectrum antibiotic is therapeutically effective against a wide range of bacteria.

**Antibody:** Substance (immunoglobulin) formed in blood or tissues that interact only with antigen that induced its synthesis (e.g., agglutinin).

**Anticoagulant:** Substance used to prevent clotting of specimens such as blood, bone marrow, and synovial fluid so that organisms do not become bound up in the clot.

**Antigen:** Molecular structure that is capable of stimulating production of antibody.

**Antimicrobial:** Chemical substance produced either by a microorganism or by synthetic means that is capable of killing or suppressing growth of microorganisms.

**Antiseptic:** Compound that stops or inhibits growth of bacteria without necessarily killing them.

**Apical:** Top.

**Apoptosis:** Programmed cell death.

**Arboviruses:** Arthropod-borne viruses.

**Arthritis, septic:** Infection of synovial tissue and joint fluid of one or more joints; characterized by joint pain, stiffness, swelling, and fever.

**Arthroconidium:** Spore formed by septation of a hypha and subsequent separation of septa.

**Ascites:** Condition in which amounts of fluids increase and accumulate in the peritoneal cavity during infection or an inflammatory process.

**Ascitic fluid:** Serous fluid in peritoneal cavity.

**Ascocarp:** A large, saclike structure that contains sexual spores of fungi.

**Aseptic meningitis:** Meningitidis characterized by an increase in lymphocytes and other mononuclear cells in the cerebrospinal fluid and negative bacterial and fungal cultures.

**Aspiration:** Inhalation of a fluid or solid.

**ASR:** Analyte specific reagent.

**Assimilation:** Utilization of nutrients. Assimilation tests are used to determine whether yeasts are able to grow with only a single carbohydrate or nitrate; these tests are useful for classification of yeasts.

**ATCC:** American Type Culture Collection.

**Autotroph:** Organism that can utilize inorganic carbon sources ($CO_2$).

**Auxotroph:** Differing from the wild strain (prototroph) by an additional nutritional requirement.

**Avid:** The property of binding strongly, such as an antibody that strongly binds to an antigen.

**Avidity:** Firmness of union of two substances; used commonly to describe union of antibody to antigen.

**B cells:** Lymphocytes involved in antibody production.

**Bacteremia:** Presence of viable organisms in blood.

**Bacterial vaginosis:** Noninflammatory condition in vagina characterized by foul-smelling vaginal discharge and presence of mixed bacteria.

**Bactericidal:** Term used to describe a drug that kills microorganisms.

**Bacteriophage:** Virus that infects a bacterial cell, sometimes bringing about its lysis.

**Bacteriostatic:** Term used to describe a drug that inhibits growth of an organism without killing it.

**Bacteriuria:** Presence of bacteria in urine.

**BCG:** Bacille Calmette-Guérin, an attenuated strain of *Mycobacterium tuberculosis* used for immunization.

**Beta-lactamases:** Enzymes that destroy penicillins and/or cephalosporins and are produced by a variety of bacteria.

**Bifurcated:** Divided into two branches.

**Biofilm:** Well-organized microcolonies of bacteria usually enclosed in polymer matrices that are separated by water channels that remove wastes and deliver nutrients.

**Biological safety cabinet:** Enclosure in which one can work with relatively dangerous organisms without risk of acquiring or spreading infection caused by them. These cabinets, also called *biosafety hoods*, vary in design according to the nature of the agents to be worked with. The simpler ones maintain a negative pressure within the work area and a laminar air curtain, both of which operate to prevent escape of organisms from the interior of hood. Air that is exhausted may be passed through a high-efficiency bacterial filter that traps all microorganisms that are anticipated or may be passed through a furnace that incinerates any organisms.

**Bioluminescence:** Light generation by living organisms.

**Biopsy:** Removal of tissue from a living body for diagnostic purposes (e.g., lymph node biopsy).

**Biotin:** Small vitamin with two binding sites, one of which can bind covalently with nucleic acid, leaving the other free to form a strong bond with the protein avidin, which, in turn, can be bound to enzymes. The system is used as a label for nucleic acid probe detection.

**Biotype:** Biologic or biochemical type of an organism. Organisms of the same biotype display identical biologic or biochemical characteristics. Certain key markers are used to define and recognize biotypes in tracing the spread of organisms in the environment and in epidemics or outbreaks.

**Blastoconidium:** A spore formed by budding, as in yeasts.

**Blepharitis:** Inflammation of eyelids.

**B lymphocytes (or B cells):** Bursa-derived lymphocytes important in humoral immunity.

**Breakpoint:** Level of an antibacterial drug achievable in: serum; organisms inhibited by this level of drug are: considered susceptible. In certain situations, clinicians strive to achieve serum or body fluid levels several times that of the breakpoint.

**Bright-field microscopy:** Conventional microscopy in which the object to be viewed is illuminated from below.

**Bronchial lavage:** Similar to bronchial washings but this term implies instillation of a larger volume of fluid before aspiration. Alveolar organisms may be present in the lavage.

**Bronchial washings:** Fluid that may be aspirated from bronchial tree during bronchoscopy.

**Bronchitis:** Inflammation of mucous membranes of bronchi; often caused by infectious agents, viruses in particular.

**Bronchoscopy:** Examination of bronchi through a bronchoscope, a tubular, illuminated instrument introduced through the trachea (windpipe).

**BSC:** Biological safety cabinet.

**Bubo:** Inflammatory enlargement of lymph node, usually in the groin or axilla.

**Buffy coat:** Layer of white blood cells and platelets above red blood cell mass when blood is sedimented.

**Bullae:** Large blebs or blisters, filled with fluid, in or just beneath the epidermal layer of skin.

**Bursitis:** Inflammation of a bursa, which is a small sac lined with synovial membrane and filled with fluid interposed between parts that move on each other.

**Butt:** Lower portion of medium in a tube in which the medium is dispensed such that the lower portion fills the tube entirely (i.e., the butt) while the upper portion is distributed in the form of a slanted surface, leaving an air space between the slant and the opposite wall of the tube.

**Butyrous:** Butterlike consistency.

**Calibrated loop:** Bacteriologic loop that is carefully calibrated to deliver a specified volume of fluid, as long as directions are followed carefully and the loop has not been damaged; used as a simple means of quantitating the number of organisms present, especially for urine culture.

**CAMP:** A diffusible extracellular protein named after Christie, Atkins, and Munch-Peterson that is produced by certain

organisms (e.g., group B streptococci) and acts synergistically with the beta lysin of *S. aureus* to cause enhanced lysis of red blood cells.

**Candle jar:** A jar with a lid providing a gas-tight seal in which a small white candle is placed and lit after the culture plates have been placed inside. Candle will burn only until the oxygen concentration has been lowered to the point at which it will no longer support the flame. Atmosphere of such a jar has a lower oxygen content than room air and a carbon dioxide content of about 3%.

**Cannula:** An artificial tube for insertion into a tube or cavity of the body.

**CAPD:** Chronic ambulatory peritoneal dialysis.

**Capnophilic:** Term used to describe microorganisms that prefer an incubation atmosphere with increased carbon dioxide concentration.

**Capsid:** Protein layer or coat surrounding viral nucleic acid core.

**Capsomere:** Protein subunits that serve as components of the viral capsid.

**Capsule:** Gelatinous material surrounding bacterial cell wall, usually of polysaccharide nature.

**Carrier:** One who harbors a pathogenic organism but is not affected by it.

**Catalase:** Bacterial enzyme that breaks down peroxides with liberation of free oxygen.

**Catheter:** Flexible tubular (rubber or plastic) instrument used for withdrawing fluids from (or introducing fluids into) a body cavity or vessel (e.g., urinary bladder catheter).

**Cation:** A positive ion.

**Cell line:** A cell culture that has been passed (subcultured) in vitro.

**Cell line, continuous:** Line of tissue cells that is maintained by serial culture of an established cell line.

**Cell line, primary:** Line of tissue cells established by cutting up fresh tissue, often kidney, into tiny pieces, trypsinizing, and putting in a flask with appropriate medium.

**Cell-mediated immunity:** Human specific immune response carried out by special lymphocytes of the T (thymus-derived) class.

**Cellulitis:** Inflammation of subcutaneous tissue.

**Cerebriform:** With brainlike folds.

**Cervical:** Pertaining either to the neck or to the cervix of the uterus.

**CF:** Complement fixation.

**CFU:** Colony-forming unit (i.e., colony count).

**Charcot-Leyden crystals:** Slender crystals shaped like a double pyramid with pointed ends, formed from the breakdown products of eosinophils and found in feces, sputum, and tissues; indicative of an immune response that may have parasitic or nonparasitic causes.

**Chemotherapeutic:** Chemical agent used to treat infections (e.g., sulfonamides).

**Chlamydospore:** Thick-walled spore formed from a vegetative cell.

**Chorioamnionitis:** Infection of the uterus and its contents during pregnancy.

**Chromatography:** Method of chemical analysis by which a mixture of substances is separated by fractional extraction or adsorption or ion exchange on a porous solid.

**Chromogen:** Bacterial species whose colonial growth is pigmented (e.g., Flavobacterium spp., yellow).

**Chromogenic:** Giving rise to color, as chromogenic substrates for colored products of biochemical reactions or chromogenic bacteria that produce pigmented colonies.

**Clavate:** Club-shaped.

**Clone:** Group of microorganisms of identical genetic makeup derived from a single common ancestor.

**CMI:** Cell-mediated immunity.

**CNS:** Central nervous system.

**Coagglutination:** Agglutination of protein A–containing cells of *Staphylococcus aureus* coated with antibody molecules when exposed to corresponding antigen.

**Coenocytic hyphae:** Sparsely septated.

**Colitis:** Inflammation of mucosa of colon.

**Colony:** Macroscopically visible growth of a microorganism on a solid culture medium.

**Commensal:** Microorganism living on or in a host but causing the host no harm.

**Community-acquired:** Pertaining to outside the hospital, such as a community-acquired infection.

**Complement fixation test:** Antigen-antibody test based on fixation of complement in the presence of both elements and use of an indicator system to determine whether complement has been fixed.

**Congenital:** Existing before or at birth.

**Conidia:** Asexual spores.

**Conjugation:** Passing genetic information between bacteria by transferring chromosomal material, often via pili.

**Conjunctivitis:** Inflammation of the conjunctivae or membranes of the eye and eyelid.

**Convalescent serum:** Serum collected later in the course of an illness than the acute serum, usually at least 2 weeks after initial collection.

**CPE:** Cytopathogenic (cytopathic) effect; visual effect of virus infection on cell culture.

**Creutzfeldt-Jakob disease:** Debilitating prion-caused disease characterized by dementia, ataxia, delirium, stupor, coma, and death; has been transmitted by organ transplant.

**Crossing point:** See "threshold cycle."

**Croup:** Inflammation of upper airways (larynx, trachea) with respiratory obstruction, often caused by virus infections in children.

**CSF:** Cerebrospinal fluid.

**Culdocentesis:** Aspiration of fluid from the cul-de-sac by puncture of the vaginal vault.

**Cystitis:** Inflammation of urinary bladder, most often caused by bacterial infection.

**Cytokine:** Group of biochemicals that is a key component of inflammation.

**Cytopathic effect (CPE):** Alteration in cell morphology resulting from viral infection of a cell culture monolayer.

**Cytotoxin:** Toxin that produces cytopathic effects in vivo or in a tissue culture system.

**Dark-field microscopy:** Technique used to visualize very small microorganisms or their characteristics by a system that permits light to be reflected or refracted from the surface of objects being viewed.

**Debridement:** Surgical or other removal of nonviable tissue.

**Decontamination:** Process of rendering an object or area safe for unprotected people by removing or making harmless biologic or chemical agents.

**Decubitus ulcer:** A craterlike defect in skin and subcutaneous tissue caused by prolonged pressure on the area. This occurs primarily over bony prominences of the lower back and hips in individuals who are unable to care for themselves well and unable to roll or move periodically; also known as a *pressure sore* or *bedsore*.

**Definitive host:** Host in which the sexual reproduction of a parasite occurs.

**Dematiaceous:** Presence of pigmentation in fungal hyphae or spores.

**Denaturation:** Process in which double-stranded DNA becomes single-stranded by heating or chemical means; also referred to as *melting*.

**Dermatophyte:** A parasitic fungus on skin, hair, or nails.

**Dermis:** Layer of skin beneath the epidermis that is composed of dense connective tissue rich in blood and nerve supply.

**Desquamation:** Shedding or scaling of skin or mucous membrane.

**DFA test:** Direct fluorescent antibody test.

**DIC:** Disseminated intravascular coagulation.

**Dichotomous:** Branching in two directions.

**Diluent:** Fluid used to dilute a substance.

**Dimorphic fungi:** Fungi with both a mold phase and a yeast phase.

**Direct wet mount:** A preparation from clinical material suspended in sterile saline or other liquid medium on a glass slide and covered with a coverslip; used for microscopic examination to detect microorganisms in clinical material and, in particular, to detect motility directly.

**Disinfectant:** Agent that destroys or inhibits microorganisms that cause disease.

**Disseminated intravascular coagulation (DIC):** Disastrous complication of sepsis.

**DNA:** Deoxyribonucleic acid, the lipoprotein molecule that contains the genetic code for most living things.

**DNA minor groove:** A location on double-stranded DNA in which the strand backbones are closer together on one side the helix than on the other.

**Droplet nucleus:** A tiny aerosolized particle that, because of its lack of mass, may stay suspended in air for extended periods.

**Duplex:** Two nucleic acid strands that have complementary base sequences that have specifically bonded with each other and formed a double-stranded molecule.

**Dx: Diagnosis.**

**Dysentery:** Inflammation of the intestinal tract, particularly the colon, with frequent bloody stools (e.g., bacillary dysentery).

**Dysgonic:** Growing poorly (bacterial cultures).

**Dysuria:** Painful or difficult urination.

**Ectoparasite:** Organism that lives on or within skin.

**Ectothrix:** Outside of hair shafts.

**Edema:** Excessive accumulation of fluid in tissue spaces.

**Effusion:** Fluid escaping into a body space or tissue (e.g., pleural effusion).

**Eh:** Oxidation-reduction potential.

**Elementary body:** The infectious stage of Chlamydia or a cellular inclusion body of a viral disease.

**ELISA:** Enzyme-linked immunosorbent assay.

**Elution:** Process of extraction by means of a solvent.

**EMB:** Eosin-methylene blue (agar plate).

**Empyema:** Accumulation of pus in a body cavity, particularly empyema of the thorax or chest.

**Encephalitis:** Inflammation of the brain.

**Endocarditis:** A serious infection of the endothelium of the heart, usually involving leaflets of the heart valves where destruction of valves or distortion of them by formation of vegetations may lead to serious physiologic disturbances and death; also, an inflammation of the endocardial surface (much less common).

**Endocervix:** Mucous membrane of the cervical canal.

**Endogenous:** Developing from within the body.

**Endoparasite:** Parasite that lives within the body.

**Endophthalmitis:** Inflammation of internal tissues of eye; may rapidly destroy the eye.

**Endothelium:** Squamous epithelium lining blood vessels.

**Endothrix:** Within the hair shaft.

**Endotoxin:** Substance containing lipopolysaccharide complexes found in the cell wall of bacteria, principally gram-negative bacteria; believed to play an important role in many of the complications of sepsis such as shock, DIC, and thrombocytopenia.

**Enteric fever:** Typhoid fever; paratyphoid fever.

**Enteroinvasive:** Capable of invading the mucosal surface and sometimes the deeper tissues of the bowel.

**Enterotoxin:** Toxin affecting the cells of the intestinal mucosa.

**Enzyme-linked immunosorbent assay (ELISA):** An immunologic assay that uses an enzyme conjugated to antibodies to produce a visible endpoint.

**Epidemiology:** The study of the occurrence and distribution of disease and factors that control presence or absence of disease.

**Epidermis:** Outermost layer of skin made of layered squamous epithelial cells.

**Epididymitis:** Inflammation of the epididymis characterized by fever and pain on one side of the scrotum; seen as a complication of prostatitis and cystitis.

**Epiglottitis:** Inflammation of the epiglottis, a structure that prevents aspirating swallowed food and fluids into the tracheobronchial tree; a serious infection because the swollen epiglottis may block the airway.

**Epithelium:** Tissue composed of contiguous cells that forms the epidermis and lines hollow organs and all passages of the respiratory, digestive, and genitourinary systems.

**Erysipelas:** An acute cellulitis caused by group A streptococci.

**Erythema:** Redness of the skin from various causes.

**Erythrasma:** A minor, superficial skin infection caused by *Corynebacterium minutissimum*.

**Eschar:** A dry scar, particularly one related to a burn.

**Etiology:** Cause or causative agent.

**Eugonic:** Growing luxuriantly (bacterial cultures).

**Eukaryotic:** Organisms with a true nucleus, in contrast to bacteria and viruses.

**Exanthem:** Skin eruption as a symptom of an acute disease, usually viral.

**Exoantigen test:** In vitro immunodiffusion test method for identifying fungal hyphae as Histoplasma, Blastomyces, or Coccidioides.

**Exoerythrocytic cycle:** Portion of the malarial life cycle occurring in the vertebrate host in which sporozoites, introduced by infected mosquitoes, penetrate the parenchymal liver cells and undergo schizogony, producing merozoites, which then initiate the erythrocytic cycle.

**Exogenous:** From outside the body.

**Exotoxin:** A toxin produced by a microorganism that is released into the surrounding environment.

**Exudate:** Fluid that has passed out of blood vessels into adjacent tissues or spaces; high protein content.

**Facultative anaerobe:** Microorganism that grows under either anaerobic or aerobic conditions.

**Fascia:** Membranous covering of muscle.

**Fermentation:** Anaerobic decomposition of carbohydrate.

**Filamentous:** Threadlike.

**Fimbriae:** Proteinaceous fingerlike surface structures of bacteria that provide for adherence to host surfaces.

**Fistula:** Abnormal communication between two surfaces or between a viscus or other hollow structure and the exterior.

**Flagella:** Complex structures mostly composed of the protein flagellin that are responsible for bacterial motility.

**Floccose:** Cottony, in tufts.

**Flocculation test:** Antigen-antibody test in which a precipitin end product forms macroscopically or microscopically visible clumps.

**Fluorescent:** Emission of light by a substance (or a microscopic preparation) while acted on by radiant energy, such as ultraviolet rays, as in the immunofluorescent procedure.

**Fluorochrome:** A dye that becomes fluorescent or self-luminous after exposure to ultraviolet light.

**Fluorophore:** A fluorescent molecule that can absorb light energy and then is elevated to an excited state that is released as fluorescence in the absence of a quencher.

**Fomite:** Any inanimate object that may be contaminated with disease-causing microorganisms and thus serves to transmit disease.

**FTA:** Fluorescent treponemal antibody.

**FTA-ABS:** Fluorescent treponemal antigen-antibody absorption: test; indirect fluorescent antibody stain used to detect antibodies directed against whole-cell antigens of *Treponema pallidum* (syphilis bacillus).

**Fungemia:** Presence of viable fungi in blood.

**FUO:** Fever of unknown origin.

**Fusiform:** Spindle-shaped, as in the anaerobe *Fusobacterium nucleatum*.

**Gamma hemolysis:** No hemolysis of red blood cells.

**Gangrene:** Death of a part of tissue resulting from disease, injury, or failure of blood supply.

**Gas-liquid chromatography (GLC):** A method for separating substances by allowing their volatile phase to flow through a heated column with a carrier gas and measuring the time required to detect their presence at the distal end of the column.

**Gastric aspirate:** Fluid that may be aspirated from the stomach via a tube placed in the stomach by way of the nose or mouth.

**Gastroenteritis:** Inflammation of the mucosa of the stomach and intestines.

**GC:** Gonococcus.

**Genotype:** Related to characteristics of an organism's genetic makeup, that is, genus and constituent nucleic acids.

**Germicide:** An agent that destroys germs; disinfectant.

**Germ tube:** Tubelike process, produced by a germinating spore that develops into mycelium.

**Glabrous:** Smooth.

**GLC:** Gas-liquid chromatography.

**Granulocytopenia:** Reduced number of granulocytic white blood cells in the blood.

**Granuloma:** Aggregation and proliferation of macrophages to form small (usually microscopic) nodules.

**HAI:** Hemagglutination inhibition.

**Halophilic:** Preferring high halide (salt) content.

**Hansen's disease:** Leprosy, a disease cause by *Mycobacterium leprae*.

**Hemadsorption:** Ability of certain virally infected cells to bind erythrocytes; mediated by glycopeptide adherence molecules (induced by viral activities within the cell) on the cell's surface.

**Hemagglutination:** Agglutination of red blood cells caused by certain antibodies, virus particles, or high molecular weight polysaccharides.

**Hematogenous:** Disseminated by the bloodstream.

**Hemolysis, alpha:** Partial destruction of, or enzymatic damage to, red blood cells in a blood agar plate, leading to greenish discoloration about the colony of the organism producing the alpha hemolysin.

**Hemolysis, beta:** Total lysis of red blood cells about a colony on a blood agar plate, leading to a completely clear zone surrounding the colony.

**Hemolysis, gamma:** No hemolysis is seen with organisms classed as gamma-hemolytic; nonhemolytic would be a better designation.

**HEPA:** High-efficiency particulate air filter; used in biological safety cabinets to trap pathogenic microorganisms.

**Herpes:** Inflammation of the skin characterized by clusters of small vesicles (e.g., caused by herpes simplex); disease caused by herpes simplex virus.

**Heterotroph:** Organism that requires an organic carbon source.

**High-pressure liquid chromatography (HPLC):** Similar to GLC but capable of higher resolution because of increased pressure of liquid carrier that runs through the column.

**HPLC:** High-pressure (or performance) liquid chromatography.

**Humoral immunity:** Immunity affected by antibody.

**Hyaline:** Colorless, transparent.

**Hybridoma:** The product of fusion of an antibody-producing cell and an immortal malignant antibody-producing cell.

**Hydrolysis:** Breakdown of a substrate by an enzyme that adds the components of water to key bonds within the substrate molecule.

**Hyperalimentation:** Process by which nutrition (literally "extra nutrition") is provided; typically administered intravenously in subjects who are not able to absorb foods well from the gut because of disease of the bowel, in subjects in whom it is desirable to put the bowel "at rest" to promote healing, and in malnourished individuals to improve their nutritional status (e.g., before surgery); usually done over an extended period and requires the use of a special-access intravenous catheter such as a Hickman catheter.

**Hyperemia:** Increased blood in a part, resulting in distention of blood vessels.

**Hypertonic:** Hyperosmotic.

**Hypertrophy:** Increased size of an organ resulting from enlargement of individual cells.

**Hypha:** Tubular cell making up the vegetative portion of mycelium of fungi.

**Hypoxia:** Decreased oxygen content of tissues.

**IFA:** Indirect fluorescent antibody; test that detects antibody by allowing an antibody to react with its substrate and adding a second fluorescein dye–labeled antibody that will bind to the first.

**Ig, IgG, IgM, etc.:** Immunoglobulin, immunoglobulin G, immunoglobulin M, etc.

**Immunodiffusion:** Detection of antigen or antibody by observing the precipitin line formed in a semisolid gel matrix when homologous antigens and antibodies are allowed to diffuse toward each other and react.

**Immunofluorescence:** Microscopic method of determining the presence or location of an antigen (or antibody) by demonstrating fluorescence when the preparation is exposed to a fluorescein-tagged antibody (or antigen) using ultraviolet radiation.

**Immunoglobulin:** Synonymous with antibody; five distinct classes have been isolated: IgG, IgM, IgA, IgE, and IgD.

**Immunoperoxidase stain:** Combination of an enzyme that catalyzes production of a colored product with an antibody to facilitate detection of certain antigens, particularly viral antigens.

**Immunosuppression:** Depression of the immune response caused by disease, irradiation, or administration of antimetabolites, antilymphocyte serum, or corticosteroids.

**Impetigo:** Acute inflammatory skin disease, caused by streptococci or staphylococci, characterized by vesicles and bullae that rupture and form yellow crusts.

**Inclusion bodies:** Microscopic bodies, usually within body cells; thought to be virus particles in morphogenesis.

**Indigenous flora:** Normal or resident flora.

**Induration:** Abnormal hardness of a tissue or part resulting from hyperemia or inflammation, as in a reactive tuberculin skin test.

**Infection:** Invasion by and multiplication of microorganisms in body tissue resulting in disease.

**Inhibitory quotient:** Ratio of the average peak achievable level of antibiotic in a body fluid from which an organism was isolated to the MIC of that organism.

**Insertion sequence:** Transposable element containing genes that encode the information required to move among plasmids and chromosomes.

**In situ hybridization:** Detection of nucleic acid of a pathogenic organism in tissue sections by separating the DNA into single-stranded molecules and allowing a labeled strand of homologous DNA to bind to the target. The target is visualized by developing the label (i.e., enzymatic precipitate, fluorescence, or radiolabel).

**Inspissation:** Process of making a liquid or semisolid medium thick by evaporation or absorption of fluid.

**Interfacing:** Communicating.

**Intermediate host:** Required host in the life cycle in which essential larval development must occur before a parasite is infective to its definitive host or to additional intermediate hosts.

**Intramuscular (intraperitoneal, intravenous):** Within the muscle (peritoneum, vein), as in intramuscular injection.

**In vitro:** Literally, within glass (i.e., in a test tube, culture plate, or other nonliving material).

**In vivo:** Within the living body.

**Involution forms:** Abnormally shaped bacterial cells occurring in an aging culture population.

**Iodine tincture:** Iodine in alcohol.

**Ion-exchange chromatography:** Separation of components of a solution by chromatography based on the reversible exchange of ions in the solution with ions present in or on an external matrix.

**Isotonic:** Of the same osmolality of body tissues, red blood cells, bacteria, etc.

**Keratitis:** Inflammation of the cornea.

**KIA:** Kligler's iron agar (tube).

**KOH:** Potassium hydroxide.

**Lag phase:** Period of slow microbial growth that occurs following inoculation of the culture medium.

**Laked blood:** Hemolyzed blood; hemolysis may be affected in various ways, but alternate freezing and thawing is a simple method.

**Laminar flow:** Nonturbulent flow of air in layers (flowing in a vertical direction in the case of a biosafety hood).

**Latent:** Not manifest; potential.

**Latex agglutination:** Agglutination of latex particles coated with antibody molecules when exposed to the corresponding antigen.

**LCR:** Ligase chain reaction.

**Lectin:** Naturally produced proteins or glycoproteins that can bind with carbohydrates or sugars to form stable complexes.

**Legionnaires' disease:** Febrile and pneumonic illness caused by Legionella species.

**Leishman-Donovan (L-D) body:** Small, round intracellular form (called amastigote or leishmanial stage) of Leishmania spp. and *Trypanosoma cruzi*.

**Leukocytosis:** Elevated white blood cell count.

**Leukopenia:** Low white blood cell count.

**LGV:** Lymphogranuloma venereum; the name for certain strains of *Chlamydia trachomatis* that cause a systemically expressed sexually transmitted disease.

**Lipopolysaccharide:** Carbohydrate-lipid complex; integral substance in gram-negative cell walls. Also known as endotoxin.

**Liposome:** Small, closed vesicle consisting of a single lipid bilayer.

**Logarithmic phase:** Period of maximal growth rate of a microorganism in a culture medium.

**LPS:** Lipopolysaccharide; see endotoxin.

**Lysis:** Disintegration or dissolution of bacteria or cells.

**Lysogeny:** Process by which a viral genome is integrated into that of its host bacterium.

**MAC:** Mycobacterium avium complex.

**Macroconidia:** Large, usually multiseptate, club- or spindle-shaped fungal spores.

**Mass spectrometry:** Method for determining composition of a substance by observing its volatile products during disintegration and comparing them with known standards.

**MBC:** Minimum bactericidal concentration.

**Media, differential:** Media that permit ready recognition of a particular organism or group of organisms by virtue of facilitating recognition of a natural product of the organism being sought or by incorporating an appropriate substrate and indicator system so that organisms possessing certain enzymes are readily recognized.

**Media, enrichment:** Media, usually liquid, that favor the growth of one or more organisms while suppressing most of the competing flora in a specimen with a mixture of organisms.

**Media, selective:** Culture media that contain inhibitory substances or unique growth factors such that one particular organism or group of organisms is conferred a real advantage over other organisms that may be found in a mixture. Efficient selective media selects out only the organism or organisms being sought, with little or no growth of other types of organisms.

**Mediastinum:** Space in the middle of the chest between the medial surfaces of the two pleurae.

**Melioidosis:** Disease caused by *Burkholderia pseudomallei*.

**Melting temperature** (Tm): The temperature at which 50% of double-stranded DNA becomes single-stranded.

**Meningitis:** Inflammation of the meninges, the membranes that cover the brain and spinal cord (e.g., bacterial meningitis).

**Meningoencephalitis:** Concomitant meningitis that occurs with encephalitis (inflammation of the brain parenchyma).

**Merozoite:** Product of schizogonic cycle in malaria that invades red blood cells.

**Mesenteric adenitis:** Inflammation of mesenteric lymph nodes.

**Mesentery:** A fold of the peritoneum that connects the intestine with the posterior abdominal wall.

**Metastatic:** Spread of an infectious (or other) process from a primary focus to a distant one via the bloodstream or lymphatic system.

**MHA-TP:** Microhemagglutination test for antibody to *Treponema pallidum*.

**MIC:** Minimum inhibitory concentration.

**Microaerobic:** Requiring a partial pressure of oxygen less than: that of atmospheric oxygen for growth. New term for "microaerophilic."

**Microaerophile, obligate:** Microorganism that grows only under reduced oxygen tension and cannot grow aerobically or anaerobically.

**Microaerophilic:** See "microaerobic."

**Microconidia:** Small, single-celled fungal spores.

**Microfilaria:** Embryos produced by filarial worms and found in the blood or tissues of individuals with filariasis.

**Miliary:** Of the size of a millet seed (0.5 to 1.0 mm); characterized by the formation of numerous lesions of the above size distributed rather uniformly throughout one or more organs.

**Minimum bactericidal concentration (MBC):** The minimum concentration of antimicrobial agent needed to yield a 99.9% reduction in viable colony-forming units of a bacterial or fungal suspension.

**Minimum inhibitory concentration (MIC):** The minimum concentration of antimicrobial agent needed to prevent visually discernible growth of a bacterial or fungal suspension.

**Mixed culture (pure culture):** More than one organism growing in or on the same culture medium, as opposed to a single organism in pure culture.

**Monoclonal antibody:** Antibody that is derived from a single cell producing one antibody molecule type that reacts with a single epitope.

**Monolayer:** A confluent layer of tissue culture cells one cell thick.

**MOTT:** Mycobacteria other than *Mycobacterium tuberculosis*.

**Mucopurulent:** Term used to describe material containing both mucus and pus (e.g., mucopurulent sputum).

**Mucosa:** A mucous membrane.

**Multiple myeloma:** Malignancy involving antibody-producing plasma cells.

**Multiplex PCR:** A PCR reaction with more than one primer pair in the reaction mixture.

**Mutation:** Change in the original nucleotide sequence of a gene or genes.

**Mycelium:** Mass of hyphae making up a colony of a fungus.

**Mycetoma:** Chronic infection, usually of feet, caused by various fungi or by Nocardia or Streptomyces, resulting in swelling and sinus tracts; pulmonary mycetoma is a mass of fungal hyphae ("fungus ball") growing in a cavity formed during previous tuberculosis infection or other pathologic condition.

**Mycoses:** Diseases caused by fungi (e.g., dermatomycosis, fungal infection of the superficial skin).

**Mycotic aneurysm:** Bacterial infection causing inflammatory damage and weakening of an arterial wall.

**Myocarditis:** Inflammation of the heart muscle.

**Myositis:** Inflammation of a muscle, sometimes caused by infection as in pyomyositis; an infection caused by *Staphylococcus aureus* that leads to small abscesses within the muscle substance.

**Nares:** External openings of nose (i.e., nostrils).

**Nasopharyngeal:** Pertaining to the part of the pharynx above the level of the soft palate.

**Necrosis:** Pathologic death of a cell or group of cells.

**Necrotizing fasciitis:** A very serious, painful infection involving the fascia (membranous covering) of one or more muscles; may spread widely in short periods since there is no anatomic barrier to spread in this type of infection.

**Neonatal:** First 4 weeks after birth.

**Nested PCR:** A PCR assay that involves the sequential use of two primer sets.

**Neurotrophic:** Having a selective affinity for nerve tissue. Rabies is caused by a neurotrophic virus.

**NGU:** Nongonococcal urethritis.

**Nick translation:** Use of enzymes to break DNA and repolymerize small sections of the molecule, usually to label the DNA with a radioactive nucleotide.

**Nomenclature:** Naming of microorganisms according to established rules and guidelines.

**Nonphotochromogens:** Slow-growing, nonpigmented mycobacteria.

**Nontuberculous mycobacteria (NTM):** All species of mycobacteria that do not belong to *M. tuberculosis* complex.

**Nosocomial:** Pertaining to or originating in a hospital, for example, nosocomial infection.

**Nucleic acid hybridization:** Process by which the single-stranded probe unites with complementary DNA.

**Nucleic acid probe:** Piece of labeled single-stranded DNA used to detect complementary DNA in clinical material or a culture that specifically identifies the presence in these materials of an organism identical to that used to make the probe.

**Nucleocapsid:** Name of viral particle that includes virus nucleic acid core enclosed in the protein capsid coat.

**O&P:** Ova and parasites.

**O-F:** Oxidation-fermentation medium.

**Octal numbers:** Numbers used in computer databases to identify biochemical profiles of organisms and thus their identification.

**Oil immersion microscopy:** Use of immersion oil to fill the space between the slide being studied and the special objective of the microscope; this keeps the light rays from dispersing and provides good resolution at high magnification (total magnification of 1000∞).

**Oncogenic:** Possessing the potential to cause normal cells to become malignant; causing cancer.

**ONPG:** o-nitrophenol-β-galactopyranoside (β-galactosidase test).

**Operculated ova:** Ova possessing a cap or lid.

**Opsonize:** To facilitate destruction of pathogens by phagocytic ingestion or lysis by complement through the action of adherent antibodies.

**Optical density:** A measurement of turbidity.

**Osteomyelitis:** Inflammation of the bone and the marrow.

**Otitis:** Inflammation of the ear from a variety of causes, including bacterial infection; otitis media is inflammation of the middle ear.

**Oxidation:** A metabolic pathway of the microorganism that involves use of oxygen as a terminal electron acceptor. This type of reaction occurs in air.

**Oxidation-reduction potential:** Electromotive force exerted by a nonreacting electrode in a solution containing the oxidized and reduced forms of a chemical, relative to a standard hydrogen electrode; the more negative the value, the more anaerobic conditions are.

**Pandemic:** Epidemic over a wide geographic area, or even worldwide.

**Paracentesis:** Surgical transcutaneous puncture of the abdominal cavity to aspirate peritoneal fluid.

**Parasite:** Organism that lives on or within and at the expense of another organism.

**Parenteral:** Route of administration of a drug other than by mouth; includes intramuscular and intravenous administration.

**Parotitis:** Inflammation of the parotid gland, the largest of the salivary glands; mumps is the most common cause of this.

**Paroxysm:** Rapid onset (or return) of symptoms; term usually applies to cyclic recurrence of malaria symptoms, which are chills, fever, and sweating.

**Pathogen:** Microorganism that causes infection and/or disease.

**Pathogenic:** Producing disease.

**Pathogenicity islands:** Stretches of DNA that contain genes that are associated with bacterial virulence and are absent in from avirulent or less virulent strains of the same species.

**Pathologic:** Caused by or involving a morbid condition, as a pathologic state.

**PCR:** Polymerase chain reaction.

**Penicillin-binding protein:** Enzymes essential for bacterial cell wall production.

**Penicillinase (b-lactamase I):** Enzyme produced by some bacterial species that inactivates the antimicrobial activity of certain penicillins (e.g., penicillin G).

**Peptidoglycan:** Bacterial cell wall or murein layer that gives the bacterial cell shape and strength to withstand changes in environmental osmotic pressures.

**Percutaneous:** Performed through the skin (e.g., percutaneous bladder aspiration).

**Pericarditis:** Inflammation of the covering of the heart (pericardium).

**Perineum:** The portion of the body bound by the pubic bone anteriorly, the coccyx posteriorly, and the bony prominences (tuberosities) of the ileum on both sides.

**Peritoneal cavity:** Space between the visceral and parietal layers of the peritoneum.

**Peritoneum:** Large, moist, continuous sheet of serous membrane lining the abdominal pelvic cavity and the outer coat of the organs contained within the cavity.

**Peritonitis:** Inflammation of the peritoneal cavity, most often caused by bacterial infection.

**Pertussis:** Upper respiratory infection caused by *Bordetella pertussis.*

**Petechiae:** Tiny hemorrhagic spots in the skin or mucous membranes.

**PFGE:** Pulsed-field gel electrophoresis.

**Phaeohyphomycosis:** Term used to describe any infection caused by a dematiaceous organism.

**Phase-contrast microscopy:** Technique for direct observation of unstained material in which light beams pass through the object to be visualized and are partially deflected by the different densities of the object. These light beams are deflected again when they impinge on a special objective lens, increasing in brightness when aligned in phase.

**Phenotype:** Related to characteristics of an organism beyond the genetic level and include readily observable features.

**Photochromogens:** Mycobacteria that produce pigment after exposure to light but whose colonies remain buff-colored in the dark.

**Phycomycosis:** Serious infection involving fungi of the zygomycete group, often beginning with necrotic lesions in the nasal mucus or palate but rapidly spreading to involve other tissues. Seen in immunocompromised patients.

**PID:** Pelvic inflammatory disease.

**Pili:** Structures in bacteria similar to fimbriae that participate in bacterial conjugation and transfer of genetic material.

**Plasma:** Fluid portion of blood; obtained by centrifuging anticoagulated blood.

**Plasmids:** Extrachromosomal DNA elements of bacteria carrying a variety of determinants that may permit survival in an adverse environment or successful competition with other microorganisms of the same or different species.

**Pleomorphic:** Having more than one form, usually widely different forms, as in pleomorphic bacteria.

**Pleura:** The serous membrane enveloping the lung and lining the internal surface of the thoracic cavity.

**PMN:** Polymorphonuclear leukocyte or neutrophil.

**Pneumonia:** Inflammation of the lungs, primarily caused by infectious agents.

**Pneumothorax:** Introduction of air (usually inadvertently) into the pleural space, leading to collapse of the lung on that side.

**Polymerase chain reaction (PCR):** A method for expanding small discrete sections of DNA by binding DNA primers to sections at the ends of the DNA to be expanded and using cycles of heat (to create single-stranded DNA) and cooler temperatures (to allow a DNA polymerase enzyme to create new sections of DNA between the primer ends).

**PPD:** Purified protein derivative (skin test antigen for tuberculosis).

**Precipitin test:** Detection of antigen by allowing specific antibody to diffuse through liquid or gel until an antigen-antibody complex forms; this complex is visualized as a line of precipitated material.

**Precision:** Reproducibility of a test when run several times.

**Prevalence:** Frequency of disease in a population at a given time.

**Prion:** Proteinaceous infectious agent associated with Creutzfeldt-Jakob disease and perhaps other chronic, debilitating central nervous system diseases.

**Proctitis:** Inflammation of the rectum.

**Prodromal:** Early manifestations of a disease before specific symptoms become evident.

**Proglottid:** Segments of the tapeworm containing male and female reproductive systems; may be immature, mature, or gravid.

**Prognosis:** Forecast as to the possible outcome of a disease.

**Prokaryotic:** Organisms without a true nucleus.

**Prophylaxis:** Preventive treatment (e.g., the use of drugs to prevent infection).

**Prostatitis:** Inflammation of the prostate gland, usually caused by infection, characterized by fever, low back or perineal pain, and at times urinary frequency and urgency; a common background factor for recurrent cystitis in males.

**Prosthesis:** An artificial part such as a hip joint or eye.

**Protein A:** A protein on the cell wall of strains of *Staphylococcus aureus* (Cowan strain) that binds the Fc portion of antibodies.

**Prototroph:** Naturally occurring or wild strain.

**Pseudomembrane:** Necrosis of mucosal surface simulating a membrane.

**Pseudomembranous colitis (PMC):** Syndrome in the large bowel characterized by a layer of necrotic tissue and dead inflammatory cells often caused by the toxin of *Clostridium difficile.*

**Psychrophilic:** Cold-loving (e.g., microorganisms that grow best at low [4° C] temperatures).

**Purulent:** Consisting of pus.

**Pus:** Product of inflammation, consisting of fluid and many white blood cells; often bacteria and cellular debris are also present.

**Pyelonephritis:** Infection of the kidney and renal pelvis and the late effects of such infection.

**Pyocin:** Pigment produced by a bacterium that has anti-bacterial properties against other strains or species of bacteria.

**Pyogenic:** Pus-producing.

**PYR test:** The enzyme, l-pyroglutamyl-amino peptidase, hydrolyzes l-pyrolidonyl-β-naphthylamide (PYR) to produce β-naphthylamine. When the β-naphthylamine combines with cinnamaldehyde reagent, a red color is produced.

**Pyuria:** Presence of eight or more leukocytes per cubic millimeter on microscopic examination of uncentrifuged urine.

**QC:** Quality control.

**QNS:** Quantity not sufficient.

**Quencher:** Molecule that can accept energy from a fluorophore and then dissipate the energy so that no fluorescence results.

**Radioisotope:** Unstable molecule that emits detectable radiation (e.g., gamma rays, X-rays) for a known period (half-life). Can be incorporated into other compounds as a label for later detection by radiographic film exposure or by measurement in a scintillation counting instrument.

**Reagin:** An antibody that reacts in various serologic tests for syphilis.

**Reservoir:** Source from which an infectious agent may be disseminated; for example, humans are the only reservoir for Mycobacterium tuberculosis.

**Resin:** Plant product composed largely of esters and ethers of organic acids and acid anhydrides.

**Restriction endonuclease:** Enzyme that breaks nucleic acid (usually DNA) at only one specific sequence of nucleotides.

**Reticulate body:** The metabolically more active form of elementary bodies of Chlamydia spp.

**Reticuloendothelial system:** Macrophage system, which includes all the phagocytic cells of the body except for the granulocytic leukocytes.

**Reverse transcription:** Synthesis of DNA from RNA by using the enzyme reverse transcriptase.

**RFLP:** Restriction fragment length polymorphism.

**Rheumatoid factor:** IgM antibodies produced by some patients against their own IgG.

**Rhinorrhea:** Runny nose.

**RNA:** Ribonucleic acid.

**RPR:** Rapid plasma reagin, nontreponemal test for antibodies developed in response to syphilis infection.

**Saccharolytic:** Capable of breaking down sugars.

**Saprophytic:** Nonpathogenic.

**Schizogony:** Stage in the asexual cycle of the malaria parasite that takes place in the red blood cells of humans.

**Schlichter test:** Synonym for the serum bactericidal level test.

**Sclerotic:** Hard, indurated.

**Scolex (pl., scolices):** Head portion of a tapeworm; may attach to the intestinal wall by suckers or hooklets.

**Scotochromogens:** Mycobacteria that are pigmented even in the absence of exposure to light.

**Sensitivity:** Ability of a test to detect all true cases of the condition being tested for; absence of false-negative results. (Also see "specificity.")

**Septate:** Having cross walls.

**Septic shock:** Acute circulatory failure caused by toxins of microorganisms; often leads to multiple organ failure and is associated with a relatively high mortality.

**Septicemia (sepsis):** Systemic disease associated with presence of pathogenic microorganisms or their toxins in the blood.

**Sereny test:** Test for bacterial invasiveness; involves applying a suspension of the organism to the conjunctiva of a small mammal and observing for development of conjunctivitis.

**Serosanguineous:** Like serous but with some blood present grossly.

**Serous:** Like serum.

**Serum:** Cell- and fibrinogen-free fluid remaining after whole blood clots.

**Serum bactericidal level:** Lowest dilution of a patient's serum that kills a standard inoculum of an organism isolated from that patient; it is related to antibiotic level achieved in the patient's serum and the bactericidal activity of the drug being used.

**Sinus:** Suppurating tract; paranasal sinus, hollows, or cavities near the nose (e.g., frontal and maxillary sinuses).

**Slant:** See definition of "butt." The slant is the upper surface of the medium in the tube described. It is exposed to air in the tube.

**Solid-phase immunosorbent assay (SPIA):** ELISA test in which the capture antigen or antibody is attached to the inside of a plastic tube, microwell, or to the outside of a plastic bead, in a filter matrix, or some other solid support. Allows faster interaction between reactants and more concentrated visual end products than ELISA tests performed in liquid.

**Somatic:** Pertaining to the body (of a cell) (e.g., the somatic antigens of Salmonella spp.).

**Southern blot:** Identification of specific genetic sequences by separating DNA fragments by gel electrophoresis and transferring them to membrane filters in situ. Labeled complementary DNA applied to the filter binds to homologous fragments, which can then be identified by detecting the presence of the labeled DNA in association with bands of certain molecular size. Named after its discoverer, E.M. Southern.

**Specificity:** Ability of a test to correctly yield a negative result when the condition being detected is absent; absence of false-positive results. (Also see "sensitivity.")

**Spore:** Reproductive cell of bacteria, fungi, or protozoa; in bacteria, may be inactive, resistant forms within the cell.

**Sporozoite:** Slender, spindle-shaped organism that is the infective stage of the malarial parasite; it is inoculated into humans by an infected mosquito and is the result of the sexual cycle of the malarial parasite in the mosquito.

**Sputum:** Material discharged from the surface of the lower respiratory tract air passages and expectorated (or swallowed).

**Standard precautions:** Infection control guidelines used in the care of all patients; they apply to blood, body fluids, and secretions and excretions except sweat.

**Stat:** Statim (Latin); immediately.

**Stationary phase:** Stage in the growth cycle of a bacterial culture in which the vegetative cell population equals the dying population.

**STD:** Sexually transmitted disease.

**Sterile (sterility):** Free of living microorganisms (the state of being sterile).

**Substrate:** A substance on which an enzyme acts.

**Sulfur granule:** Small colony of organisms with surrounding club-like material; yellow-brown; resembles grain of sulfur.

**Superantigen:** Molecules produced by microbes (viruses, bacteria, and perhaps parasites) that act independently to stimulate T-cell activities, including cytokine release. Among the most potent T-cell mitogens, superantigen stimulation can result in anergy, or alternatively, systemic immune system activation.

**Superinfection:** Strictly speaking, superinfection refers to a new infection superimposed on another being treated with an antimicrobial agent. The new infecting agent is resistant to the therapy initially used and thus survives and causes persistence of the infection (now resistant to the treatment) or a new infection at a different site. The term is also used to indicate persistence or colonization with a new organism without any evidence of resulting infection.

**Suppuration:** Formation of pus.

**Suppurative thrombophlebitis:** Inflammation of a vein wall.

**Syncytia:** Structure resulting from fusion of cell membranes of several cells to form a multinucleated cellular structure; usually the result of viral infection of the cells.

**Syndrome:** Set of symptoms occurring together (e.g., nephrotic syndrome).

**Synergism:** Combined effect of two or more agents that is greater than the sum of their individual effects.

**Synovial fluid:** Viscid fluid secreted by the synovial membrane; formed in joint cavities, bursae, and so forth.

**Tachypnea:** Rapid breathing.

**T cells:** Lymphocytes involved in cellular immunity.

**Teichoic acids:** Glycerol or ribitol phosphate polymers combined with various sugars, amino acids, and amino sugars that are in the cell wall of gram-positive bacteria.

**Teleomorph:** Sexual fungal form.

**TEM:** Transmission electron micrograph.

**Tenesmus:** Painful, unsuccessful straining in an attempt to empty the bowels.

**Therapy, antimicrobial:** Treatment of a patient to combat an infectious disease.

**Thermolabile:** Adversely affected by heat (as opposed to thermostable, not affected by heat).

**Thoracentesis:** Drainage of fluid from the pleural space.

**Thoracic:** Pertaining to the chest cavity.

**Threshold cycle** (CT): The amplification cycle number in which the fluorescent signal rises above background; also referred to as the crossing point.

**Thrush:** A form of Candida infection that typically produces white plaquelike lesions in the oral cavity.

**Tinea:** Dermatophyte infection (tinea capitis, tinea of scalp; tinea corporis, tinea of the smooth skin of the body; tinea cruris, tinea of the groin; tinea pedis, tinea of the foot).

**Titer:** Level of a substance such as antibody or toxin present in material such as serum; reciprocal of the highest dilution at which the substance can still be detected.

**T lymphocytes** (or T cells): Thymus-derived lymphocytes important in cell-mediated immunity.

**Tm:** See "melting temperature."

**Tolerance:** A form of resistance to antimicrobial drugs; of uncertain clinical importance. See "tolerant."

**Tolerant:** Characteristic of an organism that requires a great deal more antimicrobial agent to kill it than to inhibit its growth.

**TPI:** *Treponema pallidum* immobilization test, a test for antibodies against the agent of syphilis that uses live treponemes.

**Trachoma:** Serious eye infection caused by *Chlamydia trachomatis*; often leads to blindness.

**Transduction:** Moving genetic material from one prokaryote to another via a bacteriophage or viral vector.

**Transformation:** Process in which an organism takes up free DNA that is released into the environment when another organism dies and then lyses.

**Transient** bacteremia: Incidental and brief presence of bacteria in the bloodstream.

**Transmission-based precautions:** Infection control guidelines used for patients known or suspected to be infected with pathogens spread by airborne or droplet transmission or by contact with dry skin or fomites.

**Transposon:** Genetic material that can move from one genetic element to another (i.e., between plasmids or from a plasmid to a chromosome); so-called jumping genes.

**Transtracheal aspiration:** Passage of needle and plastic catheter into the trachea for obtaining lower respiratory tract secretions free of oral contamination.

**Transudate:** Similar to exudate but with low protein content.

**Trophozoite:** Feeding, motile stage of protozoa.

**Tropism:** Preferred environment or destination. In viral infection, preference for a particular tissue site (rabies viruses have a tropism for neural tissue).

**TSI:** Triple sugar iron (agar tube).

**TTA:** Transtracheal aspiration.

**Type III secretion system:** Found in many gram-negative pathogens and is responsible for secretion and injection of virulence-associated factors into the cytoplasm of host cells.

**Type IV secretion systems (bacterial):** Bacterial devices that deliver macromolecular molecules such as proteins across and into cells.

**Typing:** Methods of grouping organisms, primarily for epidemiologic purposes (e.g., biotyping, serotyping, bacteriophage typing, and the antibiogram).

**Tzanck test:** Stained smear of cells from the base of a vesicle examined for inclusions produced by herpes simplex virus or varicella-zoster virus.

**Urethritis:** Inflammation of urethra, the canal through which urine is discharged (e.g., gonococcal urethritis).

**UTI:** Urinary tract infection.

**VD:** Venereal disease.

**VDRL:** Veneral Disease Research Laboratory; classic nontreponemal serologic test for syphilis antibodies. Uses cardiolipin, lecithin, and cholesterol as cross-reactive antigen that flocculates in the presence of "reaginic" antibodies produced by patients with syphilis. Best test for cerebrospinal fluid in cases of neurosyphilis.

**Vector:** An arthropod or other agent that carries microorganisms from one infected individual to another.

**Vegetation:** In endocarditis, the aggregates of fibrin and microorganisms on the heart valves or other endocardium.

**Vesicle:** A small bulla or blister containing clear fluid.

**Villi:** Minute, elongated projections from the surface of intestinal mucosa that are important in absorption.

**Vincent's angina:** An old term, seldom used currently, referring to anaerobic tonsillitis.

**Viremia:** Presence of viruses in the bloodstream.

**Virion:** The whole viral particle, including nucleocapsid, outer membrane or envelope, and all adherence structures.

**Virulence:** Degree of pathogenicity or disease-producing ability of a microorganism.

**Viscus** (pl., viscera): Any of the organs within one of the four great body cavities (cranium, thorax, abdomen, and pelvis).

**V-P:** Voges-Proskauer.

**Western blot:** Similar to Southern blot, except that antigenic proteins of an organism are separated by gel electrophoresis and transferred to membrane filters. Antiserum is allowed to react with the filters, and specific antibody bound to its homologous antigen is detected using labeled anti-antibody detectors.

**Zoonosis:** A disease of lower animals transmissible to humans (e.g., tularemia).

**Zygomycetes:** Group of fungi with nonseptate hyphae and spores produced within a sporangium.

# Index

Page numbers followed by "f" indicate figures, "t" indicate tables, and "b" indicate boxes.

## A

Abdominal angiostrongyliasis. *See Parastrongylus costaricensis.*
*Abiotrophia* spp.
  antimicrobial therapy and susceptibility testing for, 261t-262t
  colonial appearance of, 257t
  cultivation of, 253
  direct detection of, 253, 254t
  epidemiology of, 249t
  Gram stain of, 253
  pathogenesis and spectrum of disease of, 250t-251t
Abscesses
  brain, 905
    fungal, 760, 761t
    laboratory diagnosis of, 908
  peritonsillar, 894
  specimen collection and transportation of, 54t-61t
Abstriction, 723-724
*Acanthamoeba* spp., 645-649, 646t-647t
  clinical findings in, 559t
  laboratory diagnosis of, 566t-570t, 648-649
  therapy for, 649
Accuracy of antimicrobial susceptibility testing, 188-192, 191t
Acetamide utilization, 197b
Acetate utilization, 197b
*Achromobacter denitrificans*
  antimicrobial therapy and susceptibility testing for, 364t-365t
  colonial appearance of, 362t
  identification of, 364t
  pathogenesis and spectrum of disease, 359-360, 361t
*Achromobacter faecalis*
  identification of, 363
  pathogenesis and spectrum of disease, 359-360, 361t
*Achromobacter piechaudii*
  antimicrobial therapy and susceptibility testing for, 364t-365t
  identification of, 364t
  pathogenesis and spectrum of disease, 359-360
*Achromobacter* spp.
  antimicrobial susceptibility testing and therapy for, 352-353, 352t
  epidemiology of, 348, 349t
  general characteristics of, 348
  laboratory diagnosis of, 350-352, 351t
  pathogenesis and spectrum of disease, 348-350, 349t, 359-360
  prevention of, 353
Acid-fast stains
  for bright-field microscopy, 73-76, 75f-76f, 73.e1b, 76.e1b
  fuchsin, 498
  fungal, 718t
  of mycobacteria, 497-498, 497f-498f, 499t, 498.e1b, 497.e1b
  of parasites, 566t-570t, 574b, 558.e4b
  Ziehl-Neelsen, 75f
*Acidovorax* spp.
  antimicrobial therapy and susceptibility testing for, 344t, 377t

*Acidovorax* spp. *(Continued)*
  colonial appearance of, 340t-341t, 378t
  epidemiology of, 336t, 377t
  general characteristics of, 335
  identification of, 342t, 377-378, 378t
  media for, 376-377
  pathogenesis and spectrum of disease, 337t
*Acinetobacter* spp.
  antimicrobial susceptibility testing and therapy for, 333-334, 333t
  case study of, 334b
  epidemiology of, 329, 330t
  general characteristics of, 329
  laboratory diagnosis of, 330-332, 331t-332t, 332f
  pathogenesis and spectrum of disease, 329-330, 330t
  prevention and, 334
Acquired active immunity, 142
Acquired immunodeficiency syndrome (AIDS). *See also* Human immunodeficiency virus (HIV).
  serology panels and immune status tests for, 819t
Acquired resistance, 162, 170b
*Acremonium* spp.
  direct detection of, 719t-720t
  identification of, 727t-728t, 744
  in mycetoma, 763
Acridine orange stain, 78, 78f, 78.e1b
*Actinobacillus* spp.
  colonial appearance of, 400t
  epidemiology, spectrum of disease, and antimicrobial therapy, 396-398, 397t-398t
  general characteristics of, 396
  laboratory diagnosis of, 398-401
*Actinomadura* spp.
  antimicrobial susceptibility testing and therapy for, 305t
  epidemiology and pathogenesis of, 299t
  general characteristics of, 298, 298t
  Gram-stain morphology and colonial appearance of, 302t
  laboratory diagnosis of, 300-304, 302t-304t, 303f
  spectrum of disease of, 299-300, 300t
*Actinomyces neuii*, 282t-283t
*Actinomyces* spp.
  antimicrobial therapy and susceptibility testing of, 471t
  Gram-stain morphology, colonial appearance, and other distinguishing features of, 461t-463t
  as normal flora, 474t
  pathogenesis and spectrum of disease, 475t-476t, 479
*Actinomyces viscosus*, 282t-283t
Actinomycetes
  antimicrobial susceptibility testing and therapy for, 304-305, 305t
  case study for, 305b
  epidemiology and pathogenesis of, 298, 299t
  general characteristics of, 296-298, 297b, 297t-298t
  laboratory diagnosis of, 300-304, 300f, 302f-303f, 302t-304t
  prevention of, 305
  spectrum of disease, 298-300, 299t-300t

Actinomycetoma, 299-300
Actinomycosis, 968, 968f
Acute infections, 35, 36f, 38b
Acute myeloid leukemia, 401b
Acute sera, 144
Acute urethral syndrome, 923
Additives for blood culture, 868-869
Adenine, 4, 6f
Adenosine diphosphate (ADP), 15
Adenosine triphosphate (ATP), 15-17
Adenoviruses, 821-822, 822t, 824t
  detection in hospital virology laboratory of, 793t
  electron micrographs of, 807f-808f
  isolation and identification of, 815t
  specimens of, for diagnosis, 794t-795t
Adherence, lower respiratory tract infections and, 879-880
ADP. *See* Adenosine diphosphate (ADP).
Aerobic actinomycetes
  antimicrobial susceptibility testing and therapy for, 304-305, 305t
  case study for, 305b
  epidemiology and pathogenesis of, 298, 299t
  general characteristics of, 296-298, 297b, 297t-298t
  laboratory diagnosis of, 300-304, 300f, 302f-303f, 302t-304t
  prevention of, 305
  spectrum of disease, 298-300, 299t-300t
*Aerococcus* spp.
  antimicrobial susceptibility testing and therapy for, 261t-262t
  colonial appearance of, 257t
  direct detection of, 255t-256t
  epidemiology of, 249t
  Gram stain of, 253, 255t-256t
  pathogenesis and spectrum of disease of, 250t-251t
*Aeromonas* spp.
  antimicrobial susceptibility testing and therapy for, 373, 374t
  case study for, 374b
  colonial appearance of, 370t
  epidemiology of, 367, 368t
  in gastrointestinal infections, 955t-956t
  general characteristics of, 367
  key biochemical and physiologic characteristics of, 373t
  laboratory diagnosis of, 369-373, 370t, 371f, 373t
  pathogenesis and spectrum of disease, 368-369, 369t
  prevention and, 373-374
Aerotolerance testing, 480.e1b
Affirm VP III Microbial Identification Test, 942, 942f
*Afipia felis*, 413
*Afipia* spp., 410, 413, 414b
African trypanosomiasis, 636t, 637-639
Agar, 83, 83f. *See also specific agar types.*
  blood, 64-65, 64f, 84t-86t
    anaerobic, 465t, 466, 478f
  for fungal culture, 714-717, 715t-716t
  for routine bacteriology, 84t-86t
Agar dilution testing, 173-174, 174f, 174t
  commercial systems for, 178, 179f

Agglutination assay
  direct whole pathogen, 146
  latex, 135, 135f-136f
  particle, 135-136, 135f-136f
Agglutinins, 146
*Aggregatibacter* spp.
  colonial appearance of, 400t, 407t
  epidemiology, spectrum of disease, and antimicrobial therapy, 396-398, 397t-398t
  general characteristics of, 396
  laboratory diagnosis of, 398-401, 400t
*Agrobacterium* yellow group
  colonial appearance of, 356t
  identification of, 357t
AIDS. *See* Acquired immunodeficiency syndrome (AIDS).
Airborne contact transmission, 995t
Air-handling system of laboratory, 46
*Alcaligenes faecalis*
  antimicrobial therapy and susceptibility testing for, 364t-365t
  colonial appearance of, 362t
  epidemiology of, 360t
  identification of, 364t
  pathogenesis and spectrum of disease, 361t
*Alcaligenes piechaudii*
  identification of, 363
  pathogenesis and spectrum of disease, 361t
*Alcaligenes* spp.
  antimicrobial therapy and susceptibility testing for, 363-365, 364t-365t
  epidemiology of, 359, 360t
  general characteristics of, 359
  laboratory diagnosis of, 360-363, 362t
  pathogenesis and spectrum of disease, 359-360, 361t
  prevention and, 365-366
*Alcaligenes xylosoxidans*
  antimicrobial susceptibility testing and therapy for, 352t
  colonial appearance of, 351t
  direct detection of, 350
  epidemiology of, 349t
  identification of, 351t
  media for, 350
  pathogenesis and spectrum of disease, 349t
Aleurioconidia, 743, 744f
*Alloiococcus otitidis*
  antimicrobial susceptibility testing and therapy for, 261t-262t
  epidemiology of, 249t
  pathogenesis and spectrum of disease of, 252
*Alloiococcus* spp., 247-248
  antimicrobial susceptibility testing and therapy for, 243t
  colonial appearance of, 257t
  direct detection of, 255t-256t
  epidemiology of, 249t
  pathogenesis and spectrum of disease of, 250t-251t
Alpha-hemolytic streptococci, 86f
*Alternaria* spp.
  identification of, 727t-728t, 765, 765f
  pathogenesis and spectrum of disease, 761t